User's guide to the book

This book features the following didactical elements for easy reference and quick access to structures looked for.

– Each chapter has its own **colour-code**.

– The **menu bar** located at the top of each double-page spread shows the user's present position. The sub-chapter is shown in boldface type.

– The **subject of each page** is shown in italics.

– Many figures feature a **compass rose**, whose numbers correspond to the figures of adjacent regions, so that the sequence of a structure can easily be followed over several pages.

– Small **supplement drawings** located next to complex views show visual angles and intersecting planes.

– **The colored dots placed** at the end of leader lines on topographic illustrations assist in quickly locating arteries, veins, muscles and nerves.

– Many figures are **cross-referenced**.

– Enclosed is a **separate booklet with tables** pertaining to muscles, joints and nerves, which can easily be taken along or used for quick reference. The relevant table can be placed next to a selected illustration for direct comparison.

– **Cross-references between figures and tables** enable swift correlation of illustrations and table texts.

– **A list of abbreviations, terms for anatomical directions and positions, as well as explanatory notes on information in parentheses** can be found at the end of the book.

Perfect orientation – the new Navigation System

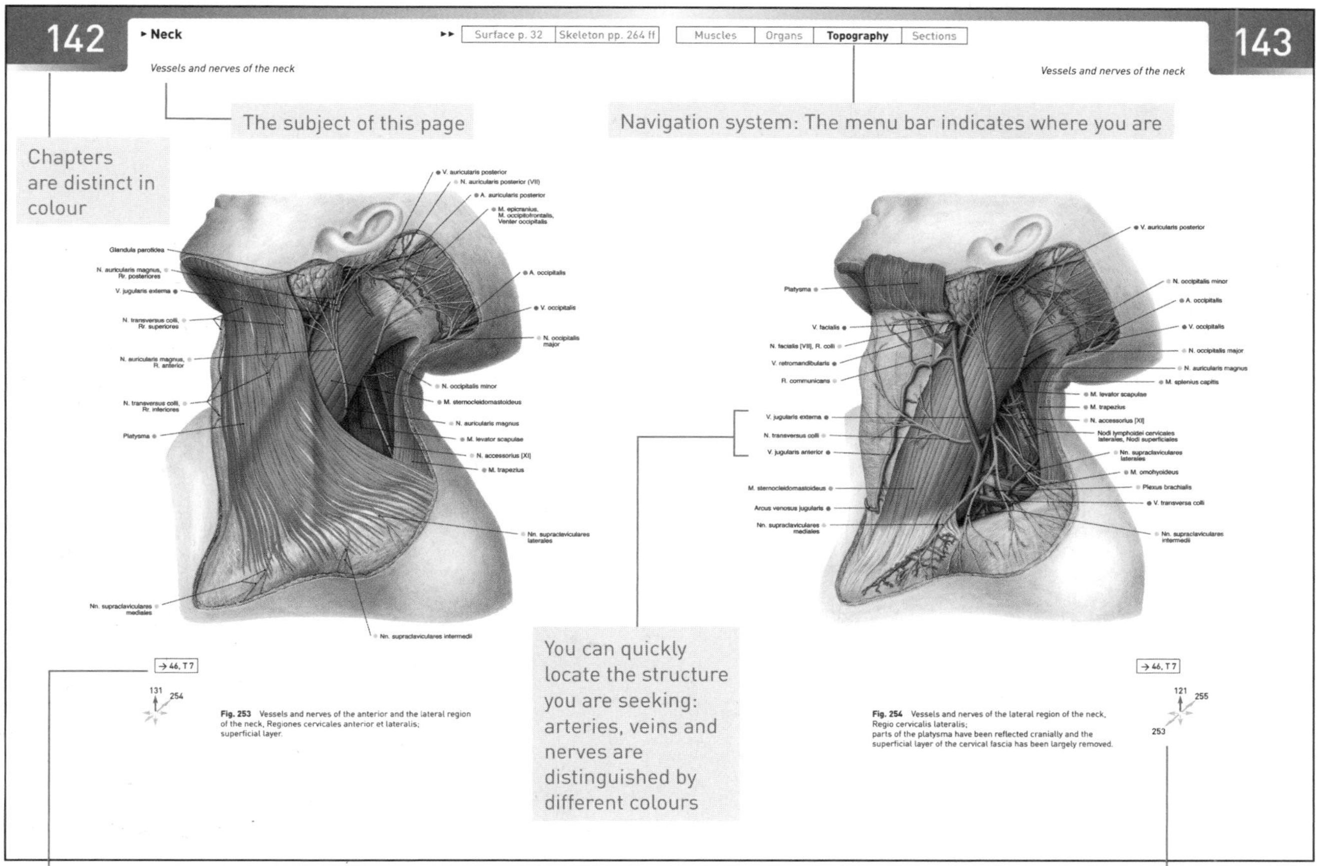

Vessels and nerves of the neck

The subject of this page

Navigation system: The menu bar indicates where you are

Chapters are distinct in colour

Fig. 253 Vessels and nerves of the anterior and the lateral region of the neck, Regiones cervicales anterior et lateralis; superficial layer.

→ 46, T 7

You can quickly locate the structure you are seeking: arteries, veins and nerves are distinguished by different colours

Vessels and nerves of the neck

Fig. 254 Vessels and nerves of the lateral region of the neck, Regio cervicalis lateralis; parts of the platysma have been reflected cranially and the superficial layer of the cervical fascia has been largely removed.

→ 46, T 7

T = Reference to the matching tables in the separate table booklet

→ 46, T 7

Cross-references to other relavant figures in the atlas

"Compass rose": Link to the figures of adjacent regions:

proximally or cranially adjacent region

deeper layer

laterally adjacent region ← → laterally adjacent region

superficial layer

distally or cranially adjacent region

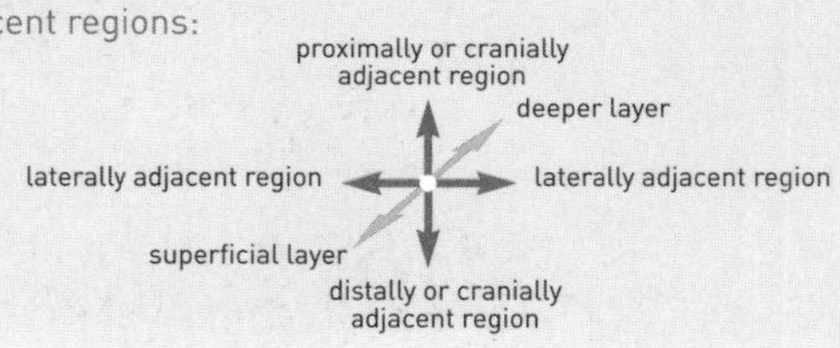

Overview

Sobotta

Atlas of Human Anatomy
One Volume Edition • Latin
Nomenclature

Edited by R. Putz and R. Pabst
In collaboration with Renate Putz

Head, Neck,
Upper Limb,
Thorax, Abdomen,
Pelvis, Lower Limb

14th edition, newly edited
1431 colour plates with 1984 figures
Booklet (tables of muscles, joints and nerves)

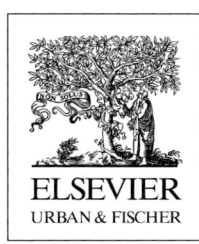

ELSEVIER
URBAN & FISCHER

URBAN & FISCHER   München

Correspondence and feedback should be addressed to:
Elsevier GmbH, Urban & Fischer Verlag, Department for Medical Student Information, Karlstraße 45, 80333 Munich, Germany
e-mail: medizinstudium@elsevier.de

Addresses of the editors:

Professor Dr. med. Reinhard Putz
Vizepräsident der
Ludwig Maximilians-Universität
Geschwister-Scholl-Platz 1
80539 München
Germany
e-mail: putz@lmu.de

Professor Dr. med. Reinhard Pabst
Leiter der Abteilung
Funktionelle und Angewandte Anatomie
Medizinische Hochschule Hannover
Carl-Neuberg-Straße 1
30625 Hannover
Germany
e-mail: pabst.reinhard@mh-hannover.de

Bibliographic information published by Die Deutsche Bibliothek

Die Deutsche Bibliothek lists this publication in the Deutsche National-bibliografie; detailed bibliographic data is available in the Internet at http://dnb.ddb.de.

The contents of this edition are identical with the 14th edition in two volumes. The order of the chapters has been changed.

Editorial staff at Elsevier: Dr. med. Dorothea Hennessen
                                Dr. med. Helmar Weiß
                                Dr. Andrea Beilmann
                                Alexandra Frntic
Editorial staff and translation: Ulrike Kriegel, buchundmehr, Munich
Illustrators: Ulrike Brugger, Munich; Rüdiger Himmelhan, Heidelberg; Horst Ruß, Munich; Henriette Rintelen, Velbert
Book production: Renate Hausdorf, buchundmehr, Munich
Composed by: Mitterweger&Partner, Plankstadt
Printed and bound by: MKT Print Ljubljana
Cover design: Carsten Tschirner, Munich
Printed on Nopacoat 115 g

Printed in Slovenija
ISBN: 978-0-7020-3483-1

This atlas was founded by Johannes Sobotta†, former Professor of Anatomy and Director of the Anatomical Institute of the University of Bonn, Germany.

German Editions:
1st Edition: 1904–1907 J. F. Lehmanns Verlag, Munich
2nd–11th Edition: 1913–1944 J. F. Lehmanns Verlag, Munich
12th–20th Edition: 1948–1993 Urban & Schwarzenberg, Munich
13th Edition: 1953, editor H. Becher
14th Edition: 1956, editor H. Becher
15th Edition: 1957, editor H. Becher
16th Edition: 1967, editor H. Becher
17th Edition: 1972, editors H. Ferner and J. Staubesand
18th Edition: 1982, editors H. Ferner and J. Staubesand
19th Edition: 1988, editor J. Staubesand
20th Edition: 1993, editors R. Putz and R. Pabst
21st Edition: 2000, editors R. Putz and R. Pabst, Urban & Fischer Verlag, Munich
22nd Edition: 2006, editors R. Putz and R. Pabst, Elsevier GmbH, Munich

Foreign Editions:
Arabic Edition
Modern Technical Center, Damascus
Chinese Edition (complex characters)
Ho-Chi Book Publishing Co, Taiwan
Chinese Edition (simplified Chinese edition)
Elsevier, Health Sciences Asia, Singapore
Croatian Edition
Naklada Slap, Jastrebarsko
Dutch Edition
Bohn Stafleu van Loghum, Houten
English Edition (with nomenclature in English)
Atlas of Human Anatomy
Lippincott Williams & Wilkins
English Edition (with nomenclature in Latin)
Atlas of Human Anatomy
Elsevier GmbH, Urban & Fischer
French Edition
Atlas d'Anatomie Humaine
Tec & Doc Lavoisier, Paris
Greek Edition (with nomenclature in Greek)
Maria G. Parissianos, Athens
Greek Edition (with nomenclature in Latin)
Maria G. Parissianos, Athens
Hungarian Edition
az ember anatómiájának atlasza
Alliter Kiadái, Budapest
Indonesian Edition
Atlas Anatomi Manusia
Penerbit Buku Kedokteran EGC, Jakarta
Italian Edition
Atlante di Anatomia Umana
UTET, Torino
Japanese Edition
Igaku Shoin Ltd., Tokyo
Korean Edition
ShingHeung MedScience, Seoul
Polish Edition
Atlas anatomii cztowieka
Urban & Partner, Wroclaw
Portuguese Edition (with nomenclature in English)
Atlas de Anatomia Humana
Editora Guanabara Koogan, Rio de Janeiro
Portuguese Edition (with nomenclature in Latin)
Atlas de Anatomia Humana
Editora Guanabara Koogan, Rio de Janeiro
Spanish Edition
Atlas de Anatomia Humana
Editorial Medica Panamericana, Buenos Aires/Madrid
Turkish Edition
Insan Anatomisi Atlasi
Beta Basim Yayim Dagitim, Istanbul

Current information by www.elsevier.com and www.elsevier.de

Contents

Preface

It was just over a hundred years ago that Johannes Sobotta set out to publish the first edition of his Atlas of Human Anatomy. Since then, this piece of work has evolved step by step as a result of the constant interaction between students, lecturers and editors. It has not only been the most modern basis for the complex subject of macroscopic anatomy throughout many generations of doctors, but has also developed into a lasting work of reference for both clinical training and advanced medical education. All in all, it has become a book for a medical doctor's life. Once again, in this new edition the additional figures have been drawn strictly on the basis of original specimens.

The 14th edition has been particularly designed to meet the demands of a reformed medical curriculum, emphasizing the integration of clinical medicine into the preclinical curriculum. For this purpose, the new edition has been extended to include the following features:
– Surface anatomy including projection of internal organs (45 colour photos)
– Anatomical diagrams next to imaging figures
– Integration of imaging techniques to a greater extent (ultrasound, X-ray, CT, MRI; 119 figures)
– Endoscopic, intraoperative colour images and figures exemplifying techniques of puncture and examination (54 figures)
– Images of patients presenting with typical palsies
– Diagrams of the most important arterial variations (93 figures)
– Frequent variations in the location of internal organs (24 figures)
– Integration of histology at low magnification of important internal organs (intestine, liver, kidney, etc.)

In order to improve the presentation of the knowledge, the following features have been introduced:
– Clear-cut arrangement of the chapters according to the different regions of the body
– Thematically corresponding figures presented on double pages
– A concise, separate booklet contains tables of muscles, joints and nerves, enabling the reader to place it next to any figure in the atlas

One particular aim of the new edition is to facilitate finding of specific structures. The SOBOTTA depicts anatomical structures precisely without the reader loosing the greater picture. Therefore, specific didactic tools have been improved and new aspects included:
– Each chapter has been allocated to a particular colour
– A "menu bar" on each double page ensures precise orientation within a given chapter
– The number of outlines depicting spatial orientation has been significantly increased (270 figures)
– Overviews of total body regions ensure general orientation

– New diagrams of particular muscles clarify their location and course (24 figures)
– Confusion is kept to a minimum by only depicting limbs of the right side of the body
– "Compass roses" point to adjacent figures, thus facilitating following a given structure over several pages
– Continuous leader lines facilitate finding of structures
– Coloured dots at the end of leader lines in topographic diagrams mark arteries, veins, nerves, and muscles
– The figures in the booklet relate directly to the figures in the atlas
– The larger dimensions of the book improve clarity

With the exception of discussions about the general concept of the atlas and mutual correction, the editors have worked separately on individual chapters, with the work divided as follows:
R. Putz: General anatomy, upper limb, brain, eye, ear, back, lower limb;
R. Pabst: Head, neck, thoracic and abdominal walls, thoracic, abdominal and pelvic viscera.

The inclusion of a large number of new figures is the result of the extraordinary capability of the following medical illustrators: Ulrike Brugger, Rüdiger Himmelhan and Horst Ruß. It is to their credit that the classic "SOBOTTA style" has been retained. Several of the diagrams have been generated on the computer by Henriette Rintelen. We also gratefully acknowledge our clinical colleagues for making clinical illustrations available to us (see picture credits). We owe a debt of gratitude to our colleagues from the institutes for their understanding and helpful suggestions. Dr. N. Sokolov and A. Buchhorn have put meticulous efforts into generating the specimen preparations. S. Fryk and G. Hoppmann have supported us in text processing.

The staff of the editorial office of Elsevier publishers, in particular Dr. D. Hennessen and A. Gattnarzik, has our sincere thanks. Some of the creative development of the work is a result of very fruitful discussions. We would also like to thank R. Hausdorf for tremendous efforts in the production of the atlas. R. Putz together with G. Meier were responsible for the proofreading and simplification of page design and legends. Our special thanks go to Dr. U. Osterkamp-Baust for generating the index, and all others involved in the corrections. With our joint efforts, the SOBOTTA has been once more modernized both in contents and design.

We have included many of the helpful suggestions made over the years by students and colleagues, and would therefore ask all readers of this edition to pass on to us any criticism or suggestions on the new format of this atlas.

Munich and Hannover, September 2005
R. Putz and R. Pabst

Picture credits

The editors sincerely thank all clinical colleagues that made ultrasound, computed tomographic and magnetic resonance images as well as endoscopic and intraoperative pictures available:

Prof. Altaras, Centre for Radiology, University of Gießen (Fig. 741, 763, 764)

Dr. Baumeister, Department of Radiology, University of Freiburg (Fig. 889)

PD Dr. Burgkardt, Orthopaedic Clinic, Technical University of Munich (Fig. 1163)

Prof. Brückmann & Dr. Linn, Neuroradiology, Institute for Diagnostic Radiology, University of Munich (Fig. 1367, 1431 a, b, 1432 a, b)

Prof. Daniel, Department of Cardiology, University of Erlangen (Fig. 631, 632, 633, 705)

Prof. Degenhardt, Bielefeld (Fig. 865, 867)

Prof. Galanski & Dr. Kirchhoff, Department of Diagnostic Radiology, Hannover Medical School (Fig. 944, 945, 994, 996)

Prof. Galanski & Dr. Schäfer, Department of Diagnostic Radiology, Hannover Medical School (Fig. 603 a, b, 659, 703, 723, 926, 936, 939, 941)

Prof. Gebel, Department of Gastroenterology, Hepatology and Endocrinology, Hannover Medical School (Fig. 242, 749, 758, 759, 770, 771, 806, 824)

Dr. Goei, Radiology, Heerlen, The Netherlands (Fig. 882, 883) (with permission from Radiology 173; 137–141: 1989)

Dr. Greeven, St.-Elizabeth-Hospital, Neuwied (Fig. 150, 970)

Prof. Hoffmann & PD Dr. Bektas, Clinic for Abdominal and Transplantation Surgery, Hannover Medical School (Fig. 772, 960)

Prof. Hohlfeld, Clinic for Pneumology, Hannover Medical School (Fig. 661, 662)

Prof. Jonas, Urology, Hannover Medical School (Fig. 834 a, b, 835)

Prof. Kampik & Prof. Müller, Ophthalmology, University of Munich (Fig. 1362)

Dr. Kirchhoff & Dr. Weidemann, Department of Diagnostic Radiology, Hannover Medical School (Fig. 773, 825, 834, 928, 930, 932, 934, 937)

Prof. Kremers, Department for Restorative Dentistry and Periodontology, University of Munich (Fig. 169)

Prof. Kunze, von Haunersches Children's Hospital, University of Munich (Fig. 327–330)

Dr. Meyer, Department of Gastroenterology, Hepatology and Endocrinology, Hannover Medical School (Fig. 676, 719 a, b, 724, 877, 878)

Prof. Müller-Vahl, Neurology, Hannover Medical School (Fig. 128 a, b)

Prof. Pfeifer, Radiology, Institute for Diagnostic Radiology, University of Munich (Fig. 293, 294, 310, 312, 449, 451, 501–504, 539–542, 987, 1018, 1019, 1049, 1050)

PD Dr. Rau, Department of Radiology, University of Freiburg (Fig. 644, 657, 658)

Prof. Ravelli †, formerly Institute of Anatomy, University of Innsbruck (Fig. 499)

PD Dr. Rieger, Radiology, Institute for Diagnostic Radiology, University of Munich (Fig. 1127)

Prof. Reich, Orofacial Surgery, University of Bonn (Fig. 113 a, b)

Prof. Reiser & Dr. Wagner, Institute for Diagnostic Radiology, University of Munich (Fig. 436, 449, 451, 453, 524, 1276, 1277, 1278, 1281, 1282)

Prof. Rudzki-Janson, Department of Orthodontics, University of Munich (Fig. 72, 73)

Dr. Scheibe, Department of Surgery, Rosman Hospital, Breisach (Fig. 1011 a–c)

Prof. Scheumann, Clinic for Abdominal and Transplantation Surgery, Hannover Medical School (Fig. 243, 244, 245)

Prof. Schillinger, Department of Gynaecology, University of Freiburg (Fig. 866)

Prof. Schliephake, Orofacial Surgery, Göttingen (Fig. 152, 196, 197)

Prof. Schlösser, Centre for Gynaecology, Hannover Medical School (Fig. 864 a, b, 872, 873, 910)

Prof. Schumacher, Neuroradiology, Department of Radiology, University of Freiburg (Fig. 1166 a, b)

Dr. Sommer & PD Dr. Bauer, Radiologists, Munich (Fig. 1022–1024, 1367)

Prof. Stotz, Paediatrics, University of Munich (Fig. 971, 972)

PD Dr. Vogl, Radiology, University of Munich (Fig. 436, 453, 1349, 1350)

Prof. Vollrath, Ear-Nose-Throat Department, Mönchengladbach (Fig. 229, 230, 231)

Prof. Wagner †, Diagnostic Radiology II, Hannover Medical School (Fig. 684, 796, 797, 801, 804, 884)

Prof. Wenz, formerly Department of Radiology, University of Freiburg (Fig. 500)

Prof. Witt, Department of Neurosurgery, University of Munich (Fig. 405)

Dr. Willführ, formerly Clinic for Abdominal and Transplantation Surgery, Hannover Medical School (Fig. 783)

PD Dr. Wimmer, Department of Radiology, University of Freiburg (Fig. 531)

Additional illustrations were obtained from the following textbooks:

Benninghoff-Drenckhahn: Anatomie, Band 1 (Drenckhahn D., Hrsg.), 16. Aufl., Urban & Fischer, München 2003 (Fig. 555, 556, 580, 581, 582)

Welsch, U.: Lehrbuch Histologie, Urban & Fischer, München 2003 (Fig. 654, 752, 829, 854, 855)

Welsch, U. (Hrsg.): Sobotta, Atlas Histologie, 6. Aufl., Urban & Fischer, München 2002 (Fig. 857 a, b, 869, 917)

Wicke, L.: Atlas der Röntgenanatomie, 3. Aufl., Urban & Schwarzenberg, München–Wien–Baltimore 1985 (Fig. 675 a, b)

Univ.-Prof. Dr. med. Reinhard Putz

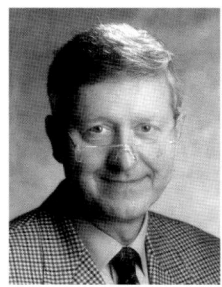

Born in Innsbruck/Austria
1962–1968	Studied medicine at the Leopold-Franzens-University of Innsbruck
1968	Received a doctorate
1968–1982	University assistant at the Institute of Anatomy at the University of Innsbruck
1978	Lecturer in anatomy
1979	Consultant for anatomy
1982–1989	Chair of the Anatomical Institute at the Albert-Ludwigs-University of Freiburg
since 1989	Chair of the Anatomical Institute at the Ludwig-Maximilians-University of Munich
1992–1994	President of the European Association of Clinical Anatomists
1993	Registration to practise medicine
1998–1999	Chairman of the Anatomical Society
1999	Member of the Akademie der Naturforscher und Ärzte (Leopoldina)
2002	Dr. h.c. of the University of Constanta, Romania
2003	Prorector I of the Ludwig-Maximilians-University of Munich

Research and fields of interest

- Functional anatomy of the passive locomotor system
- Evolution and functional anatomy of the vertebral column
- Form-function-relations of joints
- Applied anatomy (anatomical basics of orthopaedics, surgery, radiology)
- Questions about the contents and organisation of the medical curriculum
- Development of didactic training programmes at universities

Univ.-Prof. Dr. med. Reinhard Pabst

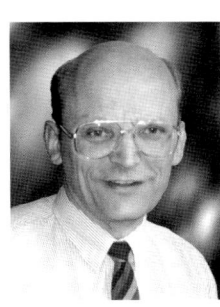

Born in Posen, grown up in Lüneburg
1965–1970	Studied medicine at the Hannover Medical School, and in Glasgow/Scotland
1970	University degree and doctorate
1971	Registration to practise medicine
1971–76	Scientific associate in the Department of Clinical Physiology, University of Ulm
1976	Lecturer for Clinical Physiology, University of Ulm, and new lectureship at the Hannover Medical School
1976–80	Senior assistant in the Department of Functional and Applied Anatomy, Hannover Medical School
1978	Extension of the Venia legendi to include anatomy
1980–1992	Head of the Department of Topographic Anatomy and Biomechanics
since 1992	Head of the Department of Functional and Applied Anatomy, Hannover Medical School
1986–1990	Prorector for studies and education, Hannover Medical School
1993–1997	Dean of the Hannover Medical School
1997–1998	Chairman of the Anatomical Society
1999–2003	Prorector of Research of the Hannover Medical School
2001	Member of the Akademie der Naturforscher und Ärzte (Leopoldina)

Research and fields of interest

- Functional anatomy of lymphatic organs
- Proliferation and migration of lymphocytes
- Development of the intestinal immune system
- Function of the pulmonary immune system
- Questions of a clinically orientated anatomy in the medical curriculum
- Evaluation of teaching

1. List of abbreviations

Singular:
A.   = Arteria
Lig. = Ligamentum
M.   = Musculus
N.   = Nervus
Proc. = Processus
R.   = Ramus
V.   = Vena

Var. = variation
r.   = right
l.   = left

Plural:
Aa.   = Arteriae
Ligg. = Ligamenta
Mm.   = Musculi

Nn.   = Nervi
Procc. = Processus
Rr.   = Rami
Vv.   = Venae

♀   = female
♂   = male

Percentages: In the light of the large variation in individual body measurements, the percentages indicating size should only be taken as approximate values.

2. General terms of direction and position

> The following terms indicate the position of organs and parts of the body in relation to each other, irrespective of the position of the body (e.g. supine or upright) or direction and position of the limbs. These terms are relevant not only for human anatomy but also for clinical medicine and comparative anatomy.

General terms

anterior – posterior = in front – behind (e.g. Arteriae tibiales anterior et posterior)
ventralis – dorsalis = towards the belly – towards the back
superior – inferior = above – below (e.g. Conchae nasales superior et inferior)
cranialis – caudalis = towards the head – towards the tail
dexter – sinister = right – left (e.g. Arteriae iliacae communes dextra et sinistra)
internus – externus = internal – external
superficialis – profundus = superficial – deep (e.g. Musculi flexores digitorum superficialis et profundus)
medius, intermedius = located between two other structures (e.g. the Concha nasalis media is located between the Concha nasalis superior and inferior)
medianus = located in the midline (Fissura mediana anterior of the spinal cord). The median plane is a sagittal plane which divides the body into right and left halves.
medialis – lateralis = located near to the midline – located away from the midline of the body (e.g. Fossae inguinales medialis et lateralis)

frontalis = located in a frontal plane, but also towards the front (e.g. Processus frontalis of the maxilla)
longitudinalis = parallel to the longitudinal axis (e.g. Musculus longitudinalis superior of the tongue)
sagittalis = located in a sagittal plane
transversalis = located in a transverse plane
transversus = transverse direction (e.g. Processus transversus of a thoracic vertebra)

Terms of direction and position for the limbs

proximalis – distalis = located towards or away from the attached end of a limb or the origin of a structure (e.g. Articulationes radioulnares proximalis et distalis)

For the upper limb:
radialis – ulnaris = on the radial side – on the ulnar side (e.g. Arteriae radialis et ulnaris)

For the hand:
palmaris – dorsalis = towards the palm of the hand – towards the back of the hand (e.g. Aponeurosis palmaris, Musculus interosseus dorsalis)

For the lower limb:
tibialis – fibularis = on the tibial side – on the fibular side (e.g. Arteria tibialis anterior)

For the foot:
plantaris – dorsalis = towards the sole of the foot – towards the back of the foot (e.g. Arteriae plantares lateralis et medialis, Arteria dorsalis pedis)

3. Use of brackets

[ ]: Latin terms in square brackets refer to alternative terms as given in the Terminologia Anatomica (1998), e.g. Ren [Nephros]. To keep the legends short, only those alternative terms have been added that differ in the root of the word and are necessary to understand clinical terms, e.g. nephrology. They are primarily used in figures in which the particular organ or structure plays a central role.

( ): Round brackets are used in different ways:
– for terms also listed in round brackets in the Terminologia Anatomica, e.g. (M. psoas minor)
– for terms not included in the official nomenclature but which the editors consider important and clinically relevant, e.g. (Crista zygomaticoalveolaris)
– to indicate the origin of a given structure, e.g. R. spinalis (A. vertebralis)
– to indicate the right (r.) or left (l.) side of the body and the approximate reduction or magnification of size, e.g. (r., 70%).

4. Orientation diagrams

Most of the topographic illustrations are supplied with "compass roses", which refer to the numbers of the illustrations of the respective adjacent regions:

proximally or cranially
adjacent region

deeper layer

laterally adjacent region ◄——►laterally adjacent region

superficial layer

distally or caudally
adjacent region

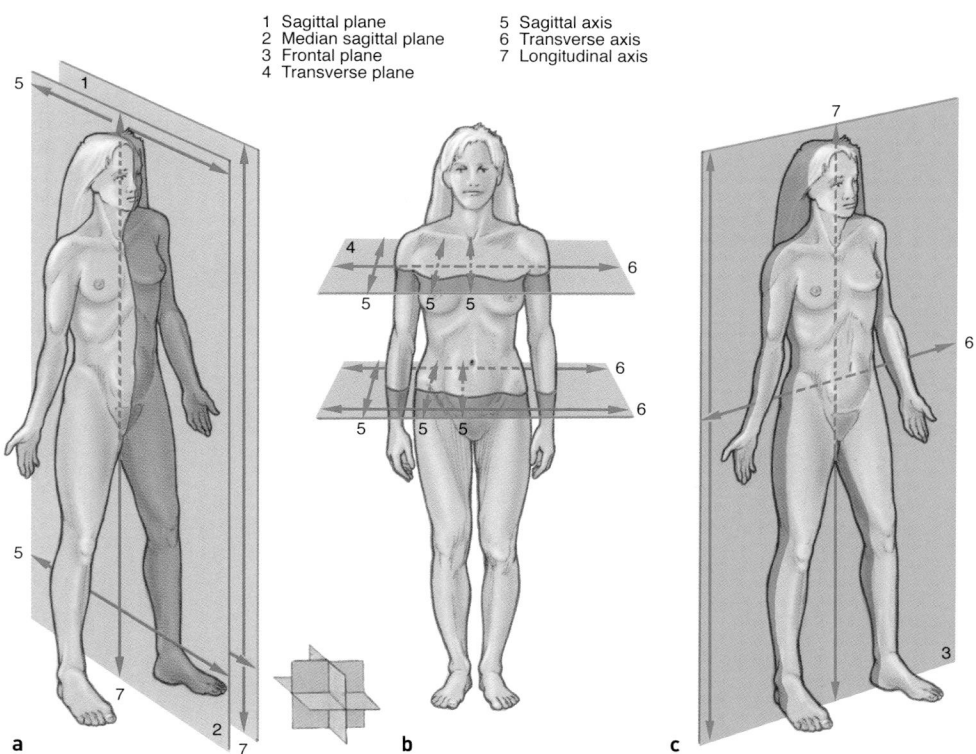

1 Sagittal plane
2 Median sagittal plane
3 Frontal plane
4 Transverse plane
5 Sagittal axis
6 Transverse axis
7 Longitudinal axis

Fig. 1 a–c   Planes and axes.
a Sagittal plane, Planum sagittale, sagittal and longitudinal axes
b Transverse plane (= horizontal plane), Planum transversale, transverse and sagittal axes
c Frontal plane (= coronal plane), Planum frontale, longitudinal and transverse axes

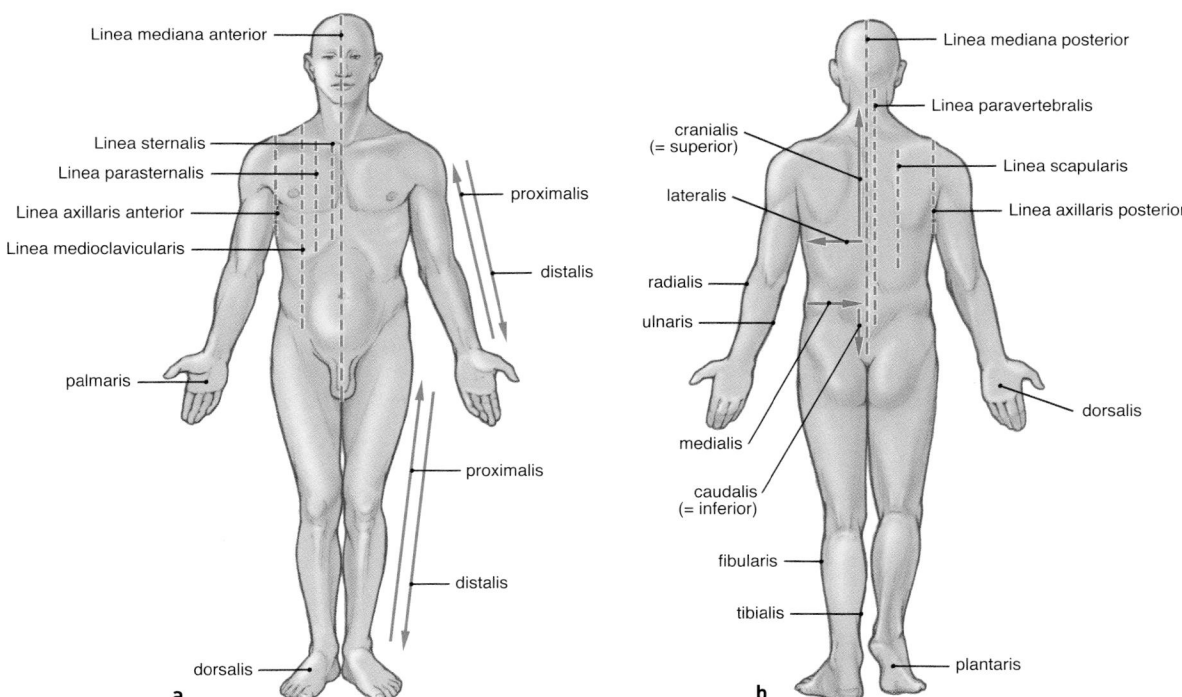

Fig. 2 a, b   Orientation lines of the human body and terms of direction and position.
a Ventral view (ventralis, anterior)
b Dorsal view (dorsalis, posterior)

Parts of the human body

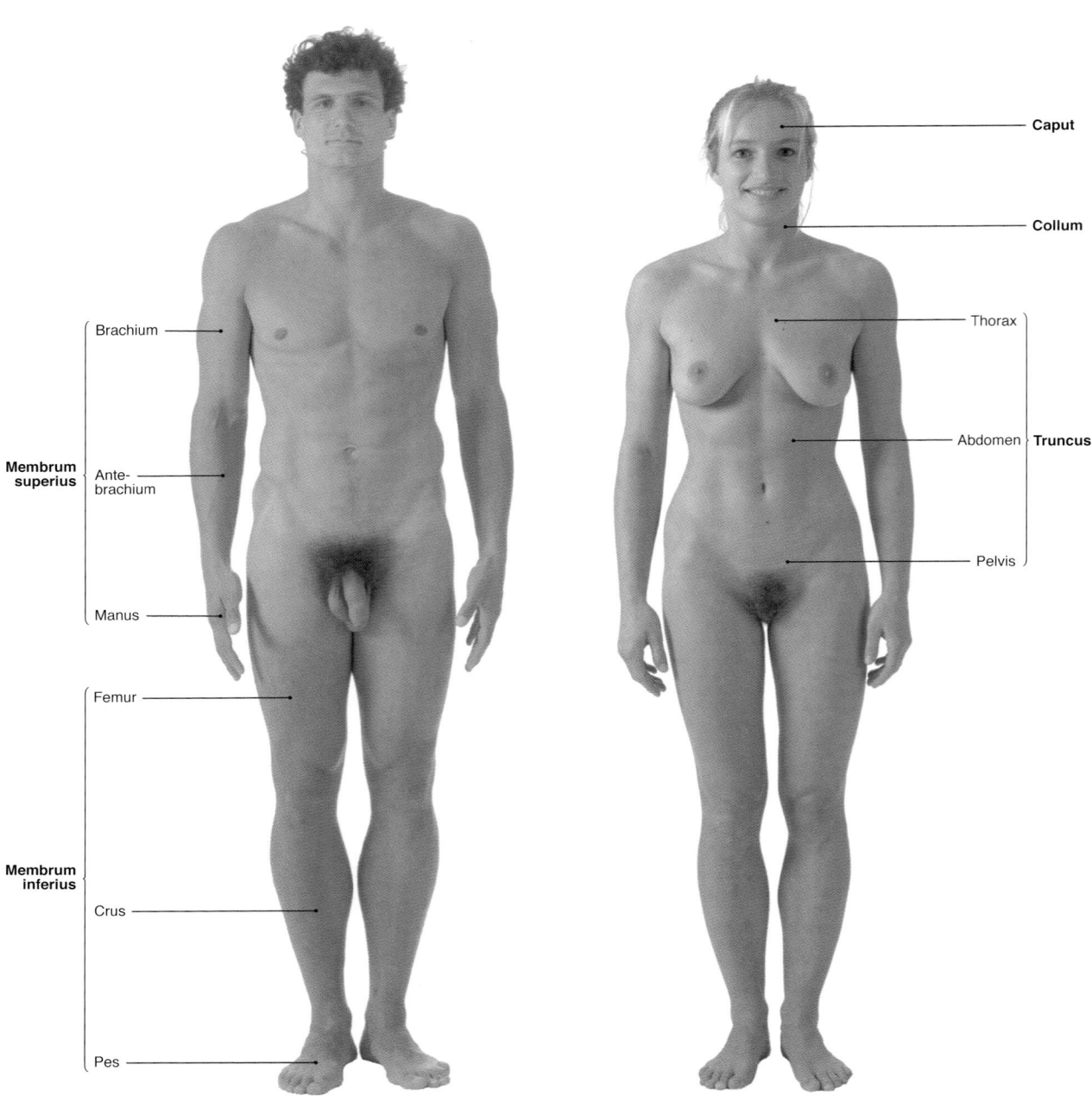

Fig. 3 Surface anatomy of the male.

Fig. 4 Surface anatomy of the female.

Parts of the human body

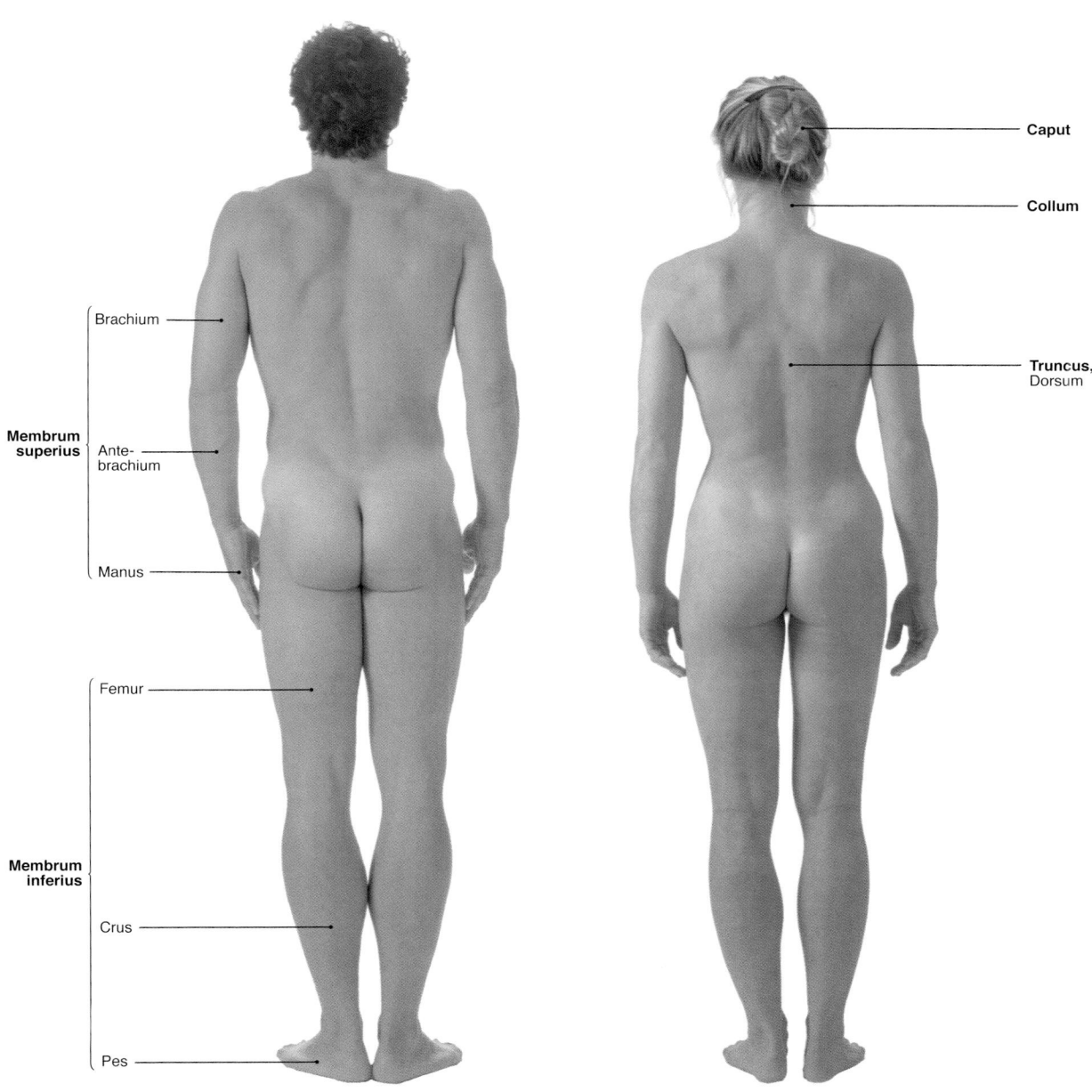

Caput

Collum

Truncus,
Dorsum

Brachium

**Membrum
superius**

Ante-
brachium

Manus

Femur

**Membrum
inferius**

Crus

Pes

Fig. 5 Surface anatomy of the male. **Fig. 6** Surface anatomy of the female.

Regions of the human body

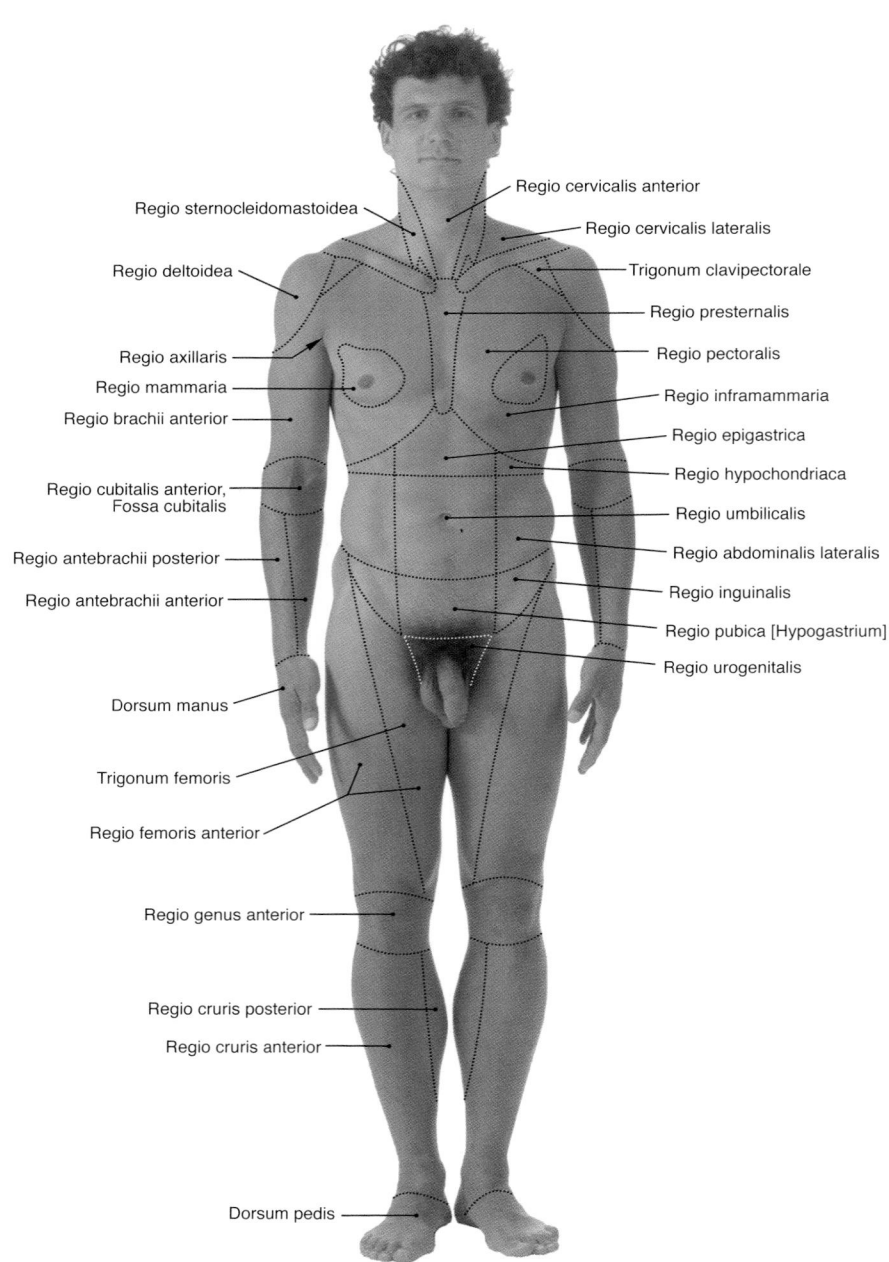

Regio sternocleidomastoidea

Regio cervicalis anterior

Regio cervicalis lateralis

Regio deltoidea

Trigonum clavipectorale

Regio presternalis

Regio axillaris

Regio pectoralis

Regio mammaria

Regio inframammaria

Regio brachii anterior

Regio epigastrica

Regio hypochondriaca

Regio cubitalis anterior,
Fossa cubitalis

Regio umbilicalis

Regio abdominalis lateralis

Regio antebrachii posterior

Regio inguinalis

Regio antebrachii anterior

Regio pubica [Hypogastrium]

Regio urogenitalis

Dorsum manus

Trigonum femoris

Regio femoris anterior

Regio genus anterior

Regio cruris posterior

Regio cruris anterior

Dorsum pedis

Fig. 7 Regions of the human body, Regiones corporis.

Regions of the human body

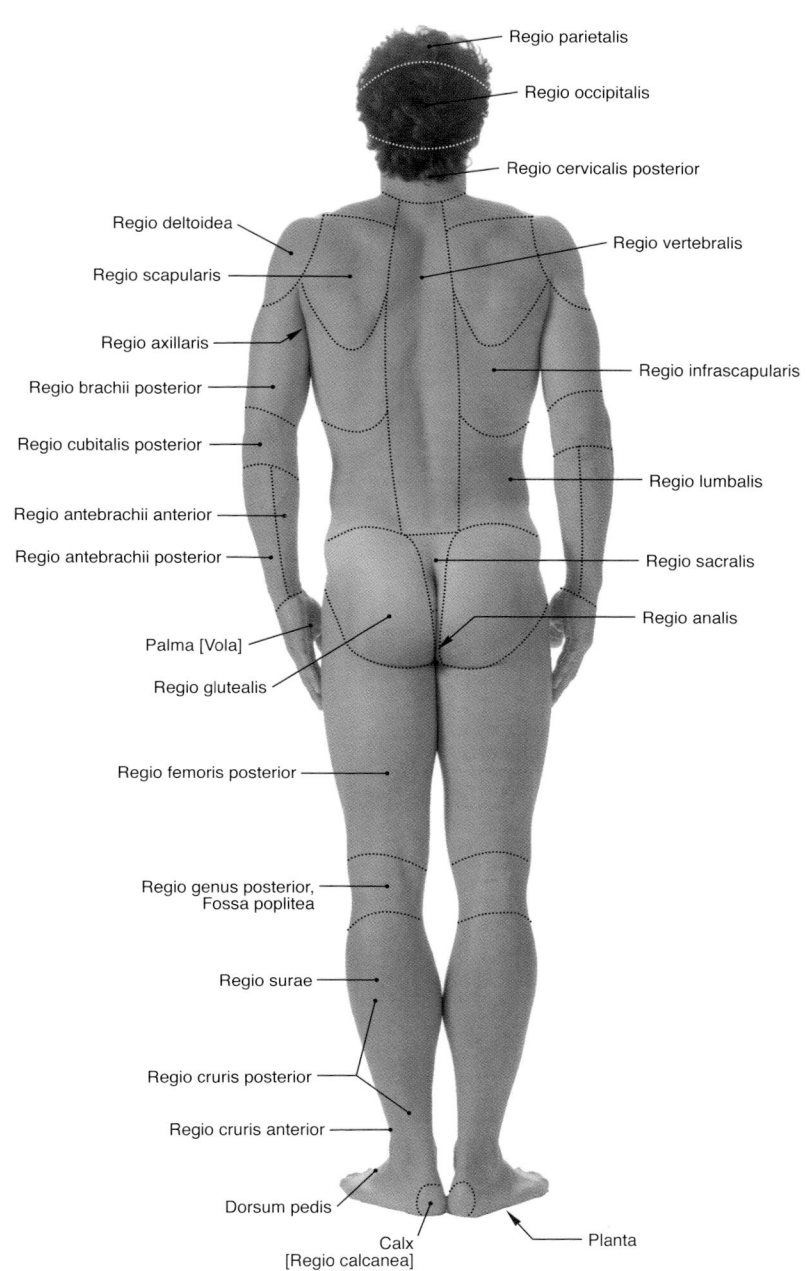

Regio parietalis

Regio occipitalis

Regio cervicalis posterior

Regio deltoidea

Regio vertebralis

Regio scapularis

Regio axillaris

Regio infrascapularis

Regio brachii posterior

Regio cubitalis posterior

Regio antebrachii anterior

Regio lumbalis

Regio antebrachii posterior

Regio sacralis

Regio analis

Palma [Vola]

Regio glutealis

Regio femoris posterior

Regio genus posterior, Fossa poplitea

Regio surae

Regio cruris posterior

Regio cruris anterior

Dorsum pedis

Planta

Calx [Regio calcanea]

Fig. 8   Regions of the human body, Regiones corporis.

Skeleton

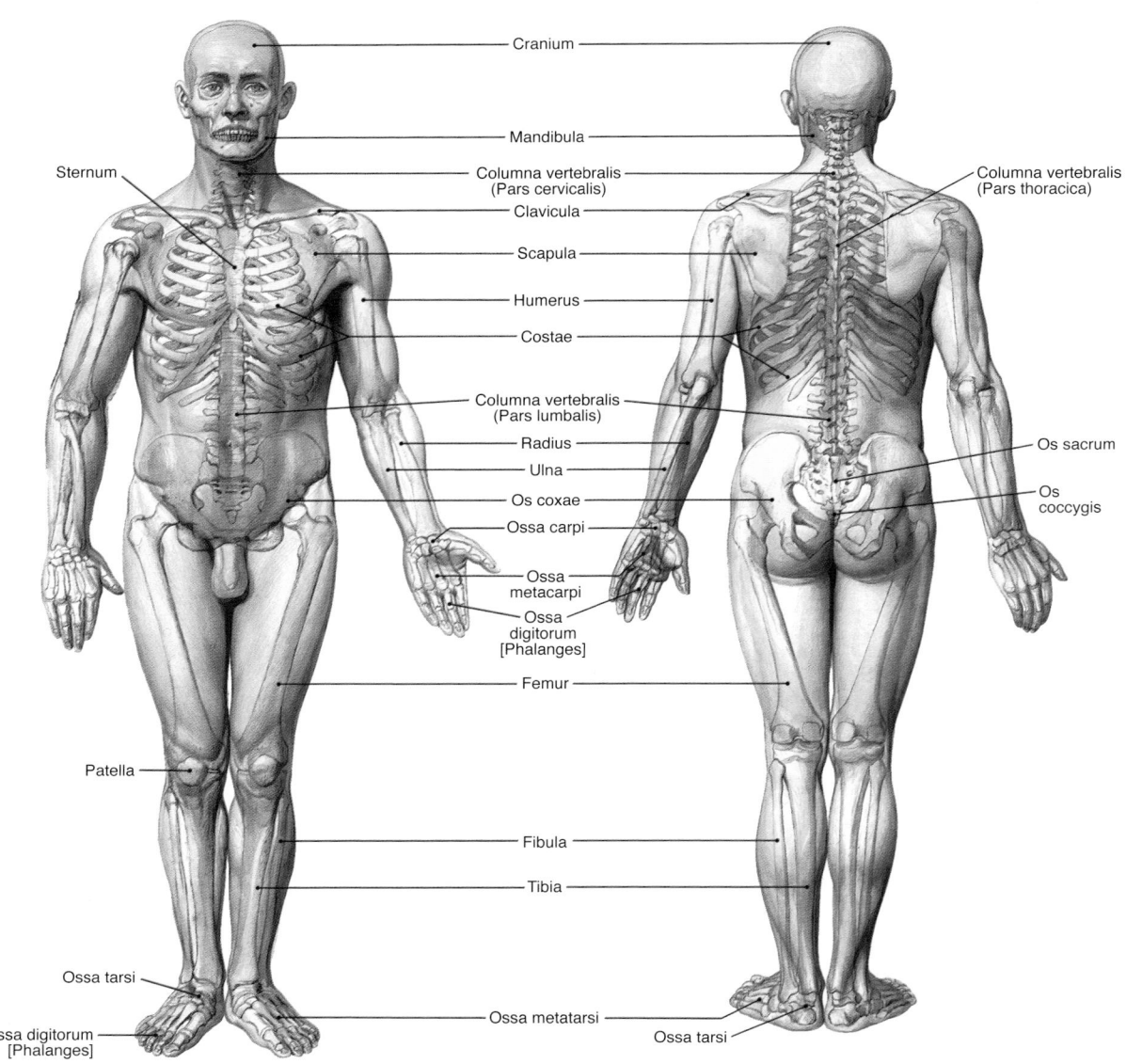

Fig. 9   Overview of the skeleton, Systema skeletale.

Fig. 10   Overview of the skeleton, Systema skeletale.

Parts of the human body

Head, Caput

Neck, Collum

Trunk, Truncus
Thorax, Thorax
Abdomen, Abdomen
Pelvis, Pelvis

Upper limb, Membrum superius
Shoulder girdle, Cingulum pectorale [Cingulum membri superioris]; Arm, Pars libera membri superioris

Lower limb, Membrum inferius
Pelvic girdle, Cingulum pelvicum [Cingulum membri inferioris]; Leg, Pars libera membri inferioris

Skeleton

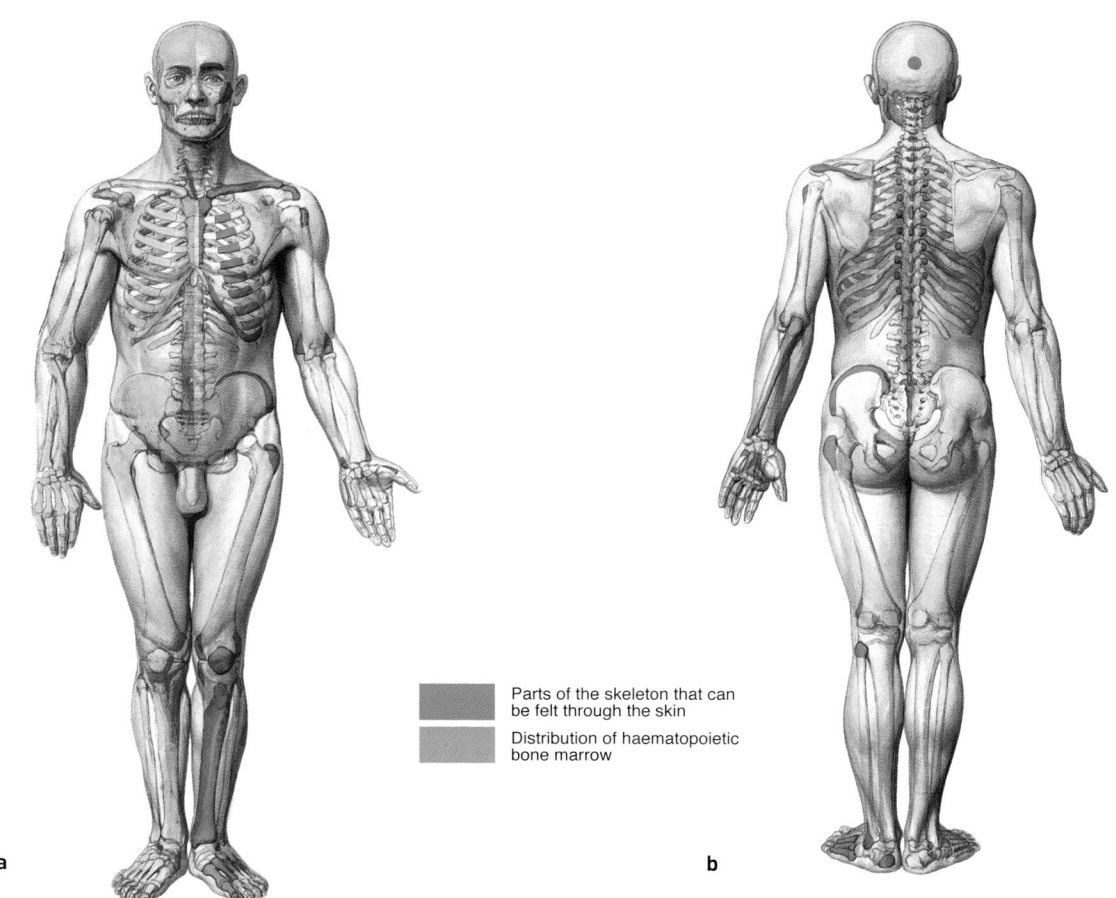

a

b

Parts of the skeleton that can be felt through the skin

Distribution of haematopoietic bone marrow

Fig. 11 a, b   Skeleton, Systema skeletale.

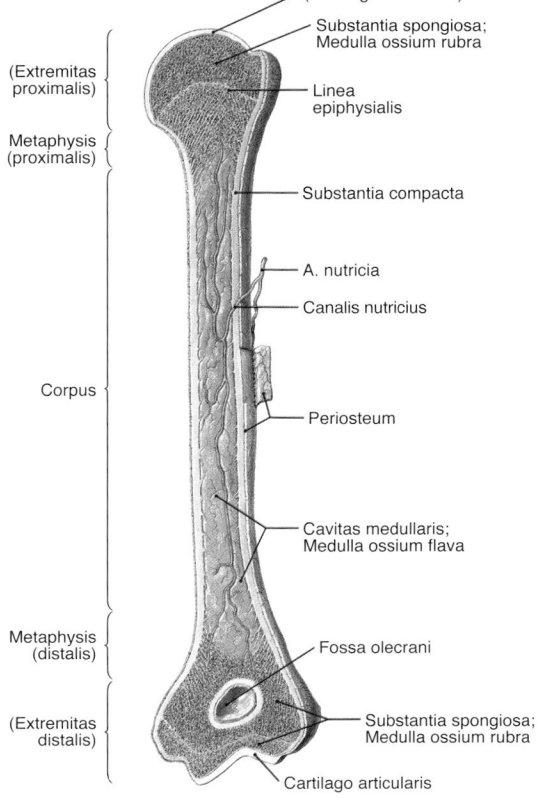

(Extremitas proximalis)

Metaphysis (proximalis)

Corpus

Metaphysis (distalis)

(Extremitas distalis)

a

(Cartilago articularis)

Substantia spongiosa; Medulla ossium rubra

Linea epiphysialis

Substantia compacta

A. nutricia

Canalis nutricius

Periosteum

Cavitas medullaris; Medulla ossium flava

Fossa olecrani

Substantia spongiosa; Medulla ossium rubra

Cartilago articularis

Epiphysis proximalis

*

Vasa nutritia

Diaphysis

Epiphysis distalis

b

Fig. 12 a, b   Structure of tubular bones, Ossa longa; longitudinal sections.
a Humerus, Humerus, of an adult
  Ossified epiphyses (epiphyseal lines) are only poorly visible.
b Humerus, Humerus, of a child
  The epiphyses consist of hyaline cartilage.
  * Epiphysis, epiphyseal plate

Bone development

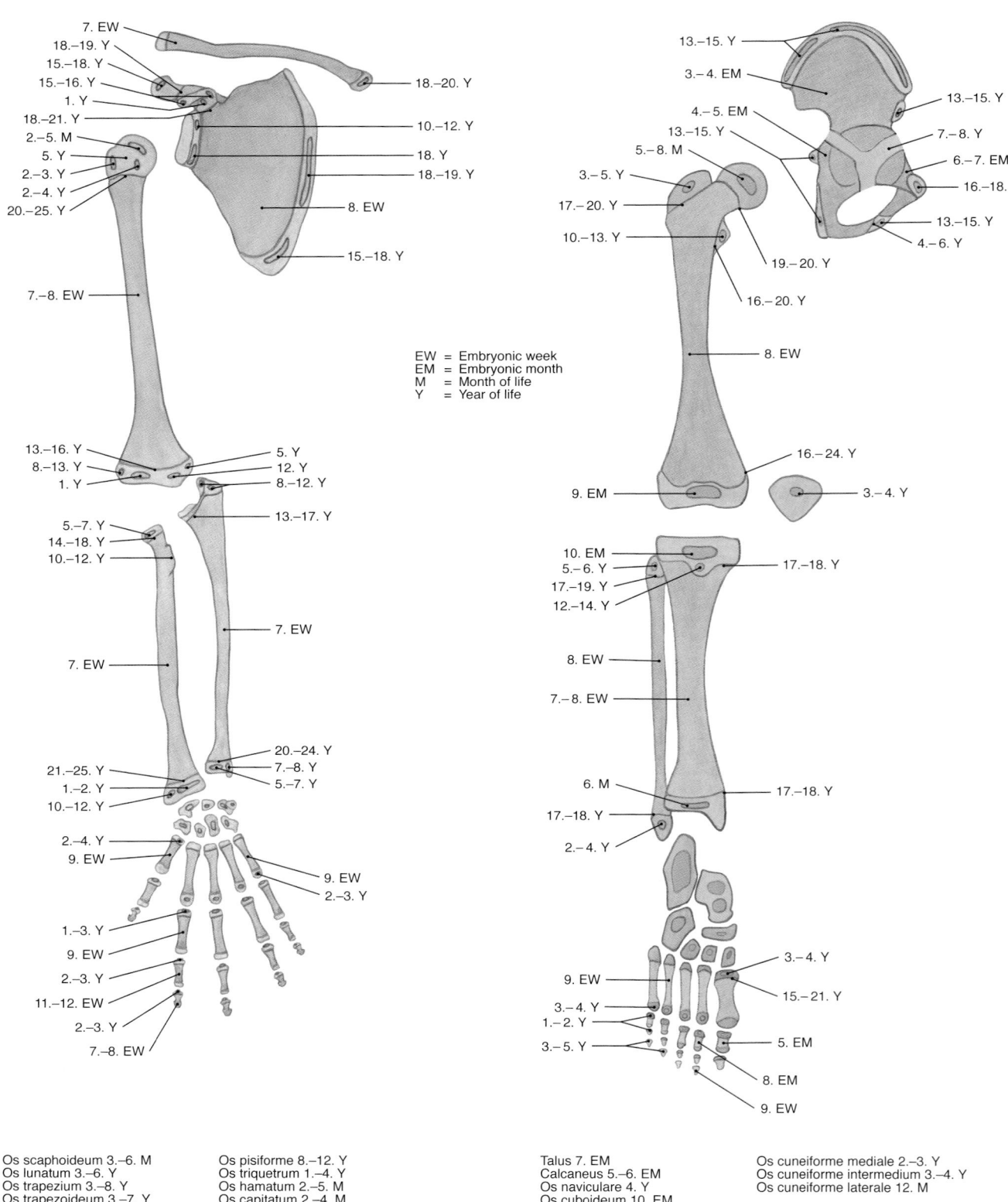

EW = Embryonic week
EM = Embryonic month
M = Month of life
Y = Year of life

Os scaphoideum 3.–6. M	Os pisiforme 8.–12. Y
Os lunatum 3.–6. Y	Os triquetrum 1.–4. Y
Os trapezium 3.–8. Y	Os hamatum 2.–5. M
Os trapezoideum 3.–7. Y	Os capitatum 2.–4. M

Talus 7. EM	Os cuneiforme mediale 2.–3. Y
Calcaneus 5.–6. EM	Os cuneiforme intermedium 3.–4. Y
Os naviculare 4. Y	Os cuneiforme laterale 12. M
Os cuboideum 10. EM	

Fig. 13 Appearance of ossification centres and synossification at the epiphyses of the upper limb (means according to v. LANZ, 1956; EXNER, 1990; HEUCK and BAST, 1994).

Fig. 14 Appearance of ossification centres and synossification at the epiphyses of the lower limb (means according to v. LANZ, 1956; EXNER, 1990; HEUCK and BAST, 1994).

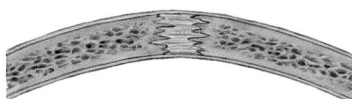

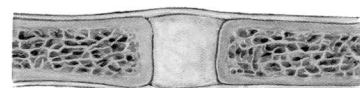

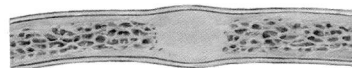

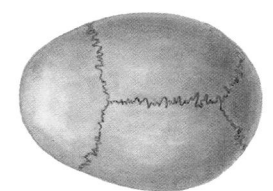

Fig. 15 Fibrous joint, Articulatio fibrosa, exemplified by the sutures of the skull.

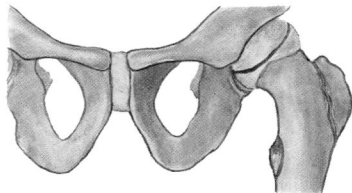

Fig. 16 Cartilaginous joint, Articulatio cartilaginea, exemplified by the pubic bone symphysis.

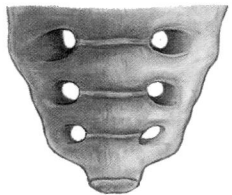

Fig. 17 Osseous joint, Articulatio ossea, exemplified by the sacrum.

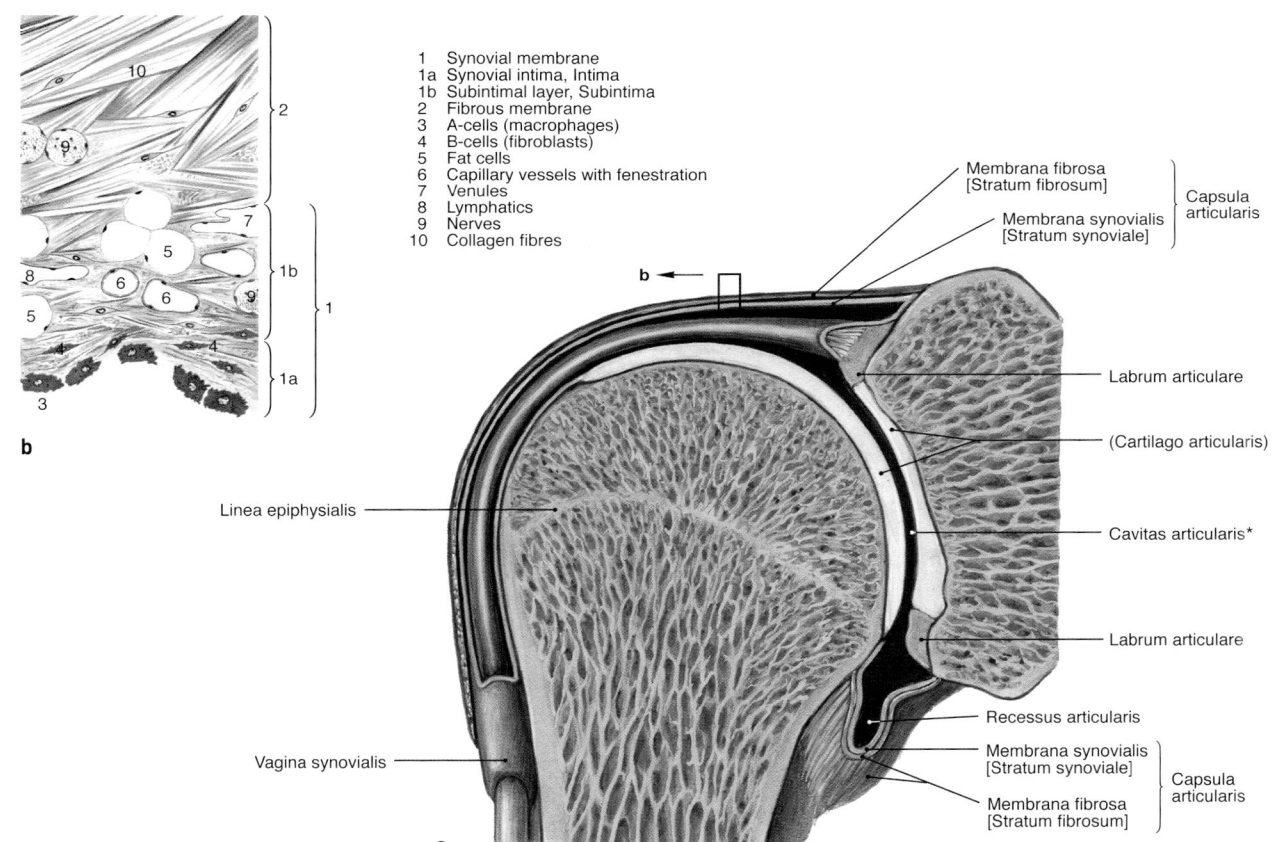

1   Synovial membrane
1a Synovial intima, Intima
1b Subintimal layer, Subintima
2   Fibrous membrane
3   A-cells (macrophages)
4   B-cells (fibroblasts)
5   Fat cells
6   Capillary vessels with fenestration
7   Venules
8   Lymphatics
9   Nerves
10 Collagen fibres

Membrana fibrosa [Stratum fibrosum]
Membrana synovialis [Stratum synoviale]
Capsula articularis

Labrum articulare

(Cartilago articularis)

Linea epiphysialis

Cavitas articularis*

Labrum articulare

Recessus articularis

Membrana synovialis [Stratum synoviale]
Membrana fibrosa [Stratum fibrosum]
Capsula articularis

Vagina synovialis

Fig. 18 a, b Synovial joint, Articulatio synovialis, exemplified by the shoulder joint.
a Section in the scapular plane
b Structure of the joint capsule
* The joint cavity, Cavitas articularis, is illustrated broader to enhance visibility.

Joints

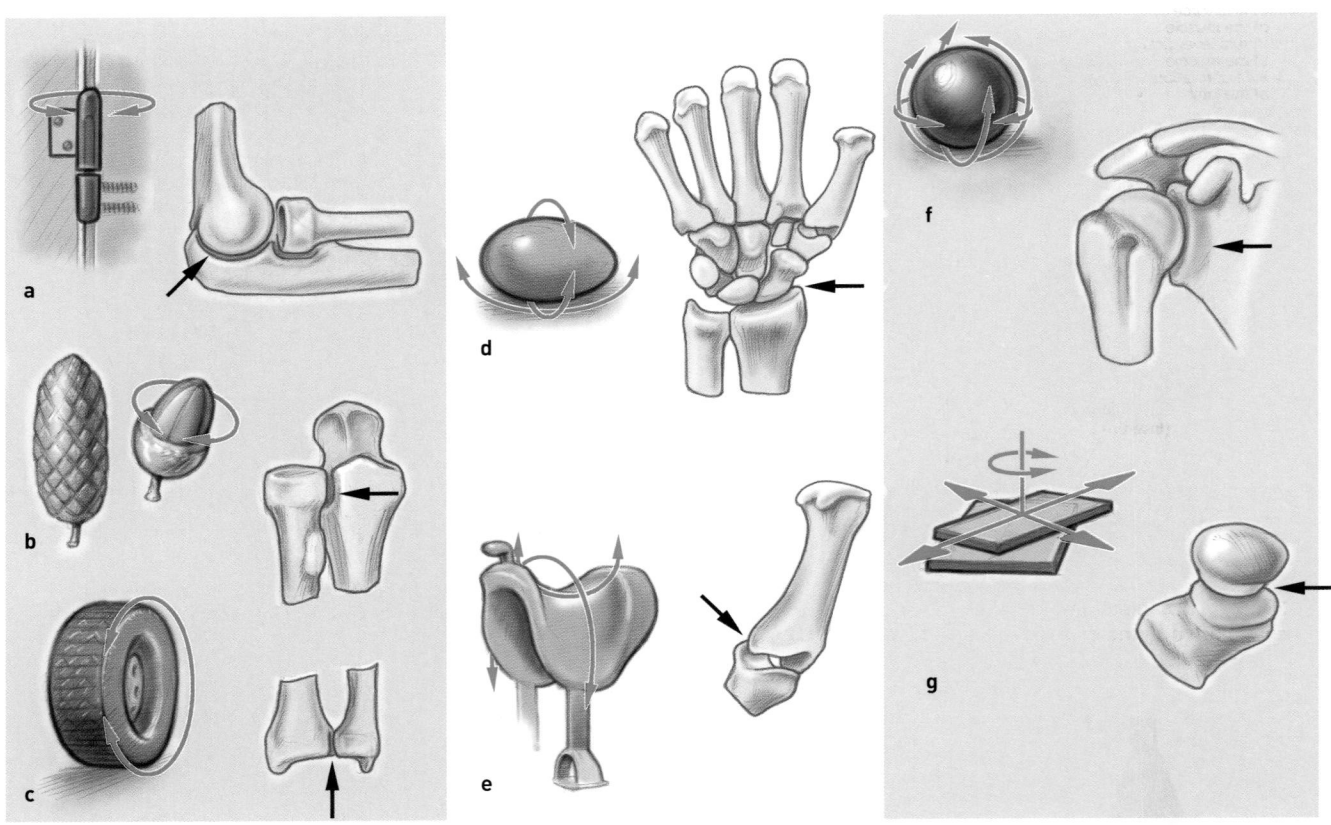

Fig. 19 a–g   Joints, Juncturae synoviales.
a Hinge joint, Articulatio cylindrica
b Conoid joint, Articulatio conoidea
c Pivot joint, Articulatio trochoidea

d Condylar joint, Articulatio ovoidea
e Saddle joint, Articulatio sellaris
f Spheroidal joint, Articulatio spheroidea
g Plane joint, Articulatio plana

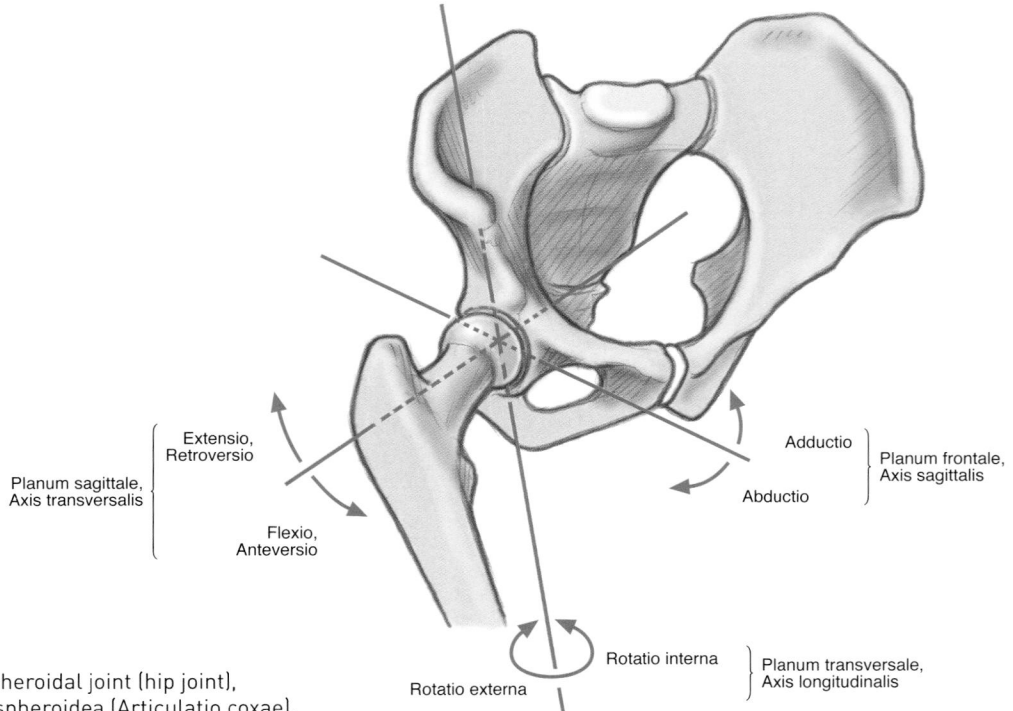

Fig. 20   Spheroidal joint (hip joint),
Articulatio spheroidea (Articulatio coxae).

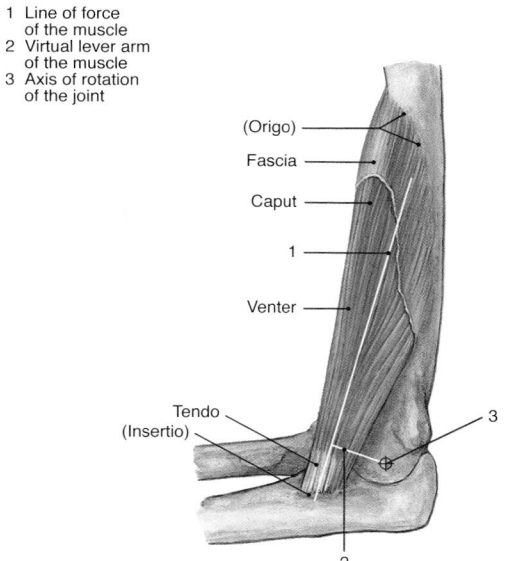

1 Line of force
  of the muscle
2 Virtual lever arm
  of the muscle
3 Axis of rotation
  of the joint

(Origo)

Fascia

Caput

1

Venter

Tendo
(Insertio)

3

2

Fig. 21 Organisation principle of skeletal muscles, exemplified by the brachial muscle, M. brachialis.

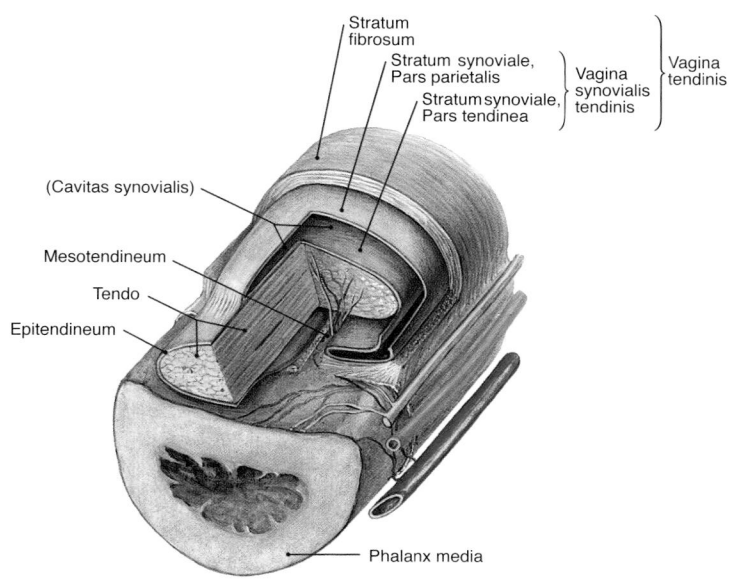

Stratum
fibrosum

Stratum synoviale,
Pars parietalis

Stratum synoviale,
Pars tendinea

Vagina
synovialis
tendinis

Vagina
tendinis

(Cavitas synovialis)

Mesotendineum

Tendo

Epitendineum

Phalanx media

Fig. 22 Structure of a tendon sheath, Vagina tendinis, exemplified by a finger.

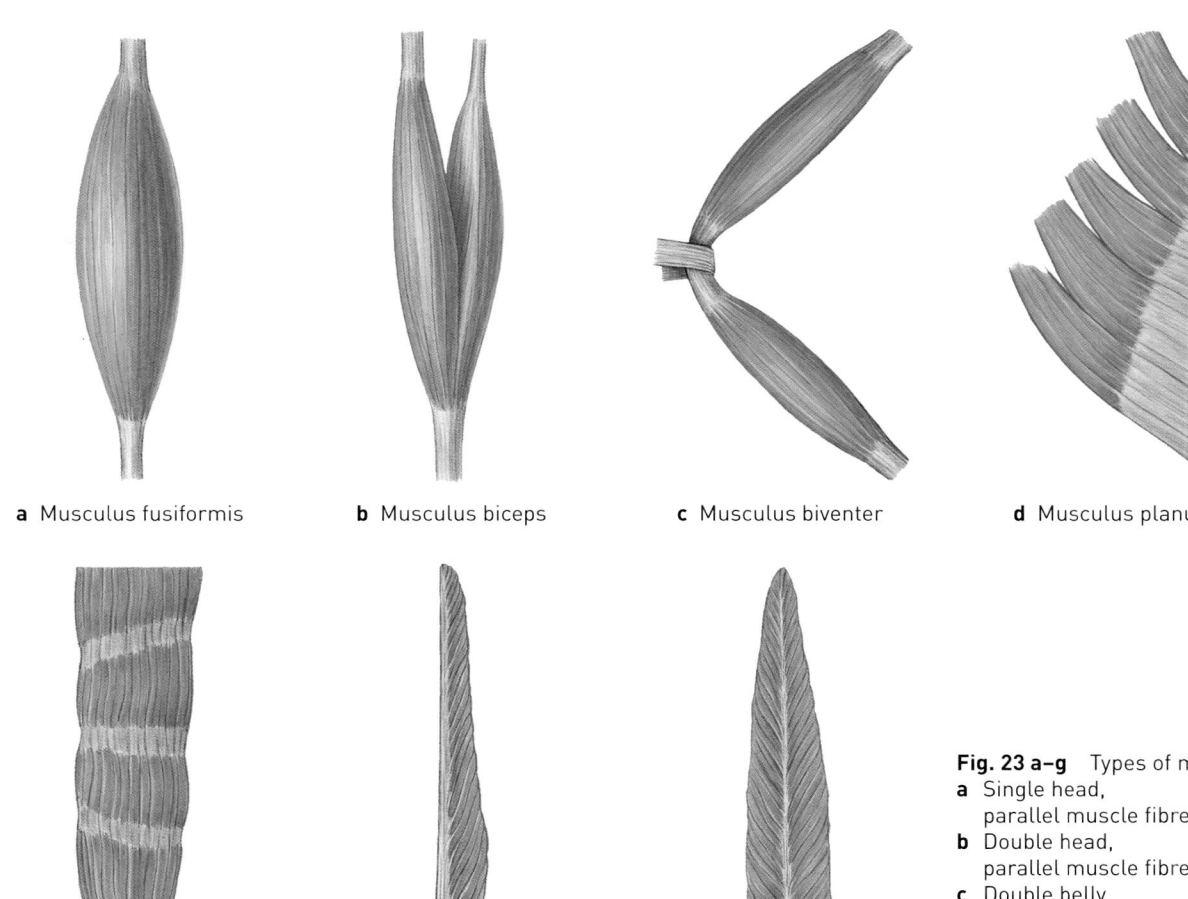

a Musculus fusiformis   **b** Musculus biceps   **c** Musculus biventer   **d** Musculus planus

e Musculus intersectus   **f** Musculus semipennatus   **g** Musculus pennatus

Fig. 23 a–g Types of muscles.
a Single head,
   parallel muscle fibres
b Double head,
   parallel muscle fibres
c Double belly,
   parallel muscle fibres
d Multi-head, flat muscle
e Multi-belly muscle with
   tendinous intersections
f Unipennate muscle
g Bipennate muscle

Skeletal muscles

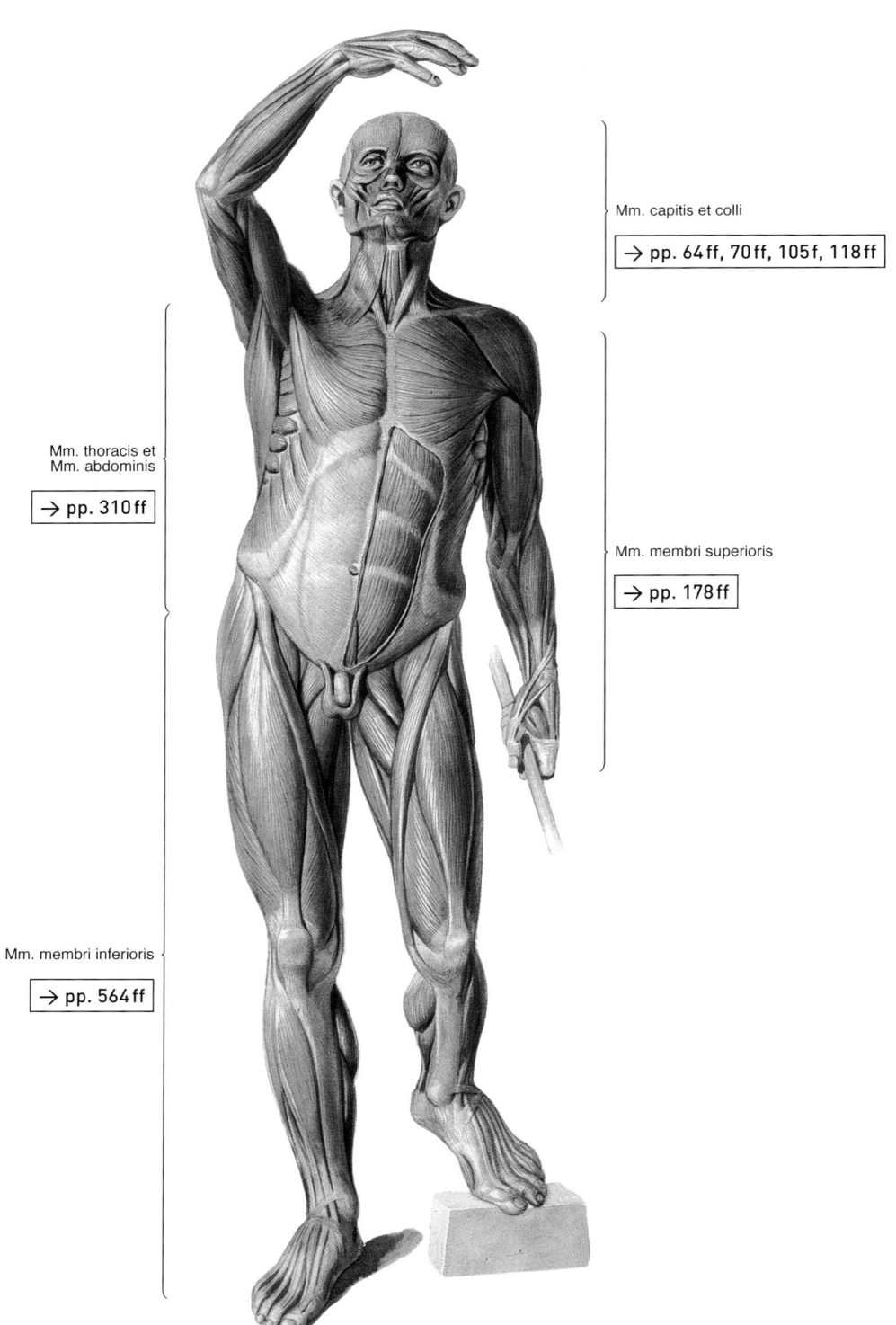

Mm. capitis et colli

→ pp. 64 ff, 70 ff, 105 f, 118 ff

Mm. thoracis et
Mm. abdominis

→ pp. 310 ff

Mm. membri superioris

→ pp. 178 ff

Mm. membri inferioris

→ pp. 564 ff

Fig. 24 Overview of the skeletal muscles.

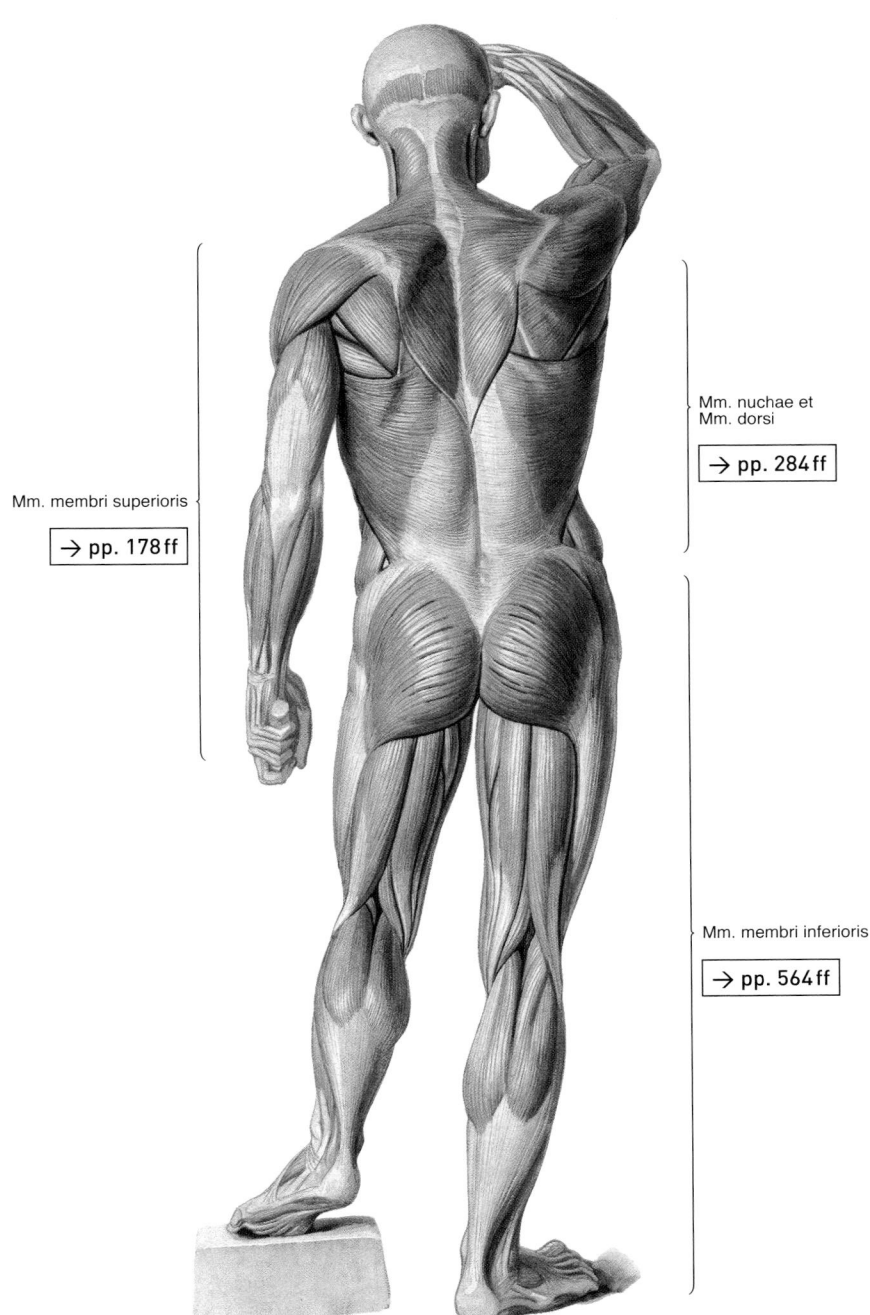

Mm. nuchae et
Mm. dorsi

→ pp. 284 ff

Mm. membri superioris

→ pp. 178 ff

Mm. membri inferioris

→ pp. 564 ff

Fig. 25 Overview of the skeletal muscles.

Digestive and respiratory system

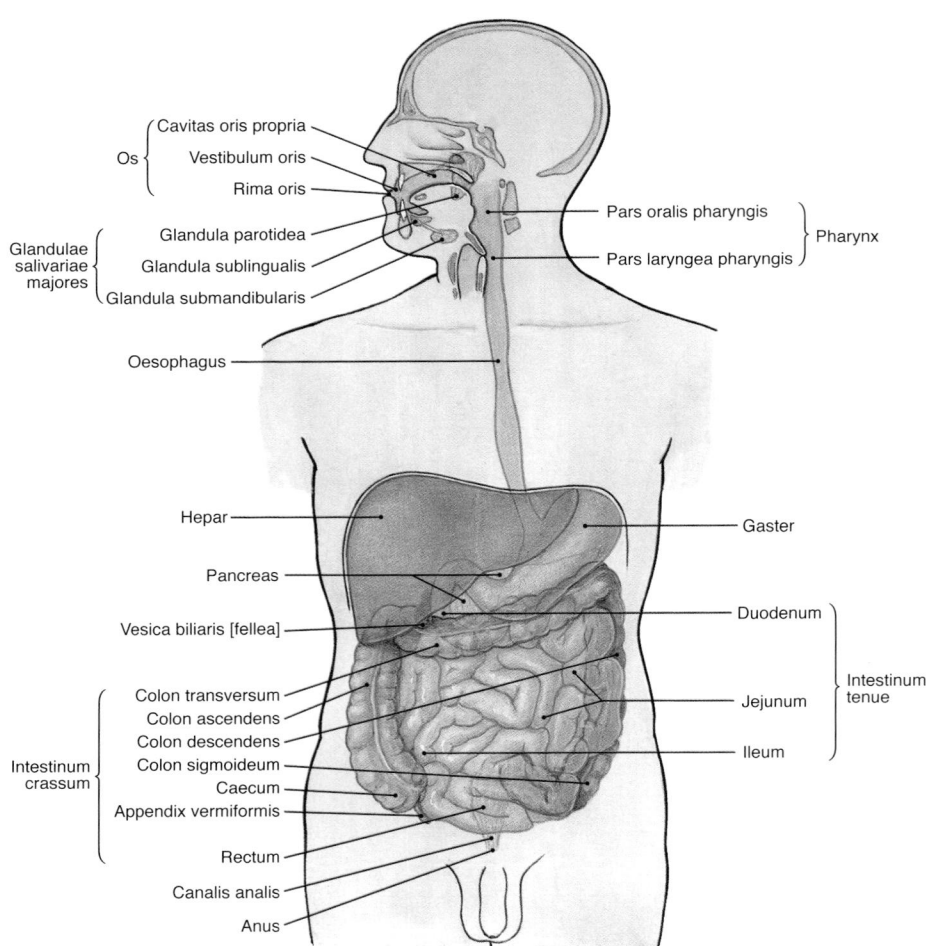

Fig. 26   Overview of the digestive system.

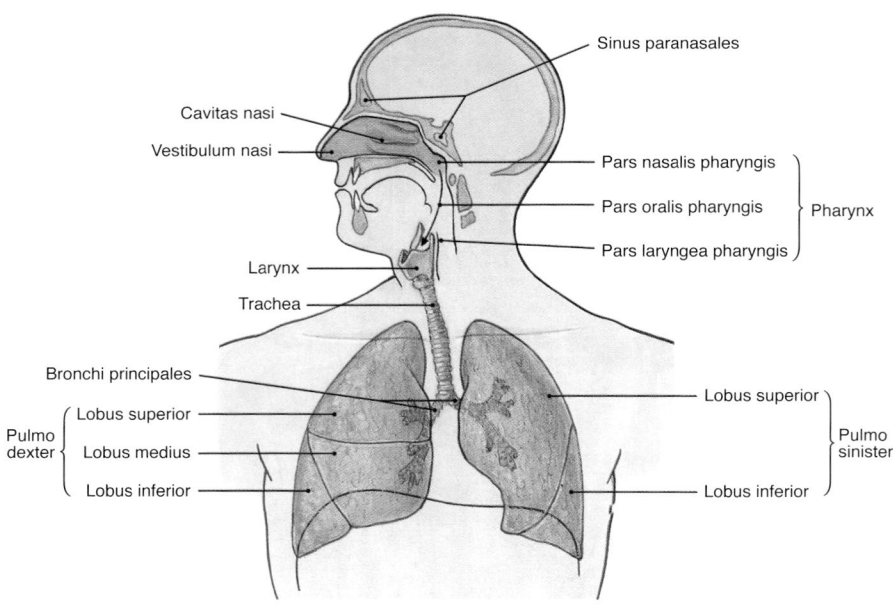

Fig. 27   Overview of the respiratory system.

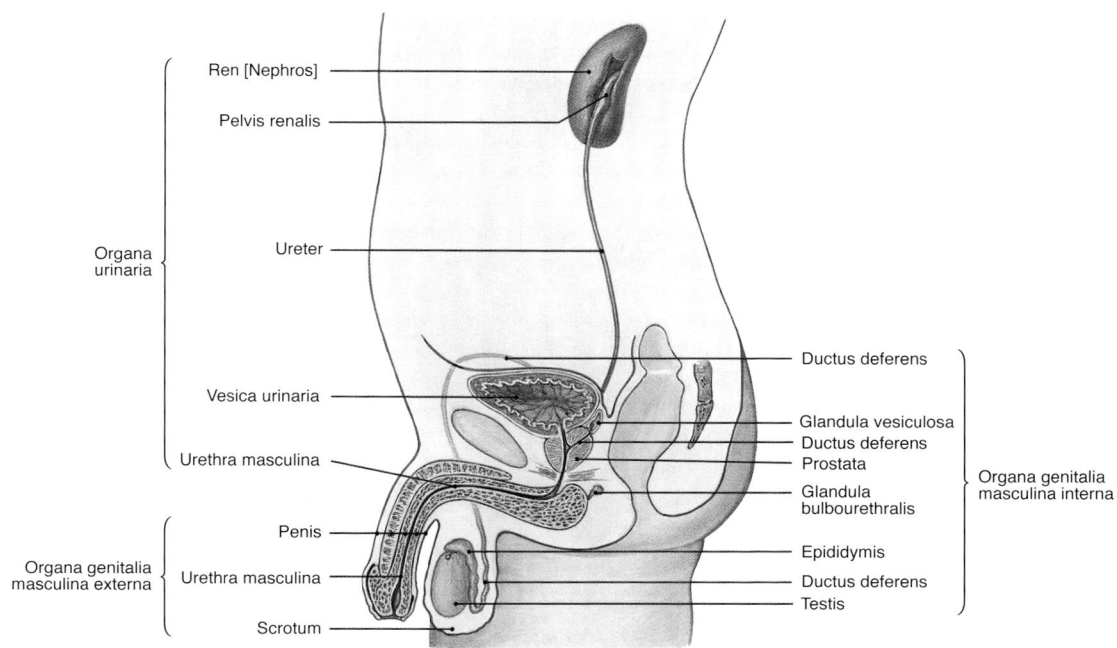

Fig. 28 Overview of the urinary and genital system of the male.

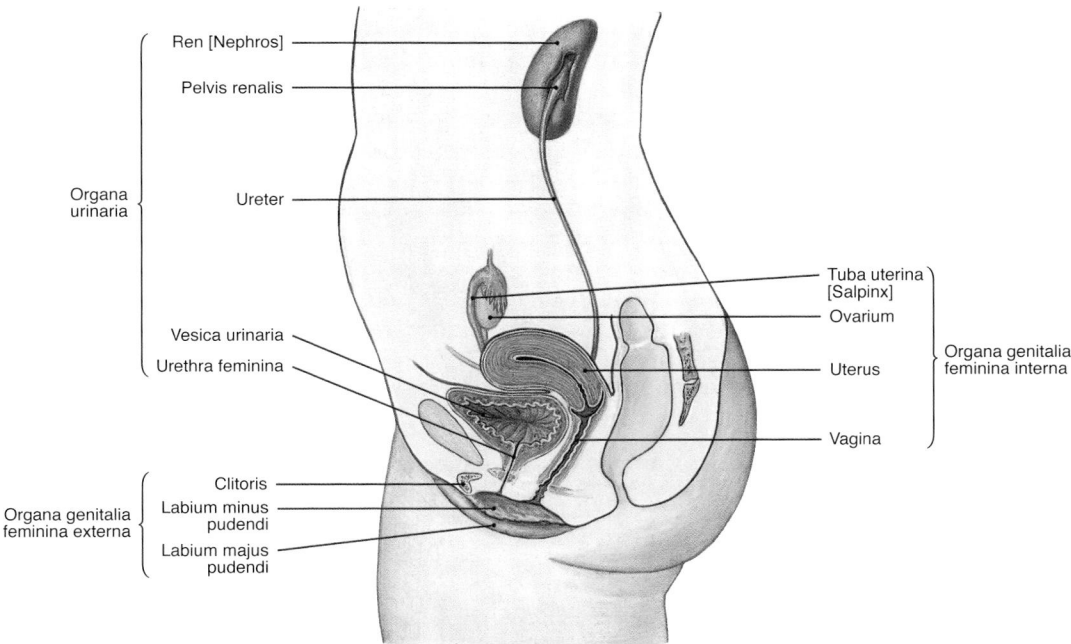

Fig. 29 Overview of the urinary and genital system of the female.

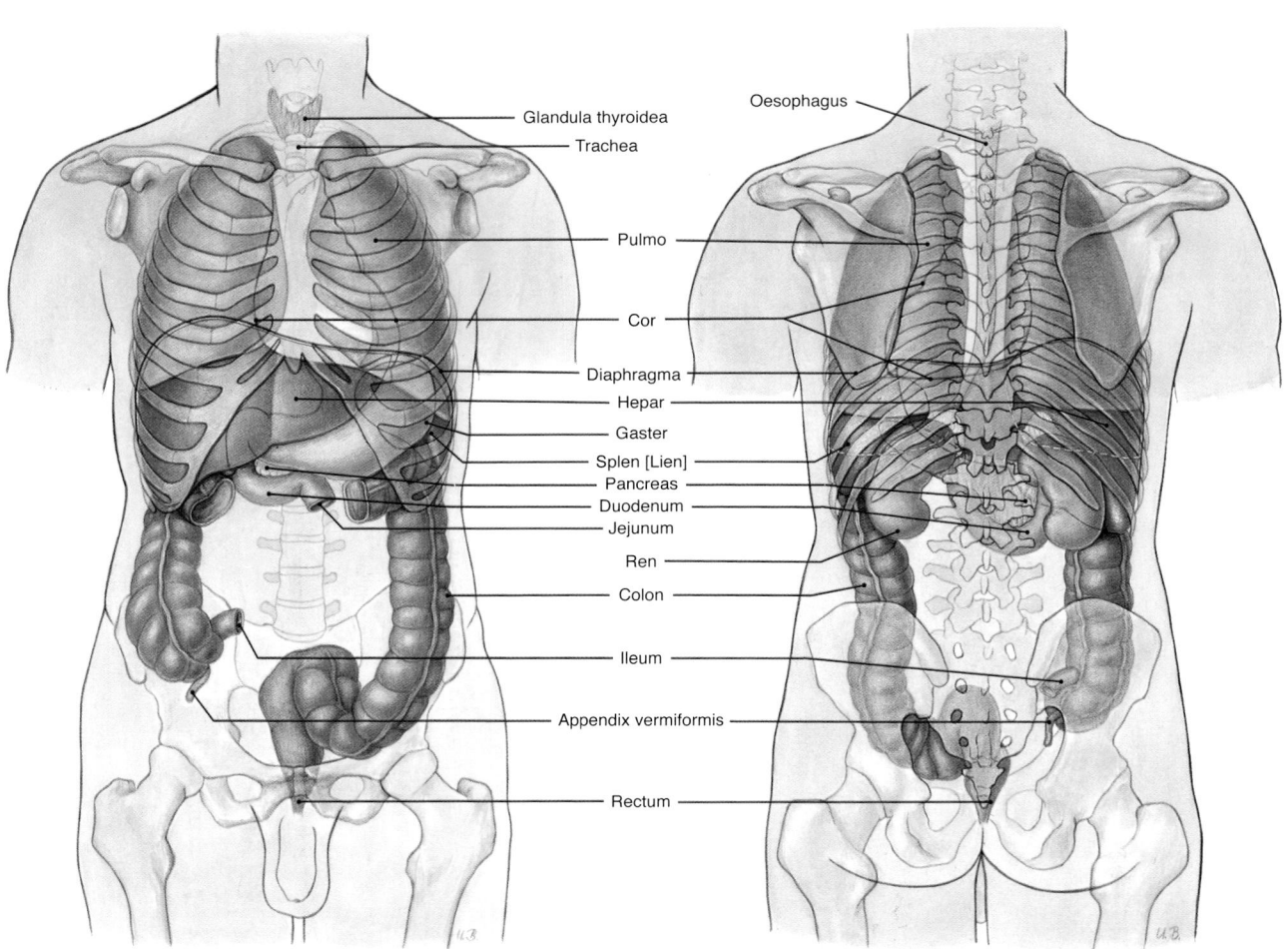

Glandula thyroidea
Trachea
Oesophagus
Pulmo
Cor
Diaphragma
Hepar
Gaster
Splen [Lien]
Pancreas
Duodenum
Jejunum
Ren
Colon
Ileum
Appendix vermiformis
Rectum

Fig. 30 Projection of the internal organs onto the surface of the body.

Fig. 31 Projection of the internal organs onto the surface of the body.

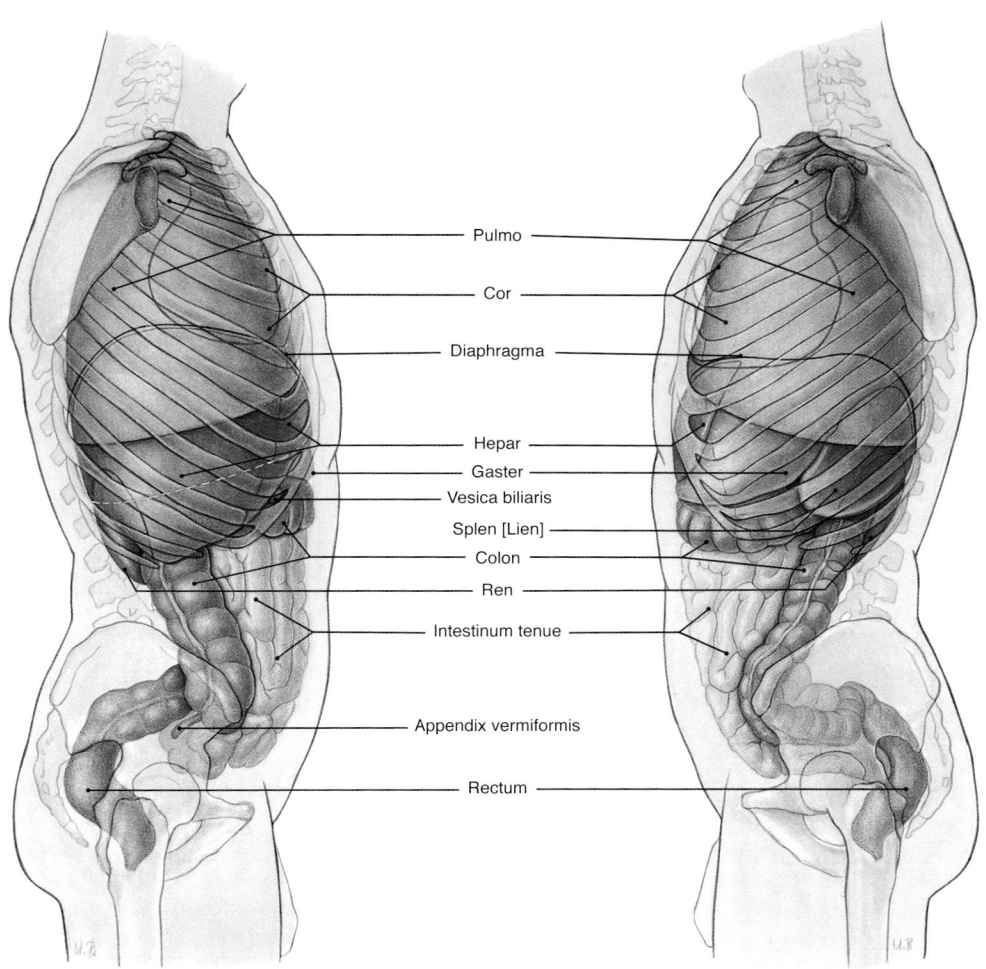

Pulmo

Cor

Diaphragma

Hepar
Gaster
Vesica biliaris
Splen [Lien]
Colon
Ren
Intestinum tenue

Appendix vermiformis

Rectum

Fig. 32   Projection of the internal organs onto the surface of the body.

Fig. 33   Projection of the internal organs onto the surface of the body.

Arteries

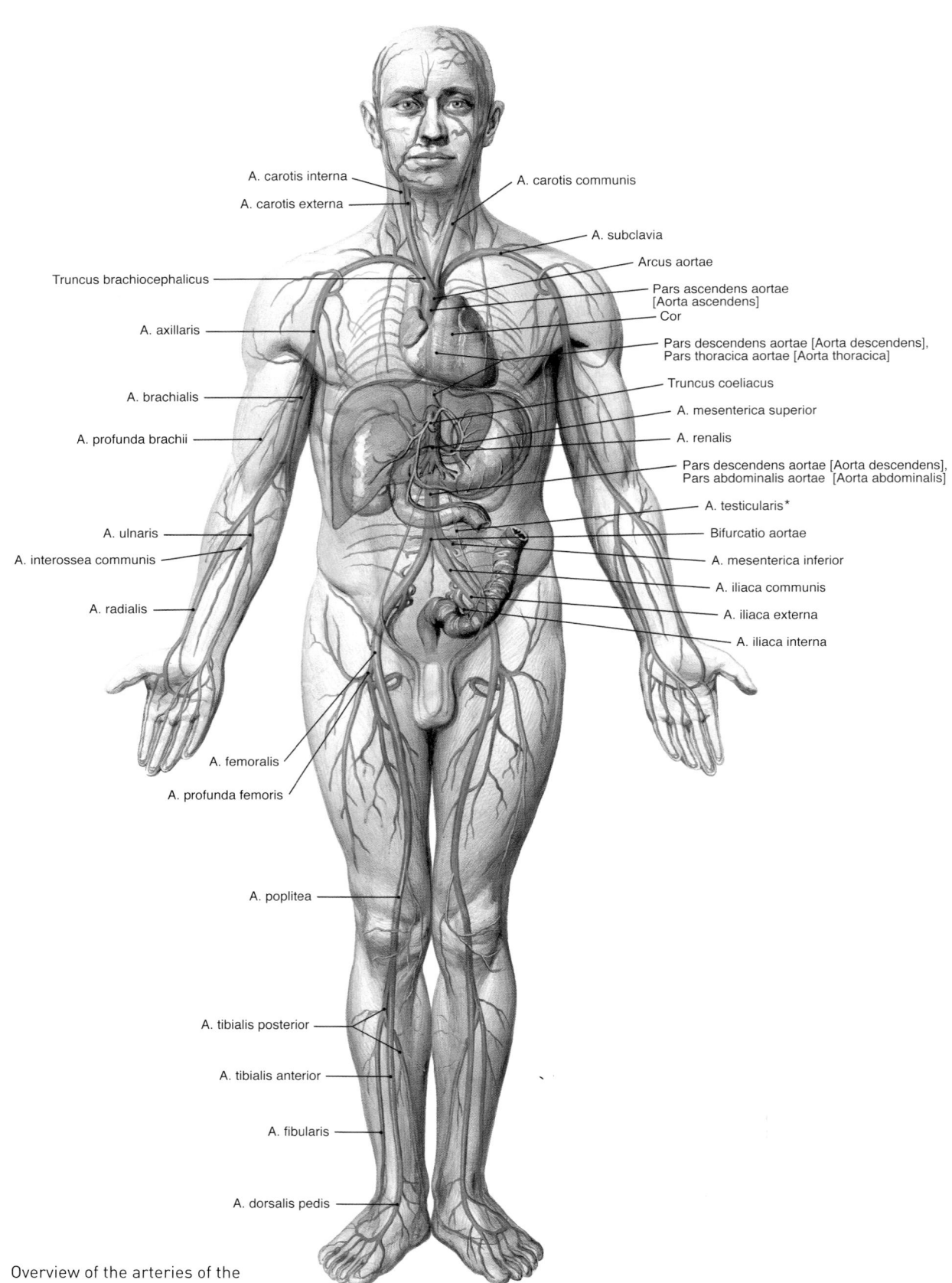

A. carotis interna

A. carotis externa

A. carotis communis

A. subclavia

Arcus aortae

Truncus brachiocephalicus

Pars ascendens aortae [Aorta ascendens]

Cor

A. axillaris

Pars descendens aortae [Aorta descendens], Pars thoracica aortae [Aorta thoracica]

Truncus coeliacus

A. brachialis

A. mesenterica superior

A. profunda brachii

A. renalis

Pars descendens aortae [Aorta descendens], Pars abdominalis aortae [Aorta abdominalis]

A. testicularis*

A. ulnaris

Bifurcatio aortae

A. interossea communis

A. mesenterica inferior

A. iliaca communis

A. radialis

A. iliaca externa

A. iliaca interna

A. femoralis

A. profunda femoris

A. poplitea

A. tibialis posterior

A. tibialis anterior

A. fibularis

A. dorsalis pedis

Fig. 34 Overview of the arteries of the systemic circulation.
* In the female: ovarian artery, A. ovarica

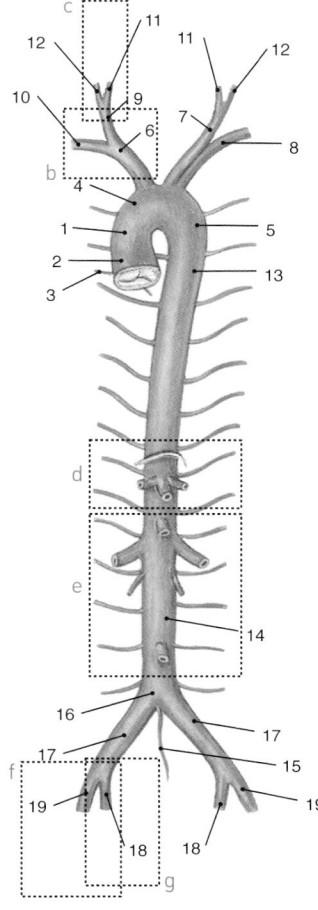

a

1 Pars ascendens aortae
2 Bulbus aortae
3 Aa. coronariae
4 Arcus aortae
5 Isthmus aortae
6 Truncus brachiocephalicus
7 A. carotis communis sinistra
8 A. subclavia sinistra
9 A. carotis communis dextra
10 A. subclavia dextra
11 A. carotis interna
12 A. carotis externa
13 Pars thoracica aortae
14 Pars abdominalis aortae
15 A. sacralis mediana
16 Bifurcatio aortae
17 A. iliaca communis
18 A. iliaca interna
19 A. iliaca externa

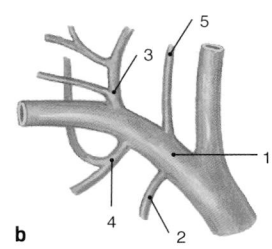

b

1 A. subclavia
2 A. thoracica interna
3 Truncus thyrocervicalis
4 Truncus costocervicalis
5 A. vertebralis

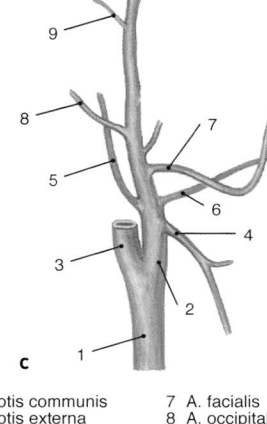

c

1 A. carotis communis
2 A. carotis externa
3 A. carotis interna
4 A. thyroidea superior
5 A. pharyngea ascendens
6 A. lingualis
7 A. facialis
8 A. occipitalis
9 A. auricularis posterior
10 A. temporalis superficialis
11 A. maxillaris

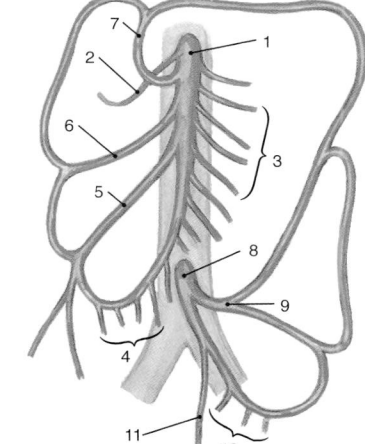

d

1 Truncus coeliacus
2 A. gastrica sinistra
3 A. hepatica communis
4 A. splenica

e

1 A. mesenterica superior
2 A. pancreatico-duodenalis inferior
3 Aa. jejunales
4 Aa. ileales
5 A. ileocolica
6 A. colica dextra
7 A. colica media
8 A. mesenterica inferior
9 A. colica sinistra
10 Aa. sigmoideae
11 A. rectalis superior

Fig. 35 a–g Aorta, Aorta, and greater arteries; schema of the branching pattern.
a Aorta, Aorta
b Subclavian artery, A. subclavia
c External carotid artery, A. carotis externa
d Coeliac trunk, Truncus coeliacus
e Superior and inferior mesenteric artery, Aa. mesentericae superior et inferior
f External iliac artery, A. iliaca externa
g Internal iliac artery, A. iliaca interna

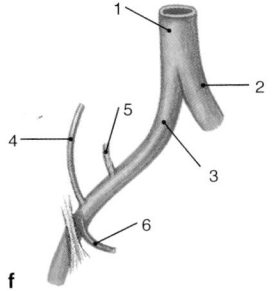

f

1 A. iliaca communis
2 A. iliaca interna
3 A. iliaca externa
4 A. epigastrica inferior
5 A. circumflexa ilium profunda
6 R. pubicus

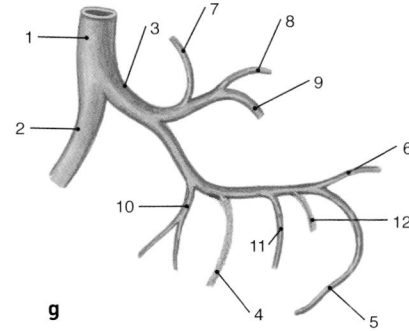

g

1 A. iliaca communis
2 A. iliaca externa
3 A. iliaca interna
4 A. obturatoria
5 A. pudenda interna
6 A. glutea inferior
7 A. iliolumbalis
8 Aa. sacrales laterales
9 A. glutea superior
10 A. umbilicalis, Pars patens
11 A. vesicalis inferior
12 A. rectalis media

Veins

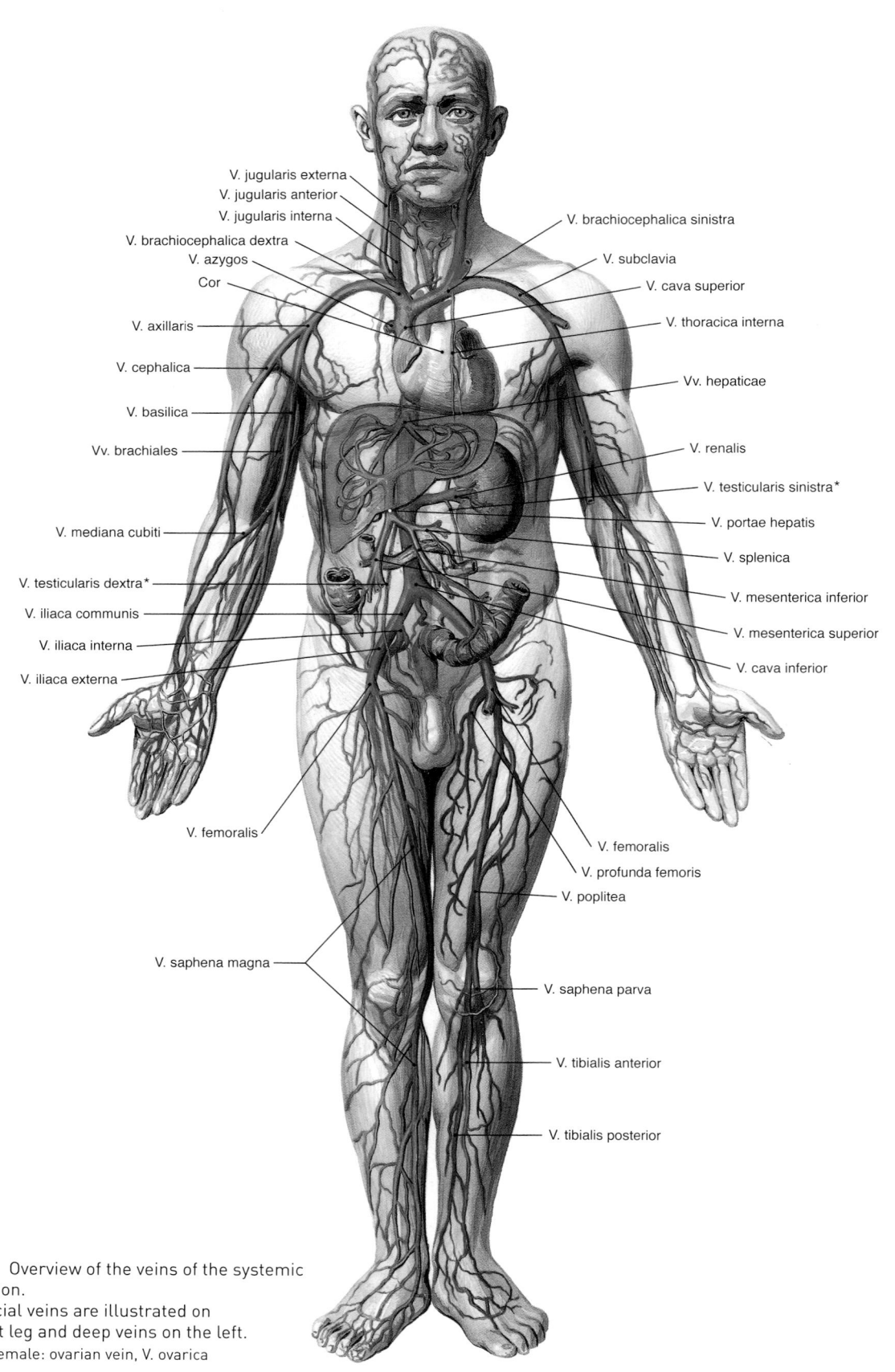

V. jugularis externa
V. jugularis anterior
V. jugularis interna
V. brachiocephalica dextra
V. azygos
Cor
V. axillaris
V. cephalica
V. basilica
Vv. brachiales
V. mediana cubiti
V. testicularis dextra*
V. iliaca communis
V. iliaca interna
V. iliaca externa
V. femoralis
V. saphena magna

V. brachiocephalica sinistra
V. subclavia
V. cava superior
V. thoracica interna
Vv. hepaticae
V. renalis
V. testicularis sinistra*
V. portae hepatis
V. splenica
V. mesenterica inferior
V. mesenterica superior
V. cava inferior
V. femoralis
V. profunda femoris
V. poplitea
V. saphena parva
V. tibialis anterior
V. tibialis posterior

Fig. 36   Overview of the veins of the systemic
circulation.
Superficial veins are illustrated on
the right leg and deep veins on the left.
* In the female: ovarian vein, V. ovarica

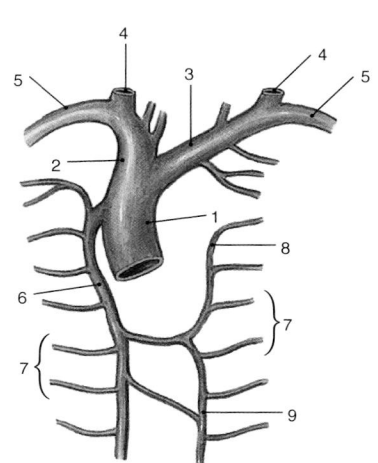

1 V. cava superior
2 V. brachiocephalica dextra
3 V. brachiocephalica sinistra
4 V. jugularis interna
5 V. subclavia

6 V. azygos
7 Vv. intercostales posteriores
8 V. hemiazygos accessoria
9 V. hemiazygos

Fig. 37 Superior vena cava, V. cava superior; schema of the tributaries.

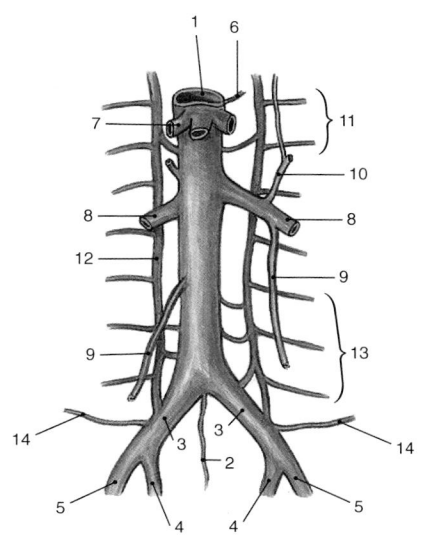

1 V. cava inferior
2 V. sacralis mediana
3 V. iliaca communis
4 V. iliaca interna
5 V. iliaca externa
6 V. phrenica inferior
7 Vv. hepaticae

8 V. renalis
9 V. testicularis/ovarica
10 V. suprarenalis
11 Vv. intercostales posteriores
12 V. lumbalis ascendens
13 Vv. lumbales
14 V. iliolumbalis

Fig. 38 Inferior vena cava, V. cava inferior; schema of the tributaries.

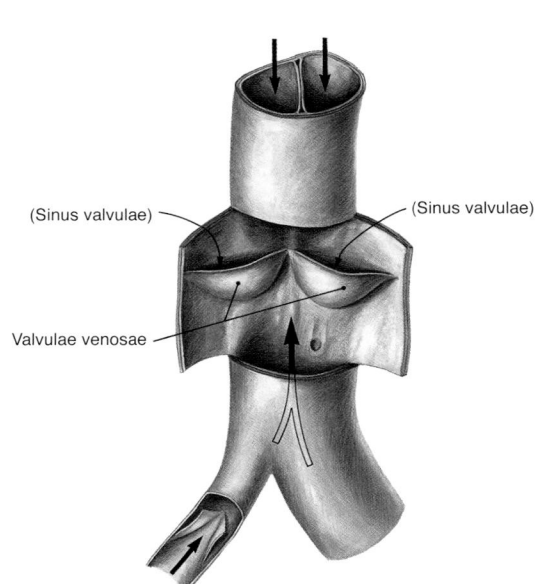

Fig. 39 Functional principle of venous valves. The arrows pointing upwards indicate the flow of blood. The valves close upon backflow of the blood (arrows pointing downwards).

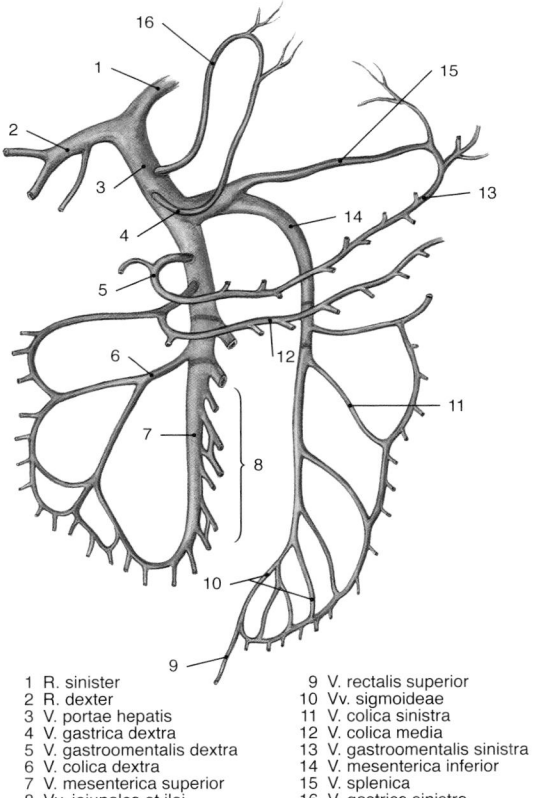

1 R. sinister
2 R. dexter
3 V. portae hepatis
4 V. gastrica dextra
5 V. gastroomentalis dextra
6 V. colica dextra
7 V. mesenterica superior
8 Vv. jejunales et ilei

9 V. rectalis superior
10 Vv. sigmoideae
11 V. colica sinistra
12 V. colica media
13 V. gastroomentalis sinistra
14 V. mesenterica inferior
15 V. splenica
16 V. gastrica sinistra

Fig. 40 Hepatic portal vein, V. portae hepatis.

Foetal circulation

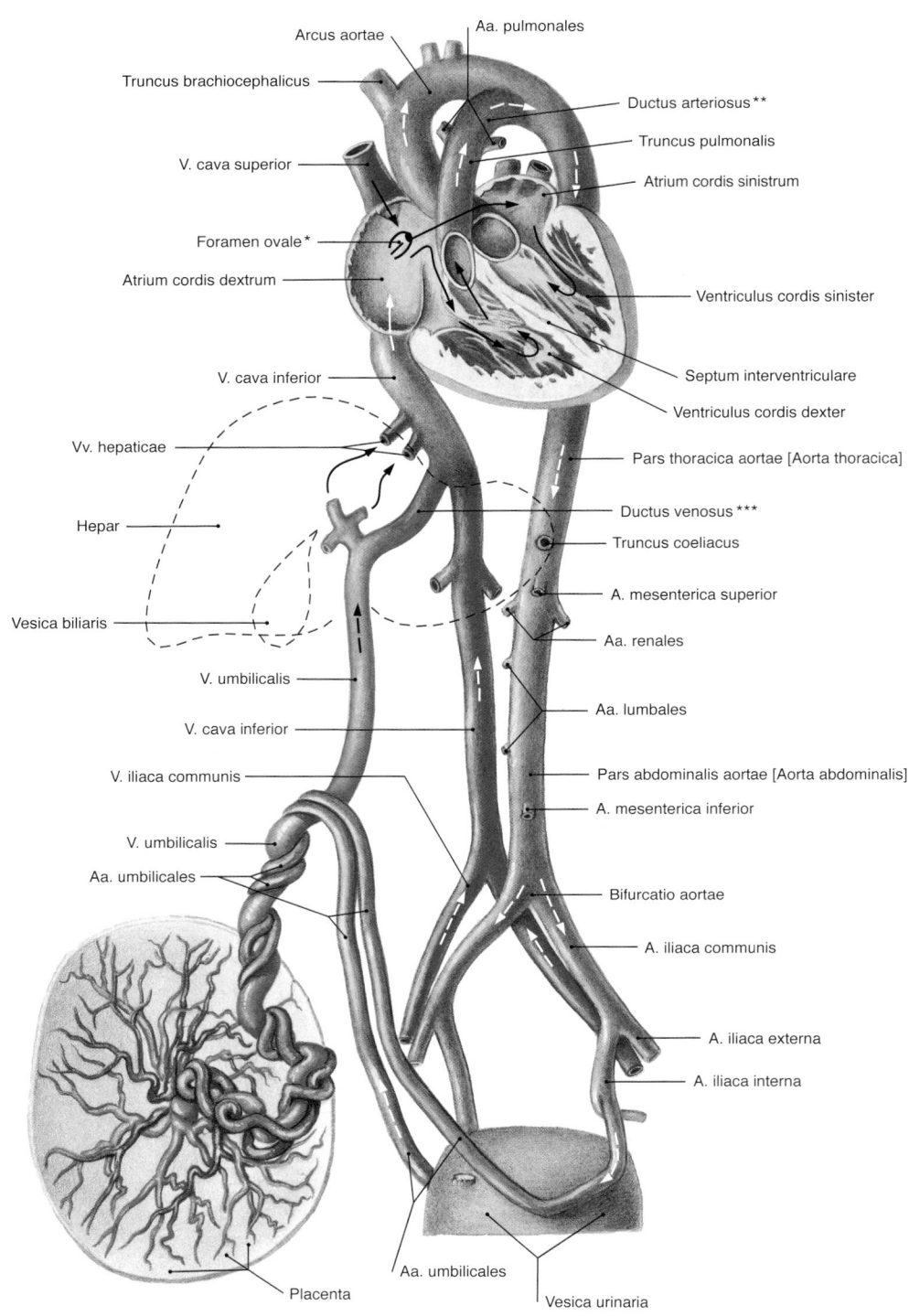

Arcus aortae
Truncus brachiocephalicus
V. cava superior
Foramen ovale *
Atrium cordis dextrum
V. cava inferior
Vv. hepaticae
Hepar
Vesica biliaris
V. umbilicalis
V. cava inferior
V. iliaca communis
V. umbilicalis
Aa. umbilicales
Placenta

Aa. pulmonales
Ductus arteriosus **
Truncus pulmonalis
Atrium cordis sinistrum
Ventriculus cordis sinister
Septum interventriculare
Ventriculus cordis dexter
Pars thoracica aortae [Aorta thoracica]
Ductus venosus ***
Truncus coeliacus
A. mesenterica superior
Aa. renales
Aa. lumbales
Pars abdominalis aortae [Aorta abdominalis]
A. mesenterica inferior
Bifurcatio aortae
A. iliaca communis
A. iliaca externa
A. iliaca interna
Aa. umbilicales
Vesica urinaria

Fig. 41 Schema of foetal circulation.
The different colours indicate the oxygen content in the blood:
red = rich in oxygen,
blue = poor in oxygen,
purple = mixed blood.
Arrows indicate the direction of the blood flow.
* Short-circuit between the right and the left atrium
** Short-circuit between the pulmonary trunk and the arch of aorta
*** Short-circuit between the umbilical vein and the inferior vena cava

Conversion from foetal to postnatal circulation:
* The valve-like connection between the right and the left atrium via the foramen ovale is passively closed at the onset of respiratory activity in the lungs.
** The ductus arteriosus (BOTALLO), on the other hand, closes only during the first months of life as its lumen gradually obliterates by epithelial proliferation and increased tension of the wall.
*** The ductus venosus (ARANTIUS) obliterates after birth and becomes the ligamentum venosum in the portal area of the liver.

Lymphatic system

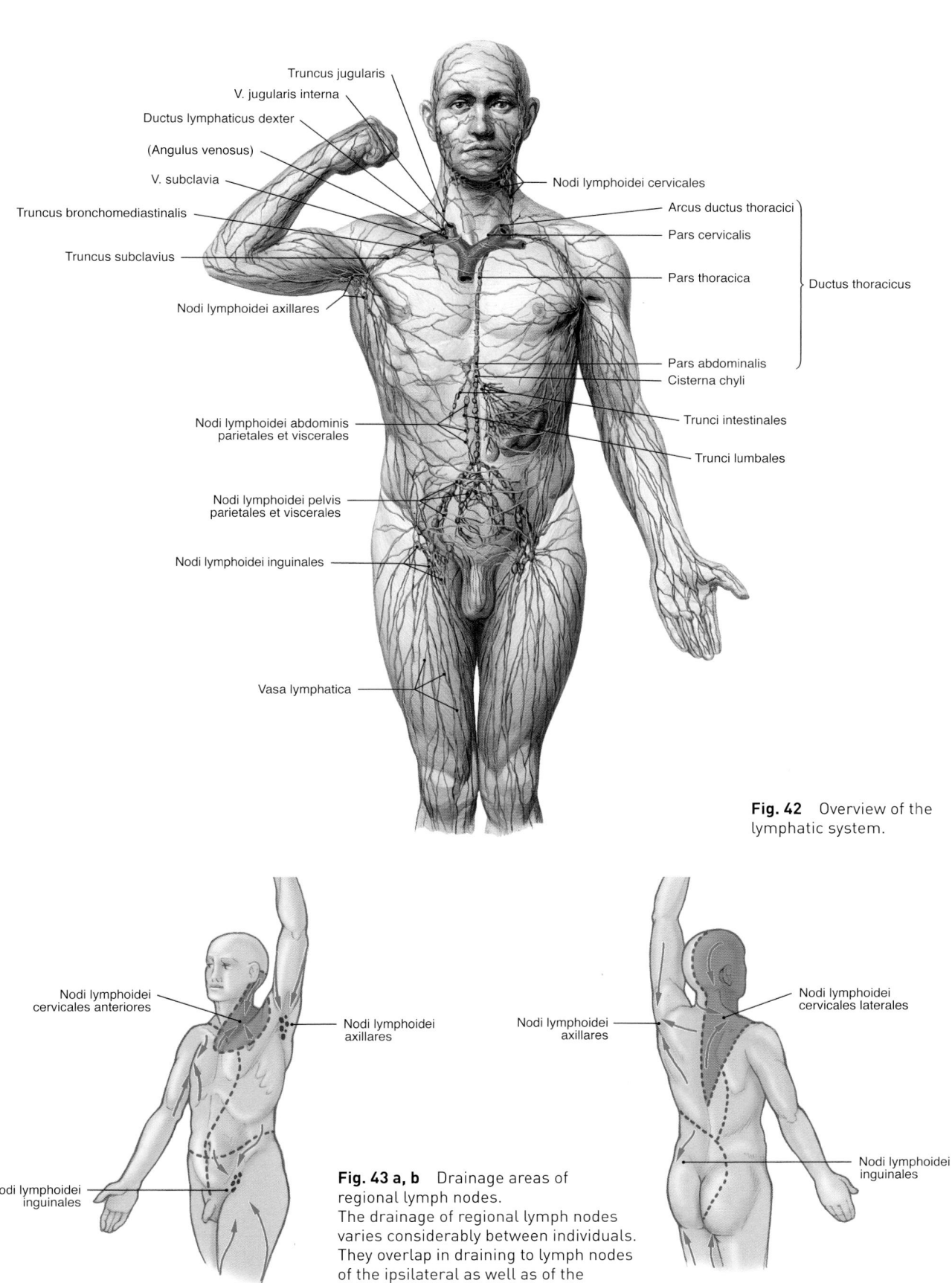

Truncus jugularis
V. jugularis interna
Ductus lymphaticus dexter
(Angulus venosus)
V. subclavia
Truncus bronchomediastinalis
Truncus subclavius
Nodi lymphoidei axillares
Nodi lymphoidei abdominis parietales et viscerales
Nodi lymphoidei pelvis parietales et viscerales
Nodi lymphoidei inguinales
Vasa lymphatica

Nodi lymphoidei cervicales
Arcus ductus thoracici
Pars cervicalis
Pars thoracica
} Ductus thoracicus
Pars abdominalis
Cisterna chyli
Trunci intestinales
Trunci lumbales

Fig. 42 Overview of the lymphatic system.

Nodi lymphoidei cervicales anteriores
Nodi lymphoidei axillares
Nodi lymphoidei inguinales

Nodi lymphoidei cervicales laterales
Nodi lymphoidei axillares
Nodi lymphoidei inguinales

Fig. 43 a, b Drainage areas of regional lymph nodes.
The drainage of regional lymph nodes varies considerably between individuals. They overlap in draining to lymph nodes of the ipsilateral as well as of the contralateral side of the body.

a

b

Nervous system

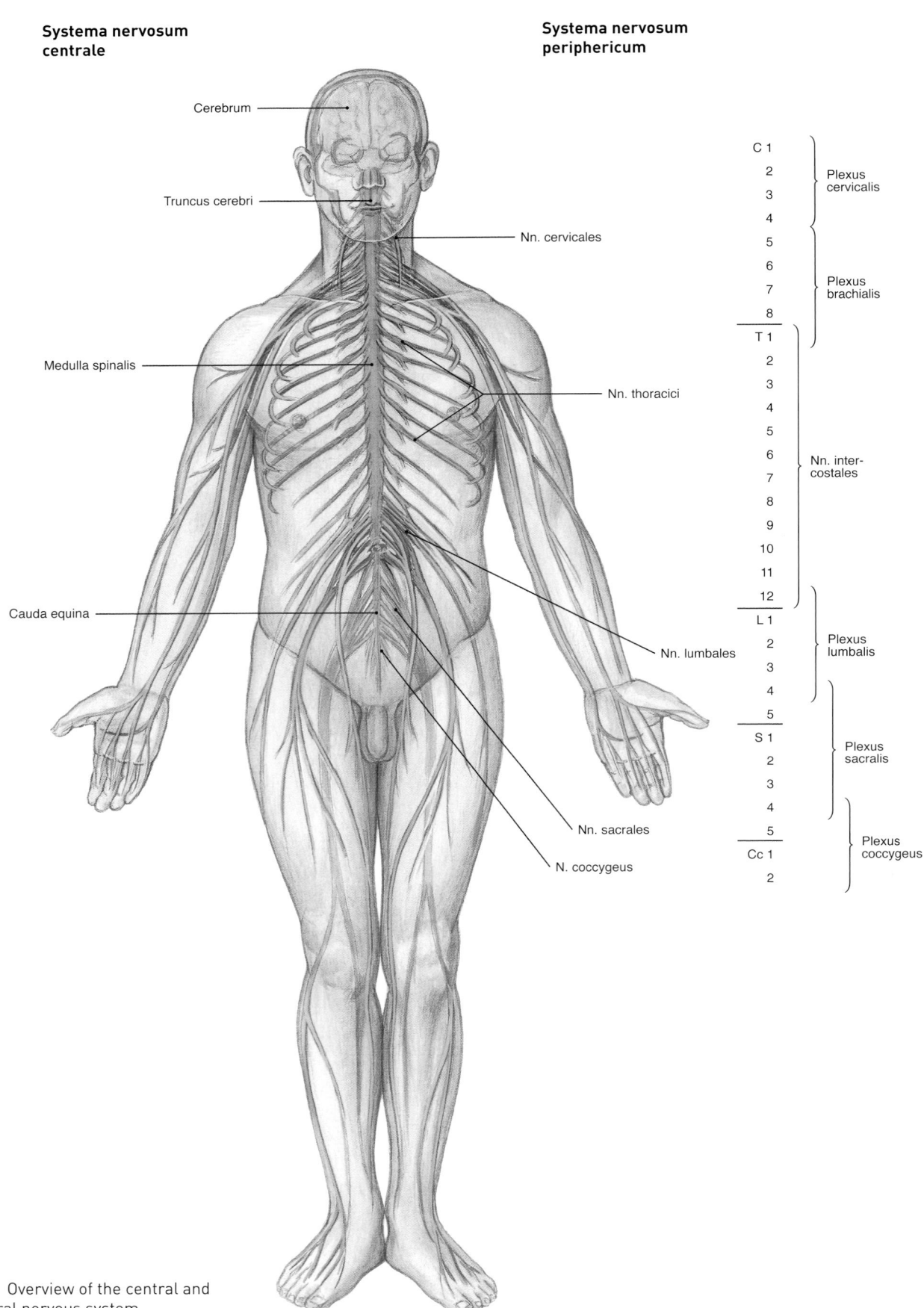

Systema nervosum centrale

Cerebrum

Truncus cerebri

Medulla spinalis

Cauda equina

Systema nervosum periphericum

Nn. cervicales

Nn. thoracici

Nn. lumbales

Nn. sacrales

N. coccygeus

C 1
2
3
4 — Plexus cervicalis

5
6
7
8 — Plexus brachialis

T 1
2
3
4
5
6
7
8
9
10
11 — Nn. inter-costales

12
L 1
2
3 — Plexus lumbalis

4
5
S 1
2
3 — Plexus sacralis

4
5
Cc 1
2 — Plexus coccygeus

Fig. 44 Overview of the central and peripheral nervous system.

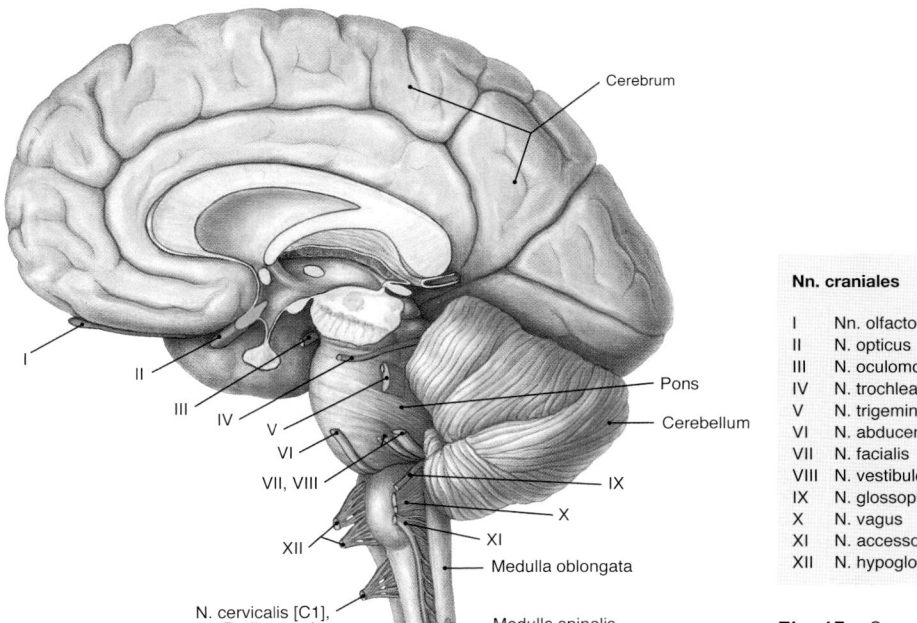

Nn. craniales

I	Nn. olfactorii
II	N. opticus
III	N. oculomotorius
IV	N. trochlearis
V	N. trigeminus
VI	N. abducens
VII	N. facialis
VIII	N. vestibulocochlearis
IX	N. glossopharyngeus
X	N. vagus
XI	N. accessorius
XII	N. hypoglossus

Fig. 45 Overview of the brain and the cranial nerves.

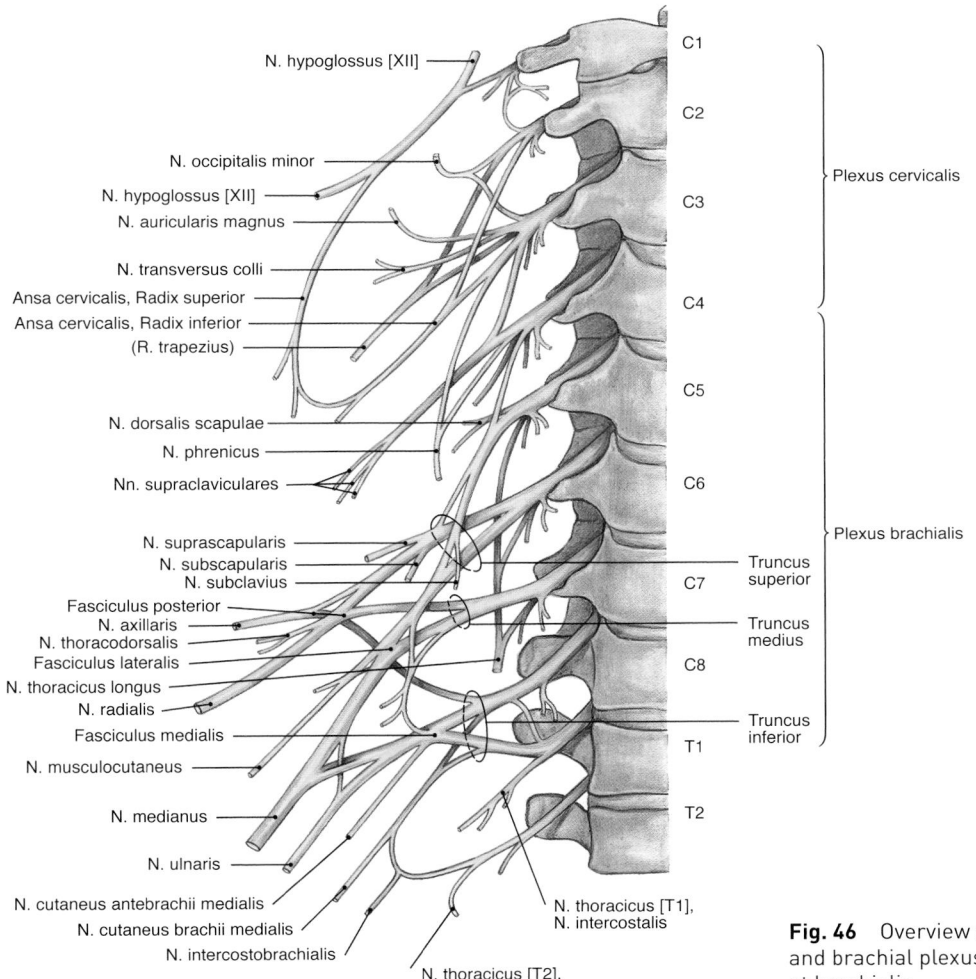

Fig. 46 Overview of the cervical and brachial plexus, Plexus cervicalis et brachialis.

Peripheral nervous system

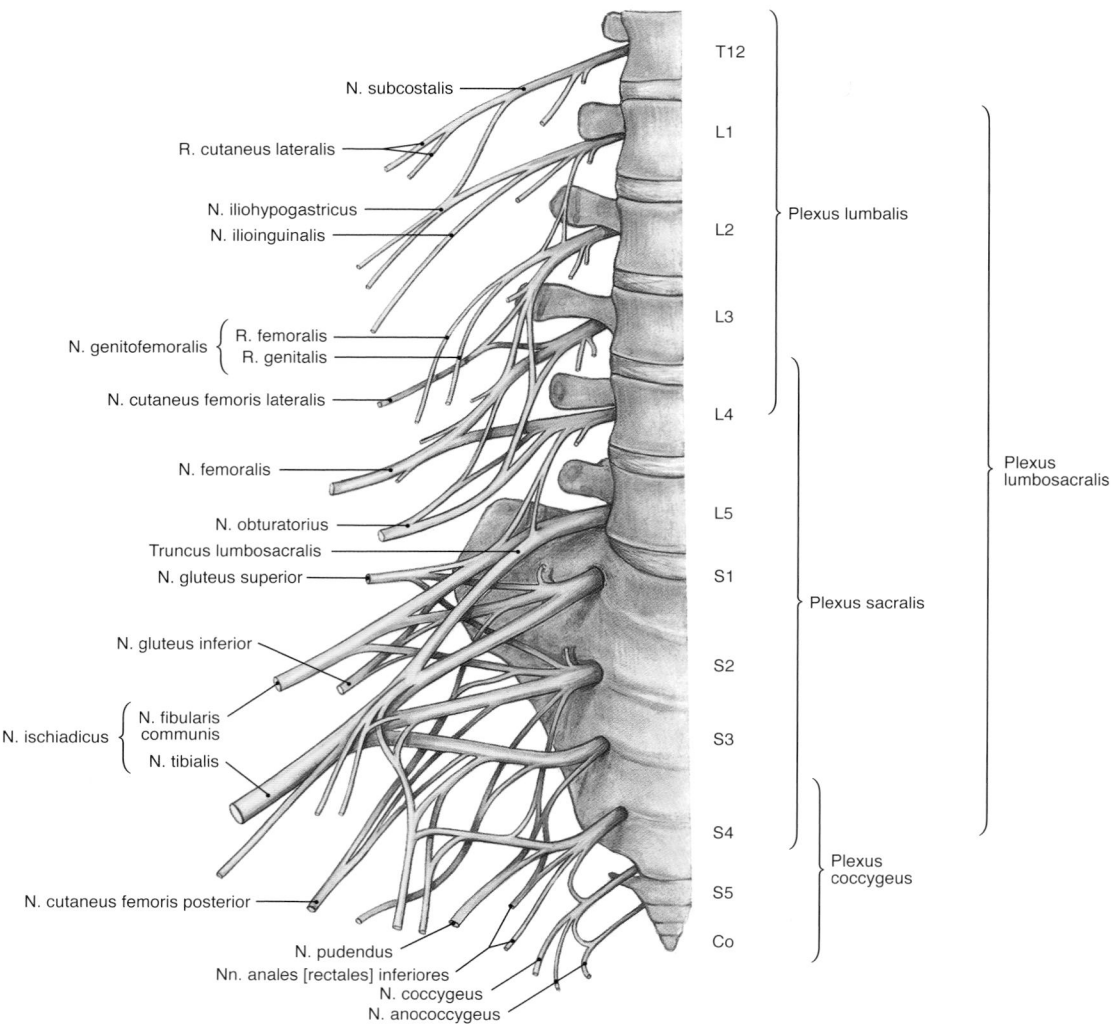

Fig. 47 Overview of the lumbosacral plexus,
Plexus lumbosacralis [Plexus lumbalis et sacralis],
and the coccygeal plexus, Plexus coccygeus.

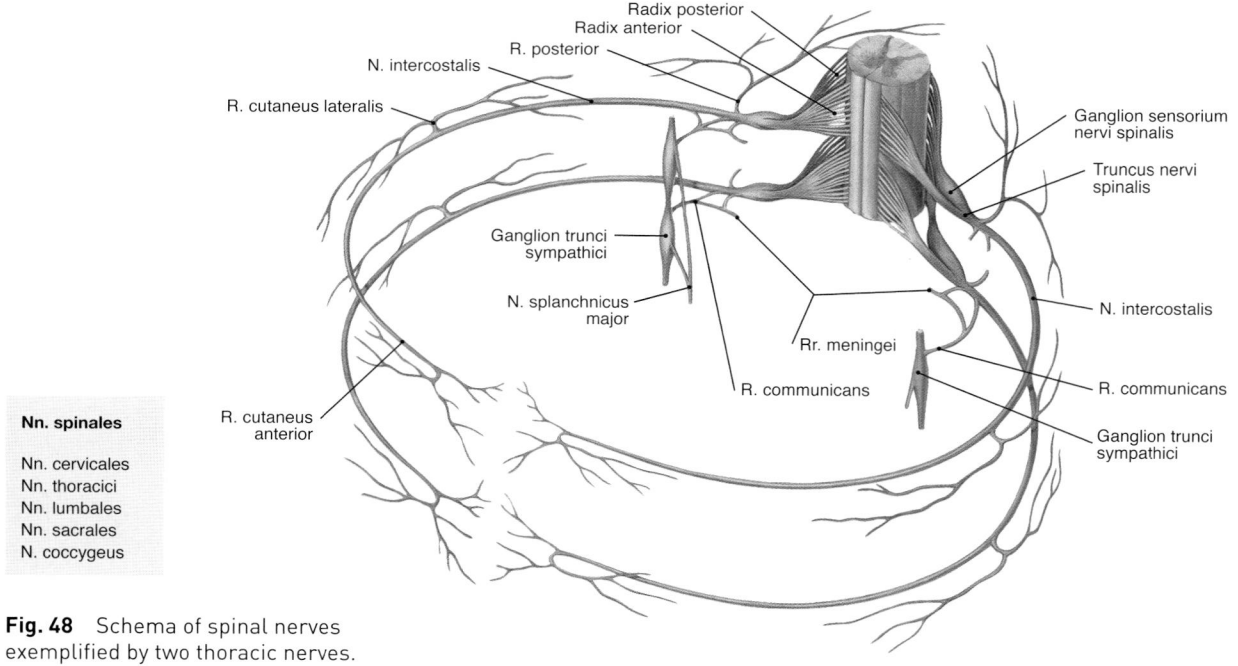

Nn. spinales

Nn. cervicales
Nn. thoracici
Nn. lumbales
Nn. sacrales
N. coccygeus

Fig. 48 Schema of spinal nerves
exemplified by two thoracic nerves.

Autonomous nervous system

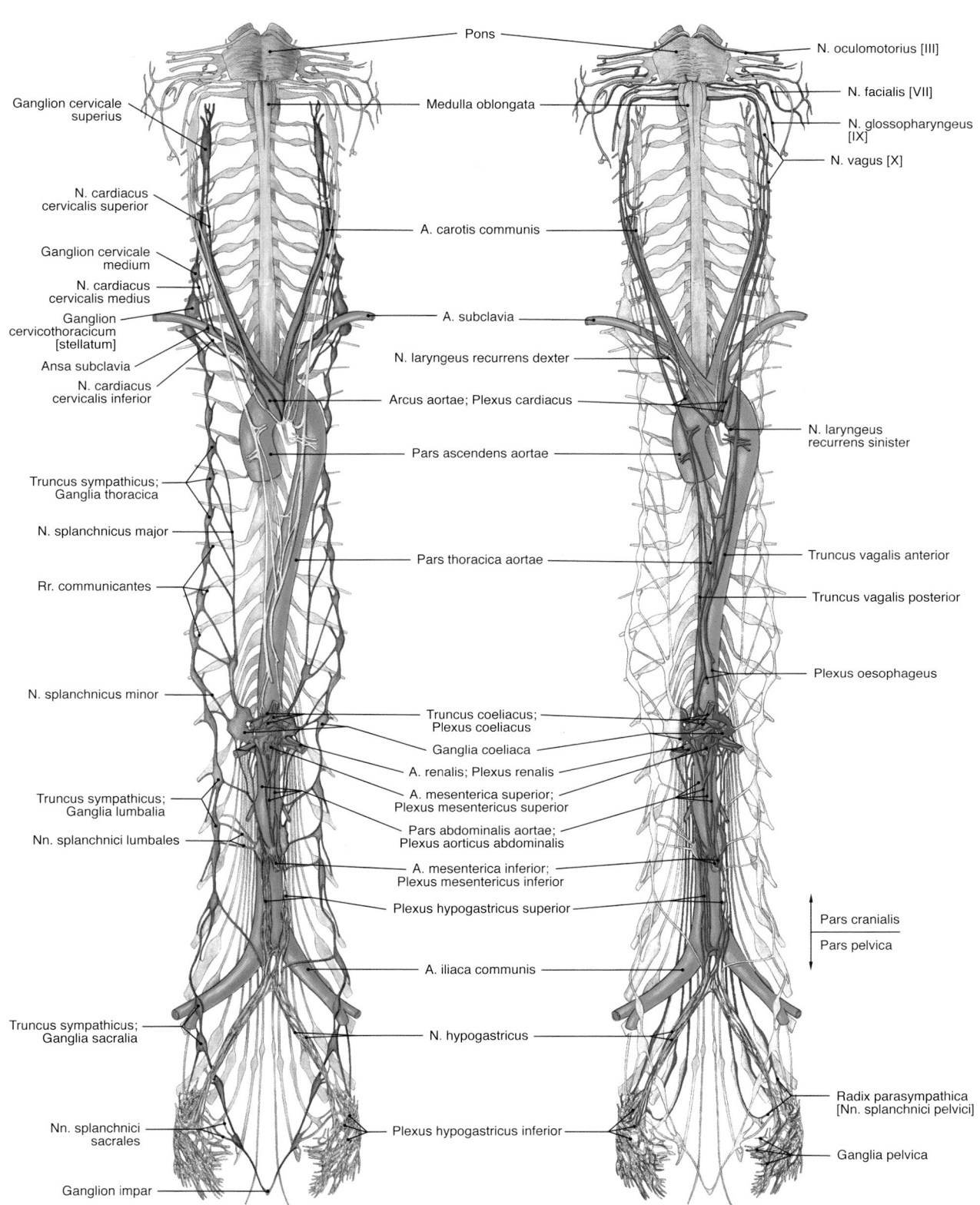

Pons

N. oculomotorius [III]

Ganglion cervicale superius

Medulla oblongata

N. facialis [VII]

N. glossopharyngeus [IX]

N. vagus [X]

N. cardiacus cervicalis superior

A. carotis communis

Ganglion cervicale medium

N. cardiacus cervicalis medius

Ganglion cervicothoracicum [stellatum]

A. subclavia

Ansa subclavia

N. laryngeus recurrens dexter

N. cardiacus cervicalis inferior

Arcus aortae; Plexus cardiacus

N. laryngeus recurrens sinister

Pars ascendens aortae

Truncus sympathicus; Ganglia thoracica

N. splanchnicus major

Pars thoracica aortae

Truncus vagalis anterior

Rr. communicantes

Truncus vagalis posterior

Plexus oesophageus

N. splanchnicus minor

Truncus coeliacus; Plexus coeliacus

Ganglia coeliaca

A. renalis; Plexus renalis

A. mesenterica superior; Plexus mesentericus superior

Truncus sympathicus; Ganglia lumbalia

Pars abdominalis aortae; Plexus aorticus abdominalis

Nn. splanchnici lumbales

A. mesenterica inferior; Plexus mesentericus inferior

Plexus hypogastricus superior

Pars cranialis

Pars pelvica

A. iliaca communis

Truncus sympathicus; Ganglia sacralia

N. hypogastricus

Radix parasympathica [Nn. splanchnici pelvici]

Nn. splanchnici sacrales

Plexus hypogastricus inferior

Ganglia pelvica

Ganglion impar

Fig. 49 Sympathetic part of the autonomous nervous system, Pars sympathica.
The entire system of sympathetic ganglia and their connections located along the vertebral column are referred to as sympathetic trunk, Truncus sympathicus (green).

Fig. 50 Parasympathetic part of the autonomous nervous system, Pars parasympathica.
Parasympathetic fibres (violet) usually travel along with other nerve fibres.

Autonomous nervous system

Pars sympathica

Pars parasympathica

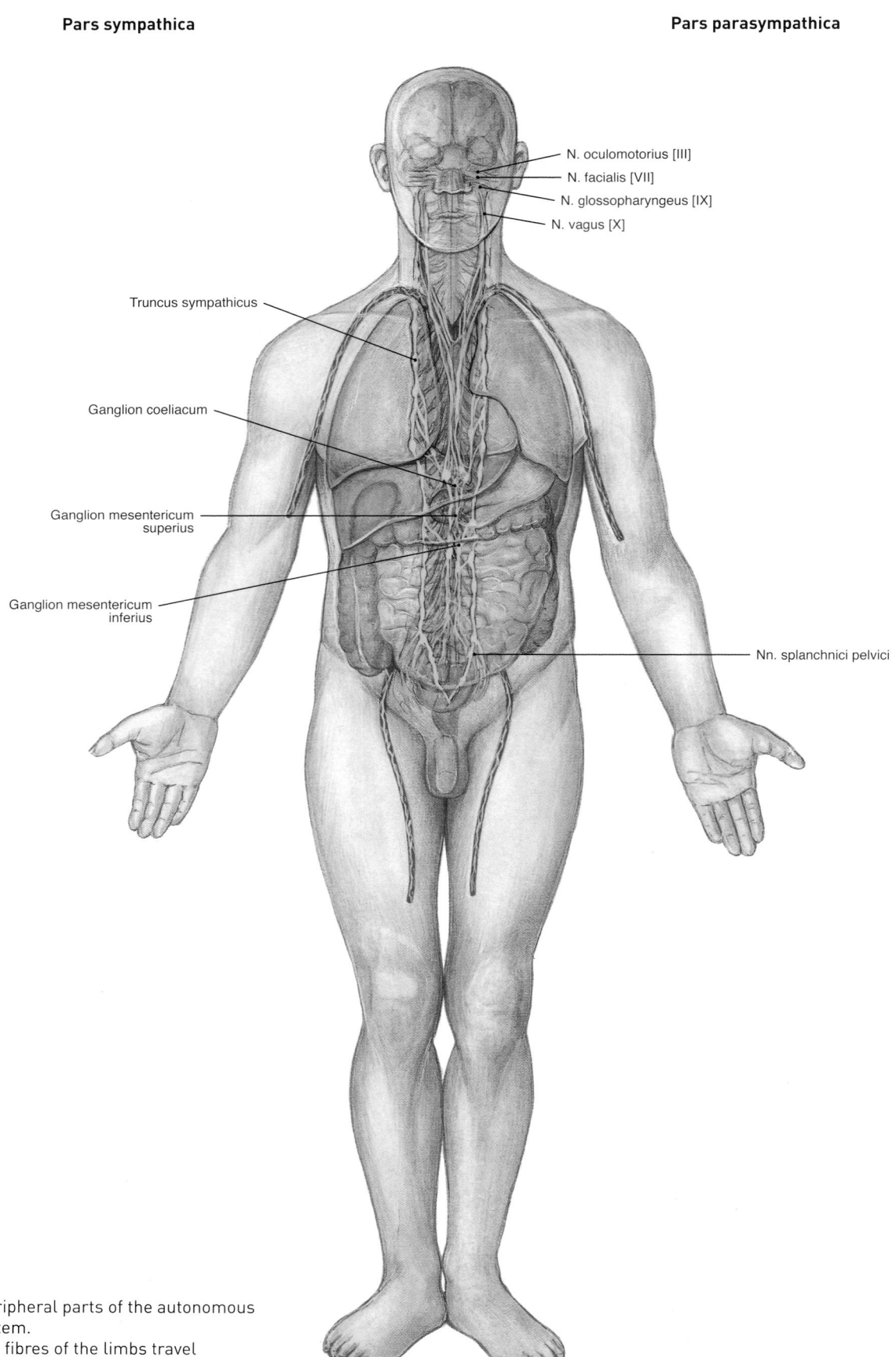

N. oculomotorius [III]

N. facialis [VII]

N. glossopharyngeus [IX]

N. vagus [X]

Truncus sympathicus

Ganglion coeliacum

Ganglion mesentericum superius

Ganglion mesentericum inferius

Nn. splanchnici pelvici

Fig. 51 Peripheral parts of the autonomous nervous system.
Sympathetic fibres of the limbs travel along with arteries.

Autonomous nervous system

Pars sympathica

Pars parasympathica

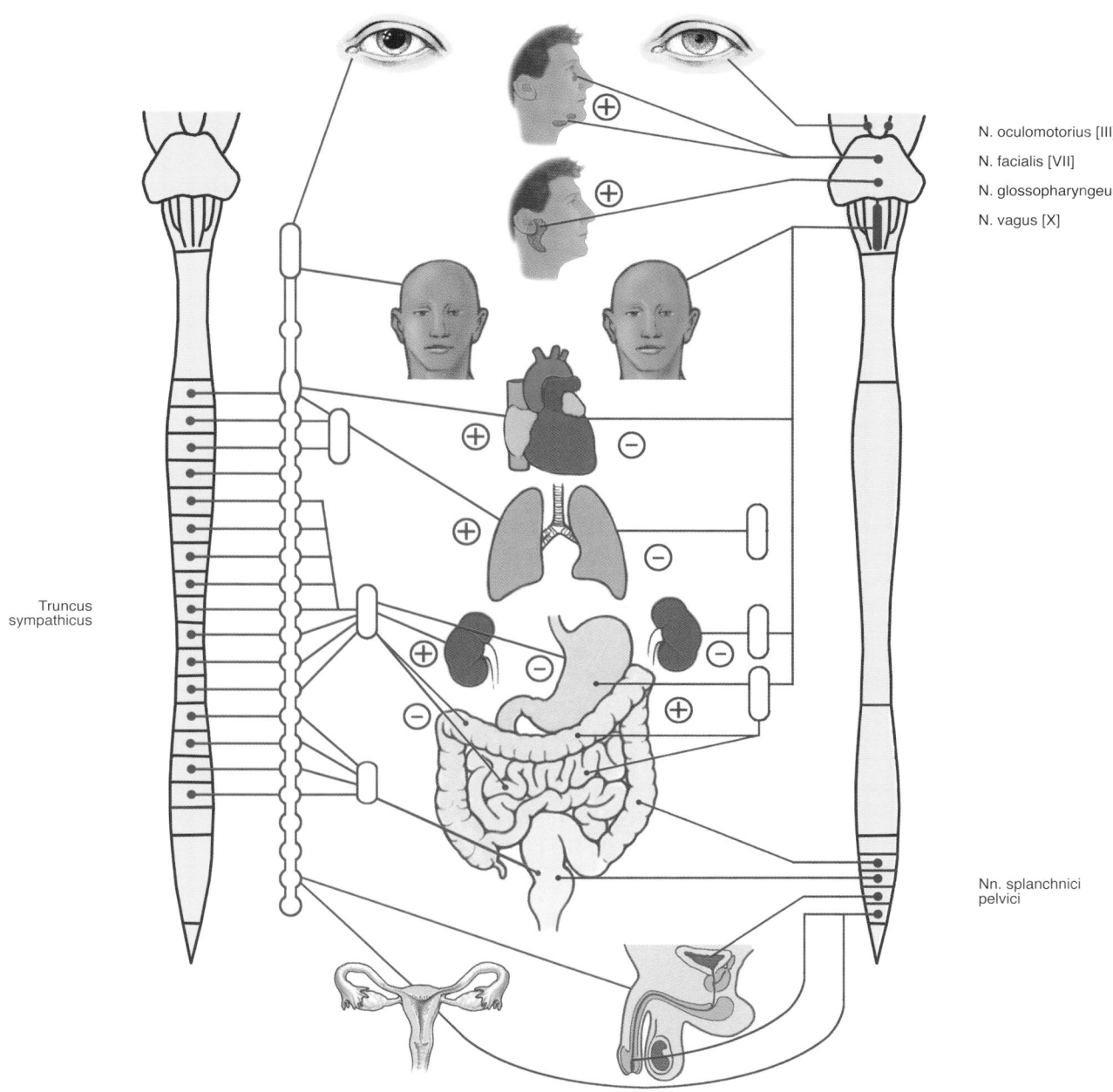

N. oculomotorius [III]

N. facialis [VII]

N. glossopharyngeus [IX]

N. vagus [X]

Truncus
sympathicus

Nn. splanchnici
pelvici

Fig. 52 Overview of the functions of the
autonomous nervous system.

Endocrine organs

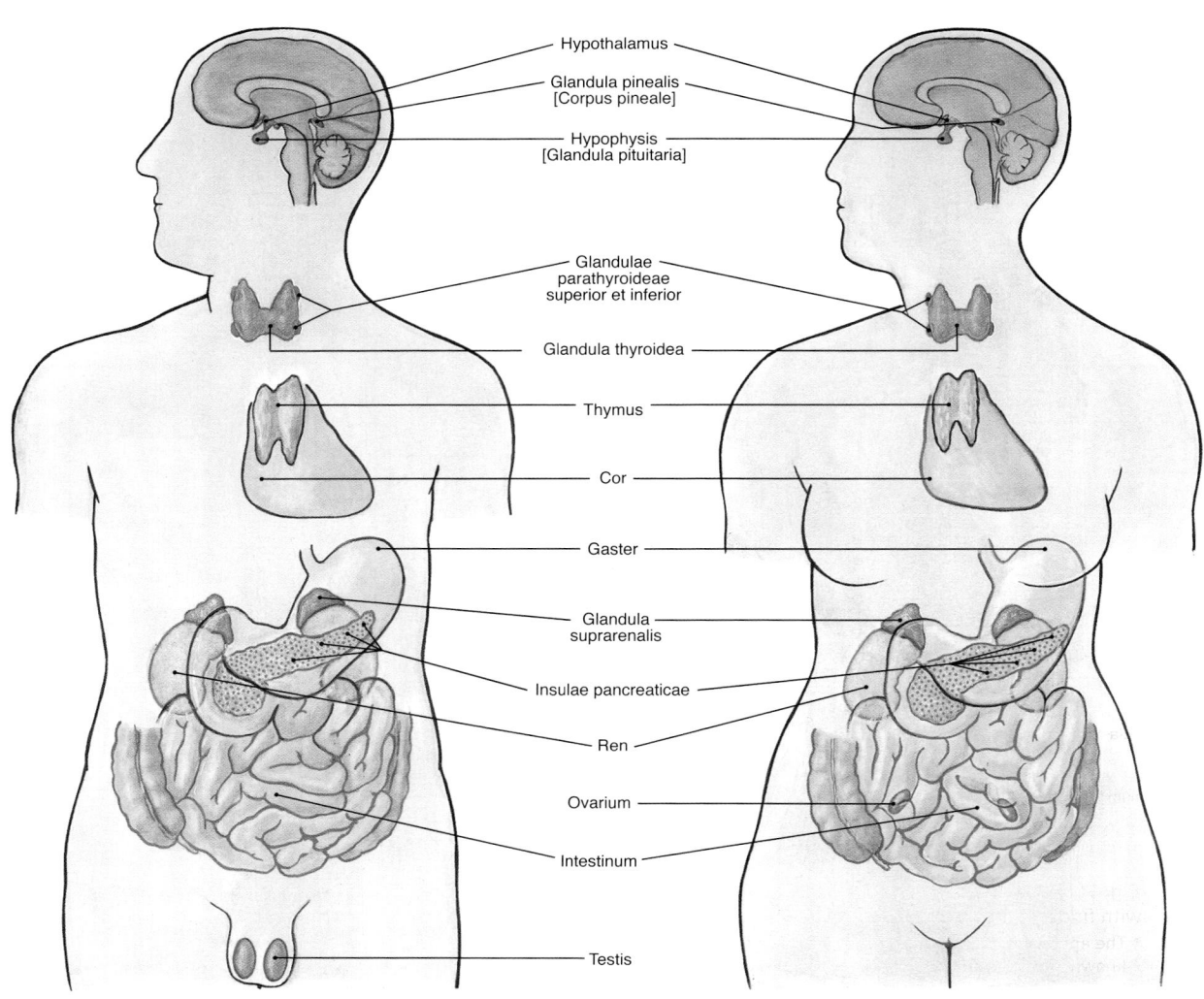

Fig. 53   Endocrine organs of the male.

Fig. 54   Endocrine organs of the female.

Skin and fingernails

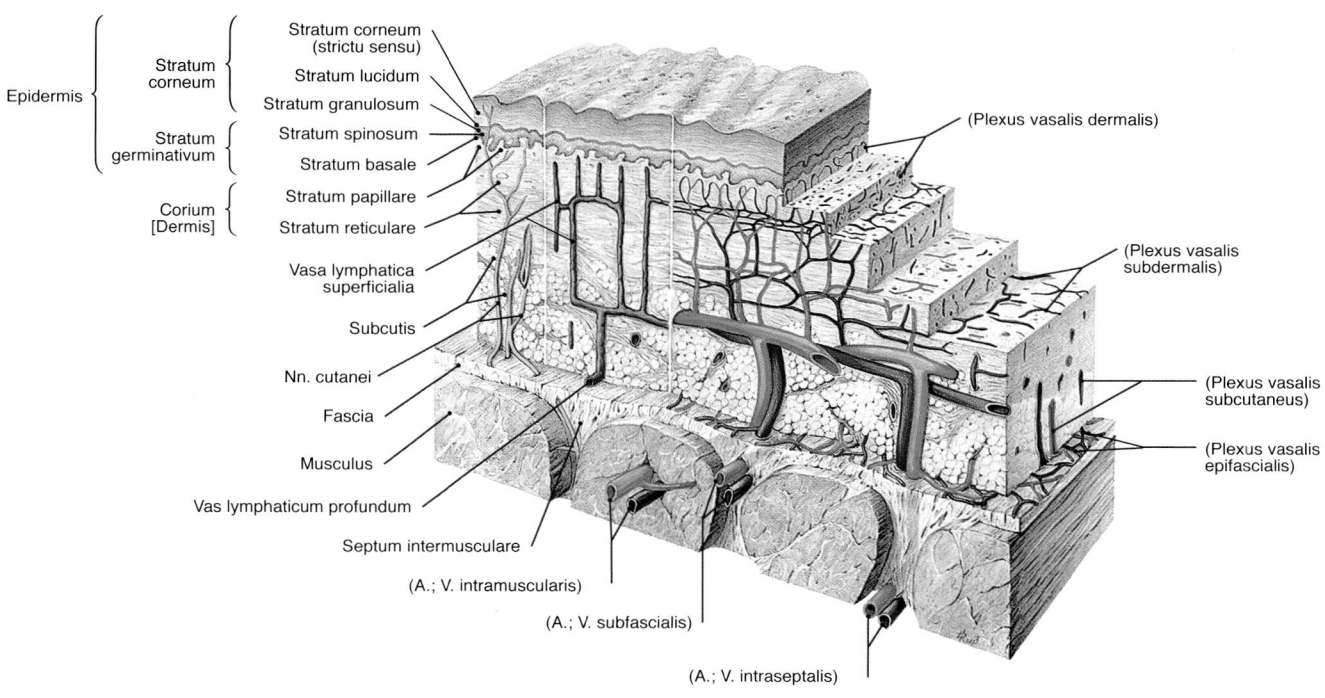

Epidermis
- Stratum corneum
  - Stratum corneum (strictu sensu)
  - Stratum lucidum
  - Stratum granulosum
- Stratum germinativum
  - Stratum spinosum
  - Stratum basale

Corium [Dermis]
- Stratum papillare
- Stratum reticulare

Vasa lymphatica superficialia
Subcutis
Nn. cutanei
Fascia
Musculus
Vas lymphaticum profundum
Septum intermusculare
(A.; V. intramuscularis)
(A.; V. subfascialis)
(A.; V. intraseptalis)

(Plexus vasalis dermalis)
(Plexus vasalis subdermalis)
(Plexus vasalis subcutaneus)
(Plexus vasalis epifascialis)

Fig. 55   Section through the skin; approximately 11-fold magnification.

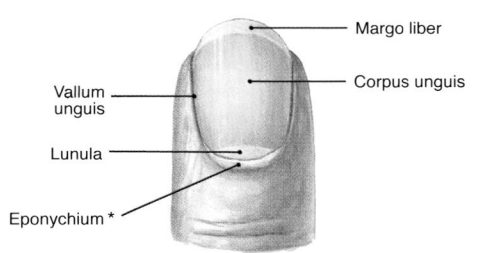

Margo liber
Vallum unguis
Corpus unguis
Lunula
Eponychium *

Fig. 56   Distal phalanx of a digit with fingernail.
* The epidermis of the nail is also known as cuticle.

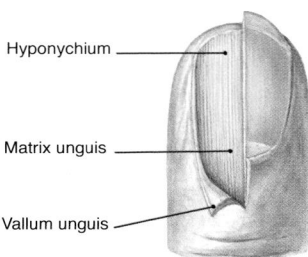

Hyponychium
Matrix unguis
Vallum unguis

Fig. 57   Distal phalanx of a digit; the nail has been partly removed.

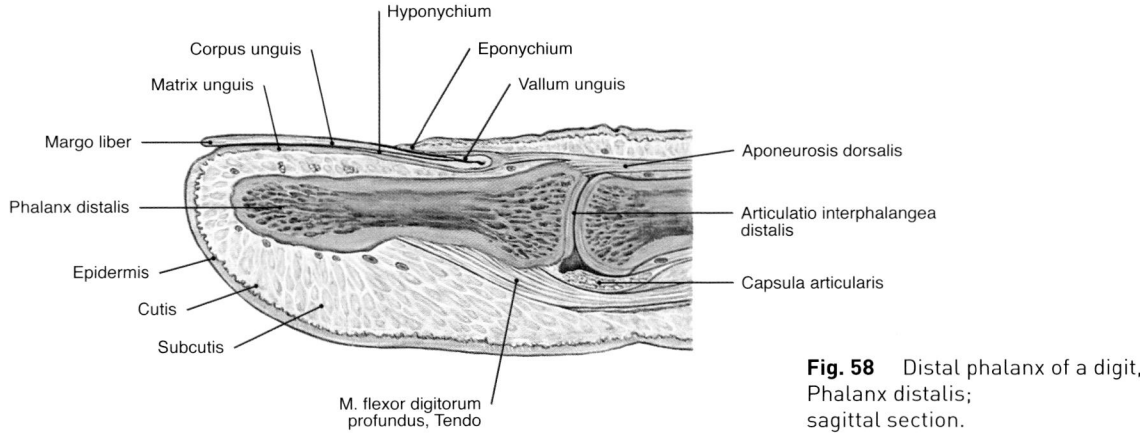

Hyponychium
Corpus unguis
Matrix unguis
Margo liber
Phalanx distalis
Epidermis
Cutis
Subcutis
M. flexor digitorum profundus, Tendo
Eponychium
Vallum unguis
Aponeurosis dorsalis
Articulatio interphalangea distalis
Capsula articularis

Fig. 58   Distal phalanx of a digit, Phalanx distalis; sagittal section.

Regions

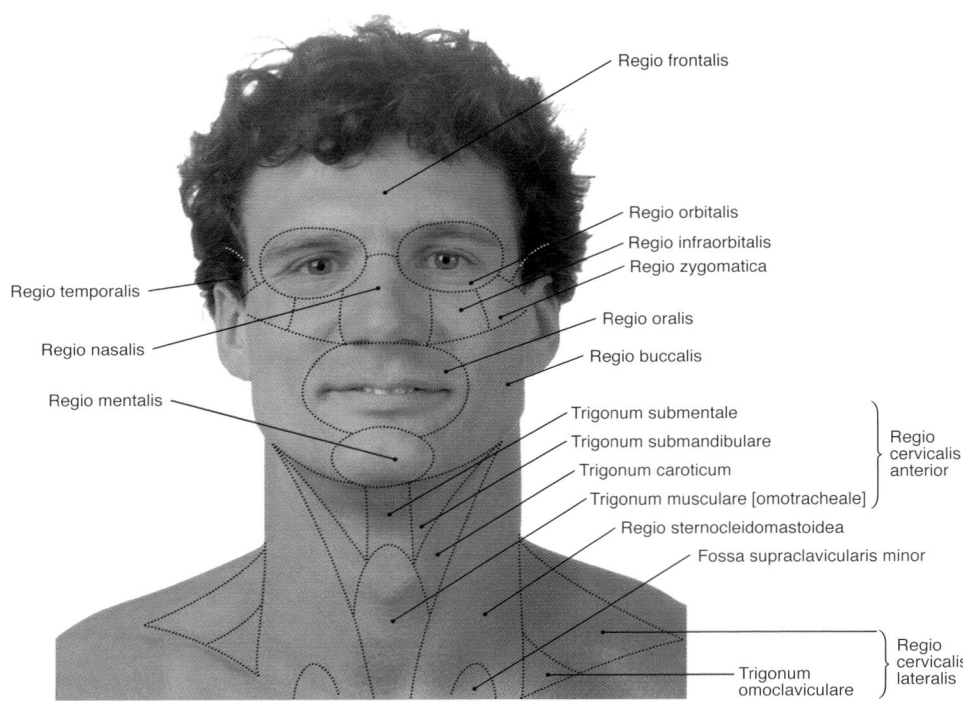

Regio frontalis
Regio orbitalis
Regio infraorbitalis
Regio zygomatica
Regio temporalis
Regio oralis
Regio nasalis
Regio buccalis
Regio mentalis
Trigonum submentale
Trigonum submandibulare
Trigonum caroticum
Regio cervicalis anterior
Trigonum musculare [omotracheale]
Regio sternocleidomastoidea
Fossa supraclavicularis minor
Regio cervicalis lateralis
Trigonum omoclaviculare

Fig. 59 Regions of the head and the neck, Regiones capitis et colli.

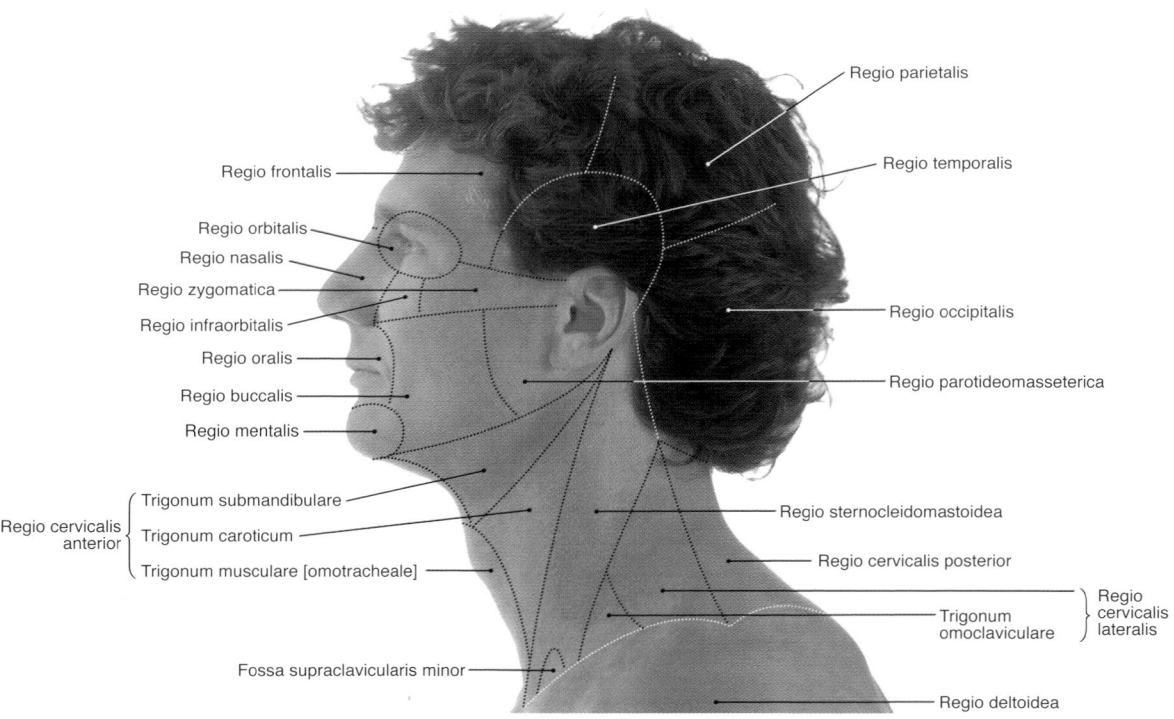

Regio parietalis
Regio frontalis
Regio temporalis
Regio orbitalis
Regio nasalis
Regio zygomatica
Regio infraorbitalis
Regio occipitalis
Regio oralis
Regio buccalis
Regio parotideomasseterica
Regio mentalis
Regio cervicalis anterior
Trigonum submandibulare
Trigonum caroticum
Regio sternocleidomastoidea
Trigonum musculare [omotracheale]
Regio cervicalis posterior
Regio cervicalis lateralis
Trigonum omoclaviculare
Fossa supraclavicularis minor
Regio deltoidea

Fig. 60 Regions of the head and the neck, Regiones capitis et colli.

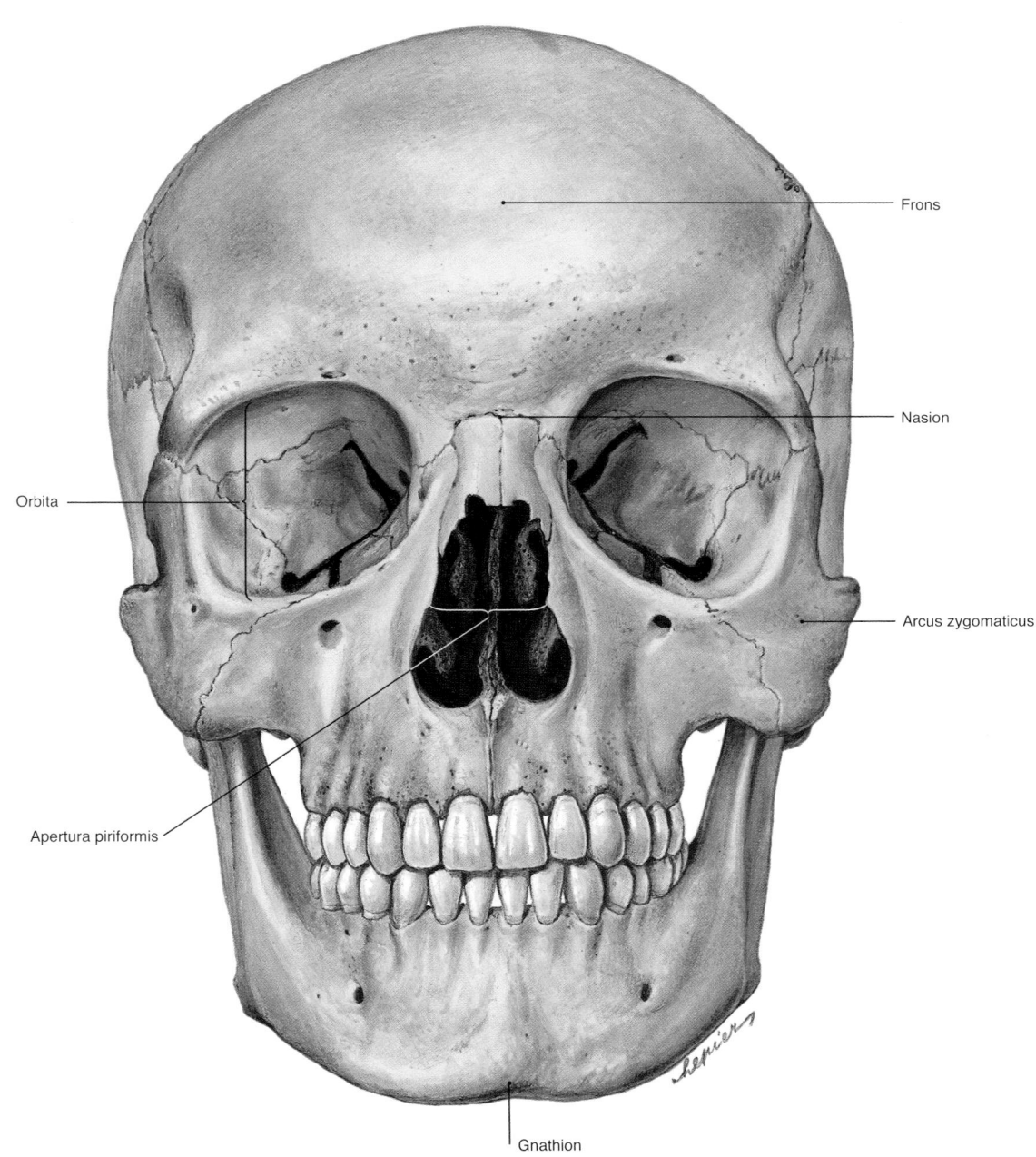

Frons

Nasion

Orbita

Arcus zygomaticus

Apertura piriformis

Gnathion

Fig. 61 Skull, Cranium.

Bones of the skull

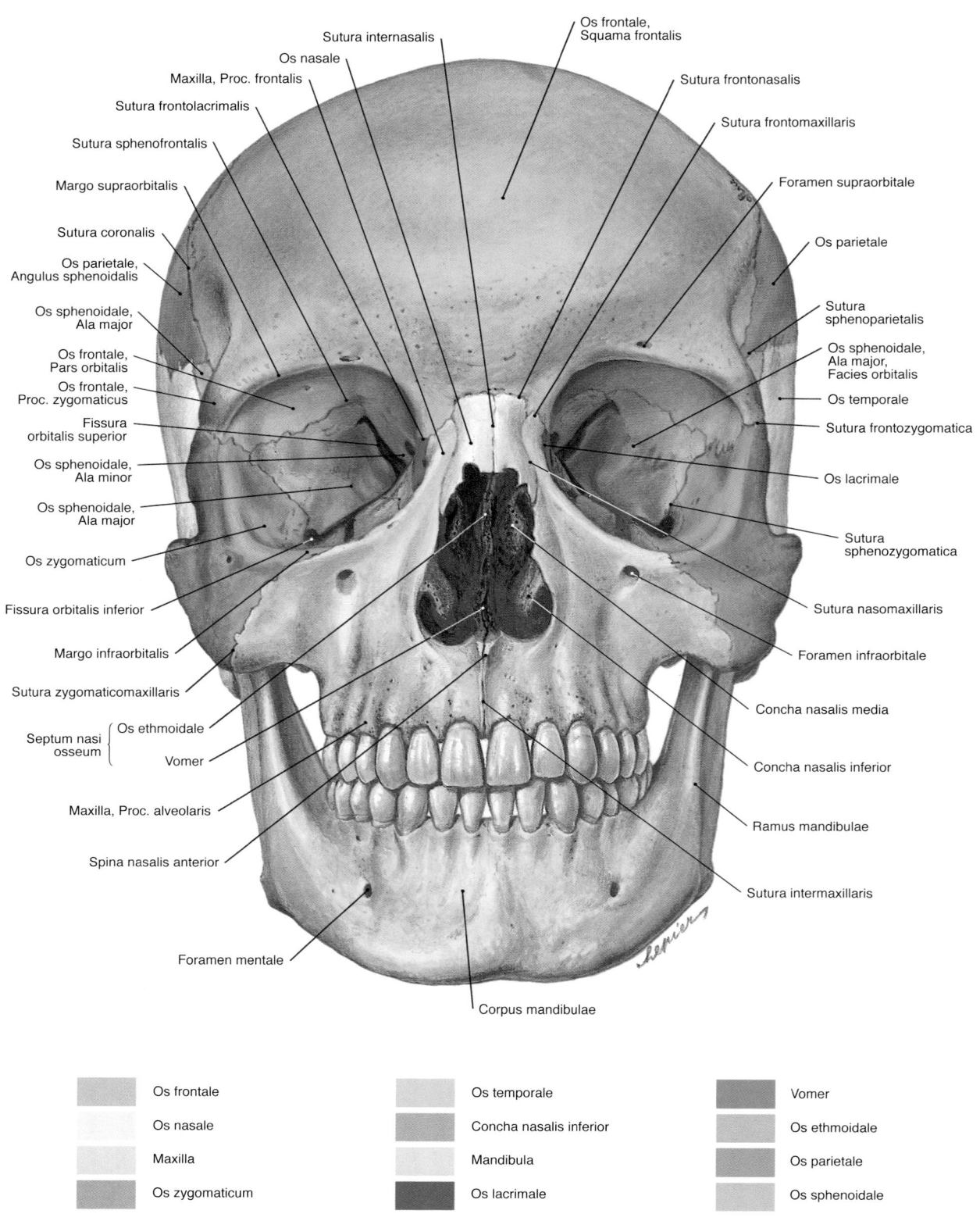

Sutura internasalis
Os nasale
Maxilla, Proc. frontalis
Sutura frontolacrimalis
Sutura sphenofrontalis
Margo supraorbitalis
Sutura coronalis
Os parietale, Angulus sphenoidalis
Os sphenoidale, Ala major
Os frontale, Pars orbitalis
Os frontale, Proc. zygomaticus
Fissura orbitalis superior
Os sphenoidale, Ala minor
Os sphenoidale, Ala major
Os zygomaticum
Fissura orbitalis inferior
Margo infraorbitalis
Sutura zygomaticomaxillaris
Septum nasi osseum { Os ethmoidale
Vomer
Maxilla, Proc. alveolaris
Spina nasalis anterior
Foramen mentale
Corpus mandibulae

Os frontale, Squama frontalis
Sutura frontonasalis
Sutura frontomaxillaris
Foramen supraorbitale
Os parietale
Sutura sphenoparietalis
Os sphenoidale, Ala major, Facies orbitalis
Os temporale
Sutura frontozygomatica
Os lacrimale
Sutura sphenozygomatica
Sutura nasomaxillaris
Foramen infraorbitale
Concha nasalis media
Concha nasalis inferior
Ramus mandibulae
Sutura intermaxillaris

Os frontale
Os nasale
Maxilla
Os zygomaticum

Os temporale
Concha nasalis inferior
Mandibula
Os lacrimale

Vomer
Os ethmoidale
Os parietale
Os sphenoidale

Fig. 62 Bones of the skull, Ossa cranii.

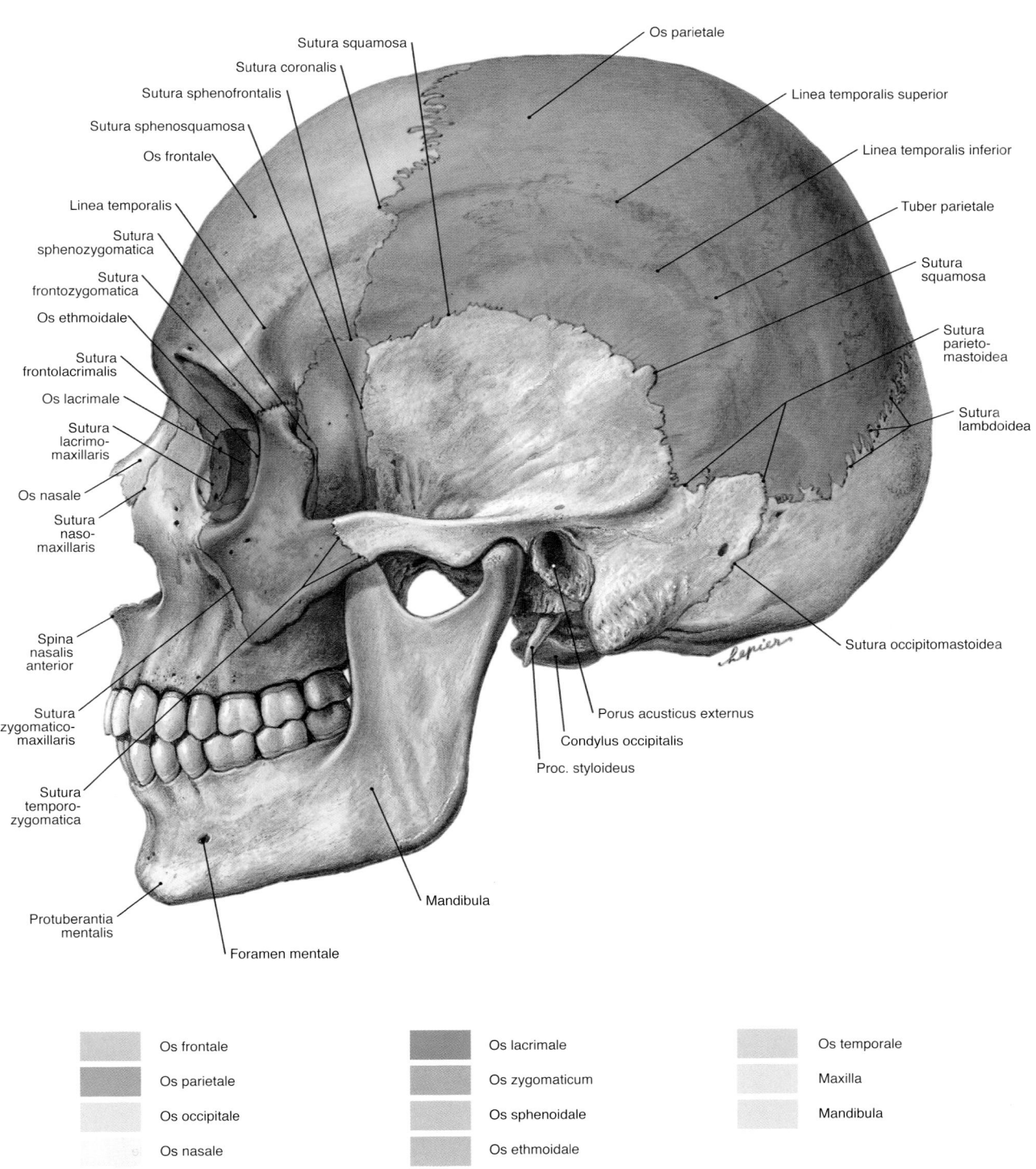

Sutura squamosa
Sutura coronalis
Sutura sphenofrontalis
Sutura sphenosquamosa
Os frontale
Linea temporalis
Sutura sphenozygomatica
Sutura frontozygomatica
Os ethmoidale
Sutura frontolacrimalis
Os lacrimale
Sutura lacrimo-maxillaris
Os nasale
Sutura naso-maxillaris
Spina nasalis anterior
Sutura zygomatico-maxillaris
Sutura temporo-zygomatica
Protuberantia mentalis
Foramen mentale

Os parietale
Linea temporalis superior
Linea temporalis inferior
Tuber parietale
Sutura squamosa
Sutura parieto-mastoidea
Sutura lambdoidea
Sutura occipitomastoidea
Porus acusticus externus
Condylus occipitalis
Proc. styloideus
Mandibula

■	Os frontale	■	Os lacrimale	■	Os temporale
■	Os parietale	■	Os zygomaticum	■	Maxilla
■	Os occipitale	■	Os sphenoidale	■	Mandibula
■	Os nasale	■	Os ethmoidale		

Fig. 63 Bones of the skull, Ossa cranii.

Bones of the skull

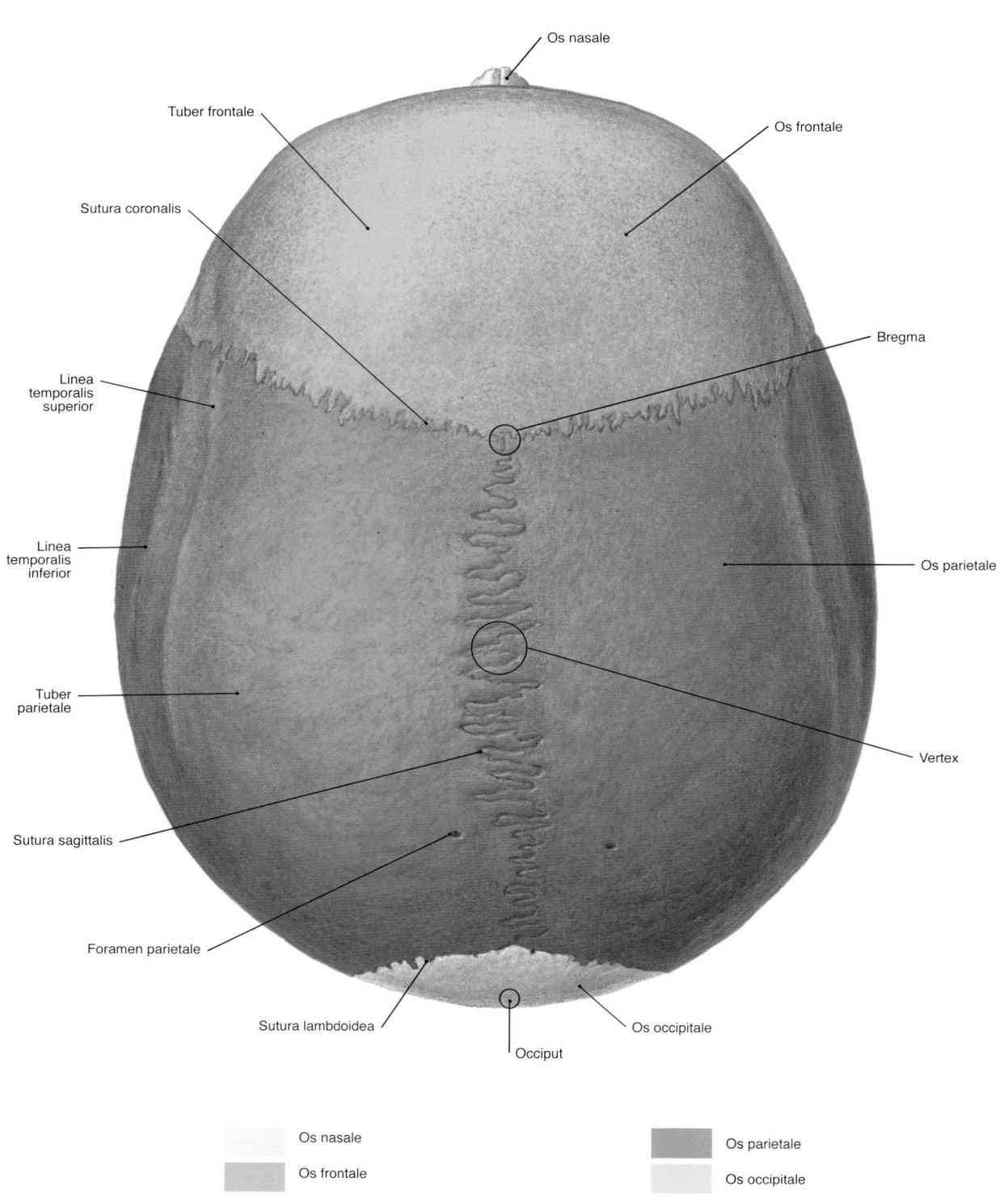

Os nasale

Tuber frontale

Os frontale

Sutura coronalis

Bregma

Linea temporalis superior

Linea temporalis inferior

Os parietale

Tuber parietale

Vertex

Sutura sagittalis

Foramen parietale

Sutura lambdoidea

Os occipitale

Occiput

Os nasale

Os frontale

Os parietale

Os occipitale

Fig. 64   Bones of the skull, Ossa cranii; superior view.

Bones of the skull

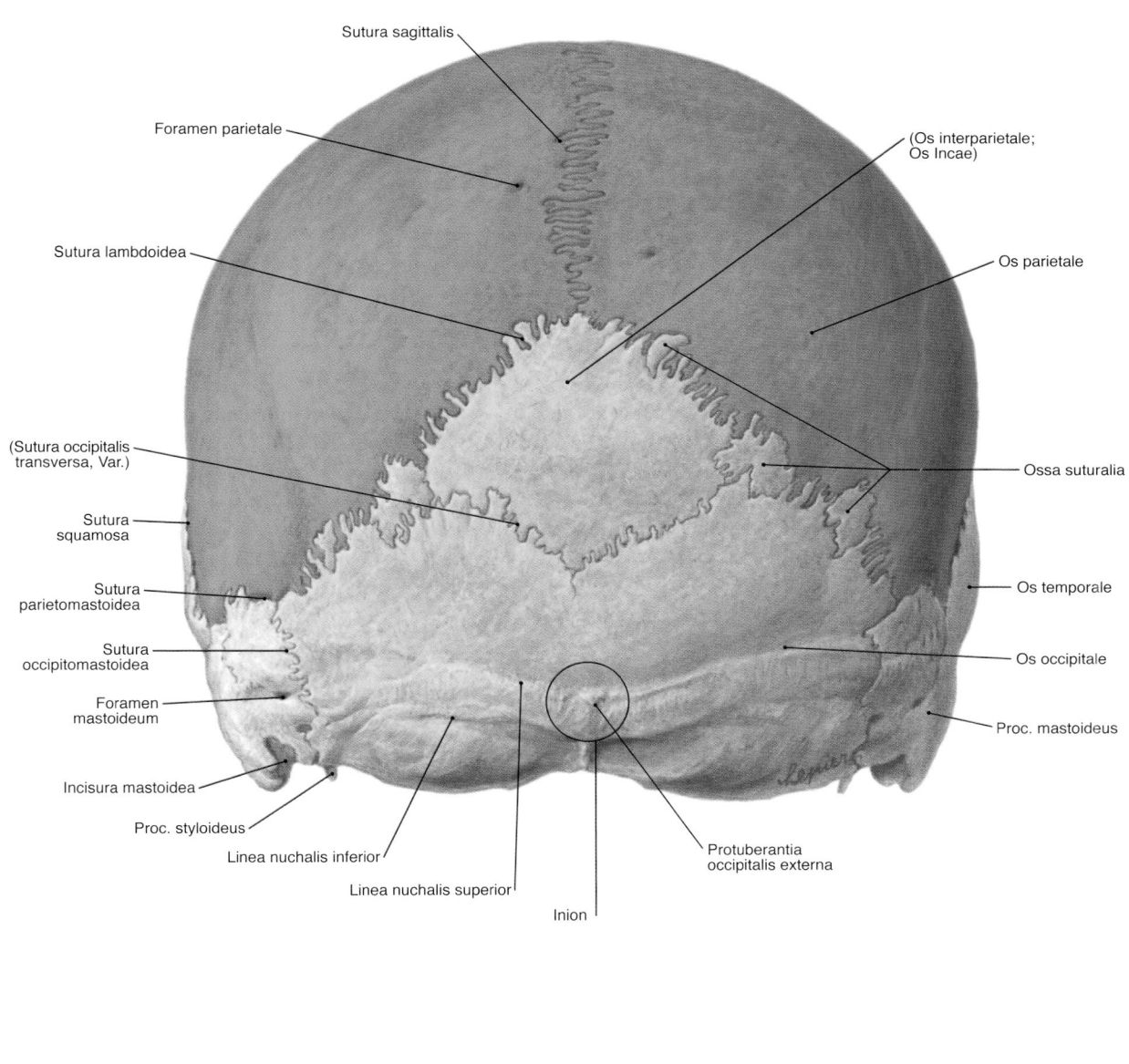

Sutura sagittalis

Foramen parietale

(Os interparietale;
Os Incae)

Sutura lambdoidea

Os parietale

(Sutura occipitalis
transversa, Var.)

Ossa suturalia

Sutura
squamosa

Sutura
parietomastoidea

Os temporale

Sutura
occipitomastoidea

Os occipitale

Foramen
mastoideum

Proc. mastoideus

Incisura mastoidea

Proc. styloideus

Linea nuchalis inferior

Linea nuchalis superior

Protuberantia
occipitalis externa

Inion

Os parietale

Os temporale

Os occipitale

Fig. 65 Bones of the skull, Ossa cranii;
posterior view.

Bones of the skull

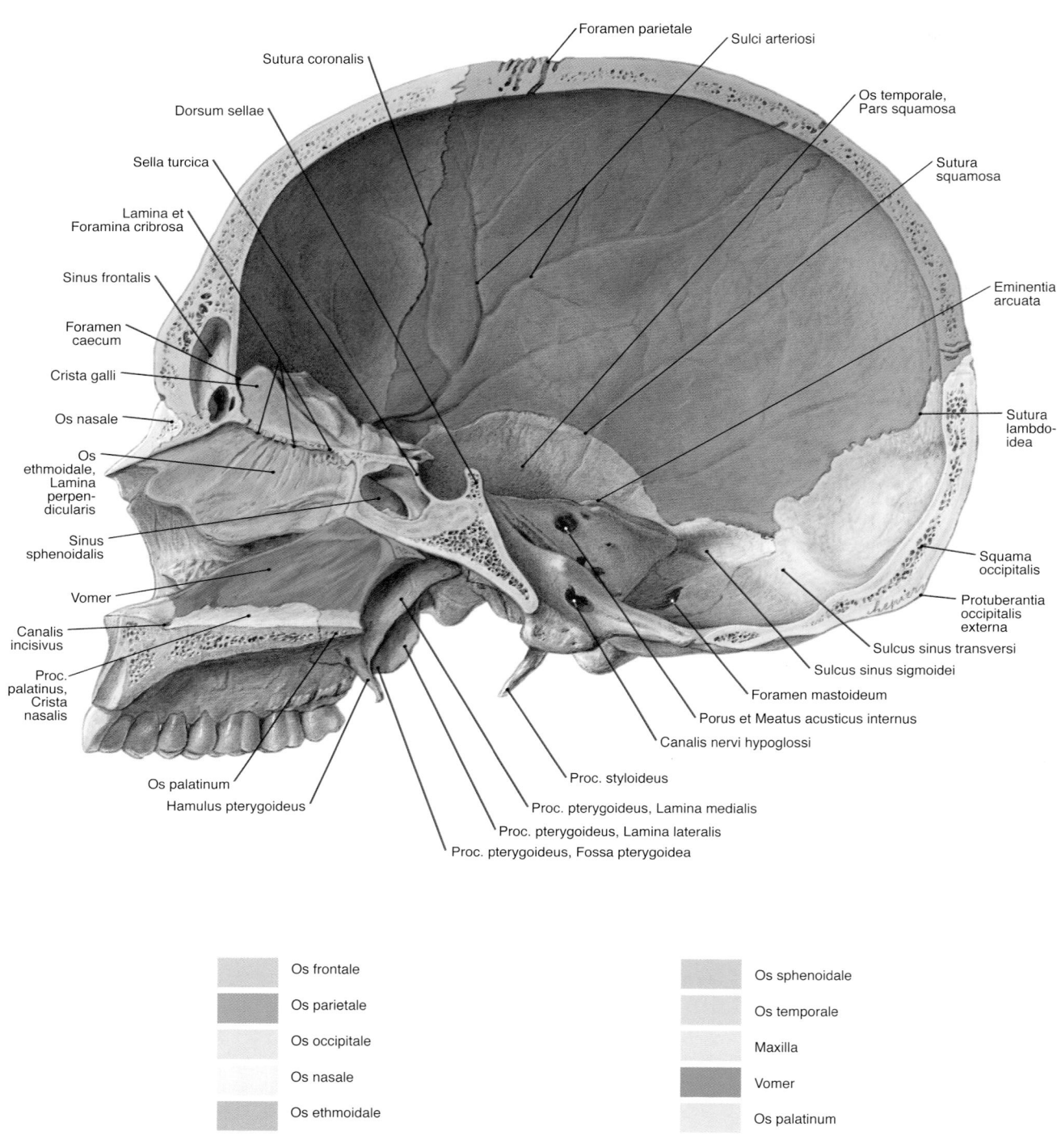

Foramen parietale
Sulci arteriosi
Sutura coronalis
Dorsum sellae
Os temporale, Pars squamosa
Sella turcica
Sutura squamosa
Lamina et Foramina cribrosa
Sinus frontalis
Eminentia arcuata
Foramen caecum
Crista galli
Os nasale
Sutura lambdoidea
Os ethmoidale, Lamina perpendicularis
Sinus sphenoidalis
Squama occipitalis
Vomer
Protuberantia occipitalis externa
Canalis incisivus
Sulcus sinus transversi
Proc. palatinus, Crista nasalis
Sulcus sinus sigmoidei
Foramen mastoideum
Porus et Meatus acusticus internus
Canalis nervi hypoglossi
Os palatinum
Hamulus pterygoideus
Proc. styloideus
Proc. pterygoideus, Lamina medialis
Proc. pterygoideus, Lamina lateralis
Proc. pterygoideus, Fossa pterygoidea

Os frontale
Os parietale
Os occipitale
Os nasale
Os ethmoidale

Os sphenoidale
Os temporale
Maxilla
Vomer
Os palatinum

Fig. 66 Bones of the skull, Ossa cranii; medial view.

Bones of the skull

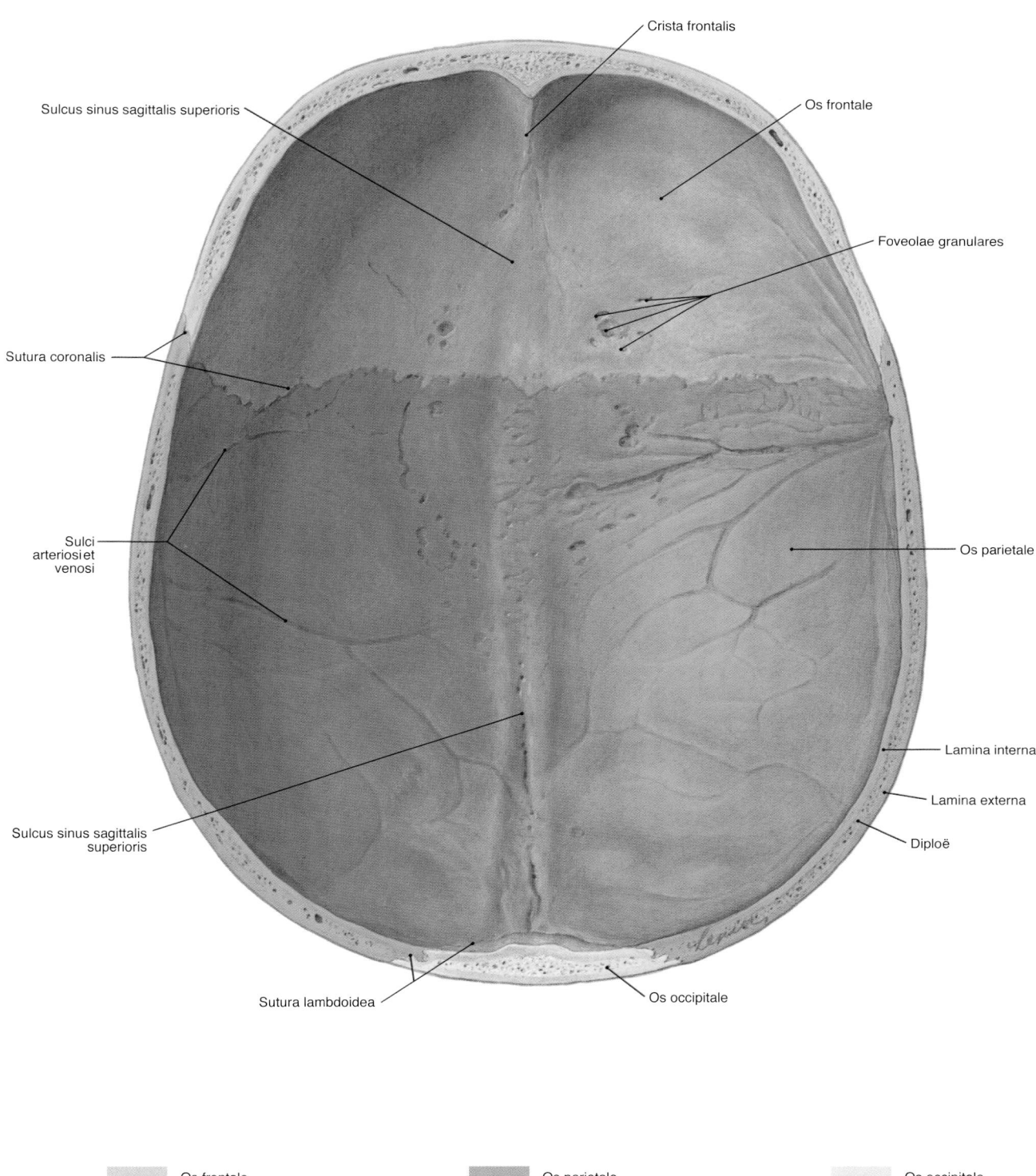

Crista frontalis

Sulcus sinus sagittalis superioris

Os frontale

Foveolae granulares

Sutura coronalis

Sulci arteriosi et venosi

Os parietale

Lamina interna

Lamina externa

Diploë

Sulcus sinus sagittalis superioris

Sutura lambdoidea

Os occipitale

Os frontale   Os parietale   Os occipitale

Fig. 67 Calvaria, Calvaria;
internal aspect.

Bones of the skull

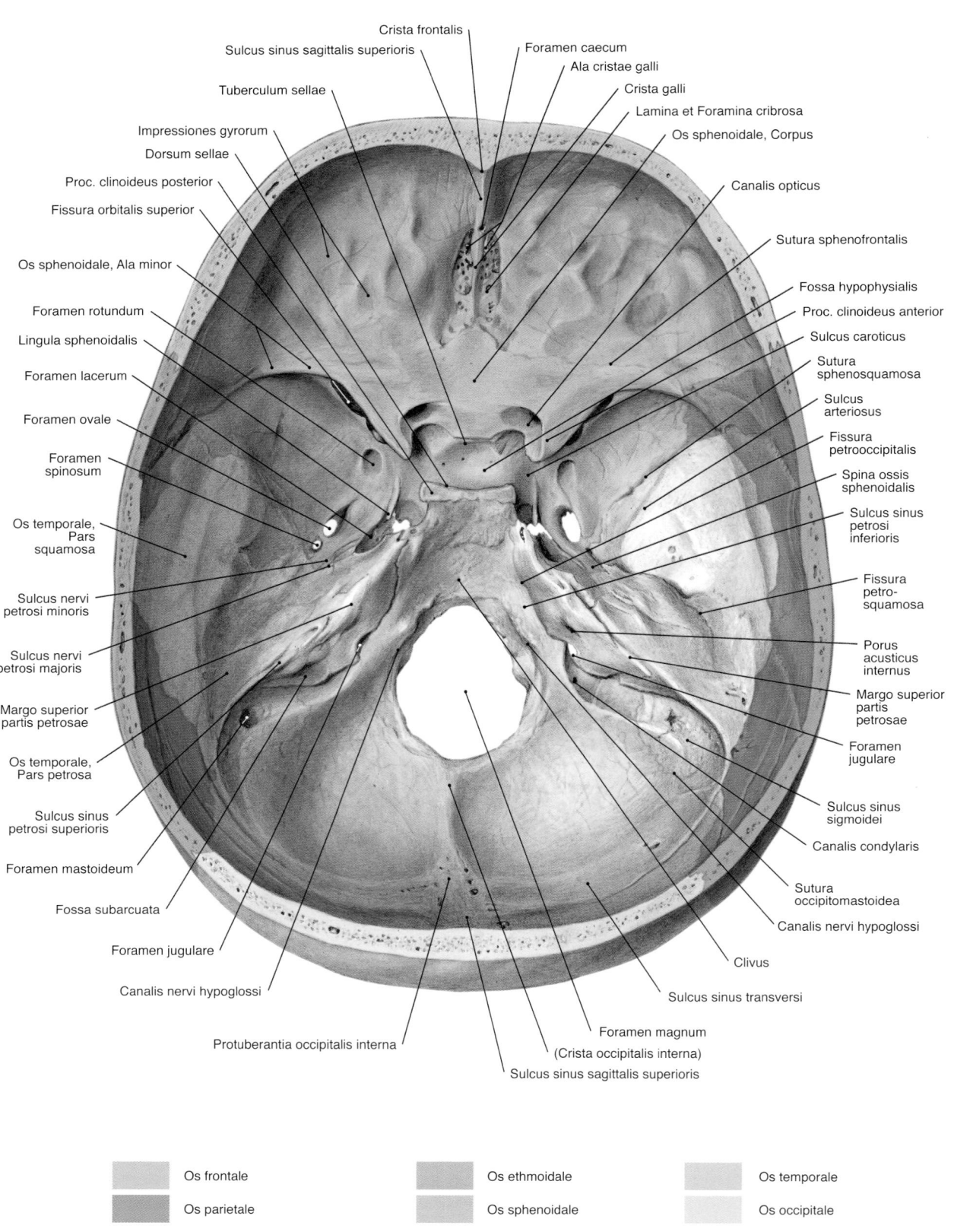

Crista frontalis
Sulcus sinus sagittalis superioris
Tuberculum sellae
Impressiones gyrorum
Dorsum sellae
Proc. clinoideus posterior
Fissura orbitalis superior
Os sphenoidale, Ala minor
Foramen rotundum
Lingula sphenoidalis
Foramen lacerum
Foramen ovale
Foramen spinosum
Os temporale, Pars squamosa
Sulcus nervi petrosi minoris
Sulcus nervi petrosi majoris
Margo superior partis petrosae
Os temporale, Pars petrosa
Sulcus sinus petrosi superioris
Foramen mastoideum
Fossa subarcuata
Foramen jugulare
Canalis nervi hypoglossi
Protuberantia occipitalis interna

Foramen caecum
Ala cristae galli
Crista galli
Lamina et Foramina cribrosa
Os sphenoidale, Corpus
Canalis opticus
Sutura sphenofrontalis
Fossa hypophysialis
Proc. clinoideus anterior
Sulcus caroticus
Sutura sphenosquamosa
Sulcus arteriosus
Fissura petrooccipitalis
Spina ossis sphenoidalis
Sulcus sinus petrosi inferioris
Fissura petro-squamosa
Porus acusticus internus
Margo superior partis petrosae
Foramen jugulare
Sulcus sinus sigmoidei
Canalis condylaris
Sutura occipitomastoidea
Canalis nervi hypoglossi
Clivus
Sulcus sinus transversi

Foramen magnum (Crista occipitalis interna)
Sulcus sinus sagittalis superioris

Os frontale
Os parietale
Os ethmoidale
Os sphenoidale
Os temporale
Os occipitale

Fig. 68 Internal surface of the base of the skull,
Basis cranii interna.

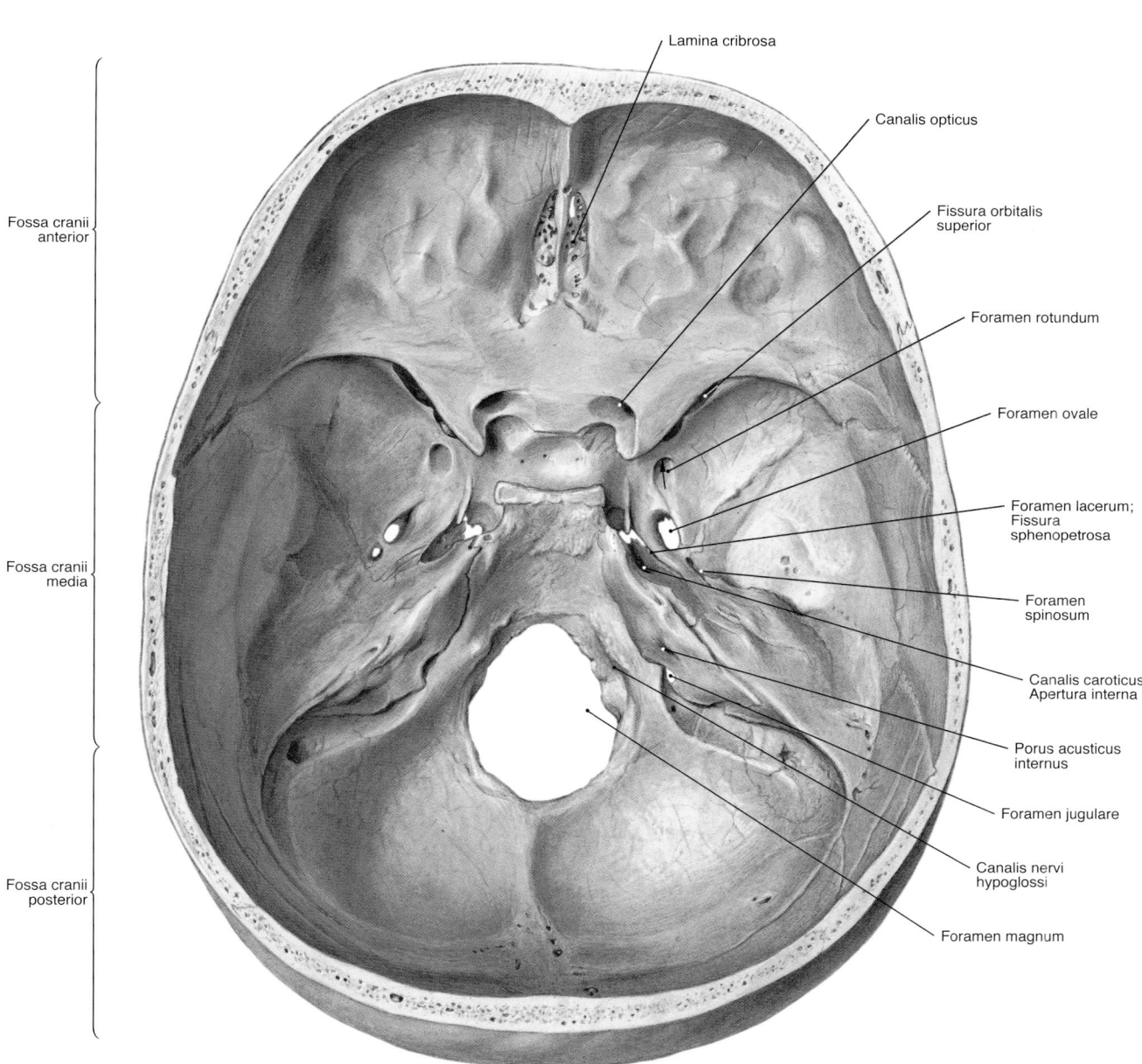

Lamina cribrosa

Canalis opticus

Fissura orbitalis superior

Foramen rotundum

Foramen ovale

Foramen lacerum; Fissura sphenopetrosa

Foramen spinosum

Canalis caroticus, Apertura interna

Porus acusticus internus

Foramen jugulare

Canalis nervi hypoglossi

Foramen magnum

Fossa cranii anterior

Fossa cranii media

Fossa cranii posterior

Fig. 69 Internal surface of the base of the skull, Basis cranii interna, and foramina, Foramina.

→ 1173

Bones of the skull

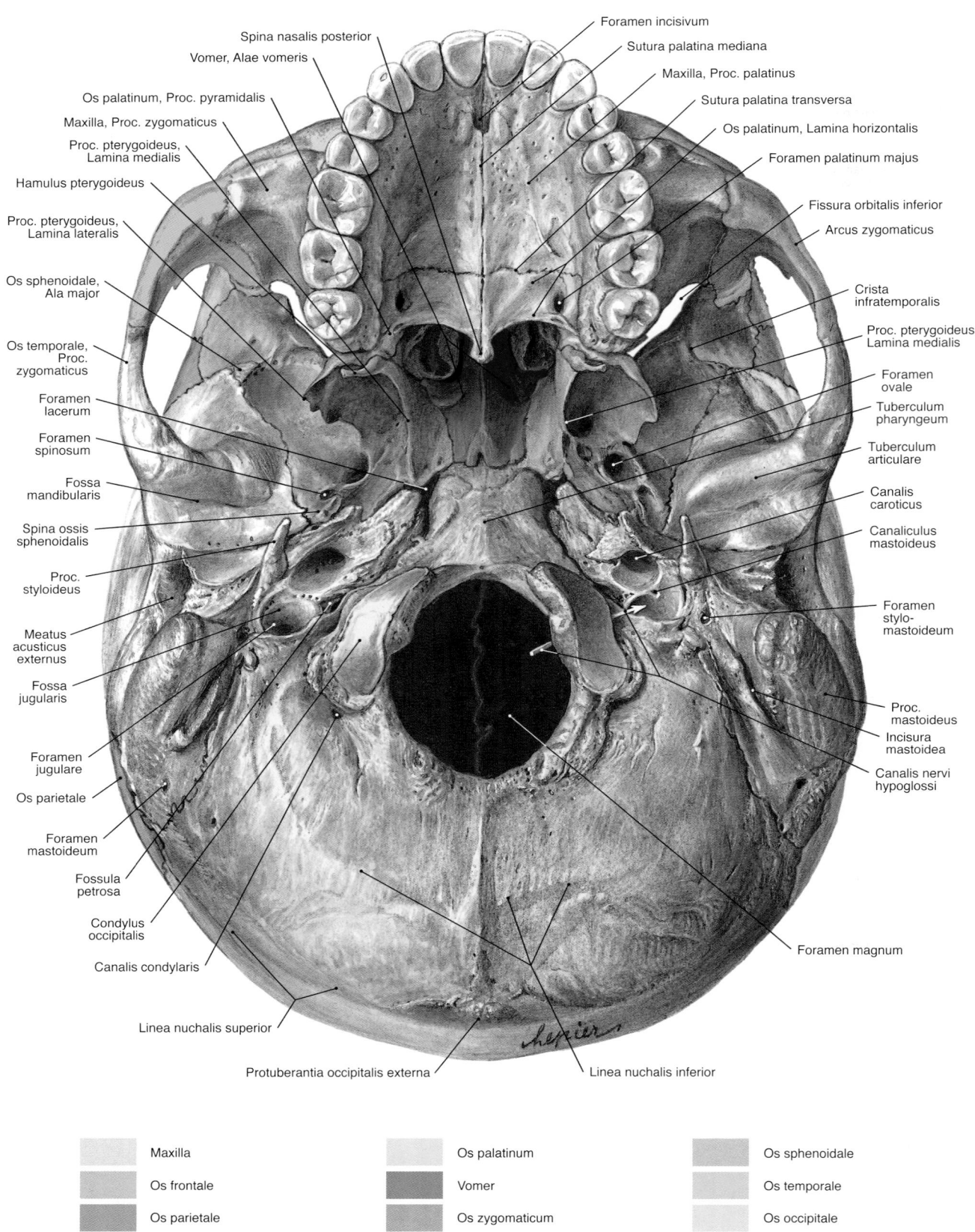

Spina nasalis posterior
Vomer, Alae vomeris
Os palatinum, Proc. pyramidalis
Maxilla, Proc. zygomaticus
Proc. pterygoideus, Lamina medialis
Hamulus pterygoideus
Proc. pterygoideus, Lamina lateralis
Os sphenoidale, Ala major
Os temporale, Proc. zygomaticus
Foramen lacerum
Foramen spinosum
Fossa mandibularis
Spina ossis sphenoidalis
Proc. styloideus
Meatus acusticus externus
Fossa jugularis
Foramen jugulare
Os parietale
Foramen mastoideum
Fossula petrosa
Condylus occipitalis
Canalis condylaris
Linea nuchalis superior
Protuberantia occipitalis externa

Foramen incisivum
Sutura palatina mediana
Maxilla, Proc. palatinus
Sutura palatina transversa
Os palatinum, Lamina horizontalis
Foramen palatinum majus
Fissura orbitalis inferior
Arcus zygomaticus
Crista infratemporalis
Proc. pterygoideus, Lamina medialis
Foramen ovale
Tuberculum pharyngeum
Tuberculum articulare
Canalis caroticus
Canaliculus mastoideus
Foramen stylomastoideum
Proc. mastoideus
Incisura mastoidea
Canalis nervi hypoglossi
Foramen magnum
Linea nuchalis inferior

Maxilla	Os palatinum	Os sphenoidale
Os frontale	Vomer	Os temporale
Os parietale	Os zygomaticum	Os occipitale

Fig. 70 External surface of the base of the skull, Basis cranii externa.

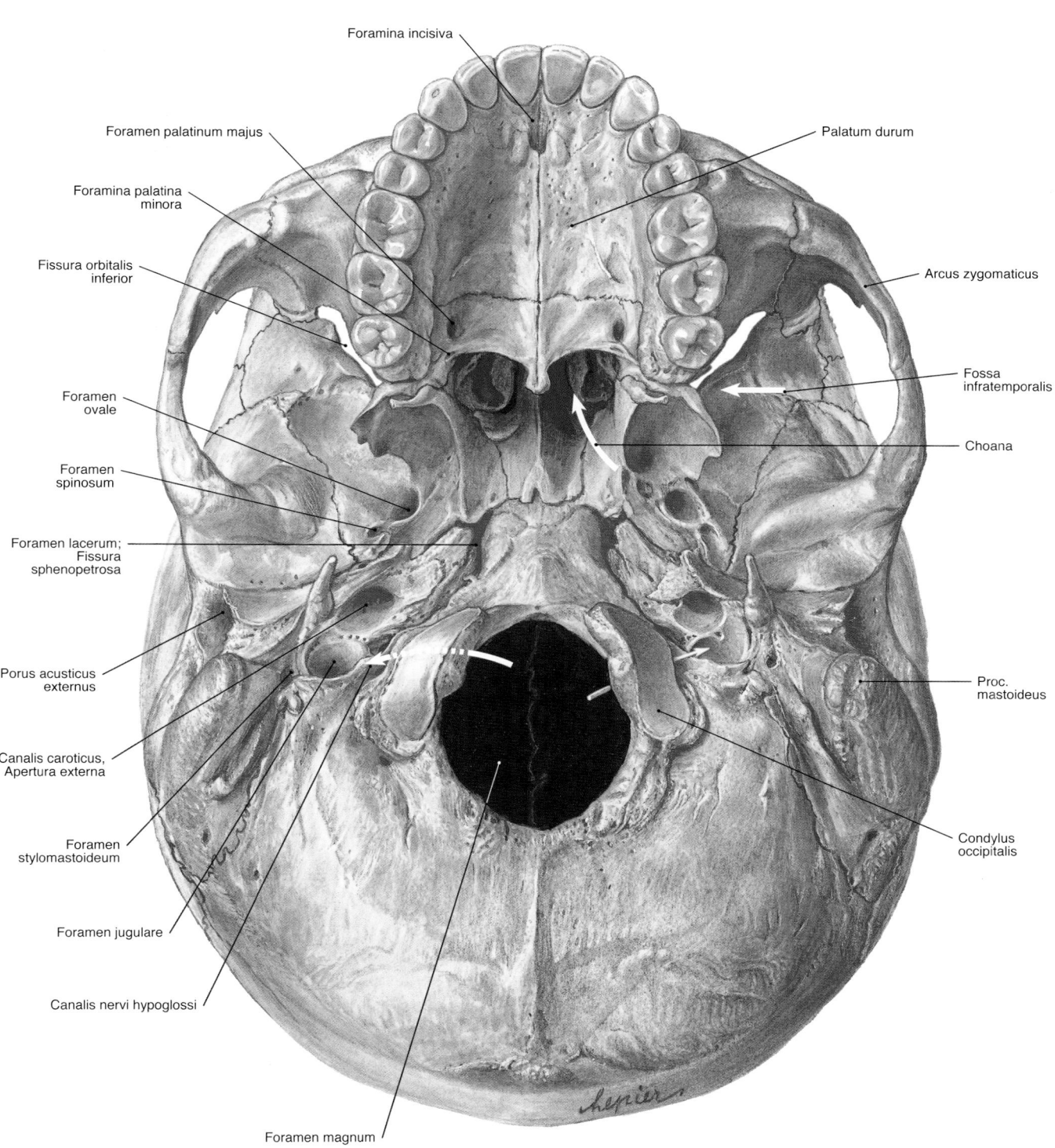

Foramina incisiva

Foramen palatinum majus

Foramina palatina minora

Fissura orbitalis inferior

Foramen ovale

Foramen spinosum

Foramen lacerum; Fissura sphenopetrosa

Porus acusticus externus

Canalis caroticus, Apertura externa

Foramen stylomastoideum

Foramen jugulare

Canalis nervi hypoglossi

Foramen magnum

Palatum durum

Arcus zygomaticus

Fossa infratemporalis

Choana

Proc. mastoideus

Condylus occipitalis

Fig. 71 External surface of the base of the skull, Basis cranii externa, and foramina, Foramina.

→ 1172

Skull, radiography

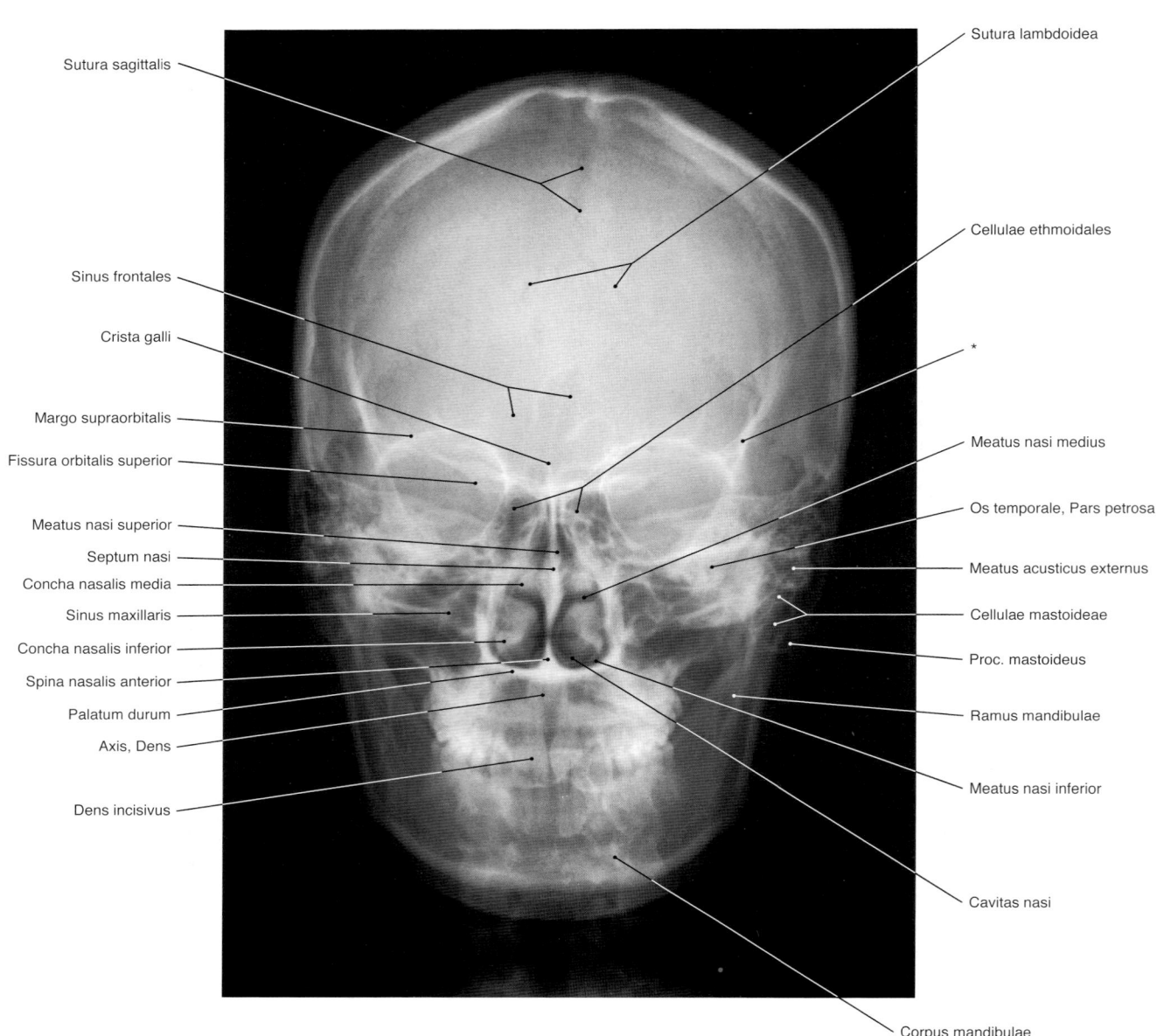

Sutura sagittalis

Sinus frontales

Crista galli

Margo supraorbitalis

Fissura orbitalis superior

Meatus nasi superior

Septum nasi

Concha nasalis media

Sinus maxillaris

Concha nasalis inferior

Spina nasalis anterior

Palatum durum

Axis, Dens

Dens incisivus

Sutura lambdoidea

Cellulae ethmoidales

*

Meatus nasi medius

Os temporale, Pars petrosa

Meatus acusticus externus

Cellulae mastoideae

Proc. mastoideus

Ramus mandibulae

Meatus nasi inferior

Cavitas nasi

Corpus mandibulae

Fig. 72 Skull, Cranium;
AP-teleradiograph.
* Innominate line, Linea innominata, a projection line
  without anatomical correlate

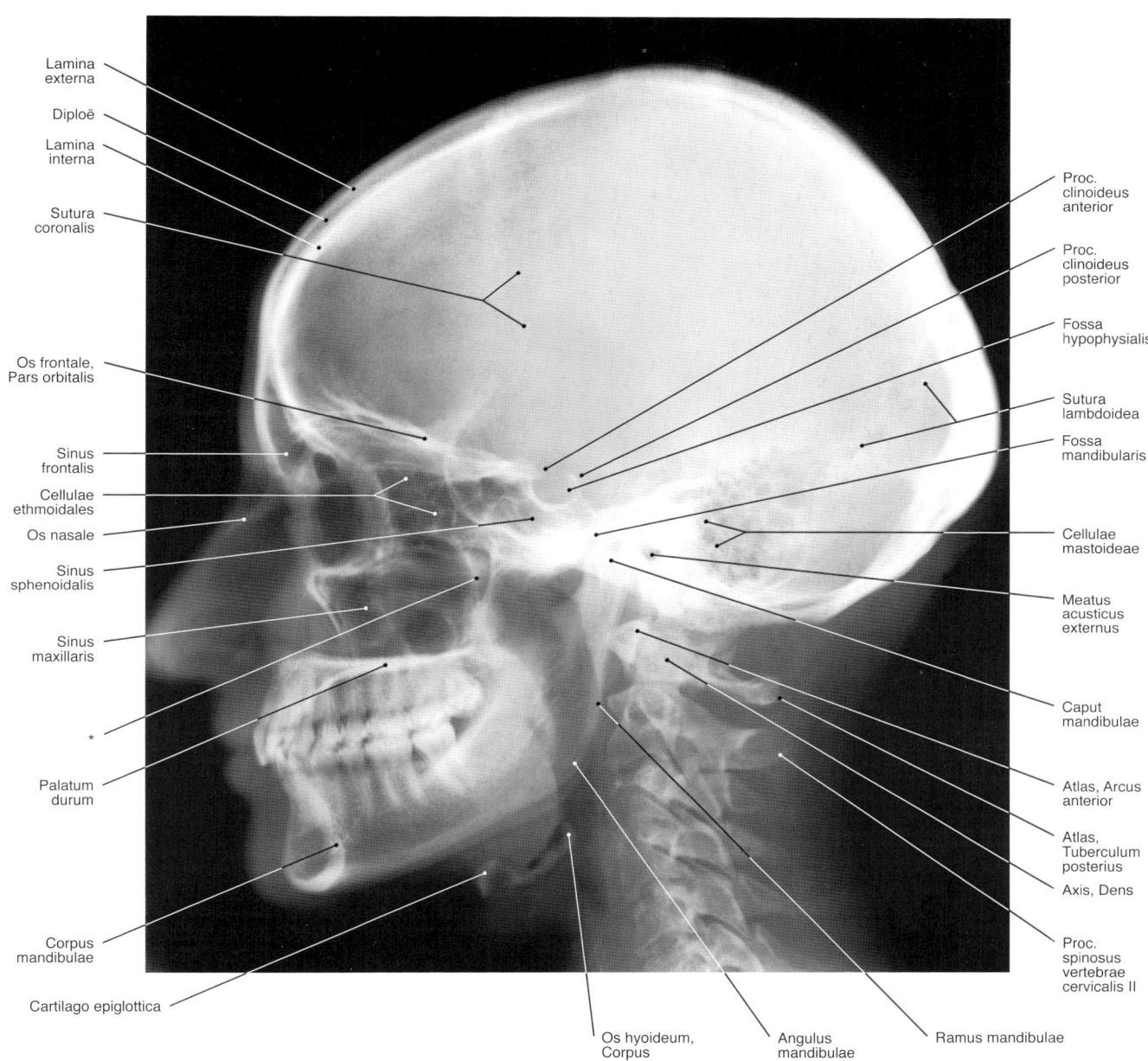

Lamina externa
Diploë
Lamina interna
Sutura coronalis
Os frontale, Pars orbitalis
Sinus frontalis
Cellulae ethmoidales
Os nasale
Sinus sphenoidalis
Sinus maxillaris
*
Palatum durum
Corpus mandibulae
Cartilago epiglottica

Proc. clinoideus anterior
Proc. clinoideus posterior
Fossa hypophysialis
Sutura lambdoidea
Fossa mandibularis
Cellulae mastoideae
Meatus acusticus externus
Caput mandibulae
Atlas, Arcus anterior
Atlas, Tuberculum posterius
Axis, Dens
Proc. spinosus vertebrae cervicalis II

Os hyoideum, Corpus
Angulus mandibulae
Ramus mandibulae

Fig. 73 Skull, Cranium; lateral teleradiograph.
* Posterior wall of the maxillary sinus

Skull, development

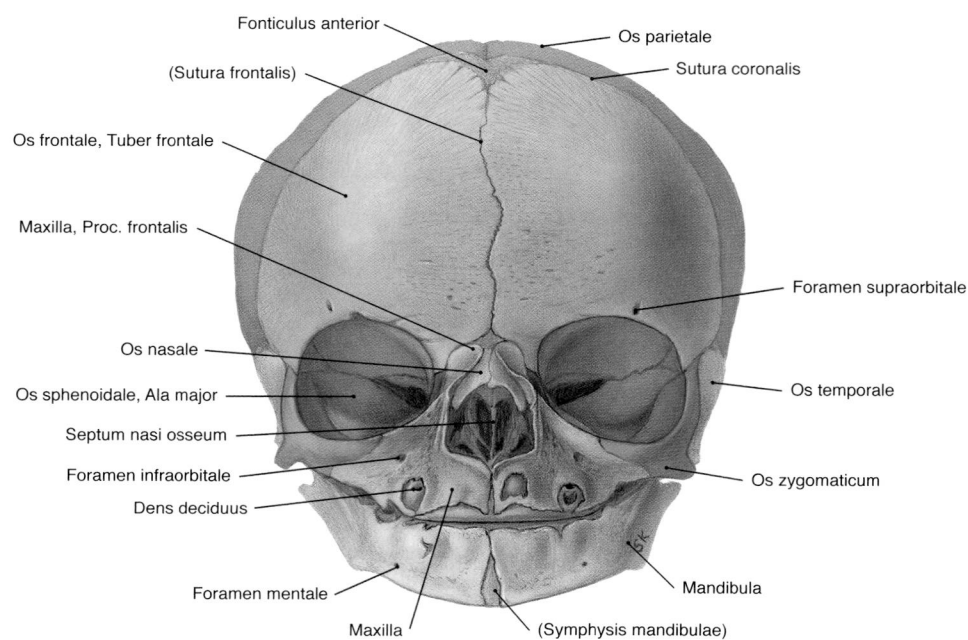

Fonticulus anterior
(Sutura frontalis)
Os frontale, Tuber frontale
Maxilla, Proc. frontalis
Os nasale
Os sphenoidale, Ala major
Septum nasi osseum
Foramen infraorbitale
Dens deciduus
Foramen mentale
Maxilla
Os parietale
Sutura coronalis
Foramen supraorbitale
Os temporale
Os zygomaticum
Mandibula
(Symphysis mandibulae)

Fig. 74 Skull, Cranium, of a neonate.

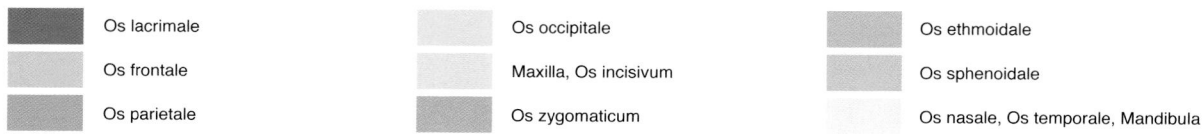

Os lacrimale
Os frontale
Os parietale

Os occipitale
Maxilla, Os incisivum
Os zygomaticum

Os ethmoidale
Os sphenoidale
Os nasale, Os temporale, Mandibula

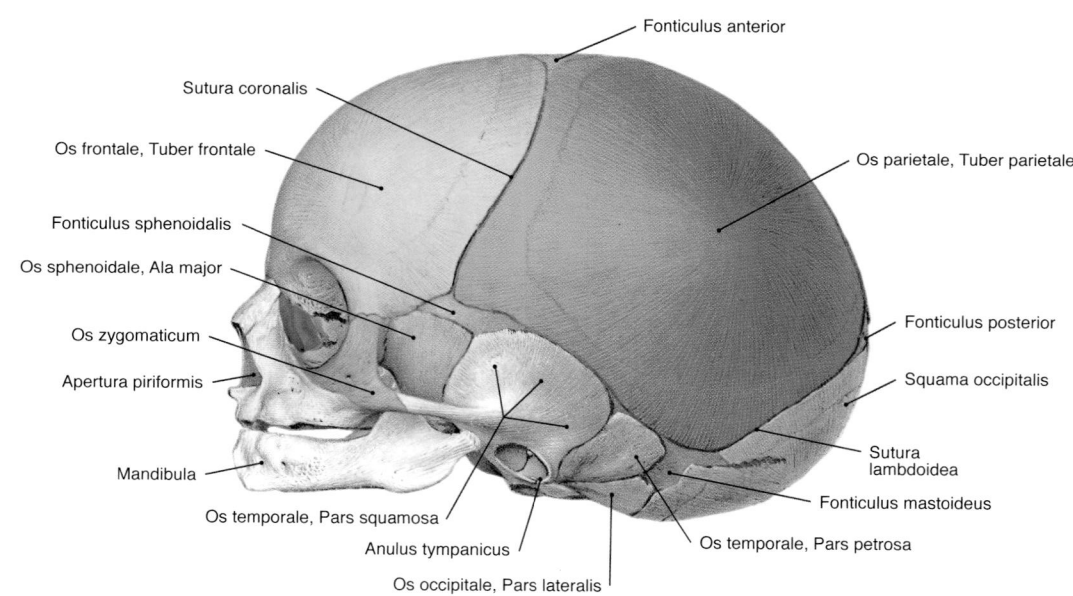

Fonticulus anterior
Sutura coronalis
Os frontale, Tuber frontale
Fonticulus sphenoidalis
Os sphenoidale, Ala major
Os zygomaticum
Apertura piriformis
Mandibula
Os temporale, Pars squamosa
Anulus tympanicus
Os occipitale, Pars lateralis
Os parietale, Tuber parietale
Fonticulus posterior
Squama occipitalis
Sutura lambdoidea
Fonticulus mastoideus
Os temporale, Pars petrosa

Fig. 75 Skull, Cranium, of a neonate.

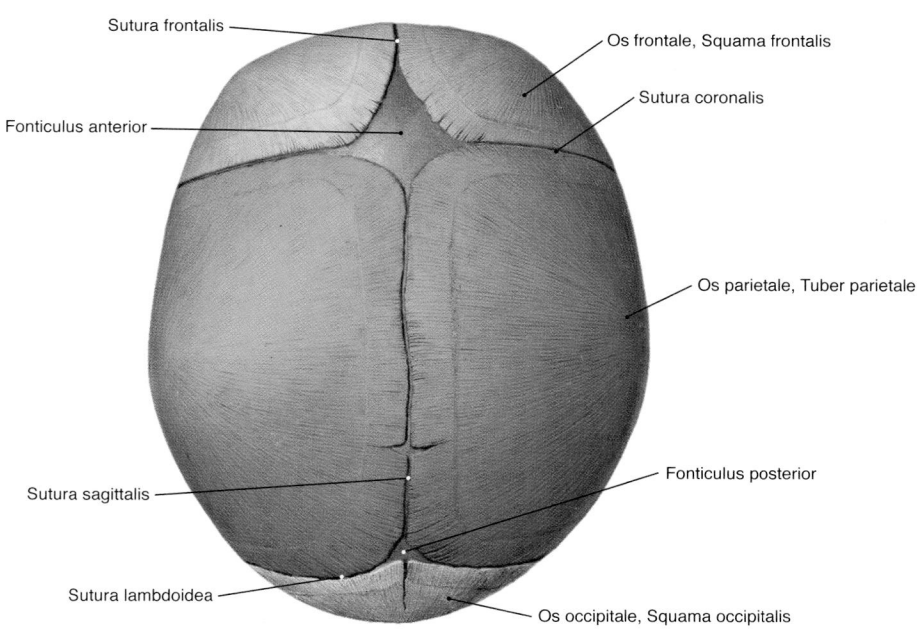

Sutura frontalis

Os frontale, Squama frontalis

Fonticulus anterior

Sutura coronalis

Os parietale, Tuber parietale

Fonticulus posterior

Sutura sagittalis

Sutura lambdoidea

Os occipitale, Squama occipitalis

Fig. 76 Skull, Cranium, of a neonate.

Vomer
Os frontale
Os parietale

Os occipitale, Os palatinum
Os temporale
Mandibula

Maxilla, Os incisivum
Os zygomaticum
Os sphenoidale

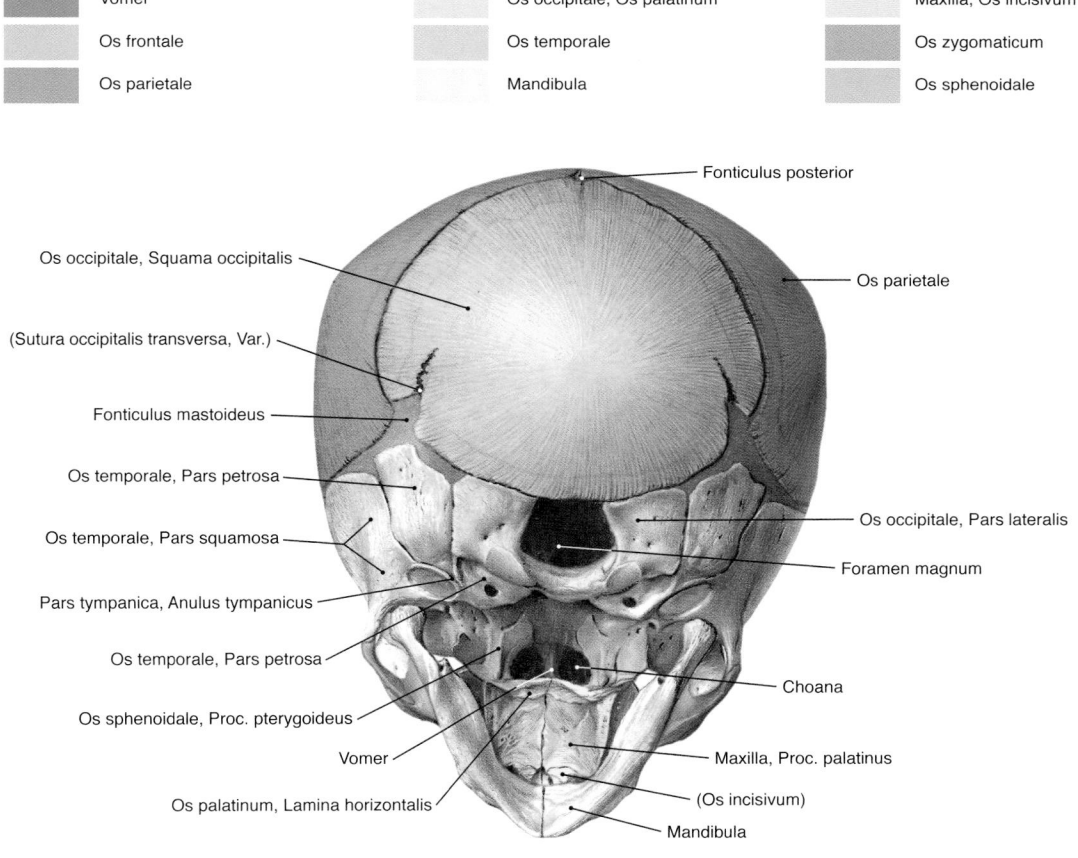

Fonticulus posterior

Os occipitale, Squama occipitalis

Os parietale

(Sutura occipitalis transversa, Var.)

Fonticulus mastoideus

Os temporale, Pars petrosa

Os occipitale, Pars lateralis

Os temporale, Pars squamosa

Foramen magnum

Pars tympanica, Anulus tympanicus

Os temporale, Pars petrosa

Os sphenoidale, Proc. pterygoideus

Choana

Vomer

Maxilla, Proc. palatinus

(Os incisivum)

Os palatinum, Lamina horizontalis

Mandibula

Fig. 77 Skull, Cranium, of a neonate.

Frontal and ethmoidal bone

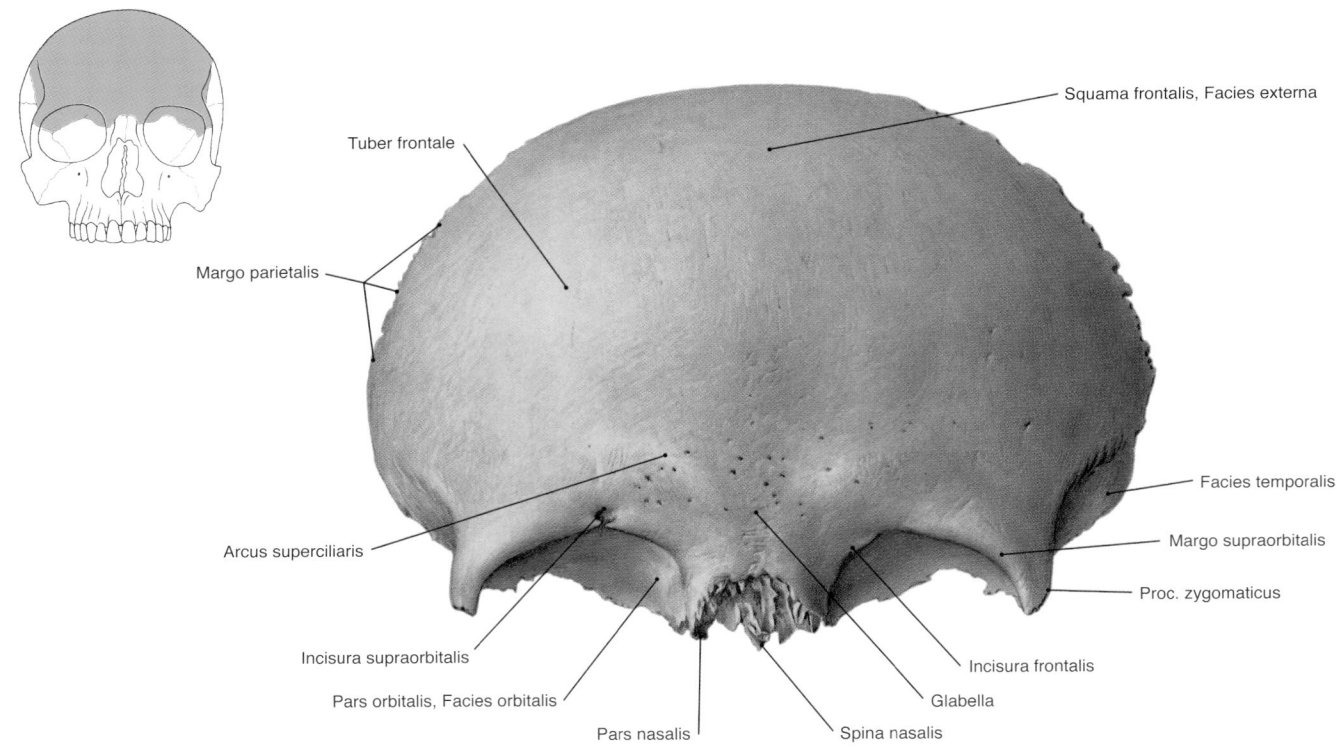

Squama frontalis, Facies externa

Tuber frontale

Margo parietalis

Facies temporalis

Margo supraorbitalis

Proc. zygomaticus

Arcus superciliaris

Incisura frontalis

Incisura supraorbitalis

Pars orbitalis, Facies orbitalis

Glabella

Pars nasalis

Spina nasalis

Fig. 78 Frontal bone, Os frontale.

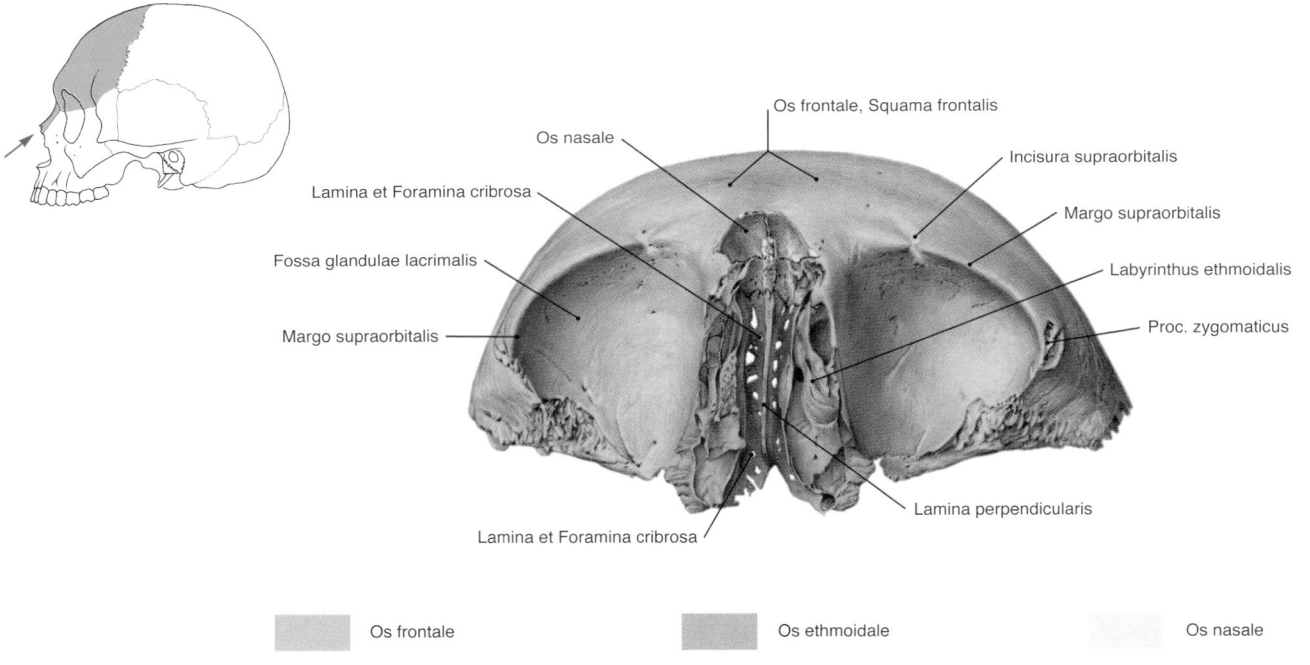

Os frontale, Squama frontalis

Os nasale

Incisura supraorbitalis

Lamina et Foramina cribrosa

Margo supraorbitalis

Fossa glandulae lacrimalis

Labyrinthus ethmoidalis

Proc. zygomaticus

Margo supraorbitalis

Lamina perpendicularis

Lamina et Foramina cribrosa

Os frontale | Os ethmoidale | Os nasale

Fig. 79 Frontal bone, Os frontale; ethmoidal bone,
Os ethmoidale, and nasal bones, Ossa nasalia.

Maxilla and palatine bone

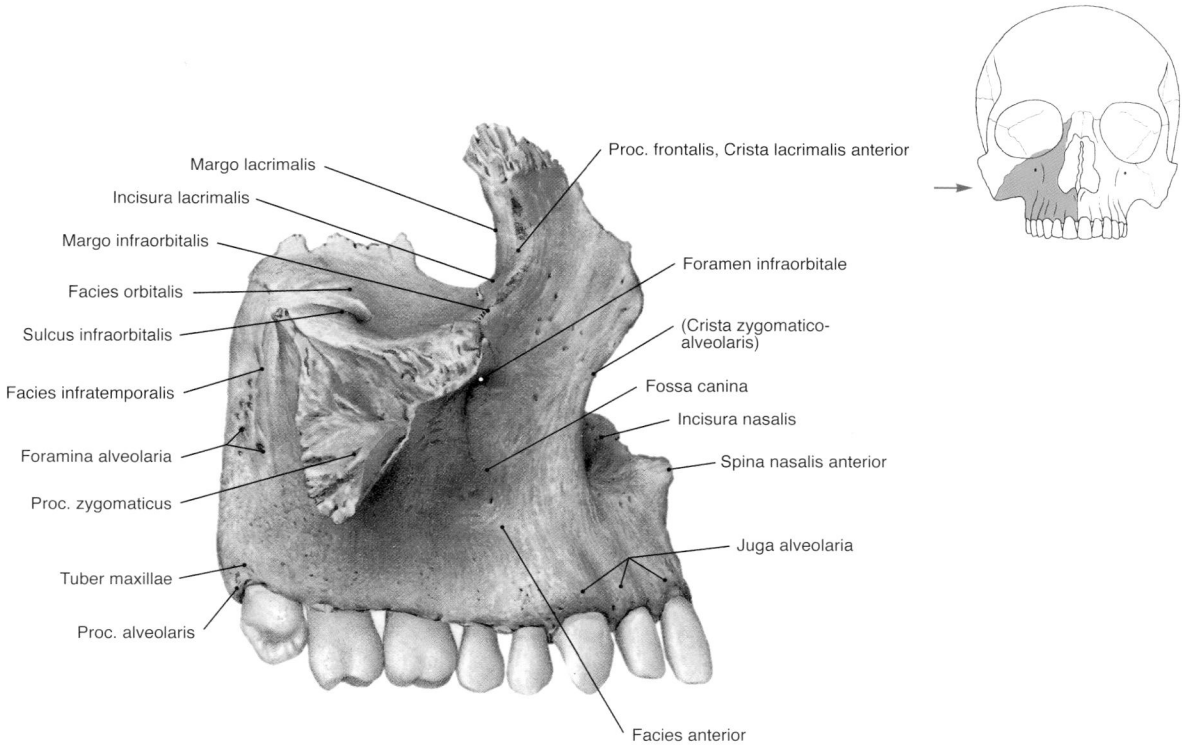

Margo lacrimalis
Incisura lacrimalis
Margo infraorbitalis
Facies orbitalis
Sulcus infraorbitalis
Facies infratemporalis
Foramina alveolaria
Proc. zygomaticus
Tuber maxillae
Proc. alveolaris

Proc. frontalis, Crista lacrimalis anterior
Foramen infraorbitale
(Crista zygomatico-alveolaris)
Fossa canina
Incisura nasalis
Spina nasalis anterior
Juga alveolaria

Facies anterior

Fig. 80 Maxilla, Maxilla.

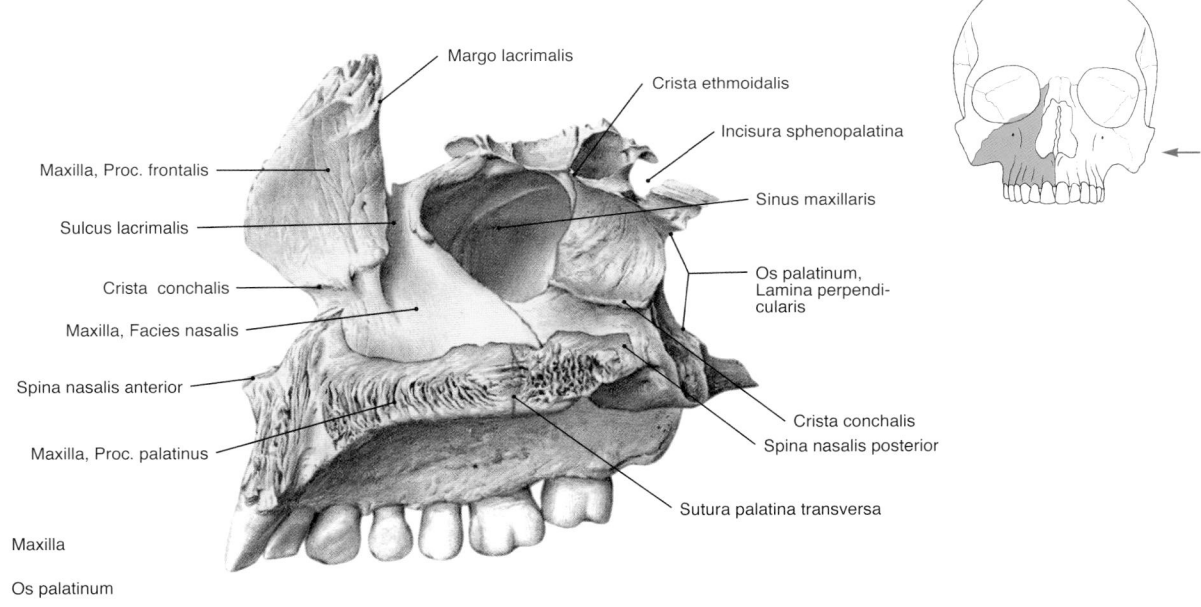

Margo lacrimalis

Maxilla, Proc. frontalis
Sulcus lacrimalis
Crista conchalis
Maxilla, Facies nasalis
Spina nasalis anterior
Maxilla, Proc. palatinus

Crista ethmoidalis
Incisura sphenopalatina
Sinus maxillaris
Os palatinum, Lamina perpendi-cularis
Crista conchalis
Spina nasalis posterior
Sutura palatina transversa

Maxilla
Os palatinum

Fig. 81 Maxilla, Maxilla, and palatine bone, Os palatinum.

Nasal cavity

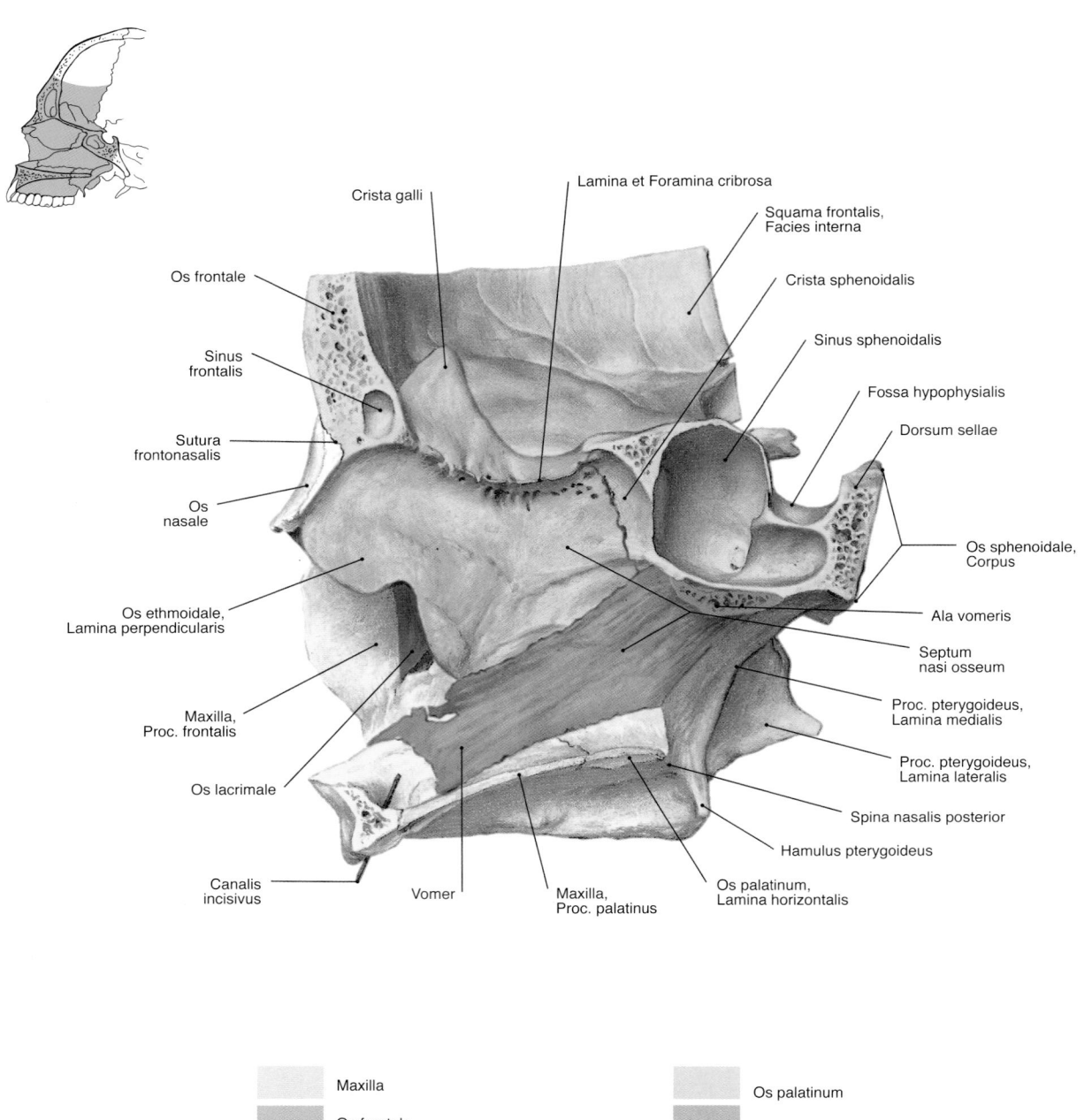

Crista galli

Lamina et Foramina cribrosa

Squama frontalis, Facies interna

Os frontale

Crista sphenoidalis

Sinus frontalis

Sinus sphenoidalis

Fossa hypophysialis

Sutura frontonasalis

Dorsum sellae

Os nasale

Os sphenoidale, Corpus

Os ethmoidale, Lamina perpendicularis

Ala vomeris

Septum nasi osseum

Maxilla, Proc. frontalis

Proc. pterygoideus, Lamina medialis

Proc. pterygoideus, Lamina lateralis

Os lacrimale

Spina nasalis posterior

Hamulus pterygoideus

Canalis incisivus

Vomer

Maxilla, Proc. palatinus

Os palatinum, Lamina horizontalis

Maxilla

Os palatinum

Os frontale

Os ethmoidale

Os nasale

Vomer

Os sphenoidale

Os lacrimale

Fig. 82 Bony nasal septum, Septum nasi osseum.

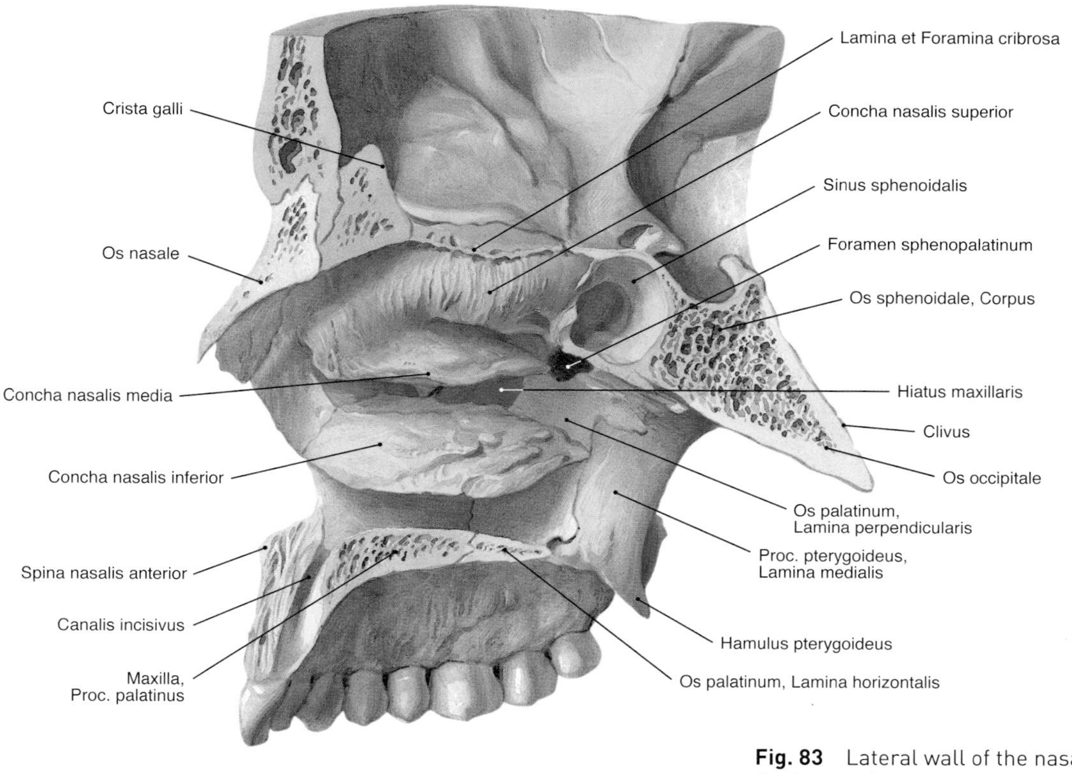

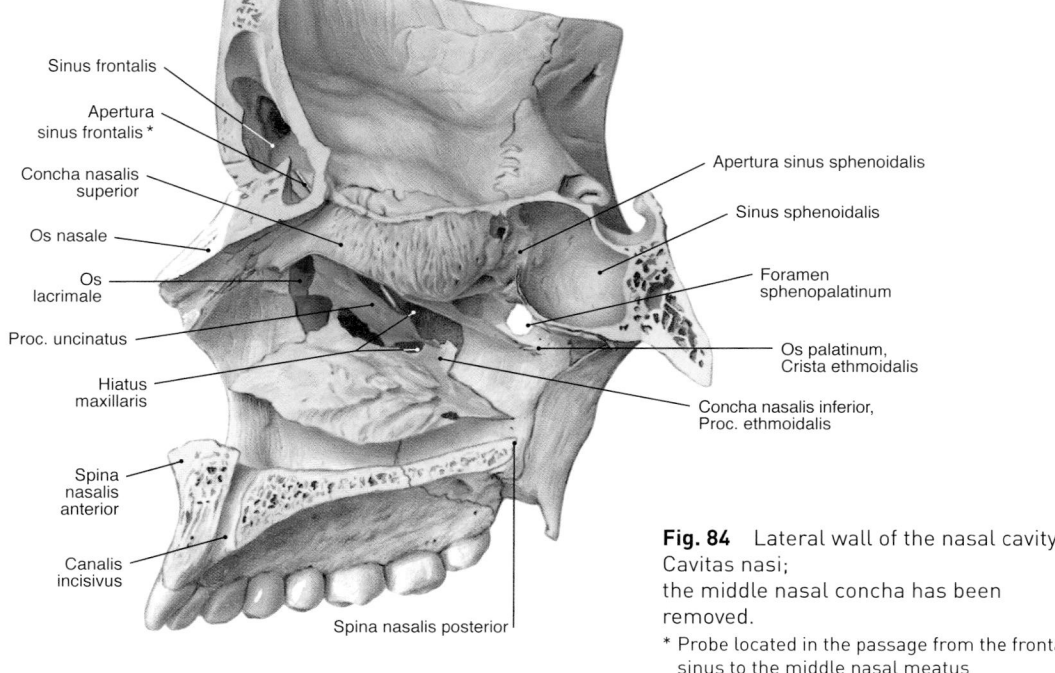

Lamina et Foramina cribrosa

Crista galli

Concha nasalis superior

Sinus sphenoidalis

Os nasale

Foramen sphenopalatinum

Os sphenoidale, Corpus

Concha nasalis media

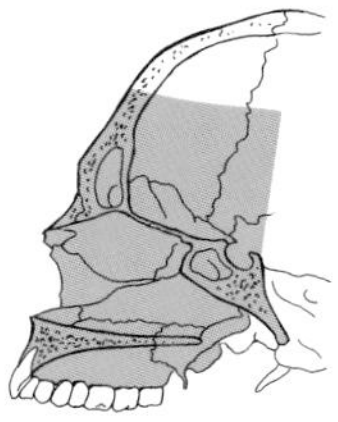

Hiatus maxillaris

Clivus

Concha nasalis inferior

Os occipitale

Os palatinum,
Lamina perpendicularis

Spina nasalis anterior

Proc. pterygoideus,
Lamina medialis

Canalis incisivus

Hamulus pterygoideus

Maxilla,
Proc. palatinus

Os palatinum, Lamina horizontalis

Fig. 83 Lateral wall of the nasal cavity,
Cavitas nasi.

Os parietale	Concha nasalis inferior
Maxilla	Os sphenoidale
Os frontale	Os occipitale
Os nasale	Os palatinum

Os ethmoidale

Os lacrimale

Sinus frontalis

Apertura
sinus frontalis *

Concha nasalis
superior

Apertura sinus sphenoidalis

Os nasale

Sinus sphenoidalis

Os
lacrimale

Foramen
sphenopalatinum

Proc. uncinatus

Os palatinum,
Crista ethmoidalis

Hiatus
maxillaris

Concha nasalis inferior,
Proc. ethmoidalis

Spina
nasalis
anterior

Canalis
incisivus

Spina nasalis posterior

Fig. 84 Lateral wall of the nasal cavity,
Cavitas nasi;
the middle nasal concha has been
removed.
* Probe located in the passage from the frontal
  sinus to the middle nasal meatus

Hard palate

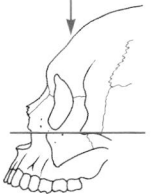

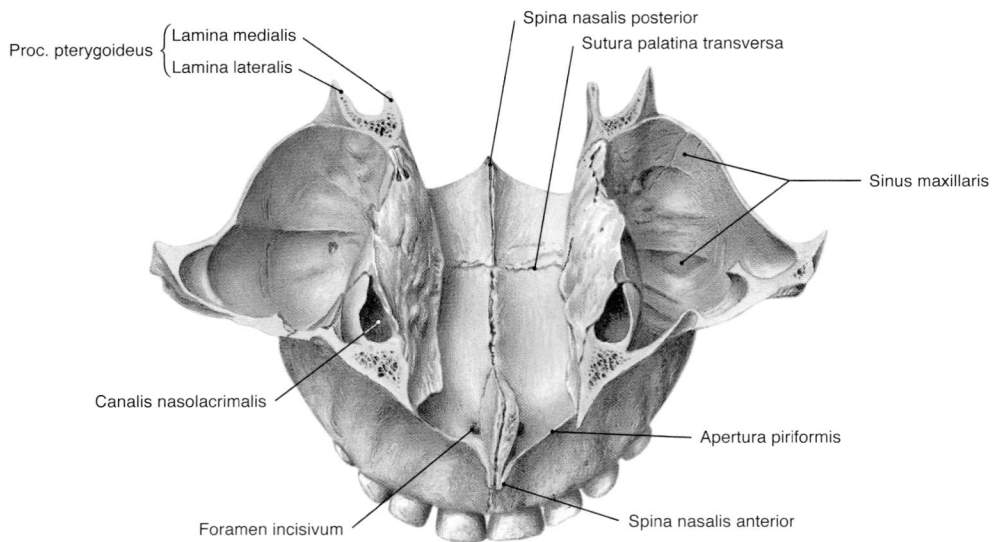

Proc. pterygoideus { Lamina medialis / Lamina lateralis

Spina nasalis posterior

Sutura palatina transversa

Sinus maxillaris

Canalis nasolacrimalis

Apertura piriformis

Foramen incisivum

Spina nasalis anterior

Fig. 85   Hard palate, Palatum durum; maxillary sinus, Sinus maxillaris, and inferior nasal concha, Concha nasalis inferior.

Maxilla

Os palatinum

Os sphenoidale

Concha nasalis inferior

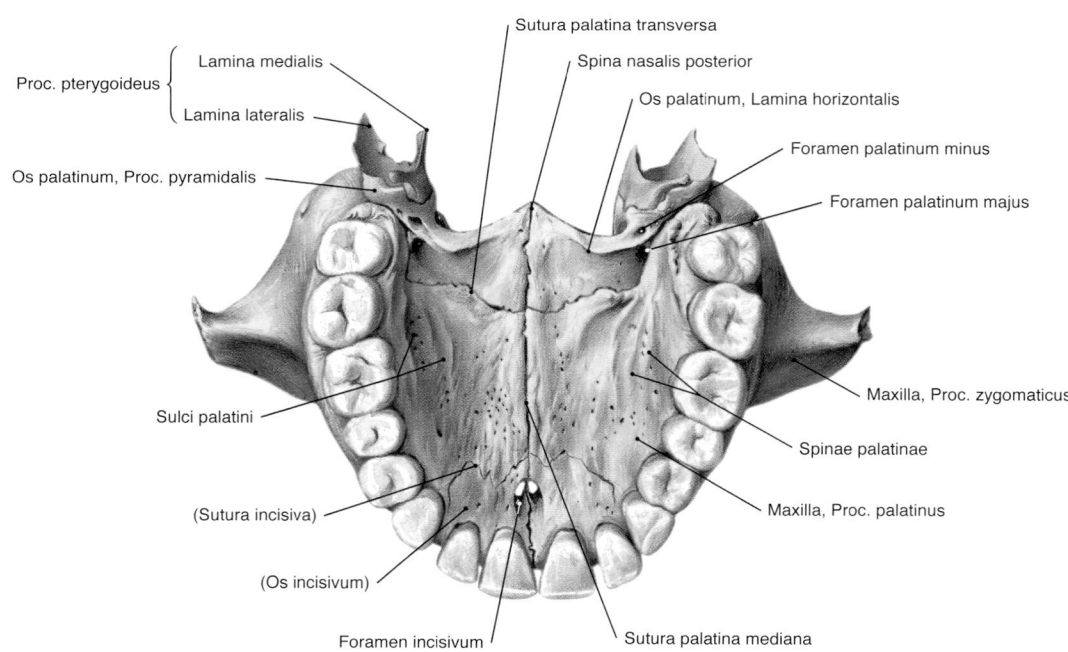

Sutura palatina transversa

Spina nasalis posterior

Proc. pterygoideus { Lamina medialis / Lamina lateralis

Os palatinum, Lamina horizontalis

Os palatinum, Proc. pyramidalis

Foramen palatinum minus

Foramen palatinum majus

Maxilla, Proc. zygomaticus

Sulci palatini

Spinae palatinae

(Sutura incisiva)

Maxilla, Proc. palatinus

(Os incisivum)

Foramen incisivum

Sutura palatina mediana

Fig. 86   Hard palate, Palatum durum.

Orbit and pterygopalatine fossa

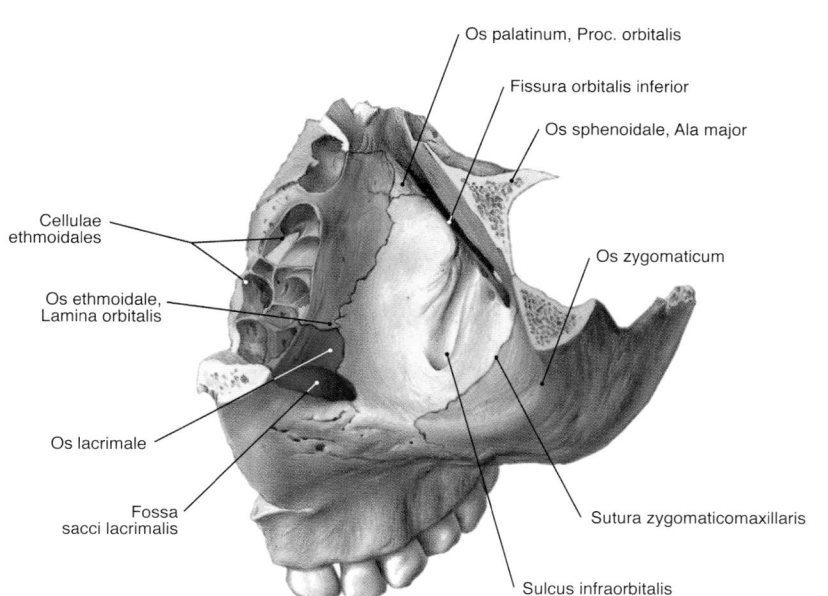
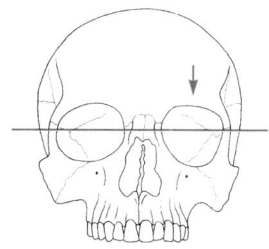

Os palatinum, Proc. orbitalis

Fissura orbitalis inferior

Os sphenoidale, Ala major

Cellulae ethmoidales

Os zygomaticum

Os ethmoidale, Lamina orbitalis

Os lacrimale

Fossa sacci lacrimalis

Sutura zygomaticomaxillaris

Sulcus infraorbitalis

Fig. 87 Base of the orbit, Orbita.

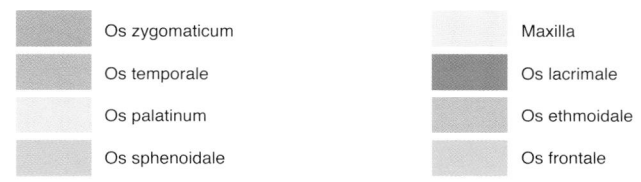

Os zygomaticum	Maxilla
Os temporale	Os lacrimale
Os palatinum	Os ethmoidale
Os sphenoidale	Os frontale

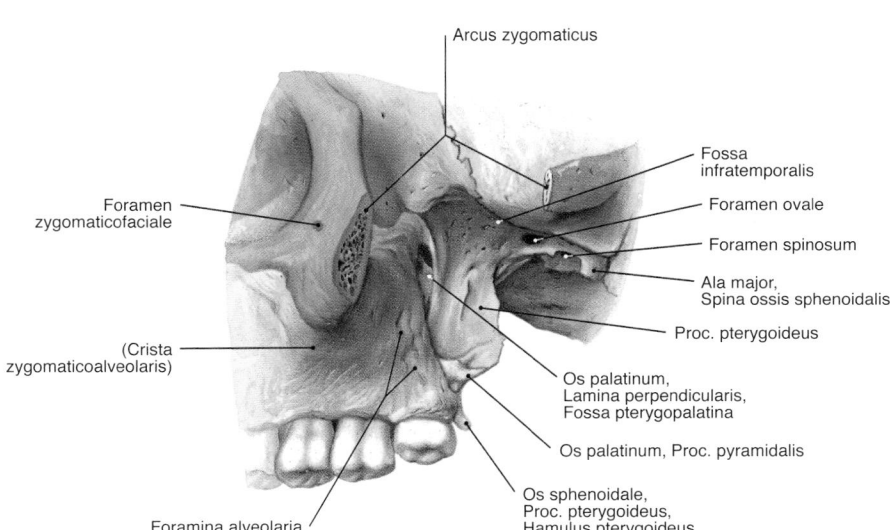
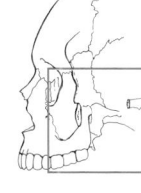

Arcus zygomaticus

Fossa infratemporalis

Foramen ovale

Foramen spinosum

Ala major, Spina ossis sphenoidalis

Proc. pterygoideus

Os palatinum, Lamina perpendicularis, Fossa pterygopalatina

Os palatinum, Proc. pyramidalis

Foramen zygomaticofaciale

(Crista zygomaticoalveolaris)

Foramina alveolaria

Os sphenoidale, Proc. pterygoideus, Hamulus pterygoideus

Fig. 88 Pterygopalatine fossa, Fossa pterygopalatina.

Orbit

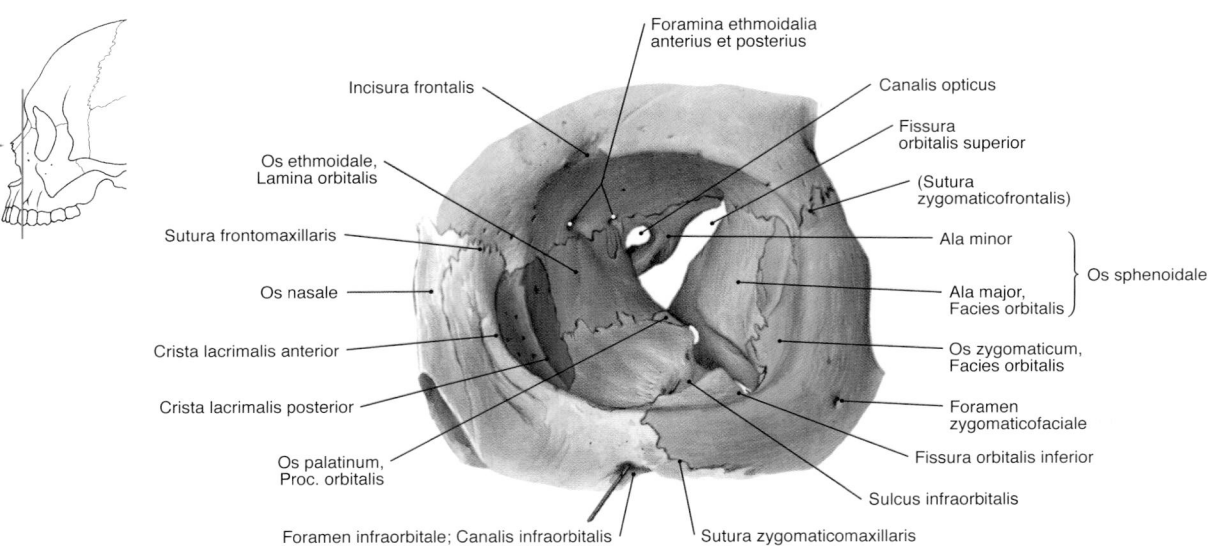

Foramina ethmoidalia
anterius et posterius

Incisura frontalis

Os ethmoidale,
Lamina orbitalis

Sutura frontomaxillaris

Os nasale

Crista lacrimalis anterior

Crista lacrimalis posterior

Os palatinum,
Proc. orbitalis

Foramen infraorbitale; Canalis infraorbitalis

Canalis opticus

Fissura
orbitalis superior

(Sutura
zygomaticofrontalis)

Ala minor

Ala major,
Facies orbitalis

} Os sphenoidale

Os zygomaticum,
Facies orbitalis

Foramen
zygomaticofaciale

Fissura orbitalis inferior

Sulcus infraorbitalis

Sutura zygomaticomaxillaris

Fig. 89 Orbit, Orbita;
probe located in the infra-orbital
canal, Canalis infraorbitalis.

Os nasale	Vomer	Os temporale
Os frontale	Os zygomaticum	Concha nasalis inferior
Os palatinum	Maxilla	Os sphenoidale
Os ethmoidale		Os lacrimale

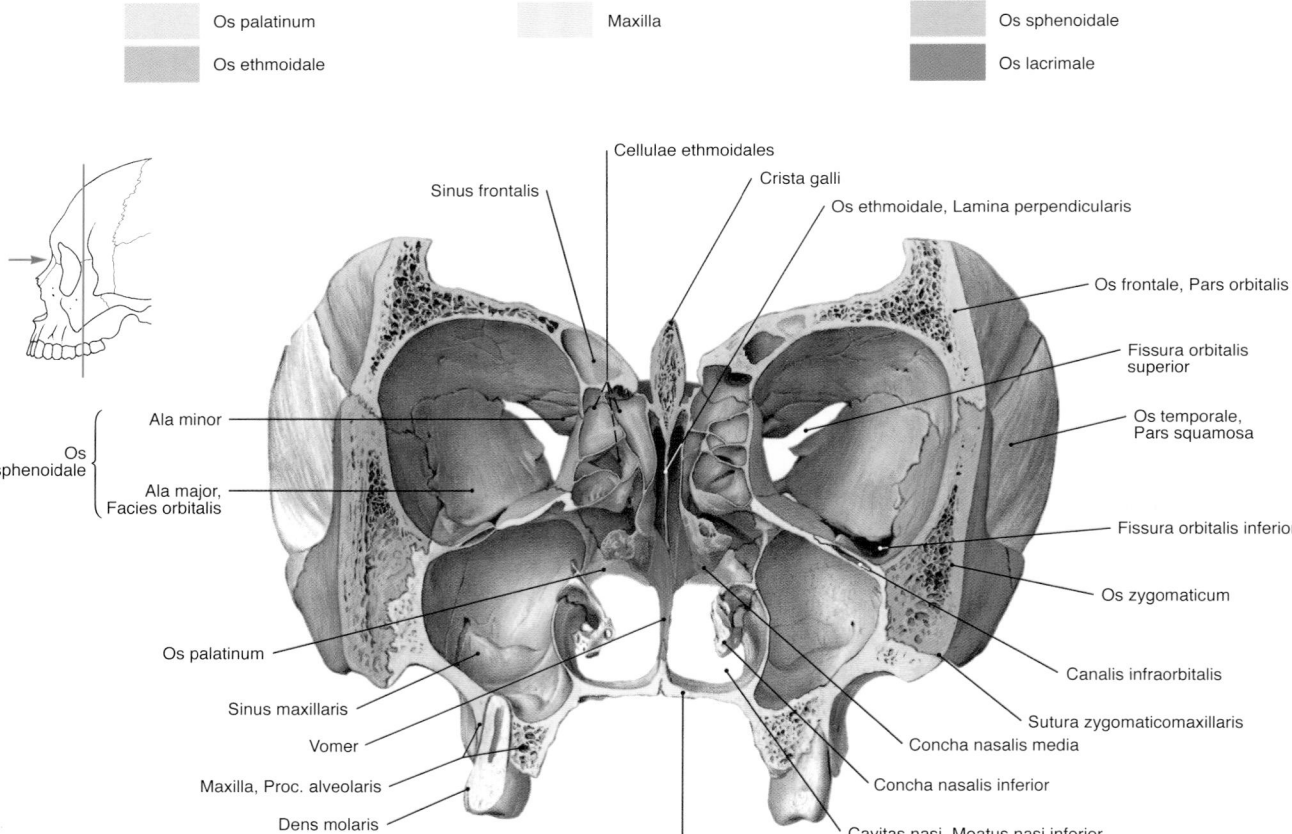

Cellulae ethmoidales

Sinus frontalis

Crista galli

Os ethmoidale, Lamina perpendicularis

Os frontale, Pars orbitalis

Fissura orbitalis
superior

Os temporale,
Pars squamosa

Fissura orbitalis inferior

Os zygomaticum

Canalis infraorbitalis

Sutura zygomaticomaxillaris

Concha nasalis media

Concha nasalis inferior

Cavitas nasi, Meatus nasi inferior

Os
sphenoidale {

Ala minor

Ala major,
Facies orbitalis

Os palatinum

Sinus maxillaris

Vomer

Maxilla, Proc. alveolaris

Dens molaris

Maxilla, Proc. palatinus

Fig. 90 Facial skeleton, Viscerocranium;
frontal section.

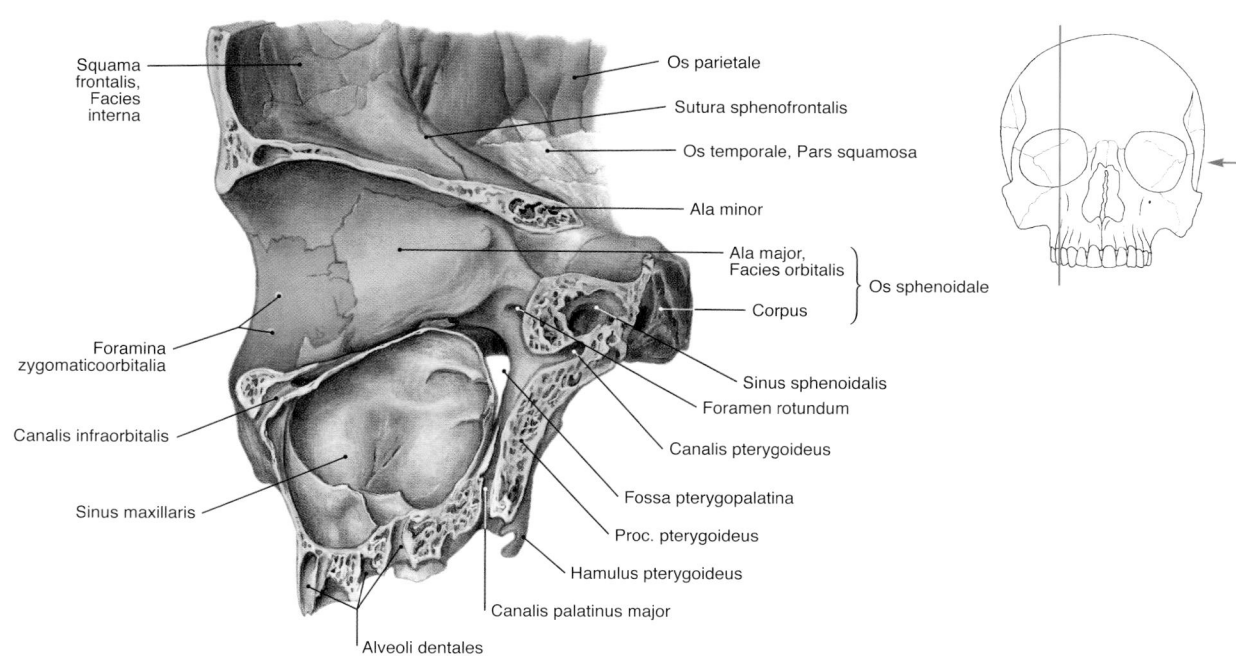

Squama frontalis, Facies interna
Os parietale
Sutura sphenofrontalis
Os temporale, Pars squamosa
Ala minor
Ala major, Facies orbitalis
Corpus
⎫ Os sphenoidale
Foramina zygomaticoorbitalia
Sinus sphenoidalis
Foramen rotundum
Canalis infraorbitalis
Canalis pterygoideus
Fossa pterygopalatina
Proc. pterygoideus
Sinus maxillaris
Hamulus pterygoideus
Canalis palatinus major
Alveoli dentales

Fig. 91 Orbit, Orbita;
lateral wall.

Os frontale	Os nasale	Maxilla
Os lacrimale	Os palatinum	Os temporale
Os sphenoidale	Os ethmoidale	Os zygomaticum

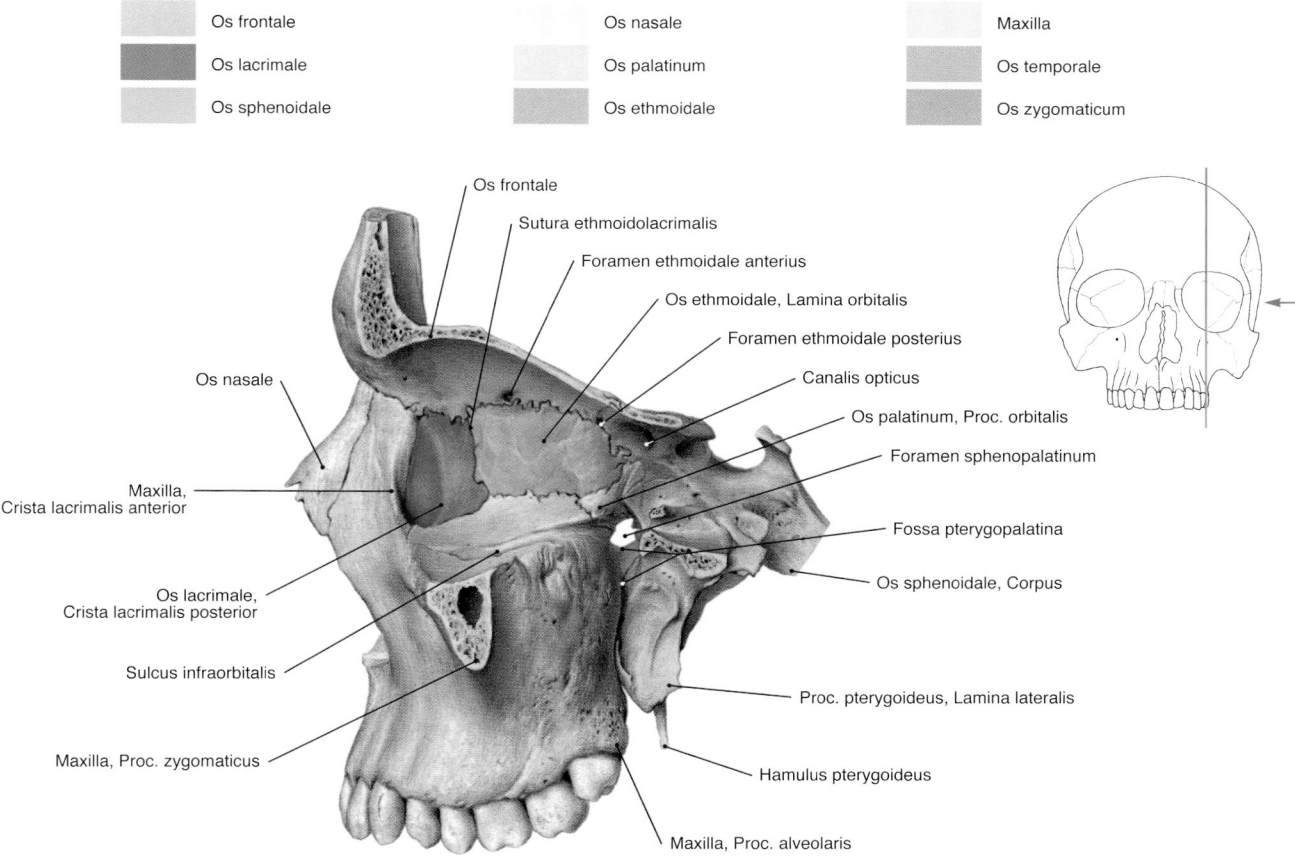

Os frontale
Sutura ethmoidolacrimalis
Foramen ethmoidale anterius
Os ethmoidale, Lamina orbitalis
Foramen ethmoidale posterius
Canalis opticus
Os nasale
Os palatinum, Proc. orbitalis
Foramen sphenopalatinum
Maxilla, Crista lacrimalis anterior
Fossa pterygopalatina
Os lacrimale, Crista lacrimalis posterior
Os sphenoidale, Corpus
Sulcus infraorbitalis
Proc. pterygoideus, Lamina lateralis
Maxilla, Proc. zygomaticus
Hamulus pterygoideus
Maxilla, Proc. alveolaris

Fig. 92 Orbit, Orbita;
medial wall.

Sphenoidal bone

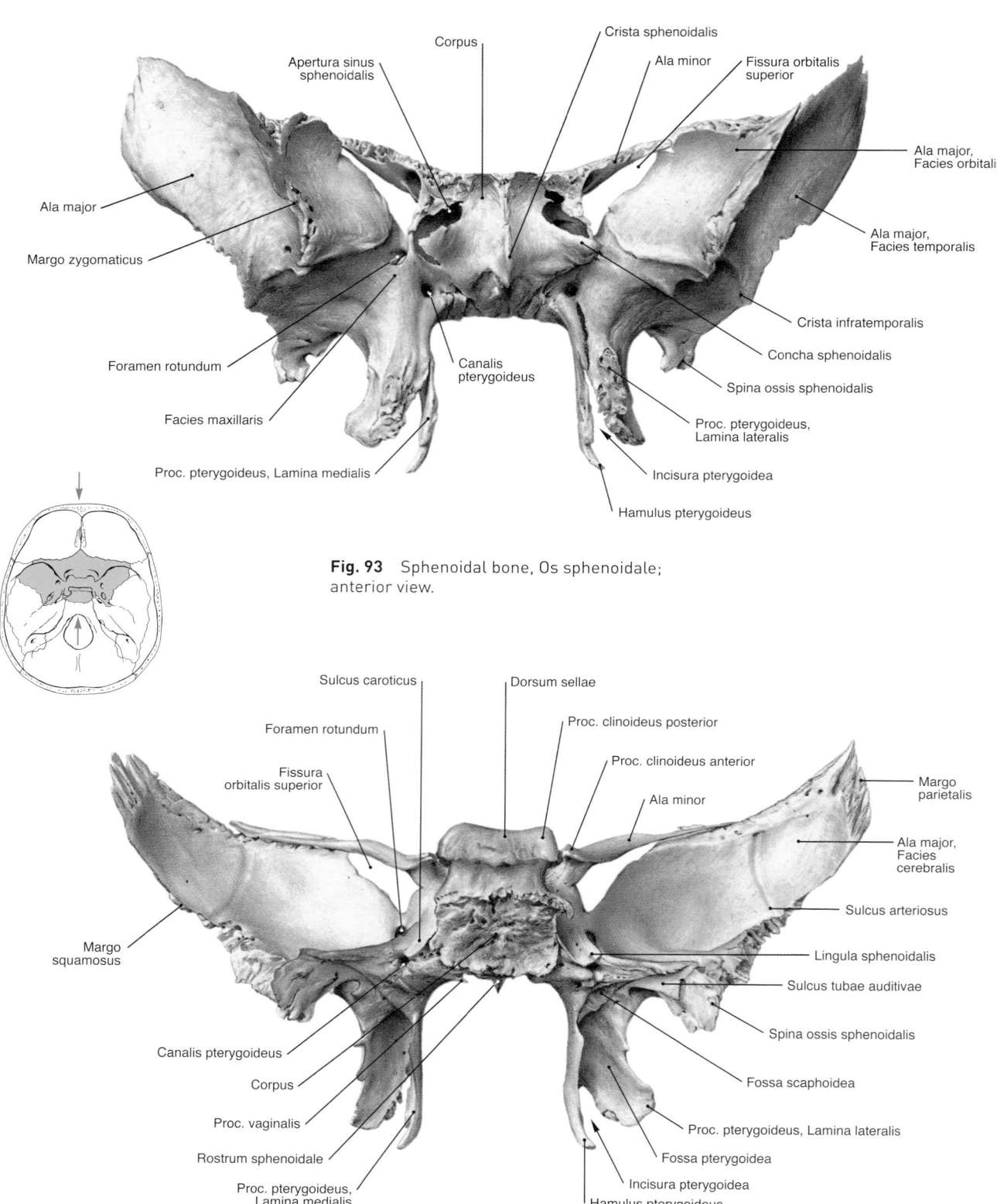

Corpus
Crista sphenoidalis
Apertura sinus sphenoidalis
Ala minor
Fissura orbitalis superior
Ala major, Facies orbitalis
Ala major
Ala major, Facies temporalis
Margo zygomaticus
Crista infratemporalis
Concha sphenoidalis
Foramen rotundum
Canalis pterygoideus
Spina ossis sphenoidalis
Facies maxillaris
Proc. pterygoideus, Lamina lateralis
Proc. pterygoideus, Lamina medialis
Incisura pterygoidea
Hamulus pterygoideus

Fig. 93 Sphenoidal bone, Os sphenoidale; anterior view.

Sulcus caroticus
Dorsum sellae
Foramen rotundum
Proc. clinoideus posterior
Fissura orbitalis superior
Proc. clinoideus anterior
Ala minor
Margo parietalis
Ala major, Facies cerebralis
Sulcus arteriosus
Margo squamosus
Lingula sphenoidalis
Sulcus tubae auditivae
Canalis pterygoideus
Spina ossis sphenoidalis
Corpus
Fossa scaphoidea
Proc. vaginalis
Proc. pterygoideus, Lamina lateralis
Rostrum sphenoidale
Fossa pterygoidea
Proc. pterygoideus, Lamina medialis
Incisura pterygoidea
Hamulus pterygoideus

Fig. 94 Sphenoidal bone, Os sphenoidale; posterior view.

Sphenoidal and occipital bone

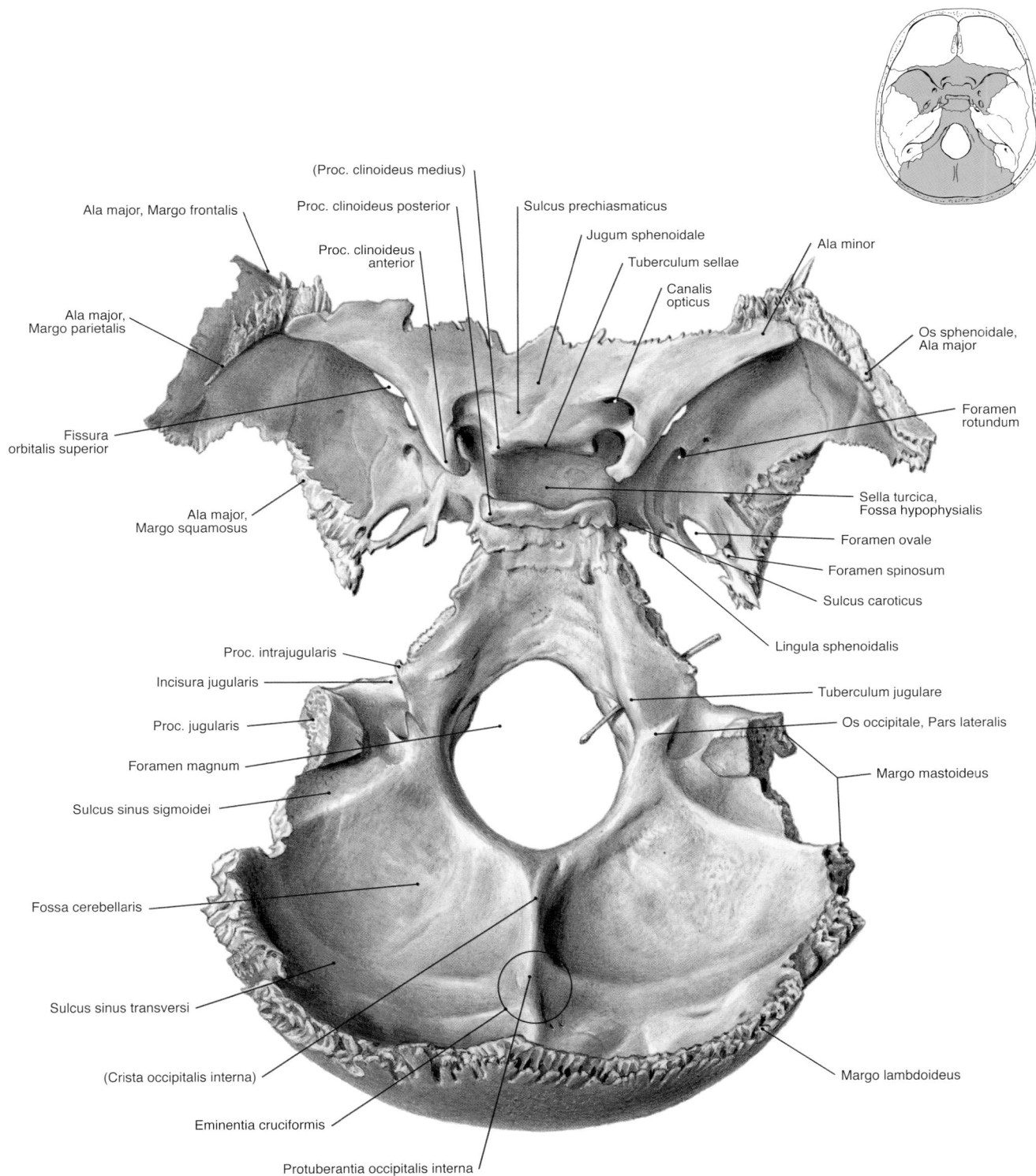

(Proc. clinoideus medius)

Proc. clinoideus posterior

Ala major, Margo frontalis

Proc. clinoideus anterior

Sulcus prechiasmaticus

Jugum sphenoidale

Tuberculum sellae

Canalis opticus

Ala minor

Ala major, Margo parietalis

Os sphenoidale, Ala major

Foramen rotundum

Fissura orbitalis superior

Sella turcica, Fossa hypophysialis

Ala major, Margo squamosus

Foramen ovale

Foramen spinosum

Sulcus caroticus

Lingula sphenoidalis

Proc. intrajugularis

Incisura jugularis

Tuberculum jugulare

Proc. jugularis

Os occipitale, Pars lateralis

Foramen magnum

Margo mastoideus

Sulcus sinus sigmoidei

Fossa cerebellaris

Sulcus sinus transversi

Margo lambdoideus

(Crista occipitalis interna)

Eminentia cruciformis

Protuberantia occipitalis interna

Fig. 95 Occipital bone, Os occipitale, and sphenoidal bone, Os sphenoidale.

Temporal bone

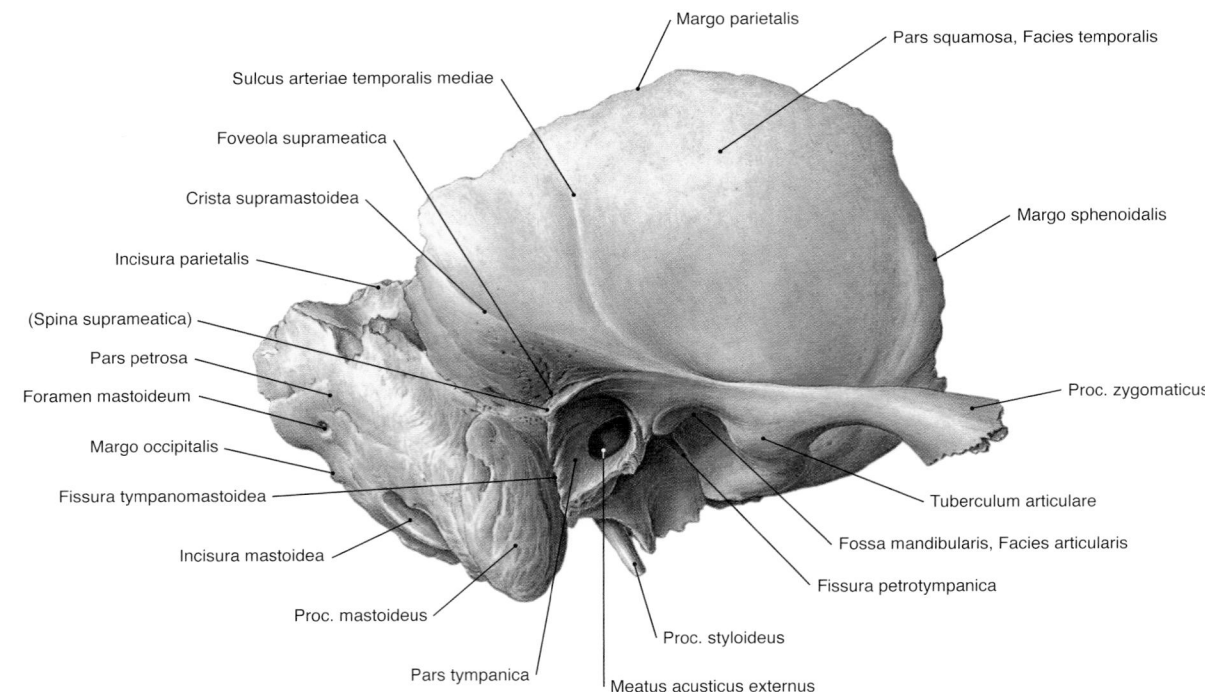

Margo parietalis
Sulcus arteriae temporalis mediae
Foveola suprameatica
Crista supramastoidea
Incisura parietalis
(Spina suprameatica)
Pars petrosa
Foramen mastoideum
Margo occipitalis
Fissura tympanomastoidea
Incisura mastoidea
Proc. mastoideus
Pars tympanica
Proc. styloideus
Meatus acusticus externus

Pars squamosa, Facies temporalis
Margo sphenoidalis
Proc. zygomaticus
Tuberculum articulare
Fossa mandibularis, Facies articularis
Fissura petrotympanica

Fig. 96   Temporal bone, Os temporale.

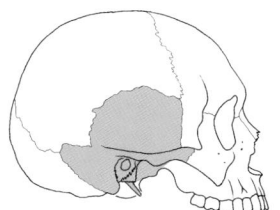

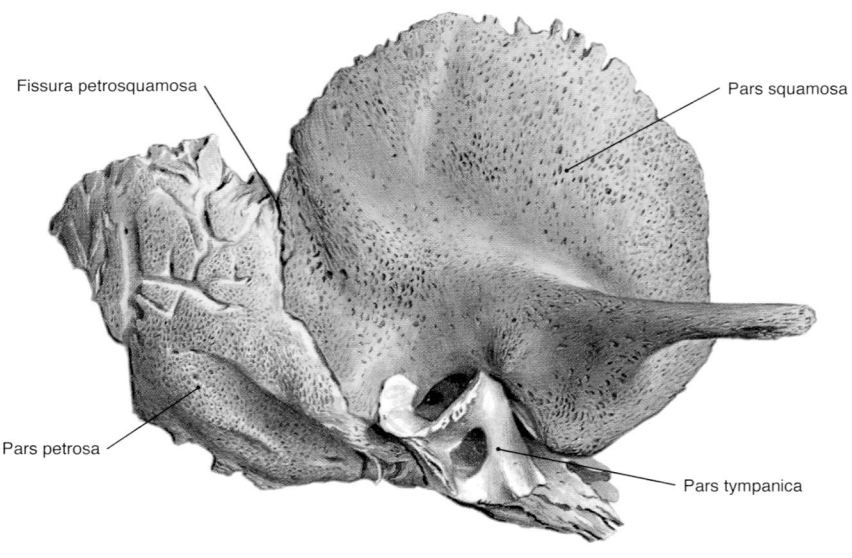

Fissura petrosquamosa
Pars petrosa
Pars squamosa
Pars tympanica

Fig. 97   Temporal bone, Os temporale, of a neonate.

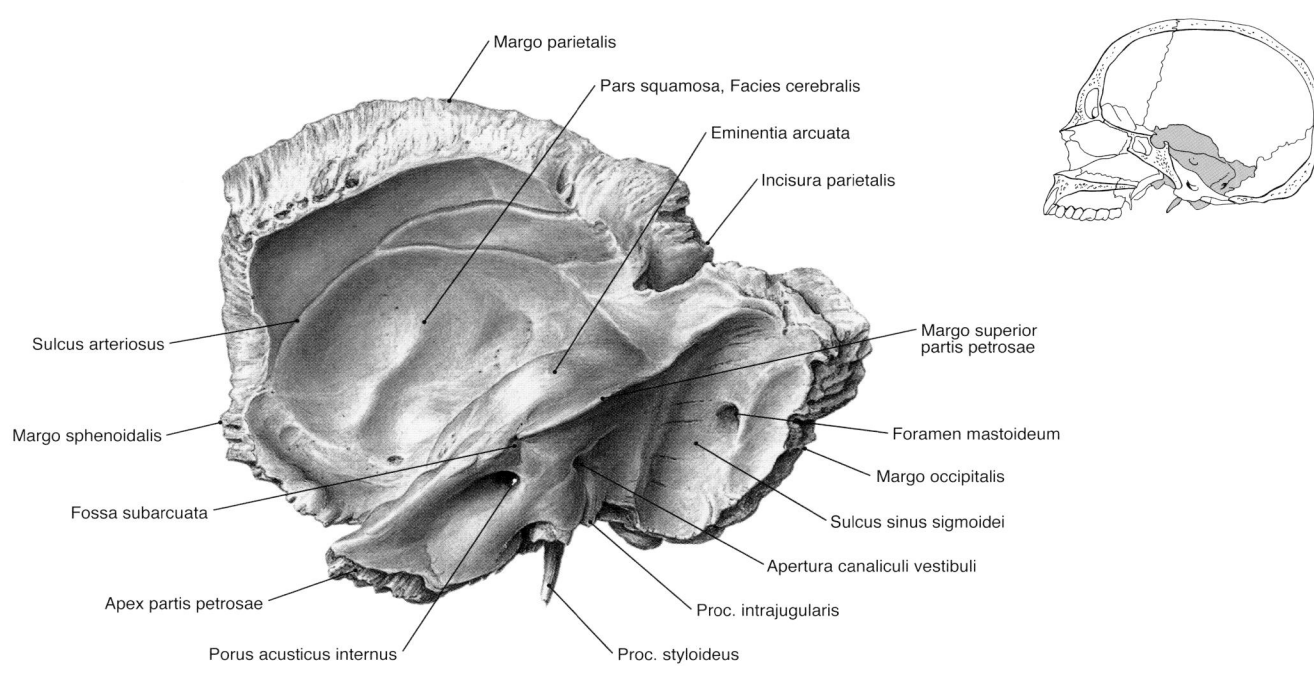

Margo parietalis
Pars squamosa, Facies cerebralis
Eminentia arcuata
Incisura parietalis
Sulcus arteriosus
Margo superior partis petrosae
Foramen mastoideum
Margo sphenoidalis
Margo occipitalis
Fossa subarcuata
Sulcus sinus sigmoidei
Apertura canaliculi vestibuli
Apex partis petrosae
Proc. intrajugularis
Porus acusticus internus
Proc. styloideus

Fig. 98   Temporal bone, Os temporale.

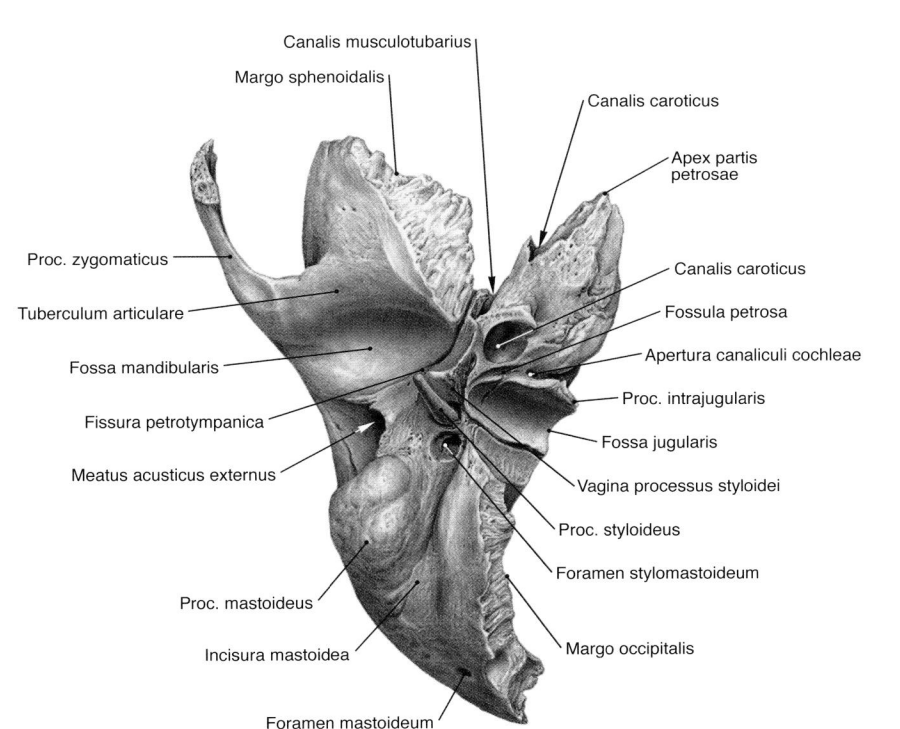

Canalis musculotubarius
Margo sphenoidalis
Canalis caroticus
Apex partis petrosae
Proc. zygomaticus
Canalis caroticus
Tuberculum articulare
Fossula petrosa
Fossa mandibularis
Apertura canaliculi cochleae
Fissura petrotympanica
Proc. intrajugularis
Meatus acusticus externus
Fossa jugularis
Vagina processus styloidei
Proc. styloideus
Foramen stylomastoideum
Proc. mastoideus
Margo occipitalis
Incisura mastoidea
Foramen mastoideum

Fig. 99   Temporal bone, Os temporale.

Mandible

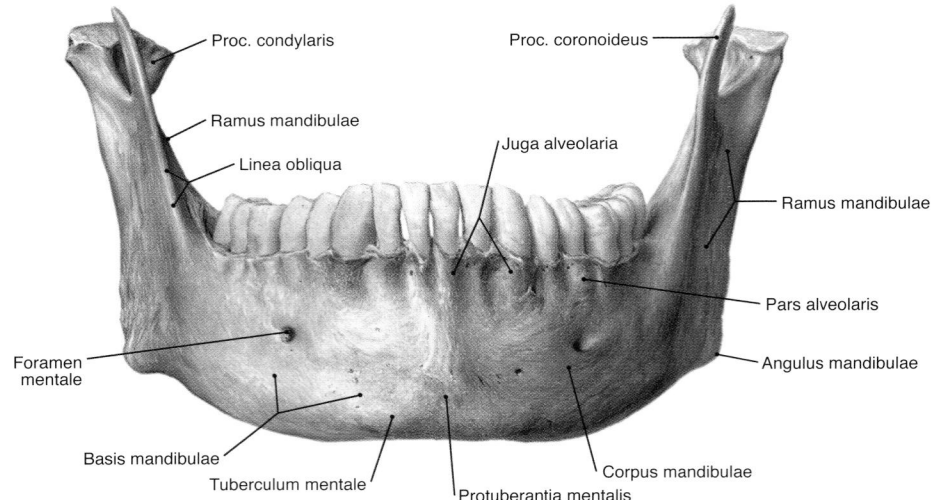

Proc. condylaris

Proc. coronoideus

Ramus mandibulae

Juga alveolaria

Linea obliqua

Ramus mandibulae

Pars alveolaris

Angulus mandibulae

Foramen mentale

Basis mandibulae

Tuberculum mentale

Protuberantia mentalis

Corpus mandibulae

Fig. 100 Mandible, Mandibula.

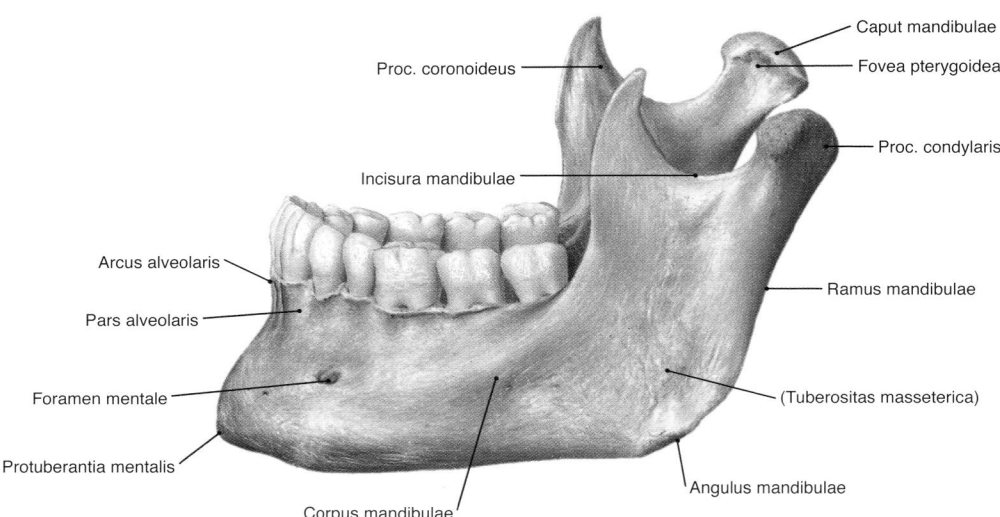

Caput mandibulae

Proc. coronoideus

Fovea pterygoidea

Incisura mandibulae

Proc. condylaris

Arcus alveolaris

Ramus mandibulae

Pars alveolaris

Foramen mentale

(Tuberositas masseterica)

Protuberantia mentalis

Angulus mandibulae

Corpus mandibulae

Fig. 101 Mandible, Mandibula.

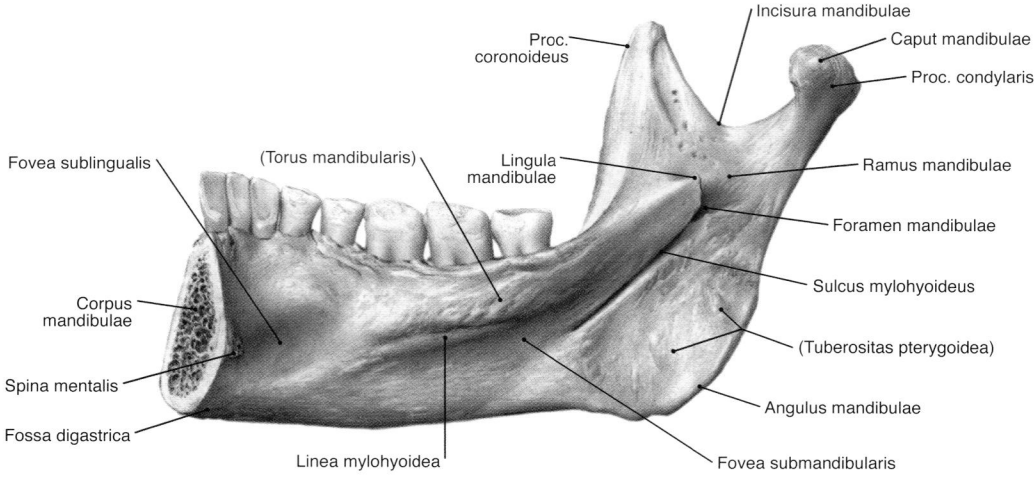

Incisura mandibulae

Proc. coronoideus

Caput mandibulae

Proc. condylaris

Fovea sublingualis

(Torus mandibularis)

Lingula mandibulae

Ramus mandibulae

Corpus mandibulae

Foramen mandibulae

Sulcus mylohyoideus

Spina mentalis

(Tuberositas pterygoidea)

Fossa digastrica

Angulus mandibulae

Linea mylohyoidea

Fovea submandibularis

Fig. 102 Mandible, Mandibula.

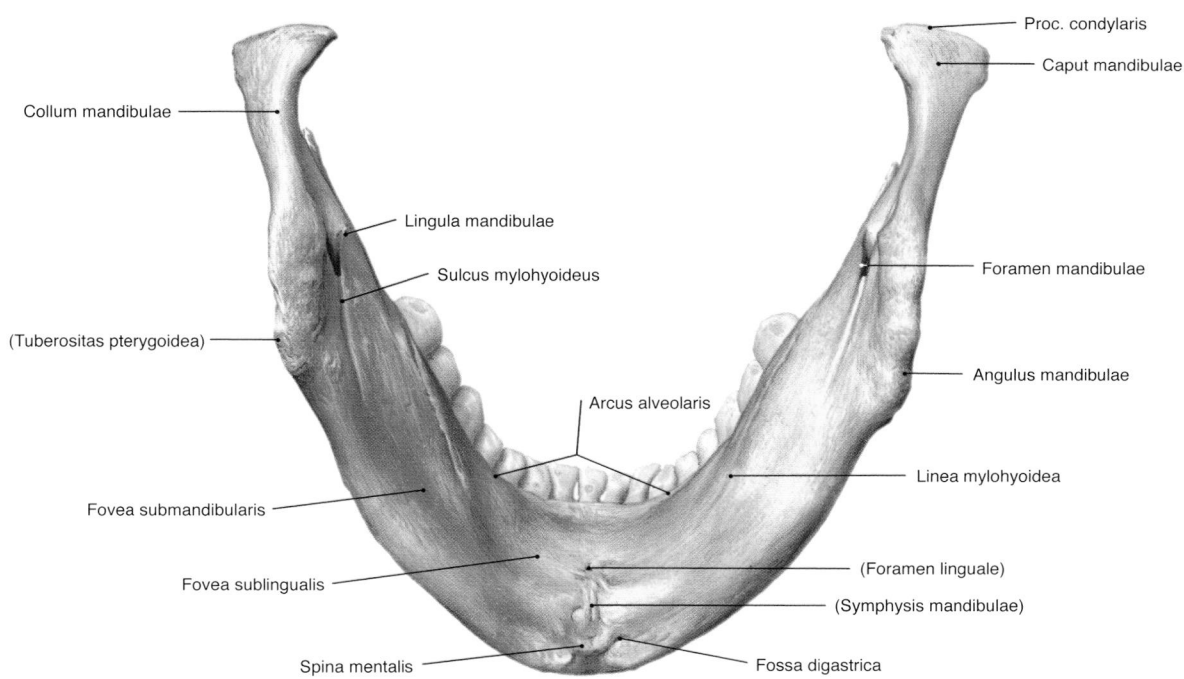

Proc. condylaris

Caput mandibulae

Collum mandibulae

Lingula mandibulae

Sulcus mylohyoideus

Foramen mandibulae

(Tuberositas pterygoidea)

Angulus mandibulae

Arcus alveolaris

Linea mylohyoidea

Fovea submandibularis

(Foramen linguale)

Fovea sublingualis

(Symphysis mandibulae)

Spina mentalis

Fossa digastrica

Fig. 103   Mandible, Mandibula.

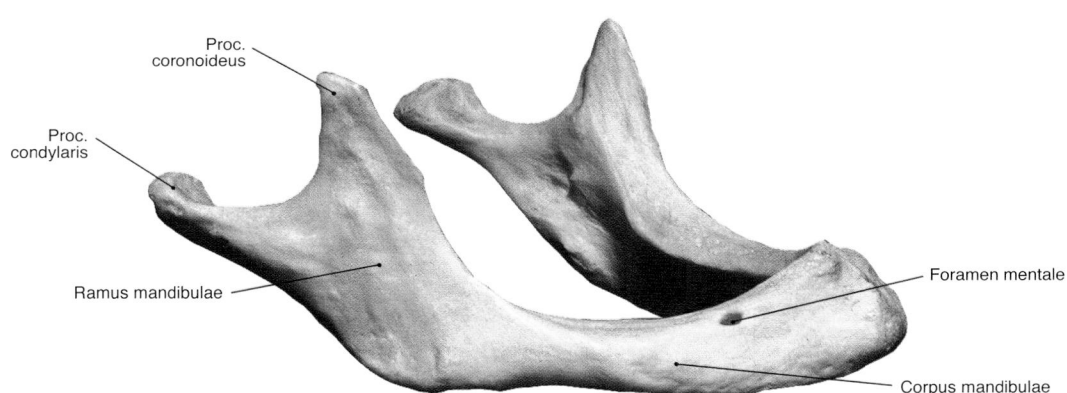

Proc. coronoideus

Proc. condylaris

Ramus mandibulae

Foramen mentale

Corpus mandibulae

Fig. 104   Mandible, Mandibula, of an elderly individual.

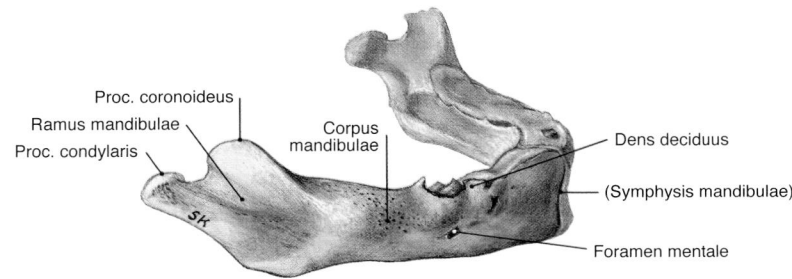

Proc. coronoideus

Ramus mandibulae

Corpus mandibulae

Proc. condylaris

Dens deciduus

(Symphysis mandibulae)

Foramen mentale

Fig. 105   Mandible, Mandibula, of a neonate.

Temporomandibular joint

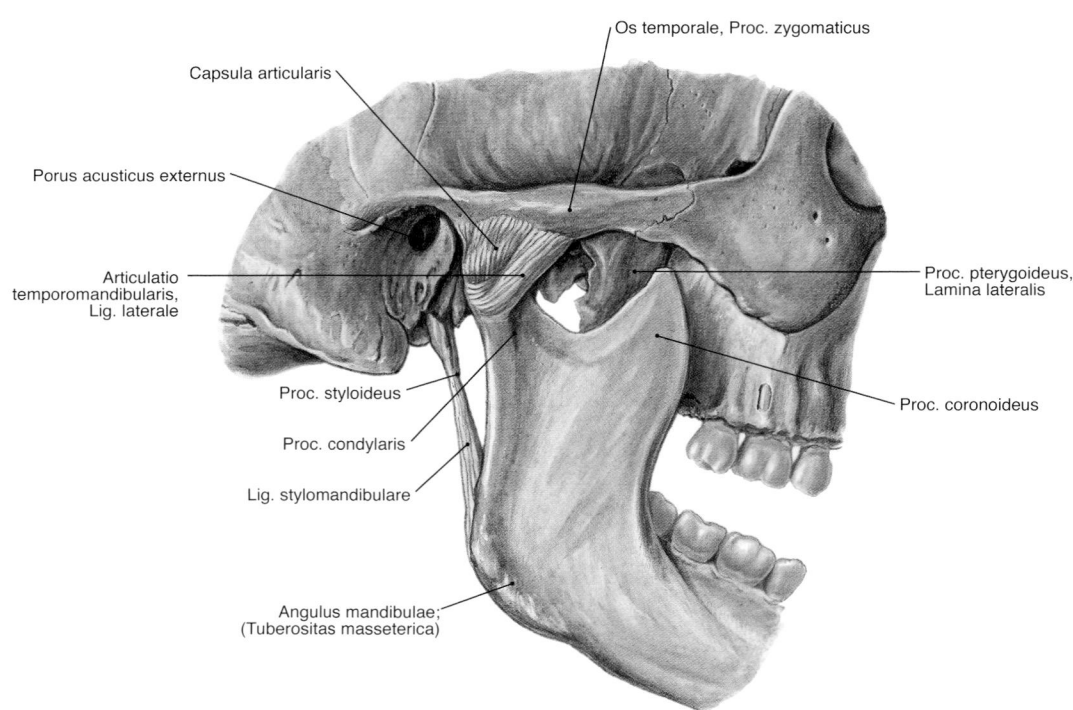

Capsula articularis

Porus acusticus externus

Articulatio temporomandibularis, Lig. laterale

Proc. styloideus

Proc. condylaris

Lig. stylomandibulare

Angulus mandibulae; (Tuberositas masseterica)

Os temporale, Proc. zygomaticus

Proc. pterygoideus, Lamina lateralis

Proc. coronoideus

Fig. 106 Temporomandibular joint, Articulatio temporomandibularis.

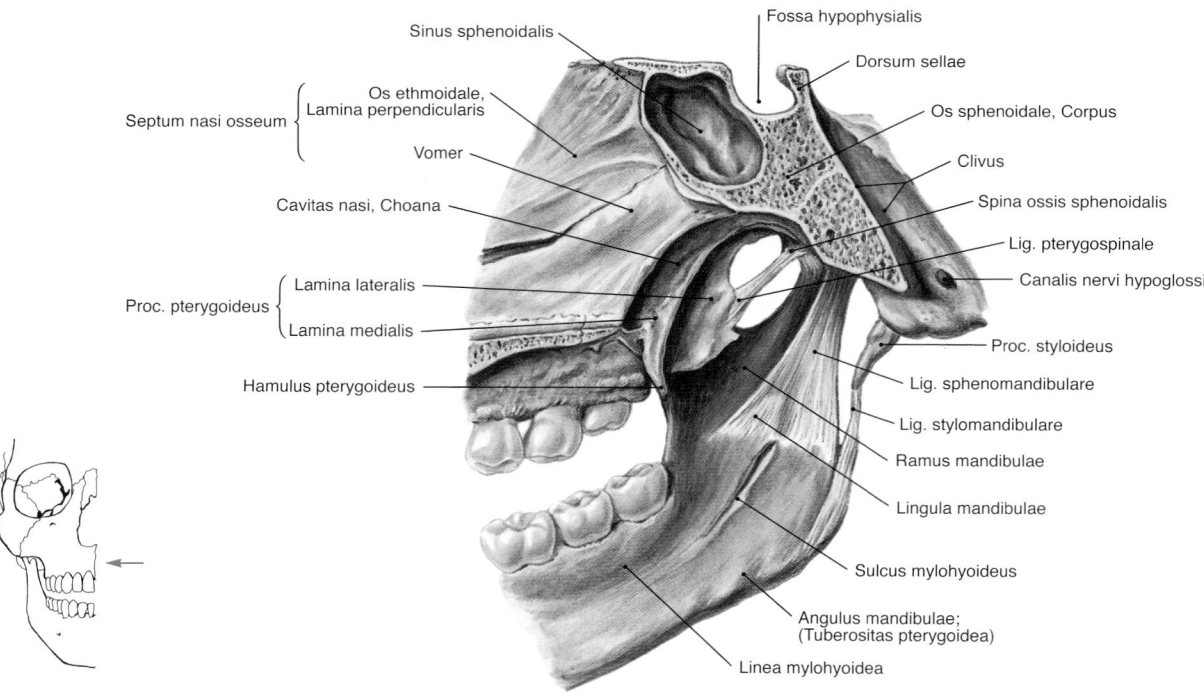

Sinus sphenoidalis

Fossa hypophysialis

Dorsum sellae

Septum nasi osseum { Os ethmoidale, Lamina perpendicularis

Os sphenoidale, Corpus

Vomer

Clivus

Cavitas nasi, Choana

Spina ossis sphenoidalis

Lig. pterygospinale

Proc. pterygoideus { Lamina lateralis

Canalis nervi hypoglossi

Lamina medialis

Proc. styloideus

Hamulus pterygoideus

Lig. sphenomandibulare

Lig. stylomandibulare

Ramus mandibulae

Lingula mandibulae

Sulcus mylohyoideus

Angulus mandibulae; (Tuberositas pterygoidea)

Linea mylohyoidea

Fig. 107 Pterygospinous and sphenomandibular ligaments, Ligg. pterygospinale et sphenomandibulare.

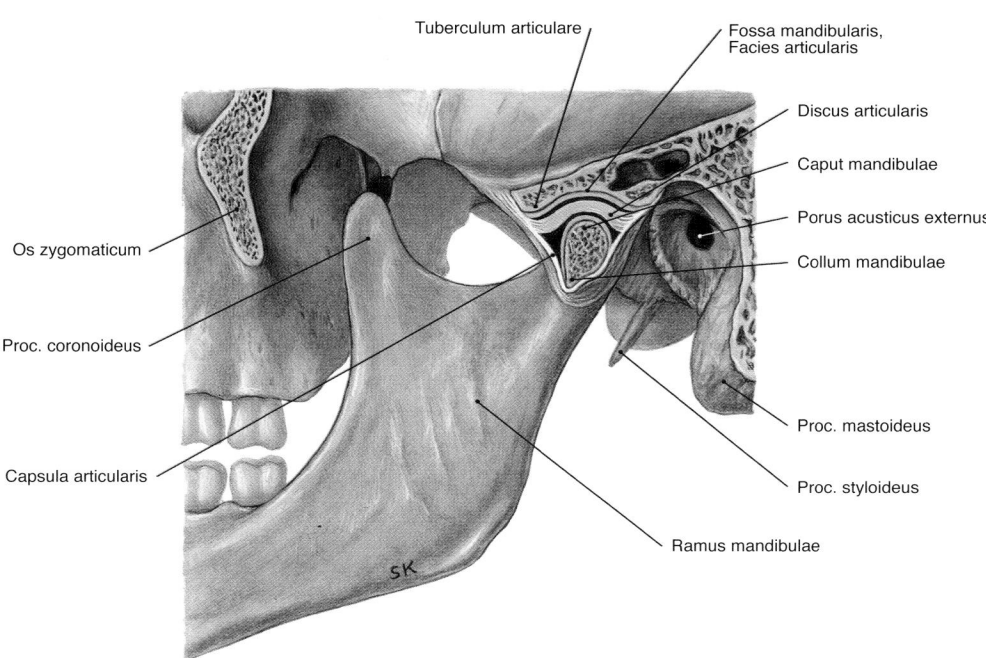

Tuberculum articulare
Fossa mandibularis, Facies articularis
Discus articularis
Caput mandibulae
Porus acusticus externus
Collum mandibulae
Os zygomaticum
Proc. coronoideus
Proc. mastoideus
Capsula articularis
Proc. styloideus
Ramus mandibulae

Fig. 108 Temporomandibular joint, Articulatio temporomandibularis; sagittal section; mouth almost closed.

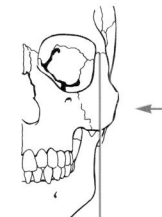

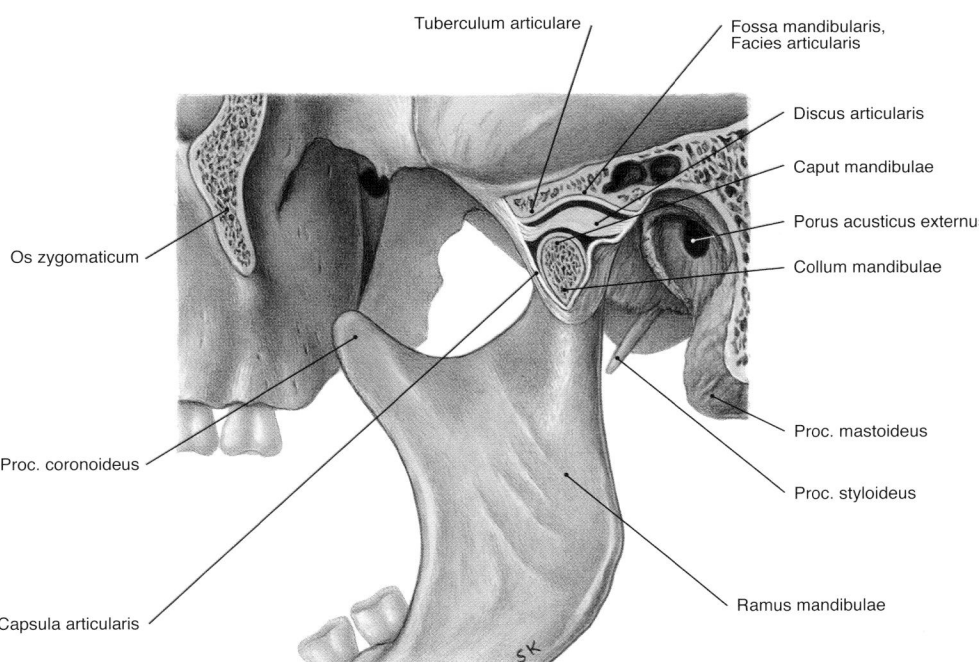

Tuberculum articulare
Fossa mandibularis, Facies articularis
Discus articularis
Caput mandibulae
Porus acusticus externus
Collum mandibulae
Os zygomaticum
Proc. coronoideus
Proc. mastoideus
Capsula articularis
Proc. styloideus
Ramus mandibulae

Fig. 109 Temporomandibular joint, Articulatio temporomandibularis; sagittal section; mouth opened.

Temporomandibular joint and masticatory muscles

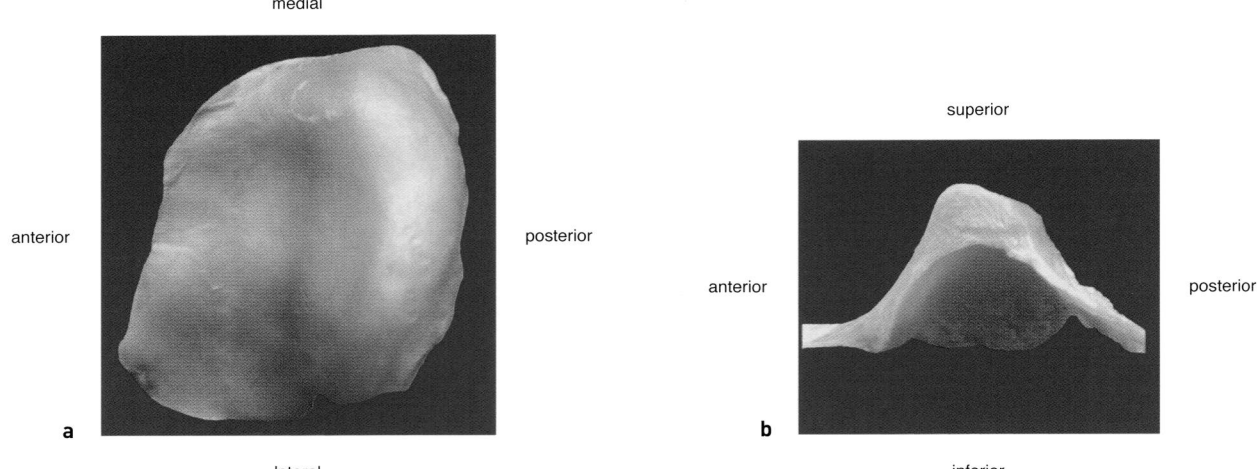

medial

anterior   posterior

a

lateral

superior

anterior   posterior

b

inferior

Fig. 110 a, b   Articular disc, Discus articularis, of the
temporomandibular joint, Articulatio temporomandibularis.
a Superior view
b Lateral view

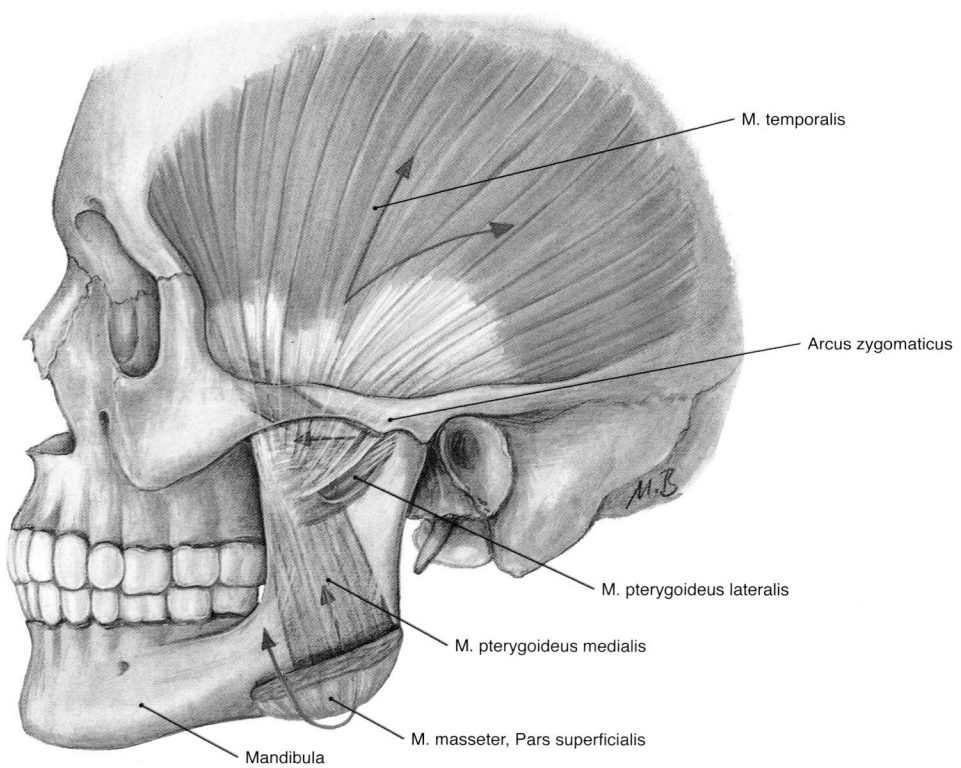

M. temporalis

Arcus zygomaticus

M. pterygoideus lateralis

M. pterygoideus medialis

M. masseter, Pars superficialis

Mandibula

→ T 4

Abb. 111   Masticatory muscles, Mm. masticatorii.
Arrows indicate the direction of muscle traction
when closing the mouth.

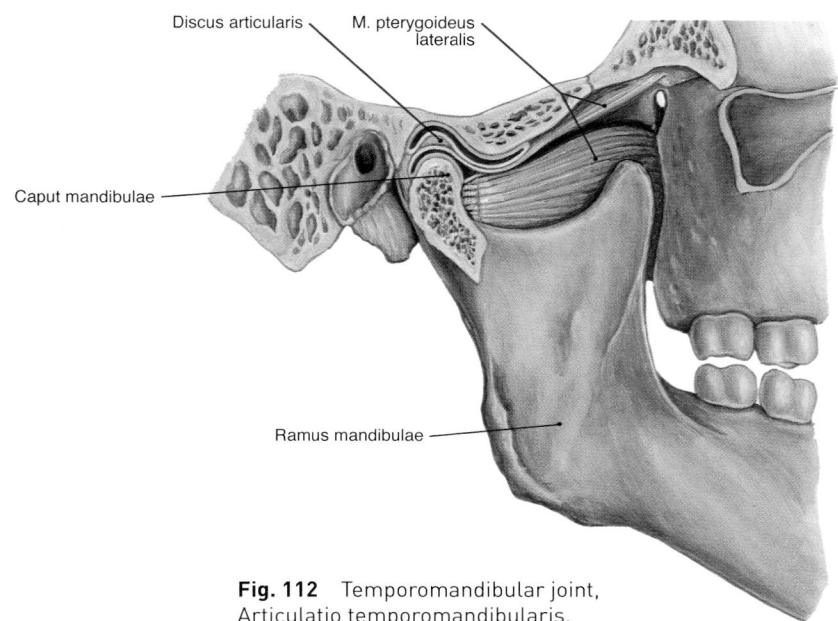

Fig. 112 Temporomandibular joint,
Articulatio temporomandibularis.

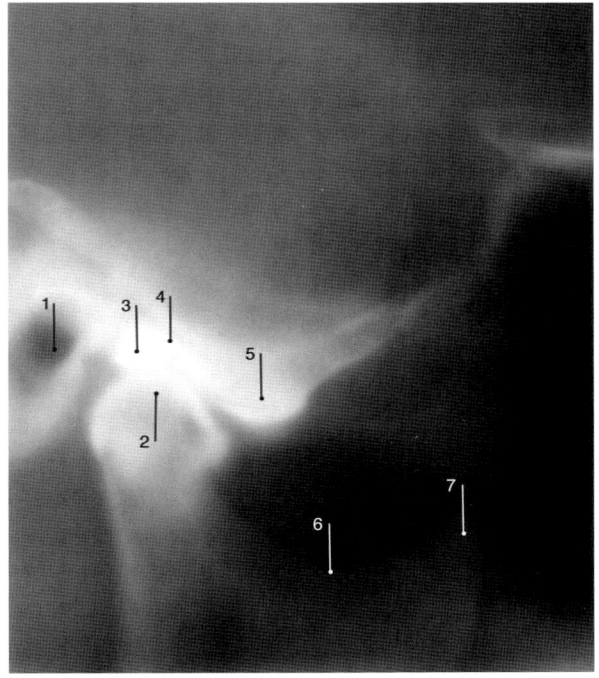

a

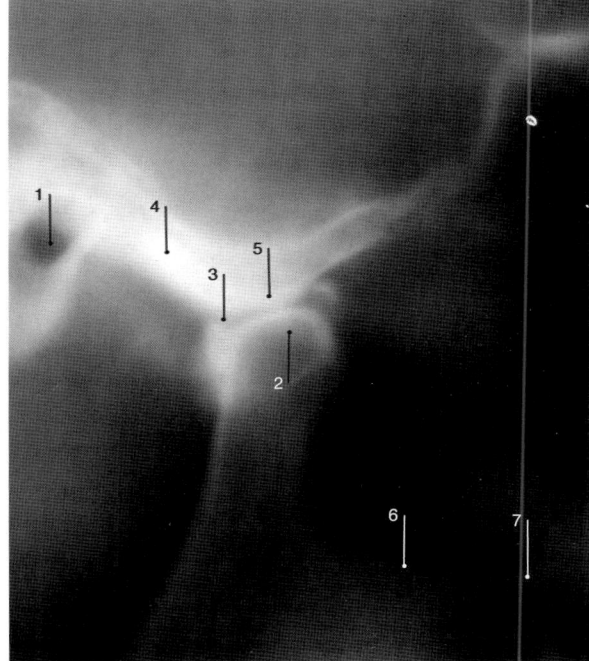

b

1 Meatus acusticus externus
2 Proc. condylaris
3 Discus articularis
4 Os temporale, Fossa mandibularis

5 Os temporale, Tuberculum articulare
6 Incisura mandibulae
7 Proc. coronoideus

Fig. 113 a, b Temporomandibular joint, Articulatio
temporomandibularis;
tomography; lateral projection after injection of a contrast
medium into the joint cavity (arthrography).
a Mouth closed
b Mouth opened

The articular disc shifts forward during opening of the mouth.

→ 108, 109

Masticatory muscles

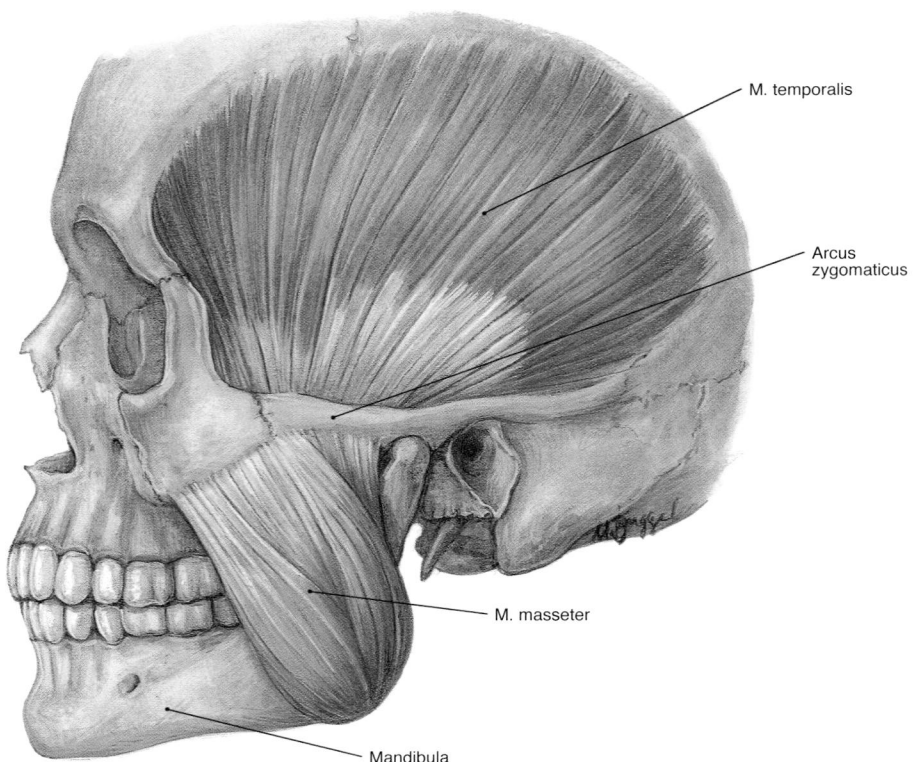

M. temporalis

Arcus
zygomaticus

M. masseter

Mandibula

→ T 4

Fig. 114 Masseter and temporal muscle,
Mm. masseter et temporalis.

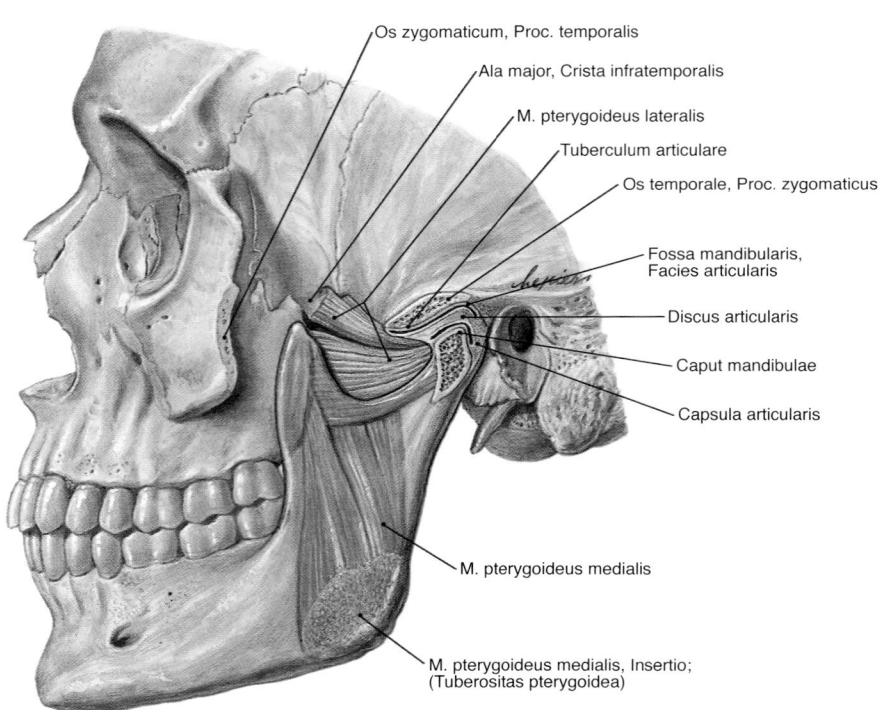

Os zygomaticum, Proc. temporalis

Ala major, Crista infratemporalis

M. pterygoideus lateralis

Tuberculum articulare

Os temporale, Proc. zygomaticus

Fossa mandibularis,
Facies articularis

Discus articularis

Caput mandibulae

Capsula articularis

M. pterygoideus medialis

M. pterygoideus medialis, Insertio;
(Tuberositas pterygoidea)

→ T 4

Fig. 115 Temporomandibular joint, Articulatio temporomandibularis;
medial and lateral pterygoid muscles,
Mm. pterygoidei medialis et lateralis.

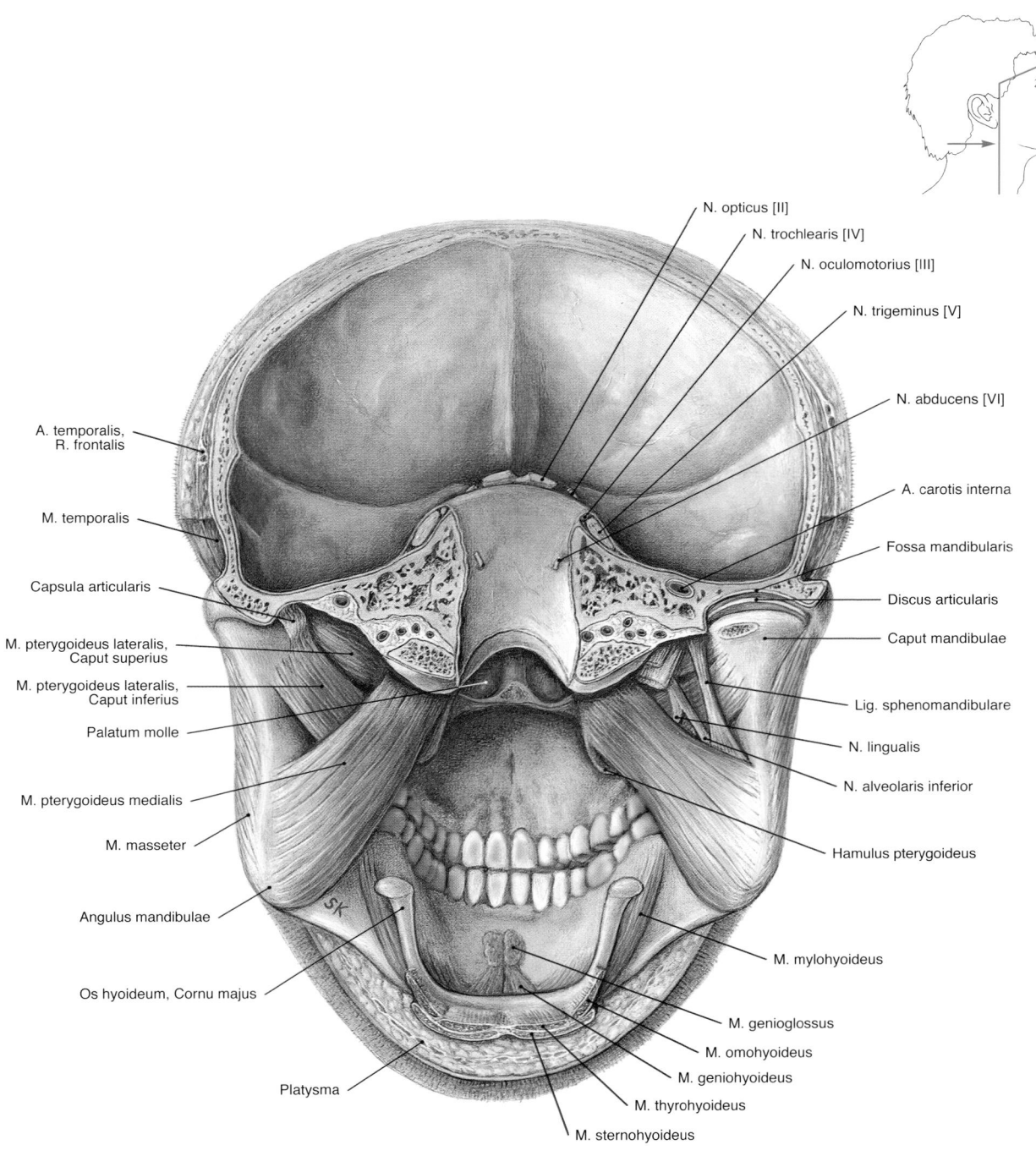

N. opticus [II]
N. trochlearis [IV]
N. oculomotorius [III]
N. trigeminus [V]
N. abducens [VI]
A. carotis interna
Fossa mandibularis
Discus articularis
Caput mandibulae
Lig. sphenomandibulare
N. lingualis
N. alveolaris inferior
Hamulus pterygoideus
M. mylohyoideus
M. genioglossus
M. omohyoideus
M. geniohyoideus
M. thyrohyoideus
M. sternohyoideus

A. temporalis, R. frontalis
M. temporalis
Capsula articularis
M. pterygoideus lateralis, Caput superius
M. pterygoideus lateralis, Caput inferius
Palatum molle
M. pterygoideus medialis
M. masseter
Angulus mandibulae
Os hyoideum, Cornu majus
Platysma

SK

Fig. 116 Masticatory muscles, Mm. masticatorii; frontal section through the temporomandibular joint and horizontal section through the calvaria; posterior view.

→ T 4

Masticatory muscles

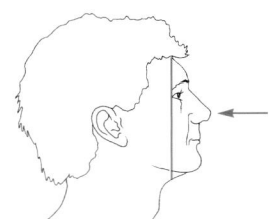

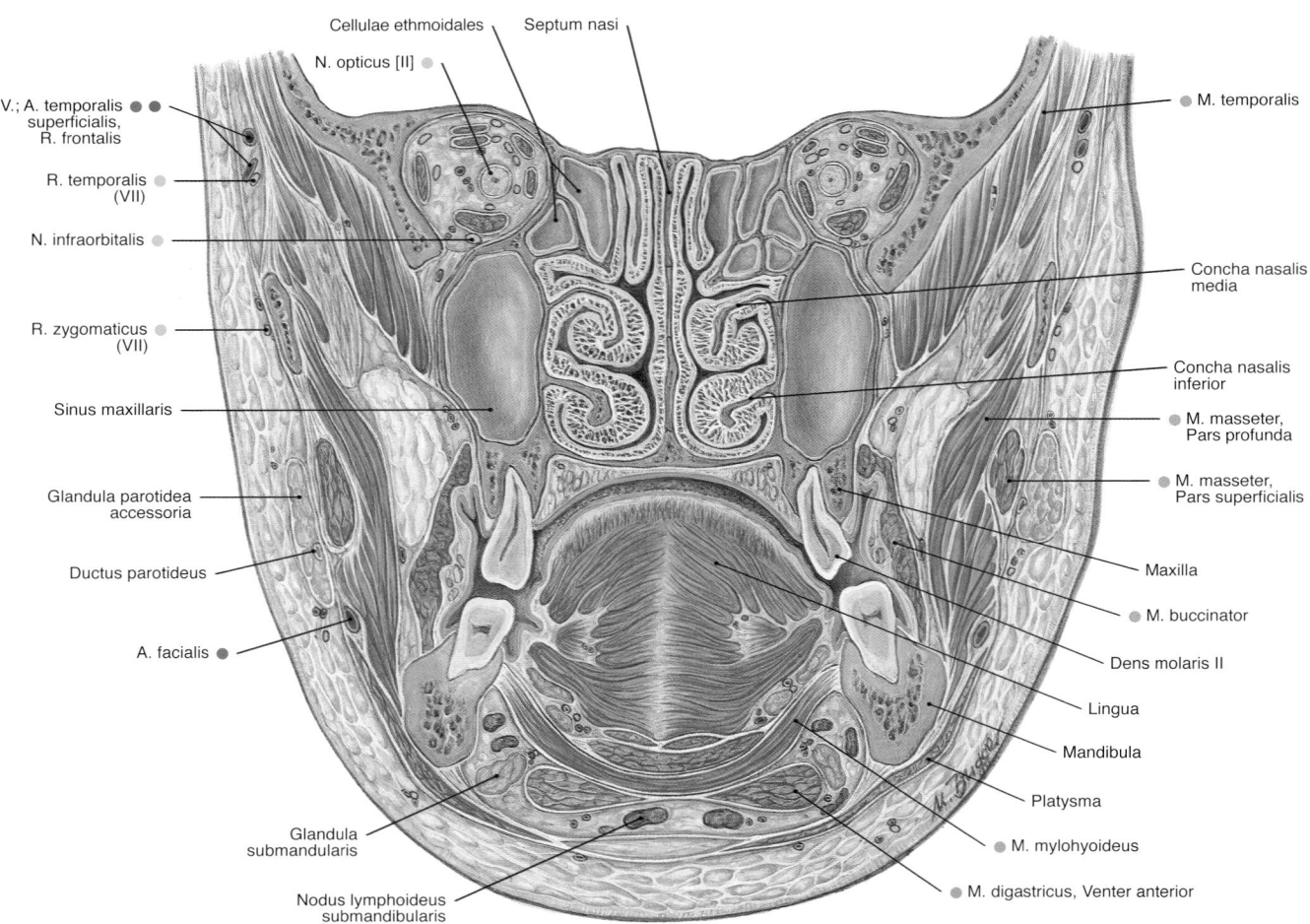

Cellulae ethmoidales — Septum nasi

N. opticus [II]

V.; A. temporalis superficialis, R. frontalis

R. temporalis (VII)

N. infraorbitalis

R. zygomaticus (VII)

Sinus maxillaris

Glandula parotidea accessoria

Ductus parotideus

A. facialis

Glandula submandularis

Nodus lymphoideus submandibularis

M. temporalis

Concha nasalis media

Concha nasalis inferior

M. masseter, Pars profunda

M. masseter, Pars superficialis

Maxilla

M. buccinator

Dens molaris II

Lingua

Mandibula

Platysma

M. mylohyoideus

M. digastricus, Venter anterior

→ T 4   **Fig. 117** Masticatory muscles, Mm. masticatorii; frontal section; anterior view.

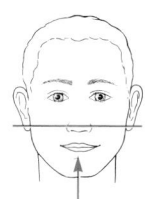

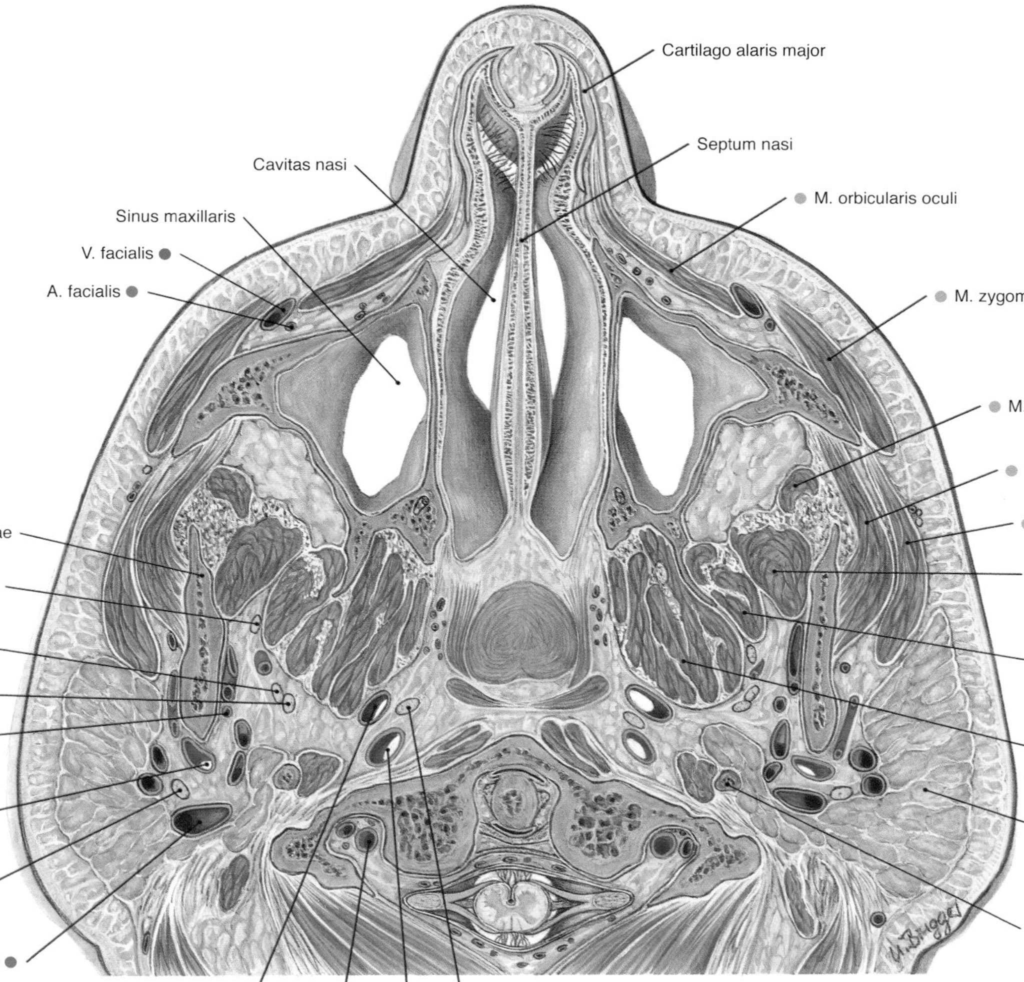

Cartilago alaris major

Septum nasi

Cavitas nasi

Sinus maxillaris

V. facialis ●

A. facialis ●

● M. orbicularis oculi

● M. zygomaticus major

● M. temporalis

● M. masseter, Pars profunda

● M. masseter, Pars superficialis

Ramus mandibulae

N. massetericus ●

N. alveolaris inferior ●

N. lingualis ●

A. alveolaris inferior ●

A. maxillaris ●

N. facialis [VII] ●

V. maxillaris ●

V. jugularis interna ●

A. vertebralis ●

● A. carotis interna

● N. vagus [X]

● M. pterygoideus lateralis, Caput inferius

● M. pterygoideus lateralis, Caput superius

● M. pterygoideus medialis

Glandula parotidea

Proc. styloideus

Fig. 118 Masticatory muscles, Mm. masticatorii; horizontal section.

→ T 4

Facial and masticatory muscles

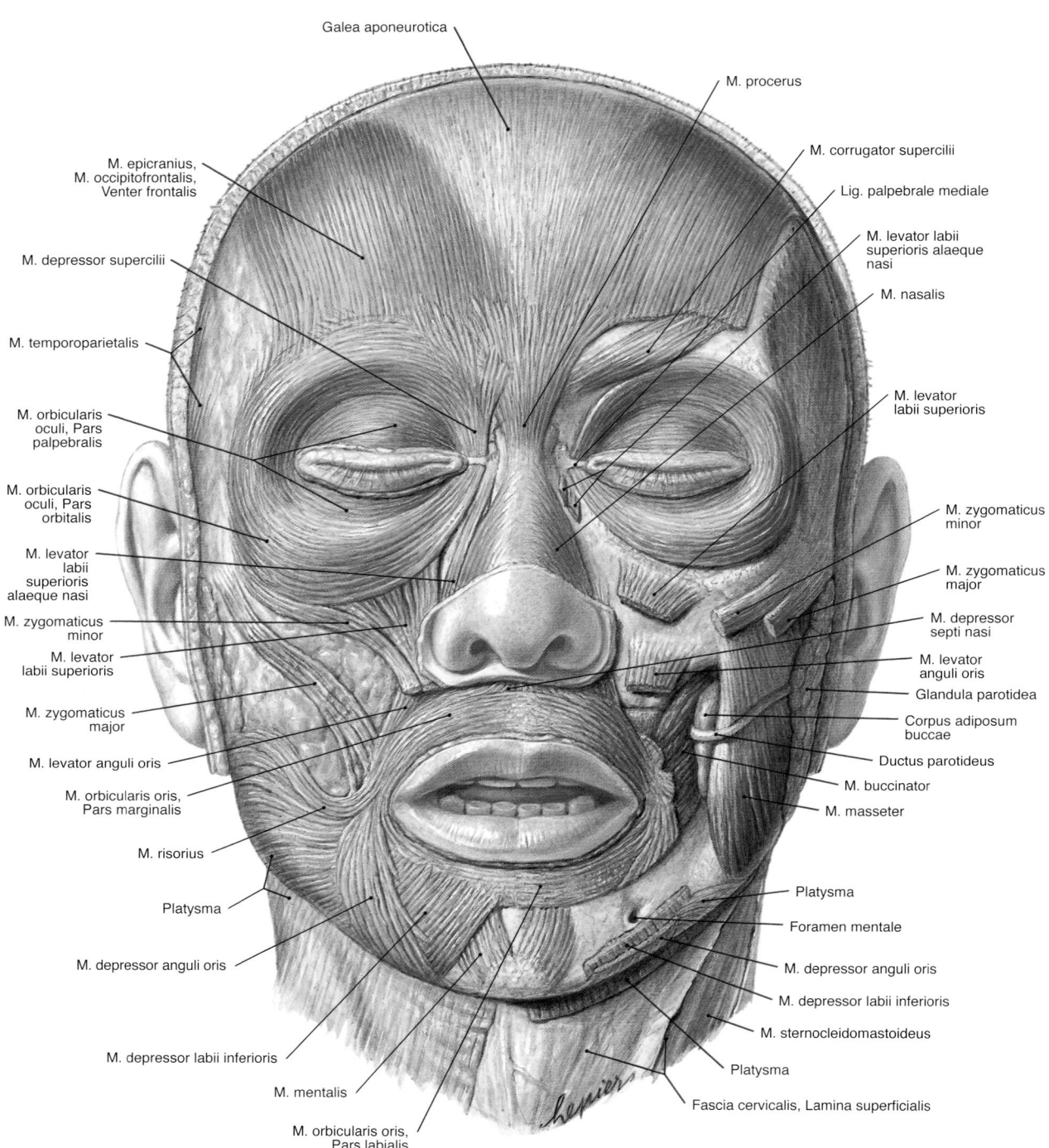

Galea aponeurotica

M. procerus

M. epicranius,
M. occipitofrontalis,
Venter frontalis

M. corrugator supercilii

Lig. palpebrale mediale

M. depressor supercilii

M. levator labii
superioris alaeque
nasi

M. nasalis

M. temporoparietalis

M. levator
labii superioris

M. orbicularis
oculi, Pars
palpebralis

M. zygomaticus
minor

M. orbicularis
oculi, Pars
orbitalis

M. zygomaticus
major

M. levator
labii
superioris
alaeque nasi

M. depressor
septi nasi

M. zygomaticus
minor

M. levator
anguli oris

M. levator
labii superioris

Glandula parotidea

M. zygomaticus
major

Corpus adiposum
buccae

M. levator anguli oris

Ductus parotideus

M. orbicularis oris,
Pars marginalis

M. buccinator

M. masseter

M. risorius

Platysma

Platysma

Foramen mentale

M. depressor anguli oris

M. depressor anguli oris

M. depressor labii inferioris

M. sternocleidomastoideus

M. depressor labii inferioris

Platysma

M. mentalis

Fascia cervicalis, Lamina superficialis

M. orbicularis oris,
Pars labialis

→ T 1 a, c–f, T 4

Fig. 119   Facial muscles, Mm. faciei,
and masticatory muscles, Mm. masticatorii.

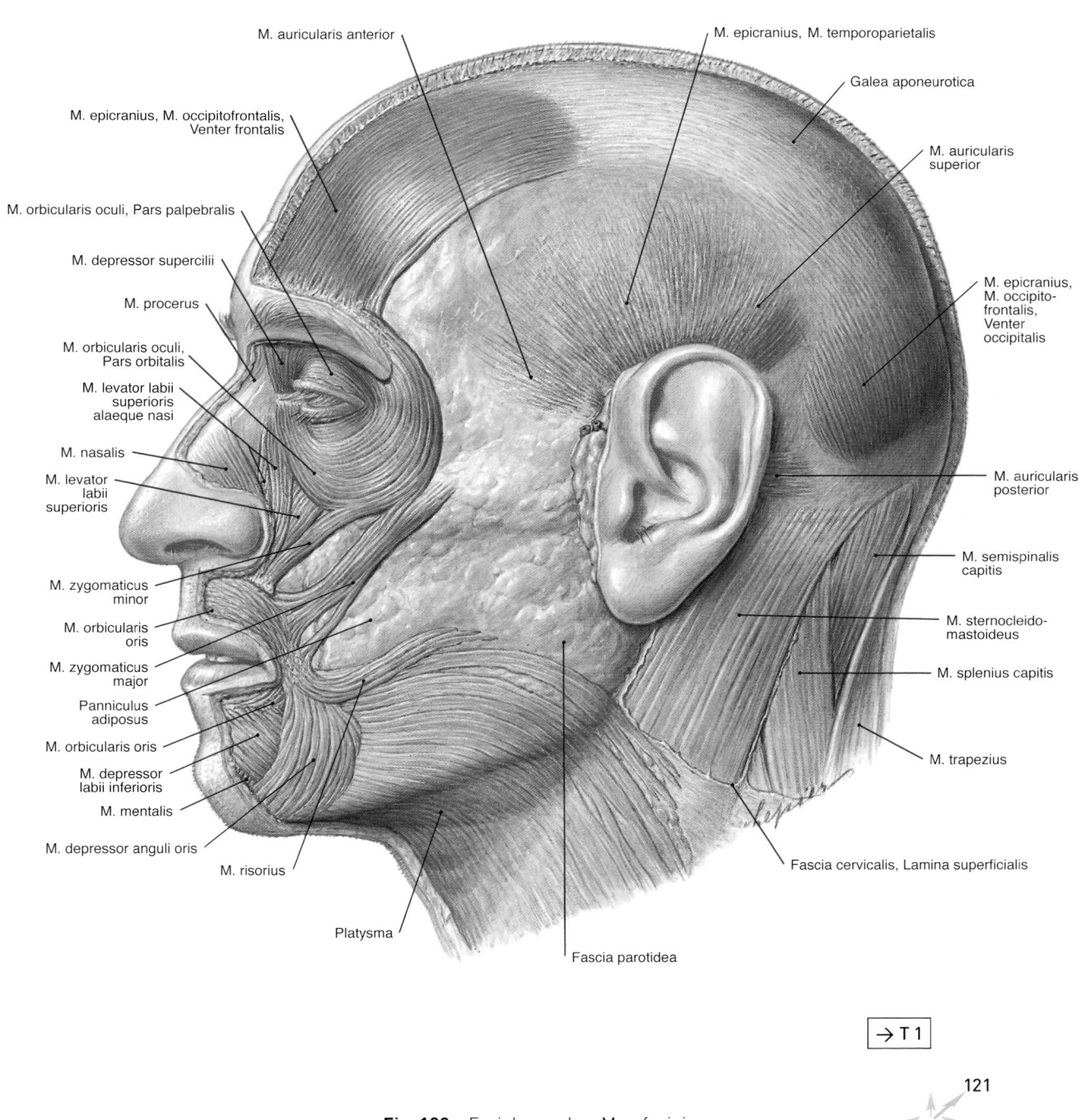

M. auricularis anterior

M. epicranius, M. temporoparietalis

Galea aponeurotica

M. epicranius, M. occipitofrontalis,
Venter frontalis

M. auricularis
superior

M. orbicularis oculi, Pars palpebralis

M. depressor supercilii

M. procerus

M. epicranius,
M. occipito-
frontalis,
Venter
occipitalis

M. orbicularis oculi,
Pars orbitalis

M. levator labii
superioris
alaeque nasi

M. nasalis

M. levator
labii
superioris

M. auricularis
posterior

M. semispinalis
capitis

M. zygomaticus
minor

M. orbicularis
oris

M. zygomaticus
major

M. sternocleido-
mastoideus

M. splenius capitis

Panniculus
adiposus

M. orbicularis oris

M. depressor
labii inferioris

M. trapezius

M. mentalis

M. depressor anguli oris

M. risorius

Platysma

Fascia cervicalis, Lamina superficialis

Fascia parotidea

→ T 1

121

253

Fig. 120 Facial muscles, Mm. faciei.

Facial and masticatory muscles

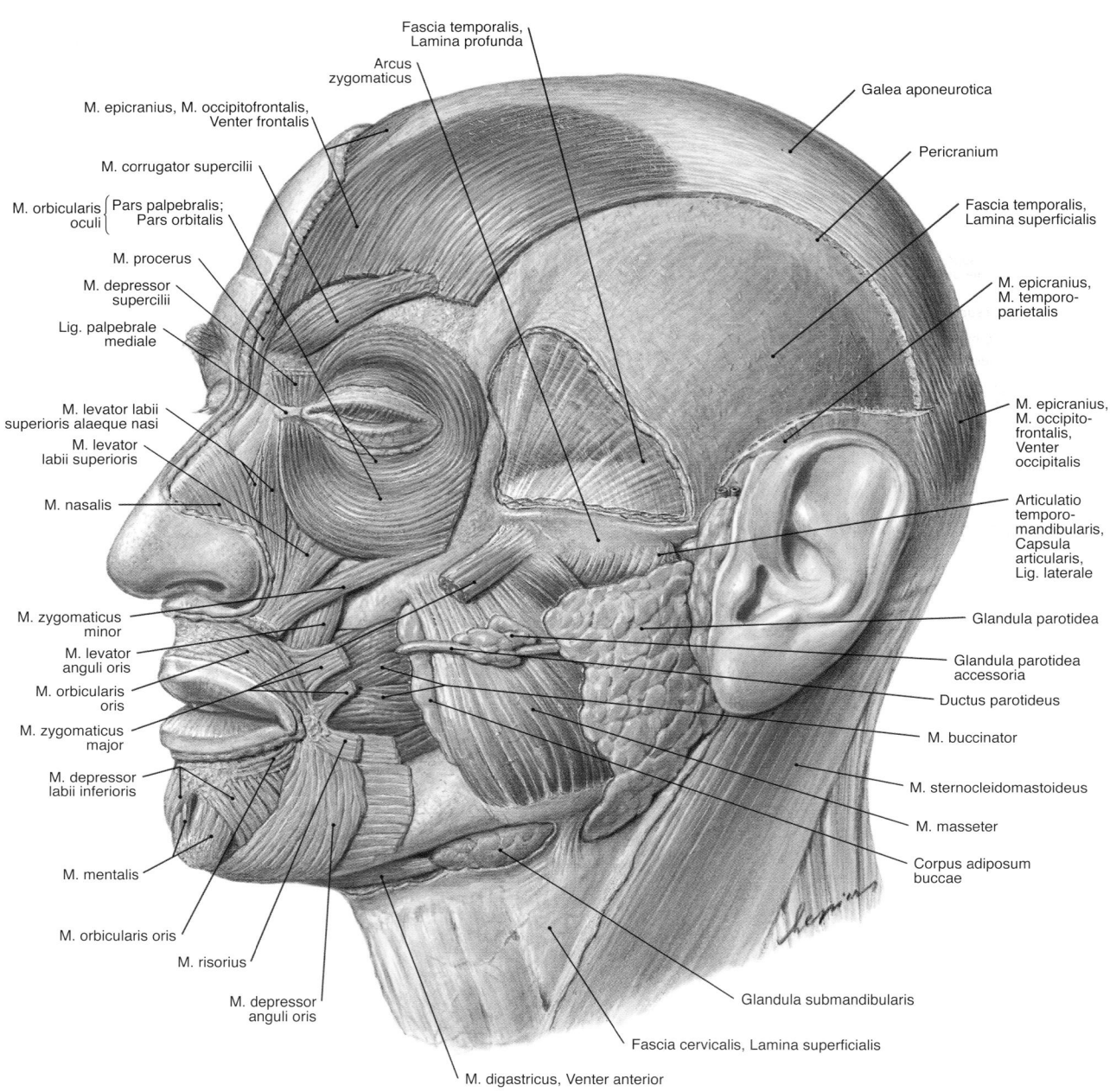

Fascia temporalis, Lamina profunda
Arcus zygomaticus
M. epicranius, M. occipitofrontalis, Venter frontalis
M. corrugator supercilii
M. orbicularis oculi { Pars palpebralis; Pars orbitalis
M. procerus
M. depressor supercilii
Lig. palpebrale mediale
M. levator labii superioris alaeque nasi
M. levator labii superioris
M. nasalis
M. zygomaticus minor
M. levator anguli oris
M. orbicularis oris
M. zygomaticus major
M. depressor labii inferioris
M. mentalis
M. orbicularis oris
M. risorius
M. depressor anguli oris

Galea aponeurotica
Pericranium
Fascia temporalis, Lamina superficialis
M. epicranius, M. temporo-parietalis
M. epicranius, M. occipito-frontalis, Venter occipitalis
Articulatio temporo-mandibularis, Capsula articularis, Lig. laterale
Glandula parotidea
Glandula parotidea accessoria
Ductus parotideus
M. buccinator
M. sternocleidomastoideus
M. masseter
Corpus adiposum buccae
Glandula submandibularis
Fascia cervicalis, Lamina superficialis
M. digastricus, Venter anterior

→ T 1, T 4

122
120   206

Fig. 121   Facial muscles, Mm. faciei, and masticatory muscles, Mm. masticatorii.

Facial and masticatory muscles

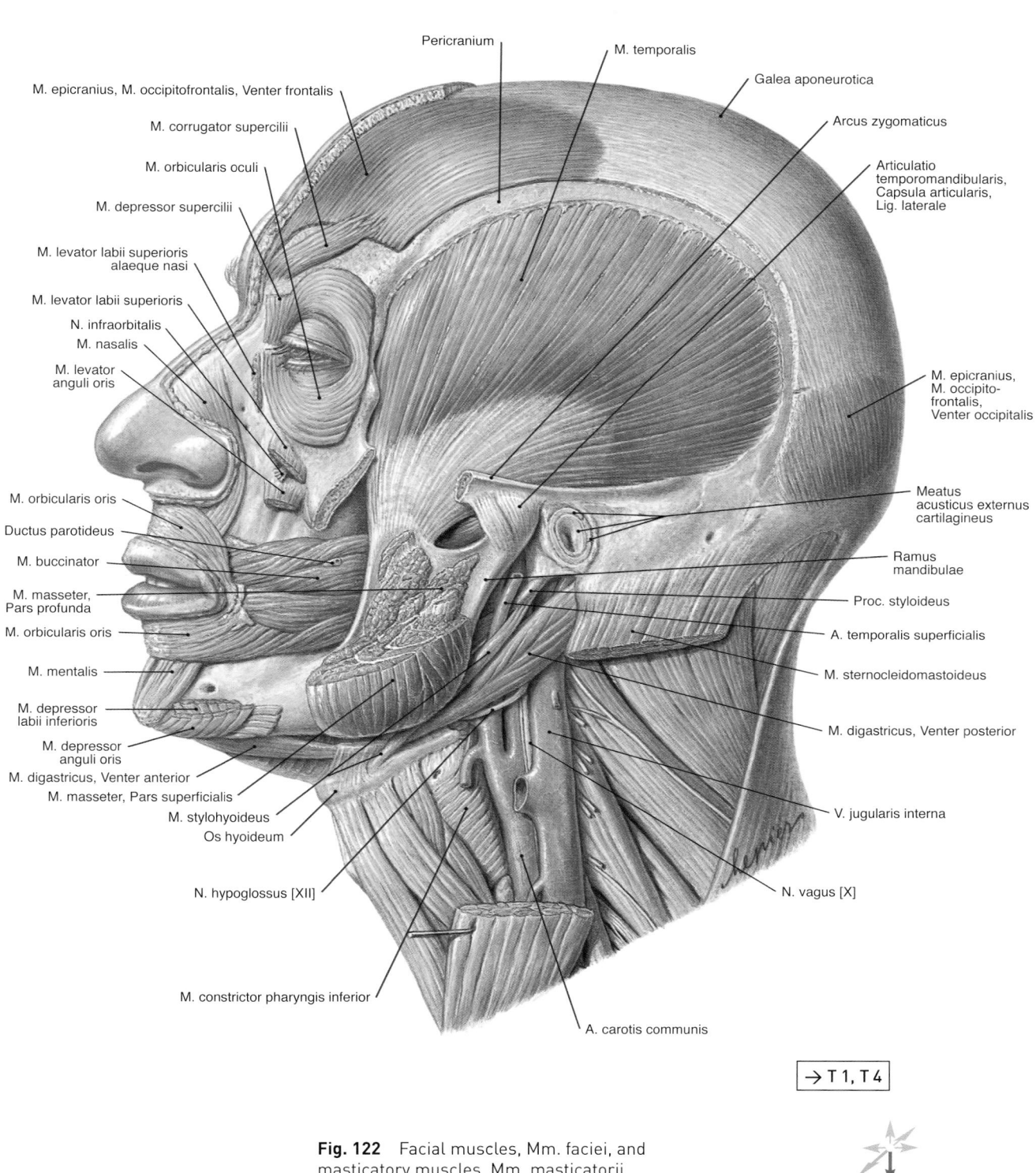

Pericranium

M. temporalis

Galea aponeurotica

M. epicranius, M. occipitofrontalis, Venter frontalis

Arcus zygomaticus

M. corrugator supercilii

Articulatio temporomandibularis, Capsula articularis, Lig. laterale

M. orbicularis oculi

M. depressor supercilii

M. levator labii superioris alaeque nasi

M. levator labii superioris

N. infraorbitalis

M. nasalis

M. levator anguli oris

M. epicranius, M. occipito-frontalis, Venter occipitalis

Meatus acusticus externus cartilagineus

M. orbicularis oris

Ductus parotideus

Ramus mandibulae

M. buccinator

Proc. styloideus

M. masseter, Pars profunda

A. temporalis superficialis

M. orbicularis oris

M. sternocleidomastoideus

M. mentalis

M. digastricus, Venter posterior

M. depressor labii inferioris

M. depressor anguli oris

M. digastricus, Venter anterior

M. masseter, Pars superficialis

V. jugularis interna

M. stylohyoideus

Os hyoideum

N. hypoglossus [XII]

N. vagus [X]

M. constrictor pharyngis inferior

A. carotis communis

→ T 1, T 4

Fig. 122 Facial muscles, Mm. faciei, and masticatory muscles, Mm. masticatorii.

121

256

Arteries of the head

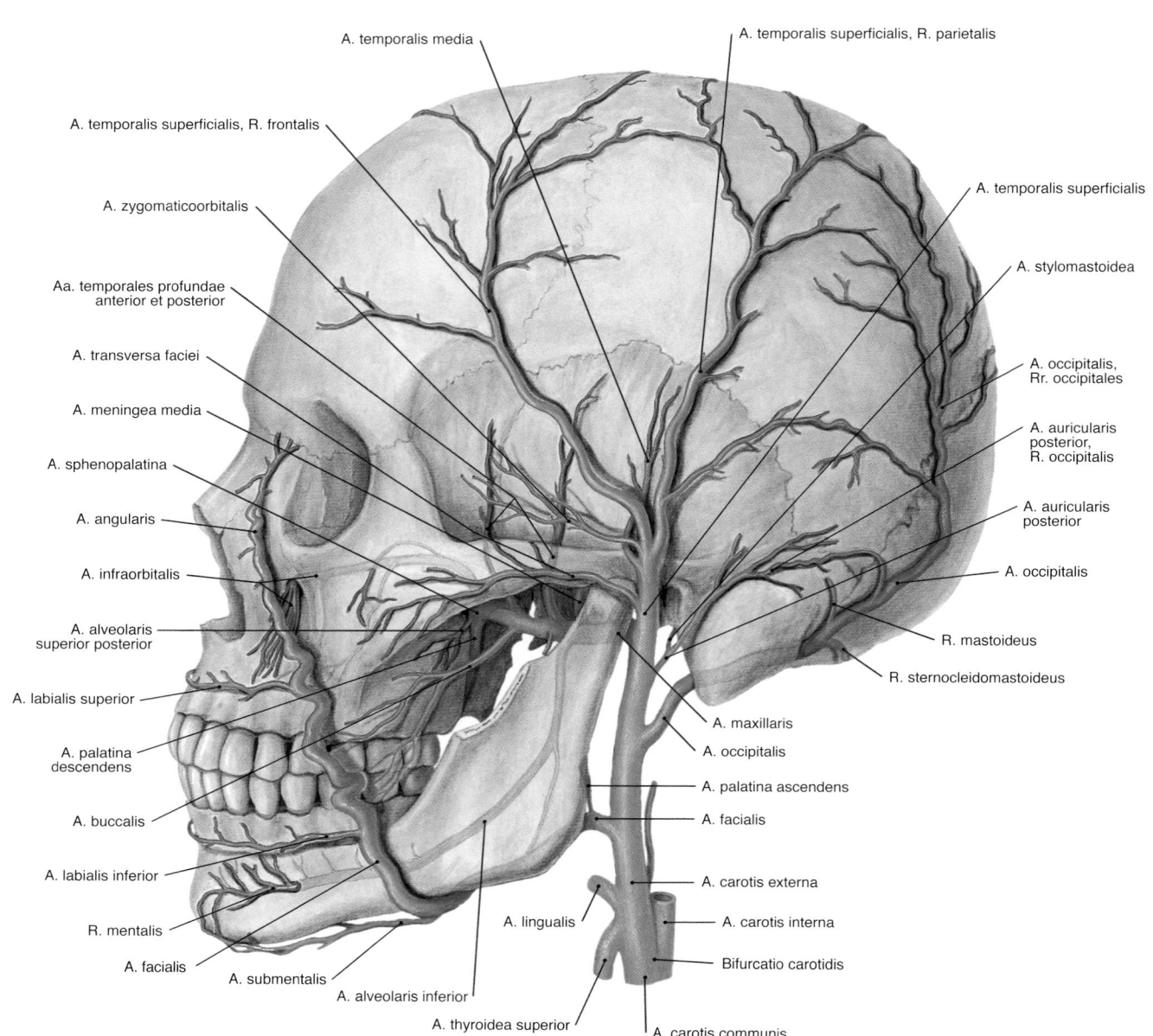

A. temporalis media

A. temporalis superficialis, R. frontalis

A. zygomaticoorbitalis

Aa. temporales profundae anterior et posterior

A. transversa faciei

A. meningea media

A. sphenopalatina

A. angularis

A. infraorbitalis

A. alveolaris superior posterior

A. labialis superior

A. palatina descendens

A. buccalis

A. labialis inferior

R. mentalis

A. facialis

A. submentalis

A. alveolaris inferior

A. thyroidea superior

A. lingualis

A. temporalis superficialis, R. parietalis

A. temporalis superficialis

A. stylomastoidea

A. occipitalis, Rr. occipitales

A. auricularis posterior, R. occipitalis

A. auricularis posterior

A. occipitalis

R. mastoideus

R. sternocleidomastoideus

A. maxillaris

A. occipitalis

A. palatina ascendens

A. facialis

A. carotis externa

A. carotis interna

Bifurcatio carotidis

A. carotis communis

→ 264

Fig. 123 External carotid artery, A. carotis externa.

Veins of the head

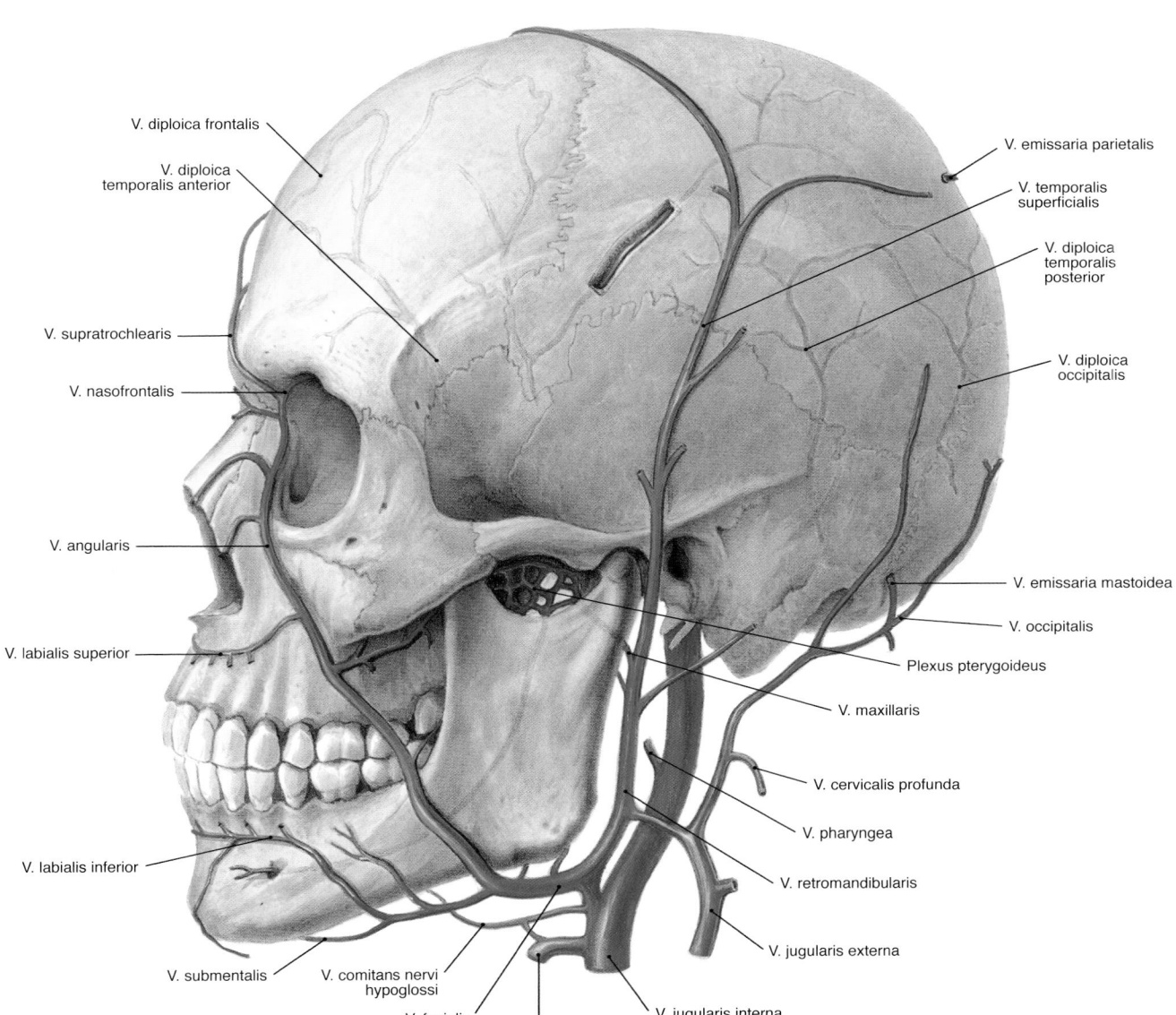

V. diploica frontalis

V. diploica temporalis anterior

V. supratrochlearis

V. nasofrontalis

V. angularis

V. labialis superior

V. labialis inferior

V. submentalis

V. comitans nervi hypoglossi

V. facialis

V. thyroidea superior

V. emissaria parietalis

V. temporalis superficialis

V. diploica temporalis posterior

V. diploica occipitalis

V. emissaria mastoidea

V. occipitalis

Plexus pterygoideus

V. maxillaris

V. cervicalis profunda

V. pharyngea

V. retromandibularis

V. jugularis externa

V. jugularis interna

Fig. 124 Internal jugular vein, V. jugularis interna.

→ 259

Lymphatics of the head and the neck

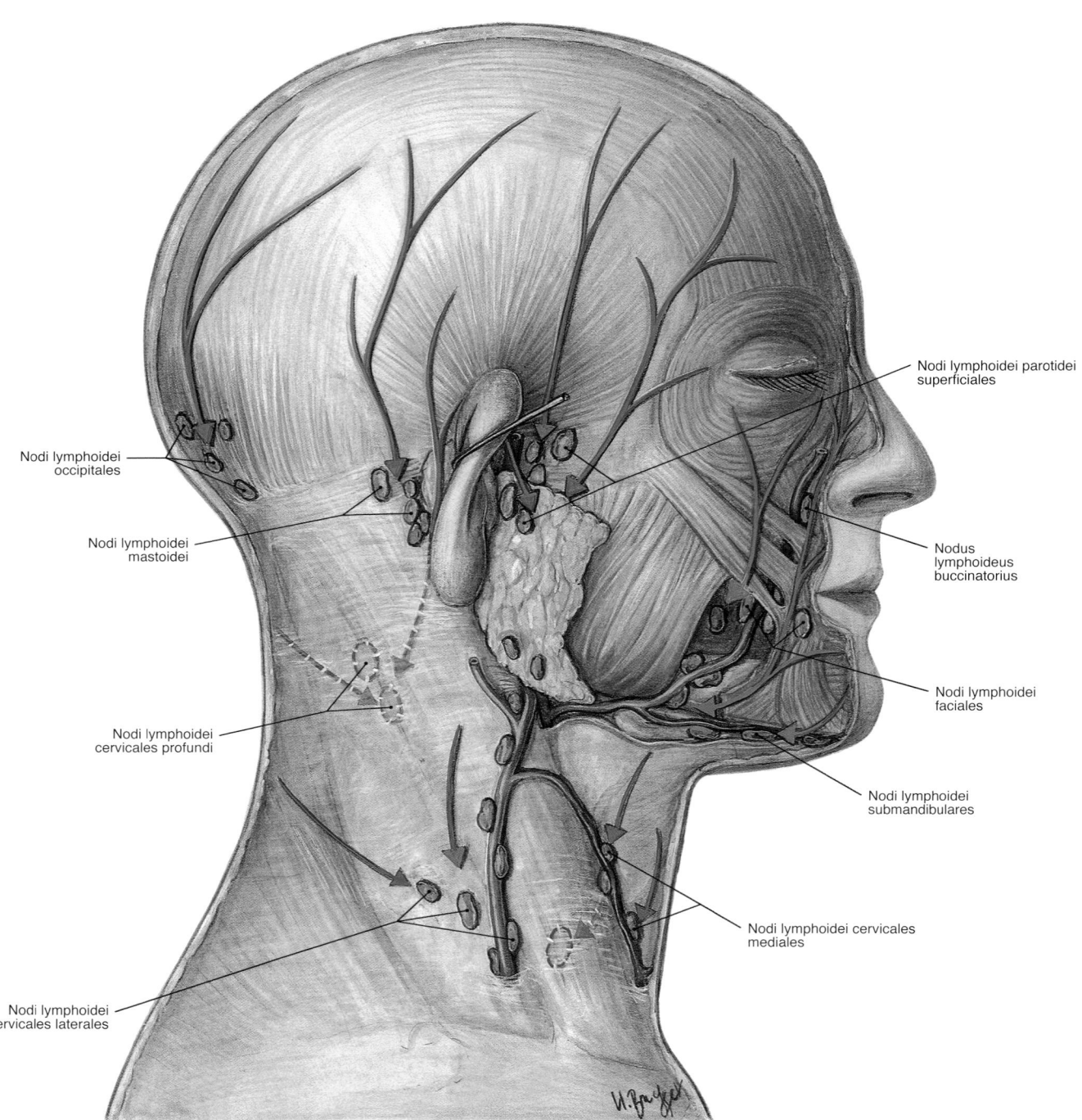

Nodi lymphoidei parotidei
superficiales

Nodi lymphoidei
occipitales

Nodi lymphoidei
mastoidei

Nodus
lymphoideus
buccinatorius

Nodi lymphoidei
cervicales profundi

Nodi lymphoidei
faciales

Nodi lymphoidei
submandibulares

Nodi lymphoidei cervicales
mediales

Nodi lymphoidei
cervicales laterales

→ 261, 414

Fig. 125 Lymph nodes and lymphatics
of the head and the neck, Nodi lymphoidei
capitis et cervicis;
arrows indicate drainage areas.

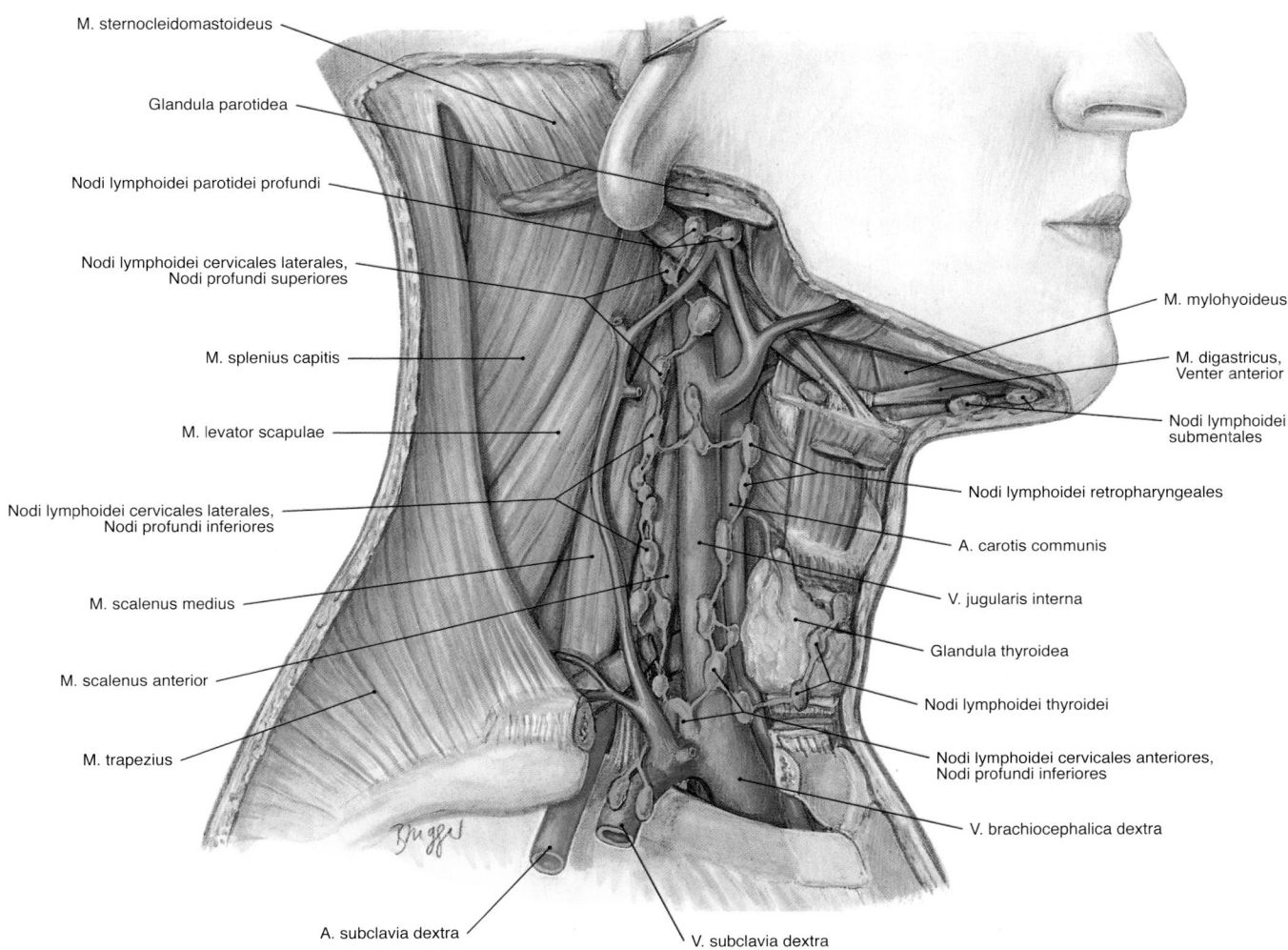

M. sternocleidomastoideus

Glandula parotidea

Nodi lymphoidei parotidei profundi

Nodi lymphoidei cervicales laterales,
Nodi profundi superiores

M. splenius capitis

M. levator scapulae

Nodi lymphoidei cervicales laterales,
Nodi profundi inferiores

M. scalenus medius

M. scalenus anterior

M. trapezius

A. subclavia dextra

V. subclavia dextra

M. mylohyoideus

M. digastricus,
Venter anterior

Nodi lymphoidei
submentales

Nodi lymphoidei retropharyngeales

A. carotis communis

V. jugularis interna

Glandula thyroidea

Nodi lymphoidei thyroidei

Nodi lymphoidei cervicales anteriores,
Nodi profundi inferiores

V. brachiocephalica dextra

Fig. 126 Deep lymph nodes of the neck,
Nodi lymphoidei cervicales profundi.

Facial nerve

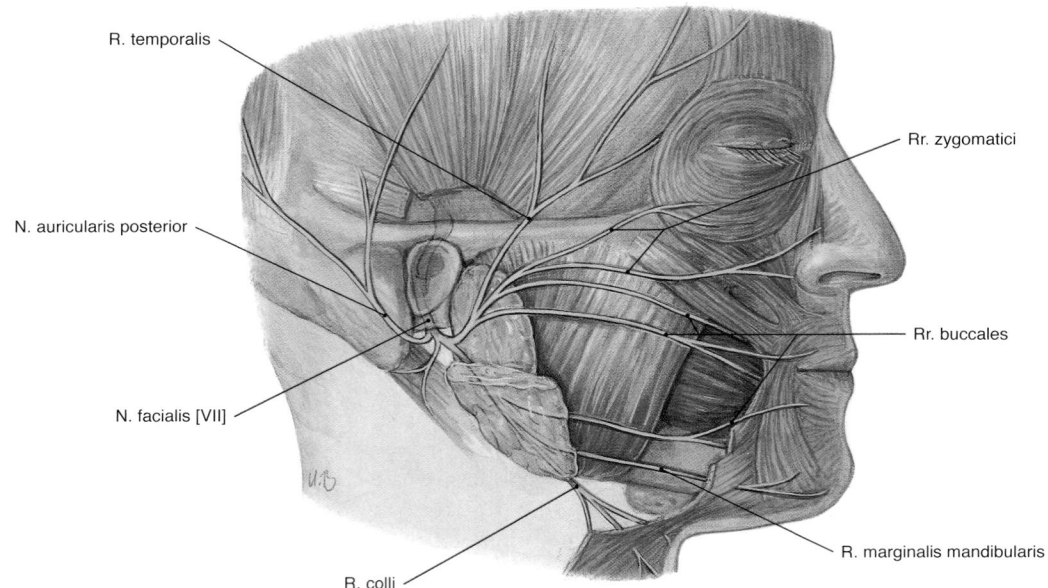

R. temporalis

N. auricularis posterior

N. facialis [VII]

R. colli

Rr. zygomatici

Rr. buccales

R. marginalis mandibularis

Fig. 127   Facial nerve, N. facialis [VII].

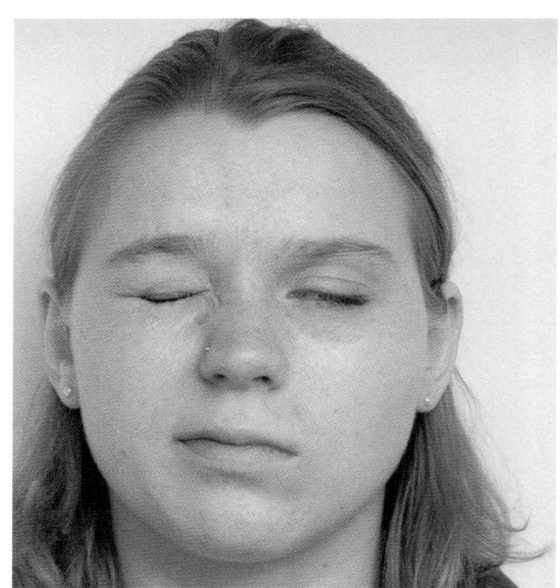

a

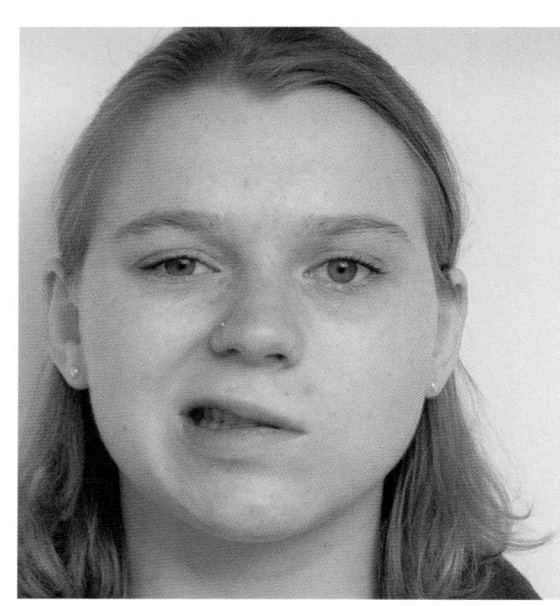

b

→ 1182

Fig. 128 a, b   Palsy of the left facial nerve, N. facialis [VII].
a The concerned eye cannot be closed upon request (lagophthalmus).
b The teeth of the concerned side cannot be shown upon request.

Cutaneous innervation

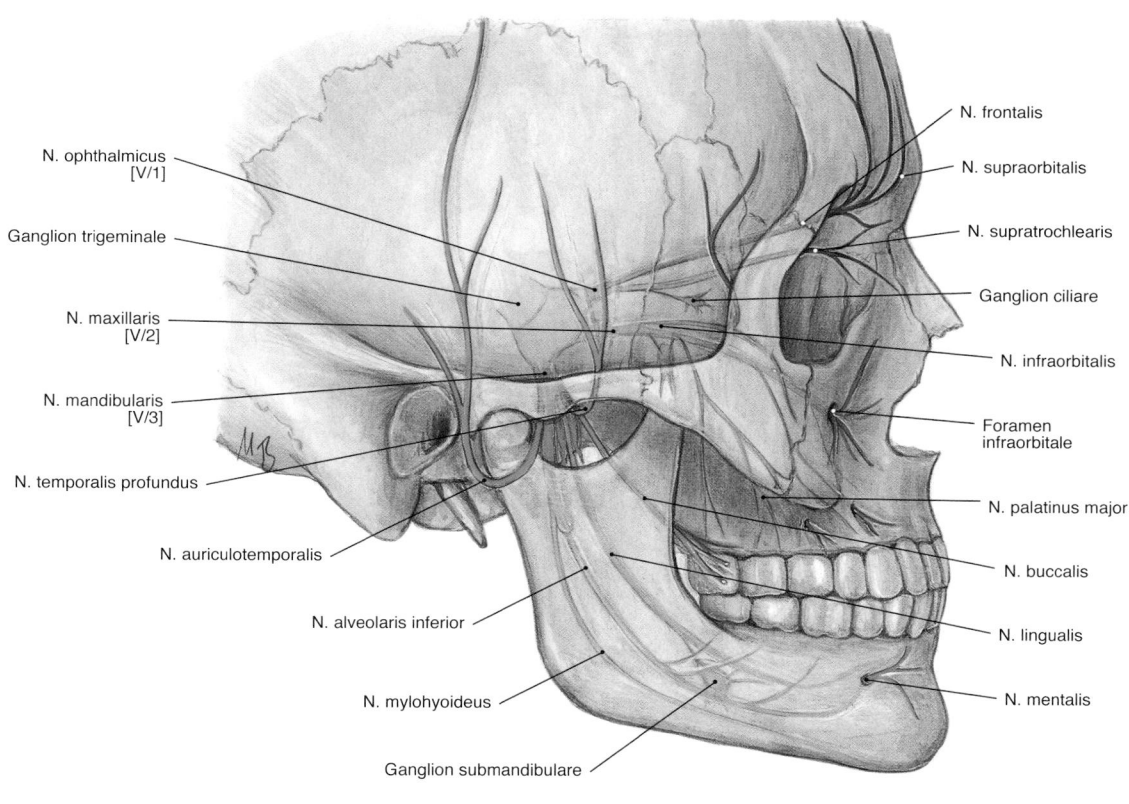

N. ophthalmicus [V/1]

Ganglion trigeminale

N. maxillaris [V/2]

N. mandibularis [V/3]

N. temporalis profundus

N. auriculotemporalis

N. alveolaris inferior

N. mylohyoideus

Ganglion submandibulare

N. frontalis

N. supraorbitalis

N. supratrochlearis

Ganglion ciliare

N. infraorbitalis

Foramen infraorbitale

N. palatinus major

N. buccalis

N. lingualis

N. mentalis

Fig. 129 Trigeminal nerve, N. trigeminus [V].

→ 472–475

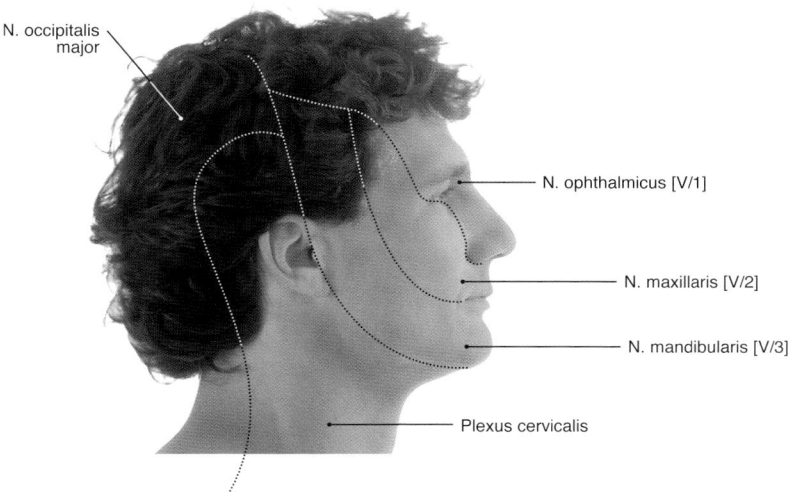

N. occipitalis major

N. ophthalmicus [V/1]

N. maxillaris [V/2]

N. mandibularis [V/3]

Plexus cervicalis

Fig. 130 Cutaneous innervation of the head and the neck.

Vessels and nerves of the head and the neck

● M. epicranius, M. occipitofrontalis

● N. supraorbitalis

A. temporalis superficialis, ●
R. frontalis

● M. orbicularis oculi

A. temporalis superficialis, ●
R. parietalis

M. temporalis ●

N. auriculotemporalis ●
(V/3)

● A. angularis

Rr. temporales ●
(VII)

● Rr. zygomatici
(VII)

Glandula parotidea

Ductus
parotideus

N. occipitalis minor, ●
(Plexus cervicalis)

● R. buccalis
(VII)

● M. masseter

V. jugularis externa ●

M. levator scapulae ●

● R. marginalis mandibularis
(VII)

N. auricularis magnus, ●
(Plexus cervicalis)

N. accessorius ●
[XI]

Platysma

M. trapezius ●

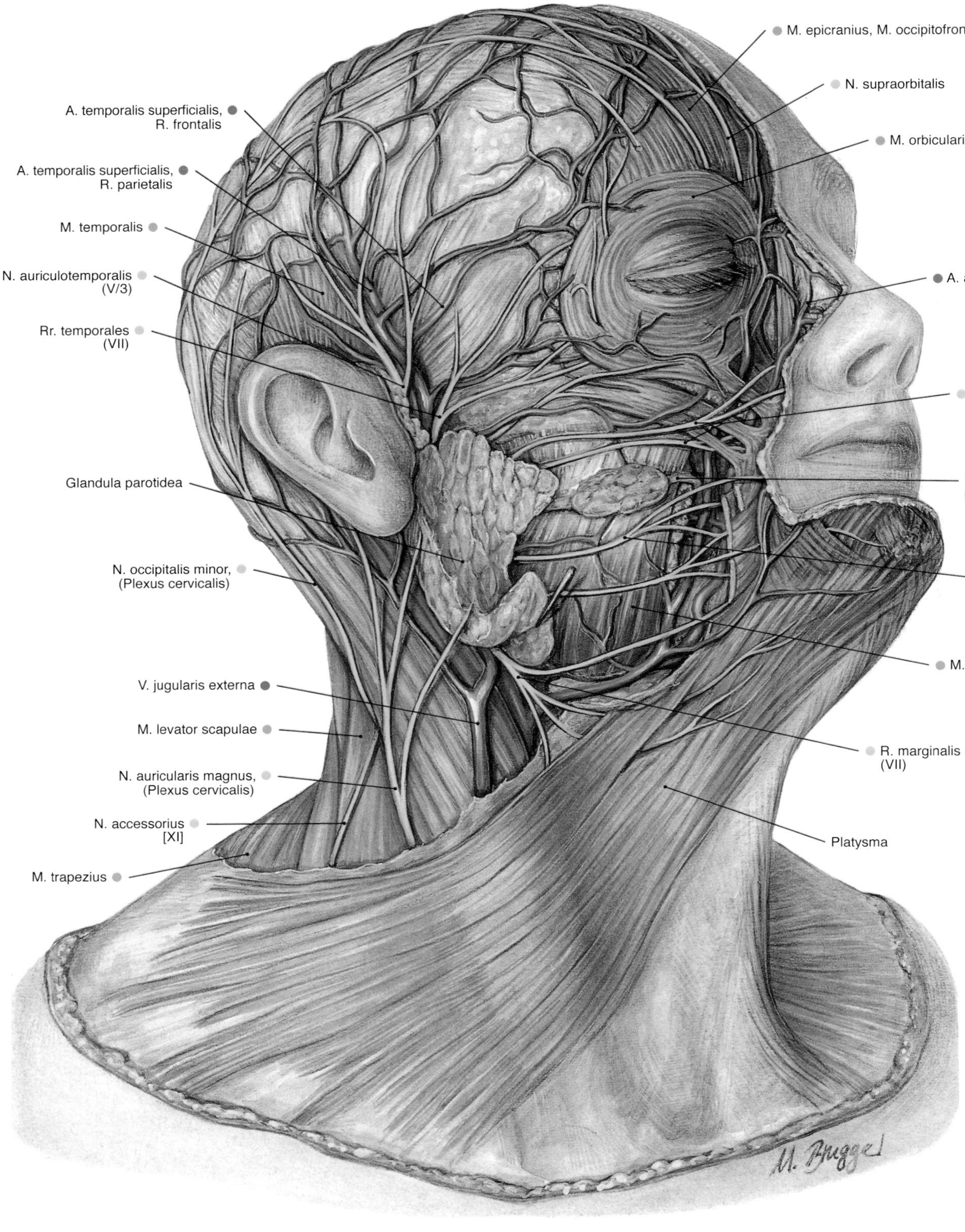

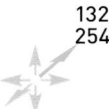

132
254

Fig. 131 Vessels and nerves of the head and the neck;
superficial lateral regions.

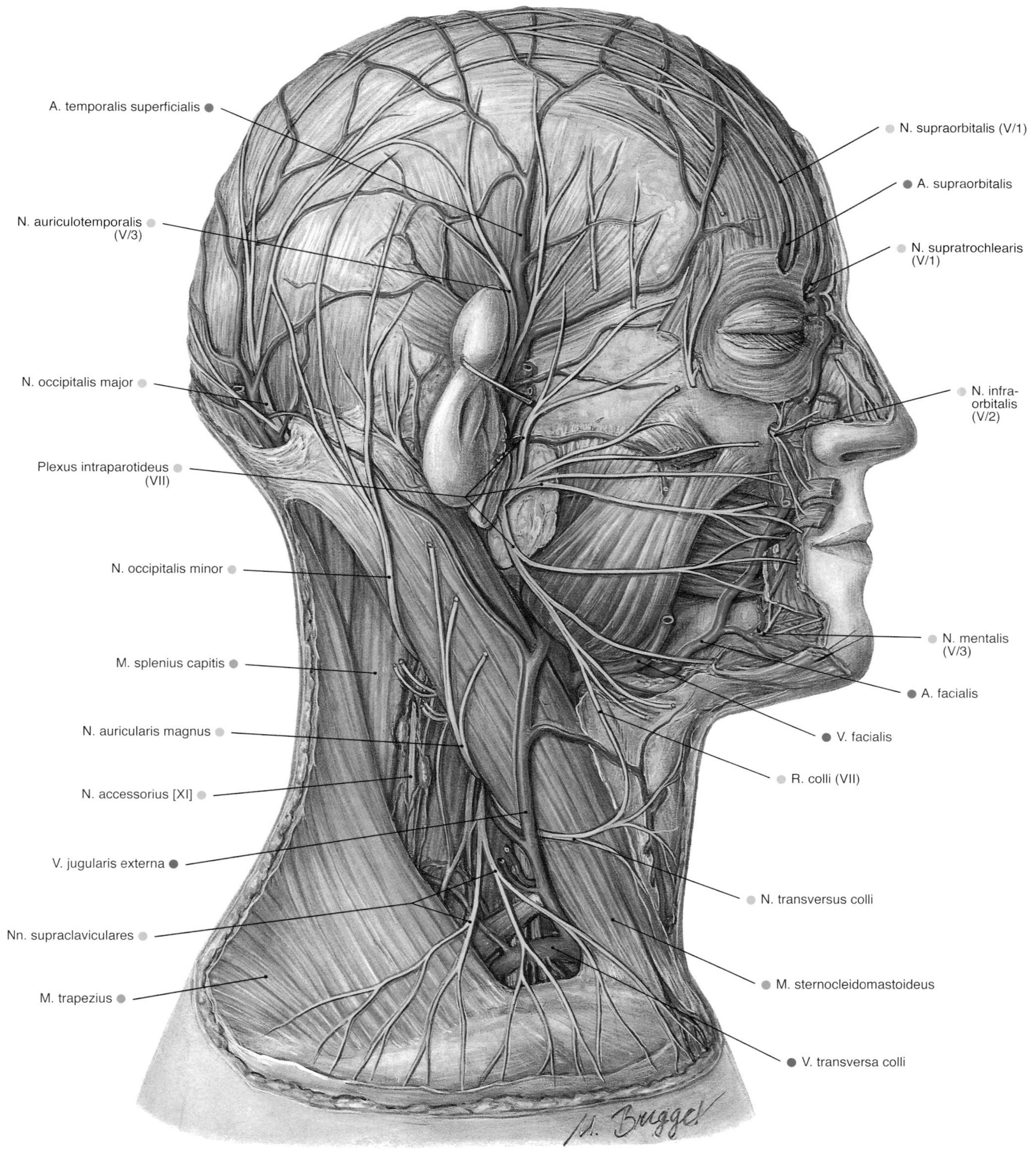

Vessels and nerves of the head and the neck

A. temporalis superficialis ●

N. auriculotemporalis ●
(V/3)

N. occipitalis major ●

Plexus intraparotideus ●
(VII)

N. occipitalis minor ●

M. splenius capitis ●

N. auricularis magnus ●

N. accessorius [XI] ●

V. jugularis externa ●

Nn. supraclaviculares ●

M. trapezius ●

● N. supraorbitalis (V/1)

● A. supraorbitalis

● N. supratrochlearis
(V/1)

● N. infra-
orbitalis
(V/2)

● N. mentalis
(V/3)

● A. facialis

● V. facialis

● R. colli (VII)

● N. transversus colli

● M. sternocleidomastoideus

● V. transversa colli

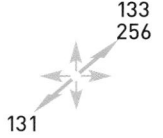

Fig. 132   Vessels and nerves of the head and the neck;
deep lateral regions.

133
256

131

Lateral region of the face

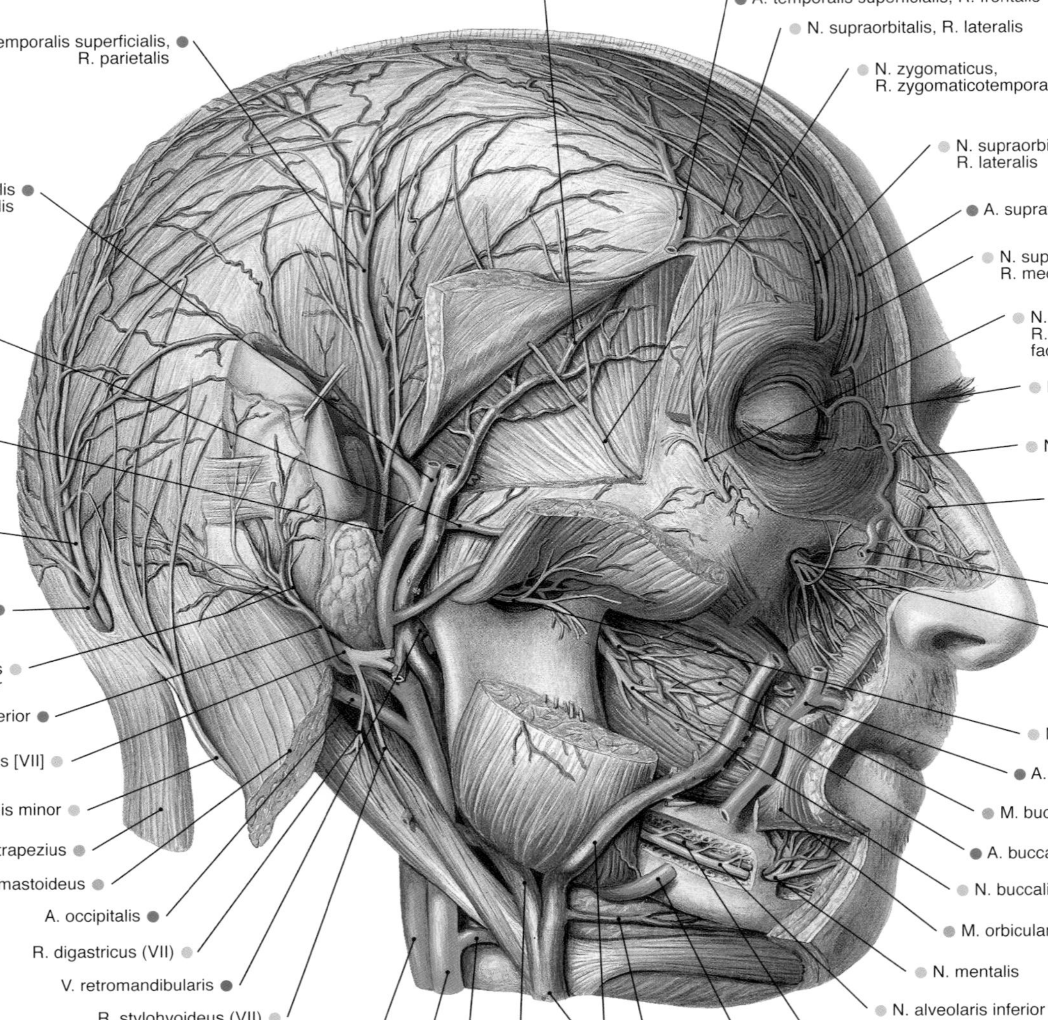

V. temporalis media ●

A. temporalis superficialis, R. frontalis ●

N. supraorbitalis, R. lateralis ●

N. zygomaticus, R. zygomaticotemporalis ●

A. temporalis superficialis, R. parietalis ●

N. supraorbitalis, R. lateralis ●

A. supratrochlearis ●

A. temporalis superficialis ●

N. supraorbitalis, R. medialis ●

A. zygomatico-orbitalis ●

N. zygomaticus, R. zygomatico-facialis ●

N. supratrochlearis ●

N. auriculo-temporalis ●

N. infratrochlearis ●

N. occipitalis major ●

N. ethmoidalis anterior, R. nasalis externus ●

A. occipitalis ●

A. angularis ●

N. auricularis posterior ●

N. infra-orbitalis ●

A. auricularis posterior ●

N. massetericus ●

N. facialis [VII] ●

A. facialis ●

N. occipitalis minor ●

M. buccinator ●

M. trapezius ●

A. buccalis ●

M. sternocleidomastoideus ●

N. buccalis ●

A. occipitalis ●

M. orbicularis oris ●

R. digastricus (VII) ●

N. mentalis ●

V. retromandibularis ●

N. alveolaris inferior ●

R. stylohyoideus (VII) ●

A. alveolaris inferior ●

A. carotis interna ●

A. carotis externa ●

A. facialis ●

A. lingualis ●

V. submentalis ●

V. retromandibularis ●

V. facialis ●

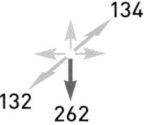

134

132 ↓ 262

Fig. 133 Vessels and nerves of the head; deep lateral regions.

Maxillary artery

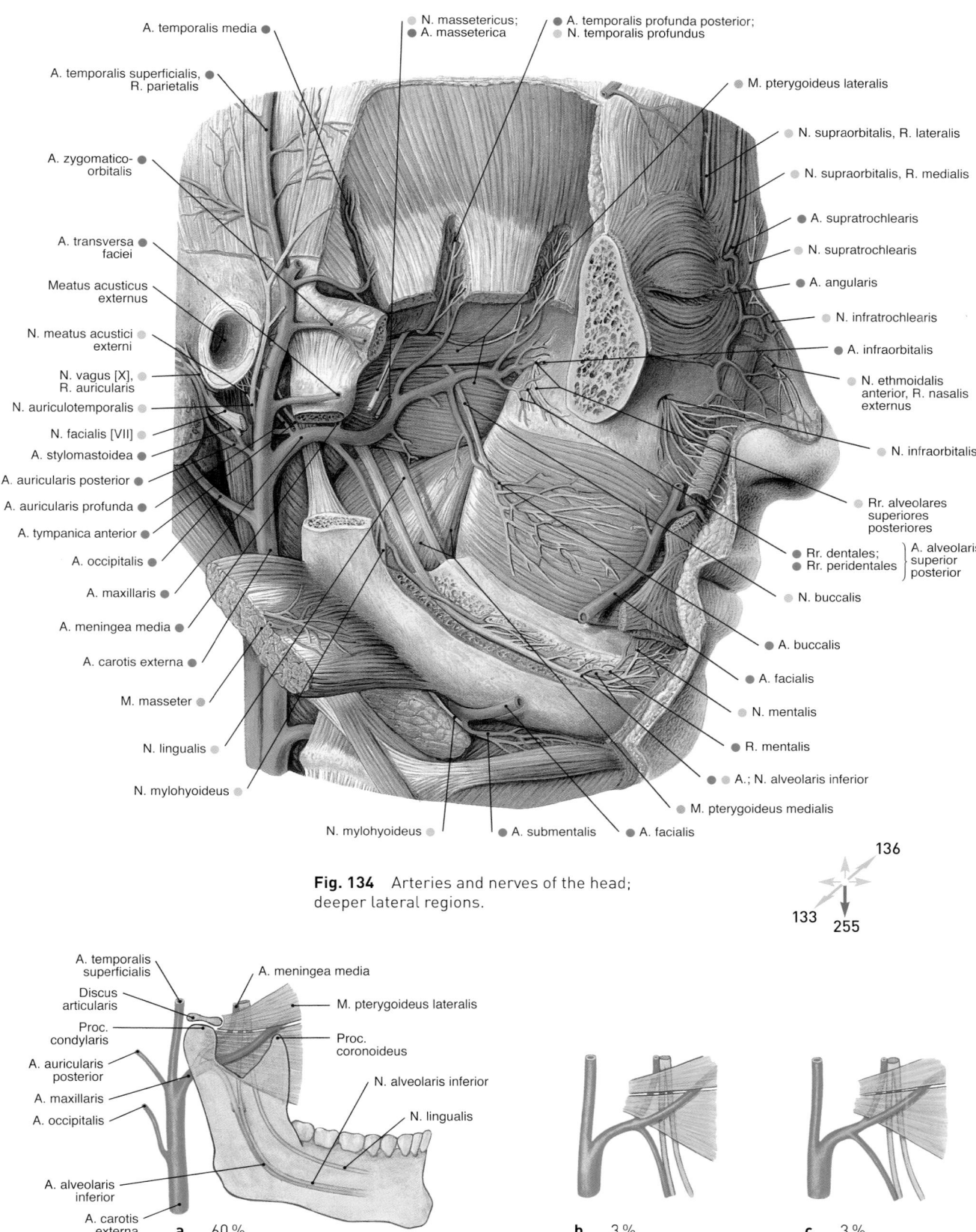

A. temporalis media

N. massetericus;
A. masseterica

A. temporalis profunda posterior;
N. temporalis profundus

A. temporalis superficialis,
R. parietalis

M. pterygoideus lateralis

A. zygomatico-
orbitalis

N. supraorbitalis, R. lateralis

N. supraorbitalis, R. medialis

A. transversa
faciei

A. supratrochlearis

N. supratrochlearis

Meatus acusticus
externus

A. angularis

N. meatus acustici
externi

N. infratrochlearis

N. vagus [X],
R. auricularis

A. infraorbitalis

N. auriculotemporalis

N. ethmoidalis
anterior, R. nasalis
externus

N. facialis [VII]

A. stylomastoidea

N. infraorbitalis

A. auricularis posterior

A. auricularis profunda

Rr. alveolares
superiores
posteriores

A. tympanica anterior

A. occipitalis

Rr. dentales;
Rr. peridentales

A. alveolaris
superior
posterior

A. maxillaris

N. buccalis

A. meningea media

A. carotis externa

A. buccalis

M. masseter

A. facialis

N. mentalis

N. lingualis

R. mentalis

N. mylohyoideus

A.; N. alveolaris inferior

M. pterygoideus medialis

N. mylohyoideus

A. submentalis

A. facialis

136

133   255

Fig. 134   Arteries and nerves of the head;
deeper lateral regions.

A. temporalis
superficialis

A. meningea media

Discus
articularis

M. pterygoideus lateralis

Proc.
condylaris

Proc.
coronoideus

A. auricularis
posterior

N. alveolaris inferior

A. maxillaris

N. lingualis

A. occipitalis

A. alveolaris
inferior

A. carotis
externa   **a**   60 %

b   3 %

c   3 %

Fig. 135 a–c   Variations of the middle
meningeal artery, A. meningea media.

a The middle meningeal artery, A. meningea media, branches off proximal to the
inferior alveolar artery, A. alveolaris inferior.

b The middle meningeal artery, A. meningea media, branches off across from the inferior
alveolar artery, A. alveolaris inferior.

c The middle meningeal artery, A. meningea media, branches off distal to the inferior
alveolar artery, A. alveolaris inferior.

Lateral region of the face

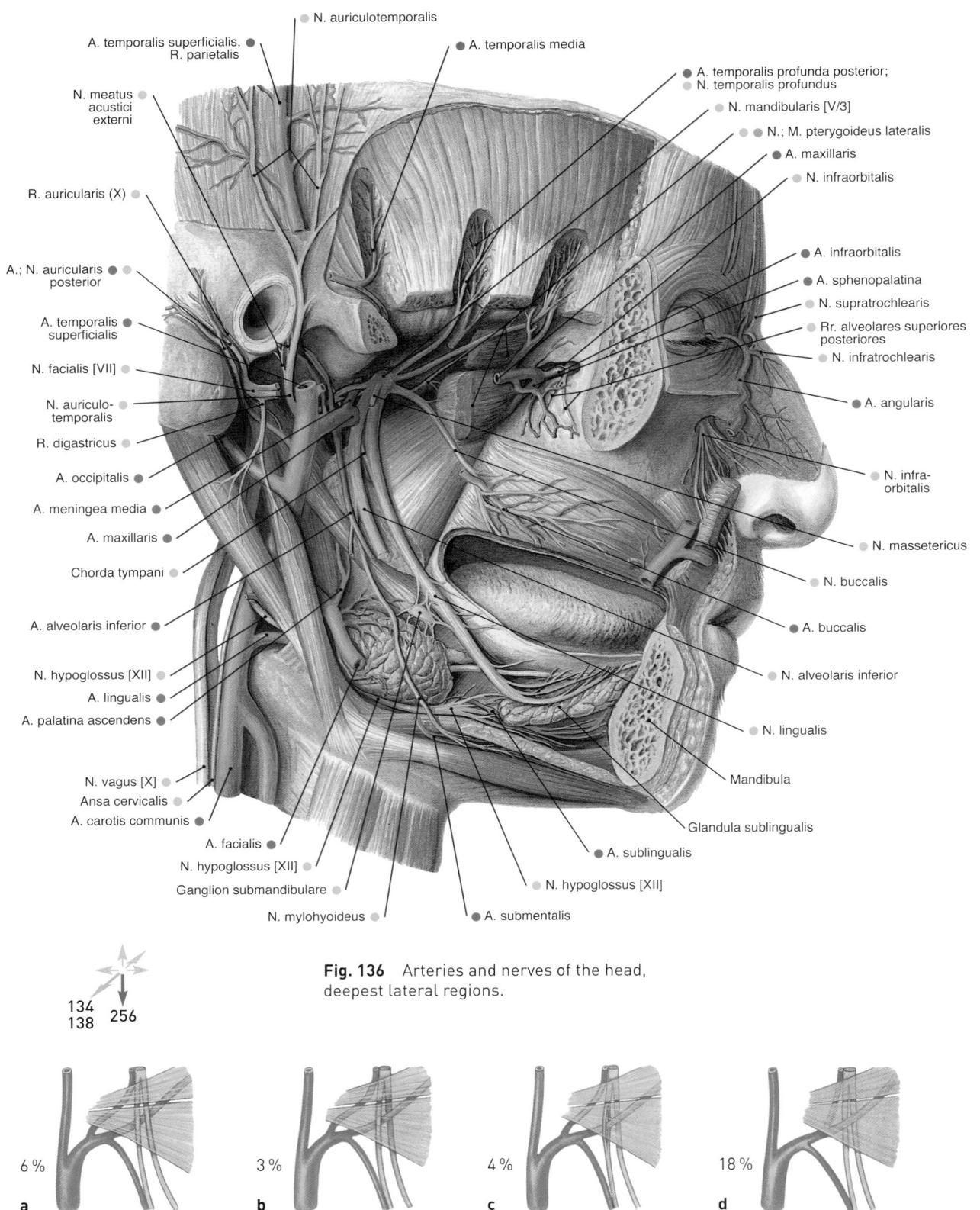

- N. auriculotemporalis
- A. temporalis superficialis, R. parietalis
- A. temporalis media
- A. temporalis profunda posterior; N. temporalis profundus
- N. meatus acustici externi
- N. mandibularis [V/3]
- N.; M. pterygoideus lateralis
- A. maxillaris
- R. auricularis (X)
- N. infraorbitalis
- A.; N. auricularis posterior
- A. infraorbitalis
- A. sphenopalatina
- N. supratrochlearis
- A. temporalis superficialis
- Rr. alveolares superiores posteriores
- N. infratrochlearis
- N. facialis [VII]
- N. auriculo-temporalis
- A. angularis
- R. digastricus
- A. occipitalis
- N. infra-orbitalis
- A. meningea media
- A. maxillaris
- N. massetericus
- Chorda tympani
- N. buccalis
- A. alveolaris inferior
- A. buccalis
- N. hypoglossus [XII]
- N. alveolaris inferior
- A. lingualis
- A. palatina ascendens
- N. lingualis
- Mandibula
- N. vagus [X]
- Ansa cervicalis
- A. carotis communis
- Glandula sublingualis
- A. facialis
- A. sublingualis
- N. hypoglossus [XII]
- Ganglion submandibulare
- N. hypoglossus [XII]
- N. mylohyoideus
- A. submentalis

Fig. 136 Arteries and nerves of the head, deepest lateral regions.

134
138 256

6 %   3 %   4 %   18 %

a   b   c   d

Fig. 137 a–d Variations in the course of the maxillary artery, A. maxillaris.

a The maxillary artery, A. maxillaris, passes medially to the lateral pterygoid muscle, M. pterygoideus lateralis, the lingual nerve, N. lingualis, and the inferior alveolar nerve, N. alveolaris inferior.

b The maxillary artery, A. maxillaris, passes between the lingual nerve, N. lingualis, and the inferior alveolar nerve, N. alveolaris inferior.

c The maxillary artery, A. maxillaris, passes through a loop formed by the inferior alveolar nerve, N. alveolaris inferior.

d The middle meningeal artery, A. meningea media, branches off distal to the inferior alveolar artery, A. alveolaris inferior.

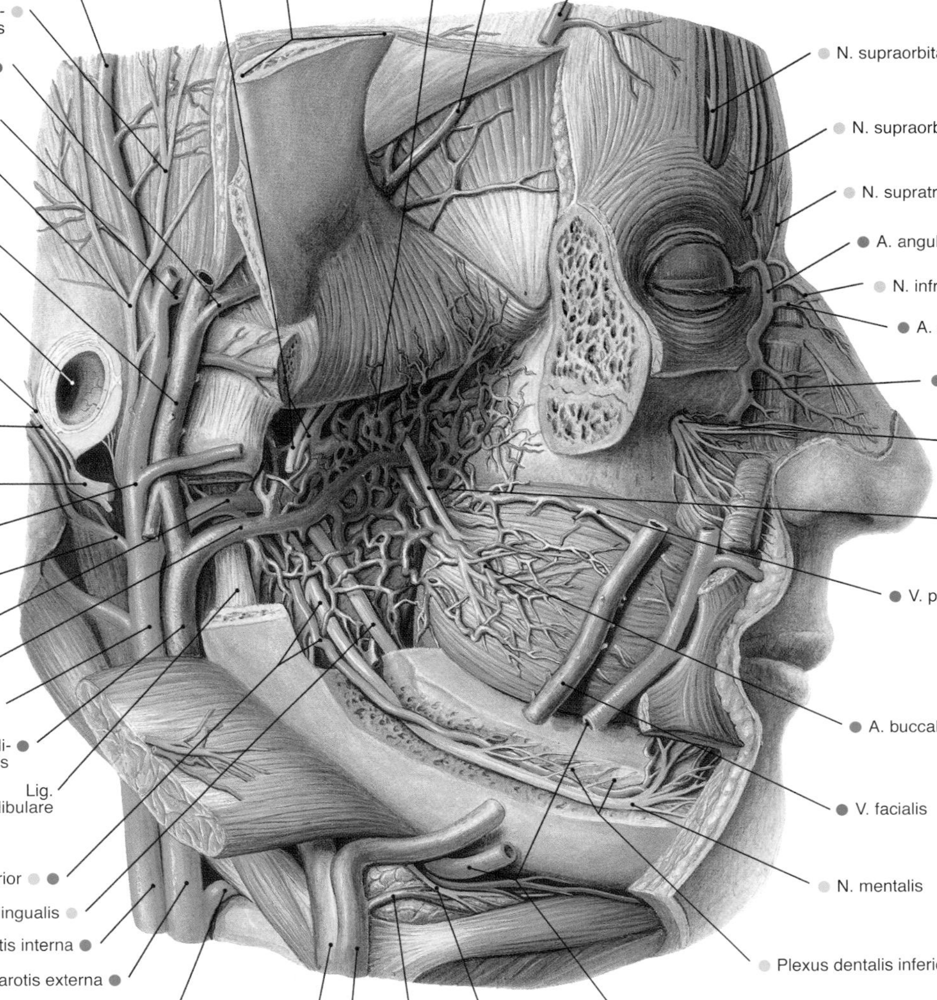

Lateral region of the face

Ramus mandibulae

N. massetericus; A. masseterica

Plexus pterygoideus

V. temporalis media

A. temporalis superficialis, R. parietalis

A. temporalis superficialis, R. frontalis

N. auriculo-temporalis

N. supraorbitalis, R. lateralis

V. temporalis media

N. supraorbitalis, R. medialis

A. temporalis media

N. supratrochlearis

N. auriculo-temporalis

A. angularis

V. temporalis superficialis

N. infratrochlearis

Meatus acusticus externus

A. dorsalis nasi

A. facialis

R. auricularis (X)

N. infraorbitalis

N. auricularis posterior

N. facialis [VII]

N. buccalis

A. temporalis superficialis

V. profunda faciei

A. auricularis posterior

A. maxillaris

V. maxillaris

A. buccalis

A. carotis externa

V. retromandibularis

V. facialis

Lig. sphenomandibulare

N. mentalis

N.; A. alveolaris inferior

N. lingualis

A. carotis interna

Plexus dentalis inferior

A. carotis externa

A. lingualis

A. facialis

V. retromandibularis

N. mylohyoideus

V. facialis

V. submentalis

Fig. 138   Vessels and nerves of the head; deeper lateral regions.

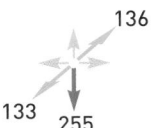

136

133   255

Skeleton of the nose

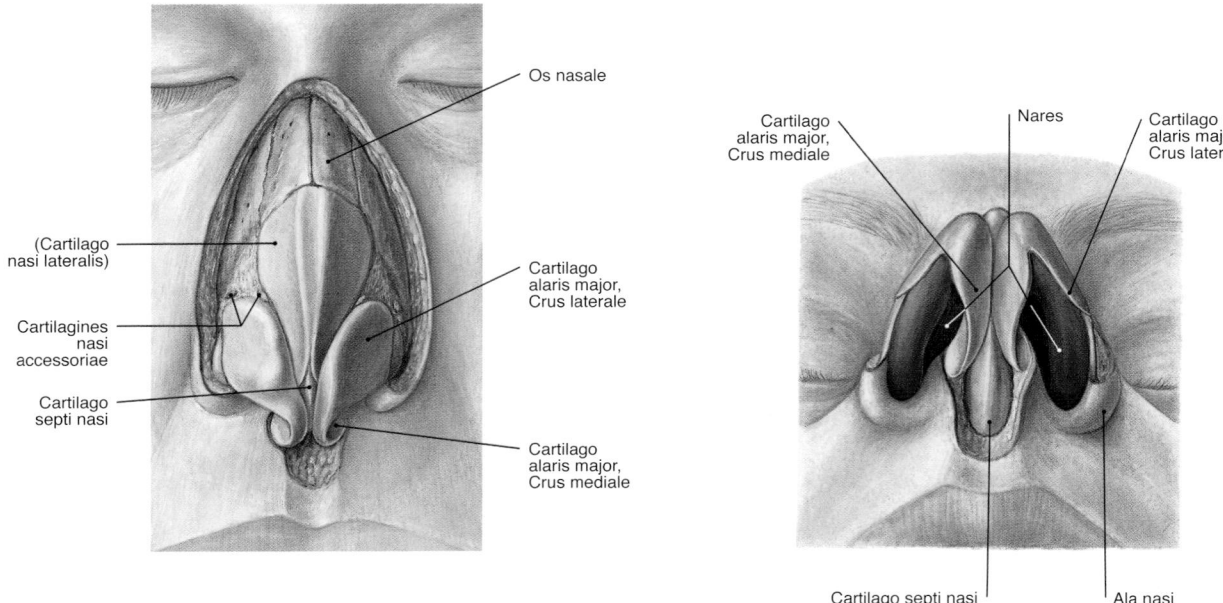

Os nasale

(Cartilago nasi lateralis)

Cartilagines nasi accessoriae

Cartilago septi nasi

Cartilago alaris major, Crus laterale

Cartilago alaris major, Crus mediale

Fig. 139 Skeleton of the nose.

Cartilago alaris major, Crus mediale

Nares

Cartilago alaris major, Crus laterale

Cartilago septi nasi

Ala nasi

Fig. 140 Nasal cartilages, Cartilagines nasi.

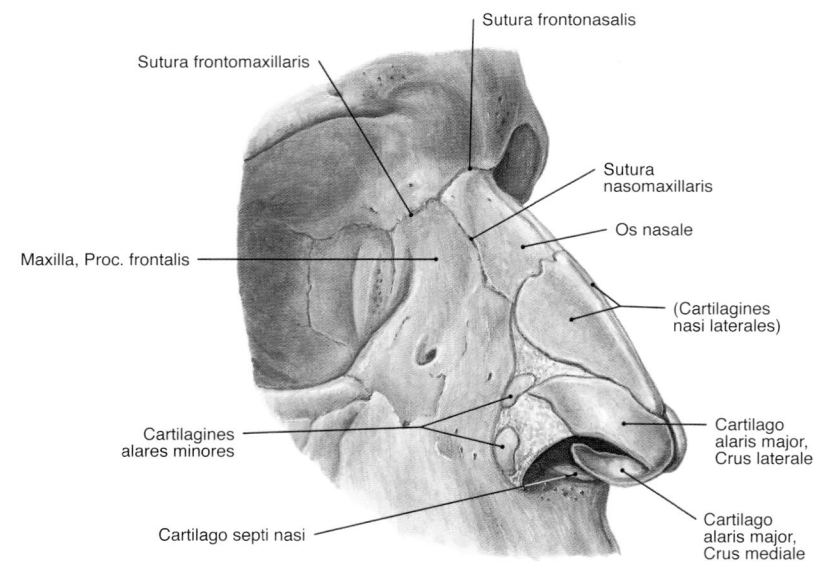

Sutura frontonasalis

Sutura frontomaxillaris

Sutura nasomaxillaris

Os nasale

Maxilla, Proc. frontalis

(Cartilagines nasi laterales)

Cartilagines alares minores

Cartilago alaris major, Crus laterale

Cartilago septi nasi

Cartilago alaris major, Crus mediale

Fig. 141 Skeleton of the nose.

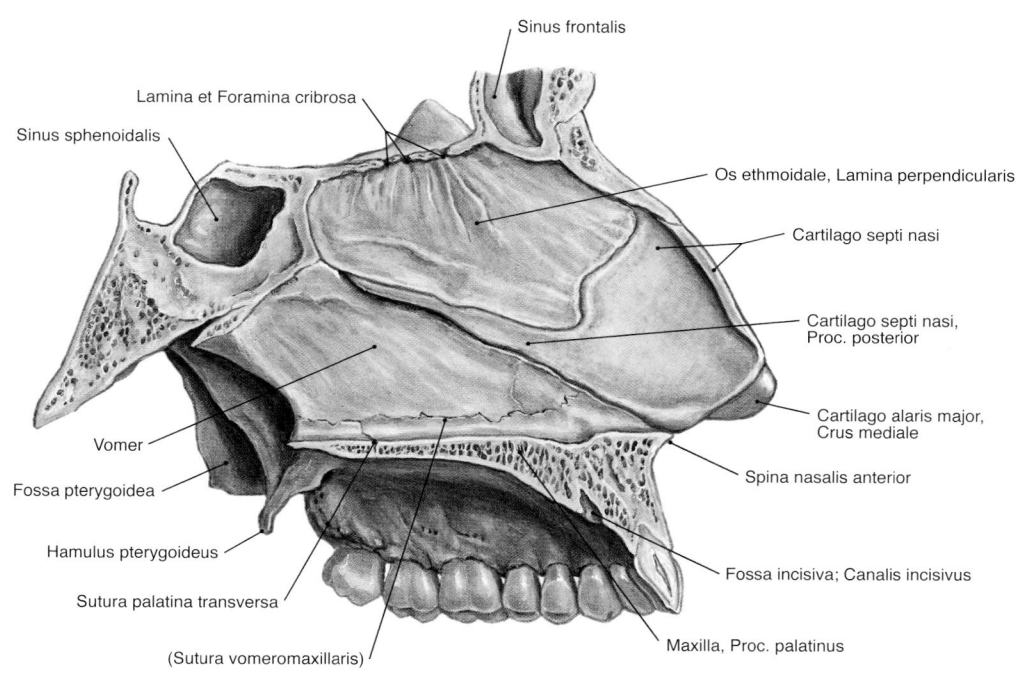

Sinus frontalis

Lamina et Foramina cribrosa

Sinus sphenoidalis

Os ethmoidale, Lamina perpendicularis

Cartilago septi nasi

Cartilago septi nasi, Proc. posterior

Cartilago alaris major, Crus mediale

Spina nasalis anterior

Vomer

Fossa pterygoidea

Hamulus pterygoideus

Sutura palatina transversa

(Sutura vomeromaxillaris)

Fossa incisiva; Canalis incisivus

Maxilla, Proc. palatinus

Fig. 142   Nasal septum, Septum nasi.

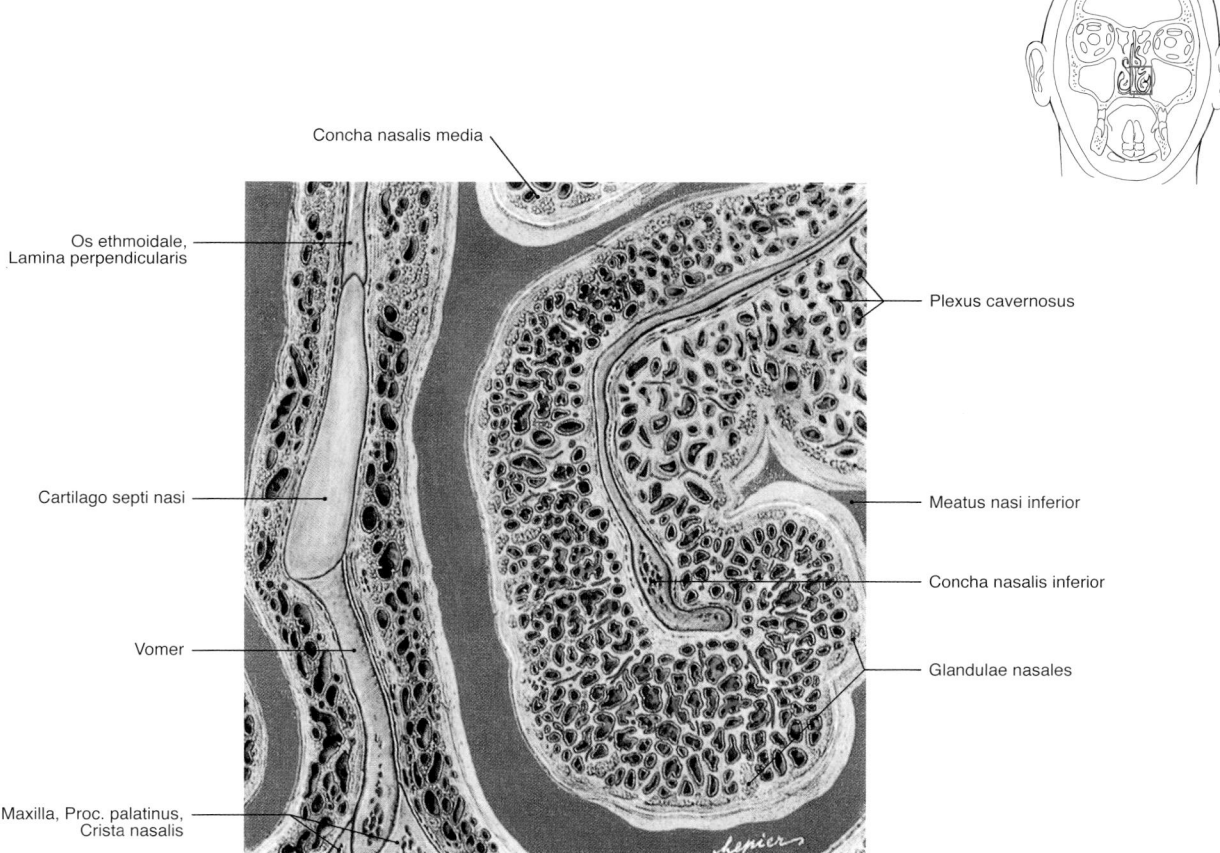

Concha nasalis media

Os ethmoidale, Lamina perpendicularis

Cartilago septi nasi

Vomer

Maxilla, Proc. palatinus, Crista nasalis

Plexus cavernosus

Meatus nasi inferior

Concha nasalis inferior

Glandulae nasales

Fig. 143   Inferior nasal concha, Concha nasalis inferior.

Nasal cavity

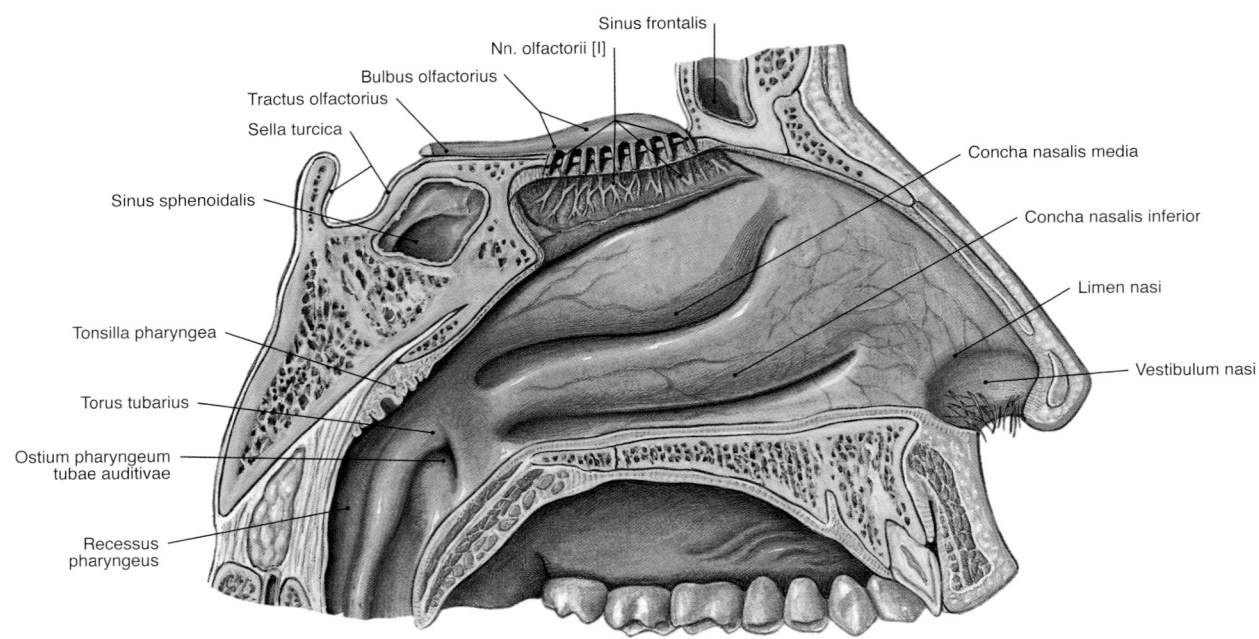

Sinus frontalis
Nn. olfactorii [I]
Bulbus olfactorius
Tractus olfactorius
Sella turcica
Sinus sphenoidalis
Tonsilla pharyngea
Torus tubarius
Ostium pharyngeum tubae auditivae
Recessus pharyngeus

Concha nasalis media
Concha nasalis inferior
Limen nasi
Vestibulum nasi

Fig. 144 Lateral wall of the nasal cavity, Cavitas nasi.

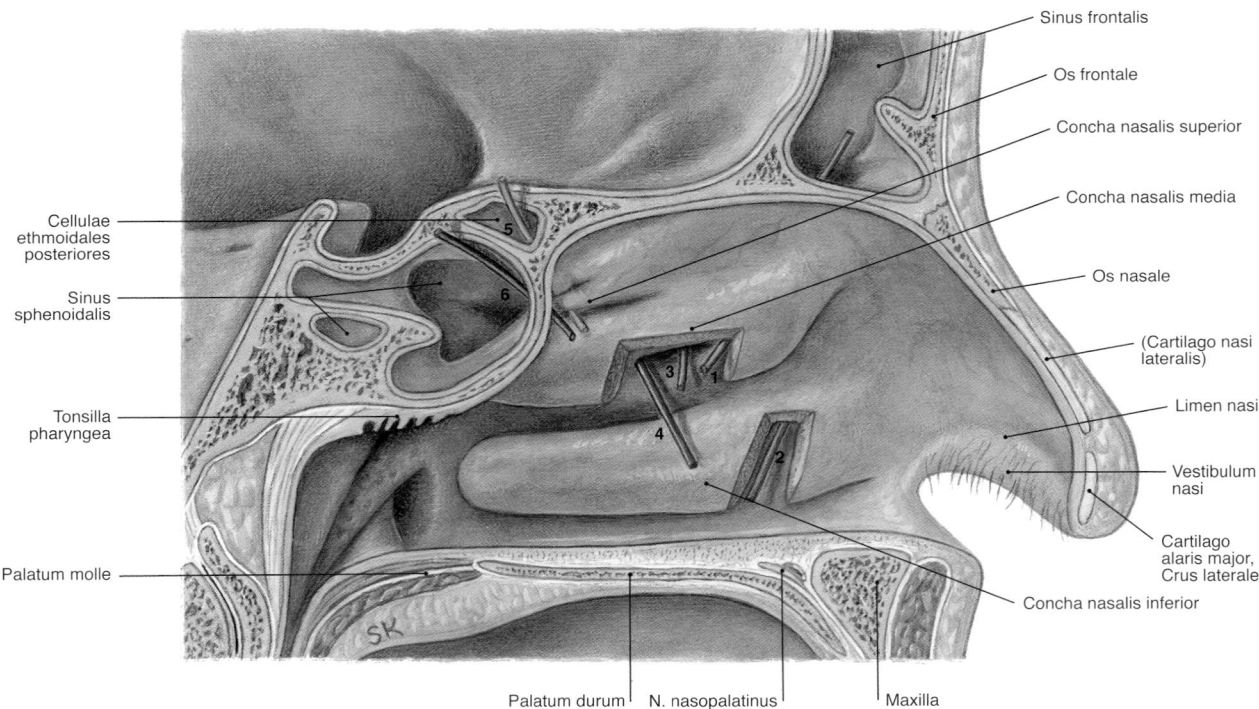

Cellulae ethmoidales posteriores
Sinus sphenoidalis
Tonsilla pharyngea
Palatum molle

Sinus frontalis
Os frontale
Concha nasalis superior
Concha nasalis media
Os nasale
(Cartilago nasi lateralis)
Limen nasi
Vestibulum nasi
Cartilago alaris major, Crus laterale
Concha nasalis inferior

Palatum durum N. nasopalatinus Maxilla

Openings of:
1 Sinus frontalis
2 Ductus nasolacrimalis
3 Cellulae ethmoidales anteriores
4 Sinus maxillaris
5 Cellulae ethmoidales posteriores
6 Sinus sphenoidalis

Fig. 145 Nasal cavity, Cavitas nasi, and openings of the paranasal sinuses, Sinus paranasales.

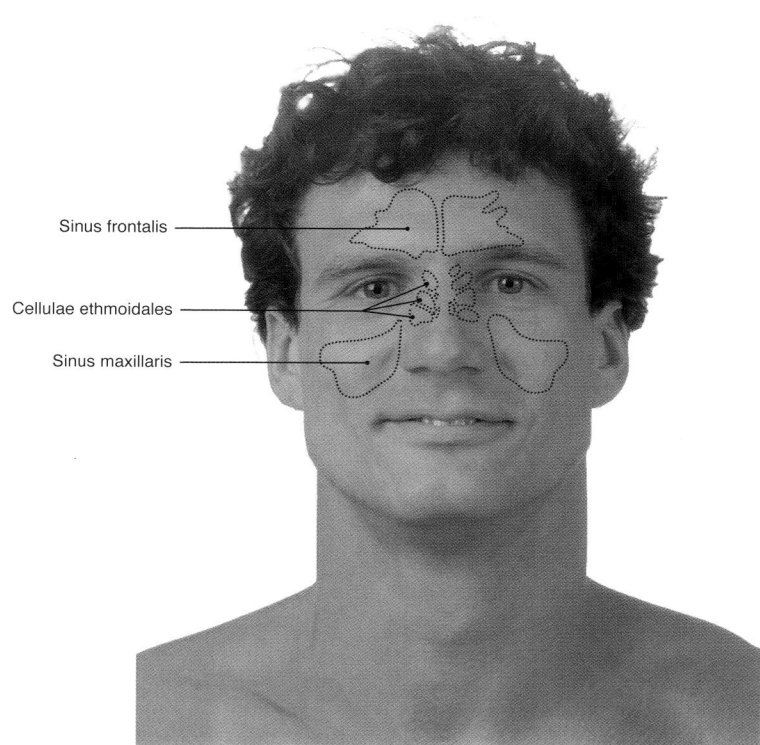

Fig. 146   Projection of the paranasal sinuses, Sinus paranasales.

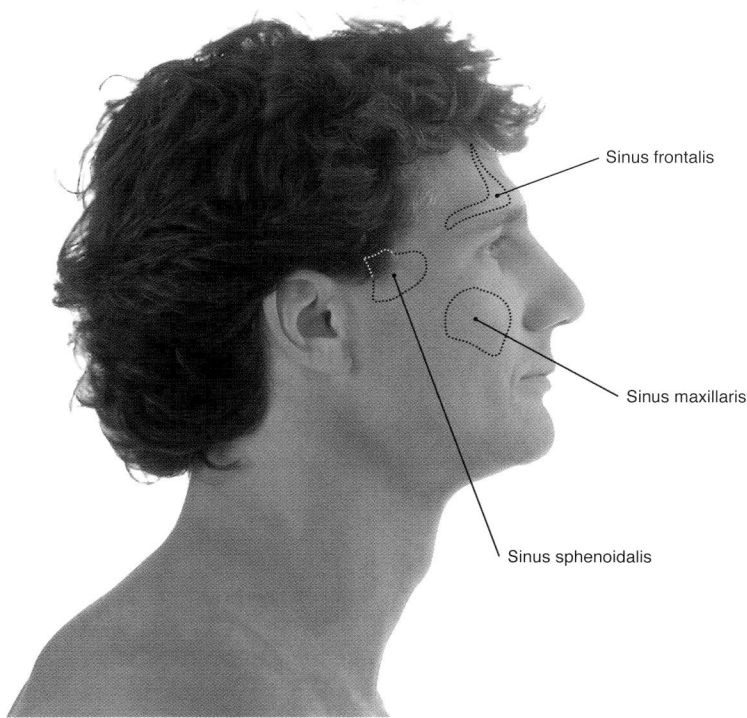

Fig. 147   Projection of the paranasal sinuses, Sinus paranasales.

Paranasal sinuses

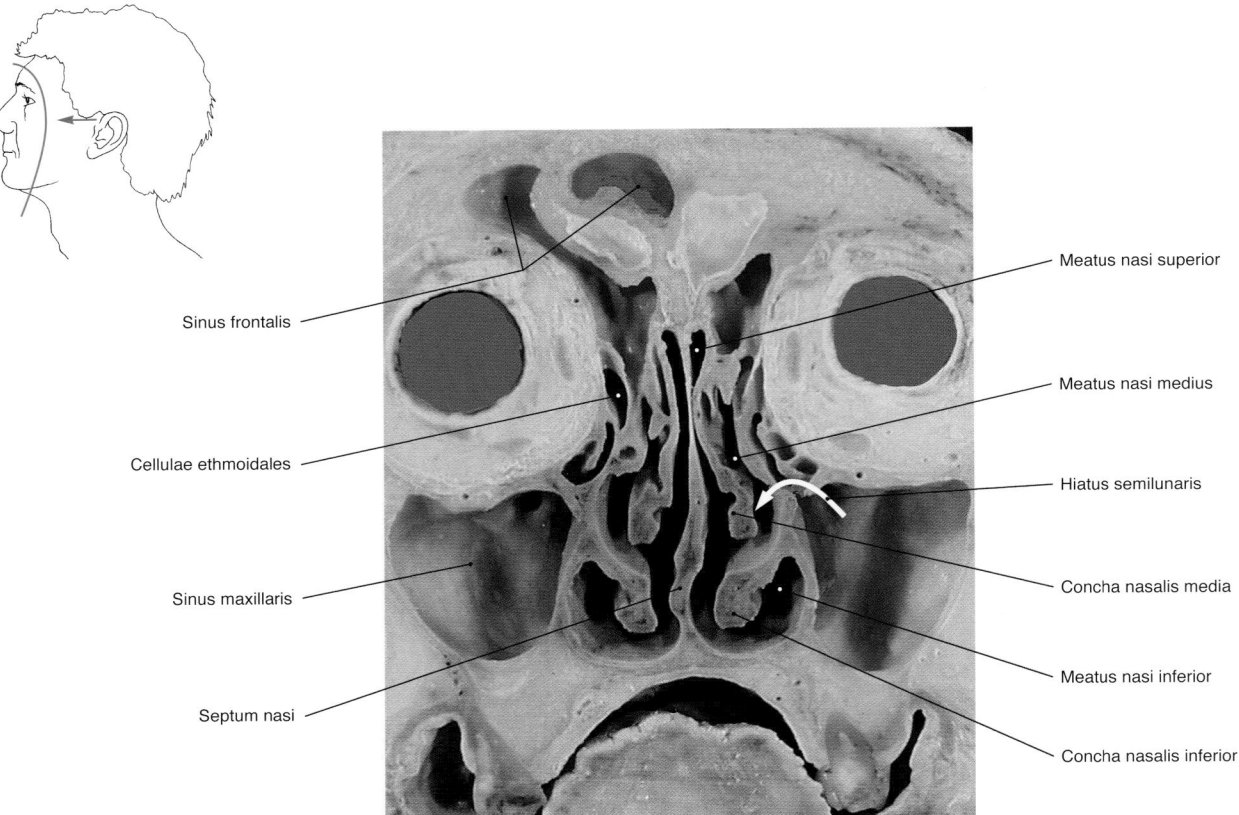

Sinus frontalis

Cellulae ethmoidales

Sinus maxillaris

Septum nasi

Meatus nasi superior

Meatus nasi medius

Hiatus semilunaris

Concha nasalis media

Meatus nasi inferior

Concha nasalis inferior

Fig. 148 Paranasal sinuses, Sinus paranasales.

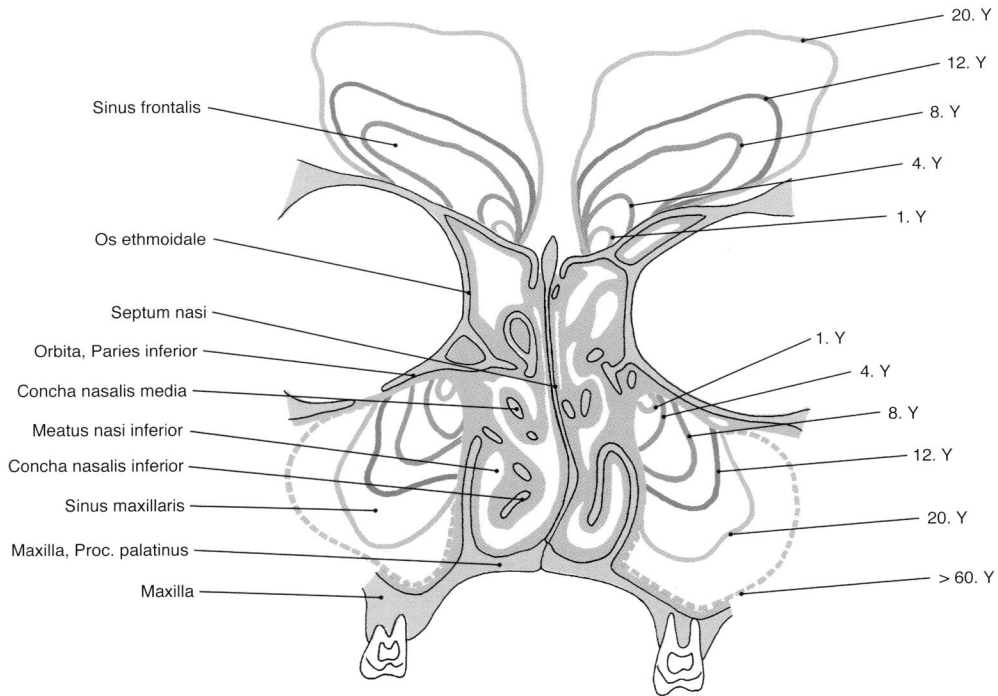

Sinus frontalis

Os ethmoidale

Septum nasi

Orbita, Paries inferior

Concha nasalis media

Meatus nasi inferior

Concha nasalis inferior

Sinus maxillaris

Maxilla, Proc. palatinus

Maxilla

20. Y

12. Y

8. Y

4. Y

1. Y

1. Y

4. Y

8. Y

12. Y

20. Y

> 60. Y

Fig. 149 Development of the maxillary and frontal sinuses.
Y – year of life

Paranasal sinuses, radiography

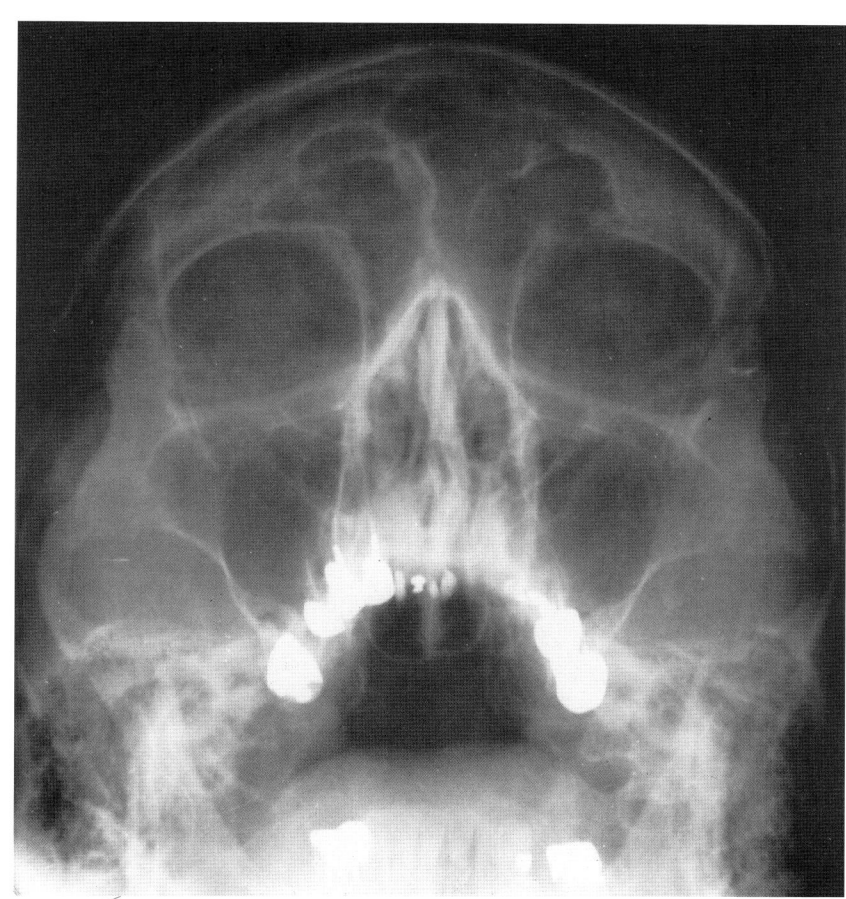

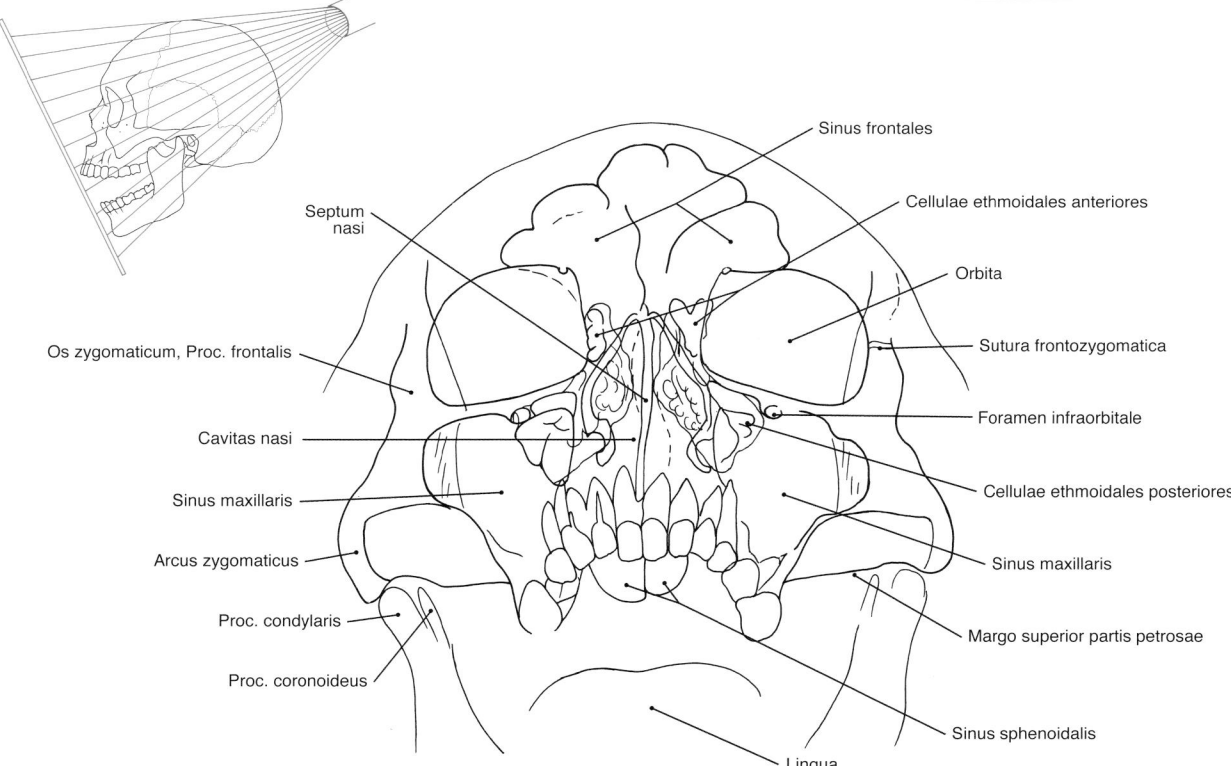

Sinus frontales

Cellulae ethmoidales anteriores

Septum nasi

Orbita

Os zygomaticum, Proc. frontalis

Sutura frontozygomatica

Foramen infraorbitale

Cavitas nasi

Cellulae ethmoidales posteriores

Sinus maxillaris

Sinus maxillaris

Arcus zygomaticus

Proc. condylaris

Margo superior partis petrosae

Proc. coronoideus

Sinus sphenoidalis

Lingua

Fig. 150   Paranasal sinuses, Sinus paranasales;
PA-radiograph.

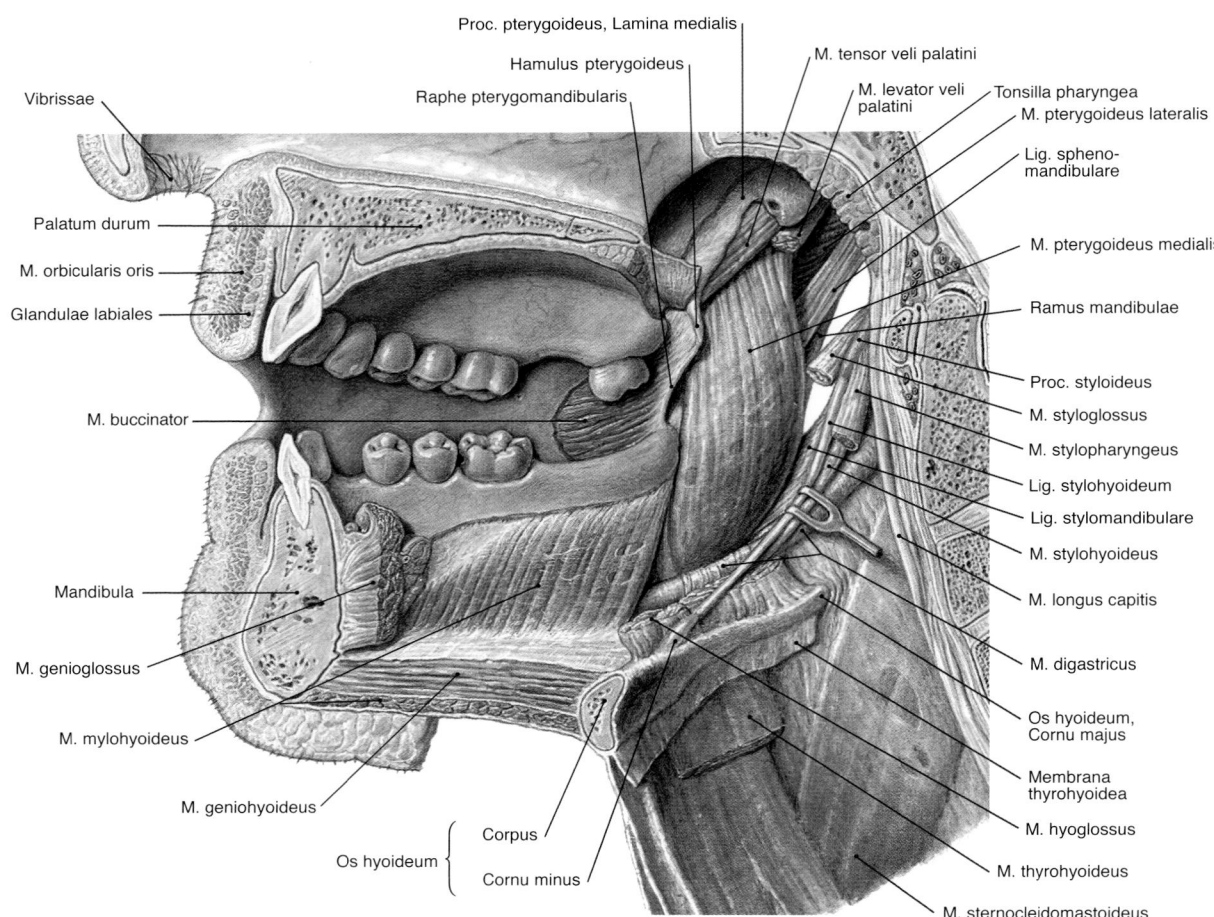

Proc. pterygoideus, Lamina medialis

Hamulus pterygoideus

Raphe pterygomandibularis

M. tensor veli palatini

M. levator veli palatini

Tonsilla pharyngea

M. pterygoideus lateralis

Lig. spheno-mandibulare

Vibrissae

Palatum durum

M. orbicularis oris

Glandulae labiales

M. buccinator

Mandibula

M. genioglossus

M. mylohyoideus

M. geniohyoideus

Os hyoideum { Corpus / Cornu minus

M. pterygoideus medialis

Ramus mandibulae

Proc. styloideus

M. styloglossus

M. stylopharyngeus

Lig. stylohyoideum

Lig. stylomandibulare

M. stylohyoideus

M. longus capitis

M. digastricus

Os hyoideum, Cornu majus

Membrana thyrohyoidea

M. hyoglossus

M. thyrohyoideus

M. sternocleidomastoideus

Fig. 151   Oral cavity, Cavitas oris.

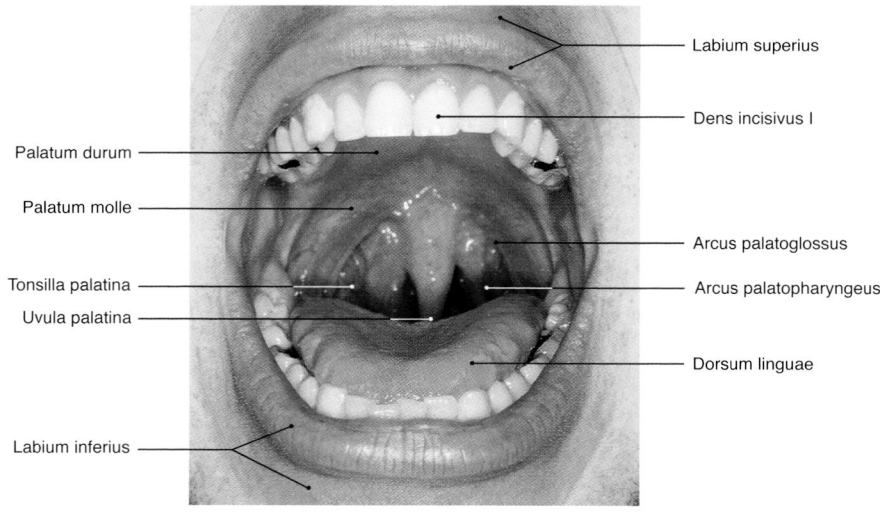

Palatum durum

Palatum molle

Tonsilla palatina

Uvula palatina

Labium inferius

Labium superius

Dens incisivus I

Arcus palatoglossus

Arcus palatopharyngeus

Dorsum linguae

Fig. 152   Oral cavity, Cavitas oris.

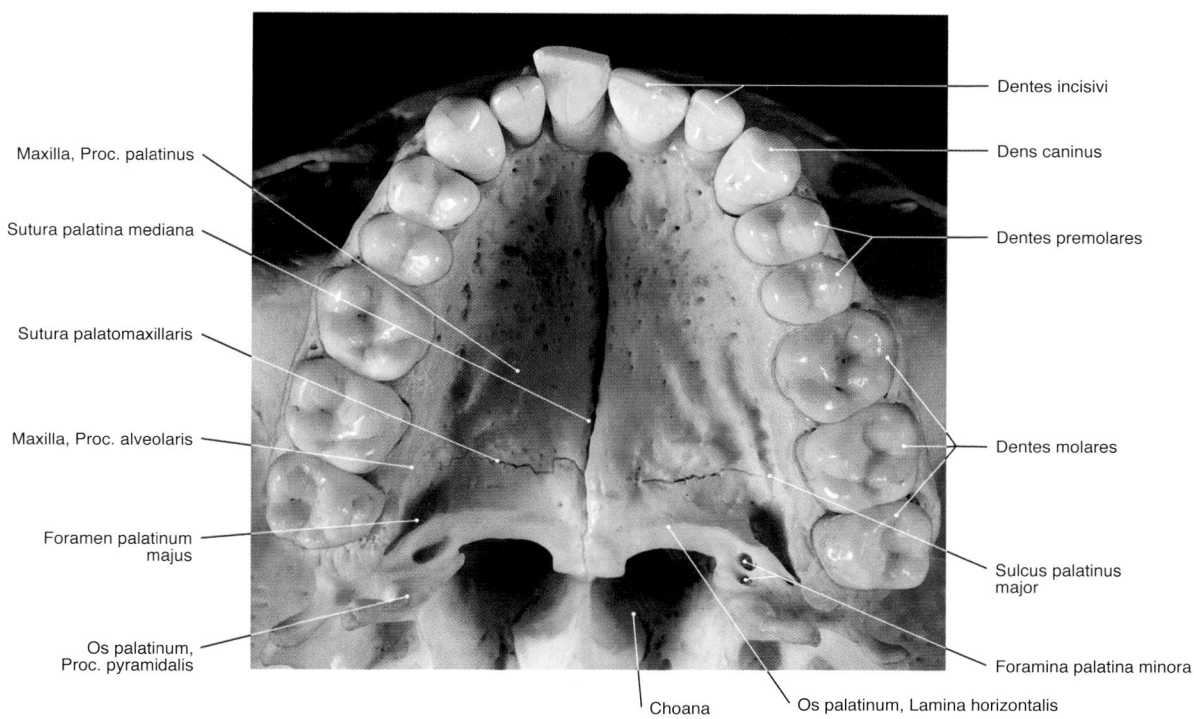

Maxilla, Proc. palatinus

Sutura palatina mediana

Sutura palatomaxillaris

Maxilla, Proc. alveolaris

Foramen palatinum majus

Os palatinum, Proc. pyramidalis

Dentes incisivi

Dens caninus

Dentes premolares

Dentes molares

Sulcus palatinus major

Foramina palatina minora

Choana

Os palatinum, Lamina horizontalis

Fig. 153   Upper dental arcade, Arcus dentalis superior, and bony palate, Palatum osseum.

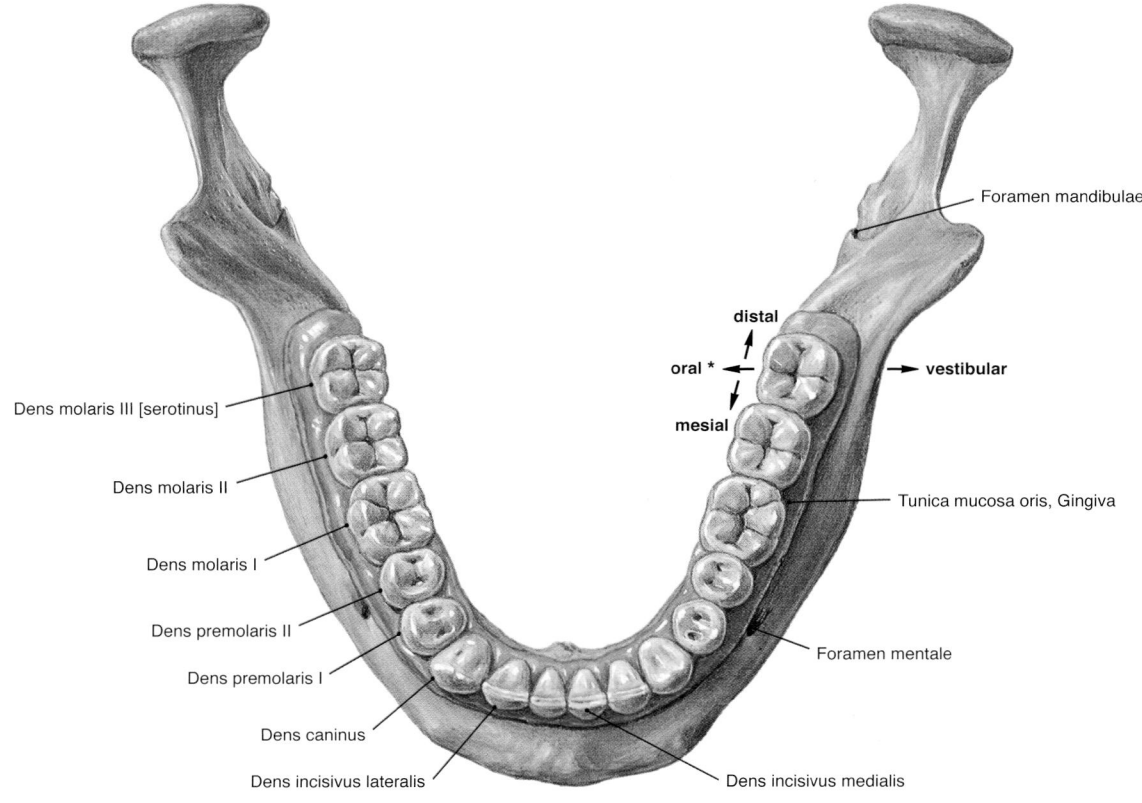

Dens molaris III [serotinus]

Dens molaris II

Dens molaris I

Dens premolaris II

Dens premolaris I

Dens caninus

Dens incisivus lateralis

Foramen mandibulae

distal

oral *

vestibular

mesial

Tunica mucosa oris, Gingiva

Foramen mentale

Dens incisivus medialis

Fig. 154   Lower dental arcade, Arcus dentalis inferior.
* In the mandible oral is synonymous with lingual, and in the maxilla it is synonymous with palatinal.

Teeth, structure

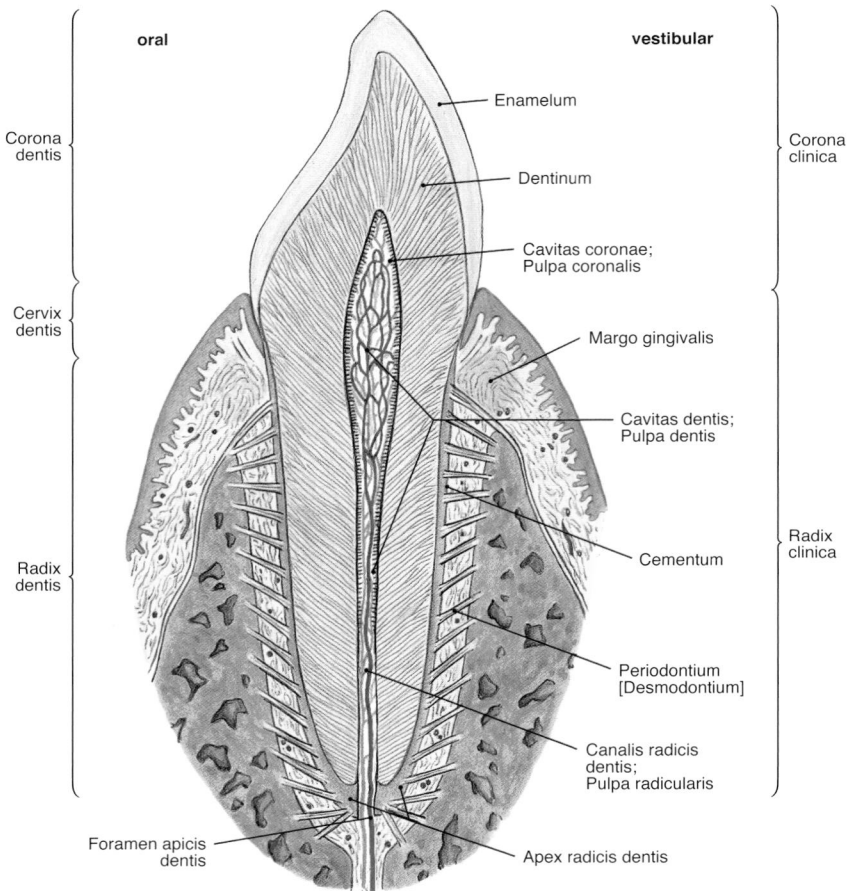

oral

vestibular

Corona dentis

Cervix dentis

Radix dentis

Enamelum

Dentinum

Cavitas coronae; Pulpa coronalis

Margo gingivalis

Cavitas dentis; Pulpa dentis

Cementum

Periodontium [Desmodontium]

Canalis radicis dentis; Pulpa radicularis

Corona clinica

Radix clinica

Foramen apicis dentis

Apex radicis dentis

Fig. 155 Incisor tooth, Dens incisivus.

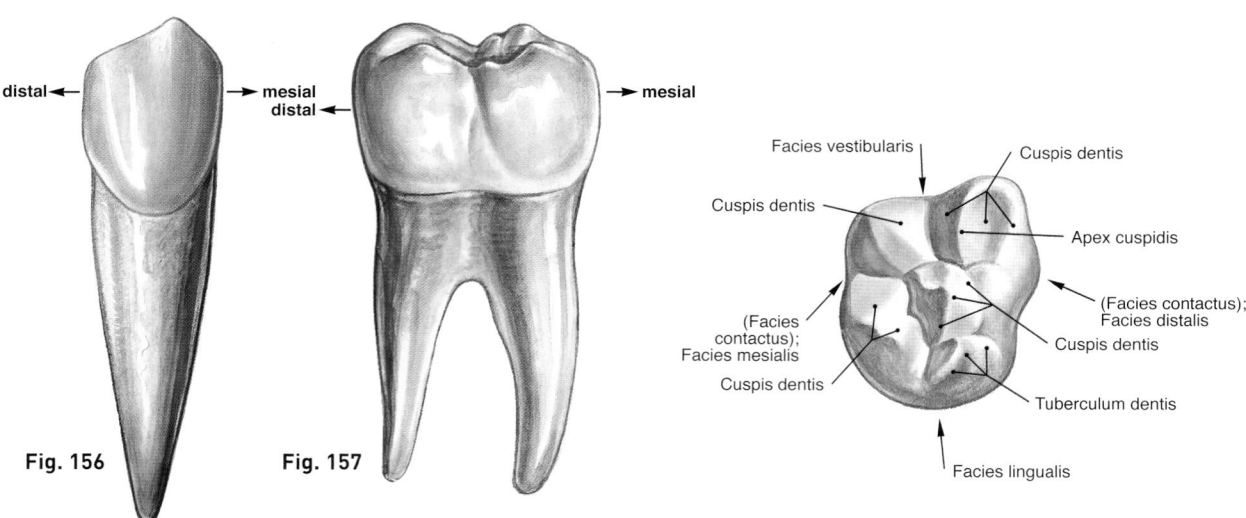

distal ← → mesial distal

mesial distal ← → mesial

Facies vestibularis

Cuspis dentis

Cuspis dentis

Apex cuspidis

(Facies contactus); Facies mesialis

(Facies contactus); Facies distalis

Cuspis dentis

Cuspis dentis

Tuberculum dentis

Facies lingualis

Fig. 156

Fig. 157

Fig. 156 Permanent lower canine tooth, Dens caninus permanens.

Fig. 157 Deciduous second molar tooth, Dens molaris deciduus.

Fig. 158 Permanent upper first molar tooth, Dens molaris primus.

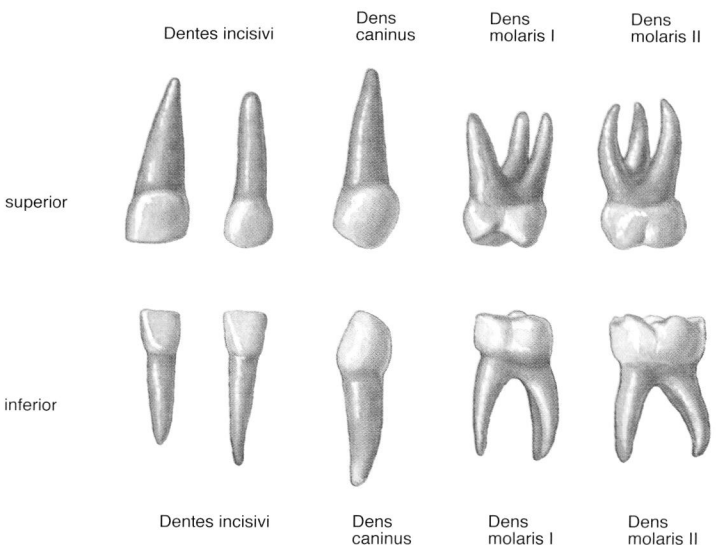

Dentes incisivi

Dens caninus

Dens molaris I

Dens molaris II

superior

inferior

Dentes incisivi

Dens caninus

Dens molaris I

Dens molaris II

Fig. 159 Deciduous teeth, Dentes decidui, of a 3-year-old child; vestibular view.

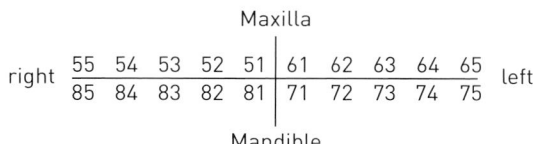

Maxilla

right $\dfrac{55 \quad 54 \quad 53 \quad 52 \quad 51 \mid 61 \quad 62 \quad 63 \quad 64 \quad 65}{85 \quad 84 \quad 83 \quad 82 \quad 81 \mid 71 \quad 72 \quad 73 \quad 74 \quad 75}$ left

Mandible

Dens incisivus lateralis

Dens caninus

Dens molaris I

Dens molaris II

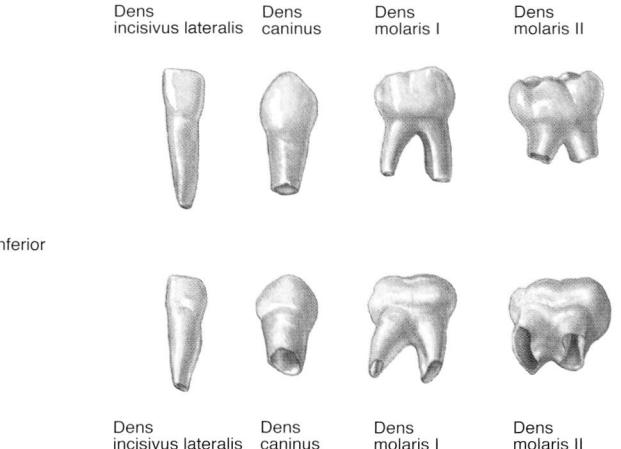

inferior

Dens incisivus lateralis

Dens caninus

Dens molaris I

Dens molaris II

Fig. 160 Deciduous teeth, Dentes decidui, of a 2-year-old child;
top row viewed from vestibular;
bottom row viewed obliquely from inferior.

Teeth

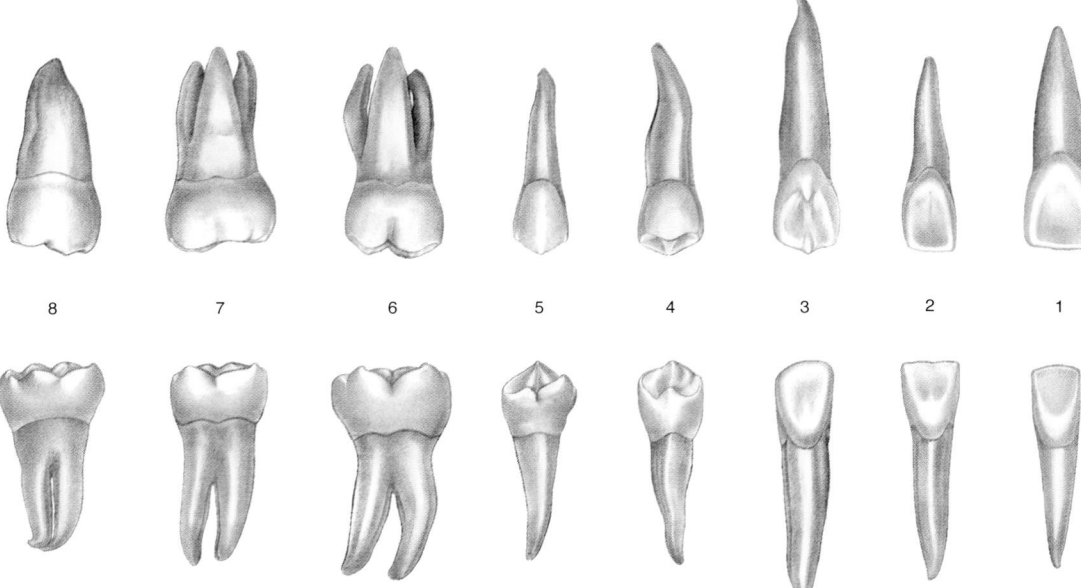

Fig. 161   Permanent teeth, Dentes permanentes;
oral view.
(See p. 97 for identification of the numbers.)

						Maxilla									
right	18	17	16	15	14	13	12	11	21	22	23	24	25	26	27	28	left
	48	47	46	45	44	43	42	41	31	32	33	34	35	36	37	38	
						Mandible									

Adult dentition

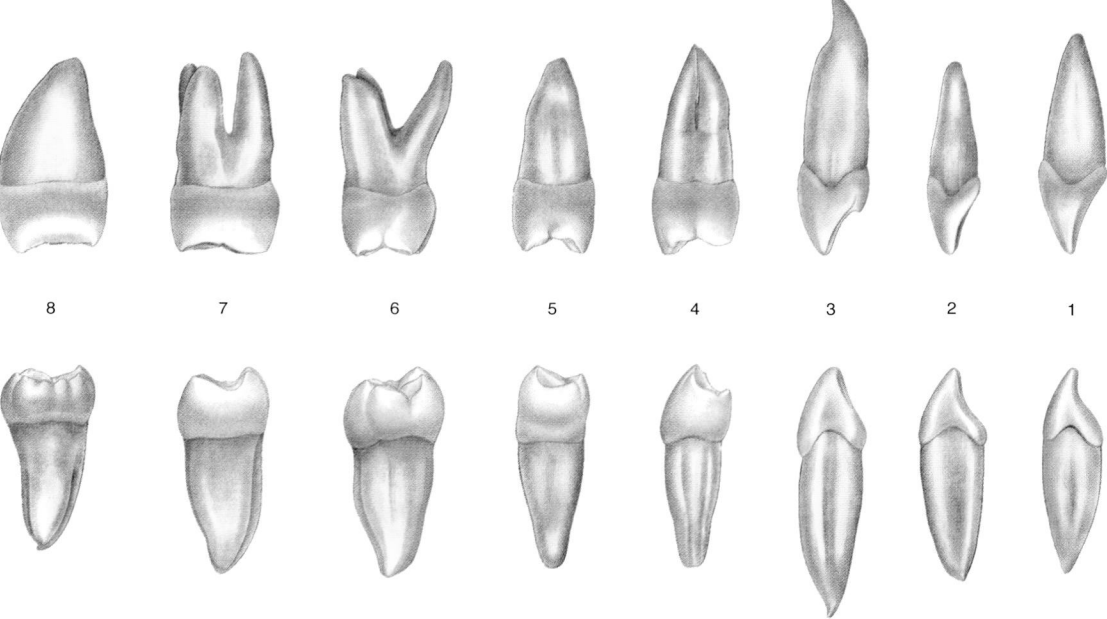

Fig. 162   Permanent teeth, Dentes permanentes;
distal view.
(See p. 97 for identification of the numbers.)

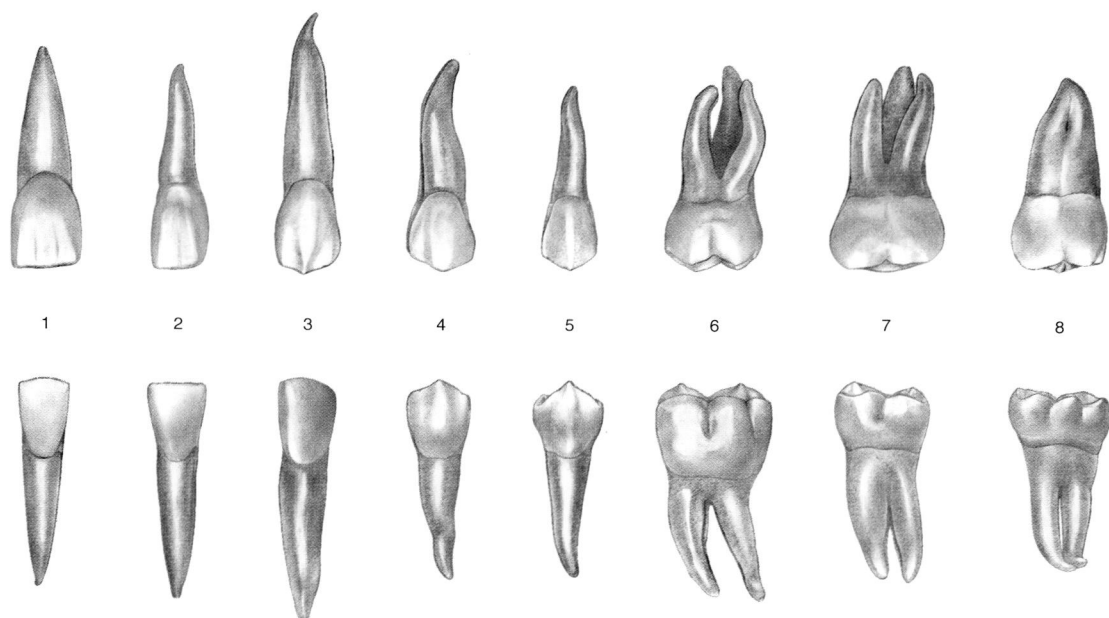

Fig. 163   Permanent teeth, Dentes permanentes; vestibular view.

1 Dens incisivus I   5 Dens premolaris II
2 Dens incisivus II   6 Dens molaris I
3 Dens caninus   7 Dens molaris II
4 Dens premolaris I   8 Dens molaris III
                               [serotinus]

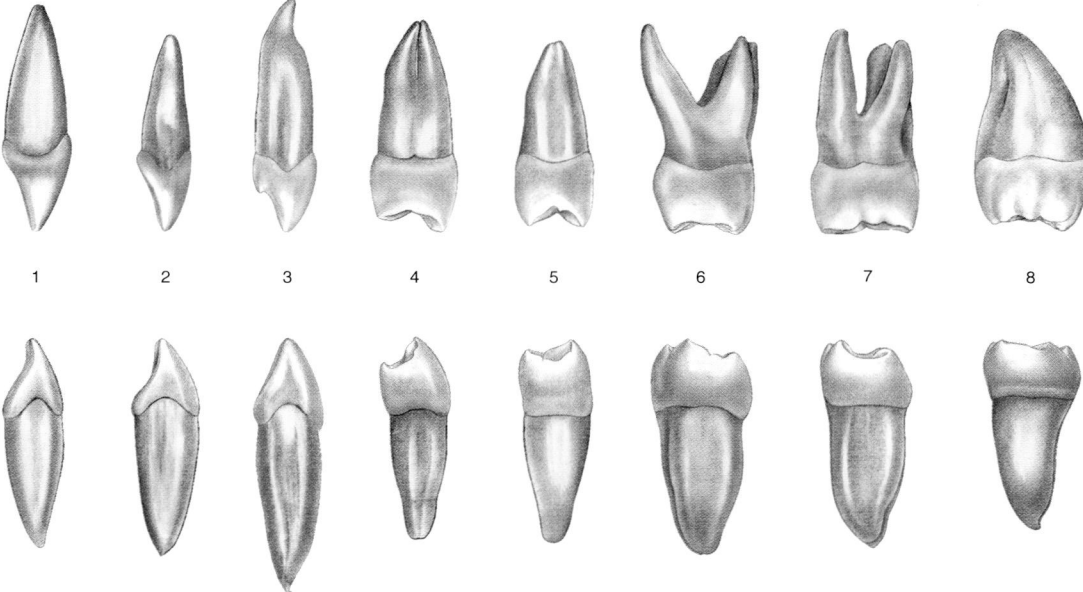

Fig. 164   Permanent teeth, Dentes permanentes; mesial view.

Teeth, development

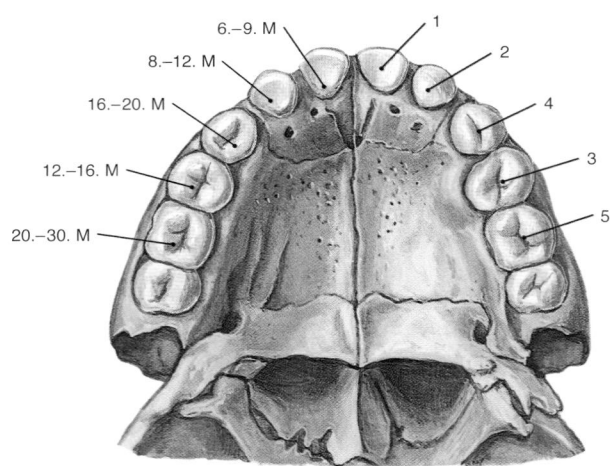

6.–9. M
8.–12. M
16.–20. M
12.–16. M
20.–30. M

1
2
4
3
5

Fig. 165 Maxilla, Maxilla, with deciduous teeth, Dentes decidui, and the first permanent tooth; left: median time of eruption in months (M); right: order of eruption.

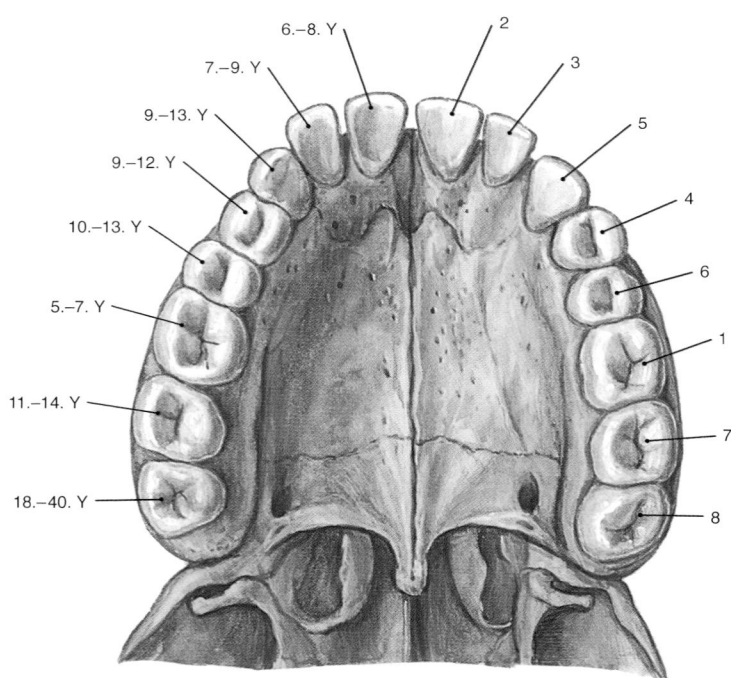

6.–8. Y
7.–9. Y
9.–13. Y
9.–12. Y
10.–13. Y
5.–7. Y
11.–14. Y
18.–40. Y

2
3
5
4
6
1
7
8

Fig. 166 Maxilla, Maxilla, with permanent teeth, Dentes permanentes; left: median time of eruption in years (Y); right: order of eruption.

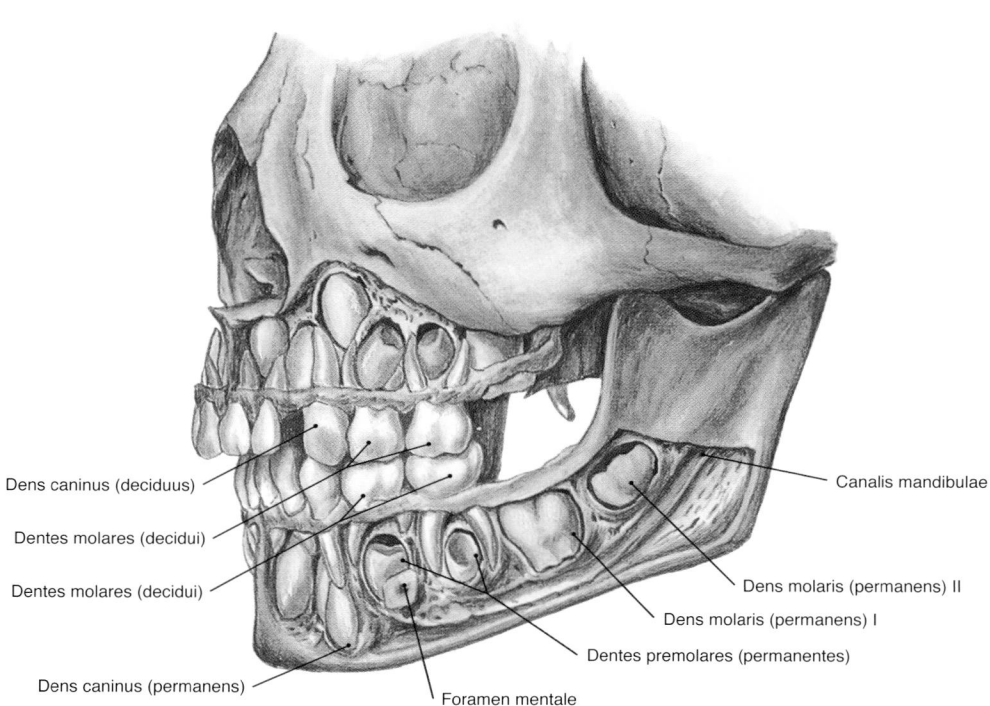

Dens caninus (deciduus)

Dentes molares (decidui)

Dentes molares (decidui)

Dens caninus (permanens)

Foramen mentale

Dentes premolares (permanentes)

Dens molaris (permanens) I

Dens molaris (permanens) II

Canalis mandibulae

Fig. 167   Maxilla, Maxilla, and mandible, Mandibula,
of a 5-year-old child;
deciduous teeth and anlage of permanent teeth.

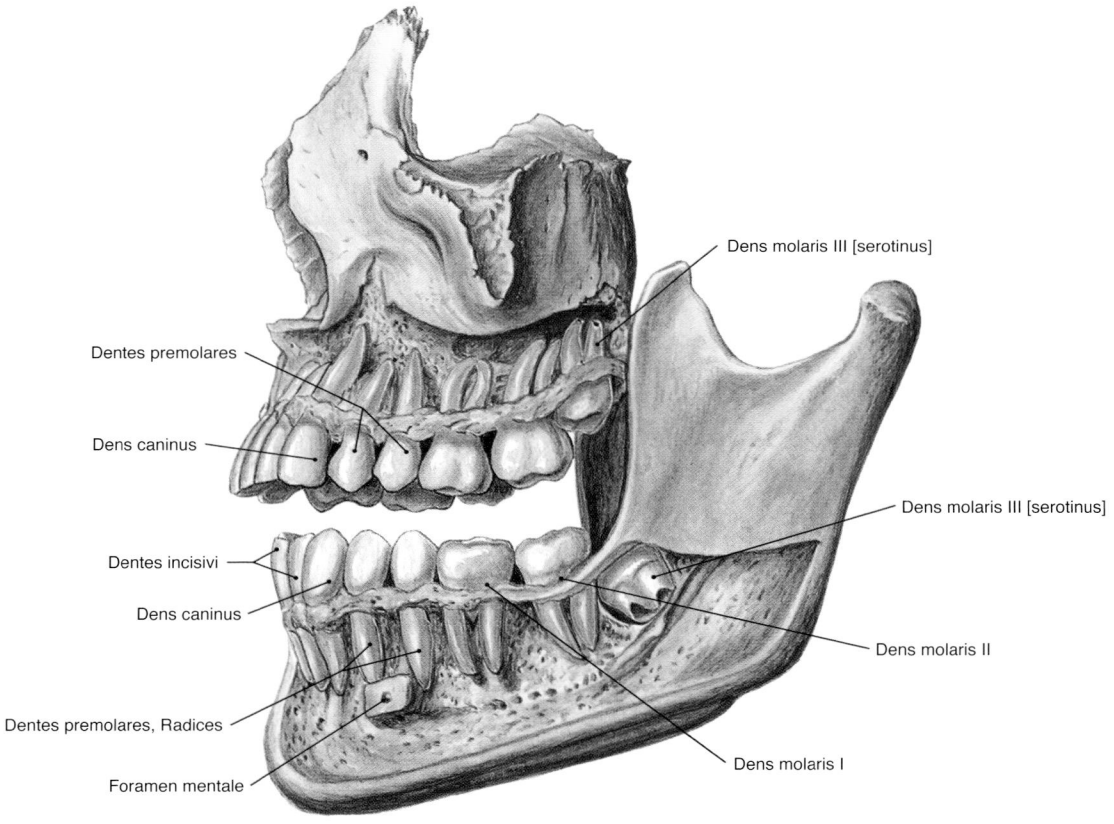

Dentes premolares

Dens caninus

Dentes incisivi

Dens caninus

Dentes premolares, Radices

Foramen mentale

Dens molaris III [serotinus]

Dens molaris III [serotinus]

Dens molaris II

Dens molaris I

Fig. 168   Maxilla, Maxilla, and mandible, Mandibula,
of a 20-year-old male.

Teeth, radiography

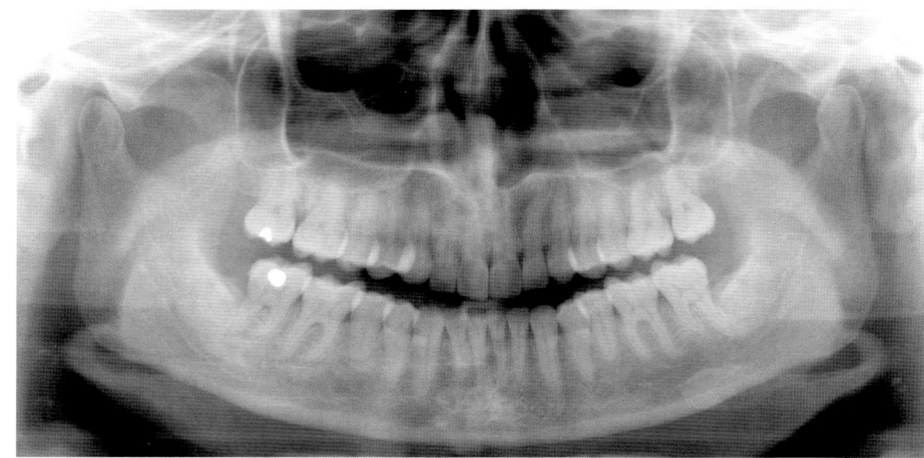

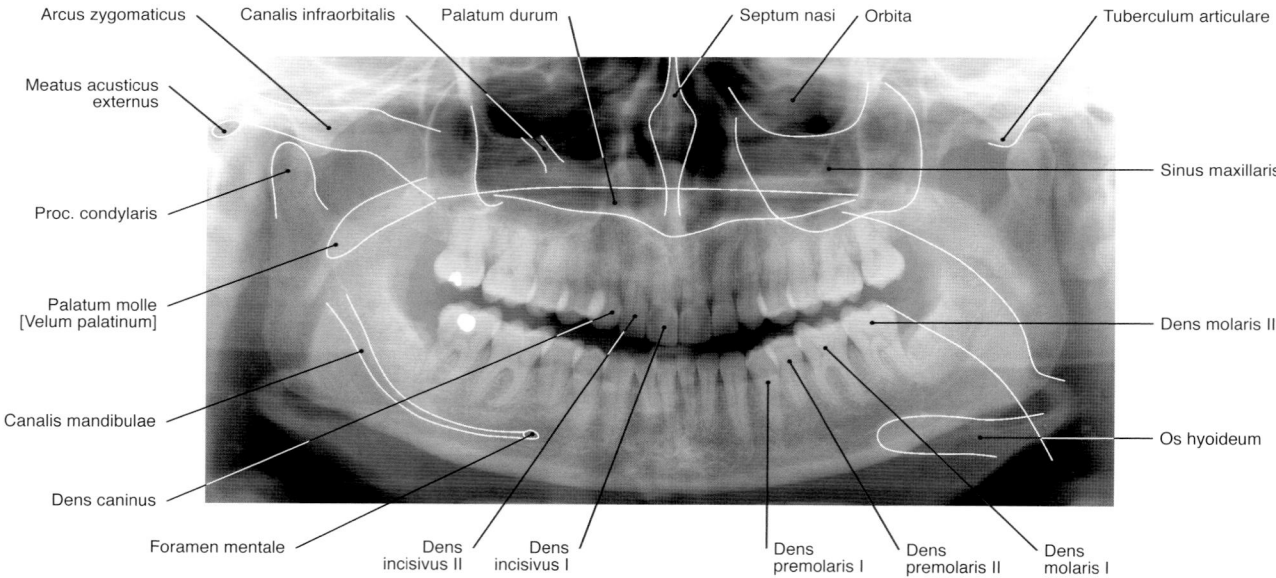

Arcus zygomaticus   Canalis infraorbitalis   Palatum durum   Septum nasi   Orbita   Tuberculum articulare

Meatus acusticus externus

Proc. condylaris

Palatum molle [Velum palatinum]

Canalis mandibulae

Dens caninus

Sinus maxillaris

Dens molaris II

Os hyoideum

Foramen mentale   Dens incisivus II   Dens incisivus I   Dens premolaris I   Dens premolaris II   Dens molaris I

Fig. 169   Maxilla, Maxilla, and mandible, Mandibula; panoramic radiograph; without wisdom teeth.

Innervation of the teeth

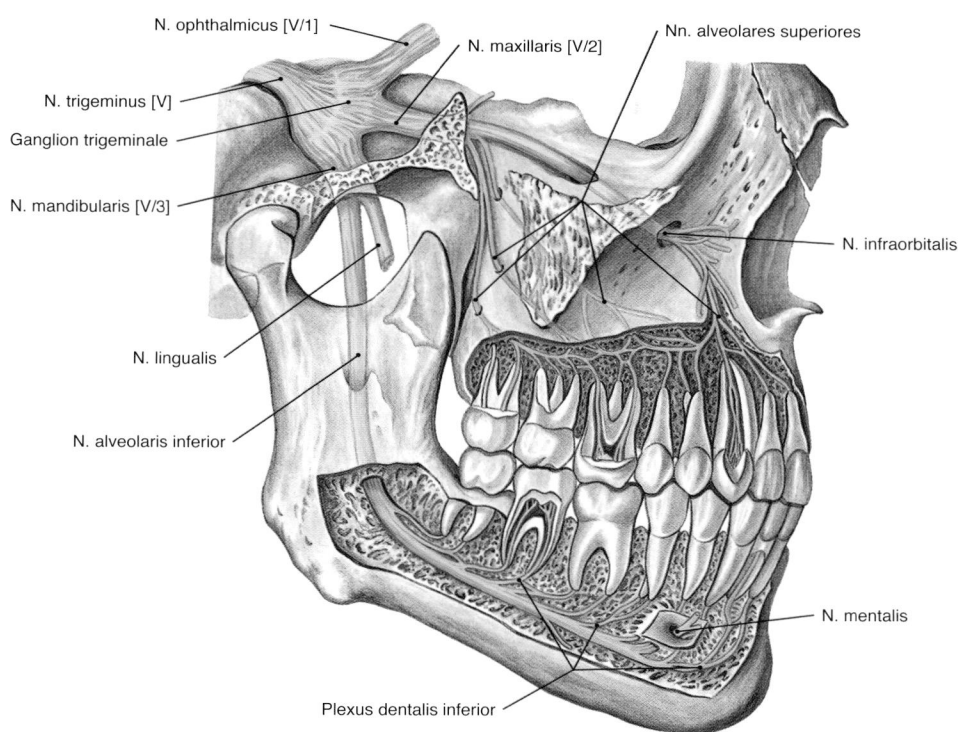

N. ophthalmicus [V/1]

N. maxillaris [V/2]

Nn. alveolares superiores

N. trigeminus [V]

Ganglion trigeminale

N. mandibularis [V/3]

N. infraorbitalis

N. lingualis

N. alveolaris inferior

N. mentalis

Plexus dentalis inferior

Fig. 170   Maxillary and mandibular nerve,
Nn. maxillaris [V/2] et mandibularis [V/3].

→ 1178, 1179

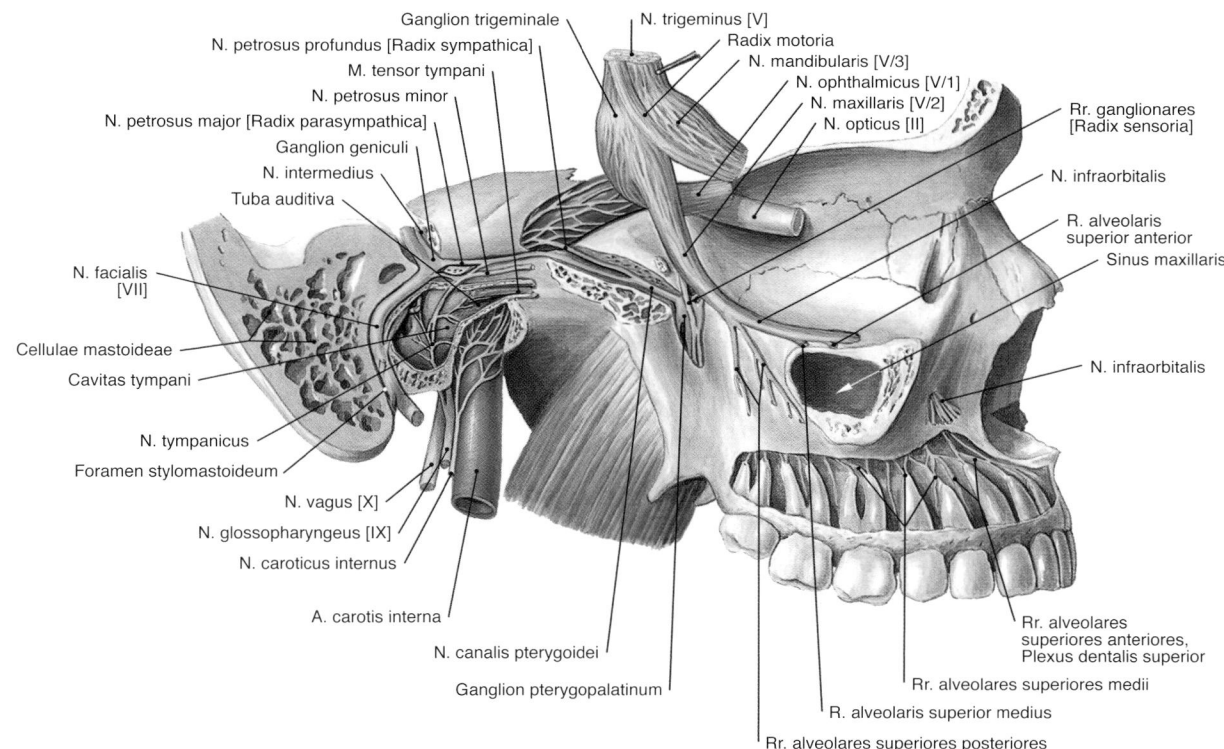

Ganglion trigeminale

N. trigeminus [V]

N. petrosus profundus [Radix sympathica]

Radix motoria

M. tensor tympani

N. mandibularis [V/3]

N. petrosus minor

N. ophthalmicus [V/1]

N. petrosus major [Radix parasympathica]

N. maxillaris [V/2]

Ganglion geniculi

N. opticus [II]

Rr. ganglionares
[Radix sensoria]

N. intermedius

Tuba auditiva

N. infraorbitalis

N. facialis
[VII]

R. alveolaris
superior anterior

Sinus maxillaris

Cellulae mastoideae

Cavitas tympani

N. infraorbitalis

N. tympanicus

Foramen stylomastoideum

N. vagus [X]

N. glossopharyngeus [IX]

N. caroticus internus

A. carotis interna

Rr. alveolares
superiores anteriores,
Plexus dentalis superior

N. canalis pterygoidei

Rr. alveolares superiores medii

Ganglion pterygopalatinum

R. alveolaris superior medius

Rr. alveolares superiores posteriores

Fig. 171   Pterygopalatine ganglion, Ganglion pterygopalatinum.

Palate

Fig. 172 Hard and soft palate,
Palatum durum et molle;
inferior view.

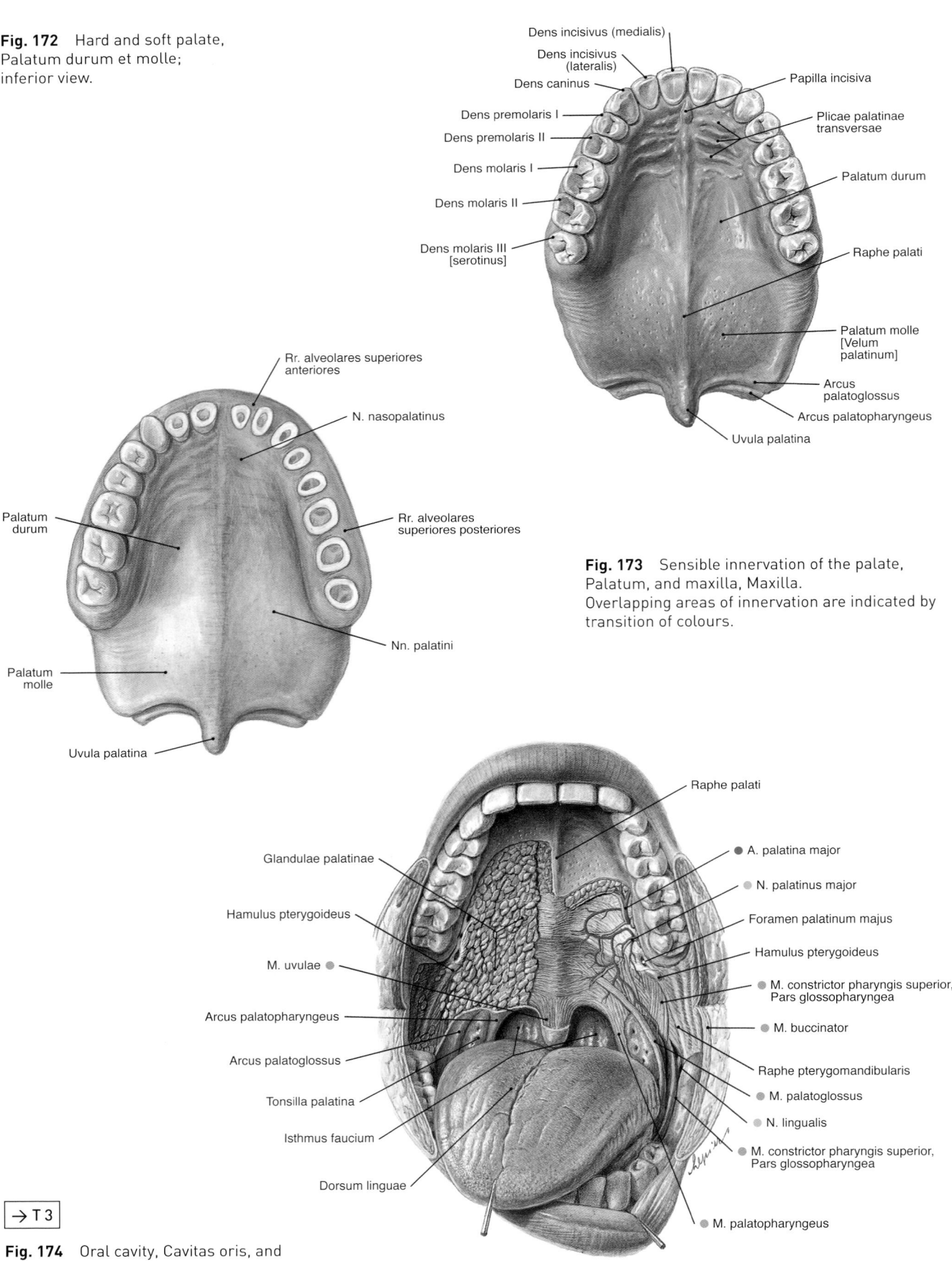

Dens incisivus (medialis)
Dens incisivus (lateralis)
Dens caninus
Dens premolaris I
Dens premolaris II
Dens molaris I
Dens molaris II
Dens molaris III [serotinus]

Papilla incisiva
Plicae palatinae transversae
Palatum durum
Raphe palati
Palatum molle [Velum palatinum]
Arcus palatoglossus
Arcus palatopharyngeus
Uvula palatina

Rr. alveolares superiores anteriores
N. nasopalatinus
Rr. alveolares superiores posteriores
Palatum durum
Nn. palatini
Palatum molle
Uvula palatina

Fig. 173 Sensible innervation of the palate,
Palatum, and maxilla, Maxilla.
Overlapping areas of innervation are indicated by
transition of colours.

Raphe palati
Glandulae palatinae
Hamulus pterygoideus
M. uvulae
Arcus palatopharyngeus
Arcus palatoglossus
Tonsilla palatina
Isthmus faucium
Dorsum linguae

● A. palatina major
● N. palatinus major
Foramen palatinum majus
Hamulus pterygoideus
● M. constrictor pharyngis superior, Pars glossopharyngea
● M. buccinator
Raphe pterygomandibularis
● M. palatoglossus
● N. lingualis
● M. constrictor pharyngis superior, Pars glossopharyngea
● M. palatopharyngeus

→ T 3

Fig. 174 Oral cavity, Cavitas oris, and
muscles of the palate, Mm. palati.

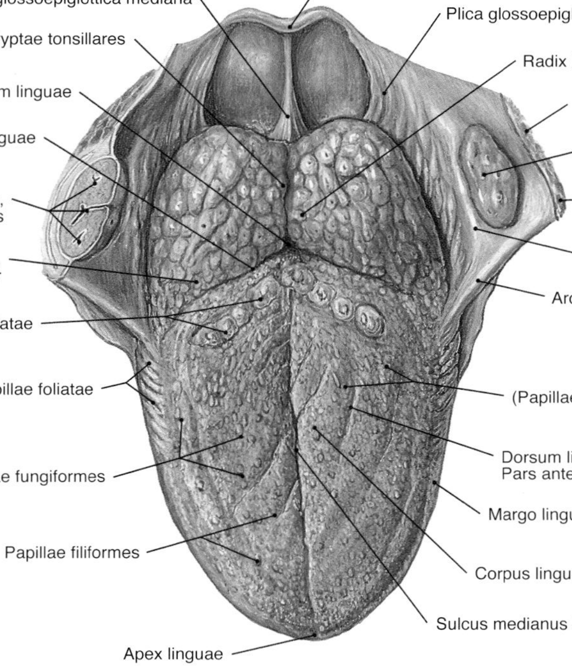

Epiglottis

Plica glossoepiglottica mediana

Plica glossoepiglottica lateralis

Tonsilla lingualis; Cryptae tonsillares

Radix linguae

Foramen caecum linguae

M. palatopharyngeus

Sulcus terminalis linguae

Tonsilla palatina

Fossulae tonsillares, Cryptae tonsillares

M. palatoglossus

Dorsum linguae, Pars posterior

(Plica triangularis)

Papillae vallatae

Arcus palatoglossus

Papillae foliatae

(Papillae conicae)

Papillae fungiformes

Dorsum linguae, Pars anterior

Papillae filiformes

Margo linguae

Corpus linguae

Sulcus medianus linguae

Apex linguae

Fig. 175   Tongue, Lingua.

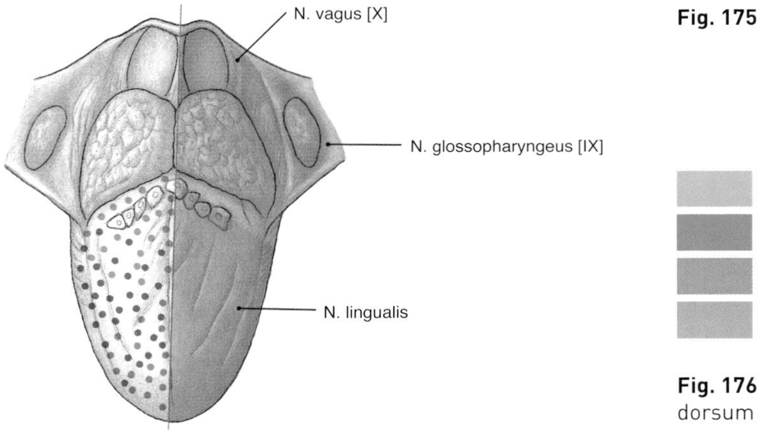

N. vagus [X]

N. glossopharyngeus [IX]

N. lingualis

Bitter

Sour

Salty

Sweet

Fig. 176   Innervation and taste categories at the dorsum of the tongue.

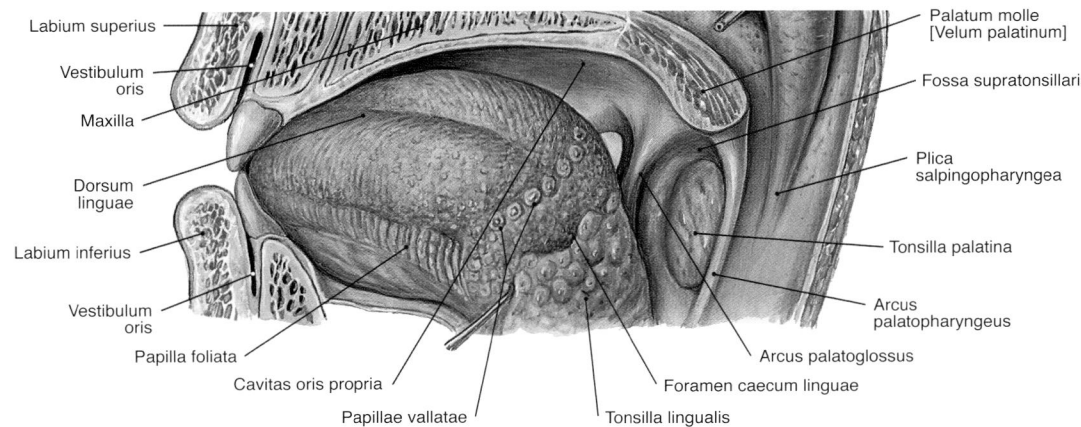

Labium superius

Palatum molle [Velum palatinum]

Vestibulum oris

Fossa supratonsillaris

Maxilla

Plica salpingopharyngea

Dorsum linguae

Labium inferius

Tonsilla palatina

Vestibulum oris

Arcus palatopharyngeus

Papilla foliata

Arcus palatoglossus

Cavitas oris propria

Foramen caecum linguae

Papillae vallatae

Tonsilla lingualis

Fig. 177   Oral cavity, Cavitas oris.

Muscles of the tongue

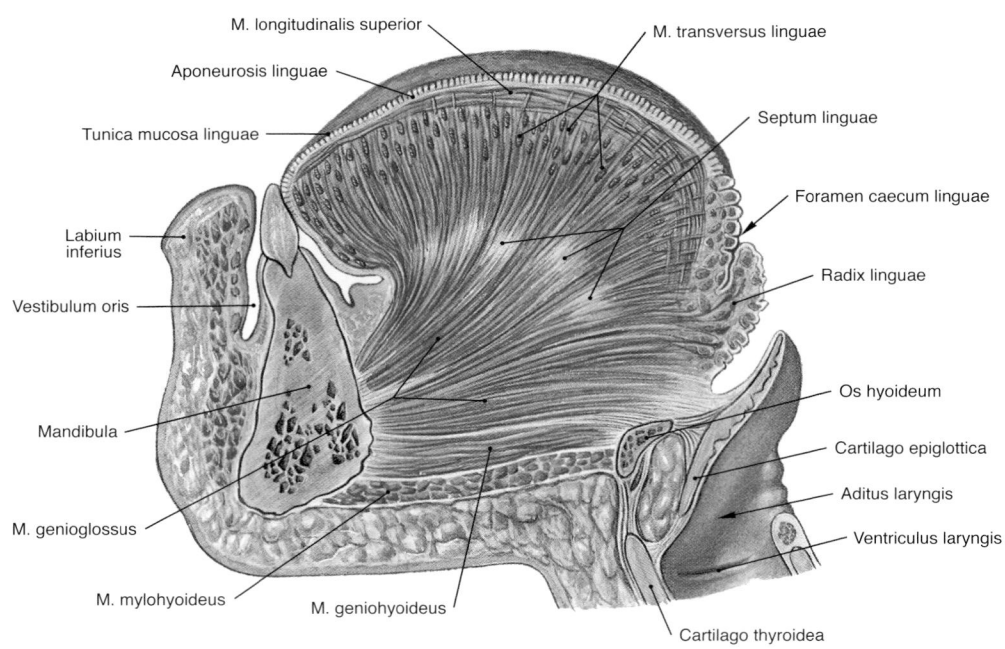

M. longitudinalis superior

Aponeurosis linguae

Tunica mucosa linguae

Labium inferius

Vestibulum oris

Mandibula

M. genioglossus

M. mylohyoideus

M. geniohyoideus

M. transversus linguae

Septum linguae

Foramen caecum linguae

Radix linguae

Os hyoideum

Cartilago epiglottica

Aditus laryngis

Ventriculus laryngis

Cartilago thyroidea

→ T 2a

Fig. 178 Tongue, Lingua, and muscles of the tongue, Mm. linguae; median section.

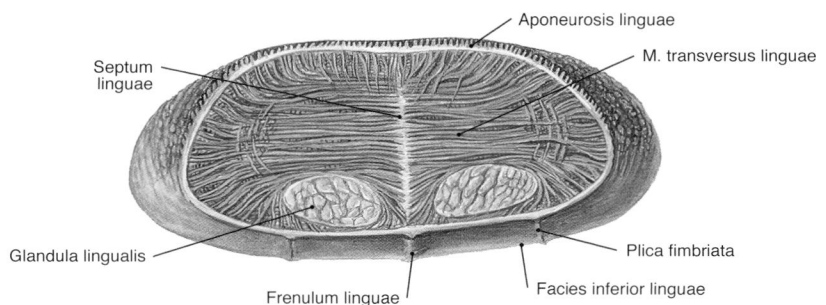

Septum linguae

Aponeurosis linguae

M. transversus linguae

Glandula lingualis

Frenulum linguae

Plica fimbriata

Facies inferior linguae

→ T 2a

Fig. 179 Tongue, Lingua, and muscles of the tongue, Mm. linguae; cross-section through the tip of the tongue.

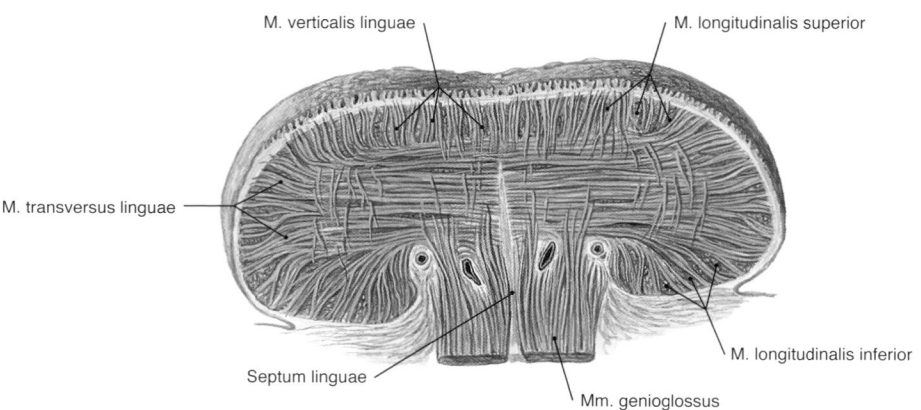

M. verticalis linguae

M. longitudinalis superior

M. transversus linguae

Septum linguae

Mm. genioglossus

M. longitudinalis inferior

→ T 2a

Fig. 180 Tongue, Lingua, and muscles of the tongue, Mm. linguae; cross-section at the level of the middle of the tongue.

Hyoid bone and infra- and suprahyoid muscles

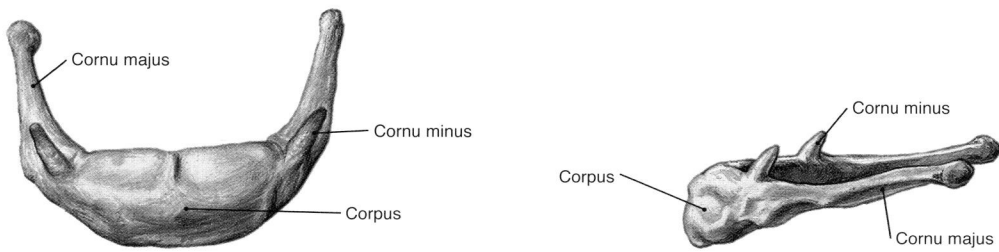

Fig. 181   Hyoid bone, Os hyoideum.

Fig. 182   Hyoid bone, Os hyoideum.

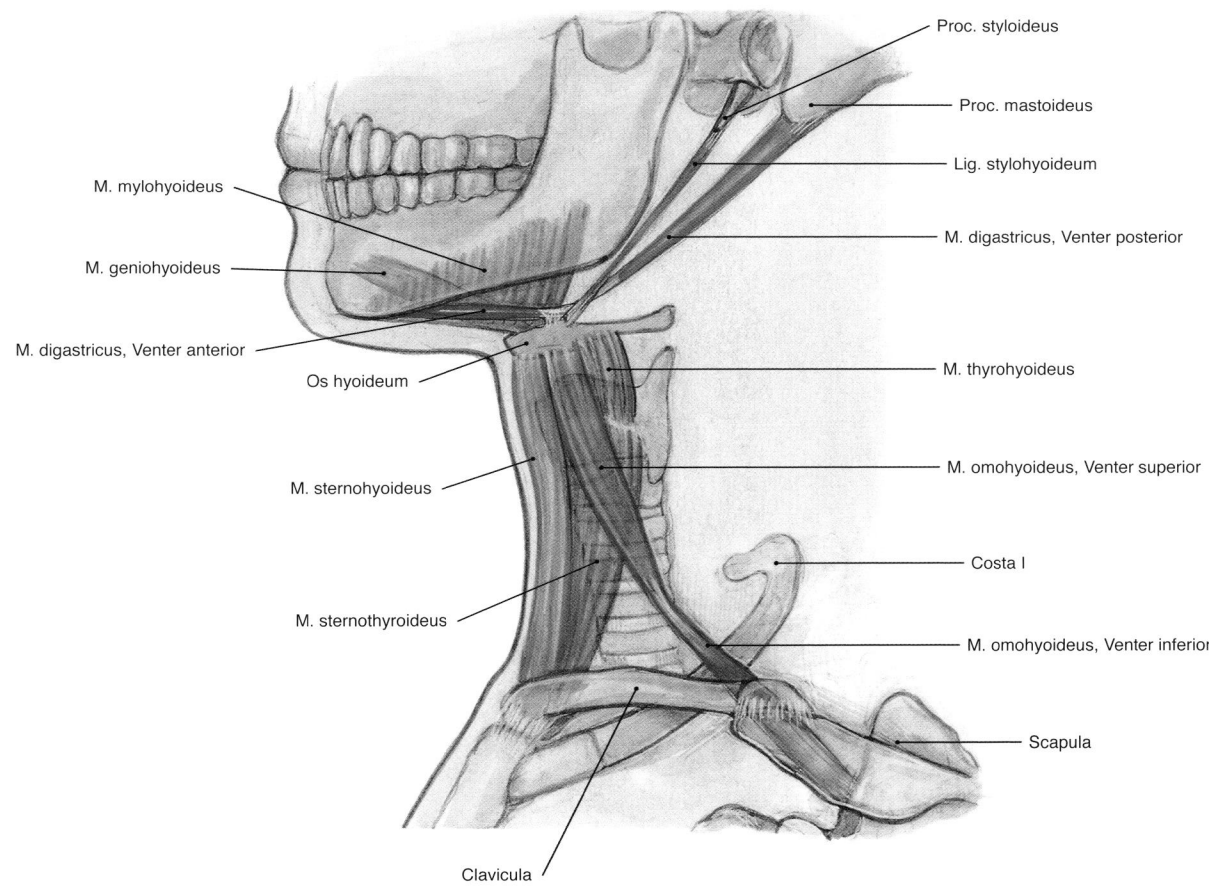

Fig. 183   Muscular suspension of the hyoid bone.

→ T9, T10

Suprahyoid muscles

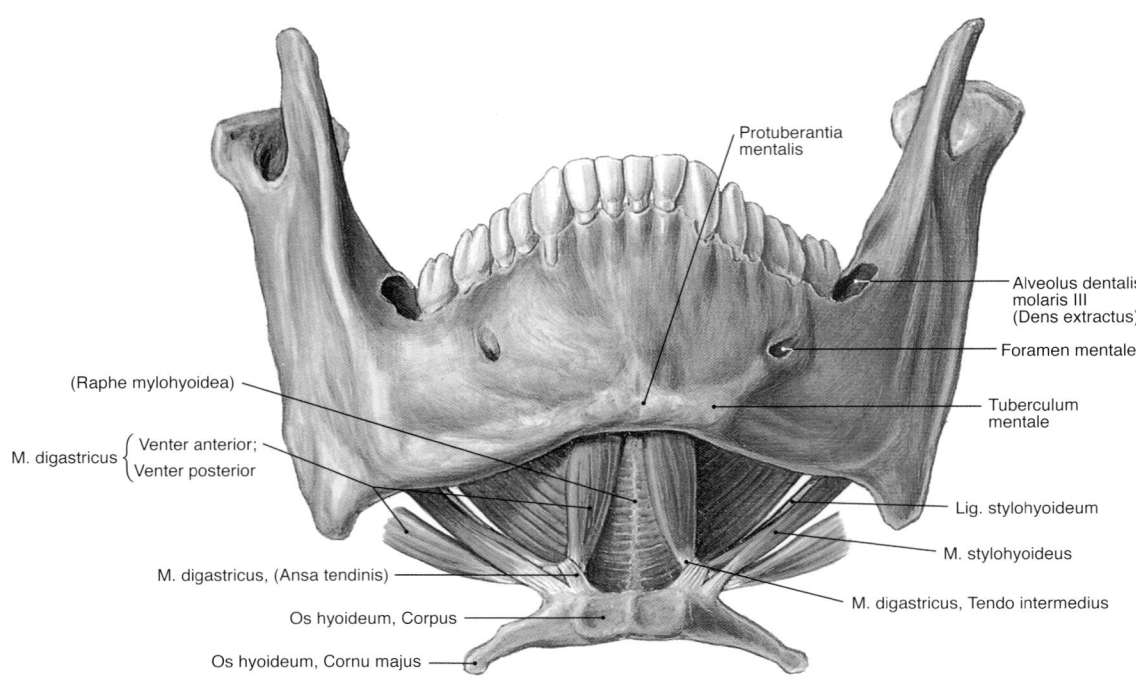

→ T 9

Fig. 184 Mandible, Mandibula, and suprahyoid muscles, Mm. suprahyoidei.

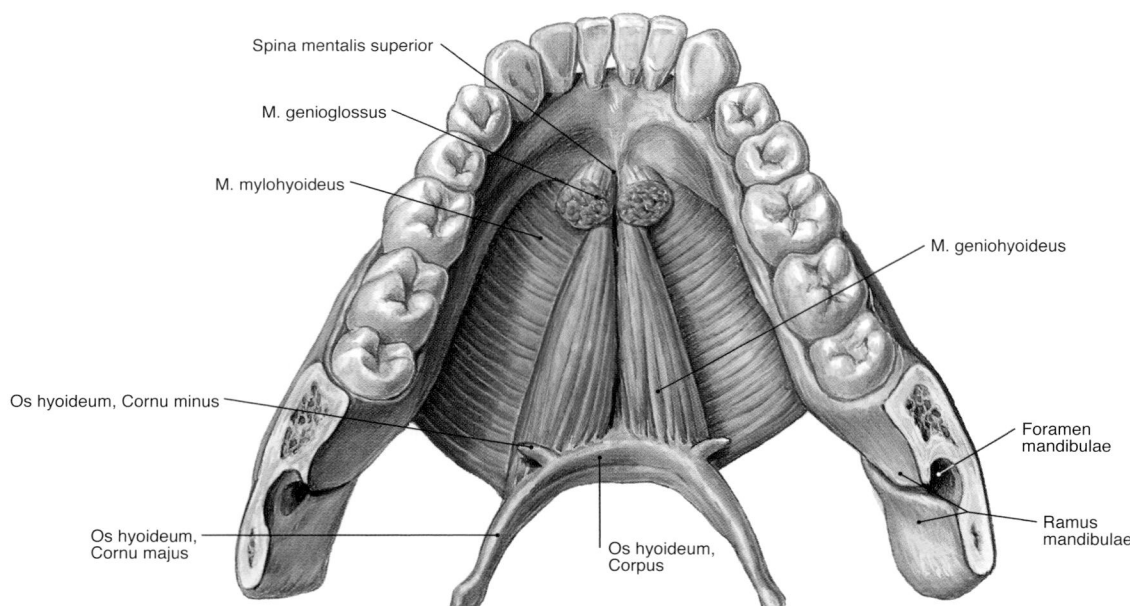

→ T 9

Fig. 185 Mandible, Mandibula; suprahyoid muscles, Mm. suprahyoidei, and hyoid bone, Os hyoideum.

Muscles of the tongue

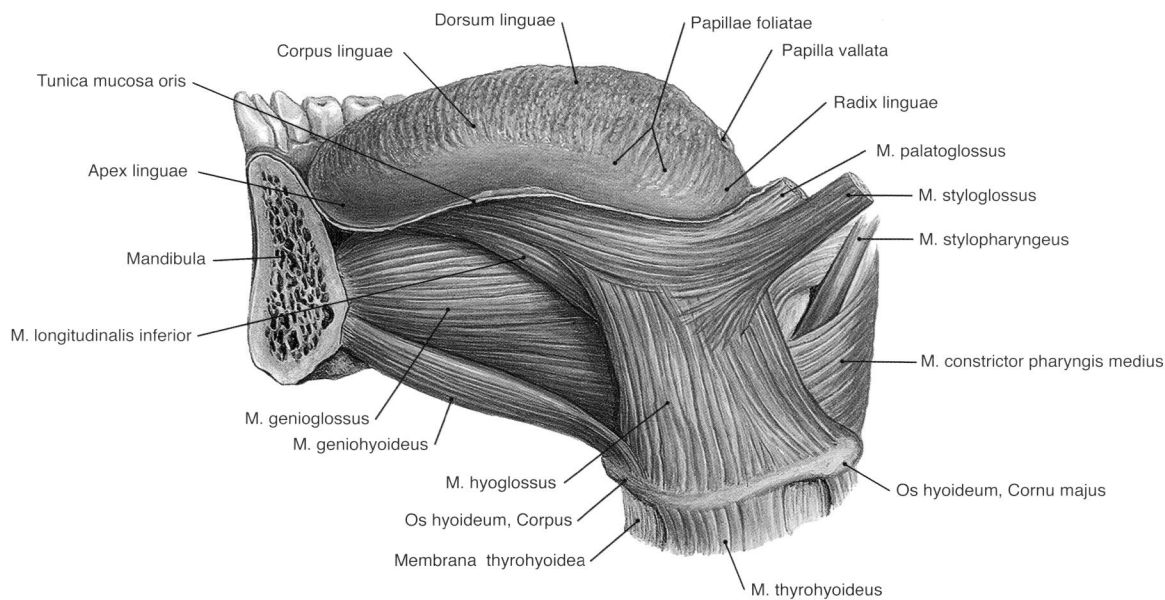

Fig. 186   Tongue, Lingua, and muscles of the
tongue, Mm. linguae.

→ T 2 b

Labels (Fig. 186):
Dorsum linguae
Corpus linguae
Papillae foliatae
Papilla vallata
Tunica mucosa oris
Radix linguae
M. palatoglossus
Apex linguae
M. styloglossus
M. stylopharyngeus
Mandibula
M. longitudinalis inferior
M. constrictor pharyngis medius
M. genioglossus
M. geniohyoideus
M. hyoglossus
Os hyoideum, Cornu majus
Os hyoideum, Corpus
Membrana thyrohyoidea
M. thyrohyoideus

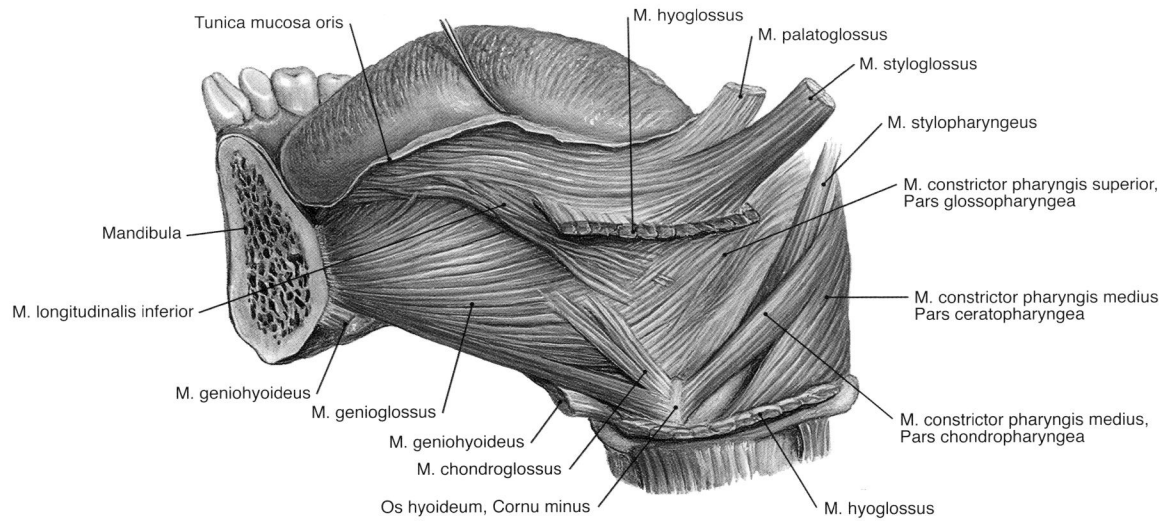

Fig. 187   Tongue, Lingua, and muscles of the
tongue, Mm. linguae.

→ T 2 b

Labels (Fig. 187):
Tunica mucosa oris
M. hyoglossus
M. palatoglossus
M. styloglossus
M. stylopharyngeus
M. constrictor pharyngis superior, Pars glossopharyngea
Mandibula
M. longitudinalis inferior
M. constrictor pharyngis medius, Pars ceratopharyngea
M. geniohyoideus
M. genioglossus
M. geniohyoideus
M. constrictor pharyngis medius, Pars chondropharyngea
M. chondroglossus
Os hyoideum, Cornu minus
M. hyoglossus

Muscles of the tongue and the pharynx

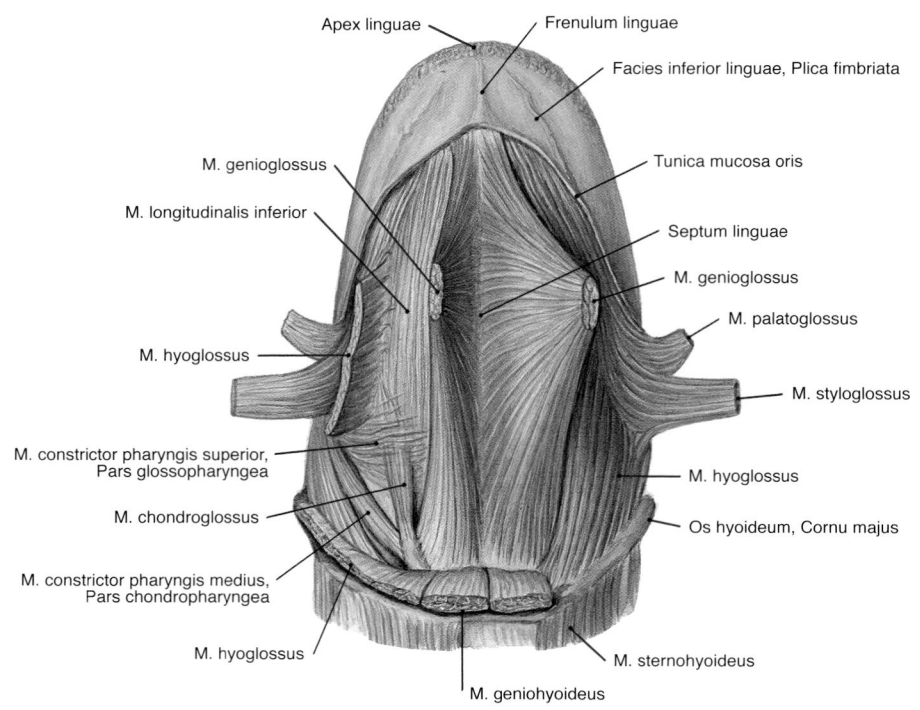

Apex linguae — Frenulum linguae

Facies inferior linguae, Plica fimbriata

M. genioglossus

Tunica mucosa oris

M. longitudinalis inferior

Septum linguae

M. genioglossus

M. palatoglossus

M. hyoglossus

M. styloglossus

M. hyoglossus

M. constrictor pharyngis superior,
Pars glossopharyngea

Os hyoideum, Cornu majus

M. chondroglossus

M. constrictor pharyngis medius,
Pars chondropharyngea

M. sternohyoideus

M. hyoglossus

M. geniohyoideus

→ T 2 b

Fig. 188 Muscles of the tongue, Mm. linguae.

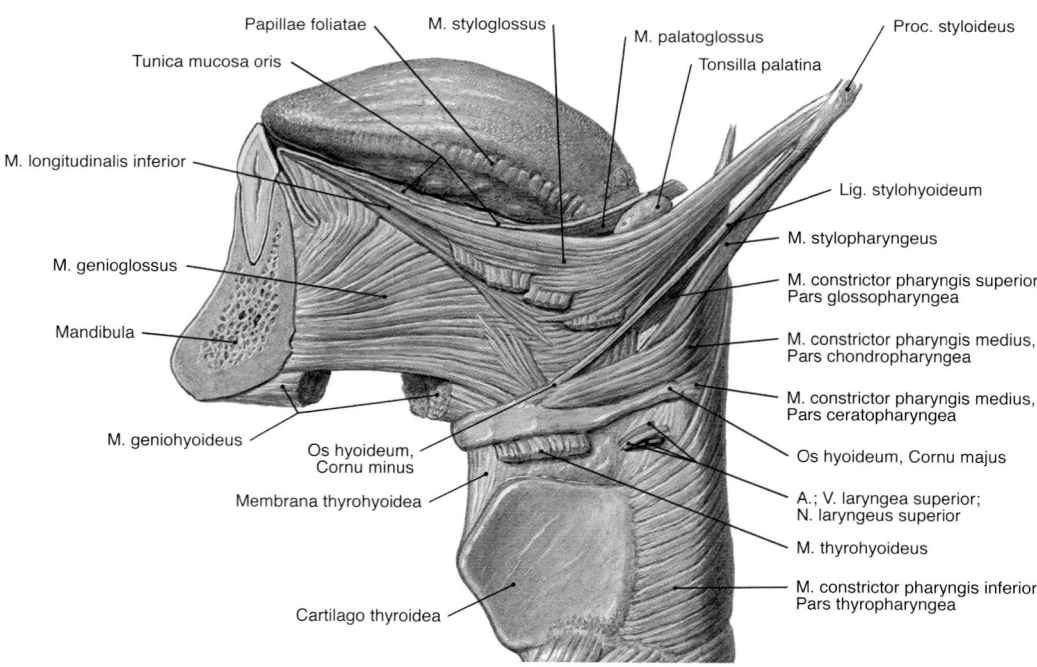

Papillae foliatae — M. styloglossus — M. palatoglossus — Proc. styloideus

Tunica mucosa oris — Tonsilla palatina

M. longitudinalis inferior

Lig. stylohyoideum

M. stylopharyngeus

M. genioglossus

M. constrictor pharyngis superior,
Pars glossopharyngea

Mandibula

M. constrictor pharyngis medius,
Pars chondropharyngea

M. constrictor pharyngis medius,
Pars ceratopharyngea

M. geniohyoideus — Os hyoideum,
Cornu minus

Os hyoideum, Cornu majus

Membrana thyrohyoidea

A.; V. laryngea superior;
N. laryngeus superior

M. thyrohyoideus

M. constrictor pharyngis inferior,
Pars thyropharyngea

Cartilago thyroidea

→ T 2 b, T 5

Fig. 189 Muscles of the tongue, Mm. linguae, and
muscles of the pharynx, Tunica muscularis pharyngis.

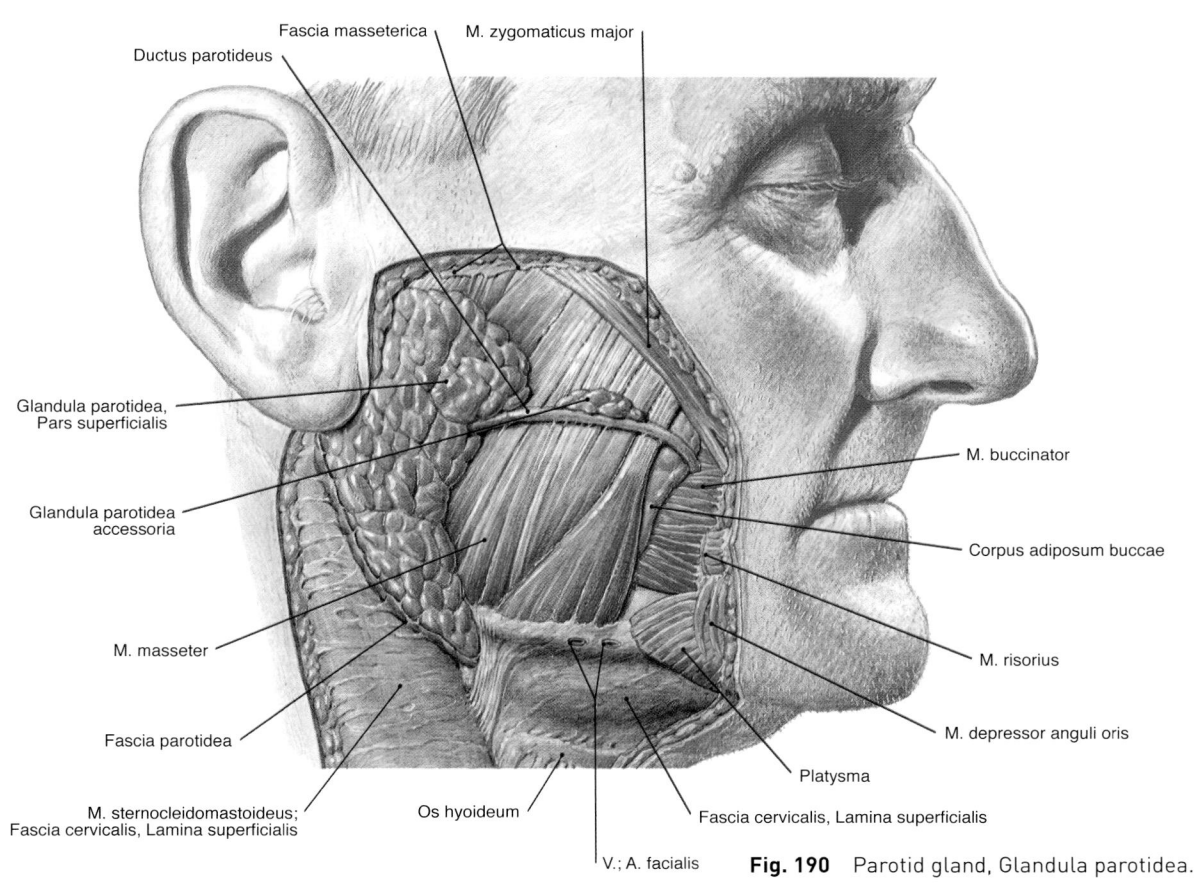

Fascia masseterica
M. zygomaticus major
Ductus parotideus
Glandula parotidea, Pars superficialis
Glandula parotidea accessoria
M. buccinator
Corpus adiposum buccae
M. masseter
M. risorius
Fascia parotidea
M. depressor anguli oris
Platysma
M. sternocleidomastoideus; Fascia cervicalis, Lamina superficialis
Os hyoideum
Fascia cervicalis, Lamina superficialis
V.; A. facialis

Fig. 190 Parotid gland, Glandula parotidea.

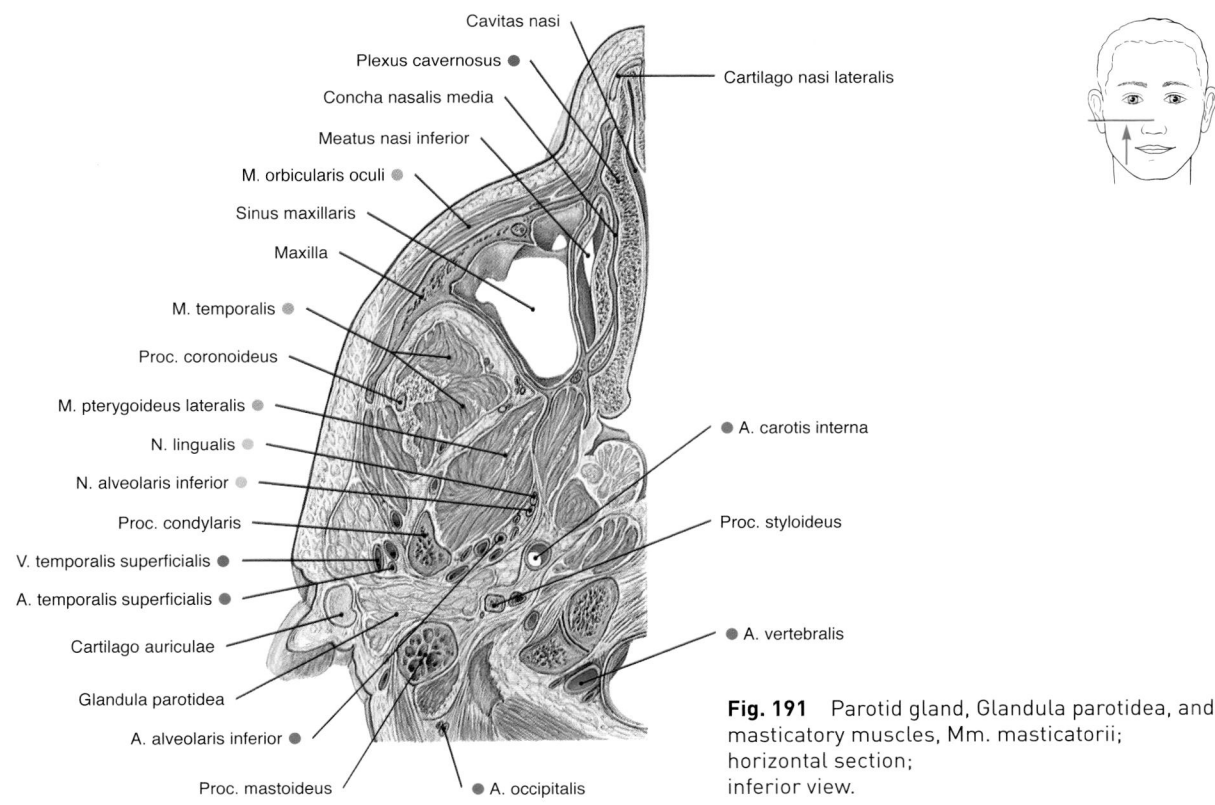

Cavitas nasi
Plexus cavernosus ●
Concha nasalis media
Cartilago nasi lateralis
Meatus nasi inferior
M. orbicularis oculi ●
Sinus maxillaris
Maxilla
M. temporalis ●
Proc. coronoideus
M. pterygoideus lateralis ●
A. carotis interna
N. lingualis ●
N. alveolaris inferior ●
Proc. condylaris
Proc. styloideus
V. temporalis superficialis ●
A. temporalis superficialis ●
Cartilago auriculae
Glandula parotidea
A. vertebralis
A. alveolaris inferior ●
Proc. mastoideus
A. occipitalis ●

Fig. 191 Parotid gland, Glandula parotidea, and masticatory muscles, Mm. masticatorii; horizontal section; inferior view.

Submandibular gland

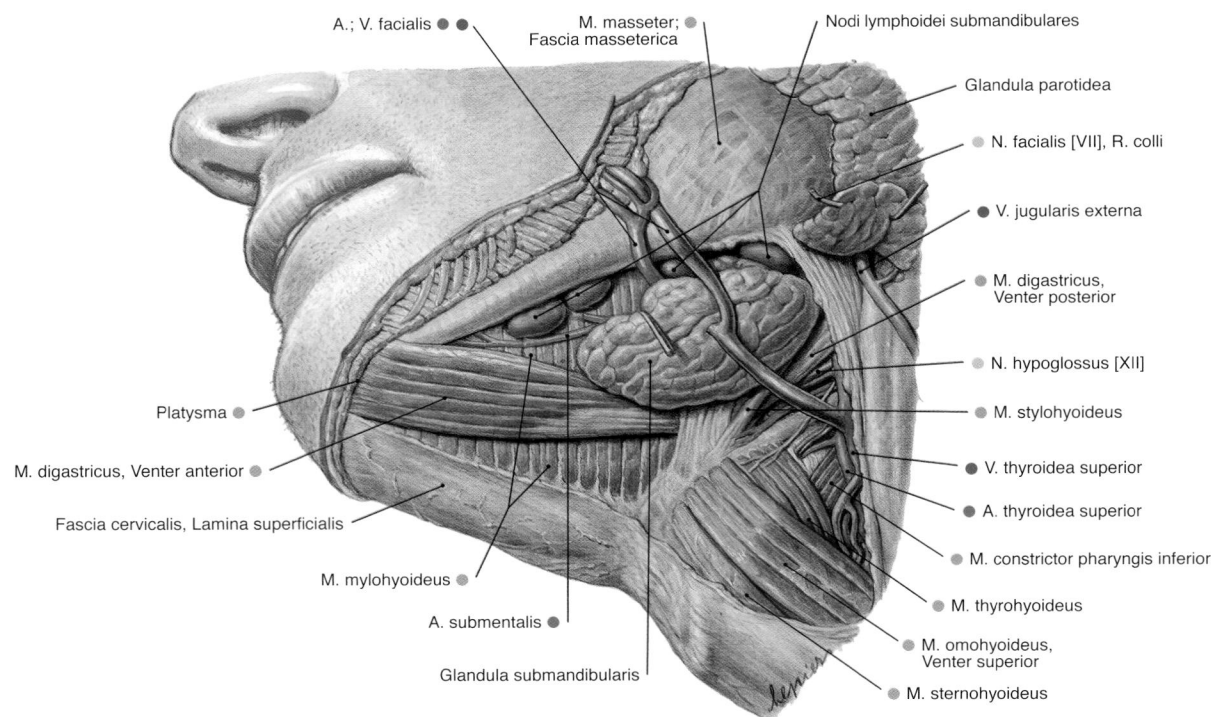

A.; V. facialis ● ●
M. masseter; ●
Fascia masseterica
Nodi lymphoidei submandibulares
Glandula parotidea
● N. facialis [VII], R. colli
● V. jugularis externa
● M. digastricus, Venter posterior
● N. hypoglossus [XII]
● M. stylohyoideus
● V. thyroidea superior
● A. thyroidea superior
● M. constrictor pharyngis inferior
● M. thyrohyoideus
● M. omohyoideus, Venter superior
● M. sternohyoideus

Platysma ●
M. digastricus, Venter anterior ●
Fascia cervicalis, Lamina superficialis
M. mylohyoideus ●
A. submentalis ●
Glandula submandibularis

Fig. 192   Submandibular gland, Glandula submandibularis.

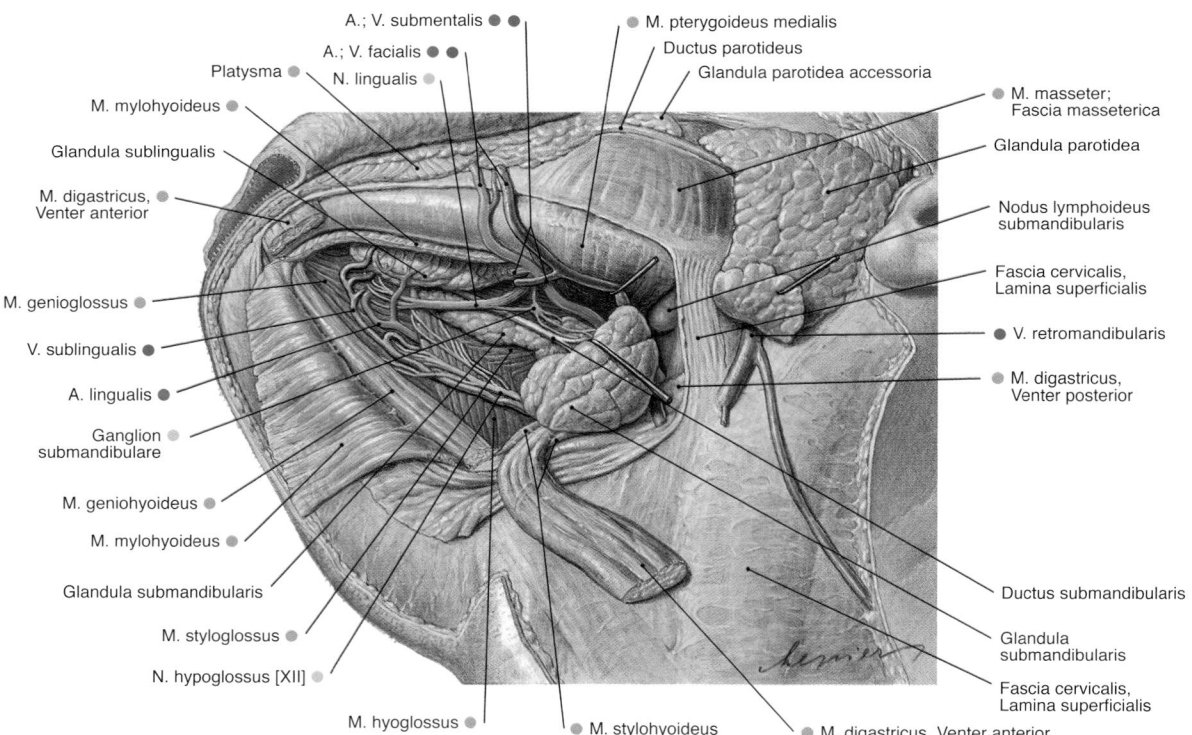

A.; V. submentalis ● ●
A.; V. facialis ● ●
Platysma ●
N. lingualis ●
M. pterygoideus medialis
Ductus parotideus
Glandula parotidea accessoria
● M. masseter; Fascia masseterica
Glandula parotidea
Nodus lymphoideus submandibularis
Fascia cervicalis, Lamina superficialis
● V. retromandibularis
● M. digastricus, Venter posterior
Ductus submandibularis
Glandula submandibularis
Fascia cervicalis, Lamina superficialis

M. mylohyoideus ●
Glandula sublingualis
M. digastricus, Venter anterior ●
M. genioglossus ●
V. sublingualis ●
A. lingualis ●
Ganglion submandibulare ●
M. geniohyoideus ●
M. mylohyoideus ●
Glandula submandibularis
M. styloglossus ●
N. hypoglossus [XII] ●
M. hyoglossus ●
M. stylohyoideus ●
M. digastricus, Venter anterior ●

Fig. 193   Major salivary glands, Glandulae salivariae majores;
inferolateral view.

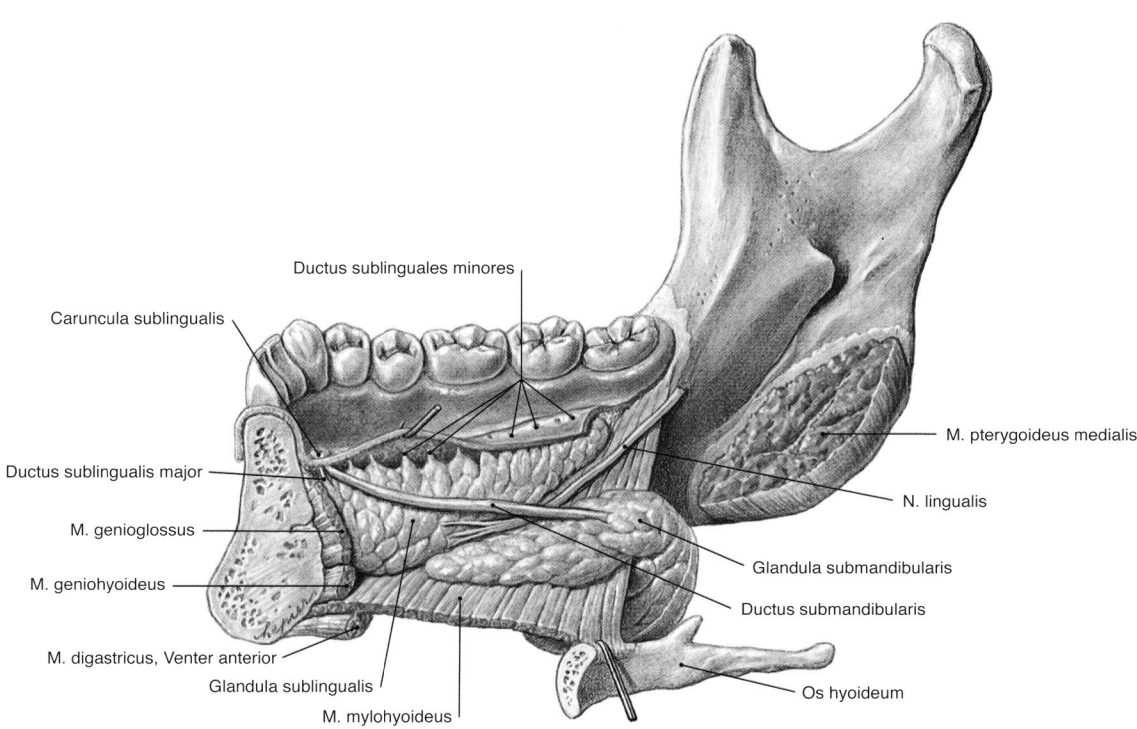

Ductus sublinguales minores

Caruncula sublingualis

Ductus sublingualis major

M. genioglossus

M. geniohyoideus

M. digastricus, Venter anterior

Glandula sublingualis

M. mylohyoideus

M. pterygoideus medialis

N. lingualis

Glandula submandibularis

Ductus submandibularis

Os hyoideum

Fig. 194   Submandibular gland, Glandula submandibularis, and sublingual gland, Glandula sublingualis.

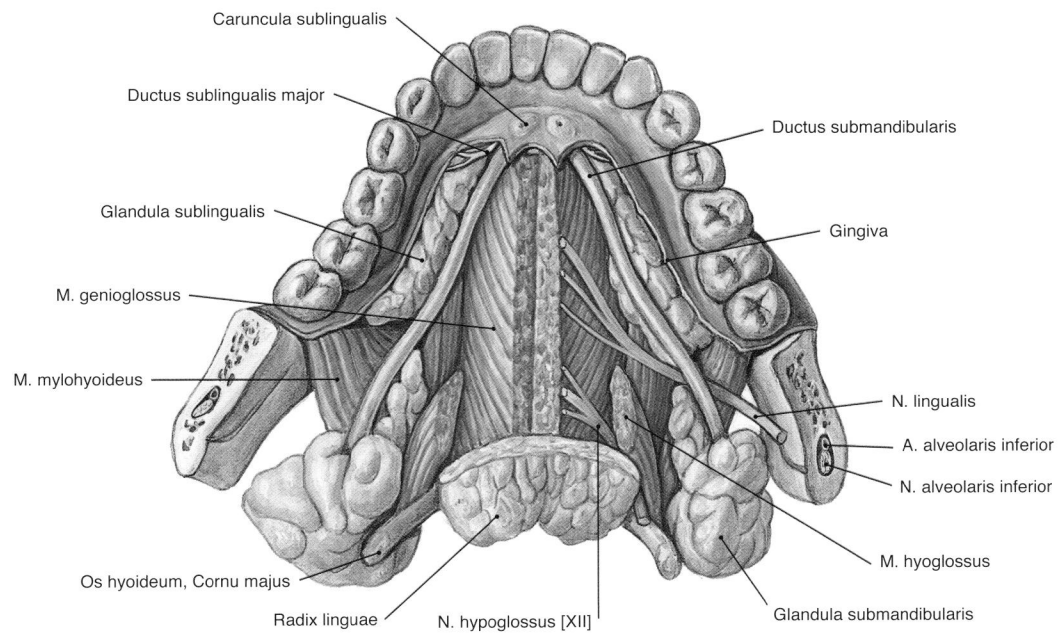

Caruncula sublingualis

Ductus sublingualis major

Glandula sublingualis

M. genioglossus

M. mylohyoideus

Os hyoideum, Cornu majus

Radix linguae

N. hypoglossus [XII]

Ductus submandibularis

Gingiva

N. lingualis

A. alveolaris inferior

N. alveolaris inferior

M. hyoglossus

Glandula submandibularis

Fig. 195   Sublingual gland, Glandula sublingualis, and submandibular gland, Glandula submandibularis; superior view.

Openings of the salivary glands

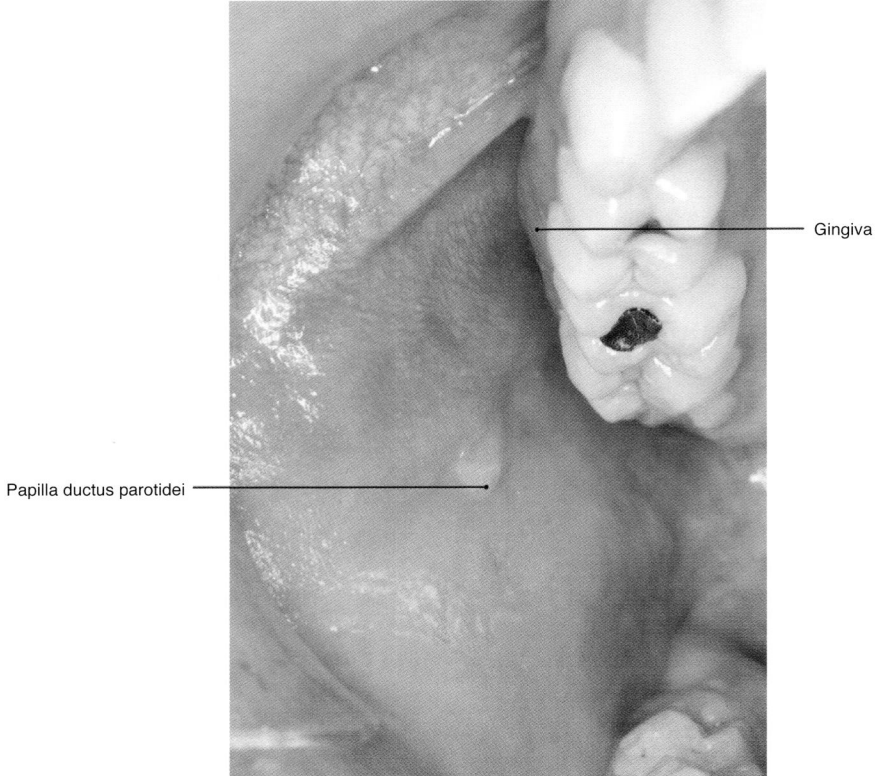

Gingiva

Papilla ductus parotidei

Fig. 196 Opening of the excretory duct of the parotid gland, Papilla ductus parotidei.

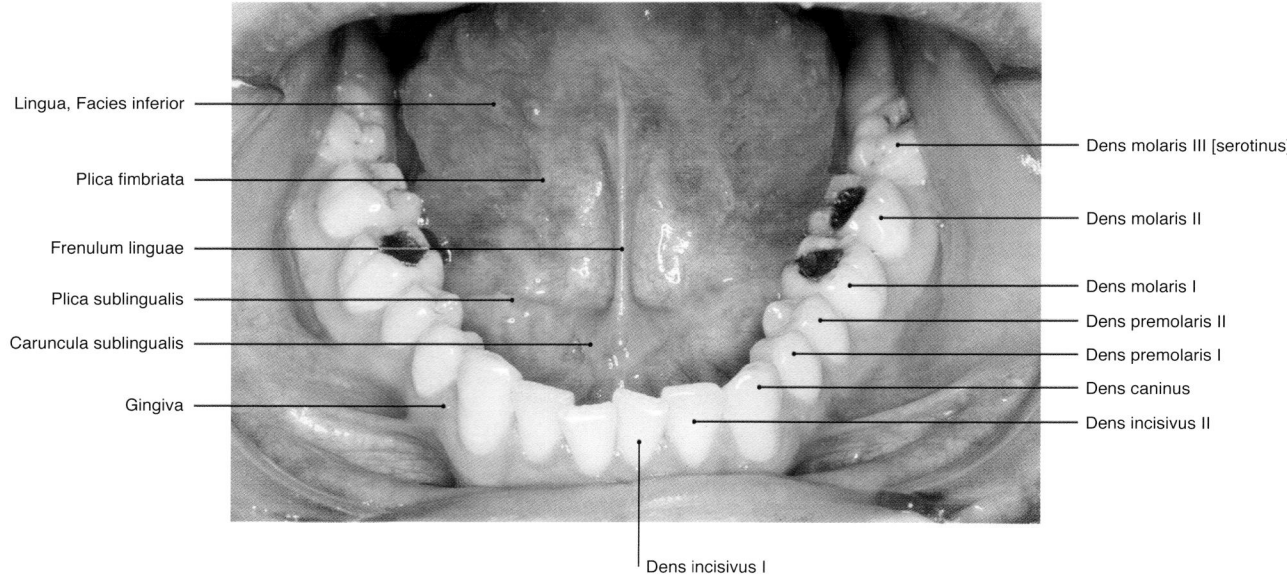

Lingua, Facies inferior

Plica fimbriata

Frenulum linguae

Plica sublingualis

Caruncula sublingualis

Gingiva

Dens molaris III [serotinus]

Dens molaris II

Dens molaris I

Dens premolaris II

Dens premolaris I

Dens caninus

Dens incisivus II

Dens incisivus I

→ 154

Fig. 197 Opening of the excretory duct of the submandibular gland, Caruncula sublingualis.

Arteries and nerves of the oral cavity

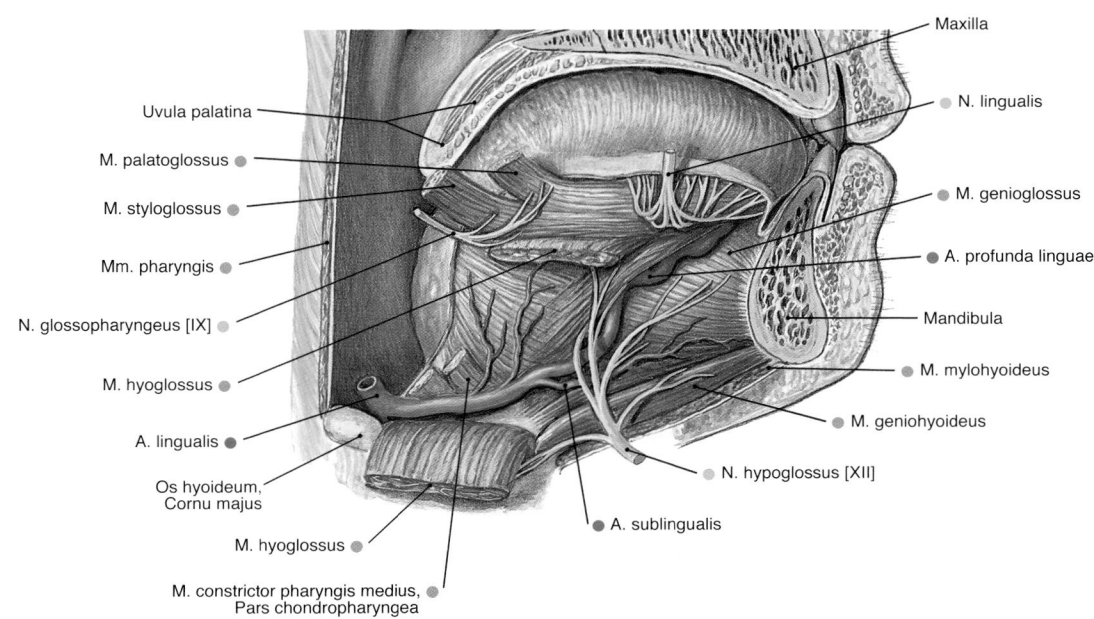

Uvula palatina

M. palatoglossus

M. styloglossus

Mm. pharyngis

N. glossopharyngeus [IX]

M. hyoglossus

A. lingualis

Os hyoideum,
Cornu majus

M. hyoglossus

M. constrictor pharyngis medius,
Pars chondropharyngea

Maxilla

N. lingualis

M. genioglossus

A. profunda linguae

Mandibula

M. mylohyoideus

M. geniohyoideus

N. hypoglossus [XII]

A. sublingualis

Fig. 198   Arteries and nerves of the tongue, Lingua;
medial view.

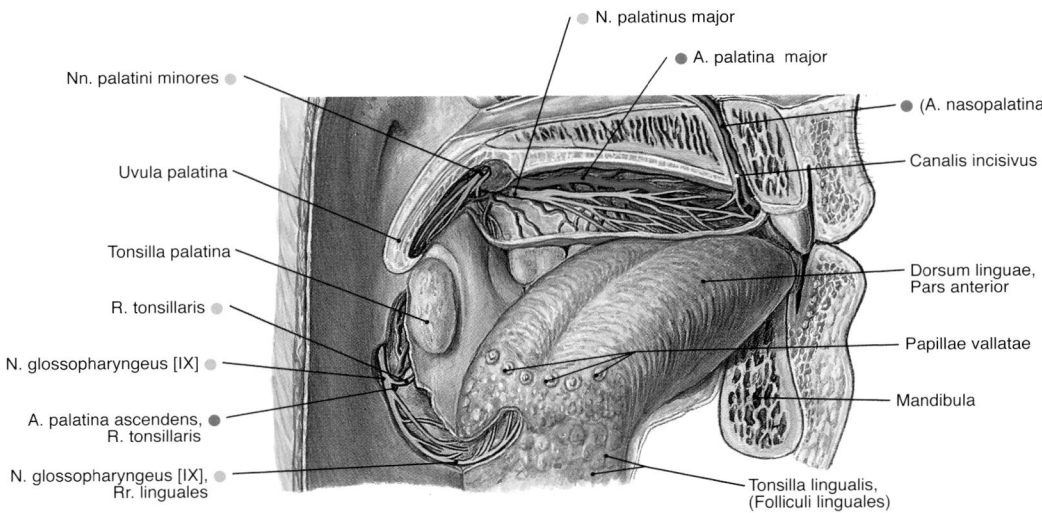

Nn. palatini minores

Uvula palatina

Tonsilla palatina

R. tonsillaris

N. glossopharyngeus [IX]

A. palatina ascendens,
R. tonsillaris

N. glossopharyngeus [IX],
Rr. linguales

N. palatinus major

A. palatina major

(A. nasopalatina)

Canalis incisivus

Dorsum linguae,
Pars anterior

Papillae vallatae

Mandibula

Tonsilla lingualis,
(Folliculi linguales)

Fig. 199   Arteries and nerves of the palate, Palatum,
and the root of the tongue, Radix linguae;
medial view.

Vessels and nerves of the tongue and the larynx

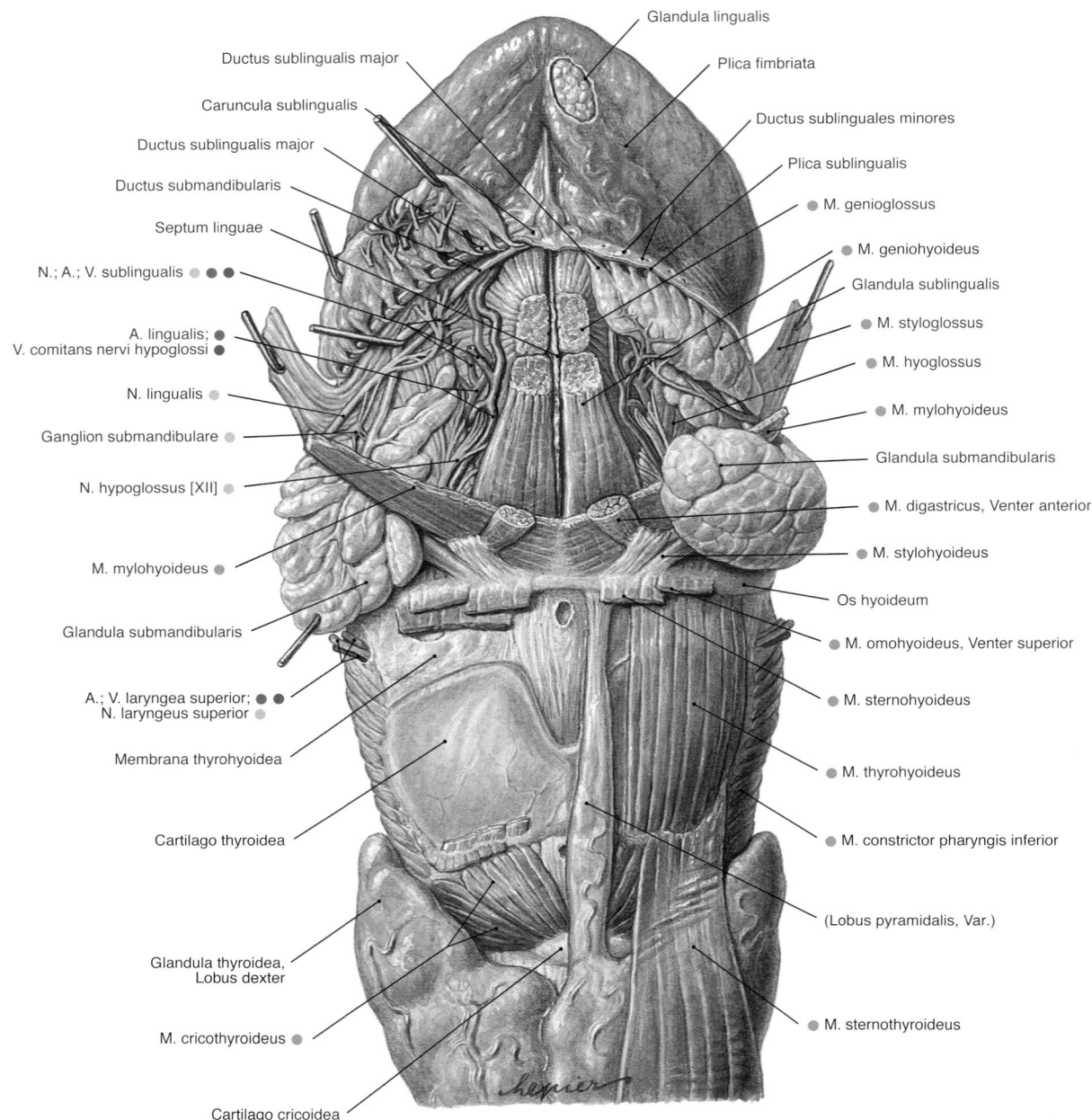

Glandula lingualis

Ductus sublingualis major

Caruncula sublingualis

Ductus sublingualis major

Ductus submandibularis

Septum linguae

N.; A.; V. sublingualis ● ● ●

A. lingualis; ●
V. comitans nervi hypoglossi ●

N. lingualis ●

Ganglion submandibulare ●

N. hypoglossus [XII] ●

M. mylohyoideus ●

Glandula submandibularis

A.; V. laryngea superior; ● ●
N. laryngeus superior ●

Membrana thyrohyoidea

Cartilago thyroidea

Glandula thyroidea,
Lobus dexter

M. cricothyroideus ●

Cartilago cricoidea

Plica fimbriata

Ductus sublinguales minores

Plica sublingualis

● M. genioglossus

● M. geniohyoideus

Glandula sublingualis

● M. styloglossus

● M. hyoglossus

● M. mylohyoideus

Glandula submandibularis

● M. digastricus, Venter anterior

● M. stylohyoideus

Os hyoideum

● M. omohyoideus, Venter superior

● M. sternohyoideus

● M. thyrohyoideus

● M. constrictor pharyngis inferior

(Lobus pyramidalis, Var.)

● M. sternothyroideus

→ 204, 218, 234, 237

Fig. 200 Vessels and nerves of the tongue, Lingua;
major salivary glands, Glandulae salivariae majores,
and larynx, Larynx;
anterior-inferior view.

Vessels and nerves of the tongue and the thyroid gland

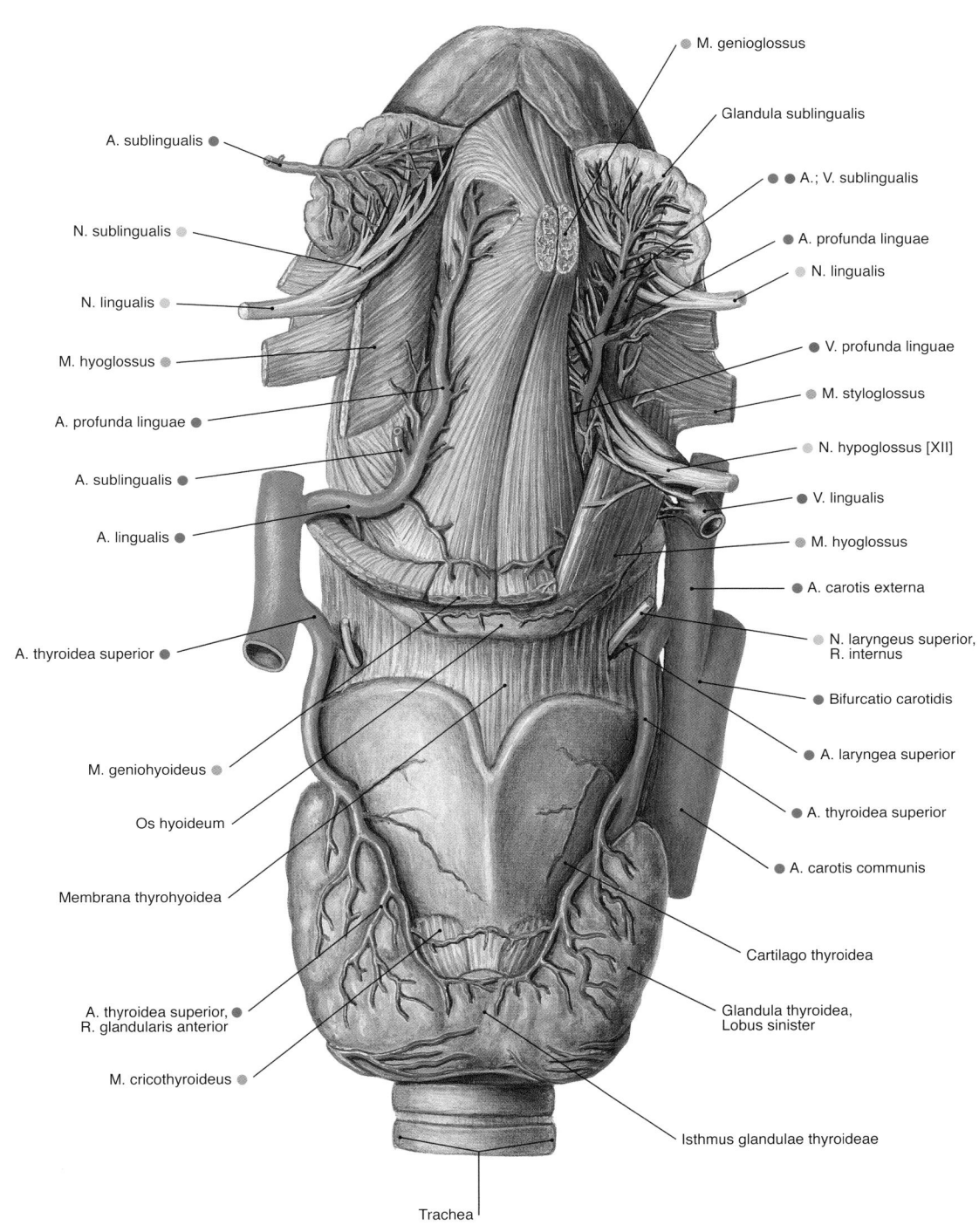

- M. genioglossus
- A. sublingualis
- Glandula sublingualis
- N. sublingualis
- A.; V. sublingualis
- N. lingualis
- A. profunda linguae
- N. lingualis
- M. hyoglossus
- V. profunda linguae
- A. profunda linguae
- M. styloglossus
- A. sublingualis
- N. hypoglossus [XII]
- A. lingualis
- V. lingualis
- M. hyoglossus
- A. carotis externa
- A. thyroidea superior
- N. laryngeus superior, R. internus
- Bifurcatio carotidis
- M. geniohyoideus
- A. laryngea superior
- Os hyoideum
- A. thyroidea superior
- A. carotis communis
- Membrana thyrohyoidea
- Cartilago thyroidea
- A. thyroidea superior, R. glandularis anterior
- Glandula thyroidea, Lobus sinister
- M. cricothyroideus
- Isthmus glandulae thyroideae
- Trachea

Fig. 201 Vessels and nerves of the tongue, Lingua, and the thyroid gland, Glandula thyroidea; anterior-inferior view.

→ 238, 264

Head, frontal section

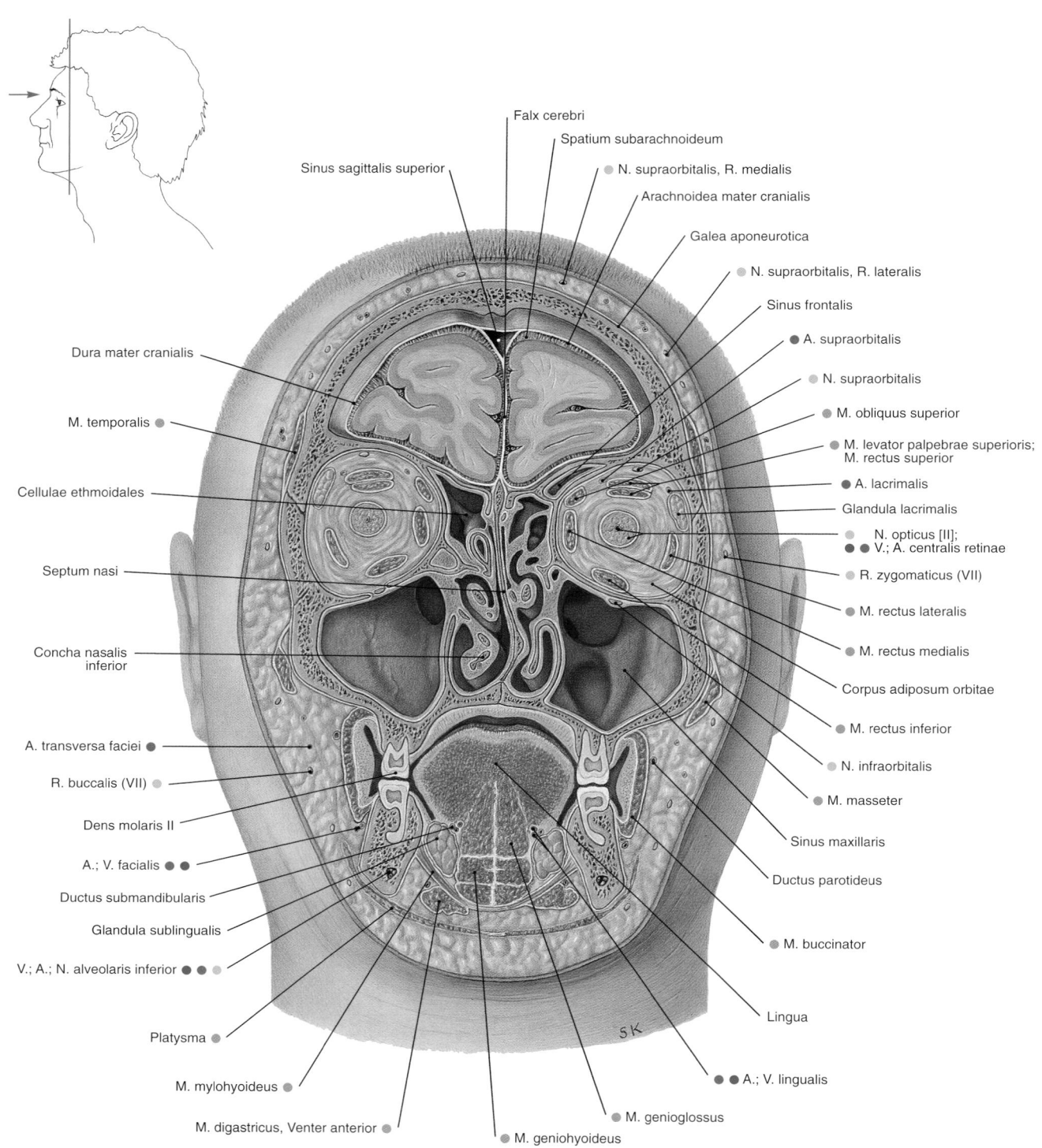

Falx cerebri
Spatium subarachnoideum
Sinus sagittalis superior
N. supraorbitalis, R. medialis
Arachnoidea mater cranialis
Galea aponeurotica
N. supraorbitalis, R. lateralis
Sinus frontalis
Dura mater cranialis
A. supraorbitalis
N. supraorbitalis
M. temporalis
M. obliquus superior
M. levator palpebrae superioris;
M. rectus superior
Cellulae ethmoidales
A. lacrimalis
Glandula lacrimalis
N. opticus [II];
V.; A. centralis retinae
Septum nasi
R. zygomaticus (VII)
M. rectus lateralis
M. rectus medialis
Concha nasalis
inferior
Corpus adiposum orbitae
M. rectus inferior
A. transversa faciei
N. infraorbitalis
R. buccalis (VII)
M. masseter
Dens molaris II
Sinus maxillaris
A.; V. facialis
Ductus parotideus
Ductus submandibularis
Glandula sublingualis
M. buccinator
V.; A.; N. alveolaris inferior
Lingua
Platysma
A.; V. lingualis
M. mylohyoideus
M. genioglossus
M. digastricus, Venter anterior
M. geniohyoideus

SK

Fig. 202 Frontal section through the head of a 48-year-old male
at the level of the second upper molar tooth;
anterior view.

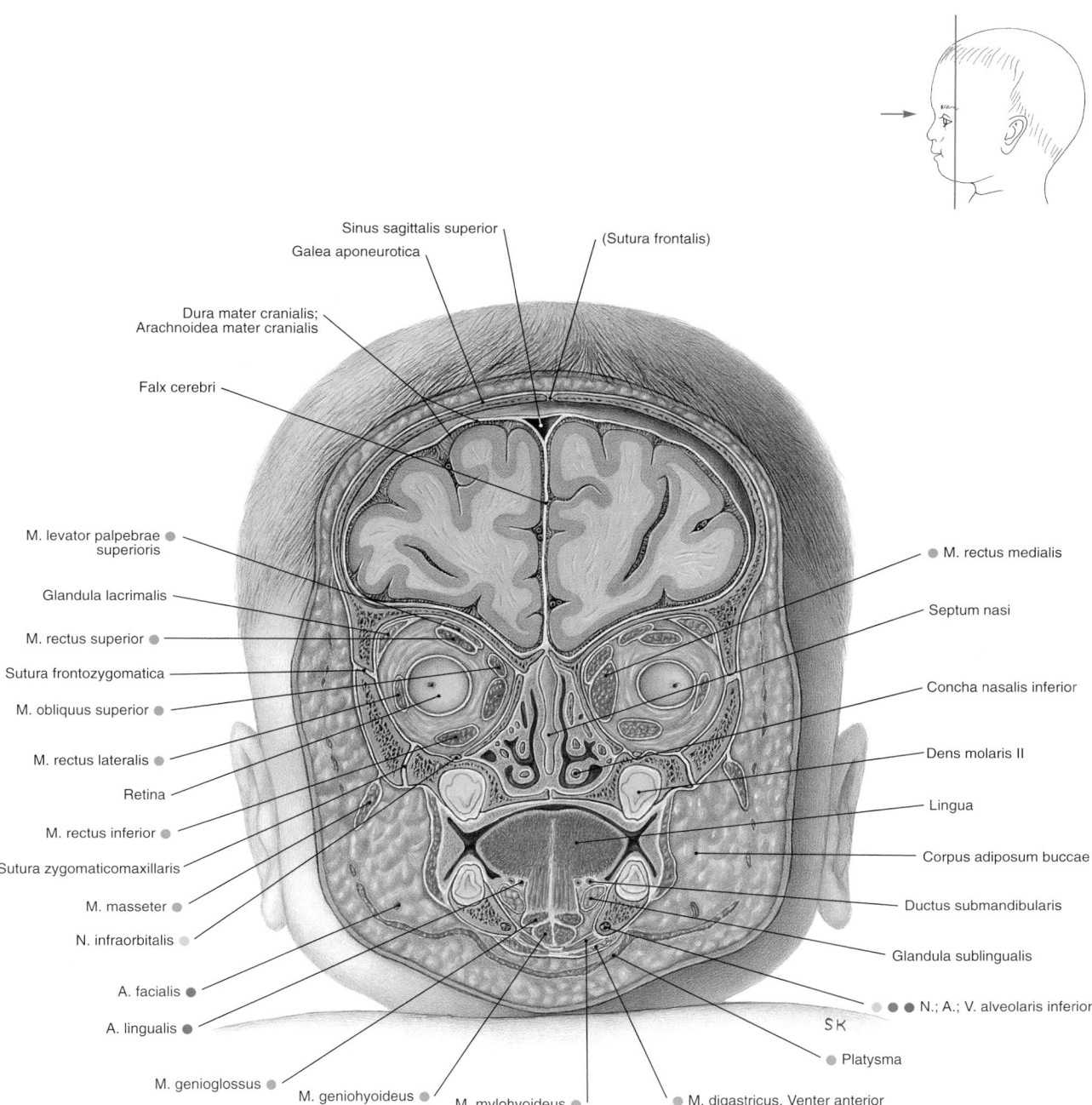

Sinus sagittalis superior

Galea aponeurotica

(Sutura frontalis)

Dura mater cranialis;
Arachnoidea mater cranialis

Falx cerebri

M. levator palpebrae
superioris

Glandula lacrimalis

M. rectus superior

Sutura frontozygomatica

M. obliquus superior

M. rectus lateralis

Retina

M. rectus inferior

Sutura zygomaticomaxillaris

M. masseter

N. infraorbitalis

A. facialis

A. lingualis

M. genioglossus

M. geniohyoideus

M. mylohyoideus

M. digastricus, Venter anterior

M. rectus medialis

Septum nasi

Concha nasalis inferior

Dens molaris II

Lingua

Corpus adiposum buccae

Ductus submandibularis

Glandula sublingualis

N.; A.; V. alveolaris inferior

Platysma

SK

Fig. 203 Frontal section through the head of a neonate
at the level of the second upper molar tooth;
anterior view.
Note the absence of the maxillary sinus and the close proximity
of the tooth anlage to the orbit.

Muscles of the neck and tracheotomy

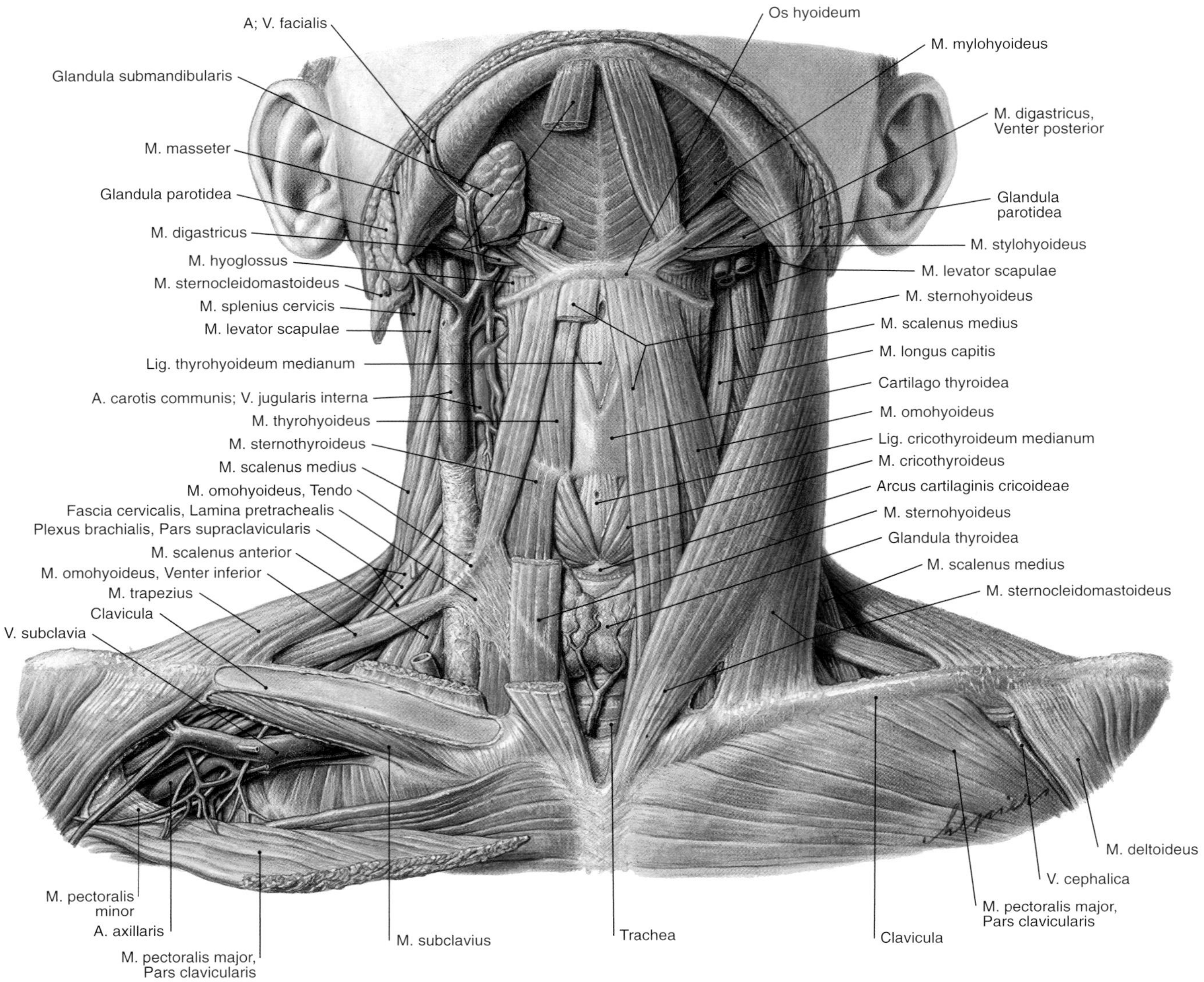

A; V. facialis

Glandula submandibularis

M. masseter

Glandula parotidea

M. digastricus

M. hyoglossus

M. sternocleidomastoideus

M. splenius cervicis

M. levator scapulae

Lig. thyrohyoideum medianum

A. carotis communis; V. jugularis interna

M. thyrohyoideus

M. sternothyroideus

M. scalenus medius

M. omohyoideus, Tendo

Fascia cervicalis, Lamina pretrachealis

Plexus brachialis, Pars supraclavicularis

M. scalenus anterior

M. omohyoideus, Venter inferior

M. trapezius

Clavicula

V. subclavia

M. pectoralis minor

A. axillaris

M. pectoralis major, Pars clavicularis

Os hyoideum

M. mylohyoideus

M. digastricus, Venter posterior

Glandula parotidea

M. stylohyoideus

M. levator scapulae

M. sternohyoideus

M. scalenus medius

M. longus capitis

Cartilago thyroidea

M. omohyoideus

Lig. cricothyroideum medianum

M. cricothyroideus

Arcus cartilaginis cricoideae

M. sternohyoideus

Glandula thyroidea

M. scalenus medius

M. sternocleidomastoideus

M. deltoideus

V. cephalica

M. pectoralis major, Pars clavicularis

Clavicula

Trachea

M. subclavius

→ T8, T9, T10, T11

Fig. 204 Muscles of the neck, Mm. colli.

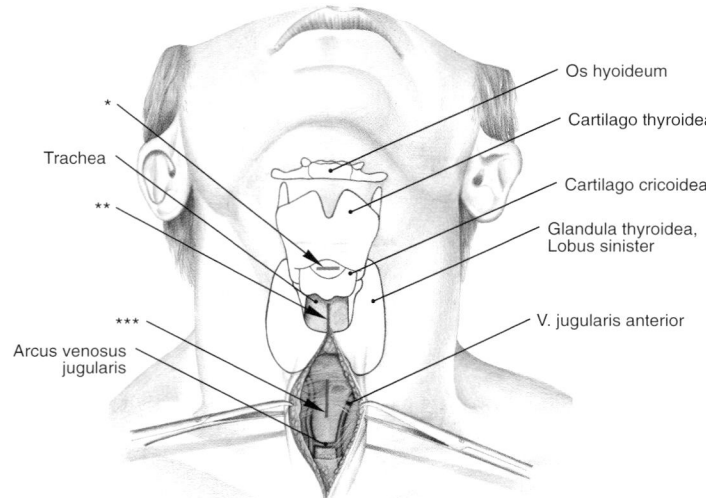

Os hyoideum

Cartilago thyroidea

Cartilago cricoidea

Glandula thyroidea, Lobus sinister

V. jugularis anterior

Trachea

*

**

***

Arcus venosus jugularis

Fig. 205 Surgical access to the trachea
with the neck hyperextended.

* Coniotomy
** Upper tracheotomy (above the isthmus of the thyroid gland)
***Lower tracheotomy (below the isthmus of the thyroid gland)

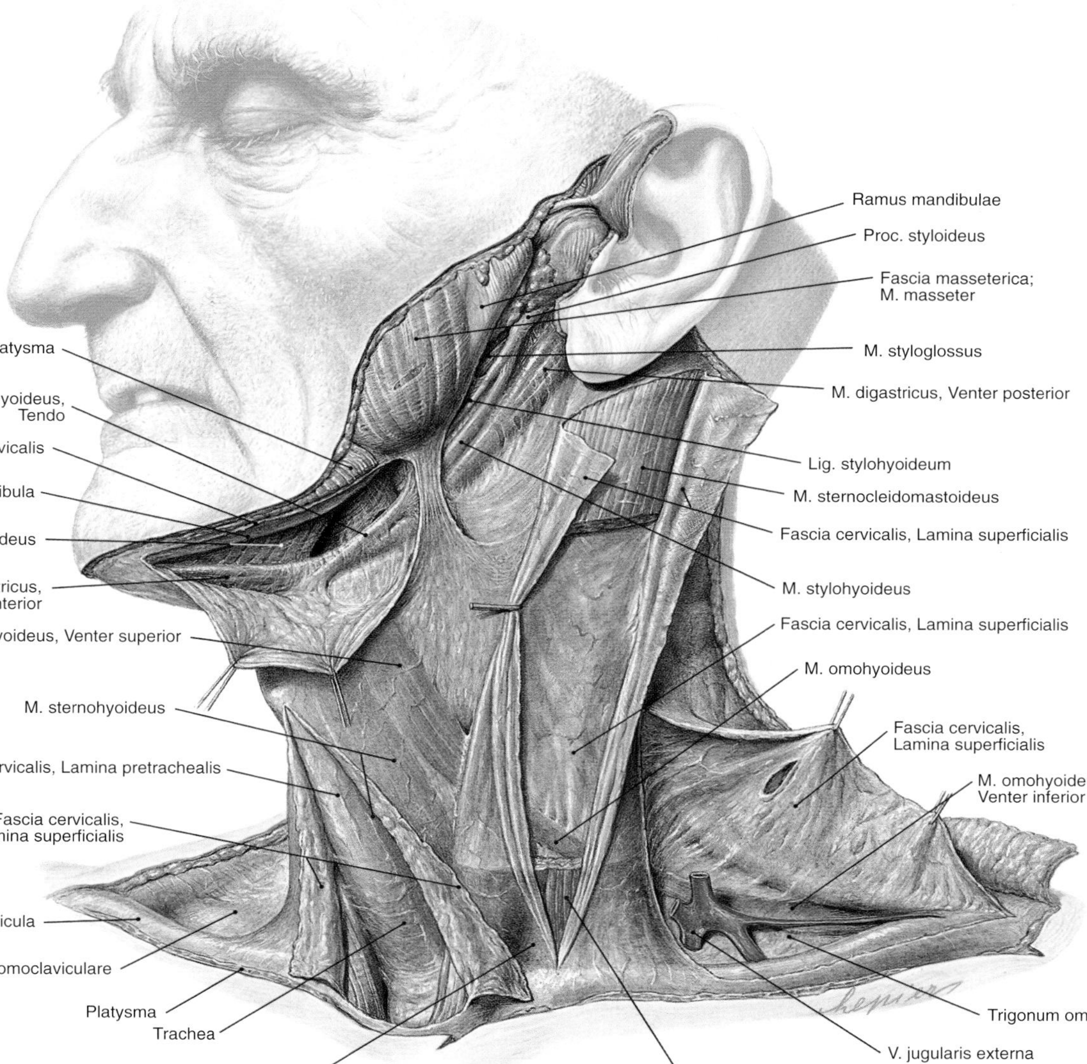

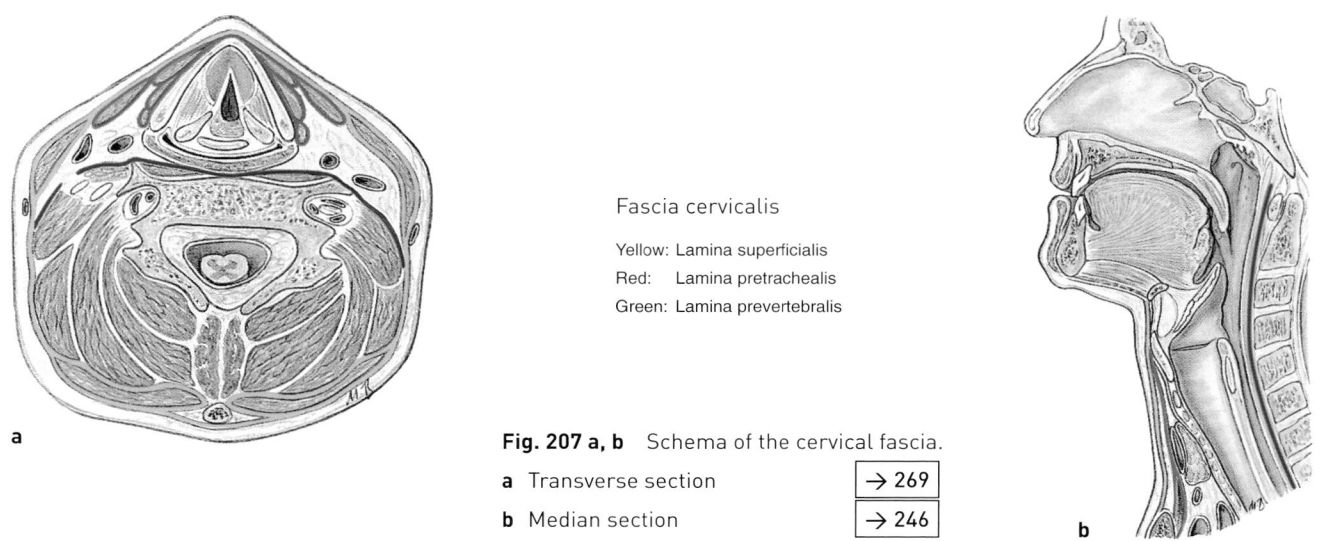

Ramus mandibulae

Proc. styloideus

Fascia masseterica;
M. masseter

Platysma

M. stylohyoideus,
Tendo

M. styloglossus

M. digastricus, Venter posterior

Fascia cervicalis

Mandibula

Lig. stylohyoideum

M. sternocleidomastoideus

M. mylohyoideus

Fascia cervicalis, Lamina superficialis

M. digastricus,
Venter anterior

M. stylohyoideus

M. omohyoideus, Venter superior

Fascia cervicalis, Lamina superficialis

M. omohyoideus

M. sternohyoideus

Fascia cervicalis,
Lamina superficialis

Fascia cervicalis, Lamina pretrachealis

M. omohyoideus,
Venter inferior

Fascia cervicalis,
Lamina superficialis

Clavicula

Trigonum omoclaviculare

Trigonum omoclaviculare

Platysma

V. jugularis externa

Trachea

M. sternocleidomastoideus

Fossa supraclavicularis minor

Fig. 206   Cervical fascia, Fascia cervicalis.

Fascia cervicalis

Yellow: Lamina superficialis
Red: Lamina pretrachealis
Green: Lamina prevertebralis

a

Fig. 207 a, b   Schema of the cervical fascia.

a Transverse section   → 269

b Median section   → 246

b

Muscles of the neck

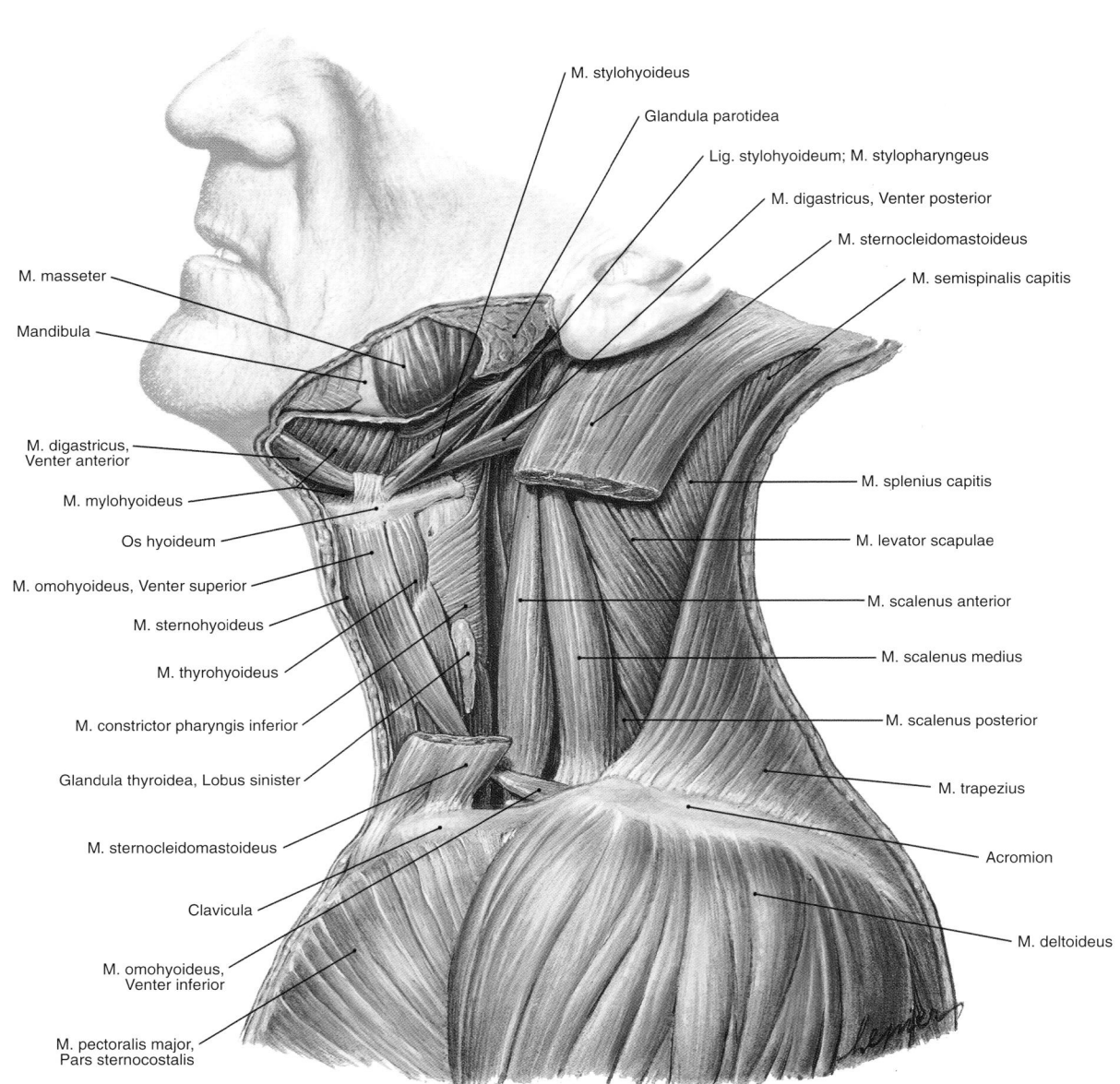

M. stylohyoideus

Glandula parotidea

Lig. stylohyoideum; M. stylopharyngeus

M. digastricus, Venter posterior

M. sternocleidomastoideus

M. semispinalis capitis

M. masseter

Mandibula

M. splenius capitis

M. digastricus, Venter anterior

M. levator scapulae

M. mylohyoideus

Os hyoideum

M. scalenus anterior

M. omohyoideus, Venter superior

M. sternohyoideus

M. scalenus medius

M. thyrohyoideus

M. scalenus posterior

M. constrictor pharyngis inferior

Glandula thyroidea, Lobus sinister

M. trapezius

M. sternocleidomastoideus

Acromion

Clavicula

M. deltoideus

M. omohyoideus, Venter inferior

M. pectoralis major, Pars sternocostalis

→ T8, T9, T10, T11

184
209
204
527

Fig. 208 Muscles of the neck, Mm. colli.

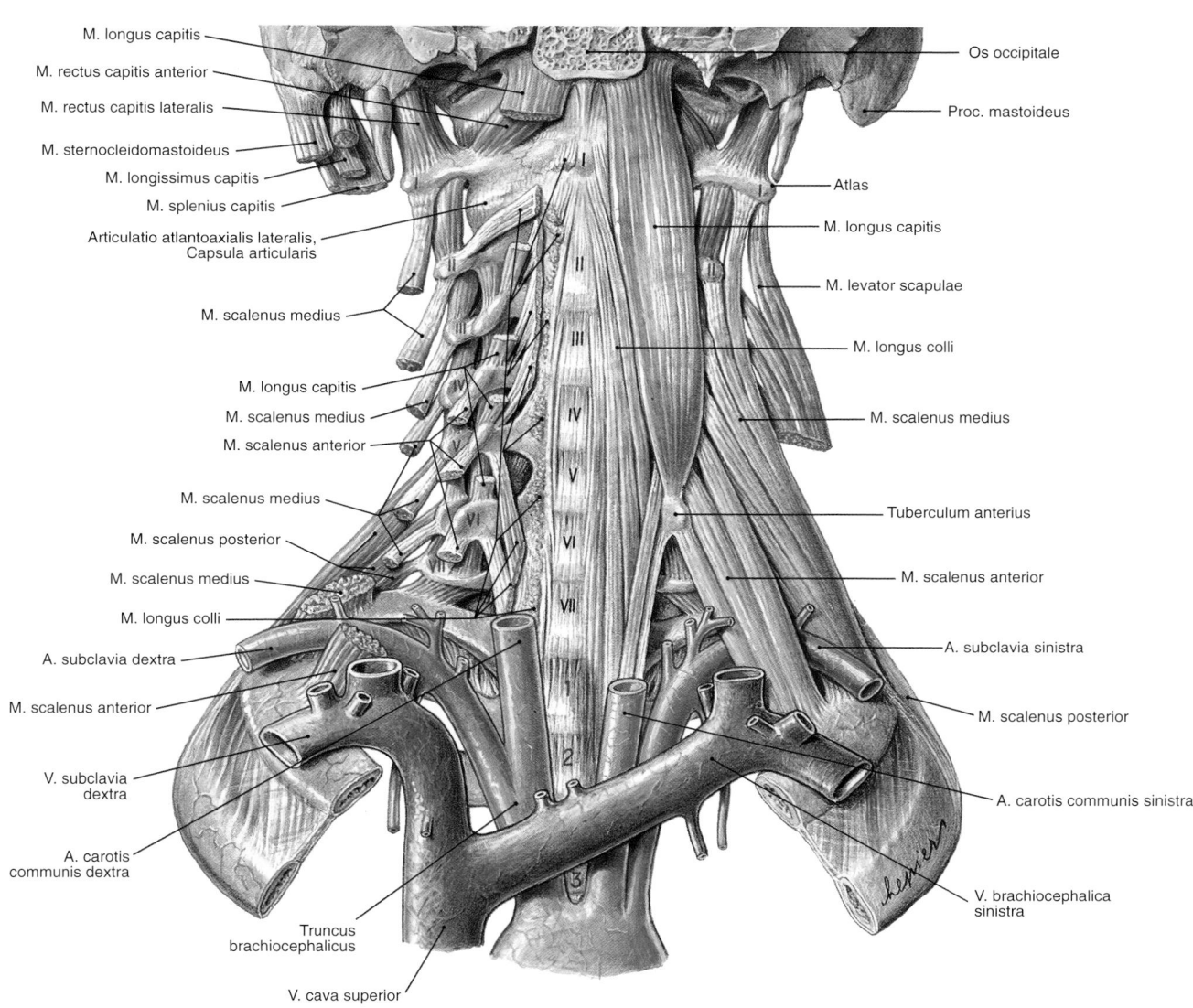

M. longus capitis

M. rectus capitis anterior

M. rectus capitis lateralis

M. sternocleidomastoideus

M. longissimus capitis

M. splenius capitis

Articulatio atlantoaxialis lateralis, Capsula articularis

M. scalenus medius

M. longus capitis

M. scalenus medius

M. scalenus anterior

M. scalenus medius

M. scalenus posterior

M. scalenus medius

M. longus colli

A. subclavia dextra

M. scalenus anterior

V. subclavia dextra

A. carotis communis dextra

Truncus brachiocephalicus

V. cava superior

Os occipitale

Proc. mastoideus

Atlas

M. longus capitis

M. levator scapulae

M. longus colli

M. scalenus medius

Tuberculum anterius

M. scalenus anterior

A. subclavia sinistra

M. scalenus posterior

A. carotis communis sinistra

V. brachiocephalica sinistra

Fig. 209 Prevertebral muscles and scalenus muscles, Mm. scaleni.
I –VII = First to seventh cervical vertebra
1 –3 = First to third thoracic vertebra

→ T 11, T 12

Skeleton of the larynx

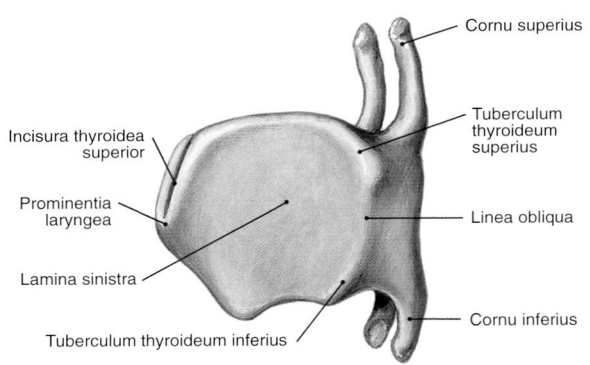

Fig. 210 Thyroid cartilage, Cartilago thyroidea; viewed from the left.

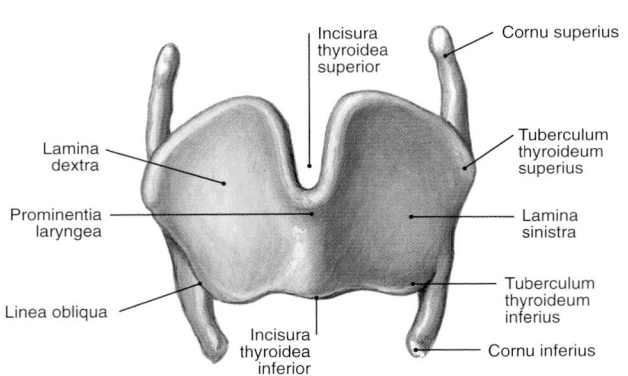

Fig. 211 Thyroid cartilage, Cartilago thyroidea; ventral view.

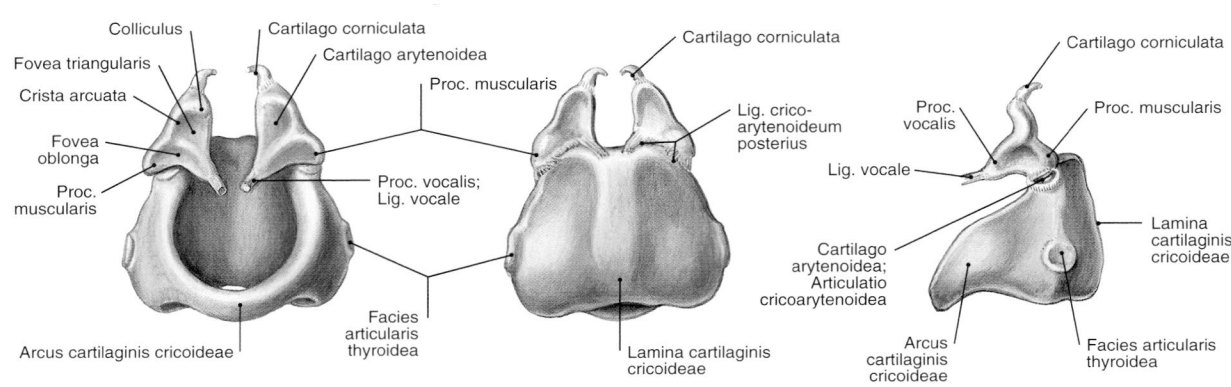

Fig. 212 Cartilages of the larynx, Cartilagines laryngis; ventrosuperior view.

Fig. 213 Cartilages of the larynx, Cartilagines laryngis; dorsal view.

Fig. 214 Cartilages of the larynx, Cartilagines laryngis; viewed from the left.

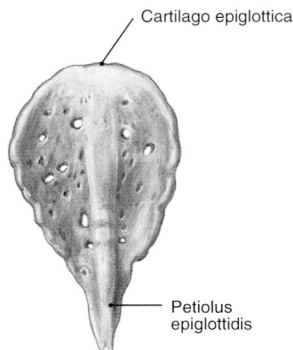

Fig. 215 Epiglottic cartilage, Cartilago epiglottica; dorsal view.

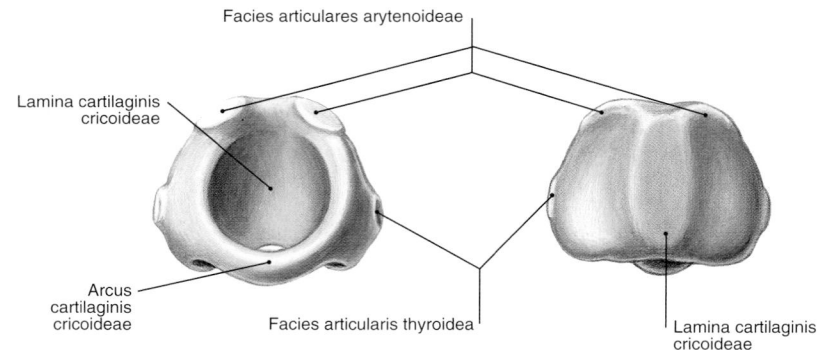

Fig. 216 Cricoid cartilage, Cartilago cricoidea; ventrosuperior view.

Fig. 217 Cricoid cartilage, Cartilago cricoidea; dorsal view.

Hyoid bone and skeleton of the larynx

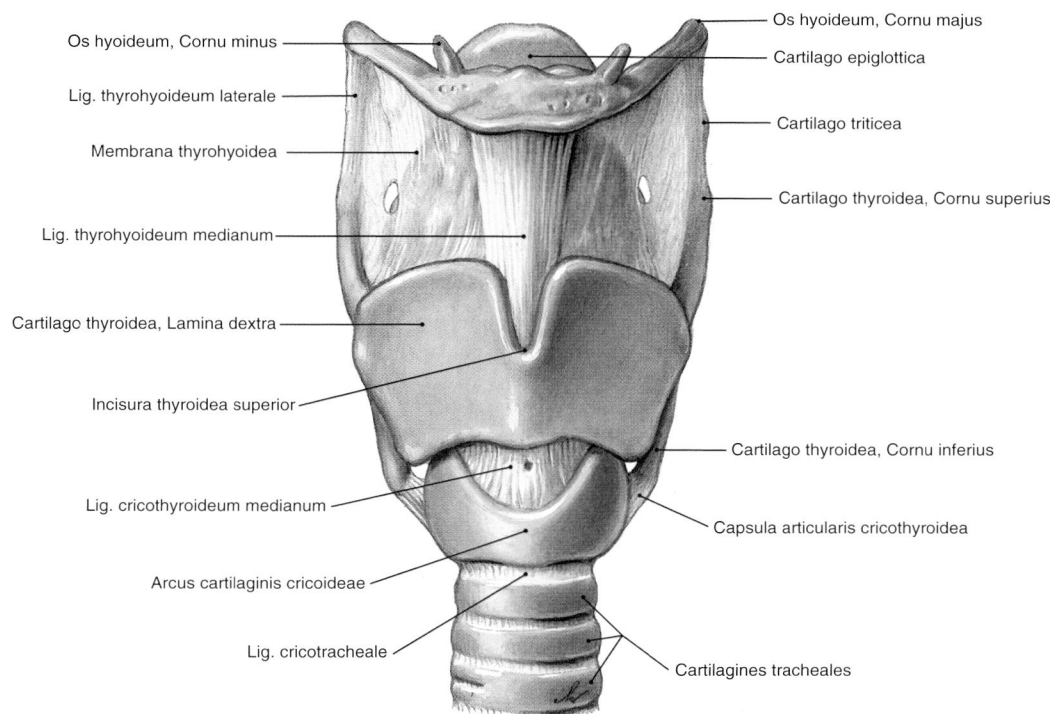

Os hyoideum, Cornu minus

Lig. thyrohyoideum laterale

Membrana thyrohyoidea

Lig. thyrohyoideum medianum

Cartilago thyroidea, Lamina dextra

Incisura thyroidea superior

Lig. cricothyroideum medianum

Arcus cartilaginis cricoideae

Lig. cricotracheale

Os hyoideum, Cornu majus

Cartilago epiglottica

Cartilago triticea

Cartilago thyroidea, Cornu superius

Cartilago thyroidea, Cornu inferius

Capsula articularis cricothyroidea

Cartilagines tracheales

Fig. 218   Larynx, Larynx,
and hyoid bone, Os hyoideum;
ventral view.

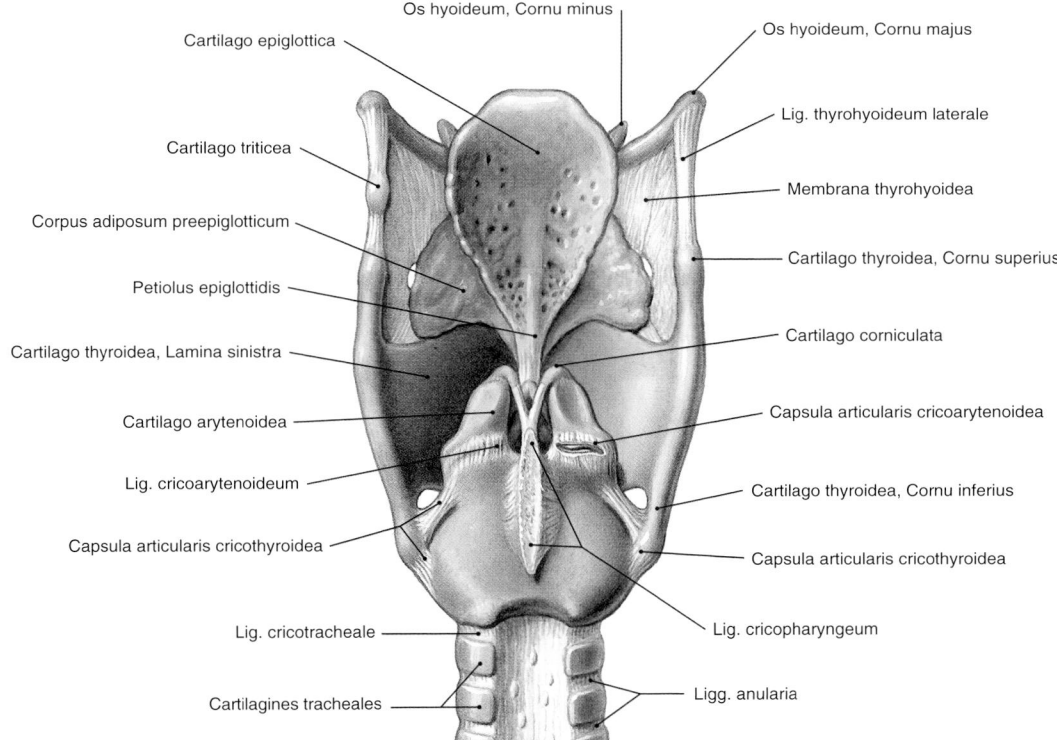

Os hyoideum, Cornu minus

Cartilago epiglottica

Cartilago triticea

Corpus adiposum preepiglotticum

Petiolus epiglottidis

Cartilago thyroidea, Lamina sinistra

Cartilago arytenoidea

Lig. cricoarytenoideum

Capsula articularis cricothyroidea

Lig. cricotracheale

Cartilagines tracheales

Os hyoideum, Cornu majus

Lig. thyrohyoideum laterale

Membrana thyrohyoidea

Cartilago thyroidea, Cornu superius

Cartilago corniculata

Capsula articularis cricoarytenoidea

Cartilago thyroidea, Cornu inferius

Capsula articularis cricothyroidea

Lig. cricopharyngeum

Ligg. anularia

Fig. 219   Cartilages of the larynx, Cartilagines laryngis,
and hyoid bone, Os hyoideum;
dorsal view.

Hyoid bone and skeleton of the larynx

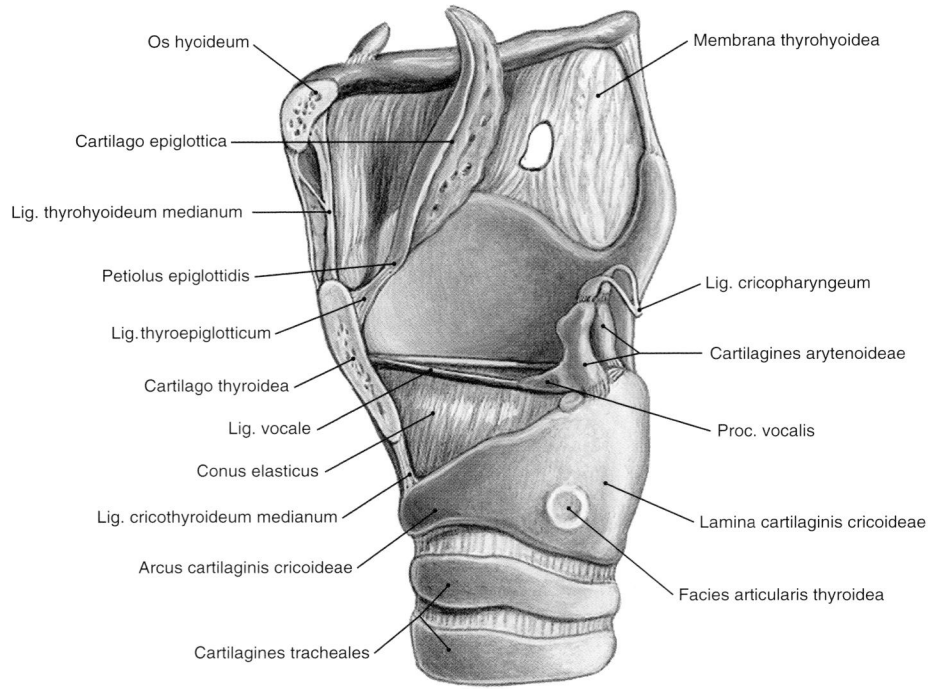

Os hyoideum

Cartilago epiglottica

Lig. thyrohyoideum medianum

Petiolus epiglottidis

Lig. thyroepiglotticum

Cartilago thyroidea

Lig. vocale

Conus elasticus

Lig. cricothyroideum medianum

Arcus cartilaginis cricoideae

Cartilagines tracheales

Membrana thyrohyoidea

Lig. cricopharyngeum

Cartilagines arytenoideae

Proc. vocalis

Lamina cartilaginis cricoideae

Facies articularis thyroidea

Fig. 220 Larynx, Larynx, and hyoid bone, Os hyoideum; viewed from the left.

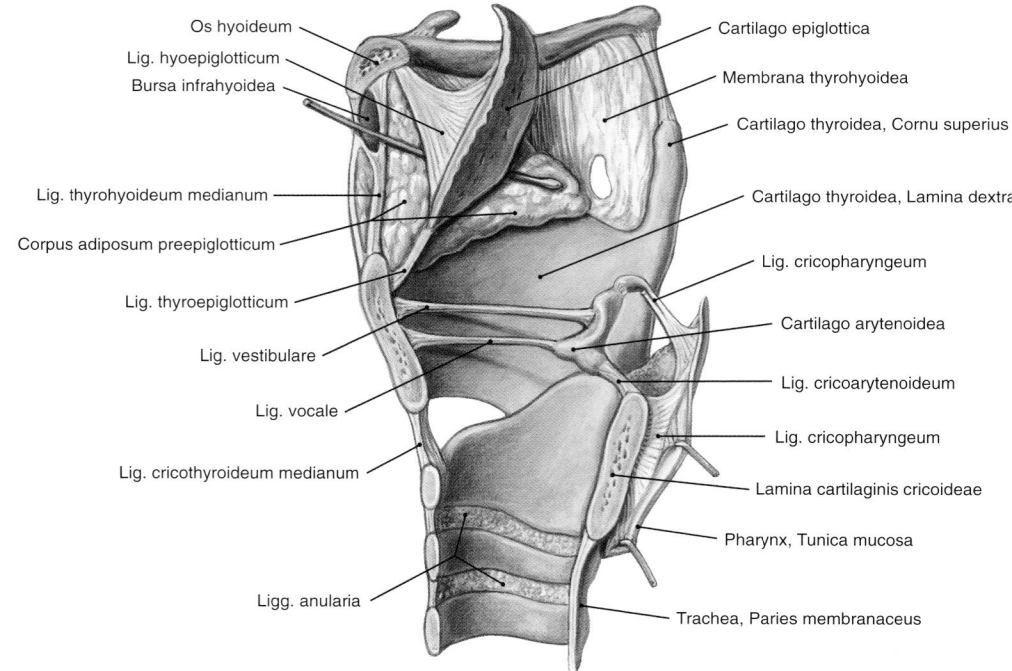

Os hyoideum

Lig. hyoepiglotticum

Bursa infrahyoidea

Lig. thyrohyoideum medianum

Corpus adiposum preepiglotticum

Lig. thyroepiglotticum

Lig. vestibulare

Lig. vocale

Lig. cricothyroideum medianum

Ligg. anularia

Cartilago epiglottica

Membrana thyrohyoidea

Cartilago thyroidea, Cornu superius

Cartilago thyroidea, Lamina dextra

Lig. cricopharyngeum

Cartilago arytenoidea

Lig. cricoarytenoideum

Lig. cricopharyngeum

Lamina cartilaginis cricoideae

Pharynx, Tunica mucosa

Trachea, Paries membranaceus

Fig. 221 Larynx, Larynx, and hyoid bone, Os hyoideum; median section; medial view.

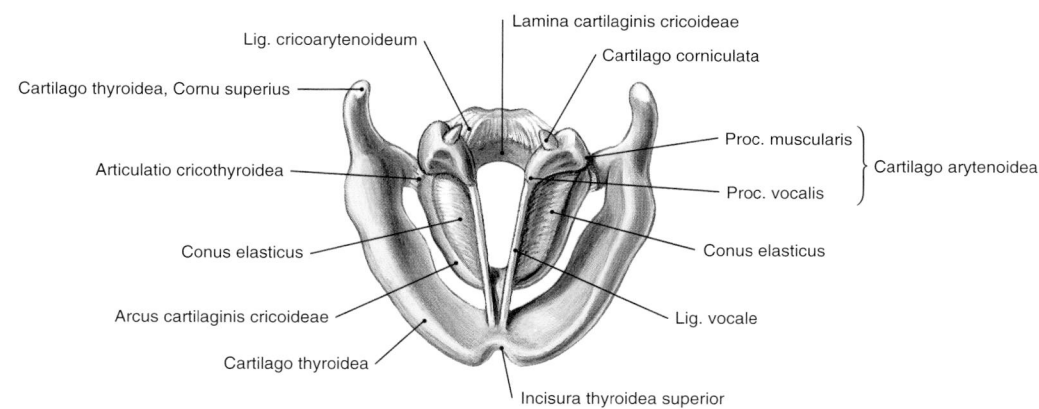

Lig. cricoarytenoideum
Lamina cartilaginis cricoideae
Cartilago corniculata
Cartilago thyroidea, Cornu superius
Proc. muscularis
Proc. vocalis
Cartilago arytenoidea
Articulatio cricothyroidea
Conus elasticus
Conus elasticus
Arcus cartilaginis cricoideae
Lig. vocale
Cartilago thyroidea
Incisura thyroidea superior

Fig. 222   Cartilages of the larynx, Cartilagines laryngis, and vocal ligament, Lig. vocale; ventrosuperior view.

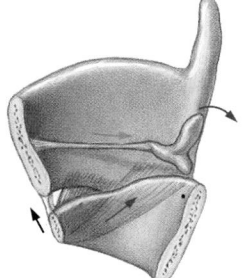

a Cricothyroid muscle, M. cricothyroideus

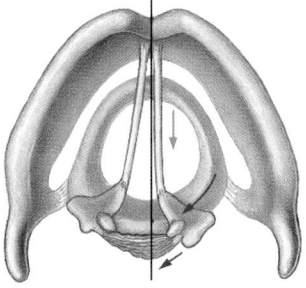

b Oblique and transverse arytenoid muscles, Mm. arytenoidei obliquus et transversus

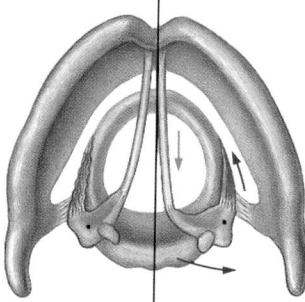

c Lateral crico-arytenoid muscle, M. cricoarytenoideus lateralis

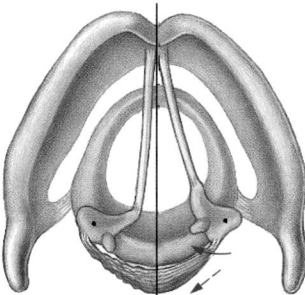

d Posterior crico-arytenoid muscle, M. cricoarytenoideus posterior

Fig. 223 a–d   Schema showing the functions of the laryngeal muscles, Mm. laryngis; yellow arrows: tension of the vocal ligament; red arrows: muscle contraction; blue arrows: direction of rotation;

the muscles on the left are relaxed; those on the right are contracted; superior view.

Laryngeal muscles

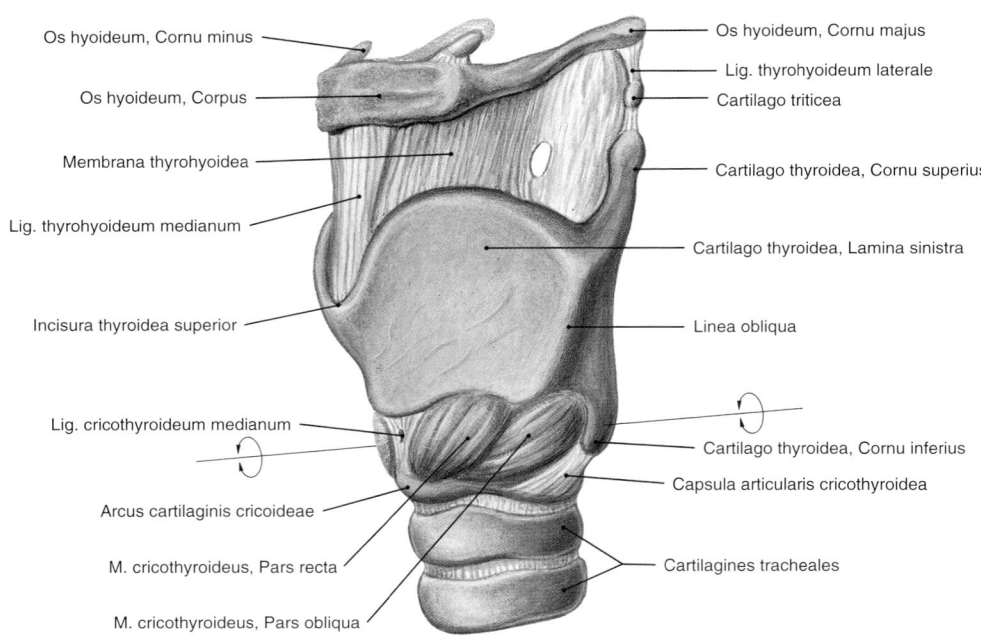

Os hyoideum, Cornu minus

Os hyoideum, Corpus

Membrana thyrohyoidea

Lig. thyrohyoideum medianum

Incisura thyroidea superior

Lig. cricothyroideum medianum

Arcus cartilaginis cricoideae

M. cricothyroideus, Pars recta

M. cricothyroideus, Pars obliqua

Os hyoideum, Cornu majus

Lig. thyrohyoideum laterale

Cartilago triticea

Cartilago thyroidea, Cornu superius

Cartilago thyroidea, Lamina sinistra

Linea obliqua

Cartilago thyroidea, Cornu inferius

Capsula articularis cricothyroidea

Cartilagines tracheales

→ T 6

Fig. 224 Cricothyroid muscle,
M. cricothyroideus;
ventral view from the left.

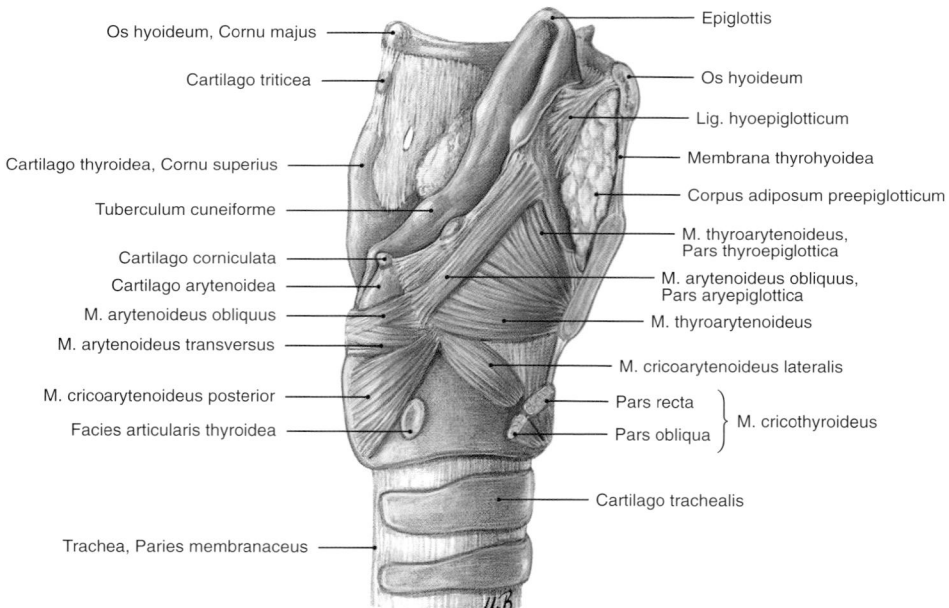

Os hyoideum, Cornu majus

Cartilago triticea

Cartilago thyroidea, Cornu superius

Tuberculum cuneiforme

Cartilago corniculata

Cartilago arytenoidea

M. arytenoideus obliquus

M. arytenoideus transversus

M. cricoarytenoideus posterior

Facies articularis thyroidea

Trachea, Paries membranaceus

Epiglottis

Os hyoideum

Lig. hyoepiglotticum

Membrana thyrohyoidea

Corpus adiposum preepiglotticum

M. thyroarytenoideus,
Pars thyroepiglottica

M. arytenoideus obliquus,
Pars aryepiglottica

M. thyroarytenoideus

M. cricoarytenoideus lateralis

Pars recta ⎫
Pars obliqua ⎭ M. cricothyroideus

Cartilago trachealis

→ T 6

Fig. 225 Laryngeal muscles, Mm. laryngis;
dorsal view from the right.

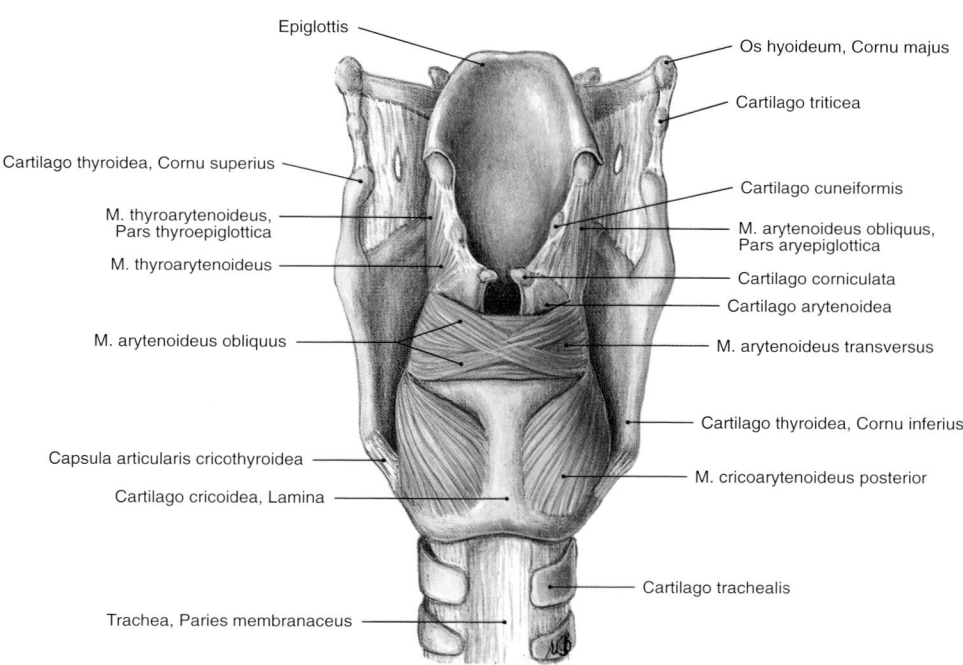

Epiglottis

Os hyoideum, Cornu majus

Cartilago triticea

Cartilago thyroidea, Cornu superius

Cartilago cuneiformis

M. thyroarytenoideus, Pars thyroepiglottica

M. arytenoideus obliquus, Pars aryepiglottica

M. thyroarytenoideus

Cartilago corniculata

Cartilago arytenoidea

M. arytenoideus obliquus

M. arytenoideus transversus

Cartilago thyroidea, Cornu inferius

Capsula articularis cricothyroidea

M. cricoarytenoideus posterior

Cartilago cricoidea, Lamina

Cartilago trachealis

Trachea, Paries membranaceus

Fig. 226   Laryngeal muscles, Mm. laryngis; dorsal view.

→ T 6

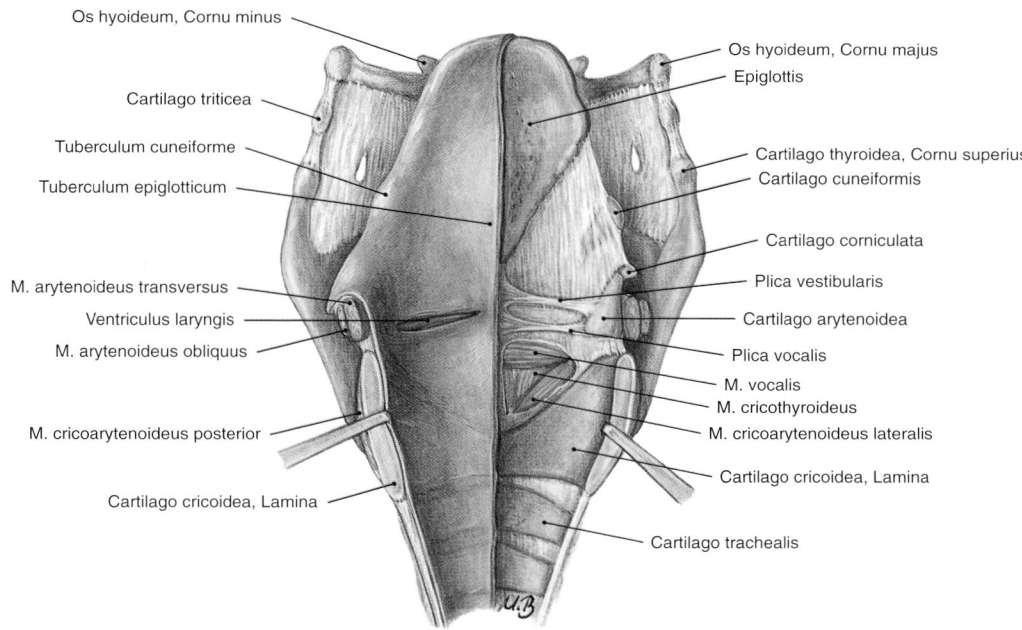

Os hyoideum, Cornu minus

Os hyoideum, Cornu majus

Epiglottis

Cartilago triticea

Tuberculum cuneiforme

Cartilago thyroidea, Cornu superius

Tuberculum epiglotticum

Cartilago cuneiformis

Cartilago corniculata

M. arytenoideus transversus

Plica vestibularis

Ventriculus laryngis

Cartilago arytenoidea

M. arytenoideus obliquus

Plica vocalis

M. vocalis

M. cricothyroideus

M. cricoarytenoideus posterior

M. cricoarytenoideus lateralis

Cartilago cricoidea, Lamina

Cartilago cricoidea, Lamina

Cartilago trachealis

Fig. 227   Larynx, Larynx; sectioned from dorsal in the median plane and separated with hooks; dorsal view.

→ T 6

Laryngoscopy

Fig. 228 a, b Laryngoscopy.
a Indirect laryngoscopy
b Direct, endoscopic laryngoscopy

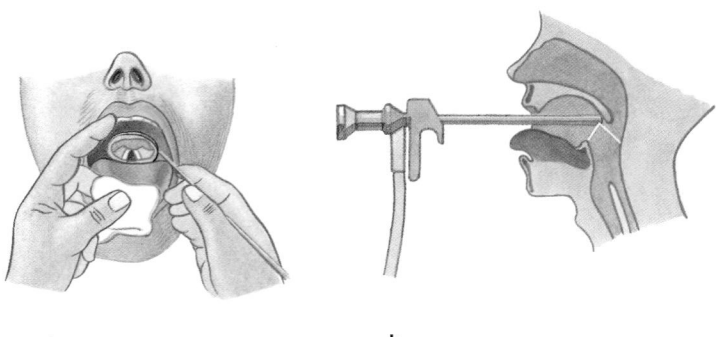

a   b

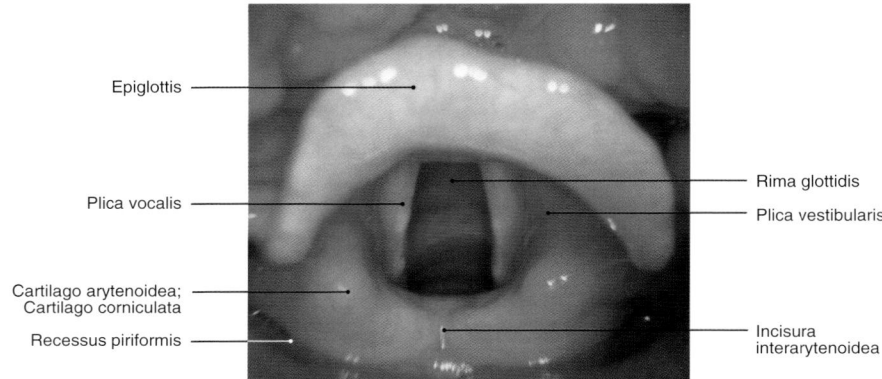

Epiglottis

Plica vocalis

Cartilago arytenoidea;
Cartilago corniculata

Recessus piriformis

Rima glottidis

Plica vestibularis

Incisura
interarytenoidea

Fig. 229 Direct laryngoscopy;
respiratory position.

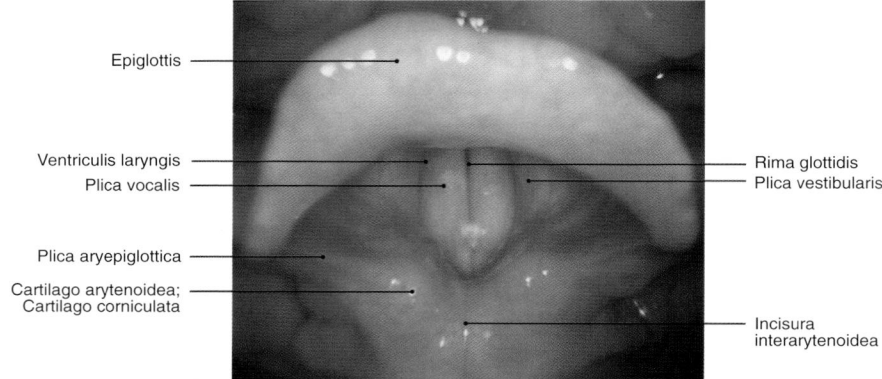

Epiglottis

Ventriculis laryngis
Plica vocalis

Plica aryepiglottica

Cartilago arytenoidea;
Cartilago corniculata

Rima glottidis
Plica vestibularis

Incisura
interarytenoidea

Fig. 230 Direct laryngoscopy;
phonation position.

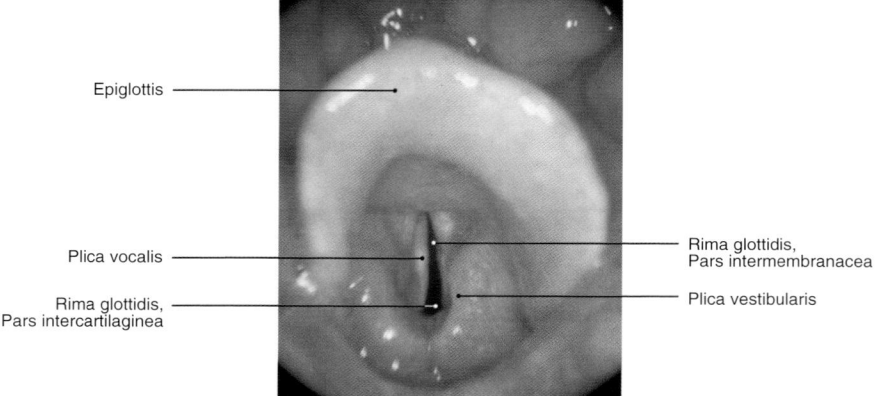

Epiglottis

Plica vocalis

Rima glottidis,
Pars intercartilaginea

Rima glottidis,
Pars intermembranacea

Plica vestibularis

Fig. 231 Direct laryngoscopy;
whispering position.

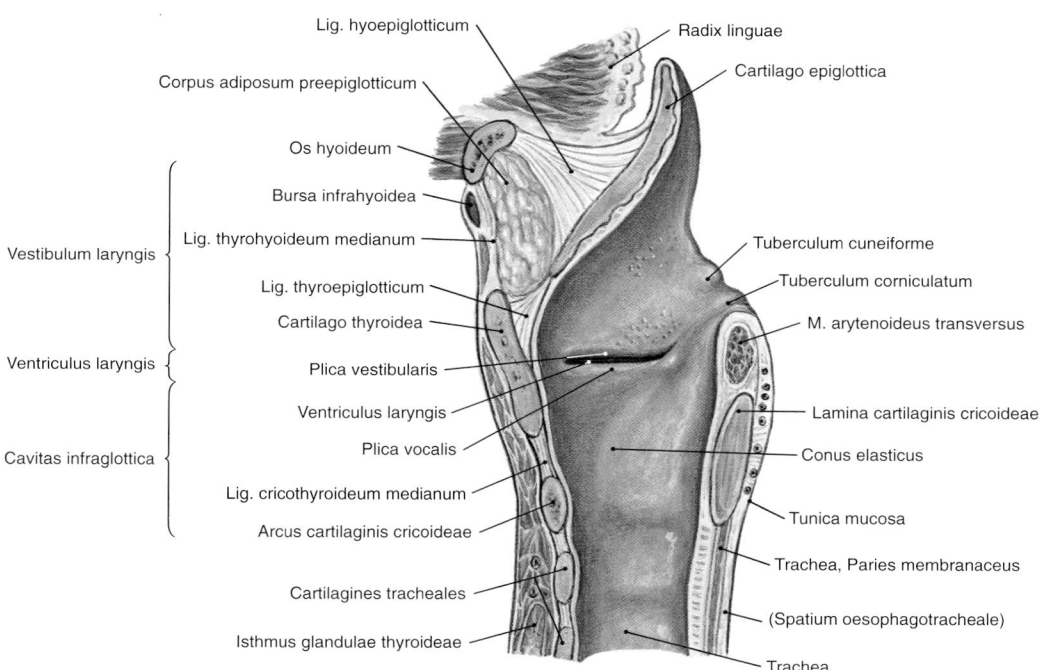

Lig. hyoepiglotticum
Radix linguae
Corpus adiposum preepiglotticum
Cartilago epiglottica
Os hyoideum
Bursa infrahyoidea
Vestibulum laryngis
Lig. thyrohyoideum medianum
Tuberculum cuneiforme
Tuberculum corniculatum
Lig. thyroepiglotticum
M. arytenoideus transversus
Cartilago thyroidea
Ventriculus laryngis
Plica vestibularis
Ventriculus laryngis
Lamina cartilaginis cricoideae
Plica vocalis
Conus elasticus
Cavitas infraglottica
Lig. cricothyroideum medianum
Tunica mucosa
Arcus cartilaginis cricoideae
Trachea, Paries membranaceus
Cartilagines tracheales
(Spatium oesophagotracheale)
Isthmus glandulae thyroideae
Trachea

Fig. 232   Larynx, Larynx.

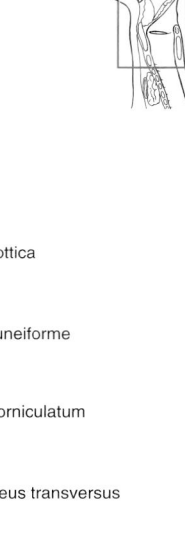

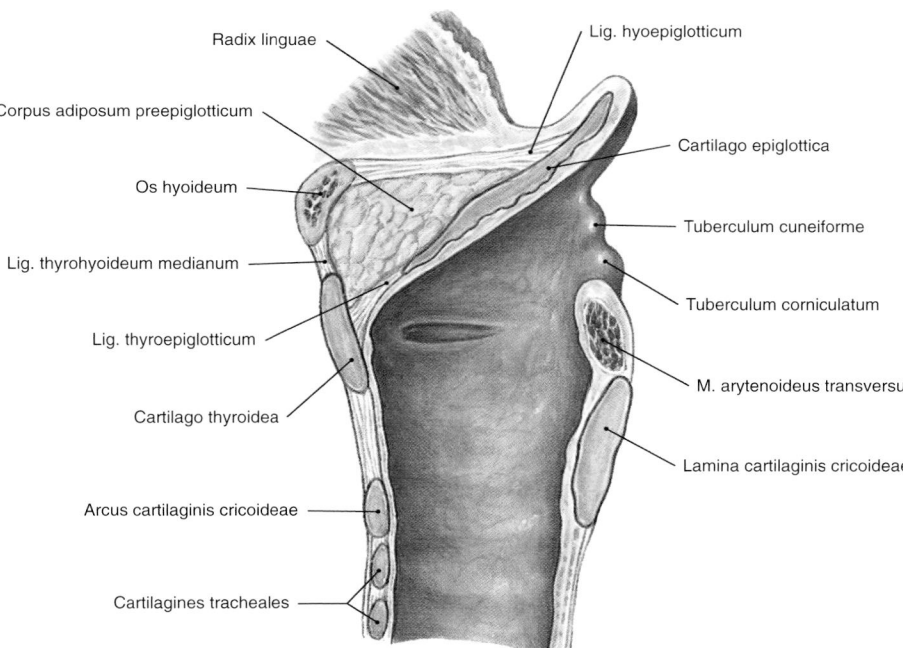

Radix linguae
Lig. hyoepiglotticum
Corpus adiposum preepiglotticum
Cartilago epiglottica
Os hyoideum
Lig. thyrohyoideum medianum
Tuberculum cuneiforme
Lig. thyroepiglotticum
Tuberculum corniculatum
Cartilago thyroidea
M. arytenoideus transversus
Lamina cartilaginis cricoideae
Arcus cartilaginis cricoideae
Cartilagines tracheales

Fig. 233   Larynx, Larynx;
position of the epiglottis during swallowing.

Arteries and nerves of the larynx

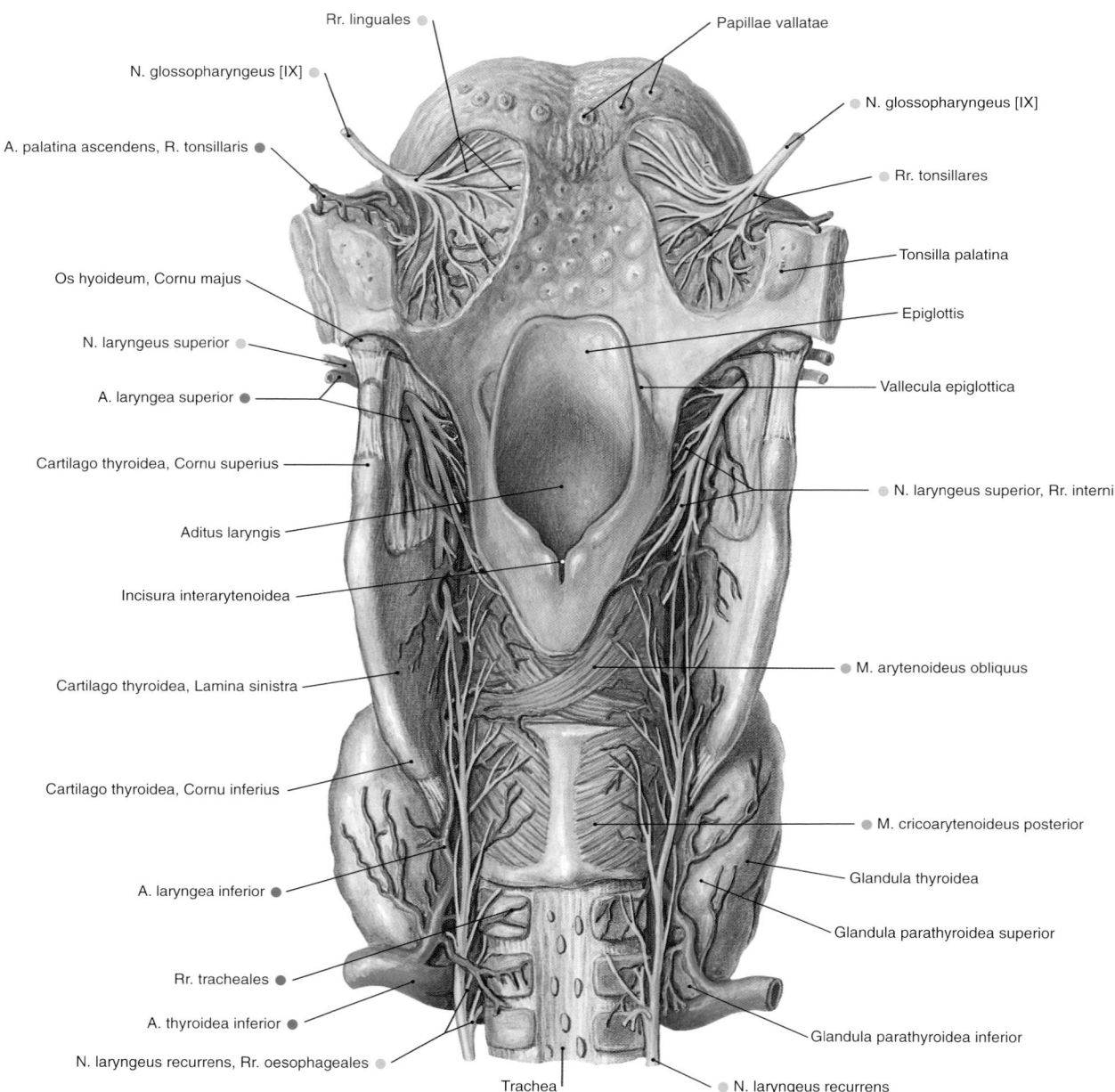

Rr. linguales

N. glossopharyngeus [IX]

A. palatina ascendens, R. tonsillaris

Os hyoideum, Cornu majus

N. laryngeus superior

A. laryngea superior

Cartilago thyroidea, Cornu superius

Aditus laryngis

Incisura interarytenoidea

Cartilago thyroidea, Lamina sinistra

Cartilago thyroidea, Cornu inferius

A. laryngea inferior

Rr. tracheales

A. thyroidea inferior

N. laryngeus recurrens, Rr. oesophageales

Trachea

Papillae vallatae

N. glossopharyngeus [IX]

Rr. tonsillares

Tonsilla palatina

Epiglottis

Vallecula epiglottica

N. laryngeus superior, Rr. interni

M. arytenoideus obliquus

M. cricoarytenoideus posterior

Glandula thyroidea

Glandula parathyroidea superior

Glandula parathyroidea inferior

N. laryngeus recurrens

→ 252

Fig. 234   Arteries and nerves of the larynx, Larynx, and the root of the tongue, Radix linguae.

Larynx, transverse sections

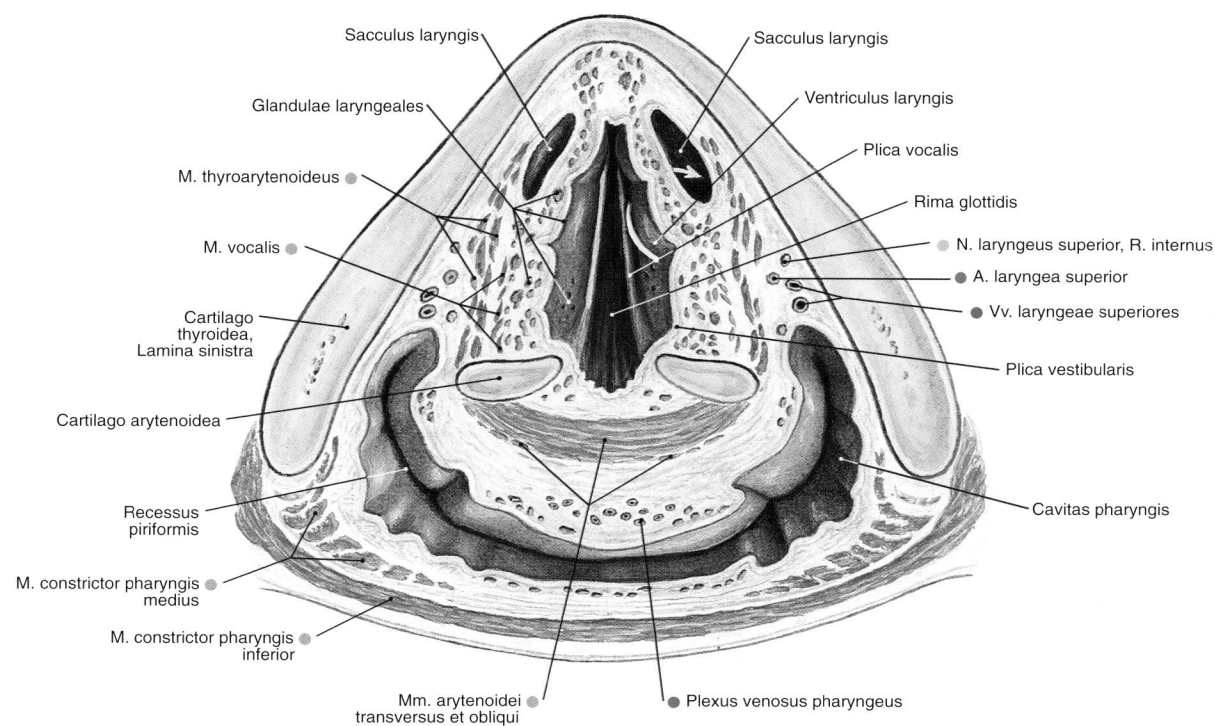

Sacculus laryngis
Glandulae laryngeales
M. thyroarytenoideus
M. vocalis
Cartilago thyroidea, Lamina sinistra
Cartilago arytenoidea
Recessus piriformis
M. constrictor pharyngis medius
M. constrictor pharyngis inferior
Mm. arytenoidei transversus et obliqui
Sacculus laryngis
Ventriculus laryngis
Plica vocalis
Rima glottidis
N. laryngeus superior, R. internus
A. laryngea superior
Vv. laryngeae superiores
Plica vestibularis
Cavitas pharyngis
Plexus venosus pharyngeus

Fig. 235   Larynx, Larynx.
The white arrow indicates the connection between the laryngeal ventricle and the laryngeal saccule.

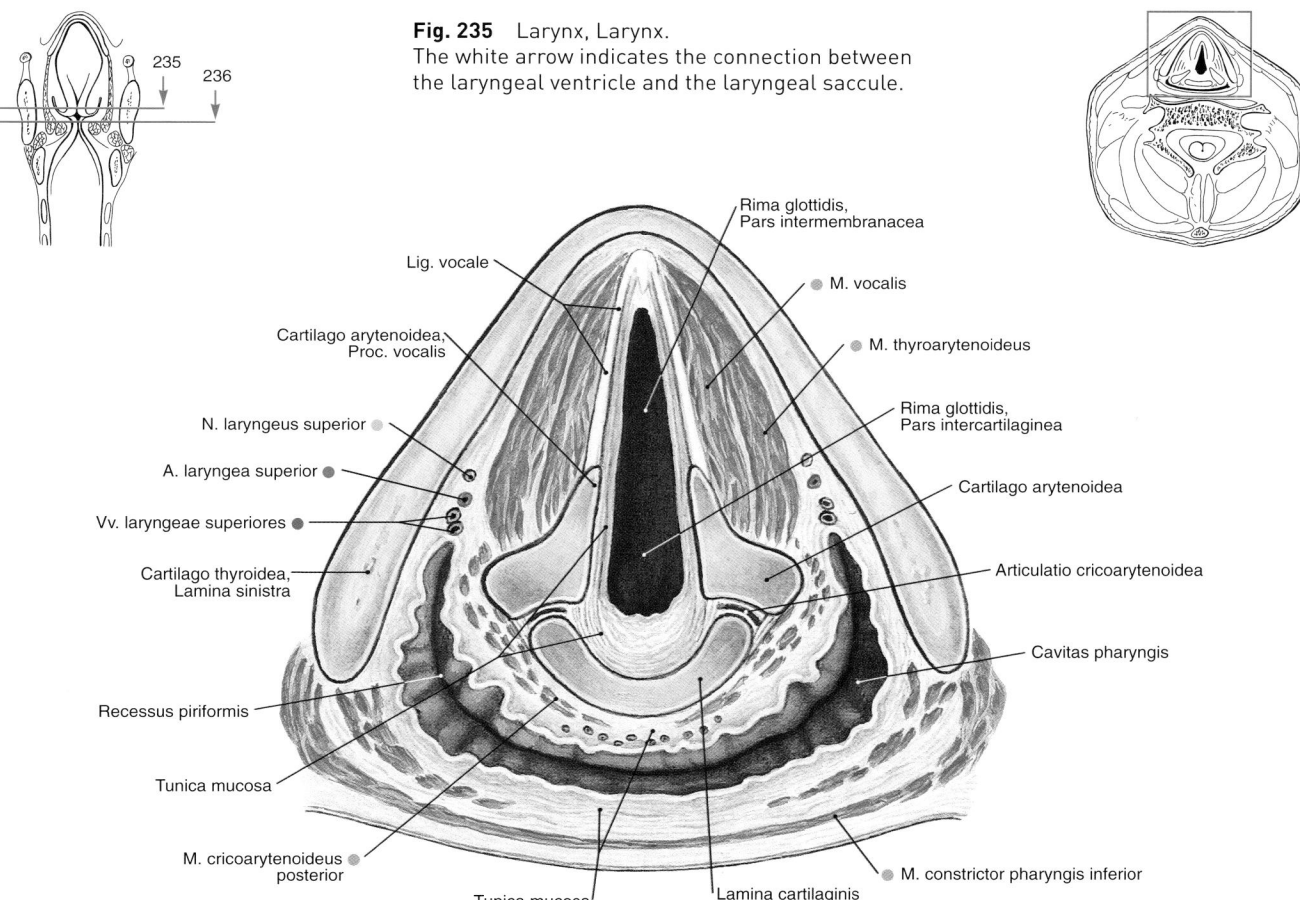

Rima glottidis, Pars intermembranacea
Lig. vocale
Cartilago arytenoidea, Proc. vocalis
N. laryngeus superior
A. laryngea superior
Vv. laryngeae superiores
Cartilago thyroidea, Lamina sinistra
Recessus piriformis
Tunica mucosa
M. cricoarytenoideus posterior
Tunica mucosa
Lamina cartilaginis cricoideae
M. vocalis
M. thyroarytenoideus
Rima glottidis, Pars intercartilaginea
Cartilago arytenoidea
Articulatio cricoarytenoidea
Cavitas pharyngis
M. constrictor pharyngis inferior

Fig. 236   Larynx, Larynx.

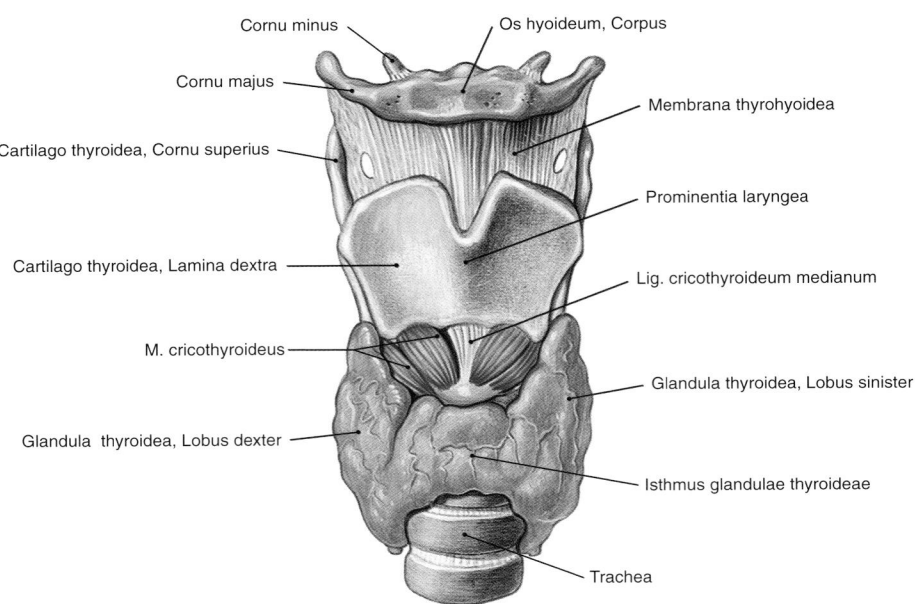

→ 205

Fig. 237 Thyroid gland, Glandula thyroidea, and larynx, Larynx.

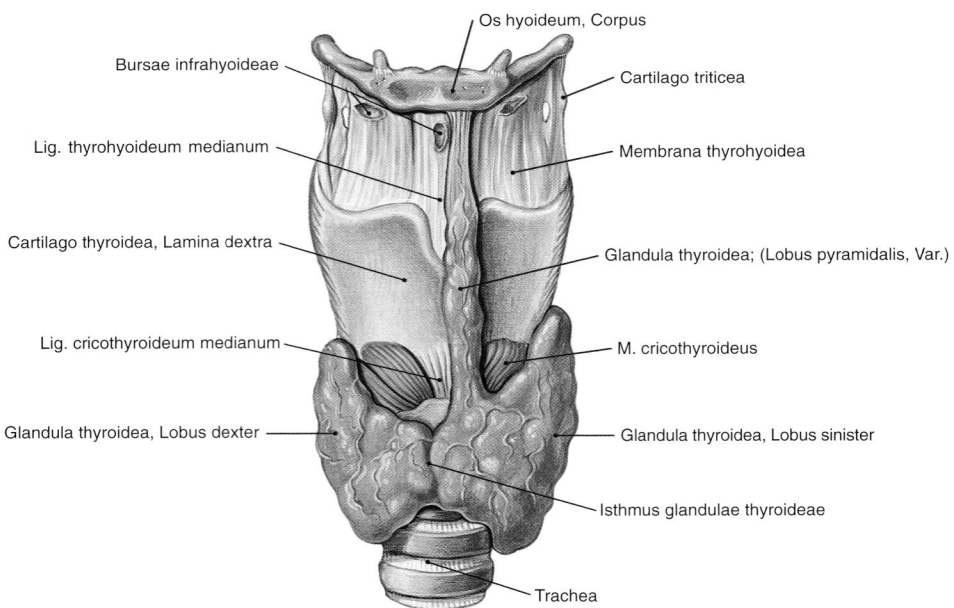

Fig. 238 Thyroid gland, Glandula thyroidea, and larynx, Larynx.

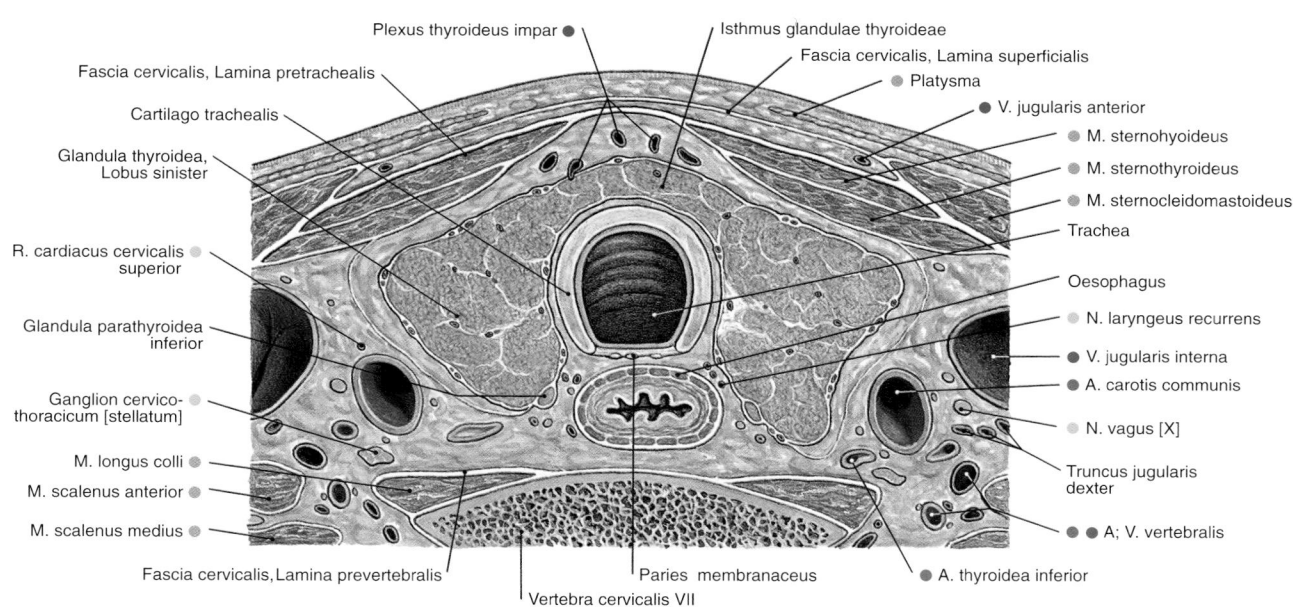

Plexus thyroideus impar ●
Fascia cervicalis, Lamina pretrachealis
Cartilago trachealis
Glandula thyroidea, Lobus sinister
R. cardiacus cervicalis ● superior
Glandula parathyroidea inferior
Ganglion cervico- ● thoracicum [stellatum]
M. longus colli ●
M. scalenus anterior ●
M. scalenus medius ●
Fascia cervicalis, Lamina prevertebralis
Vertebra cervicalis VII

Isthmus glandulae thyroideae
Fascia cervicalis, Lamina superficialis
● Platysma
● V. jugularis anterior
● M. sternohyoideus
● M. sternothyroideus
● M. sternocleidomastoideus
Trachea
Oesophagus
● N. laryngeus recurrens
● V. jugularis interna
● A. carotis communis
● N. vagus [X]
Truncus jugularis dexter
● ● A; V. vertebralis
● A. thyroidea inferior
Paries membranaceus

Fig. 239 Thyroid gland, Glandula thyroidea; horizontal section.

239 ↓   ←240

Cartilago epiglottica
Os hyoideum
Membrana thyrohyoidea
Membrana quadrangularis
Fascia cervicalis, Lamina pretrachealis
Lig. vestibulare
Rima vestibuli
Ventriculus laryngis
Cartilago thyroidea
Lig. vocale
A; V. thyroidea superior
Rima glottidis
Cavitas infraglottica
Cartilago cricoidea
Lig. cricotracheale
Cartilago trachealis

Vestibulum laryngis
M. arytenoideus obliquus, Pars aryepiglottica
Sacculus laryngis
M. thyrohyoideus
Plica vestibularis
Plica vocalis
M. constrictor pharyngis inferior, Pars thyropharyngea
M. sternothyroideus
M. cricoarytenoideus lateralis
M. vocalis
M. cricothyroideus
Conus elasticus
Glandula thyroidea
Trachea
Glandula parathyroidea inferior

Fig. 240 Thyroid gland, Glandula thyroidea; frontal section.

Arterial supply of the thyroid gland

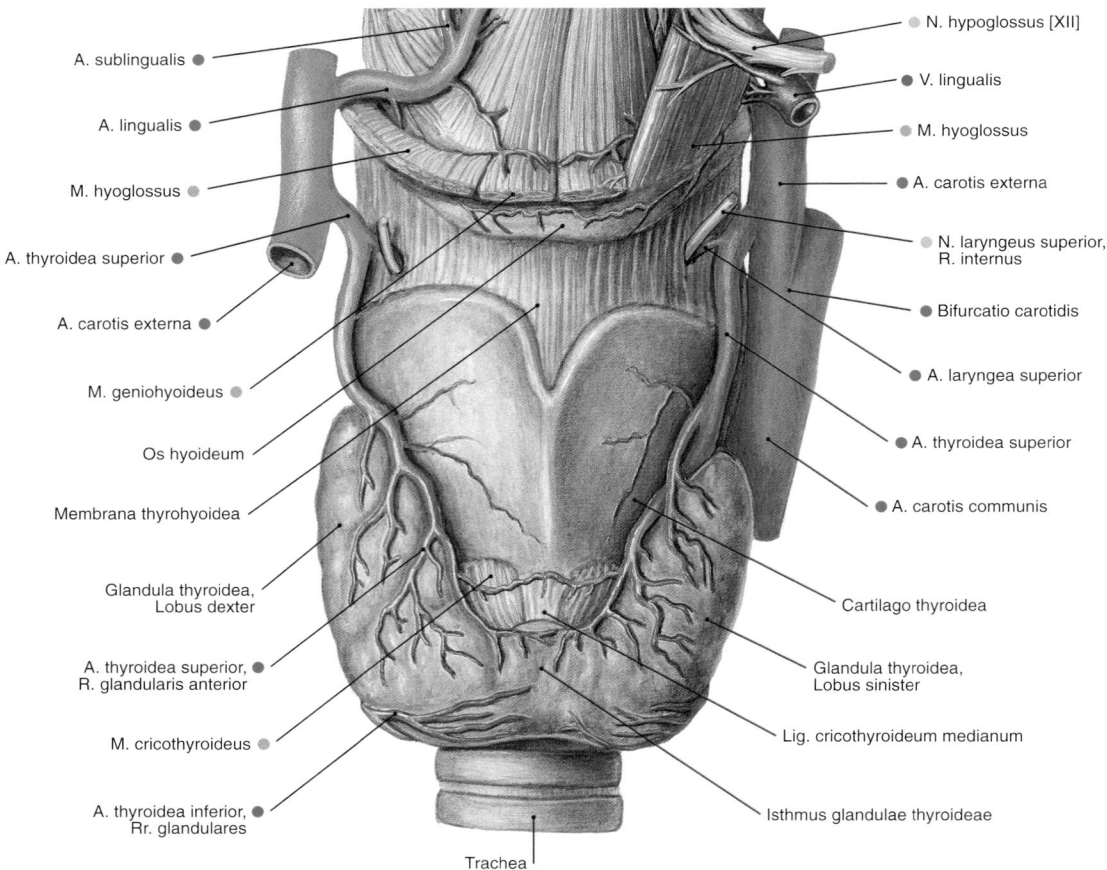

A. sublingualis ●

A. lingualis ●

M. hyoglossus ●

A. thyroidea superior ●

A. carotis externa ●

M. geniohyoideus ●

Os hyoideum

Membrana thyrohyoidea

Glandula thyroidea,
Lobus dexter

A. thyroidea superior, ●
R. glandularis anterior

M. cricothyroideus ●

A. thyroidea inferior, ●
Rr. glandulares

Trachea

● N. hypoglossus [XII]

● V. lingualis

● M. hyoglossus

● A. carotis externa

● N. laryngeus superior,
R. internus

● Bifurcatio carotidis

● A. laryngea superior

● A. thyroidea superior

● A. carotis communis

Cartilago thyroidea

Glandula thyroidea,
Lobus sinister

Lig. cricothyroideum medianum

Isthmus glandulae thyroideae

Fig. 241 Vessels and nerves of the thyroid gland,
Glandula thyroidea, and the larynx, Larynx.

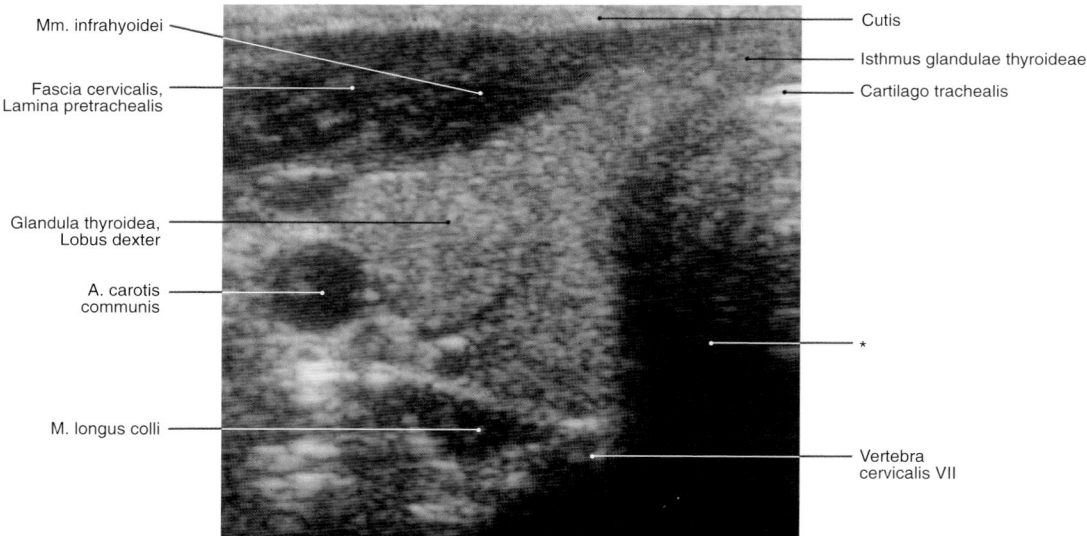

Mm. infrahyoidei

Fascia cervicalis,
Lamina pretrachealis

Glandula thyroidea,
Lobus dexter

A. carotis
communis

M. longus colli

Cutis

Isthmus glandulae thyroideae

Cartilago trachealis

*

Vertebra
cervicalis VII

Fig. 242 Thyroid gland, Glandula thyroidea;
oblique ultrasound image in ventrodorsal direction;
inferior view (right, 200%).
* Ultrasound shadow of the trachea

Pathological enlargement of the thyroid gland

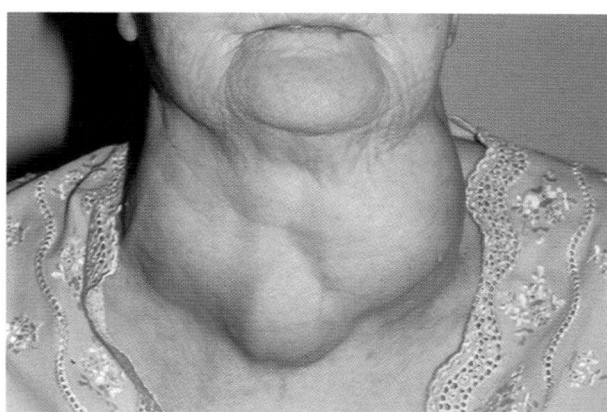

Fig. 243 Thyroid gland, Glandula thyroidea;
enlargement of the thyroid gland with three obvious nodes, Struma nodosa.

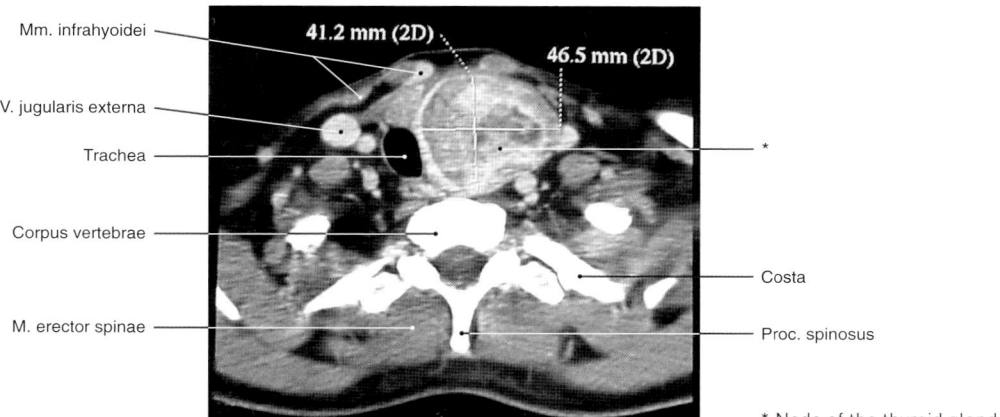

Mm. infrahyoidei

41.2 mm (2D)

46.5 mm (2D)

V. jugularis externa

Trachea

Corpus vertebrae

M. erector spinae

*

Costa

Proc. spinosus

* Node of the thyroid gland

Fig. 244 Neck, Collum;
computed tomographic (CT) section;
inferior view.
The trachea is displaced towards the right by a pathologically enlarged
node of the thyroid gland.

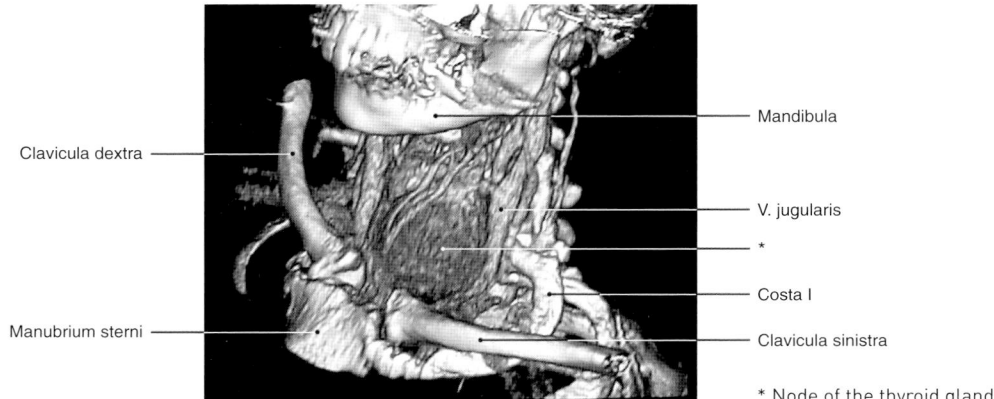

Clavicula dextra

Manubrium sterni

Mandibula

V. jugularis

*

Costa I

Clavicula sinistra

* Node of the thyroid gland

Fig. 245 Neck, Collum;
3-dimensional reconstruction from computed tomographic (CT) sections
showing a heavily enlarged left lobe of the thyroid gland;
same patient as in Fig. 244.

Nasal and pharyngeal cavity, paramedian section

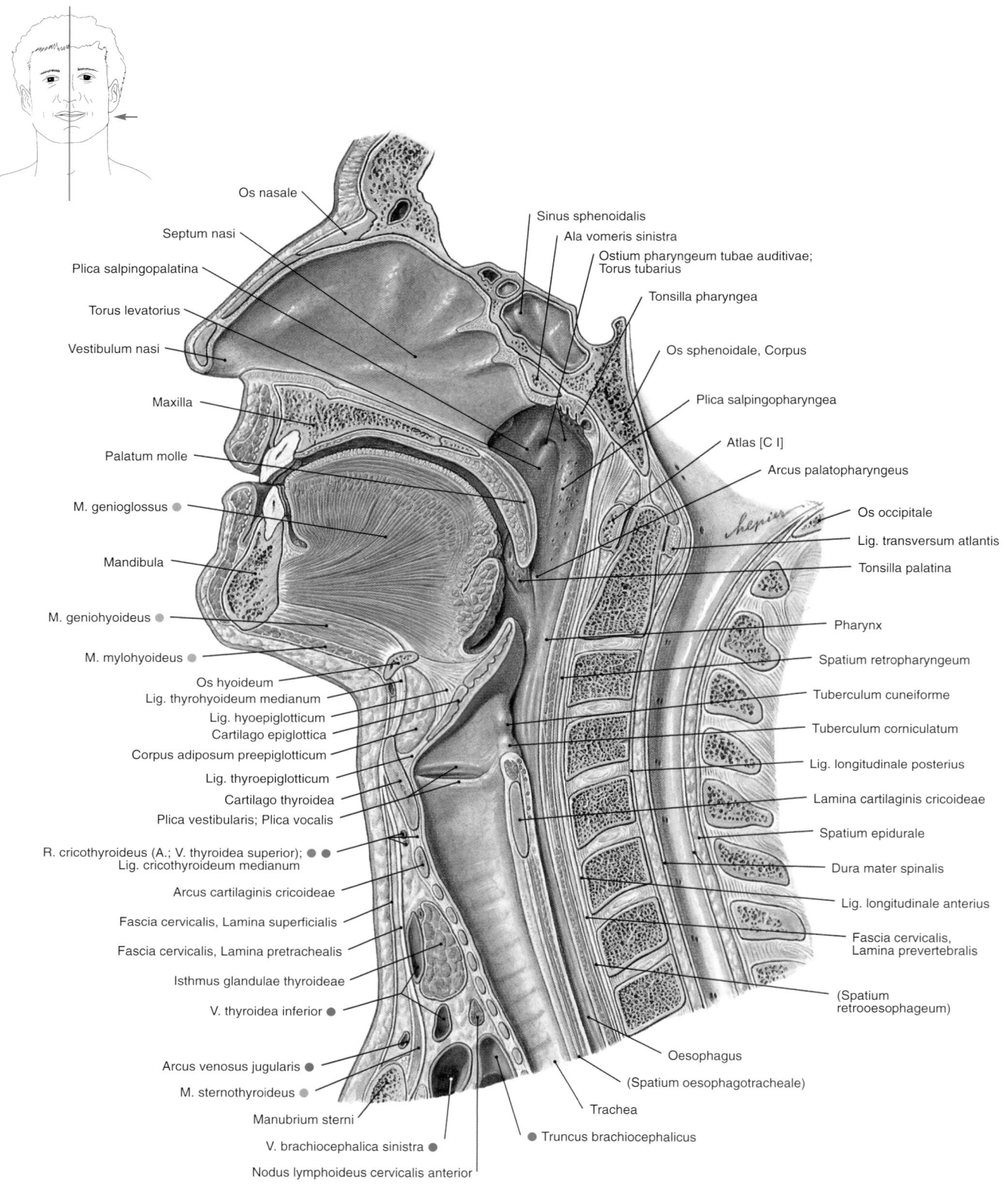

Os nasale

Septum nasi

Plica salpingopalatina

Torus levatorius

Vestibulum nasi

Maxilla

Palatum molle

M. genioglossus ●

Mandibula

M. geniohyoideus ●

M. mylohyoideus ●

Os hyoideum
Lig. thyrohyoideum medianum
Lig. hyoepiglotticum
Cartilago epiglottica
Corpus adiposum preepiglotticum
Lig. thyroepiglotticum
Cartilago thyroidea
Plica vestibularis; Plica vocalis

R. cricothyroideus (A.; V. thyroidea superior); ● ●
Lig. cricothyroideum medianum

Arcus cartilaginis cricoideae

Fascia cervicalis, Lamina superficialis

Fascia cervicalis, Lamina pretrachealis

Isthmus glandulae thyroideae

V. thyroidea inferior ●

Arcus venosus jugularis ●

M. sternothyroideus ●

Manubrium sterni

V. brachiocephalica sinistra ●

Nodus lymphoideus cervicalis anterior

Sinus sphenoidalis

Ala vomeris sinistra

Ostium pharyngeum tubae auditivae;
Torus tubarius

Tonsilla pharyngea

Os sphenoidale, Corpus

Plica salpingopharyngea

Atlas [C I]

Arcus palatopharyngeus

Os occipitale

Lig. transversum atlantis

Tonsilla palatina

Pharynx

Spatium retropharyngeum

Tuberculum cuneiforme

Tuberculum corniculatum

Lig. longitudinale posterius

Lamina cartilaginis cricoideae

Spatium epidurale

Dura mater spinalis

Lig. longitudinale anterius

Fascia cervicalis,
Lamina prevertebralis

(Spatium
retrooesophageum)

Oesophagus

(Spatium oesophagotracheale)

Trachea

● Truncus brachiocephalicus

→ 271

Fig. 246 Nasal cavity, Cavitas nasi;
oral cavity, Cavitas oris; pharynx, Pharynx,
and larynx, Larynx;
paramedian section.

Pharyngeal muscles

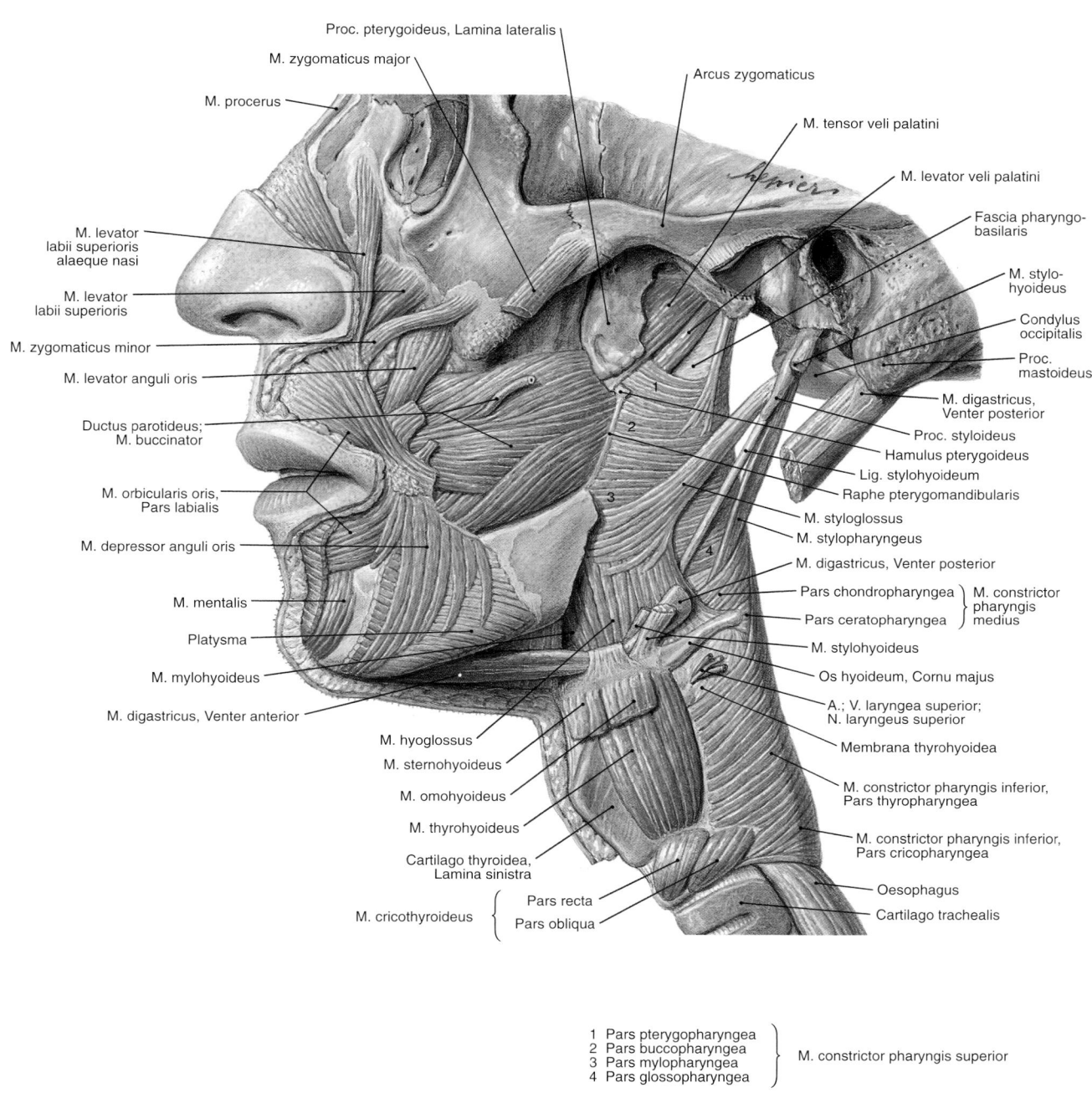

Proc. pterygoideus, Lamina lateralis

M. zygomaticus major

M. procerus

Arcus zygomaticus

M. tensor veli palatini

M. levator veli palatini

Fascia pharyngo-basilaris

M. levator labii superioris alaeque nasi

M. stylo-hyoideus

M. levator labii superioris

Condylus occipitalis

M. zygomaticus minor

Proc. mastoideus

M. levator anguli oris

M. digastricus, Venter posterior

Ductus parotideus; M. buccinator

Proc. styloideus

Hamulus pterygoideus

Lig. stylohyoideum

M. orbicularis oris, Pars labialis

Raphe pterygomandibularis

M. styloglossus

M. stylopharyngeus

M. depressor anguli oris

M. digastricus, Venter posterior

Pars chondropharyngea | M. constrictor pharyngis medius

M. mentalis

Pars ceratopharyngea

Platysma

M. stylohyoideus

M. mylohyoideus

Os hyoideum, Cornu majus

M. digastricus, Venter anterior

A.; V. laryngea superior; N. laryngeus superior

M. hyoglossus

Membrana thyrohyoidea

M. sternohyoideus

M. omohyoideus

M. constrictor pharyngis inferior, Pars thyropharyngea

M. thyrohyoideus

M. constrictor pharyngis inferior, Pars cricopharyngea

Cartilago thyroidea, Lamina sinistra

Oesophagus

Pars recta

M. cricothyroideus

Cartilago trachealis

Pars obliqua

1 Pars pterygopharyngea
2 Pars buccopharyngea
3 Pars mylopharyngea   M. constrictor pharyngis superior
4 Pars glossopharyngea

Fig. 247 Pharyngeal muscles, Mm. pharyngis, and facial muscles, Mm. faciei.

→ T 1 e, f, T 5

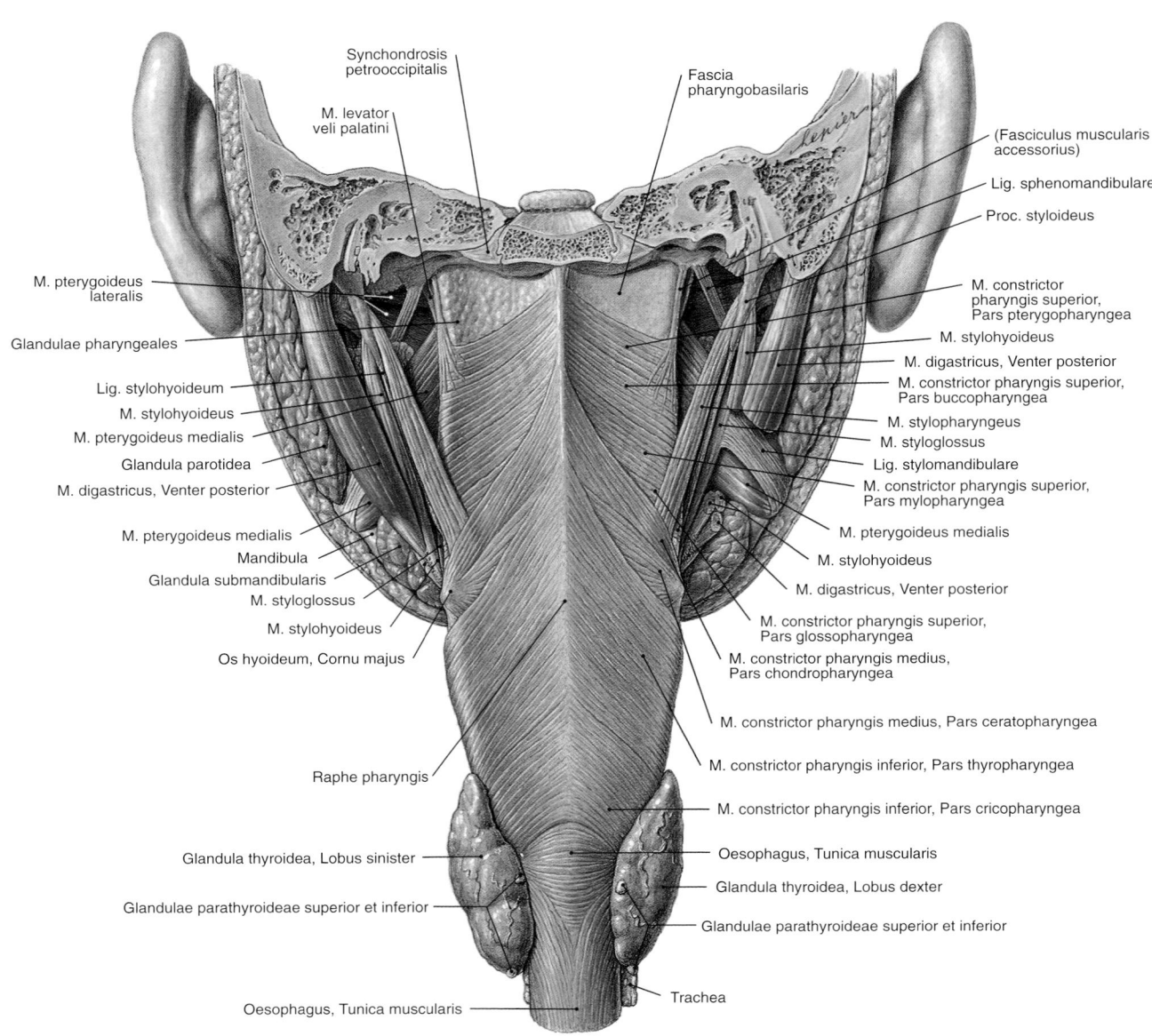

Synchondrosis petrooccipitalis

Fascia pharyngobasilaris

M. levator veli palatini

(Fasciculus muscularis accessorius)

Lig. sphenomandibulare

Proc. styloideus

M. pterygoideus lateralis

M. constrictor pharyngis superior, Pars pterygopharyngea

Glandulae pharyngeales

M. stylohyoideus

M. digastricus, Venter posterior

Lig. stylohyoideum

M. constrictor pharyngis superior, Pars buccopharyngea

M. stylohyoideus

M. stylopharyngeus

M. pterygoideus medialis

M. styloglossus

Glandula parotidea

Lig. stylomandibulare

M. digastricus, Venter posterior

M. constrictor pharyngis superior, Pars mylopharyngea

M. pterygoideus medialis

M. pterygoideus medialis

Mandibula

M. stylohyoideus

Glandula submandibularis

M. digastricus, Venter posterior

M. styloglossus

M. constrictor pharyngis superior, Pars glossopharyngea

M. stylohyoideus

M. constrictor pharyngis medius, Pars chondropharyngea

Os hyoideum, Cornu majus

M. constrictor pharyngis medius, Pars ceratopharyngea

M. constrictor pharyngis inferior, Pars thyropharyngea

Raphe pharyngis

M. constrictor pharyngis inferior, Pars cricopharyngea

Glandula thyroidea, Lobus sinister

Oesophagus, Tunica muscularis

Glandula thyroidea, Lobus dexter

Glandulae parathyroideae superior et inferior

Glandulae parathyroideae superior et inferior

Trachea

Oesophagus, Tunica muscularis

→ T 5   **Fig. 248**   Pharyngeal muscles, Mm. pharyngis.

Inner contour of the pharynx

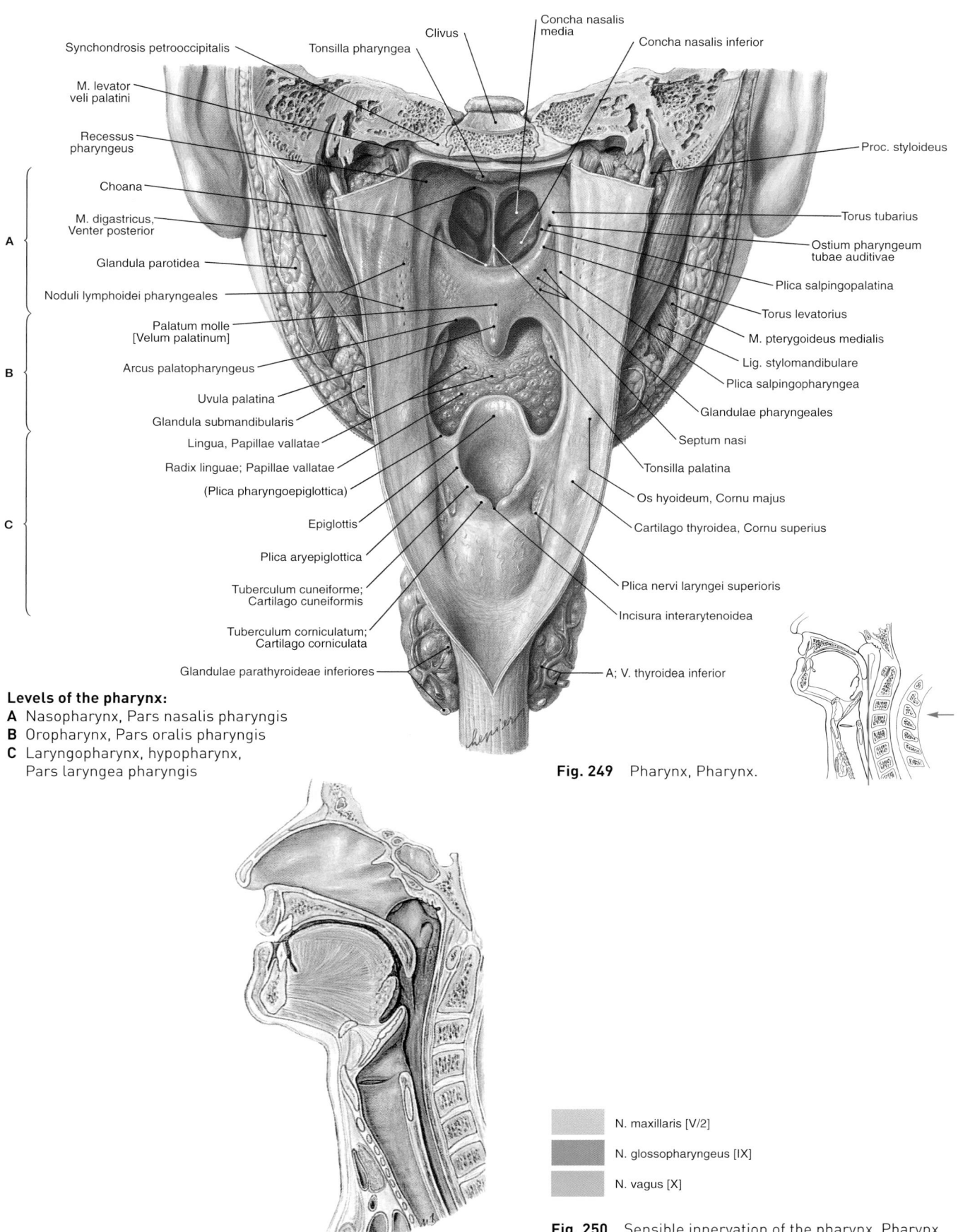

Synchondrosis petrooccipitalis

Tonsilla pharyngea

Clivus

Concha nasalis media

Concha nasalis inferior

M. levator veli palatini

Recessus pharyngeus

Proc. styloideus

Choana

Torus tubarius

M. digastricus, Venter posterior

Ostium pharyngeum tubae auditivae

Glandula parotidea

Plica salpingopalatina

Noduli lymphoidei pharyngeales

Torus levatorius

Palatum molle [Velum palatinum]

M. pterygoideus medialis

Arcus palatopharyngeus

Lig. stylomandibulare

Uvula palatina

Plica salpingopharyngea

Glandula submandibularis

Glandulae pharyngeales

Lingua, Papillae vallatae

Septum nasi

Radix linguae; Papillae vallatae

Tonsilla palatina

(Plica pharyngoepiglottica)

Os hyoideum, Cornu majus

Epiglottis

Cartilago thyroidea, Cornu superius

Plica aryepiglottica

Plica nervi laryngei superioris

Tuberculum cuneiforme; Cartilago cuneiformis

Incisura interarytenoidea

Tuberculum corniculatum; Cartilago corniculata

Glandulae parathyroideae inferiores

A; V. thyroidea inferior

Levels of the pharynx:
A Nasopharynx, Pars nasalis pharyngis
B Oropharynx, Pars oralis pharyngis
C Laryngopharynx, hypopharynx, Pars laryngea pharyngis

Fig. 249 Pharynx, Pharynx.

N. maxillaris [V/2]

N. glossopharyngeus [IX]

N. vagus [X]

Fig. 250 Sensible innervation of the pharynx, Pharynx.

Vessels and nerves of the parapharyngeal space

N. vagus [X]

N. glossopharyngeus [IX]

N. accessorius [XI], R. internus

M. constrictor pharyngis superior

Bulbus superior venae jugularis

Vv. pharyngeae

Foramen jugulare

Sinus transversus

Sinus sigmoideus

Os temporale

Ganglion superius

A. meningea posterior

A. carotis interna

N. caroticus internus

R. auricularis

Ganglion inferius (IX)

Proc. mastoideus

N. accessorius [XI], R. externus

A. carotis interna

Proc. styloideus

Ganglion inferius (X)

N. hypoglossus [XII]

N. jugularis (Truncus sympathicus)

M. stylopharyngeus

Ramus mandibulae

N. glossopharyngeus [IX]

Ganglion cervicale superius (Truncus sympathicus)

R. pharyngealis

A. pharyngea ascendens

M. digastricus, Venter posterior

N. glossopharyngeus [IX]

N. laryngeus superior

A. palatina ascendens

A. carotis externa

A. facialis

R. pharyngealis

A. lingualis

A. facialis

A. carotis externa

A. lingualis

N. laryngeus superior, R. externus

A. thyroidea superior

N. laryngeus superior, R. internus

N. cardiacus cervicalis superior (Truncus sympathicus)

M. constrictor pharyngis medius

A. thyroidea superior

V. jugularis interna

Rr. pharyngeales

R. pharyngealis

N. vagus [X]

M. constrictor pharyngis inferior

A. carotis communis

Plexus caroticus communis

Truncus sympathicus

Glandula thyroidea

Bulbus inferior venae jugularis

R. pharyngealis

Ganglion cervicale medium

A. thyroidea inferior

Ganglion cervicothoracicum [stellatum]

R. cardiacus cervicalis superior

N. cardiacus cervicalis medius (Truncus sympathicus)

Oesophagus

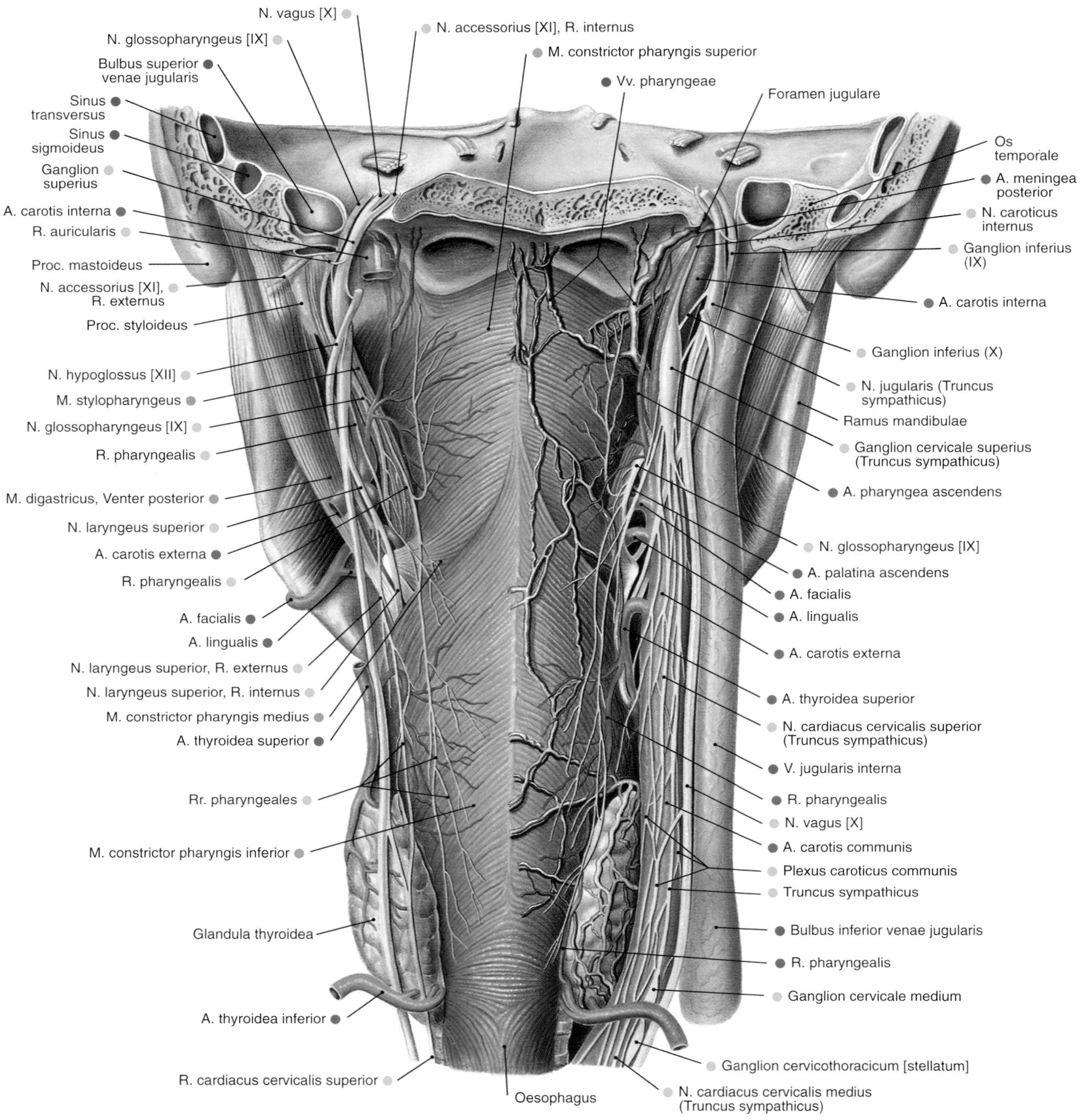

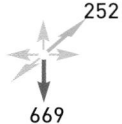

252

669

Fig. 251 Vessels and nerves of the pharynx, Pharynx, and the parapharyngeal space, Spatium lateropharyngeum.

Vessels and nerves of the parapharyngeal space

Truncus nervi accessorii, R. internus
N. vagus [X]
N. glossopharyngeus [IX]
Sinus transversus
Sinus sigmoideus
Ganglion inferius (X)
N. hypoglossus [XII]
Torus tubarius
M. digastricus, Venter posterior
M. uvulae
Plica salpingopharyngea
Tonsilla palatina
Arcus palatopharyngeus
Plica aryepiglottica
Cartilago thyroidea, Cornu superius
Tuberculum cuneiforme
Tuberculum corniculatum
Recessus piriformis, Plica nervi laryngei superioris
N. vagus [X]
Oesophagus, Tunica muscularis
Ganglion cervicale medium
A. thyroidea inferior
Bulbus inferior venae jugularis
Truncus thyrocervicalis
Ganglion cervicothoracicum [stellatum]
A.; V. subclavia
V. brachiocephalica sinistra
A. carotis communis
N. laryngeus recurrens
N. vagus [X]
Pars descendens aortae

Tonsilla pharyngea
Fascia pharyngobasilaris
Cartilago tubae auditivae; Ostium pharyngeum tubae auditivae
N. hypoglossus [XII]

N. vagus [X]
N. accessorius [XI]
Bulbus superior venae jugularis
A. carotis interna
N. accessorius [XI], R. externus
A. occipitalis
Proc. mastoideus
Ganglion cervicale superius (Truncus sympathicus)
M. tensor veli palatini
M. constrictor pharyngis superior
M. salpingopharyngeus
M. palatopharyngeus
Sulcus terminalis
Dorsum linguae, Pars posterior
Epiglottis
N. laryngeus superior; A.; V. laryngea superior
N. vagus [X]
M. arytenoideus transversus; M. arytenoideus obliquus
M. cricoarytenoideus posterior
Truncus sympathicus, Plexus caroticus communis
Glandula thyroidea
Glandula parathyroidea inferior
Truncus thyrocervicalis
N. vagus [X], R. cardiacus cervicalis superior
Bulbus inferior venae jugularis
A. subclavia
V. subclavia
N. vagus [X]
N. laryngeus recurrens
V. brachiocephalica dextra
Trachea, Paries membranaceus
Truncus brachiocephalicus
V. cava superior

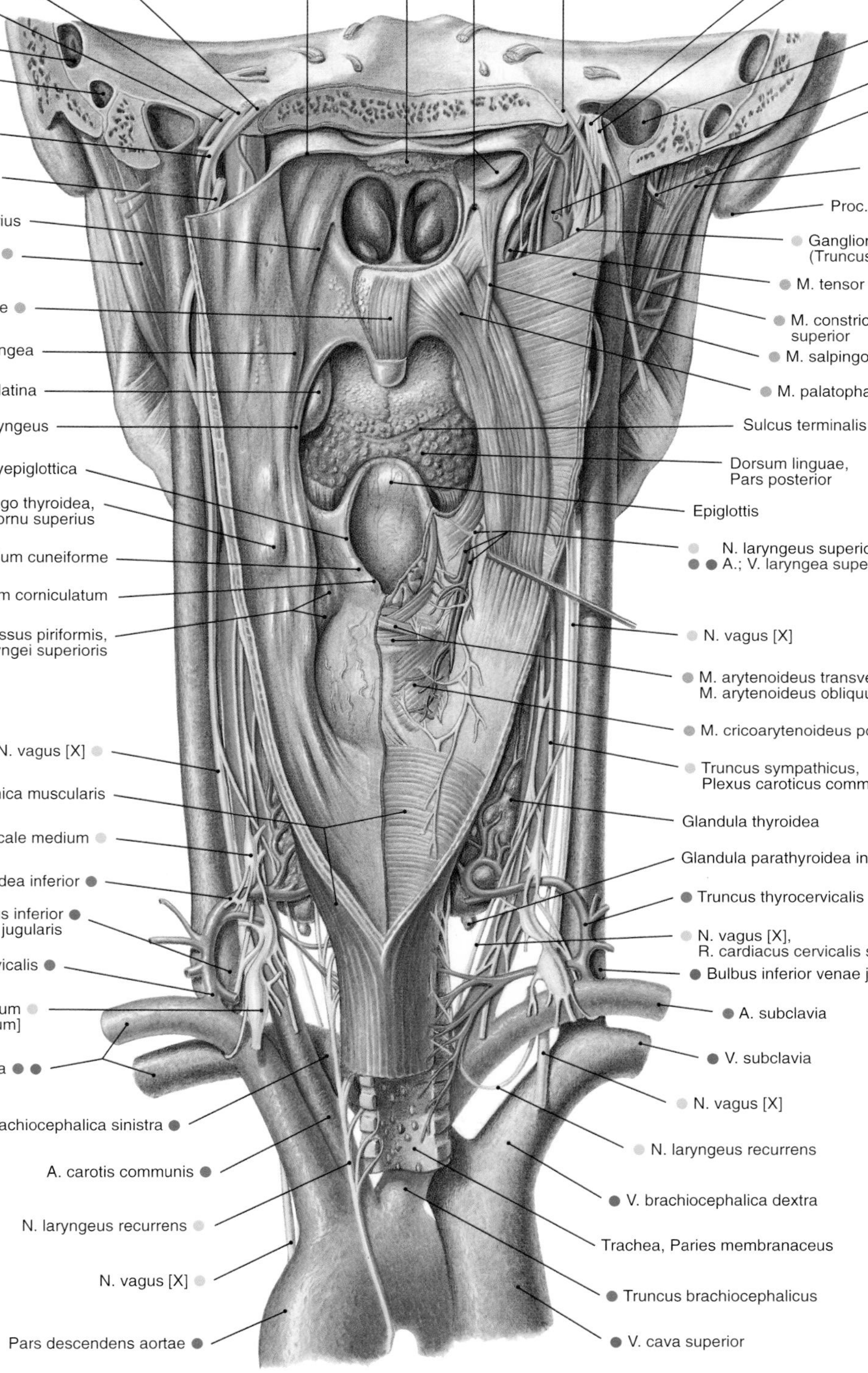

Fig. 252 Vessels and nerves of the pharynx, Pharynx, and the parapharyngeal space, Spatium lateropharyngeum.

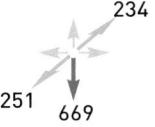

234
251 669

Vessels and nerves of the neck

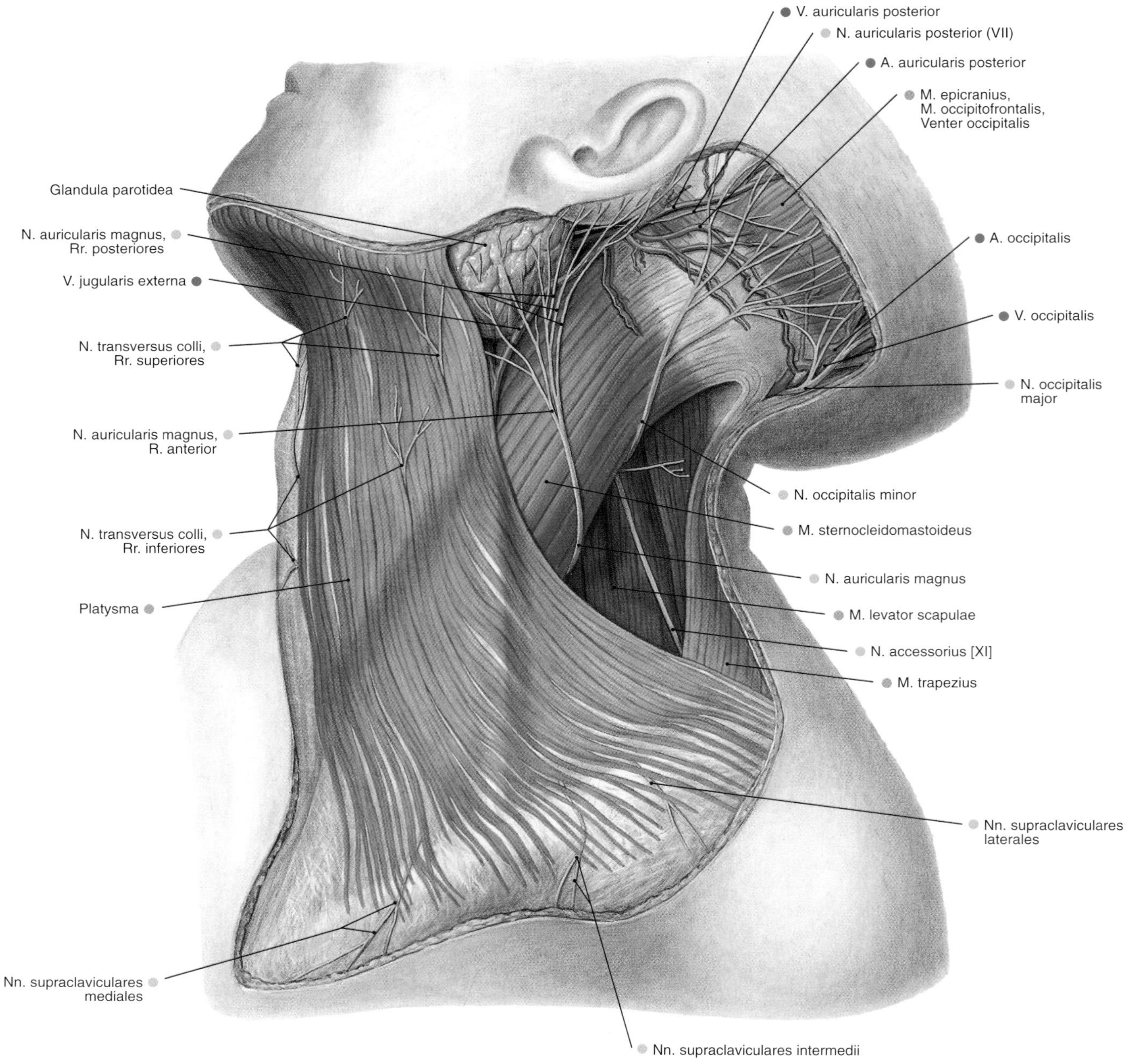

● V. auricularis posterior
● N. auricularis posterior (VII)
● A. auricularis posterior
● M. epicranius,
M. occipitofrontalis,
Venter occipitalis

Glandula parotidea

N. auricularis magnus, ●
Rr. posteriores

V. jugularis externa ●

N. transversus colli, ●
Rr. superiores

N. auricularis magnus, ●
R. anterior

● A. occipitalis

● V. occipitalis

● N. occipitalis
major

● N. occipitalis minor

● M. sternocleidomastoideus

● N. auricularis magnus

● M. levator scapulae

● N. accessorius [XI]

● M. trapezius

N. transversus colli, ●
Rr. inferiores

Platysma ●

● Nn. supraclaviculares
laterales

Nn. supraclaviculares ●
mediales

● Nn. supraclaviculares intermedii

→ 46, T 7

131
254

Fig. 253 Vessels and nerves of the anterior and the lateral region
of the neck, Regiones cervicales anterior et lateralis;
superficial layer.

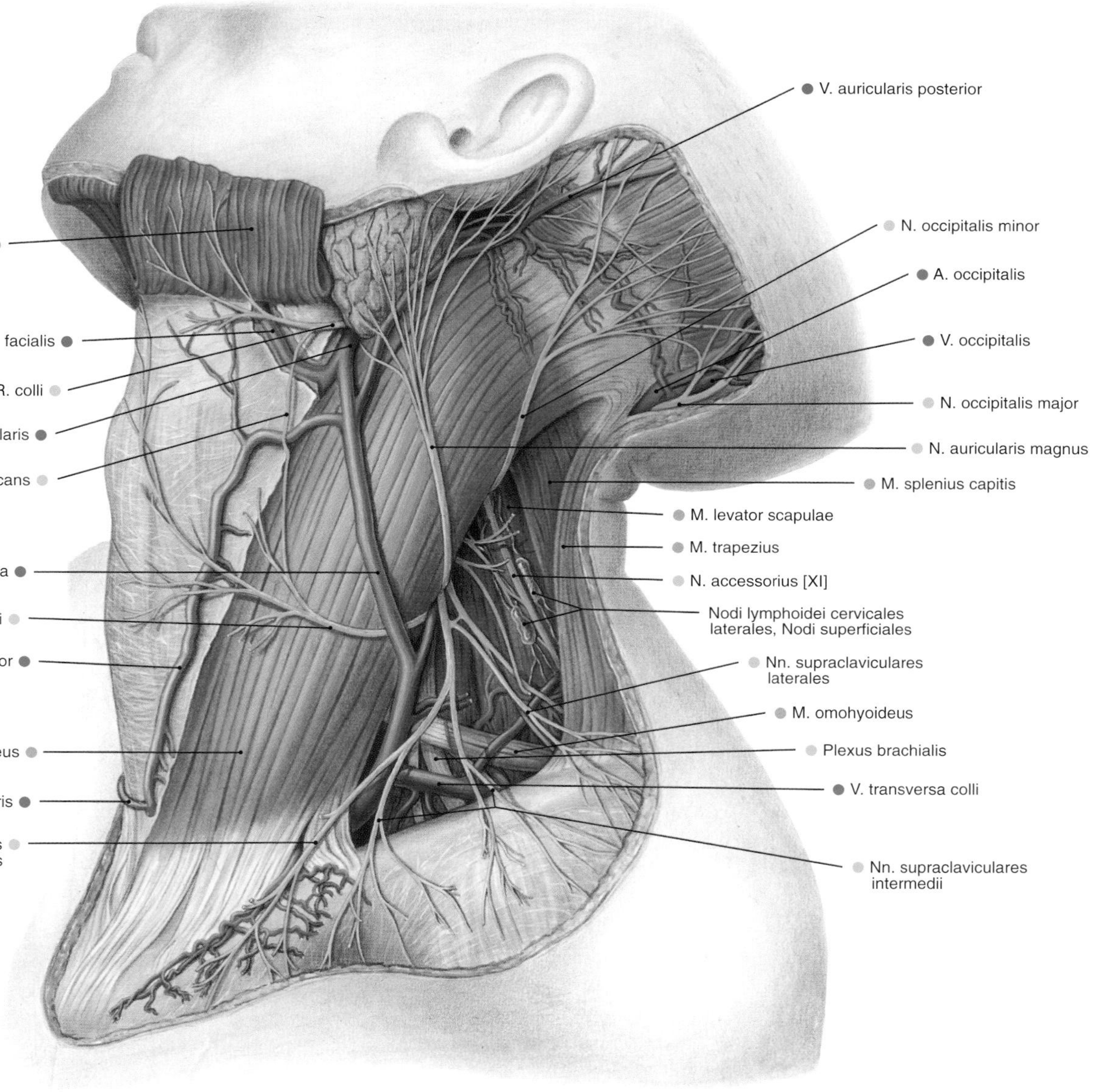

● V. auricularis posterior

● N. occipitalis minor

● A. occipitalis

● V. occipitalis

● N. occipitalis major

● N. auricularis magnus

● M. splenius capitis

● M. levator scapulae

● M. trapezius

● N. accessorius [XI]

Nodi lymphoidei cervicales laterales, Nodi superficiales

● Nn. supraclaviculares laterales

● M. omohyoideus

● Plexus brachialis

● V. transversa colli

● Nn. supraclaviculares intermedii

Platysma ●

V. facialis ●

N. facialis [VII], R. colli ●

V. retromandibularis ●

R. communicans ●

V. jugularis externa ●

N. transversus colli ●

V. jugularis anterior ●

M. sternocleidomastoideus ●

Arcus venosus jugularis ●

Nn. supraclaviculares mediales ●

→ 46, T 7

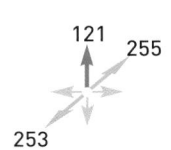

121
255
253

Fig. 254   Vessels and nerves of the lateral region of the neck,
Regio cervicalis lateralis;
parts of the platysma have been reflected cranially and the
superficial layer of the cervical fascia has been largely removed.

Vessels and nerves of the neck

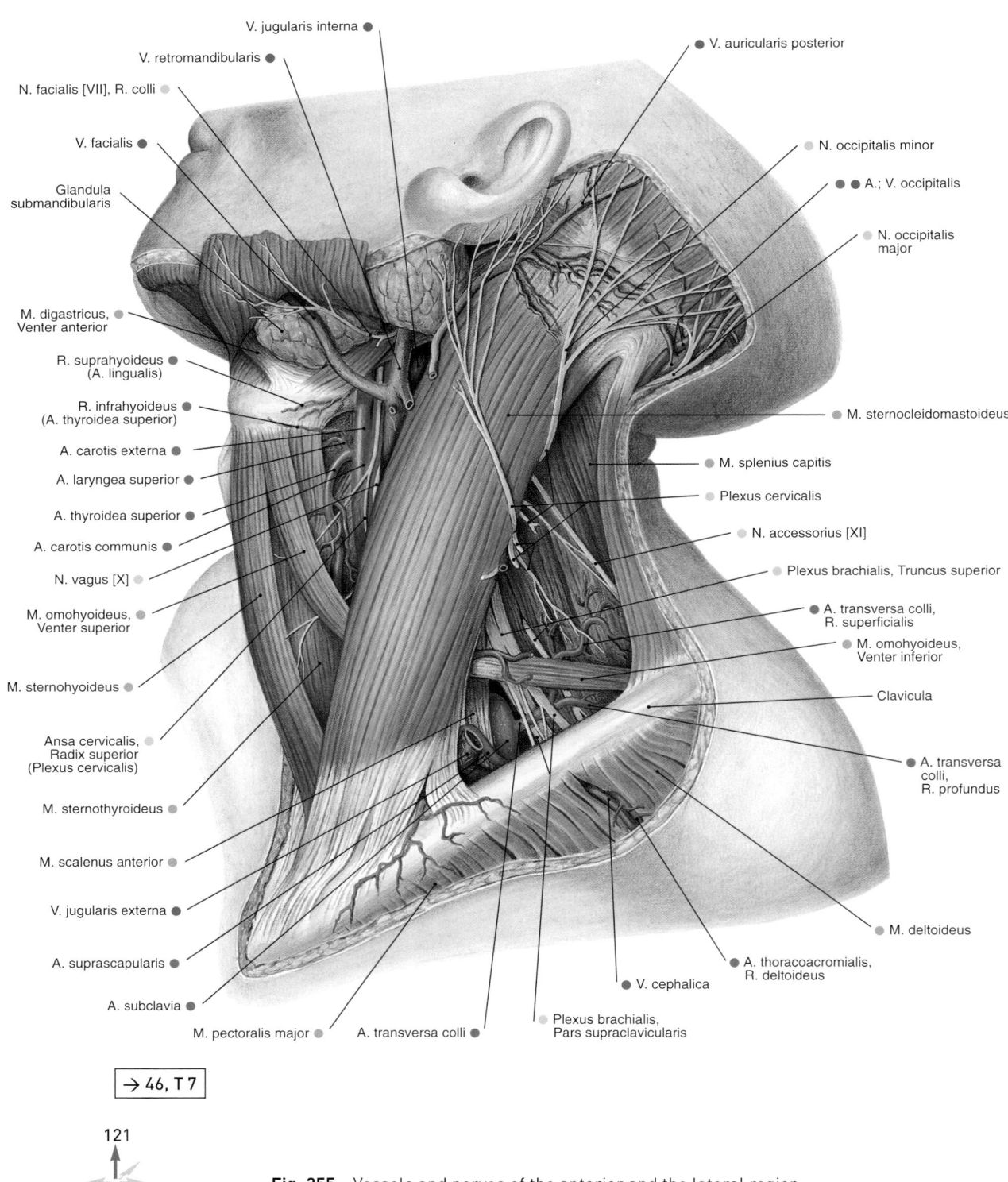

V. jugularis interna ●

V. retromandibularis ●

N. facialis [VII], R. colli ●

V. facialis ●

Glandula submandibularis

M. digastricus, ● Venter anterior

R. suprahyoideus ● (A. lingualis)

R. infrahyoideus ● (A. thyroidea superior)

A. carotis externa ●

A. laryngea superior ●

A. thyroidea superior ●

A. carotis communis ●

N. vagus [X] ●

M. omohyoideus, ● Venter superior

M. sternohyoideus ●

Ansa cervicalis, ● Radix superior (Plexus cervicalis)

M. sternothyroideus ●

M. scalenus anterior ●

V. jugularis externa ●

A. suprascapularis ●

A. subclavia ●

M. pectoralis major ●   A. transversa colli ●

● V. auricularis posterior

● N. occipitalis minor

● ● A.; V. occipitalis

● N. occipitalis major

● M. sternocleidomastoideus

● M. splenius capitis

● Plexus cervicalis

● N. accessorius [XI]

● Plexus brachialis, Truncus superior

● A. transversa colli, R. superficialis

● M. omohyoideus, Venter inferior

● Clavicula

● A. transversa colli, R. profundus

● M. deltoideus

● A. thoracoacromialis, R. deltoideus

● V. cephalica

Plexus brachialis, Pars supraclavicularis

→ 46, T 7

121
↑

254

Fig. 255 Vessels and nerves of the anterior and the lateral region of the neck, Regiones cervicales anterior et lateralis; the superficial and the middle layer of the cervical fascia have been removed.

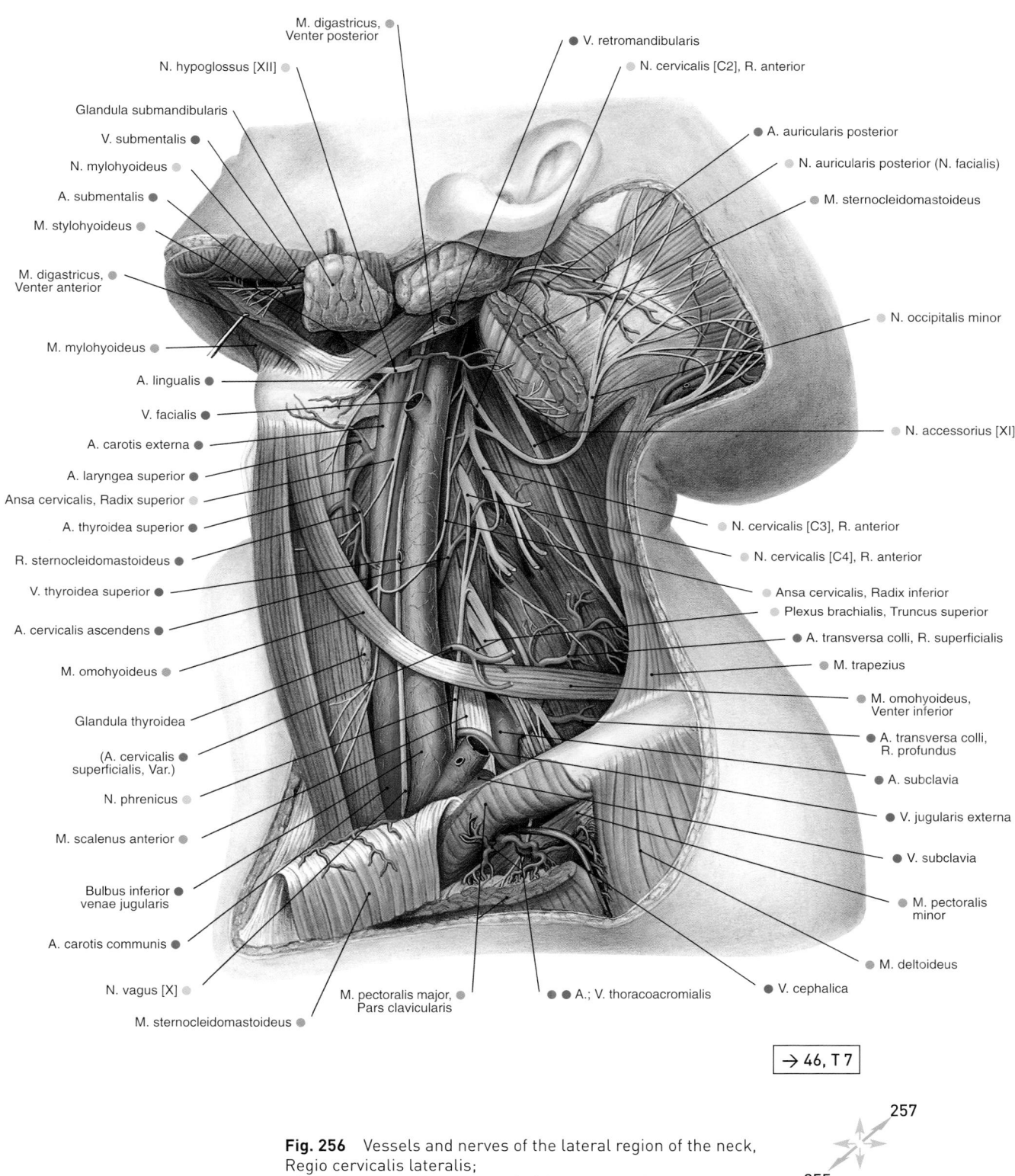

M. digastricus,
Venter posterior

N. hypoglossus [XII]

Glandula submandibularis

V. submentalis

N. mylohyoideus

A. submentalis

M. stylohyoideus

M. digastricus,
Venter anterior

M. mylohyoideus

A. lingualis

V. facialis

A. carotis externa

A. laryngea superior

Ansa cervicalis, Radix superior

A. thyroidea superior

R. sternocleidomastoideus

V. thyroidea superior

A. cervicalis ascendens

M. omohyoideus

Glandula thyroidea

(A. cervicalis
superficialis, Var.)

N. phrenicus

M. scalenus anterior

Bulbus inferior
venae jugularis

A. carotis communis

N. vagus [X]

M. sternocleidomastoideus

M. pectoralis major,
Pars clavicularis

V. retromandibularis

N. cervicalis [C2], R. anterior

A. auricularis posterior

N. auricularis posterior (N. facialis)

M. sternocleidomastoideus

N. occipitalis minor

N. accessorius [XI]

N. cervicalis [C3], R. anterior

N. cervicalis [C4], R. anterior

Ansa cervicalis, Radix inferior

Plexus brachialis, Truncus superior

A. transversa colli, R. superficialis

M. trapezius

M. omohyoideus,
Venter inferior

A. transversa colli,
R. profundus

A. subclavia

V. jugularis externa

V. subclavia

M. pectoralis
minor

M. deltoideus

V. cephalica

A.; V. thoracoacromialis

→ 46, T 7

Fig. 256 Vessels and nerves of the lateral region of the neck,
Regio cervicalis lateralis;
after almost complete removal of the sternocleidomastoid
muscle.

257

255

Vessels and nerves of the neck

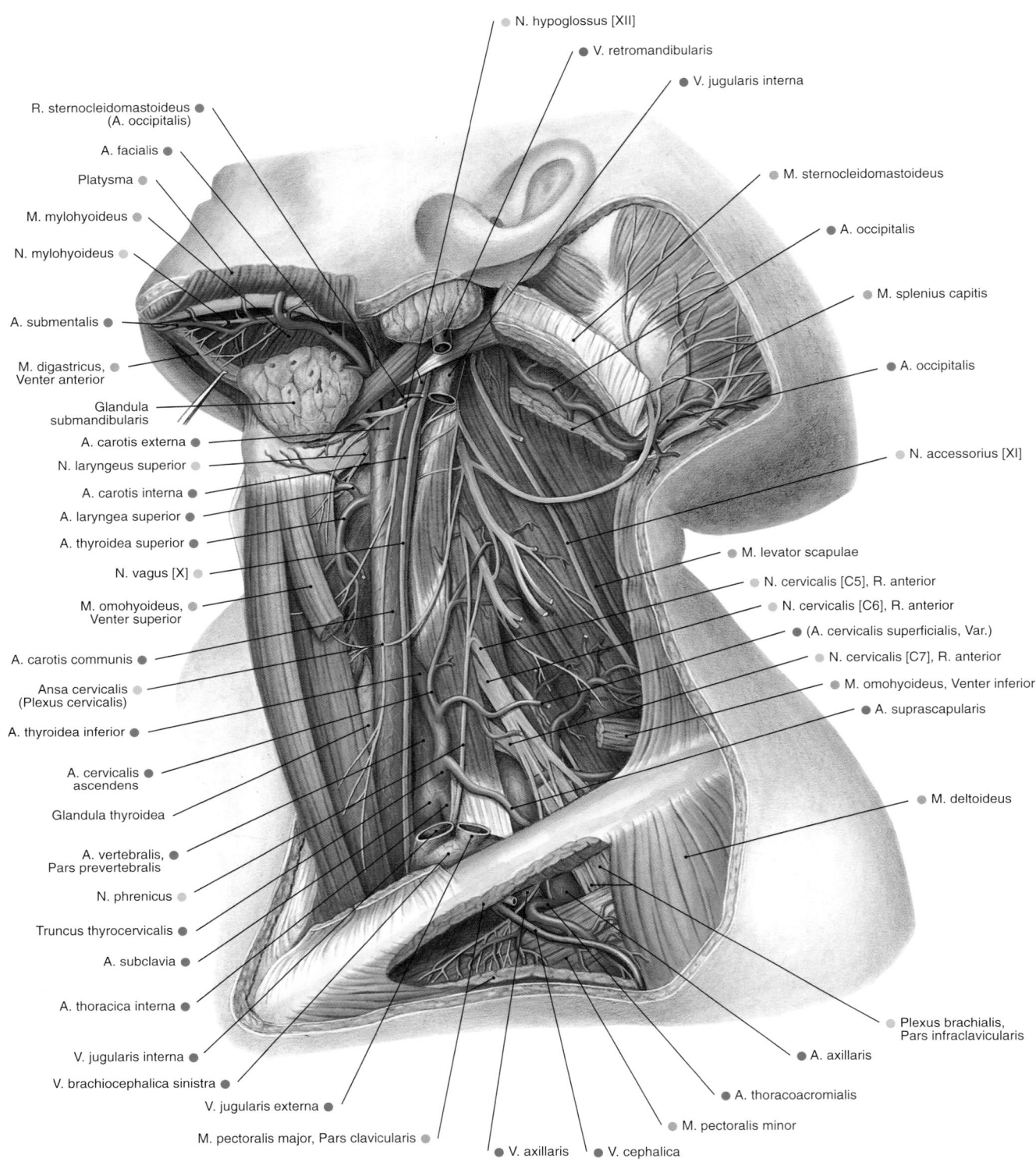

- N. hypoglossus [XII]
- V. retromandibularis
- V. jugularis interna
- R. sternocleidomastoideus (A. occipitalis)
- A. facialis
- Platysma
- M. mylohyoideus
- N. mylohyoideus
- A. submentalis
- M. digastricus, Venter anterior
- Glandula submandibularis
- A. carotis externa
- N. laryngeus superior
- A. carotis interna
- A. laryngea superior
- A. thyroidea superior
- N. vagus [X]
- M. omohyoideus, Venter superior
- A. carotis communis
- Ansa cervicalis (Plexus cervicalis)
- A. thyroidea inferior
- A. cervicalis ascendens
- Glandula thyroidea
- A. vertebralis, Pars prevertebralis
- N. phrenicus
- Truncus thyrocervicalis
- A. subclavia
- A. thoracica interna
- V. jugularis interna
- V. brachiocephalica sinistra
- V. jugularis externa
- M. pectoralis major, Pars clavicularis
- V. axillaris
- V. cephalica
- M. sternocleidomastoideus
- A. occipitalis
- M. splenius capitis
- A. occipitalis
- N. accessorius [XI]
- M. levator scapulae
- N. cervicalis [C5], R. anterior
- N. cervicalis [C6], R. anterior
- (A. cervicalis superficialis, Var.)
- N. cervicalis [C7], R. anterior
- M. omohyoideus, Venter inferior
- A. suprascapularis
- M. deltoideus
- Plexus brachialis, Pars infraclavicularis
- A. axillaris
- A. thoracoacromialis
- M. pectoralis minor

→ 46, T 7

258
256

Fig. 257 Vessels and nerves of the lateral region of the neck, Regio cervicalis lateralis; deep layer.

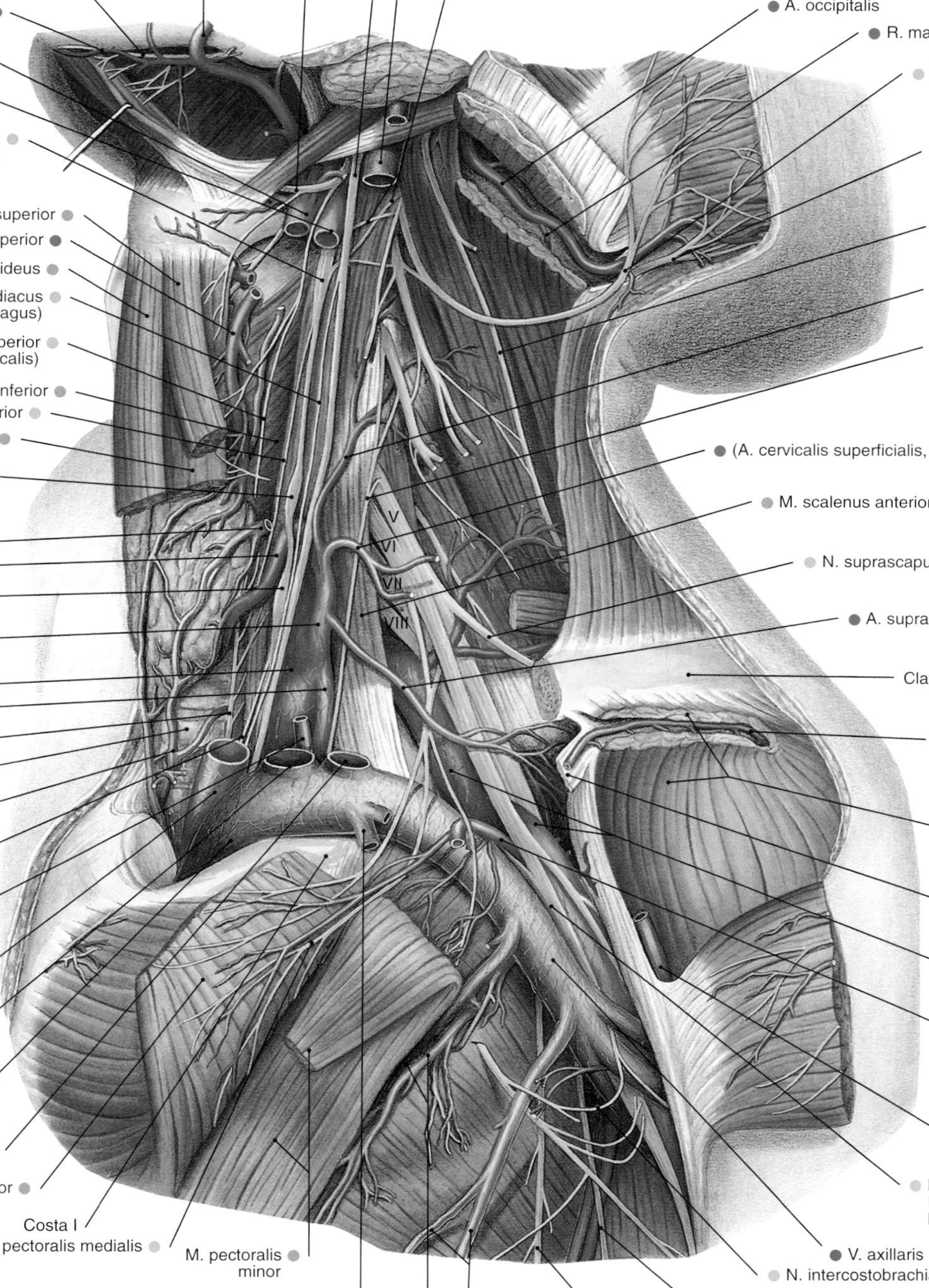

Vessels and nerves of the neck and the axilla

N. vagus [X]

N. hypoglossus [XII]

N. mylohyoideus

A. facialis

V. jugularis interna

Rr. communicantes (Truncus sympathicus)

A. submentalis

A. occipitalis

A. carotis externa

R. mastoideus

A. carotis interna

N. occipitalis minor

Ganglion cervicale superius
(Truncus sympathicus)

N. occipitalis
major

M. omohyoideus, Venter superior

A. thyroidea superior

N. accessorius
[XI]

M. sternohyoideus

A. cervicalis
ascendens

R. cardiacus
cervicalis superior (N. vagus)

N. phrenicus

Ansa cervicalis, Radix superior
(Plexus cervicalis)

M. constrictor pharyngis inferior

N. cardiacus cervicalis superior

M. sternothyroideus

(A. cervicalis superficialis, Var.)

(Ganglion
sympathicum
accessorium)

M. scalenus anterior

V. thyroidea superior

N. suprascapularis

A. thyroidea inferior

Ganglion
cervicale medium

A. suprascapularis

Truncus
thyrocervicalis

Clavicula

A. subclavia

A. thoracica interna

R. acromialis
(A. thoracoacromialis)

N. laryngeus recurrens

Trachea

M. deltoideus

V. thyroidea inferior

N. cardiacus cervicalis
medius (Truncus
sympathicus)

M. pectoralis
minor, Tendo

V. vertebralis,
Pars
prevertebralis

A. axillaris

A. carotis communis

A. thoraco-
acromialis

V. jugularis interna

V. brachio-
cephalica sinistra

V. cephalica

V. jugularis externa

Plexus brachialis,
Pars infraclavicularis,
Fasciculus medialis

M. pectoralis major

V. axillaris

Costa I
N. pectoralis medialis

N. intercostobrachialis

M. pectoralis
minor

N. thoracodorsalis

V. cephalica

N. thoracicus longus

A.; V. thoracica lateralis

Vv. thoracoepigastricae

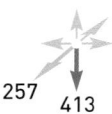

→ 46, T 7

Fig. 258 Vessels and nerves of the lateral region of the neck,
Regio cervicalis lateralis, and the axillary region, Regio axillaris.
The numbers V–VIII indicate ventral branches of the
corresponding cervical nerves.

257   413

Veins of the neck

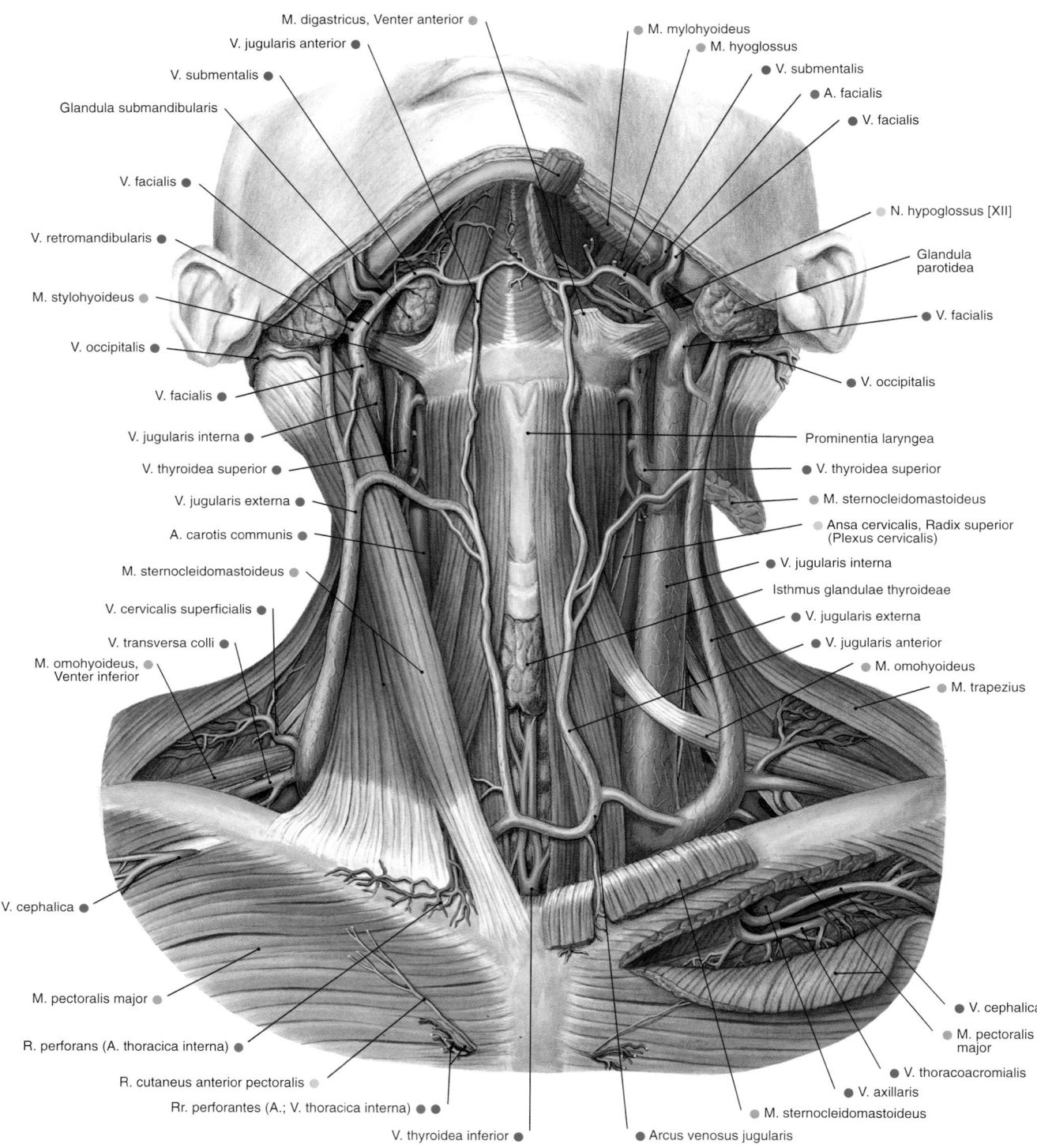

M. digastricus, Venter anterior ●
V. jugularis anterior ●
V. submentalis ●
Glandula submandibularis ●
V. facialis ●
V. retromandibularis ●
M. stylohyoideus ●
V. occipitalis ●
V. facialis ●
V. jugularis interna ●
V. thyroidea superior ●
V. jugularis externa ●
A. carotis communis ●
M. sternocleidomastoideus ●
V. cervicalis superficialis ●
V. transversa colli ●
M. omohyoideus, Venter inferior ●
V. cephalica ●
M. pectoralis major ●
R. perforans (A. thoracica interna) ●
R. cutaneus anterior pectoralis ●
Rr. perforantes (A.; V. thoracica interna) ● ●
V. thyroidea inferior ●

M. mylohyoideus ●
M. hyoglossus ●
V. submentalis ●
A. facialis ●
V. facialis ●
N. hypoglossus [XII] ●
Glandula parotidea
V. facialis ●
V. occipitalis ●
Prominentia laryngea
V. thyroidea superior ●
M. sternocleidomastoideus ●
Ansa cervicalis, Radix superior (Plexus cervicalis) ●
V. jugularis interna ●
Isthmus glandulae thyroideae
V. jugularis externa ●
V. jugularis anterior ●
M. omohyoideus ●
M. trapezius ●
V. cephalica ●
M. pectoralis major ●
V. thoracoacromialis ●
V. axillaris ●
M. sternocleidomastoideus ●
Arcus venosus jugularis ●

124
260
254

Fig. 259   Veins of the neck, Collum.

Vessels and nerves of the neck and the upper thoracic aperture

M. digastricus, Venter anterior

M. mylohyoideus

Os hyoideum

M. hyoglossus

N. lingualis

M. digastricus, Venter anterior

V. retromandibularis

A. facialis

V. facialis

N. hypoglossus [XII]

V. occipitalis

Glandula parotidea

M. sternohyoideus

V. thyroidea superior

M. thyrohyoideus

M. sternocleidomastoideus

M. omohyoideus

A. thyroidea superior

Ansa cervicalis,
Radix superior
(Plexus cervicalis)

Cartilago thyroidea

N. vagus [X]

V. jugularis externa

V. thyroidea media

Glandula thyroidea

N. accessorius [XI]

Plexus thyroideus impar

N. phrenicus

N. vagus [X]

Plexus
brachialis,
Pars supra-
clavicularis

A. transversa
colli

V. transversa
colli

M. omo-
hyoideus

Clavicula

V. jugularis
anterior

A. subclavia;
V. jugularis
externa

A. subclavia

V. subclavia

V. subclavia

V. cephalica

V. brachio-
cephalica
dextra

V. jugularis
interna

V. thyroidea
inferior

M. pectoralis major

V. thoracica interna

Costa I

V. cava superior

A. carotis communis;
N. laryngeus recurrens
sinister

V. brachiocephalica sinistra

N. vagus [X]

Pars ascendens aortae

N. laryngeus
recurrens sinister

Vv. thymicae

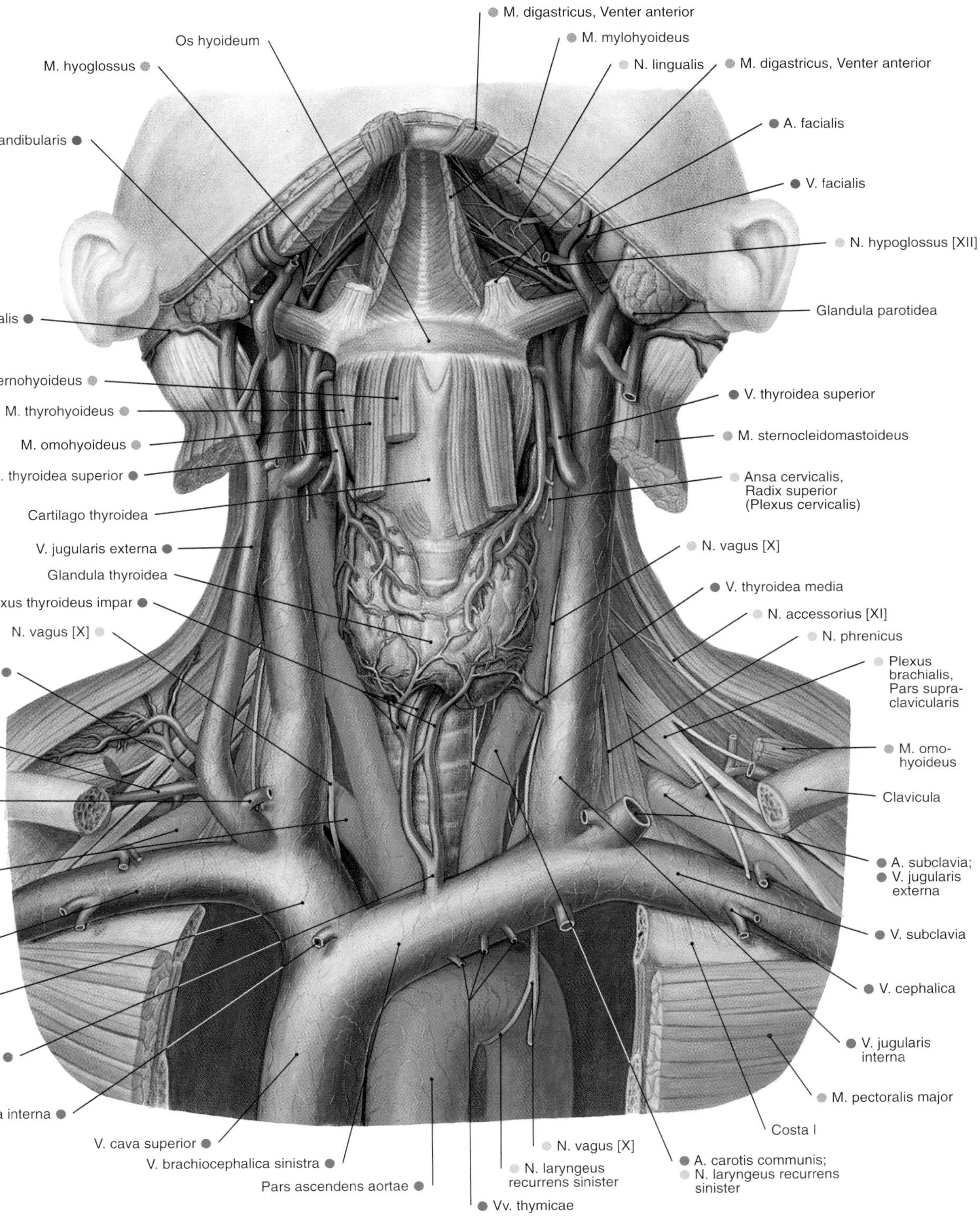

Fig. 260 Vessels and nerves of the neck, Collum, and
the upper thoracic aperture, Apertura thoracis superior.

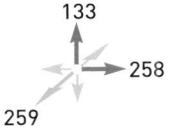

133

258

259

Lymphatics of the neck

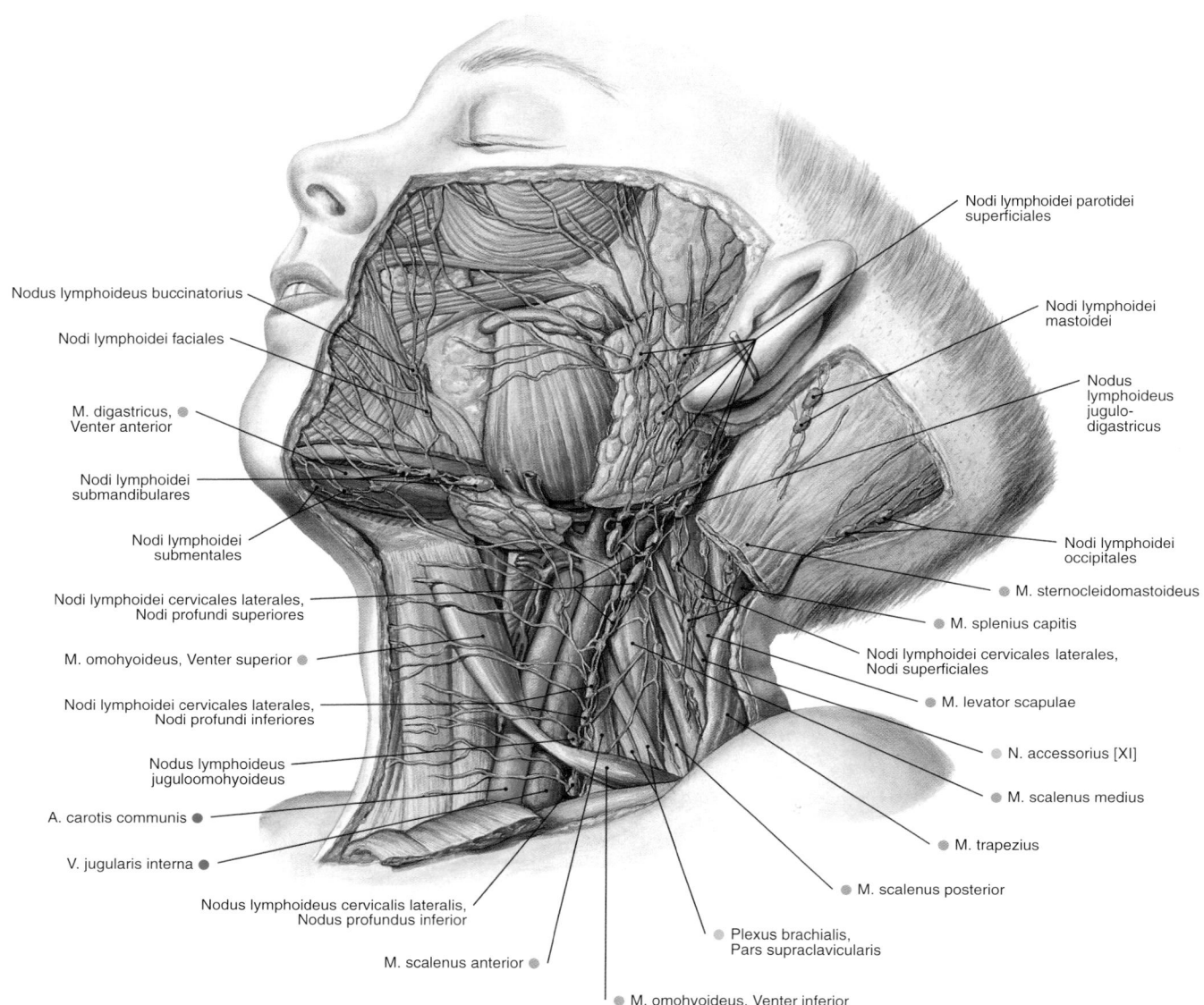

Nodi lymphoidei parotidei
superficiales

Nodi lymphoidei
mastoidei

Nodus
lymphoideus
jugulo-
digastricus

Nodi lymphoidei
occipitales

● M. sternocleidomastoideus

● M. splenius capitis

Nodi lymphoidei cervicales laterales,
Nodi superficiales

● M. levator scapulae

● N. accessorius [XI]

● M. scalenus medius

● M. trapezius

● M. scalenus posterior

Nodus lymphoideus buccinatorius

Nodi lymphoidei faciales

M. digastricus, ●
Venter anterior

Nodi lymphoidei
submandibulares

Nodi lymphoidei
submentales

Nodi lymphoidei cervicales laterales,
Nodi profundi superiores

M. omohyoideus, Venter superior ●

Nodi lymphoidei cervicales laterales,
Nodi profundi inferiores

Nodus lymphoideus
juguloomohyoideus

A. carotis communis ●

V. jugularis interna ●

Nodus lymphoideus cervicalis lateralis,
Nodus profundus inferior

M. scalenus anterior ●

● Plexus brachialis,
Pars supraclavicularis

● M. omohyoideus, Venter inferior

→ 125, 126

Fig. 261 Superficial lymphatics, Vasa lymphatica
superficialia, and lymph nodes, Nodi lymphoidei, of the
head and the neck of an 8-year-old child.

Vessels and nerves of the submandibular triangle

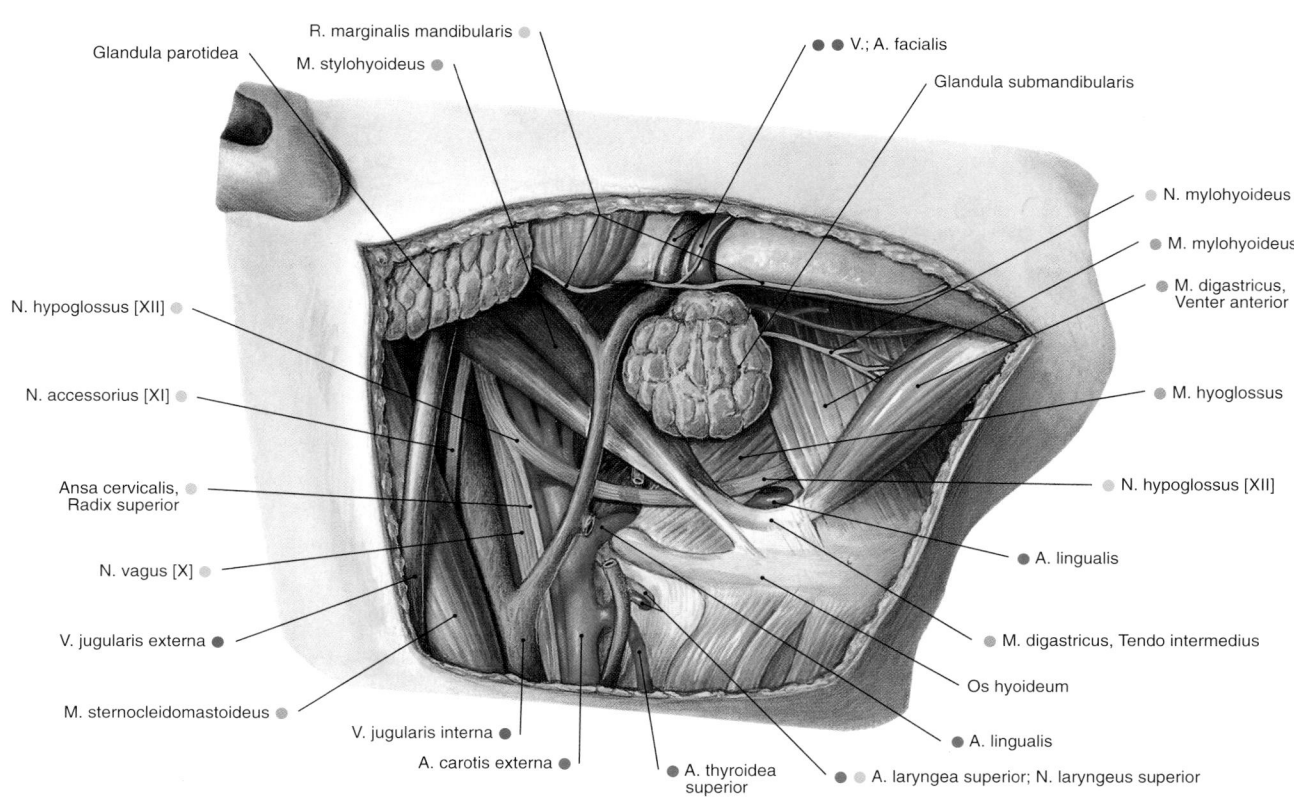

Glandula parotidea

R. marginalis mandibularis

M. stylohyoideus

V.; A. facialis

Glandula submandibularis

N. mylohyoideus

M. mylohyoideus

M. digastricus, Venter anterior

N. hypoglossus [XII]

N. accessorius [XI]

M. hyoglossus

Ansa cervicalis, Radix superior

N. hypoglossus [XII]

N. vagus [X]

A. lingualis

V. jugularis externa

M. digastricus, Tendo intermedius

M. sternocleidomastoideus

Os hyoideum

V. jugularis interna

A. lingualis

A. carotis externa

A. thyroidea superior

A. laryngea superior; N. laryngeus superior

Fig. 262 Vessels and nerves of the submandibular triangle, Trigonum submandibulare.

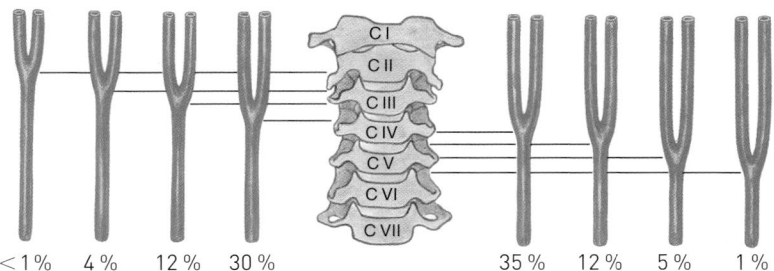

C I
C II
C III
C IV
C V
C VI
C VII

<1 %   4 %   12 %   30 %   35 %   12 %   5 %   1 %

Fig. 263 Level of the bifurcation of the common carotid artery, A. carotis communis, in relation to the cervical vertebrae.

Subclavian artery

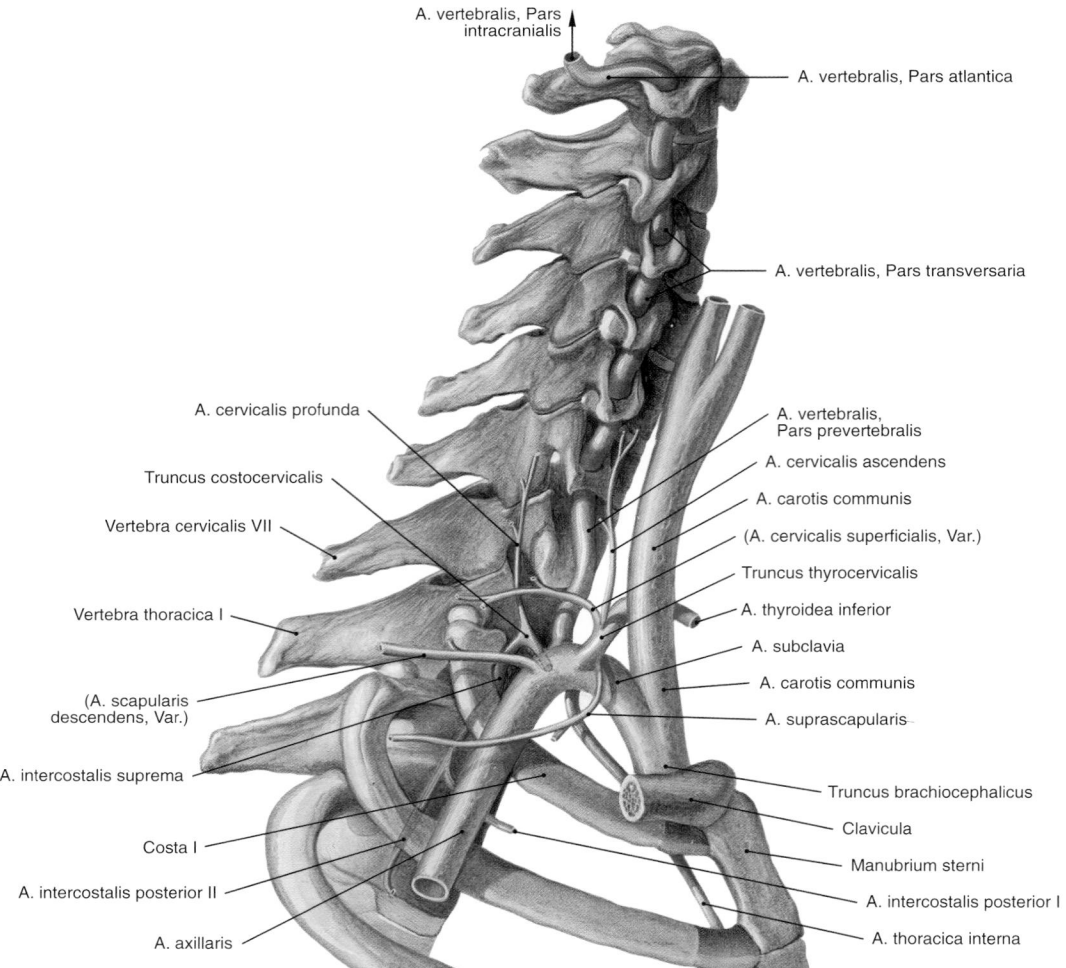

A. vertebralis, Pars intracranialis

A. vertebralis, Pars atlantica

A. vertebralis, Pars transversaria

A. cervicalis profunda

Truncus costocervicalis

Vertebra cervicalis VII

Vertebra thoracica I

(A. scapularis descendens, Var.)

A. intercostalis suprema

Costa I

A. intercostalis posterior II

A. axillaris

A. vertebralis, Pars prevertebralis

A. cervicalis ascendens

A. carotis communis

(A. cervicalis superficialis, Var.)

Truncus thyrocervicalis

A. thyroidea inferior

A. subclavia

A. carotis communis

A. suprascapularis

Truncus brachiocephalicus

Clavicula

Manubrium sterni

A. intercostalis posterior I

A. thoracica interna

Fig. 264 Subclavian artery, A. subclavia.

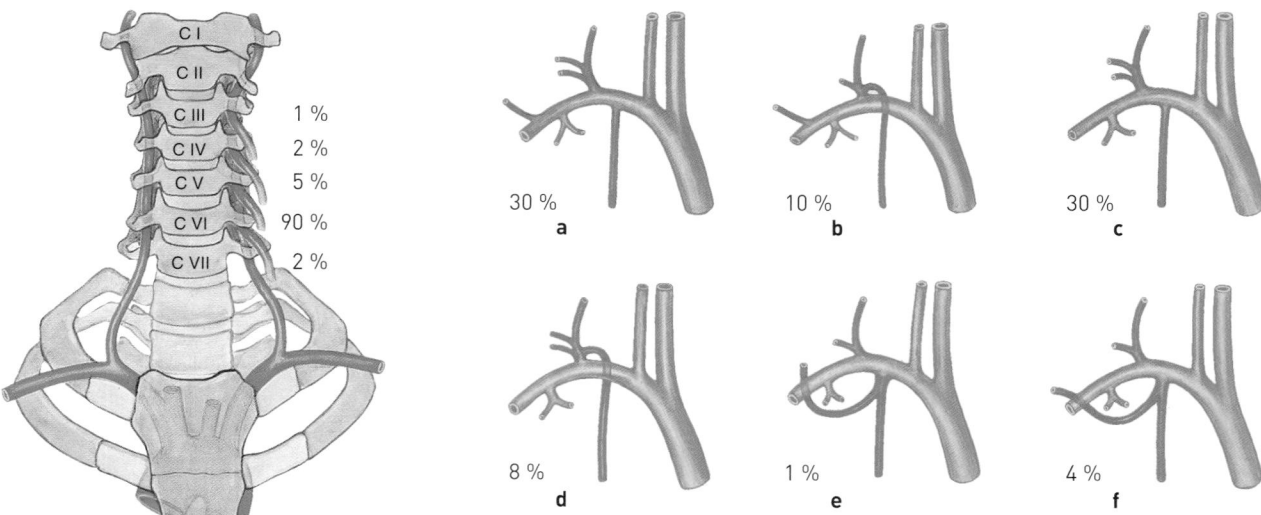

C I
C II
C III — 1 %
C IV — 2 %
C V — 5 %
C VI — 90 %
C VII — 2 %

30 % a

10 % b

30 % c

8 % d

1 % e

4 % f

Fig. 265 Level of the entry of the vertebral artery, A. vertebralis, into the transverse foramina, Foramina transversaria.

Fig. 266 a–f Variations in the truncus formed by the inferior thyroid artery, A. thyroidea inferior, the suprascapular artery, A. suprascapularis, the transverse cervical artery, A. transversa colli, and the internal thoracic artery, A. thoracica interna, when the vertebral artery, A. vertebralis, branches off separately from the costocervical truncus, Truncus costocervicalis.

Vessels and nerves of the neck and the upper thoracic aperture

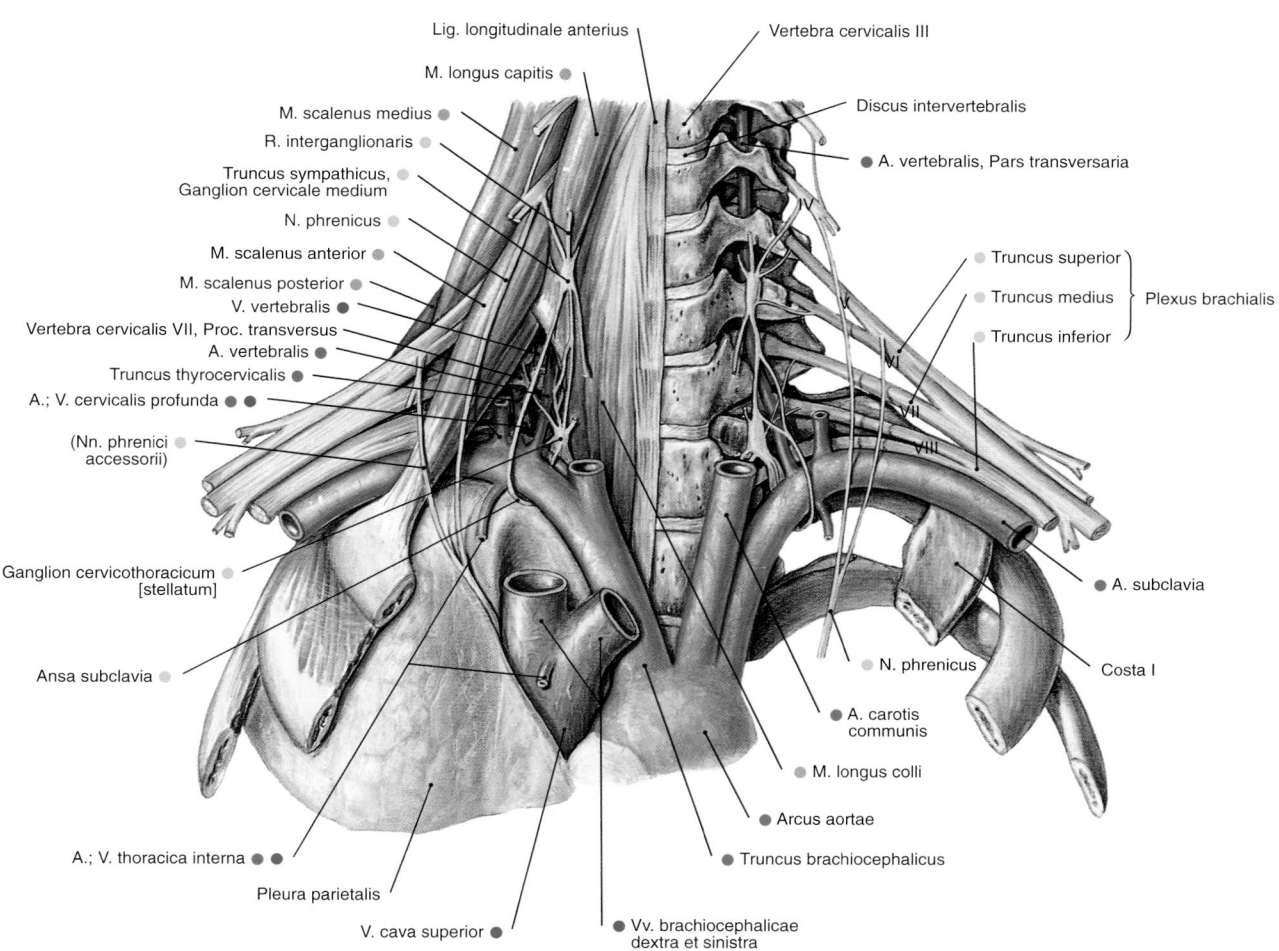

Lig. longitudinale anterius

Vertebra cervicalis III

M. longus capitis ●

M. scalenus medius ●

R. interganglionaris ●

Truncus sympathicus, ●
Ganglion cervicale medium

N. phrenicus ●

M. scalenus anterior ●

M. scalenus posterior ●

V. vertebralis ●

Vertebra cervicalis VII, Proc. transversus

A. vertebralis ●

Truncus thyrocervicalis ●

A.; V. cervicalis profunda ● ●

(Nn. phrenici ●
accessorii)

Ganglion cervicothoracicum ●
[stellatum]

Ansa subclavia ●

A.; V. thoracica interna ● ●

Pleura parietalis

V. cava superior ●

Discus intervertebralis

● A. vertebralis, Pars transversaria

○ Truncus superior ⎫
○ Truncus medius ⎬ Plexus brachialis
○ Truncus inferior ⎭

● A. subclavia

Costa I

○ N. phrenicus

● A. carotis
communis

● M. longus colli

● Arcus aortae

● Truncus brachiocephalicus

● Vv. brachiocephalicae
dextra et sinistra

Fig. 267 Vessels and nerves at the transition
from the neck to the thorax.
The numbers IV–VIII indicate ventral branches of the
corresponding spinal nerves.

→ 46, 386, T 7, T 24

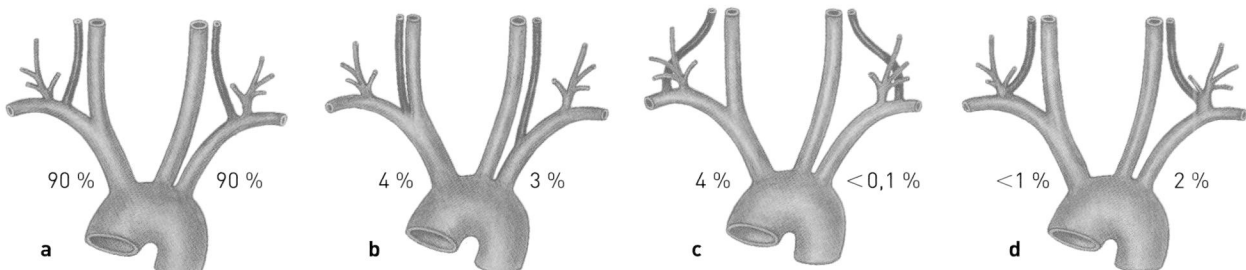

90 %   90 %   4 %   3 %   4 %   <0,1 %   <1 %   2 %

a   b   c   d

Fig. 268 a–d Variations in the origin of the vertebral artery,
A. vertebralis.

Neck, transverse section

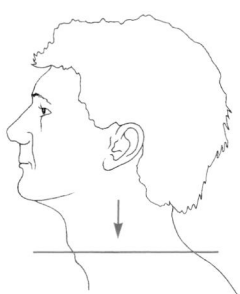

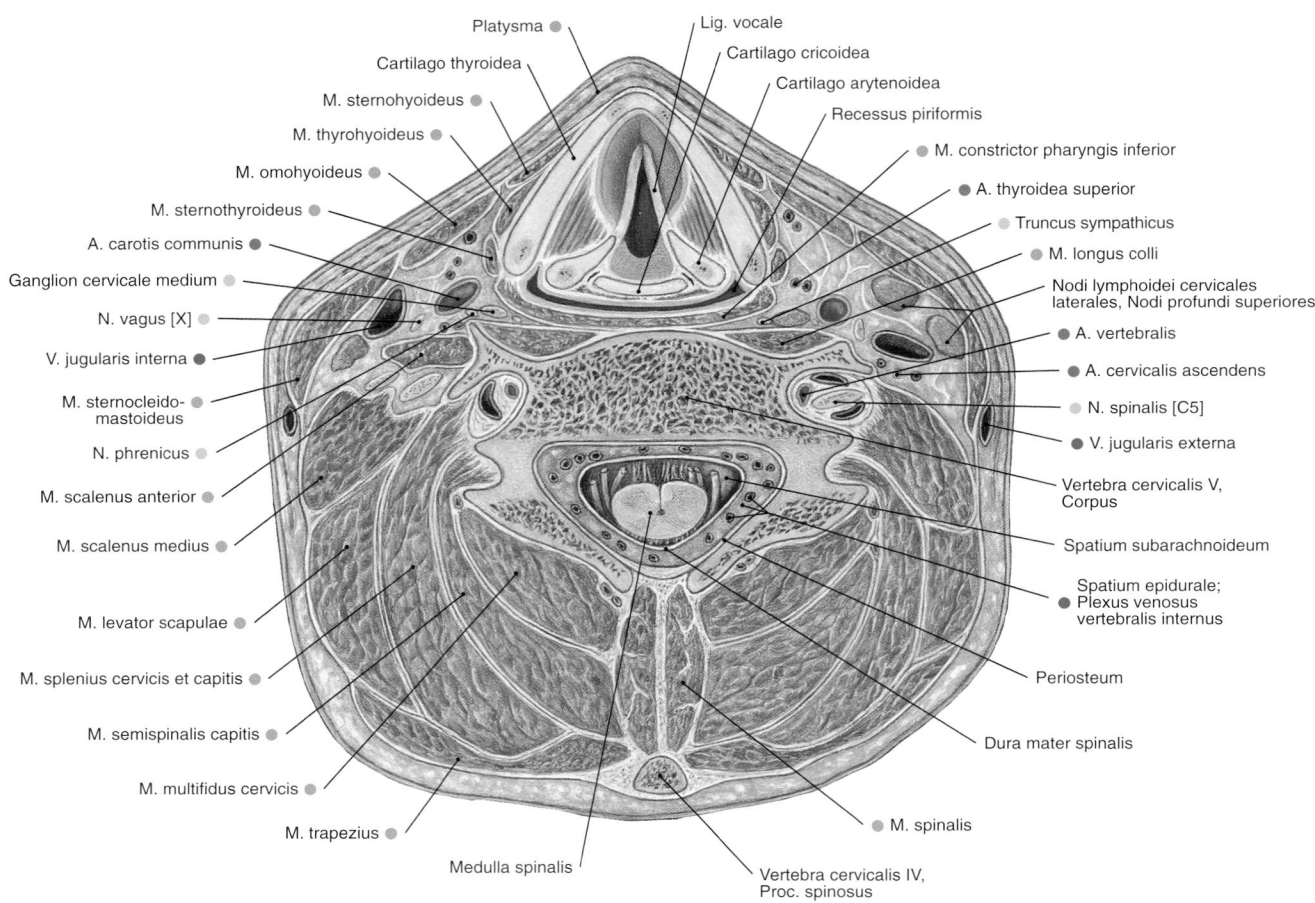

Platysma ●
Cartilago thyroidea
M. sternohyoideus ●
M. thyrohyoideus ●
M. omohyoideus ●
M. sternothyroideus ●
A. carotis communis ●
Ganglion cervicale medium ●
N. vagus [X] ●
V. jugularis interna ●
M. sternocleido-
mastoideus
N. phrenicus ●
M. scalenus anterior ●
M. scalenus medius ●
M. levator scapulae ●
M. splenius cervicis et capitis ●
M. semispinalis capitis ●
M. multifidus cervicis ●
M. trapezius ●
Medulla spinalis

Lig. vocale
Cartilago cricoidea
Cartilago arytenoidea
Recessus piriformis
● M. constrictor pharyngis inferior
● A. thyroidea superior
● Truncus sympathicus
● M. longus colli
Nodi lymphoidei cervicales
laterales, Nodi profundi superiores
● A. vertebralis
● A. cervicalis ascendens
● N. spinalis [C5]
● V. jugularis externa
Vertebra cervicalis V,
Corpus
Spatium subarachnoideum
Spatium epidurale;
● Plexus venosus
vertebralis internus
Periosteum
Dura mater spinalis
● M. spinalis
Vertebra cervicalis IV,
Proc. spinosus

→ 236

Fig. 269   Neck, Collum;
transverse section at the level of the vocal cord.

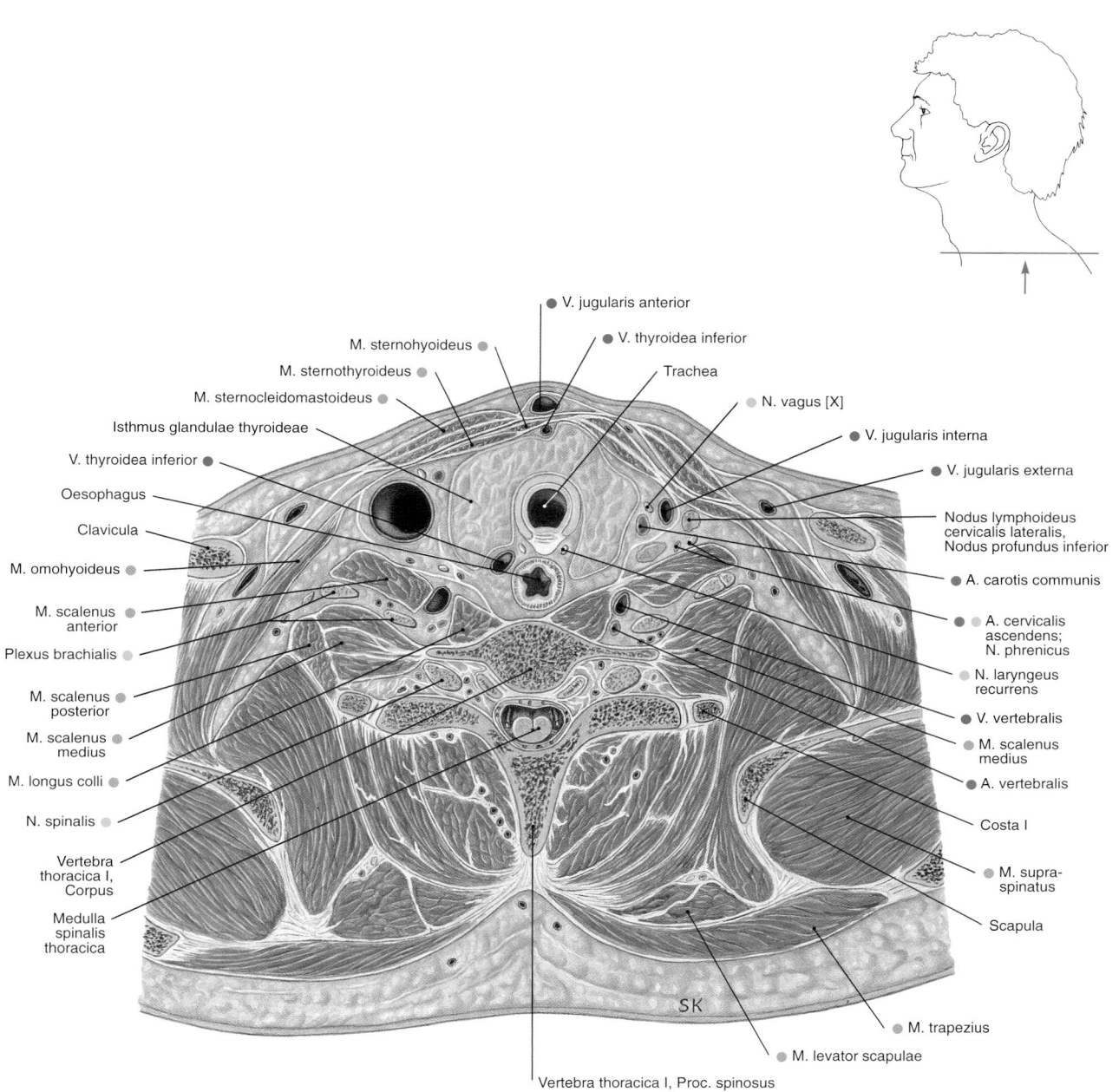

V. jugularis anterior

M. sternohyoideus

V. thyroidea inferior

M. sternothyroideus

Trachea

M. sternocleidomastoideus

N. vagus [X]

Isthmus glandulae thyroideae

V. jugularis interna

V. thyroidea inferior

V. jugularis externa

Oesophagus

Nodus lymphoideus cervicalis lateralis, Nodus profundus inferior

Clavicula

M. omohyoideus

A. carotis communis

M. scalenus anterior

A. cervicalis ascendens; N. phrenicus

Plexus brachialis

N. laryngeus recurrens

M. scalenus posterior

V. vertebralis

M. scalenus medius

M. scalenus medius

M. longus colli

A. vertebralis

N. spinalis

Costa I

Vertebra thoracica I, Corpus

M. supra-spinatus

Medulla spinalis thoracica

Scapula

SK

M. trapezius

M. levator scapulae

Vertebra thoracica I, Proc. spinosus

Fig. 270   Neck, Collum;
transverse section at the level of the first thoracic vertebra.

→ 239

Oral cavity and pharynx, median section

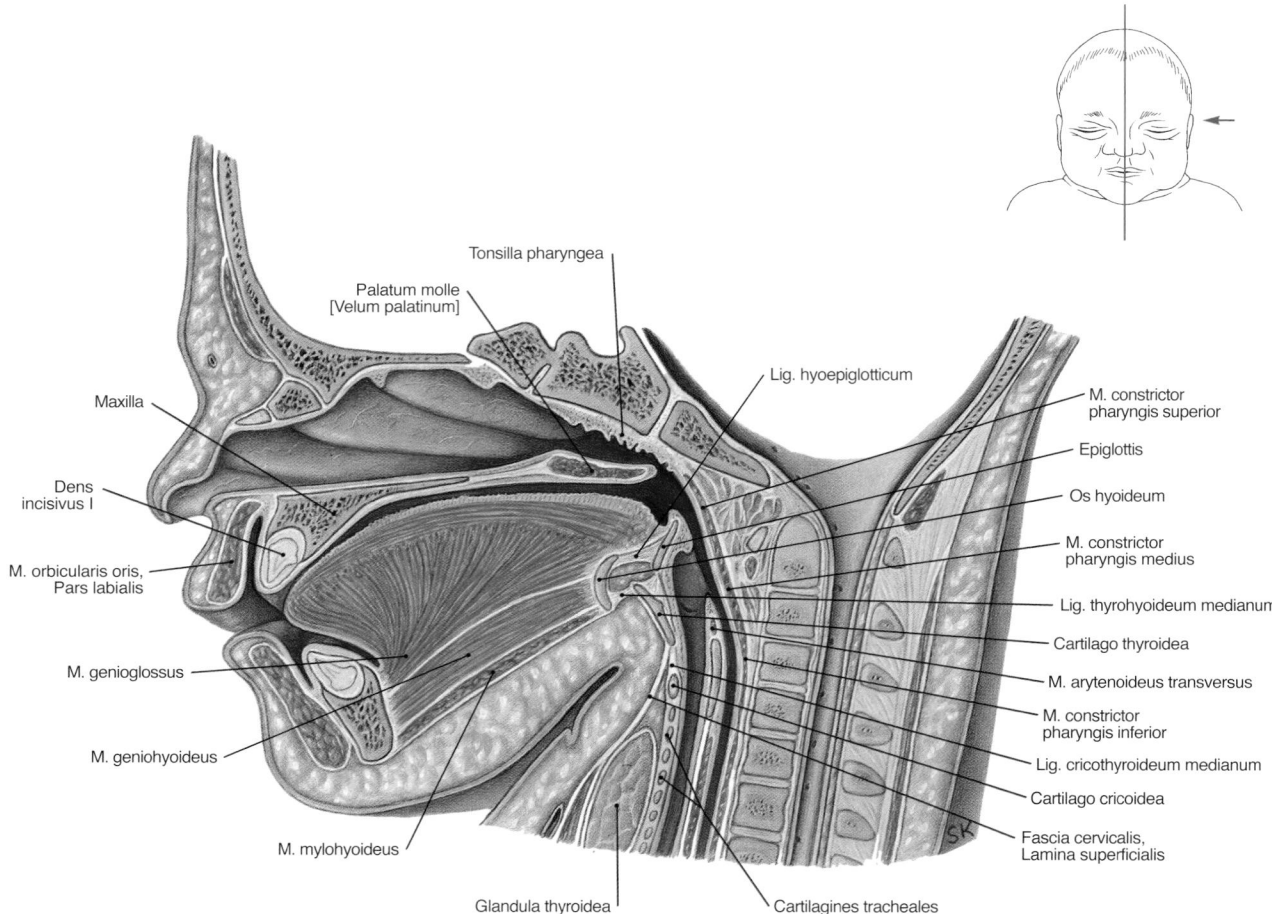

Tonsilla pharyngea

Palatum molle
[Velum palatinum]

Maxilla

Dens
incisivus I

M. orbicularis oris,
Pars labialis

M. genioglossus

M. geniohyoideus

M. mylohyoideus

Glandula thyroidea

Lig. hyoepiglotticum

M. constrictor
pharyngis superior

Epiglottis

Os hyoideum

M. constrictor
pharyngis medius

Lig. thyrohyoideum medianum

Cartilago thyroidea

M. arytenoideus transversus

M. constrictor
pharyngis inferior

Lig. cricothyroideum medianum

Cartilago cricoidea

Fascia cervicalis,
Lamina superficialis

Cartilagines tracheales

→ 246

Fig. 271 Facial part of the head, Caput, and neck, Collum;
median section through the head of a neonate.

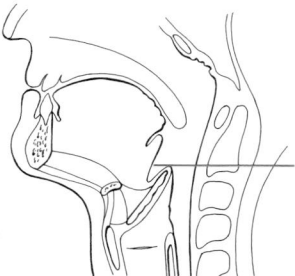

Fig. 272 Schema illustrating the distance between
the root of the tongue, Radix linguae, and the epiglottis,
Epiglottis, in the adult.

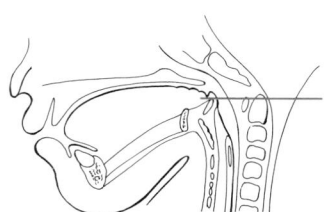

Fig. 273 Schema illustrating that the larynx in
the neonate is positioned considerably higher than
in the adult.

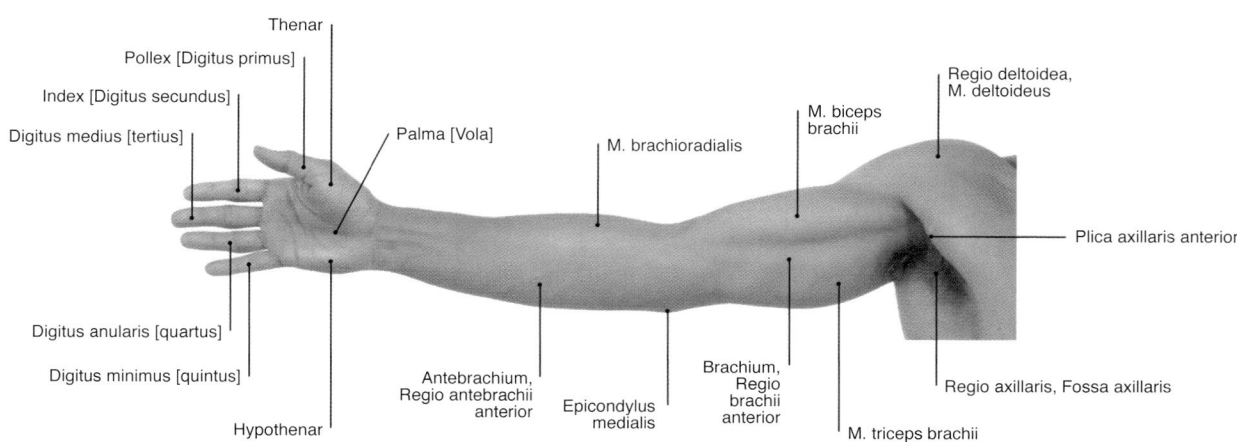

Thenar

Pollex [Digitus primus]

Index [Digitus secundus]

Digitus medius [tertius]

Palma [Vola]

M. brachioradialis

M. biceps brachii

Regio deltoidea, M. deltoideus

Plica axillaris anterior

Digitus anularis [quartus]

Digitus minimus [quintus]

Antebrachium, Regio antebrachii anterior

Epicondylus medialis

Brachium, Regio brachii anterior

Regio axillaris, Fossa axillaris

Hypothenar

M. triceps brachii

Fig. 274 Upper limb, Membrum superius.

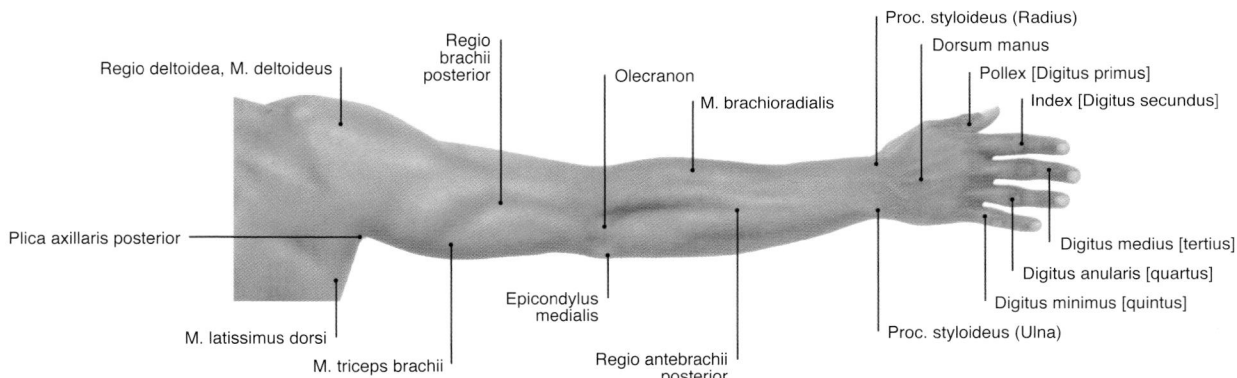

Regio deltoidea, M. deltoideus

Regio brachii posterior

Olecranon

M. brachioradialis

Proc. styloideus (Radius)

Dorsum manus

Pollex [Digitus primus]

Index [Digitus secundus]

Plica axillaris posterior

Digitus medius [tertius]

Digitus anularis [quartus]

Digitus minimus [quintus]

Proc. styloideus (Ulna)

M. latissimus dorsi

M. triceps brachii

Epicondylus medialis

Regio antebrachii posterior

Fig. 275 Upper limb, Membrum superius.

Skeleton of the upper limb

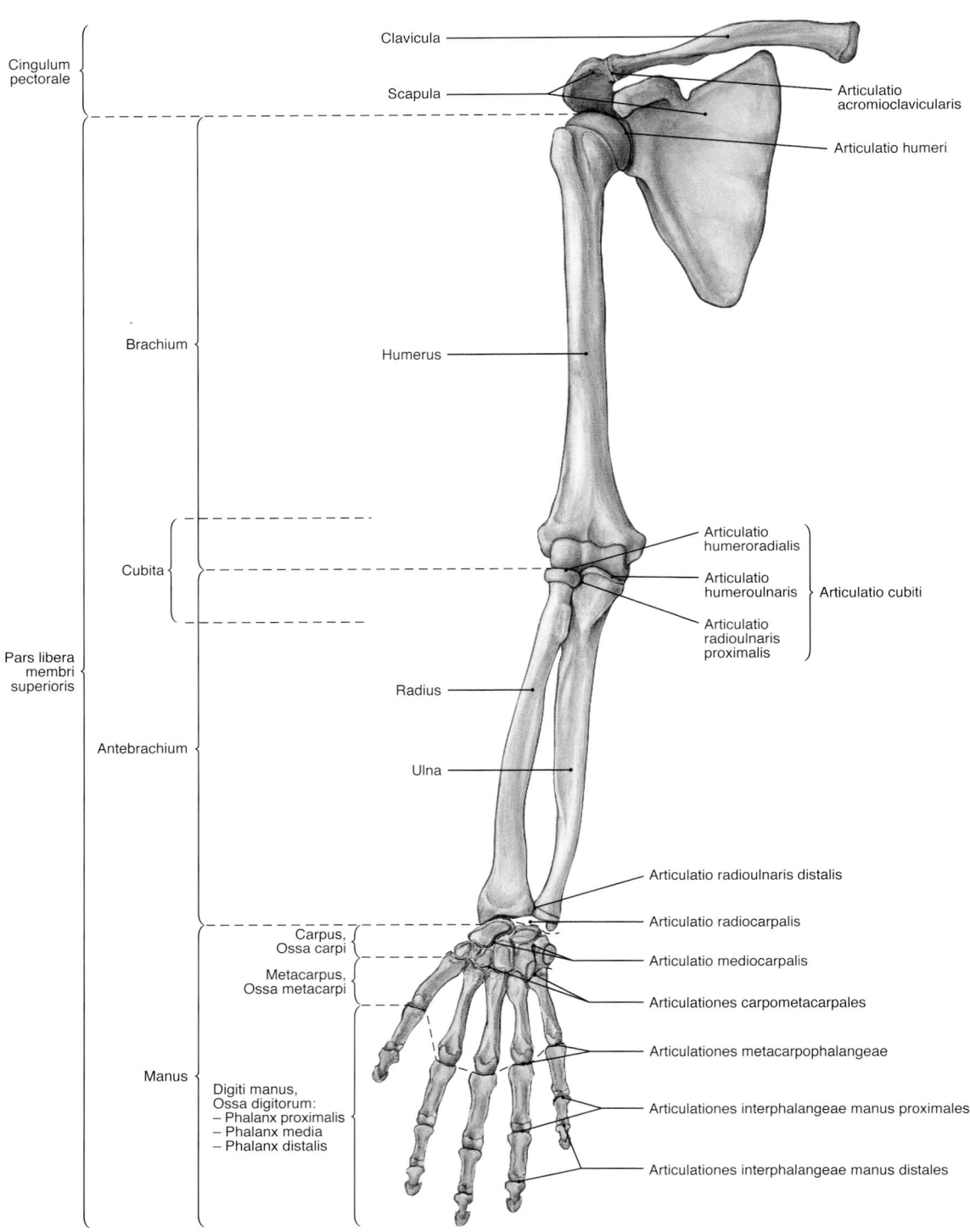

Cingulum pectorale

Brachium

Cubita

Pars libera membri superioris

Antebrachium

Manus

Clavicula

Scapula

Articulatio acromioclavicularis

Articulatio humeri

Humerus

Articulatio humeroradialis

Articulatio humeroulnaris

Articulatio radioulnaris proximalis

Articulatio cubiti

Radius

Ulna

Articulatio radioulnaris distalis

Articulatio radiocarpalis

Carpus, Ossa carpi

Articulatio mediocarpalis

Metacarpus, Ossa metacarpi

Articulationes carpometacarpales

Articulationes metacarpophalangeae

Digiti manus,
Ossa digitorum:
– Phalanx proximalis
– Phalanx media
– Phalanx distalis

Articulationes interphalangeae manus proximales

Articulationes interphalangeae manus distales

Fig. 276 Upper limb, Membrum superius; overview, bones and joints.

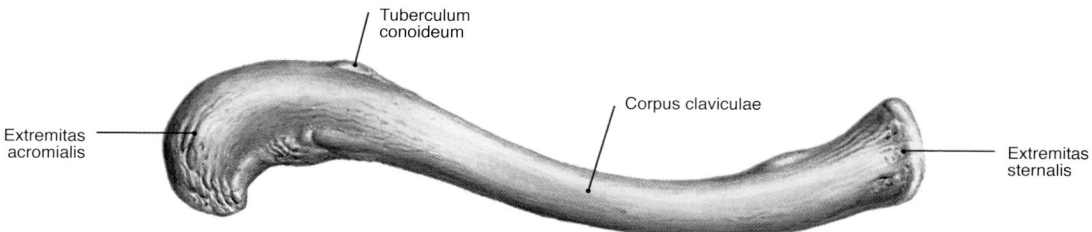

Fig. 277 Clavicle, Clavicula;
superior view.

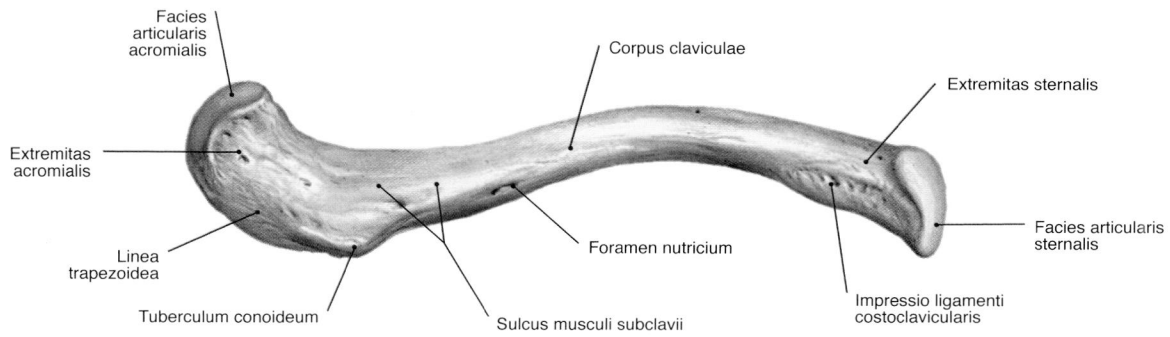

Fig. 278 Clavicle, Clavicula;
inferior view.

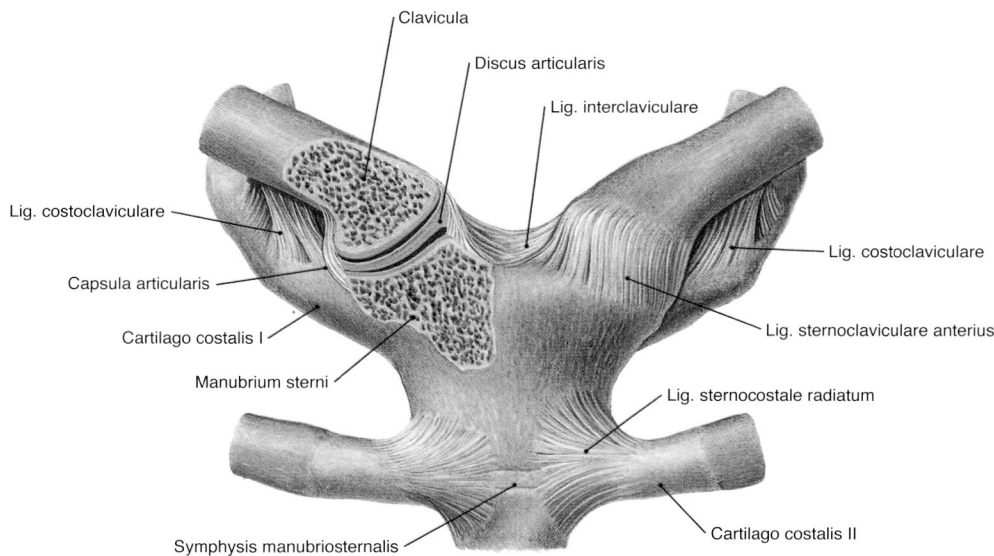

Fig. 279 Sternoclavicular joint,
Articulatio sternoclavicularis;
ventral view.

Scapula

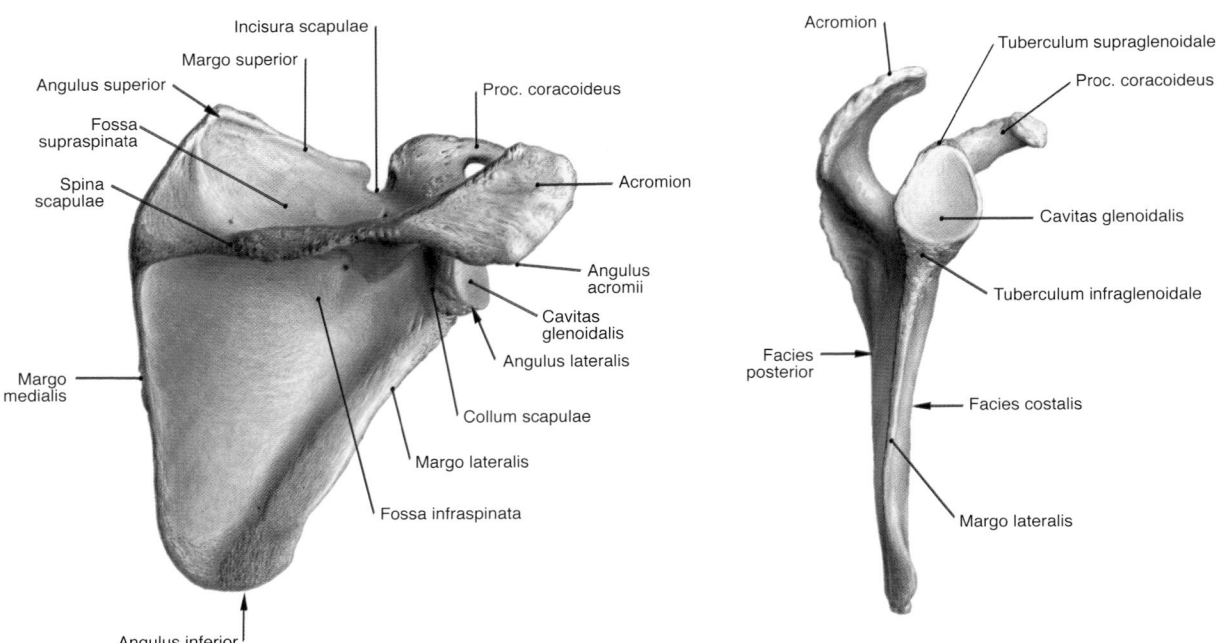

Incisura scapulae
Margo superior
Angulus superior
Fossa supraspinata
Spina scapulae
Margo medialis
Proc. coracoideus
Acromion
Angulus acromii
Cavitas glenoidalis
Angulus lateralis
Collum scapulae
Margo lateralis
Fossa infraspinata
Angulus inferior

Acromion
Tuberculum supraglenoidale
Proc. coracoideus
Cavitas glenoidalis
Tuberculum infraglenoidale
Facies posterior
Facies costalis
Margo lateralis

Fig. 280 Scapula, Scapula; dorsal view.

Fig. 281 Scapula, Scapula; lateral view.

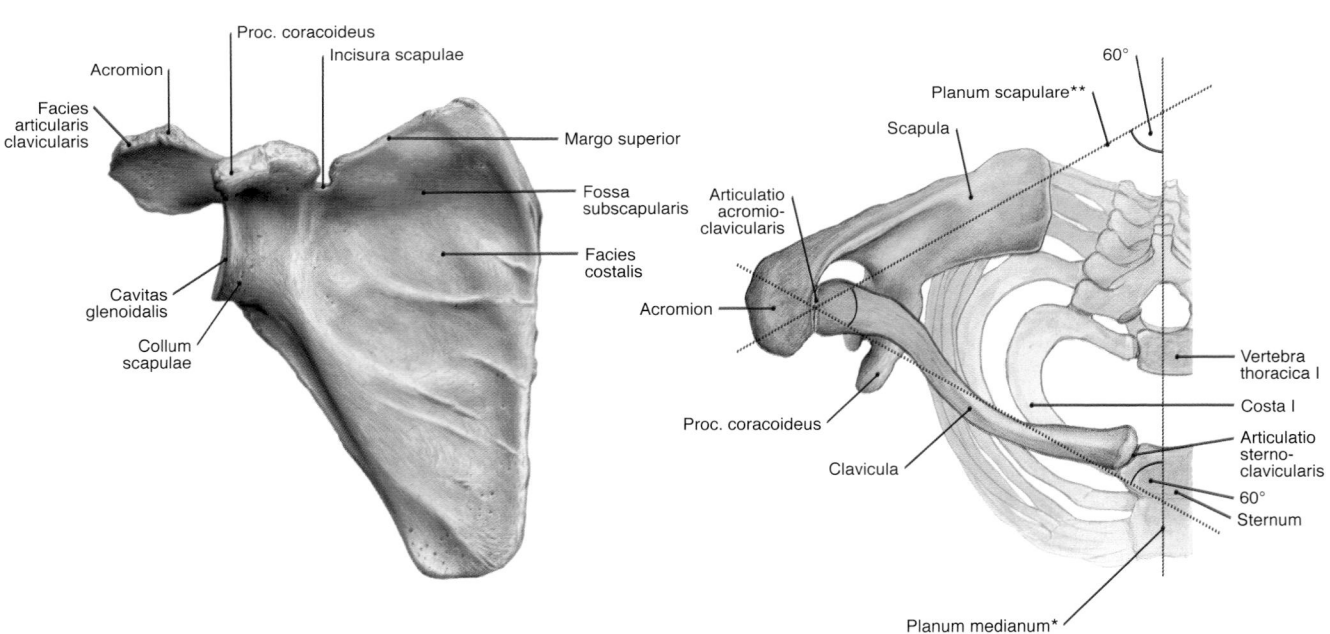

Proc. coracoideus
Incisura scapulae
Acromion
Facies articularis clavicularis
Margo superior
Fossa subscapularis
Facies costalis
Cavitas glenoidalis
Collum scapulae

60°
Planum scapulare**
Scapula
Articulatio acromio-clavicularis
Acromion
Proc. coracoideus
Clavicula
Vertebra thoracica I
Costa I
Articulatio sterno-clavicularis
60°
Sternum
Planum medianum*

Fig. 282 Scapula, Scapula; ventral view.

Fig. 283 Shoulder girdle, Cingulum pectorale; superior view.
The angles refer to the average relations in the adult.
* Median plane
** Scapular plane

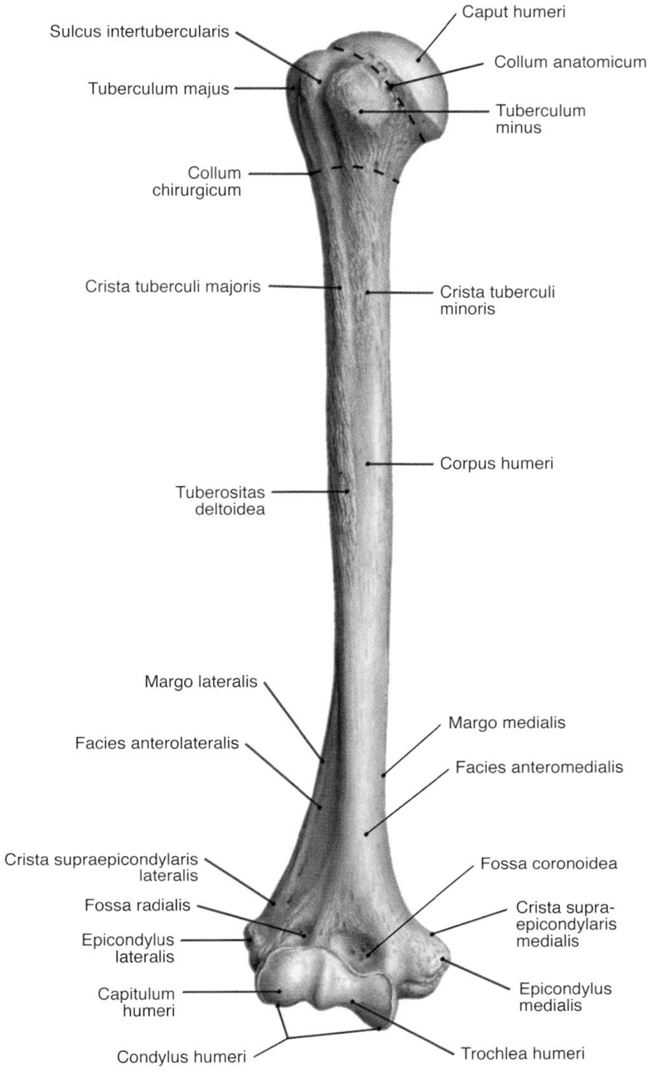

Sulcus intertubercularis
Tuberculum majus
Collum chirurgicum
Crista tuberculi majoris
Tuberositas deltoidea
Margo lateralis
Facies anterolateralis
Crista supraepicondylaris lateralis
Fossa radialis
Epicondylus lateralis
Capitulum humeri
Condylus humeri

Caput humeri
Collum anatomicum
Tuberculum minus
Crista tuberculi minoris
Corpus humeri
Margo medialis
Facies anteromedialis
Fossa coronoidea
Crista supra-epicondylaris medialis
Epicondylus medialis
Trochlea humeri

Fig. 284 Humerus, Humerus; ventral view.

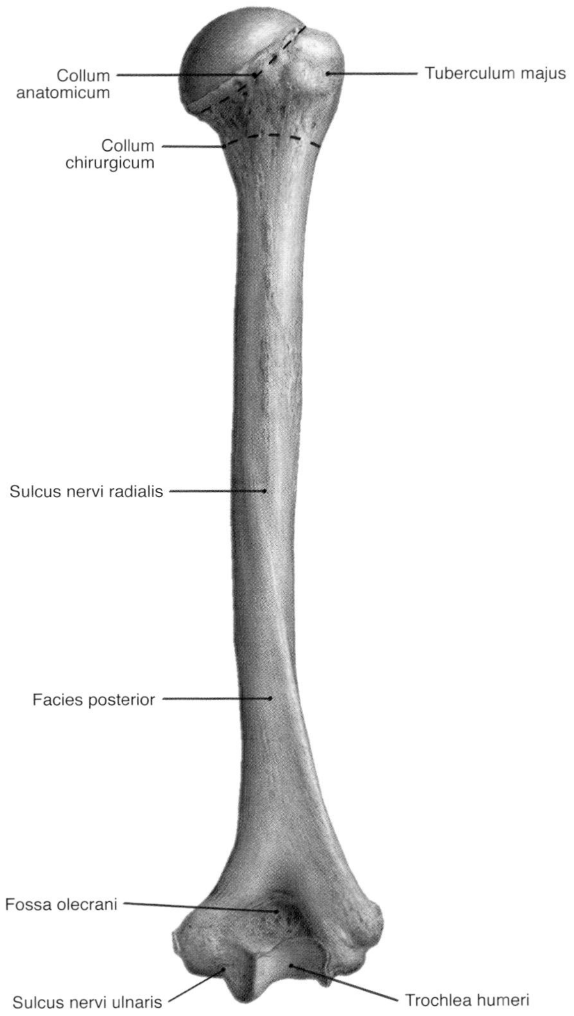

Collum anatomicum
Collum chirurgicum
Sulcus nervi radialis
Facies posterior
Fossa olecrani
Sulcus nervi ulnaris

Tuberculum majus
Trochlea humeri

Fig. 285 Humerus, Humerus; dorsal view.

Insertions of the tendons of:
1 M. supraspinatus
2 M. infraspinatus
3 M. teres minor

Tuberculum minus
Collum anatomicum
Caput humeri

Sulcus intertubercularis
1
2
3
Tuberculum majus

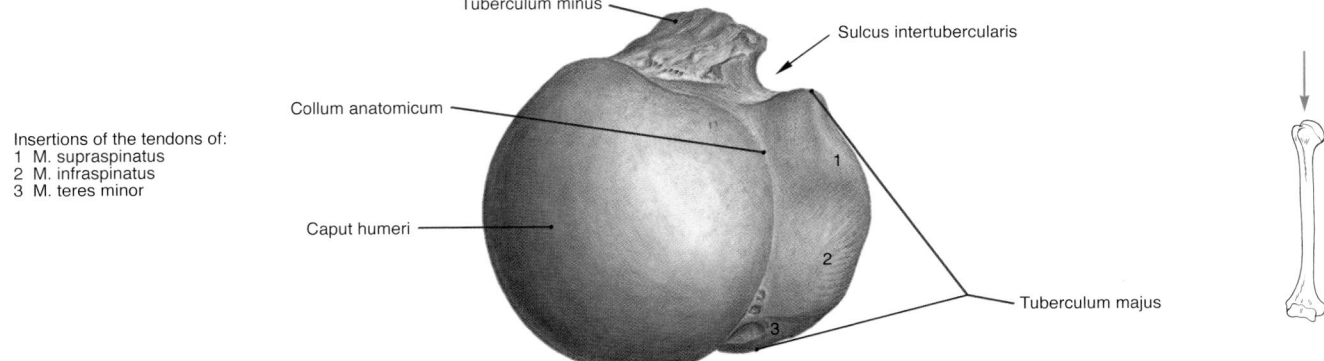

Fig. 286 Humerus, Humerus; proximal view.

Shoulder joint

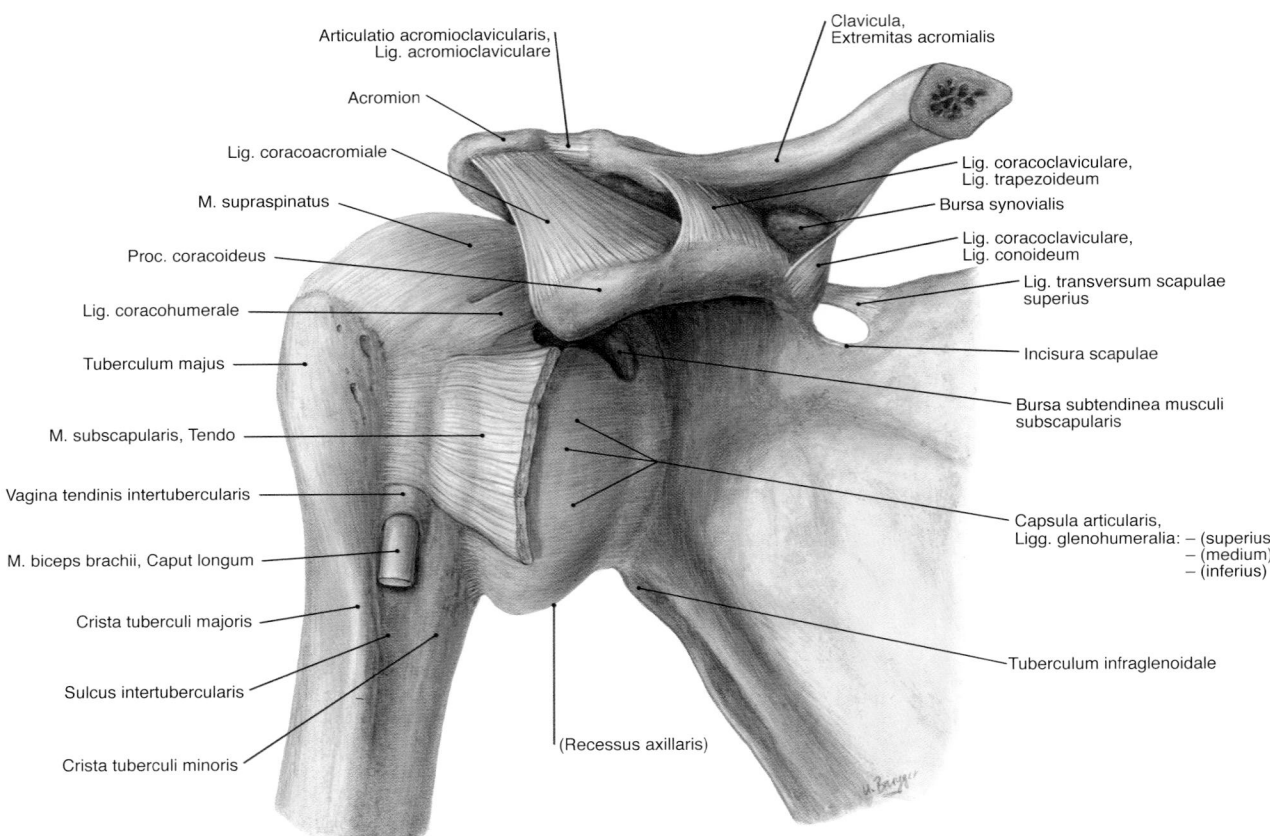

Articulatio acromioclavicularis, Lig. acromioclaviculare

Acromion

Lig. coracoacromiale

M. supraspinatus

Proc. coracoideus

Lig. coracohumerale

Tuberculum majus

M. subscapularis, Tendo

Vagina tendinis intertubercularis

M. biceps brachii, Caput longum

Crista tuberculi majoris

Sulcus intertubercularis

Crista tuberculi minoris

Clavicula, Extremitas acromialis

Lig. coracoclaviculare, Lig. trapezoideum

Bursa synovialis

Lig. coracoclaviculare, Lig. conoideum

Lig. transversum scapulae superius

Incisura scapulae

Bursa subtendinea musculi subscapularis

Capsula articularis, Ligg. glenohumeralia: − (superius)
− (medium)
− (inferius)

Tuberculum infraglenoidale

(Recessus axillaris)

Fig. 287 Shoulder joint, Articulatio humeri; ventral view.

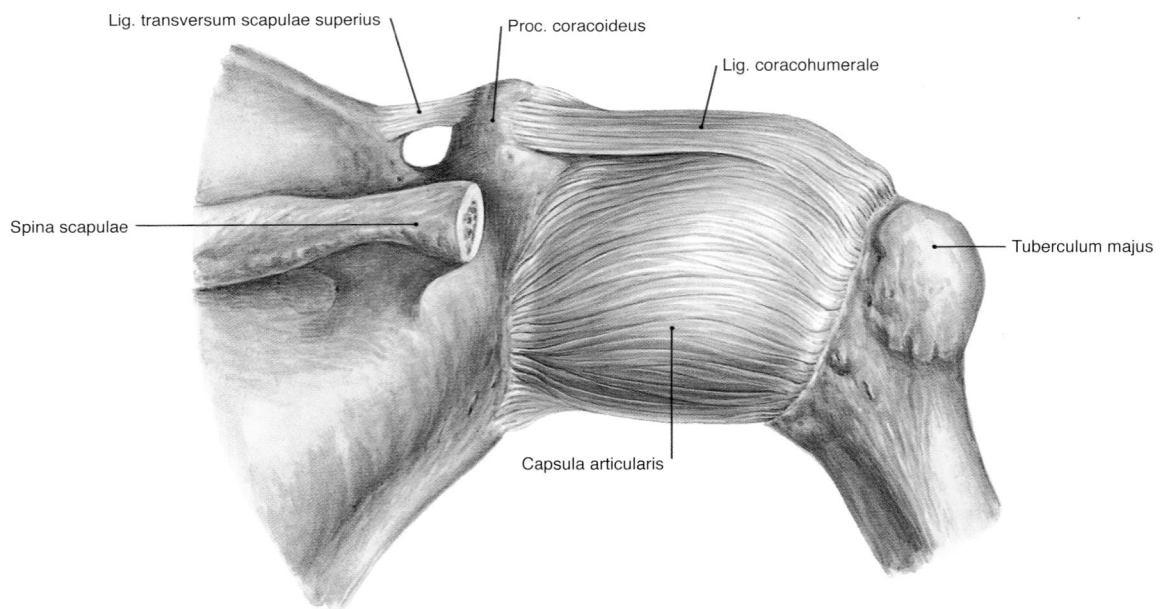

Lig. transversum scapulae superius

Proc. coracoideus

Lig. coracohumerale

Spina scapulae

Tuberculum majus

Capsula articularis

Fig. 288 Shoulder joint, Articulatio humeri; the acromion has been removed; dorsal view.

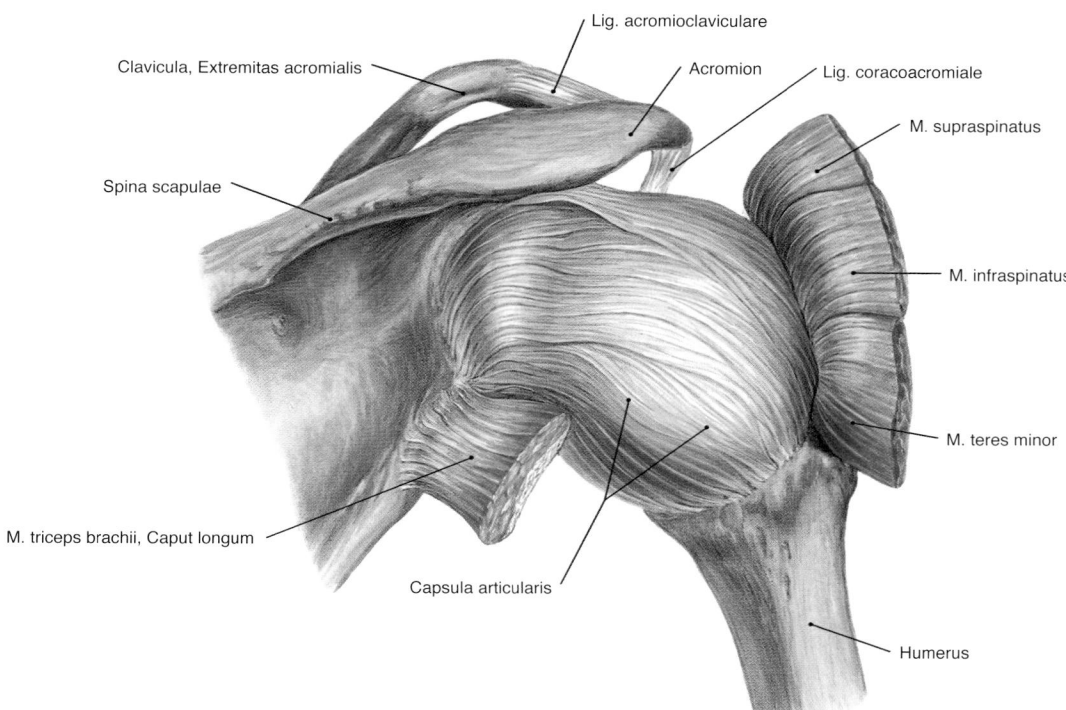

Clavicula, Extremitas acromialis
Spina scapulae
M. triceps brachii, Caput longum
Capsula articularis
Lig. acromioclaviculare
Acromion
Lig. coracoacromiale
M. supraspinatus
M. infraspinatus
M. teres minor
Humerus

Fig. 289 Shoulder joint, Articulatio humeri; dorsal view.

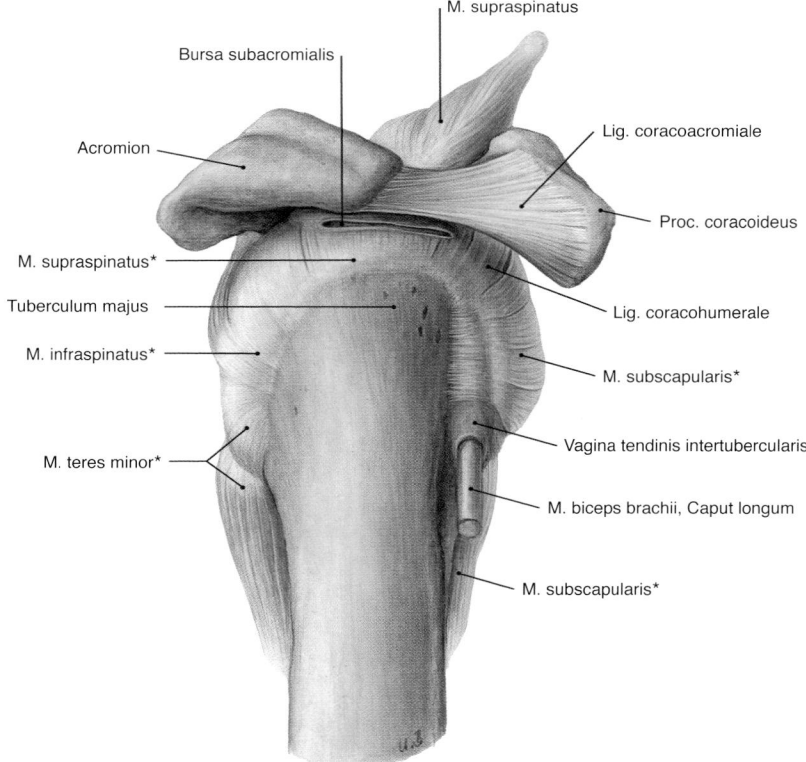

Bursa subacromialis
Acromion
M. supraspinatus*
Tuberculum majus
M. infraspinatus*
M. teres minor*
M. supraspinatus
Lig. coracoacromiale
Proc. coracoideus
Lig. coracohumerale
M. subscapularis*
Vagina tendinis intertubercularis
M. biceps brachii, Caput longum
M. subscapularis*

Fig. 290 Shoulder joint, Articulatio humeri; lateral view.

Together, the muscle tendons marked with * form the so-called rotator cuff.

Shoulder joint

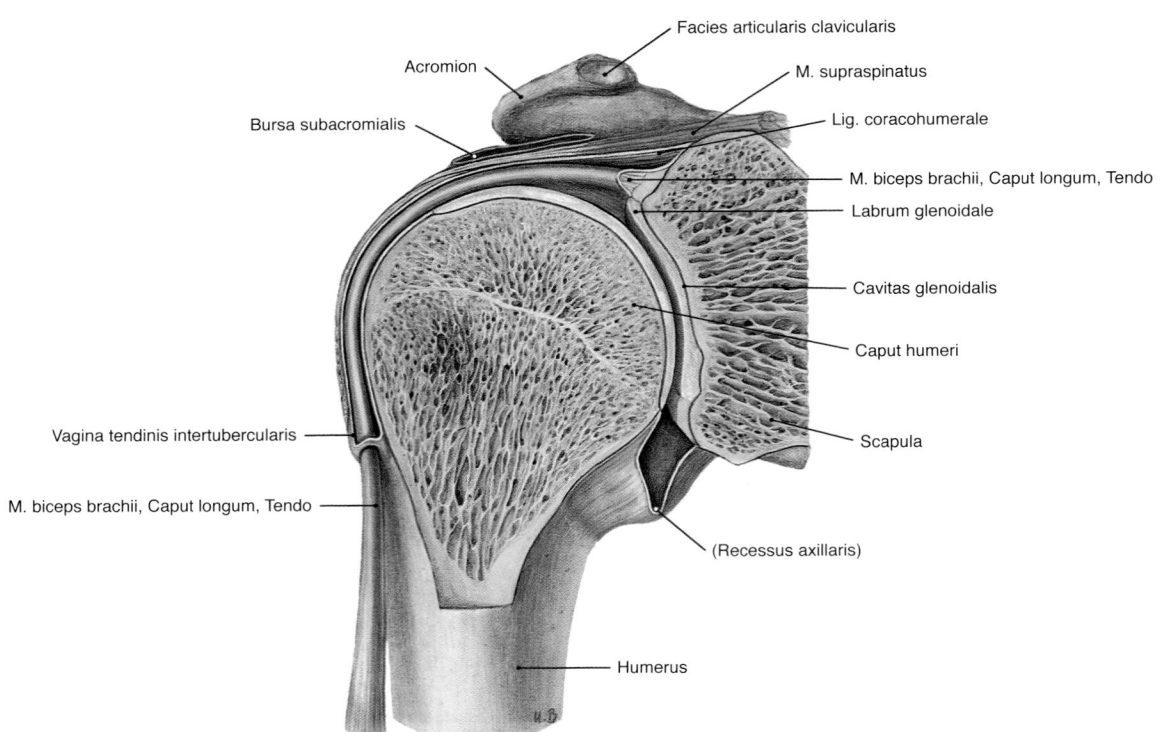

Fig. 291 Shoulder joint, Articulatio humeri; section at the level of the scapula; ventral view.

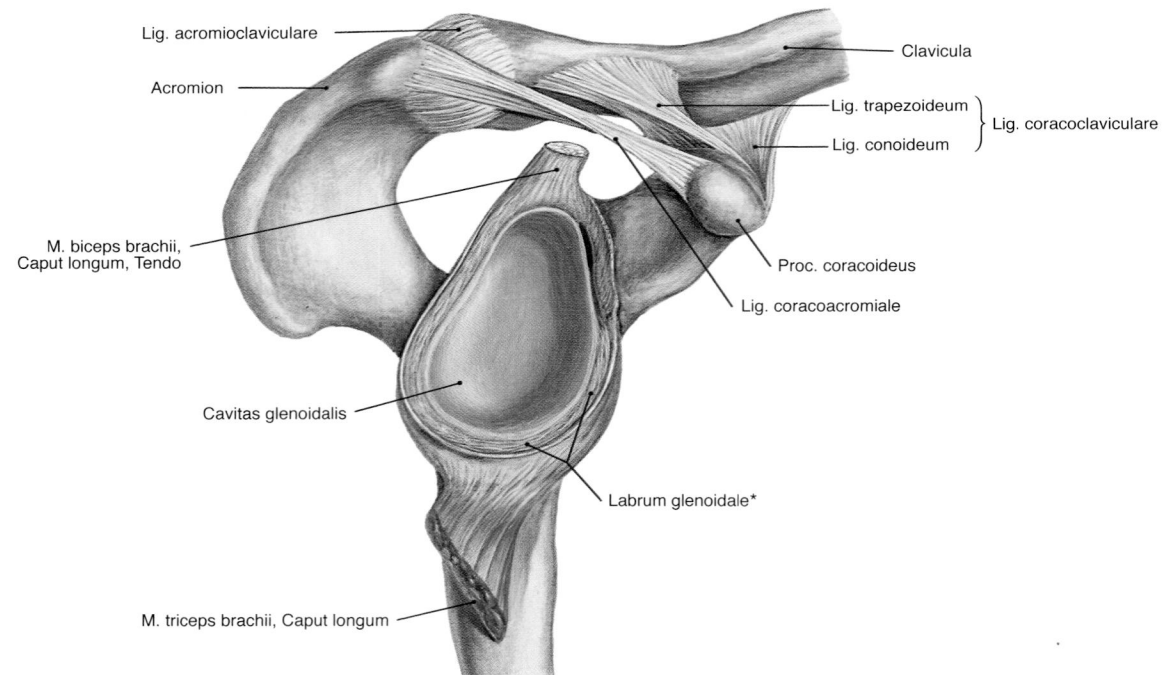

Fig. 292 Shoulder joint, Articulatio humeri; lateral view.
Next to its origin at the supraglenoidal tubercle, the tendon of the biceps muscle is predominantly attached to the glenoid labrum.
* It forms a fibrocartilaginous collar around the glenoid cavity.

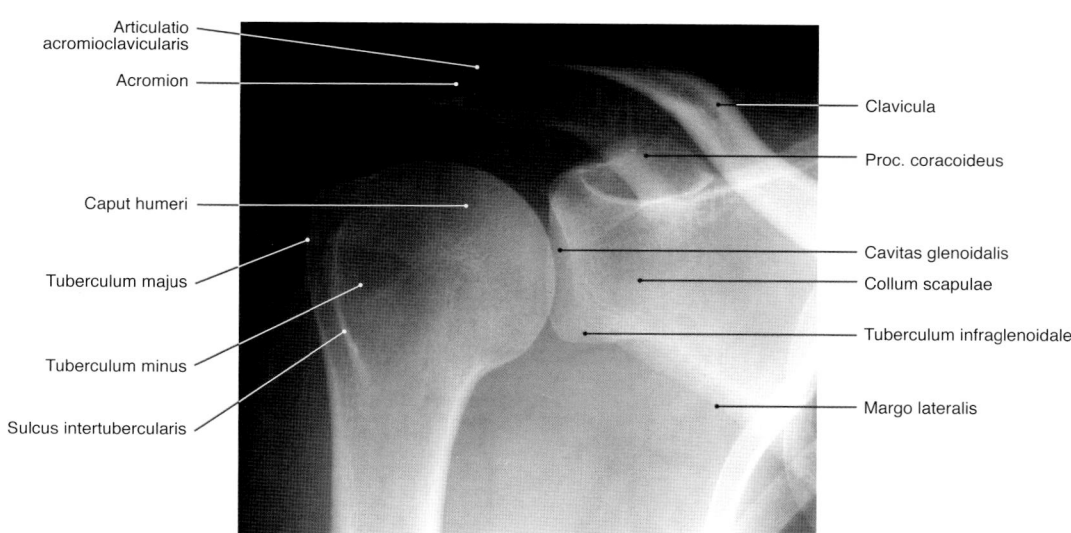

Articulatio acromioclavicularis

Acromion

Caput humeri

Tuberculum majus

Tuberculum minus

Sulcus intertubercularis

Clavicula

Proc. coracoideus

Cavitas glenoidalis
Collum scapulae

Tuberculum infraglenoidale

Margo lateralis

Fig. 293 Shoulder joint, Articulatio humeri; AP-radiograph.

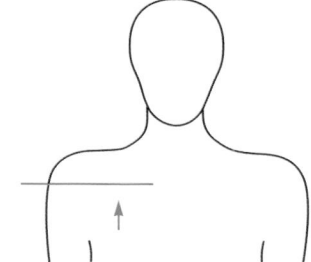

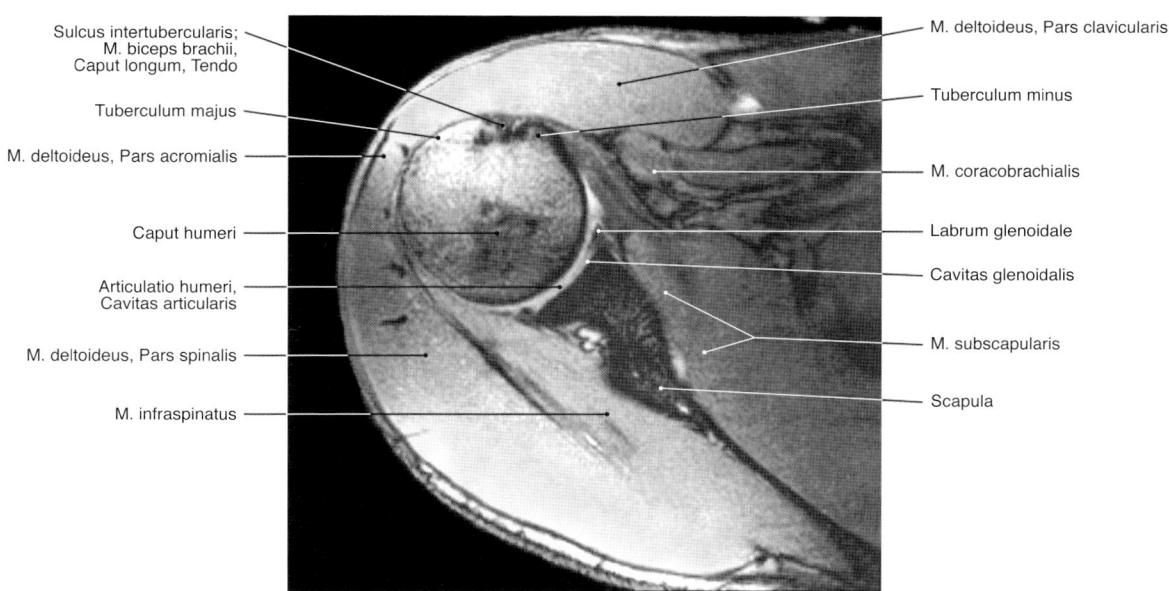

Sulcus intertubercularis; M. biceps brachii, Caput longum, Tendo

Tuberculum majus

M. deltoideus, Pars acromialis

Caput humeri

Articulatio humeri, Cavitas articularis

M. deltoideus, Pars spinalis

M. infraspinatus

M. deltoideus, Pars clavicularis

Tuberculum minus

M. coracobrachialis

Labrum glenoidale

Cavitas glenoidalis

M. subscapularis

Scapula

Fig. 294 Shoulder joint, Articulatio humeri; computed tomographic (CT) cross-section; the joint cavity is filled with air (pneumo-CT); inferior view.

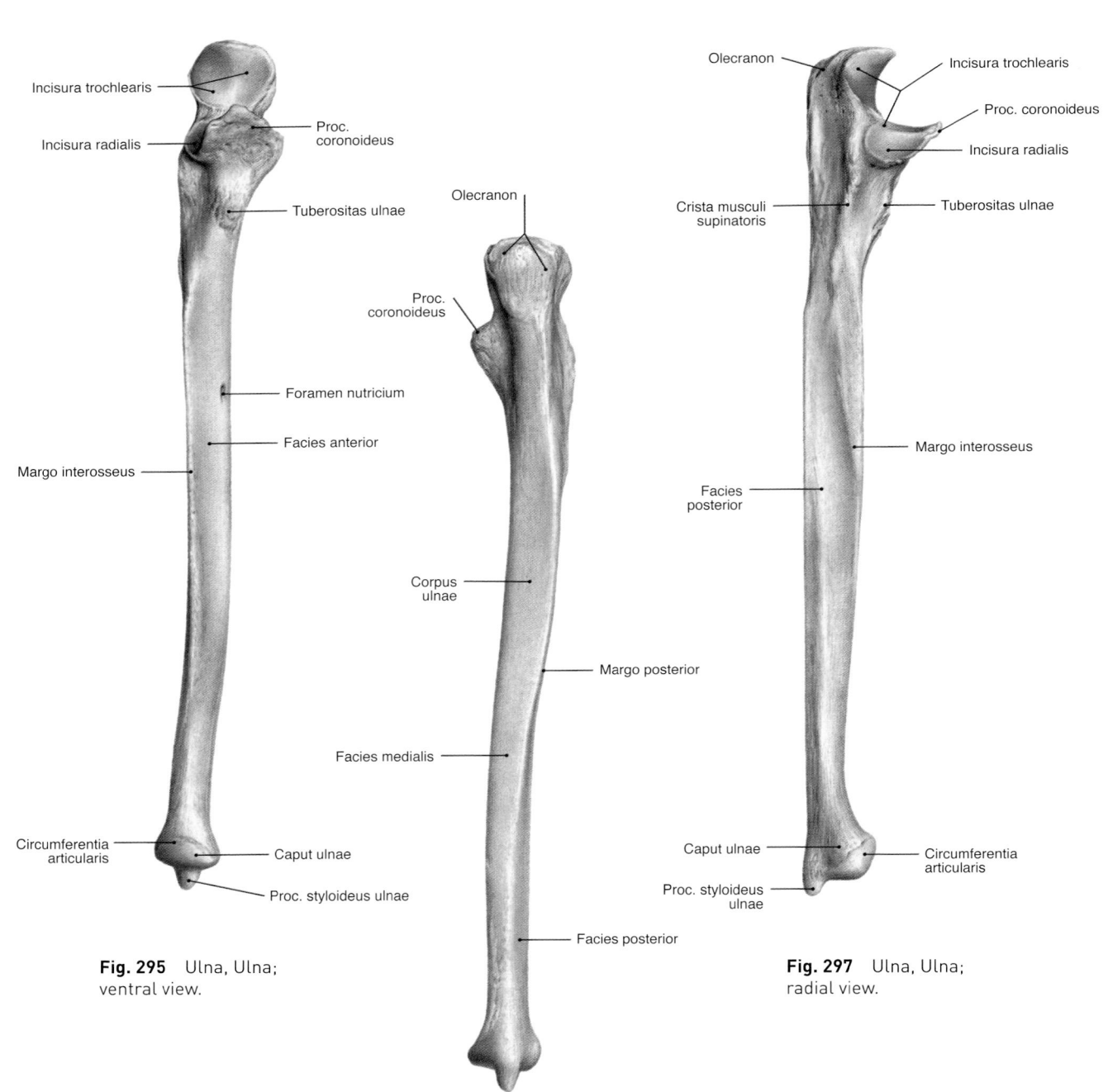

Incisura trochlearis

Incisura radialis

Proc. coronoideus

Tuberositas ulnae

Foramen nutricium

Facies anterior

Margo interosseus

Circumferentia articularis

Caput ulnae

Proc. styloideus ulnae

Fig. 295 Ulna, Ulna; ventral view.

Olecranon

Proc. coronoideus

Corpus ulnae

Margo posterior

Facies medialis

Facies posterior

Fig. 296 Ulna, Ulna; dorsal view.

Olecranon

Incisura trochlearis

Proc. coronoideus

Incisura radialis

Crista musculi supinatoris

Tuberositas ulnae

Margo interosseus

Facies posterior

Caput ulnae

Circumferentia articularis

Proc. styloideus ulnae

Fig. 297 Ulna, Ulna; radial view.

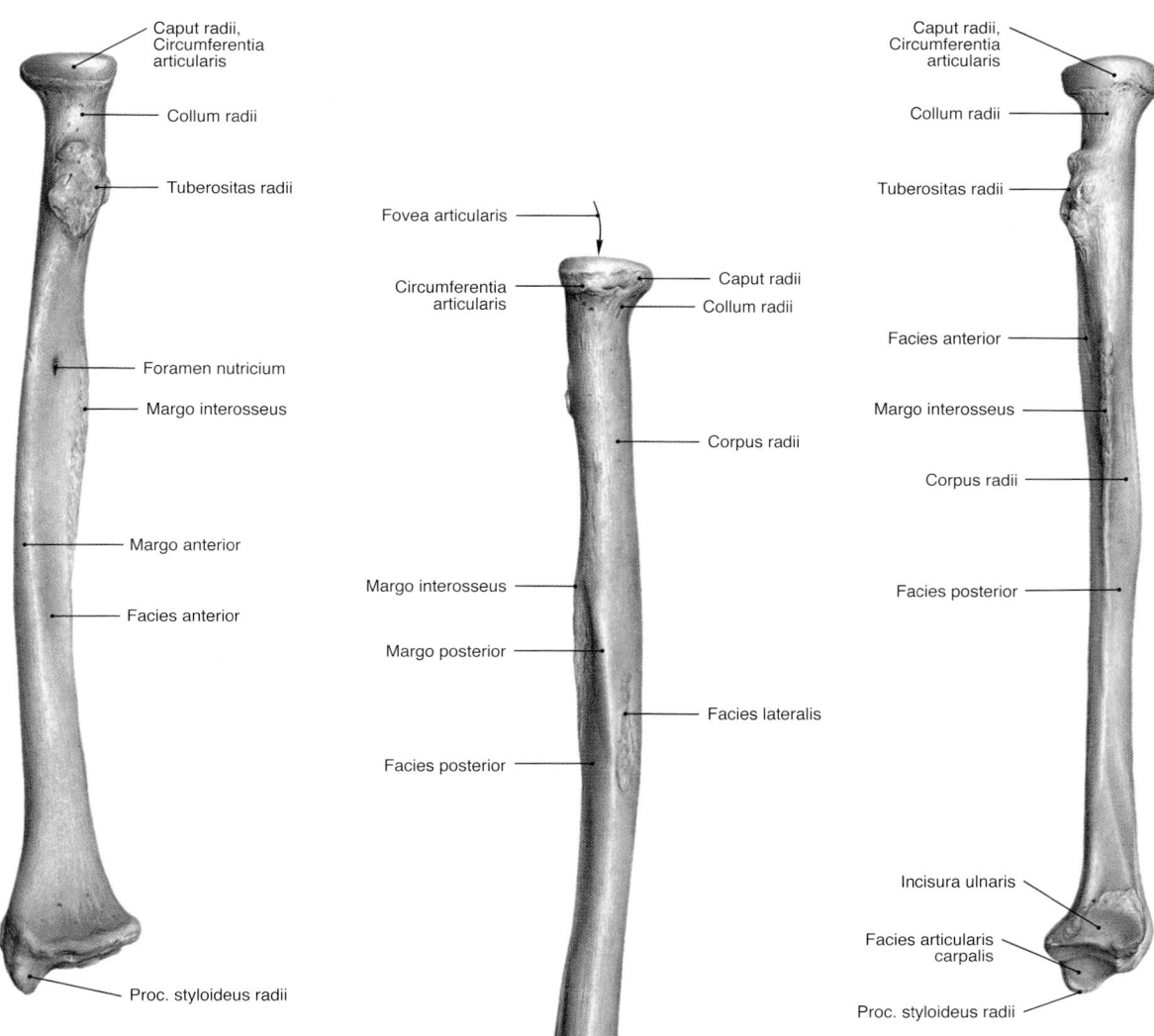

Caput radii,
Circumferentia
articularis

Collum radii

Tuberositas radii

Foramen nutricium

Margo interosseus

Margo anterior

Facies anterior

Proc. styloideus radii

Fig. 298 Radius, Radius;
ventral view.

Fovea articularis

Circumferentia
articularis

Caput radii

Collum radii

Corpus radii

Margo interosseus

Margo posterior

Facies lateralis

Facies posterior

Tuberculum dorsale

*

Fig. 299 Radius, Radius;
dorsal view.

* Grooves and crests for the
attachment of the extensor
tendons

Caput radii,
Circumferentia
articularis

Collum radii

Tuberositas radii

Facies anterior

Margo interosseus

Corpus radii

Facies posterior

Incisura ulnaris

Facies articularis
carpalis

Proc. styloideus radii

Fig. 300 Radius, Radius;
ulnar view.

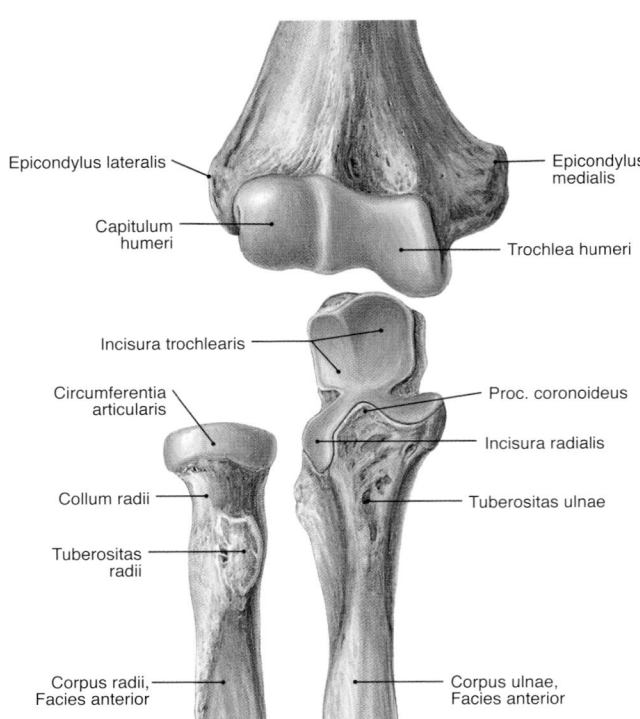

Epicondylus lateralis
Epicondylus medialis
Capitulum humeri
Trochlea humeri
Incisura trochlearis
Circumferentia articularis
Proc. coronoideus
Incisura radialis
Collum radii
Tuberositas ulnae
Tuberositas radii
Corpus radii, Facies anterior
Corpus ulnae, Facies anterior

Fig. 301 Elbow joint, Articulatio cubiti; ventral view.

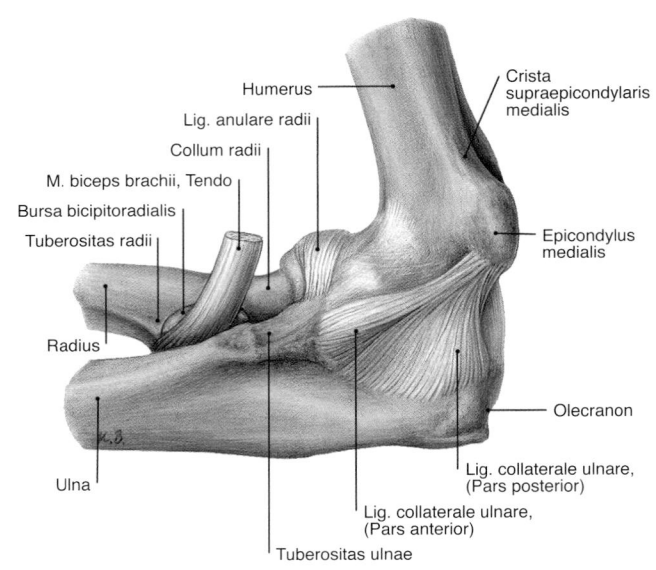

Humerus
Crista supraepicondylaris medialis
Lig. anulare radii
Collum radii
M. biceps brachii, Tendo
Bursa bicipitoradialis
Tuberositas radii
Epicondylus medialis
Radius
Ulna
Olecranon
Lig. collaterale ulnare, (Pars posterior)
Lig. collaterale ulnare, (Pars anterior)
Tuberositas ulnae

Fig. 302 Elbow joint, Articulatio cubiti, in 90° flexion and 90° supination; medial view.

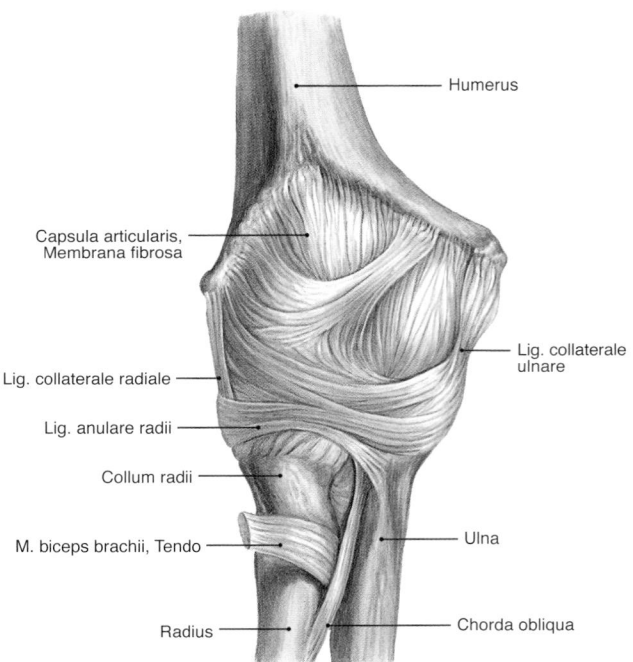

Humerus
Capsula articularis, Membrana fibrosa
Lig. collaterale ulnare
Lig. collaterale radiale
Lig. anulare radii
Collum radii
M. biceps brachii, Tendo
Ulna
Radius
Chorda obliqua

Fig. 303 Elbow joint, Articulatio cubiti; ventral view.

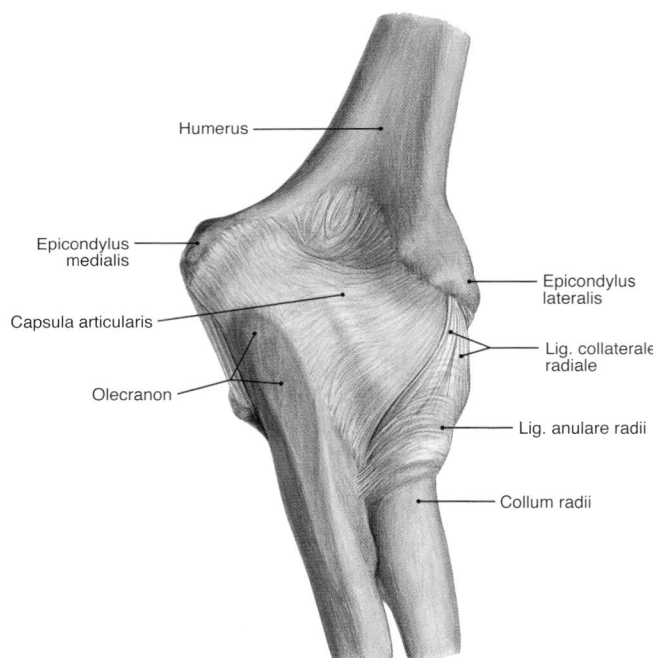

Humerus
Epicondylus medialis
Epicondylus lateralis
Capsula articularis
Lig. collaterale radiale
Olecranon
Lig. anulare radii
Collum radii

Fig. 304 Elbow joint, Articulatio cubiti; dorsal view.

Junctions of the bones of the forearm

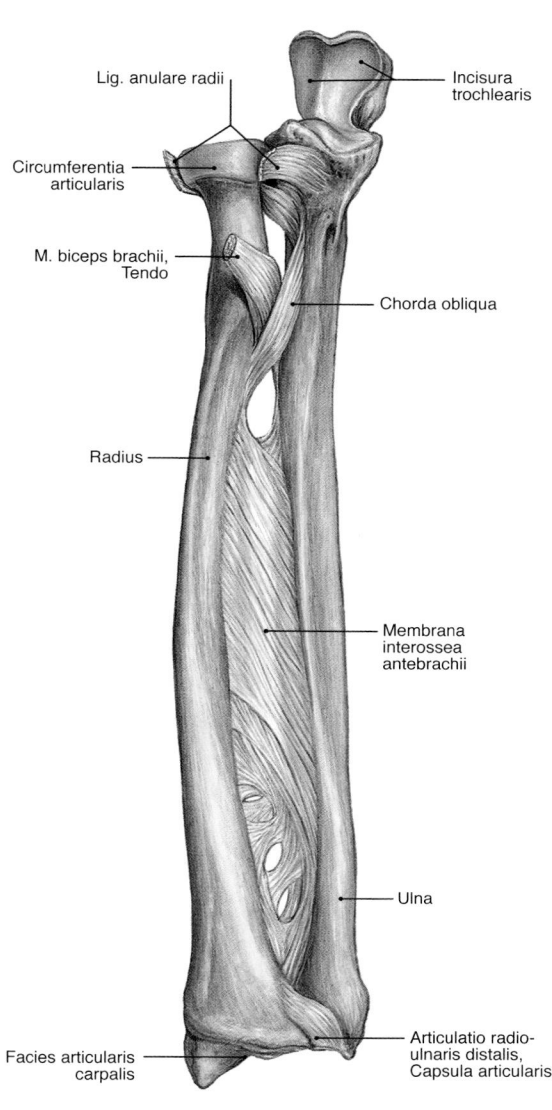

Lig. anulare radii

Incisura trochlearis

Circumferentia articularis

M. biceps brachii, Tendo

Chorda obliqua

Radius

Membrana interossea antebrachii

Ulna

Facies articularis carpalis

Articulatio radio-ulnaris distalis, Capsula articularis

Fig. 305   Junctions of the bones of the forearm; in supination; ventral view.

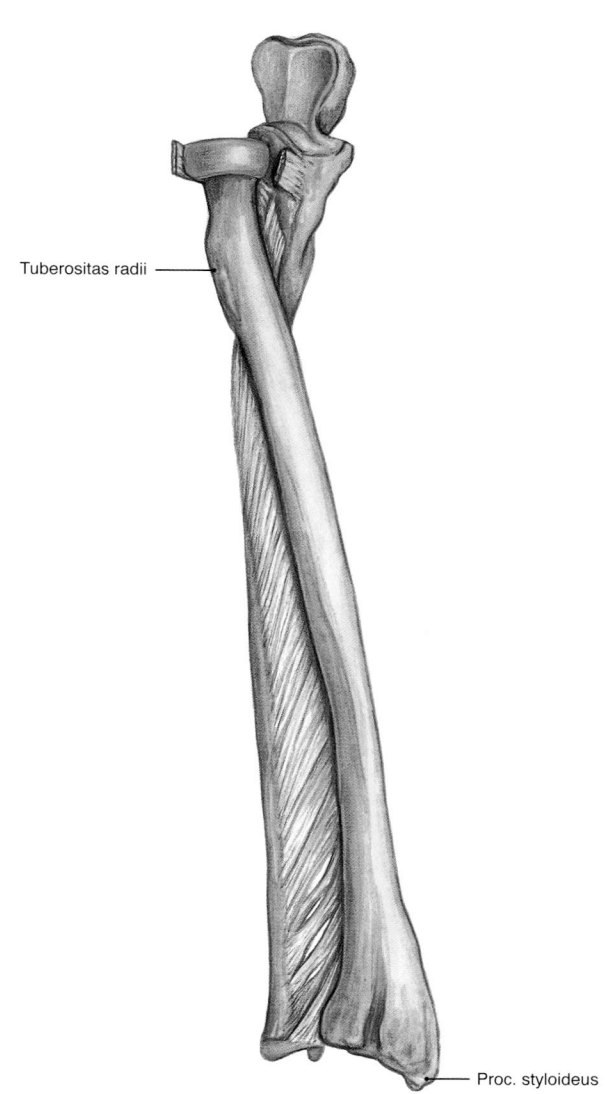

Tuberositas radii

Proc. styloideus

Fig. 306   Junctions of the bones of the forearm; in pronation; ventral view of the ulna, dorsal view of the radius.

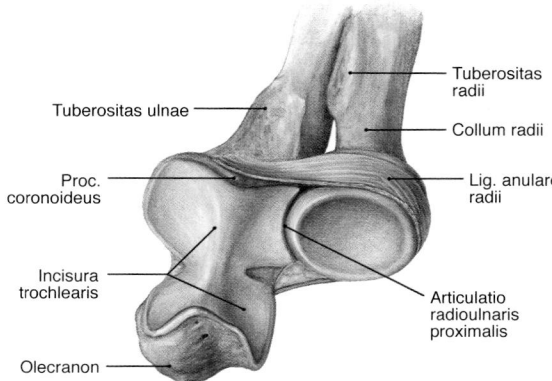

Tuberositas ulnae

Proc. coronoideus

Incisura trochlearis

Olecranon

Tuberositas radii

Collum radii

Lig. anulare radii

Articulatio radioulnaris proximalis

Fig. 307   Proximal radio-ulnar joint, Articulatio radio-ulnaris proximalis; ventroproximal view.

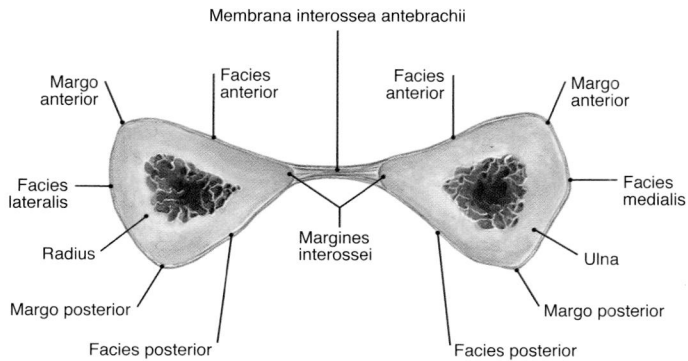

Membrana interossea antebrachii

Margo anterior

Facies anterior

Facies anterior

Margo anterior

Facies lateralis

Facies medialis

Radius

Margines interossei

Ulna

Margo posterior

Facies posterior

Facies posterior

Margo posterior

Fig. 308   Cross-section through the bones of the forearm; distal view.

Elbow joint, sections and radiography

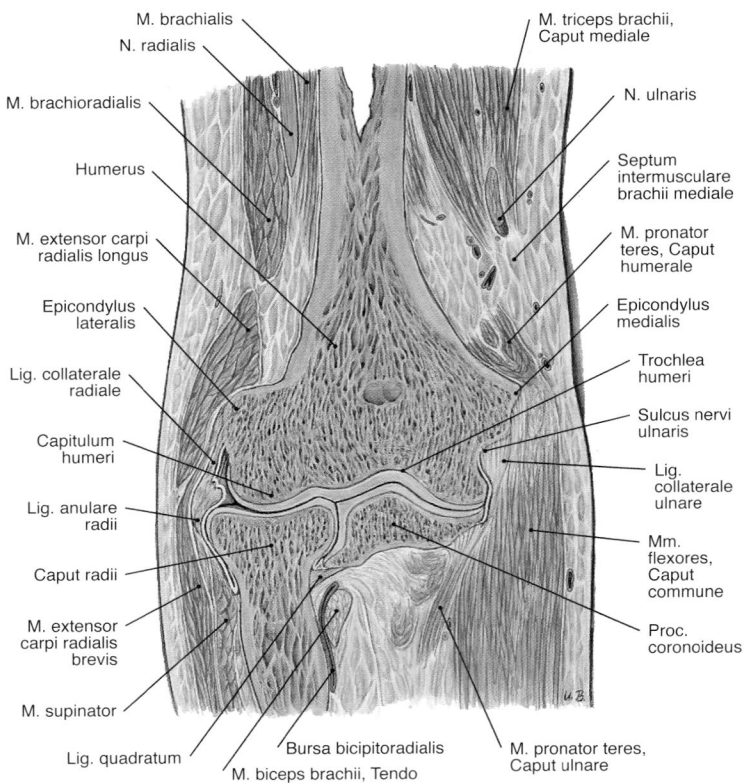

M. brachialis
N. radialis
M. brachioradialis
Humerus
M. extensor carpi radialis longus
Epicondylus lateralis
Lig. collaterale radiale
Capitulum humeri
Lig. anulare radii
Caput radii
M. extensor carpi radialis brevis
M. supinator
Lig. quadratum
Bursa bicipitoradialis
M. biceps brachii, Tendo

M. triceps brachii, Caput mediale
N. ulnaris
Septum intermusculare brachii mediale
M. pronator teres, Caput humerale
Epicondylus medialis
Trochlea humeri
Sulcus nervi ulnaris
Lig. collaterale ulnare
Mm. flexores, Caput commune
Proc. coronoideus
M. pronator teres, Caput ulnare

Fig. 309 Elbow joint, Articulatio cubiti; frontal section.

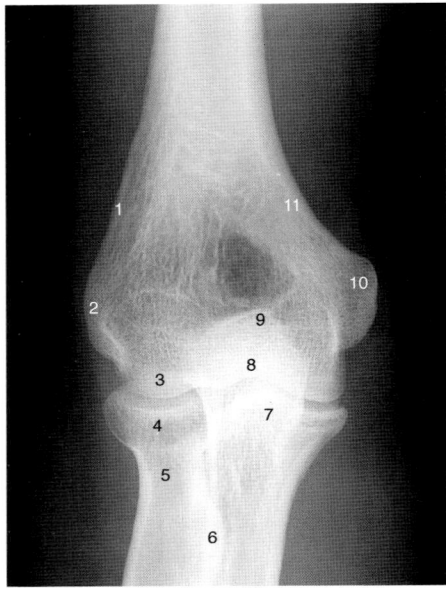

1 Crista supraepicondylaris lateralis	6 Tuberositas radii
2 Epicondylus lateralis	7 Proc. coronoideus
3 Capitulum humeri	8 Trochlea humeri
4 Caput radii	9 Olecranon
5 Collum radii	10 Epicondylus medialis
	11 Crista supraepicondylaris medialis

Fig. 310 Elbow joint, Articulatio cubiti; AP-radiograph.

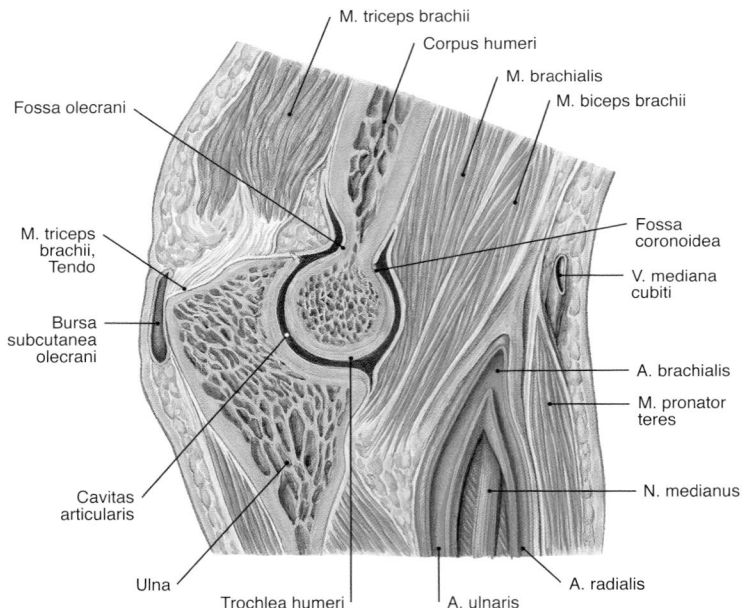

Fossa olecrani
M. triceps brachii, Tendo
Bursa subcutanea olecrani
Cavitas articularis
Ulna
Trochlea humeri
A. ulnaris

M. triceps brachii
Corpus humeri
M. brachialis
M. biceps brachii
Fossa coronoidea
V. mediana cubiti
A. brachialis
M. pronator teres
N. medianus
A. radialis

Fig. 311 Elbow joint, Articulatio cubiti; sagittal section.

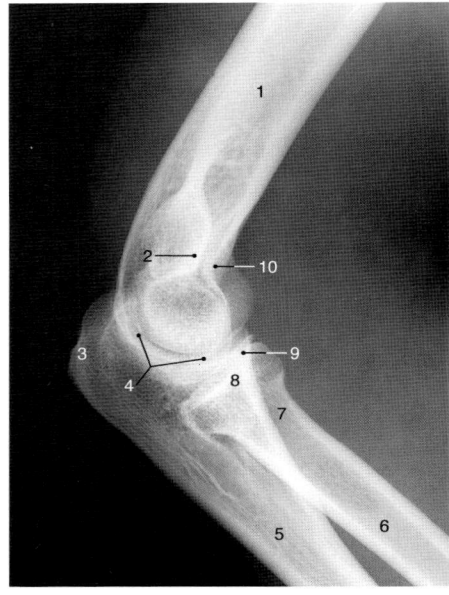

1 Humerus	6 Radius
2 Fossa olecrani	7 Collum radii
3 Olecranon	8 Caput radii
4 Incisura trochlearis	9 Proc. coronoideus
5 Ulna	10 Fossa coronoidea

Fig. 312 Elbow joint, Articulatio cubiti; lateral radiograph.

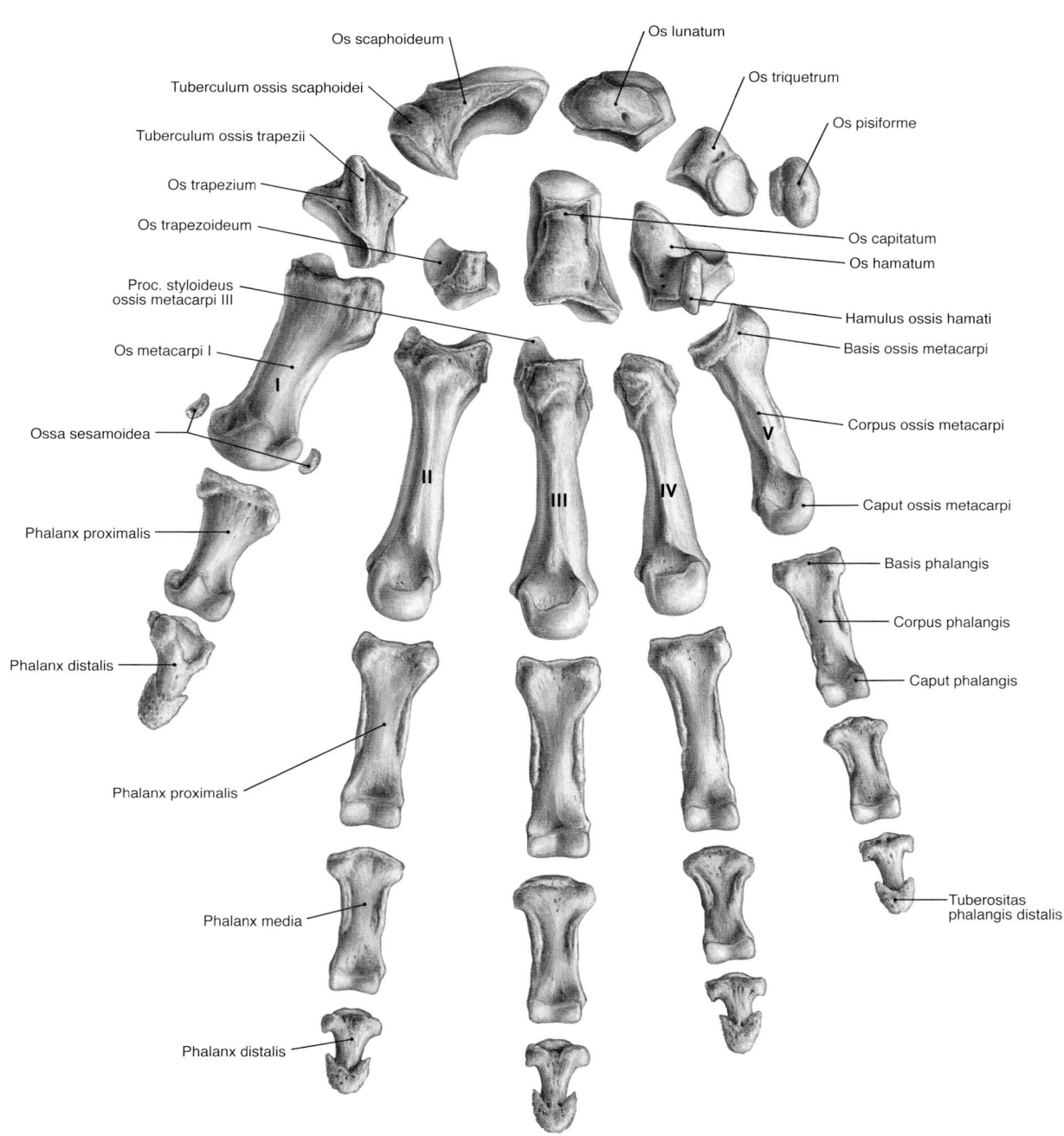

Os scaphoideum
Os lunatum
Tuberculum ossis scaphoidei
Os triquetrum
Tuberculum ossis trapezii
Os pisiforme
Os trapezium
Os trapezoideum
Os capitatum
Os hamatum
Proc. styloideus ossis metacarpi III
Hamulus ossis hamati
Os metacarpi I
Basis ossis metacarpi
Ossa sesamoidea
Corpus ossis metacarpi
Phalanx proximalis
Caput ossis metacarpi
Basis phalangis
Corpus phalangis
Phalanx distalis
Caput phalangis
Phalanx proximalis
Phalanx media
Tuberositas phalangis distalis
Phalanx distalis

I   Pollex [Digitus primus]
II Index [Digitus secundus]
III Digitus medius [Digitus tertius]
IV Digitus anularis [Digitus quartus]
V   Digitus minimus [Digitus quintus]

Fig. 313   Bones of the hand, Ossa manus; palmar view.

Skeleton of the hand

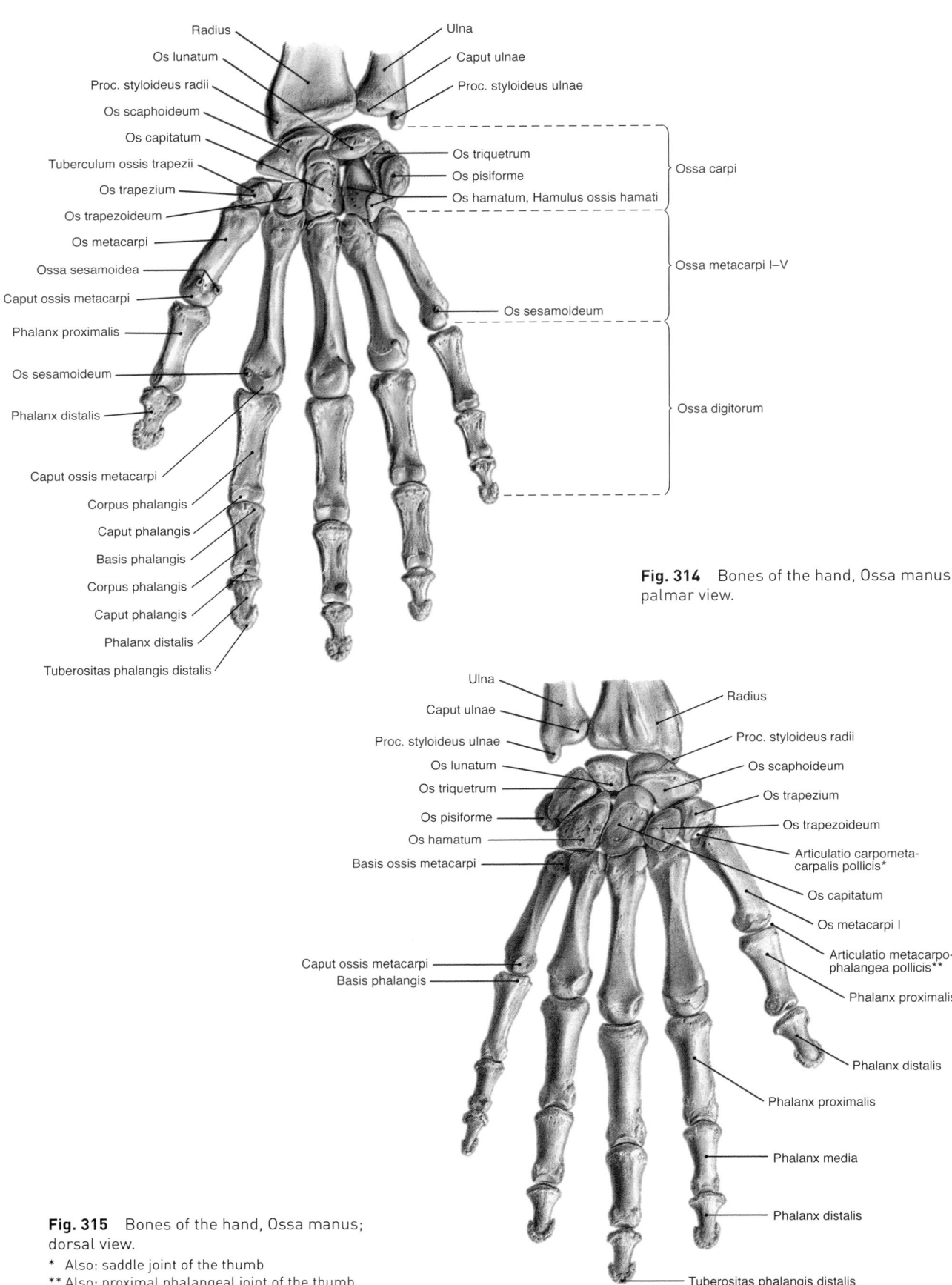

Radius
Os lunatum
Proc. styloideus radii
Os scaphoideum
Os capitatum
Tuberculum ossis trapezii
Os trapezium
Os trapezoideum
Os metacarpi
Ossa sesamoidea
Caput ossis metacarpi
Phalanx proximalis
Os sesamoideum
Phalanx distalis
Caput ossis metacarpi
Corpus phalangis
Caput phalangis
Basis phalangis
Corpus phalangis
Caput phalangis
Phalanx distalis
Tuberositas phalangis distalis

Ulna
Caput ulnae
Proc. styloideus ulnae
Os triquetrum
Os pisiforme
Os hamatum, Hamulus ossis hamati
Ossa carpi
Ossa metacarpi I–V
Os sesamoideum
Ossa digitorum

Fig. 314 Bones of the hand, Ossa manus; palmar view.

Ulna
Caput ulnae
Proc. styloideus ulnae
Os lunatum
Os triquetrum
Os pisiforme
Os hamatum
Basis ossis metacarpi
Caput ossis metacarpi
Basis phalangis

Radius
Proc. styloideus radii
Os scaphoideum
Os trapezium
Os trapezoideum
Articulatio carpometacarpalis pollicis*
Os capitatum
Os metacarpi I
Articulatio metacarpophalangea pollicis**
Phalanx proximalis
Phalanx distalis
Phalanx proximalis
Phalanx media
Phalanx distalis
Tuberositas phalangis distalis

Fig. 315 Bones of the hand, Ossa manus; dorsal view.
* Also: saddle joint of the thumb
** Also: proximal phalangeal joint of the thumb

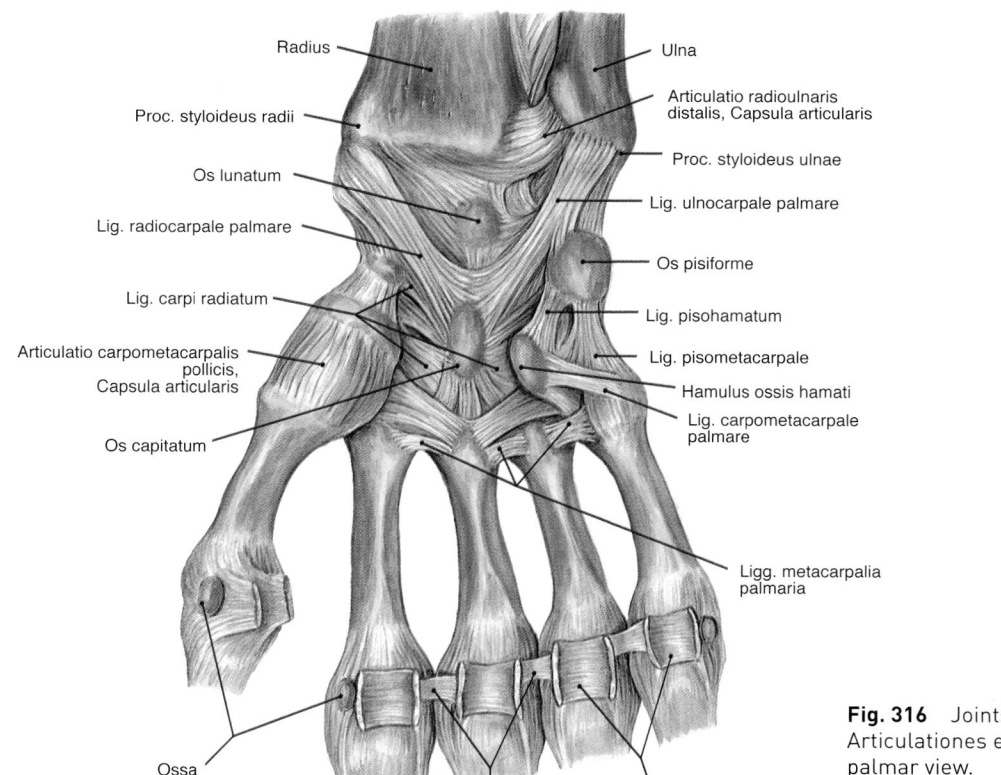

Radius
Ulna
Proc. styloideus radii
Articulatio radioulnaris distalis, Capsula articularis
Os lunatum
Proc. styloideus ulnae
Lig. radiocarpale palmare
Lig. ulnocarpale palmare
Lig. carpi radiatum
Os pisiforme
Articulatio carpometacarpalis pollicis, Capsula articularis
Lig. pisohamatum
Lig. pisometacarpale
Os capitatum
Hamulus ossis hamati
Lig. carpometacarpale palmare
Ligg. metacarpalia palmaria
Ossa sesamoidea
Ligg. metacarpalia transversa profunda
Ligg. palmaria

Fig. 316 Joints and ligaments of the hand, Articulationes et Ligamenta manus; palmar view.

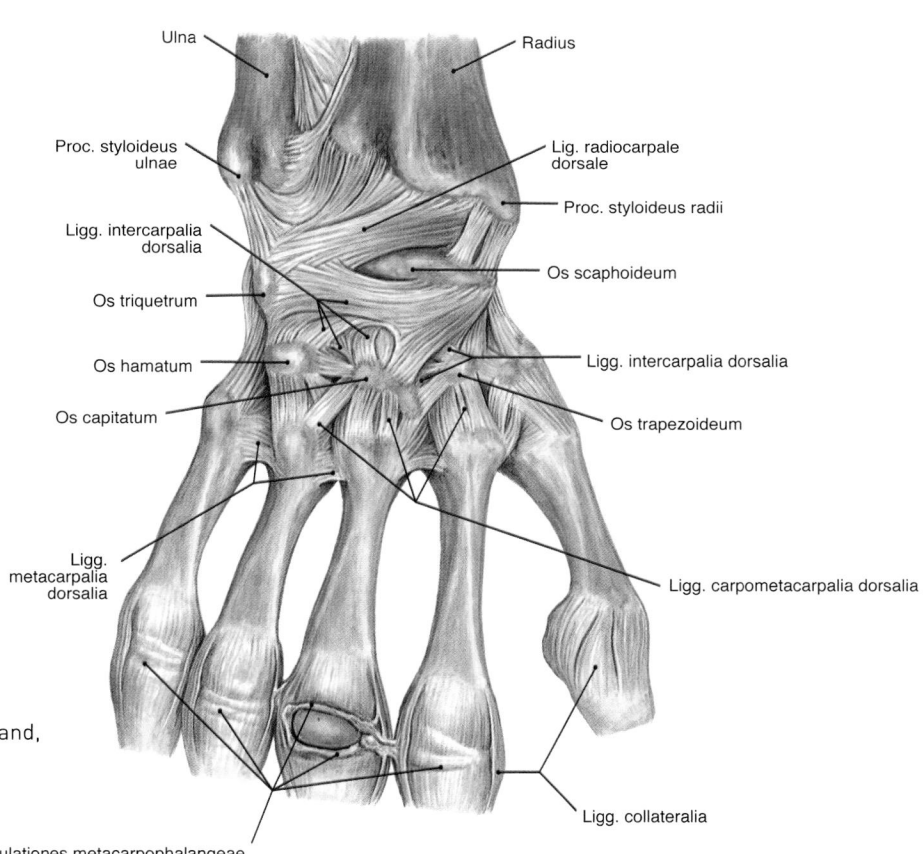

Ulna
Radius
Proc. styloideus ulnae
Lig. radiocarpale dorsale
Proc. styloideus radii
Ligg. intercarpalia dorsalia
Os scaphoideum
Os triquetrum
Os hamatum
Ligg. intercarpalia dorsalia
Os capitatum
Os trapezoideum
Ligg. metacarpalia dorsalia
Ligg. carpometacarpalia dorsalia
Ligg. collateralia

Fig. 317 Joints and ligaments of the hand, Articulationes et Ligamenta manus; dorsal view.

Articulationes metacarpophalangeae, Capsulae articulares

Joints of the hand

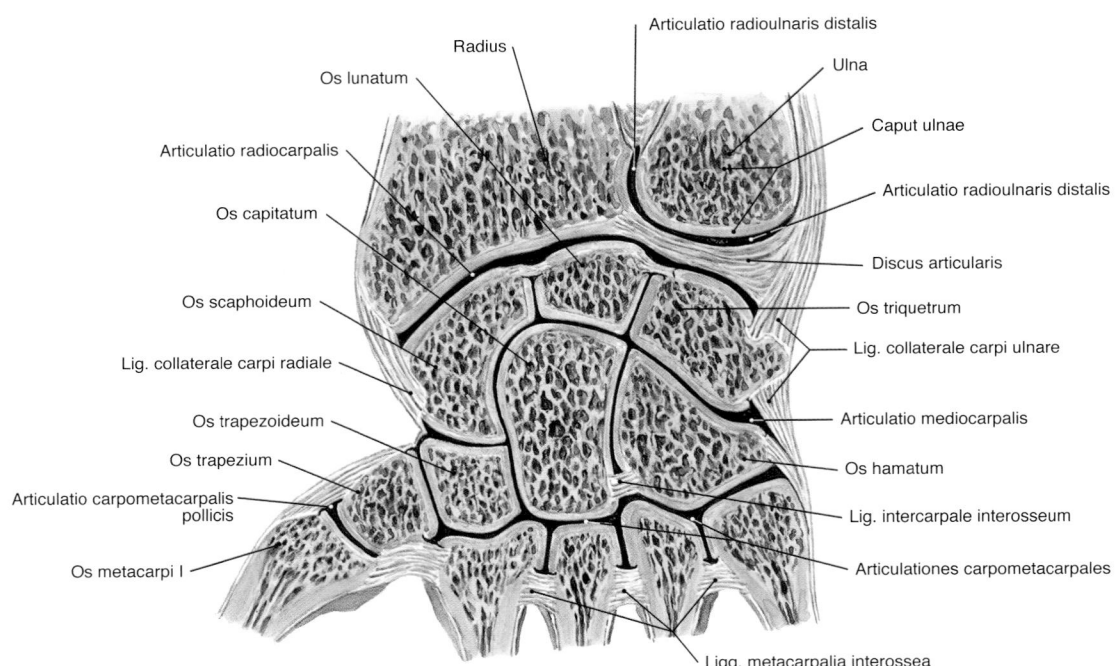

Fig. 318 Carpal joints, Articulationes carpi;
longitudinal section parallel to the dorsum of the hand.

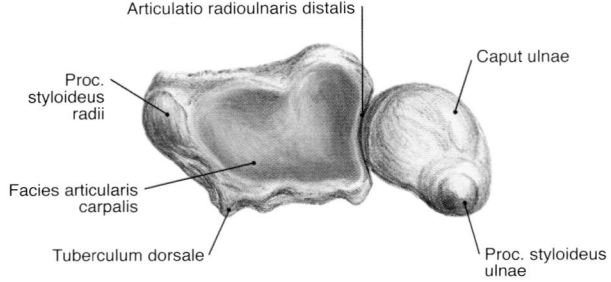

Fig. 319 Ulna and radius, Ulna et Radius;
distal view.

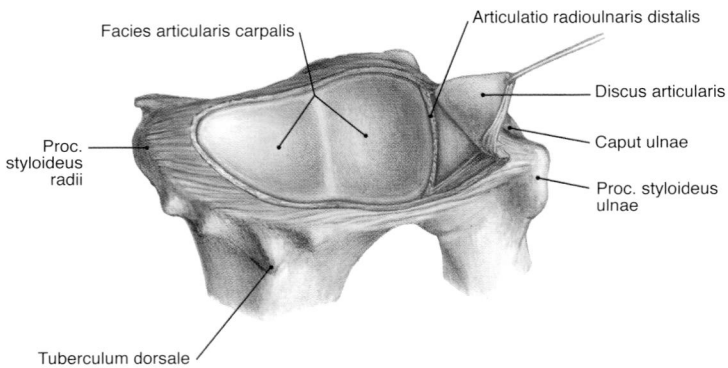

Fig. 320 Distal radio-ulnar joint,
Articulatio radioulnaris distalis;
distal-dorsal view.

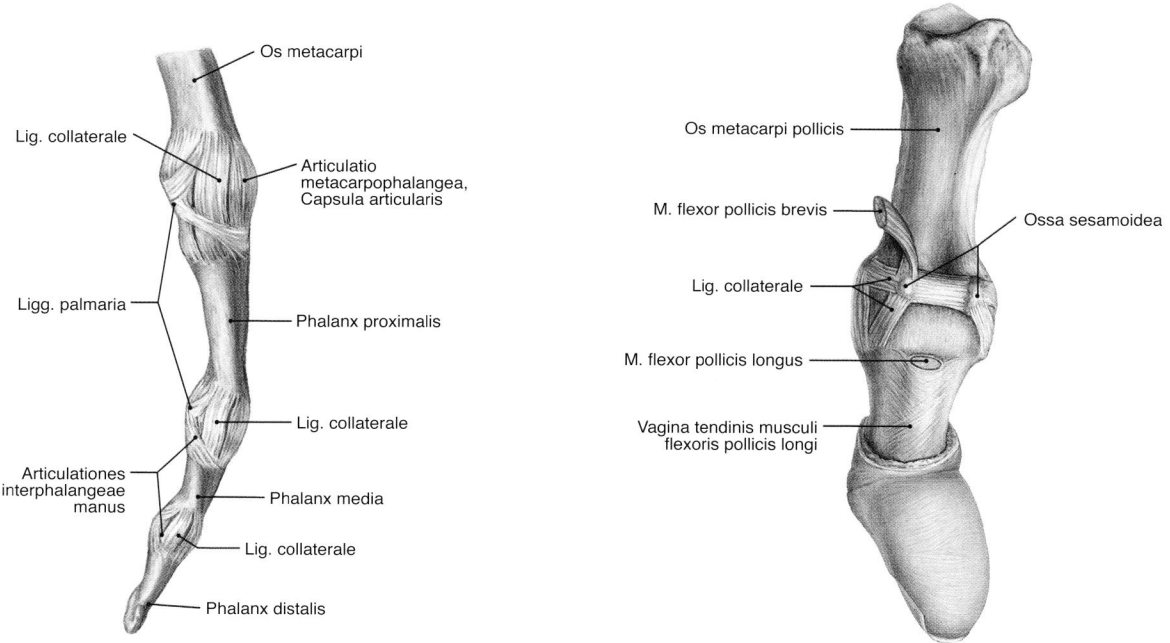

Fig. 321 Finger joints, Articulationes digiti; lateral view.

Fig. 322 Metacarpophalangeal joint of the thumb, Articulatio metacarpophalangea pollicis; radial-palmar view.

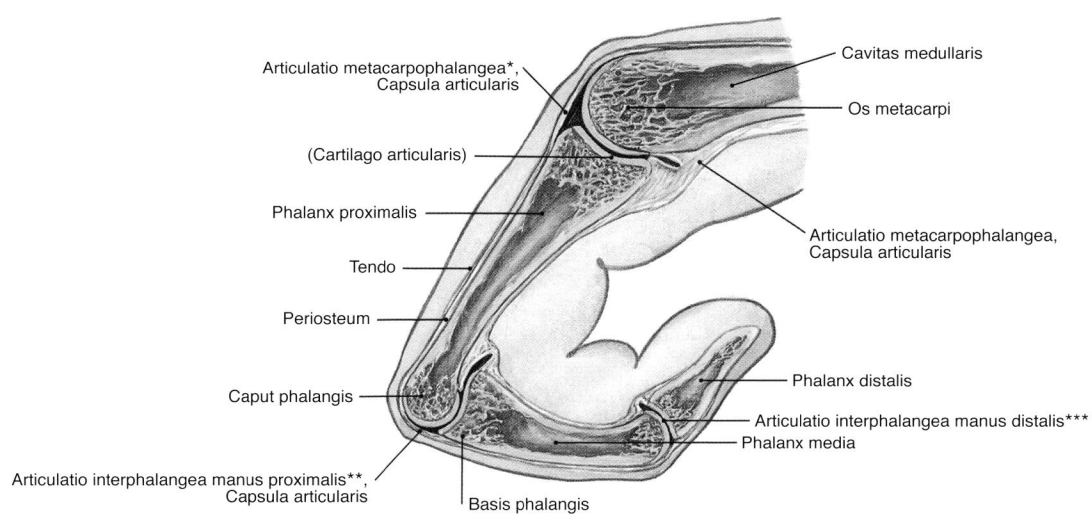

Fig. 323 Finger joints, Articulationes digiti; sagittal section; lateral view.

*   Clinical term: **MP** (= **m**etacarpo**p**halangeal joint)
**   Clinical term: **PIP** (= **p**roximal **i**nter**p**halangeal joint)
***Clinical term: **DIP** (= **d**istal **i**nter**p**halangeal joint)

Wrist, radiography

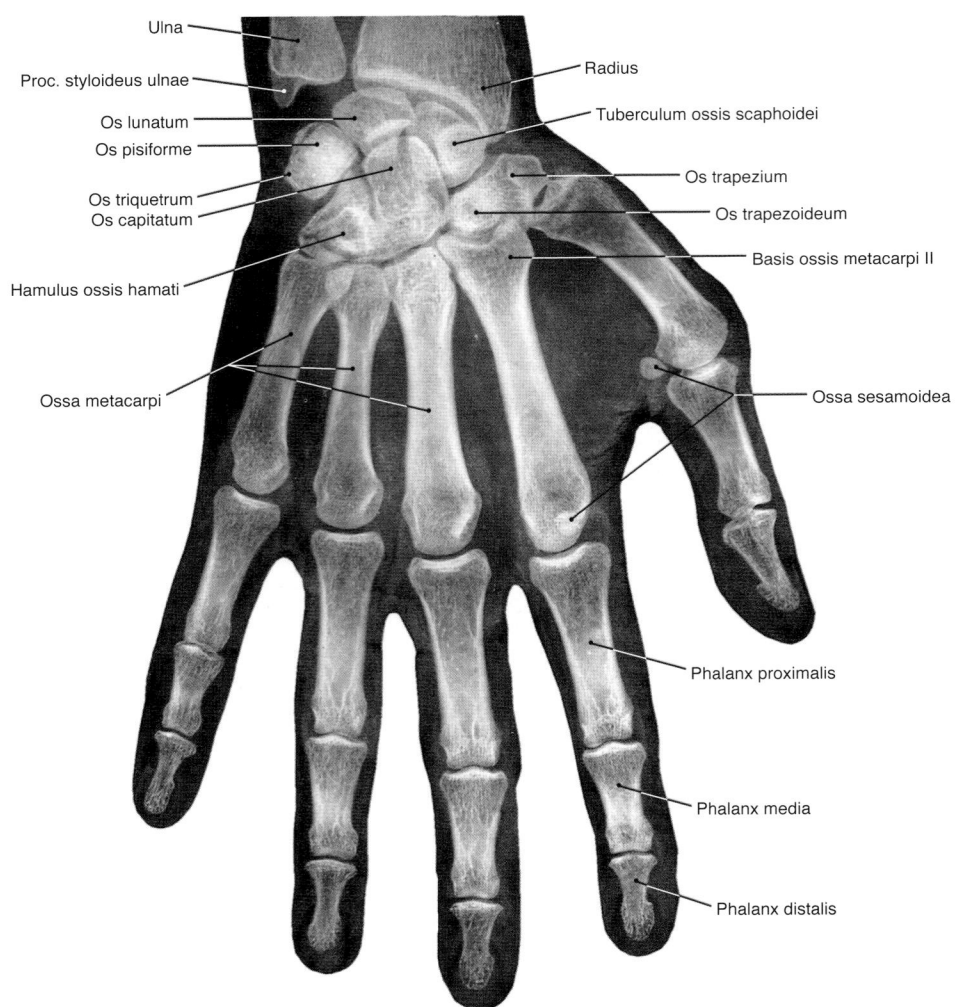

Ulna
Proc. styloideus ulnae
Os lunatum
Os pisiforme
Os triquetrum
Os capitatum
Hamulus ossis hamati
Ossa metacarpi

Radius
Tuberculum ossis scaphoidei
Os trapezium
Os trapezoideum
Basis ossis metacarpi II
Ossa sesamoidea

Phalanx proximalis

Phalanx media

Phalanx distalis

Fig. 324 Hand, Manus;
PA-radiograph.
Note: The pisiform bone is projected onto
the triquetral bone.

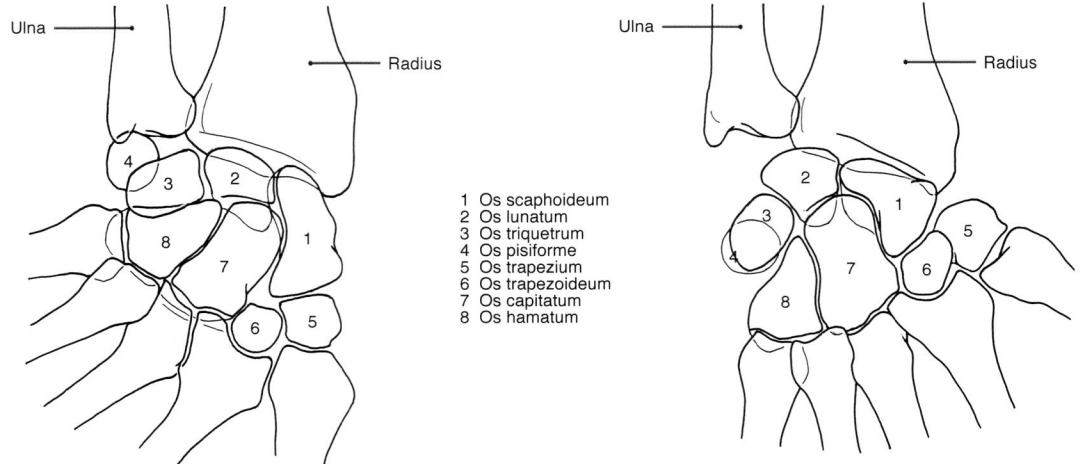

Ulna
Radius

Ulna
Radius

1 Os scaphoideum
2 Os lunatum
3 Os triquetrum
4 Os pisiforme
5 Os trapezium
6 Os trapezoideum
7 Os capitatum
8 Os hamatum

Fig. 325 Ulnar abduction of the hand;
schema of a PA-radiograph.

Fig. 326 Radial abduction of the hand;
schema of a PA-radiograph.

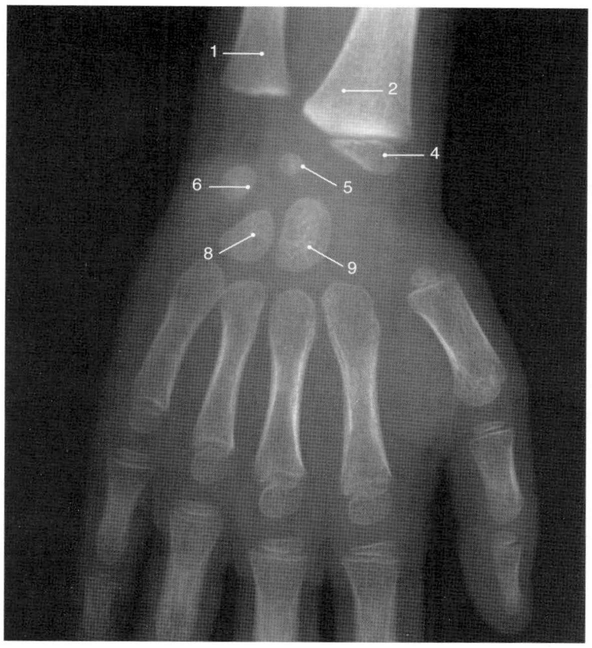

Wrist, development

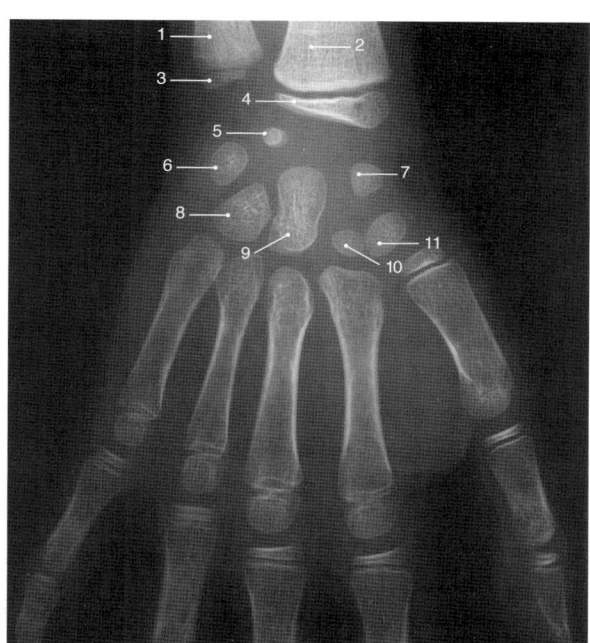

Fig. 327 PA-radiograph of the hand of a 4½-year-old boy.

Fig. 328 PA-radiograph of the hand of a 7-year-old boy.

1 Ulna, Diaphysis	4 Radius, Epiphysis distalis
2 Radius, Diaphysis	5 Os lunatum
3 Ulna, Epiphysis distalis	6 Os triquetrum

7 Os scaphoideum	10 Os trapezoideum
8 Os hamatum	11 Os trapezium
9 Os capitatum	12 Os pisiforme

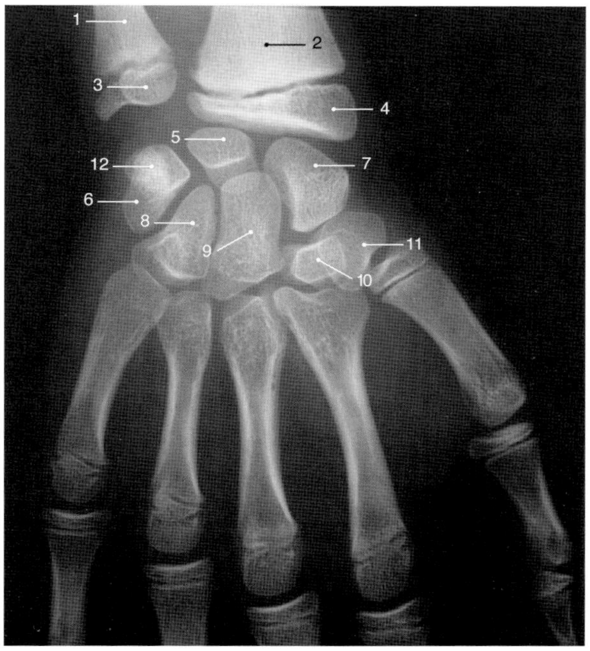

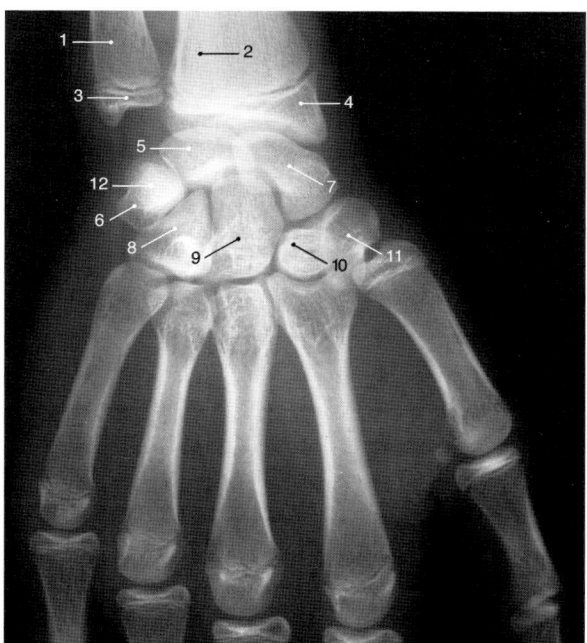

Fig. 329 PA-radiograph of the hand of an 11-year-old boy.

Fig. 330 PA-radiograph of the hand of a 13-year-old boy.

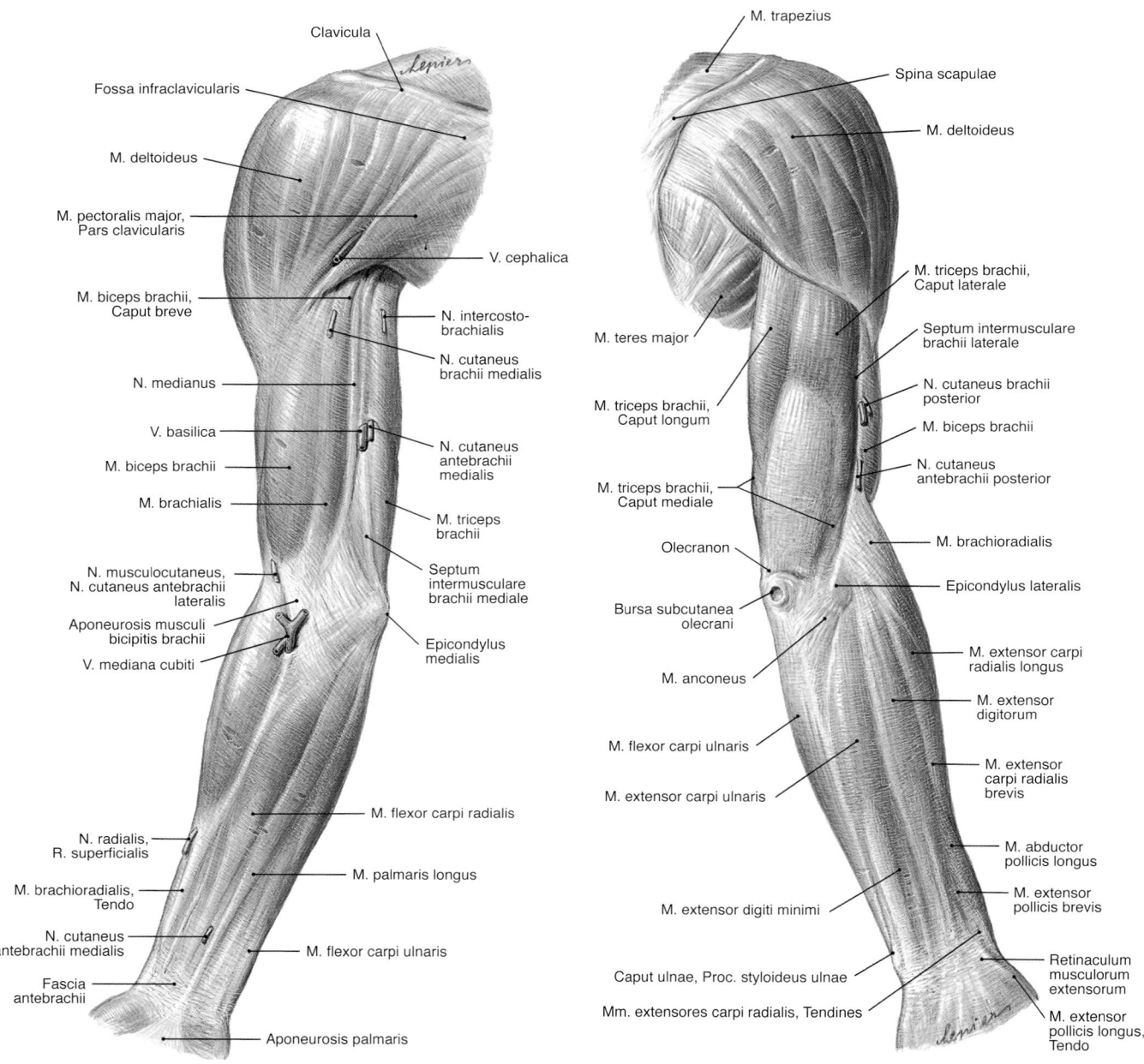

Fig. 331 Fascia of the flexor aspect of the upper limb.

Fig. 332 Fascia of the extensor aspect of the upper limb.

Muscles of the upper limb

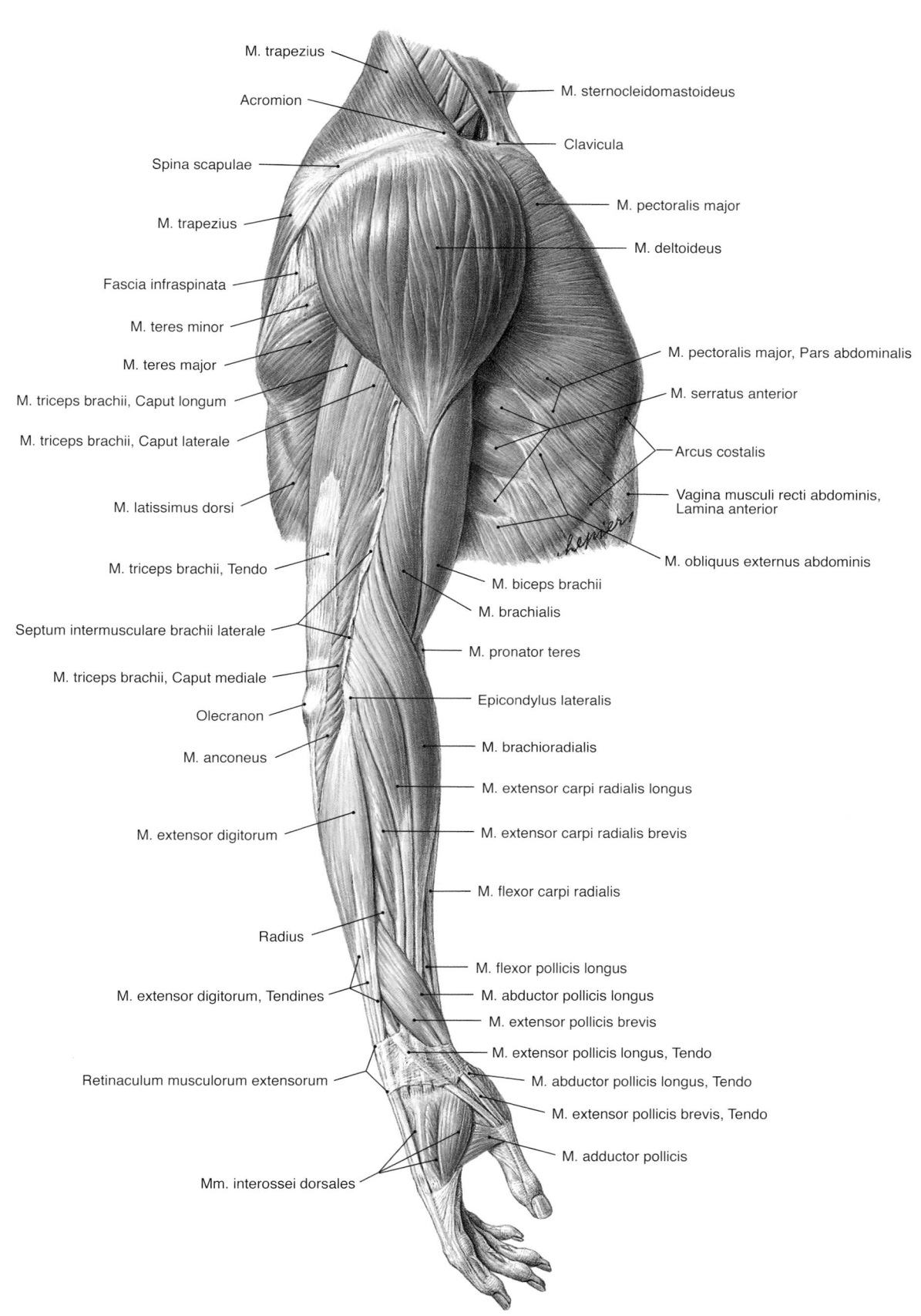

M. trapezius

Acromion

Spina scapulae

M. trapezius

Fascia infraspinata

M. teres minor

M. teres major

M. triceps brachii, Caput longum

M. triceps brachii, Caput laterale

M. latissimus dorsi

M. triceps brachii, Tendo

Septum intermusculare brachii laterale

M. triceps brachii, Caput mediale

Olecranon

M. anconeus

M. extensor digitorum

Radius

M. extensor digitorum, Tendines

Retinaculum musculorum extensorum

Mm. interossei dorsales

M. sternocleidomastoideus

Clavicula

M. pectoralis major

M. deltoideus

M. pectoralis major, Pars abdominalis

M. serratus anterior

Arcus costalis

Vagina musculi recti abdominis,
Lamina anterior

M. obliquus externus abdominis

M. biceps brachii

M. brachialis

M. pronator teres

Epicondylus lateralis

M. brachioradialis

M. extensor carpi radialis longus

M. extensor carpi radialis brevis

M. flexor carpi radialis

M. flexor pollicis longus

M. abductor pollicis longus

M. extensor pollicis brevis

M. extensor pollicis longus, Tendo

M. abductor pollicis longus, Tendo

M. extensor pollicis brevis, Tendo

M. adductor pollicis

Fig. 333 Muscles of the upper limb, the thorax and
the inferior region of the neck.

→ T 26–T 38

Muscles of the upper limb

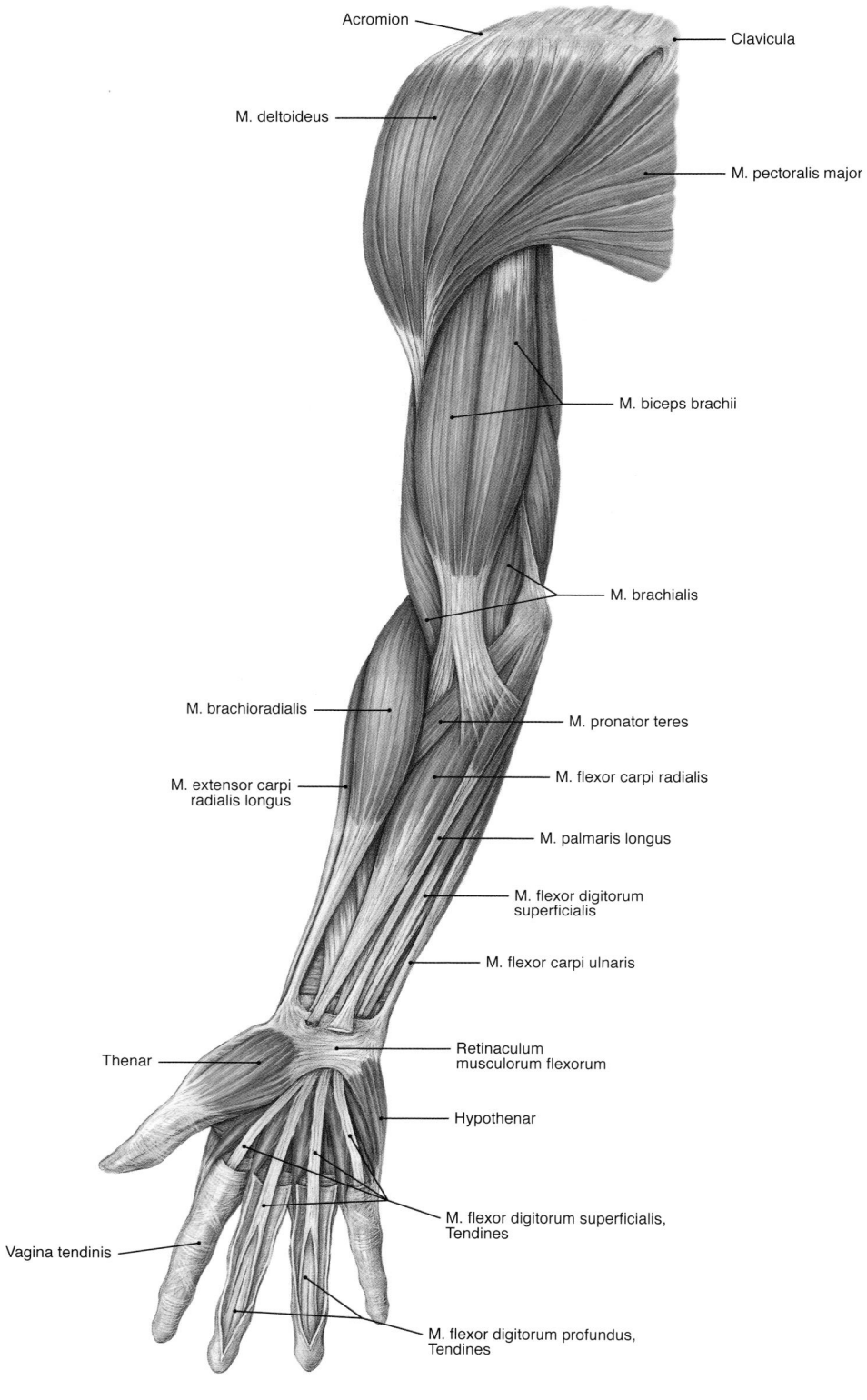

Acromion

Clavicula

M. deltoideus

M. pectoralis major

M. biceps brachii

M. brachialis

M. brachioradialis

M. pronator teres

M. extensor carpi radialis longus

M. flexor carpi radialis

M. palmaris longus

M. flexor digitorum superficialis

M. flexor carpi ulnaris

Thenar

Retinaculum musculorum flexorum

Hypothenar

M. flexor digitorum superficialis, Tendines

Vagina tendinis

M. flexor digitorum profundus, Tendines

→ T 26–T 38

Fig. 334 Muscles of the flexor aspect of the upper limb.

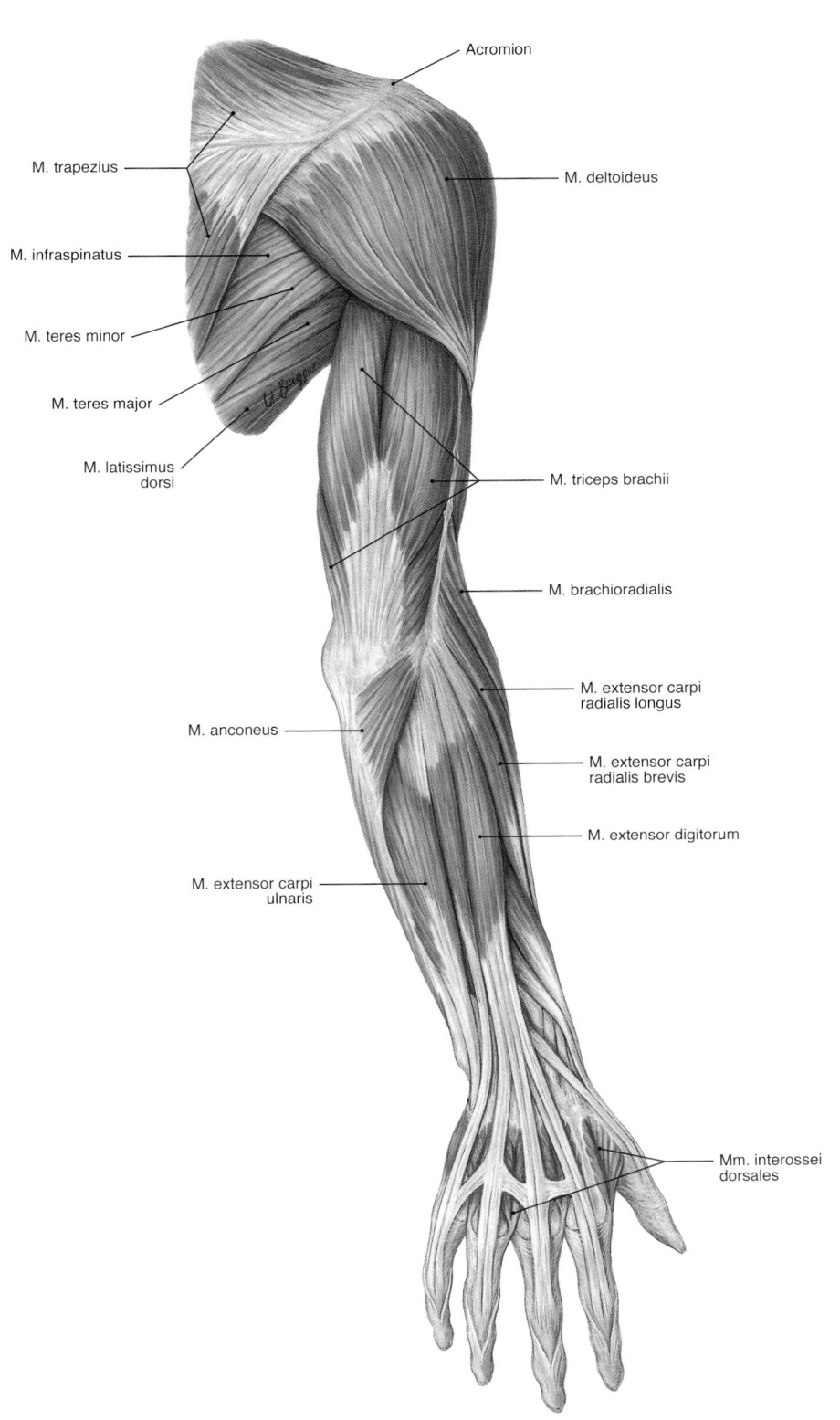

Acromion

M. trapezius

M. deltoideus

M. infraspinatus

M. teres minor

M. teres major

M. triceps brachii

M. latissimus
dorsi

M. brachioradialis

M. extensor carpi
radialis longus

M. anconeus

M. extensor carpi
radialis brevis

M. extensor digitorum

M. extensor carpi
ulnaris

Mm. interossei
dorsales

Fig. 335 Muscles of the extensor aspect of the upper limb.

→ T 26–T 38

Muscles of the shoulder

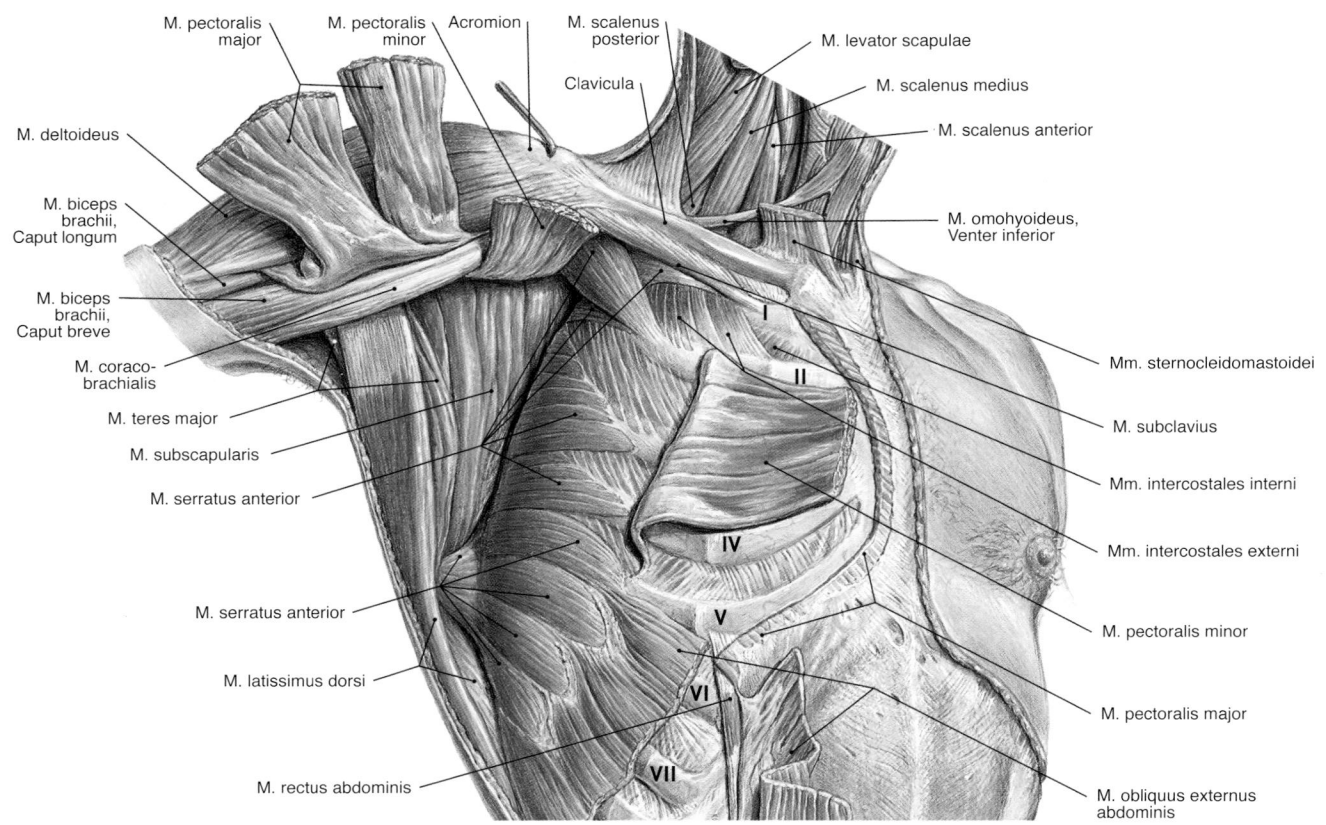

M. pectoralis major
M. pectoralis minor
Acromion
M. scalenus posterior
Clavicula
M. levator scapulae
M. scalenus medius
M. scalenus anterior
M. deltoideus
M. biceps brachii, Caput longum
M. omohyoideus, Venter inferior
M. biceps brachii, Caput breve
M. coraco-brachialis
I
II
Mm. sternocleidomastoidei
M. subclavius
M. teres major
M. subscapularis
M. serratus anterior
IV
Mm. intercostales interni
Mm. intercostales externi
M. serratus anterior
V
M. pectoralis minor
M. latissimus dorsi
VI
M. pectoralis major
M. rectus abdominis
VII
M. obliquus externus abdominis

→ 204, 570, 571

Fig. 336 Muscles of the arm, the thorax and the inferior region of the neck.
I, II, IV–VII indicate the corresponding ribs.

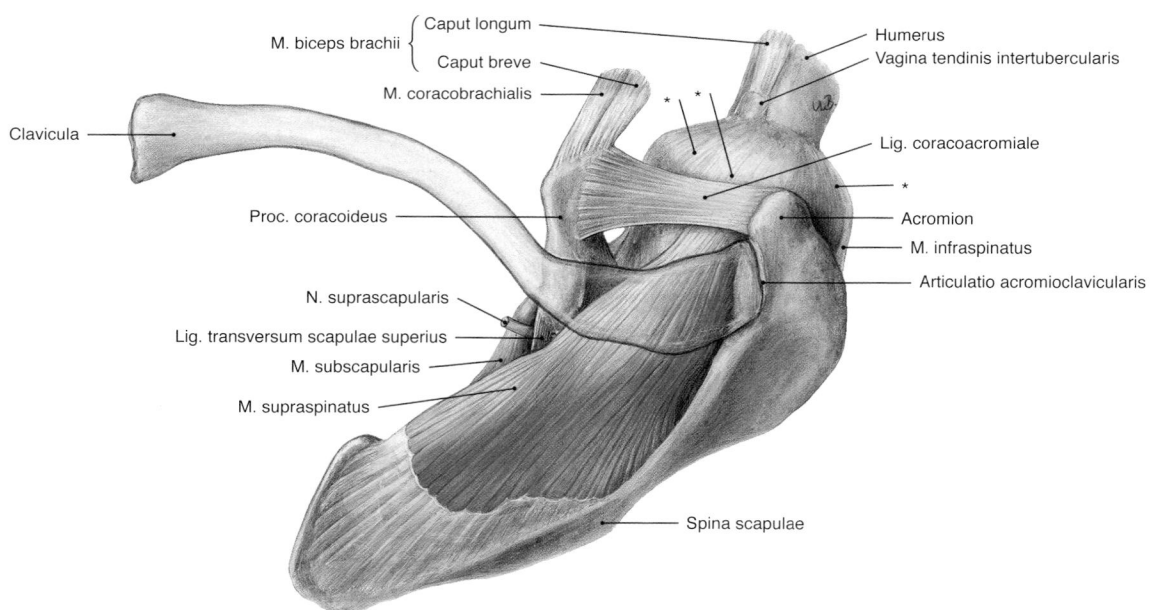

M. biceps brachii { Caput longum
Caput breve
M. coracobrachialis
Humerus
Vagina tendinis intertubercularis
Clavicula
* *
Lig. coracoacromiale
Proc. coracoideus
*
Acromion
N. suprascapularis
M. infraspinatus
Lig. transversum scapulae superius
Articulatio acromioclavicularis
M. subscapularis
M. supraspinatus
Spina scapulae

→ T 27

Fig. 337 Shoulder and muscles of the shoulder.
Together, the muscle tendons marked with * form
the so-called rotator cuff.

Muscles of the shoulder

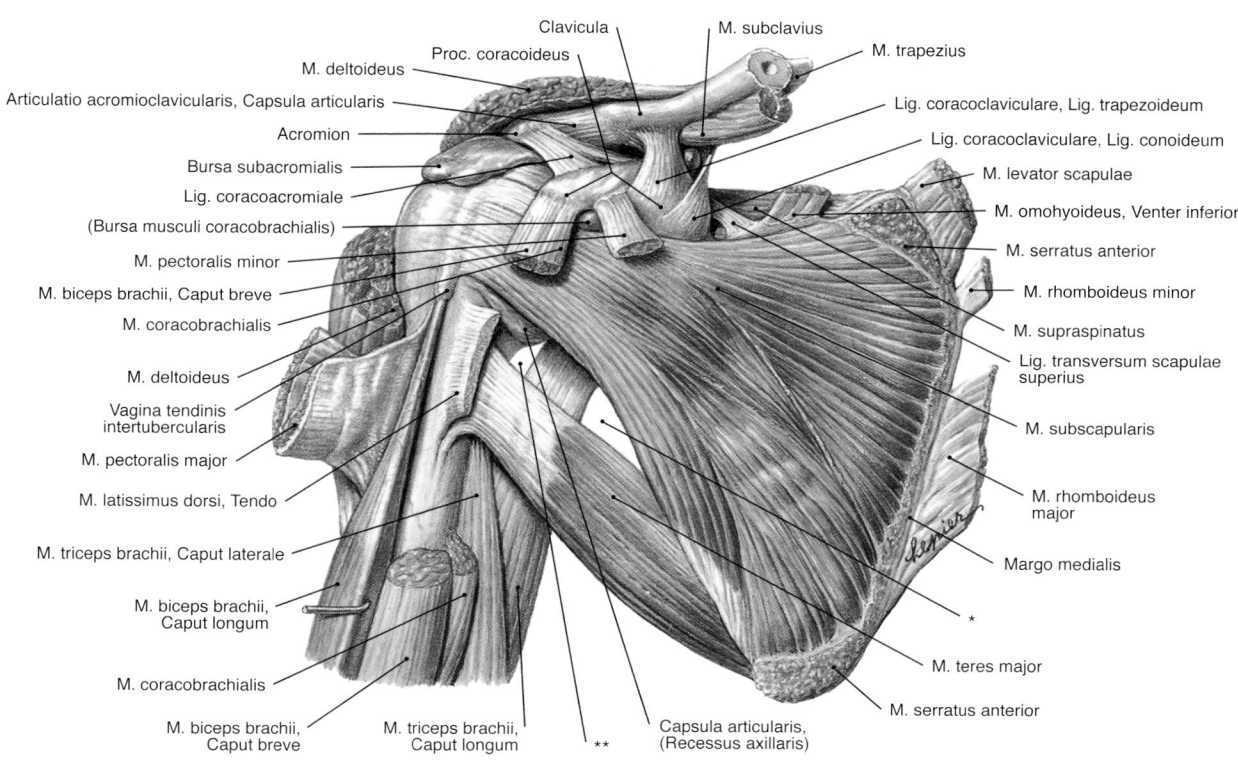

Clavicula
Proc. coracoideus
M. subclavius
M. trapezius
M. deltoideus
Articulatio acromioclavicularis, Capsula articularis
Acromion
Bursa subacromialis
Lig. coracoacromiale
(Bursa musculi coracobrachialis)
M. pectoralis minor
M. biceps brachii, Caput breve
M. coracobrachialis
M. deltoideus
Vagina tendinis intertubercularis
M. pectoralis major
M. latissimus dorsi, Tendo
M. triceps brachii, Caput laterale
M. biceps brachii, Caput longum
M. coracobrachialis
M. biceps brachii, Caput breve
M. triceps brachii, Caput longum
**
Capsula articularis, (Recessus axillaris)
Lig. coracoclaviculare, Lig. trapezoideum
Lig. coracoclaviculare, Lig. conoideum
M. levator scapulae
M. omohyoideus, Venter inferior
M. serratus anterior
M. rhomboideus minor
M. supraspinatus
Lig. transversum scapulae superius
M. subscapularis
M. rhomboideus major
Margo medialis
M. teres major
M. serratus anterior

Fig. 338 Shoulder and muscles of the shoulder.
* Triangular space, Spatium axillare mediale
** Quadrangular space, Spatium axillare laterale

→ T26

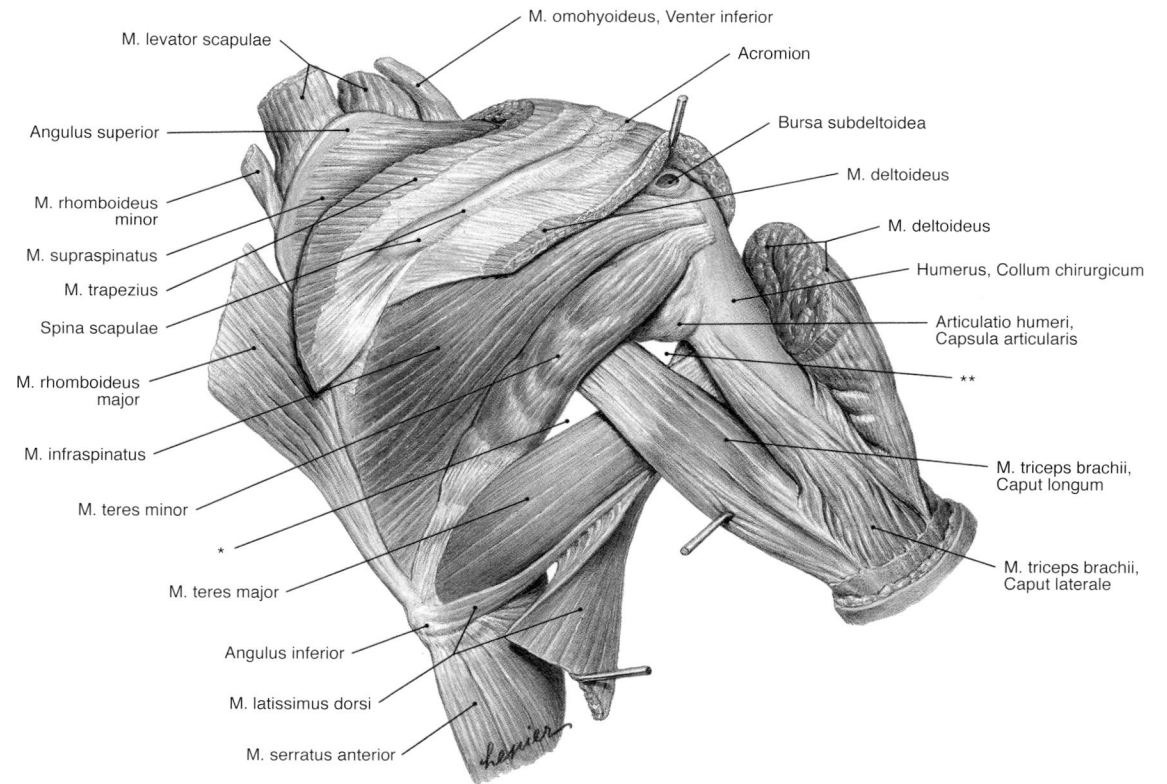

M. omohyoideus, Venter inferior
M. levator scapulae
Acromion
Angulus superior
M. rhomboideus minor
M. supraspinatus
M. trapezius
Spina scapulae
M. rhomboideus major
M. infraspinatus
M. teres minor
*
M. teres major
Angulus inferior
M. latissimus dorsi
M. serratus anterior
Bursa subdeltoidea
M. deltoideus
M. deltoideus
Humerus, Collum chirurgicum
Articulatio humeri, Capsula articularis
**
M. triceps brachii, Caput longum
M. triceps brachii, Caput laterale

Fig. 339 Shoulder and muscles of the shoulder.
* Triangular space, Spatium axillare mediale
** Quadrangular space, Spatium axillare laterale

→ T28

Muscles of the shoulder

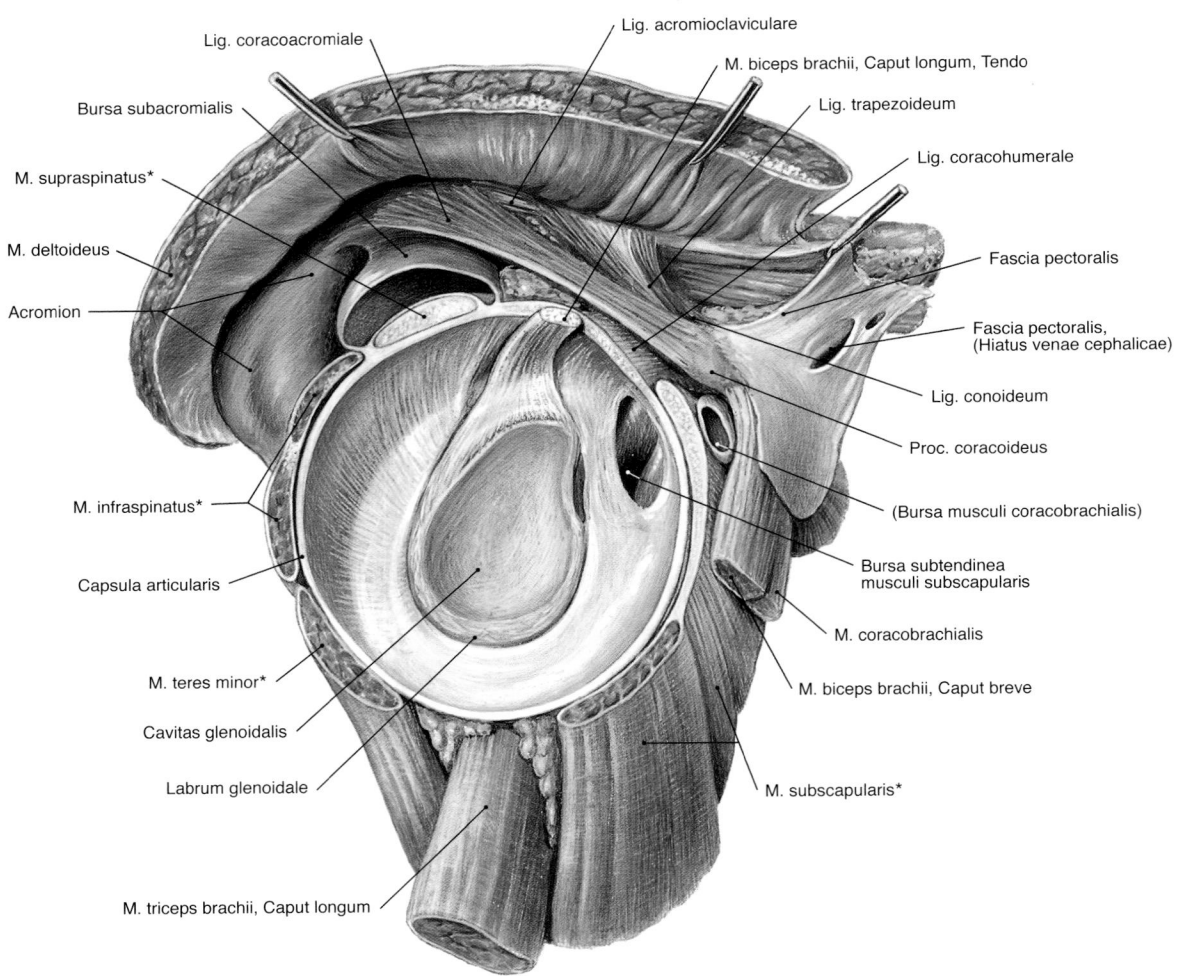

Lig. coracoacromiale

Lig. acromioclaviculare

M. biceps brachii, Caput longum, Tendo

Lig. trapezoideum

Bursa subacromialis

Lig. coracohumerale

M. supraspinatus*

Fascia pectoralis

M. deltoideus

Acromion

Fascia pectoralis, (Hiatus venae cephalicae)

Lig. conoideum

Proc. coracoideus

M. infraspinatus*

(Bursa musculi coracobrachialis)

Capsula articularis

Bursa subtendinea musculi subscapularis

M. coracobrachialis

M. teres minor*

M. biceps brachii, Caput breve

Cavitas glenoidalis

Labrum glenoidale

M. subscapularis*

M. triceps brachii, Caput longum

→ T 26–T 28

Fig. 340 Shoulder joint, Articulatio humeri; lateral view.
Together, the muscle tendons marked with * form the so-called rotator cuff.

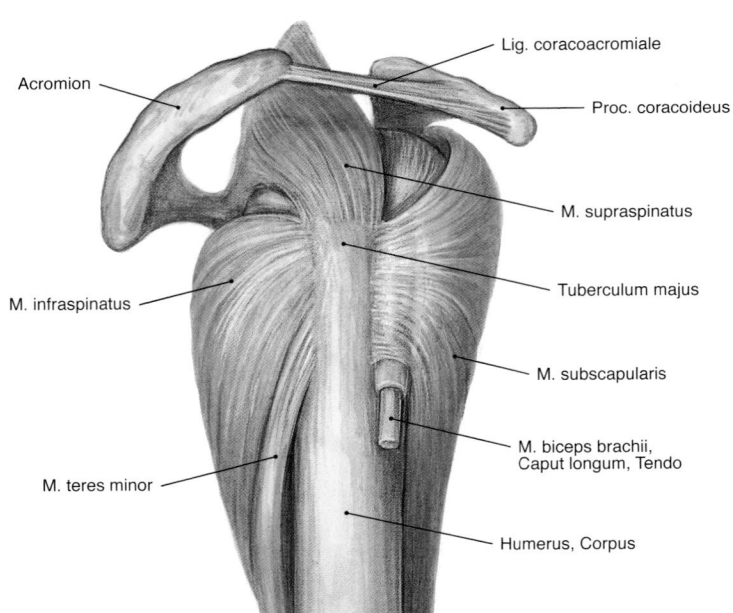

Acromion

Lig. coracoacromiale

Proc. coracoideus

M. supraspinatus

M. infraspinatus

Tuberculum majus

M. subscapularis

M. biceps brachii, Caput longum, Tendo

M. teres minor

Humerus, Corpus

→ T 26–T 28

Fig. 341 Muscles of the so-called rotator cuff; lateral view.

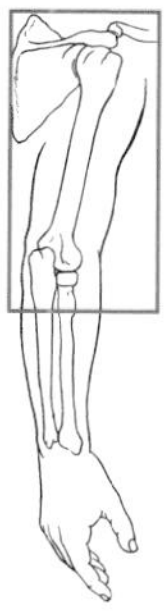

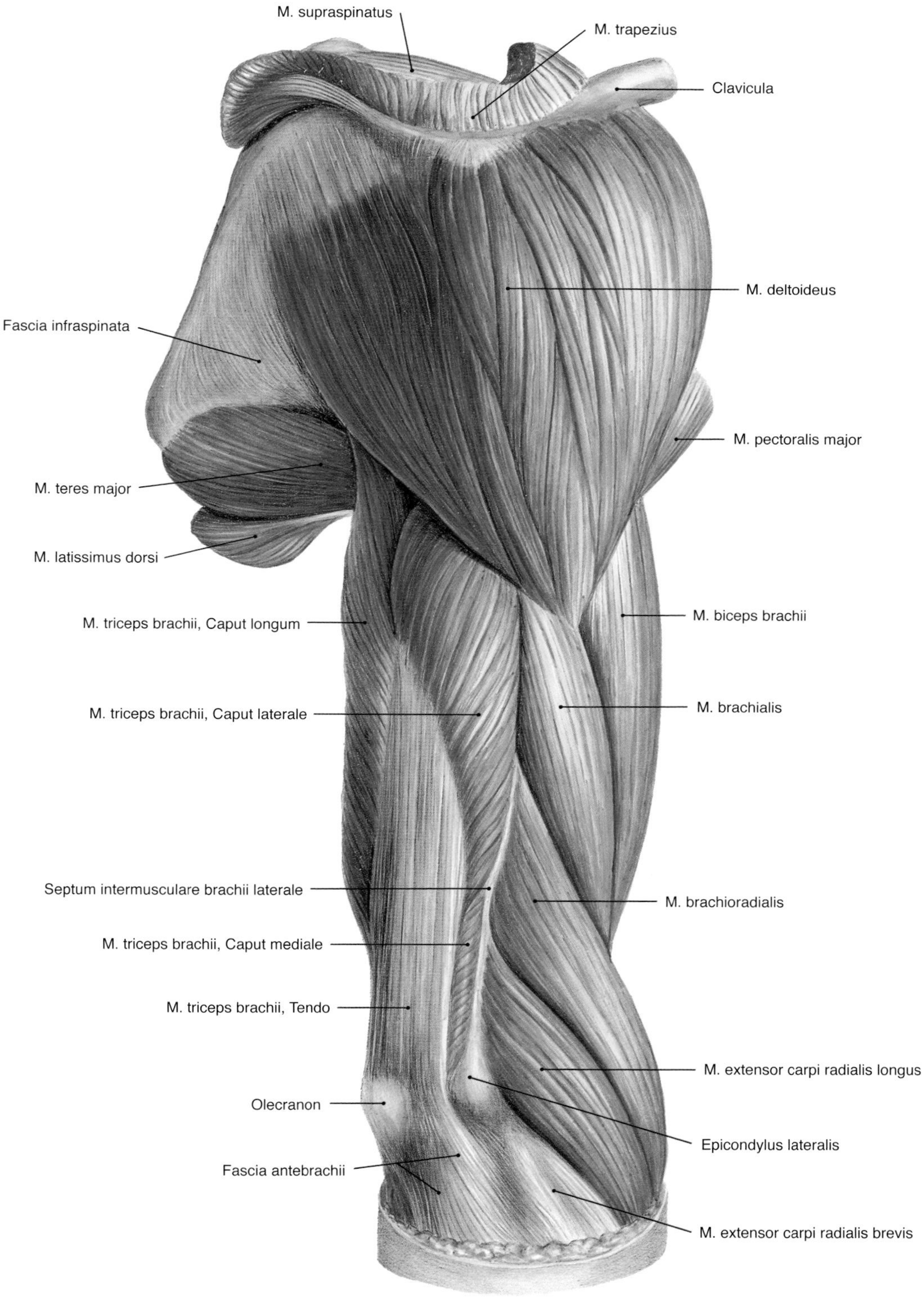

Muscles of the arm

M. supraspinatus

M. trapezius

Clavicula

M. deltoideus

Fascia infraspinata

M. pectoralis major

M. teres major

M. latissimus dorsi

M. biceps brachii

M. triceps brachii, Caput longum

M. brachialis

M. triceps brachii, Caput laterale

Septum intermusculare brachii laterale

M. brachioradialis

M. triceps brachii, Caput mediale

M. triceps brachii, Tendo

M. extensor carpi radialis longus

Olecranon

Epicondylus lateralis

Fascia antebrachii

M. extensor carpi radialis brevis

Fig. 342   Muscles of the arm;
superficial layer;
dorsolateral view.

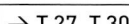 → T 27, T 30

Origins and insertions of the muscles of the shoulder and the arm

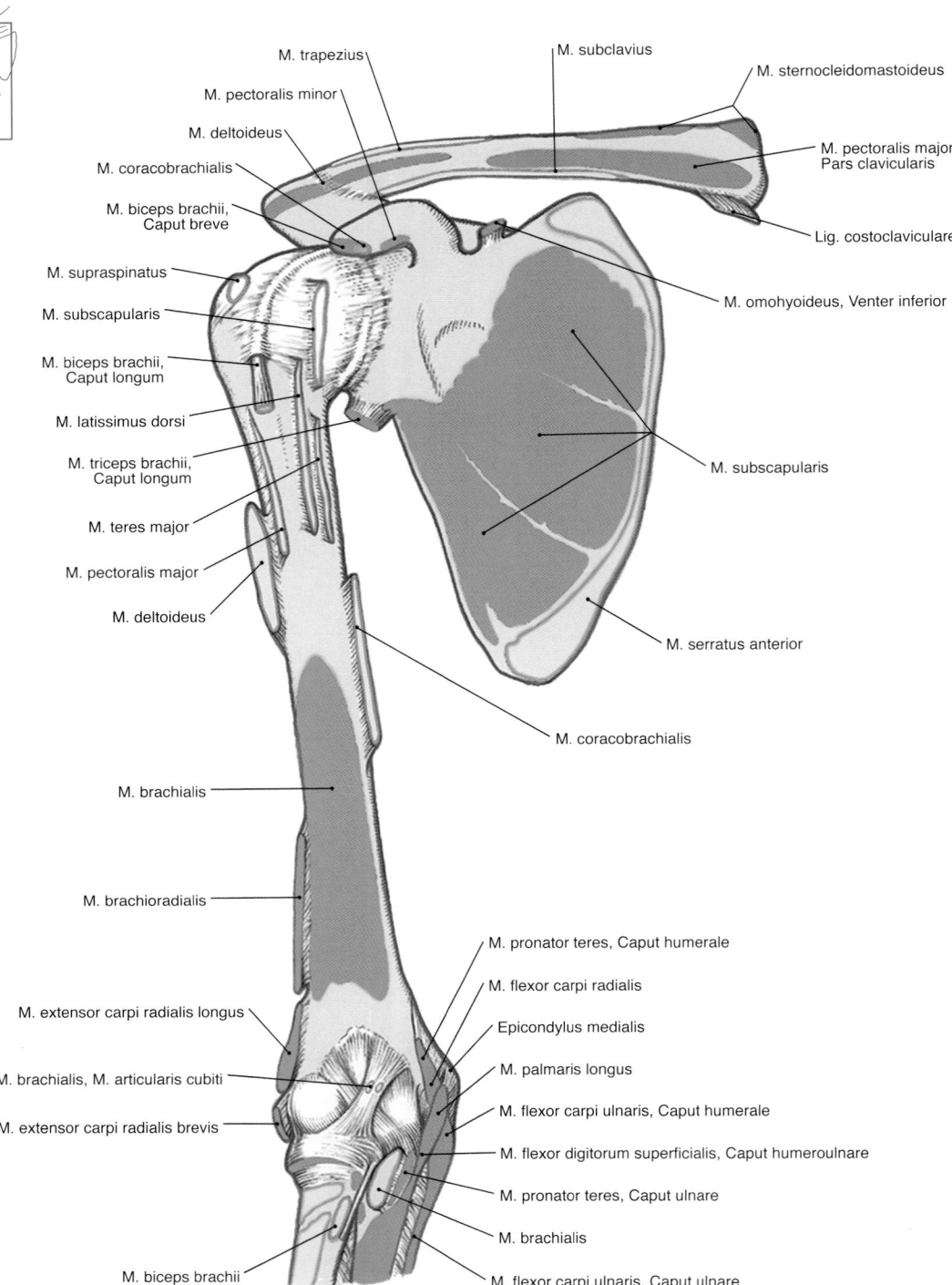

M. trapezius

M. pectoralis minor

M. deltoideus

M. coracobrachialis

M. biceps brachii, Caput breve

M. supraspinatus

M. subscapularis

M. biceps brachii, Caput longum

M. latissimus dorsi

M. triceps brachii, Caput longum

M. teres major

M. pectoralis major

M. deltoideus

M. brachialis

M. brachioradialis

M. extensor carpi radialis longus

M. brachialis, M. articularis cubiti

M. extensor carpi radialis brevis

M. biceps brachii

M. subclavius

M. sternocleidomastoideus

M. pectoralis major, Pars clavicularis

Lig. costoclaviculare

M. omohyoideus, Venter inferior

M. subscapularis

M. serratus anterior

M. coracobrachialis

M. pronator teres, Caput humerale

M. flexor carpi radialis

Epicondylus medialis

M. palmaris longus

M. flexor carpi ulnaris, Caput humerale

M. flexor digitorum superficialis, Caput humeroulnare

M. pronator teres, Caput ulnare

M. brachialis

M. flexor carpi ulnaris, Caput ulnare

→ T 26–T 30

Fig. 343 Origins and insertions of the muscles at the clavicle, Clavicula, the scapula, Scapula, and the humerus, Humerus (as well as ulnar origins of multi-head muscles).

Origins and insertions of the muscles of the shoulder and the arm

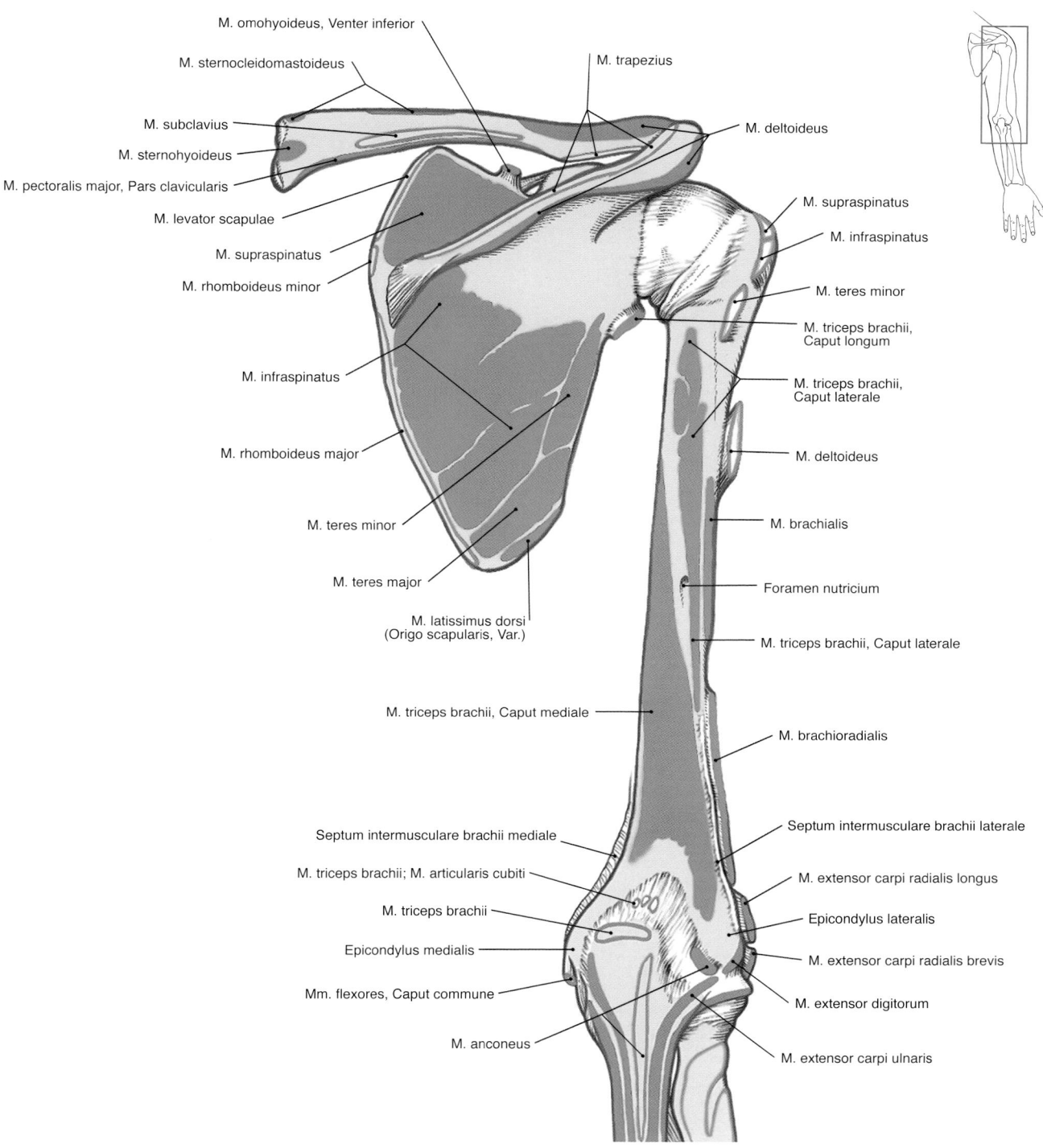

M. omohyoideus, Venter inferior

M. sternocleidomastoideus

M. subclavius

M. sternohyoideus

M. pectoralis major, Pars clavicularis

M. levator scapulae

M. supraspinatus

M. rhomboideus minor

M. infraspinatus

M. rhomboideus major

M. teres minor

M. teres major

M. latissimus dorsi
(Origo scapularis, Var.)

M. triceps brachii, Caput mediale

Septum intermusculare brachii mediale

M. triceps brachii; M. articularis cubiti

M. triceps brachii

Epicondylus medialis

Mm. flexores, Caput commune

M. anconeus

M. trapezius

M. deltoideus

M. supraspinatus

M. infraspinatus

M. teres minor

M. triceps brachii, Caput longum

M. triceps brachii, Caput laterale

M. deltoideus

M. brachialis

Foramen nutricium

M. triceps brachii, Caput laterale

M. brachioradialis

Septum intermusculare brachii laterale

M. extensor carpi radialis longus

Epicondylus lateralis

M. extensor carpi radialis brevis

M. extensor digitorum

M. extensor carpi ulnaris

Fig. 344   Origins and insertions of the muscles at the clavicle,
Clavicula, the scapula, Scapula, and the humerus, Humerus
(as well as ulnar origins of multi-head muscles).

→ T 26–T 30

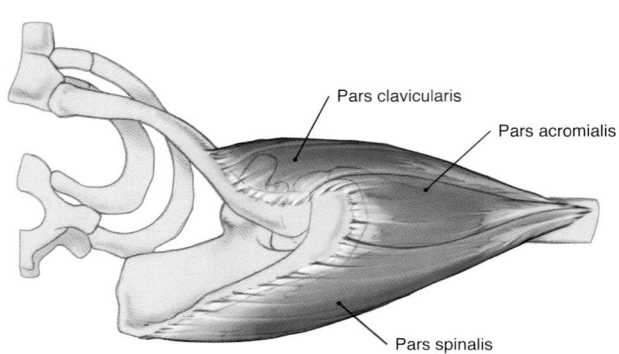

Fig. 345 Deltoid muscle, M. deltoideus.

→ T 27

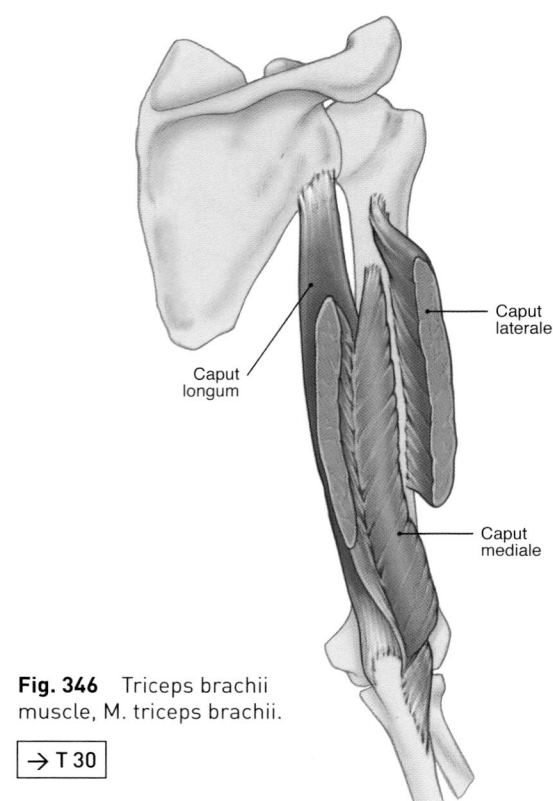

Fig. 346 Triceps brachii muscle, M. triceps brachii.

→ T 30

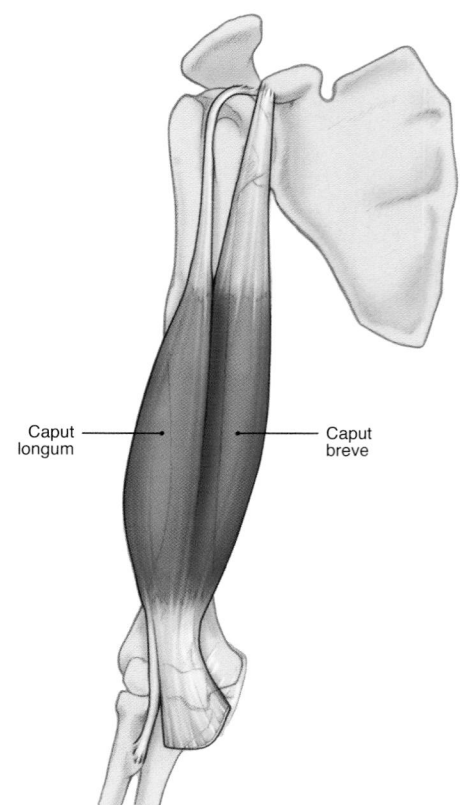

Fig. 347 Biceps brachii muscle, M. biceps brachii.

→ T 29

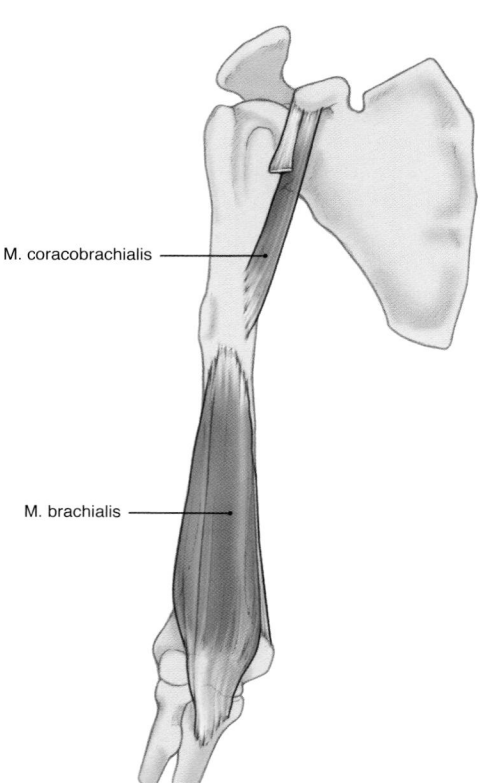

Fig. 348 Brachial and coracobrachial muscles, Mm. brachialis et coracobrachialis.

→ T 29

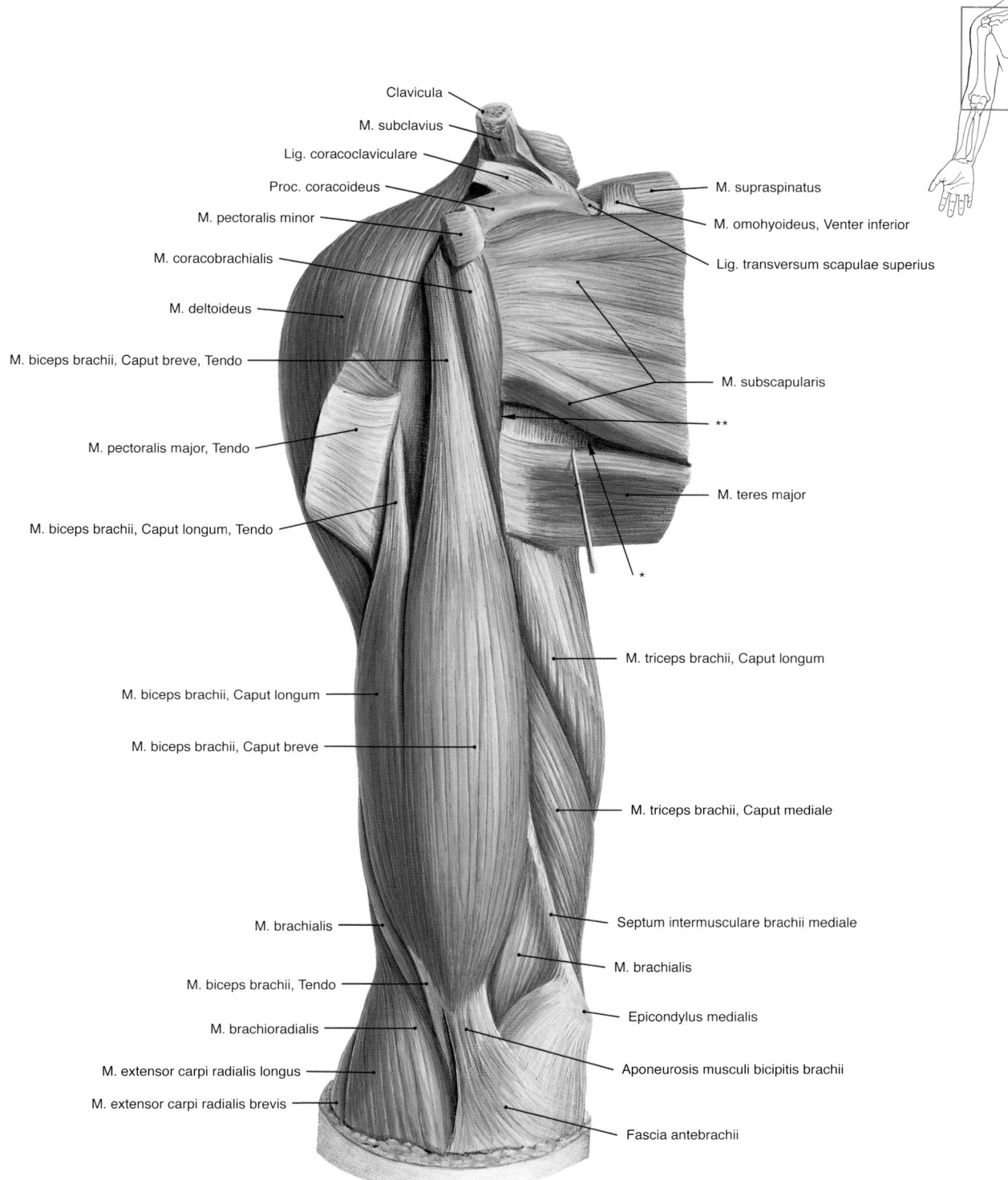

Clavicula
M. subclavius
Lig. coracoclaviculare
Proc. coracoideus
M. pectoralis minor
M. coracobrachialis
M. deltoideus
M. biceps brachii, Caput breve, Tendo
M. pectoralis major, Tendo
M. biceps brachii, Caput longum, Tendo
M. biceps brachii, Caput longum
M. biceps brachii, Caput breve
M. brachialis
M. biceps brachii, Tendo
M. brachioradialis
M. extensor carpi radialis longus
M. extensor carpi radialis brevis

M. supraspinatus
M. omohyoideus, Venter inferior
Lig. transversum scapulae superius
M. subscapularis
**
M. teres major
*
M. triceps brachii, Caput longum
M. triceps brachii, Caput mediale
Septum intermusculare brachii mediale
M. brachialis
Epicondylus medialis
Aponeurosis musculi bicipitis brachii
Fascia antebrachii

Fig. 349 Muscles of the arm;
flexor aspect, superficial layer.
* Triangular space, Spatium axillare mediale
** Quadrangular space, Spatium axillare laterale

→ T 29

Muscles of the arm

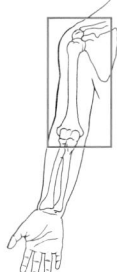

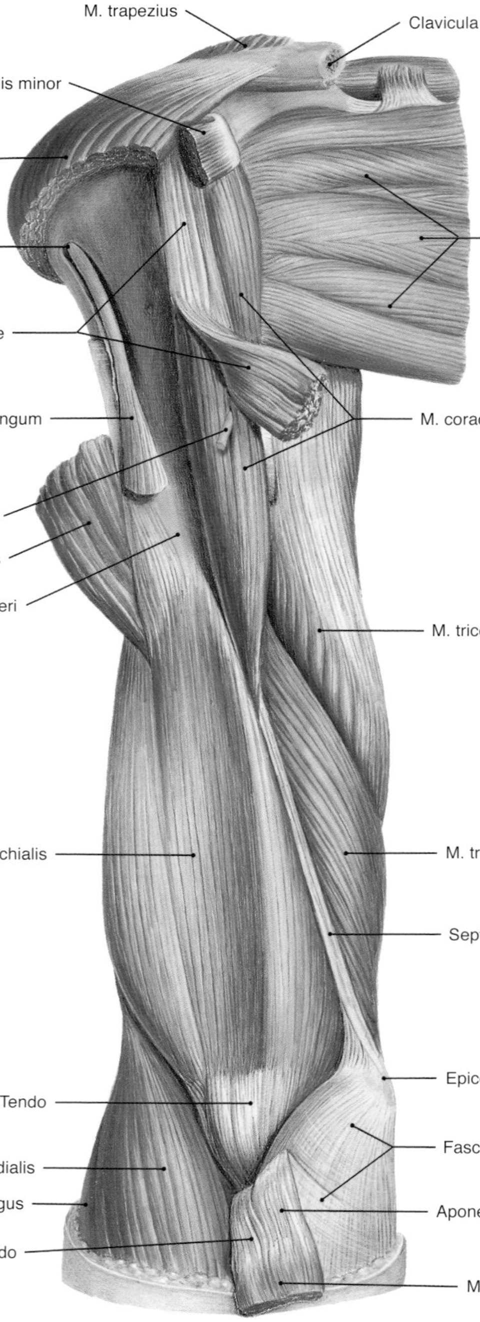

M. trapezius
Clavicula
M. pectoralis minor
M. deltoideus
M. subscapularis
Vagina tendinis intertubercularis
M. biceps brachii, Caput breve
M. biceps brachii, Caput longum
M. coracobrachialis
N. musculocutaneus
M. deltoideus
Corpus humeri
M. triceps brachii, Caput longum
M. brachialis
M. triceps brachii, Caput mediale
Septum intermusculare brachii mediale
Epicondylus medialis
M. brachialis, Tendo
Fascia antebrachii
M. brachioradialis
Aponeurosis musculi bicipitis brachii
M. extensor carpi radialis longus
M. biceps brachii, Tendo
M. biceps brachii

→ T 29

Fig. 350 Muscles of the arm;
flexor aspect, deep layer.

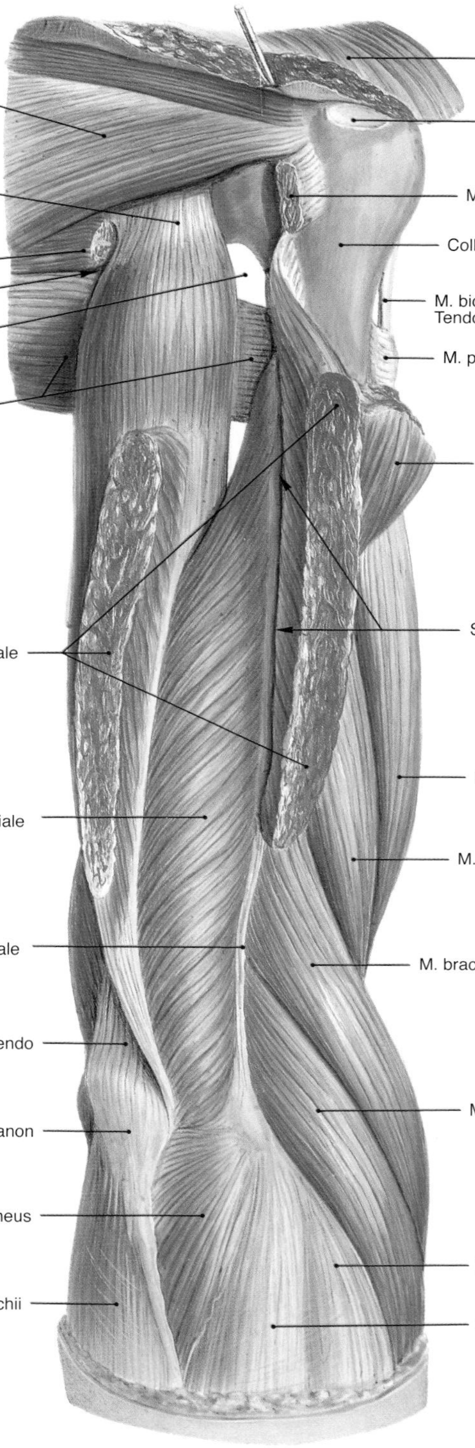

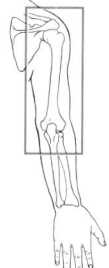

M. deltoideus

M. infraspinatus

Bursa subdeltoidea

M. triceps brachii,
Caput longum

M. teres minor

M. teres minor

Collum chirurgicum

*

M. biceps brachii, Caput longum,
Tendo

**

M. pectoralis major, Tendo

M. teres major

M. deltoideus

M. triceps brachii, Caput laterale

Sulcus nervi radialis

M. triceps brachii, Caput mediale

M. biceps brachii

M. brachialis

Septum intermusculare brachii laterale

M. brachioradialis

M. triceps brachii, Tendo

M. extensor carpi radialis longus

Olecranon

M. anconeus

M. extensor carpi radialis brevis

Fascia antebrachii

M. extensor digitorum

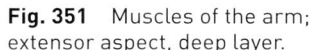

Fig. 351   Muscles of the arm;
extensor aspect, deep layer.

→ T 30

*   Triangular space, Spatium axillare mediale
** Quadrangular space, Spatium axillare laterale

Origins and insertions of the ventral muscles of the forearm

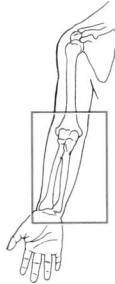

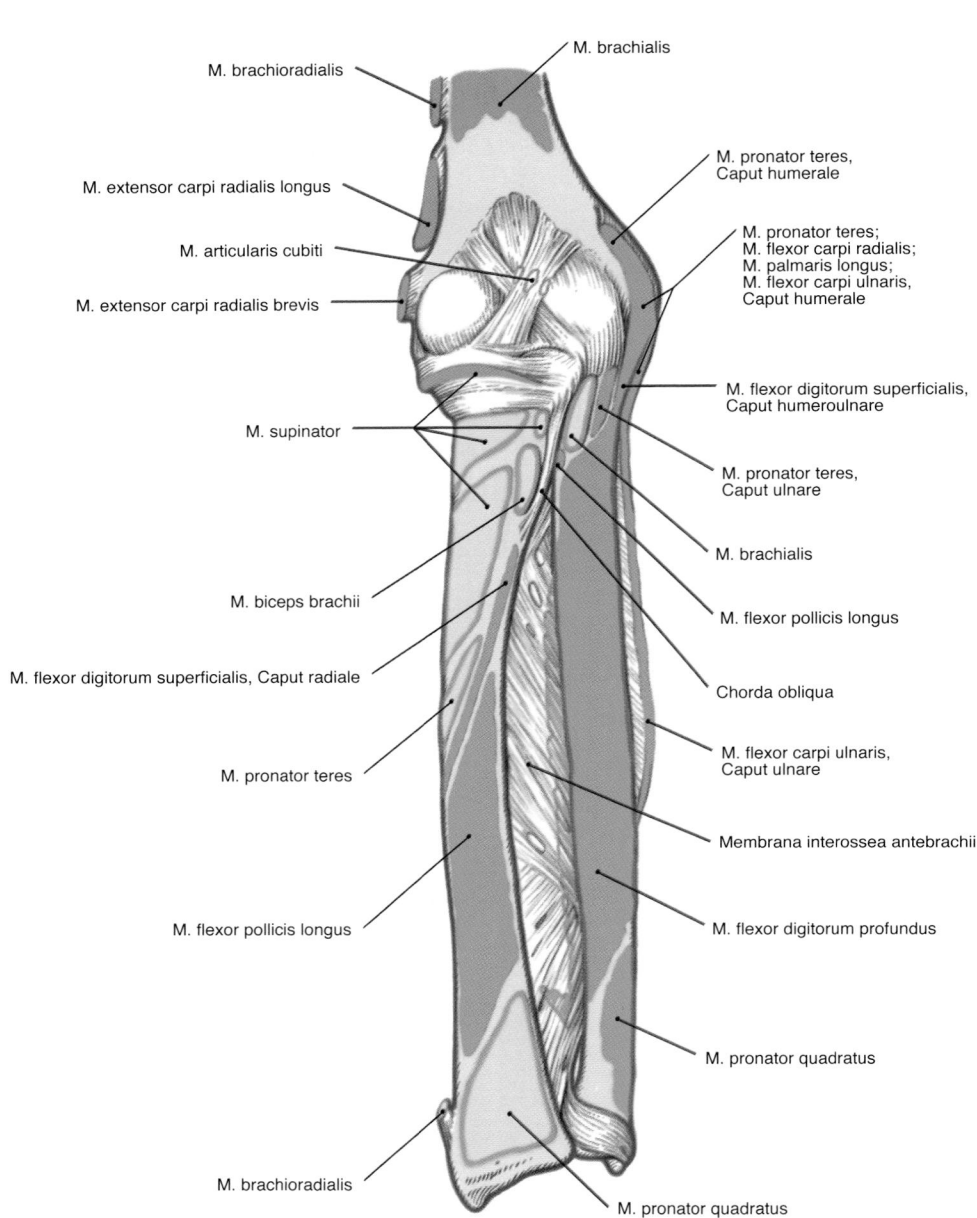

M. brachialis

M. brachioradialis

M. pronator teres,
Caput humerale

M. extensor carpi radialis longus

M. pronator teres;
M. flexor carpi radialis;
M. palmaris longus;
M. flexor carpi ulnaris,
Caput humerale

M. articularis cubiti

M. extensor carpi radialis brevis

M. flexor digitorum superficialis,
Caput humeroulnare

M. supinator

M. pronator teres,
Caput ulnare

M. brachialis

M. biceps brachii

M. flexor pollicis longus

M. flexor digitorum superficialis, Caput radiale

Chorda obliqua

M. flexor carpi ulnaris,
Caput ulnare

M. pronator teres

Membrana interossea antebrachii

M. flexor pollicis longus

M. flexor digitorum profundus

M. pronator quadratus

M. brachioradialis

M. pronator quadratus

→ T 31–T 33

Fig. 352 Origins and insertions of the muscles
at the radius, Radius, the ulna, Ulna, and the
distal part of the humerus, Humerus.

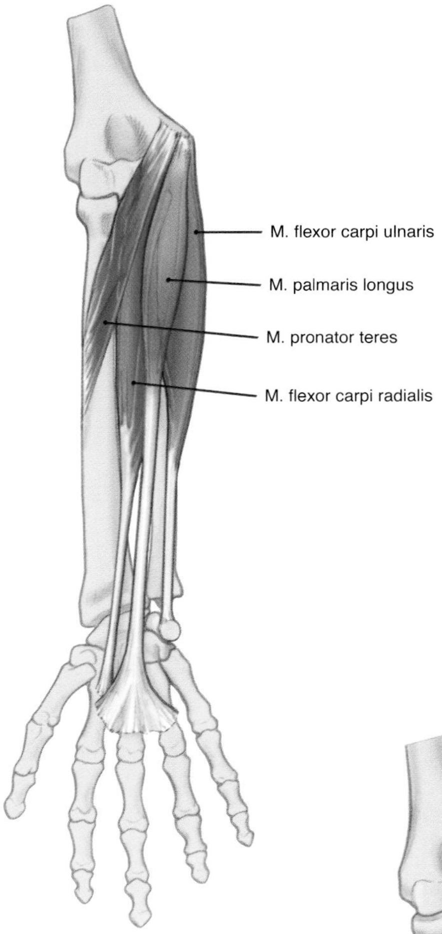

Muscles of the forearm

M. flexor carpi ulnaris

M. palmaris longus

M. pronator teres

M. flexor carpi radialis

M. flexor digitorum superficialis

Fig. 353 Ventral muscles of the forearm; superficial layer.

→ T 31

Fig. 354 Ventral muscles of the forearm; middle layer.

→ T 32

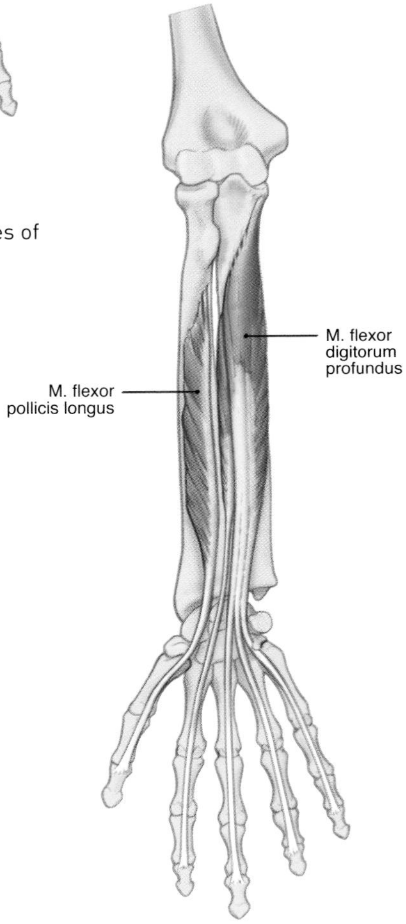

M. flexor digitorum profundus

M. flexor pollicis longus

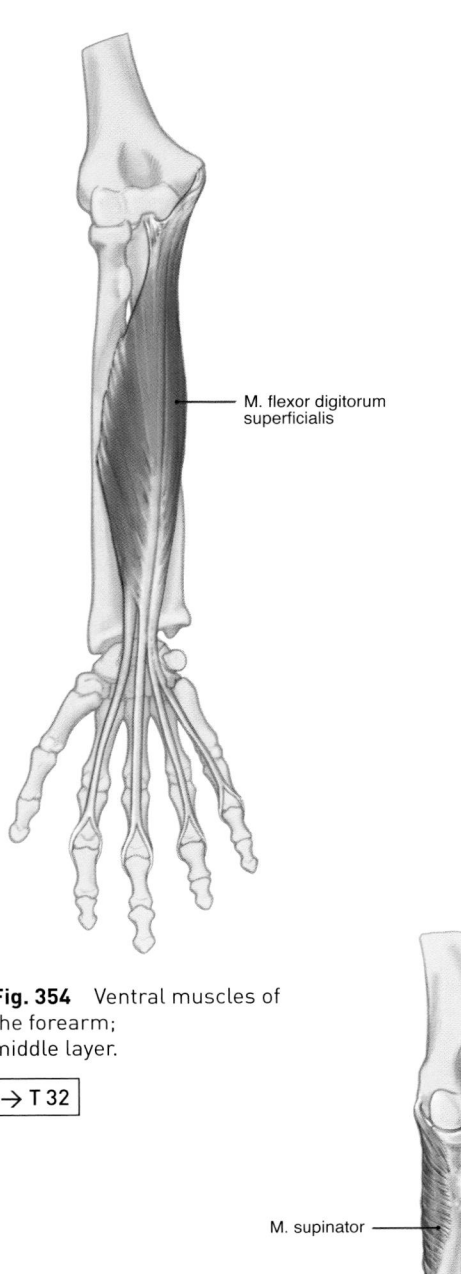

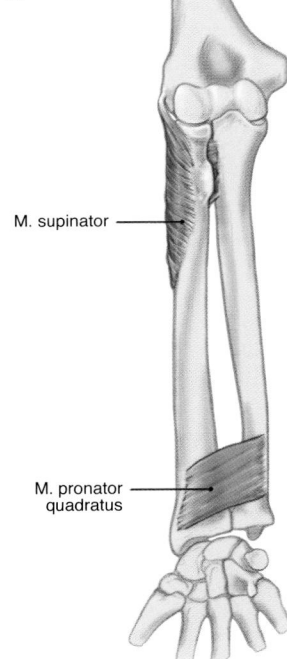

M. supinator

M. pronator quadratus

Fig. 355 Ventral muscles of the forearm; deep layer.

→ T 31, T 32

Fig. 356 Ventral muscles of the forearm; deepest layer.

→ T 31, T 35

Muscles of the forearm

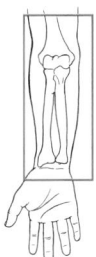

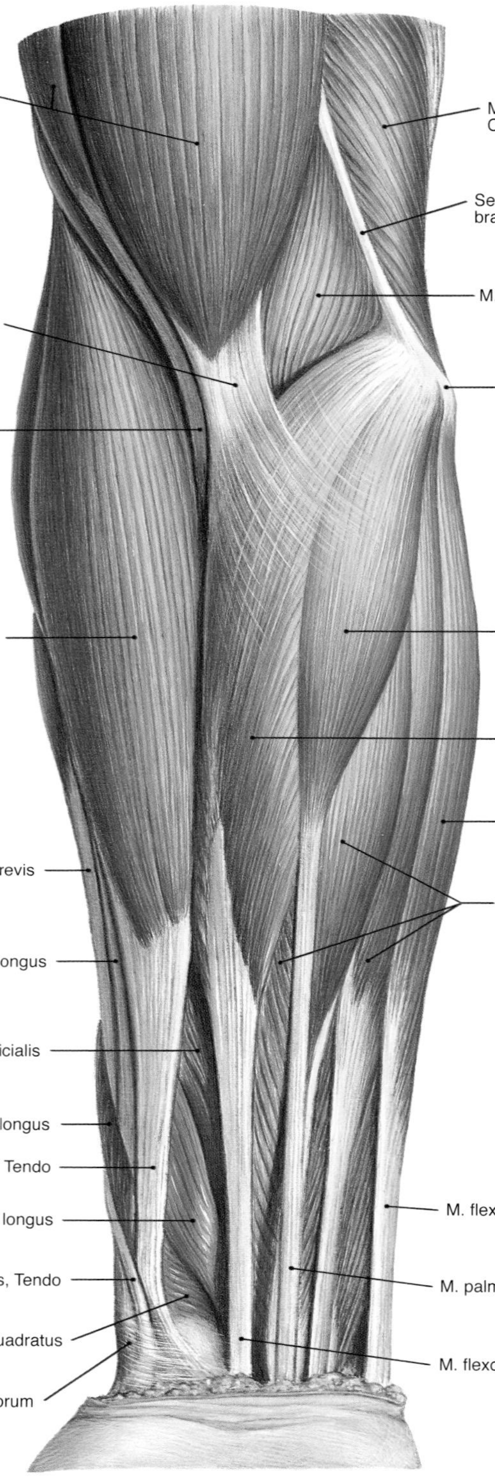

M. biceps brachii

Aponeurosis musculi bicipitis brachii

M. biceps brachii, Tendo

M. brachioradialis

M. extensor carpi radialis brevis

M. extensor carpi radialis longus

M. flexor digitorum superficialis

M. abductor pollicis longus

M. brachioradialis, Tendo

M. flexor pollicis longus

M. abductor pollicis longus, Tendo

M. pronator quadratus

Retinaculum musculorum extensorum

M. triceps brachii, Caput mediale

Septum intermusculare brachii mediale

M. brachialis

Epicondylus medialis

M. palmaris longus

M. flexor carpi radialis

M. flexor carpi ulnaris

M. flexor digitorum superficialis

M. flexor carpi ulnaris, Tendo

M. palmaris longus, Tendo

M. flexor carpi radialis, Tendo

→ T 31

Fig. 357 Muscles of the forearm; flexor aspect, superficial layer.

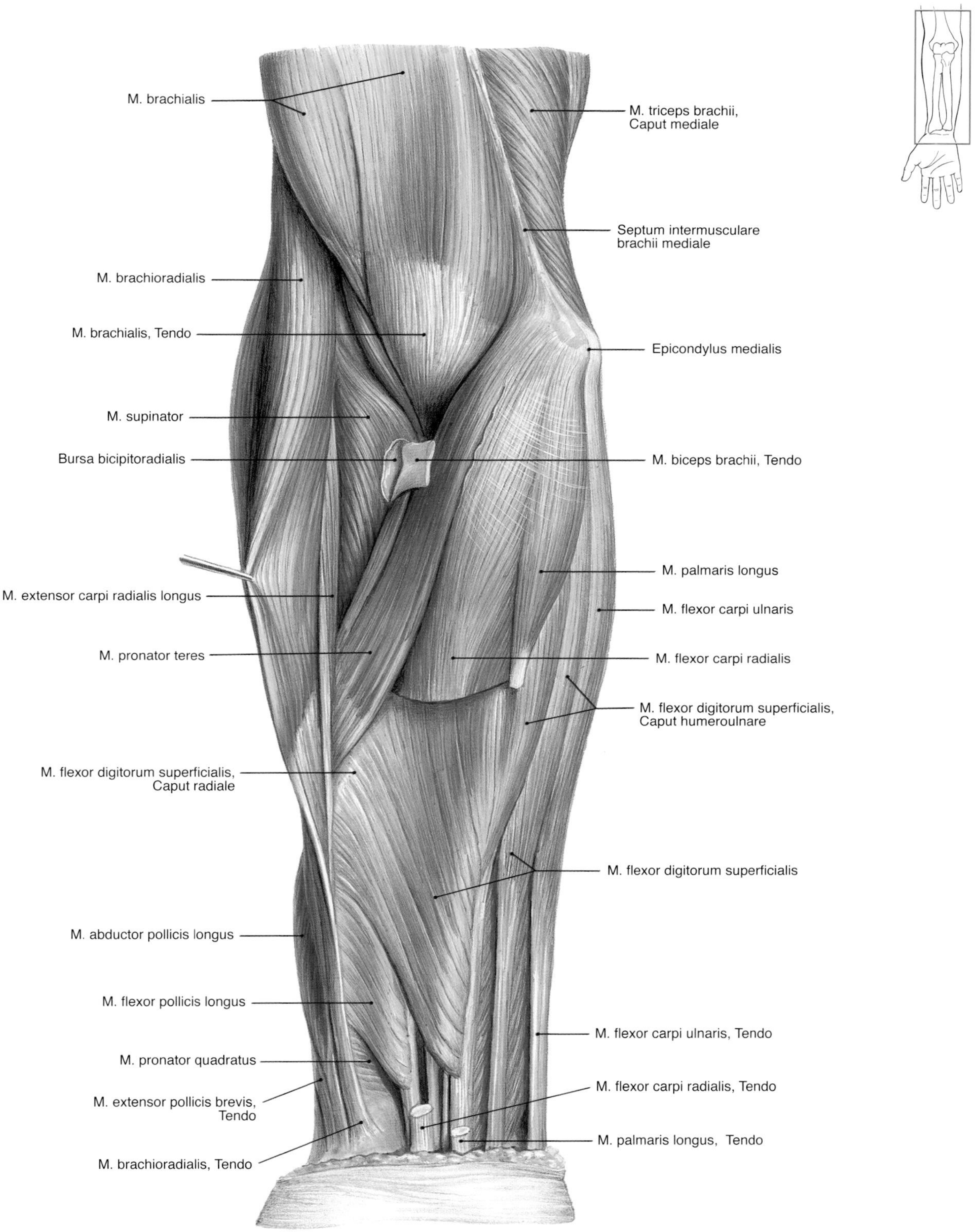

Muscles of the forearm

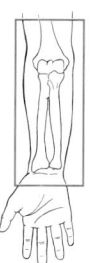

M. brachialis

M. triceps brachii, Caput mediale

Septum intermusculare brachii mediale

M. brachioradialis

M. brachialis, Tendo

Epicondylus medialis

M. supinator

Bursa bicipitoradialis

M. biceps brachii, Tendo

M. palmaris longus

M. flexor carpi ulnaris

M. extensor carpi radialis longus

M. pronator teres

M. flexor carpi radialis

M. flexor digitorum superficialis, Caput humeroulnare

M. flexor digitorum superficialis, Caput radiale

M. flexor digitorum superficialis

M. abductor pollicis longus

M. flexor pollicis longus

M. flexor carpi ulnaris, Tendo

M. pronator quadratus

M. flexor carpi radialis, Tendo

M. extensor pollicis brevis, Tendo

M. palmaris longus, Tendo

M. brachioradialis, Tendo

Fig. 358   Muscles of the forearm;
flexor aspect, middle layer.

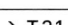 → T31

Muscles of the forearm

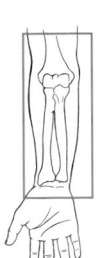

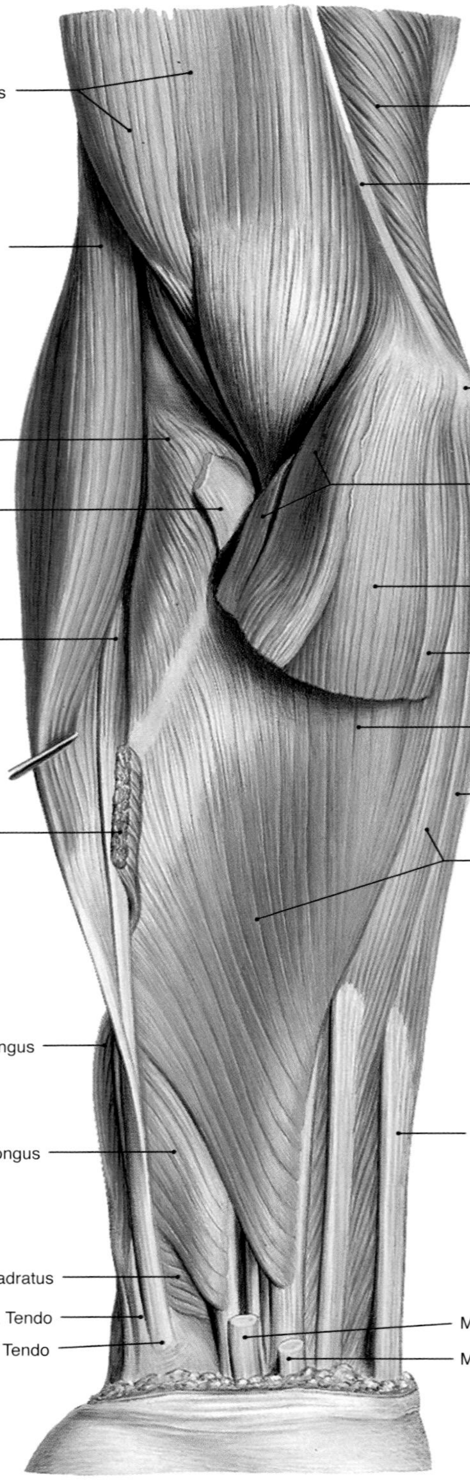

M. brachialis

M. triceps brachii, Caput mediale

Septum intermusculare brachii mediale

M. brachioradialis

Epicondylus medialis

M. supinator

M. pronator teres

M. biceps brachii, Tendo

M. flexor carpi radialis

M. extensor carpi radialis longus

M. palmaris longus

Mm. flexores, Caput commune

M. flexor carpi ulnaris

M. pronator teres

M. flexor digitorum superficialis

M. abductor pollicis longus

M. flexor carpi ulnaris, Tendo

M. flexor pollicis longus

M. pronator quadratus

M. abductor pollicis longus, Tendo

M. flexor carpi radialis, Tendo

M. brachioradialis, Tendo

M. palmaris longus, Tendo

→ T 31, T 32

Fig. 359 Muscles of the forearm; flexor aspect, middle layer after section of the pronator teres muscle.

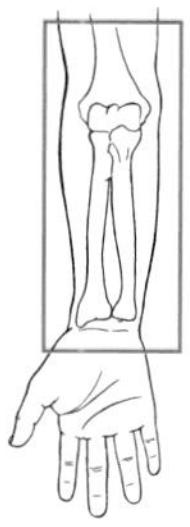

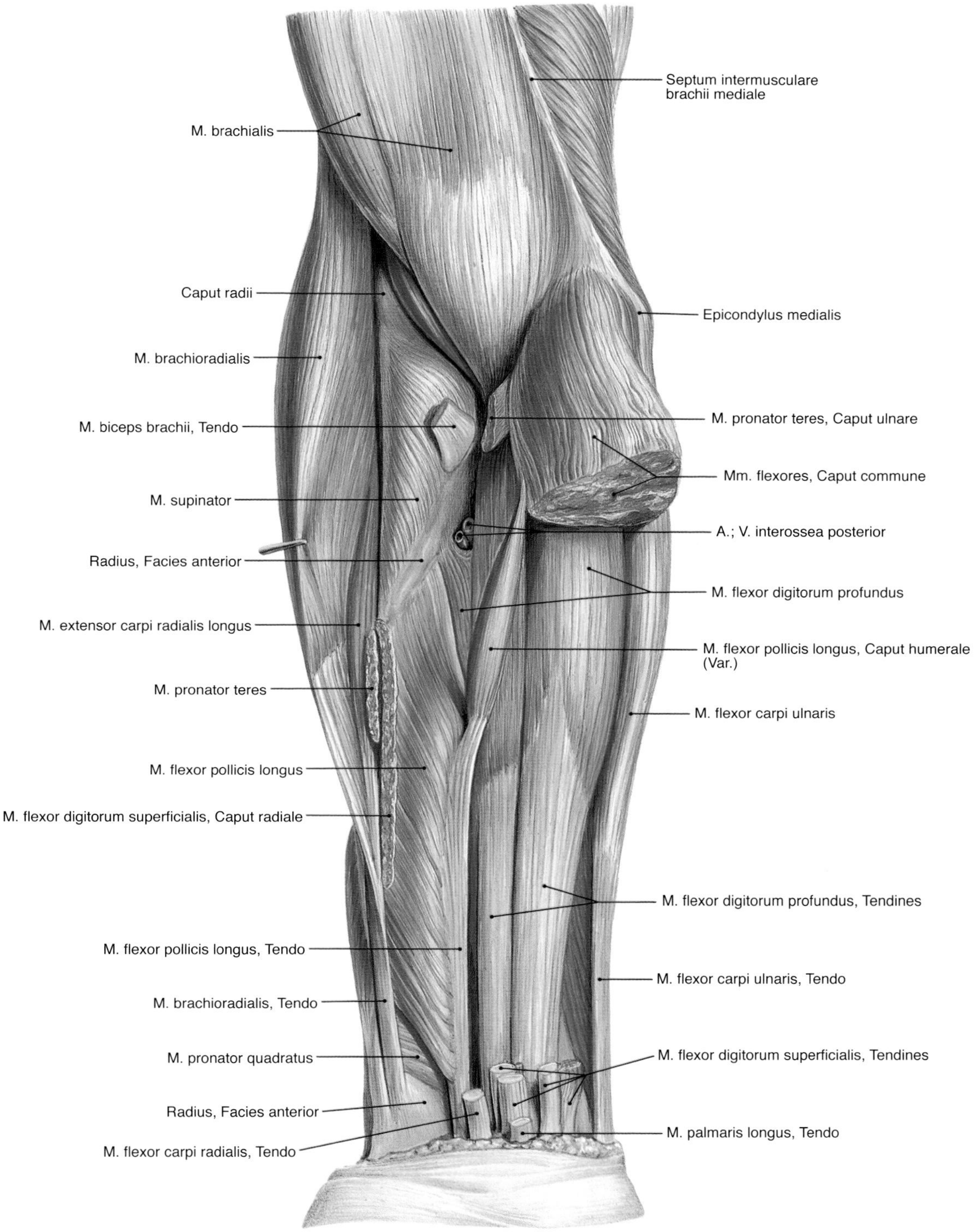

M. brachialis

Caput radii

M. brachioradialis

M. biceps brachii, Tendo

M. supinator

Radius, Facies anterior

M. extensor carpi radialis longus

M. pronator teres

M. flexor pollicis longus

M. flexor digitorum superficialis, Caput radiale

M. flexor pollicis longus, Tendo

M. brachioradialis, Tendo

M. pronator quadratus

Radius, Facies anterior

M. flexor carpi radialis, Tendo

Septum intermusculare brachii mediale

Epicondylus medialis

M. pronator teres, Caput ulnare

Mm. flexores, Caput commune

A.; V. interossea posterior

M. flexor digitorum profundus

M. flexor pollicis longus, Caput humerale (Var.)

M. flexor carpi ulnaris

M. flexor digitorum profundus, Tendines

M. flexor carpi ulnaris, Tendo

M. flexor digitorum superficialis, Tendines

M. palmaris longus, Tendo

Fig. 360   Muscles of the forearm; flexor aspect, deep layer.

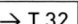 → T 32

Origins and insertions of the dorsal muscles of the forearm

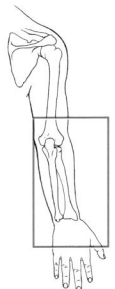

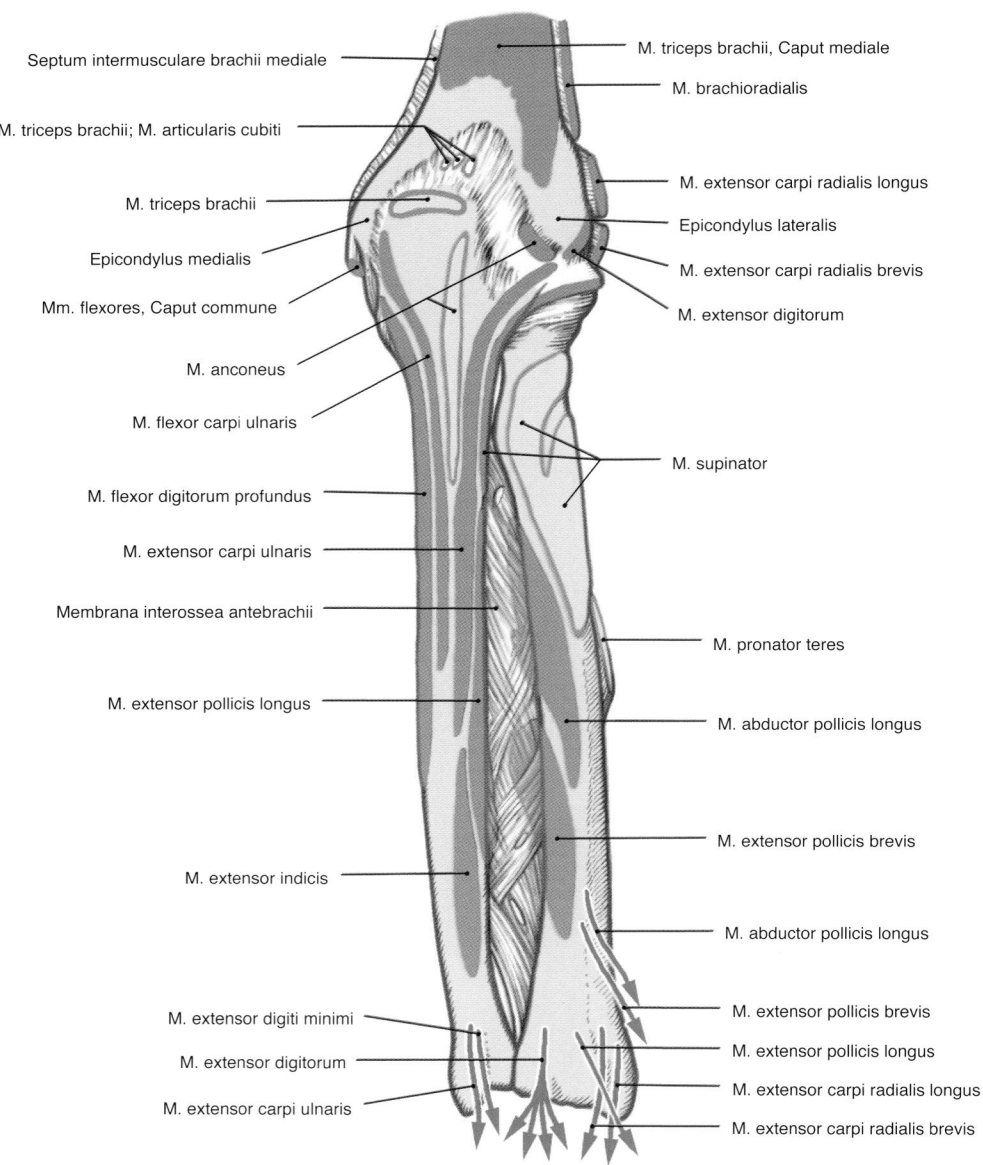

Septum intermusculare brachii mediale

M. triceps brachii; M. articularis cubiti

M. triceps brachii

Epicondylus medialis

Mm. flexores, Caput commune

M. anconeus

M. flexor carpi ulnaris

M. flexor digitorum profundus

M. extensor carpi ulnaris

Membrana interossea antebrachii

M. extensor pollicis longus

M. extensor indicis

M. extensor digiti minimi

M. extensor digitorum

M. extensor carpi ulnaris

M. triceps brachii, Caput mediale

M. brachioradialis

M. extensor carpi radialis longus

Epicondylus lateralis

M. extensor carpi radialis brevis

M. extensor digitorum

M. supinator

M. pronator teres

M. abductor pollicis longus

M. extensor pollicis brevis

M. abductor pollicis longus

M. extensor pollicis brevis

M. extensor pollicis longus

M. extensor carpi radialis longus

M. extensor carpi radialis brevis

→ T 34, T 35

Fig. 361   Origins and insertions of the muscles
at the radius, Radius, the ulna, Ulna, and the
distal part of the humerus, Humerus.

Muscles of the forearm

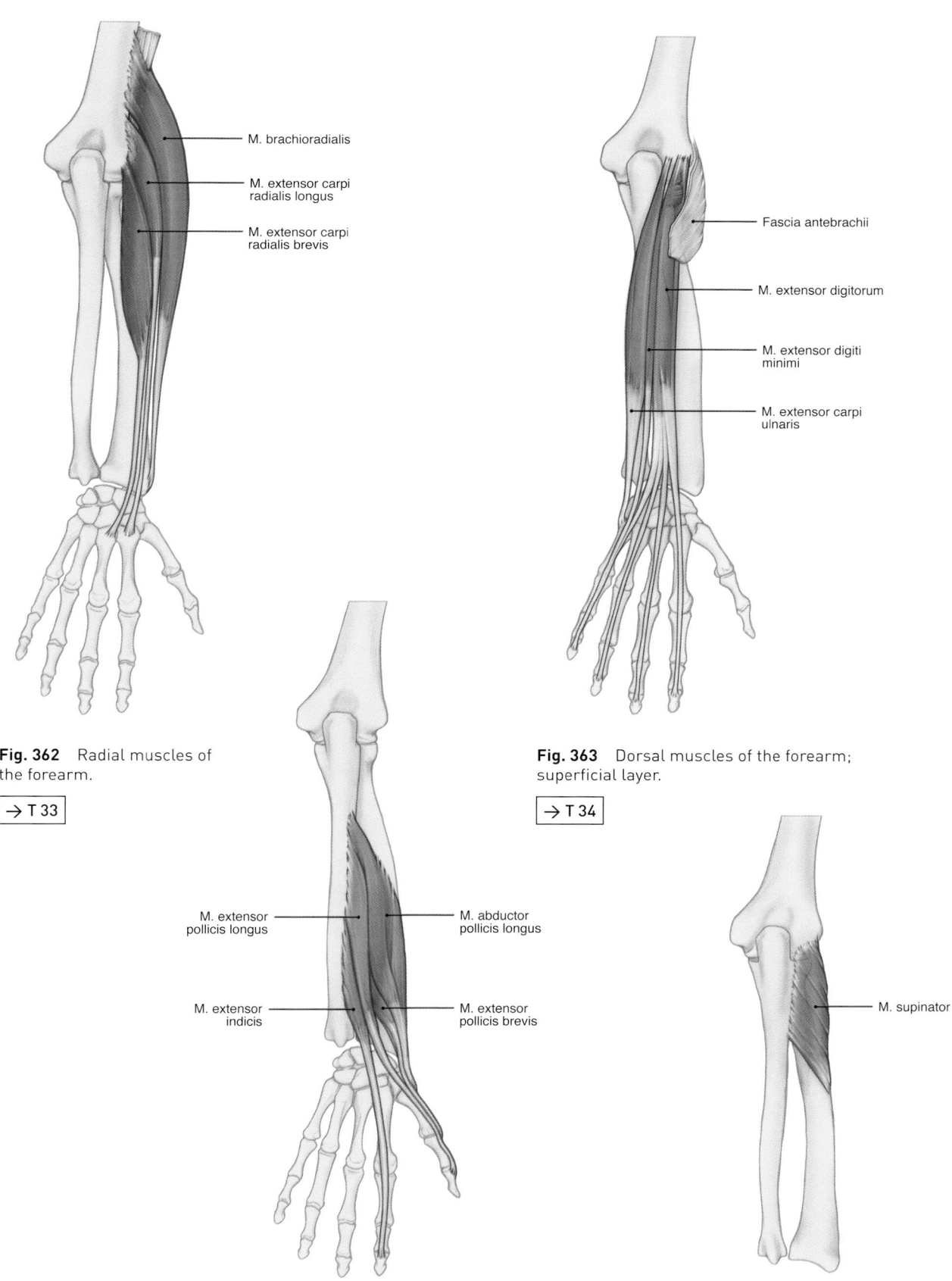

M. brachioradialis

M. extensor carpi
radialis longus

M. extensor carpi
radialis brevis

Fig. 362 Radial muscles of
the forearm.

→ T 33

Fascia antebrachii

M. extensor digitorum

M. extensor digiti
minimi

M. extensor carpi
ulnaris

Fig. 363 Dorsal muscles of the forearm;
superficial layer.

→ T 34

M. extensor
pollicis longus

M. extensor
indicis

M. abductor
pollicis longus

M. extensor
pollicis brevis

Fig. 364 Dorsal muscles of the forearm;
middle layer.

→ T 35

M. supinator

Fig. 365 Dorsal muscles of the forearm;
deep layer.

→ T 35

Muscles of the forearm

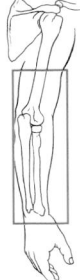

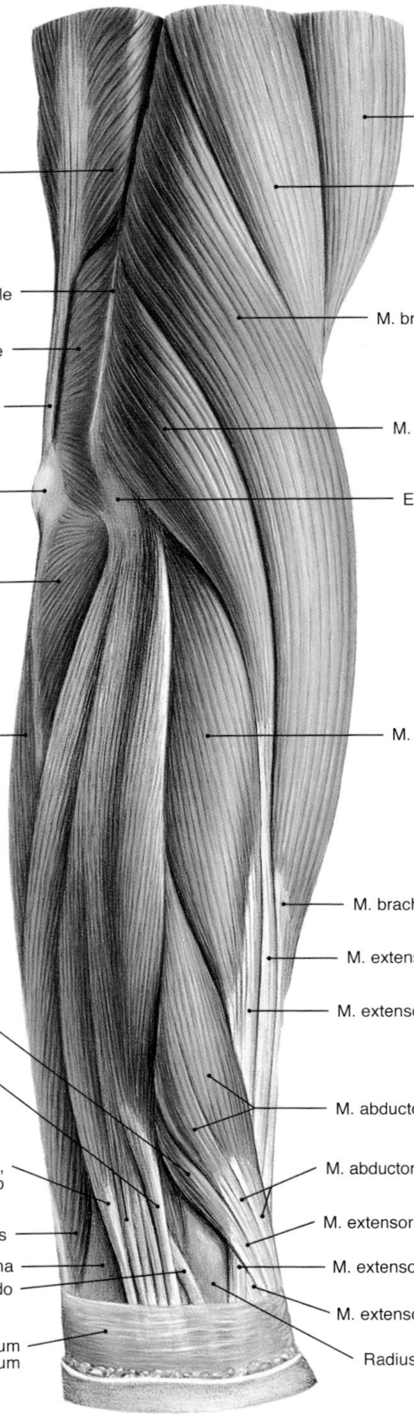

M. triceps brachii, Caput laterale ——

Septum intermusculare brachii laterale ——

M. triceps brachii, Caput mediale ——

M. triceps brachii, Tendo ——

Olecranon ——

M. anconeus ——

M. flexor carpi ulnaris ——

M. extensor pollicis brevis ——

M. extensor digitorum, Tendines ——

M. extensor digiti minimi, Tendo ——

M. extensor carpi ulnaris ——

Ulna ——

M. extensor pollicis longus, Tendo ——

Retinaculum musculorum extensorum ——

—— M. biceps brachii

—— M. brachialis

—— M. brachioradialis

—— M. extensor carpi radialis longus

—— Epicondylus lateralis

—— M. extensor carpi radialis brevis

—— M. brachioradialis, Tendo

—— M. extensor carpi radialis longus, Tendo

—— M. extensor carpi radialis brevis, Tendo

—— M. abductor pollicis longus

—— M. abductor pollicis longus, Tendo

—— M. extensor pollicis brevis, Tendo

—— M. extensor carpi radialis brevis, Tendo

—— M. extensor carpi radialis longus, Tendo

Radius

→ T 33

Fig. 366 Muscles of the forearm and
the distal part of the arm;
lateral view;
intermediate position of the forearm between
supination and pronation.

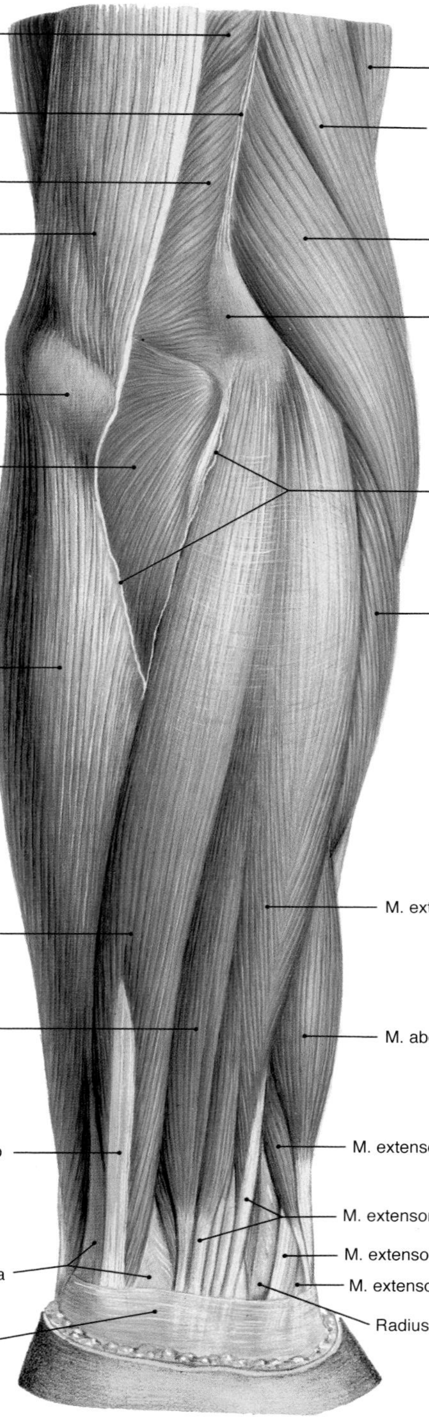

M. triceps brachii, Caput laterale

Septum intermusculare brachii laterale

M. triceps brachii, Caput mediale

M. triceps brachii, Tendo

Olecranon

M. anconeus

M. flexor carpi ulnaris

M. extensor carpi ulnaris

M. extensor digiti minimi

M. extensor carpi ulnaris, Tendo

Ulna

Retinaculum musculorum extensorum

M. brachialis

M. brachioradialis

M. extensor carpi radialis longus

Epicondylus lateralis

Fascia antebrachii

M. extensor carpi radialis brevis

M. extensor digitorum

M. abductor pollicis longus

M. extensor pollicis brevis

M. extensor digitorum, Tendines

M. extensor carpi radialis brevis, Tendo

M. extensor carpi radialis longus, Tendo

Radius

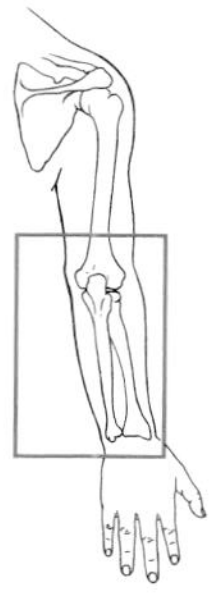

Fig. 367   Muscles of the forearm and the distal part of the arm; extensor aspect, superficial layer; intermediate position of the forearm between supination and pronation.

 → T 34

Muscles of the forearm

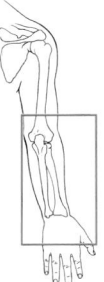

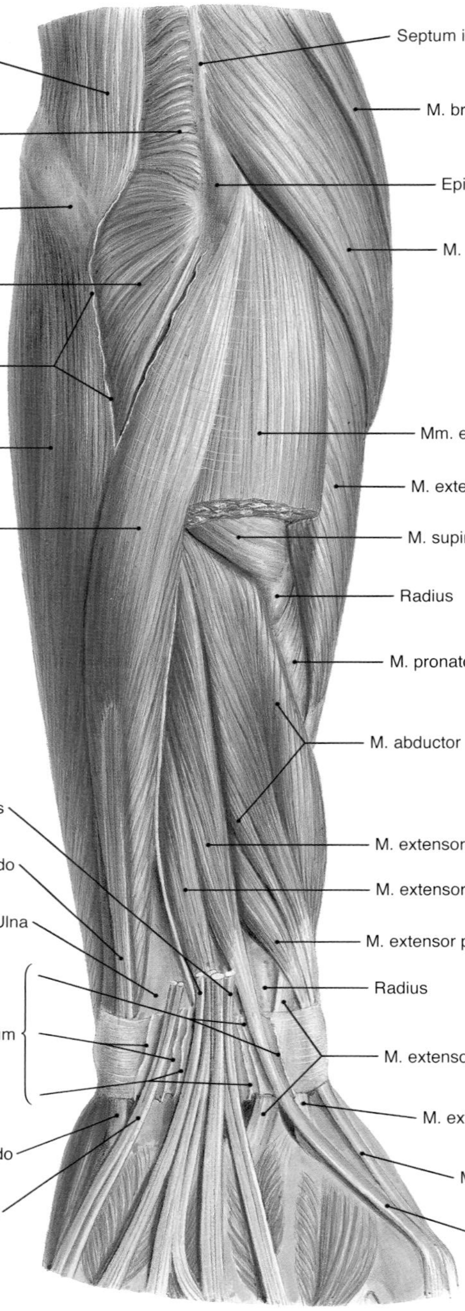

M. triceps brachii, Tendo

M. triceps brachii, Caput mediale

Olecranon

M. anconeus

Fascia antebrachii

M. flexor carpi ulnaris

M. extensor carpi ulnaris

M. extensor digitorum, Tendines

M. extensor carpi ulnaris, Tendo

Ulna

Retinaculum musculorum extensorum

M. extensor carpi ulnaris, Tendo

M. extensor digiti minimi, Tendo

Septum intermusculare brachii laterale

M. brachioradialis

Epicondylus lateralis

M. extensor carpi radialis longus

Mm. extensores digitorum et digiti minimi

M. extensor carpi radialis brevis

M. supinator

Radius

M. pronator teres, Tendo

M. abductor pollicis longus

M. extensor pollicis longus

M. extensor indicis

M. extensor pollicis brevis

Radius

M. extensor carpi radialis brevis, Tendo

M. extensor carpi radialis longus, Tendo

M. extensor pollicis brevis, Tendo

M. extensor pollicis longus, Tendo

→ T 34, T 35

Fig. 368 Muscles of the forearm;
extensor aspect, middle layer;
intermediate position of the forearm between
supination and pronation.

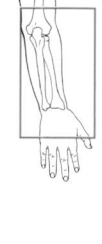

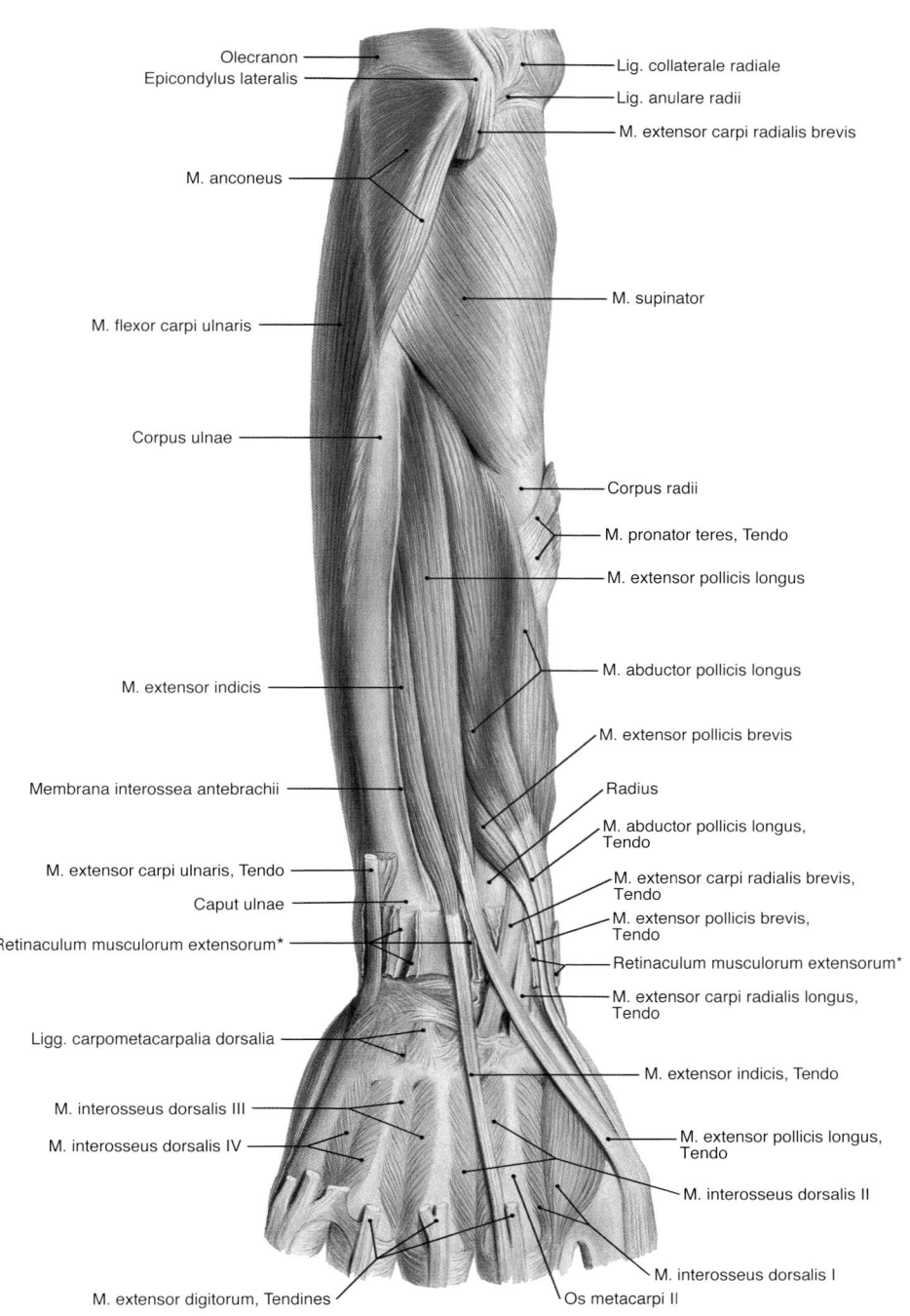

Olecranon
Epicondylus lateralis

M. anconeus

M. flexor carpi ulnaris

Corpus ulnae

M. extensor indicis

Membrana interossea antebrachii

M. extensor carpi ulnaris, Tendo

Caput ulnae

Retinaculum musculorum extensorum*

Ligg. carpometacarpalia dorsalia

M. interosseus dorsalis III

M. interosseus dorsalis IV

M. extensor digitorum, Tendines

Lig. collaterale radiale
Lig. anulare radii
M. extensor carpi radialis brevis

M. supinator

Corpus radii

M. pronator teres, Tendo

M. extensor pollicis longus

M. abductor pollicis longus

M. extensor pollicis brevis

Radius

M. abductor pollicis longus, Tendo

M. extensor carpi radialis brevis, Tendo

M. extensor pollicis brevis, Tendo

Retinaculum musculorum extensorum*

M. extensor carpi radialis longus, Tendo

M. extensor indicis, Tendo

M. extensor pollicis longus, Tendo

M. interosseus dorsalis II

M. interosseus dorsalis I

Os metacarpi II

Fig. 369   Muscles of the forearm and the hand;
extensor aspect, deep layer;
intermediate position of the forearm between
supination and pronation.
* The tendon compartments formed by the extensor retinaculum
  have been opened longitudinally.

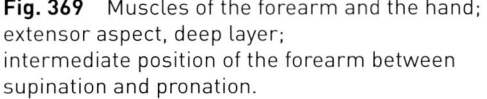

→ T 35

Muscles of the forearm

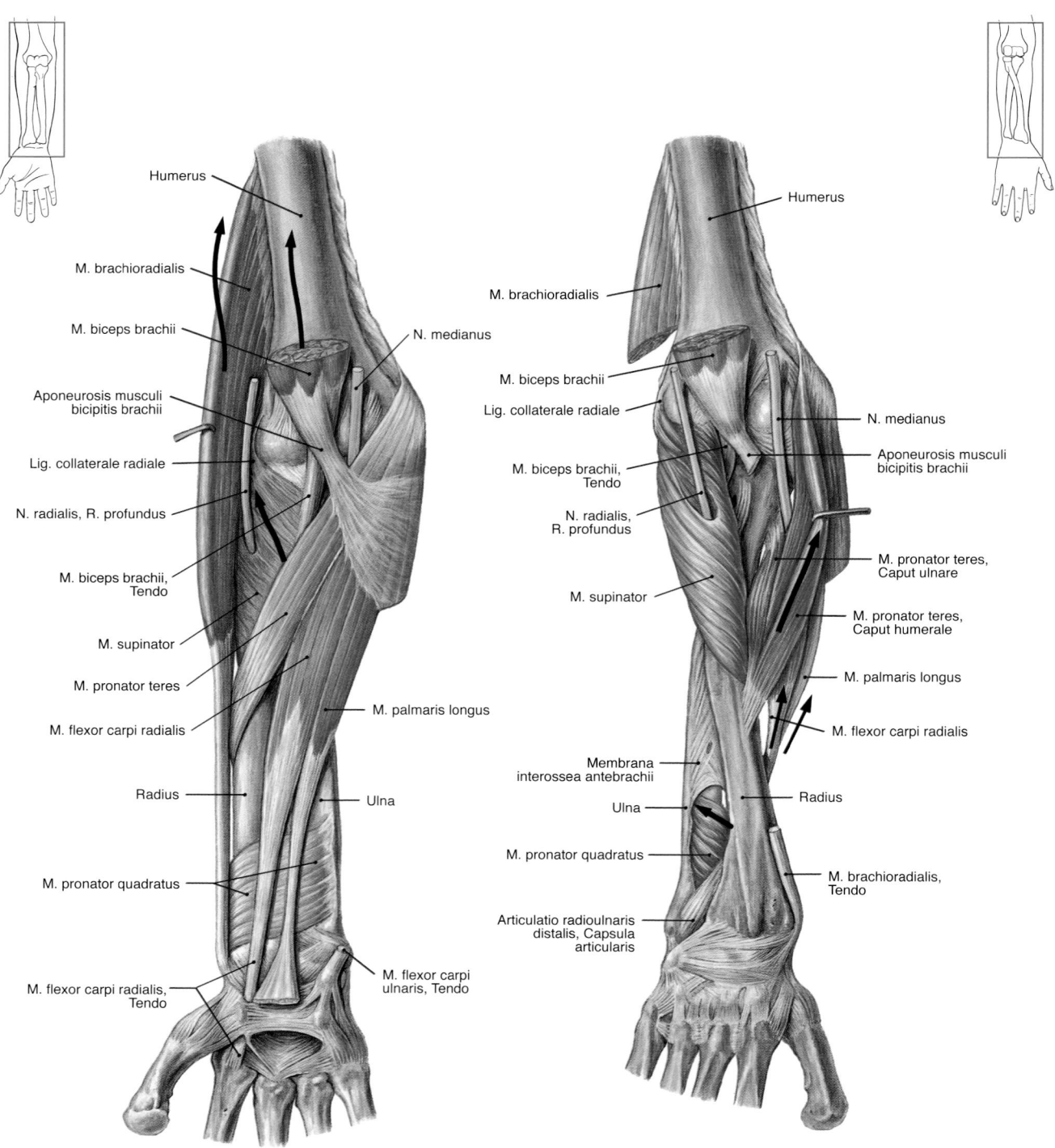

Fig. 370 Forearm in supination;
ventropalmar view.
Arrows indicate the direction of force generated
by the main supinator muscles.

→ T 32, T 33, T 35

Fig. 371 Forearm in pronation;
ventral view of the elbow region, dorsal view of the
dorsum of the hand.
Arrows indicate the direction of force generated
by the main pronator muscles.

→ T 32, T 33, T 35

Origins and insertions of the muscles of the hand

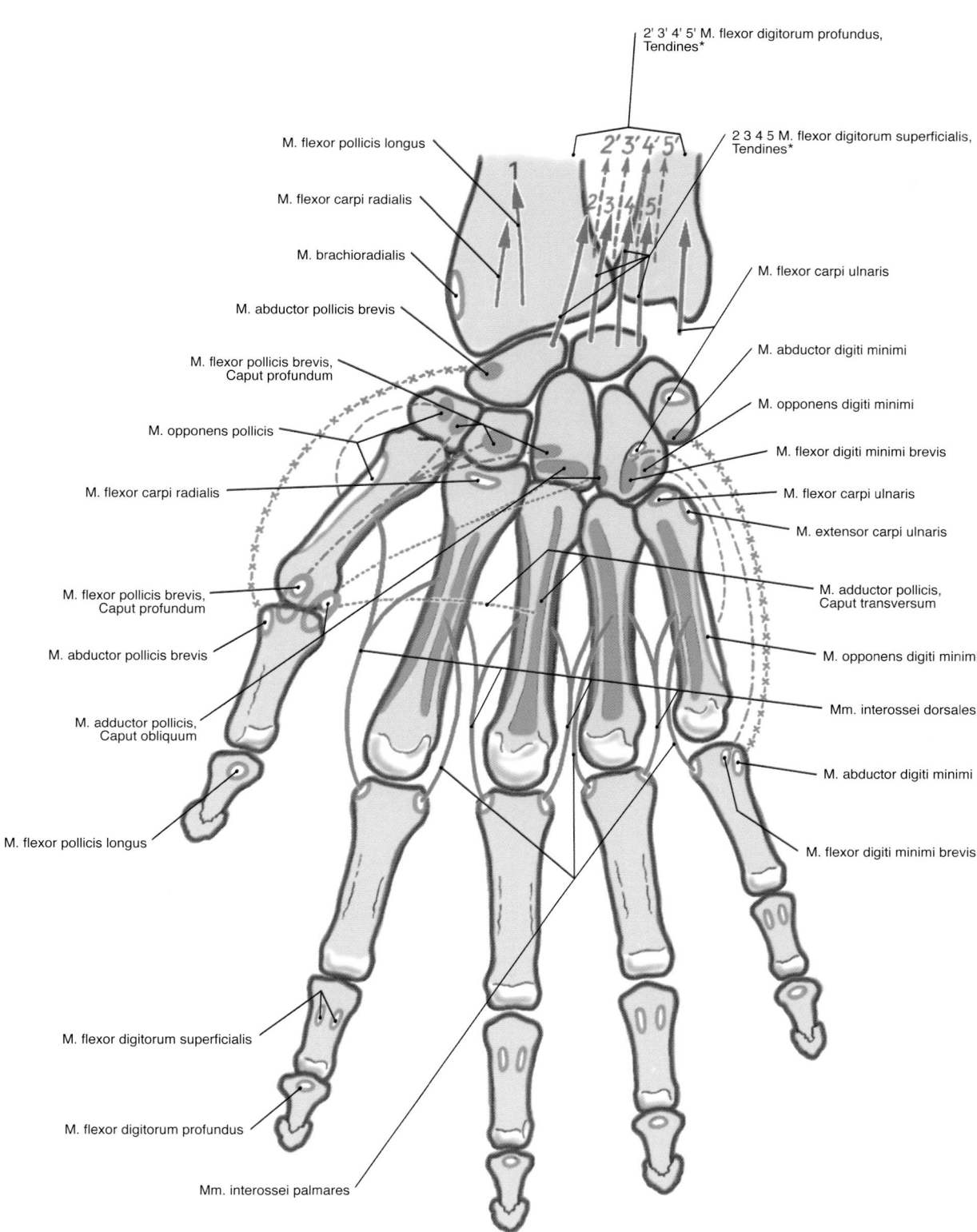

2' 3' 4' 5' M. flexor digitorum profundus, Tendines*

M. flexor pollicis longus

2 3 4 5 M. flexor digitorum superficialis, Tendines*

M. flexor carpi radialis

M. brachioradialis

M. flexor carpi ulnaris

M. abductor pollicis brevis

M. abductor digiti minimi

M. flexor pollicis brevis, Caput profundum

M. opponens digiti minimi

M. opponens pollicis

M. flexor digiti minimi brevis

M. flexor carpi radialis

M. flexor carpi ulnaris

M. extensor carpi ulnaris

M. flexor pollicis brevis, Caput profundum

M. adductor pollicis, Caput transversum

M. abductor pollicis brevis

M. opponens digiti minimi

M. adductor pollicis, Caput obliquum

Mm. interossei dorsales

M. abductor digiti minimi

M. flexor pollicis longus

M. flexor digiti minimi brevis

M. flexor digitorum superficialis

M. flexor digitorum profundus

Mm. interossei palmares

Fig. 372   Origins and insertions of the muscles of the hand at the bones of the hand.
* The flexors insert at the second to fifth digit.

→ T 36–T 38

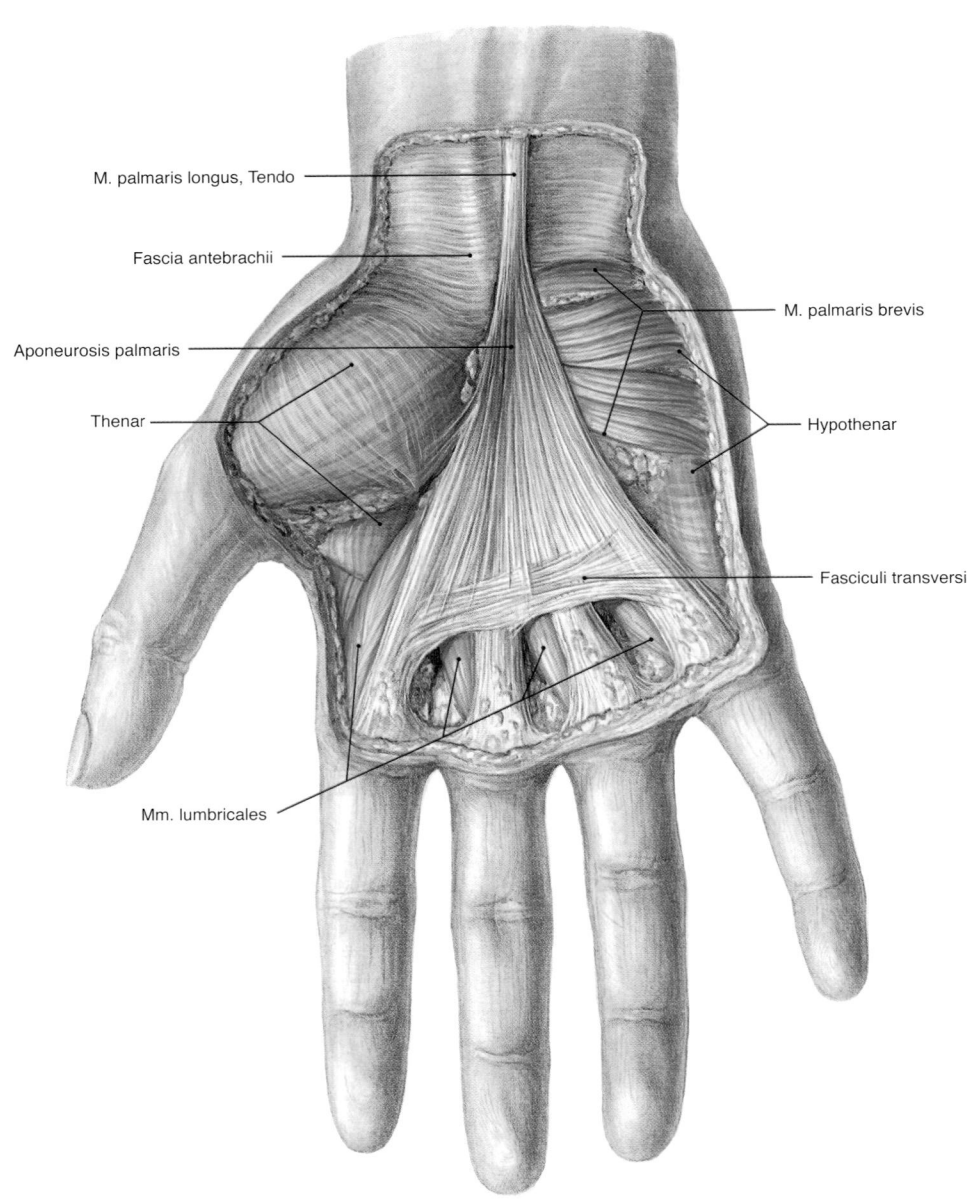

M. palmaris longus, Tendo

Fascia antebrachii

Aponeurosis palmaris

Thenar

Mm. lumbricales

M. palmaris brevis

Hypothenar

Fasciculi transversi

→ T 31, T 36–T 38

Fig. 373 Muscles of the palm;
superficial layer.

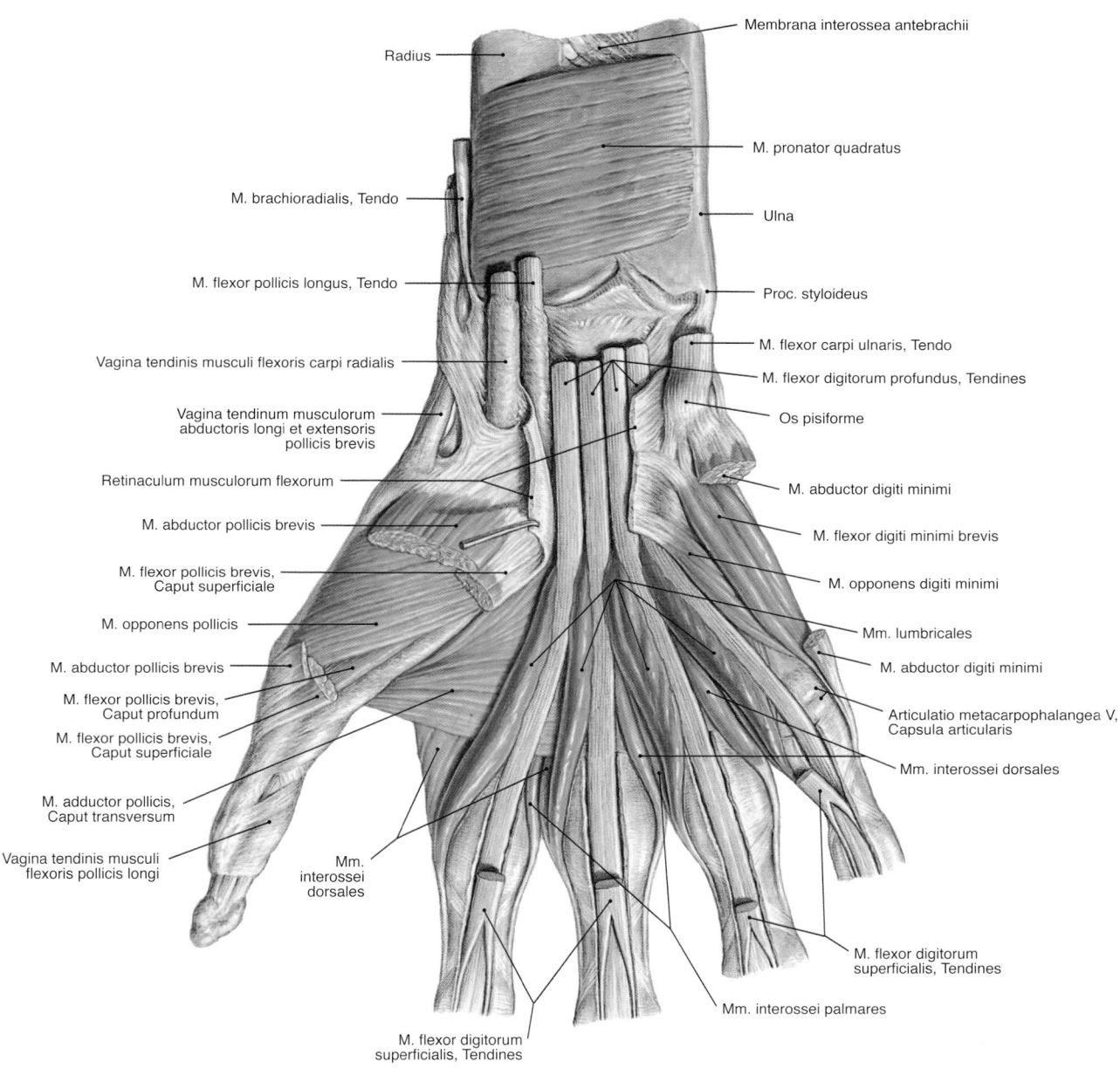

Radius

Membrana interossea antebrachii

M. pronator quadratus

M. brachioradialis, Tendo

Ulna

M. flexor pollicis longus, Tendo

Proc. styloideus

Vagina tendinis musculi flexoris carpi radialis

M. flexor carpi ulnaris, Tendo

M. flexor digitorum profundus, Tendines

Vagina tendinum musculorum abductoris longi et extensoris pollicis brevis

Os pisiforme

Retinaculum musculorum flexorum

M. abductor digiti minimi

M. abductor pollicis brevis

M. flexor digiti minimi brevis

M. flexor pollicis brevis, Caput superficiale

M. opponens digiti minimi

M. opponens pollicis

Mm. lumbricales

M. abductor pollicis brevis

M. abductor digiti minimi

M. flexor pollicis brevis, Caput profundum

Articulatio metacarpophalangea V, Capsula articularis

M. flexor pollicis brevis, Caput superficiale

Mm. interossei dorsales

M. adductor pollicis, Caput transversum

Vagina tendinis musculi flexoris pollicis longi

Mm. interossei dorsales

M. flexor digitorum superficialis, Tendines

Mm. interossei palmares

M. flexor digitorum superficialis, Tendines

Fig. 374 Muscles of the palm; middle layer.

→ T 32, T 36–T 38

Tendon sheaths of the hand

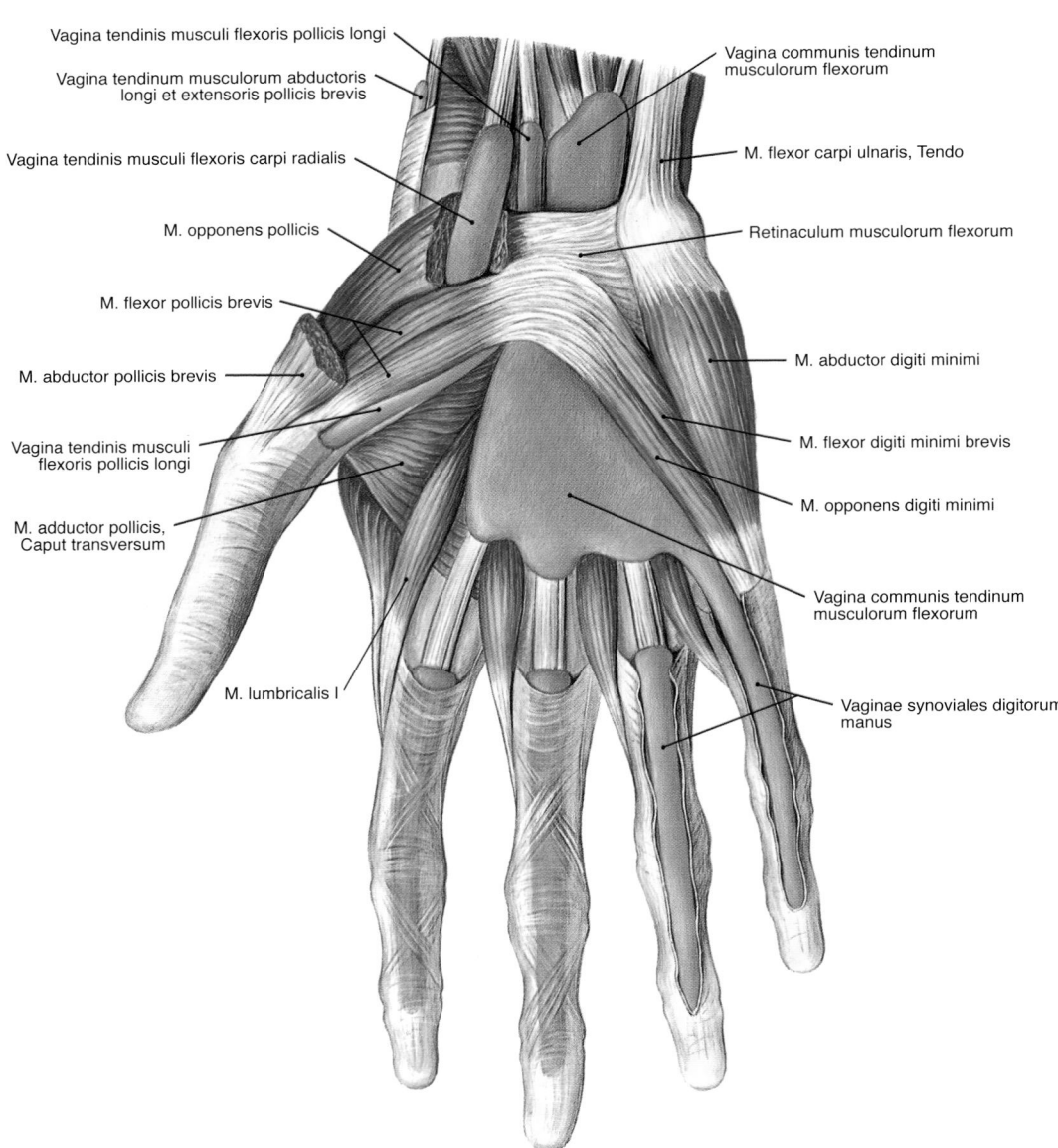

Vagina tendinis musculi flexoris pollicis longi

Vagina tendinum musculorum abductoris longi et extensoris pollicis brevis

Vagina tendinis musculi flexoris carpi radialis

M. opponens pollicis

M. flexor pollicis brevis

M. abductor pollicis brevis

Vagina tendinis musculi flexoris pollicis longi

M. adductor pollicis, Caput transversum

M. lumbricalis I

Vagina communis tendinum musculorum flexorum

M. flexor carpi ulnaris, Tendo

Retinaculum musculorum flexorum

M. abductor digiti minimi

M. flexor digiti minimi brevis

M. opponens digiti minimi

Vagina communis tendinum musculorum flexorum

Vaginae synoviales digitorum manus

Fig. 375 Tendon sheaths, Vaginae tendinum, of the hand.

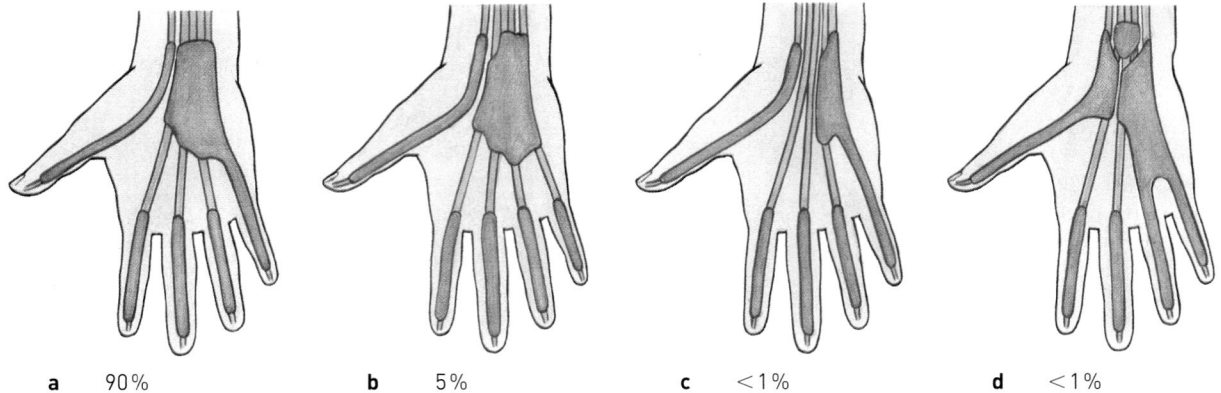

a 90%   b 5%   c <1%   d <1%

Fig. 376 a–d Frequent variations of the palmar tendon sheaths.

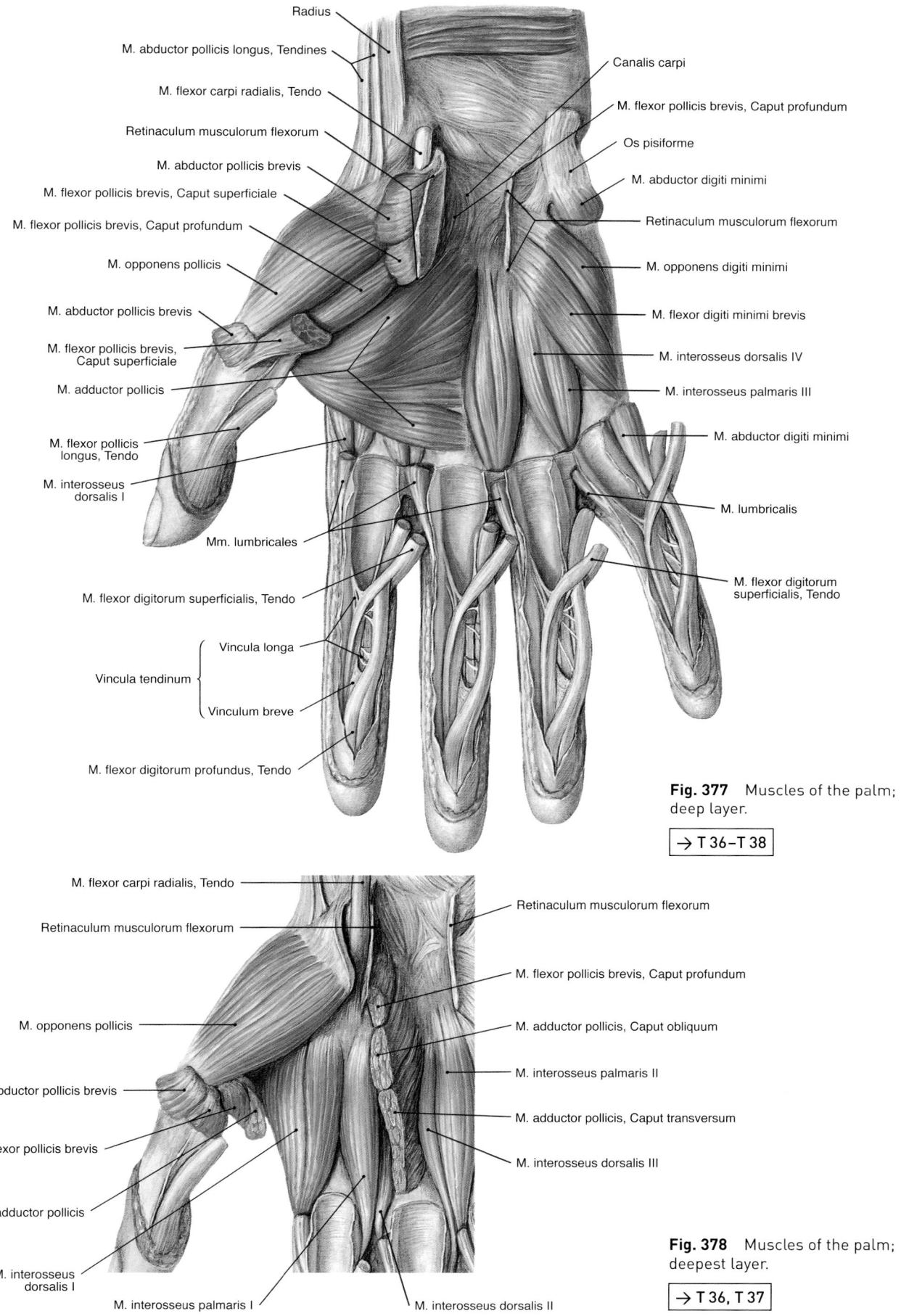

Radius

M. abductor pollicis longus, Tendines

Canalis carpi

M. flexor carpi radialis, Tendo

M. flexor pollicis brevis, Caput profundum

Retinaculum musculorum flexorum

Os pisiforme

M. abductor pollicis brevis

M. abductor digiti minimi

M. flexor pollicis brevis, Caput superficiale

Retinaculum musculorum flexorum

M. flexor pollicis brevis, Caput profundum

M. opponens digiti minimi

M. opponens pollicis

M. flexor digiti minimi brevis

M. abductor pollicis brevis

M. interosseus dorsalis IV

M. flexor pollicis brevis, Caput superficiale

M. interosseus palmaris III

M. adductor pollicis

M. abductor digiti minimi

M. flexor pollicis longus, Tendo

M. interosseus dorsalis I

M. lumbricalis

Mm. lumbricales

M. flexor digitorum superficialis, Tendo

M. flexor digitorum superficialis, Tendo

Vincula longa

Vincula tendinum {

Vinculum breve

M. flexor digitorum profundus, Tendo

Fig. 377 Muscles of the palm; deep layer.

→ T 36–T 38

M. flexor carpi radialis, Tendo

Retinaculum musculorum flexorum

Retinaculum musculorum flexorum

M. flexor pollicis brevis, Caput profundum

M. opponens pollicis

M. adductor pollicis, Caput obliquum

M. interosseus palmaris II

M. abductor pollicis brevis

M. adductor pollicis, Caput transversum

M. flexor pollicis brevis

M. interosseus dorsalis III

M. adductor pollicis

M. interosseus dorsalis I

Fig. 378 Muscles of the palm; deepest layer.

→ T 36, T 37

M. interosseus palmaris I

M. interosseus dorsalis II

Muscles of the hand

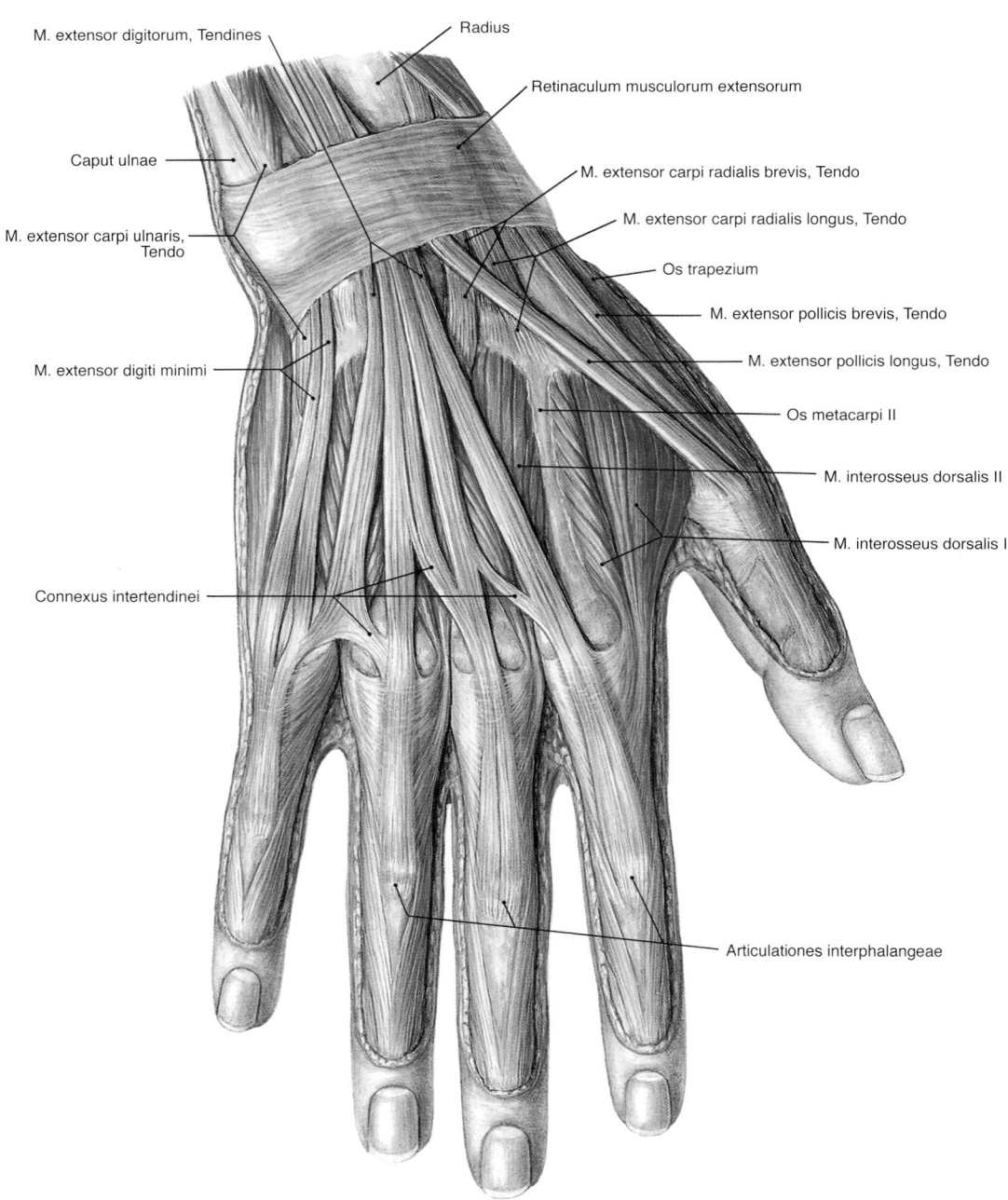

M. extensor digitorum, Tendines

Radius

Retinaculum musculorum extensorum

Caput ulnae

M. extensor carpi radialis brevis, Tendo

M. extensor carpi ulnaris, Tendo

M. extensor carpi radialis longus, Tendo

Os trapezium

M. extensor pollicis brevis, Tendo

M. extensor pollicis longus, Tendo

M. extensor digiti minimi

Os metacarpi II

M. interosseus dorsalis II

M. interosseus dorsalis I

Connexus intertendinei

Articulationes interphalangeae

→ T 34, T 35, T 37

Fig. 379   Muscles of the dorsum of the hand.

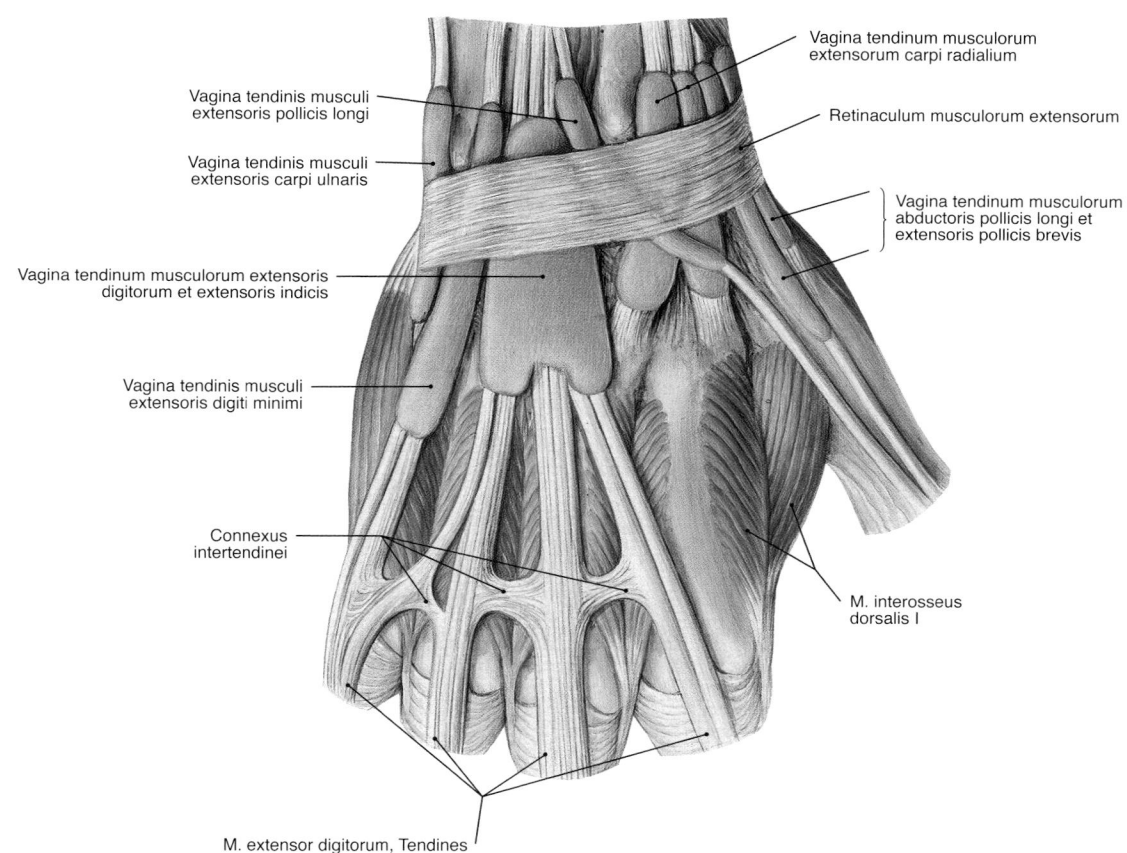

Vagina tendinum musculorum extensorum carpi radialium

Vagina tendinis musculi extensoris pollicis longi

Retinaculum musculorum extensorum

Vagina tendinis musculi extensoris carpi ulnaris

Vagina tendinum musculorum abductoris pollicis longi et extensoris pollicis brevis

Vagina tendinum musculorum extensoris digitorum et extensoris indicis

Vagina tendinis musculi extensoris digiti minimi

Connexus intertendinei

M. interosseus dorsalis I

M. extensor digitorum, Tendines

Fig. 380   Dorsal carpal tendon sheaths.

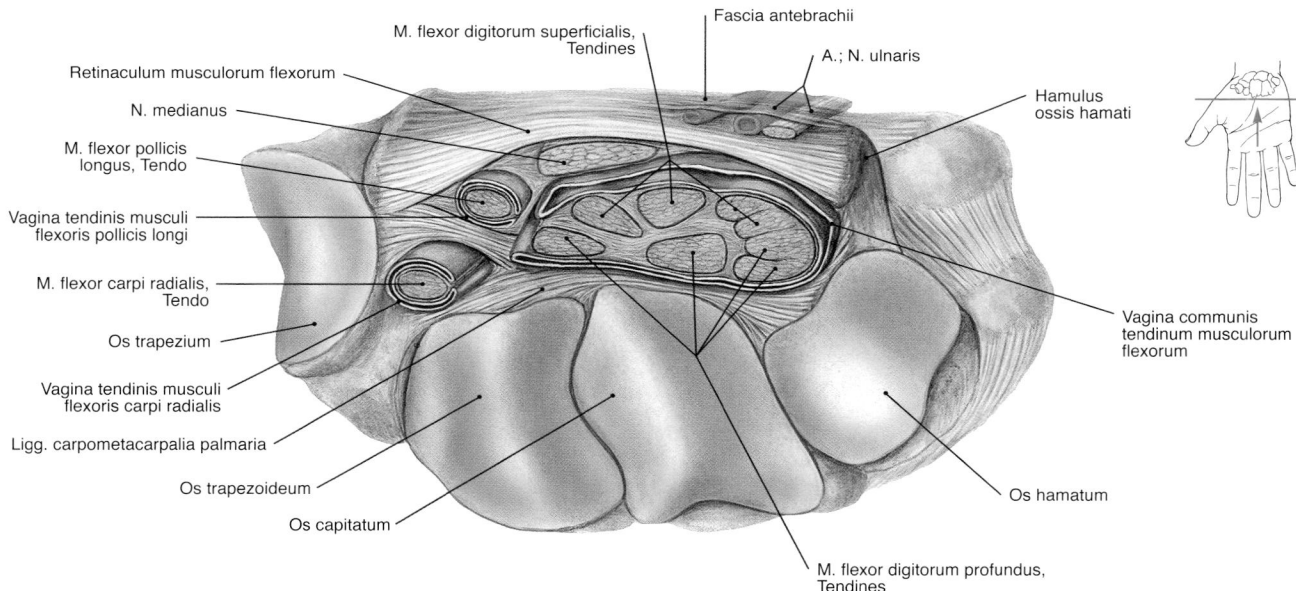

M. flexor digitorum superficialis, Tendines

Fascia antebrachii

A.; N. ulnaris

Retinaculum musculorum flexorum

N. medianus

Hamulus ossis hamati

M. flexor pollicis longus, Tendo

Vagina tendinis musculi flexoris pollicis longi

M. flexor carpi radialis, Tendo

Os trapezium

Vagina communis tendinum musculorum flexorum

Vagina tendinis musculi flexoris carpi radialis

Ligg. carpometacarpalia palmaria

Os trapezoideum

Os capitatum

Os hamatum

M. flexor digitorum profundus, Tendines

Fig. 381   Palmar carpal tendon sheaths; transverse section.

The compression of the median nerve in the carpal tunnel is known as "carpal tunnel syndrome".

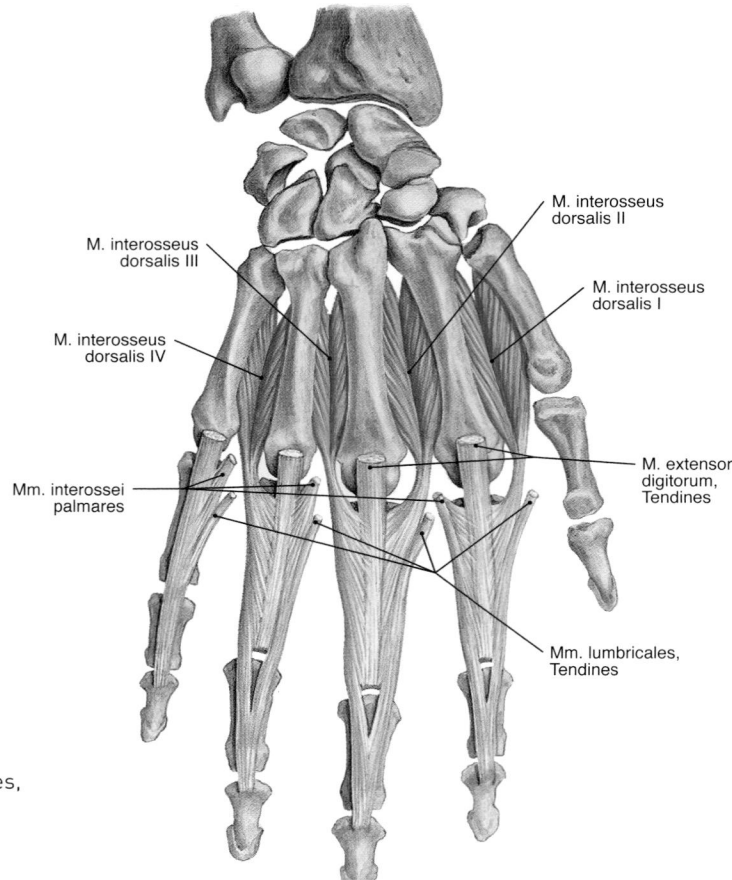

M. interosseus
dorsalis II

M. interosseus
dorsalis III

M. interosseus
dorsalis I

M. interosseus
dorsalis IV

M. extensor
digitorum,
Tendines

Mm. interossei
palmares

Mm. lumbricales,
Tendines

Fig. 382 Dorsal interosseous muscles,
Mm. interossei dorsales;
dorsal view.

→ T 37

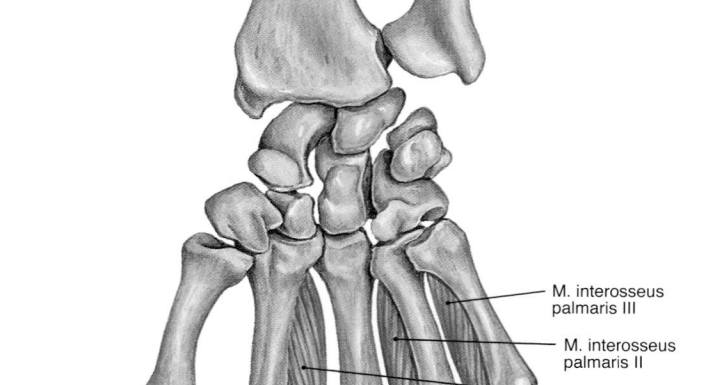

M. interosseus
palmaris III

M. interosseus
palmaris II

M. interosseus
palmaris I

Fig. 383 Palmar interosseous muscles,
Mm. interossei palmares;
palmar view.
The tendons of the interosseous and the
lumbrical muscles radiate into the so-called
dorsal aponeurosis of the fingers (arrows).

→ T37

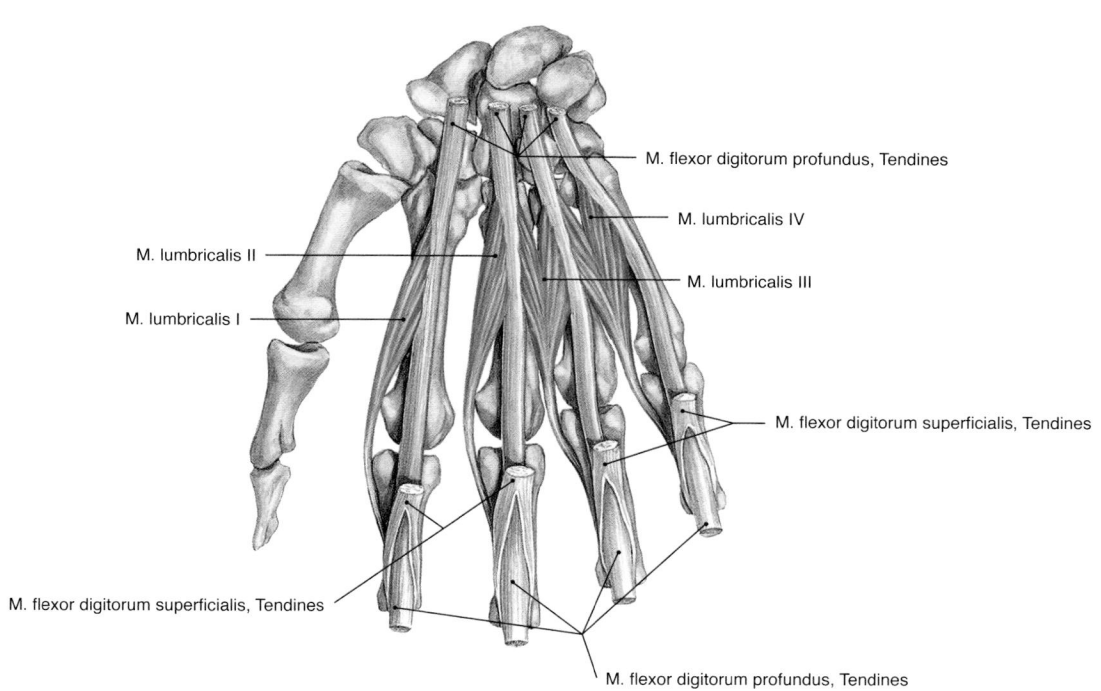

M. flexor digitorum profundus, Tendines

M. lumbricalis IV

M. lumbricalis II

M. lumbricalis III

M. lumbricalis I

M. flexor digitorum superficialis, Tendines

M. flexor digitorum superficialis, Tendines

M. flexor digitorum profundus, Tendines

Fig. 384 Lumbrical muscles,
Mm. lumbricales;
palmar view.

→ T 37

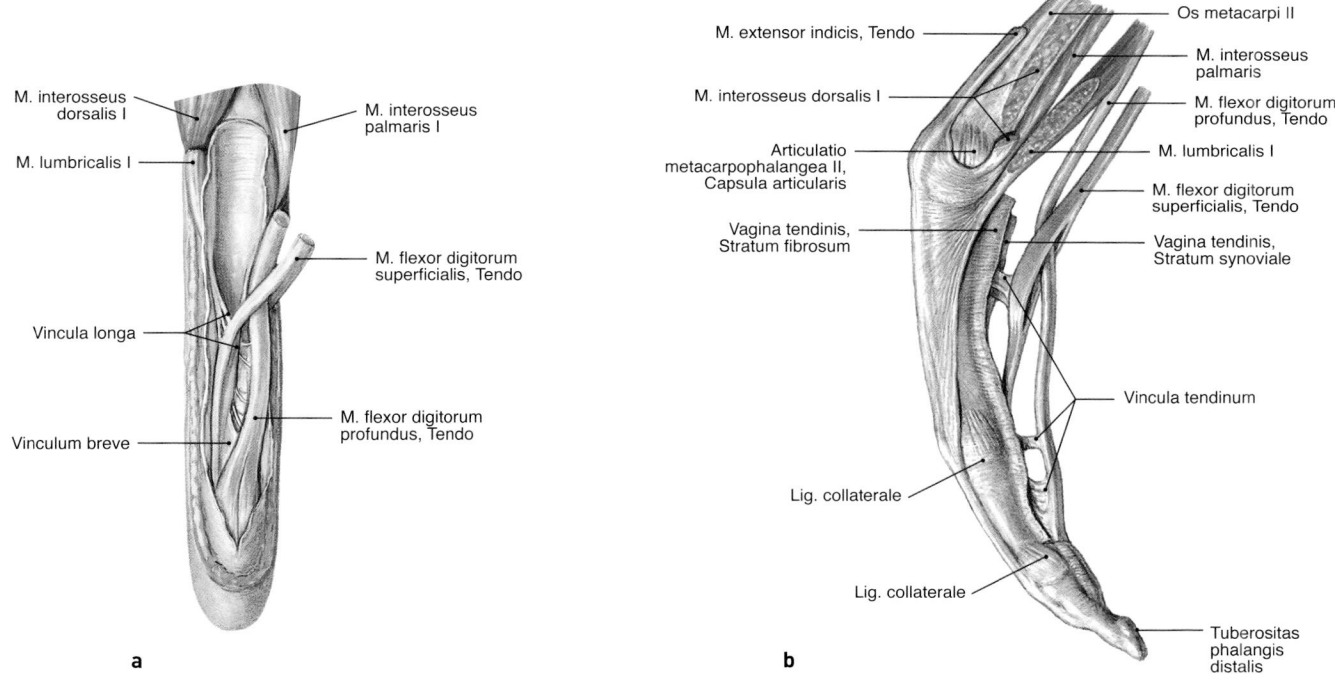

M. interosseus
dorsalis I

M. interosseus
palmaris I

M. lumbricalis I

M. flexor digitorum
superficialis, Tendo

Vincula longa

Vinculum breve

M. flexor digitorum
profundus, Tendo

M. extensor indicis, Tendo

Os metacarpi II

M. interosseus
palmaris

M. interosseus dorsalis I

M. flexor digitorum
profundus, Tendo

Articulatio
metacarpophalangea II,
Capsula articularis

M. lumbricalis I

M. flexor digitorum
superficialis, Tendo

Vagina tendinis,
Stratum fibrosum

Vagina tendinis,
Stratum synoviale

Vincula tendinum

Lig. collaterale

Lig. collaterale

Tuberositas
phalangis
distalis

a

b

Fig. 385 a, b   Tendon insertions at the index;
the tendons of both flexors have been dissected from
the tendon sheath.
a Palmar view
b Lateral view

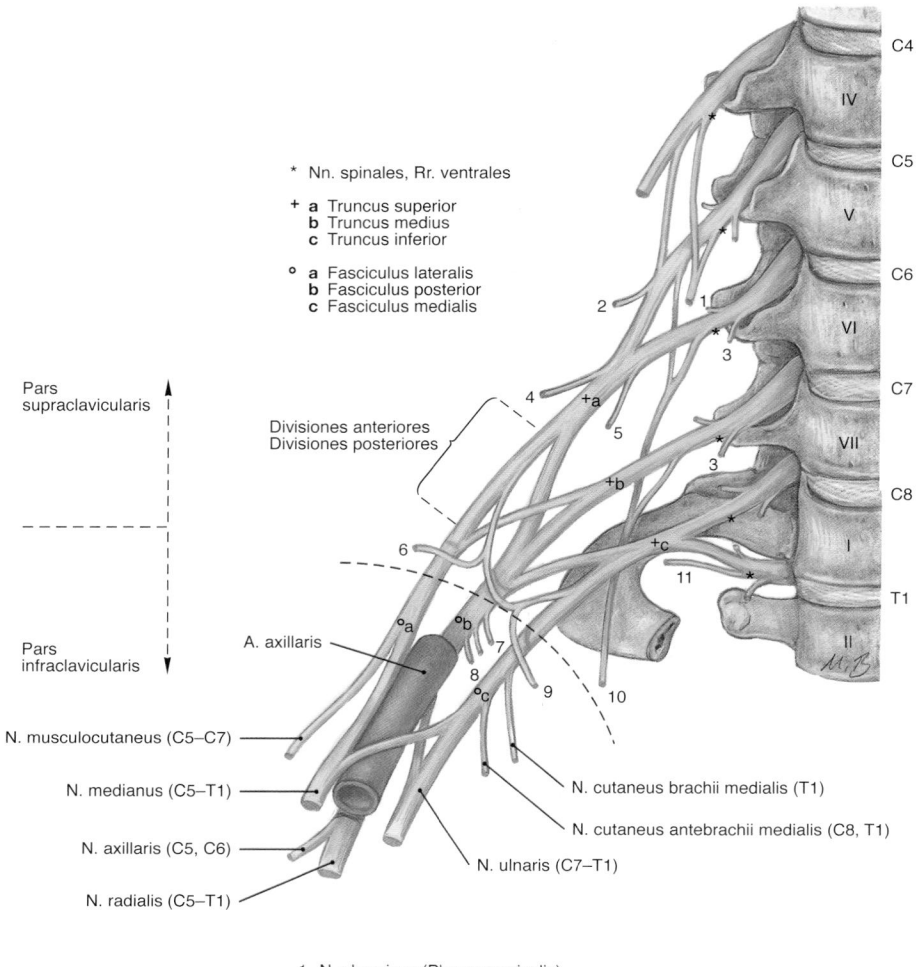

* Nn. spinales, Rr. ventrales

+ **a** Truncus superior
  b Truncus medius
  c Truncus inferior

° **a** Fasciculus lateralis
  b Fasciculus posterior
  c Fasciculus medialis

Pars
supraclavicularis

Divisiones anteriores
Divisiones posteriores

Pars
infraclavicularis

A. axillaris

N. musculocutaneus (C5–C7)

N. medianus (C5–T1)

N. axillaris (C5, C6)

N. radialis (C5–T1)

N. cutaneus brachii medialis (T1)

N. cutaneus antebrachii medialis (C8, T1)

N. ulnaris (C7–T1)

C4
IV
C5
V
C6
VI
C7
VII
C8
I
T1
II

1 N. phrenicus (Plexus cervicalis)
2 N. dorsalis scapulae (C5)
3 Rr. musculares
4 N. suprascapularis (C5, C6)
5 N. subclavius (C5, C6)
6 N. pectoralis lateralis (C5–C7)
7 N. subscapularis (C5–C7)
8 N. thoracodorsalis (C6–C8)
9 N. pectoralis medialis (C8, T1)
10 N. thoracicus longus (C5–C7)
11 N. intercostalis (T1)

→ T 24, T 25

Fig. 386 Brachial plexus, Plexus brachialis.

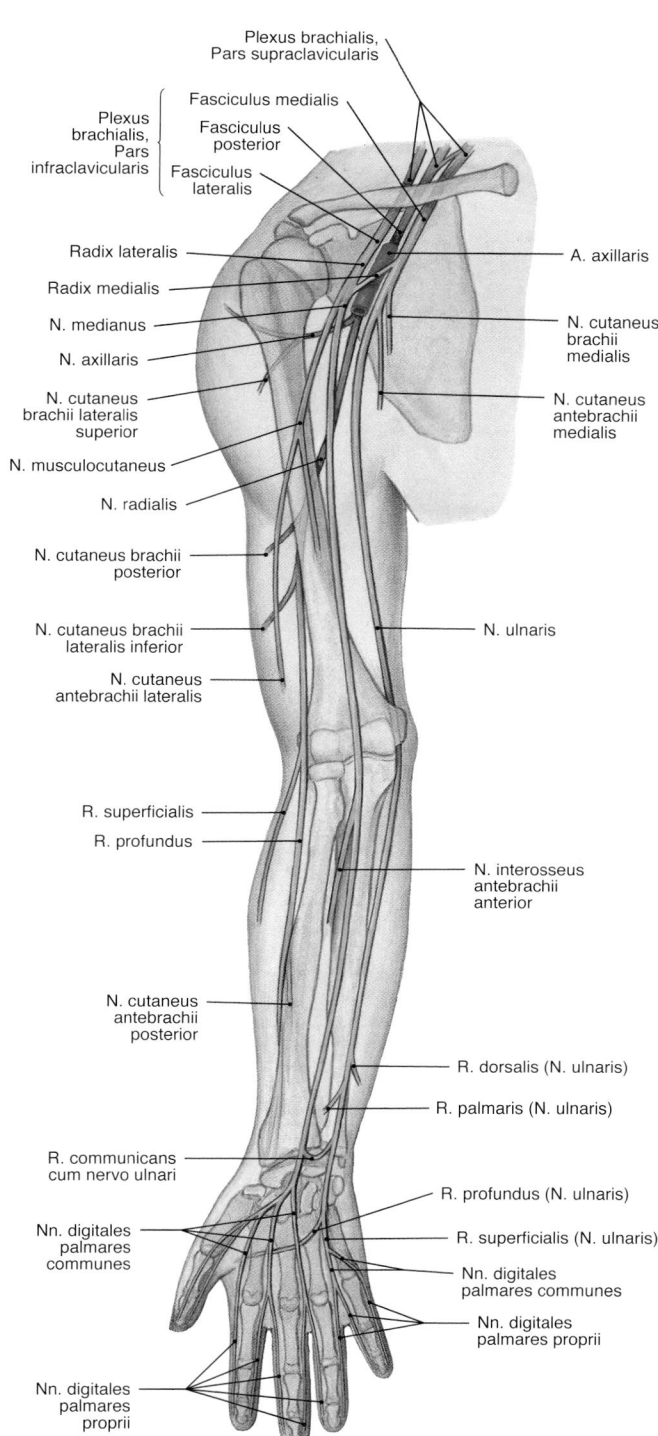

Plexus brachialis,
Pars supraclavicularis

Plexus
brachialis,
Pars
infraclavicularis
{
Fasciculus medialis
Fasciculus posterior
Fasciculus lateralis

Radix lateralis

Radix medialis

N. medianus

N. axillaris

N. cutaneus brachii lateralis superior

N. musculocutaneus

N. radialis

N. cutaneus brachii posterior

N. cutaneus brachii lateralis inferior

N. cutaneus antebrachii lateralis

R. superficialis

R. profundus

N. cutaneus antebrachii posterior

R. communicans cum nervo ulnari

Nn. digitales palmares communes

Nn. digitales palmares proprii

A. axillaris

N. cutaneus brachii medialis

N. cutaneus antebrachii medialis

N. ulnaris

N. interosseus antebrachii anterior

R. dorsalis (N. ulnaris)

R. palmaris (N. ulnaris)

R. profundus (N. ulnaris)

R. superficialis (N. ulnaris)

Nn. digitales palmares communes

Nn. digitales palmares proprii

Fig. 387   Nerves of the upper limb;
overview.

→ T 24, T 25

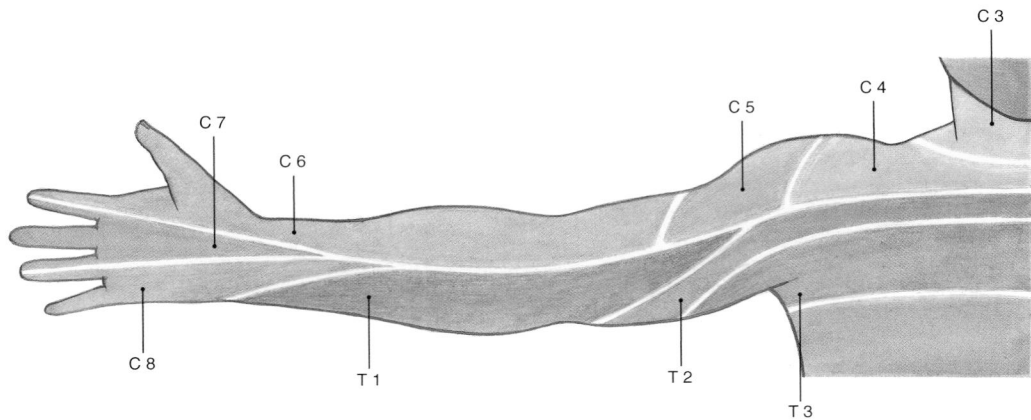

→ T 24   **Fig. 388** Segmental cutaneous innervation (dermatomes) of the upper limb.

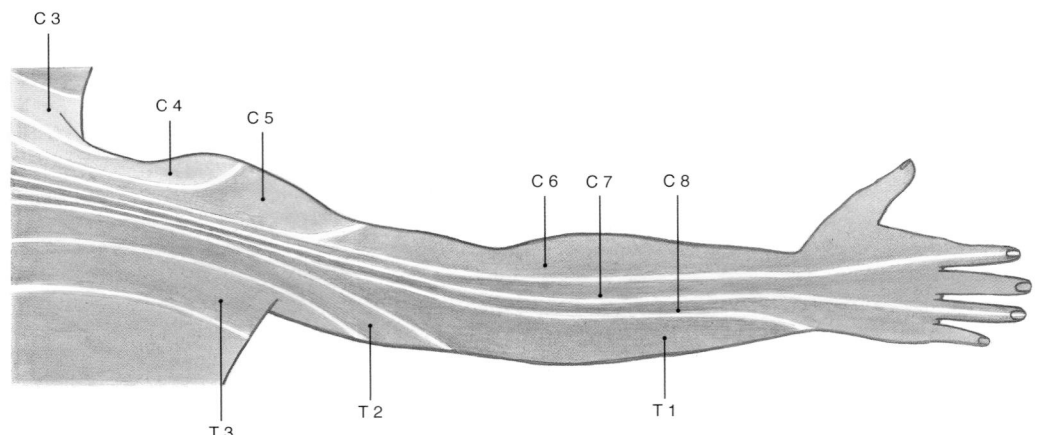

→ T 24   **Fig. 389** Segmental cutaneous innervation (dermatomes) of the upper limb.

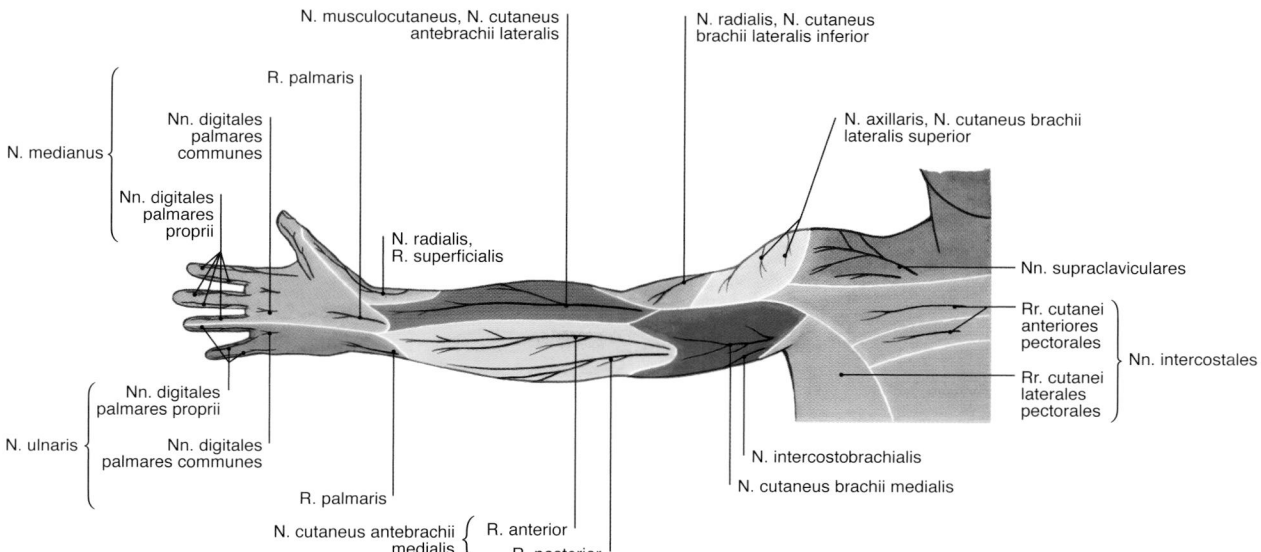

N. medianus
- Nn. digitales palmares communes
- Nn. digitales palmares proprii

N. ulnaris
- Nn. digitales palmares proprii
- Nn. digitales palmares communes

R. palmaris

R. palmaris

N. cutaneus antebrachii medialis
- R. anterior
- R. posterior

N. musculocutaneus, N. cutaneus antebrachii lateralis

N. radialis, R. superficialis

N. radialis, N. cutaneus brachii lateralis inferior

N. axillaris, N. cutaneus brachii lateralis superior

Nn. supraclaviculares

Nn. intercostales
- Rr. cutanei anteriores pectorales
- Rr. cutanei laterales pectorales

N. intercostobrachialis

N. cutaneus brachii medialis

Fig. 390 Cutaneous nerves of the upper limb.

→ T 24

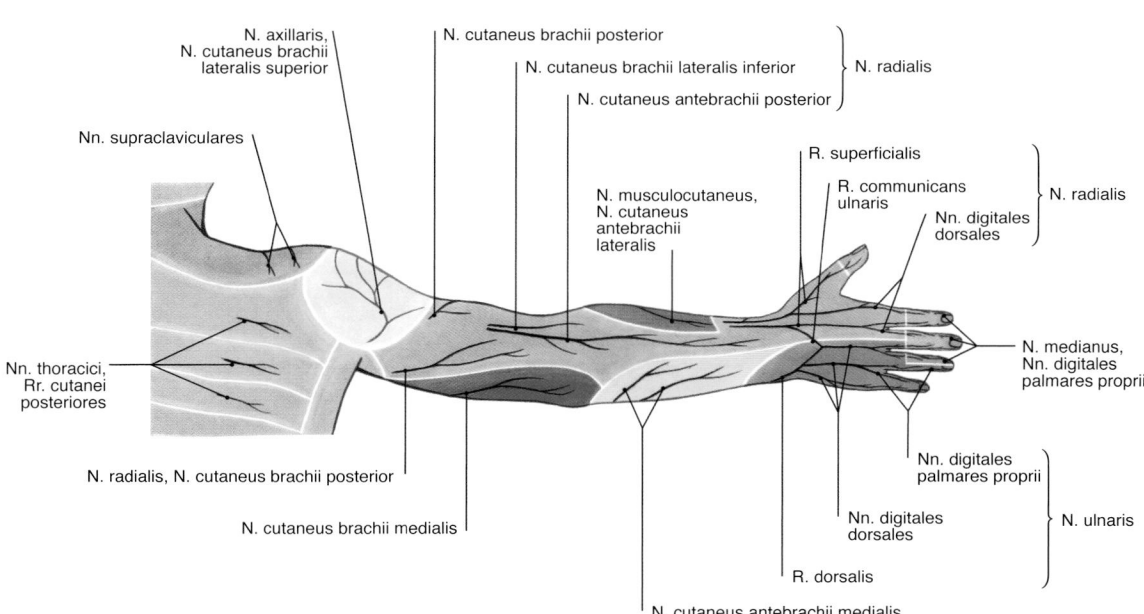

N. axillaris, N. cutaneus brachii lateralis superior

Nn. supraclaviculares

Nn. thoracici, Rr. cutanei posteriores

N. radialis, N. cutaneus brachii posterior

N. cutaneus brachii medialis

N. cutaneus brachii posterior

N. cutaneus brachii lateralis inferior

N. cutaneus antebrachii posterior

N. radialis

N. musculocutaneus, N. cutaneus antebrachii lateralis

R. superficialis

R. communicans ulnaris

Nn. digitales dorsales

N. radialis

N. medianus, Nn. digitales palmares proprii

Nn. digitales palmares proprii

Nn. digitales dorsales

N. ulnaris

R. dorsalis

N. cutaneus antebrachii medialis

Fig. 391 Cutaneous nerves of the upper limb.

→ T 24

Musculocutaneous nerve

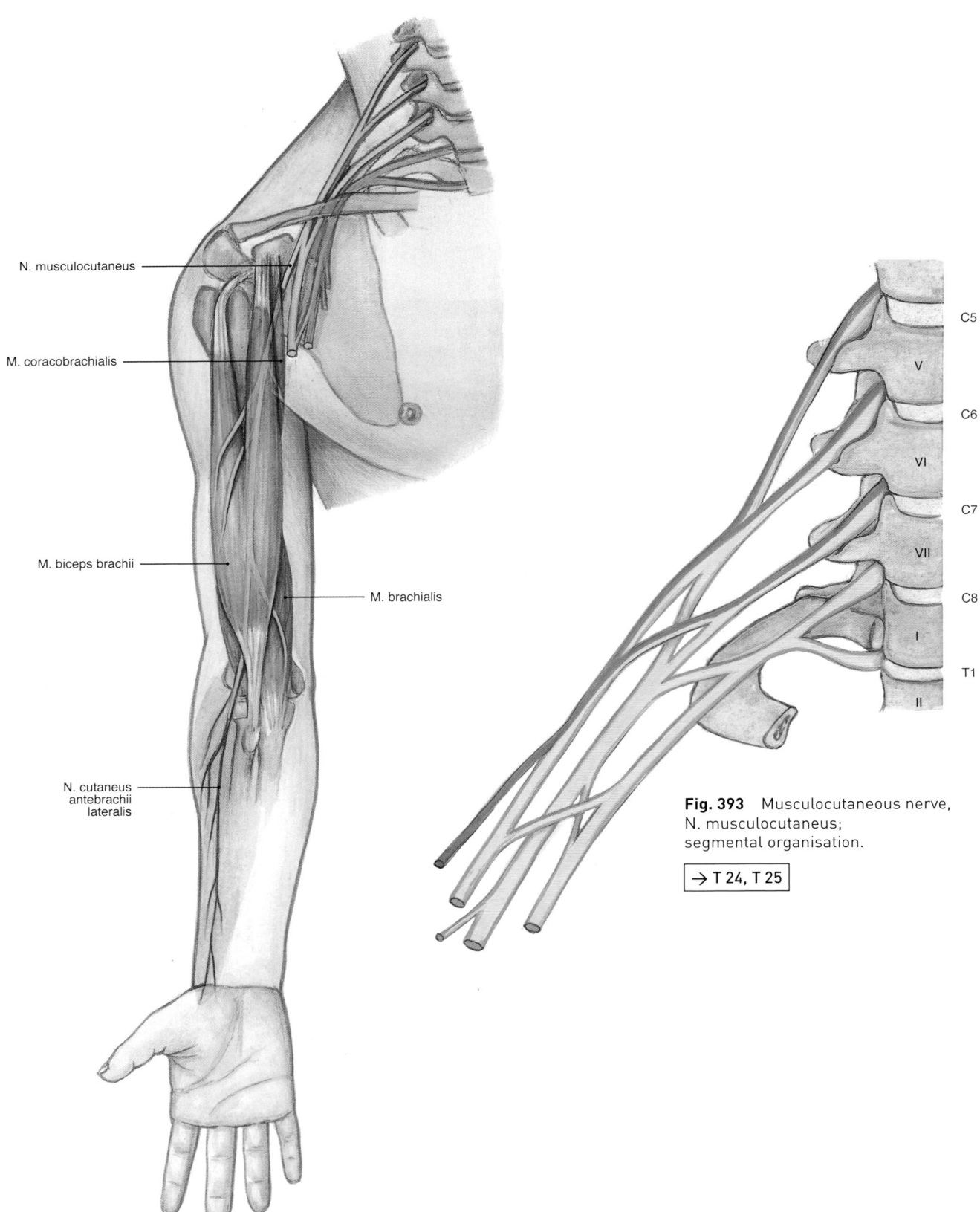

N. musculocutaneus

M. coracobrachialis

M. biceps brachii

M. brachialis

N. cutaneus antebrachii lateralis

C5

V

C6

VI

C7

VII

C8

I

T1

II

Fig. 393 Musculocutaneous nerve, N. musculocutaneus; segmental organisation.

→ T 24, T 25

Fig. 392 Musculocutaneous nerve, N. musculocutaneus; supplying areas. The skin branches and the cutaneous innervation are illustrated in blue.

→ 46, 386, T 24, T 25

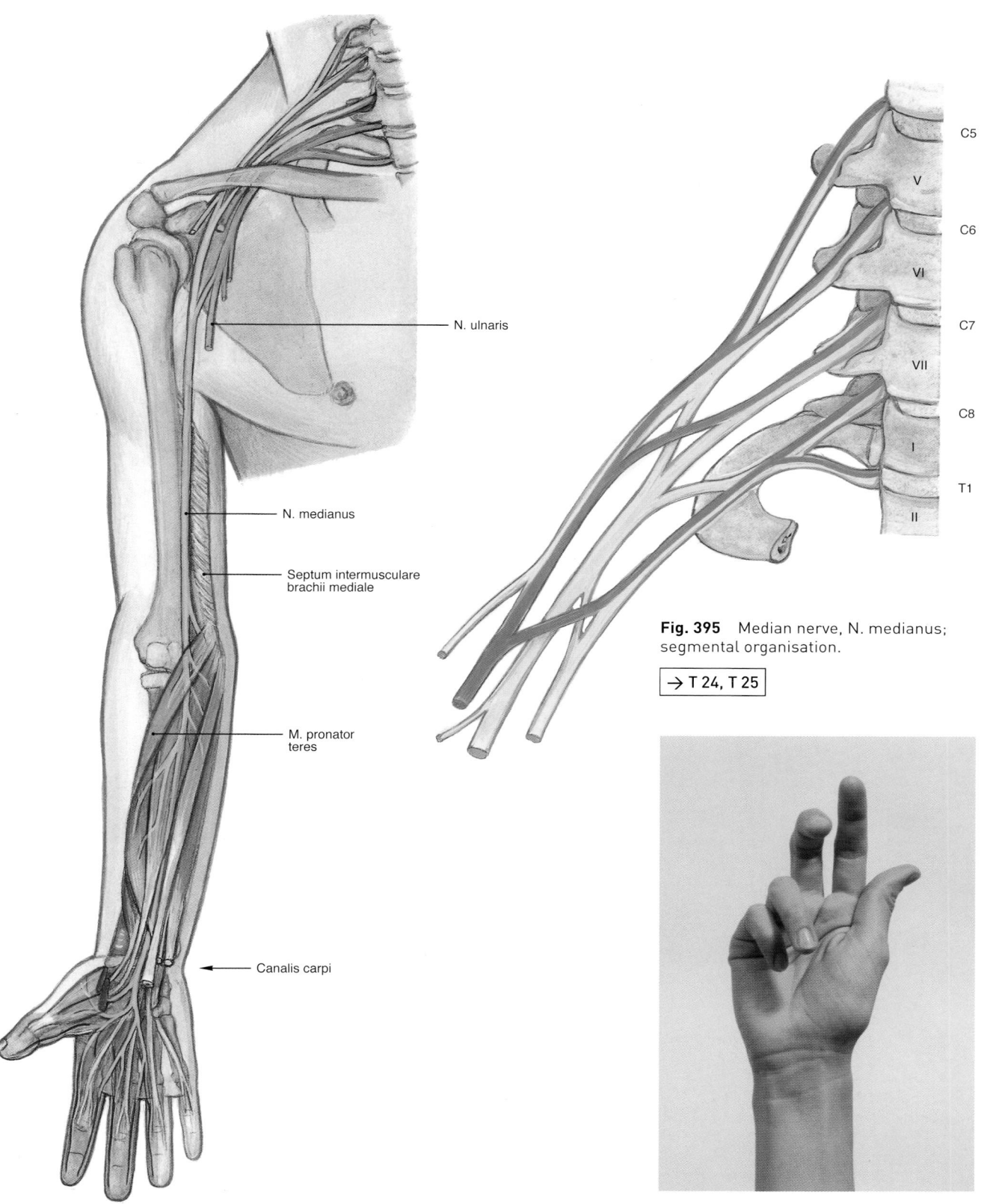

N. ulnaris

N. medianus

Septum intermusculare
brachii mediale

M. pronator
teres

Canalis carpi

C5

V

C6

VI

C7

VII

C8

I

T1

II

Fig. 395   Median nerve, N. medianus;
segmental organisation.

→ T 24, T 25

Fig. 394   Median nerve,
N. medianus;
supplying areas.

→ 46, 386, T 24, T 25

Fig. 396   Median nerve, N. medianus;
proximal palsy: typical posture.

Ulnar nerve

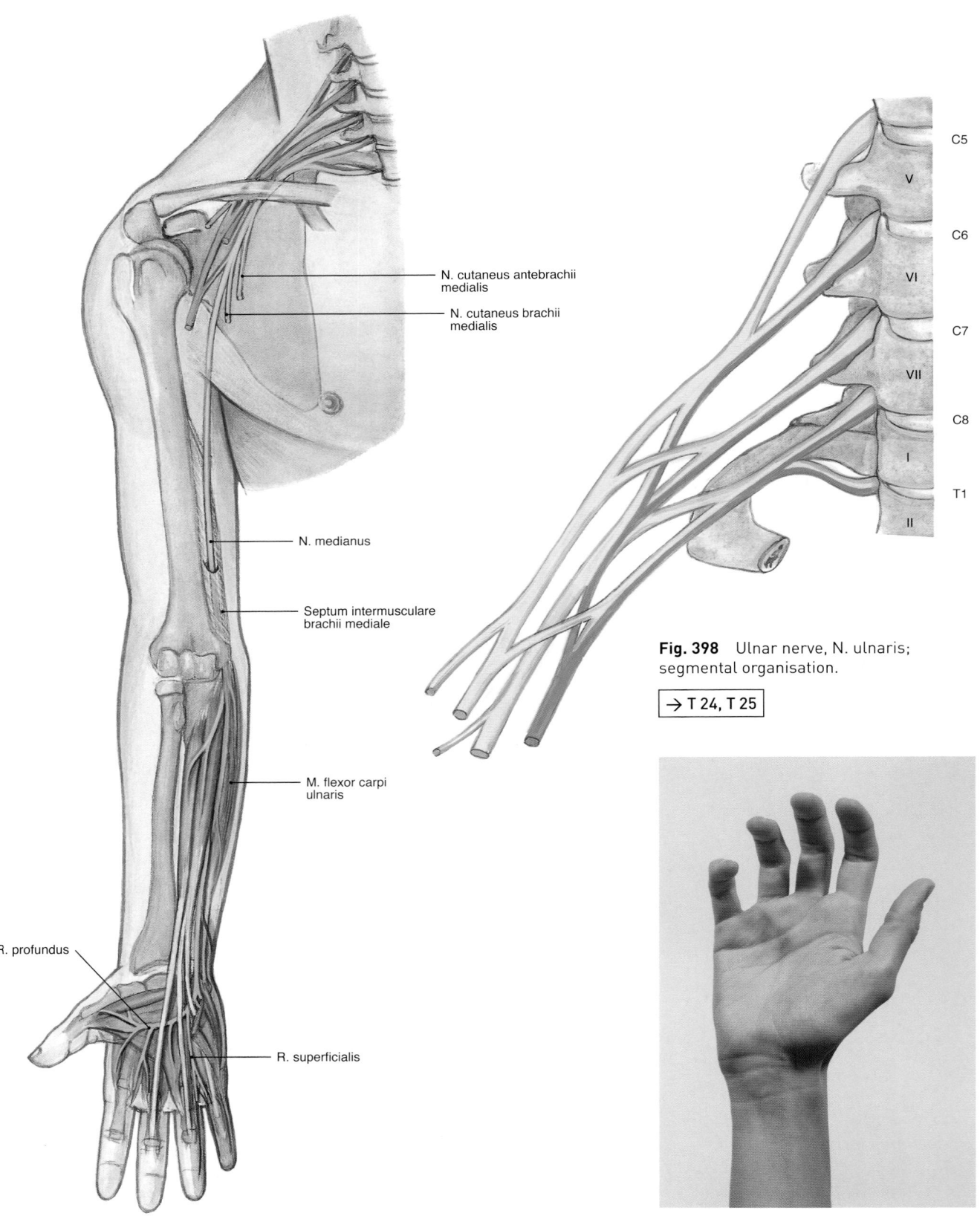

N. cutaneus antebrachii medialis

N. cutaneus brachii medialis

N. medianus

Septum intermusculare brachii mediale

M. flexor carpi ulnaris

R. profundus

R. superficialis

C5

V

C6

VI

C7

VII

C8

I

T1

II

Fig. 398 Ulnar nerve, N. ulnaris; segmental organisation.

→ T 24, T 25

Fig. 397 Ulnar nerve, N. ulnaris; supplying areas.

→ 46, 386, T 24, T 25

Fig. 399 Ulnar nerve, N. ulnaris; proximal palsy.

Radial nerve

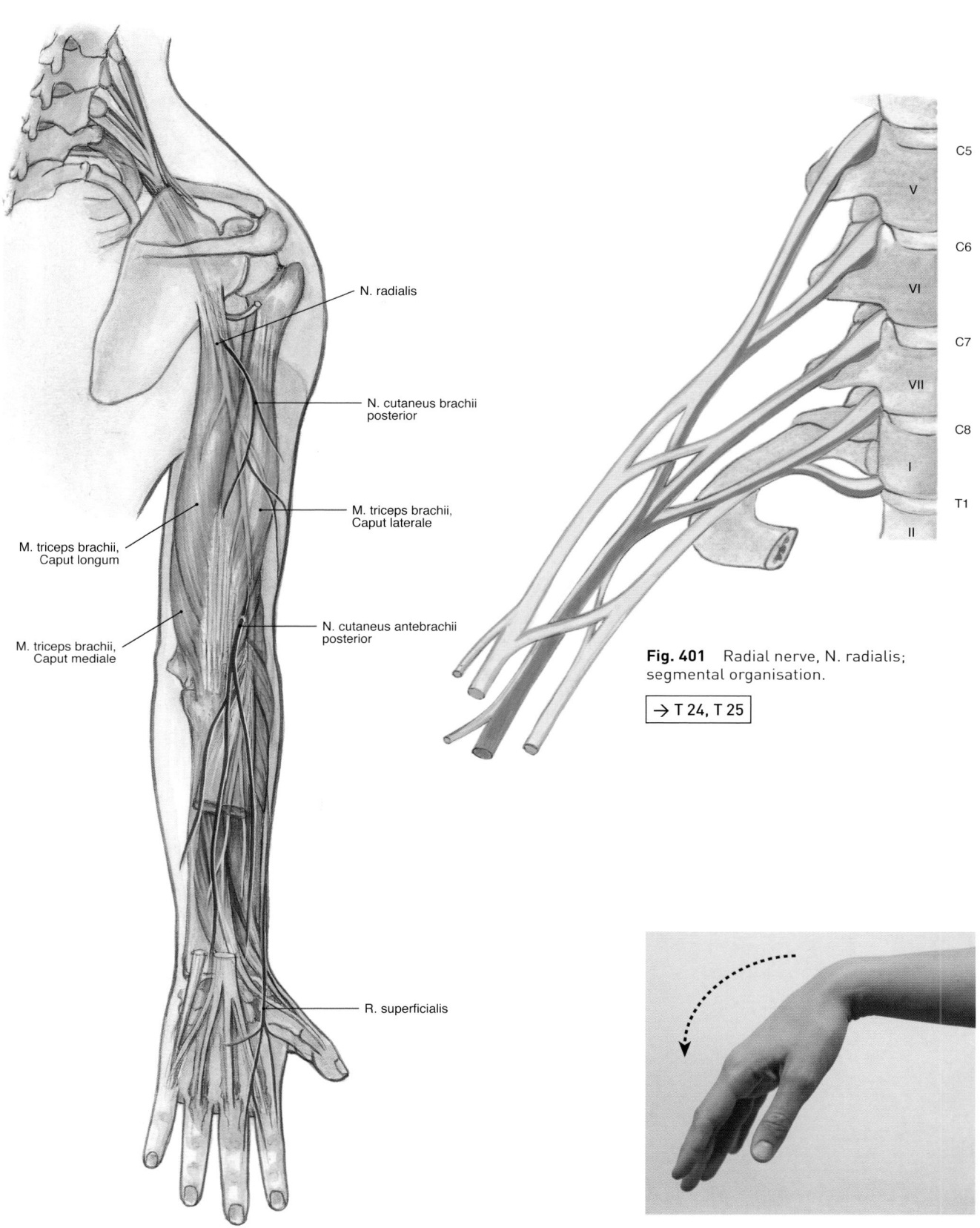

N. radialis

N. cutaneus brachii
posterior

M. triceps brachii,
Caput laterale

M. triceps brachii,
Caput longum

M. triceps brachii,
Caput mediale

N. cutaneus antebrachii
posterior

R. superficialis

Fig. 400   Radial nerve,
N. radialis;
supplying areas.

→ 46, 386, T 24, T 25

C5

V

C6

VI

C7

VII

C8

I

T1

II

Fig. 401   Radial nerve, N. radialis;
segmental organisation.

→ T 24, T 25

Fig. 402   Radial nerve,
N. radialis;
proximal palsy.

Axillary nerve

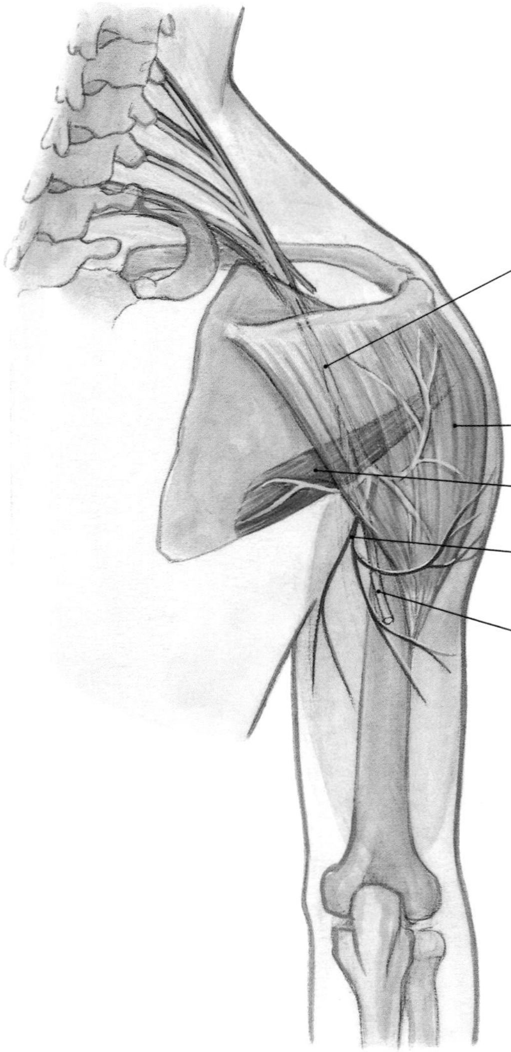

N. axillaris

M. deltoideus

M. teres major

N. cutaneus brachii
lateralis superior

N. radialis

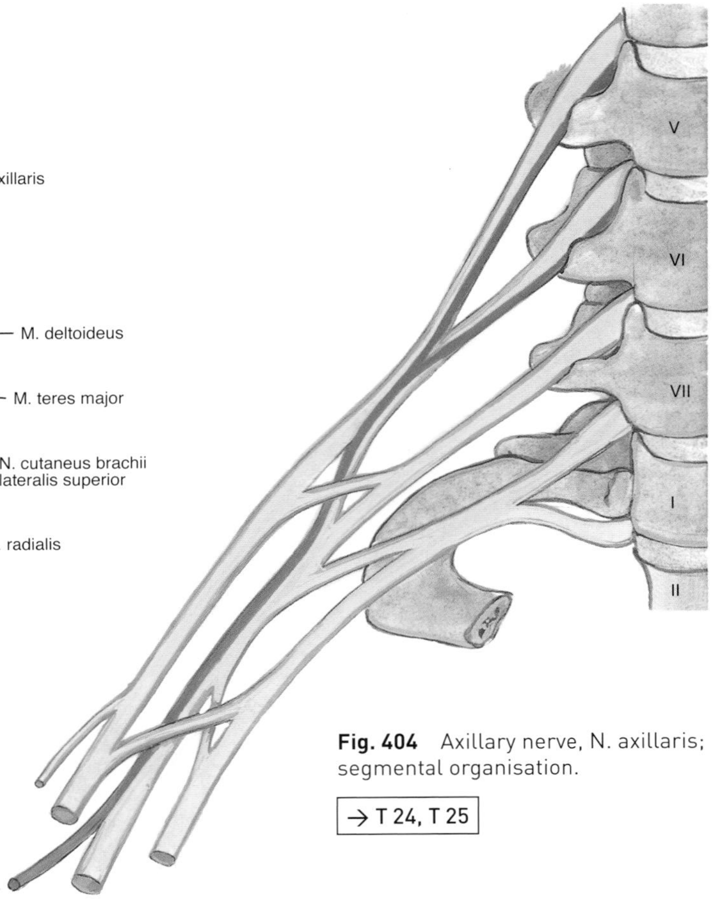

C5

V

C6

VI

C7

VII

C8

I

T1

II

Fig. 404 Axillary nerve, N. axillaris;
segmental organisation.

→ T 24, T 25

Fig. 403 Axillary nerve, N. axillaris;
supplying areas.
The axillary nerve passes to the
dorsal side of the arm through the
quadrangular space along with the
posterior circumflex humeral artery.

→ 46, 386, T 24, T 25

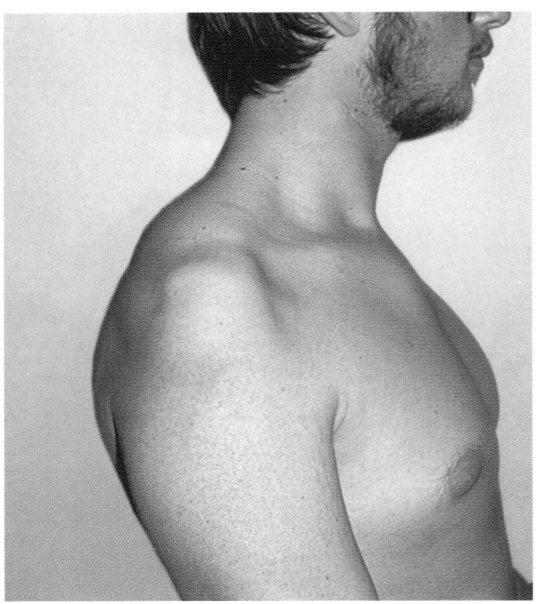

Fig. 405 Axillary nerve,
N. axillaris;
palsy: deltoid muscle atrophy.

Arteries of the upper limb

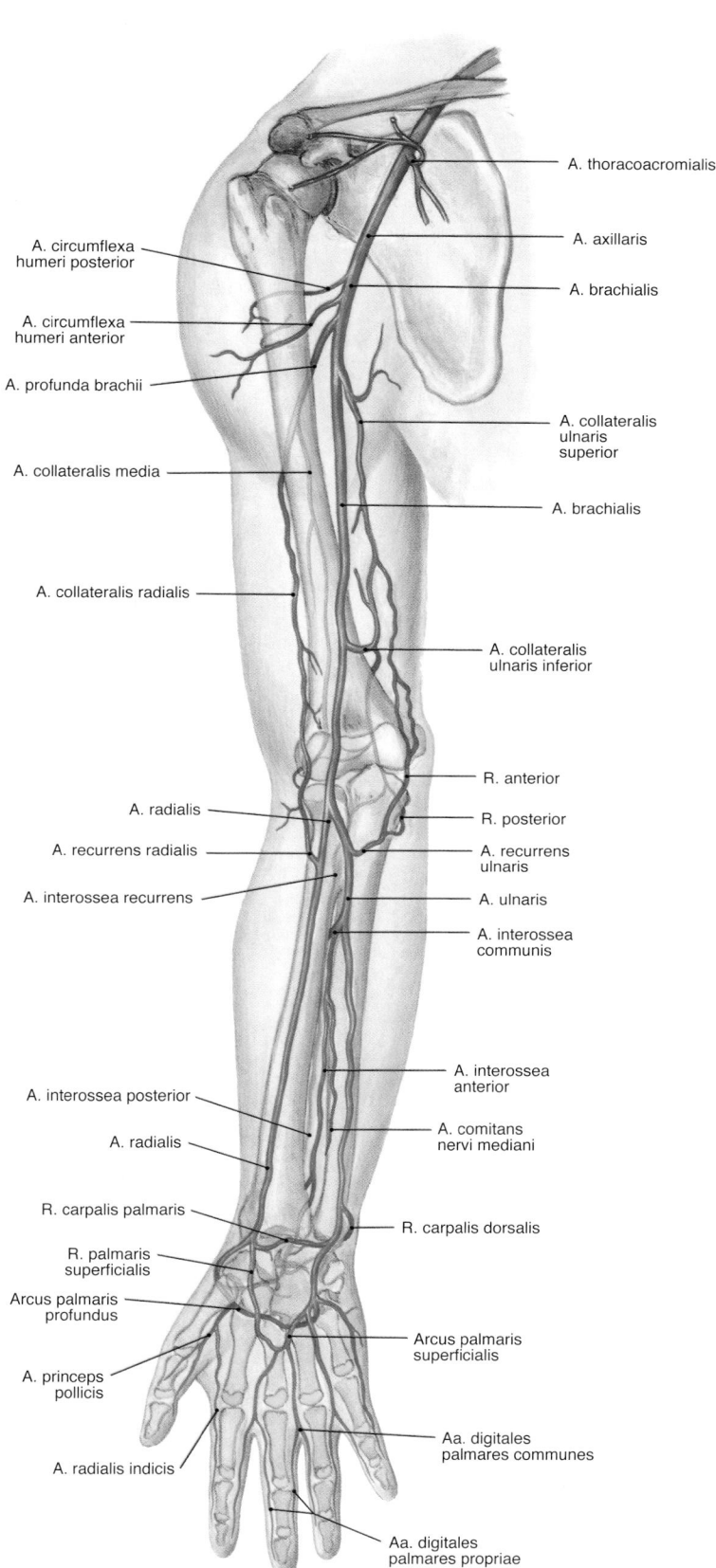

A. thoracoacromialis

A. axillaris

A. brachialis

A. circumflexa humeri posterior

A. circumflexa humeri anterior

A. profunda brachii

A. collateralis ulnaris superior

A. collateralis media

A. brachialis

A. collateralis radialis

A. collateralis ulnaris inferior

R. anterior

A. radialis

R. posterior

A. recurrens radialis

A. recurrens ulnaris

A. interossea recurrens

A. ulnaris

A. interossea communis

A. interossea anterior

A. interossea posterior

A. radialis

A. comitans nervi mediani

R. carpalis palmaris

R. carpalis dorsalis

R. palmaris superficialis

Arcus palmaris profundus

Arcus palmaris superficialis

A. princeps pollicis

Aa. digitales palmares communes

A. radialis indicis

Aa. digitales palmares propriae

Fig. 406   Arteries of the upper limb; overview.
Arteries adjacent to the elbow joint form the cubital anastomosis.

→ 264

Lymphatics of the axilla

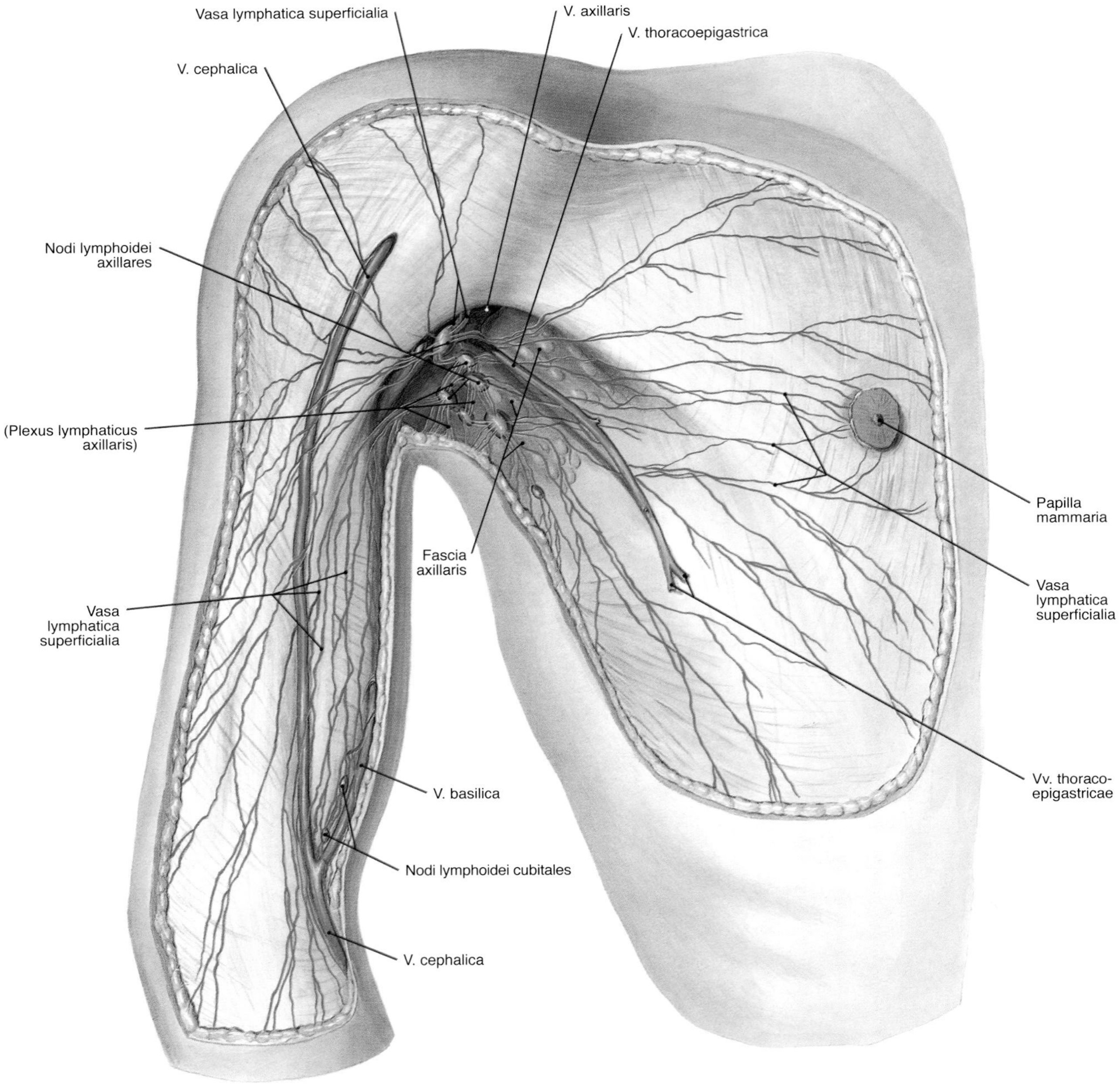

Vasa lymphatica superficialia

V. cephalica

V. axillaris

V. thoracoepigastrica

Nodi lymphoidei axillares

(Plexus lymphaticus axillaris)

Papilla mammaria

Fascia axillaris

Vasa lymphatica superficialia

Vasa lymphatica superficialia

V. basilica

Vv. thoracoepigastricae

Nodi lymphoidei cubitales

V. cephalica

→ 42

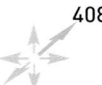

408

Fig. 407 Superficial lymphatics, lymph nodes and vein trunks in the regions of the arm, the lateral thoracic wall and the axilla.

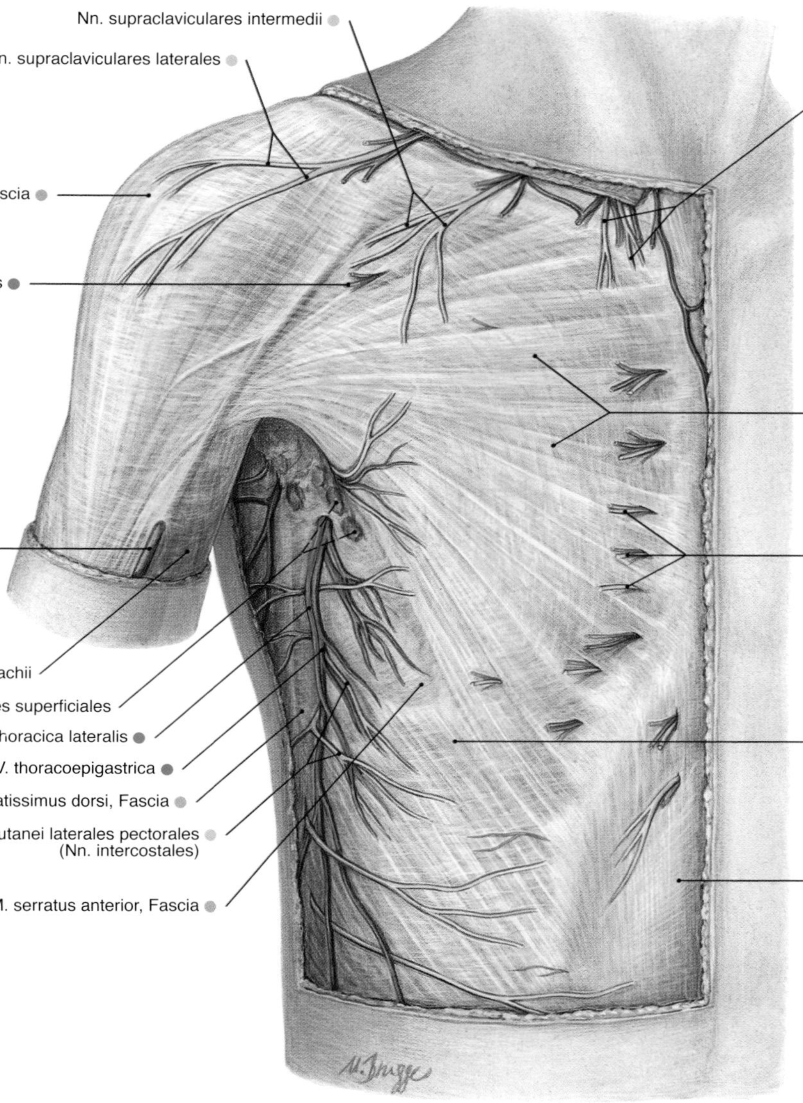

Fascia of the chest, the shoulder and the axilla

Nn. supraclaviculares intermedii ●

Nn. supraclaviculares laterales ●

Nn. supraclaviculares mediales ●

M. deltoideus, Fascia ●

A. thoracoacromialis, R. pectoralis ●

M. pectoralis major, Fascia ●

Rr. cutanei anteriores pectorales (Nn. intercostales) ●

V. cephalica ●

Fascia brachii

Nodi lymphoidei axillares superficiales

A. thoracica lateralis ●

V. thoracoepigastrica ●

M. latissimus dorsi, Fascia ●

Rr. cutanei laterales pectorales (Nn. intercostales) ●

M. serratus anterior, Fascia ●

M. obliquus abdominis externus, Fascia ●

Vagina musculi recti abdominis

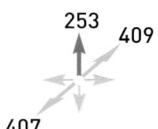

Fig. 408 Vessels and nerves in the regions of
the upper arm as well as the shoulder, and the
clavipectoral triangle, Trigonum clavipectorale.

253
409

407

Clavipectoral triangle

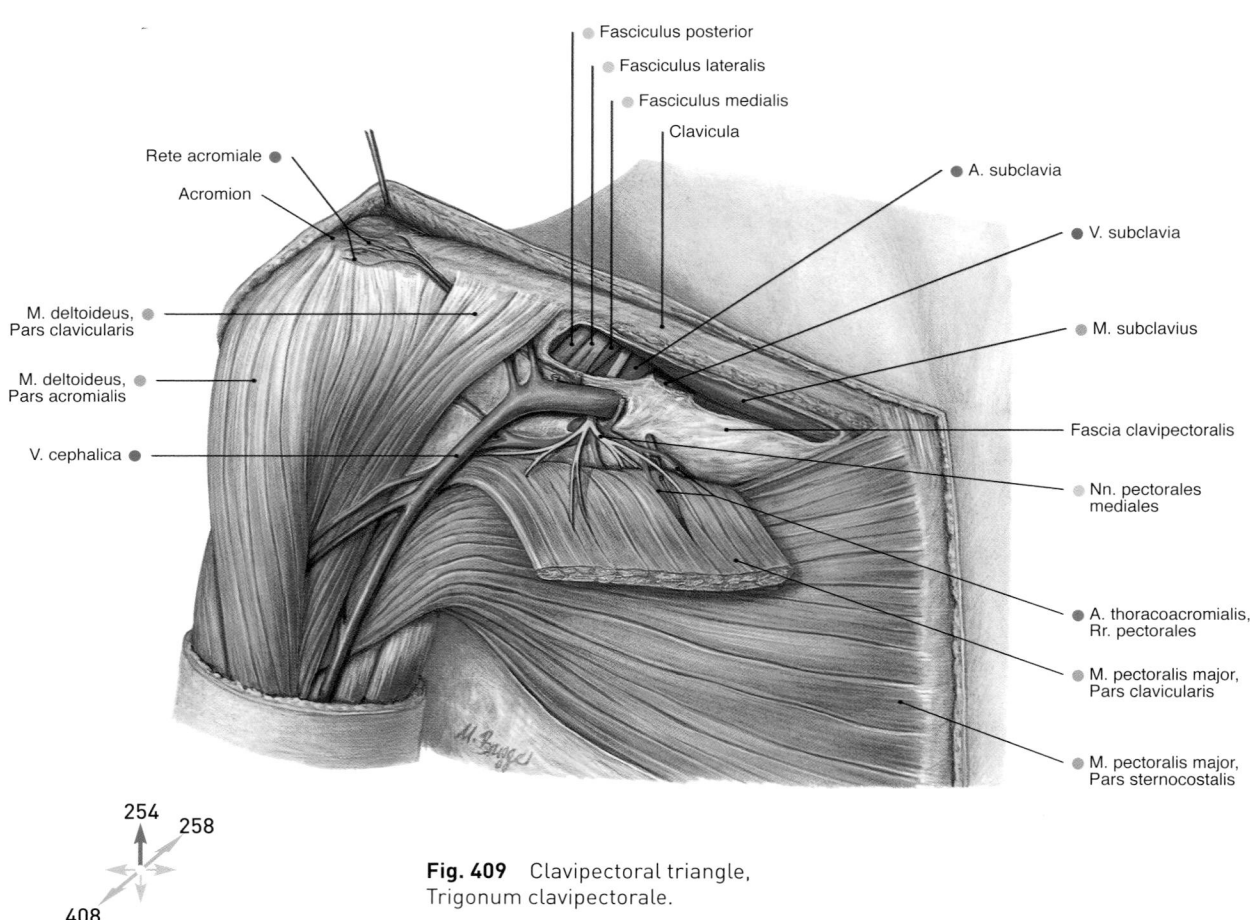

Fasciculus posterior
Fasciculus lateralis
Fasciculus medialis
Clavicula
A. subclavia
V. subclavia
M. subclavius
Fascia clavipectoralis
Nn. pectorales mediales
A. thoracoacromialis, Rr. pectorales
M. pectoralis major, Pars clavicularis
M. pectoralis major, Pars sternocostalis

Rete acromiale
Acromion
M. deltoideus, Pars clavicularis
M. deltoideus, Pars acromialis
V. cephalica

254
258
408

Fig. 409 Clavipectoral triangle, Trigonum clavipectorale.

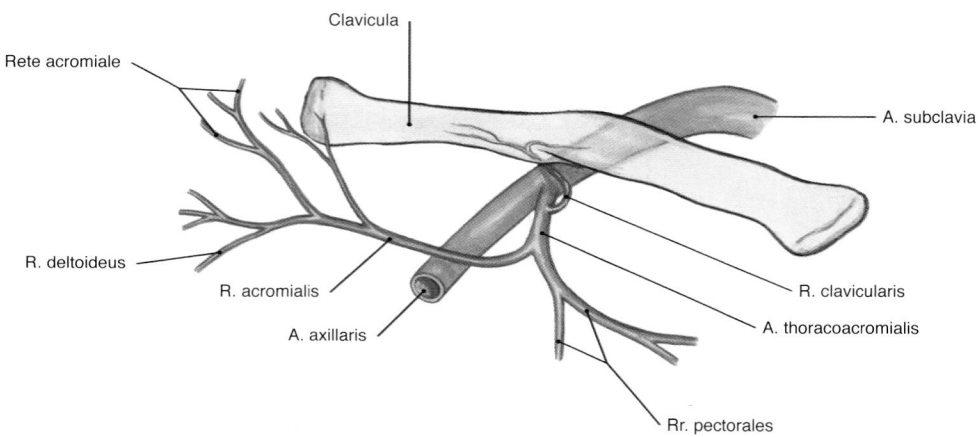

Clavicula
Rete acromiale
A. subclavia
R. deltoideus
R. acromialis
R. clavicularis
A. thoracoacromialis
A. axillaris
Rr. pectorales

Fig. 410 Branching pattern of the thoraco-acromial artery, A. thoracoacromialis.

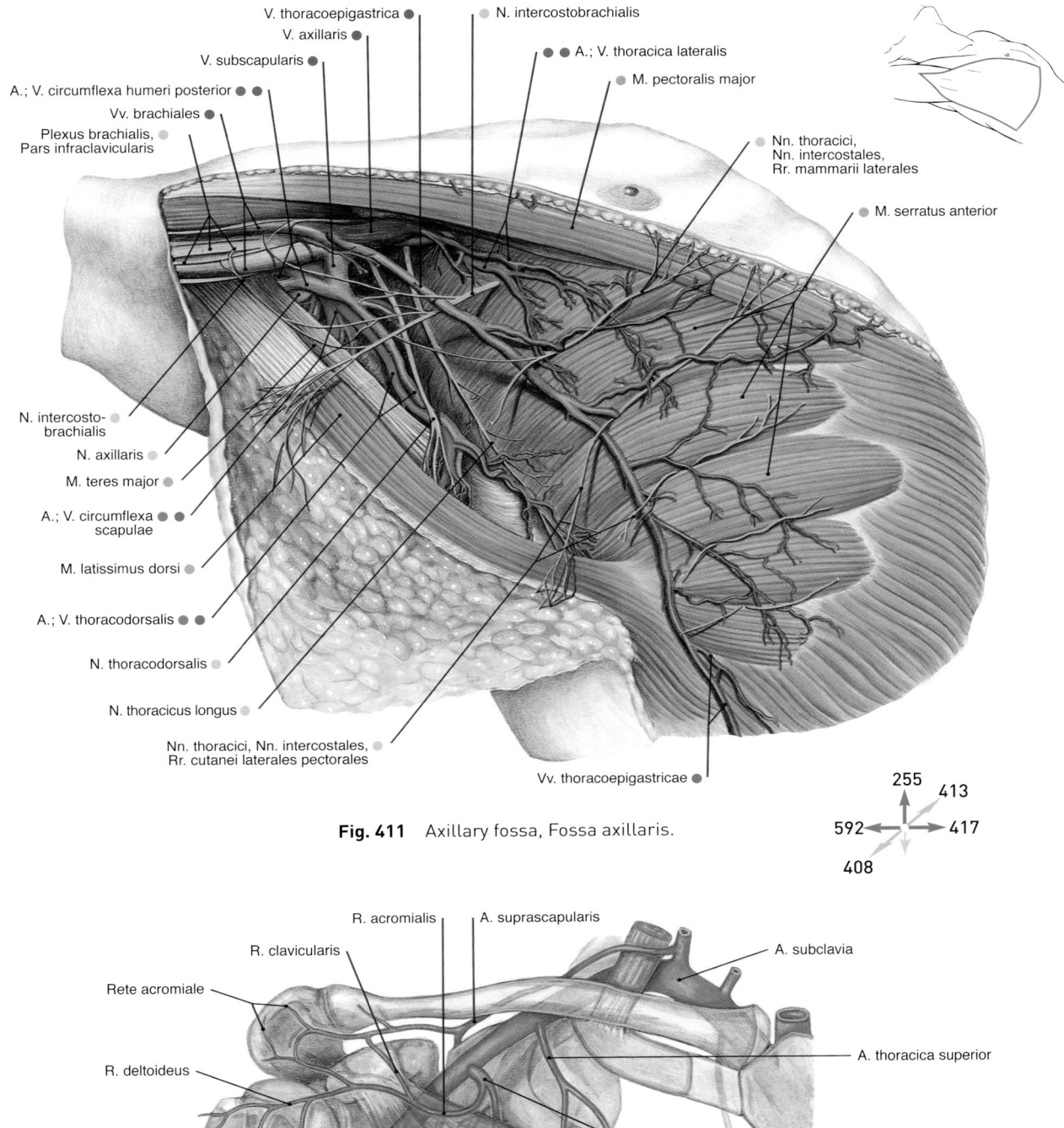

V. thoracoepigastrica
V. axillaris
V. subscapularis
A.; V. circumflexa humeri posterior
Vv. brachiales
Plexus brachialis, Pars infraclavicularis

N. intercostobrachialis
A.; V. thoracica lateralis
M. pectoralis major
Nn. thoracici, Nn. intercostales, Rr. mammarii laterales
M. serratus anterior

N. intercosto-brachialis
N. axillaris
M. teres major
A.; V. circumflexa scapulae
M. latissimus dorsi
A.; V. thoracodorsalis
N. thoracodorsalis
N. thoracicus longus
Nn. thoracici, Nn. intercostales, Rr. cutanei laterales pectorales
Vv. thoracoepigastricae

255
413
592
417
408

Fig. 411   Axillary fossa, Fossa axillaris.

R. acromialis
R. clavicularis
Rete acromiale
R. deltoideus
A. circumflexa humeri posterior
A. circumflexa humeri anterior
A. thoracica lateralis
A. subscapularis
A. brachialis
A. profunda brachii

A. suprascapularis
A. subclavia
A. thoracica superior
A. thoracoacromialis

Fig. 412   Arteries of the shoulder region.

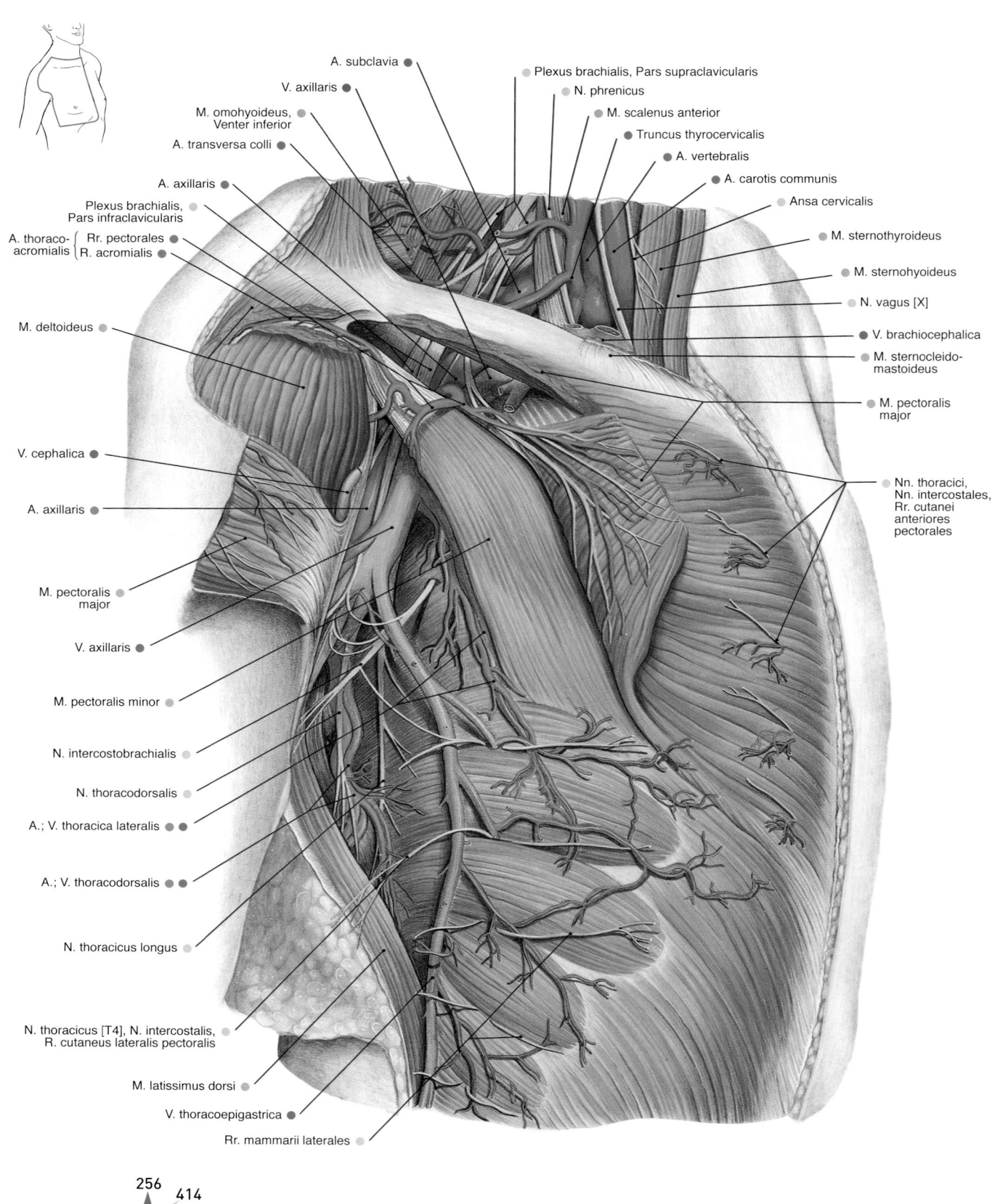

A. subclavia ●
V. axillaris ●
M. omohyoideus, ●
Venter inferior
A. transversa colli ●
A. axillaris ●
Plexus brachialis, ●
Pars infraclavicularis
A. thoraco- ⎰ Rr. pectorales ●
acromialis ⎱ R. acromialis ●
M. deltoideus ●
V. cephalica ●
A. axillaris ●
M. pectoralis ●
major
V. axillaris ●
M. pectoralis minor ●
N. intercostobrachialis ●
N. thoracodorsalis ●
A.; V. thoracica lateralis ● ●
A.; V. thoracodorsalis ● ●
N. thoracicus longus ●
N. thoracicus [T4], N. intercostalis,
R. cutaneus lateralis pectoralis ●
M. latissimus dorsi ●
V. thoracoepigastrica ●
Rr. mammarii laterales ●

Plexus brachialis, Pars supraclavicularis
N. phrenicus
M. scalenus anterior
Truncus thyrocervicalis
A. vertebralis
A. carotis communis
Ansa cervicalis
M. sternothyroideus
M. sternohyoideus
N. vagus [X]
V. brachiocephalica
M. sternocleido-mastoideus
M. pectoralis major
Nn. thoracici,
Nn. intercostales,
Rr. cutanei
anteriores
pectorales

256
414
411
417

Fig. 413 Lateral thoracic wall; infraclavicular fossa, Fossa infraclavicularis, and axillary fossa, Fossa axillaris.

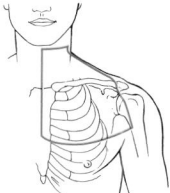

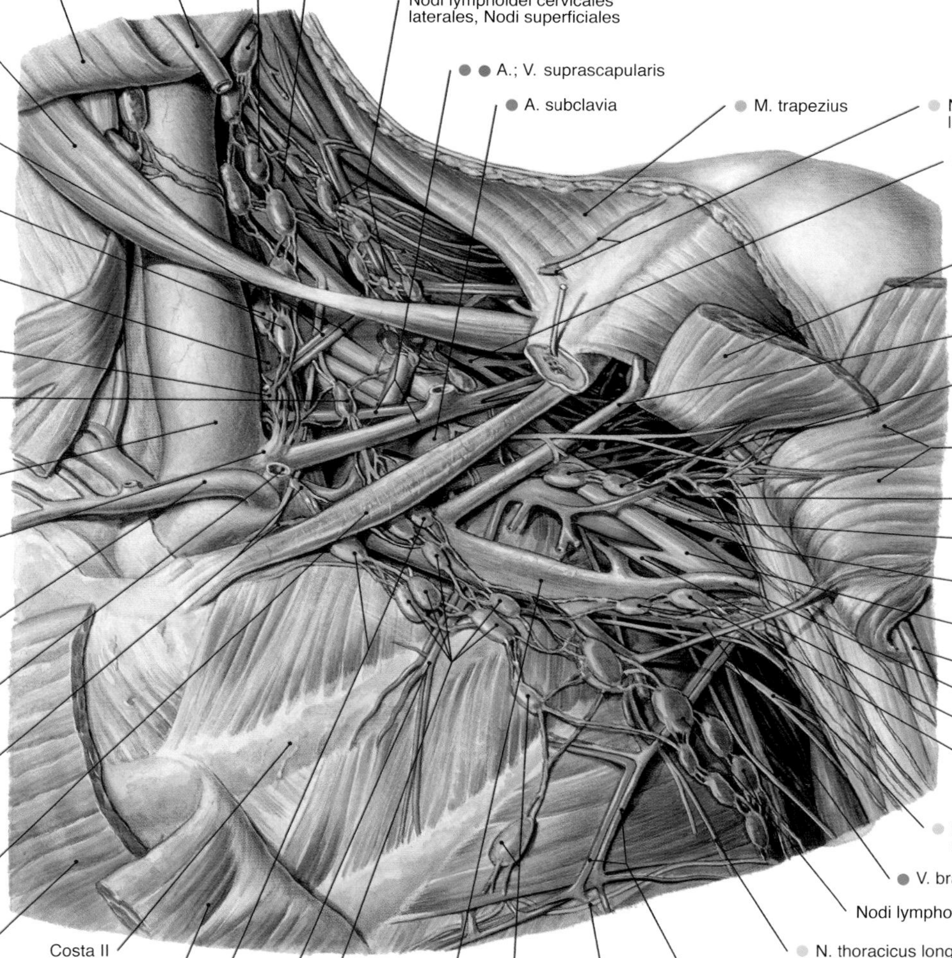

Nodi lymphoidei cervicales anteriores,
Nodi superficiales et profundi

V. jugularis externa ●

M. sternocleidomastoideus ●

M. omohyoideus,
Venter superior ●

A.; V. transversa ● ●
colli,
R. superficialis

Nodi lymphoidei
cervicales ant.
superfic. et prof.

M. scalenus ●
anterior

Truncus
jugularis sinister

Nodus lymphoideus
cervicalis lateralis,
Nodus profundus
inferior

Bulbus inferior ●
venae jugularis

Ductus
thoracicus,
Pars cervicalis

Arcus ●
venosus jugularis

V. jugularis externa ●

Trunci subclavius
et bronchomediasti-
nalis sinister

M. subclavius ●

M. pectoralis major ●

Costa II

M. pectoralis minor ●

Nodi lymphoidei deltopectorales

A. thoracica superior ●

Nodi lymphoidei axillares centrales

● M. scalenus medius

Nodi lymphoidei cervicales
laterales, Nodi superficiales

● ● A.; V. suprascapularis

● A. subclavia

● M. trapezius

V. axillaris ●

Nodi lymphoidei
pectorales

● ● A.; V. thoracica lateralis

● N. intercostobrachialis

● N. thoracicus longus

● V. brachialis

Nodi lymphoidei intercostales

● N. cutaneus brachii
medialis

Nodi lymphoidei
axillares laterales

● N. ulnaris

● V. brachialis

● V. cephalica

● N. medianus

● A. circumflexa
humeri posterior

● N. musculo-
cutaneus

● N. radialis

● M. pectoralis
major

Nodi lymphoidei
subscapulares

● V. cephalica

● M. pectoralis
minor

● N. suprascapularis

Nn. supraclaviculares
laterales

Fig. 414   Axillary fossa, Fossa axillaris, and
deep cervical region;
exemplary illustration of lymphatics and lymph
nodes.

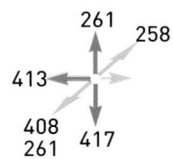

261   258
413
408   417
261

Vessels and nerves of the arm

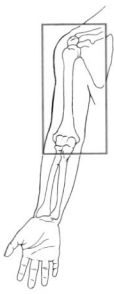

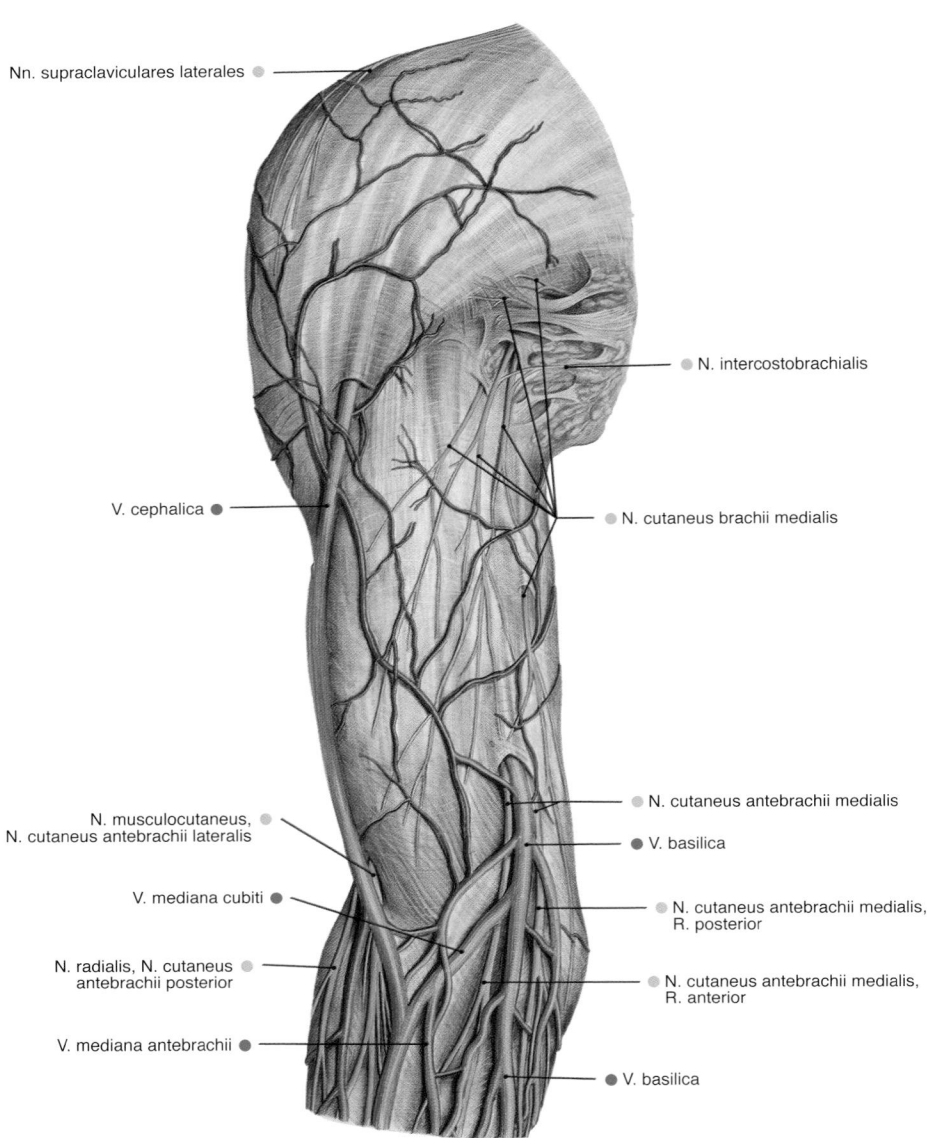

Nn. supraclaviculares laterales ●

● N. intercostobrachialis

V. cephalica ●

● N. cutaneus brachii medialis

N. musculocutaneus, ●
N. cutaneus antebrachii lateralis

● N. cutaneus antebrachii medialis

● V. basilica

V. mediana cubiti ●

● N. cutaneus antebrachii medialis,
R. posterior

N. radialis, N. cutaneus ●
antebrachii posterior

● N. cutaneus antebrachii medialis,
R. anterior

V. mediana antebrachii ●

● V. basilica

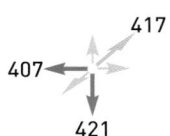

417

407 ← → 421

Fig. 415   Epifascial vessels and nerves of the shoulder,
Regio deltoidea, the anterior region of the arm,
Regio brachii anterior, and the anterior region
of the elbow, Regio cubitalis anterior.

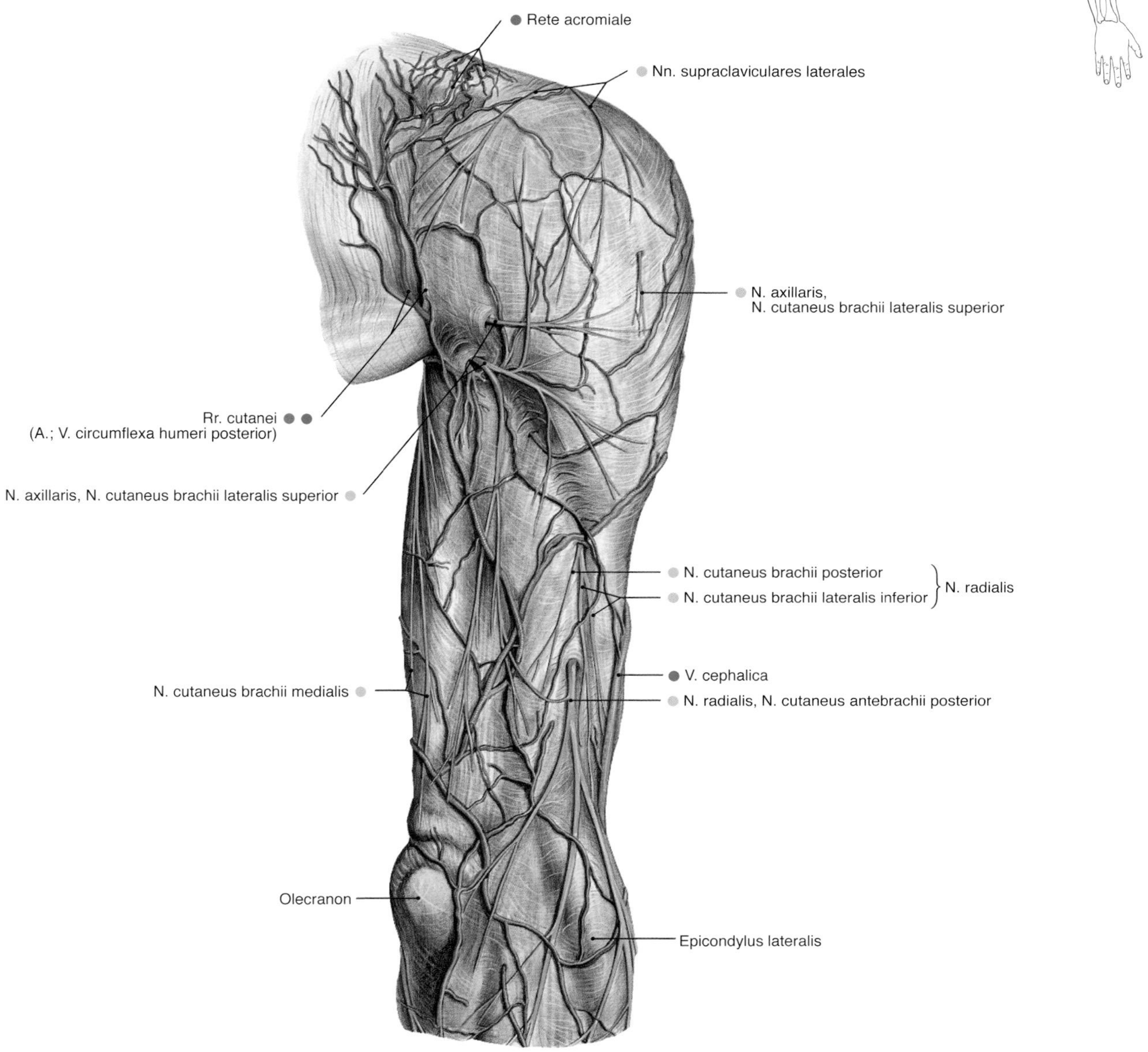

Vessels and nerves of the arm

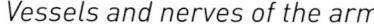

● Rete acromiale

● Nn. supraclaviculares laterales

● N. axillaris,
N. cutaneus brachii lateralis superior

Rr. cutanei ● ●
(A.; V. circumflexa humeri posterior)

N. axillaris, N. cutaneus brachii lateralis superior ●

● N. cutaneus brachii posterior ⎫ N. radialis
● N. cutaneus brachii lateralis inferior ⎭

● V. cephalica

N. cutaneus brachii medialis ●

● N. radialis, N. cutaneus antebrachii posterior

Olecranon

Epicondylus lateralis

Fig. 416   Epifascial vessels and nerves of the shoulder,
Regio deltoidea, the posterior region of the arm,
Regio brachii posterior, and the posterior region
of the elbow, Regio cubitalis posterior.

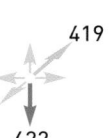

419

422

Vessels and nerves of the arm

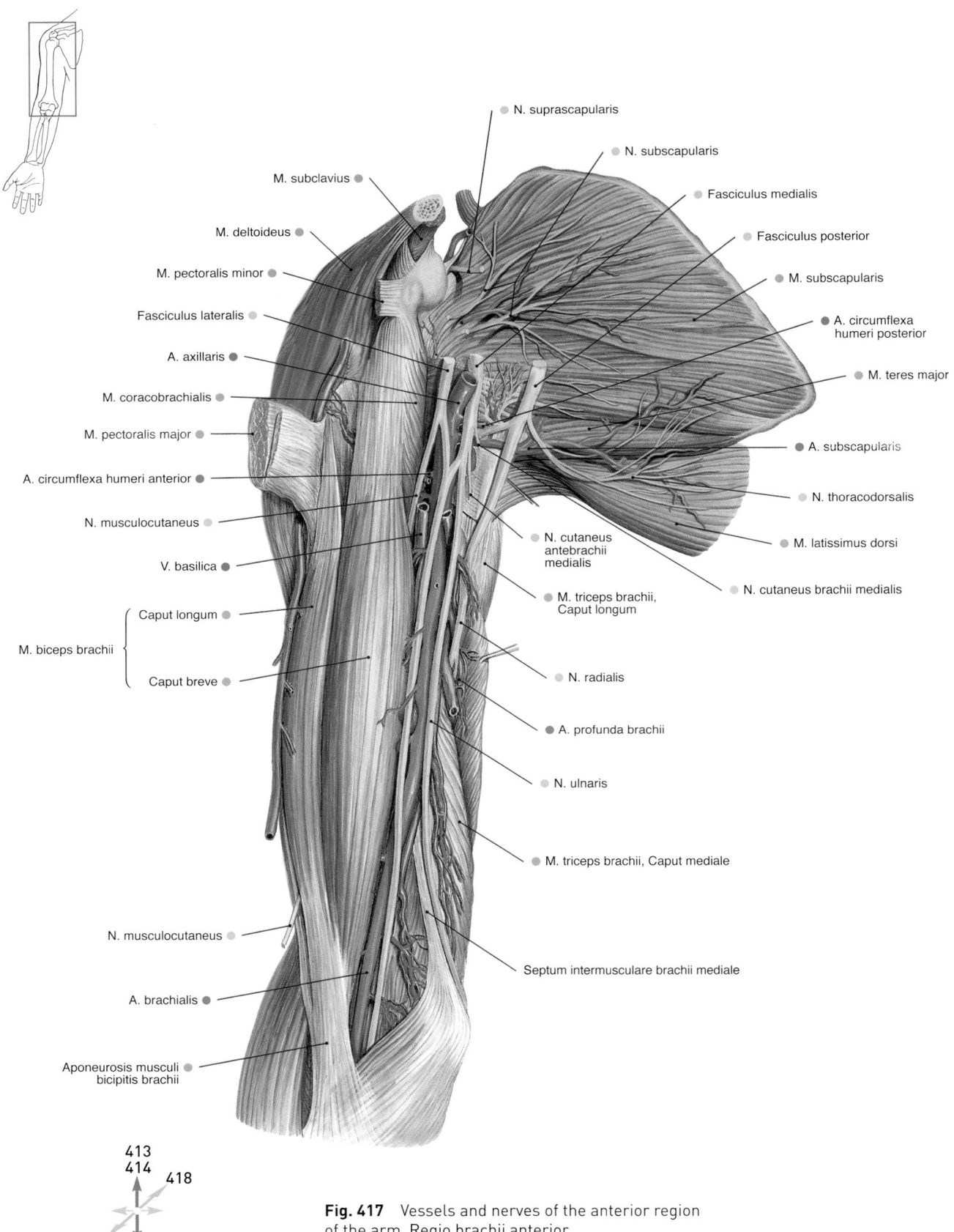

N. suprascapularis

N. subscapularis

Fasciculus medialis

Fasciculus posterior

M. subscapularis

A. circumflexa humeri posterior

M. teres major

A. subscapularis

N. thoracodorsalis

M. latissimus dorsi

N. cutaneus brachii medialis

M. subclavius

M. deltoideus

M. pectoralis minor

Fasciculus lateralis

A. axillaris

M. coracobrachialis

M. pectoralis major

A. circumflexa humeri anterior

N. musculocutaneus

V. basilica

Caput longum

M. biceps brachii

Caput breve

N. cutaneus antebrachii medialis

M. triceps brachii, Caput longum

N. radialis

A. profunda brachii

N. ulnaris

M. triceps brachii, Caput mediale

N. musculocutaneus

A. brachialis

Aponeurosis musculi bicipitis brachii

Septum intermusculare brachii mediale

413
414
418
415
424

Fig. 417 Vessels and nerves of the anterior region of the arm, Regio brachii anterior.

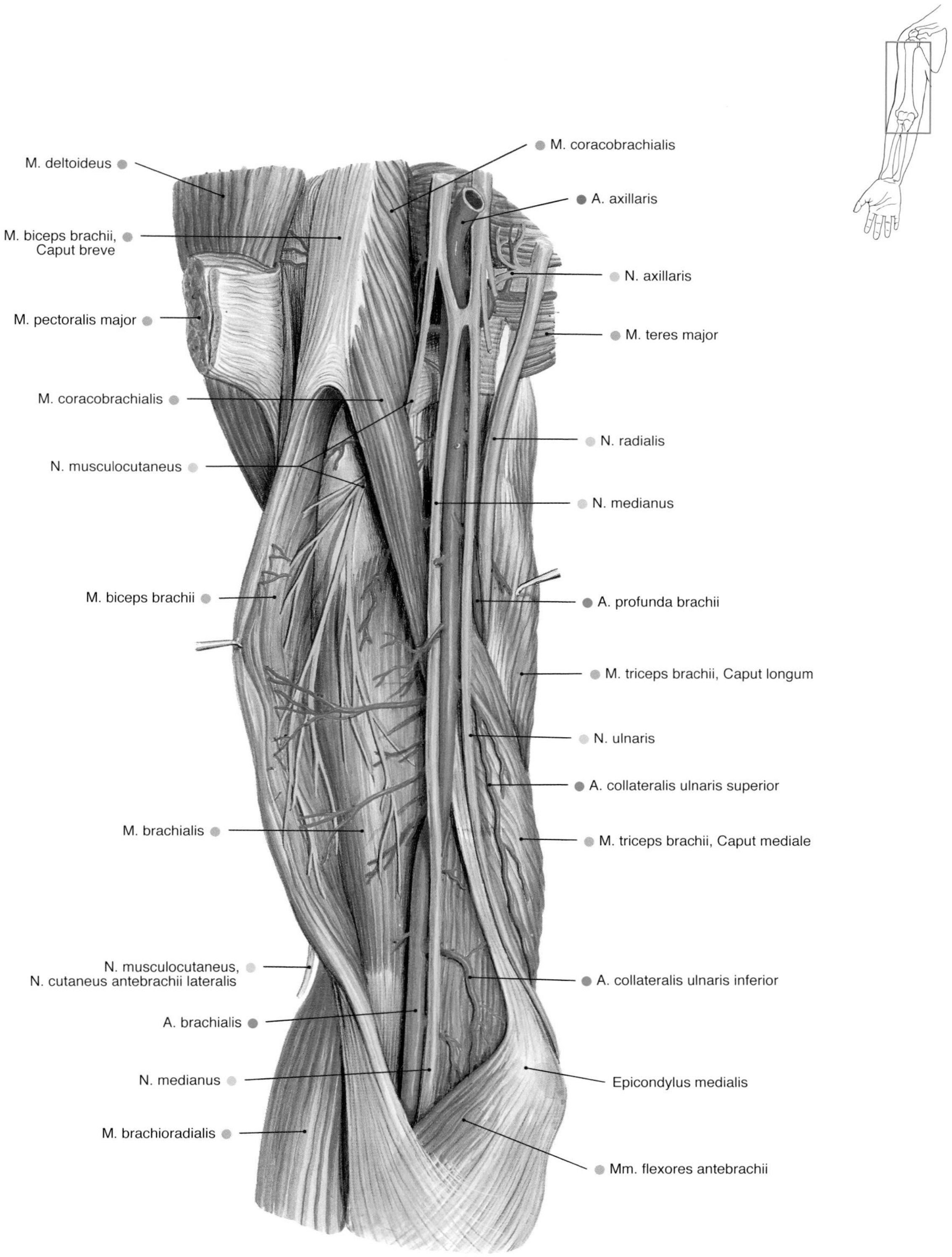

Arteries and nerves of the arm

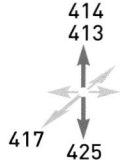

M. deltoideus ●

M. biceps brachii, ●
Caput breve

M. pectoralis major ●

M. coracobrachialis ●

N. musculocutaneus ●

M. biceps brachii ●

M. brachialis ●

N. musculocutaneus, ●
N. cutaneus antebrachii lateralis

A. brachialis ●

N. medianus ●

M. brachioradialis ●

● M. coracobrachialis

● A. axillaris

● N. axillaris

● M. teres major

● N. radialis

● N. medianus

● A. profunda brachii

● M. triceps brachii, Caput longum

● N. ulnaris

● A. collateralis ulnaris superior

● M. triceps brachii, Caput mediale

● A. collateralis ulnaris inferior

● Epicondylus medialis

● Mm. flexores antebrachii

Fig. 418 Arteries and nerves of the anterior region
of the arm, Regio brachii anterior.

414
413

417   425

Arteries and nerves of the arm

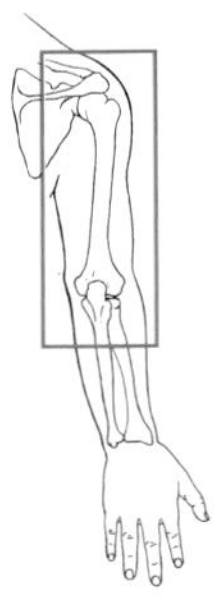

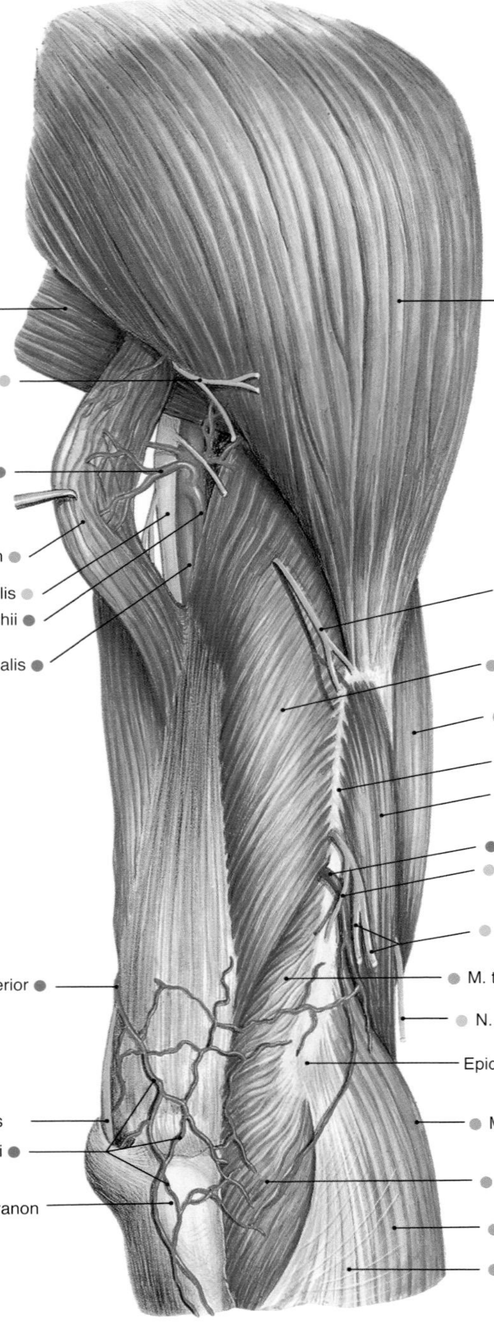

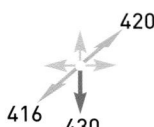

M. teres major ●

N. axillaris, N. cutaneus brachii ● lateralis superior

A. profunda brachii, R. deltoideus ●

M. triceps brachii, Caput longum ●

N. radialis ●
A. profunda brachii ●

A. brachialis ●

A. collateralis ulnaris inferior ●

● N. ulnaris
Rete articulare cubiti ●

Olecranon

● M. deltoideus

● N. radialis, N. cutaneus brachii posterior

● M. triceps brachii, Caput laterale

● M. biceps brachii

Septum intermusculare brachii laterale

● M. brachialis

● A. collateralis radialis
● N. cutaneus brachii lateralis inferior

● N. radialis, N. cutaneus antebrachii posterior

● M. triceps brachii, Caput mediale

● N. musculocutaneus, N. cutaneus antebrachii lateralis

Epicondylus lateralis

● M. brachioradialis

● M. anconeus

● M. extensor carpi radialis longus

● M. extensor carpi radialis brevis

420

416 430

Fig. 419   Arteries and nerves of the posterior region of the arm, Regio brachii posterior.

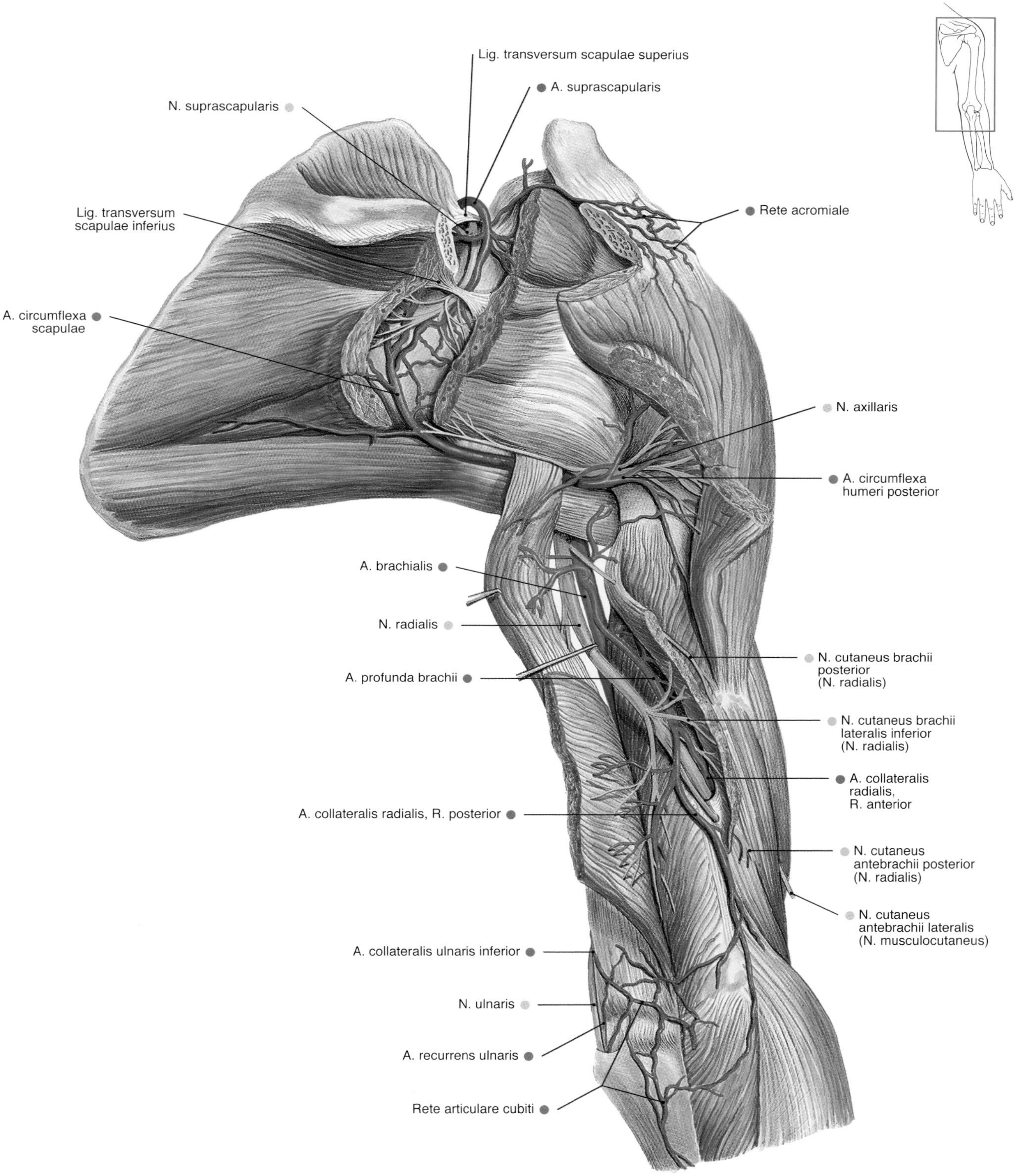

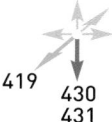

Lig. transversum scapulae superius

● A. suprascapularis

N. suprascapularis ●

Lig. transversum
scapulae inferius

● Rete acromiale

A. circumflexa ●
scapulae

● N. axillaris

● A. circumflexa
humeri posterior

A. brachialis ●

N. radialis ●

● N. cutaneus brachii
posterior
(N. radialis)

A. profunda brachii ●

● N. cutaneus brachii
lateralis inferior
(N. radialis)

● A. collateralis
radialis,
R. anterior

A. collateralis radialis, R. posterior ●

● N. cutaneus
antebrachii posterior
(N. radialis)

● N. cutaneus
antebrachii lateralis
(N. musculocutaneus)

A. collateralis ulnaris inferior ●

N. ulnaris ●

A. recurrens ulnaris ●

Rete articulare cubiti ●

Fig. 420   Arteries and nerves of the scapular region,
Regio scapularis, and the posterior region
of the arm, Regio brachii posterior.

419
430
431

Veins and nerves of the forearm

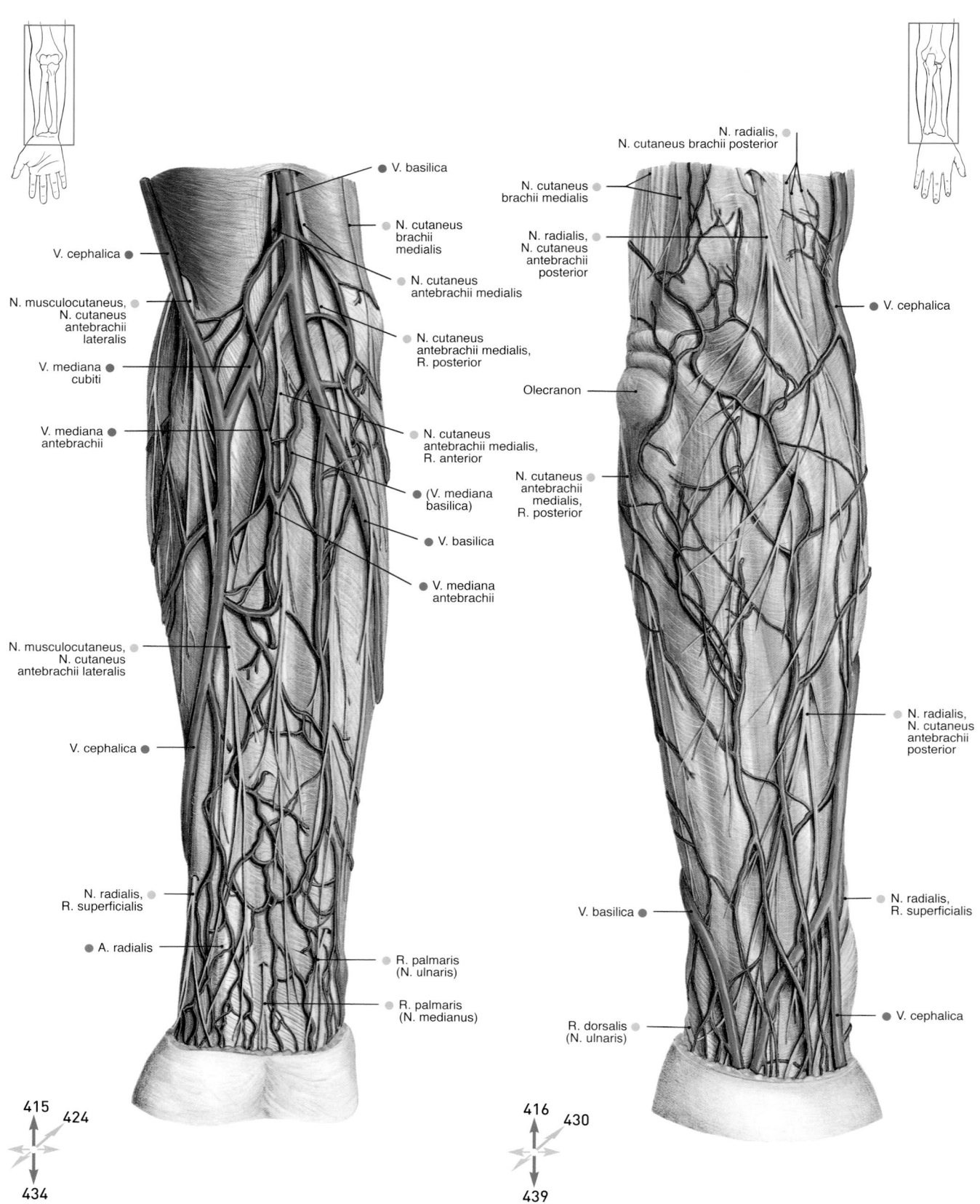

● V. basilica

● N. cutaneus
brachii
medialis

● N. cutaneus
antebrachii medialis

V. cephalica ●

N. musculocutaneus, ●
N. cutaneus
antebrachii
lateralis

● N. cutaneus
antebrachii medialis,
R. posterior

V. mediana ●
cubiti

V. mediana ●
antebrachii

● N. cutaneus
antebrachii medialis,
R. anterior

● (V. mediana
basilica)

● V. basilica

● V. mediana
antebrachii

N. musculocutaneus, ●
N. cutaneus
antebrachii lateralis

V. cephalica ●

N. radialis, ●
R. superficialis

● A. radialis

● R. palmaris
(N. ulnaris)

● R. palmaris
(N. medianus)

N. radialis, ●
N. cutaneus brachii posterior

N. cutaneus ●
brachii medialis

N. radialis, ●
N. cutaneus
antebrachii
posterior

● V. cephalica

Olecranon

N. cutaneus ●
antebrachii
medialis,
R. posterior

● N. radialis,
N. cutaneus
antebrachii
posterior

V. basilica ●

● N. radialis,
R. superficialis

R. dorsalis ●
(N. ulnaris)

● V. cephalica

415
424
434

416
430
439

Fig. 421 Veins and nerves of the anterior region
of the forearm, Regio antebrachii anterior;
epifascial layer.

Fig. 422 Veins and nerves of the posterior region
of the forearm, Regio antebrachii posterior;
epifascial layer.

Veins of the cubital fossa

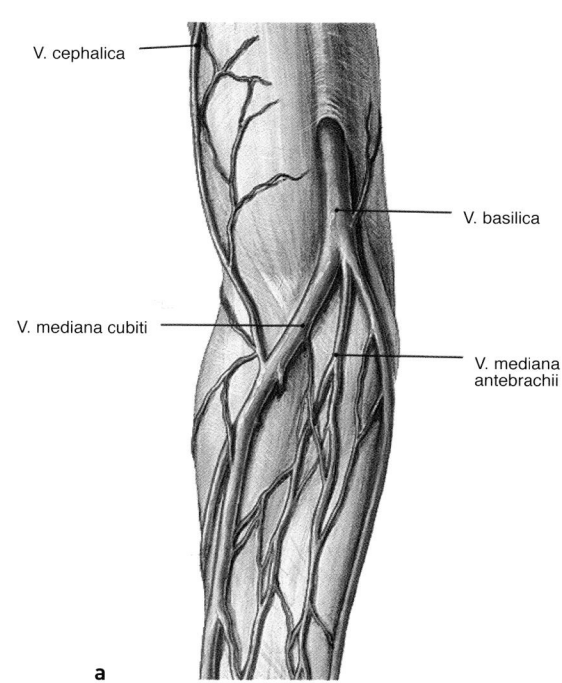

V. cephalica

V. basilica

V. mediana cubiti

V. mediana antebrachii

a

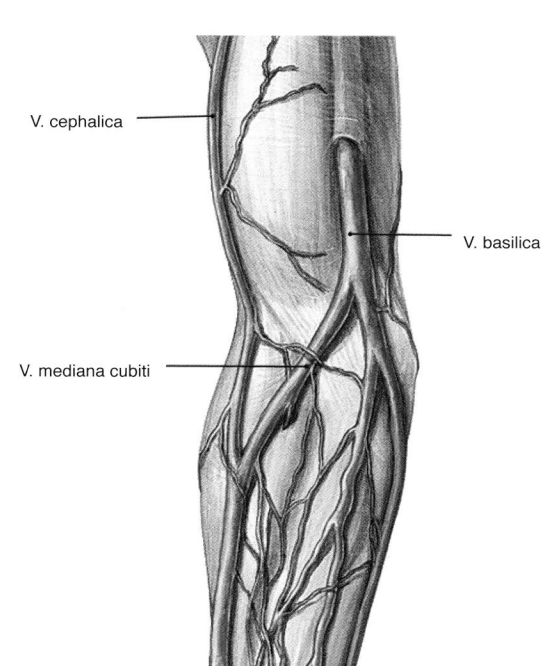

V. cephalica

V. basilica

V. mediana cubiti

b

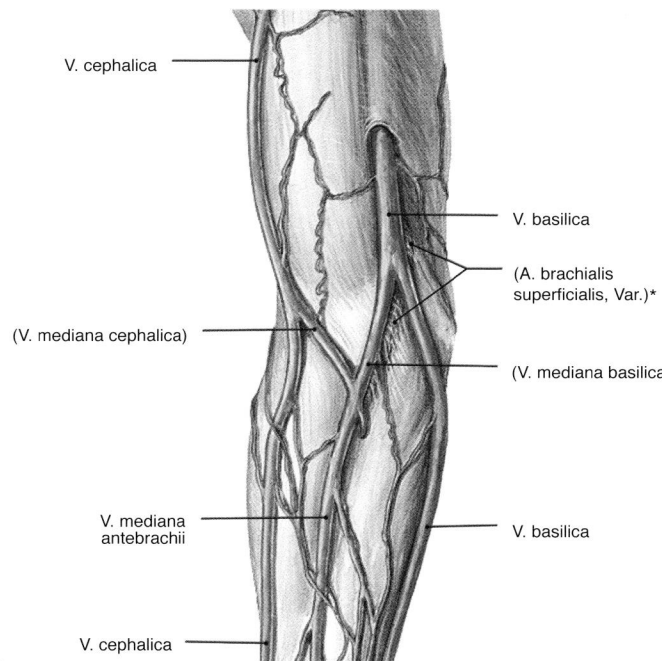

V. cephalica

V. basilica

(A. brachialis superficialis, Var.)*

(V. mediana cephalica)

(V. mediana basilica)

V. mediana antebrachii

V. basilica

V. cephalica

c

Fig. 423 a–c Variations in the epifascial veins of the cubital fossa.

* With regard to intravenous injections, this rare variation is particularly important, as a supposedly intravenous injection can mistakenly become intra-arterial.

Arteries and nerves of the forearm

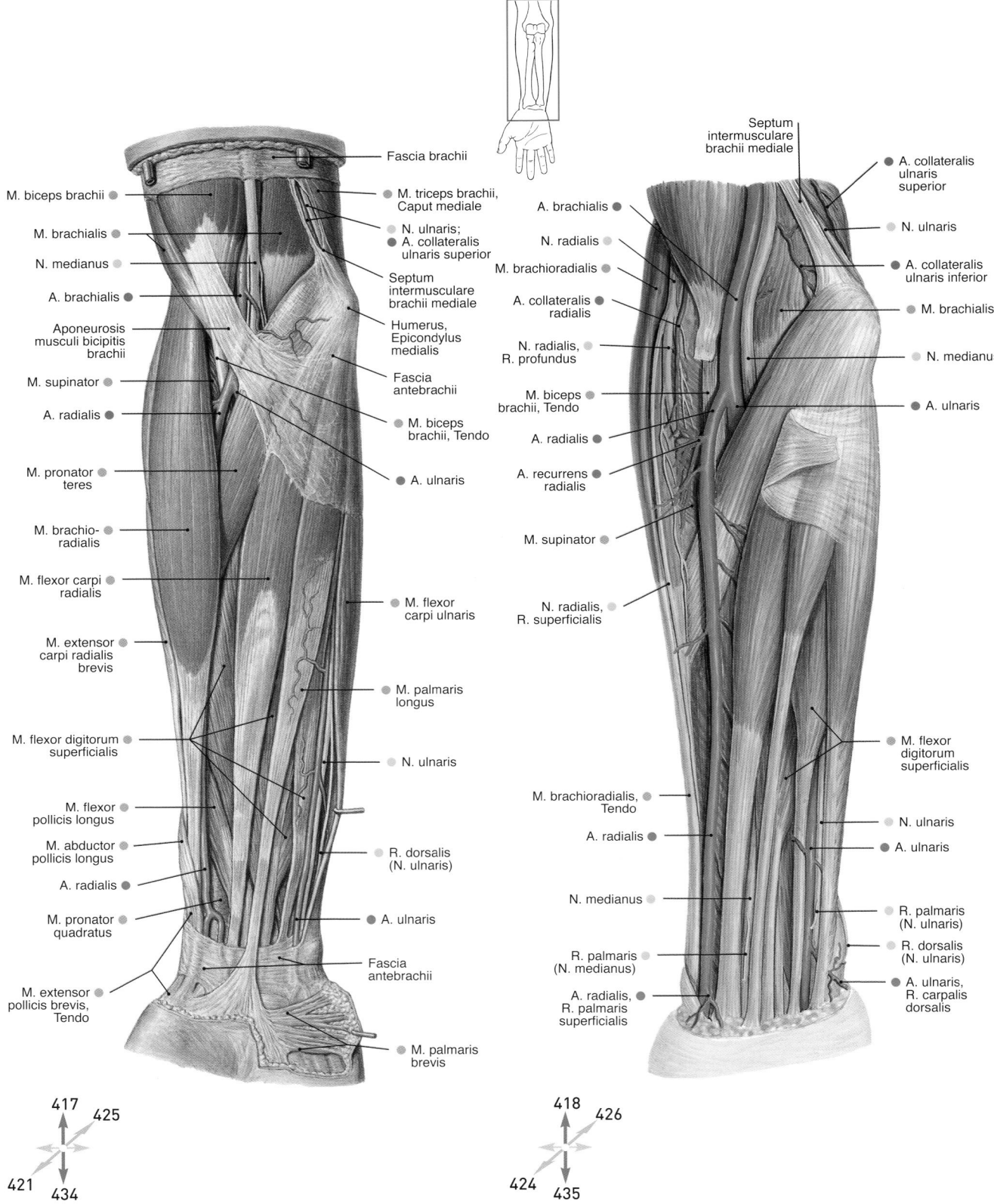

Fascia brachii

M. biceps brachii ●
M. brachialis ●
N. medianus ●
A. brachialis ●
Aponeurosis musculi bicipitis brachii
M. supinator ●
A. radialis ●
M. pronator teres ●
M. brachio-radialis ●
M. flexor carpi radialis ●
M. extensor carpi radialis brevis ●
M. flexor digitorum superficialis ●
M. flexor pollicis longus ●
M. abductor pollicis longus ●
A. radialis ●
M. pronator quadratus ●
M. extensor pollicis brevis, Tendo ●

● M. triceps brachii, Caput mediale
● N. ulnaris; ● A. collateralis ulnaris superior
Septum intermusculare brachii mediale
Humerus, Epicondylus medialis
Fascia antebrachii
● M. biceps brachii, Tendo
● A. ulnaris
● M. flexor carpi ulnaris
● M. palmaris longus
● N. ulnaris
● R. dorsalis (N. ulnaris)
● A. ulnaris
Fascia antebrachii
● M. palmaris brevis

417 425
421 434

Septum intermusculare brachii mediale

A. brachialis ●
N. radialis ●
M. brachioradialis ●
A. collateralis ● radialis
N. radialis, R. profundus ●
M. biceps brachii, Tendo ●
A. radialis ●
A. recurrens ● radialis
M. supinator ●
N. radialis, R. superficialis ●
M. brachioradialis, ● Tendo
A. radialis ●
N. medianus ●
R. palmaris ● (N. medianus)
A. radialis, ● R. palmaris superficialis

● A. collateralis ulnaris superior
● N. ulnaris
● A. collateralis ulnaris inferior
● M. brachialis
● N. medianus
● A. ulnaris
● M. flexor digitorum superficialis
● N. ulnaris
● A. ulnaris
● R. palmaris (N. ulnaris)
● R. dorsalis (N. ulnaris)
● A. ulnaris, R. carpalis dorsalis

418 426
424 435

Fig. 424 Arteries and nerves of the anterior region of the forearm, Regio antebrachii anterior; subfascial layer.

Fig. 425 Arteries and nerves of the anterior region of the forearm, Regio antebrachii anterior; course of the radial artery, A. radialis.

Arteries and nerves of the forearm

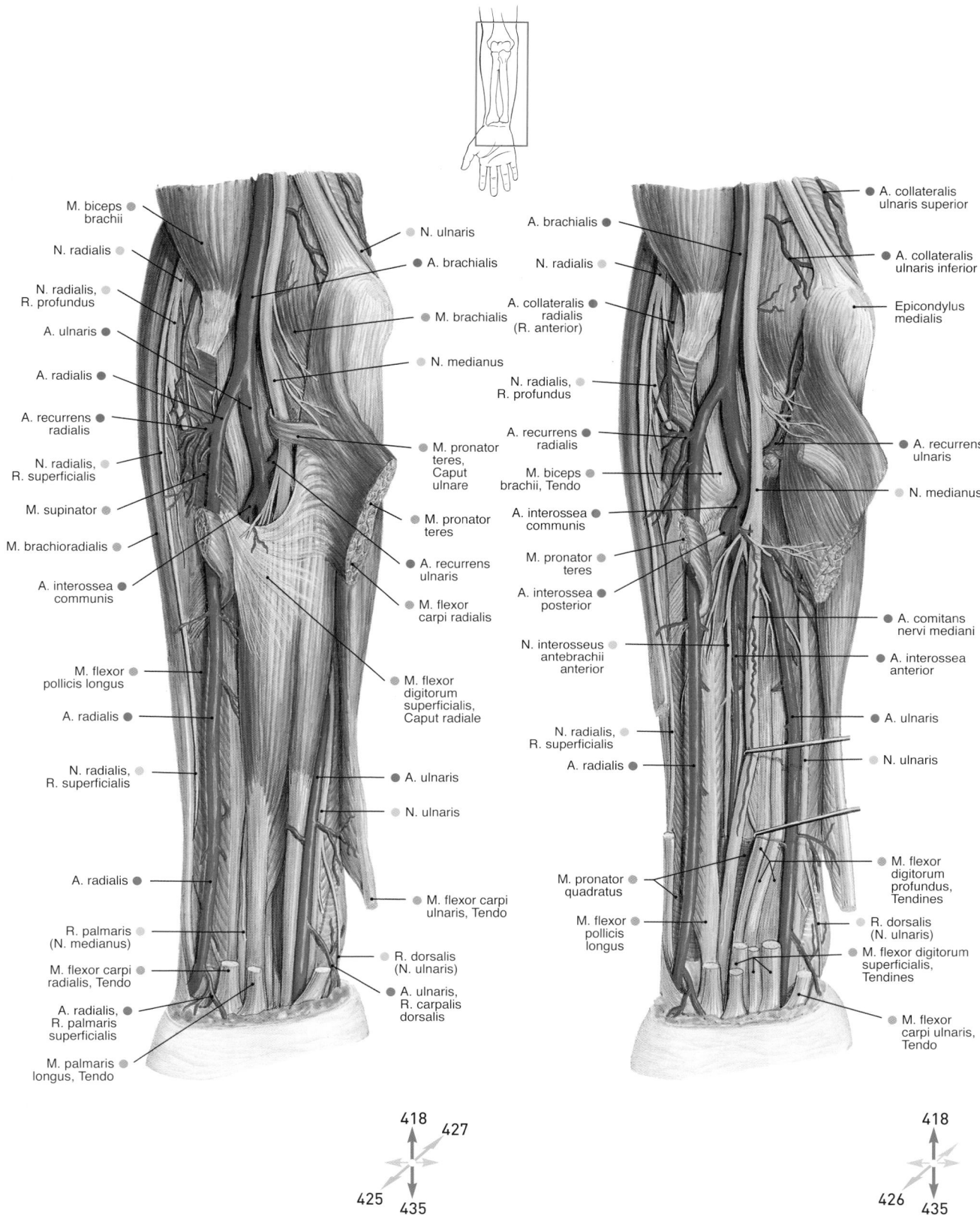

M. biceps brachii

N. radialis

N. radialis, R. profundus

A. ulnaris

A. radialis

A. recurrens radialis

N. radialis, R. superficialis

M. supinator

M. brachioradialis

A. interossea communis

M. flexor pollicis longus

A. radialis

N. radialis, R. superficialis

A. radialis

R. palmaris (N. medianus)

M. flexor carpi radialis, Tendo

A. radialis, R. palmaris superficialis

M. palmaris longus, Tendo

N. ulnaris

A. brachialis

M. brachialis

N. medianus

M. pronator teres, Caput ulnare

M. pronator teres

A. recurrens ulnaris

M. flexor carpi radialis

M. flexor digitorum superficialis, Caput radiale

A. ulnaris

N. ulnaris

M. flexor carpi ulnaris, Tendo

R. dorsalis (N. ulnaris)

A. ulnaris, R. carpalis dorsalis

A. brachialis

N. radialis

A. collateralis radialis (R. anterior)

N. radialis, R. profundus

A. recurrens radialis

M. biceps brachii, Tendo

A. interossea communis

M. pronator teres

A. interossea posterior

N. interosseus antebrachii anterior

N. radialis, R. superficialis

A. radialis

M. pronator quadratus

M. flexor pollicis longus

A. collateralis ulnaris superior

A. collateralis ulnaris inferior

Epicondylus medialis

A. recurrens ulnaris

N. medianus

A. comitans nervi mediani

A. interossea anterior

A. ulnaris

N. ulnaris

M. flexor digitorum profundus, Tendines

R. dorsalis (N. ulnaris)

M. flexor digitorum superficialis, Tendines

M. flexor carpi ulnaris, Tendo

418
427
425
435

418
426
435

Fig. 426 Arteries and nerves of the anterior region of the forearm, Regio antebrachii anterior; deep layer.

Fig. 427 Arteries and nerves of the anterior region of the forearm, Regio antebrachii anterior; deep layer after partial removal of the flexor digitorum superficialis muscle.

Arteries and nerves of the cubital fossa

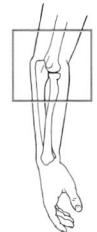

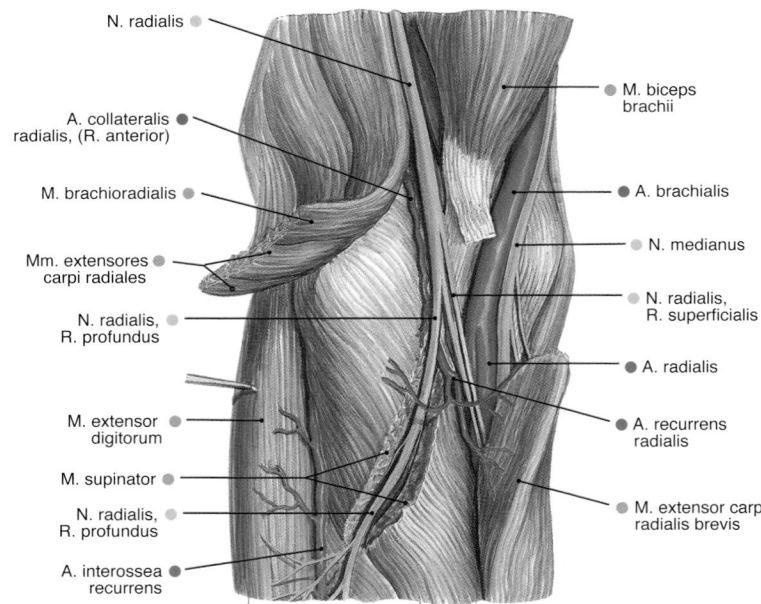

N. radialis

A. collateralis radialis, (R. anterior)

M. brachioradialis

Mm. extensores carpi radiales

N. radialis, R. profundus

M. extensor digitorum

M. supinator

N. radialis, R. profundus

A. interossea recurrens

M. biceps brachii

A. brachialis

N. medianus

N. radialis, R. superficialis

A. radialis

A. recurrens radialis

M. extensor carpi radialis brevis

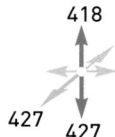

418

427   427

Fig. 428   Arteries and nerves of the anterior region of the elbow, Regio cubitalis anterior; after removal of the radial muscles of the forearm; lateral (radial) view.

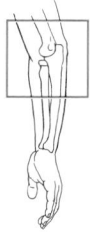

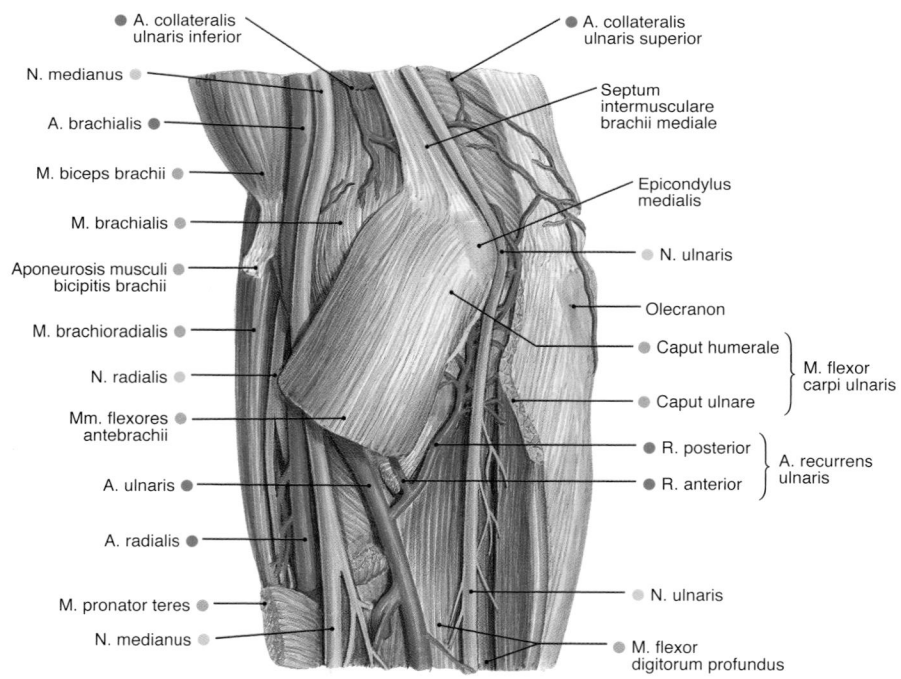

A. collateralis ulnaris inferior

N. medianus

A. brachialis

M. biceps brachii

M. brachialis

Aponeurosis musculi bicipitis brachii

M. brachioradialis

N. radialis

Mm. flexores antebrachii

A. ulnaris

A. radialis

M. pronator teres

N. medianus

A. collateralis ulnaris superior

Septum intermusculare brachii mediale

Epicondylus medialis

N. ulnaris

Olecranon

Caput humerale ⎫
                ⎬ M. flexor
Caput ulnare ⎭ carpi ulnaris

R. posterior ⎫
             ⎬ A. recurrens
R. anterior ⎭ ulnaris

N. ulnaris

M. flexor digitorum profundus

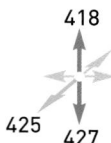

418

425   427

Fig. 429   Arteries and nerves of the anterior region of the elbow, Regio cubitalis anterior; after partial removal of the flexor muscles of the forearm; medial (ulnar) view.

Arteries and nerves of the forearm

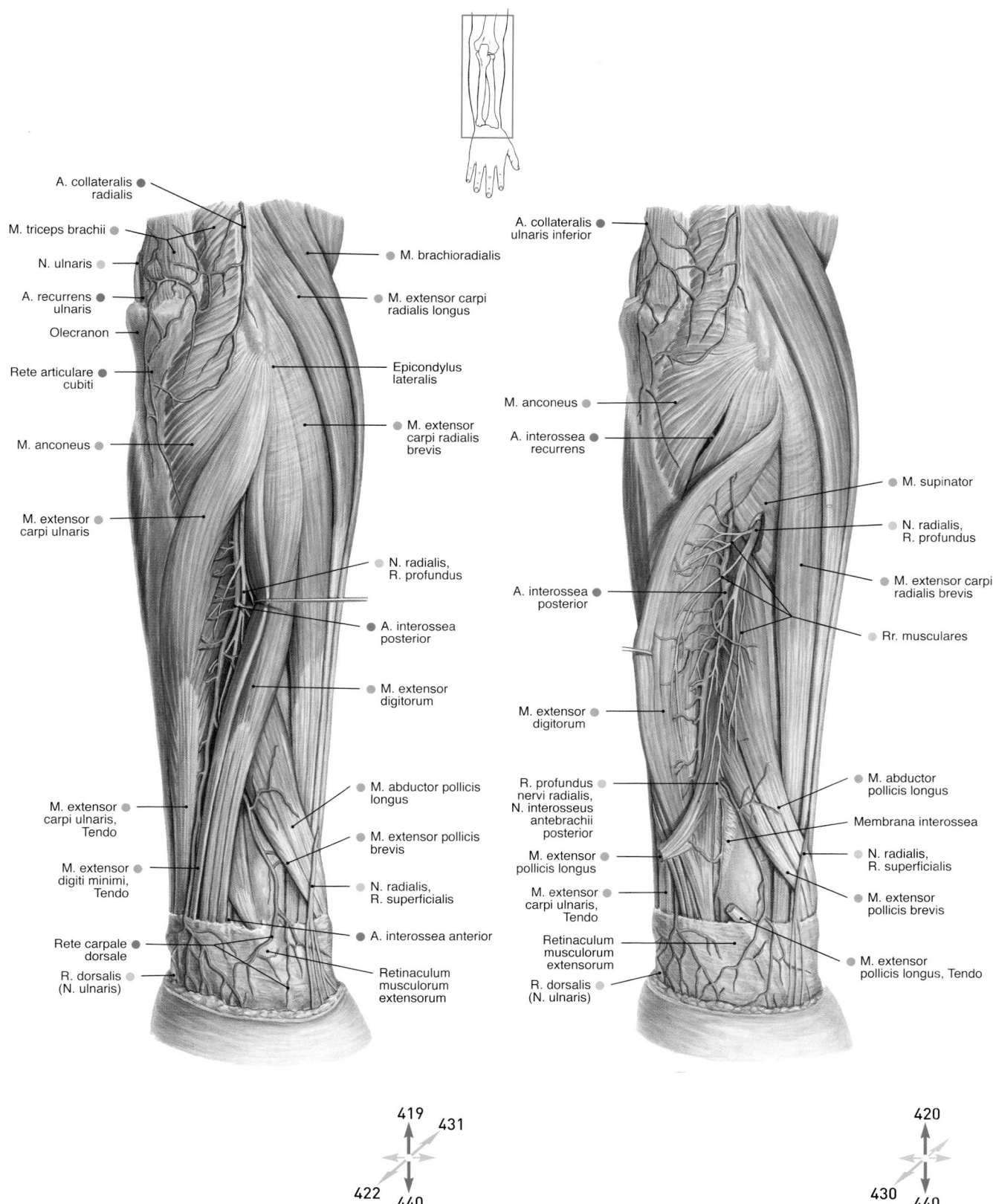

A. collateralis
radialis

M. triceps brachii

N. ulnaris

A. recurrens
ulnaris

Olecranon

Rete articulare
cubiti

M. anconeus

M. extensor
carpi ulnaris

M. extensor
carpi ulnaris,
Tendo

M. extensor
digiti minimi,
Tendo

Rete carpale
dorsale

R. dorsalis
(N. ulnaris)

M. brachioradialis

M. extensor carpi
radialis longus

Epicondylus
lateralis

M. extensor
carpi radialis
brevis

N. radialis,
R. profundus

A. interossea
posterior

M. extensor
digitorum

M. abductor pollicis
longus

M. extensor pollicis
brevis

N. radialis,
R. superficialis

A. interossea anterior

Retinaculum
musculorum
extensorum

A. collateralis
ulnaris inferior

M. anconeus

A. interossea
recurrens

A. interossea
posterior

M. extensor
digitorum

R. profundus
nervi radialis,
N. interosseus
antebrachii
posterior

M. extensor
pollicis longus

M. extensor
carpi ulnaris,
Tendo

Retinaculum
musculorum
extensorum

R. dorsalis
(N. ulnaris)

M. supinator

N. radialis,
R. profundus

M. extensor carpi
radialis brevis

Rr. musculares

M. abductor
pollicis longus

Membrana interossea

N. radialis,
R. superficialis

M. extensor
pollicis brevis

M. extensor
pollicis longus, Tendo

419
431

422
440

420

430
440

Fig. 430 Arteries and nerves of the posterior region
of the forearm, Regio antebrachii posterior;
superficial layer.

Fig. 431 Arteries and nerves of the posterior region
of the forearm, Regio antebrachii posterior;
deep layer.

Arteries of the hand

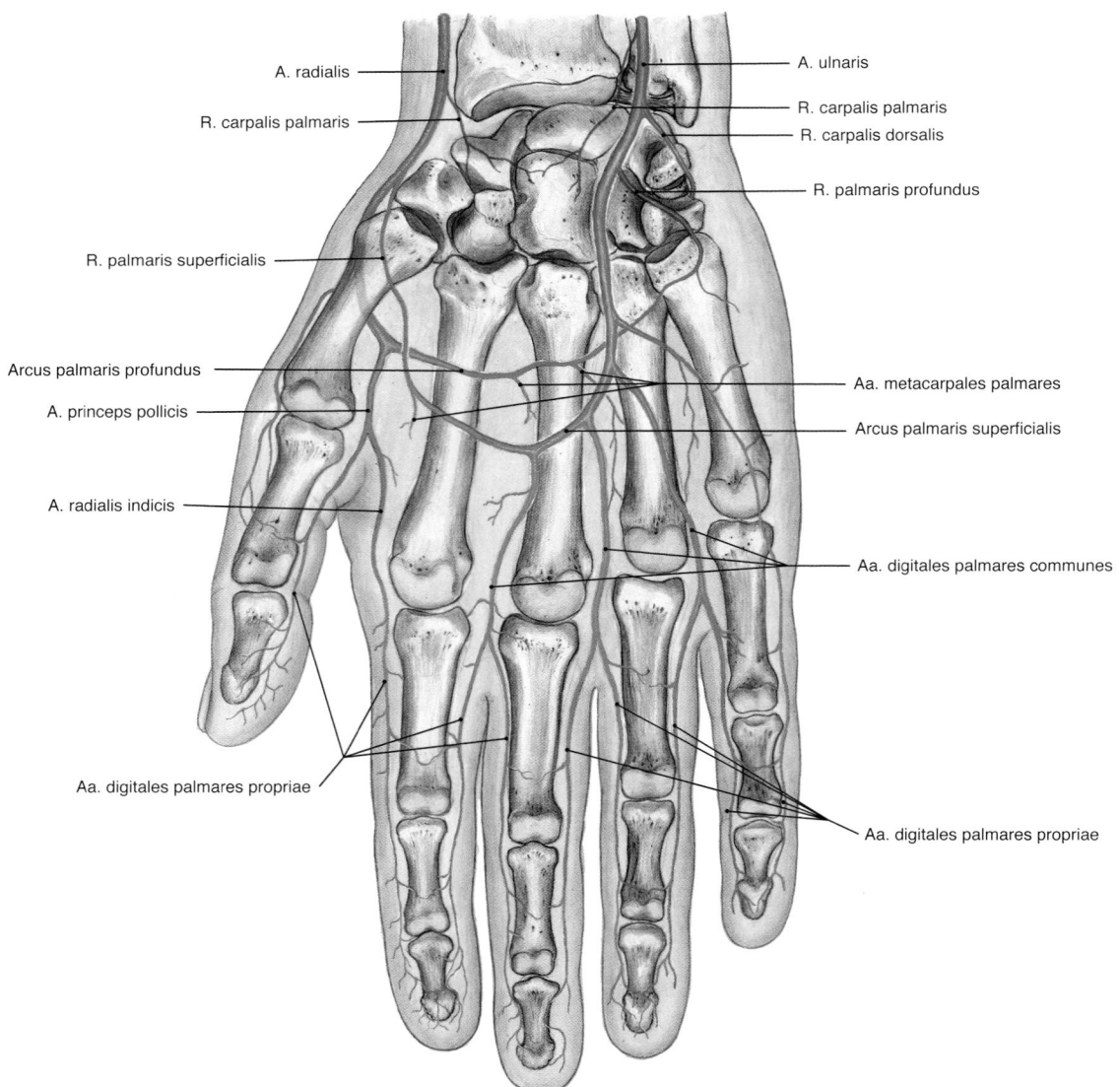

A. radialis
R. carpalis palmaris
R. palmaris superficialis
Arcus palmaris profundus
A. princeps pollicis
A. radialis indicis
Aa. digitales palmares propriae

A. ulnaris
R. carpalis palmaris
R. carpalis dorsalis
R. palmaris profundus
Aa. metacarpales palmares
Arcus palmaris superficialis
Aa. digitales palmares communes
Aa. digitales palmares propriae

Fig. 432 Arteries of the palm, Palma; overview.

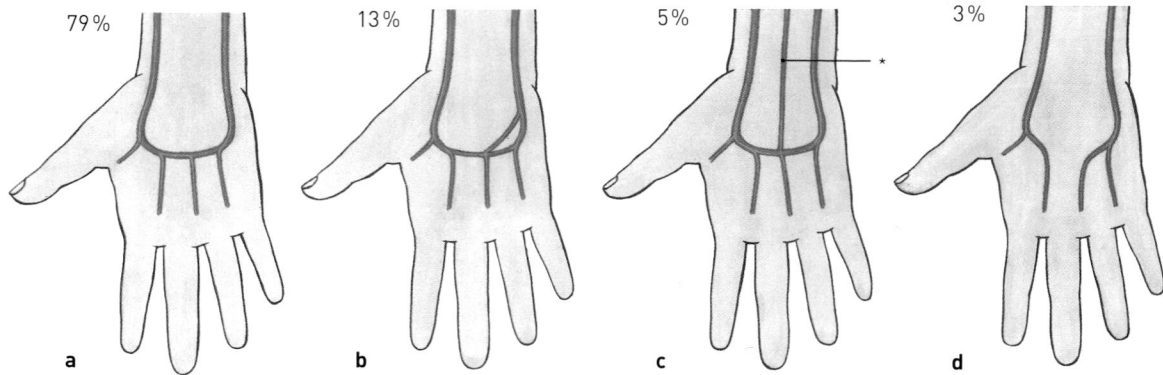

79%
13%
5%
3%

a
b
c
d

Fig. 433 a–d Variations of the deep palmar arch, Arcus palmaris profundus.
a "Textbook case", simple, closed arch
b Doubling of the ulnar part

c Anastomosis with the anterior interosseous artery, A. interossea anterior (*)
d The radial artery, A. radialis, supplies both radial fingers, whereas the ulnar artery, A. ulnaris, supplies the three ulnar fingers.

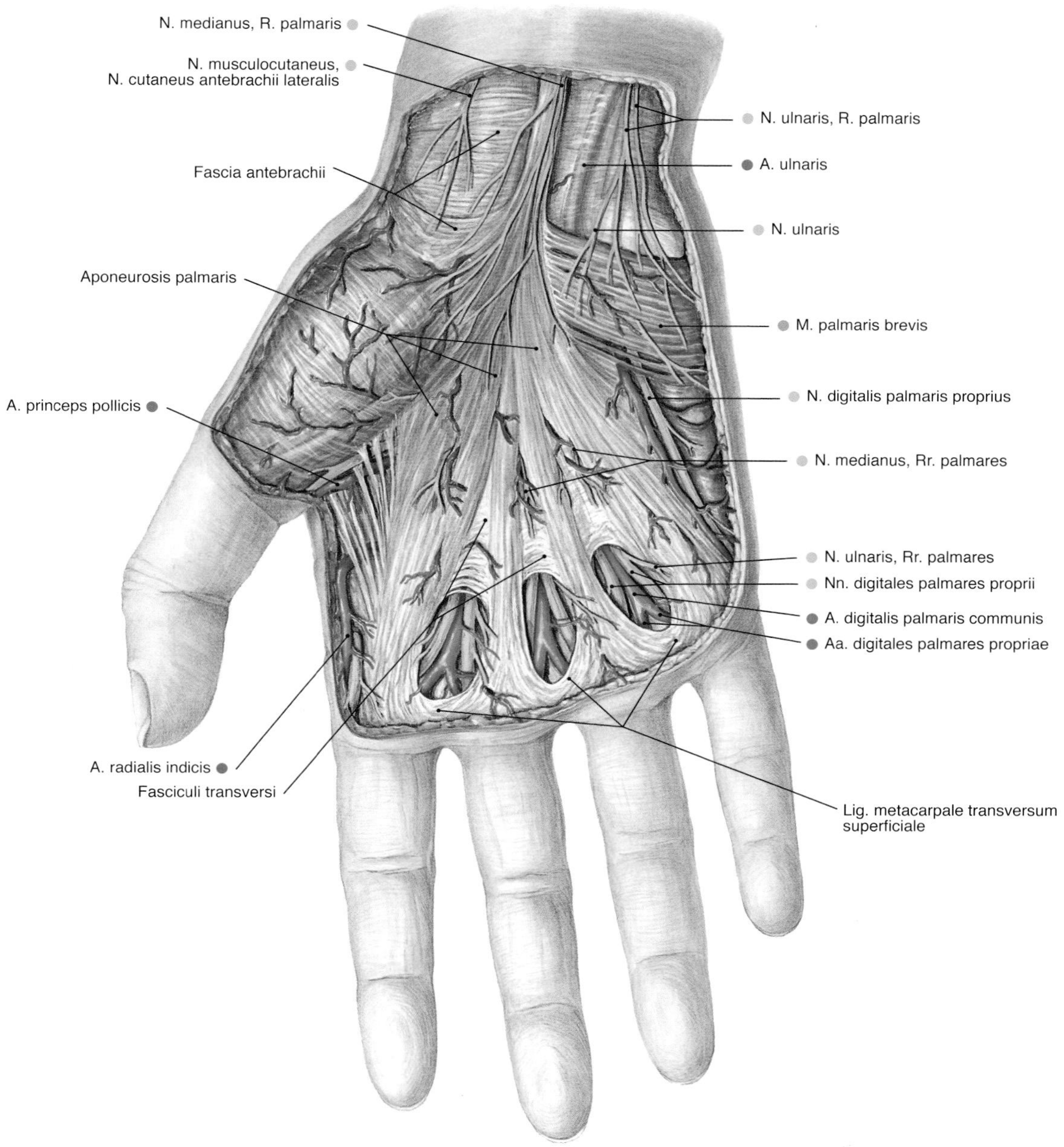

N. medianus, R. palmaris ●

N. musculocutaneus, ●
N. cutaneus antebrachii lateralis

Fascia antebrachii

Aponeurosis palmaris

A. princeps pollicis ●

A. radialis indicis ●
Fasciculi transversi

● N. ulnaris, R. palmaris

● A. ulnaris

● N. ulnaris

● M. palmaris brevis

● N. digitalis palmaris proprius

● N. medianus, Rr. palmares

● N. ulnaris, Rr. palmares
● Nn. digitales palmares proprii
● A. digitalis palmaris communis
● Aa. digitales palmares propriae

Lig. metacarpale transversum
superficiale

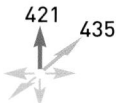

Fig. 434 Arteries and nerves of the palm, Palma;
superficial layer.

Arteries and nerves of the hand

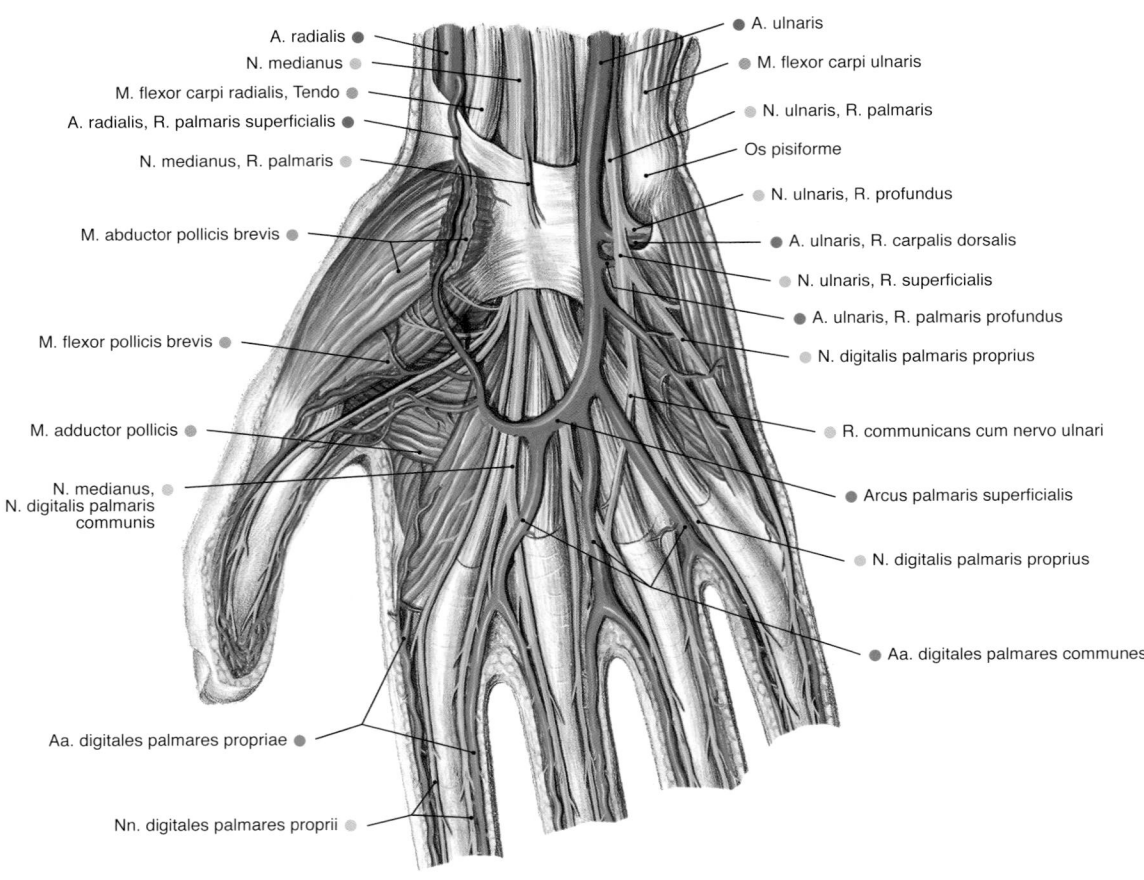

A. radialis ●
N. medianus ●
M. flexor carpi radialis, Tendo ●
A. radialis, R. palmaris superficialis ●
N. medianus, R. palmaris ●
M. abductor pollicis brevis ●
M. flexor pollicis brevis ●
M. adductor pollicis ●
N. medianus, N. digitalis palmaris communis ●
Aa. digitales palmares propriae ●
Nn. digitales palmares proprii ●

● A. ulnaris
● M. flexor carpi ulnaris
● N. ulnaris, R. palmaris
Os pisiforme
● N. ulnaris, R. profundus
● A. ulnaris, R. carpalis dorsalis
● N. ulnaris, R. superficialis
● A. ulnaris, R. palmaris profundus
● N. digitalis palmaris proprius
● R. communicans cum nervo ulnari
● Arcus palmaris superficialis
● N. digitalis palmaris proprius
● Aa. digitales palmares communes

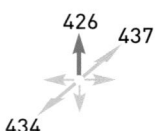

Fig. 435 Arteries and nerves of the palm, Palma; middle layer.

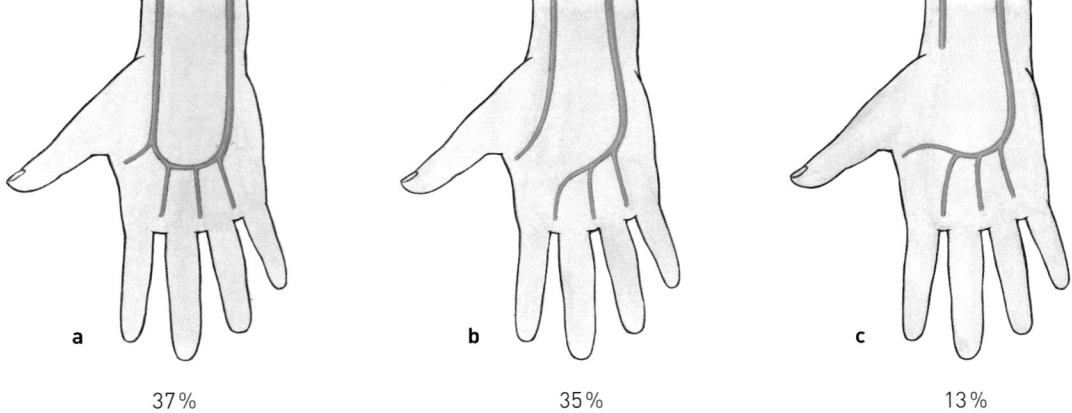

a   37%

b   35%

c   13%

Fig. 436a–c Variations of the superficial palmar arch, Arcus palmaris superficialis.
a "Textbook case", closed arch
b The ulnar artery, A. ulnaris, supplies the three ulnar fingers.
c All fingers are supplied by the ulnar artery, A. ulnaris.

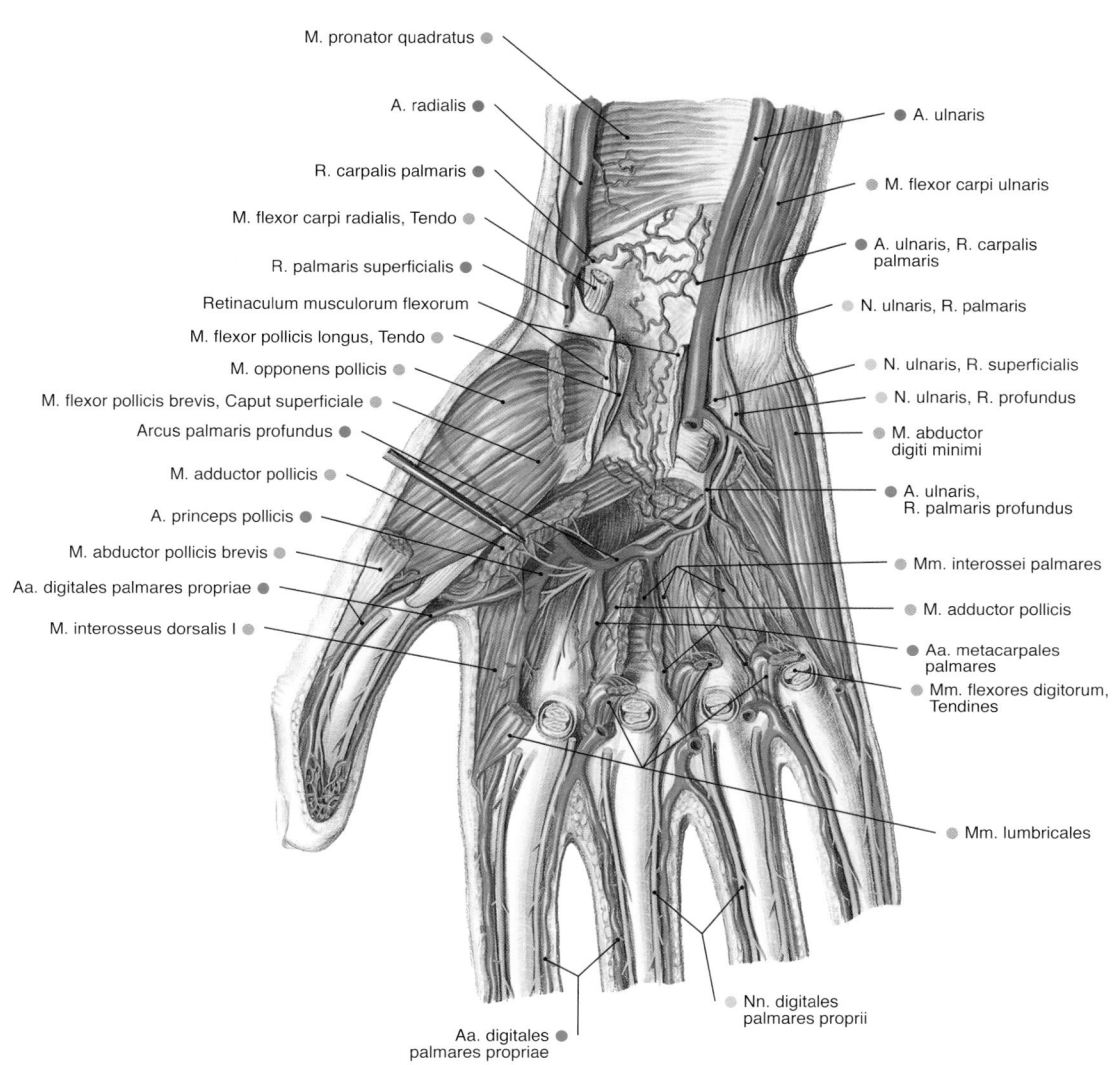

M. pronator quadratus ●

A. radialis ●

R. carpalis palmaris ●

M. flexor carpi radialis, Tendo ●

R. palmaris superficialis ●

Retinaculum musculorum flexorum

M. flexor pollicis longus, Tendo ●

M. opponens pollicis ●

M. flexor pollicis brevis, Caput superficiale ●

Arcus palmaris profundus ●

M. adductor pollicis ●

A. princeps pollicis ●

M. abductor pollicis brevis ●

Aa. digitales palmares propriae ●

M. interosseus dorsalis I ●

● A. ulnaris

● M. flexor carpi ulnaris

● A. ulnaris, R. carpalis palmaris

● N. ulnaris, R. palmaris

● N. ulnaris, R. superficialis

● N. ulnaris, R. profundus

● M. abductor digiti minimi

● A. ulnaris, R. palmaris profundus

● Mm. interossei palmares

● M. adductor pollicis

● Aa. metacarpales palmares

● Mm. flexores digitorum, Tendines

● Mm. lumbricales

Nn. digitales palmares proprii ●

Aa. digitales ● palmares propriae

Fig. 437   Arteries and nerves of the palm, Palma; deep layer.

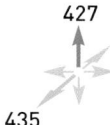

427

435

Arteries and nerves of the hand

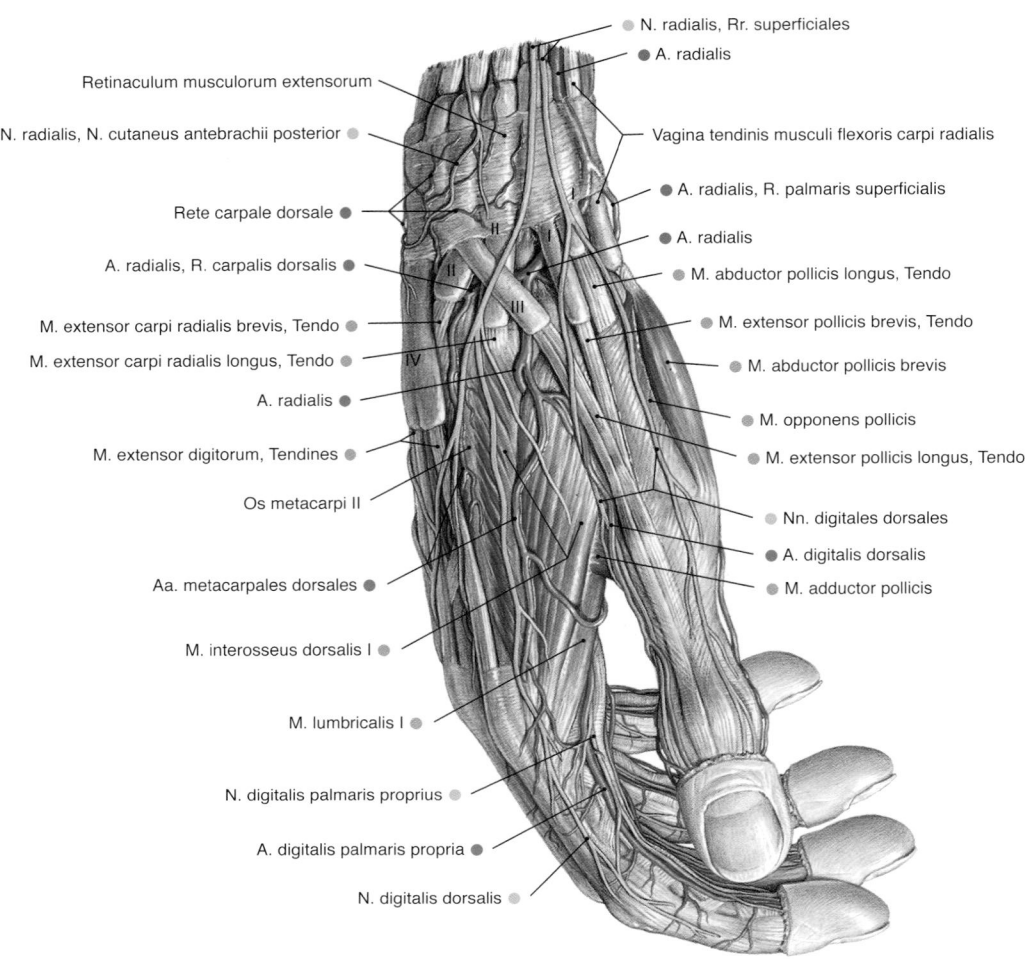

N. radialis, Rr. superficiales

A. radialis

Retinaculum musculorum extensorum

N. radialis, N. cutaneus antebrachii posterior

Vagina tendinis musculi flexoris carpi radialis

A. radialis, R. palmaris superficialis

Rete carpale dorsale

A. radialis

A. radialis, R. carpalis dorsalis

M. abductor pollicis longus, Tendo

M. extensor carpi radialis brevis, Tendo

M. extensor pollicis brevis, Tendo

M. extensor carpi radialis longus, Tendo

M. abductor pollicis brevis

A. radialis

M. opponens pollicis

M. extensor digitorum, Tendines

M. extensor pollicis longus, Tendo

Os metacarpi II

Nn. digitales dorsales

A. digitalis dorsalis

Aa. metacarpales dorsales

M. adductor pollicis

M. interosseus dorsalis I

M. lumbricalis I

N. digitalis palmaris proprius

A. digitalis palmaris propria

N. digitalis dorsalis

I–IV Vaginae tendinum musculorum extensorum:
I   Vagina tendinum musculorum abductoris longi
     et extensoris pollicis brevis
II   Vagina tendinum musculorum extensorum carpi radialium
III Vagina tendinis musculi extensoris pollicis longi
IV   Vagina tendinum musculorum extensoris digitorum
     et extensoris indicis

430
440 ← → 434

Fig. 438   Arteries and nerves of the hand.

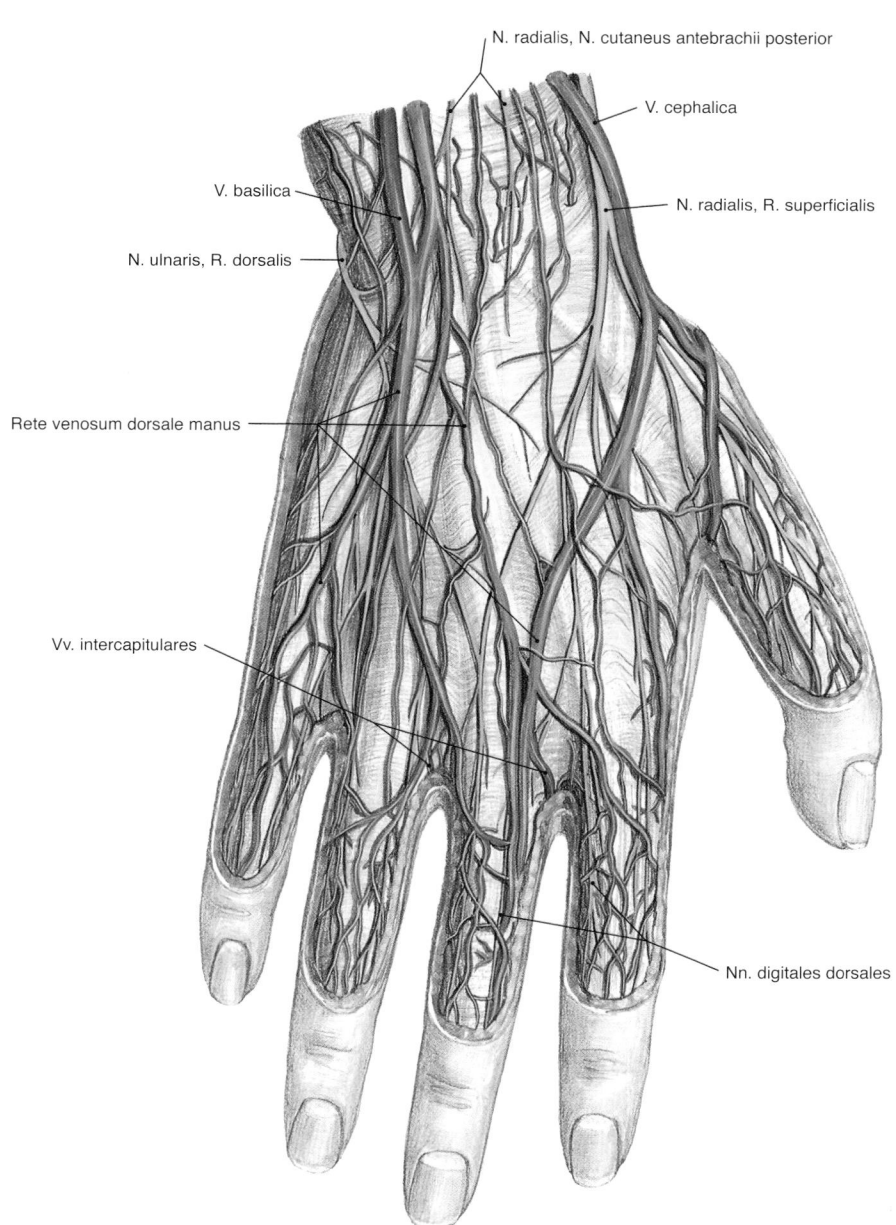

N. radialis, N. cutaneus antebrachii posterior

V. cephalica

V. basilica

N. radialis, R. superficialis

N. ulnaris, R. dorsalis

Rete venosum dorsale manus

Vv. intercapitulares

Nn. digitales dorsales

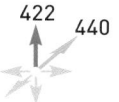

422   440

Fig. 439   Vessels and nerves of the dorsum of
the hand, Dorsum manus;
superficial layer.

Arteries and nerves of the hand

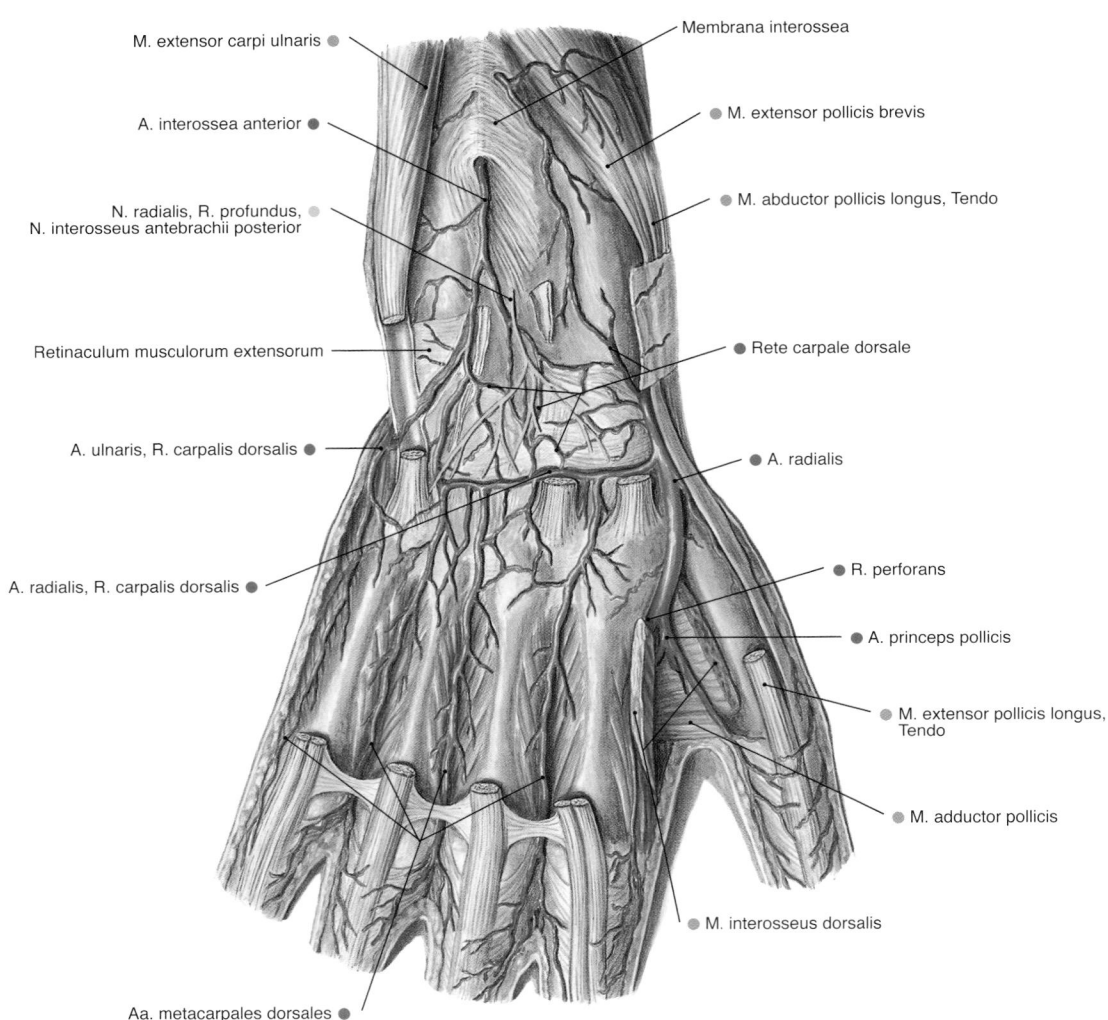

M. extensor carpi ulnaris ●

A. interossea anterior ●

N. radialis, R. profundus, ●
N. interosseus antebrachii posterior

Retinaculum musculorum extensorum

A. ulnaris, R. carpalis dorsalis ●

A. radialis, R. carpalis dorsalis ●

Aa. metacarpales dorsales ●

Membrana interossea

● M. extensor pollicis brevis

● M. abductor pollicis longus, Tendo

● Rete carpale dorsale

● A. radialis

● R. perforans

● A. princeps pollicis

● M. extensor pollicis longus, Tendo

● M. adductor pollicis

● M. interosseus dorsalis

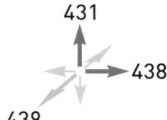

Fig. 440   Arteries and nerves of the dorsum of the hand, Dorsum manus; deep layer.

Topographic spaces of the hand

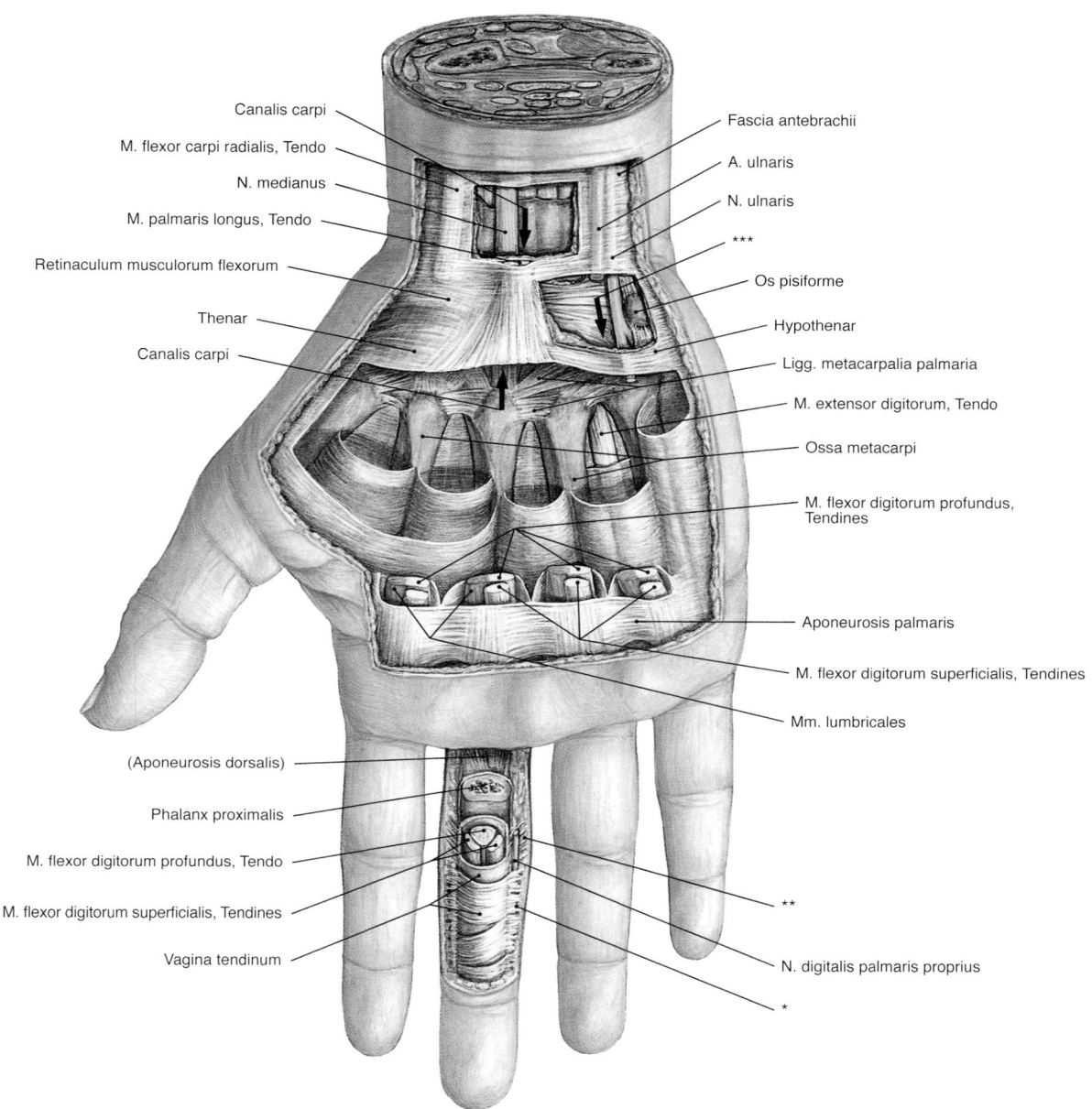

Canalis carpi

M. flexor carpi radialis, Tendo

N. medianus

M. palmaris longus, Tendo

Retinaculum musculorum flexorum

Thenar

Canalis carpi

Fascia antebrachii

A. ulnaris

N. ulnaris

***

Os pisiforme

Hypothenar

Ligg. metacarpalia palmaria

M. extensor digitorum, Tendo

Ossa metacarpi

M. flexor digitorum profundus, Tendines

Aponeurosis palmaris

M. flexor digitorum superficialis, Tendines

Mm. lumbricales

(Aponeurosis dorsalis)

Phalanx proximalis

M. flexor digitorum profundus, Tendo

M. flexor digitorum superficialis, Tendines

Vagina tendinum

**

N. digitalis palmaris proprius

*

Fig. 441   Fascial compartments of the hand.
*   Clinical term: ligament of GRAYSON
**   Clinical term: ligament of CLELAND
***Clinical term: ulnar canal, Canalis ulnocarpalis (loge de GUYON)

Hand, sagittal section

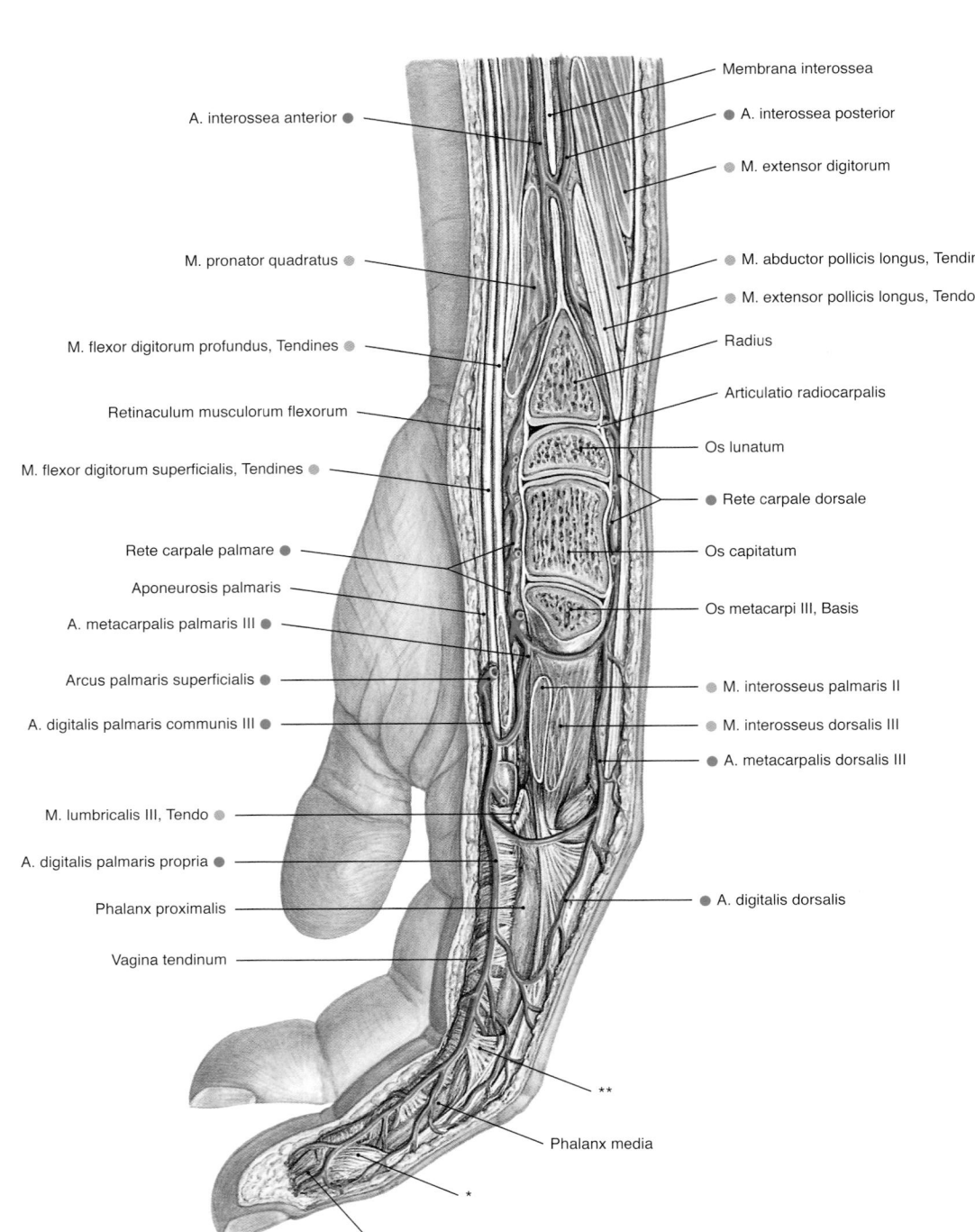

A. interossea anterior ●

M. pronator quadratus ●

M. flexor digitorum profundus, Tendines ●

Retinaculum musculorum flexorum

M. flexor digitorum superficialis, Tendines ●

Rete carpale palmare ●

Aponeurosis palmaris

A. metacarpalis palmaris III ●

Arcus palmaris superficialis ●

A. digitalis palmaris communis III ●

M. lumbricalis III, Tendo ●

A. digitalis palmaris propria ●

Phalanx proximalis

Vagina tendinum

Membrana interossea

● A. interossea posterior

● M. extensor digitorum

● M. abductor pollicis longus, Tendines

● M. extensor pollicis longus, Tendo

Radius

Articulatio radiocarpalis

Os lunatum

● Rete carpale dorsale

Os capitatum

Os metacarpi III, Basis

● M. interosseus palmaris II

● M. interosseus dorsalis III

● A. metacarpalis dorsalis III

● A. digitalis dorsalis

**

Phalanx media

*

Phalanx distalis

Fig. 442   Hand, Manus;
sagittal section at the level of the ulnar plane of the middle finger.
*   Clinical term: ligament of CLELAND
** Clinical term: ligament of GRAYSON

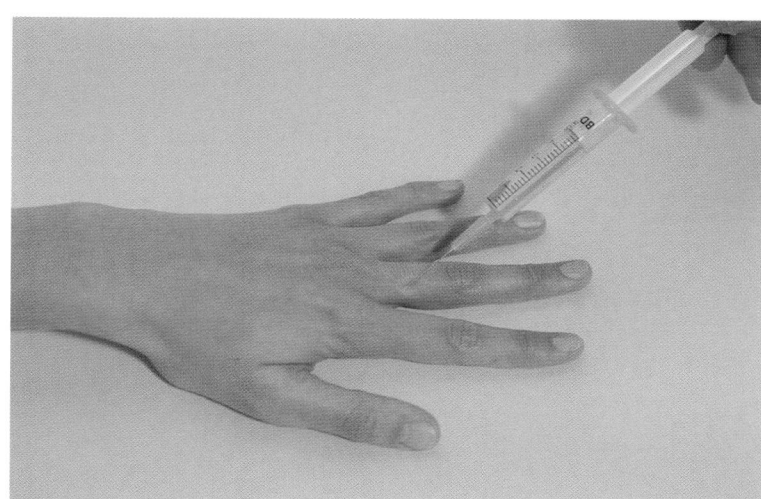

Fig. 443   Points of injection for regional
conduction anaesthesia at the middle finger.

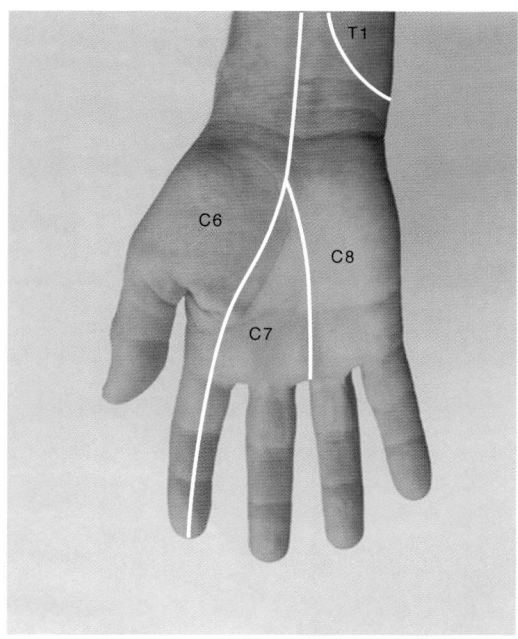

Fig. 444   Palm, Palma;
segmental cutaneous innervation.

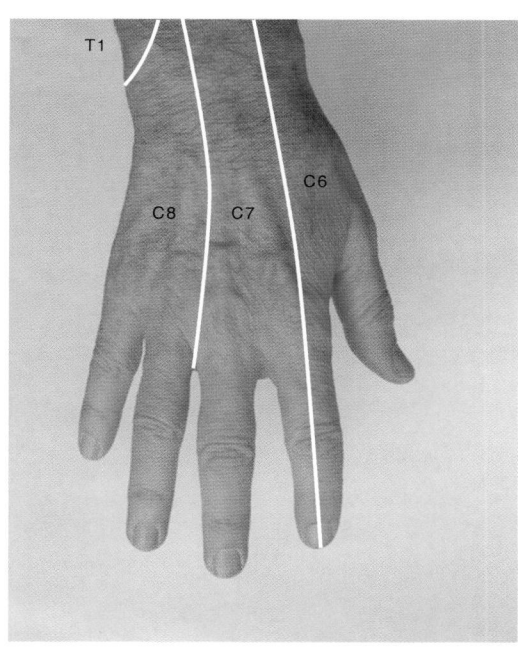

Fig. 445   Dorsum of the hand, Dorsum manus;
segmental cutaneous innervation.

Arm, transverse sections

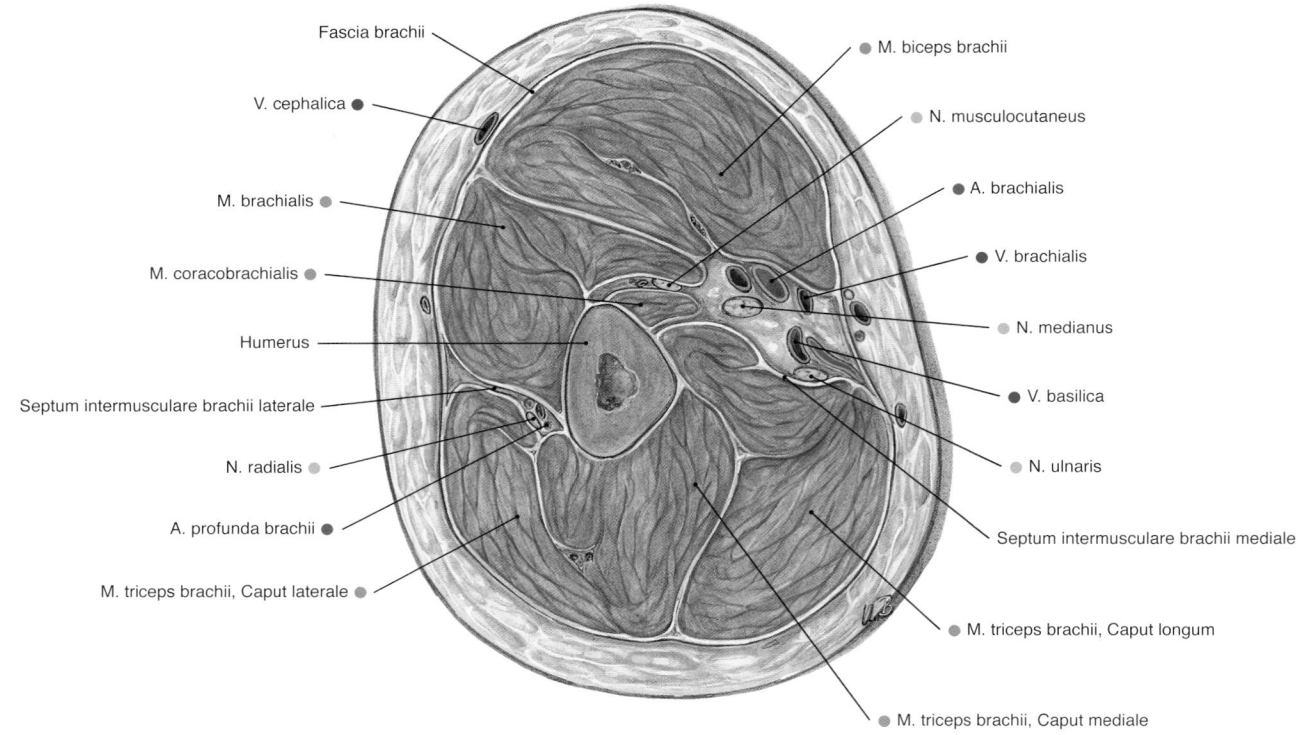

Fig. 446   Arm, Brachium;
transverse section.

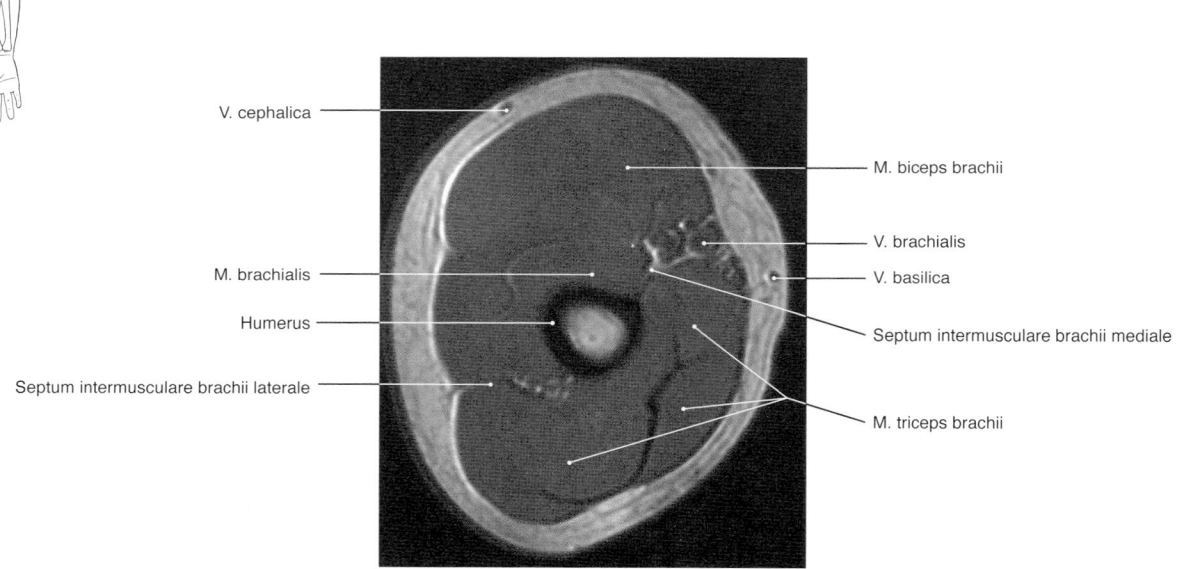

Fig. 447   Arm, Brachium;
magnetic resonance tomographic image (MRI);
cross-section at the level of the middle of the arm;
distal view.

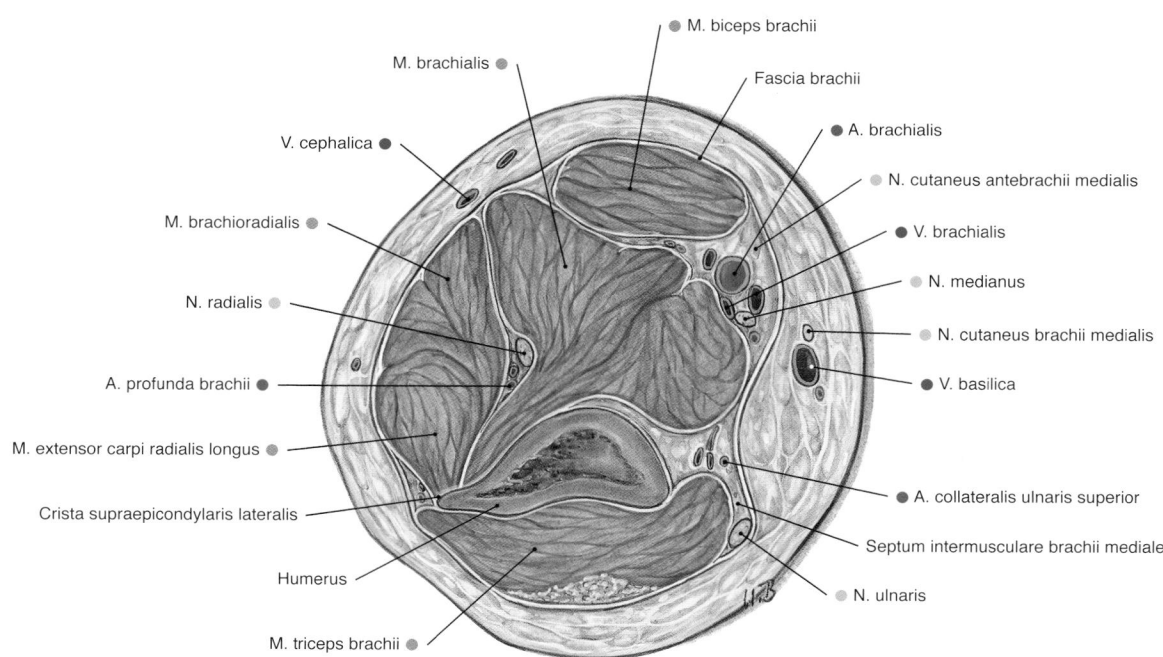

M. biceps brachii

M. brachialis ●

Fascia brachii

V. cephalica ●

● A. brachialis

● N. cutaneus antebrachii medialis

M. brachioradialis ●

● V. brachialis

N. radialis ●

● N. medianus

● N. cutaneus brachii medialis

A. profunda brachii ●

● V. basilica

M. extensor carpi radialis longus ●

Crista supraepicondylaris lateralis

● A. collateralis ulnaris superior

Septum intermusculare brachii mediale

Humerus

● N. ulnaris

M. triceps brachii ●

Fig. 448   Arm, Brachium;
transverse section through the lower third
of the arm.

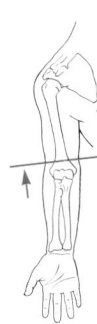

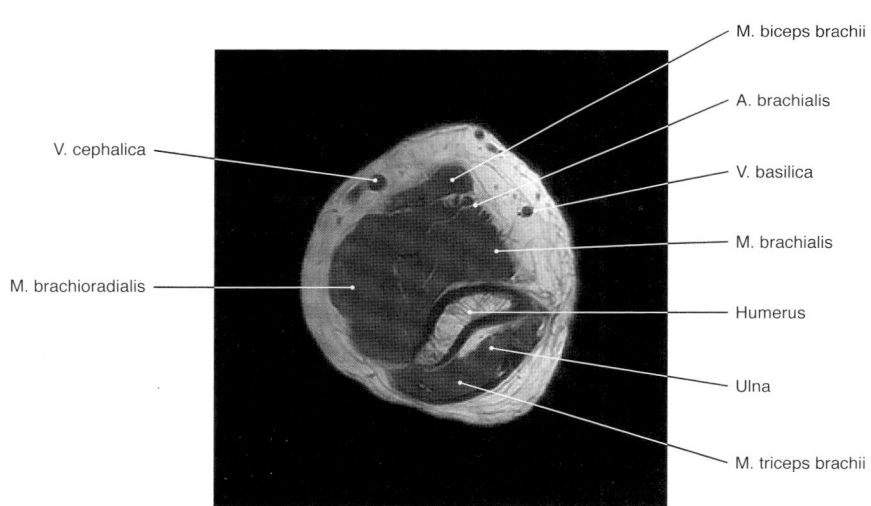

M. biceps brachii

A. brachialis

V. cephalica

V. basilica

M. brachialis

M. brachioradialis

Humerus

Ulna

M. triceps brachii

Fig. 449   Arm, Brachium;
magnetic resonance tomographic image (MRI);
cross-section at the level of the lower third of the arm;
distal view.

Forearm, transverse sections

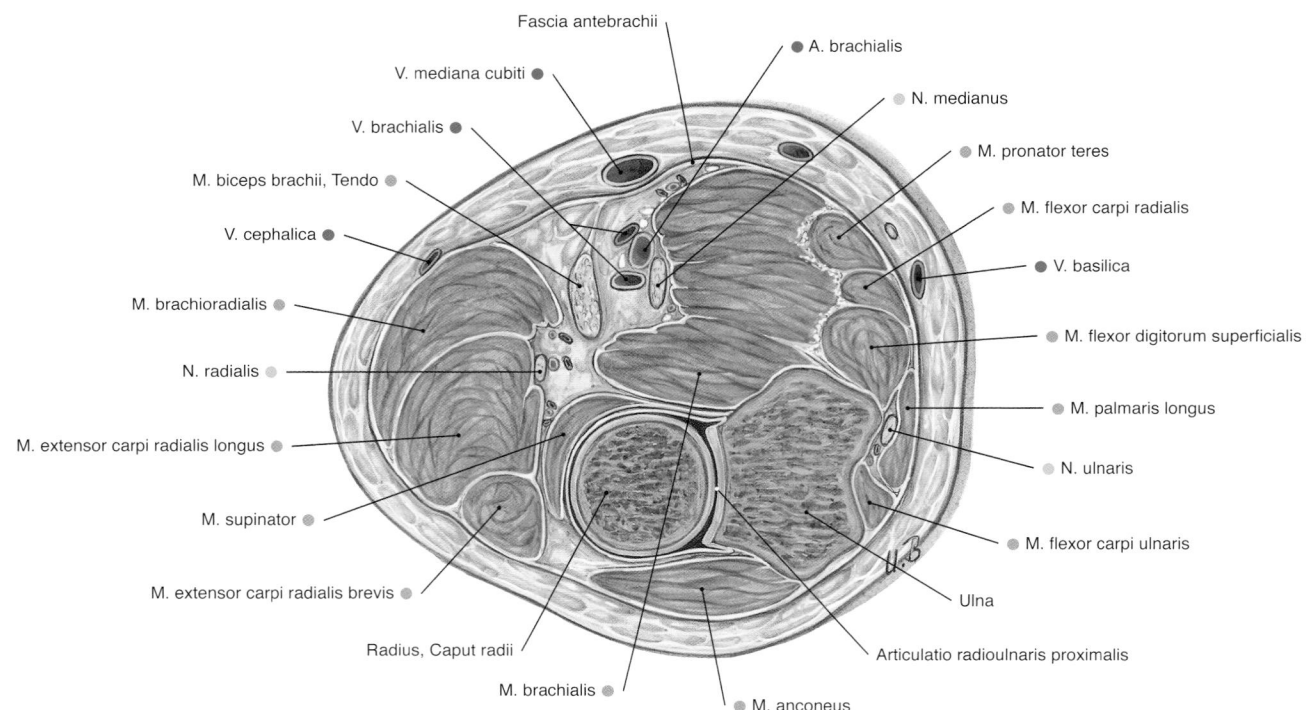

Fascia antebrachii
V. mediana cubiti ●
V. brachialis ●
M. biceps brachii, Tendo ●
V. cephalica ●
M. brachioradialis ●
N. radialis ●
M. extensor carpi radialis longus ●
M. supinator ●
M. extensor carpi radialis brevis ●
Radius, Caput radii
M. brachialis ●
M. anconeus ●

● A. brachialis
● N. medianus
● M. pronator teres
● M. flexor carpi radialis
● V. basilica
● M. flexor digitorum superficialis
● M. palmaris longus
● N. ulnaris
● M. flexor carpi ulnaris
Ulna
Articulatio radioulnaris proximalis

Fig. 450   Forearm, Antebrachium;
transverse section at the level of the
proximal radio-ulnar joint.

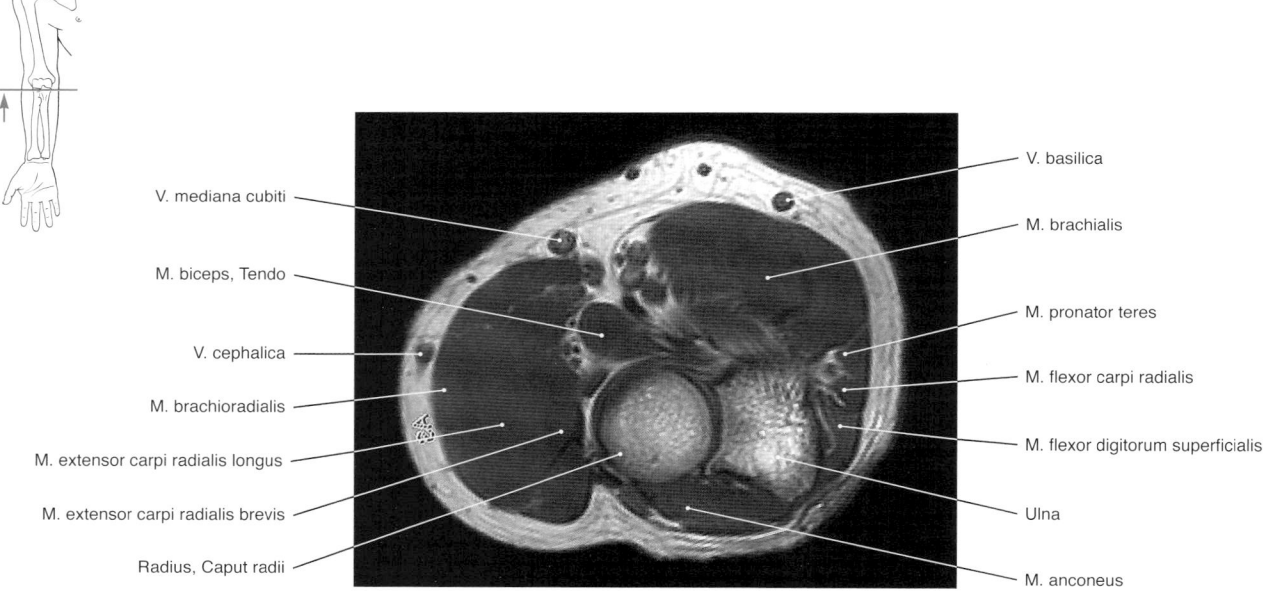

V. mediana cubiti
M. biceps, Tendo
V. cephalica
M. brachioradialis
M. extensor carpi radialis longus
M. extensor carpi radialis brevis
Radius, Caput radii

V. basilica
M. brachialis
M. pronator teres
M. flexor carpi radialis
M. flexor digitorum superficialis
Ulna
M. anconeus

Fig. 451   Forearm, Antebrachium;
magnetic resonance tomographic image (MRI);
cross-section at the level of the elbow joint;
distal view.

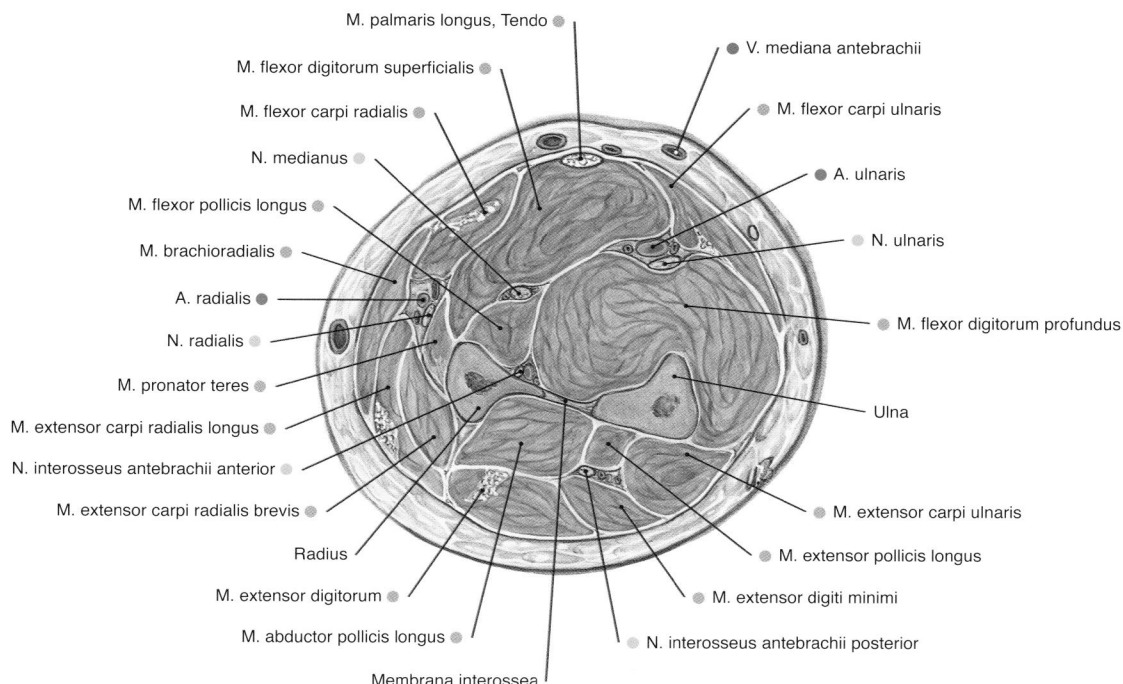

M. palmaris longus, Tendo ●

● V. mediana antebrachii

M. flexor digitorum superficialis ●

M. flexor carpi radialis ●

● M. flexor carpi ulnaris

N. medianus ●

● A. ulnaris

M. flexor pollicis longus ●

● N. ulnaris

M. brachioradialis ●

A. radialis ●

● M. flexor digitorum profundus

N. radialis ●

M. pronator teres ●

M. extensor carpi radialis longus ●

Ulna

N. interosseus antebrachii anterior ●

M. extensor carpi radialis brevis ●

● M. extensor carpi ulnaris

Radius

● M. extensor pollicis longus

M. extensor digitorum ●

● M. extensor digiti minimi

M. abductor pollicis longus ●

● N. interosseus antebrachii posterior

Membrana interossea

Fig. 452   Forearm, Antebrachium;
transverse section through the lower third of
the forearm.

453
452

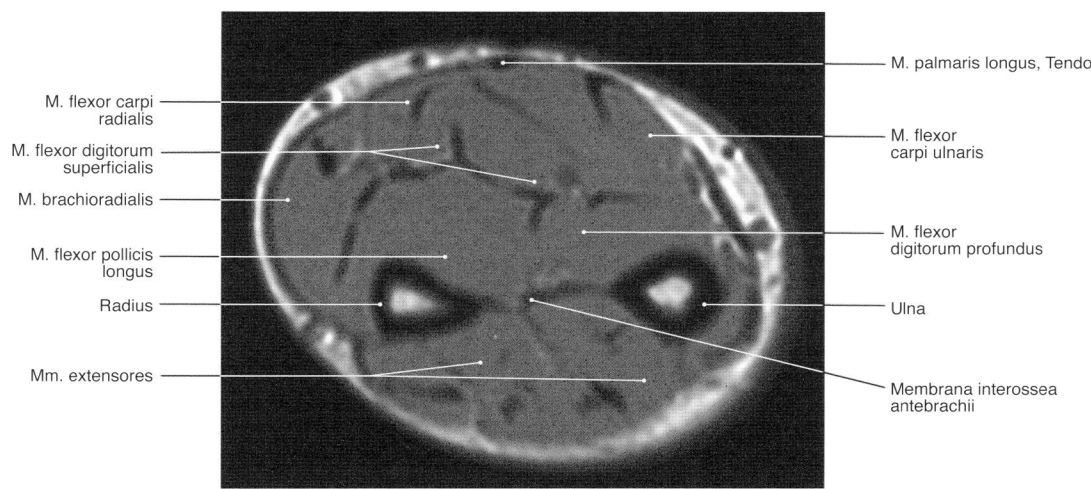

M. flexor carpi radialis

M. palmaris longus, Tendo

M. flexor digitorum superficialis

M. flexor carpi ulnaris

M. brachioradialis

M. flexor pollicis longus

M. flexor digitorum profundus

Radius

Ulna

Mm. extensores

Membrana interossea antebrachii

Fig. 453   Forearm, Antebrachium;
magnetic resonance tomographic image (MRI);
cross-section at the level of the middle of the forearm;
distal view.

Forearm and hand, transverse sections

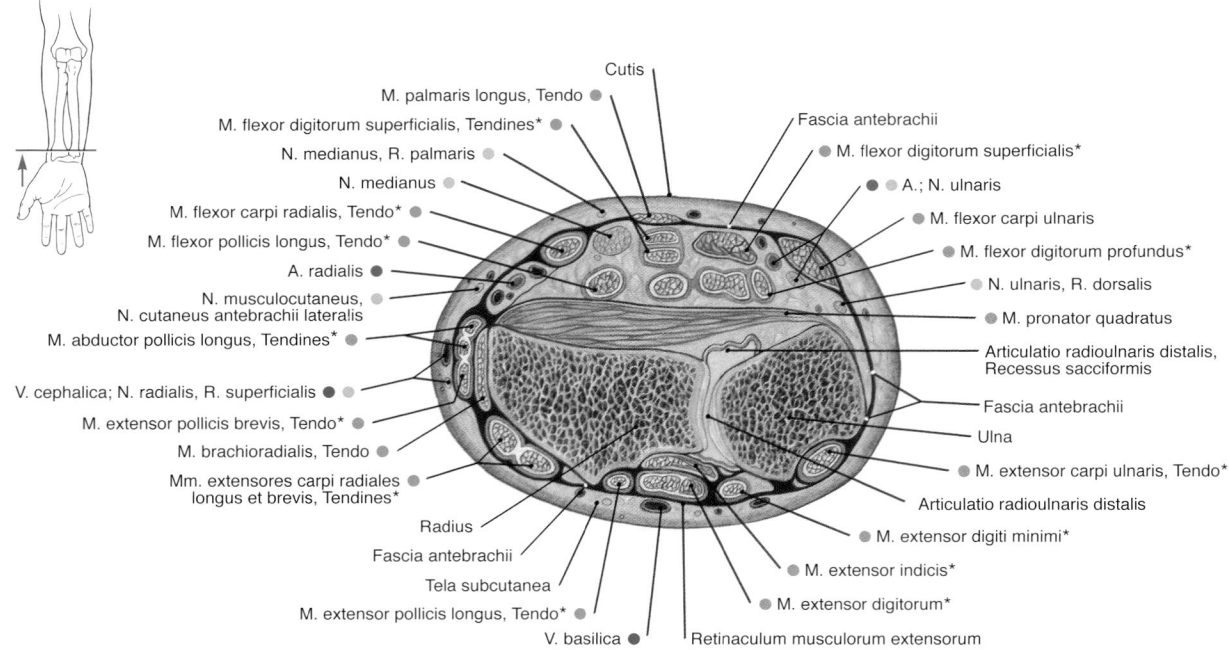

Cutis
M. palmaris longus, Tendo ●
M. flexor digitorum superficialis, Tendines* ●
N. medianus, R. palmaris ●
N. medianus ●
M. flexor carpi radialis, Tendo* ●
M. flexor pollicis longus, Tendo* ●
A. radialis ●
N. musculocutaneus,
N. cutaneus antebrachii lateralis
M. abductor pollicis longus, Tendines* ●

V. cephalica; N. radialis, R. superficialis ● ●
M. extensor pollicis brevis, Tendo* ●
M. brachioradialis, Tendo ●
Mm. extensores carpi radiales
longus et brevis, Tendines* ●
Radius
Fascia antebrachii
Tela subcutanea
M. extensor pollicis longus, Tendo* ●
V. basilica ●

Fascia antebrachii
● M. flexor digitorum superficialis*
● ● A.; N. ulnaris
● M. flexor carpi ulnaris
● M. flexor digitorum profundus*
● N. ulnaris, R. dorsalis
● M. pronator quadratus
Articulatio radioulnaris distalis,
Recessus sacciformis
Fascia antebrachii
Ulna
● M. extensor carpi ulnaris, Tendo*
Articulatio radioulnaris distalis
● M. extensor digiti minimi*
● M. extensor indicis*
● M. extensor digitorum*
Retinaculum musculorum extensorum

Fig. 454 Forearm, Antebrachium;
transverse section at the level of the distal radio-ulnar joint.
At this level, the muscle tendons marked with * run within
tendon sheaths, Vaginae tendinum.

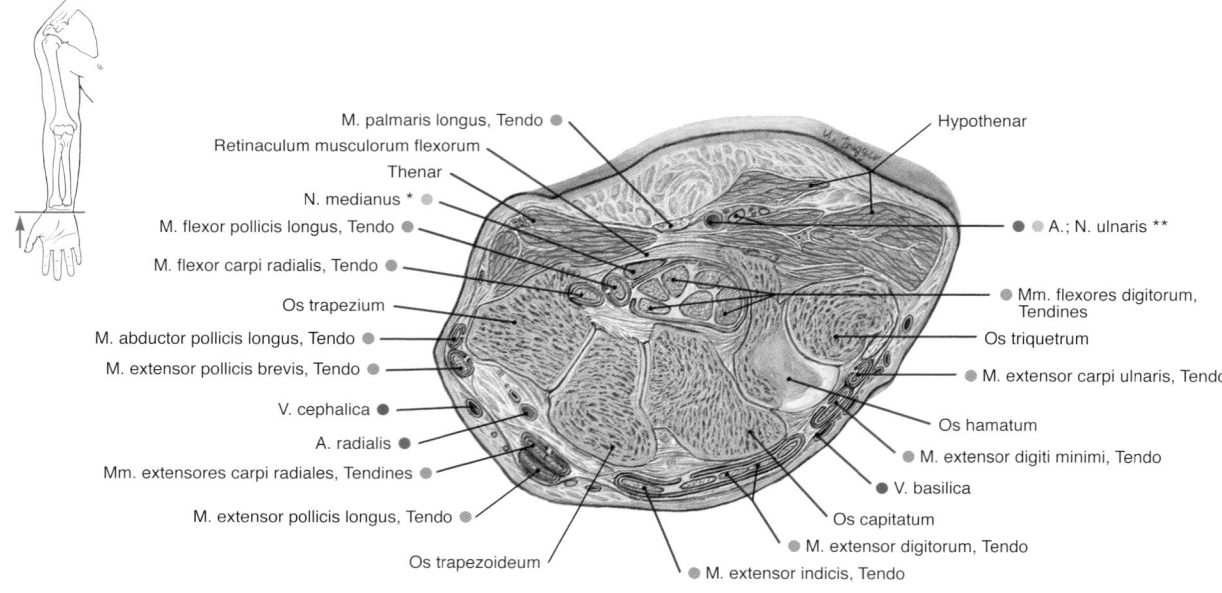

M. palmaris longus, Tendo ●
Retinaculum musculorum flexorum
Thenar
N. medianus * ●
M. flexor pollicis longus, Tendo ●
M. flexor carpi radialis, Tendo ●
Os trapezium
M. abductor pollicis longus, Tendo ●
M. extensor pollicis brevis, Tendo ●
V. cephalica ●
A. radialis ●
Mm. extensores carpi radiales, Tendines ●
M. extensor pollicis longus, Tendo ●
Os trapezoideum

Hypothenar
● ● A.; N. ulnaris **
● Mm. flexores digitorum,
Tendines
Os triquetrum
● M. extensor carpi ulnaris, Tendo
Os hamatum
● M. extensor digiti minimi, Tendo
● V. basilica
Os capitatum
● M. extensor digitorum, Tendo
● M. extensor indicis, Tendo

Fig. 455 Wrist, Carpus;
transverse section at the level of the hook of the hamate
bone, Hamulus ossis hamati.
* Carpal tunnel
** ulnar canal (loge de GUYON)

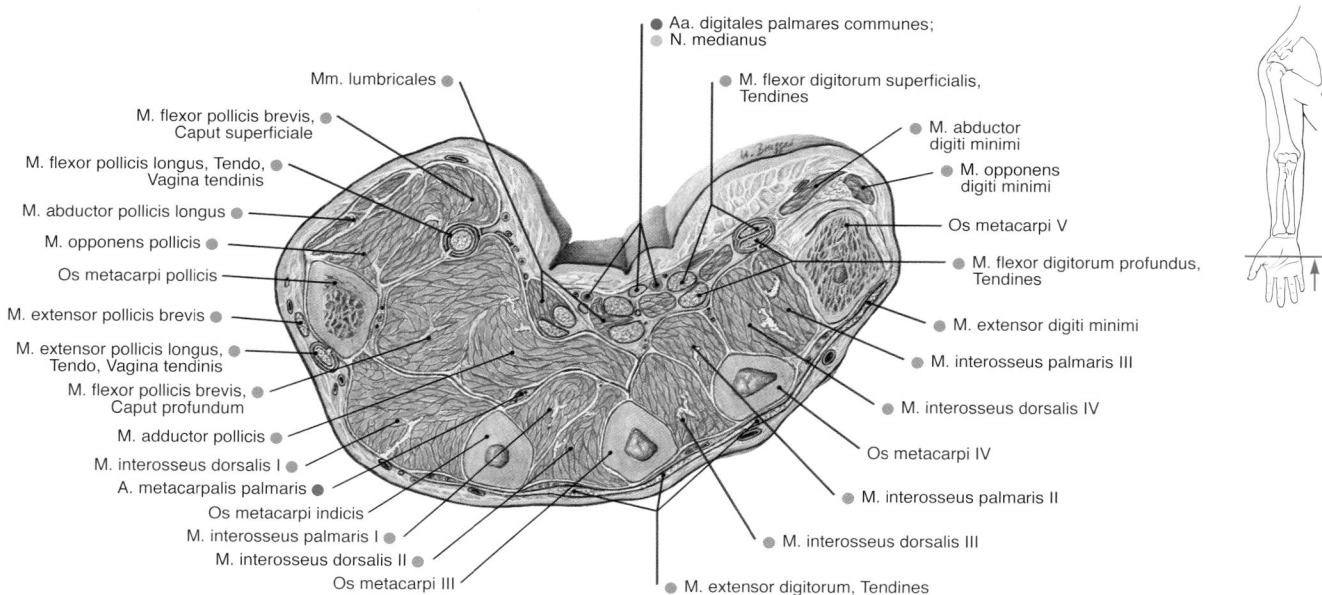

Aa. digitales palmares communes;
N. medianus

Mm. lumbricales

M. flexor pollicis brevis,
Caput superficiale

M. flexor pollicis longus, Tendo,
Vagina tendinis

M. abductor pollicis longus

M. opponens pollicis

Os metacarpi pollicis

M. extensor pollicis brevis

M. extensor pollicis longus,
Tendo, Vagina tendinis

M. flexor pollicis brevis,
Caput profundum

M. adductor pollicis

M. interosseus dorsalis I

A. metacarpalis palmaris

Os metacarpi indicis

M. interosseus palmaris I

M. interosseus dorsalis II

Os metacarpi III

M. flexor digitorum superficialis,
Tendines

M. abductor digiti minimi

M. opponens digiti minimi

Os metacarpi V

M. flexor digitorum profundus,
Tendines

M. extensor digiti minimi

M. interosseus palmaris III

M. interosseus dorsalis IV

Os metacarpi IV

M. interosseus palmaris II

M. interosseus dorsalis III

M. extensor digitorum, Tendines

Fig. 456   Metacarpus, Metacarpus; transverse section at the level of the third metacarpal bone.

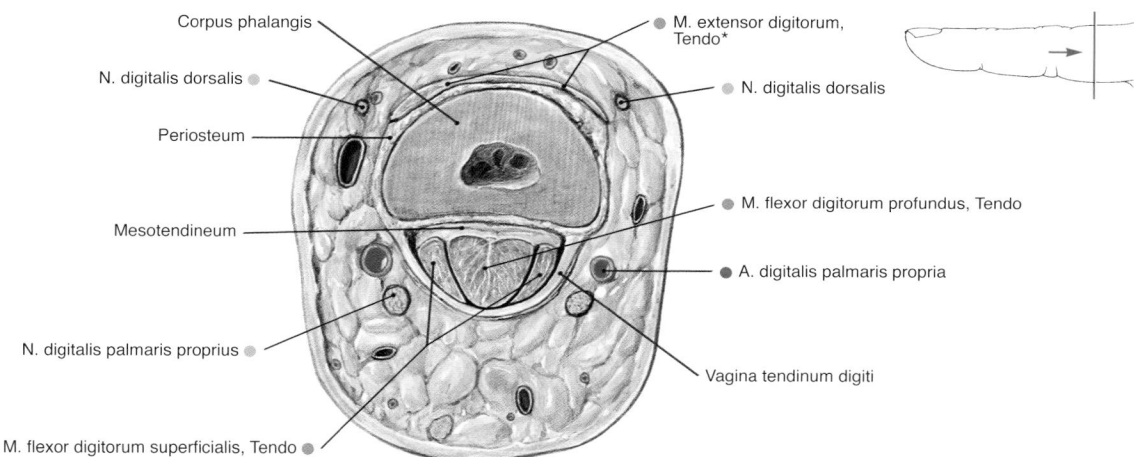

Corpus phalangis

N. digitalis dorsalis

Periosteum

Mesotendineum

N. digitalis palmaris proprius

M. flexor digitorum superficialis, Tendo

M. extensor digitorum,
Tendo*

N. digitalis dorsalis

M. flexor digitorum profundus, Tendo

A. digitalis palmaris propria

Vagina tendinum digiti

Fig. 457   Middle finger, Digitus medius [III];
transverse section through the shaft of the proximal phalanx.

* So-called dorsal aponeurosis into which the branching tendon
of the extensor digitorum muscle, as well as the tendons of the
interosseous and lumbrical muscles radiate

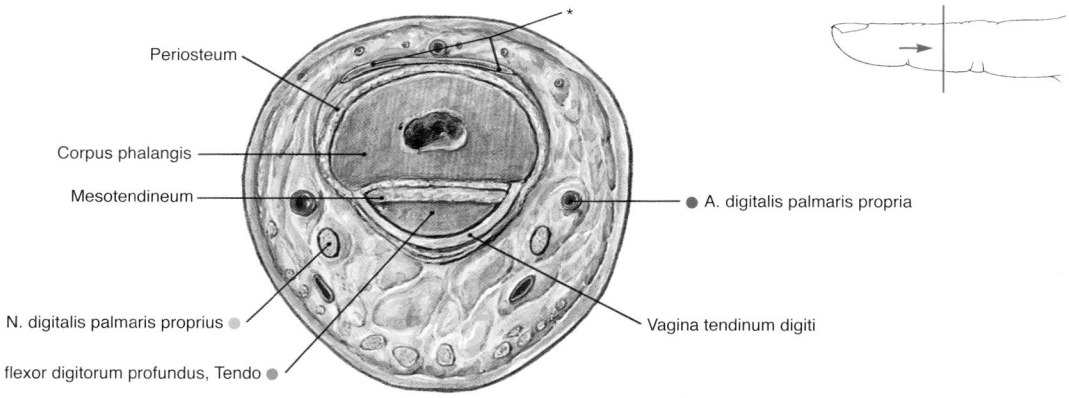

Periosteum

Corpus phalangis

Mesotendineum

N. digitalis palmaris proprius

M. flexor digitorum profundus, Tendo

A. digitalis palmaris propria

Vagina tendinum digiti

Fig. 458   Middle finger, Digitus medius [III];
transverse section through the shaft of the middle phalanx.

* So-called dorsal aponeurosis

Regions

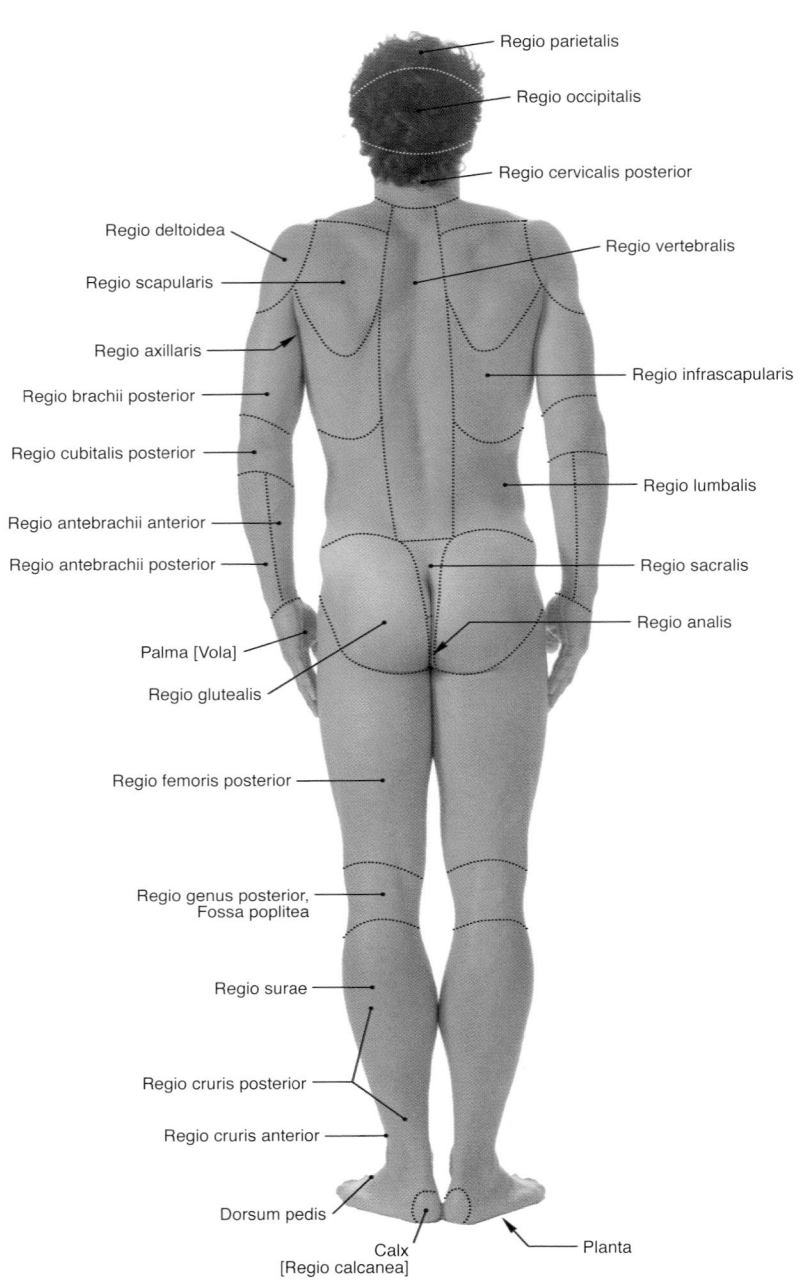

Regio parietalis

Regio occipitalis

Regio cervicalis posterior

Regio deltoidea

Regio scapularis

Regio vertebralis

Regio axillaris

Regio brachii posterior

Regio infrascapularis

Regio cubitalis posterior

Regio antebrachii anterior

Regio antebrachii posterior

Regio lumbalis

Regio sacralis

Palma [Vola]

Regio analis

Regio glutealis

Regio femoris posterior

Regio genus posterior,
Fossa poplitea

Regio surae

Regio cruris posterior

Regio cruris anterior

Dorsum pedis

Calx
[Regio calcanea]

Planta

Fig. 459   Regions of the human body, Regiones corporis.

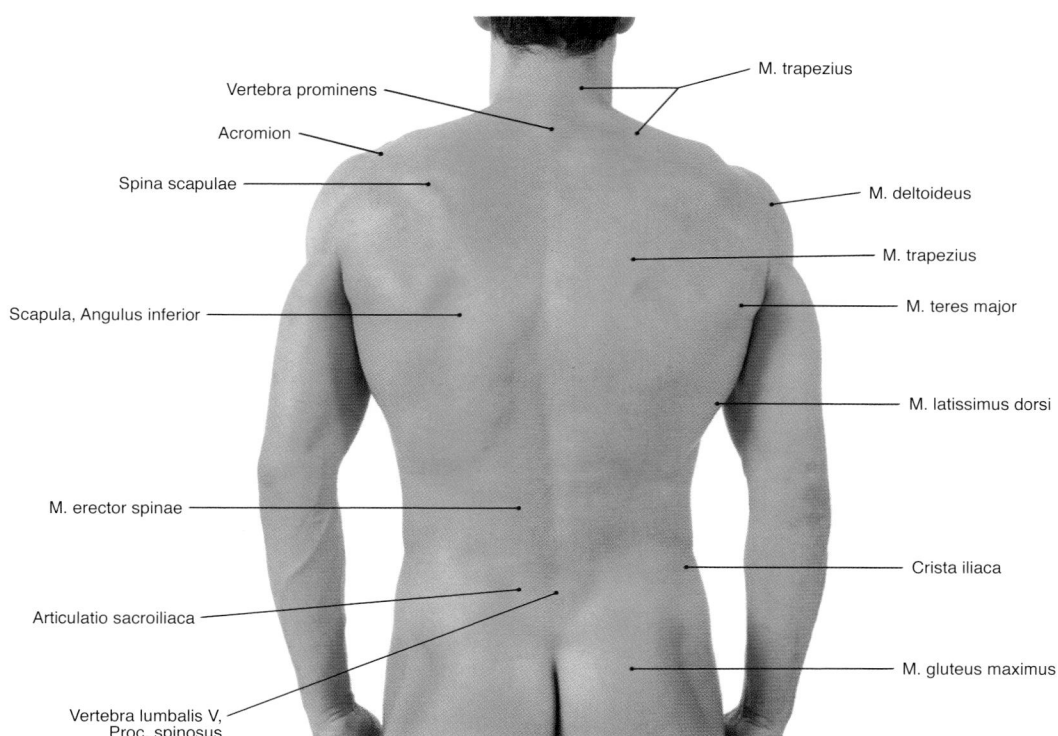

Vertebra prominens

Acromion

Spina scapulae

Scapula, Angulus inferior

M. erector spinae

Articulatio sacroiliaca

Vertebra lumbalis V, Proc. spinosus

M. trapezius

M. deltoideus

M. trapezius

M. teres major

M. latissimus dorsi

Crista iliaca

M. gluteus maximus

Fig. 460 Back, Dorsum; surface anatomy.

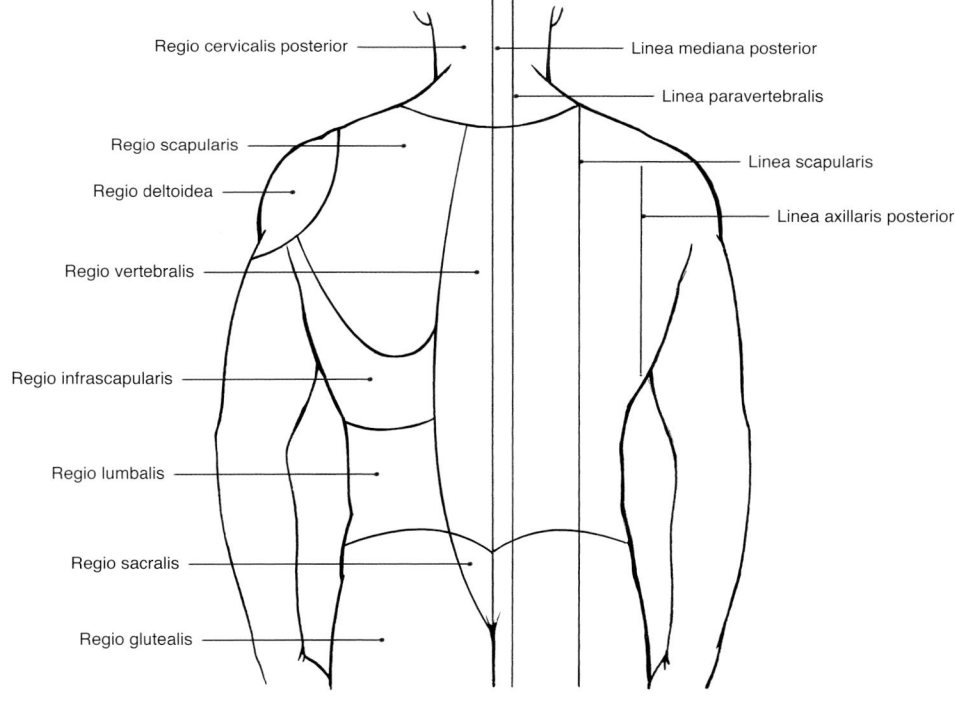

Regio cervicalis posterior

Regio scapularis

Regio deltoidea

Regio vertebralis

Regio infrascapularis

Regio lumbalis

Regio sacralis

Regio glutealis

Linea mediana posterior

Linea paravertebralis

Linea scapularis

Linea axillaris posterior

Fig. 461 Regions and orientation lines of the back.

Skeleton of the trunk

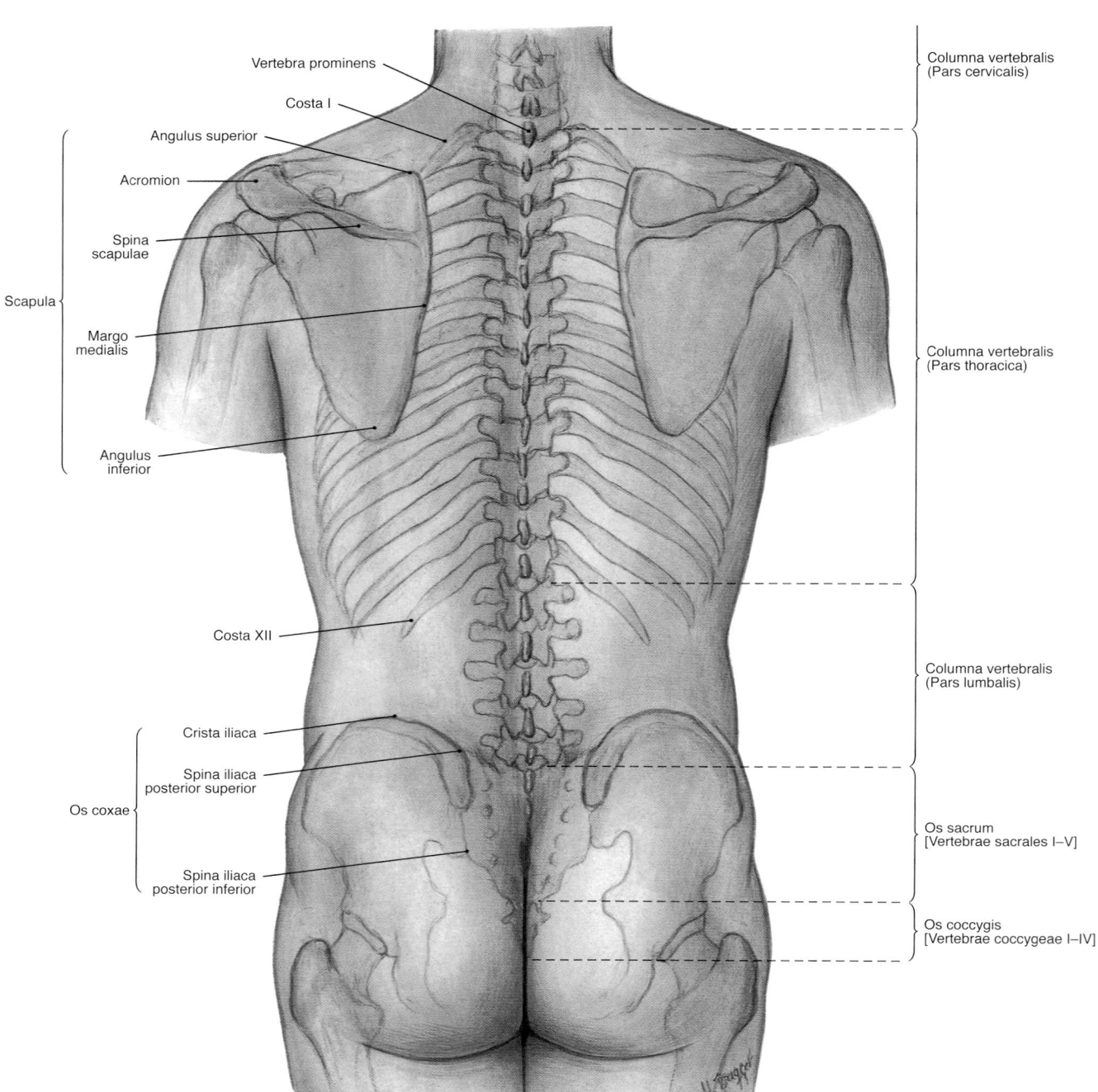

Vertebra prominens

Costa I

Angulus superior

Acromion

Spina scapulae

Scapula

Margo medialis

Angulus inferior

Costa XII

Crista iliaca

Spina iliaca posterior superior

Os coxae

Spina iliaca posterior inferior

Columna vertebralis (Pars cervicalis)

Columna vertebralis (Pars thoracica)

Columna vertebralis (Pars lumbalis)

Os sacrum [Vertebrae sacrales I–V]

Os coccygis [Vertebrae coccygeae I–IV]

Fig. 462 Skeletal system, Systema skeletale, of the trunk.

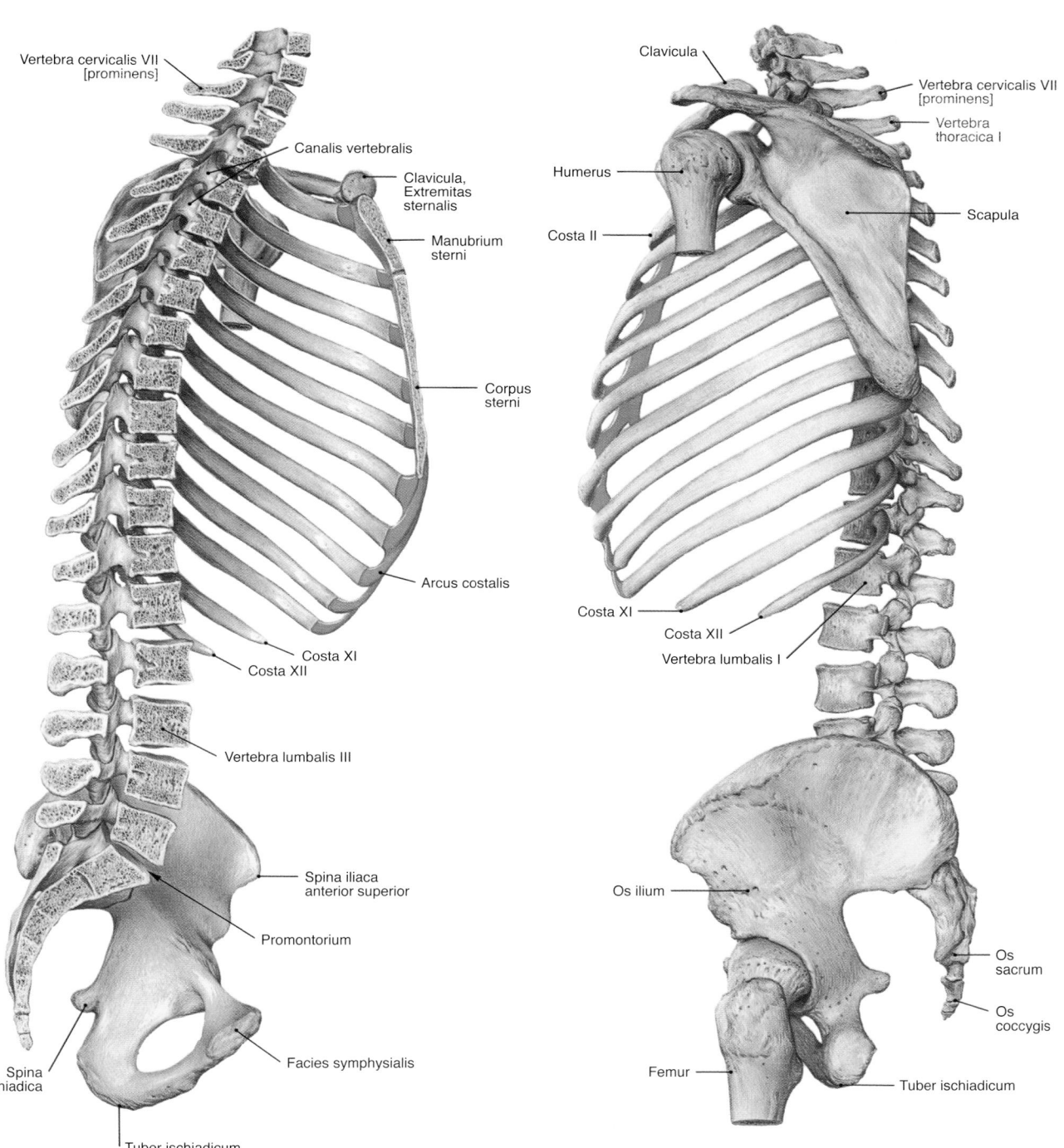

Vertebra cervicalis VII [prominens]

Canalis vertebralis

Clavicula, Extremitas sternalis

Manubrium sterni

Corpus sterni

Arcus costalis

Costa XI
Costa XII

Vertebra lumbalis III

Spina iliaca anterior superior

Promontorium

Spina ischiadica

Facies symphysialis

Tuber ischiadicum

Clavicula

Vertebra cervicalis VII [prominens]

Vertebra thoracica I

Humerus

Costa II

Scapula

Costa XI

Costa XII

Vertebra lumbalis I

Os ilium

Os sacrum

Os coccygis

Femur

Tuber ischiadicum

Fig. 463 Vertebral column, Columna vertebralis; pectoral girdle, Cingulum pectorale, and pelvic girdle, Cingulum pelvicum; median section through the vertebral column; medial view.

Fig. 464 Vertebral column, Columna vertebralis; pectoral girdle, Cingulum pectorale, and pelvic girdle, Cingulum pelvicum; median section through the vertebral column; viewed from the left.

Vertebral column

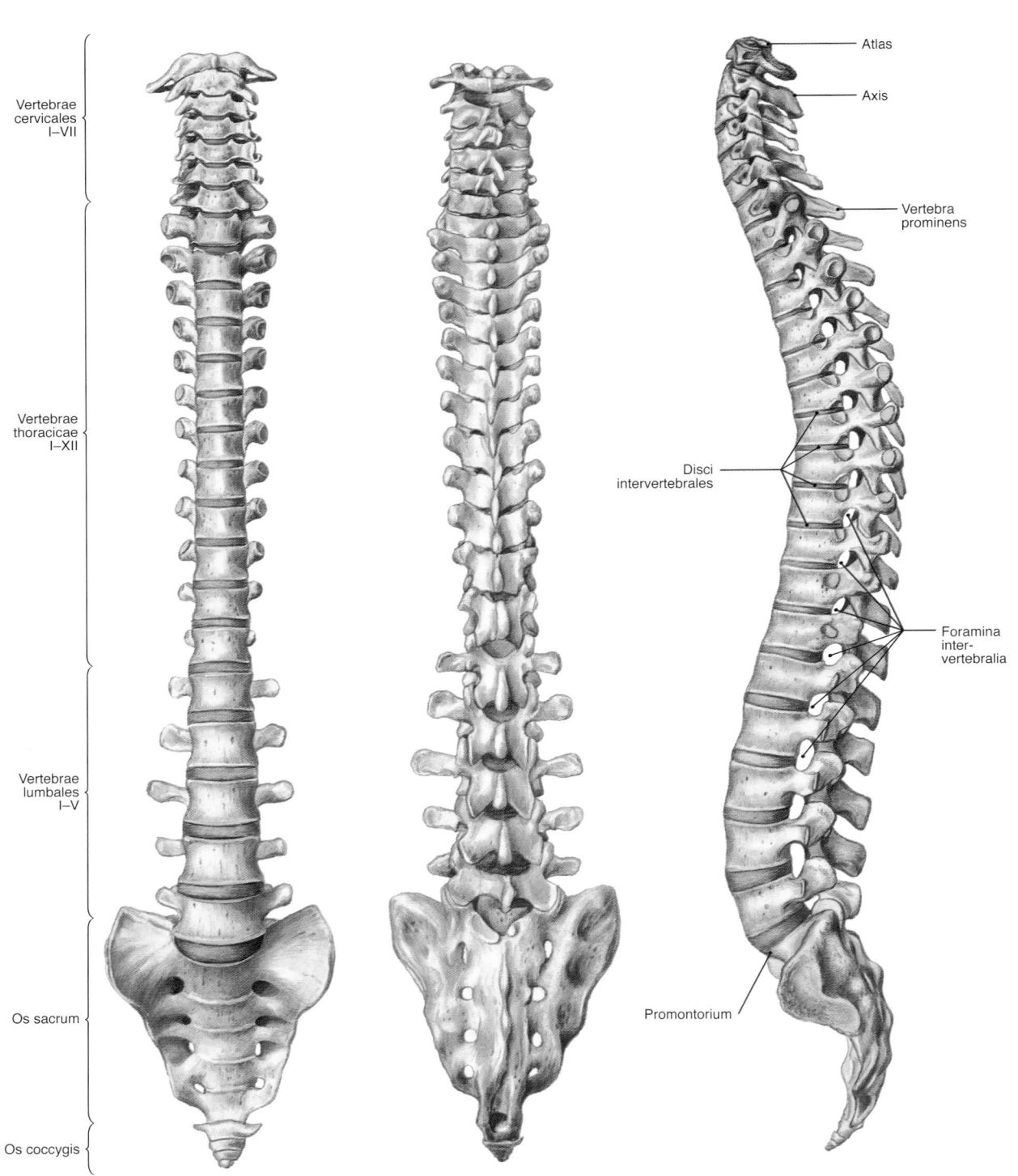

Vertebrae
cervicales
I–VII

Vertebrae
thoracicae
I–XII

Vertebrae
lumbales
I–V

Os sacrum

Os coccygis

Atlas

Axis

Vertebra
prominens

Disci
intervertebrales

Foramina
inter-
vertebralia

Promontorium

Fig. 465 Vertebral column,
Columna vertebralis;
ventral view.

Fig. 466 Vertebral column,
Columna vertebralis;
dorsal view.

Fig. 467 Vertebral column,
Columna vertebralis;
viewed from the left.

Vertebral column, development

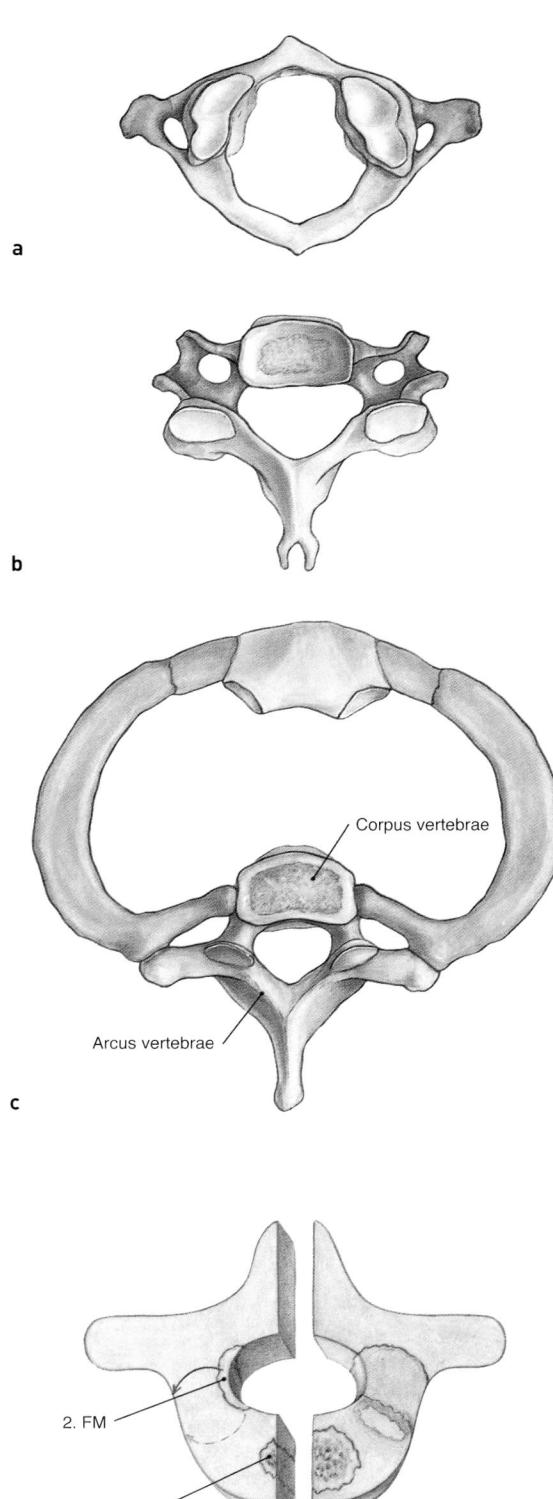

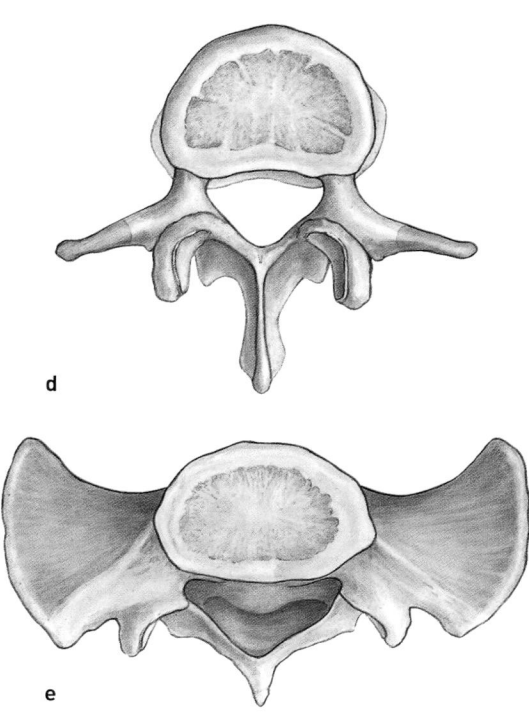

Corpus vertebrae

Arcus vertebrae

Fig. 468 a–e Regional characteristics of the vertebrae. Only in the thoracic region of the vertebral column do the lateral parts (labelled in red) remain separated and form ribs.

a First cervical vertebra, Atlas
b Fourth cervical vertebra, Vertebra cervicalis IV
c First thoracic vertebra, Vertebra thoracica I, with corresponding ribs, Costae, and sternum, Sternum
d Third lumbar vertebra, Vertebra lumbalis III
e Sacrum, Os sacrum

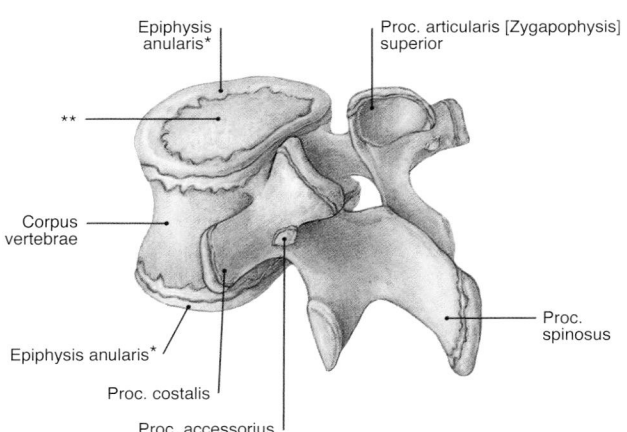

Epiphysis anularis*

Proc. articularis [Zygapophysis] superior

**

Corpus vertebrae

Proc. spinosus

Epiphysis anularis*

Proc. costalis

Proc. accessorius

2. FM

3.–6. FM

Fig. 469 Vertebral development.
Demonstration of the appearance of primary ossification centres in a lumbar vertebra (pedicle: second foetal month; corpus: third to sixth foetal month).
Synostosis of the ossification centres of the vertebral arch with those of the corpus occurs between the third and the sixth year of life.

Fig. 470 Vertebral development.
Circular ossification centres (= rims*) appear in the epiphyses of the vertebrae during the eighth year of life and fuse with the vertebral bodies until the eighteenth year of life.
The central portions of the epiphyses remain as hyaline cartilaginous laminae ** throughout life.
Secondary ossification centres (apophyses) develop at the processes.

Atlas and axis

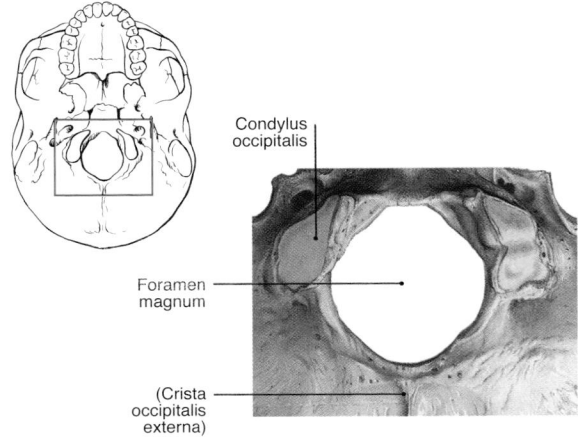

Condylus occipitalis

Foramen magnum

(Crista occipitalis externa)

Fig. 471 Occipital bone, Os occipitale; section illustrating the foramen magnum and the articular surfaces of the atlanto-occipital joint; inferior view.

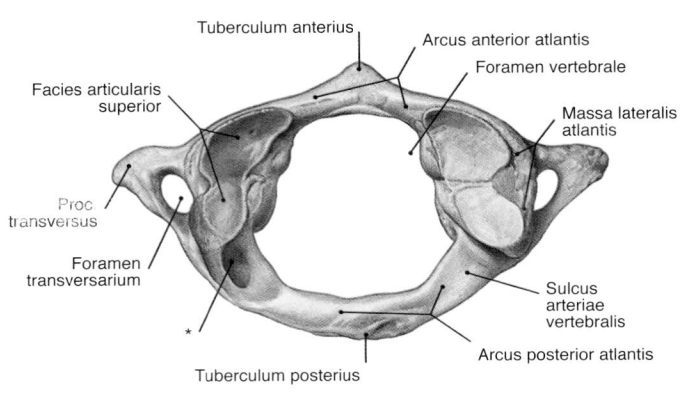

Tuberculum anterius

Arcus anterior atlantis

Foramen vertebrale

Facies articularis superior

Massa lateralis atlantis

Proc. transversus

Foramen transversarium

Sulcus arteriae vertebralis

*

Arcus posterior atlantis

Tuberculum posterius

Fig. 472 First cervical vertebra, Atlas; superior view.
The superior articular surfaces of the atlas are frequently divided.
* Canalis arteriae vertebralis as a variation

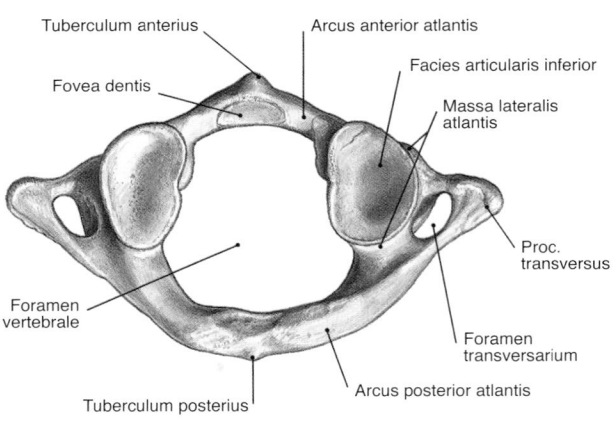

Tuberculum anterius

Arcus anterior atlantis

Fovea dentis

Facies articularis inferior

Massa lateralis atlantis

Proc. transversus

Foramen vertebrale

Foramen transversarium

Tuberculum posterius

Arcus posterior atlantis

Fig. 473 First cervical vertebra, Atlas; inferior view.

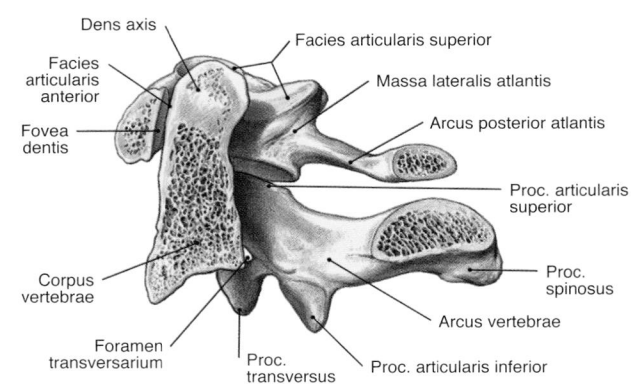

Dens axis

Facies articularis superior

Facies articularis anterior

Massa lateralis atlantis

Fovea dentis

Arcus posterior atlantis

Proc. articularis superior

Corpus vertebrae

Proc. spinosus

Arcus vertebrae

Foramen transversarium

Proc. transversus

Proc. articularis inferior

Fig. 474 First and second cervical vertebrae, Atlas et Axis; median section.

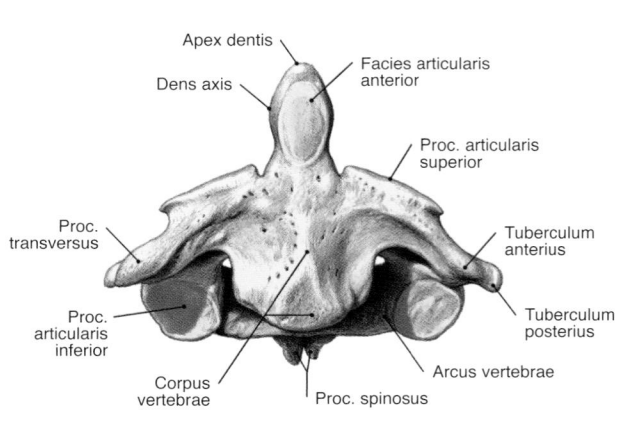

Apex dentis

Dens axis

Facies articularis anterior

Proc. articularis superior

Tuberculum anterius

Proc. transversus

Tuberculum posterius

Proc. articularis inferior

Corpus vertebrae

Proc. spinosus

Arcus vertebrae

Fig. 475 Second cervical vertebra, Axis; ventral view.

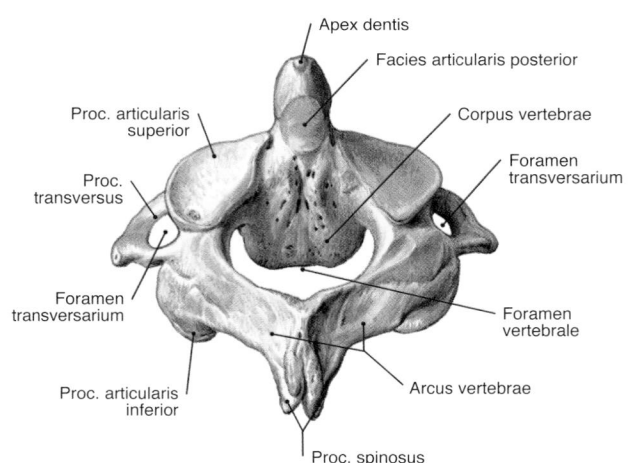

Apex dentis

Facies articularis posterior

Proc. articularis superior

Corpus vertebrae

Proc. transversus

Foramen transversarium

Foramen transversarium

Foramen vertebrale

Proc. articularis inferior

Arcus vertebrae

Proc. spinosus

Fig. 476 Second cervical vertebra, Axis; dorsosuperior view.

Cervical vertebrae

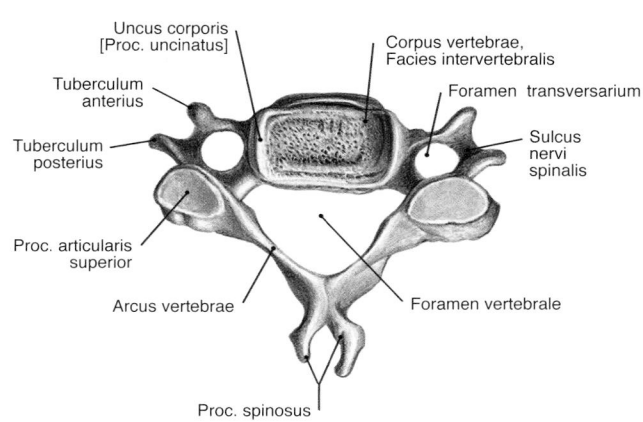

Fig. 477   Fifth cervical vertebra, Vertebra cervicalis V; superior view.
The tips of the spinous processes of the cervical vertebrae II–VI are frequently divided.

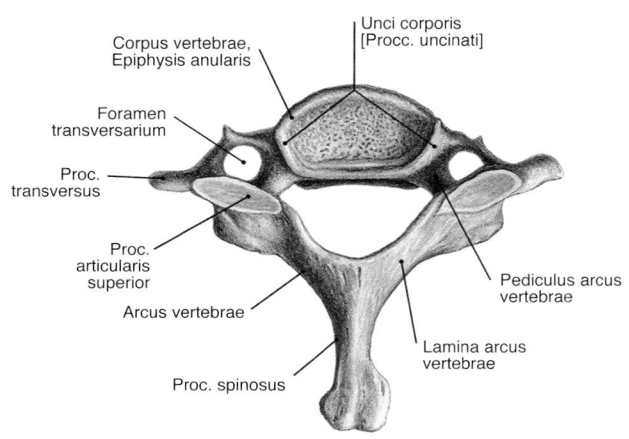

Fig. 478   Seventh cervical vertebra, Vertebra cervicalis VII; superior view.
In general the seventh cervical vertebra can be easily identified by its protruding spinous process and is referred to as vertebra prominens. In fact, the spinous process of the first thoracic vertebra often protrudes even further.

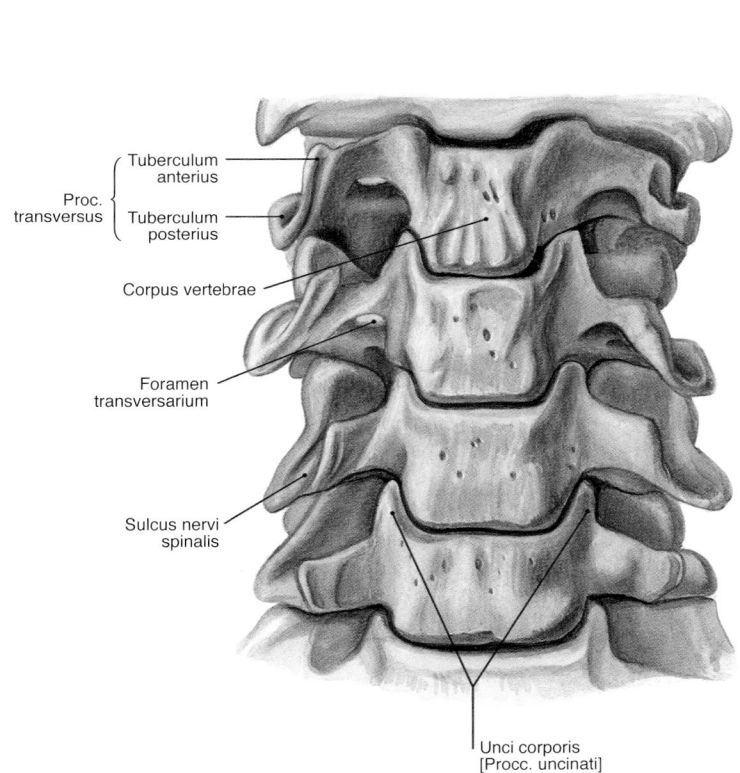

Fig. 479   Second to seventh cervical vertebrae, Vertebrae cervicales II–VII; ventral view.

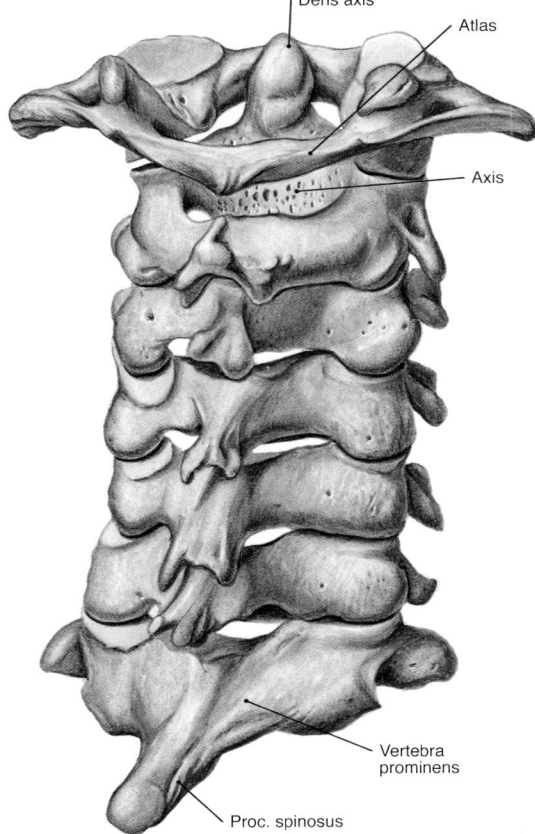

Fig. 480   First to seventh cervical vertebrae, Vertebrae cervicales I–VII; dorsolateral view.

Thoracic and lumbar vertebrae

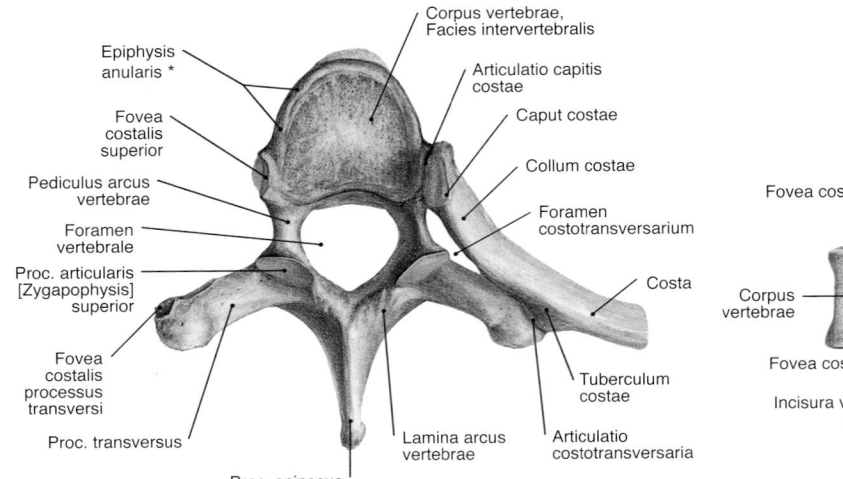

Corpus vertebrae, Facies intervertebralis
Epiphysis anularis *
Articulatio capitis costae
Fovea costalis superior
Caput costae
Pediculus arcus vertebrae
Collum costae
Foramen vertebrale
Foramen costotransversarium
Proc. articularis [Zygapophysis] superior
Costa
Fovea costalis processus transversi
Tuberculum costae
Proc. transversus
Lamina arcus vertebrae
Articulatio costotransversaria
Proc. spinosus

Fig. 481 Vertebra, Vertebra;
typical structural features exemplified by the
fifth thoracic vertebra;
superior view.
* Also: rim of vertebral body

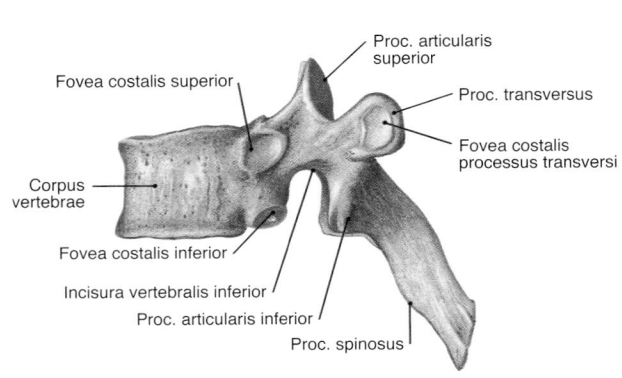

Fovea costalis superior
Proc. articularis superior
Proc. transversus
Corpus vertebrae
Fovea costalis processus transversi
Fovea costalis inferior
Incisura vertebralis inferior
Proc. articularis inferior
Proc. spinosus

Fig. 482 Sixth thoracic vertebra, Vertebra thoracica VI;
viewed from the left.

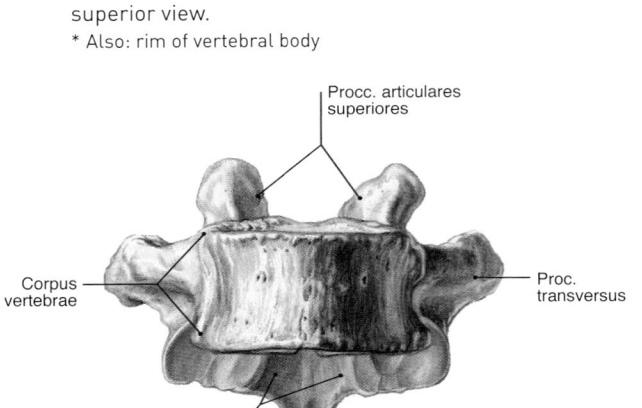

Procc. articulares superiores
Corpus vertebrae
Proc. transversus
Arcus vertebrae
Proc. spinosus

Fig. 483 Tenth thoracic vertebra, Vertebra thoracica X;
ventral view.

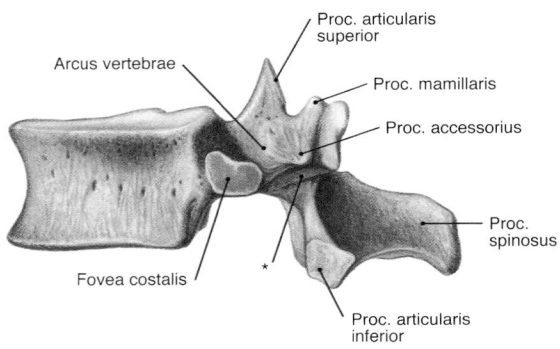

Proc. articularis superior
Arcus vertebrae
Proc. mamillaris
Proc. accessorius
Proc. spinosus
Fovea costalis
Proc. articularis inferior

Fig. 484 Twelfth thoracic vertebra, Vertebra thoracica XII;
viewed from the left.
* Region of the vertebral arch between the superior and
inferior articular processes
("isthmus" = interarticular portion)

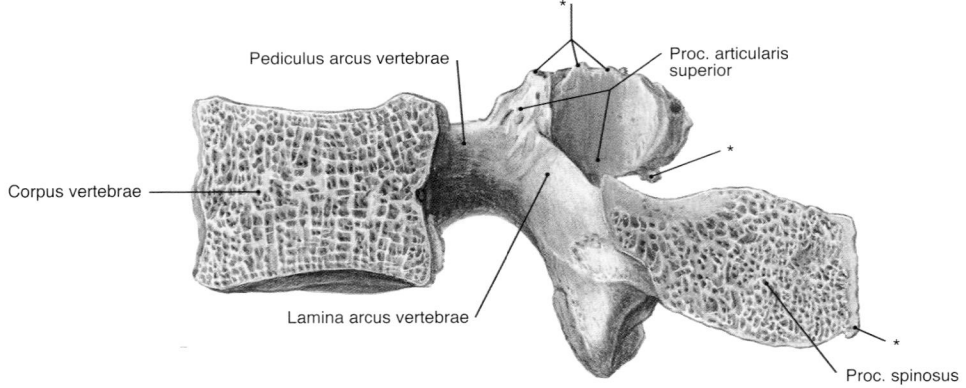

Pediculus arcus vertebrae
Proc. articularis superior
Corpus vertebrae
Lamina arcus vertebrae
Proc. spinosus

Fig. 485 Third lumbar vertebra, Vertebra lumbalis III;
median section; specimen of an older individual.
* Ossification of the ligamentous insertions

Thoracic and lumbar vertebrae

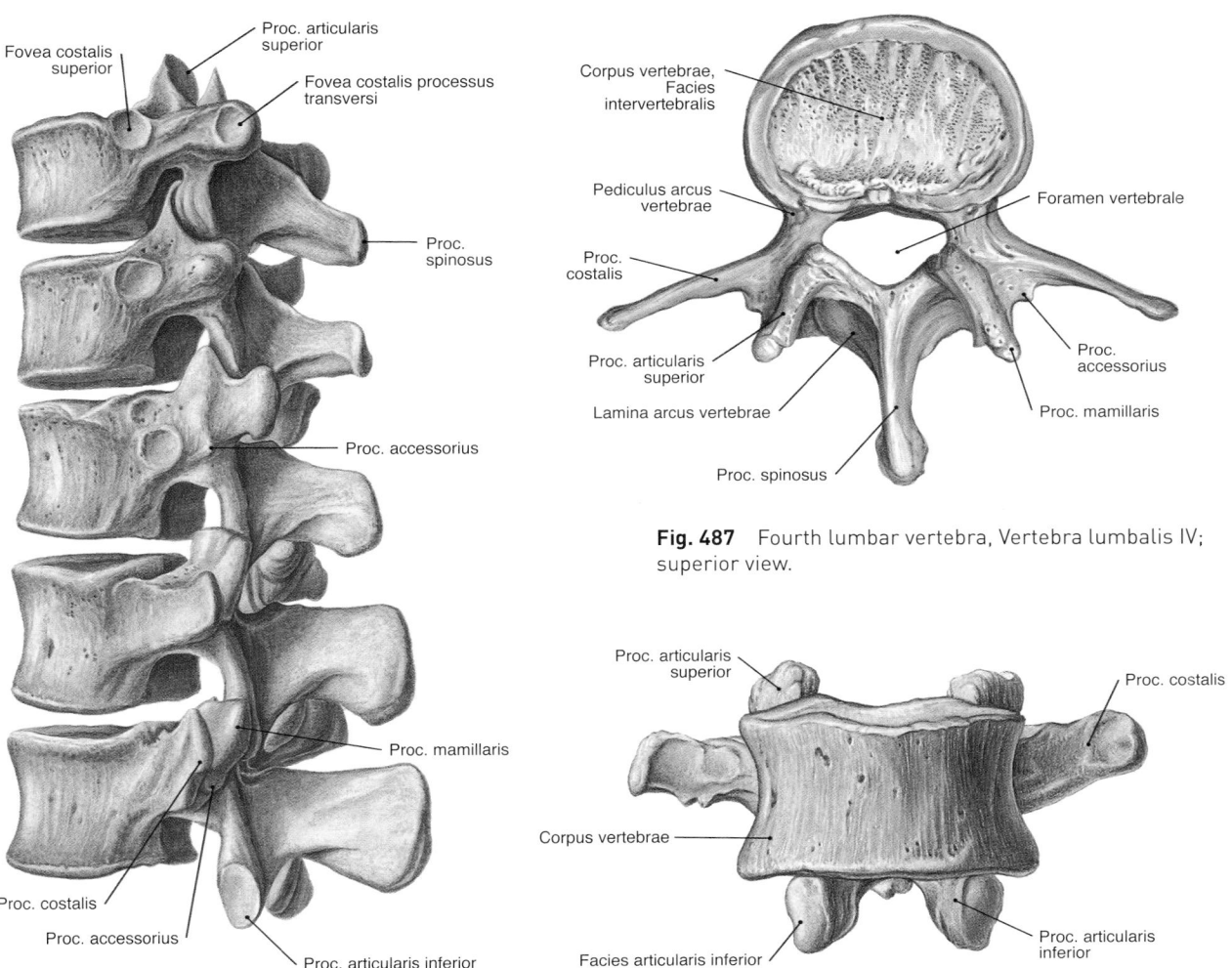

Proc. articularis superior

Fovea costalis superior

Fovea costalis processus transversi

Proc. spinosus

Proc. accessorius

Proc. mamillaris

Proc. costalis

Proc. accessorius

Proc. articularis inferior

Corpus vertebrae, Facies intervertebralis

Pediculus arcus vertebrae

Foramen vertebrale

Proc. costalis

Proc. articularis superior

Lamina arcus vertebrae

Proc. accessorius

Proc. mamillaris

Proc. spinosus

Fig. 487   Fourth lumbar vertebra, Vertebra lumbalis IV; superior view.

Proc. articularis superior

Proc. costalis

Corpus vertebrae

Facies articularis inferior

Proc. articularis inferior

Fig. 486   Tenth to twelfth thoracic vertebrae, Vertebrae thoracicae X–XII, and first to second lumbar vertebrae, Vertebrae lumbales I–II; dorsal view from the left.

Fig. 488   Fourth lumbar vertebra, Vertebra lumbalis IV; ventral view.

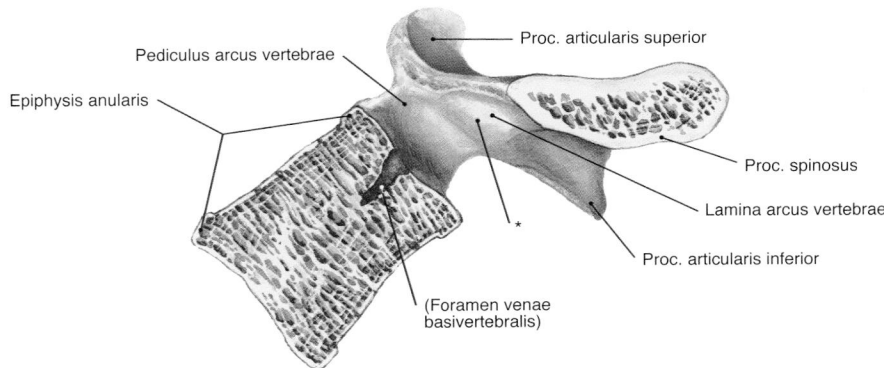

Pediculus arcus vertebrae

Epiphysis anularis

Proc. articularis superior

Proc. spinosus

Lamina arcus vertebrae

*

Proc. articularis inferior

(Foramen venae basivertebralis)

Fig. 489   Fifth lumbar vertebra, Vertebra lumbalis V; median section.
Note the characteristic wedge-shape of the body of the fifth lumbar vertebra.

* Region of the vertebral arch between the superior and inferior articular process. Here in the fifth and less frequently in the fourth lumbar vertebra a cleft, bridged by connective tissue (spondylolysis) can be formed. This is probably caused by local bending stress. As a consequence, the superior vertebra may slip (olisthesis) onto the inferior vertebra (spondylolisthesis).

Sacrum

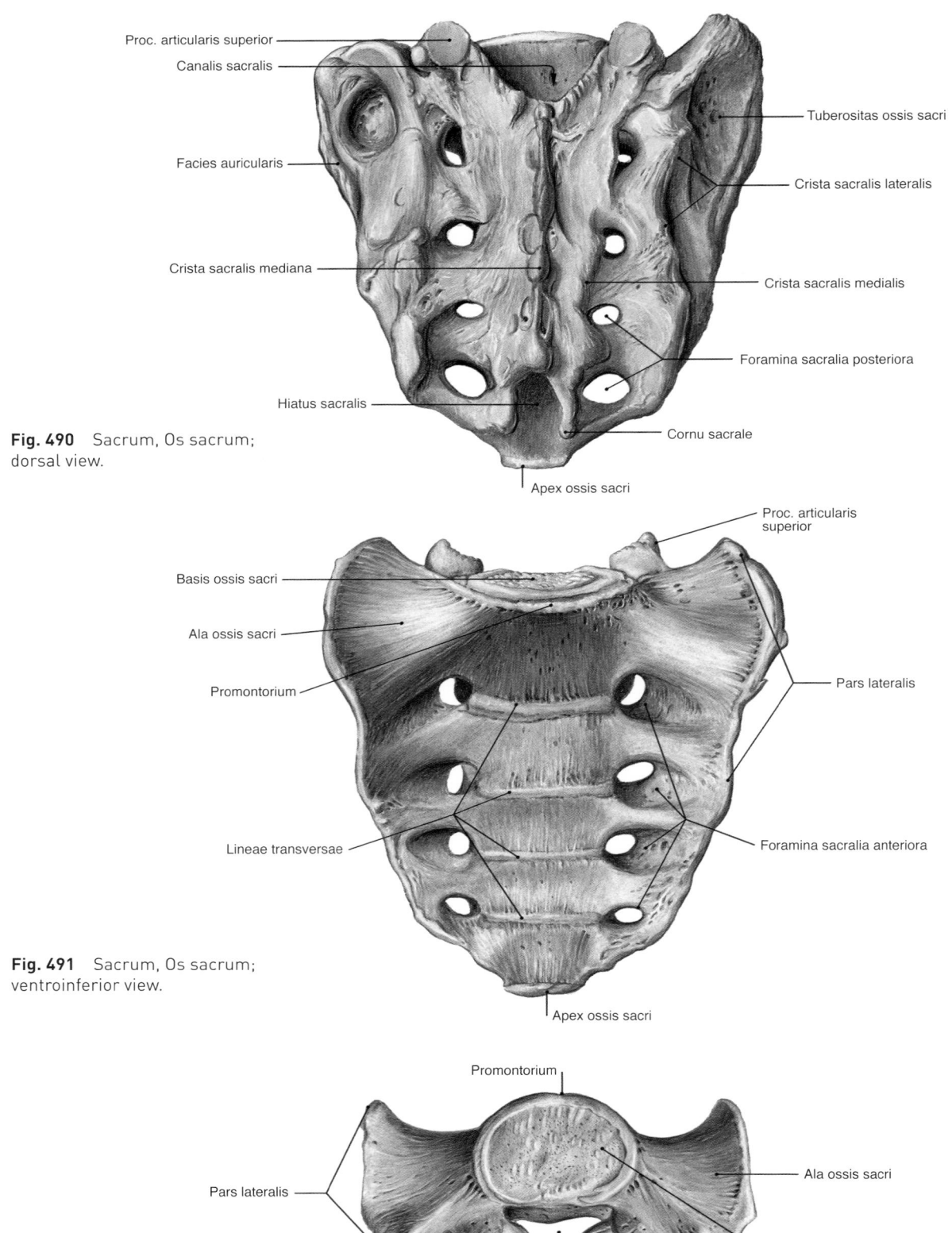

Proc. articularis superior
Canalis sacralis
Tuberositas ossis sacri
Facies auricularis
Crista sacralis lateralis
Crista sacralis mediana
Crista sacralis medialis
Foramina sacralia posteriora
Hiatus sacralis
Cornu sacrale
Apex ossis sacri

Fig. 490 Sacrum, Os sacrum; dorsal view.

Proc. articularis superior
Basis ossis sacri
Ala ossis sacri
Promontorium
Pars lateralis
Lineae transversae
Foramina sacralia anteriora
Apex ossis sacri

Fig. 491 Sacrum, Os sacrum; ventroinferior view.

Promontorium
Ala ossis sacri
Pars lateralis
Basis ossis sacri
Proc. articularis superior
Crista sacralis medialis
Canalis sacralis
Crista sacralis mediana

Fig. 492 Sacrum, Os sacrum; the bone has been sectioned at the level of the second sacral vertebra; superior view.

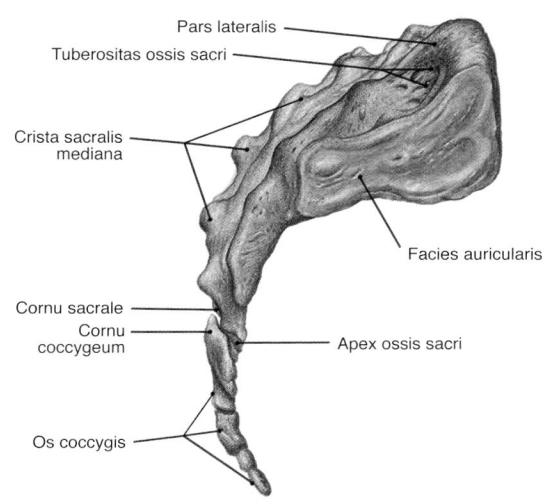

Pars lateralis
Tuberositas ossis sacri
Crista sacralis mediana
Cornu sacrale
Cornu coccygeum
Os coccygis
Facies auricularis
Apex ossis sacri

Fig. 493   Sacrum, Os sacrum; viewed from the right.

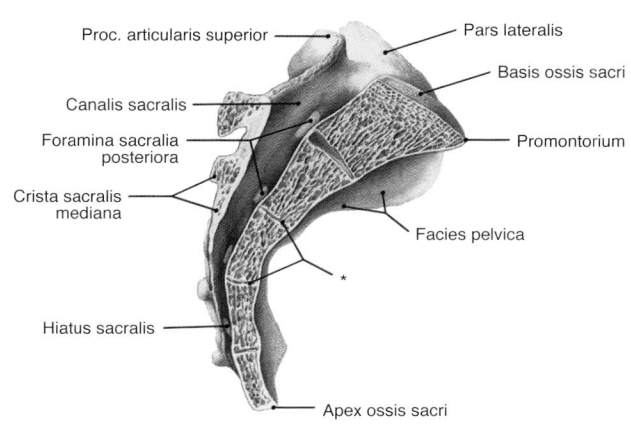

Proc. articularis superior
Canalis sacralis
Foramina sacralia posteriora
Crista sacralis mediana
Hiatus sacralis
Pars lateralis
Basis ossis sacri
Promontorium
Facies pelvica
*
Apex ossis sacri

Fig. 494   Sacrum, Os sacrum; median section.
* Remnants of intervertebral disc tissue persist even in the adult.

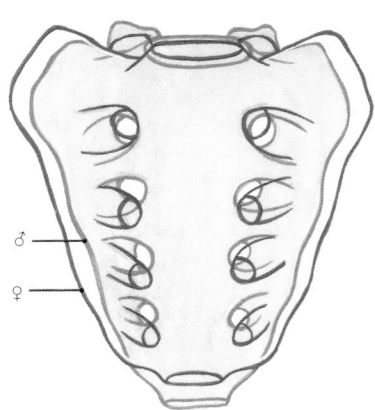

♂
♀

Fig. 495   Sacrum, Os sacrum; gender differences.

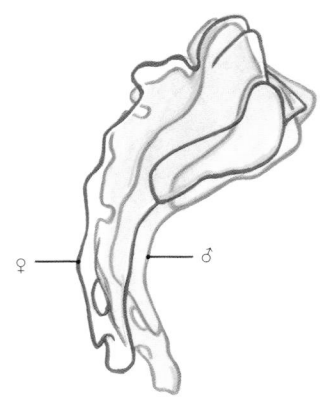

♀   ♂

Fig. 496   Sacrum, Os sacrum; gender differences.

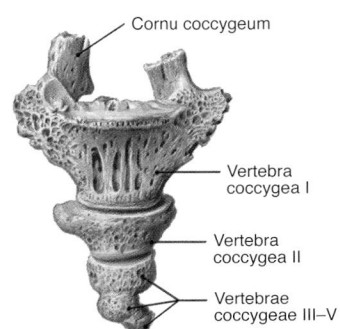

Cornu coccygeum
Vertebra coccygea I
Vertebra coccygea II
Vertebrae coccygeae III–V

Fig. 497   Coccyx, Os coccygis; ventrosuperior view.

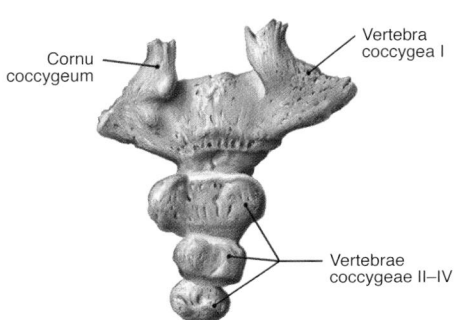

Cornu coccygeum
Vertebra coccygea I
Vertebrae coccygeae II–IV

Fig. 498   Coccyx, Os coccygis; dorsoinferior view.

Cervical part of the vertebral column, radiography

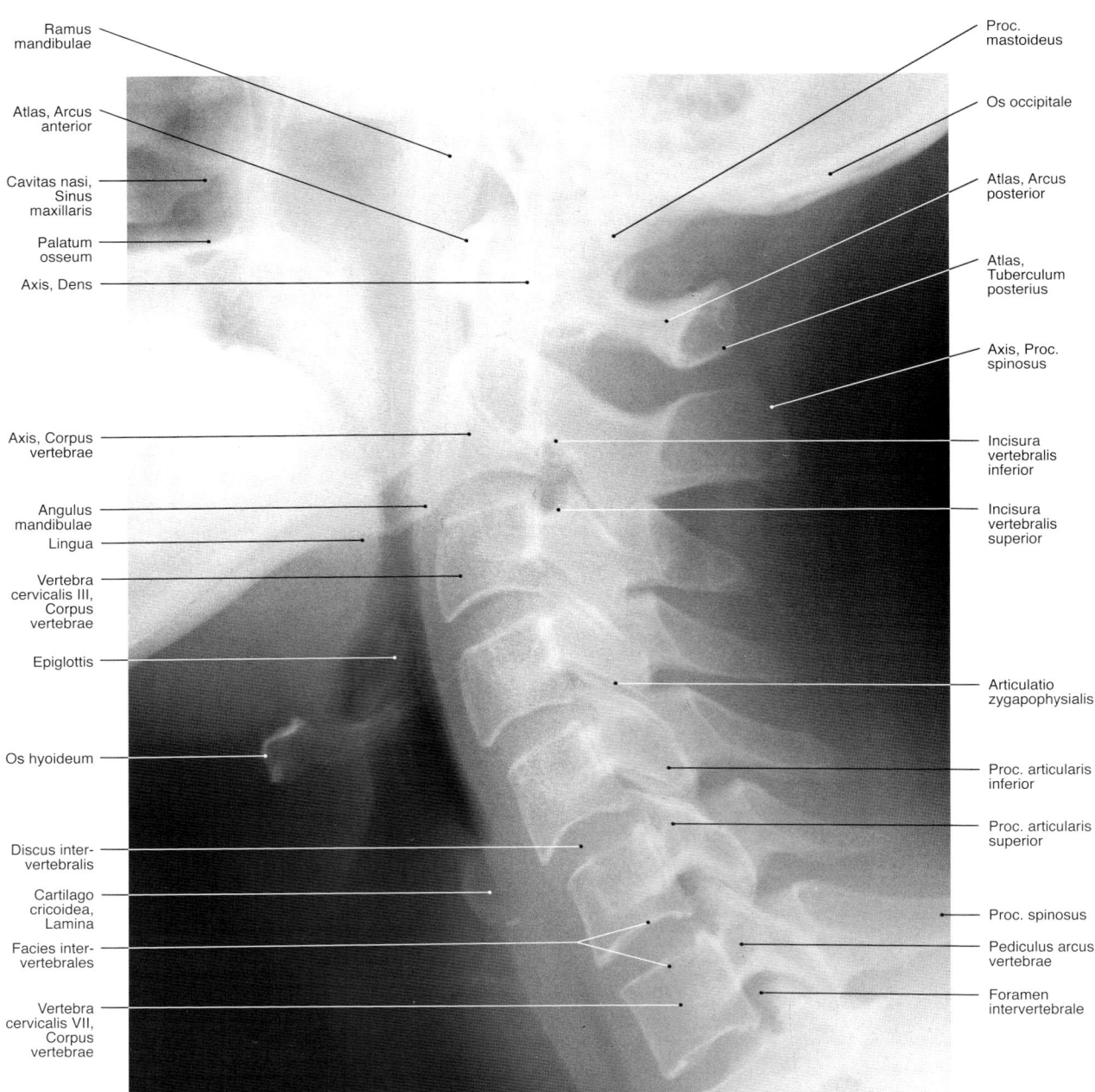

Ramus
mandibulae

Atlas, Arcus
anterior

Cavitas nasi,
Sinus
maxillaris

Palatum
osseum

Axis, Dens

Axis, Corpus
vertebrae

Angulus
mandibulae

Lingua

Vertebra
cervicalis III,
Corpus
vertebrae

Epiglottis

Os hyoideum

Discus inter-
vertebralis

Cartilago
cricoidea,
Lamina

Facies inter-
vertebrales

Vertebra
cervicalis VII,
Corpus
vertebrae

Proc.
mastoideus

Os occipitale

Atlas, Arcus
posterior

Atlas,
Tuberculum
posterius

Axis, Proc.
spinosus

Incisura
vertebralis
inferior

Incisura
vertebralis
superior

Articulatio
zygapophysialis

Proc. articularis
inferior

Proc. articularis
superior

Proc. spinosus

Pediculus arcus
vertebrae

Foramen
intervertebrale

Fig. 499 Cervical vertebrae, Vertebrae cervicales;
lateral radiograph of the cervical part of the vertebral column;
upright position; the central beam is directed
onto the third cervical vertebra;
shoulders are pulled downwards.

Cervical part of the vertebral column, radiography

Proc. spinosus ——

Proc. transversus ——

Unci corporum
[Procc. uncinati]

Vertebra cervicalis VI, ——
Corpus vertebrae

*

Trachea ——

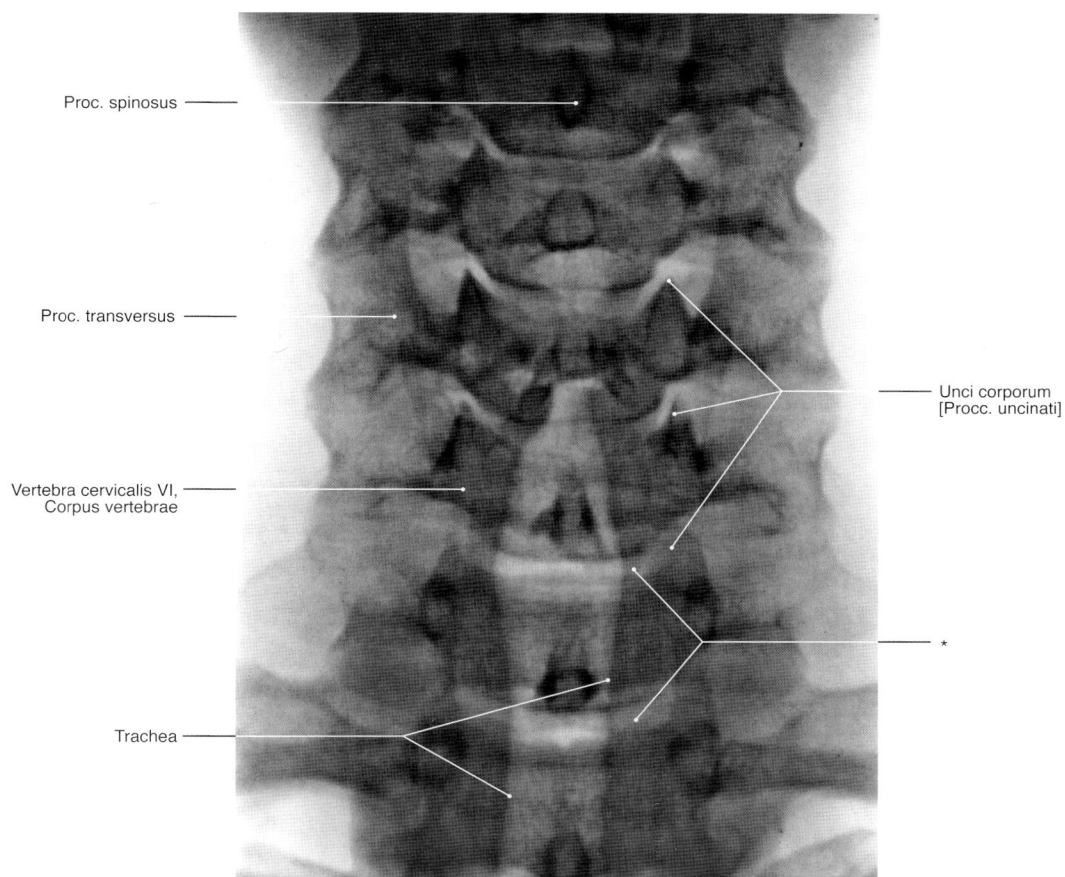

Fig. 500 Cervical vertebrae, Vertebrae cervicales;
AP-radiograph of the cervical part of the vertebral column;
upright position; the central beam is directed
onto the third cervical vertebra.
* Intervertebral disc spaces

Thoracic part of the vertebral column, radiography

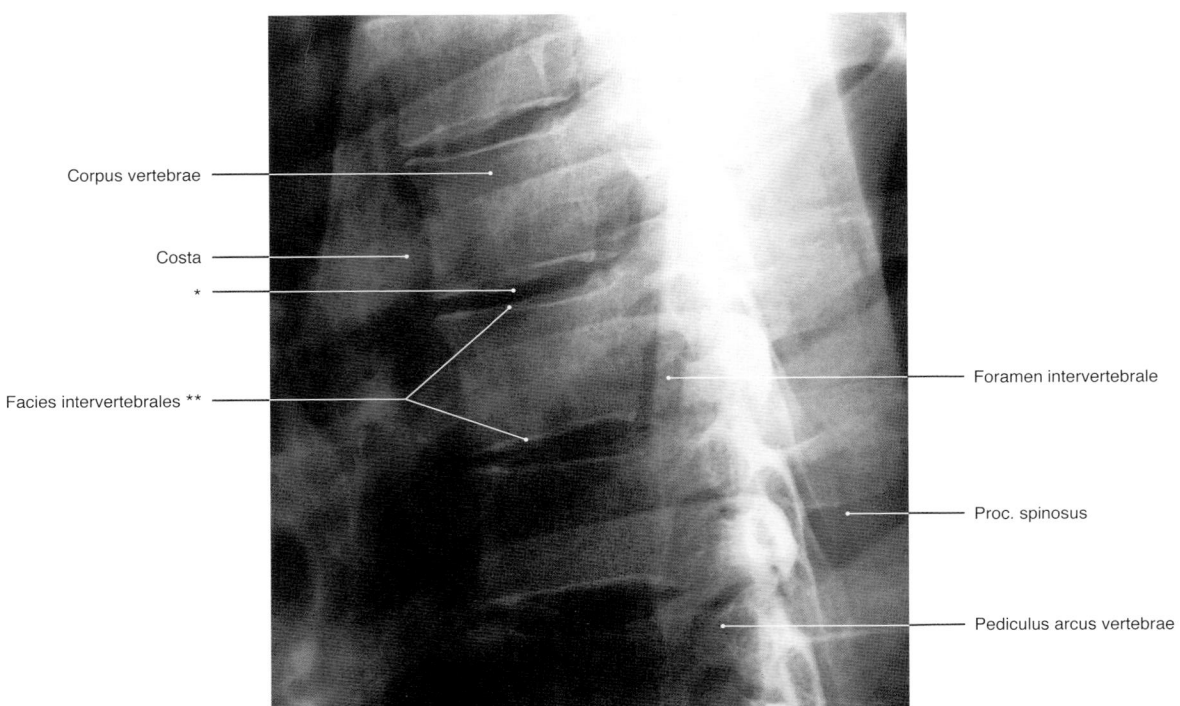

Corpus vertebrae

Costa

*

Facies intervertebrales **

Foramen intervertebrale

Proc. spinosus

Pediculus arcus vertebrae

Fig. 501   Thoracic vertebrae, Vertebrae thoracicae;
lateral radiograph of the thoracic part of the vertebral column;
upright position with the thorax in inspiration;
the central beam is directed onto the sixth thoracic vertebra.

*   Intervertebral disc space
** Clinical term: end-plates

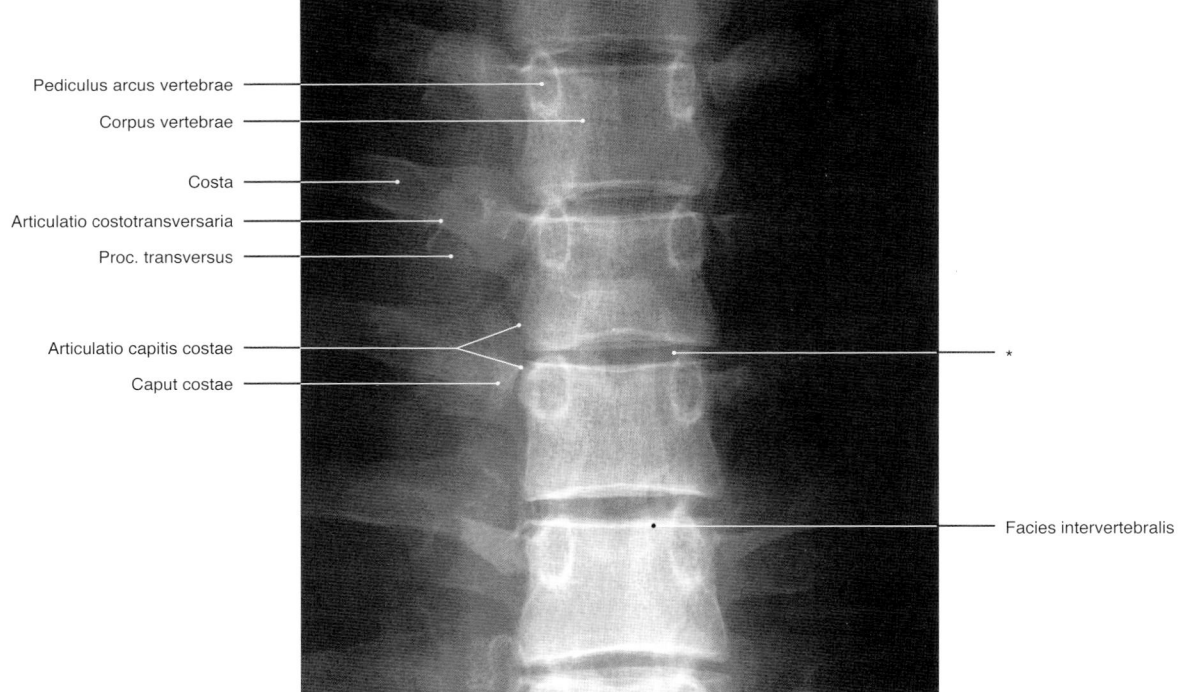

Pediculus arcus vertebrae

Corpus vertebrae

Costa

Articulatio costotransversaria

Proc. transversus

Articulatio capitis costae

Caput costae

*

Facies intervertebralis

Fig. 502   Thoracic vertebrae, Vertebrae thoracicae;
AP-radiograph of the thoracic part of the vertebral column;
upright position with the thorax in inspiration;
the central beam is directed onto the sixth thoracic vertebra.

* Intervertebral disc space

Lumbar part of the vertebral column, radiography

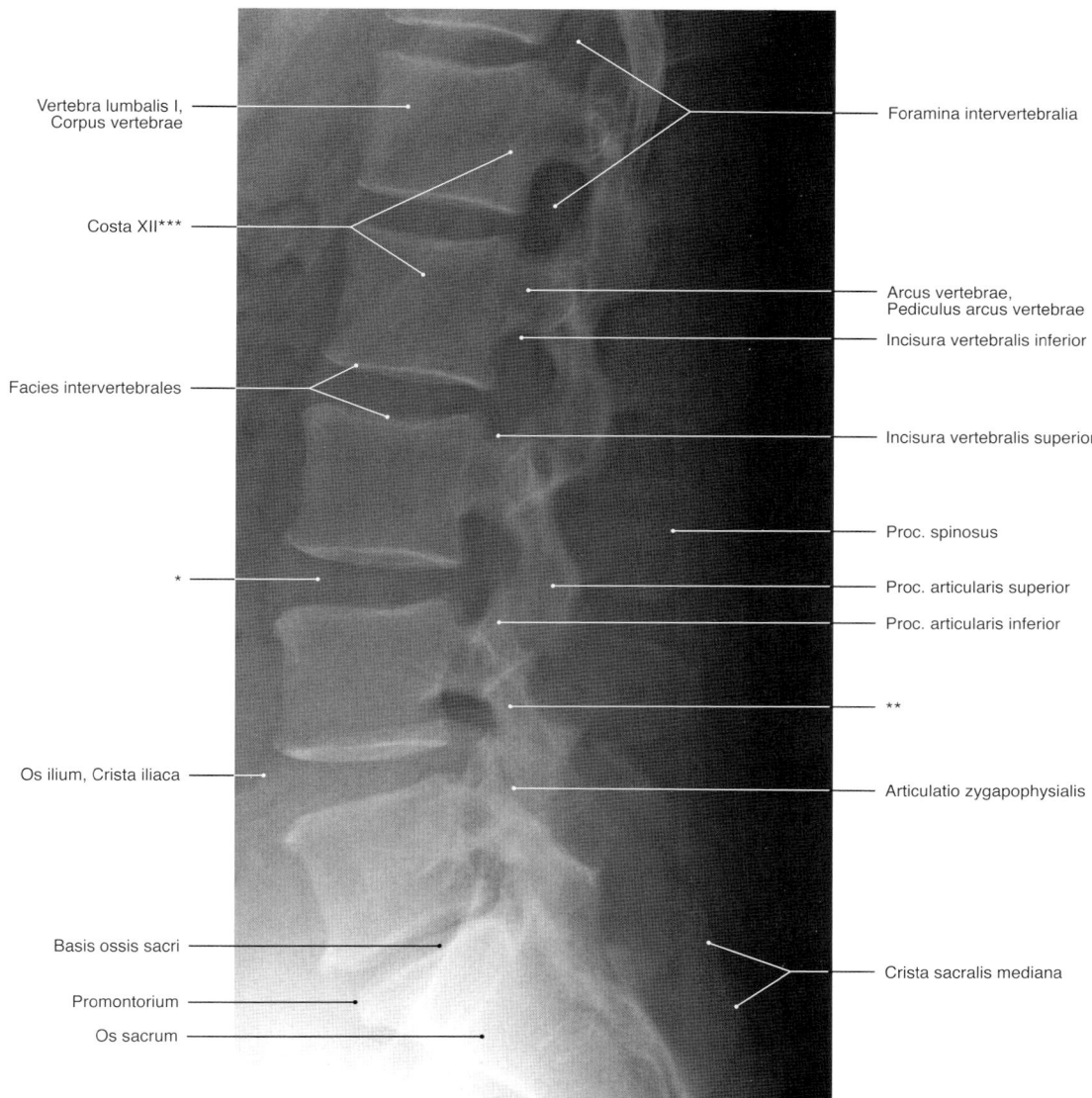

Vertebra lumbalis I, Corpus vertebrae

Costa XII***

Facies intervertebrales

*

Os ilium, Crista iliaca

Basis ossis sacri

Promontorium

Os sacrum

Foramina intervertebralia

Arcus vertebrae, Pediculus arcus vertebrae

Incisura vertebralis inferior

Incisura vertebralis superior

Proc. spinosus

Proc. articularis superior

Proc. articularis inferior

**

Articulatio zygapophysialis

Crista sacralis mediana

Fig. 503 Lumbar vertebrae, Vertebrae lumbales;
lateral radiograph of the lumbar part of the vertebral column;
upright position;
the central beam is directed onto the second lumbar vertebra.
In this case, the anterior edges of the lower lumbar vertebrae
are oblique due to pathological alterations.

* Intervertebral disc space
** Region of the vertebral arch between the superior and inferior
articular processes ("isthmus" = interarticular portion)
***The marks indicate the position of the twelfth rib, which is poorly
visible in this copy of the radiograph.

Lumbar part of the vertebral column, radiography

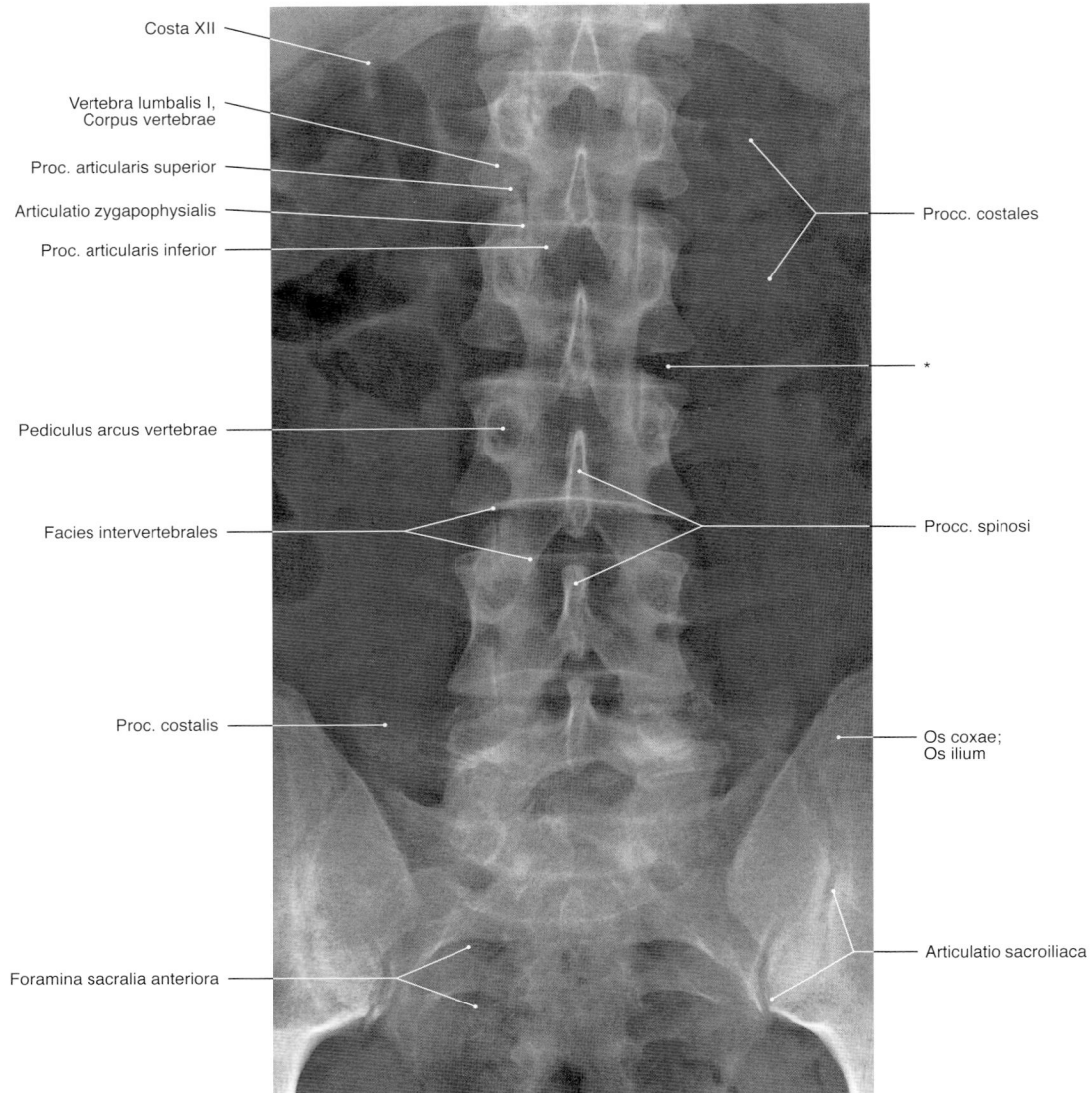

Costa XII

Vertebra lumbalis I,
Corpus vertebrae

Proc. articularis superior

Articulatio zygapophysialis

Proc. articularis inferior

Pediculus arcus vertebrae

Facies intervertebrales

Proc. costalis

Foramina sacralia anteriora

Procc. costales

*

Procc. spinosi

Os coxae;
Os ilium

Articulatio sacroiliaca

Fig. 504 Lumbar vertebrae, Vertebrae lumbales;
AP-radiograph of the lumbar part of the vertebral column
and the sacrum;
upright position; the central beam is directed onto the second
lumbar vertebra.
* Intervertebral disc space

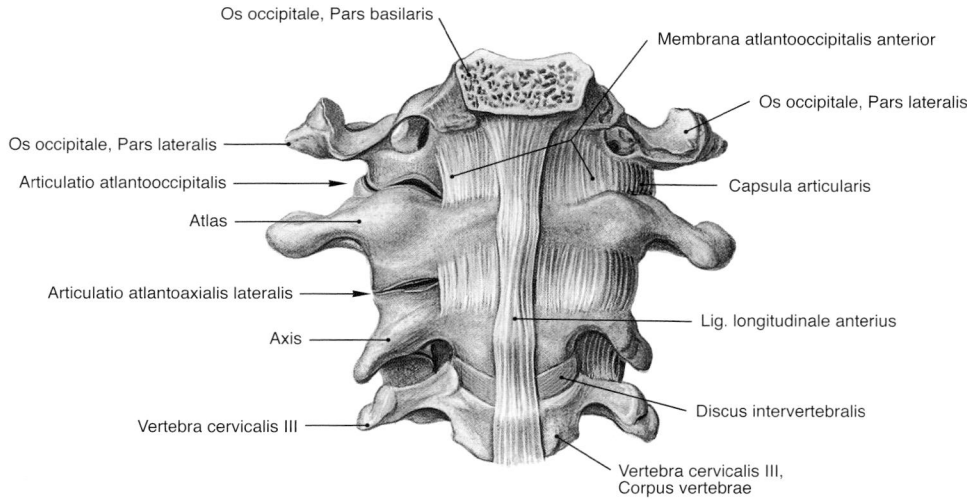

Os occipitale, Pars basilaris

Membrana atlantooccipitalis anterior

Os occipitale, Pars lateralis

Os occipitale, Pars lateralis

Articulatio atlantooccipitalis

Capsula articularis

Atlas

Articulatio atlantoaxialis lateralis

Axis

Lig. longitudinale anterius

Vertebra cervicalis III

Discus intervertebralis

Vertebra cervicalis III, Corpus vertebrae

Fig. 505 Craniocervical junctions and the upper cervical part of the vertebral column; ventral view.

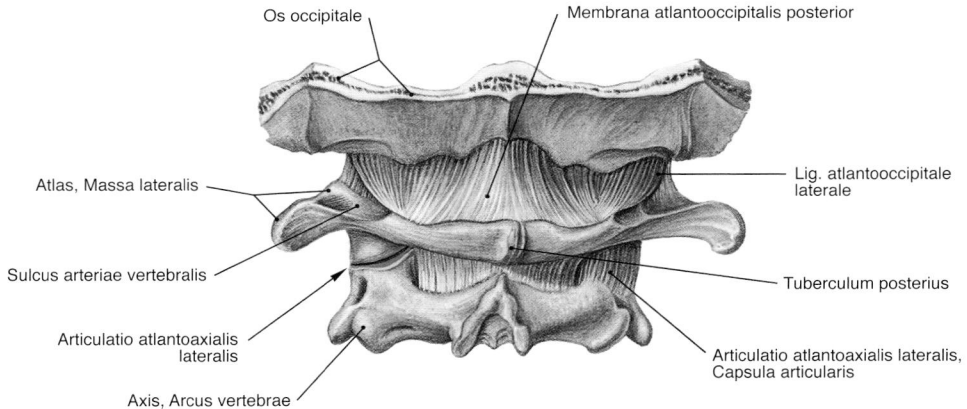

Os occipitale

Membrana atlantooccipitalis posterior

Atlas, Massa lateralis

Lig. atlantooccipitale laterale

Sulcus arteriae vertebralis

Tuberculum posterius

Articulatio atlantoaxialis lateralis

Articulatio atlantoaxialis lateralis, Capsula articularis

Axis, Arcus vertebrae

Fig. 506 Craniocervical junctions; dorsal view.

Craniocervical junctions

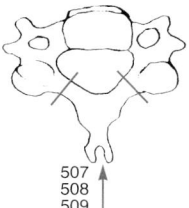

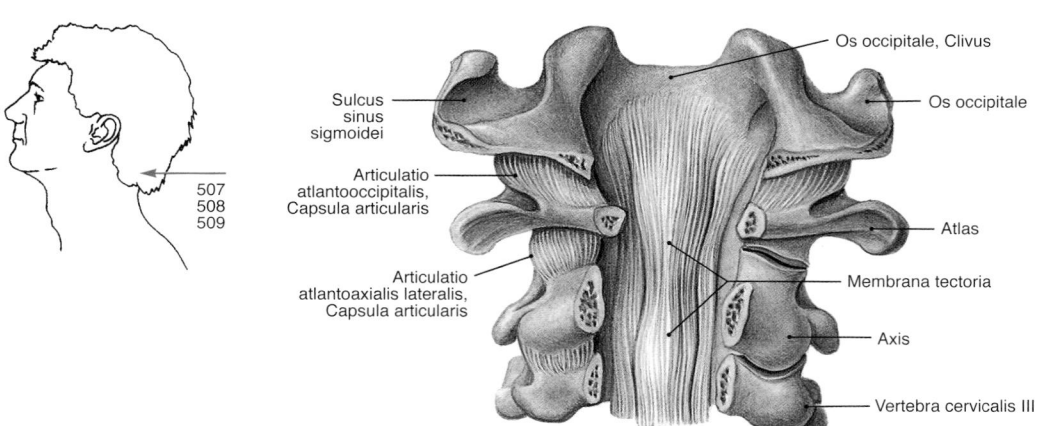

Os occipitale, Clivus

Sulcus sinus sigmoidei

Os occipitale

Articulatio atlantooccipitalis, Capsula articularis

Atlas

Articulatio atlantoaxialis lateralis, Capsula articularis

Membrana tectoria

Axis

Vertebra cervicalis III

507
508
509

Fig. 507 Craniocervical junctions, deep ligaments; dorsal view.

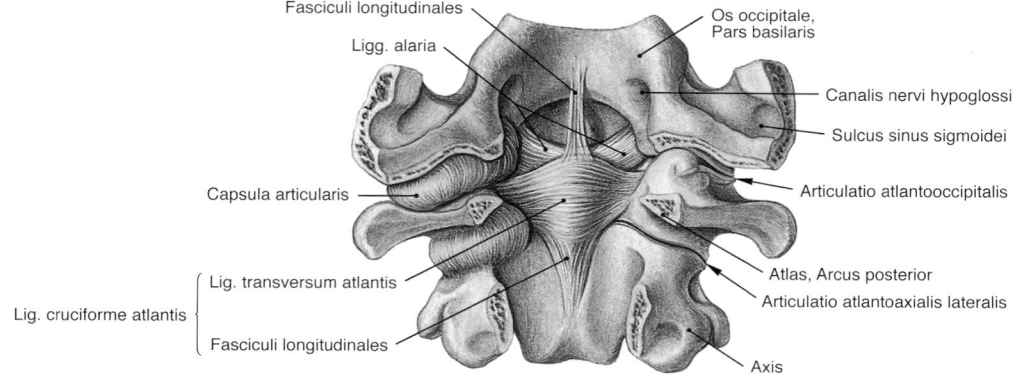

Fasciculi longitudinales

Ligg. alaria

Os occipitale, Pars basilaris

Canalis nervi hypoglossi

Sulcus sinus sigmoidei

Capsula articularis

Articulatio atlantooccipitalis

Lig. transversum atlantis

Lig. cruciforme atlantis {

Fasciculi longitudinales

Atlas, Arcus posterior

Articulatio atlantoaxialis lateralis

Axis

Fig. 508 Craniocervical junctions, deep ligaments; dorsal view.

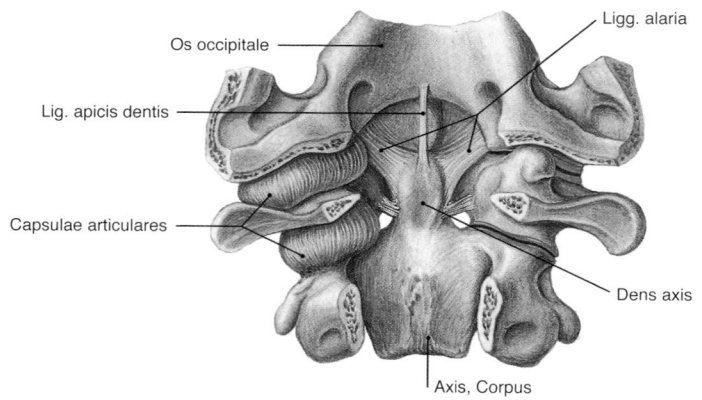

Os occipitale

Ligg. alaria

Lig. apicis dentis

Capsulae articulares

Dens axis

Axis, Corpus

Fig. 509 Craniocervical junctions, deep ligaments; dorsal view.
The alar ligaments frequently extend to the lateral masses of the atlas.

Craniocervical junctions

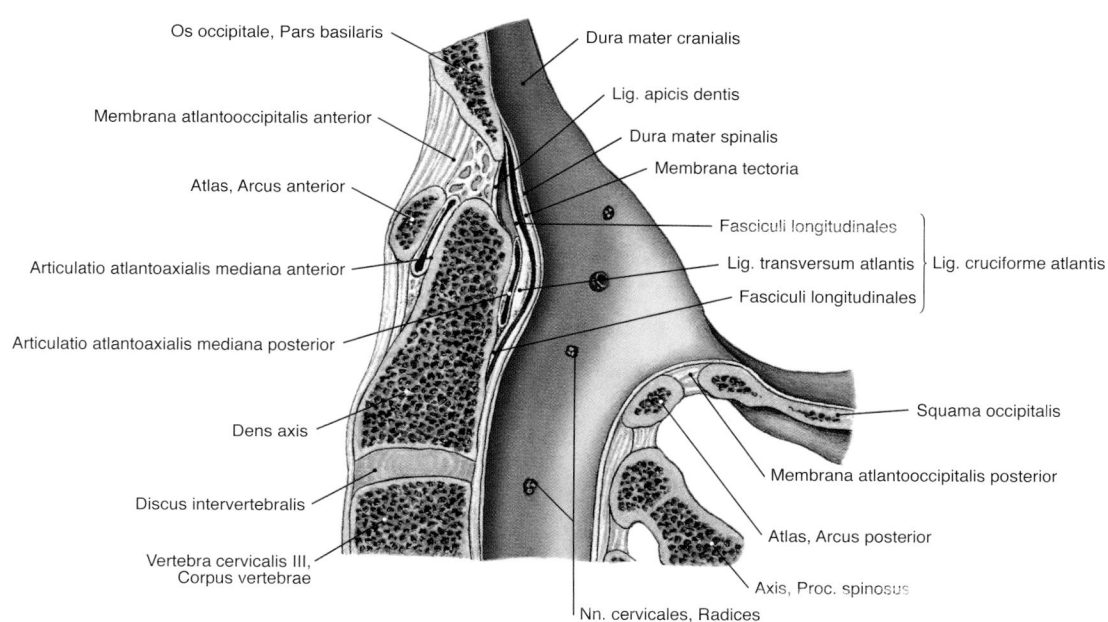

Os occipitale, Pars basilaris

Membrana atlantooccipitalis anterior

Atlas, Arcus anterior

Articulatio atlantoaxialis mediana anterior

Articulatio atlantoaxialis mediana posterior

Dens axis

Discus intervertebralis

Vertebra cervicalis III, Corpus vertebrae

Dura mater cranialis

Lig. apicis dentis

Dura mater spinalis

Membrana tectoria

Fasciculi longitudinales

Lig. transversum atlantis } Lig. cruciforme atlantis

Fasciculi longitudinales

Squama occipitalis

Membrana atlantooccipitalis posterior

Atlas, Arcus posterior

Axis, Proc. spinosus

Nn. cervicales, Radices

Fig. 510 Craniocervical junctions; median section.

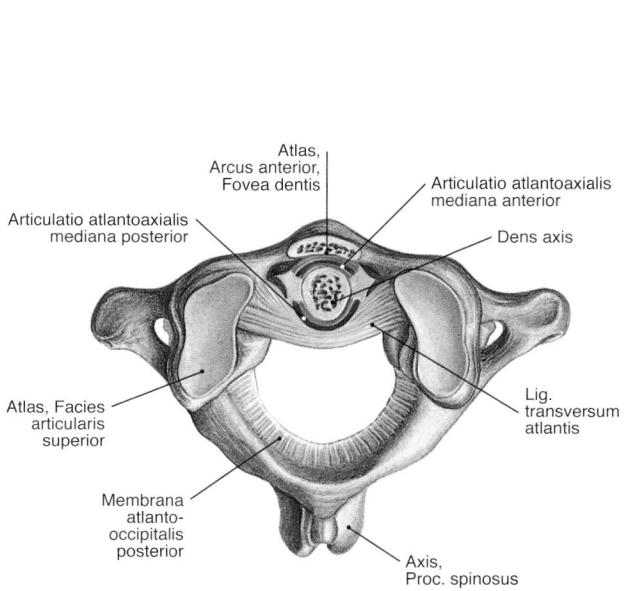

Atlas, Arcus anterior, Fovea dentis

Articulatio atlantoaxialis mediana posterior

Articulatio atlantoaxialis mediana anterior

Dens axis

Atlas, Facies articularis superior

Lig. transversum atlantis

Membrana atlanto-occipitalis posterior

Axis, Proc. spinosus

Fig. 511 Craniocervical junctions; superior view.

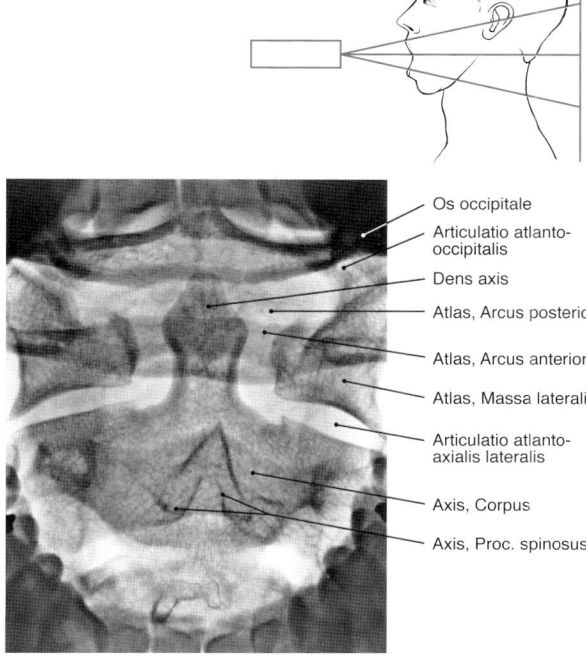

Os occipitale

Articulatio atlanto-occipitalis

Dens axis

Atlas, Arcus posterior

Atlas, Arcus anterior

Atlas, Massa lateralis

Articulatio atlanto-axialis lateralis

Axis, Corpus

Axis, Proc. spinosus

Fig. 512 Craniocervical junctions; AP-radiograph.

Ligaments of the vertebral column

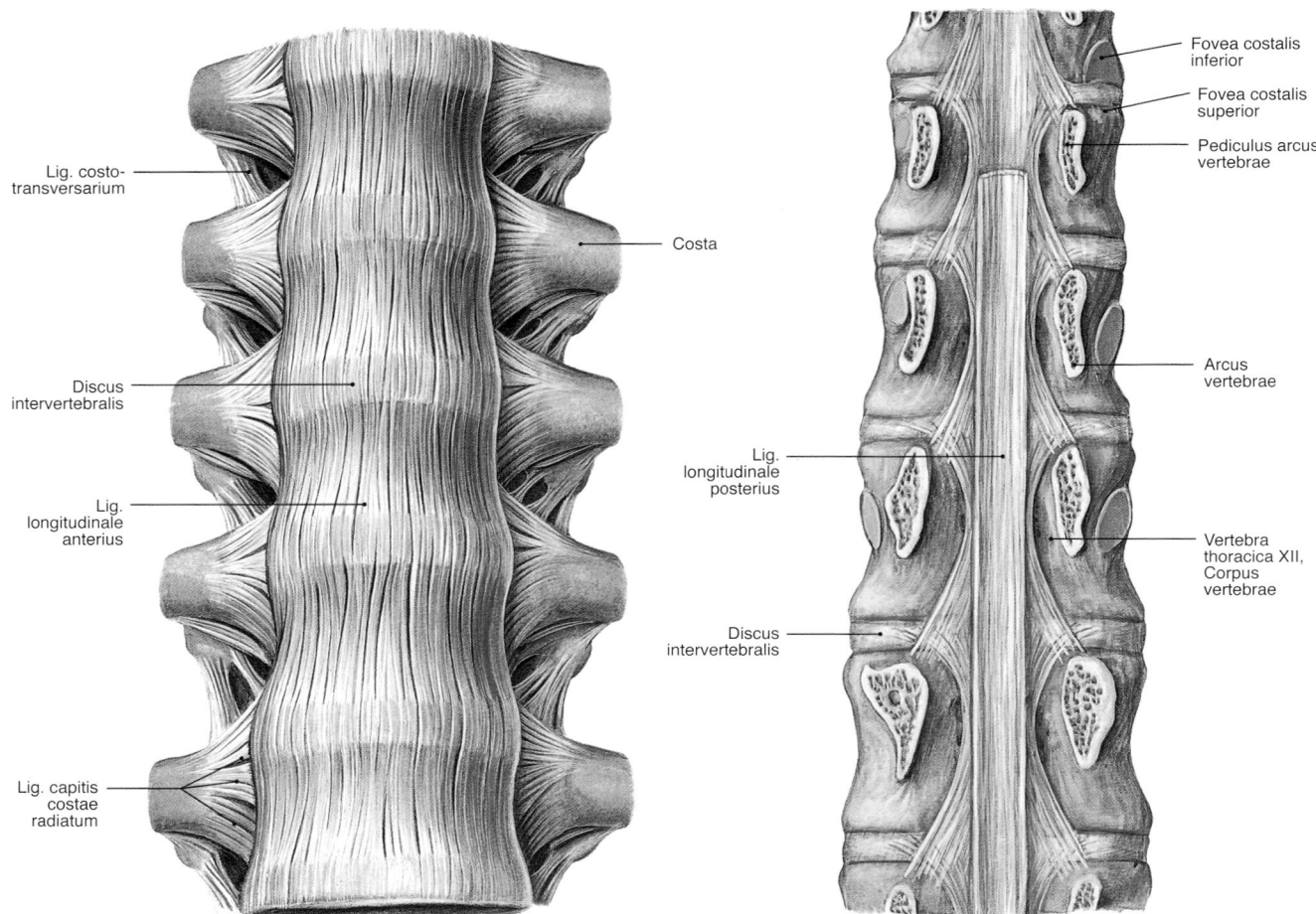

Lig. costo-transversarium

Discus intervertebralis

Lig. longitudinale anterius

Lig. capitis costae radiatum

Costa

Fovea costalis inferior

Fovea costalis superior

Pediculus arcus vertebrae

Arcus vertebrae

Lig. longitudinale posterius

Vertebra thoracica XII, Corpus vertebrae

Discus intervertebralis

Fig. 513 Ligaments of the vertebral column; exemplified by the lower thoracic part of the vertebral column; ventral view.

Fig. 514 Ligaments of the vertebral column; exemplified by the lower thoracic and the upper lumbar part of the vertebral column; dorsal view.

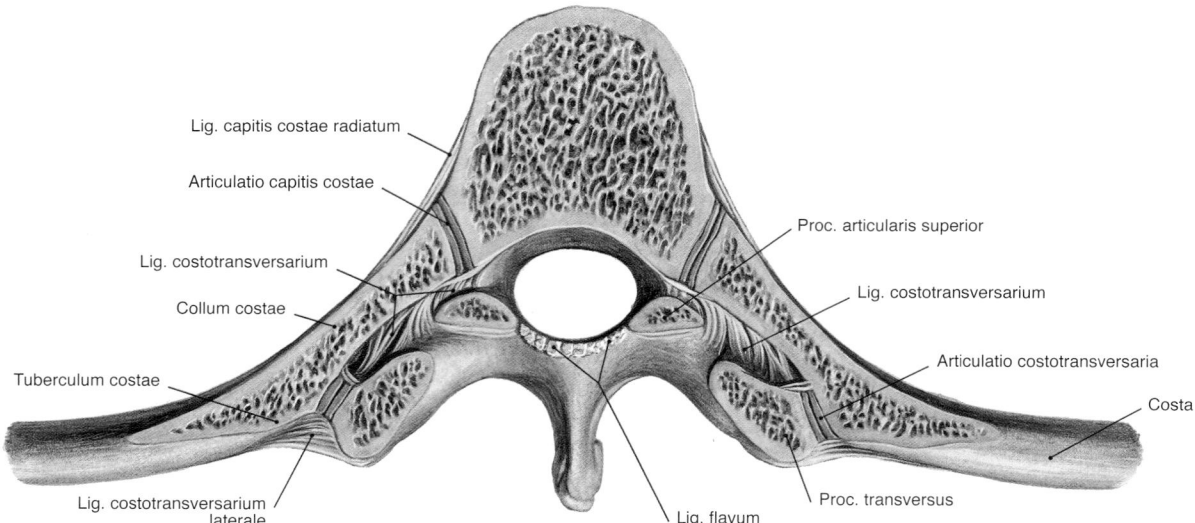

Lig. capitis costae radiatum

Articulatio capitis costae

Lig. costotransversarium

Collum costae

Tuberculum costae

Lig. costotransversarium laterale

Proc. articularis superior

Lig. costotransversarium

Articulatio costotransversaria

Costa

Proc. transversus

Lig. flavum

Fig. 515 Costovertebral joints, Articulationes costovertebrales; cross-section at the level of the lower part of the joint at a head of a rib; superior view.

Ligaments of the vertebral column

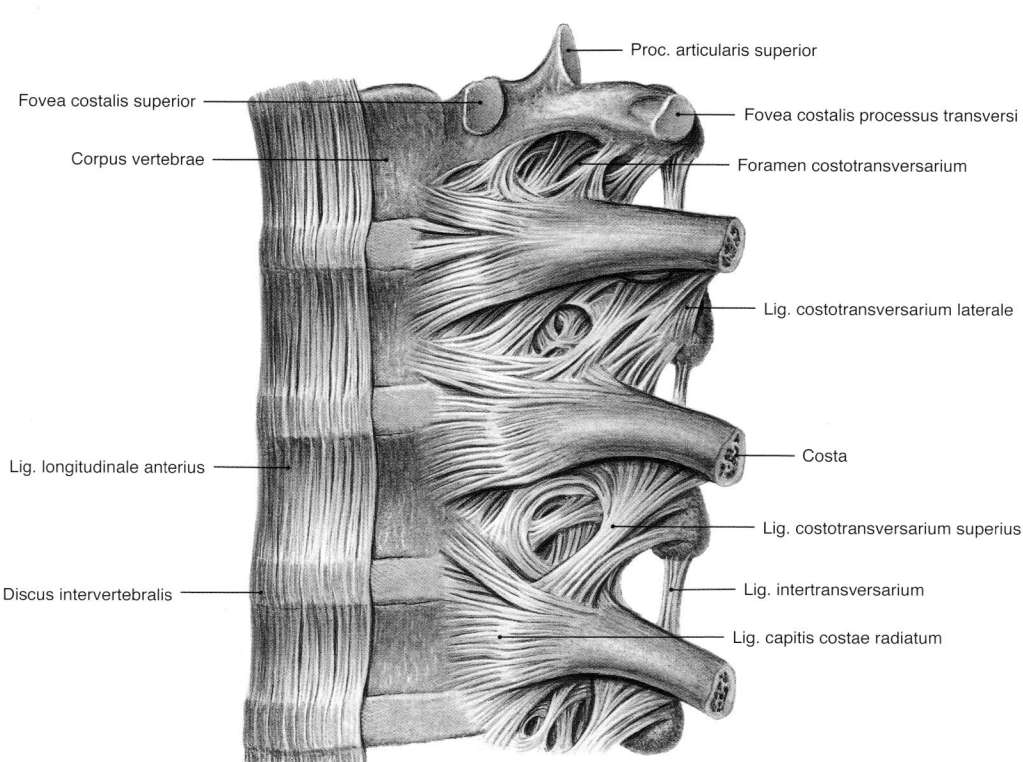

Proc. articularis superior

Fovea costalis superior

Corpus vertebrae

Fovea costalis processus transversi

Foramen costotransversarium

Lig. costotransversarium laterale

Lig. longitudinale anterius

Costa

Lig. costotransversarium superius

Lig. intertransversarium

Discus intervertebralis

Lig. capitis costae radiatum

Fig. 516 Ligaments of the vertebral column and the costovertebral joints, Articulationes costovertebrales; lateral parts of the anterior longitudinal ligament have been removed; viewed from the left.

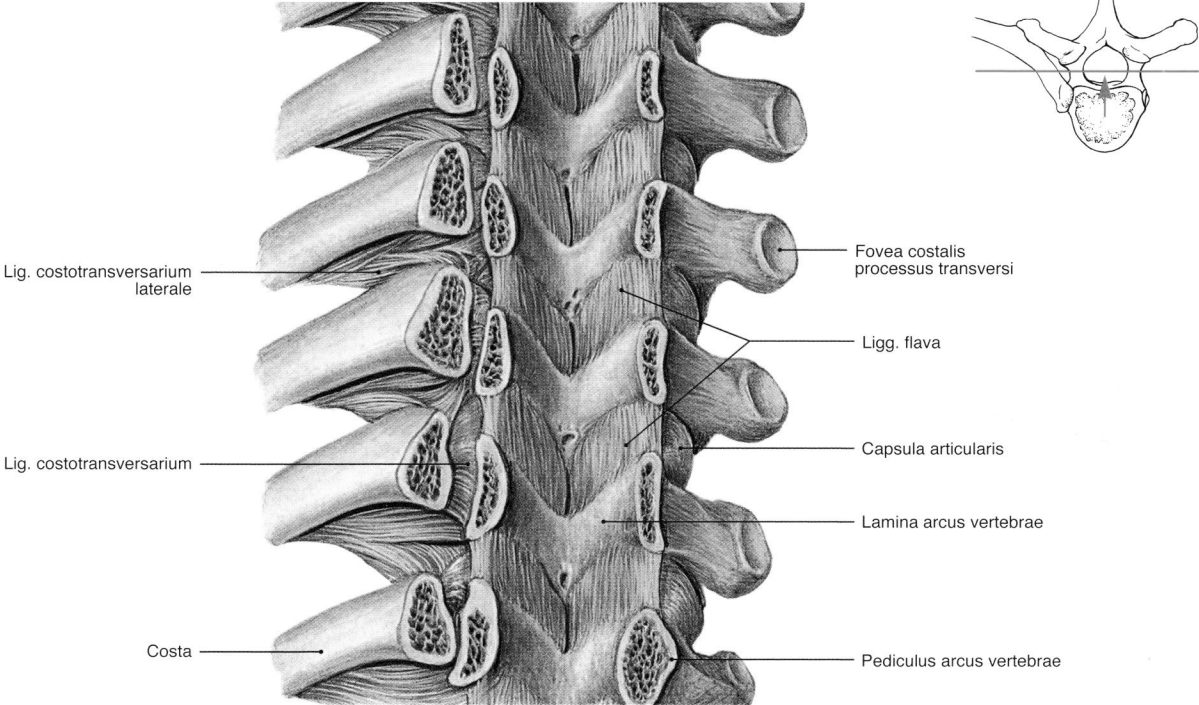

Lig. costotransversarium laterale

Fovea costalis processus transversi

Ligg. flava

Lig. costotransversarium

Capsula articularis

Lamina arcus vertebrae

Costa

Pediculus arcus vertebrae

Fig. 517 Junctions between the vertebral arches; ventral view.

Costovertebral joints

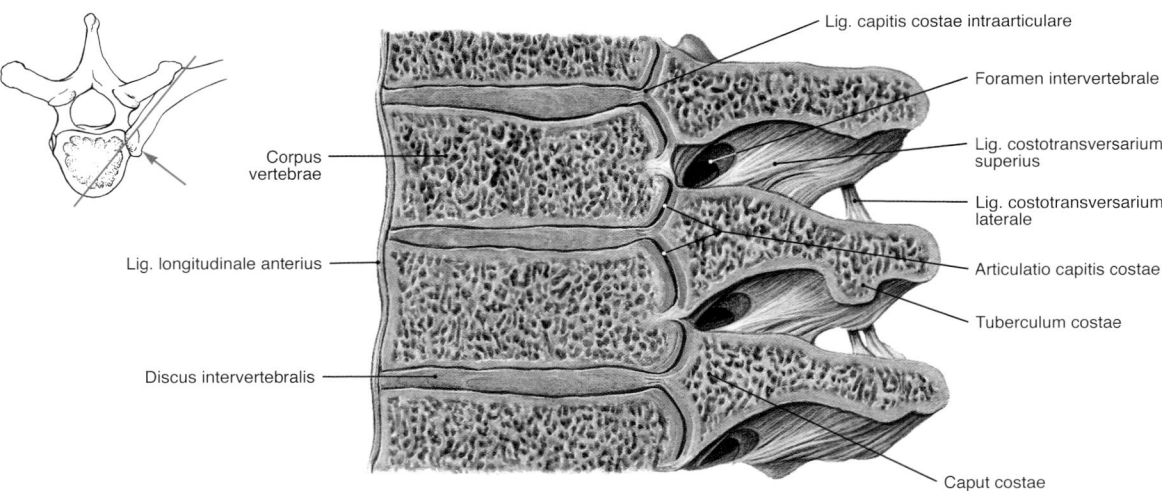

Lig. capitis costae intraarticulare

Foramen intervertebrale

Corpus vertebrae

Lig. costotransversarium superius

Lig. costotransversarium laterale

Lig. longitudinale anterius

Articulatio capitis costae

Tuberculum costae

Discus intervertebralis

Caput costae

Fig. 518   Costovertebral joints, Articulationes costovertebrales;
ventral view from the left.

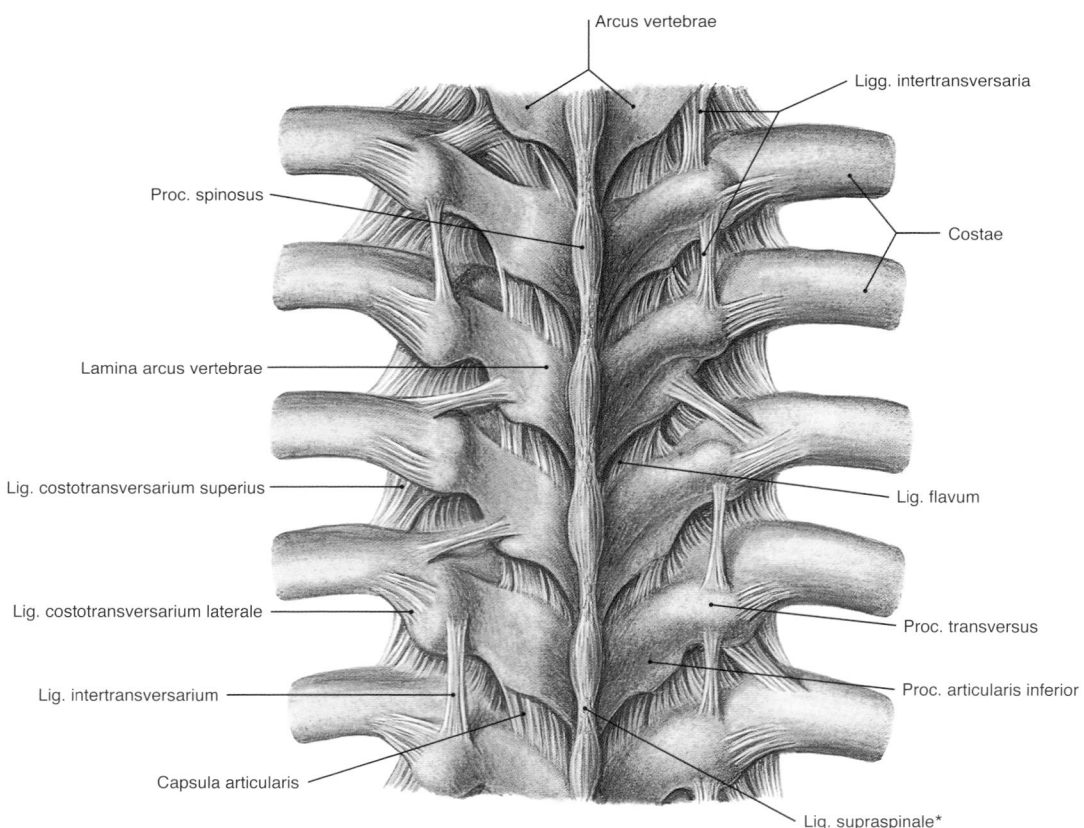

Arcus vertebrae

Ligg. intertransversaria

Proc. spinosus

Costae

Lamina arcus vertebrae

Lig. costotransversarium superius

Lig. flavum

Lig. costotransversarium laterale

Proc. transversus

Lig. intertransversarium

Proc. articularis inferior

Capsula articularis

Lig. supraspinale*

Fig. 519   Ligaments of the vertebral arches and the
costovertebral joints, Articulationes costovertebrales;
dorsal view.
* The median portion of the thoracolumbar fascia is referred
  to as supraspinous ligament.

Ligaments of the lumbar part of the vertebral column

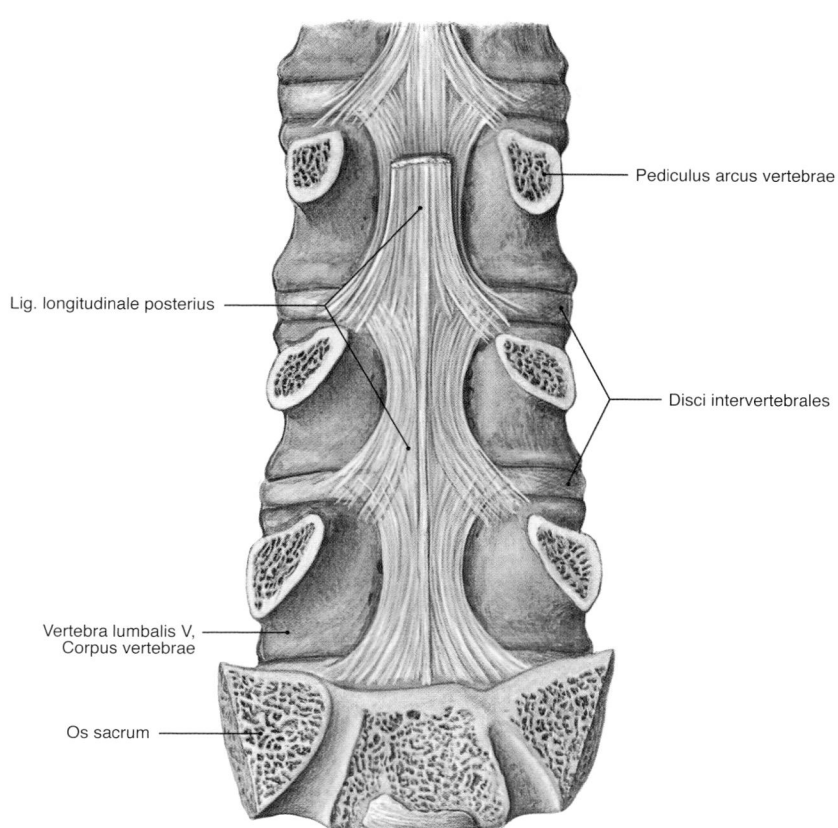

Pediculus arcus vertebrae

Lig. longitudinale posterius

Disci intervertebrales

Vertebra lumbalis V,
Corpus vertebrae

Os sacrum

Fig. 520   Ligaments of the lumbar part
of the vertebral column.

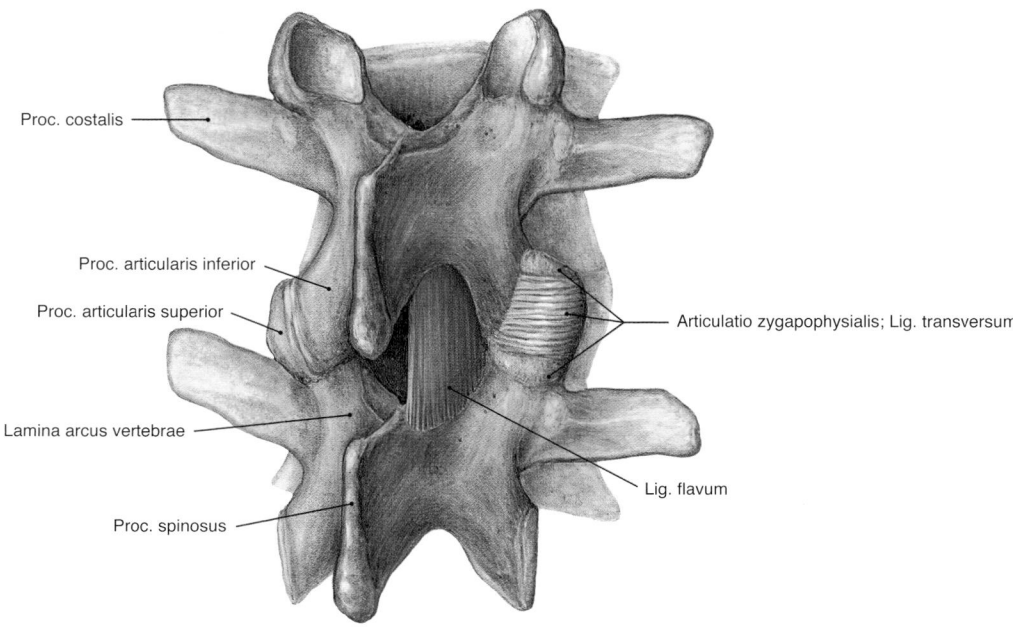

Proc. costalis

Proc. articularis inferior

Proc. articularis superior

Articulatio zygapophysialis; Lig. transversum

Lamina arcus vertebrae

Lig. flavum

Proc. spinosus

Fig. 521   Vertebral joints of the lumbar part of the vertebral
column, Articulationes zygapophysiales lumbales;
dorsal view from the right.

Reinforcement of the interarticular joints by strong and
transverse fibres (Ligg. transversa) is restricted to the lumbar
part of the vertebral column.

Intervertebral discs

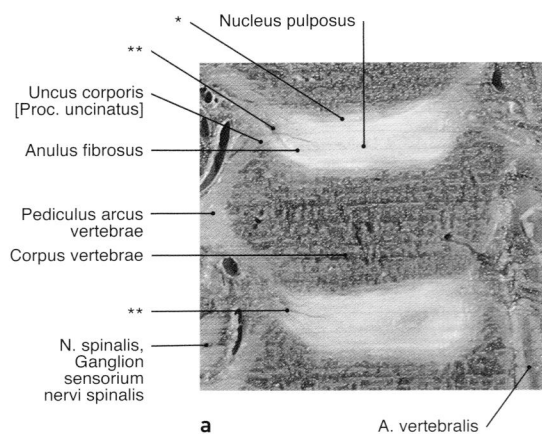

Nucleus pulposus

Uncus corporis [Proc. uncinatus]

Anulus fibrosus

Pediculus arcus vertebrae

Corpus vertebrae

N. spinalis, Ganglion sensorium nervi spinalis

A. vertebralis

a

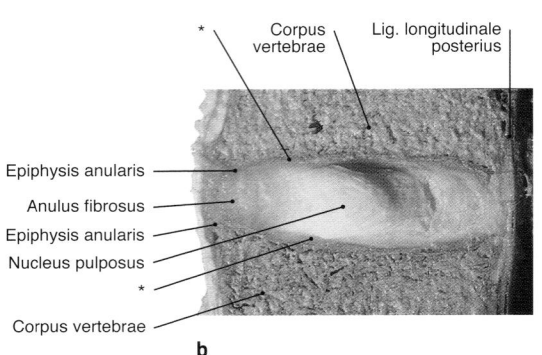

Corpus vertebrae

Lig. longitudinale posterius

Epiphysis anularis

Anulus fibrosus

Epiphysis anularis

Nucleus pulposus

Corpus vertebrae

b

Fig. 522 a, b Intervertebral discs, Disci intervertebrales.
a Cervical intervertebral discs, Disci intervertebrales cervicales;
frontal section
b Lumbar intervertebral disc, Discus intervertebralis lumbalis;
median section

* Hyaline cartilaginous covering of the end-plates of the vertebral bodies reflecting the non-ossified portion of the epiphyses
** In the first decade of life, so-called uncovertebral clefts develop in the lateral zones of the cervical intervertebral discs, which can progress further towards the middle in the following decades.

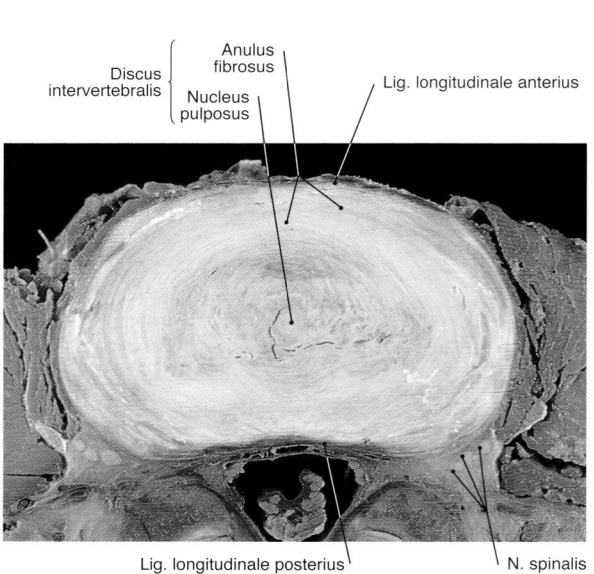

Discus intervertebralis
Anulus fibrosus
Nucleus pulposus
Lig. longitudinale anterius

Lig. longitudinale posterius

N. spinalis

Fig. 523 Lumbar intervertebral disc,
Discus intervertebralis lumbalis;
superior view.

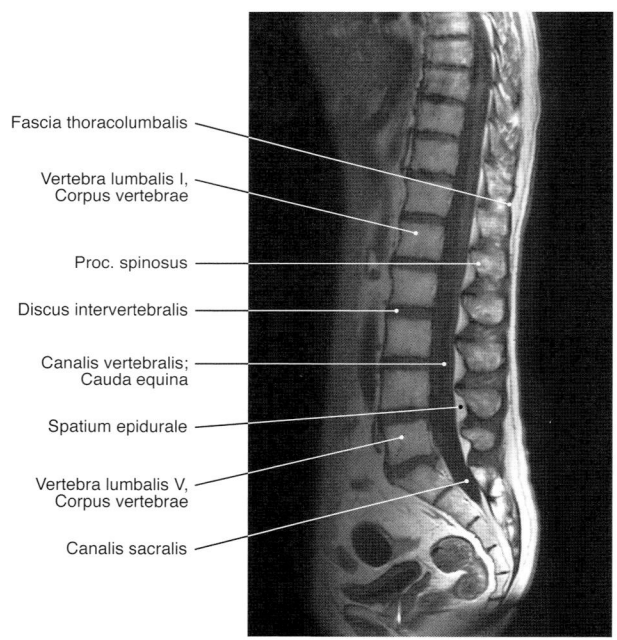

Fascia thoracolumbalis

Vertebra lumbalis I, Corpus vertebrae

Proc. spinosus

Discus intervertebralis

Canalis vertebralis; Cauda equina

Spatium epidurale

Vertebra lumbalis V, Corpus vertebrae

Canalis sacralis

Fig. 524 Lumbar parts of the vertebral column;
magnetic resonance tomographic image (MRI);
median section.

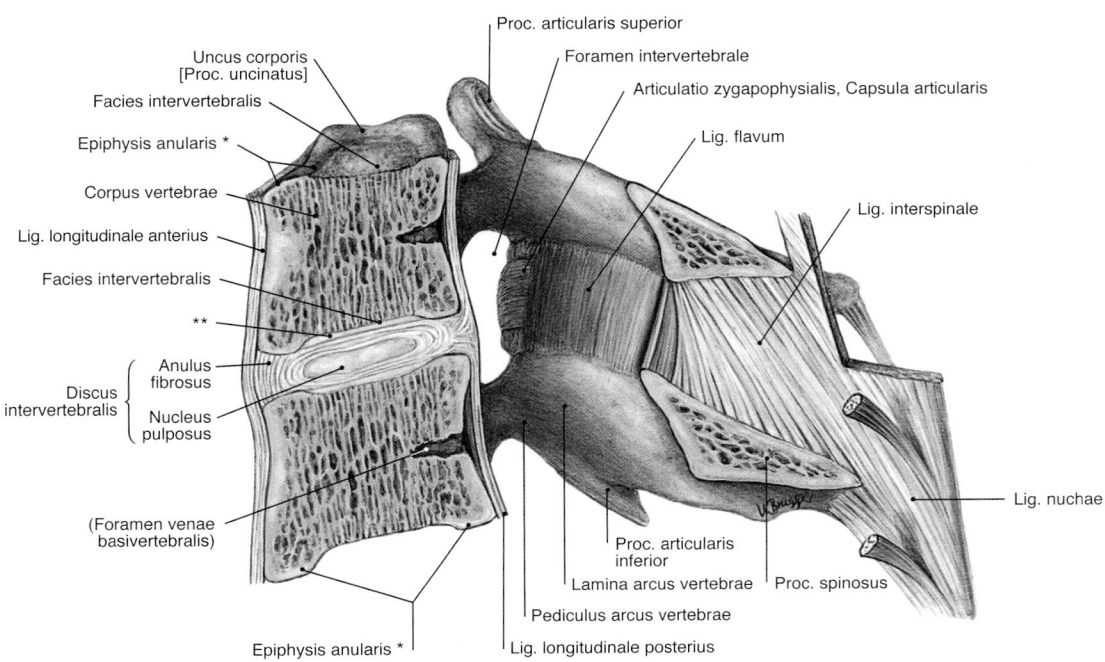

Proc. articularis superior

Foramen intervertebrale

Articulatio zygapophysialis, Capsula articularis

Lig. flavum

Lig. interspinale

Uncus corporis [Proc. uncinatus]

Facies intervertebralis

Epiphysis anularis *

Corpus vertebrae

Lig. longitudinale anterius

Facies intervertebralis

**

Discus intervertebralis { Anulus fibrosus / Nucleus pulposus

Lig. nuchae

(Foramen venae basivertebralis)

Proc. articularis inferior

Lamina arcus vertebrae

Proc. spinosus

Pediculus arcus vertebrae

Epiphysis anularis *

Lig. longitudinale posterius

Fig. 525 Cervical motion segment; schematic median section.

* Also: rim of vertebral body
** Hyaline cartilaginous covering of the end-plate of the vertebral body reflecting the non-ossified portion of the epiphysis

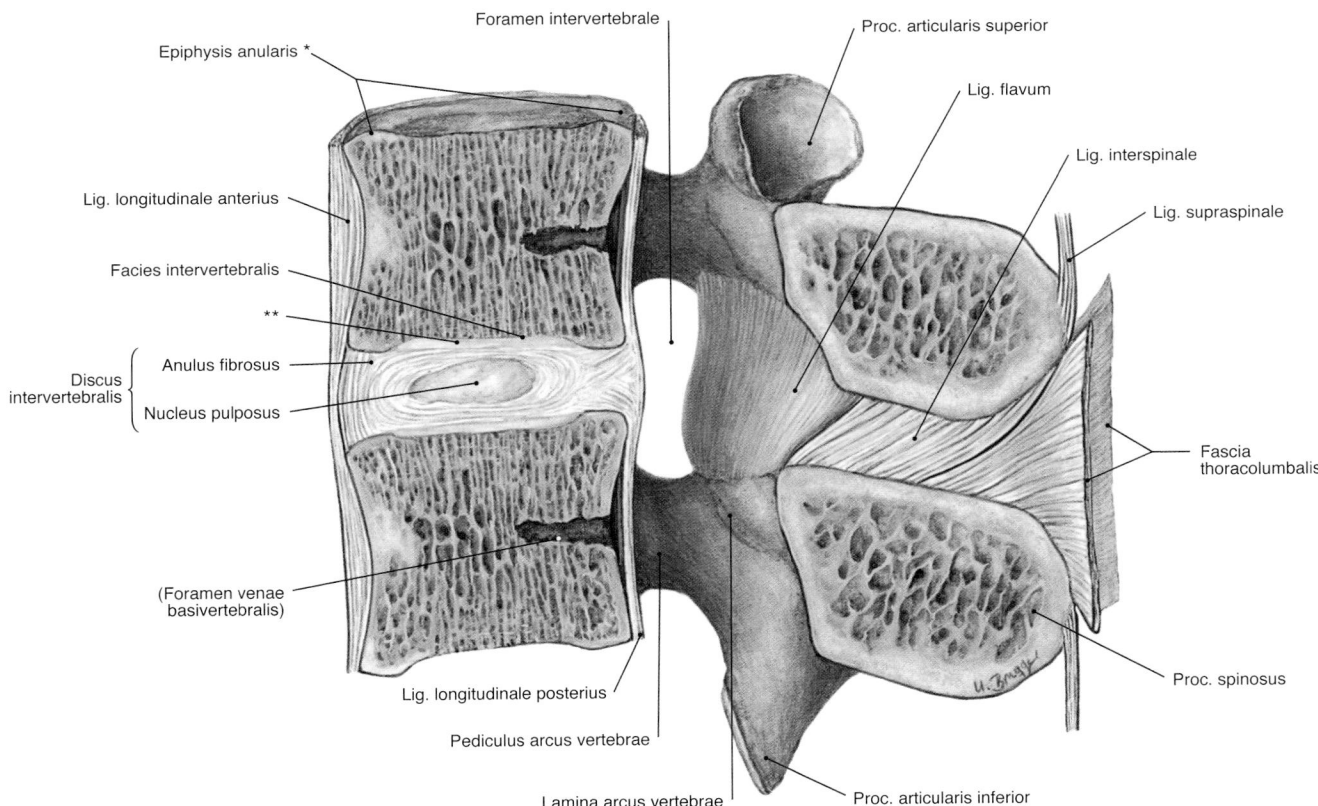

Foramen intervertebrale

Proc. articularis superior

Epiphysis anularis *

Lig. flavum

Lig. interspinale

Lig. supraspinale

Lig. longitudinale anterius

Facies intervertebralis

**

Discus intervertebralis { Anulus fibrosus / Nucleus pulposus

Fascia thoracolumbalis

(Foramen venae basivertebralis)

Proc. spinosus

Lig. longitudinale posterius

Pediculus arcus vertebrae

Lamina arcus vertebrae

Proc. articularis inferior

Fig. 526 Lumbar motion segment; schematic median section.

* Also: rim of vertebral body
** Hyaline cartilaginous covering of the end-plate of the vertebral body reflecting the non-ossified portion of the epiphysis

Superficial muscles of the back

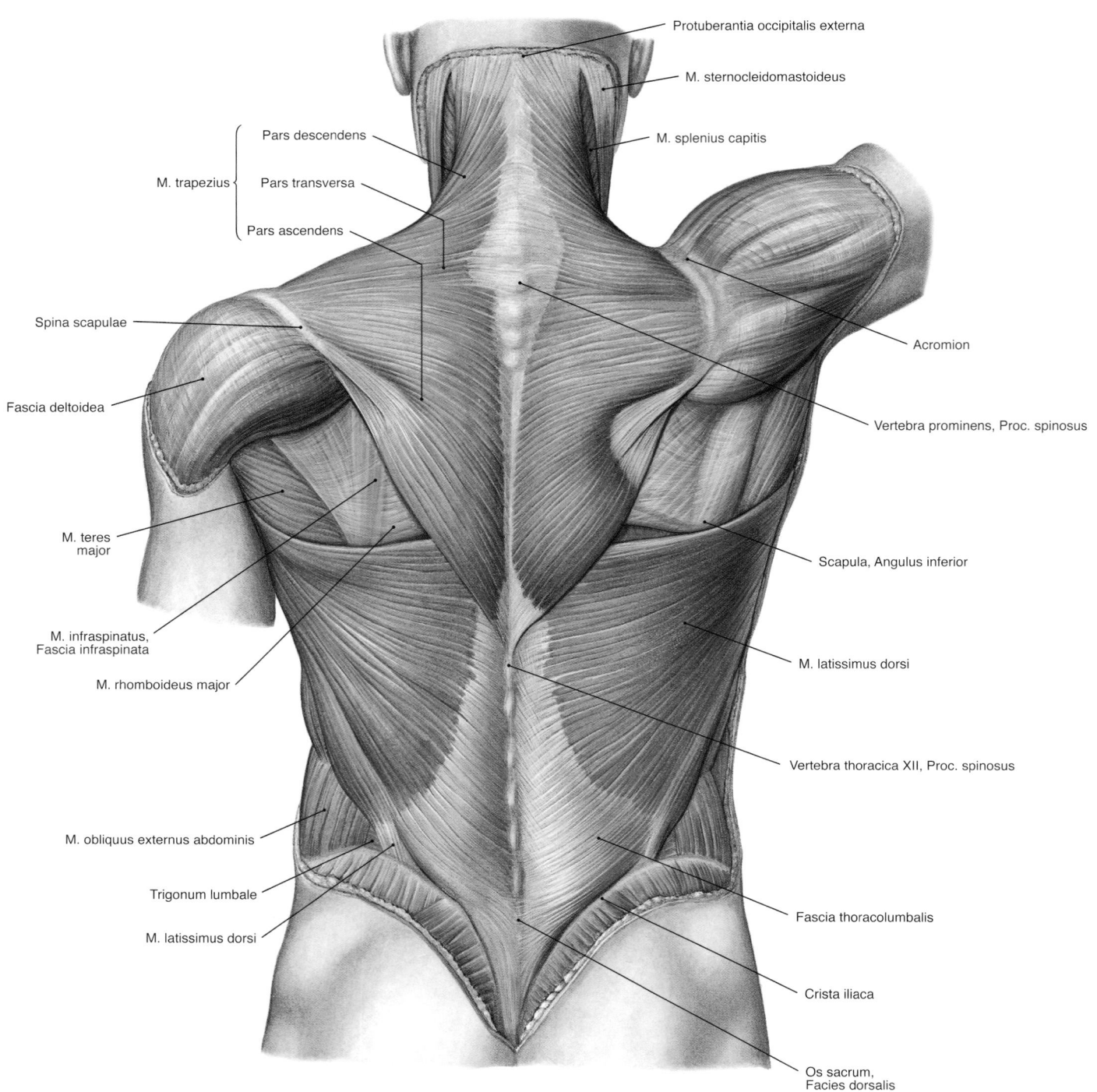

Protuberantia occipitalis externa

M. sternocleidomastoideus

M. splenius capitis

M. trapezius
{ Pars descendens
Pars transversa
Pars ascendens }

Spina scapulae

Fascia deltoidea

M. teres major

M. infraspinatus, Fascia infraspinata

M. rhomboideus major

M. obliquus externus abdominis

Trigonum lumbale

M. latissimus dorsi

Acromion

Vertebra prominens, Proc. spinosus

Scapula, Angulus inferior

M. latissimus dorsi

Vertebra thoracica XII, Proc. spinosus

Fascia thoracolumbalis

Crista iliaca

Os sacrum, Facies dorsalis

→ T 17, T 18

Fig. 527 Muscles of the back, Mm. dorsi; superficial layer of the trunk-arm and trunk-shoulder girdle muscles.

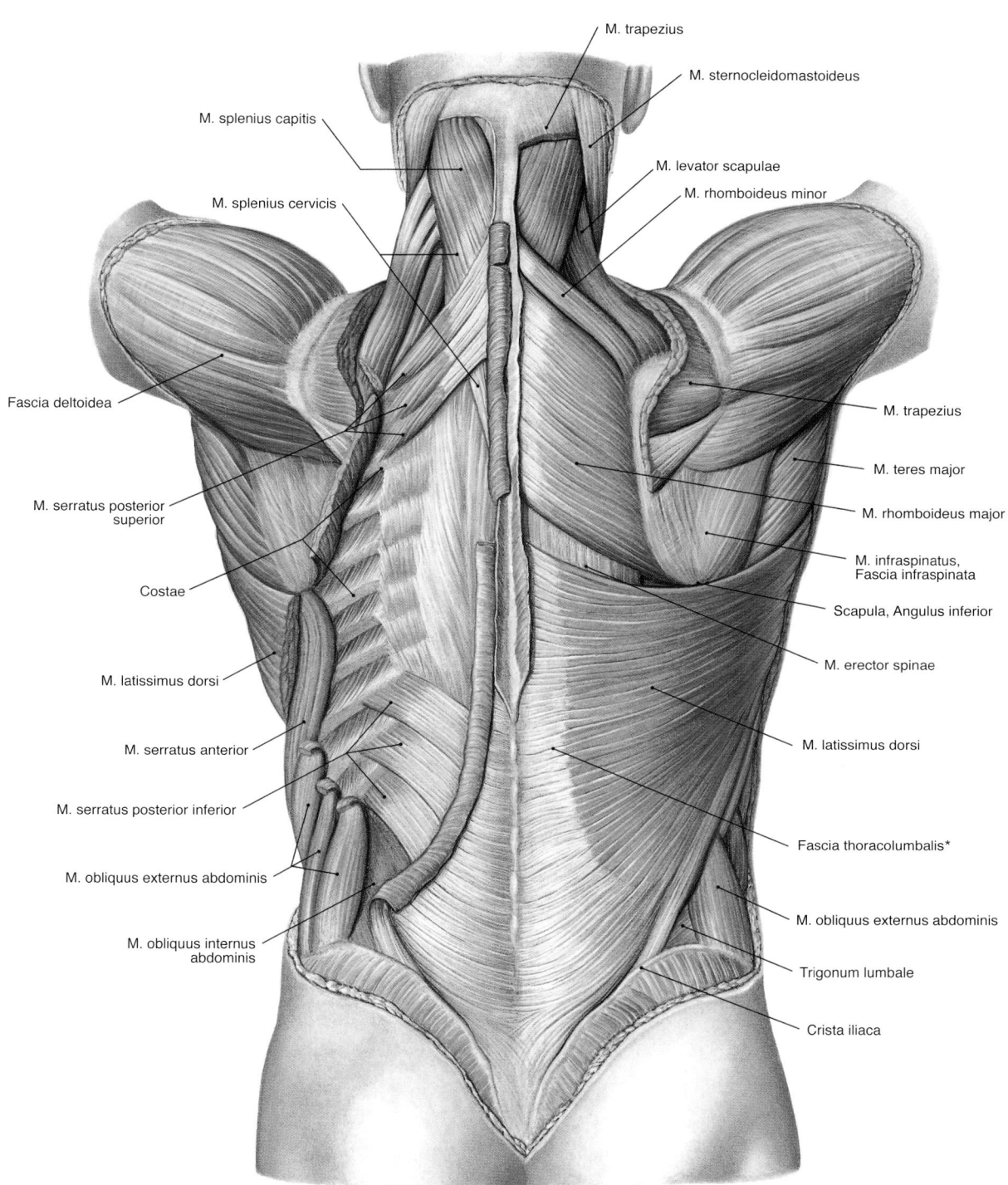

M. trapezius

M. sternocleidomastoideus

M. splenius capitis

M. levator scapulae

M. splenius cervicis

M. rhomboideus minor

Fascia deltoidea

M. trapezius

M. teres major

M. serratus posterior superior

M. rhomboideus major

Costae

M. infraspinatus, Fascia infraspinata

Scapula, Angulus inferior

M. latissimus dorsi

M. erector spinae

M. serratus anterior

M. latissimus dorsi

M. serratus posterior inferior

M. obliquus externus abdominis

Fascia thoracolumbalis*

M. obliquus externus abdominis

M. obliquus internus abdominis

Trigonum lumbale

Crista iliaca

Fig. 528 Muscles of the back, Mm. dorsi; deep layer of the trunk-arm and trunk-shoulder girdle muscles.

* The so-called thoracolumbar fascia forms a dense aponeurosis.

→ T 17–T 19

Deep muscles of the back

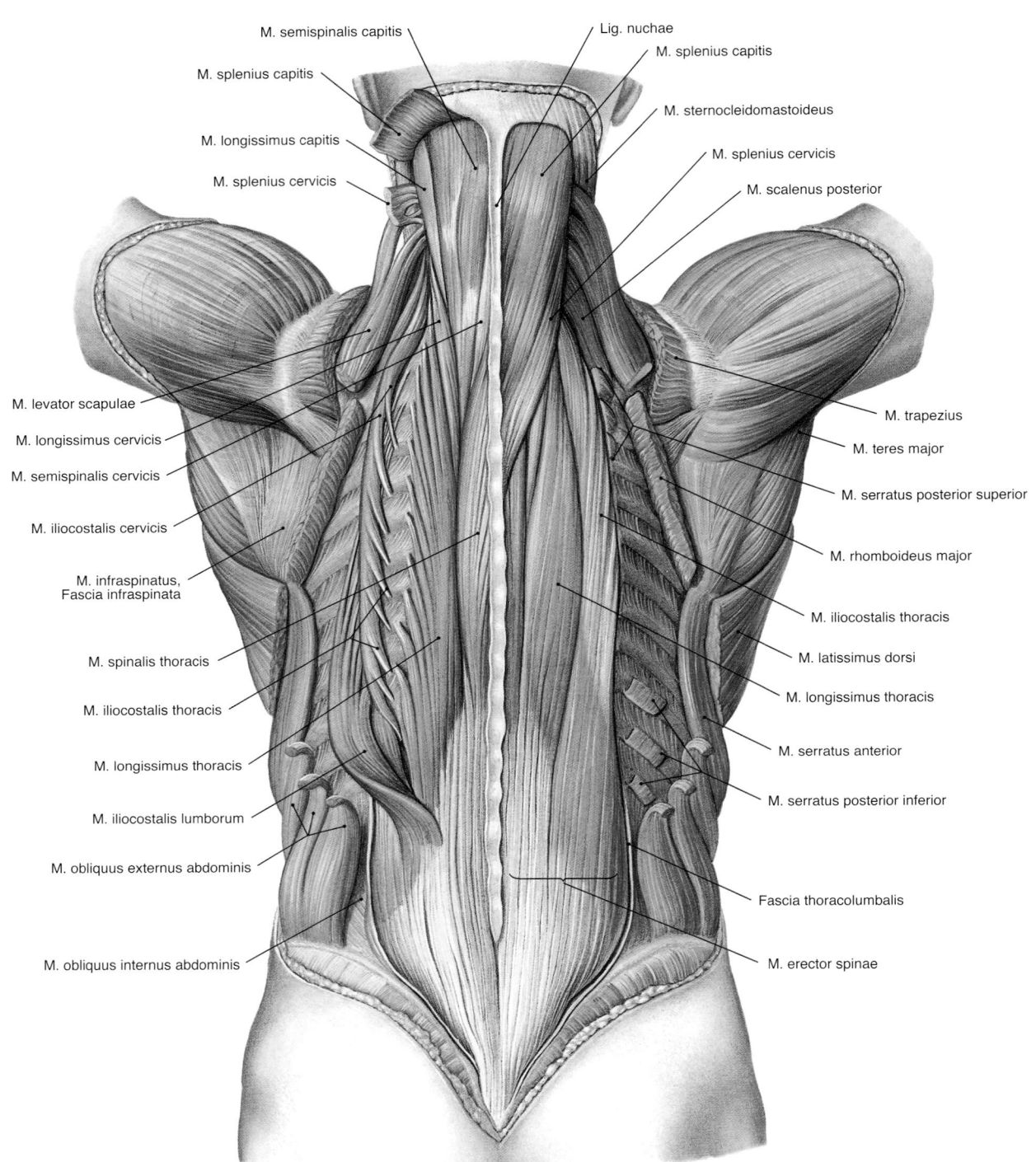

M. semispinalis capitis
M. splenius capitis
M. longissimus capitis
M. splenius cervicis

Lig. nuchae
M. splenius capitis
M. sternocleidomastoideus
M. splenius cervicis
M. scalenus posterior

M. levator scapulae
M. longissimus cervicis
M. semispinalis cervicis
M. iliocostalis cervicis
M. infraspinatus, Fascia infraspinata
M. spinalis thoracis
M. iliocostalis thoracis
M. longissimus thoracis
M. iliocostalis lumborum
M. obliquus externus abdominis
M. obliquus internus abdominis

M. trapezius
M. teres major
M. serratus posterior superior
M. rhomboideus major
M. iliocostalis thoracis
M. latissimus dorsi
M. longissimus thoracis
M. serratus anterior
M. serratus posterior inferior
Fascia thoracolumbalis
M. erector spinae

→ T 20 a, b

Fig. 529   Muscles of the back, Mm. dorsi;
superficial layer of the deep (autochthonous) muscles.

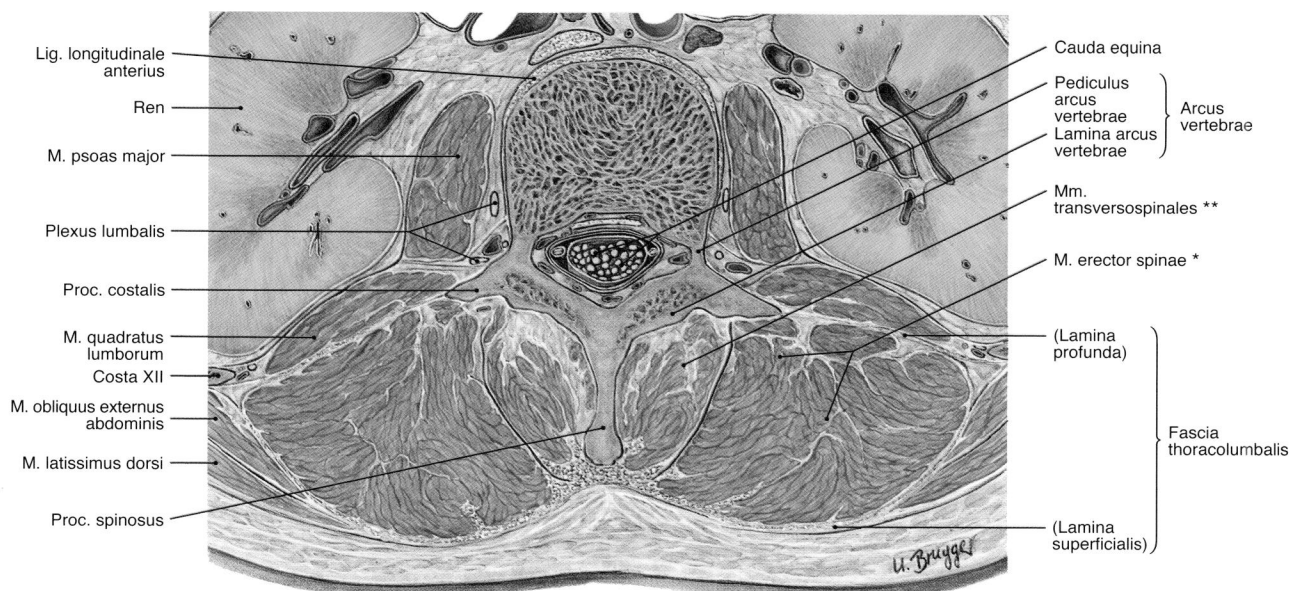

Lig. longitudinale anterius
Ren
M. psoas major
Plexus lumbalis
Proc. costalis
M. quadratus lumborum
Costa XII
M. obliquus externus abdominis
M. latissimus dorsi
Proc. spinosus

Cauda equina
Pediculus arcus vertebrae
Lamina arcus vertebrae
} Arcus vertebrae
Mm. transversospinales **
M. erector spinae *
(Lamina profunda)
(Lamina superficialis)
} Fascia thoracolumbalis

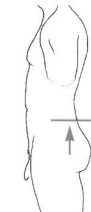

Fig. 530 Muscles of the back, Mm. dorsi;
cross-section at the level of the second lumbar vertebra;
inferior view.
The deep (autochthonous) muscles of the back lie within an osteofibrous tube formed by dorsal parts of the vertebrae and the surrounding aponeurotic thoracolumbar fascia. The muscles are divided into a lateral * and a medial ** tract.

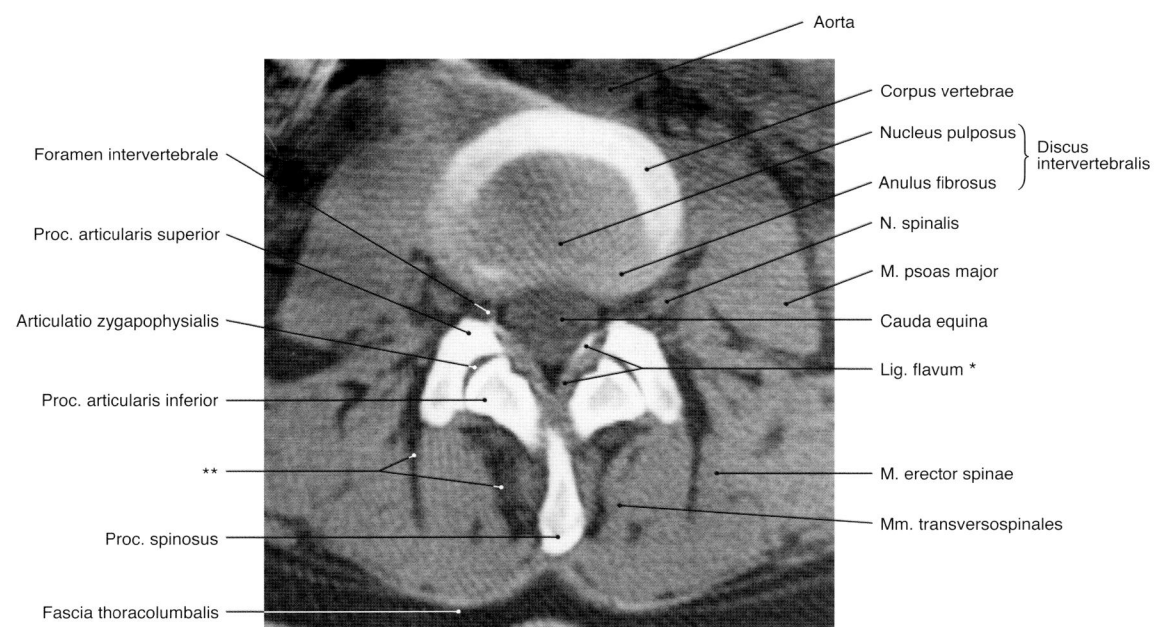

Aorta
Corpus vertebrae
Nucleus pulposus
Anulus fibrosus
} Discus intervertebralis
N. spinalis
M. psoas major
Cauda equina
Lig. flavum *
M. erector spinae
Mm. transversospinales

Foramen intervertebrale
Proc. articularis superior
Articulatio zygapophysialis
Proc. articularis inferior
**
Proc. spinosus
Fascia thoracolumbalis

Fig. 531 Muscles of the back, Mm. dorsi;
computed tomographic cross-section (CT) at the level of the intervertebral disc between the third and the fourth lumbar vertebra;
inferior view.

* Calcification or ossification frequently occurs at the sites of insertion of the ligamenta flava, even in younger individuals.

** Adipose tissue deposits

Deep muscles of the back

Tract	Longitudinal system		Oblique system	Tract

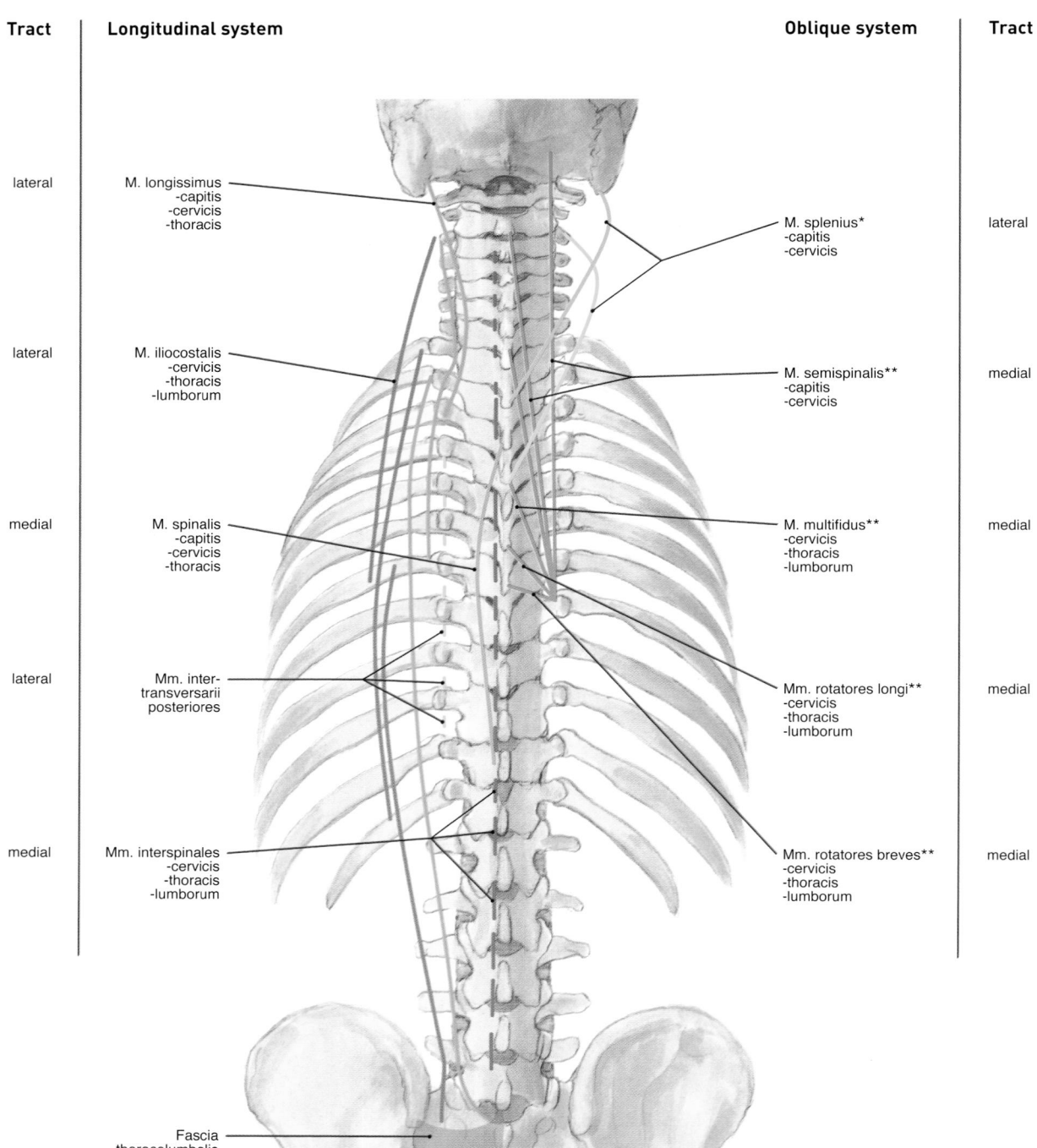

lateral — M. longissimus -capitis -cervicis -thoracis

lateral — M. iliocostalis -cervicis -thoracis -lumborum

medial — M. spinalis -capitis -cervicis -thoracis

lateral — Mm. inter-transversarii posteriores

medial — Mm. interspinales -cervicis -thoracis -lumborum

Fascia thoracolumbalis

M. splenius* -capitis -cervicis — **lateral**

M. semispinalis** -capitis -cervicis — **medial**

M. multifidus** -cervicis -thoracis -lumborum — **medial**

Mm. rotatores longi** -cervicis -thoracis -lumborum — **medial**

Mm. rotatores breves** -cervicis -thoracis -lumborum — **medial**

Fig. 532 Deep (autochthonous) muscles of the back; diagram of the different groups of muscles.
The deep (autochthonous) muscles of the back can be divided into a longitudinal and an oblique system, as well as into a medial and a lateral tract.
* Spinotransverse
** Transversospinal

Deep muscles of the back

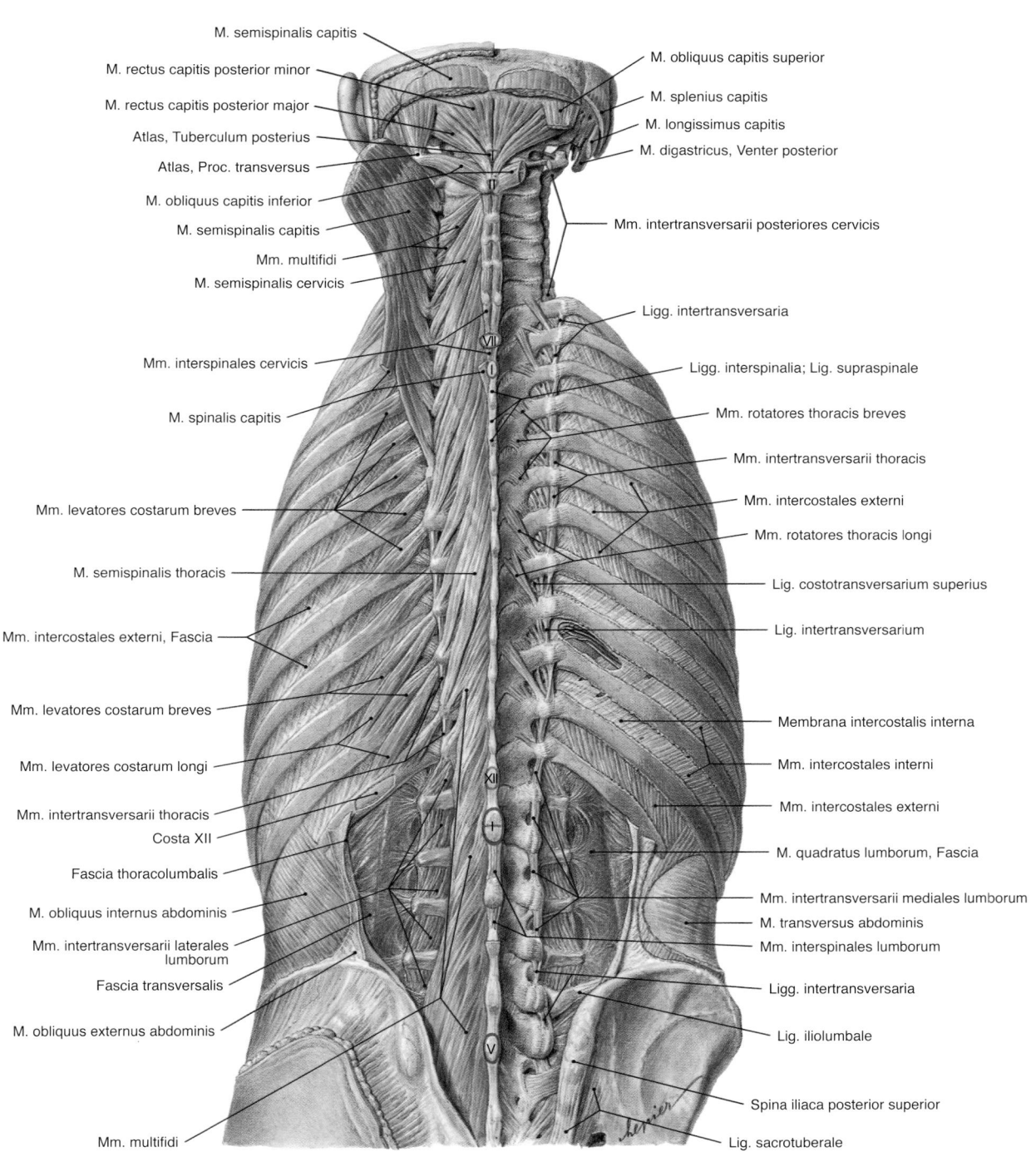

M. semispinalis capitis

M. rectus capitis posterior minor

M. rectus capitis posterior major

Atlas, Tuberculum posterius

Atlas, Proc. transversus

M. obliquus capitis inferior

M. semispinalis capitis

Mm. multifidi

M. semispinalis cervicis

Mm. interspinales cervicis

M. spinalis capitis

Mm. levatores costarum breves

M. semispinalis thoracis

Mm. intercostales externi, Fascia

Mm. levatores costarum breves

Mm. levatores costarum longi

Mm. intertransversarii thoracis

Costa XII

Fascia thoracolumbalis

M. obliquus internus abdominis

Mm. intertransversarii laterales lumborum

Fascia transversalis

M. obliquus externus abdominis

Mm. multifidi

M. obliquus capitis superior

M. splenius capitis

M. longissimus capitis

M. digastricus, Venter posterior

Mm. intertransversarii posteriores cervicis

Ligg. intertransversaria

Ligg. interspinalia; Lig. supraspinale

Mm. rotatores thoracis breves

Mm. intertransversarii thoracis

Mm. intercostales externi

Mm. rotatores thoracis longi

Lig. costotransversarium superius

Lig. intertransversarium

Membrana intercostalis interna

Mm. intercostales interni

Mm. intercostales externi

M. quadratus lumborum, Fascia

Mm. intertransversarii mediales lumborum

M. transversus abdominis

Mm. interspinales lumborum

Ligg. intertransversaria

Lig. iliolumbale

Spina iliaca posterior superior

Lig. sacrotuberale

Fig. 533   Muscles of the back, Mm. dorsi, and suboccipital muscles, Mm. suboccipitales.

→ T 20 b, c

Deep muscles of the back

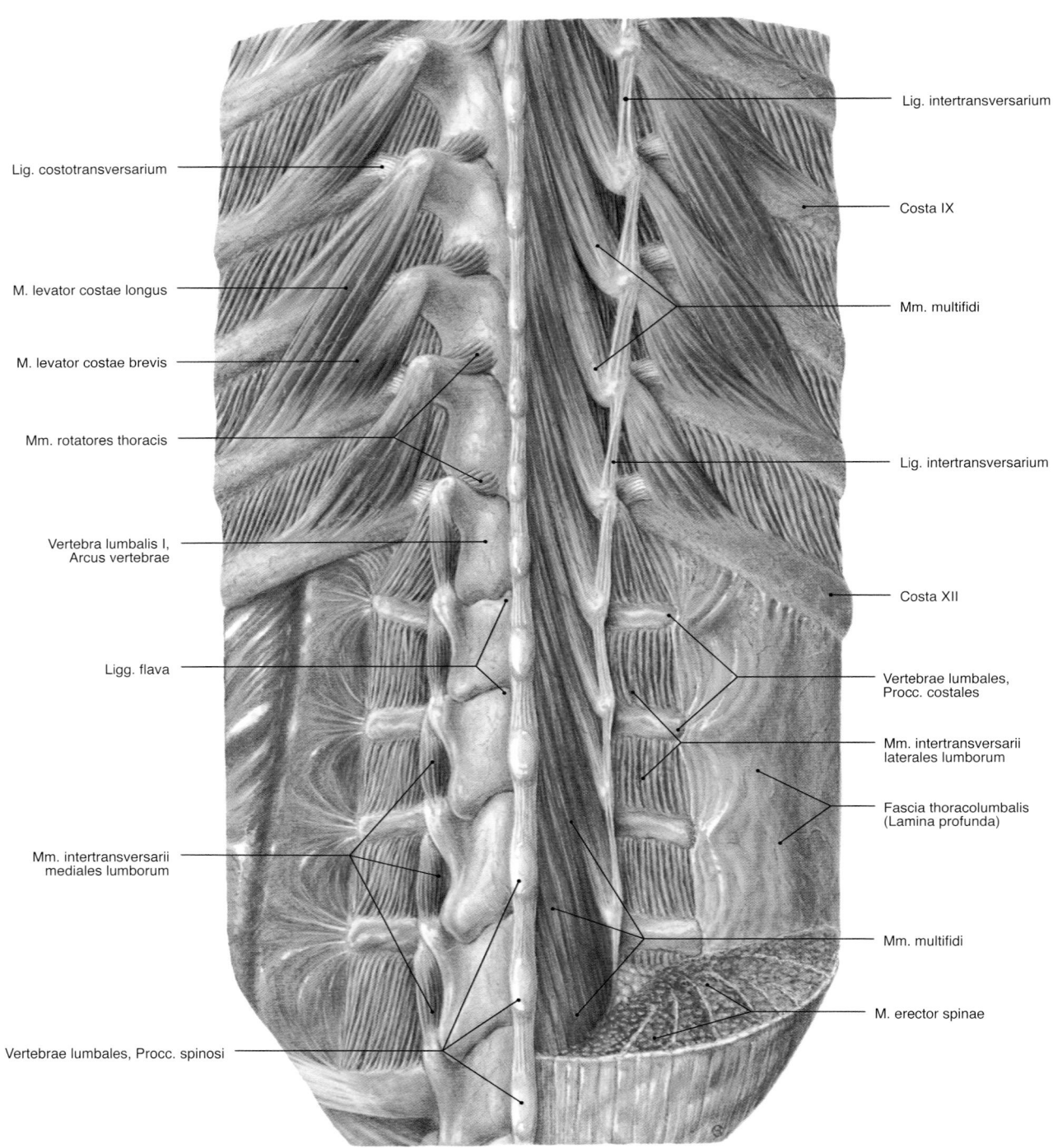

Lig. costotransversarium

M. levator costae longus

M. levator costae brevis

Mm. rotatores thoracis

Vertebra lumbalis I,
Arcus vertebrae

Ligg. flava

Mm. intertransversarii
mediales lumborum

Vertebrae lumbales, Procc. spinosi

Lig. intertransversarium

Costa IX

Mm. multifidi

Lig. intertransversarium

Costa XII

Vertebrae lumbales,
Procc. costales

Mm. intertransversarii
laterales lumborum

Fascia thoracolumbalis
(Lamina profunda)

Mm. multifidi

M. erector spinae

→ T 20 a, b

Fig. 534 Muscles of the back, Mm. dorsi;
deepest layer in the region of the lower thoracic and the lumbar
part of the vertebral column.

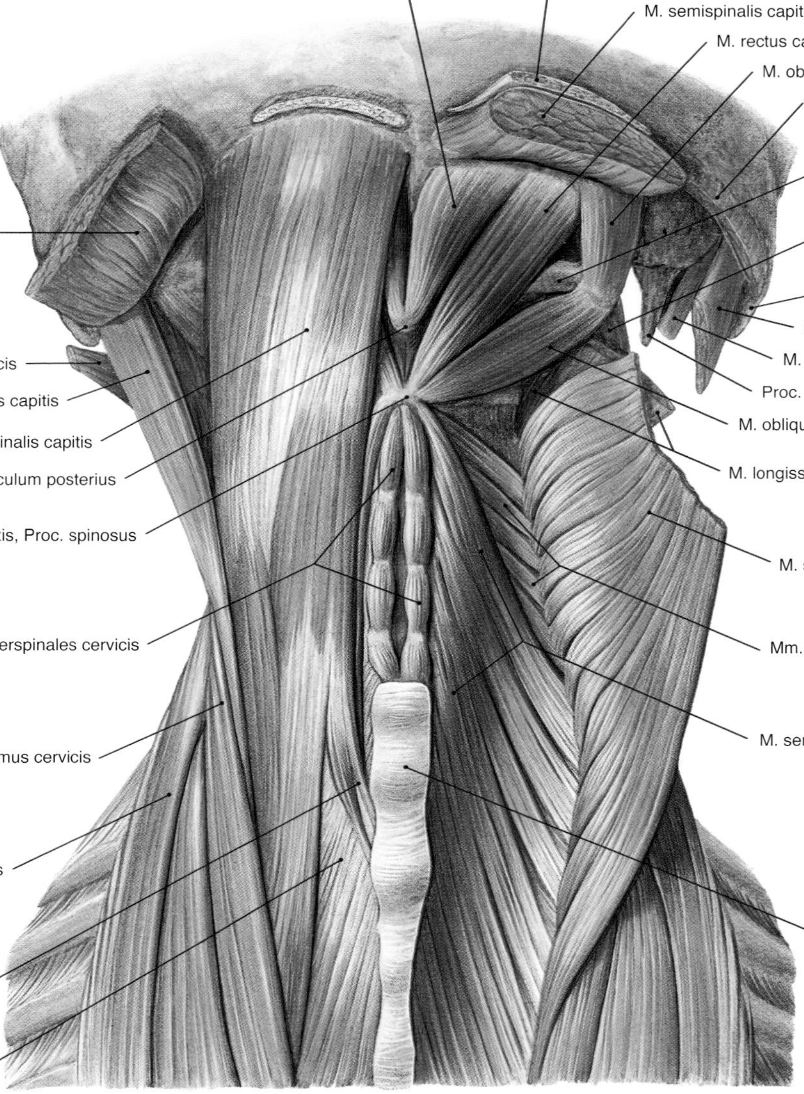

Suboccipital muscles

M. rectus capitis posterior minor

M. trapezius

M. semispinalis capitis

M. rectus capitis posterior major

M. obliquus capitis superior

M. splenius capitis

Atlas, Arcus posterior

M. splenius capitis

M. splenius cervicis

M. splenius cervicis

Proc. mastoideus

M. longissimus capitis

M. longissimus capitis

M. digastricus, Venter posterior

M. semispinalis capitis

Proc. styloideus

Atlas, Tuberculum posterius

M. obliquus capitis inferior

Axis, Proc. spinosus

M. longissimus capitis

M. semispinalis capitis

Mm. interspinales cervicis

Mm. multifidi

M. longissimus cervicis

M. semispinalis cervicis

M. iliocostalis cervicis

M. semispinalis capitis

Lig. supraspinale

M. semispinalis thoracis

Fig. 535 Muscles of the back, Mm. dorsi, and suboccipital muscles, Mm. suboccipitales.

→ T 20 b, c

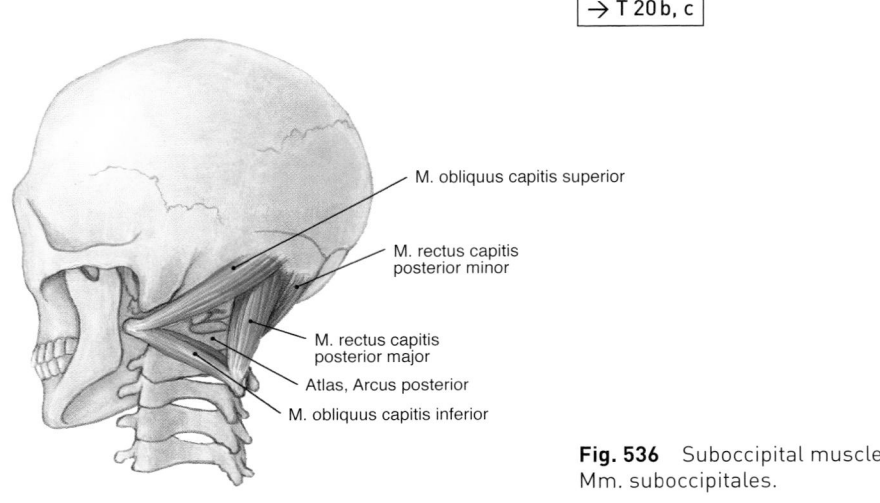

M. obliquus capitis superior

M. rectus capitis posterior minor

M. rectus capitis posterior major

Atlas, Arcus posterior

M. obliquus capitis inferior

Fig. 536 Suboccipital muscles, Mm. suboccipitales.

→ T 20 c

Suboccipital muscles

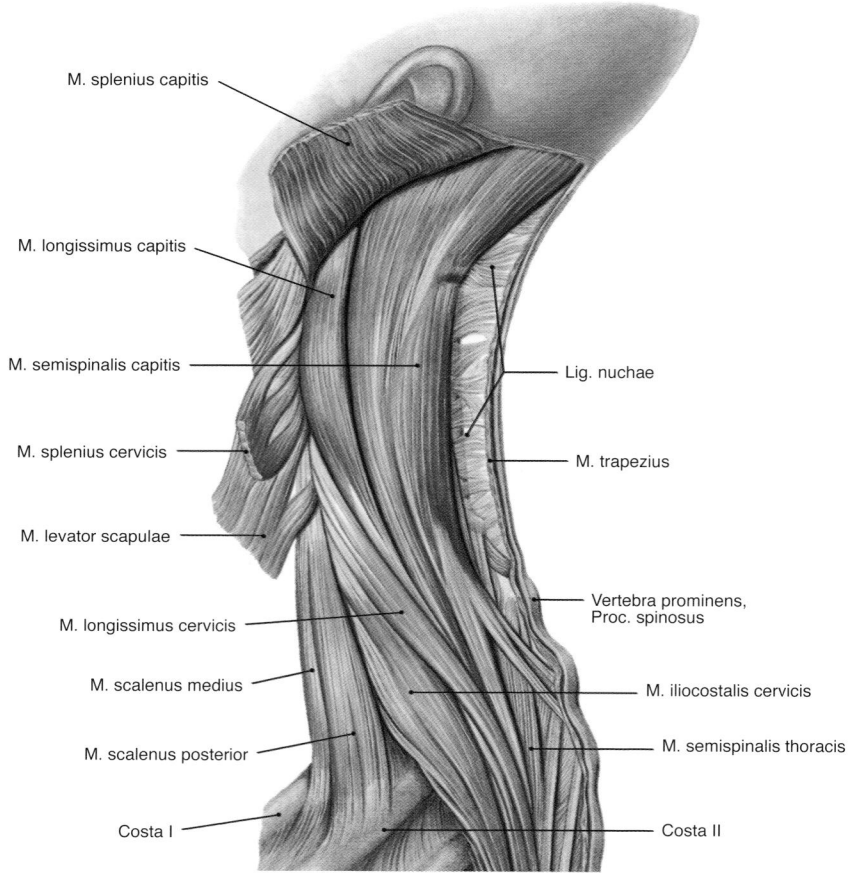

M. splenius capitis

M. longissimus capitis

M. semispinalis capitis

M. splenius cervicis

M. levator scapulae

M. longissimus cervicis

M. scalenus medius

M. scalenus posterior

Costa I

Lig. nuchae

M. trapezius

Vertebra prominens, Proc. spinosus

M. iliocostalis cervicis

M. semispinalis thoracis

Costa II

→ T 20 a, b

Fig. 537 Muscles of the back, Mm. dorsi, and muscles of the neck, Mm. colli.

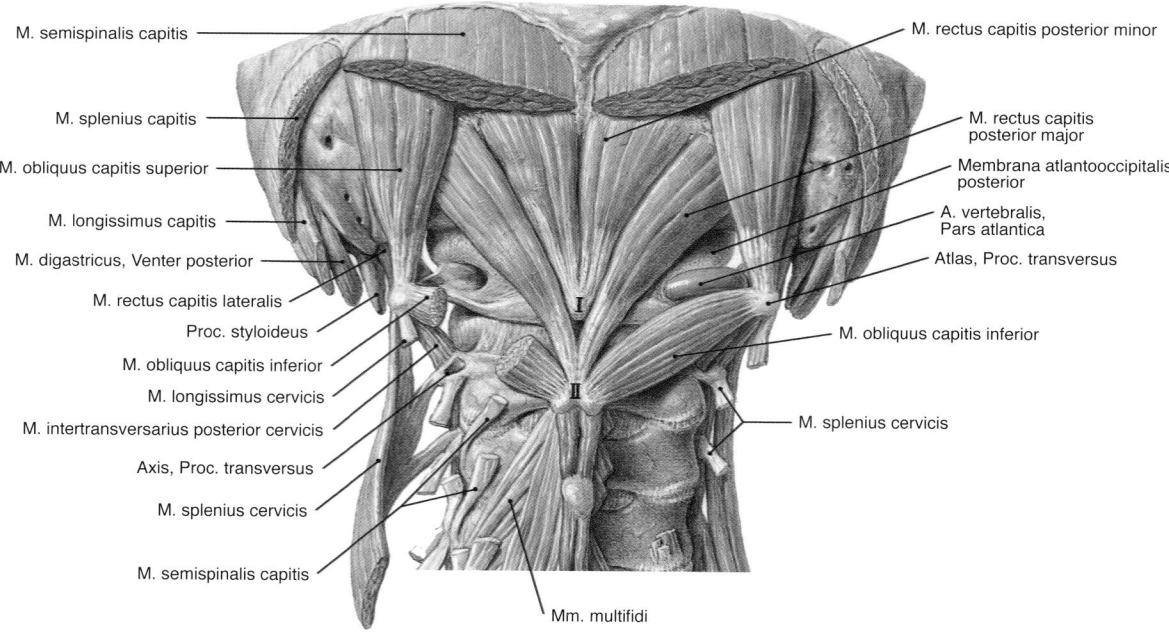

M. semispinalis capitis

M. splenius capitis

M. obliquus capitis superior

M. longissimus capitis

M. digastricus, Venter posterior

M. rectus capitis lateralis

Proc. styloideus

M. obliquus capitis inferior

M. longissimus cervicis

M. intertransversarius posterior cervicis

Axis, Proc. transversus

M. splenius cervicis

M. semispinalis capitis

Mm. multifidi

M. rectus capitis posterior minor

M. rectus capitis posterior major

Membrana atlantooccipitalis posterior

A. vertebralis, Pars atlantica

Atlas, Proc. transversus

M. obliquus capitis inferior

M. splenius cervicis

→ T 20 c

Fig. 538 Suboccipital muscles, Mm. suboccipitales.

I = Posterior tubercle of the atlas
II = Spinous process of the axis

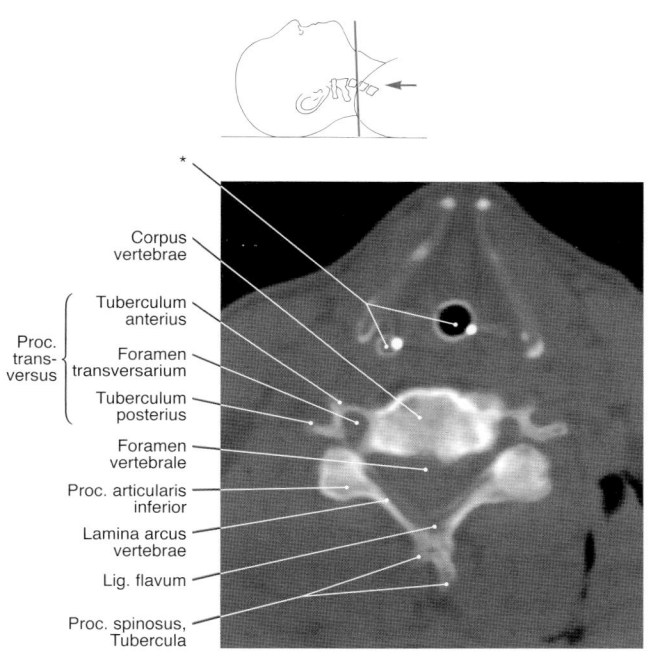

Fig. 539 Cervical part of the vertebral column; computed tomographic cross-section (CT) at the level of the intervertebral disc between the fourth and the fifth cervical vertebra.

* Endotracheal tube and endoscope

Corpus vertebrae
Proc. trans-versus {
Tuberculum anterius
Foramen transversarium
Tuberculum posterius
}
Foramen vertebrale
Proc. articularis inferior
Lamina arcus vertebrae
Lig. flavum
Proc. spinosus, Tubercula

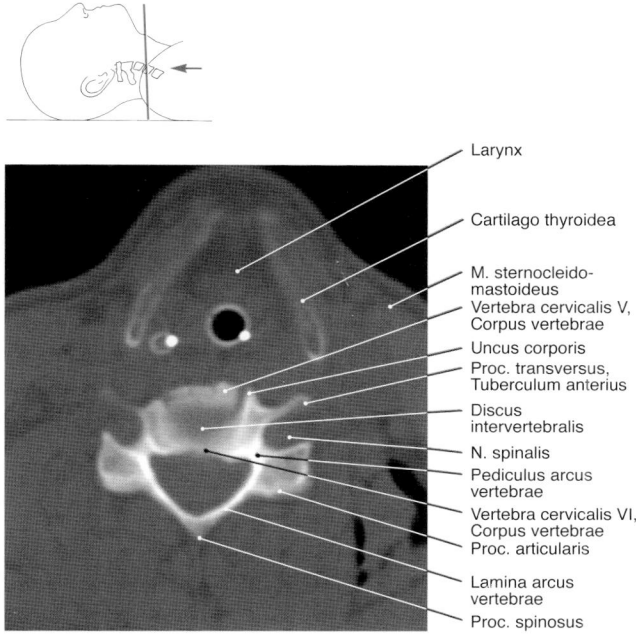

Fig. 540 Cervical part of the vertebral column; computed tomographic cross-section (CT) at the level of the fifth and the sixth cervical vertebra.

Larynx
Cartilago thyroidea
M. sternocleido-mastoideus
Vertebra cervicalis V, Corpus vertebrae
Uncus corporis
Proc. transversus, Tuberculum anterius
Discus intervertebralis
N. spinalis
Pediculus arcus vertebrae
Vertebra cervicalis VI, Corpus vertebrae
Proc. articularis
Lamina arcus vertebrae
Proc. spinosus

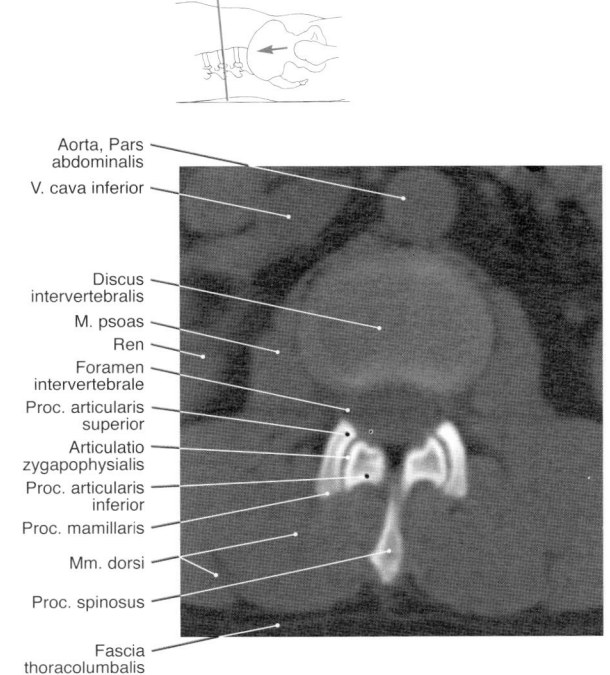

Fig. 541 Lumbar part of the vertebral column; computed tomographic cross-section (CT) at the level of the intervertebral disc between the second and the third lumbar vertebra.

Aorta, Pars abdominalis
V. cava inferior
Discus intervertebralis
M. psoas
Ren
Foramen intervertebrale
Proc. articularis superior
Articulatio zygapophysialis
Proc. articularis inferior
Proc. mamillaris
Mm. dorsi
Proc. spinosus
Fascia thoracolumbalis

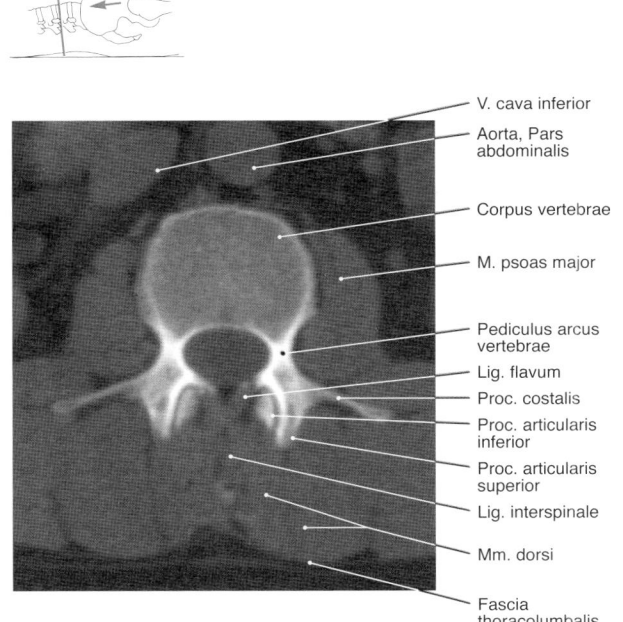

Fig. 542 Lumbar part of the vertebral column; computed tomographic cross-section (CT) at the level of the pedicles of the third lumbar vertebra.

V. cava inferior
Aorta, Pars abdominalis
Corpus vertebrae
M. psoas major
Pediculus arcus vertebrae
Lig. flavum
Proc. costalis
Proc. articularis inferior
Proc. articularis superior
Lig. interspinale
Mm. dorsi
Fascia thoracolumbalis

Cutaneous innervation

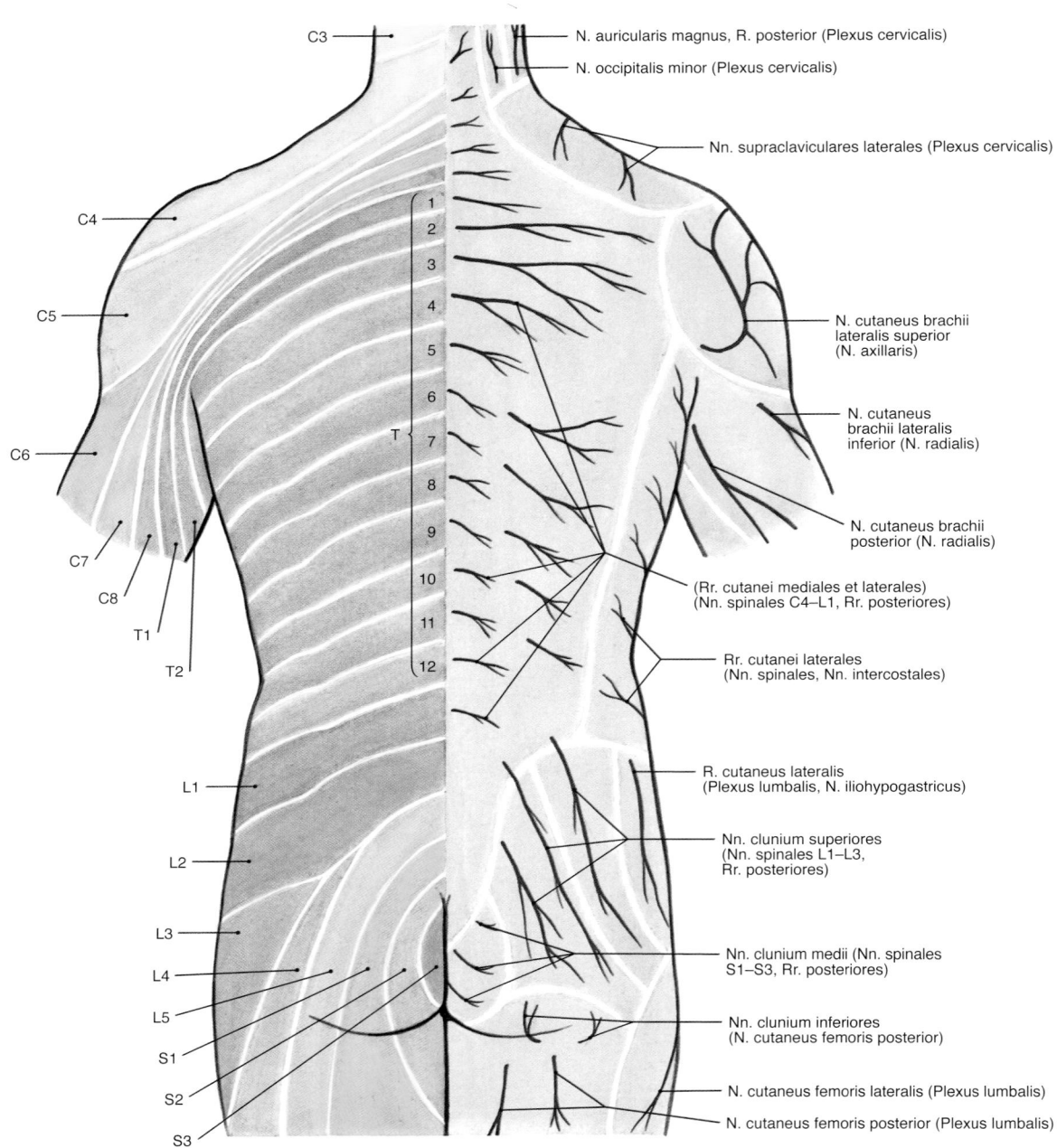

C3 — N. auricularis magnus, R. posterior (Plexus cervicalis)

N. occipitalis minor (Plexus cervicalis)

Nn. supraclaviculares laterales (Plexus cervicalis)

C4

C5

N. cutaneus brachii lateralis superior (N. axillaris)

N. cutaneus brachii lateralis inferior (N. radialis)

C6

N. cutaneus brachii posterior (N. radialis)

C7

C8

(Rr. cutanei mediales et laterales) (Nn. spinales C4–L1, Rr. posteriores)

T1

T2

Rr. cutanei laterales (Nn. spinales, Nn. intercostales)

L1

R. cutaneus lateralis (Plexus lumbalis, N. iliohypogastricus)

Nn. clunium superiores (Nn. spinales L1–L3, Rr. posteriores)

L2

L3

Nn. clunium medii (Nn. spinales S1–S3, Rr. posteriores)

L4

L5

Nn. clunium inferiores (N. cutaneus femoris posterior)

S1

N. cutaneus femoris lateralis (Plexus lumbalis)

S2

N. cutaneus femoris posterior (Plexus lumbalis)

S3

T 1 2 3 4 5 6 7 8 9 10 11 12

Fig. 543 Segmental cutaneous innervation (dermatomes) and cutaneous nerves of the back.

Vessels and nerves of the back

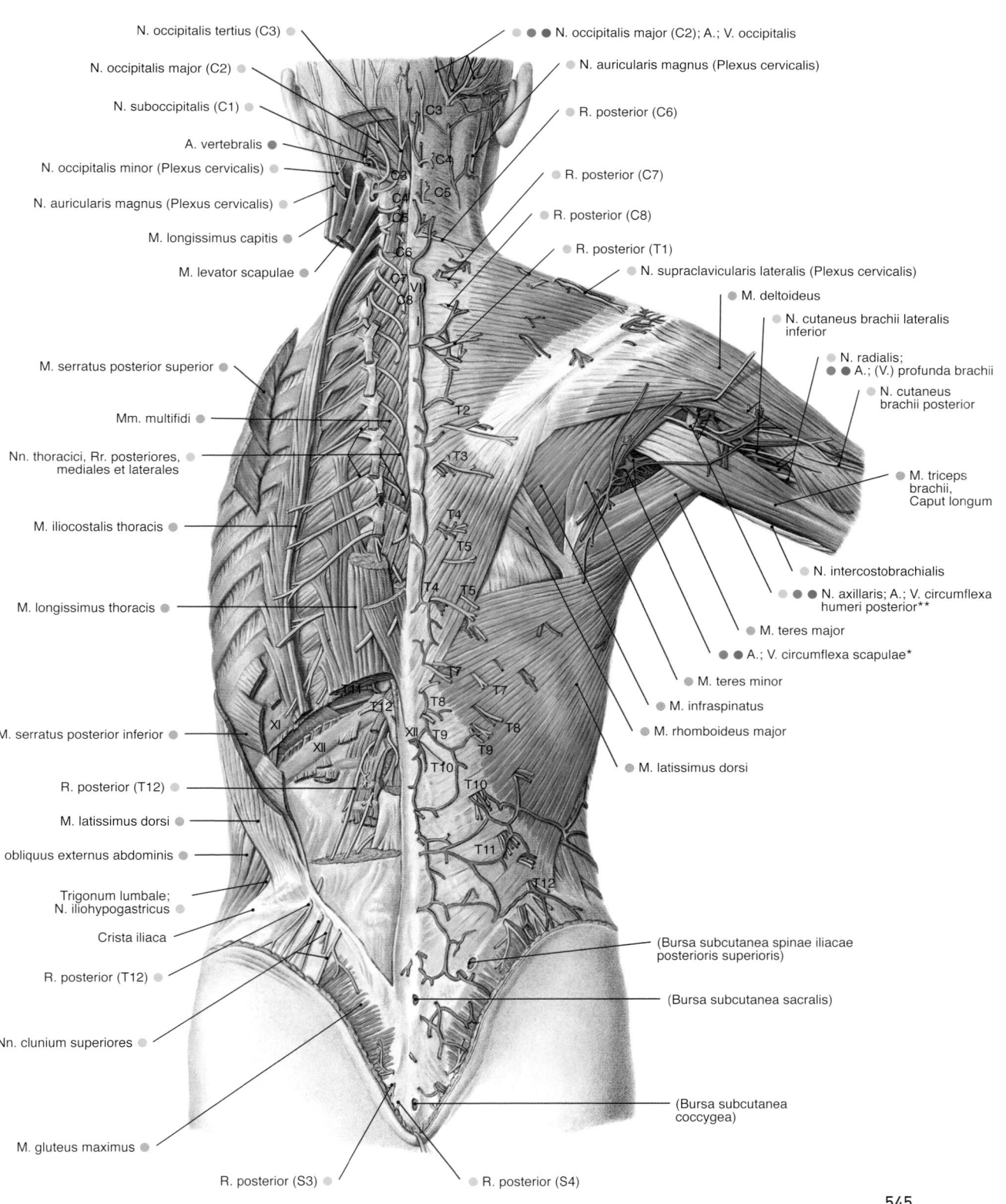

N. occipitalis tertius (C3)
N. occipitalis major (C2)
N. suboccipitalis (C1)
A. vertebralis
N. occipitalis minor (Plexus cervicalis)
N. auricularis magnus (Plexus cervicalis)
M. longissimus capitis
M. levator scapulae

M. serratus posterior superior

Mm. multifidi

Nn. thoracici, Rr. posteriores, mediales et laterales

M. iliocostalis thoracis

M. longissimus thoracis

M. serratus posterior inferior

R. posterior (T12)

M. latissimus dorsi

M. obliquus externus abdominis

Trigonum lumbale; N. iliohypogastricus

Crista iliaca

R. posterior (T12)

Nn. clunium superiores

M. gluteus maximus

R. posterior (S3)

N. occipitalis major (C2); A.; V. occipitalis
N. auricularis magnus (Plexus cervicalis)
R. posterior (C6)
R. posterior (C7)
R. posterior (C8)
R. posterior (T1)
N. supraclavicularis lateralis (Plexus cervicalis)
M. deltoideus
N. cutaneus brachii lateralis inferior
N. radialis; A.; (V.) profunda brachii
N. cutaneus brachii posterior
M. triceps brachii, Caput longum
N. intercostobrachialis
N. axillaris; A.; V. circumflexa humeri posterior**
M. teres major
A.; V. circumflexa scapulae*
M. teres minor
M. infraspinatus
M. rhomboideus major
M. latissimus dorsi

(Bursa subcutanea spinae iliacae posterioris superioris)
(Bursa subcutanea sacralis)
(Bursa subcutanea coccygea)

R. posterior (S4)

545
546

Fig. 544 Vessels and nerves of the back.
* Vessels and nerves of the triangular space
** Vessels and nerves of the quadrangular space

Vessels and nerves of the posterior cervical region

N. occipitalis major ●

M. semispinalis capitis ●

A; V. occipitalis ● ●

A. occipitalis ●

V. auricularis posterior ●

A. occipitalis, ●
R. mastoideus

N. occipitalis minor ●

M. longissimus capitis ●

N accessorius [XI] ●

M. splenius capitis ●

M. levator scapulae ●

N. dorsalis scapulae ●

R. profundus ●
(A. transversa colli)

M. levator scapulae ●

V. transversa ●
colli

M. rhomboideus ●
minor

M. trapezius ●

M. rhomboideus ●
major

M. latissimus dorsi ●

● A. occipitalis, Rr. occipitales

● A. occipitalis

● N. occipitalis major

● V. occipitalis

● N. occipitalis minor

● N. auricularis magnus

● A. auricularis posterior, R. occipitalis

● M. splenius capitis

● M. sternocleidomastoideus

● V. jugularis externa

● Rr. cutanei posteriores (Nn. cervicales et
thoracici, Rr. posteriores)

● M. trapezius

● Rr. cutanei posteriores
(Nn. thoracici,
Rr. posteriores)

● Rr. cutanei laterales
pectorales (Nn. thoracici,
Nn. intercostales)

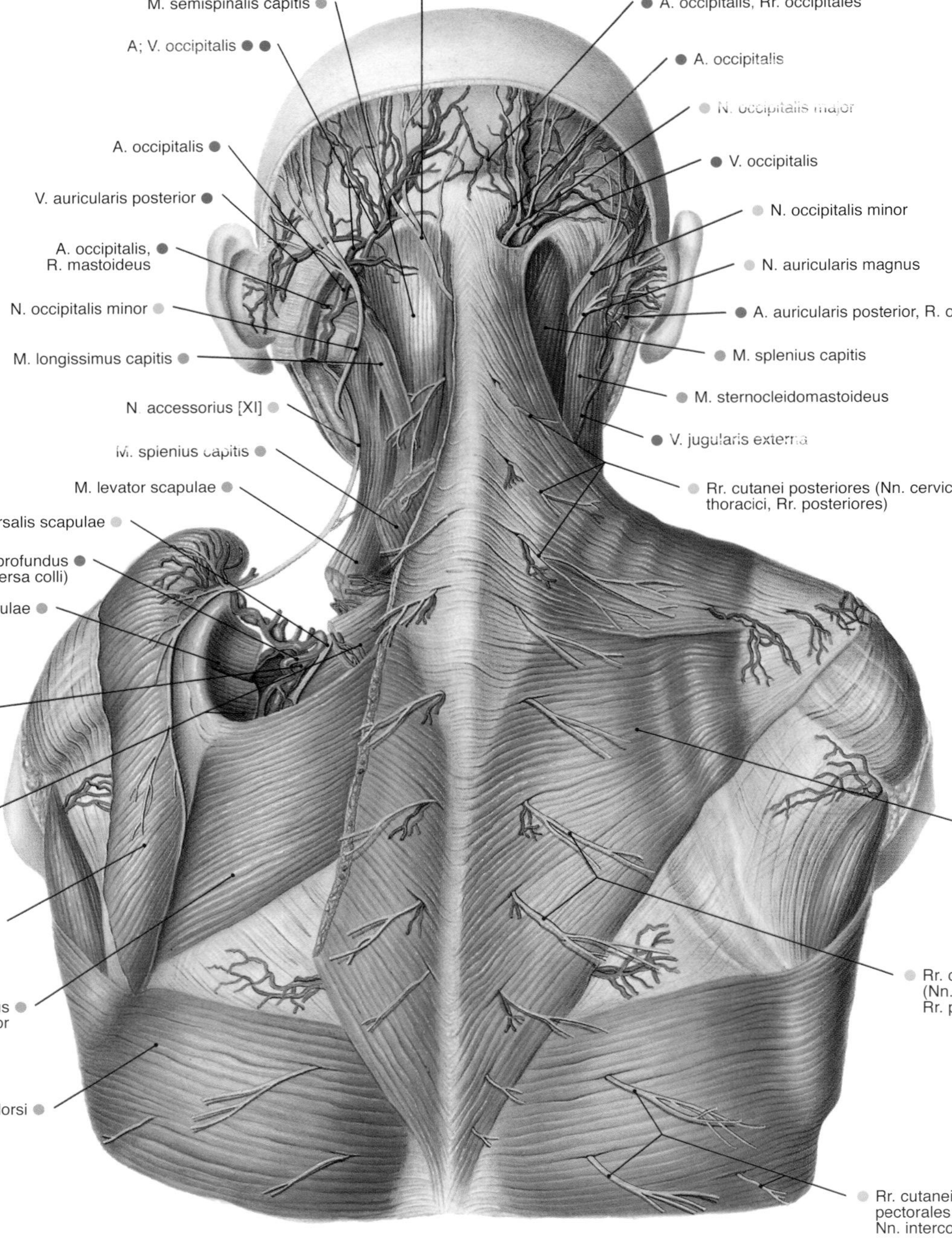

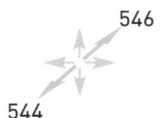

546

544 ◄

Fig. 545   Vessels and nerves of the occipital region,
Regio occipitalis, the posterior cervical region,
Regio cervicalis posterior, and the upper back.

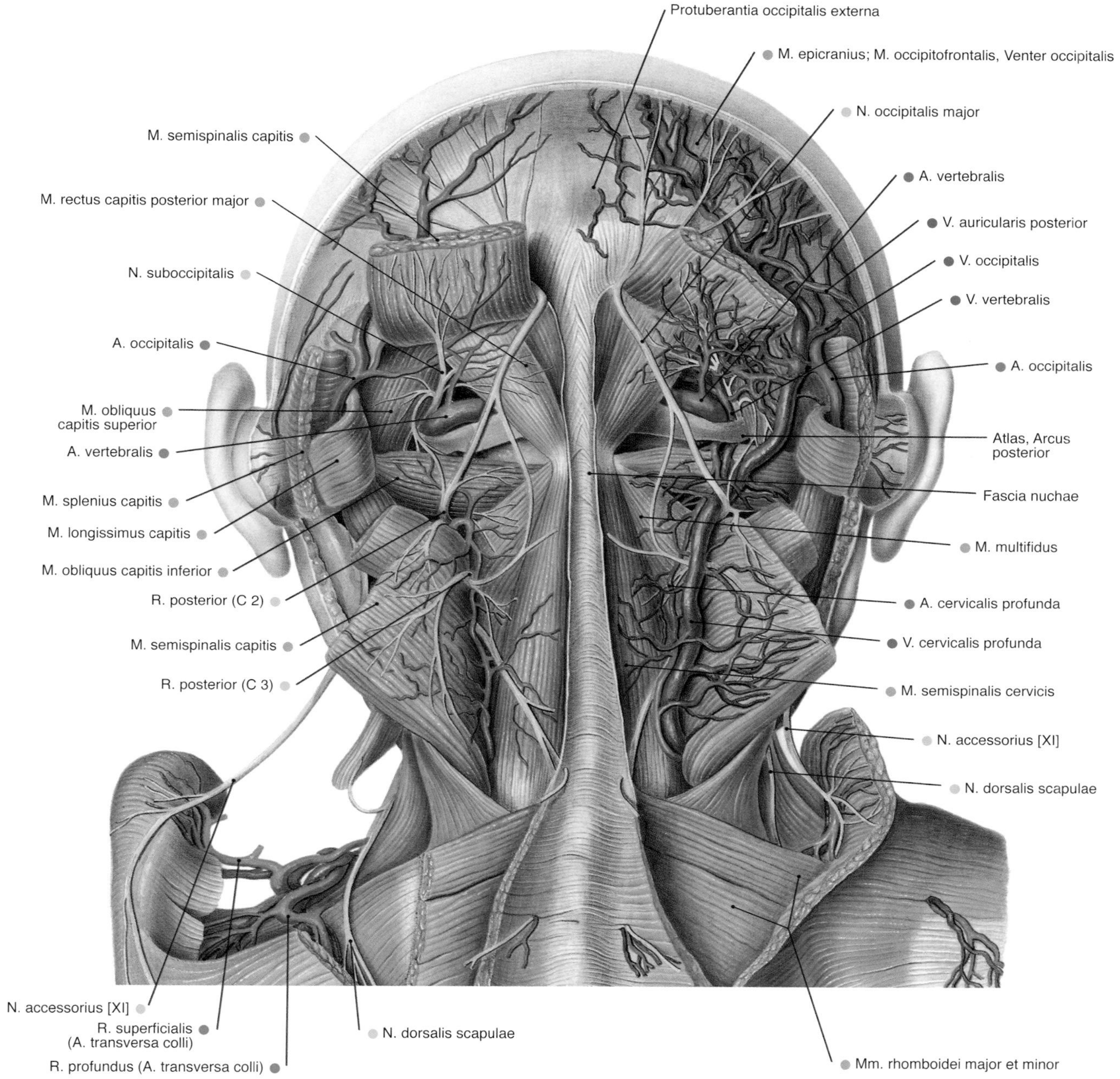

Vessels and nerves of the posterior cervical region

Protuberantia occipitalis externa

M. epicranius; M. occipitofrontalis, Venter occipitalis

N. occipitalis major

M. semispinalis capitis

A. vertebralis

M. rectus capitis posterior major

V. auricularis posterior

N. suboccipitalis

V. occipitalis

V. vertebralis

A. occipitalis

A. occipitalis

M. obliquus capitis superior

Atlas, Arcus posterior

A. vertebralis

Fascia nuchae

M. splenius capitis

M. longissimus capitis

M. multifidus

M. obliquus capitis inferior

R. posterior (C 2)

A. cervicalis profunda

M. semispinalis capitis

V. cervicalis profunda

R. posterior (C 3)

M. semispinalis cervicis

N. accessorius [XI]

N. dorsalis scapulae

N. accessorius [XI]

R. superficialis (A. transversa colli)

N. dorsalis scapulae

R. profundus (A. transversa colli)

Mm. rhomboidei major et minor

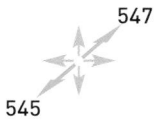
547
545

Fig. 546 Vessels and nerves of the occipital region,
Regio occipitalis, and the posterior cervical region,
Regio cervicalis posterior.

Cervical part of the vertebral canal

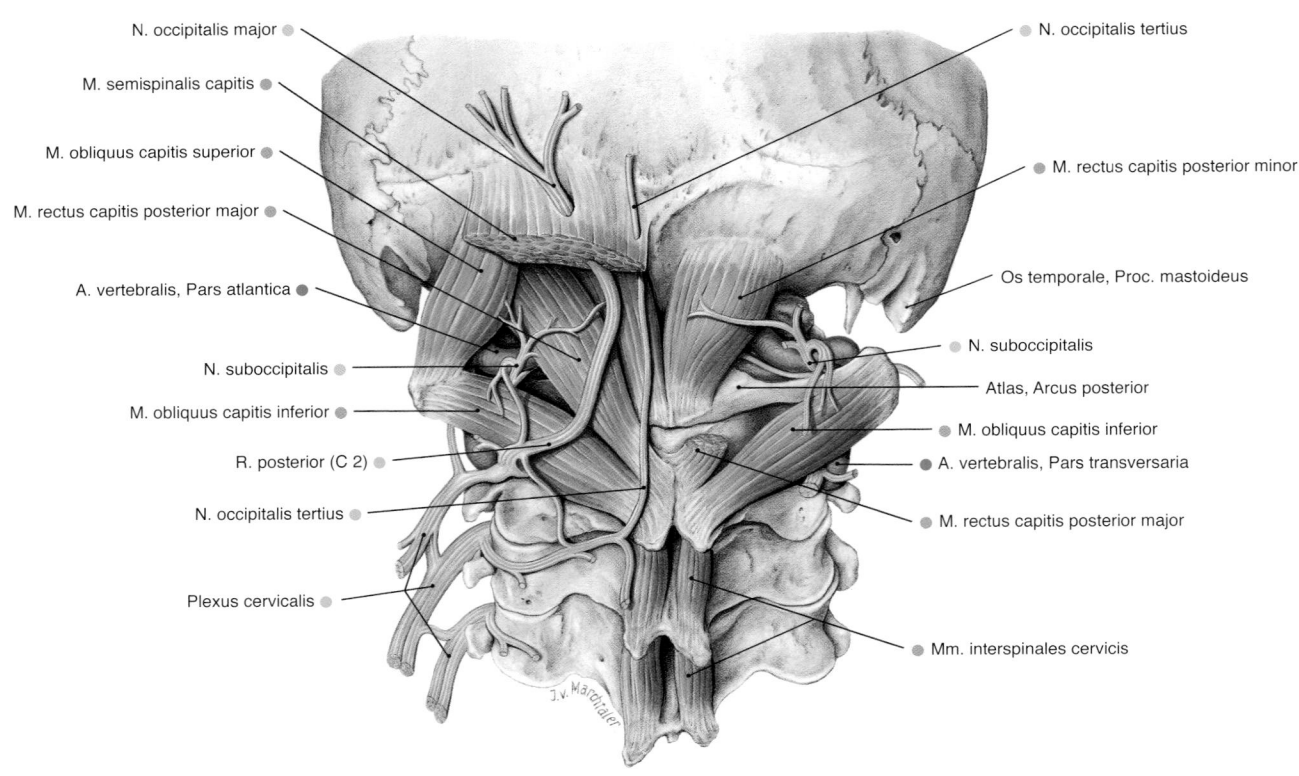

N. occipitalis major ●

M. semispinalis capitis ●

M. obliquus capitis superior ●

M. rectus capitis posterior major ●

A. vertebralis, Pars atlantica ●

N. suboccipitalis ●

M. obliquus capitis inferior ●

R. posterior (C 2) ●

N. occipitalis tertius ●

Plexus cervicalis ●

● N. occipitalis tertius

● M. rectus capitis posterior minor

Os temporale, Proc. mastoideus

● N. suboccipitalis

Atlas, Arcus posterior

● M. obliquus capitis inferior

● A. vertebralis, Pars transversaria

● M. rectus capitis posterior major

● Mm. interspinales cervicis

Fig. 547 Nerves of the posterior cervical region, Regio cervicalis posterior, and the vertebral artery, A. vertebralis.

546

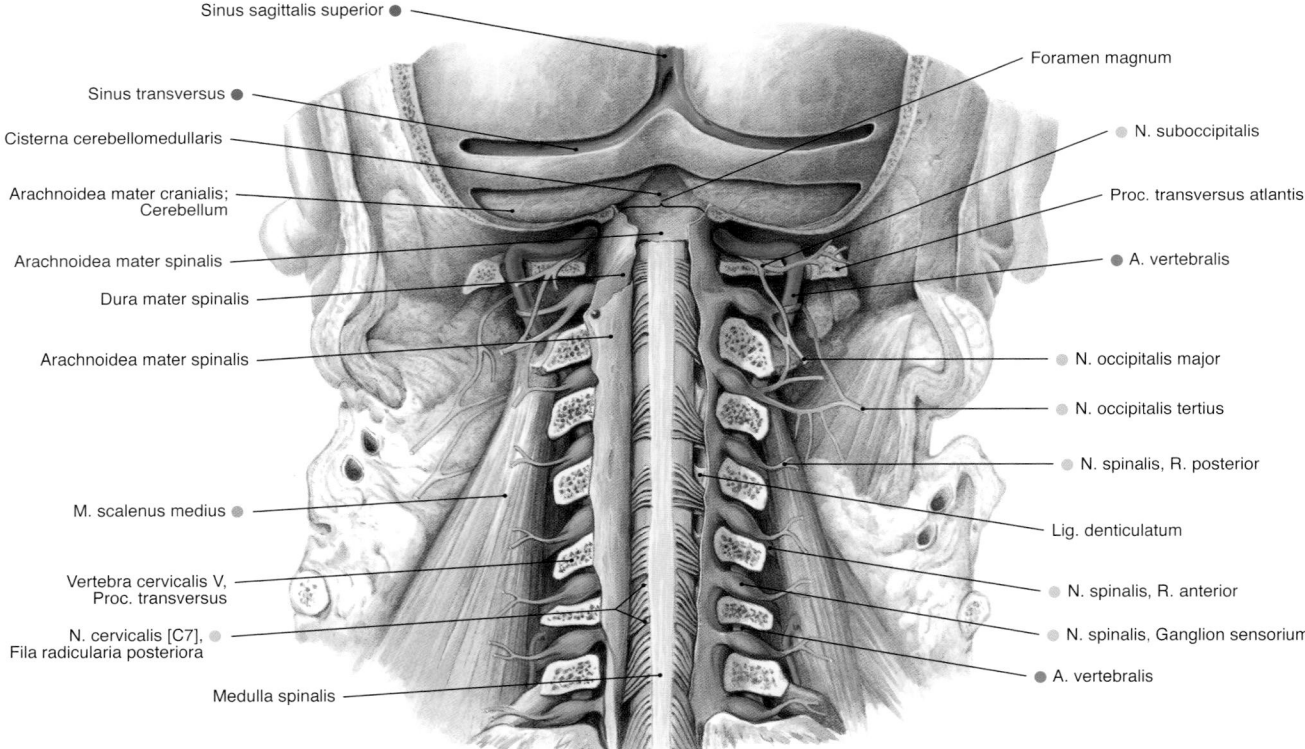

Sinus sagittalis superior ●

Sinus transversus ●

Cisterna cerebellomedullaris ●

Arachnoidea mater cranialis;
Cerebellum

Arachnoidea mater spinalis ●

Dura mater spinalis ●

Arachnoidea mater spinalis ●

M. scalenus medius ●

Vertebra cervicalis V,
Proc. transversus

N. cervicalis [C7], ●
Fila radicularia posteriora

Medulla spinalis ●

Foramen magnum

● N. suboccipitalis

Proc. transversus atlantis

● A. vertebralis

● N. occipitalis major

● N. occipitalis tertius

● N. spinalis, R. posterior

Lig. denticulatum

● N. spinalis, R. anterior

● N. spinalis, Ganglion sensorium

● A. vertebralis

Fig. 548 Vessels and nerves of the deep posterior cervical region, Regio cervicalis posterior, and the content of the vertebral canal.

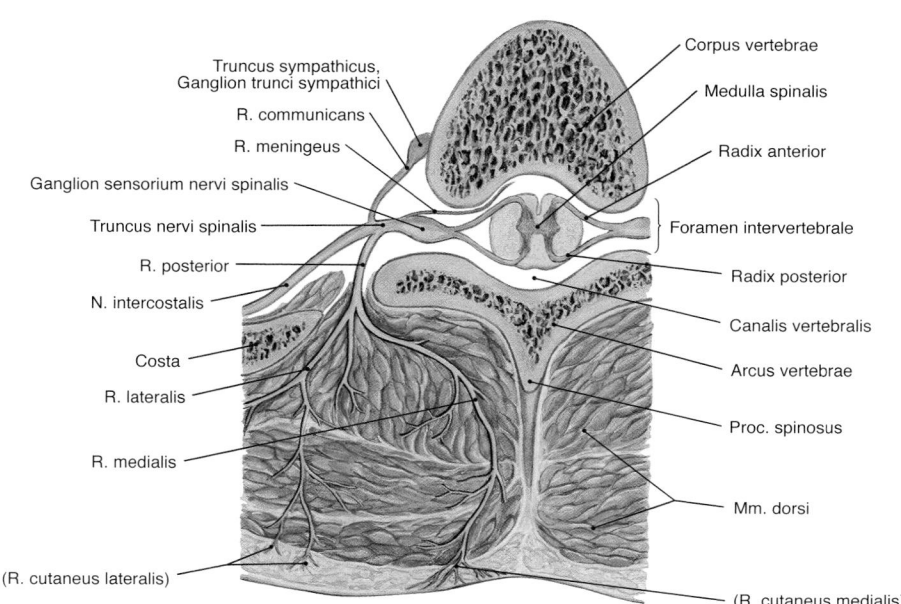

Truncus sympathicus, Ganglion trunci sympathici
R. communicans
R. meningeus
Ganglion sensorium nervi spinalis
Truncus nervi spinalis
R. posterior
N. intercostalis
Costa
R. lateralis
R. medialis
(R. cutaneus lateralis)

Corpus vertebrae
Medulla spinalis
Radix anterior
Foramen intervertebrale
Radix posterior
Canalis vertebralis
Arcus vertebrae
Proc. spinosus
Mm. dorsi
(R. cutaneus medialis)

Fig. 549 Spinal nerve, N. spinalis; in the thoracic region.

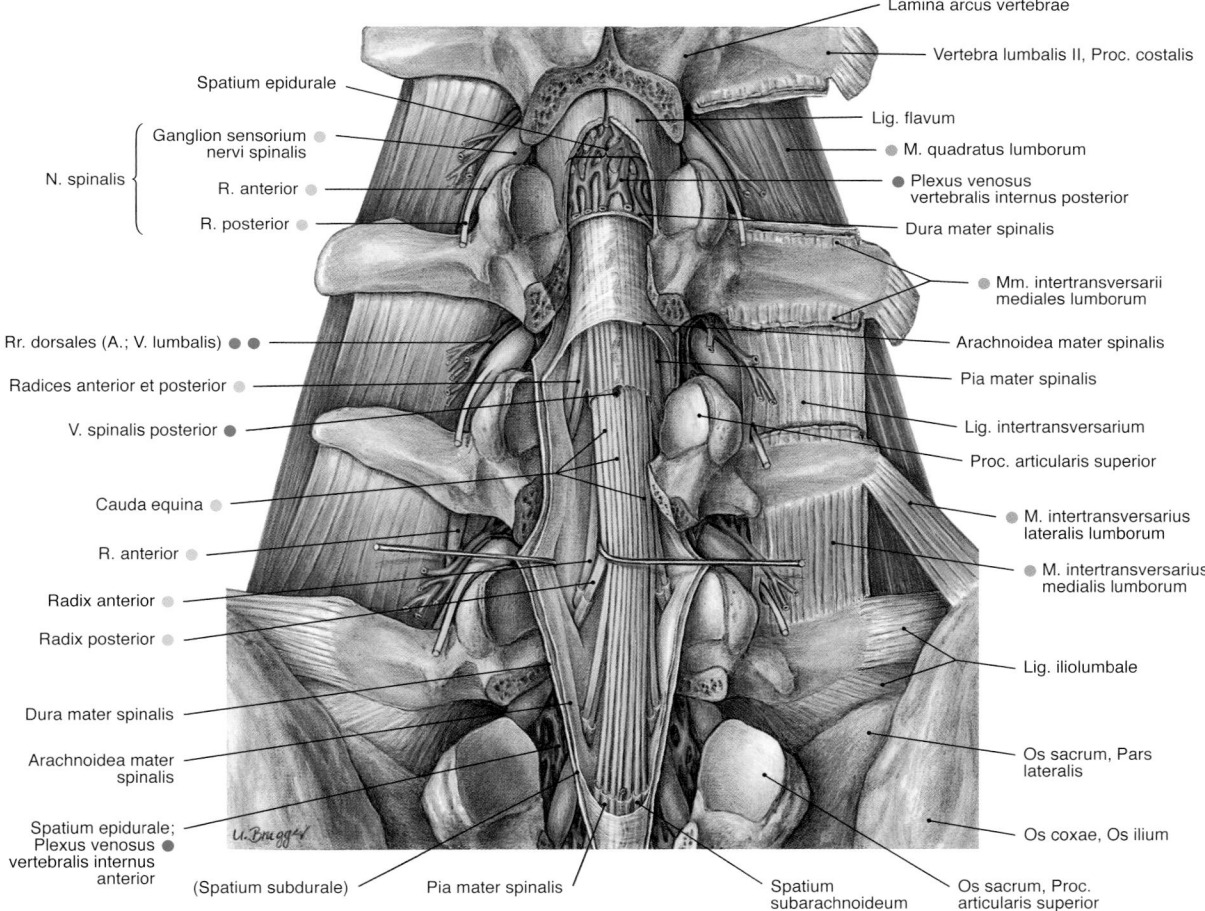

Spatium epidurale
N. spinalis {
Ganglion sensorium nervi spinalis
R. anterior
R. posterior
}
Rr. dorsales (A.; V. lumbalis)
Radices anterior et posterior
V. spinalis posterior
Cauda equina
R. anterior
Radix anterior
Radix posterior
Dura mater spinalis
Arachnoidea mater spinalis
Spatium epidurale; Plexus venosus vertebralis internus anterior
(Spatium subdurale)
Pia mater spinalis

Lamina arcus vertebrae
Vertebra lumbalis II, Proc. costalis
Lig. flavum
M. quadratus lumborum
Plexus venosus vertebralis internus posterior
Dura mater spinalis
Mm. intertransversarii mediales lumborum
Arachnoidea mater spinalis
Pia mater spinalis
Lig. intertransversarium
Proc. articularis superior
M. intertransversarius lateralis lumborum
M. intertransversarius medialis lumborum
Lig. iliolumbale
Os sacrum, Pars lateralis
Os coxae, Os ilium
Os sacrum, Proc. articularis superior
Spatium subarachnoideum

Fig. 550 Vessels and nerves of the lumbar part of the vertebral canal, Regio lumbalis.

Veins and nerves of the lumbar part of the vertebral column

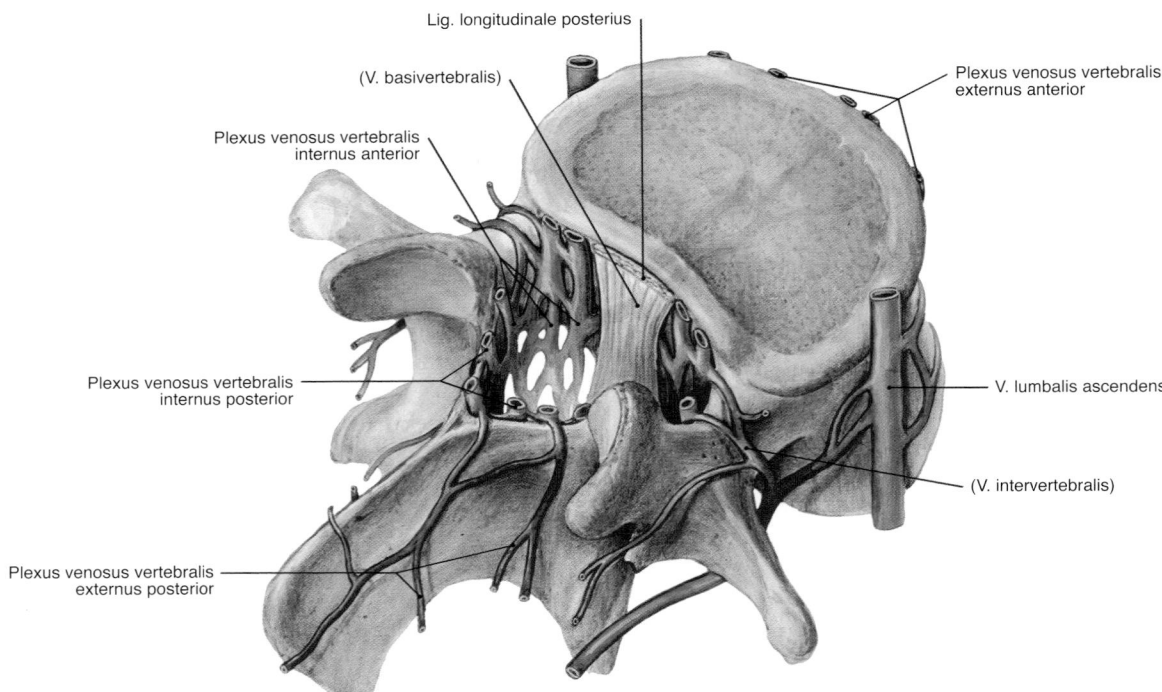

Lig. longitudinale posterius

(V. basivertebralis)

Plexus venosus vertebralis internus anterior

Plexus venosus vertebralis externus anterior

Plexus venosus vertebralis internus posterior

V. lumbalis ascendens

(V. intervertebralis)

Plexus venosus vertebralis externus posterior

Fig. 551 Veins of the vertebral canal, Canalis vertebralis; venous plexus.

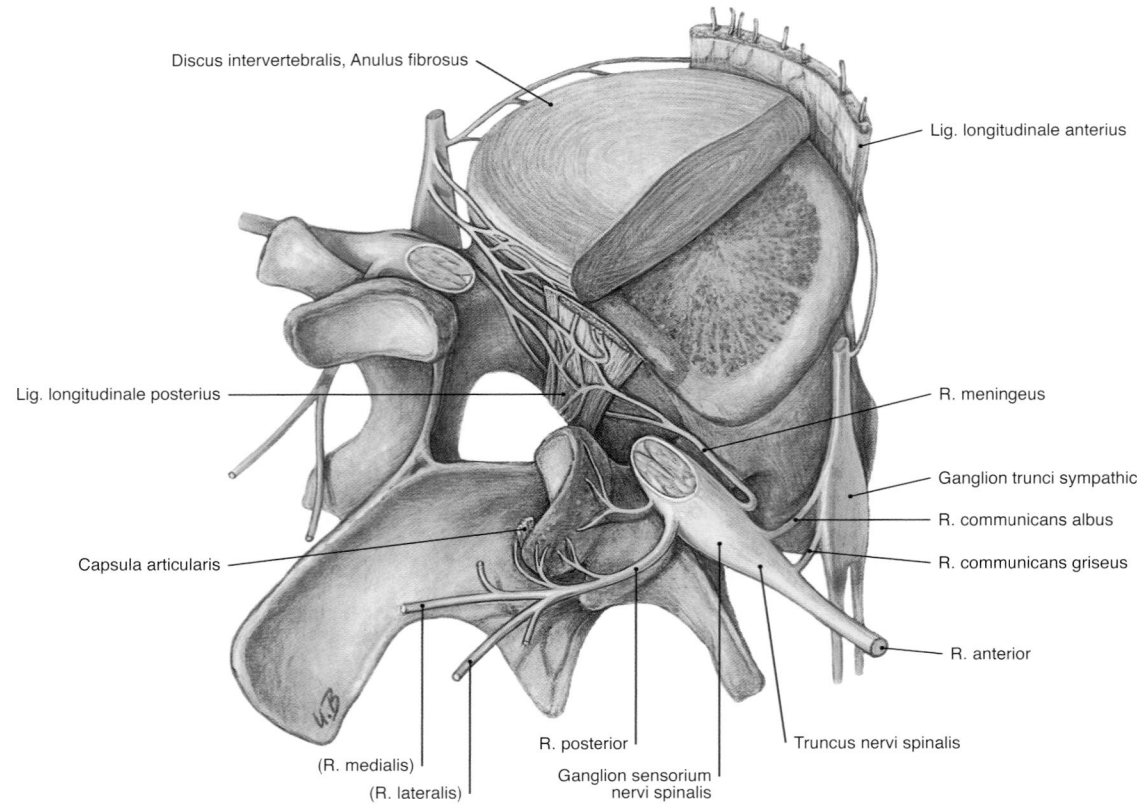

Discus intervertebralis, Anulus fibrosus

Lig. longitudinale anterius

Lig. longitudinale posterius

R. meningeus

Ganglion trunci sympathici

R. communicans albus

R. communicans griseus

Capsula articularis

R. anterior

(R. medialis)

R. posterior

Truncus nervi spinalis

(R. lateralis)

Ganglion sensorium nervi spinalis

Fig. 552 Nerves of the vertebral column, Columna vertebralis; somatic and autonomous innervation.

Vessels and nerves of the vertebral canal

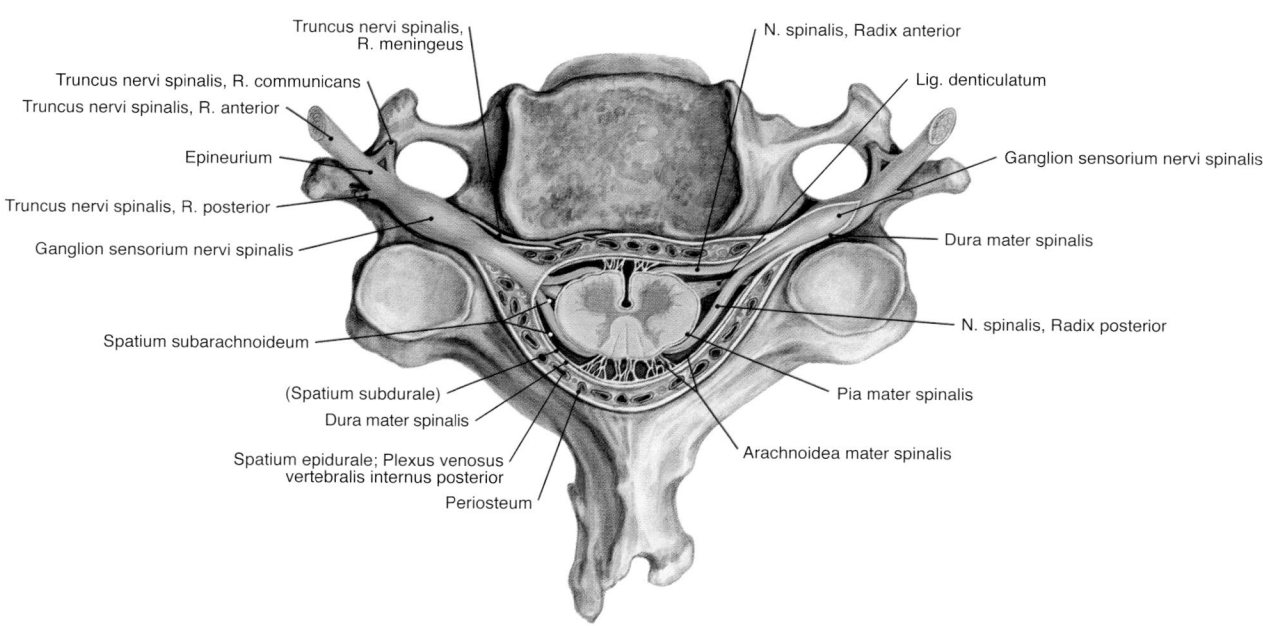

Truncus nervi spinalis, R. meningeus
Truncus nervi spinalis, R. communicans
Truncus nervi spinalis, R. anterior
Epineurium
Truncus nervi spinalis, R. posterior
Ganglion sensorium nervi spinalis
Spatium subarachnoideum
(Spatium subdurale)
Dura mater spinalis
Spatium epidurale; Plexus venosus vertebralis internus posterior
Periosteum

N. spinalis, Radix anterior
Lig. denticulatum
Ganglion sensorium nervi spinalis
Dura mater spinalis
N. spinalis, Radix posterior
Pia mater spinalis
Arachnoidea mater spinalis

Fig. 553 Content of the vertebral canal, Canalis vertebralis; cross-section at the level of the fifth cervical vertebra.

→ 1304 ff

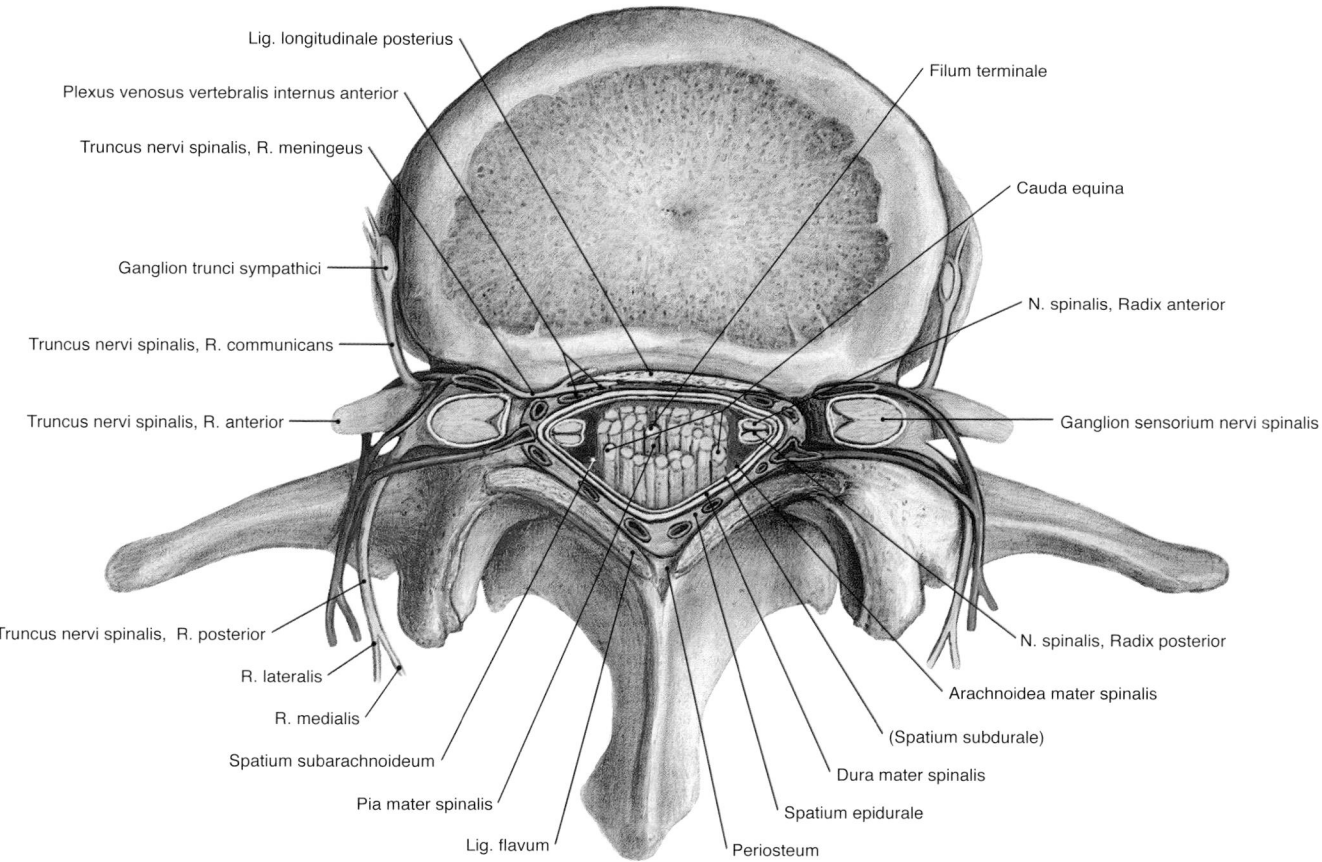

Lig. longitudinale posterius
Plexus venosus vertebralis internus anterior
Truncus nervi spinalis, R. meningeus
Ganglion trunci sympathici
Truncus nervi spinalis, R. communicans
Truncus nervi spinalis, R. anterior
Truncus nervi spinalis, R. posterior
R. lateralis
R. medialis
Spatium subarachnoideum
Pia mater spinalis
Lig. flavum

Filum terminale
Cauda equina
N. spinalis, Radix anterior
Ganglion sensorium nervi spinalis
N. spinalis, Radix posterior
Arachnoidea mater spinalis
(Spatium subdurale)
Dura mater spinalis
Spatium epidurale
Periosteum

Fig. 554 Content of the vertebral canal, Canalis vertebralis; cross-section at the level of the third lumbar vertebra.

→ 1304 ff

Lumbar and sacral puncture

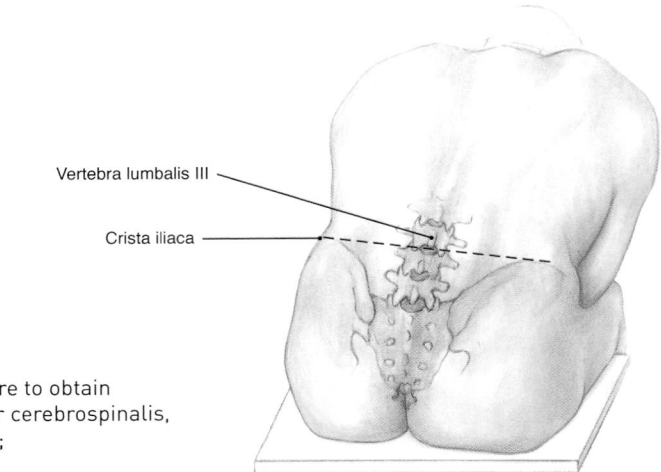

Vertebra lumbalis III

Crista iliaca

Fig. 555 Lumbar puncture to obtain
cerebrospinal fluid, Liquor cerebrospinalis,
or for lumbal anaesthesia;
position of the patient.

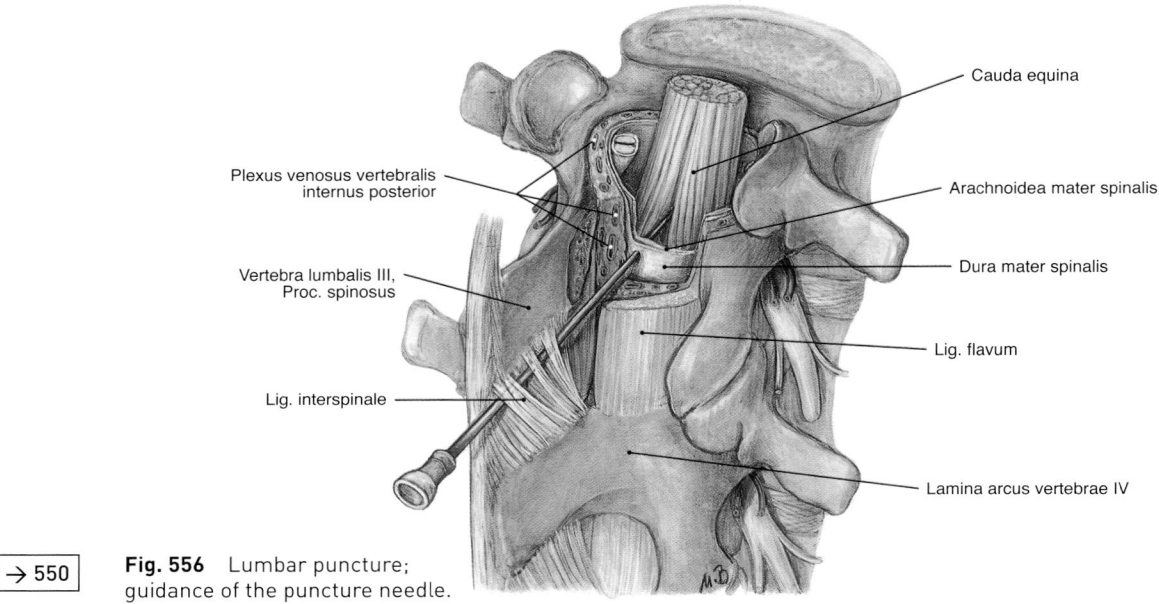

Cauda equina

Plexus venosus vertebralis
internus posterior

Arachnoidea mater spinalis

Vertebra lumbalis III,
Proc. spinosus

Dura mater spinalis

Lig. flavum

Lig. interspinale

Lamina arcus vertebrae IV

→ 550

Fig. 556 Lumbar puncture;
guidance of the puncture needle.

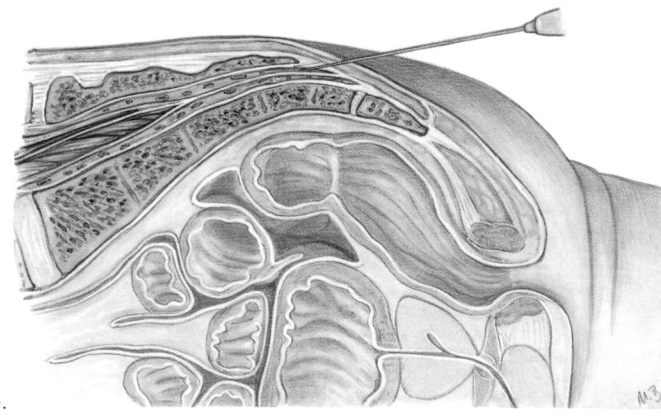

Fig. 557 Sacral puncture;
guidance of the puncture needle.

Vessels and nerves of the vertebral canal

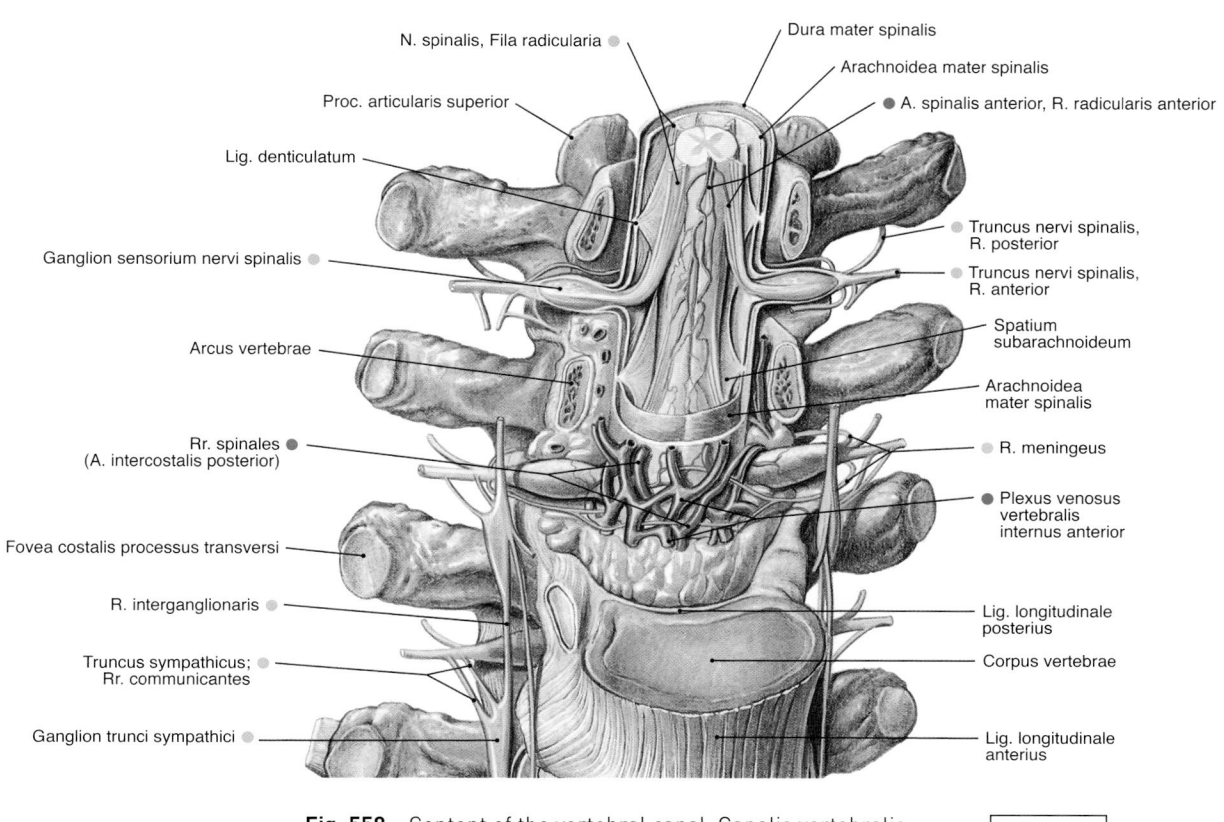

N. spinalis, Fila radicularia ●

Proc. articularis superior

Lig. denticulatum

Ganglion sensorium nervi spinalis ●

Arcus vertebrae

Rr. spinales ●
(A. intercostalis posterior)

Fovea costalis processus transversi

R. interganglionaris ●

Truncus sympathicus;
Rr. communicantes ●

Ganglion trunci sympathici ●

Dura mater spinalis

Arachnoidea mater spinalis

● A. spinalis anterior, R. radicularis anterior

Truncus nervi spinalis,
R. posterior ●

Truncus nervi spinalis,
R. anterior ●

Spatium
subarachnoideum

Arachnoidea
mater spinalis

● R. meningeus

● Plexus venosus
vertebralis
internus anterior

Lig. longitudinale
posterius

Corpus vertebrae

Lig. longitudinale
anterius

Fig. 558 Content of the vertebral canal, Canalis vertebralis; thoracic portion after stepwise exposure; ventral view.

→ 1304 ff

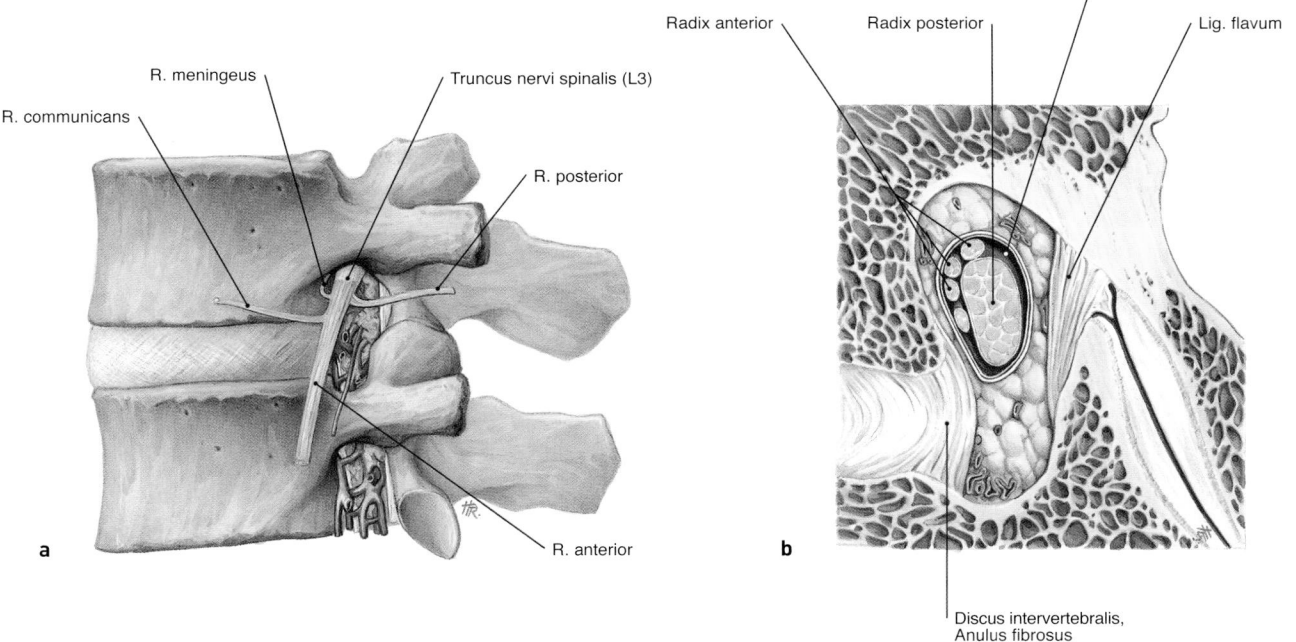

R. communicans

R. meningeus

Truncus nervi spinalis (L3)

R. posterior

R. anterior

a

Radix anterior

Radix posterior

Spatium subarachnoideum

Lig. flavum

Discus intervertebralis,
Anulus fibrosus

b

Fig. 559 a, b Intervertebral foramina, Foramina intervertebralia; lumbar part of the vertebral column.

a Viewed from the left
b Sagittal section

Surface anatomy

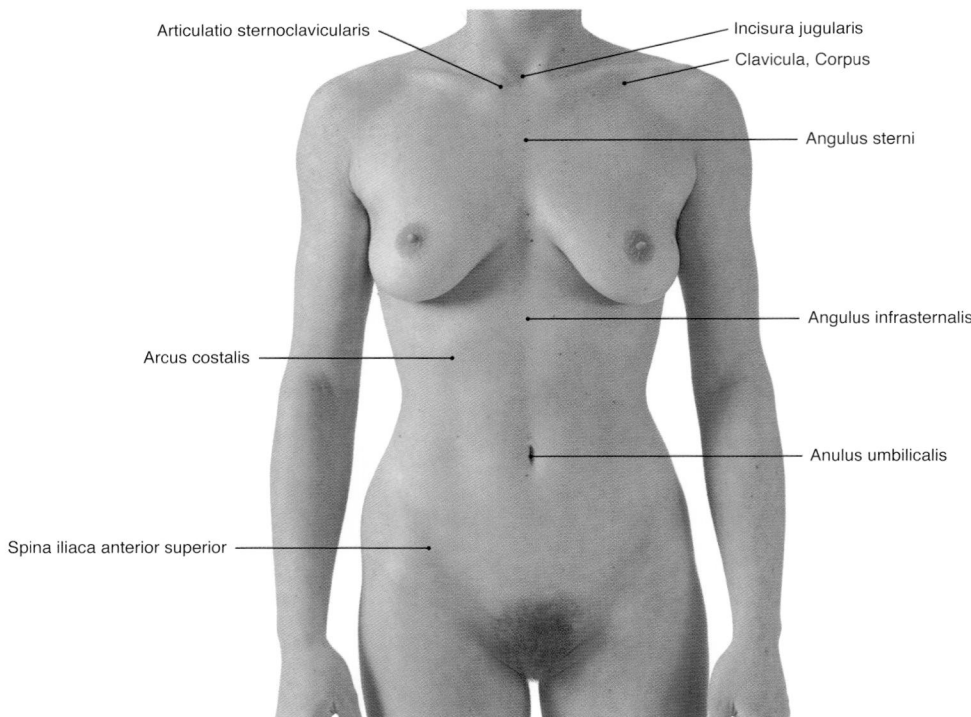

Articulatio sternoclavicularis
Incisura jugularis
Clavicula, Corpus
Angulus sterni
Angulus infrasternalis
Arcus costalis
Anulus umbilicalis
Spina iliaca anterior superior

Fig. 560 Surface anatomy of the thoracic and abdominal wall of a young woman.

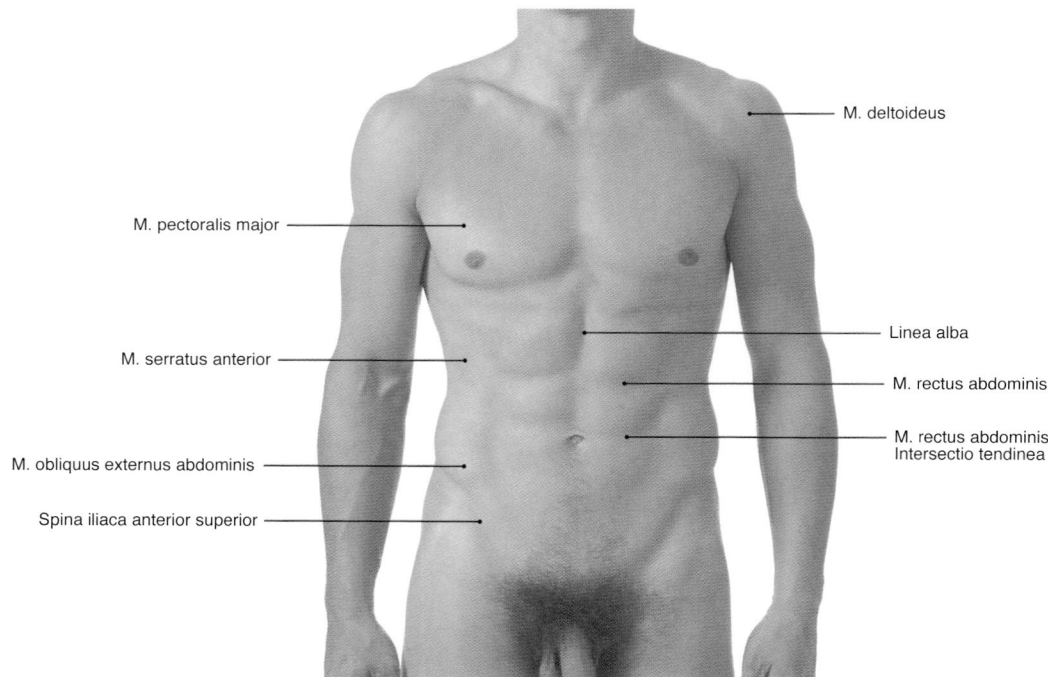

M. deltoideus
M. pectoralis major
Linea alba
M. serratus anterior
M. rectus abdominis
M. rectus abdominis, Intersectio tendinea
M. obliquus externus abdominis
Spina iliaca anterior superior

Fig. 561 Surface anatomy of the thoracic and abdominal wall of a young man.

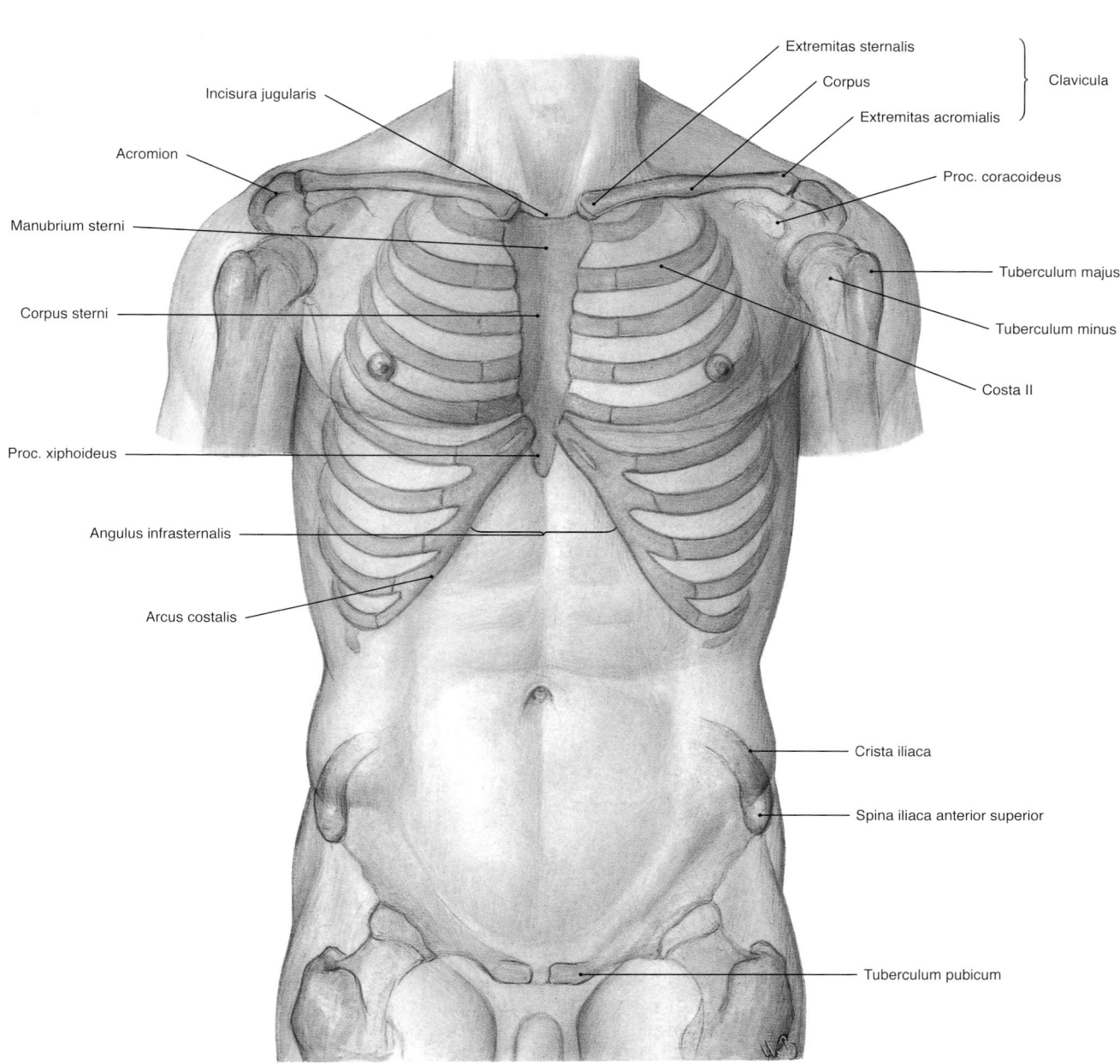

Incisura jugularis

Acromion

Manubrium sterni

Corpus sterni

Proc. xiphoideus

Angulus infrasternalis

Arcus costalis

Extremitas sternalis

Corpus

Extremitas acromialis

Clavicula

Proc. coracoideus

Tuberculum majus

Tuberculum minus

Costa II

Crista iliaca

Spina iliaca anterior superior

Tuberculum pubicum

Fig. 562 Projection of the skeleton onto the thoracic and abdominal wall.

Skeleton of the trunk

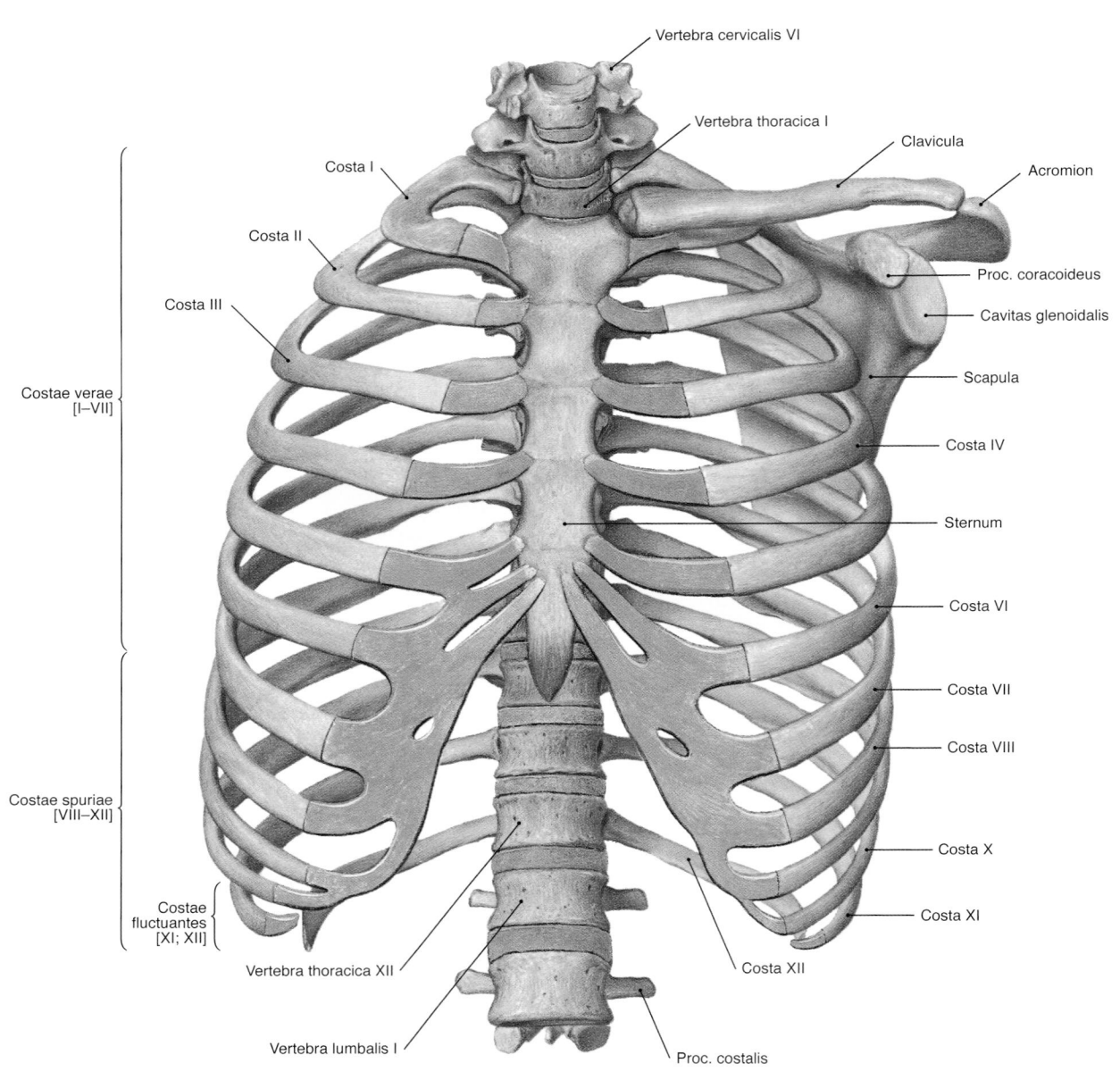

Fig. 563   Thoracic cage, Cavea thoracis, and left shoulder girdle, Cingulum pectorale.

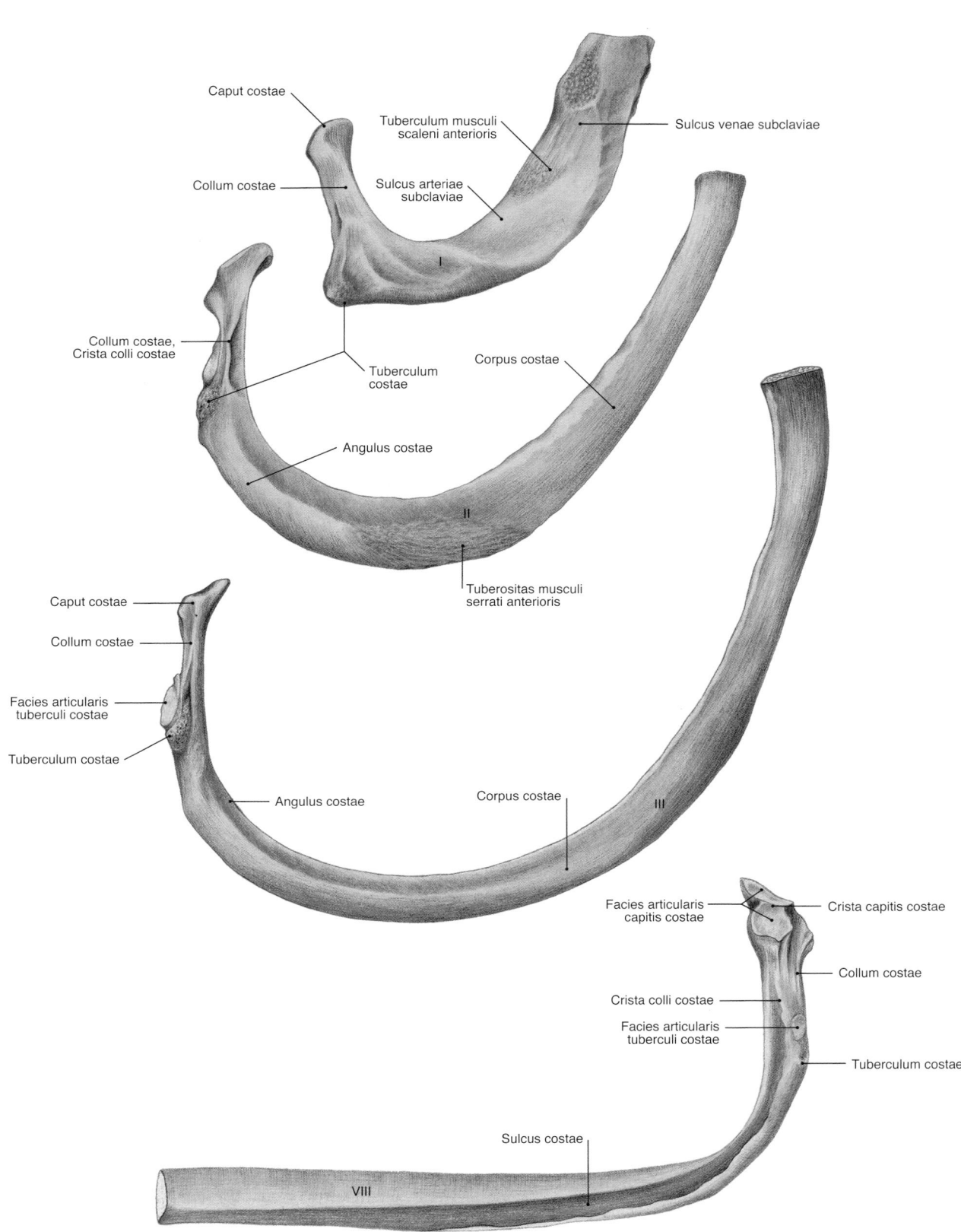

Caput costae

Tuberculum musculi
scaleni anterioris

Sulcus venae subclaviae

Collum costae

Sulcus arteriae
subclaviae

I

Collum costae,
Crista colli costae

Tuberculum
costae

Corpus costae

Angulus costae

II

Tuberositas musculi
serrati anterioris

Caput costae

Collum costae

Facies articularis
tuberculi costae

Tuberculum costae

Angulus costae

Corpus costae

III

Facies articularis
capitis costae

Crista capitis costae

Collum costae

Crista colli costae

Facies articularis
tuberculi costae

Tuberculum costae

Sulcus costae

VIII

Fig. 564 Ribs, Costae;
I.–III. rib, superior view;
VIII. rib, inferior view.

Sternum

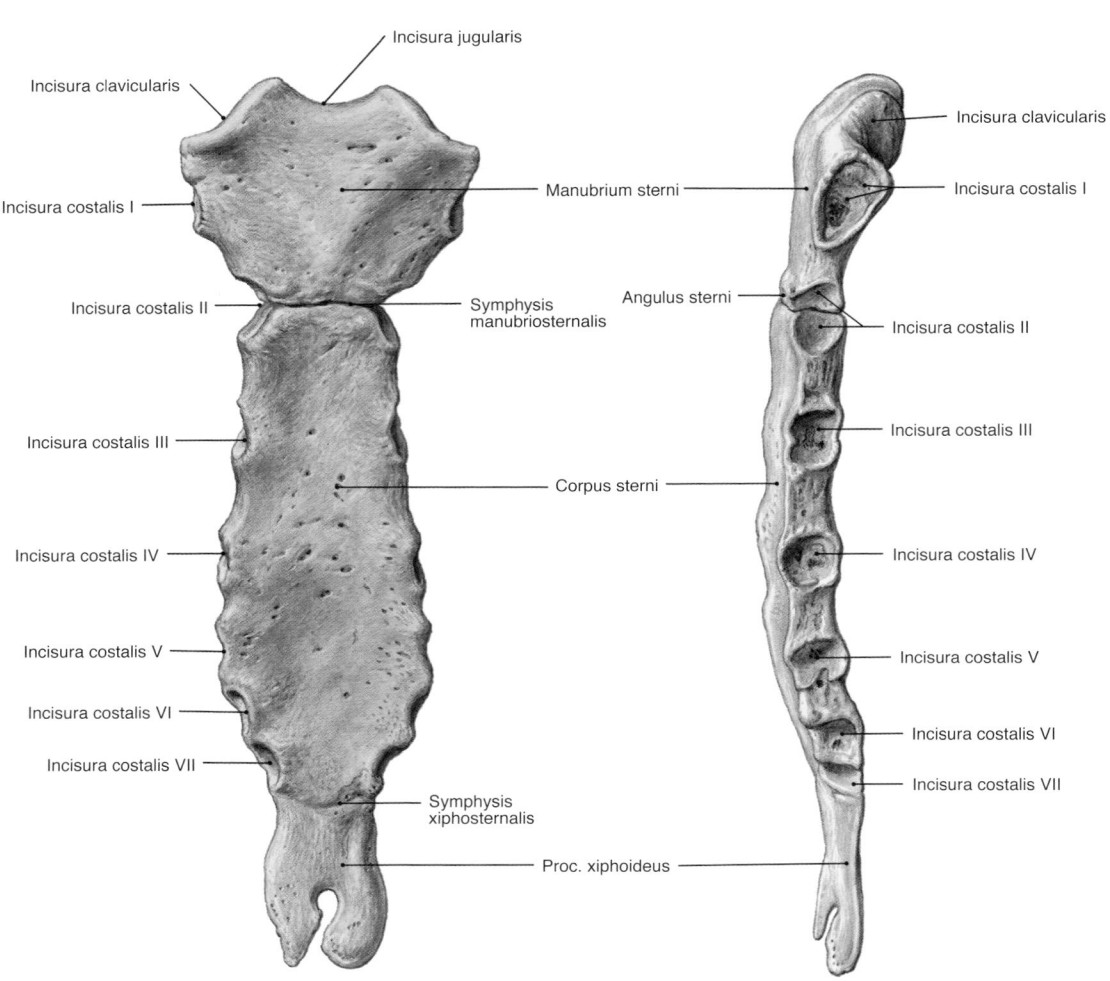

Incisura jugularis

Incisura clavicularis

Incisura costalis I

Manubrium sterni

Incisura costalis II

Symphysis manubriosternalis

Incisura costalis III

Corpus sterni

Incisura costalis IV

Incisura costalis V

Incisura costalis VI

Incisura costalis VII

Symphysis xiphosternalis

Proc. xiphoideus

Incisura clavicularis

Incisura costalis I

Angulus sterni

Incisura costalis II

Incisura costalis III

Incisura costalis IV

Incisura costalis V

Incisura costalis VI

Incisura costalis VII

Fig. 565 Sternum, Sternum.   **Fig. 566** Sternum, Sternum.

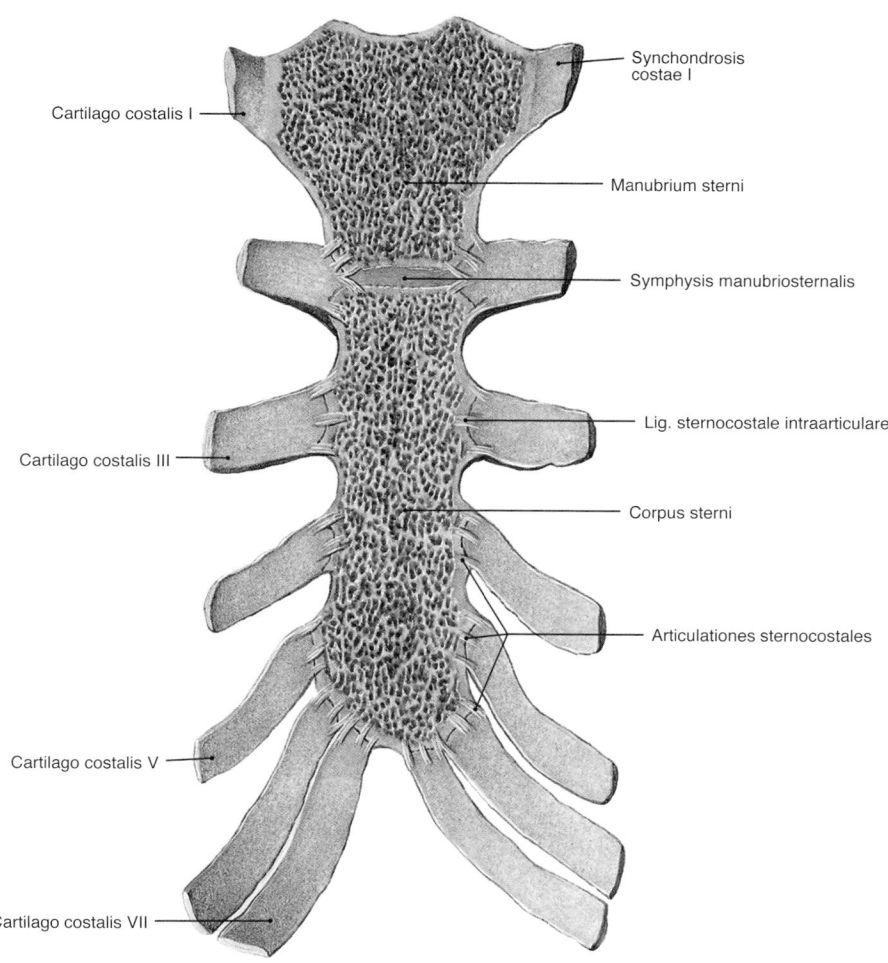

Synchondrosis costae I

Cartilago costalis I

Manubrium sterni

Symphysis manubriosternalis

Lig. sternocostale intraarticulare

Cartilago costalis III

Corpus sterni

Articulationes sternocostales

Cartilago costalis V

Cartilago costalis VII

Fig. 567 Sternum, Sternum, and costal cartilages, Cartilagines costales; section.

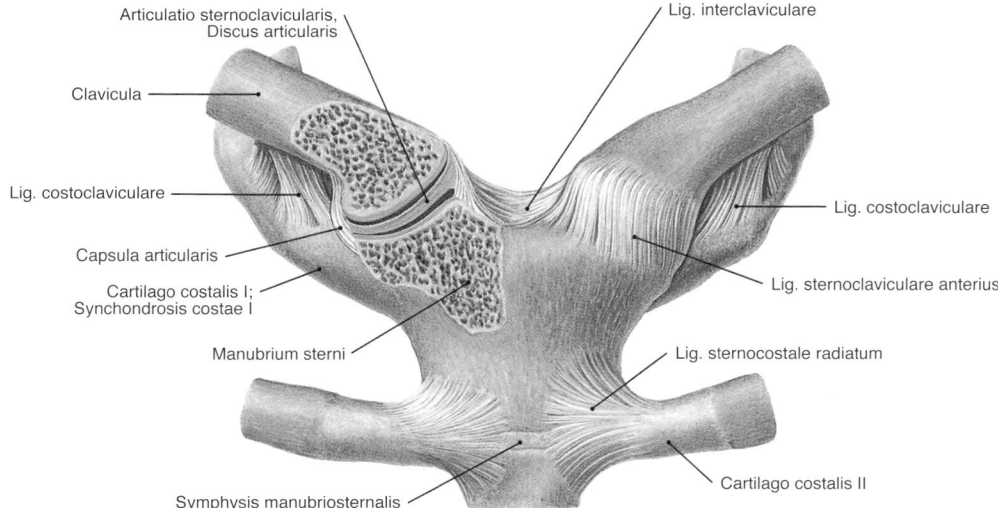

Articulatio sternoclavicularis, Discus articularis

Lig. interclaviculare

Clavicula

Lig. costoclaviculare

Lig. costoclaviculare

Capsula articularis

Lig. sternoclaviculare anterius

Cartilago costalis I; Synchondrosis costae I

Manubrium sterni

Lig. sternocostale radiatum

Symphysis manubriosternalis

Cartilago costalis II

Fig. 568 Sternoclavicular joint, Articulatio sternoclavicularis.

Muscles of the thoracic and the abdominal wall

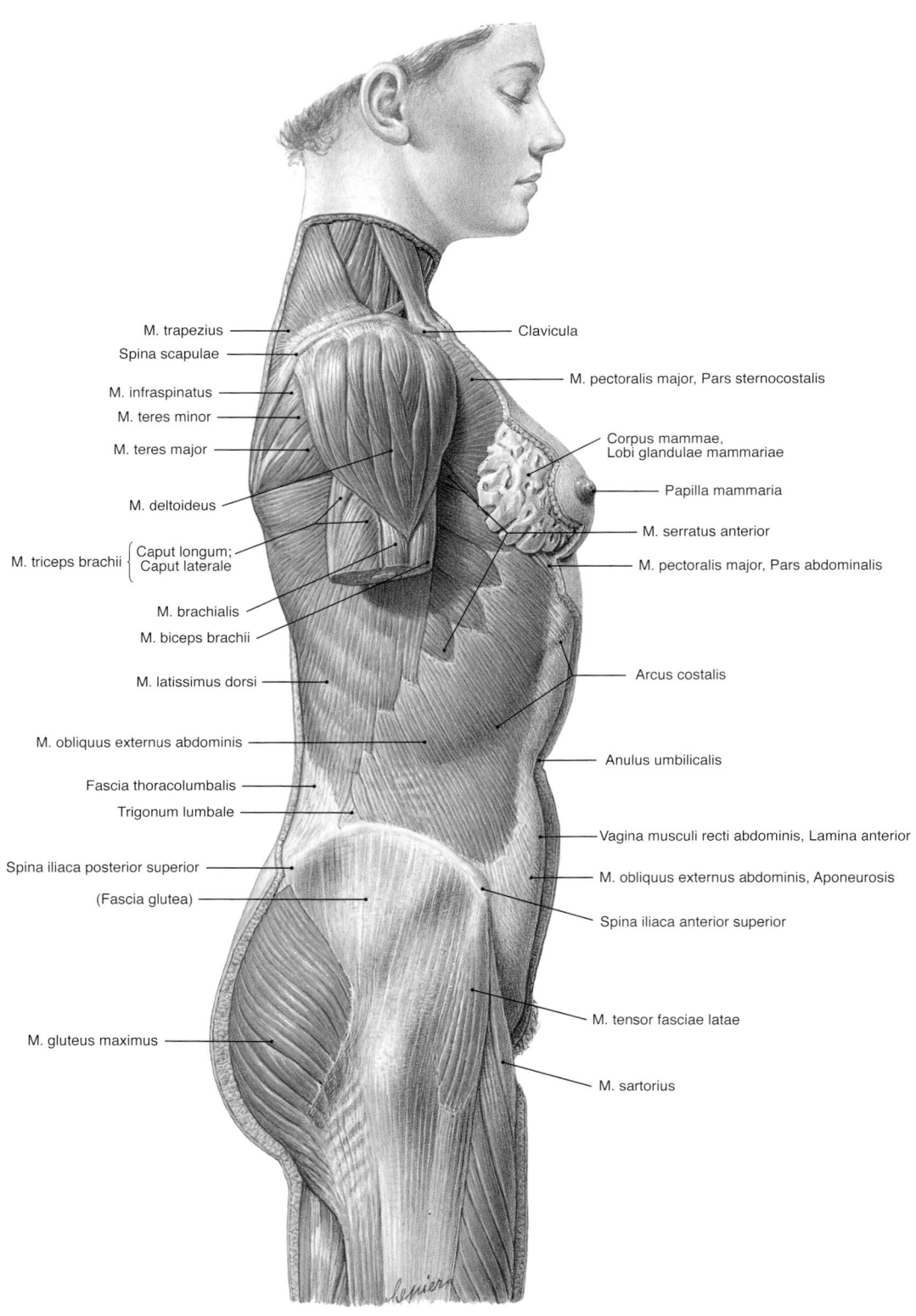

M. trapezius
Spina scapulae
M. infraspinatus
M. teres minor
M. teres major
M. deltoideus
M. triceps brachii { Caput longum; Caput laterale
M. brachialis
M. biceps brachii
M. latissimus dorsi
M. obliquus externus abdominis
Fascia thoracolumbalis
Trigonum lumbale
Spina iliaca posterior superior
(Fascia glutea)
M. gluteus maximus

Clavicula
M. pectoralis major, Pars sternocostalis
Corpus mammae, Lobi glandulae mammariae
Papilla mammaria
M. serratus anterior
M. pectoralis major, Pars abdominalis
Arcus costalis
Anulus umbilicalis
Vagina musculi recti abdominis, Lamina anterior
M. obliquus externus abdominis, Aponeurosis
Spina iliaca anterior superior
M. tensor fasciae latae
M. sartorius

→ T 15, T 17, T 18, T 26

Fig. 569 Muscles of the thoracic and the abdominal wall, Mm. thoracis et abdominis.

Muscles of the thoracic and the abdominal wall

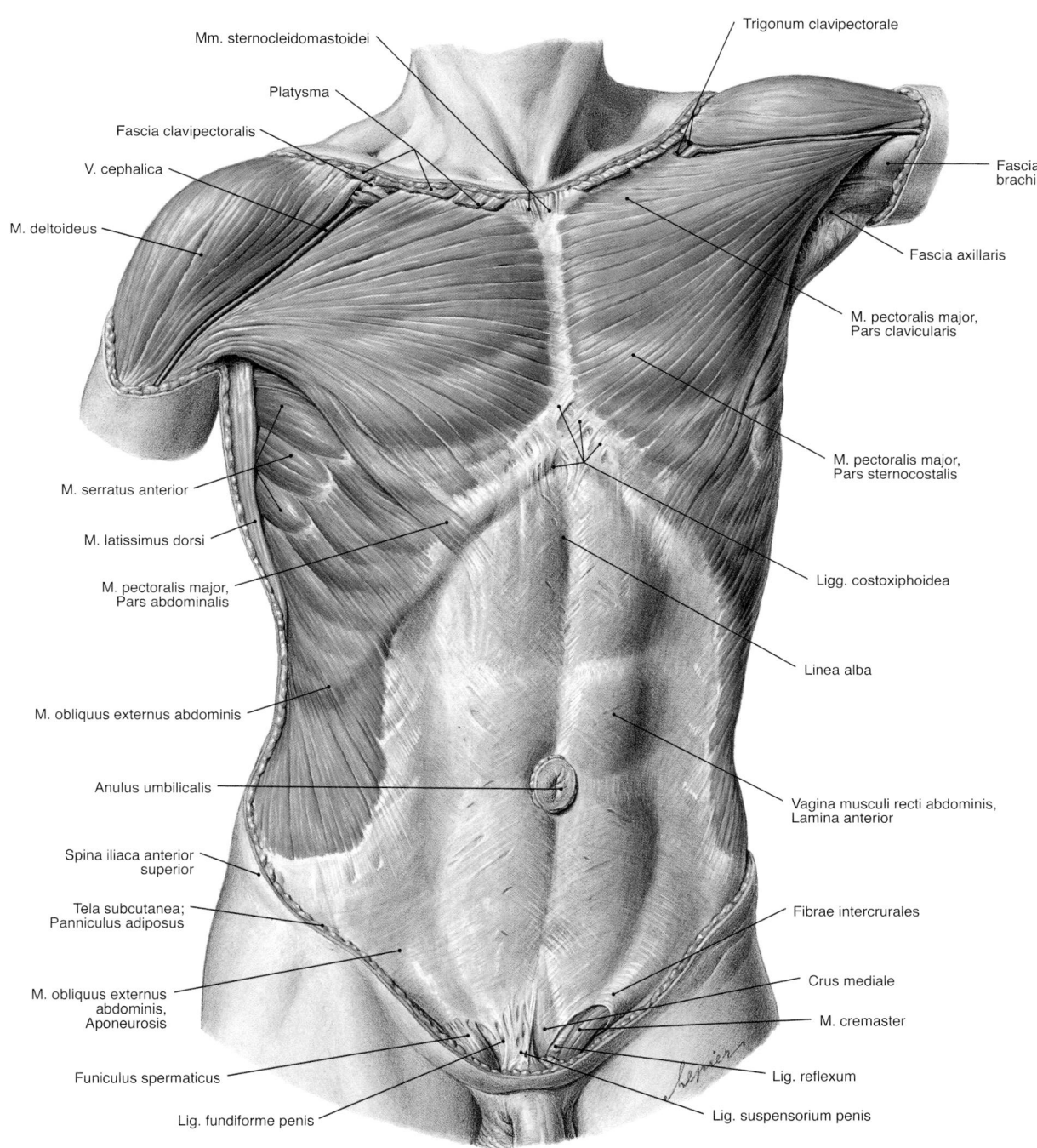

Mm. sternocleidomastoidei

Platysma

Fascia clavipectoralis

V. cephalica

M. deltoideus

M. serratus anterior

M. latissimus dorsi

M. pectoralis major,
Pars abdominalis

M. obliquus externus abdominis

Anulus umbilicalis

Spina iliaca anterior
superior

Tela subcutanea;
Panniculus adiposus

M. obliquus externus
abdominis,
Aponeurosis

Funiculus spermaticus

Lig. fundiforme penis

Trigonum clavipectorale

Fascia
brachii

Fascia axillaris

M. pectoralis major,
Pars clavicularis

M. pectoralis major,
Pars sternocostalis

Ligg. costoxiphoidea

Linea alba

Vagina musculi recti abdominis,
Lamina anterior

Fibrae intercrurales

Crus mediale

M. cremaster

Lig. reflexum

Lig. suspensorium penis

Fig. 570 Muscles of the thoracic and the abdominal wall;
superficial layer.

→ T 15, T 17, T 18, T 26

Muscles of the thoracic and the abdominal wall

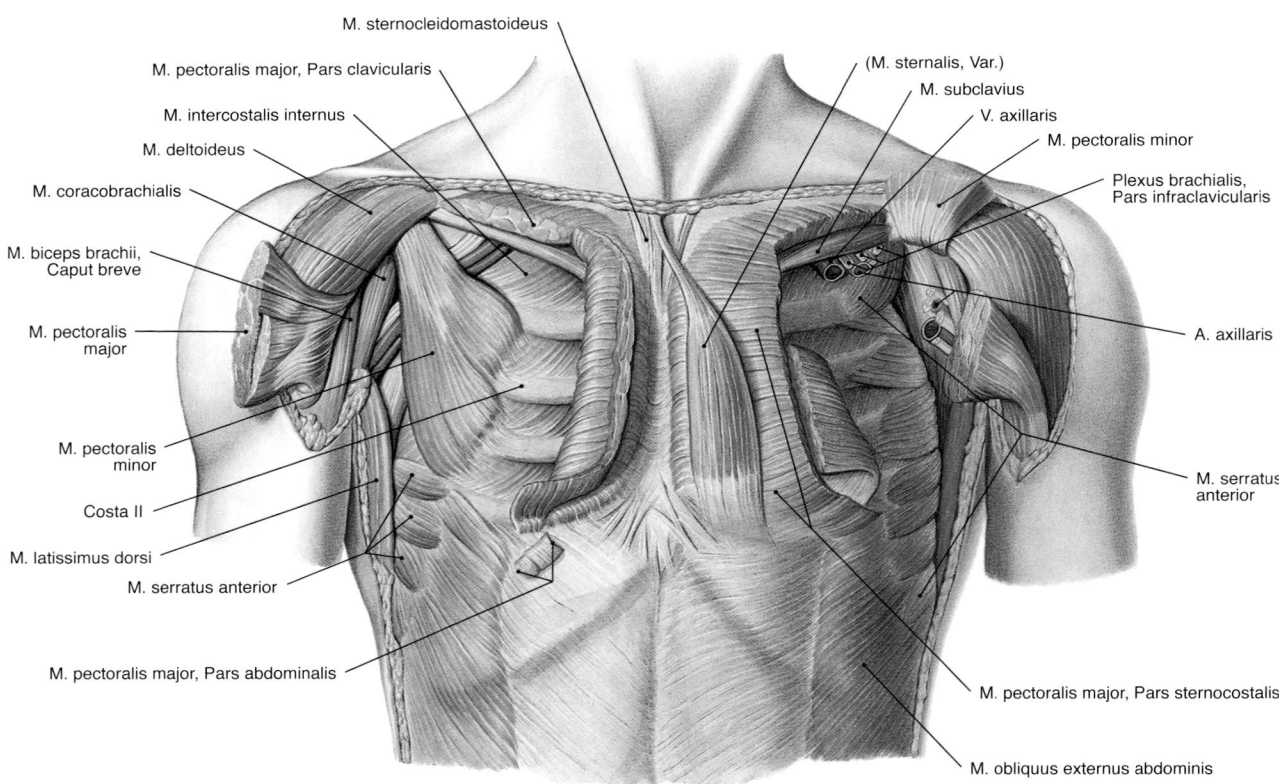

M. sternocleidomastoideus

M. pectoralis major, Pars clavicularis

M. intercostalis internus

M. deltoideus

M. coracobrachialis

M. biceps brachii, Caput breve

M. pectoralis major

M. pectoralis minor

Costa II

M. latissimus dorsi

M. serratus anterior

M. pectoralis major, Pars abdominalis

(M. sternalis, Var.)

M. subclavius

V. axillaris

M. pectoralis minor

Plexus brachialis, Pars infraclavicularis

A. axillaris

M. serratus anterior

M. pectoralis major, Pars sternocostalis

M. obliquus externus abdominis

→ T 13, T 15, T 26

Fig. 571   Muscles of the thoracic wall, Mm. thoracis.

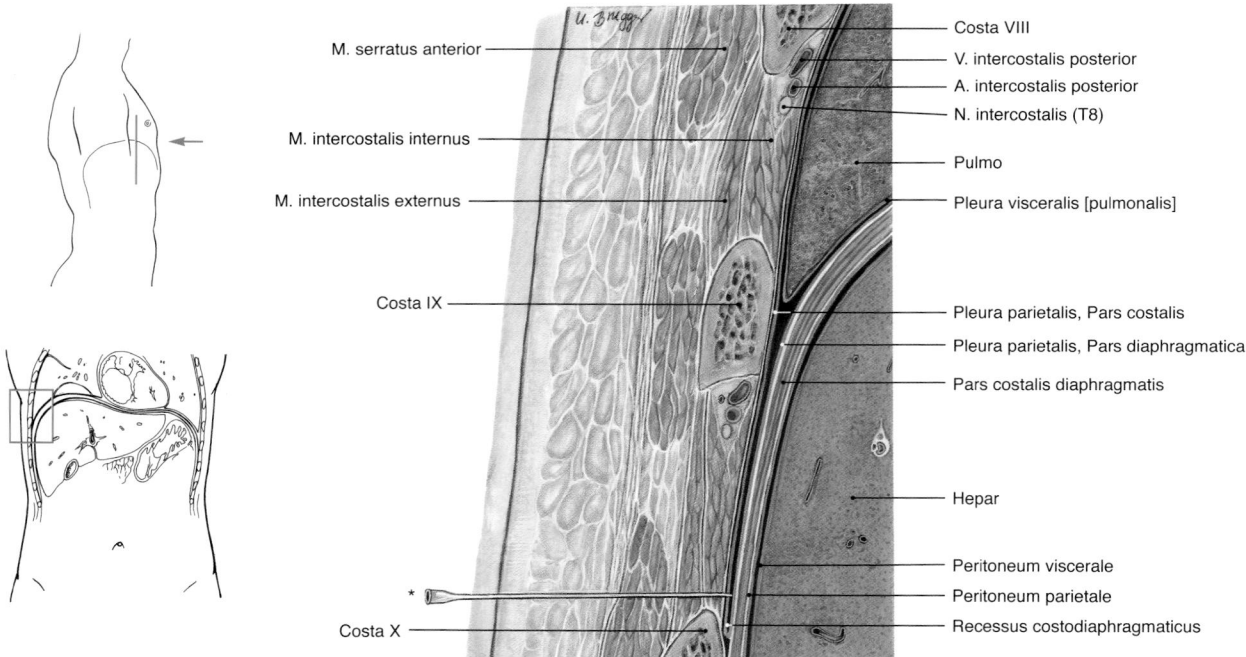

M. serratus anterior

M. intercostalis internus

M. intercostalis externus

Costa IX

Costa X

Costa VIII

V. intercostalis posterior

A. intercostalis posterior

N. intercostalis (T8)

Pulmo

Pleura visceralis [pulmonalis]

Pleura parietalis, Pars costalis

Pleura parietalis, Pars diaphragmatica

Pars costalis diaphragmatis

Hepar

Peritoneum viscerale

Peritoneum parietale

Recessus costodiaphragmaticus

→ T 13

Fig. 572   Muscles of the thoracic wall, Mm. thoracis; frontal section.

* Position of the needle for puncture of the pleural cavity (pleurocentesis)

Muscles of the thoracic wall

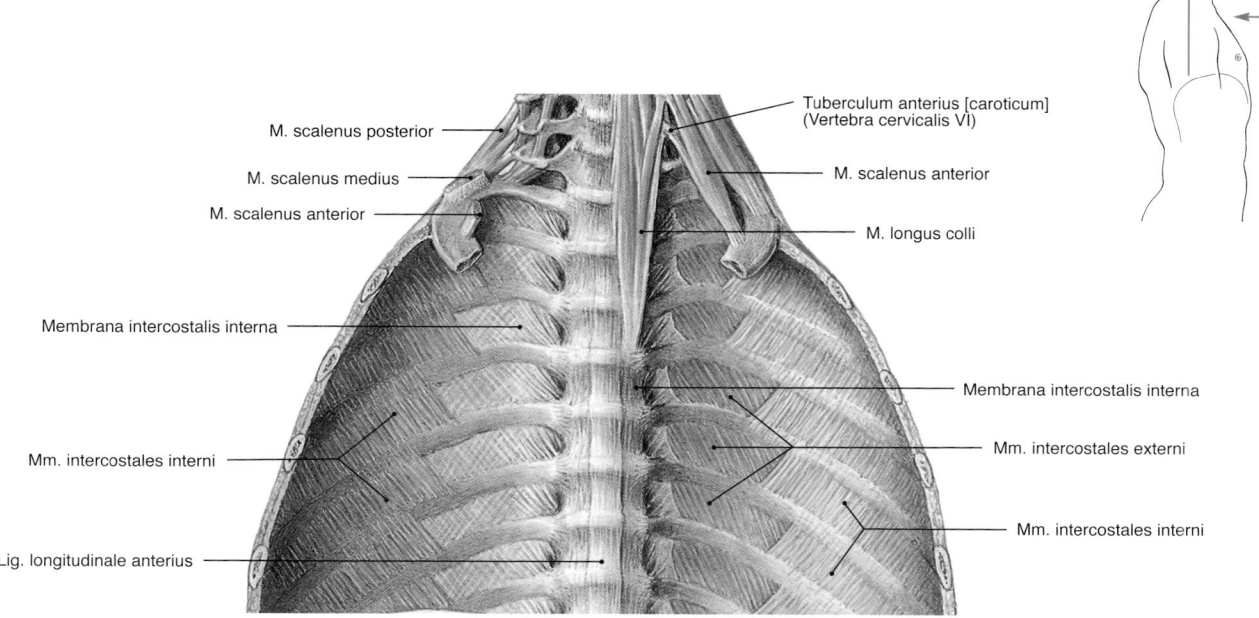

M. scalenus posterior
M. scalenus medius
M. scalenus anterior
Membrana intercostalis interna
Mm. intercostales interni
Lig. longitudinale anterius

Tuberculum anterius [caroticum]
(Vertebra cervicalis VI)
M. scalenus anterior
M. longus colli
Membrana intercostalis interna
Mm. intercostales externi
Mm. intercostales interni

Fig. 573 Thoracic cage, Cavea thoracis;
posterior wall.

→ T 11–T 13

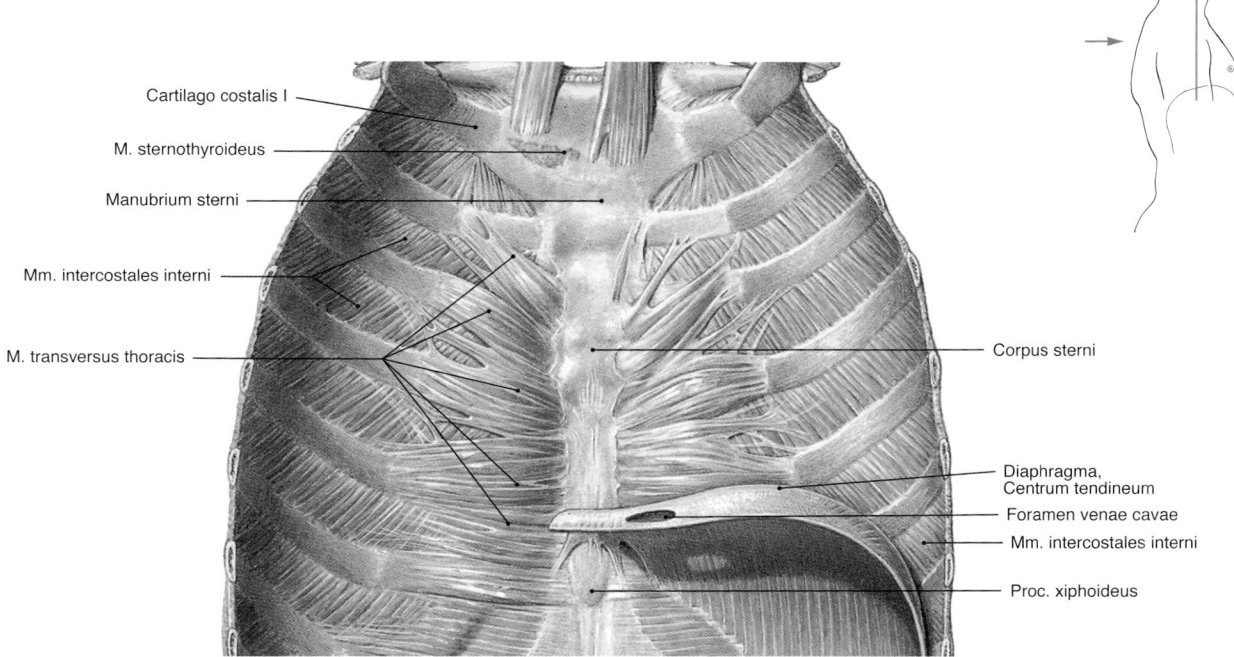

Cartilago costalis I
M. sternothyroideus
Manubrium sterni
Mm. intercostales interni
M. transversus thoracis

Corpus sterni

Diaphragma,
Centrum tendineum
Foramen venae cavae
Mm. intercostales interni
Proc. xiphoideus

Fig. 574 Thoracic cage, Cavea thoracis;
anterior wall.

→ T 13

Abdominal muscles

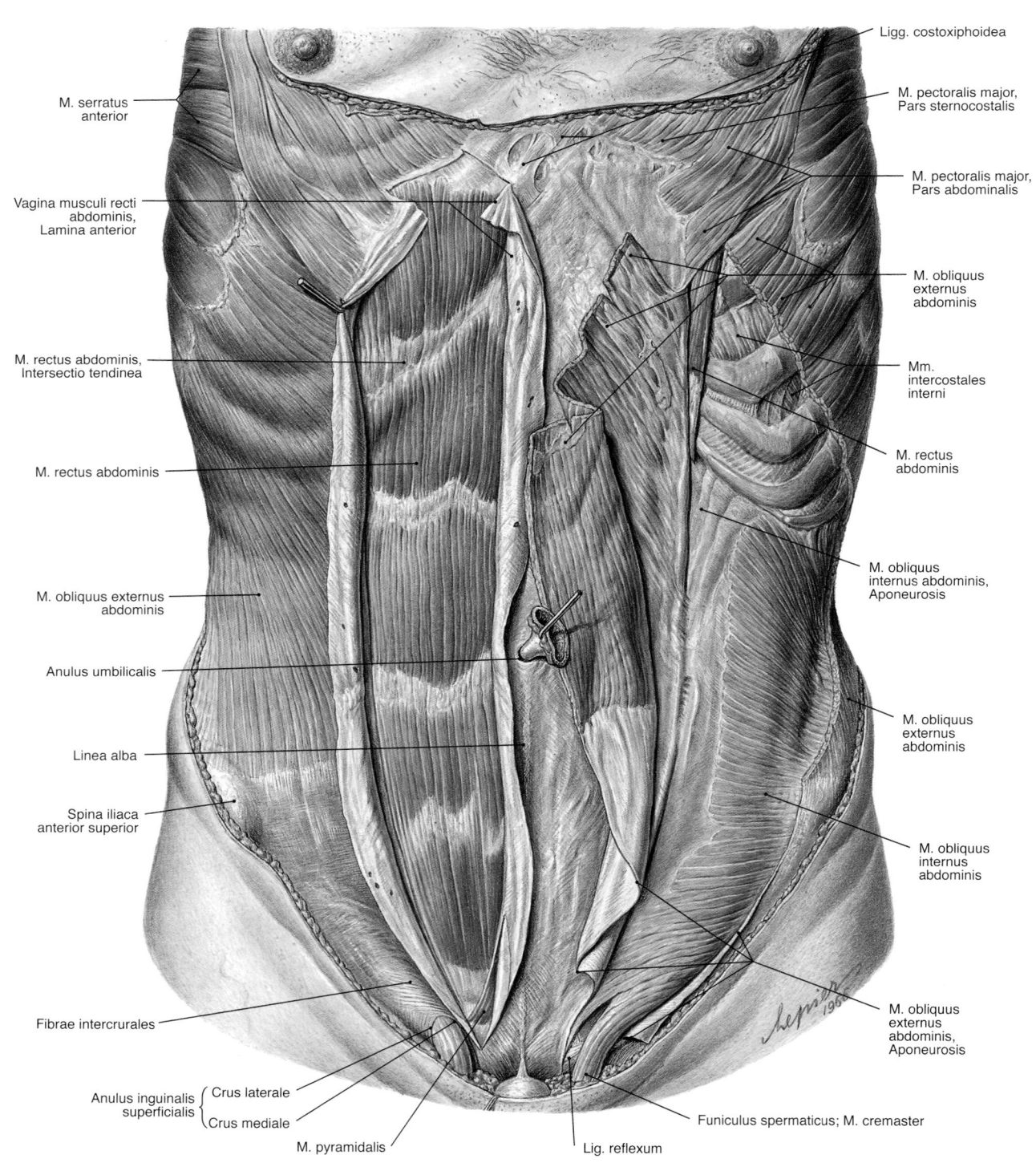

Ligg. costoxiphoidea

M. serratus anterior

M. pectoralis major, Pars sternocostalis

Vagina musculi recti abdominis, Lamina anterior

M. pectoralis major, Pars abdominalis

M. rectus abdominis, Intersectio tendinea

M. obliquus externus abdominis

M. rectus abdominis

Mm. intercostales interni

M. rectus abdominis

M. obliquus externus abdominis

M. obliquus internus abdominis, Aponeurosis

Anulus umbilicalis

Linea alba

M. obliquus externus abdominis

Spina iliaca anterior superior

M. obliquus internus abdominis

Fibrae intercrurales

M. obliquus externus abdominis, Aponeurosis

Anulus inguinalis superficialis { Crus laterale / Crus mediale

Funiculus spermaticus; M. cremaster

M. pyramidalis

Lig. reflexum

→ T 13–T 15, T 17, T 26

Fig. 575 Muscles of the abdominal wall, Mm. abdominis; superficial and middle layer.

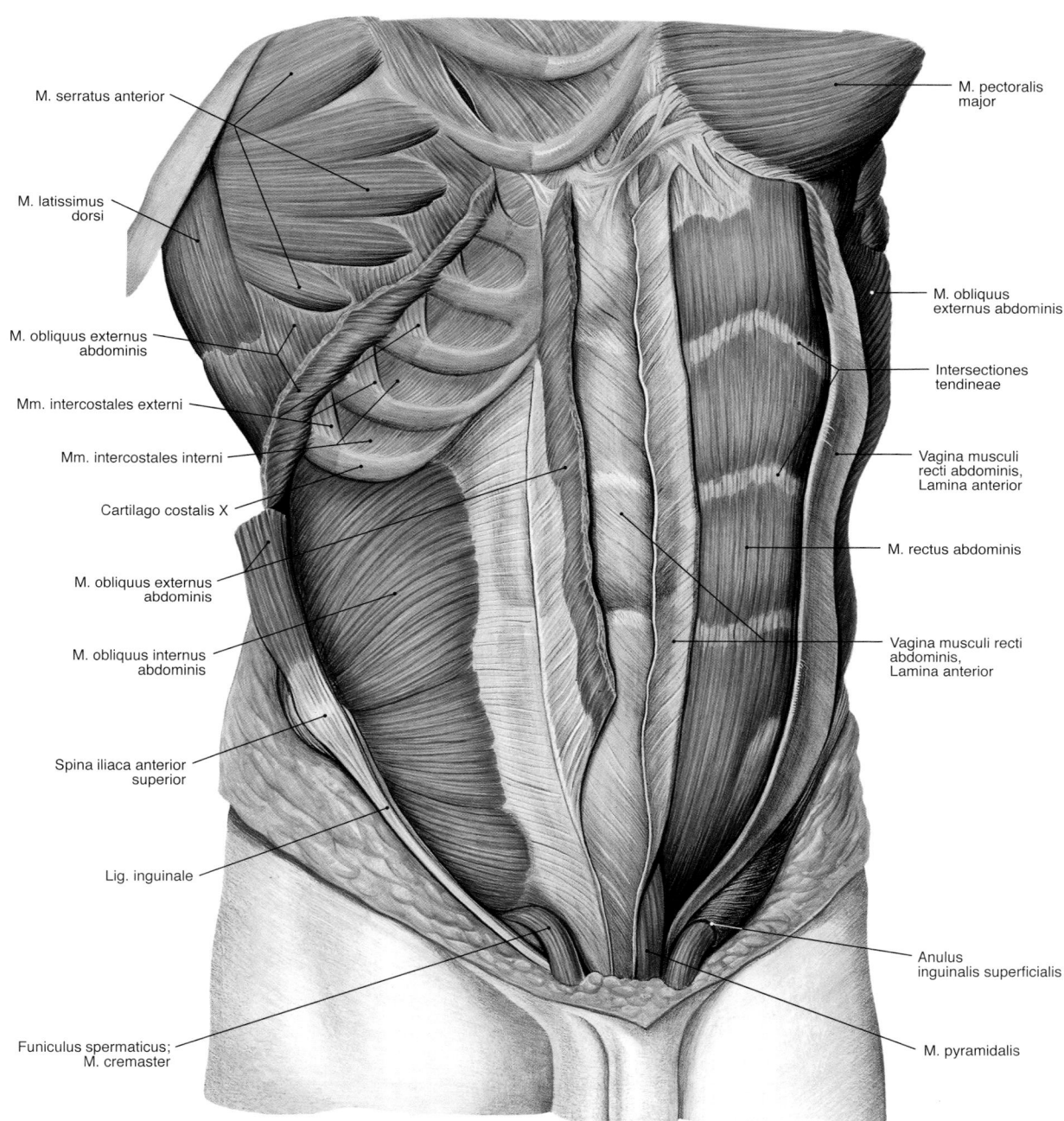

M. serratus anterior

M. latissimus dorsi

M. obliquus externus abdominis

Mm. intercostales externi

Mm. intercostales interni

Cartilago costalis X

M. obliquus externus abdominis

M. obliquus internus abdominis

Spina iliaca anterior superior

Lig. inguinale

Funiculus spermaticus; M. cremaster

M. pectoralis major

M. obliquus externus abdominis

Intersectiones tendineae

Vagina musculi recti abdominis, Lamina anterior

M. rectus abdominis

Vagina musculi recti abdominis, Lamina anterior

Anulus inguinalis superficialis

M. pyramidalis

Fig. 576 Muscles of the abdominal wall, Mm. abdominis; middle layer.

→ T 13–T 15, T 17

Abdominal muscles

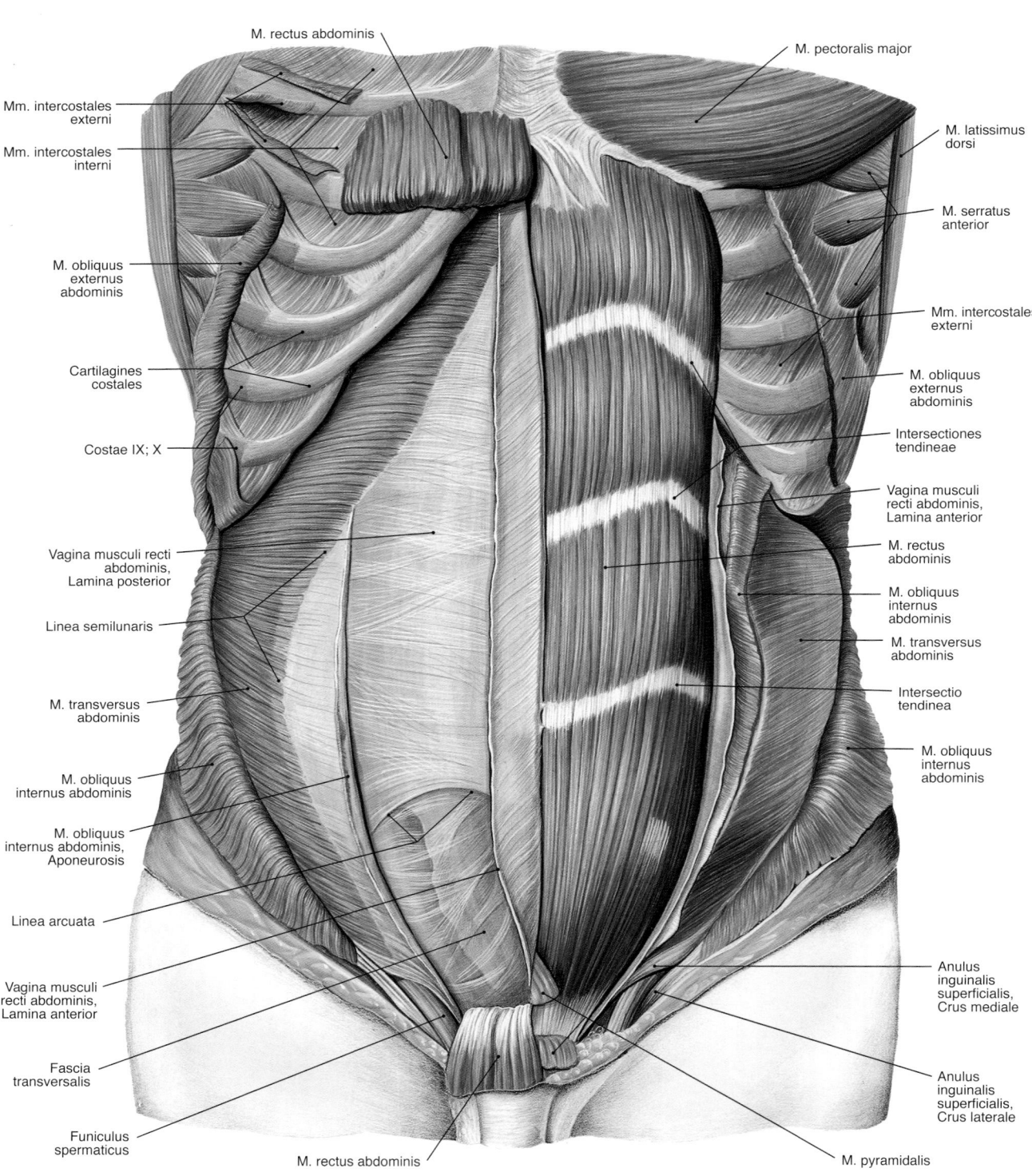

M. rectus abdominis

Mm. intercostales externi

Mm. intercostales interni

M. obliquus externus abdominis

Cartilagines costales

Costae IX; X

Vagina musculi recti abdominis, Lamina posterior

Linea semilunaris

M. transversus abdominis

M. obliquus internus abdominis

M. obliquus internus abdominis, Aponeurosis

Linea arcuata

Vagina musculi recti abdominis, Lamina anterior

Fascia transversalis

Funiculus spermaticus

M. rectus abdominis

M. pectoralis major

M. latissimus dorsi

M. serratus anterior

Mm. intercostales externi

M. obliquus externus abdominis

Intersectiones tendineae

Vagina musculi recti abdominis, Lamina anterior

M. rectus abdominis

M. obliquus internus abdominis

M. transversus abdominis

Intersectio tendinea

M. obliquus internus abdominis

Anulus inguinalis superficialis, Crus mediale

Anulus inguinalis superficialis, Crus laterale

M. pyramidalis

→ T 13–T 15

Fig. 577 Muscles of the abdominal wall, Mm. abdominis; deep layer.

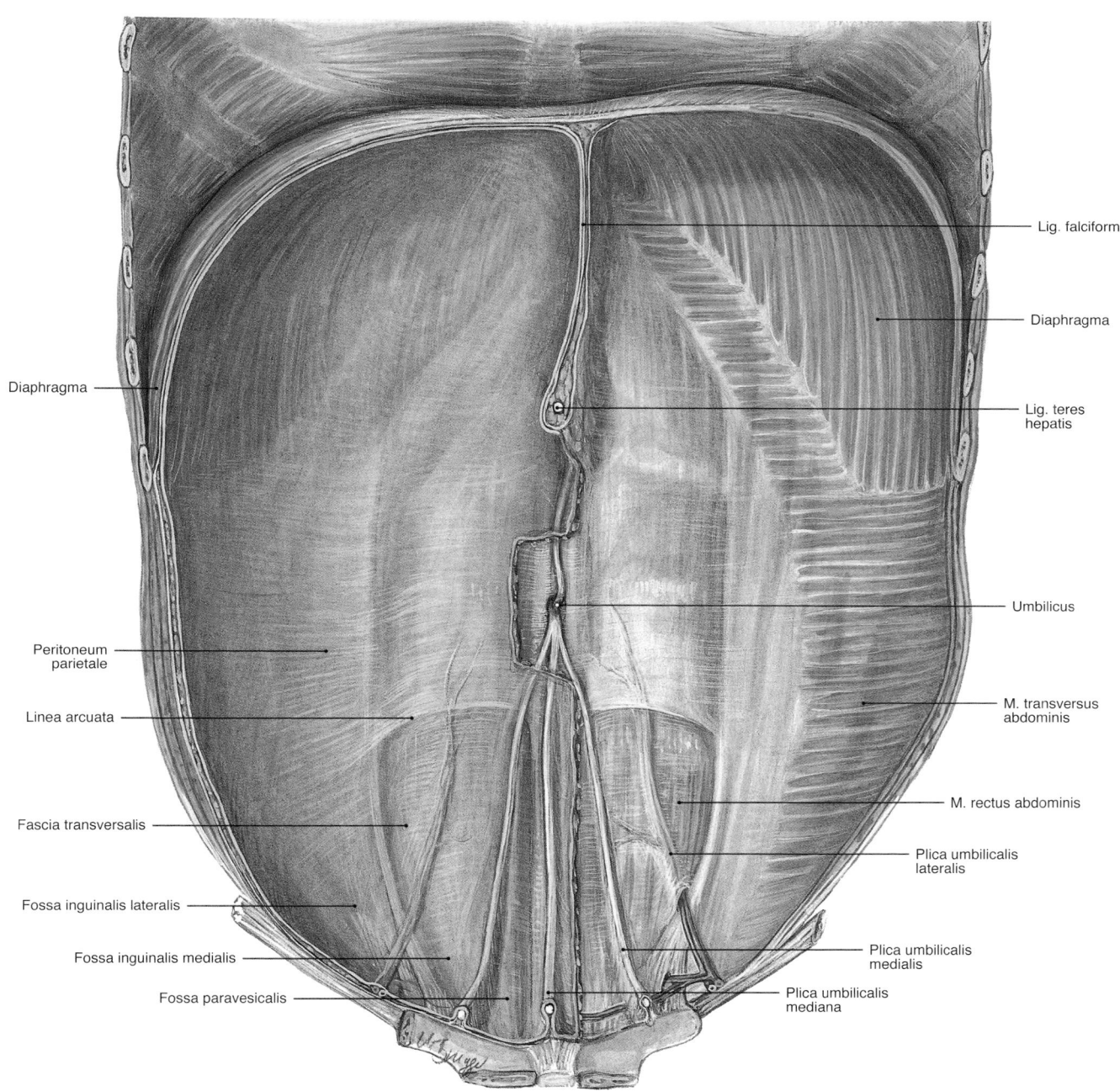

Lig. falciforme

Diaphragma

Diaphragma

Lig. teres hepatis

Umbilicus

Peritoneum parietale

M. transversus abdominis

Linea arcuata

M. rectus abdominis

Fascia transversalis

Plica umbilicalis lateralis

Fossa inguinalis lateralis

Fossa inguinalis medialis

Plica umbilicalis medialis

Fossa paravesicalis

Plica umbilicalis mediana

Fig. 578 Internal surface of the anterior abdominal wall.

→ T 14, T 15, T 21

Inguinal canal

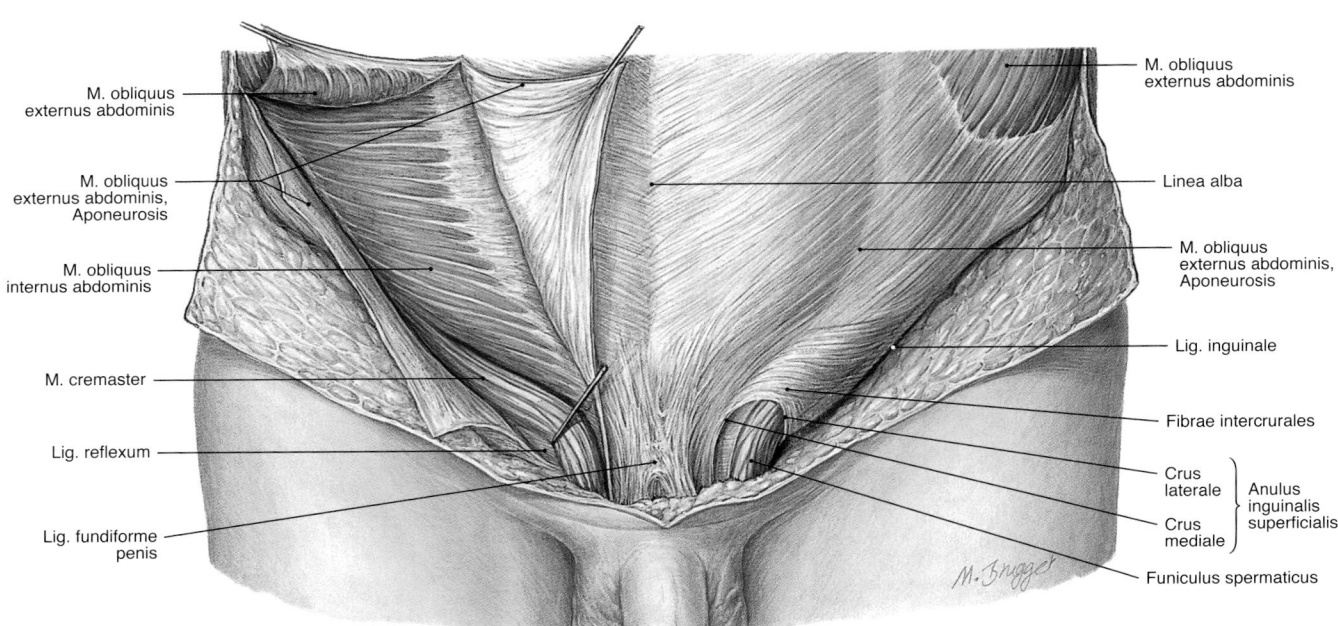

M. obliquus
externus abdominis

M. obliquus
externus abdominis,
Aponeurosis

M. obliquus
internus abdominis

M. cremaster

Lig. reflexum

Lig. fundiforme
penis

M. obliquus
externus abdominis

Linea alba

M. obliquus
externus abdominis,
Aponeurosis

Lig. inguinale

Fibrae intercrurales

Crus
laterale } Anulus
inguinalis
superficialis
Crus
mediale

Funiculus spermaticus

Fig. 579   Superficial inguinal ring, Anulus inguinalis superficialis.

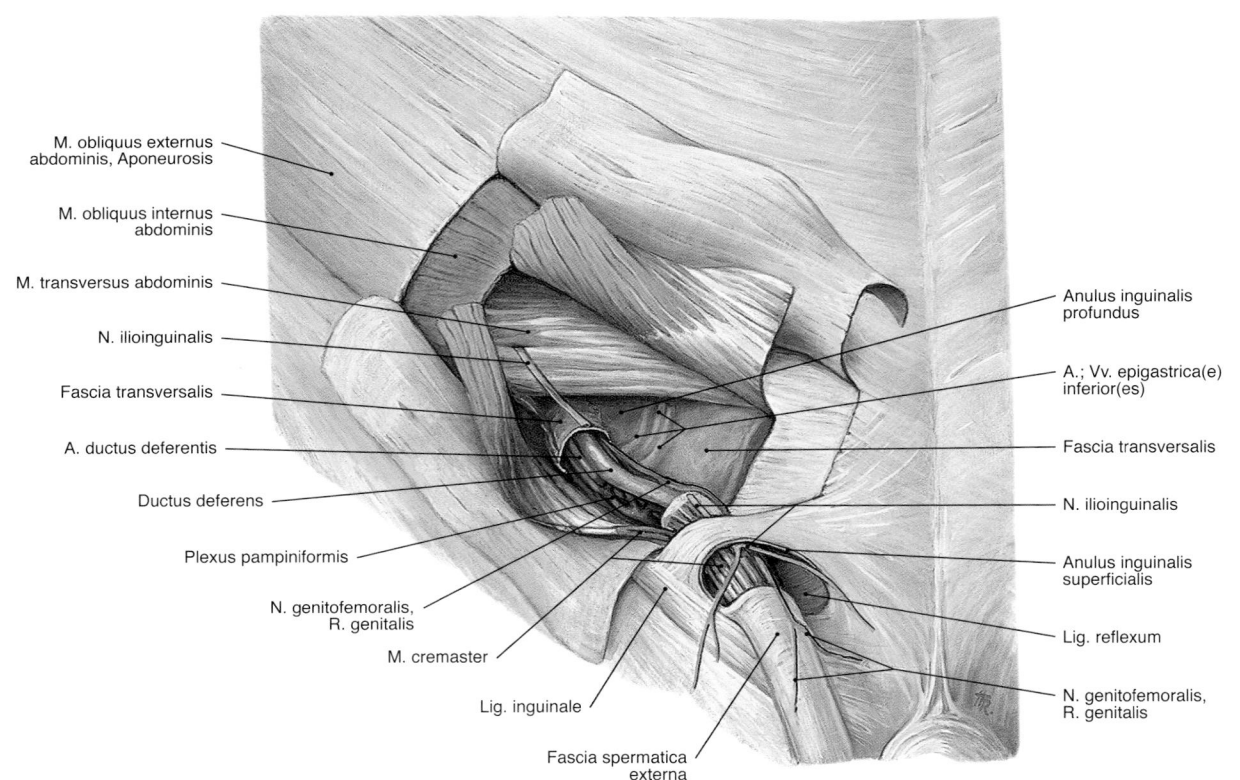

M. obliquus externus
abdominis, Aponeurosis

M. obliquus internus
abdominis

M. transversus abdominis

N. ilioinguinalis

Fascia transversalis

A. ductus deferentis

Ductus deferens

Plexus pampiniformis

N. genitofemoralis,
R. genitalis

M. cremaster

Lig. inguinale

Fascia spermatica
externa

Anulus inguinalis
profundus

A.; Vv. epigastrica(e)
inferior(es)

Fascia transversalis

N. ilioinguinalis

Anulus inguinalis
superficialis

Lig. reflexum

N. genitofemoralis,
R. genitalis

Fig. 580   Walls of the inguinal canal.

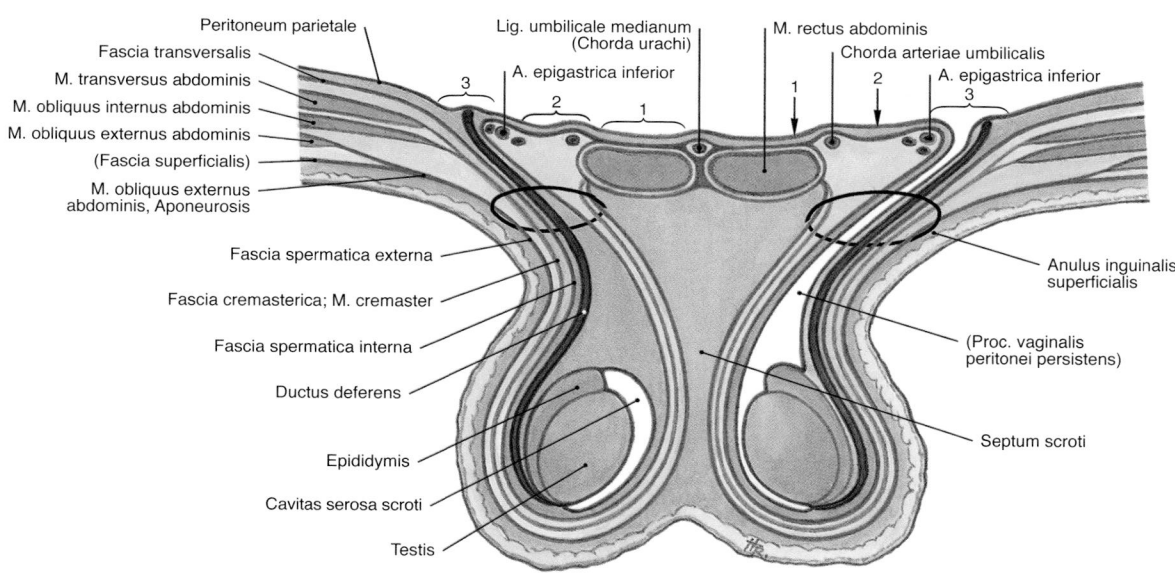

Peritoneum parietale
Fascia transversalis
M. transversus abdominis
M. obliquus internus abdominis
M. obliquus externus abdominis
(Fascia superficialis)
M. obliquus externus abdominis, Aponeurosis

Lig. umbilicale medianum (Chorda urachi)
A. epigastrica inferior

M. rectus abdominis
Chorda arteriae umbilicalis
A. epigastrica inferior

Fascia spermatica externa
Fascia cremasterica; M. cremaster
Fascia spermatica interna
Ductus deferens
Epididymis
Cavitas serosa scroti
Testis

Anulus inguinalis superficialis
(Proc. vaginalis peritonei persistens)
Septum scroti

Fig. 581 Diagram of the inguinal canal.
The inguinal canal, the spermatic cord and the scrotum are
illustrated in the same plane for didactical reasons.

1 Fossa supravesicalis
2 Fossa inguinalis medialis
3 Fossa inguinalis lateralis

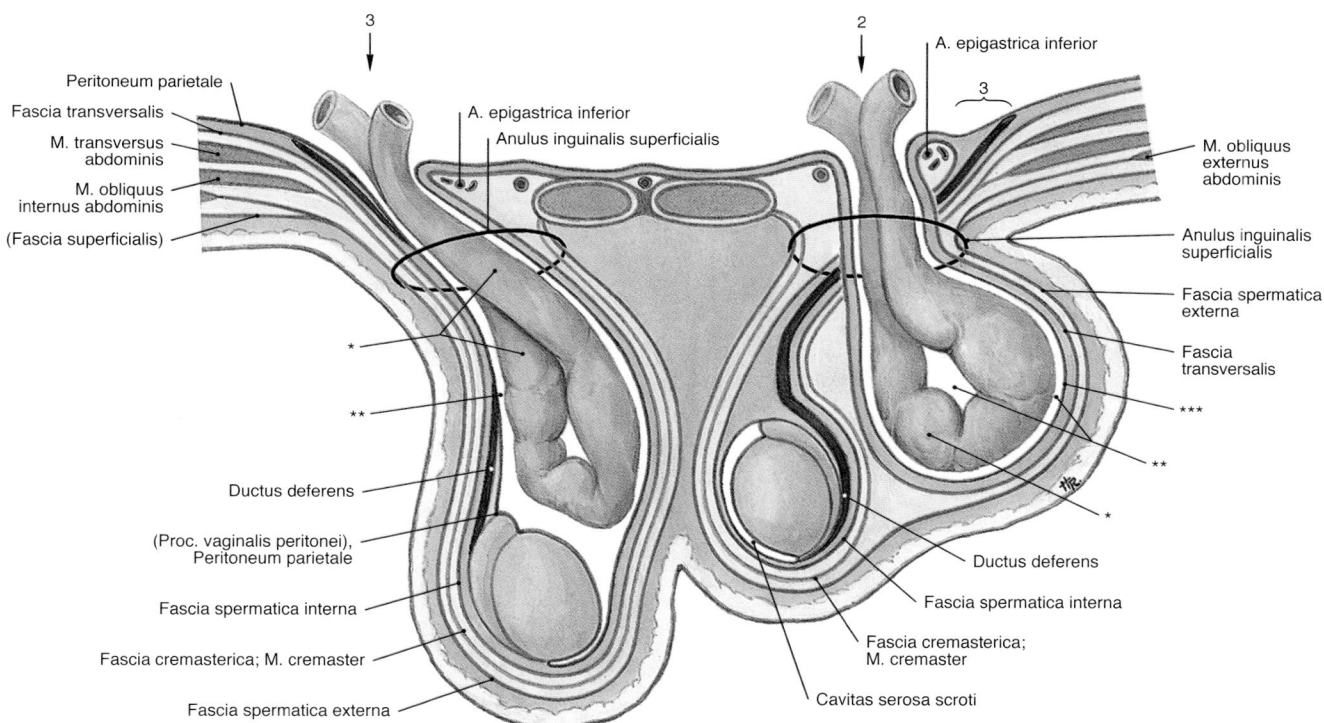

Peritoneum parietale
Fascia transversalis
M. transversus abdominis
M. obliquus internus abdominis
(Fascia superficialis)

A. epigastrica inferior
Anulus inguinalis superficialis

A. epigastrica inferior

M. obliquus externus abdominis
Anulus inguinalis superficialis
Fascia spermatica externa
Fascia transversalis

Ductus deferens
(Proc. vaginalis peritonei), Peritoneum parietale
Fascia spermatica interna
Fascia cremasterica; M. cremaster
Fascia spermatica externa

Ductus deferens
Fascia spermatica interna
Fascia cremasterica; M. cremaster
Cavitas serosa scroti

Fig. 582 Diagram of inguinal hernias;
left side: lateral, indirect hernia;
right side: medial, direct hernia.

* Hernial sac with an intestinal loop
** Peritoneal space
***Newly formed peritoneal hernial sac

Diaphragm and posterior abdominal wall

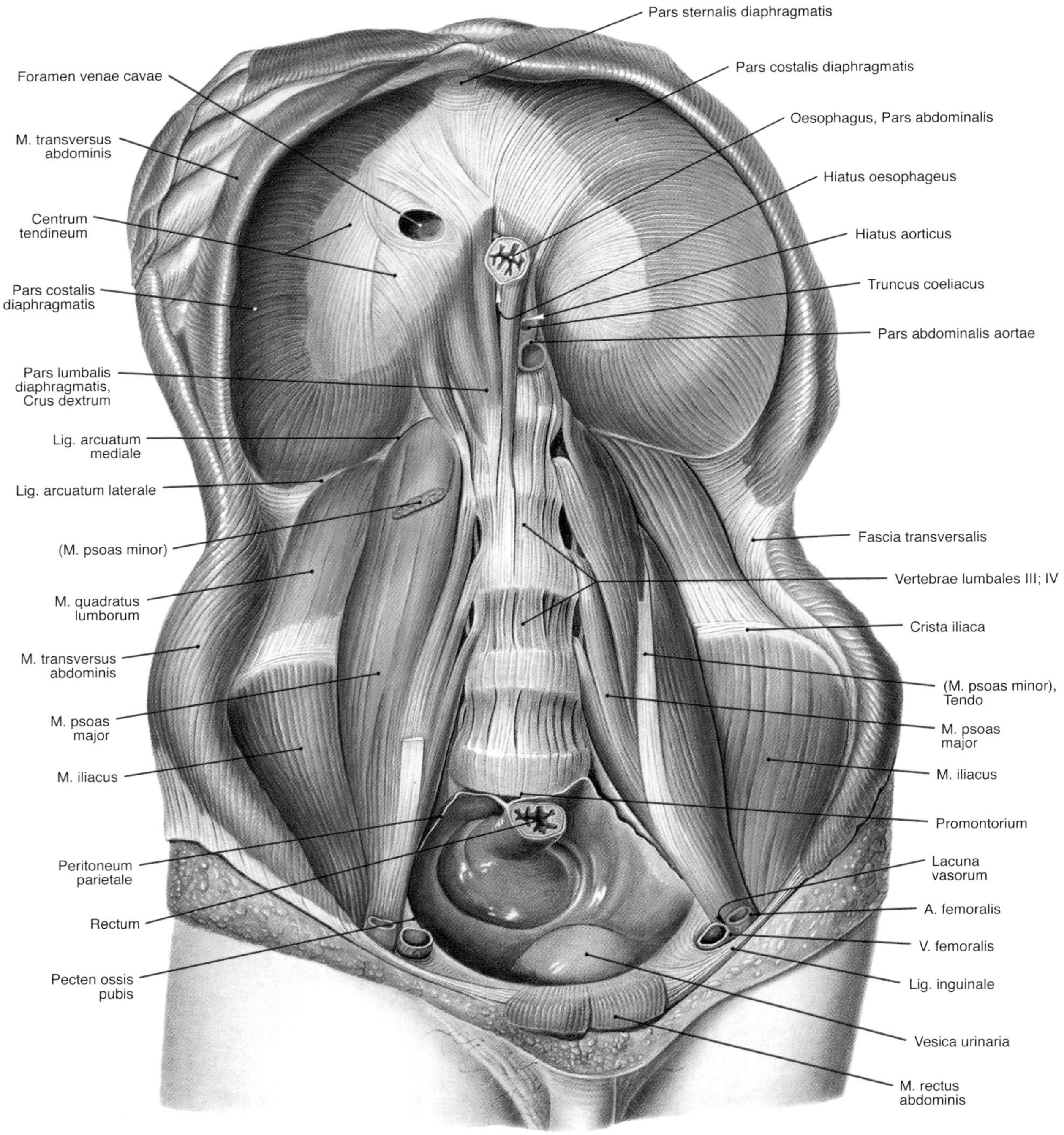

Pars sternalis diaphragmatis

Foramen venae cavae

Pars costalis diaphragmatis

Oesophagus, Pars abdominalis

M. transversus abdominis

Hiatus oesophageus

Centrum tendineum

Hiatus aorticus

Truncus coeliacus

Pars costalis diaphragmatis

Pars abdominalis aortae

Pars lumbalis diaphragmatis, Crus dextrum

Lig. arcuatum mediale

Lig. arcuatum laterale

Fascia transversalis

Vertebrae lumbales III; IV

(M. psoas minor)

M. quadratus lumborum

Crista iliaca

M. transversus abdominis

(M. psoas minor), Tendo

M. psoas major

M. psoas major

M. iliacus

M. iliacus

Promontorium

Peritoneum parietale

Lacuna vasorum

Rectum

A. femoralis

Pecten ossis pubis

V. femoralis

Lig. inguinale

Vesica urinaria

M. rectus abdominis

→ T 15, T 16, T 21, T 42

Fig. 583 Diaphragm, Diaphragma, and muscles of the abdominal wall, Mm. abdominis.

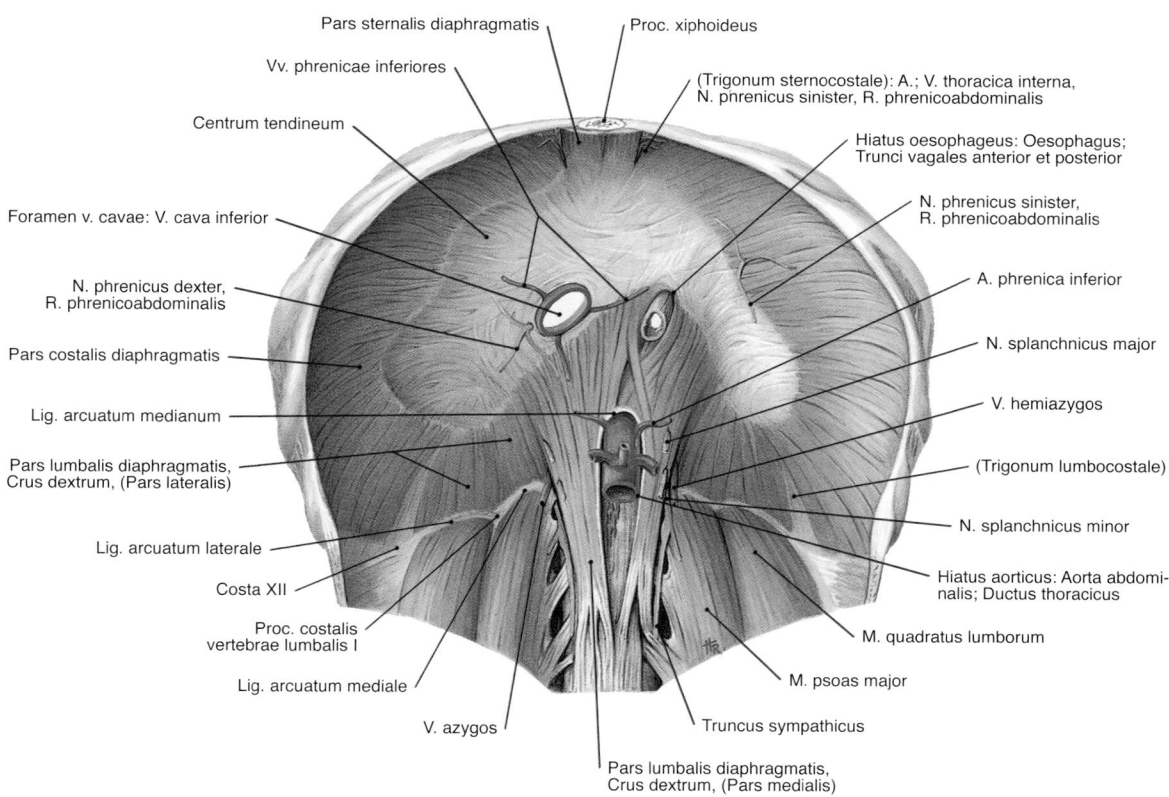

Pars sternalis diaphragmatis
Proc. xiphoideus
Vv. phrenicae inferiores
Centrum tendineum
(Trigonum sternocostale): A.; V. thoracica interna, N. pnrenicus sinister, R. phrenicoabdominalis
Hiatus oesophageus: Oesophagus; Trunci vagales anterior et posterior
Foramen v. cavae: V. cava inferior
N. phrenicus sinister, R. phrenicoabdominalis
N. phrenicus dexter, R. phrenicoabdominalis
A. phrenica inferior
Pars costalis diaphragmatis
N. splanchnicus major
Lig. arcuatum medianum
V. hemiazygos
Pars lumbalis diaphragmatis, Crus dextrum, (Pars lateralis)
(Trigonum lumbocostale)
N. splanchnicus minor
Lig. arcuatum laterale
Hiatus aorticus: Aorta abdominalis; Ductus thoracicus
Costa XII
M. quadratus lumborum
Proc. costalis vertebrae lumbalis I
M. psoas major
Lig. arcuatum mediale
V. azygos
Truncus sympathicus
Pars lumbalis diaphragmatis, Crus dextrum, (Pars medialis)

Fig. 584 Diaphragm, Diaphragma. → T 21

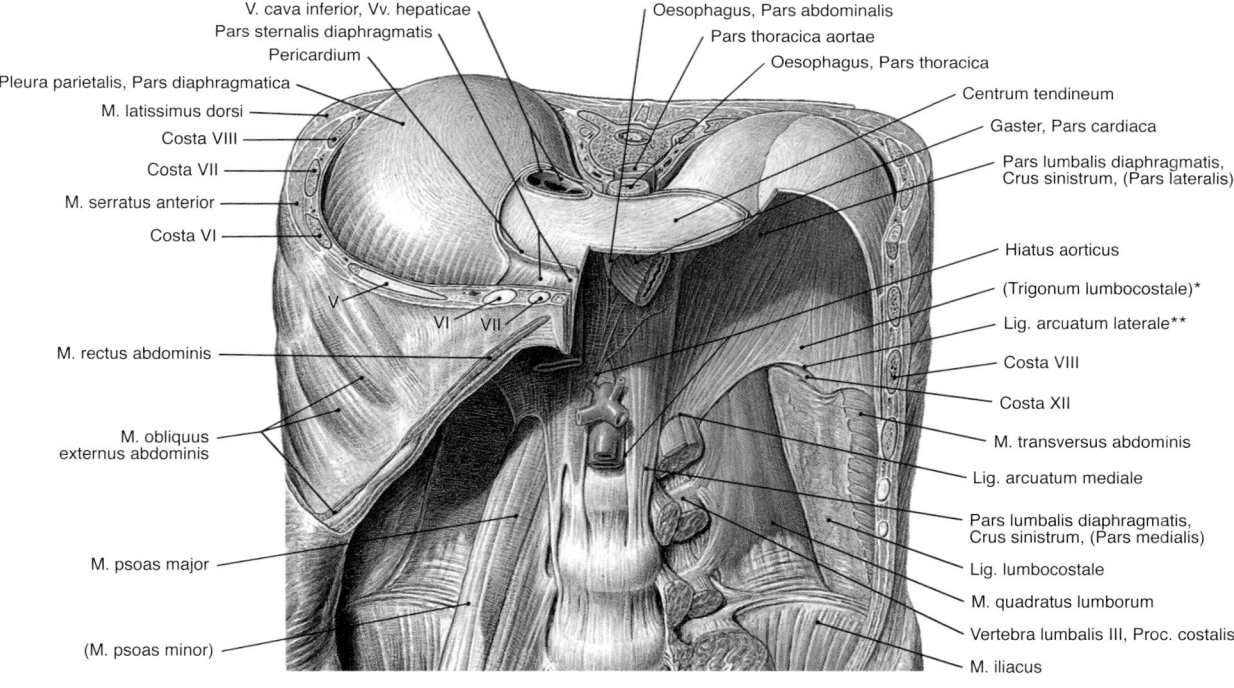

V. cava inferior, Vv. hepaticae
Oesophagus, Pars abdominalis
Pars sternalis diaphragmatis
Pars thoracica aortae
Pericardium
Oesophagus, Pars thoracica
Pleura parietalis, Pars diaphragmatica
Centrum tendineum
M. latissimus dorsi
Gaster, Pars cardiaca
Costa VIII
Pars lumbalis diaphragmatis, Crus sinistrum, (Pars lateralis)
Costa VII
M. serratus anterior
Hiatus aorticus
Costa VI
(Trigonum lumbocostale)*
Lig. arcuatum laterale**
M. rectus abdominis
Costa VIII
Costa XII
M. transversus abdominis
M. obliquus externus abdominis
Lig. arcuatum mediale
Pars lumbalis diaphragmatis, Crus sinistrum, (Pars medialis)
M. psoas major
Lig. lumbocostale
M. quadratus lumborum
Vertebra lumbalis III, Proc. costalis
(M. psoas minor)
M. iliacus

Fig. 585 Diaphragm, Diaphragma, with apertures and muscles of the posterior abdominal wall. → T 21
* Clinical term: BOCHDALEK's triangle
** Psoas arcade

Breast

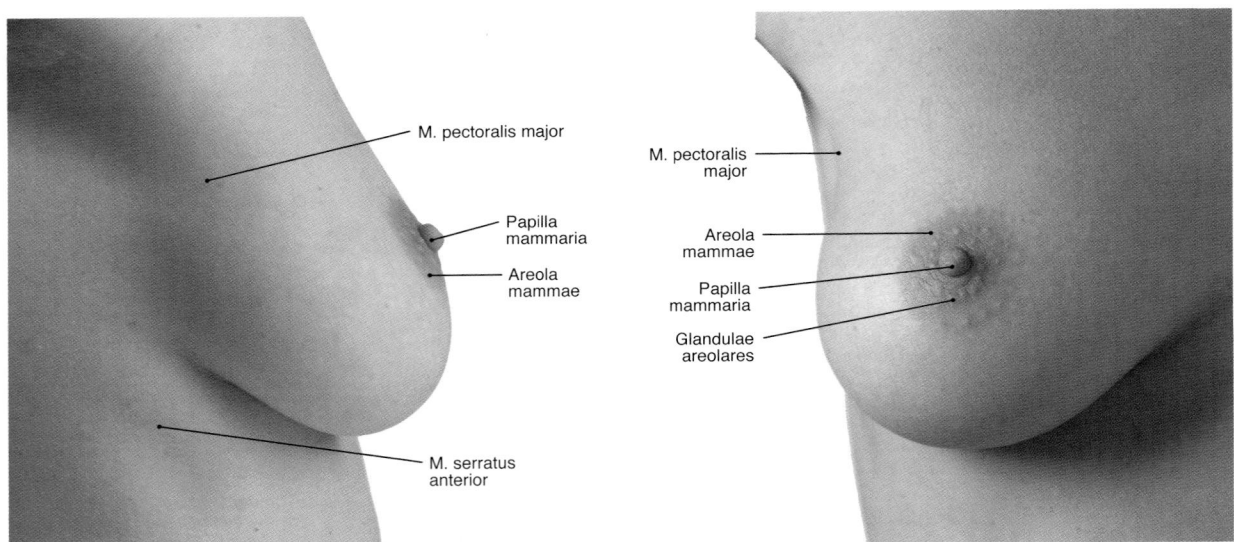

Fig. 586   Breast, Mamma.

Fig. 587   Breast, Mamma.

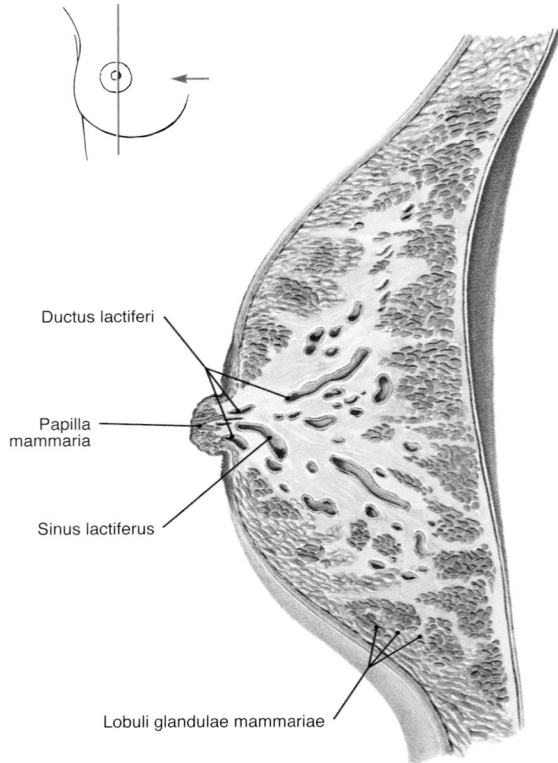

Fig. 588   Breast, Mamma, of a pregnant woman.

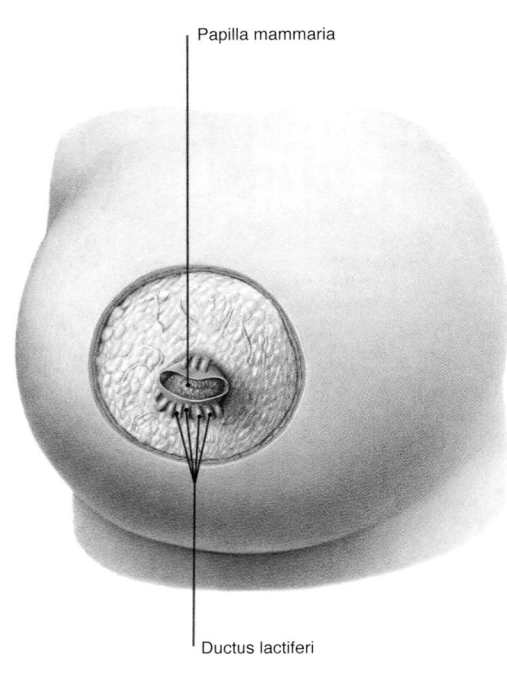

Fig. 589   Breast, Mamma, of a pregnant woman.

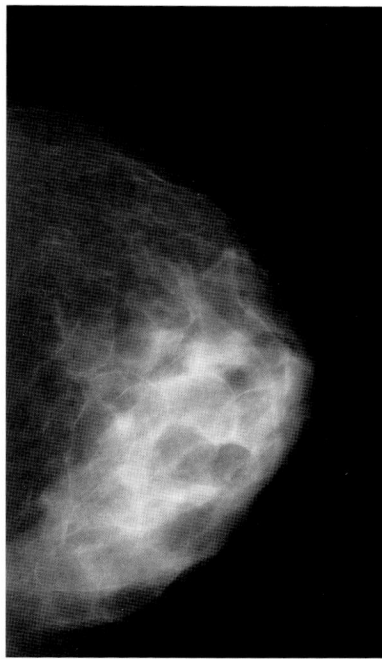

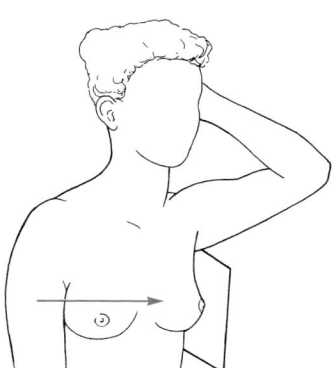

Fig. 590 Radiograph of the breast, mammography, of a 47-year-old woman.

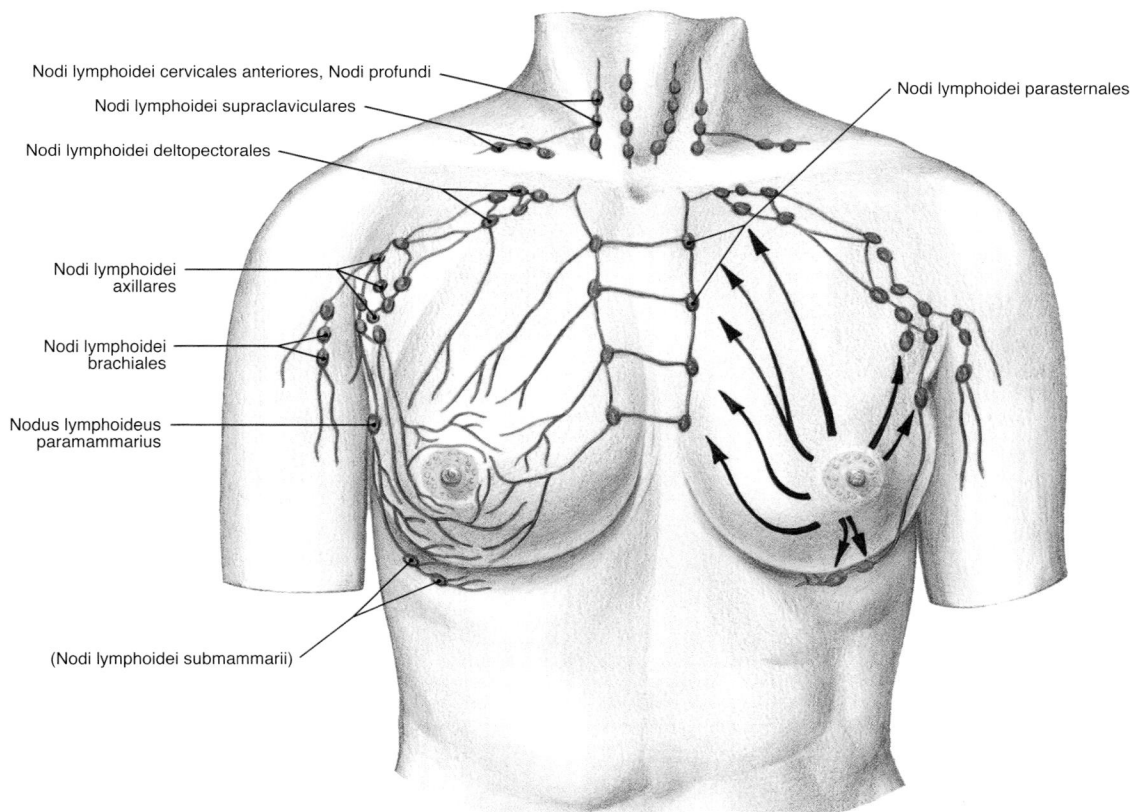

Nodi lymphoidei cervicales anteriores, Nodi profundi

Nodi lymphoidei supraclaviculares

Nodi lymphoidei deltopectorales

Nodi lymphoidei axillares

Nodi lymphoidei brachiales

Nodus lymphoideus paramammarius

(Nodi lymphoidei submammarii)

Nodi lymphoidei parasternales

Fig. 591 Lymphatic drainage of the breast and location of the regional lymph nodes.

Vessels and nerves of the wall of the trunk

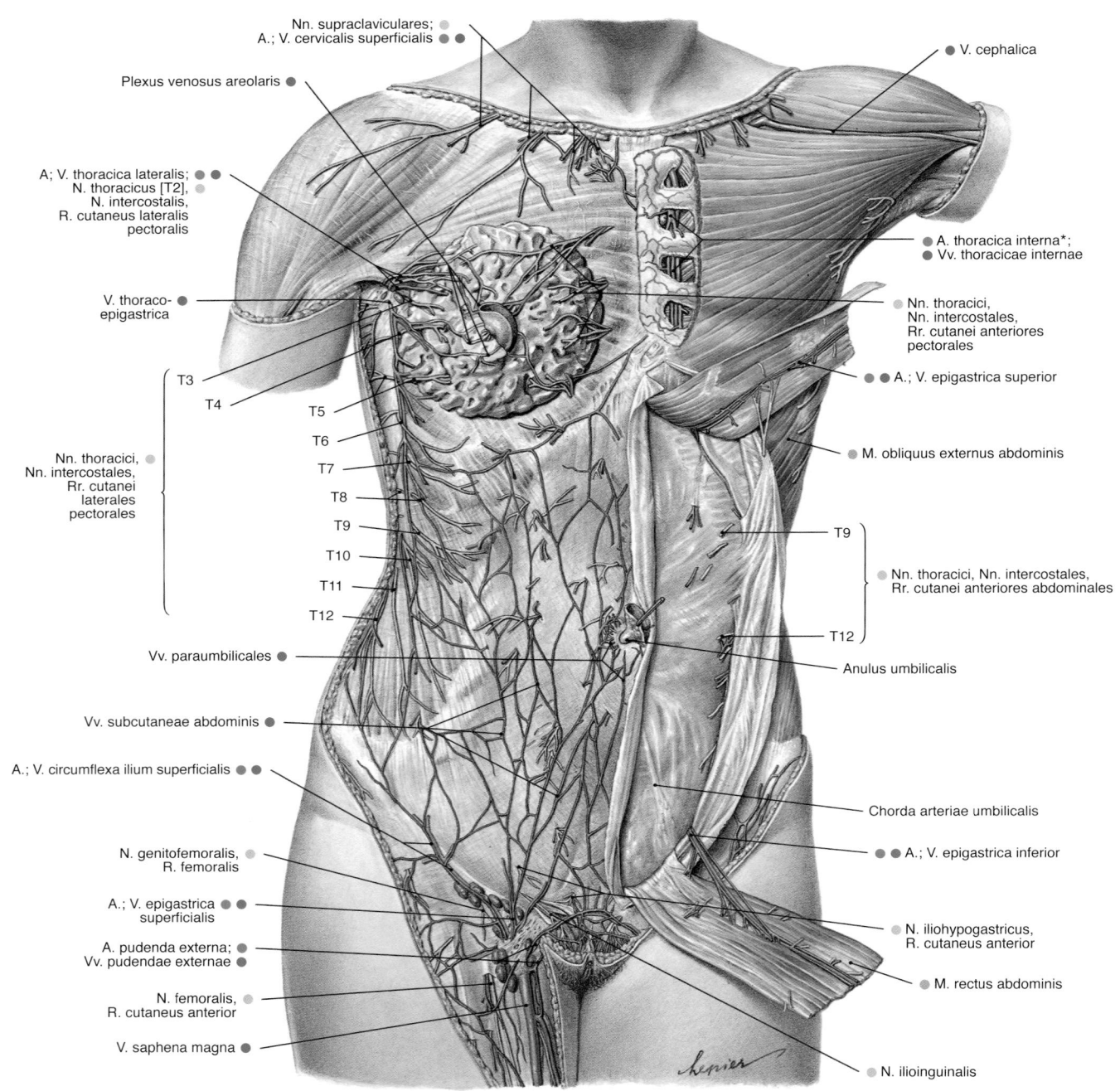

Nn. supraclaviculares;
A.; V. cervicalis superficialis

Plexus venosus areolaris

A; V. thoracica lateralis;
N. thoracicus [T2],
N. intercostalis,
R. cutaneus lateralis
pectoralis

V. thoraco-
epigastrica

T3
T4
T5
T6
T7
T8
T9
T10
T11
T12

Nn. thoracici,
Nn. intercostales,
Rr. cutanei
laterales
pectorales

Vv. paraumbilicales

Vv. subcutaneae abdominis

A.; V. circumflexa ilium superficialis

N. genitofemoralis,
R. femoralis

A.; V. epigastrica
superficialis

A. pudenda externa;
Vv. pudendae externae

N. femoralis,
R. cutaneus anterior

V. saphena magna

V. cephalica

A. thoracica interna*;
Vv. thoracicae internae

Nn. thoracici,
Nn. intercostales,
Rr. cutanei anteriores
pectorales

A.; V. epigastrica superior

M. obliquus externus abdominis

T9

Nn. thoracici, Nn. intercostales,
Rr. cutanei anteriores abdominales

T12

Anulus umbilicalis

Chorda arteriae umbilicalis

A.; V. epigastrica inferior

N. iliohypogastricus,
R. cutaneus anterior

M. rectus abdominis

N. ilioinguinalis

Fig. 592 Vessels and nerves of the thoracic and the abdominal wall.
* Clinical term: internal mammary artery

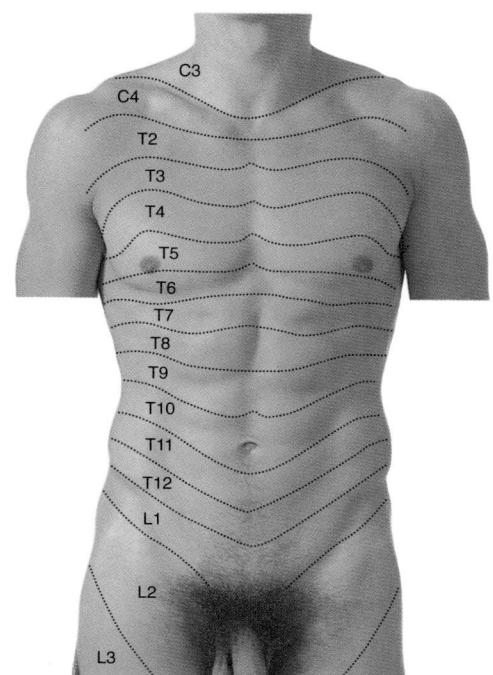

Fig. 593 Segmental sensory innervation of the anterior thoracic and abdominal wall (dermatomes).

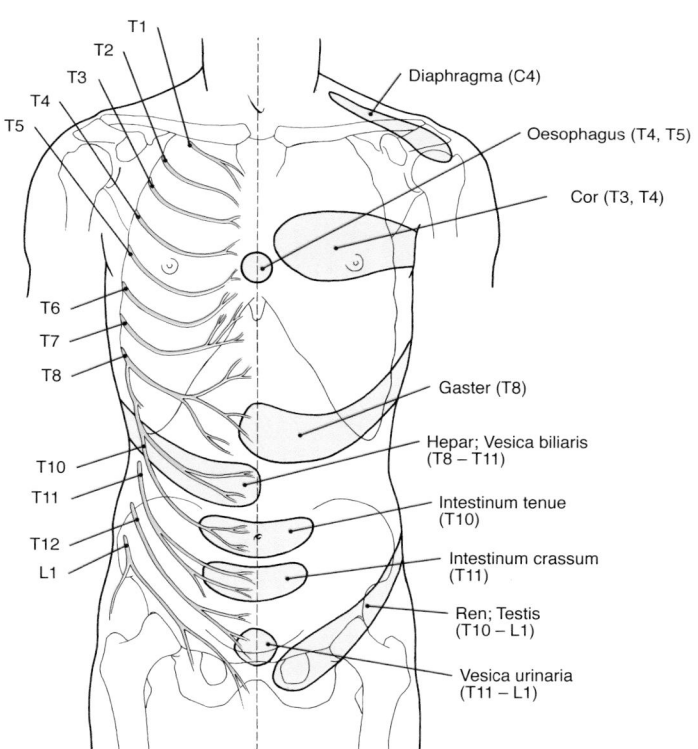

Diaphragma (C4)

Oesophagus (T4, T5)

Cor (T3, T4)

Gaster (T8)

Hepar; Vesica biliaris (T8 – T11)

Intestinum tenue (T10)

Intestinum crassum (T11)

Ren; Testis (T10 – L1)

Vesica urinaria (T11 – L1)

Fig. 594 Segmental sensory innervation of the anterior thoracic and abdominal wall.
Regions to which pain from diseased viscera (zones of HEAD) is referred to are indicated in grey.

Lumbosacral plexus

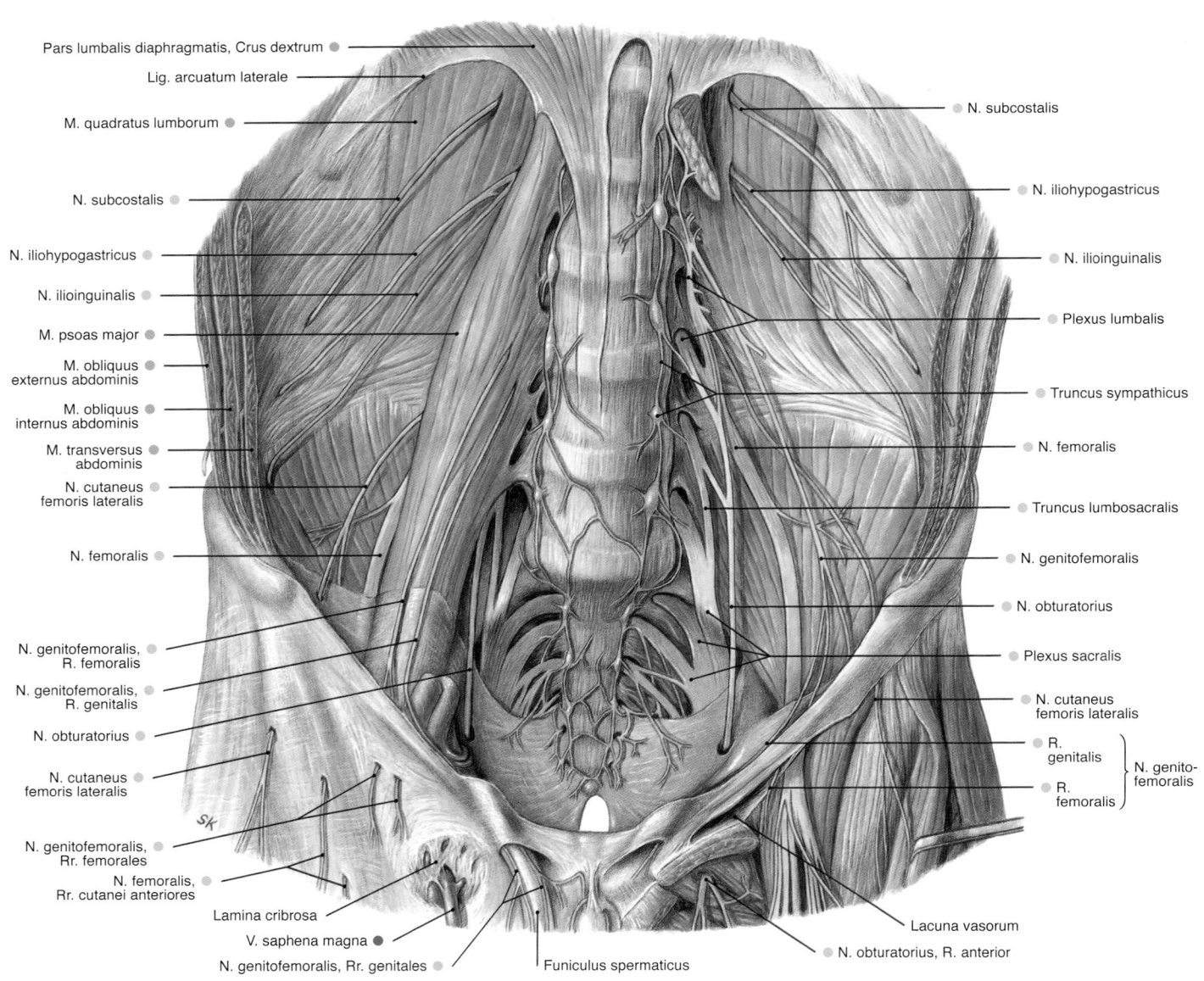

Pars lumbalis diaphragmatis, Crus dextrum ●
Lig. arcuatum laterale
M. quadratus lumborum ●

N. subcostalis ●

N. iliohypogastricus ●
N. ilioinguinalis ●
M. psoas major ●
M. obliquus externus abdominis ●
M. obliquus internus abdominis ●
M. transversus abdominis ●
N. cutaneus femoris lateralis ●

N. femoralis ●

N. genitofemoralis, R. femoralis ●
N. genitofemoralis, R. genitalis ●
N. obturatorius ●
N. cutaneus femoris lateralis ●

N. genitofemoralis, Rr. femorales ●
N. femoralis, Rr. cutanei anteriores ●
Lamina cribrosa
V. saphena magna ●
N. genitofemoralis, Rr. genitales ●

● N. subcostalis

● N. iliohypogastricus

● N. ilioinguinalis

● Plexus lumbalis

● Truncus sympathicus

● N. femoralis

● Truncus lumbosacralis

● N. genitofemoralis

● N. obturatorius

● Plexus sacralis

● N. cutaneus femoris lateralis

● R. genitalis } N. genito-
● R. femoralis } femoralis

Lacuna vasorum
● N. obturatorius, R. anterior

Funiculus spermaticus

Fig. 595 Lumbosacral plexus, Plexus lumbosacralis.

→ 47, 1102, T 40

Vessels of the anterior wall of the trunk

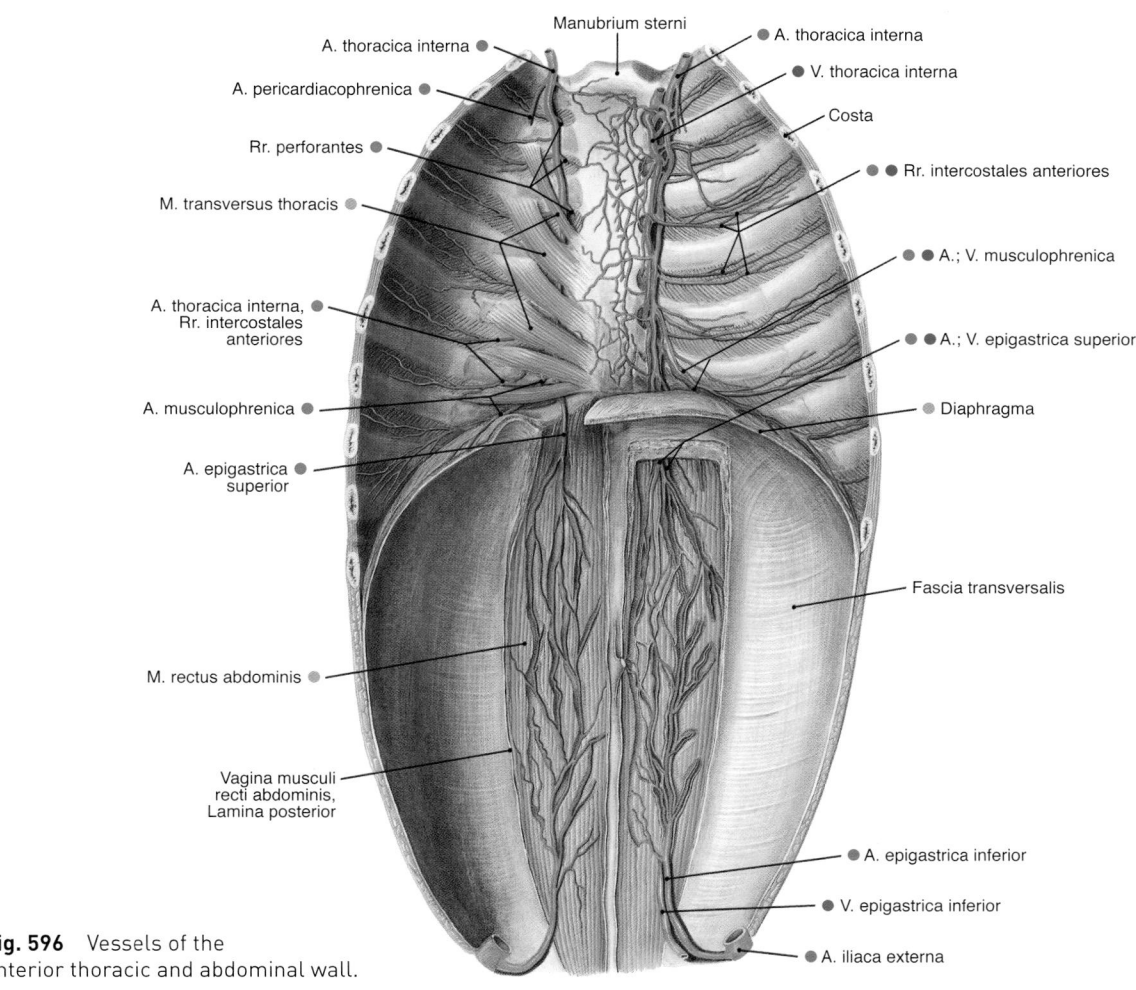

A. thoracica interna ●
A. pericardiacophrenica ●
Rr. perforantes ●
M. transversus thoracis ●
A. thoracica interna, ●
Rr. intercostales
anteriores
A. musculophrenica ●
A. epigastrica ●
superior
M. rectus abdominis ●
Vagina musculi
recti abdominis,
Lamina posterior

Manubrium sterni

● A. thoracica interna
● V. thoracica interna
Costa
● ● Rr. intercostales anteriores
● ● A.; V. musculophrenica
● ● A.; V. epigastrica superior
● Diaphragma
Fascia transversalis

● A. epigastrica inferior
● V. epigastrica inferior
● A. iliaca externa

Fig. 596 Vessels of the
anterior thoracic and abdominal wall.

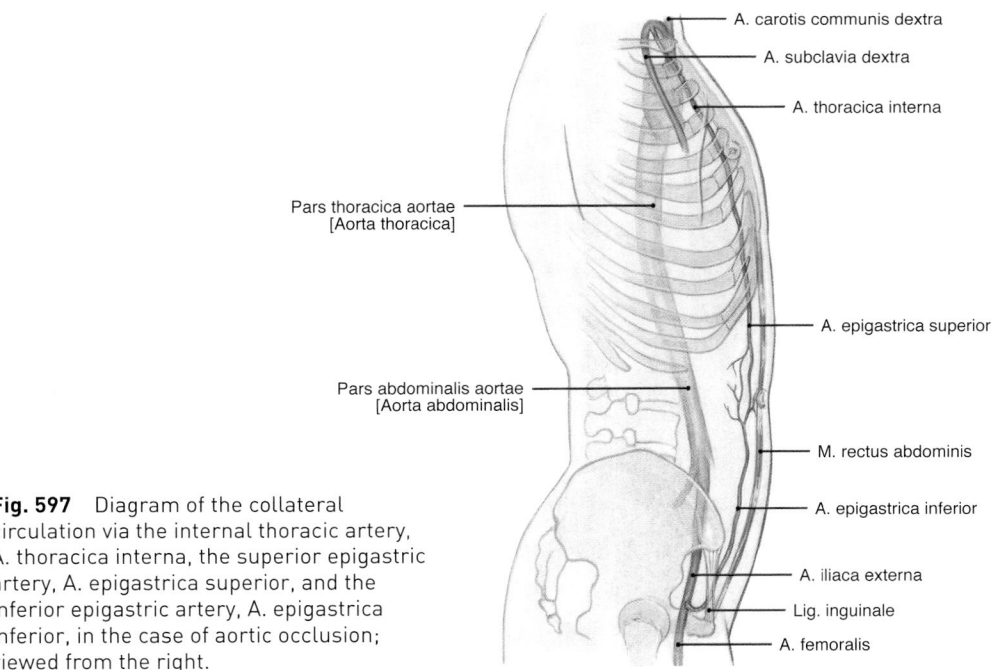

A. carotis communis dextra
A. subclavia dextra
A. thoracica interna
Pars thoracica aortae
[Aorta thoracica]
A. epigastrica superior
Pars abdominalis aortae
[Aorta abdominalis]
M. rectus abdominis
A. epigastrica inferior
A. iliaca externa
Lig. inguinale
A. femoralis

Fig. 597 Diagram of the collateral
circulation via the internal thoracic artery,
A. thoracica interna, the superior epigastric
artery, A. epigastrica superior, and the
inferior epigastric artery, A. epigastrica
inferior, in the case of aortic occlusion;
viewed from the right.

Abdominal wall of a neonate

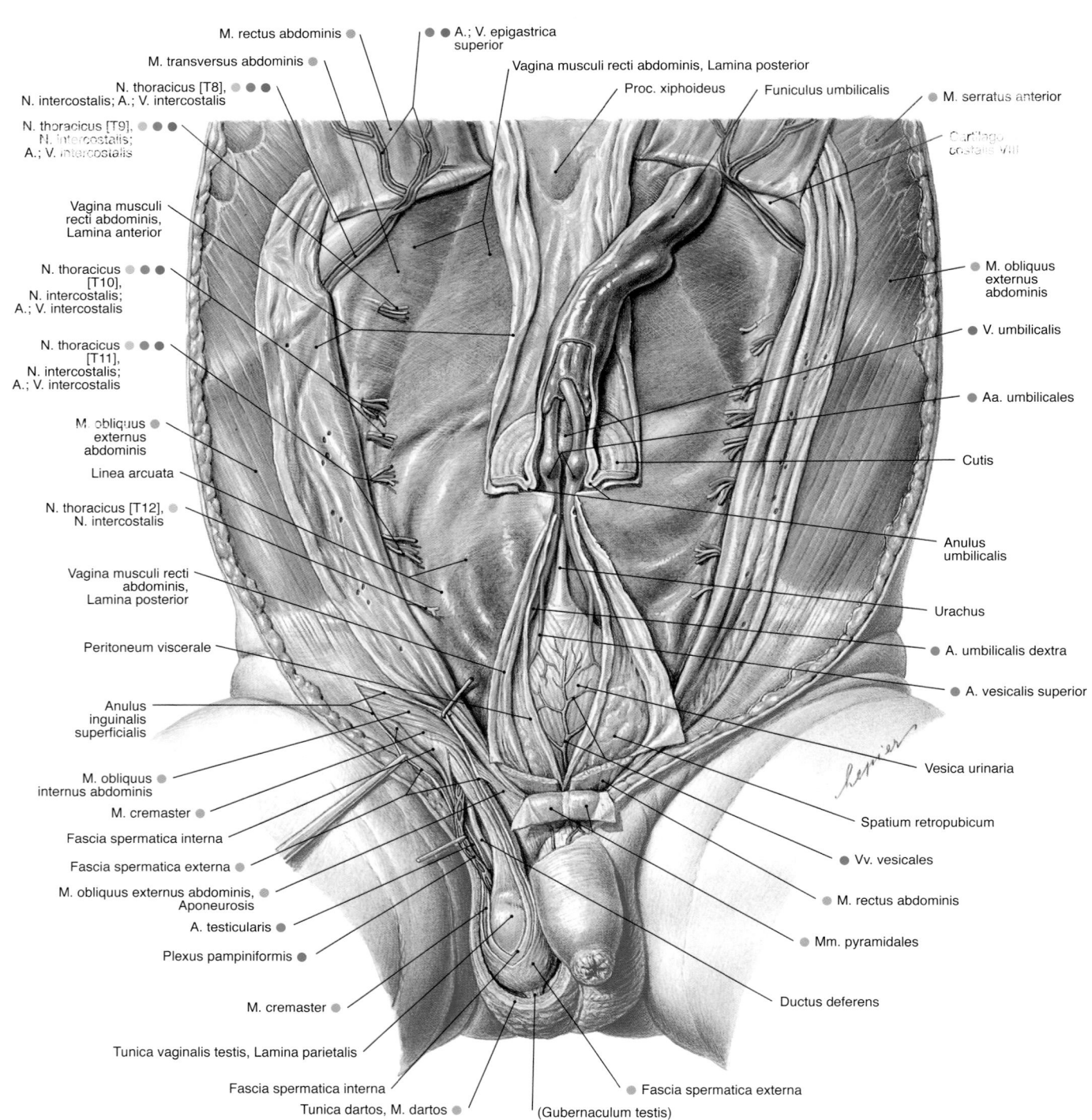

M. rectus abdominis

A.; V. epigastrica superior

M. transversus abdominis

Vagina musculi recti abdominis, Lamina posterior

N. thoracicus [T8],
N. intercostalis; A.; V. intercostalis

Proc. xiphoideus

Funiculus umbilicalis

M. serratus anterior

N. thoracicus [T9],
N. intercostalis;
A.; V. intercostalis

Cartilago costalis VIII

Vagina musculi recti abdominis, Lamina anterior

M. obliquus externus abdominis

N. thoracicus [T10],
N. intercostalis;
A.; V. intercostalis

V. umbilicalis

N. thoracicus [T11],
N. intercostalis;
A.; V. intercostalis

Aa. umbilicales

M. obliquus externus abdominis

Cutis

Linea arcuata

N. thoracicus [T12],
N. intercostalis

Anulus umbilicalis

Vagina musculi recti abdominis, Lamina posterior

Urachus

Peritoneum viscerale

A. umbilicalis dextra

A. vesicalis superior

Anulus inguinalis superficialis

Vesica urinaria

M. obliquus internus abdominis

Spatium retropubicum

M. cremaster

Vv. vesicales

Fascia spermatica interna

M. rectus abdominis

Fascia spermatica externa

M. obliquus externus abdominis, Aponeurosis

Mm. pyramidales

A. testicularis

Plexus pampiniformis

Ductus deferens

M. cremaster

Tunica vaginalis testis, Lamina parietalis

Fascia spermatica interna

Fascia spermatica externa

Tunica dartos, M. dartos

(Gubernaculum testis)

Fig. 598   Anterior abdominal wall of a neonate.

Inner contour of the anterior abdominal wall

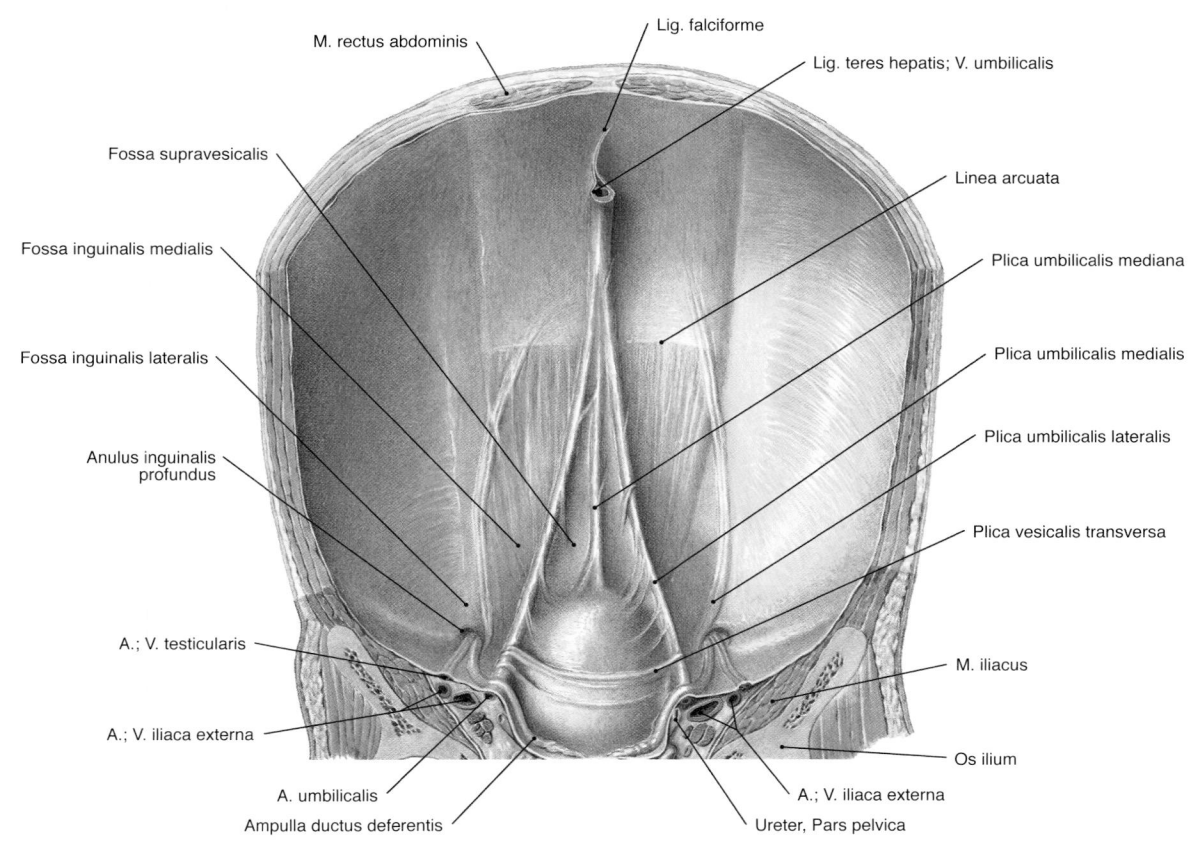

M. rectus abdominis

Lig. falciforme

Lig. teres hepatis; V. umbilicalis

Fossa supravesicalis

Linea arcuata

Fossa inguinalis medialis

Plica umbilicalis mediana

Fossa inguinalis lateralis

Plica umbilicalis medialis

Anulus inguinalis profundus

Plica umbilicalis lateralis

Plica vesicalis transversa

A.; V. testicularis

M. iliacus

A.; V. iliaca externa

Os ilium

A. umbilicalis

A.; V. iliaca externa

Ampulla ductus deferentis

Ureter, Pars pelvica

Fig. 599   Anterior abdominal wall of a neonate.

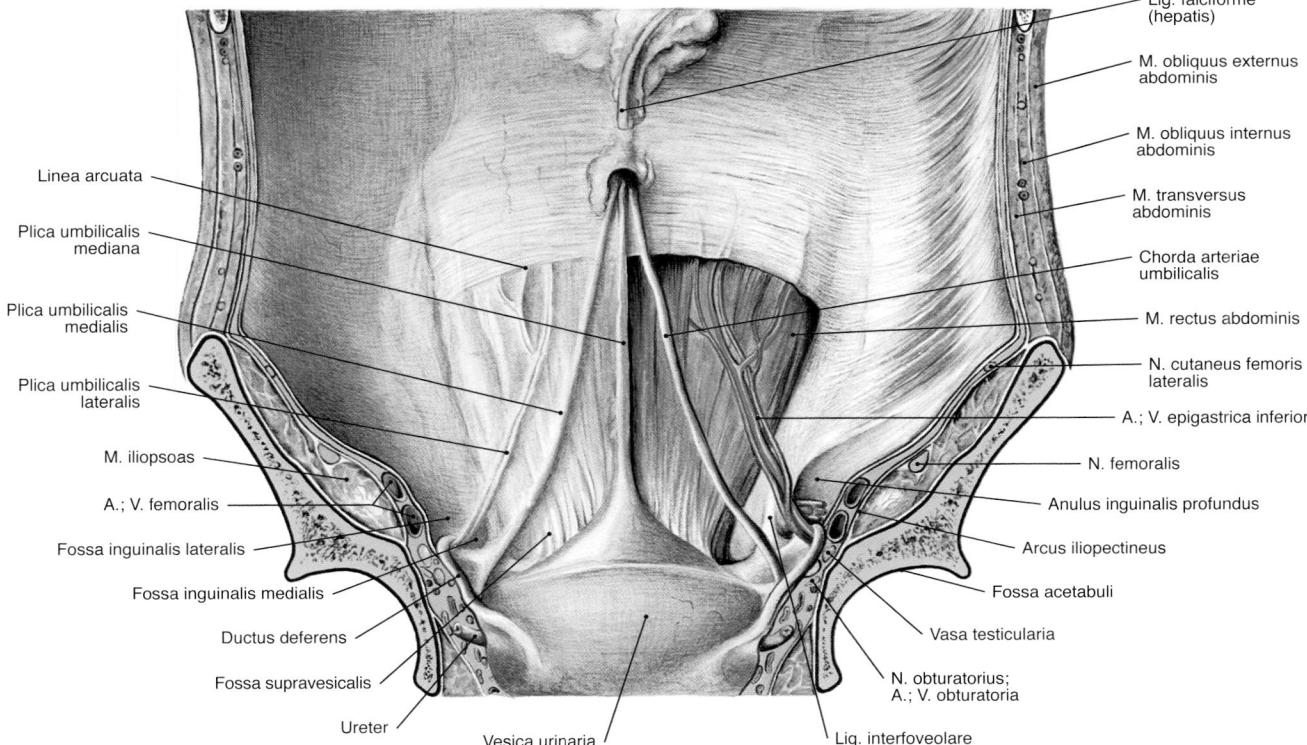

Lig. falciforme (hepatis)

M. obliquus externus abdominis

M. obliquus internus abdominis

Linea arcuata

M. transversus abdominis

Plica umbilicalis mediana

Chorda arteriae umbilicalis

Plica umbilicalis medialis

M. rectus abdominis

Plica umbilicalis lateralis

N. cutaneus femoris lateralis

M. iliopsoas

A.; V. epigastrica inferior

A.; V. femoralis

N. femoralis

Fossa inguinalis lateralis

Anulus inguinalis profundus

Fossa inguinalis medialis

Arcus iliopectineus

Ductus deferens

Fossa acetabuli

Fossa supravesicalis

Vasa testicularia

Ureter

N. obturatorius; A.; V. obturatoria

Vesica urinaria

Lig. interfoveolare

Fig. 600   Anterior abdominal wall, internal aspect.

Abdominal wall, sections

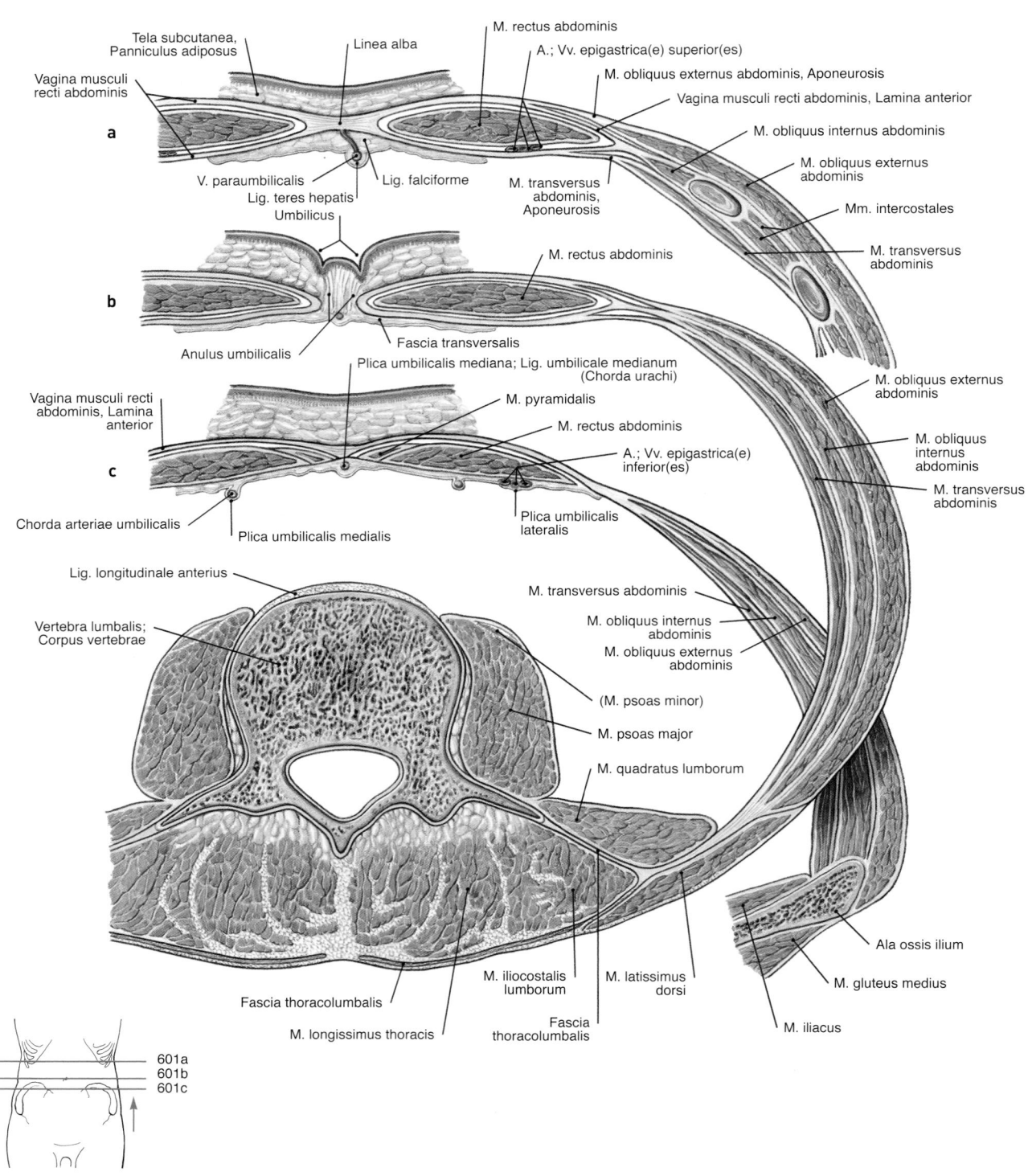

Tela subcutanea, Panniculus adiposus
Linea alba
M. rectus abdominis
A.; Vv. epigastrica(e) superior(es)
Vagina musculi recti abdominis
M. obliquus externus abdominis, Aponeurosis
Vagina musculi recti abdominis, Lamina anterior
M. obliquus internus abdominis
M. obliquus externus abdominis
Mm. intercostales
M. transversus abdominis

a

V. paraumbilicalis
Lig. teres hepatis
Umbilicus
Lig. falciforme
M. transversus abdominis, Aponeurosis

M. rectus abdominis

b

Anulus umbilicalis
Fascia transversalis
M. obliquus externus abdominis

Plica umbilicalis mediana; Lig. umbilicale medianum (Chorda urachi)
Vagina musculi recti abdominis, Lamina anterior
M. pyramidalis
M. rectus abdominis
A.; Vv. epigastrica(e) inferior(es)
M. obliquus internus abdominis
M. transversus abdominis

c

Chorda arteriae umbilicalis
Plica umbilicalis medialis
Plica umbilicalis lateralis

Lig. longitudinale anterius
Vertebra lumbalis; Corpus vertebrae
M. transversus abdominis
M. obliquus internus abdominis
M. obliquus externus abdominis
(M. psoas minor)
M. psoas major
M. quadratus lumborum

Fascia thoracolumbalis
M. longissimus thoracis
M. iliocostalis lumborum
M. latissimus dorsi
Fascia thoracolumbalis
M. iliacus
M. gluteus medius
Ala ossis ilium

601a
601b
601c

→ T 14–T 16, T 20a, b, T 42

Fig. 601a–c Muscles of the abdominal wall, Mm. abdominis; horizontal sections.

Abdominal wall, sections

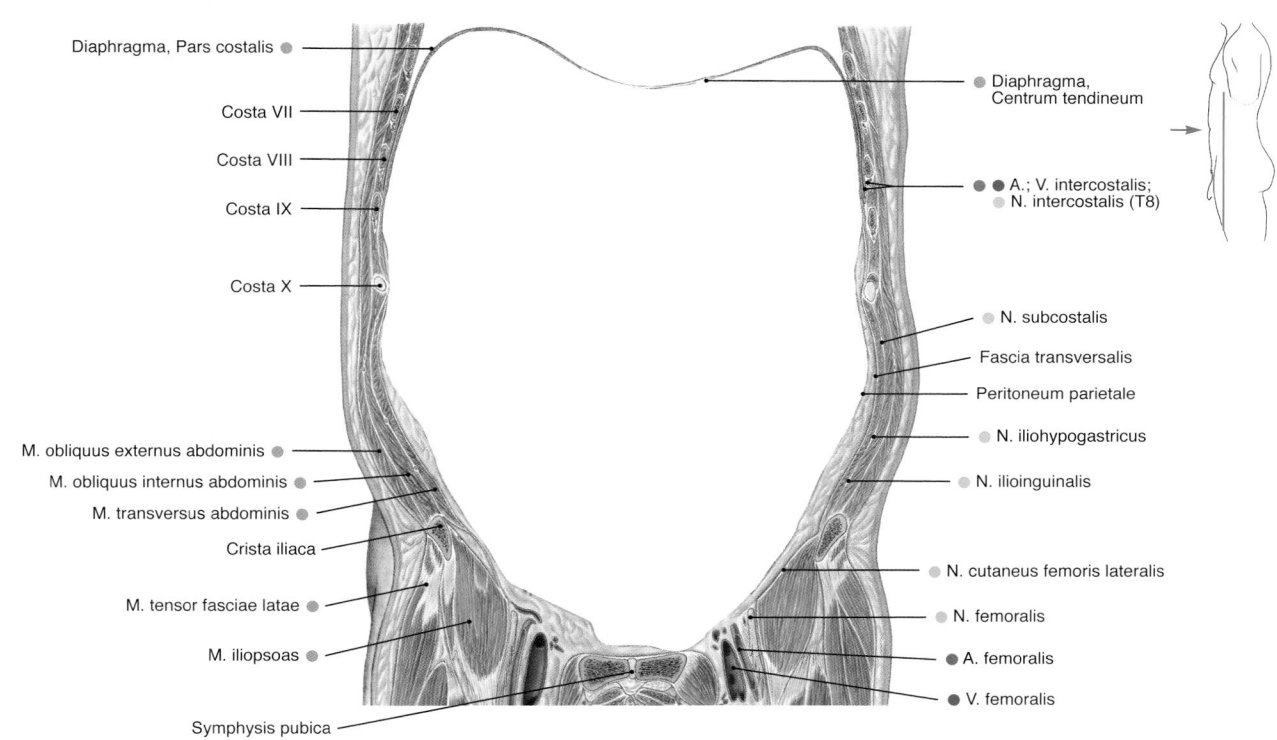

Diaphragma, Pars costalis ●

Costa VII

Costa VIII

Costa IX

Costa X

M. obliquus externus abdominis ●

M. obliquus internus abdominis ●

M. transversus abdominis ●

Crista iliaca

M. tensor fasciae latae ●

M. iliopsoas ●

Symphysis pubica

● Diaphragma, Centrum tendineum

● ● A.; V. intercostalis; ● N. intercostalis (T8)

● N. subcostalis

Fascia transversalis

Peritoneum parietale

● N. iliohypogastricus

● N. ilioinguinalis

● N. cutaneus femoris lateralis

● N. femoralis

● A. femoralis

● V. femoralis

Fig. 602 Muscles of the abdominal wall, Mm. abdominis; frontal section.

603a
603b

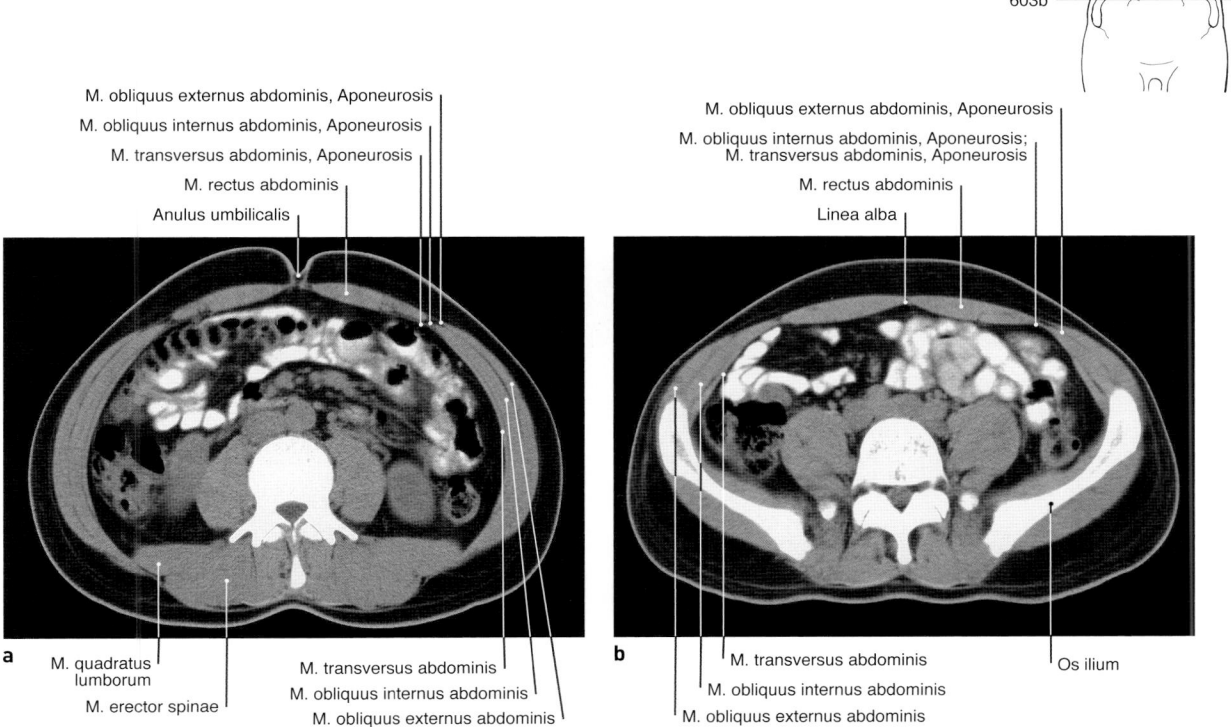

M. obliquus externus abdominis, Aponeurosis

M. obliquus internus abdominis, Aponeurosis

M. transversus abdominis, Aponeurosis

M. rectus abdominis

Anulus umbilicalis

M. obliquus externus abdominis, Aponeurosis

M. obliquus internus abdominis, Aponeurosis; M. transversus abdominis, Aponeurosis

M. rectus abdominis

Linea alba

a M. quadratus lumborum

M. erector spinae

M. transversus abdominis

M. obliquus internus abdominis

M. obliquus externus abdominis

b M. transversus abdominis

M. obliquus internus abdominis

M. obliquus externus abdominis

Os ilium

Fig. 603 a, b Muscles of the abdominal wall, Mm. abdominis; computed tomographic cross-sections (CT).

Heart

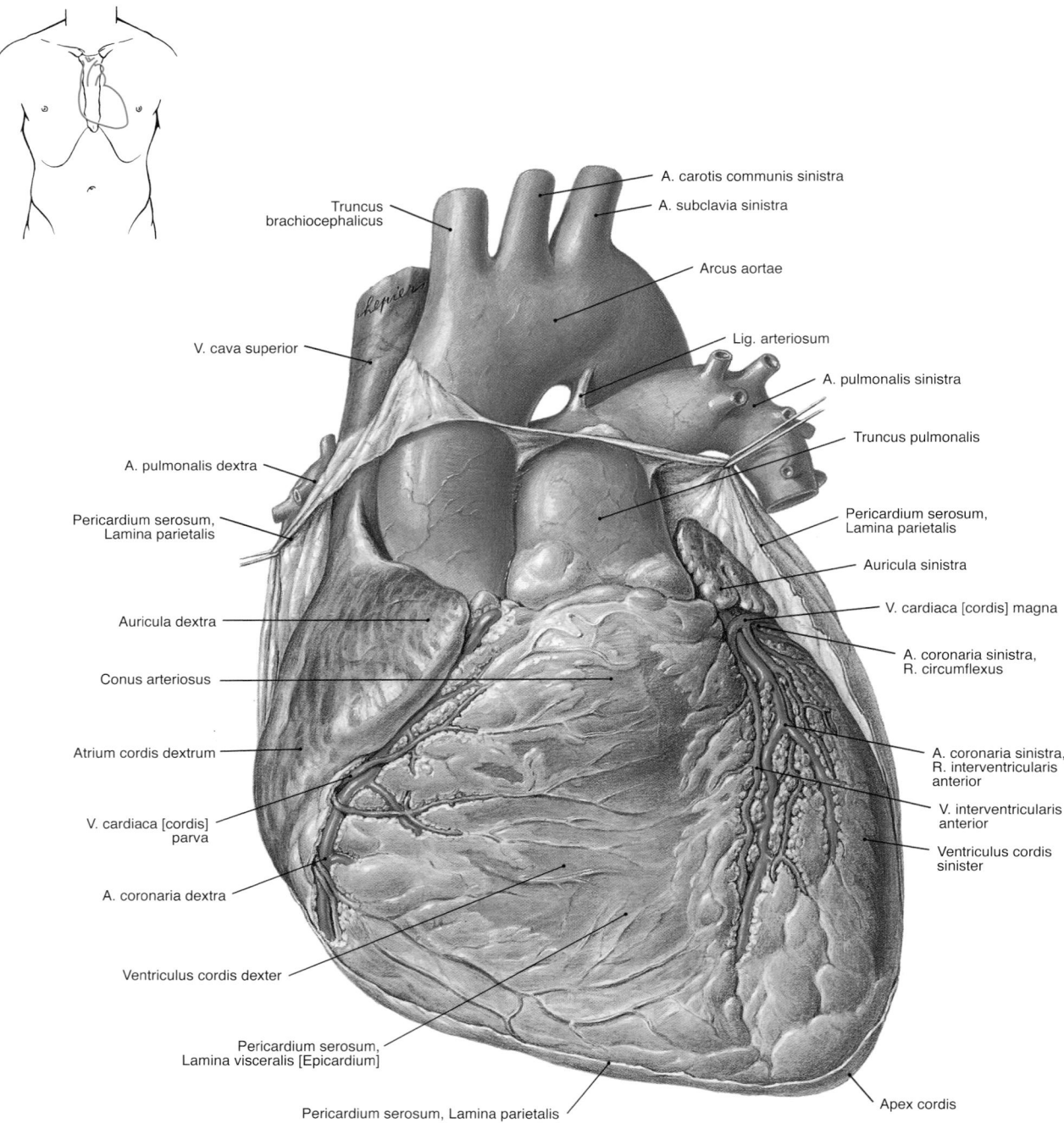

A. carotis communis sinistra

A. subclavia sinistra

Arcus aortae

Truncus
brachiocephalicus

Lig. arteriosum

V. cava superior

A. pulmonalis sinistra

Truncus pulmonalis

A. pulmonalis dextra

Pericardium serosum,
Lamina parietalis

Pericardium serosum,
Lamina parietalis

Auricula sinistra

Auricula dextra

V. cardiaca [cordis] magna

Conus arteriosus

A. coronaria sinistra,
R. circumflexus

Atrium cordis dextrum

A. coronaria sinistra,
R. interventricularis
anterior

V. interventricularis
anterior

V. cardiaca [cordis]
parva

Ventriculus cordis
sinister

A. coronaria dextra

Ventriculus cordis dexter

Pericardium serosum,
Lamina visceralis [Epicardium]

Apex cordis

Pericardium serosum, Lamina parietalis

Abb. 604   Heart, Cor.

Pericardium fibrosum
Pericardium serosum   } Pericardium
Lamina parietalis
Lamina visceralis   =   Epicardium

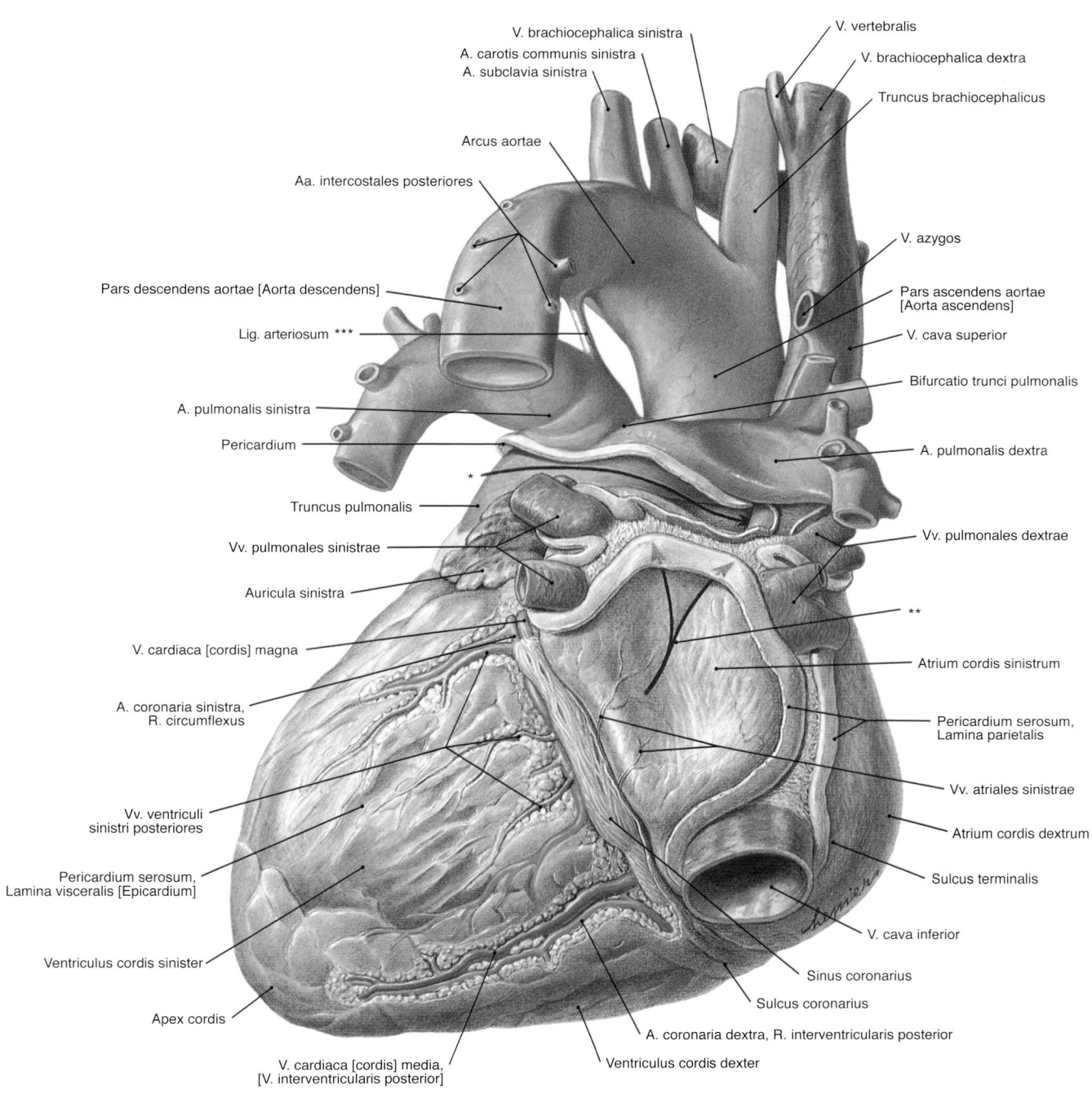

V. brachiocephalica sinistra
A. carotis communis sinistra
A. subclavia sinistra
V. vertebralis
V. brachiocephalica dextra
Truncus brachiocephalicus
Arcus aortae
Aa. intercostales posteriores
V. azygos
Pars descendens aortae [Aorta descendens]
Pars ascendens aortae [Aorta ascendens]
Lig. arteriosum ***
V. cava superior
Bifurcatio trunci pulmonalis
A. pulmonalis sinistra
Pericardium
A. pulmonalis dextra
*
Truncus pulmonalis
Vv. pulmonales sinistrae
Vv. pulmonales dextrae
Auricula sinistra
**
V. cardiaca [cordis] magna
Atrium cordis sinistrum
A. coronaria sinistra, R. circumflexus
Pericardium serosum, Lamina parietalis
Vv. ventriculi sinistri posteriores
Vv. atriales sinistrae
Pericardium serosum, Lamina visceralis [Epicardium]
Atrium cordis dextrum
Sulcus terminalis
Ventriculus cordis sinister
V. cava inferior
Sinus coronarius
Apex cordis
Sulcus coronarius
A. coronaria dextra, R. interventricularis posterior
V. cardiaca [cordis] media, [V. interventricularis posterior]
Ventriculus cordis dexter

Fig. 605 Heart, Cor, and great vessels; dorsal view.

* Arrow in the transverse pericardial sinus
** Double arrows in the oblique pericardial sinus
*** Remnants of the foetal ductus arteriosus (BOTALLO's ligament)

Myocardium

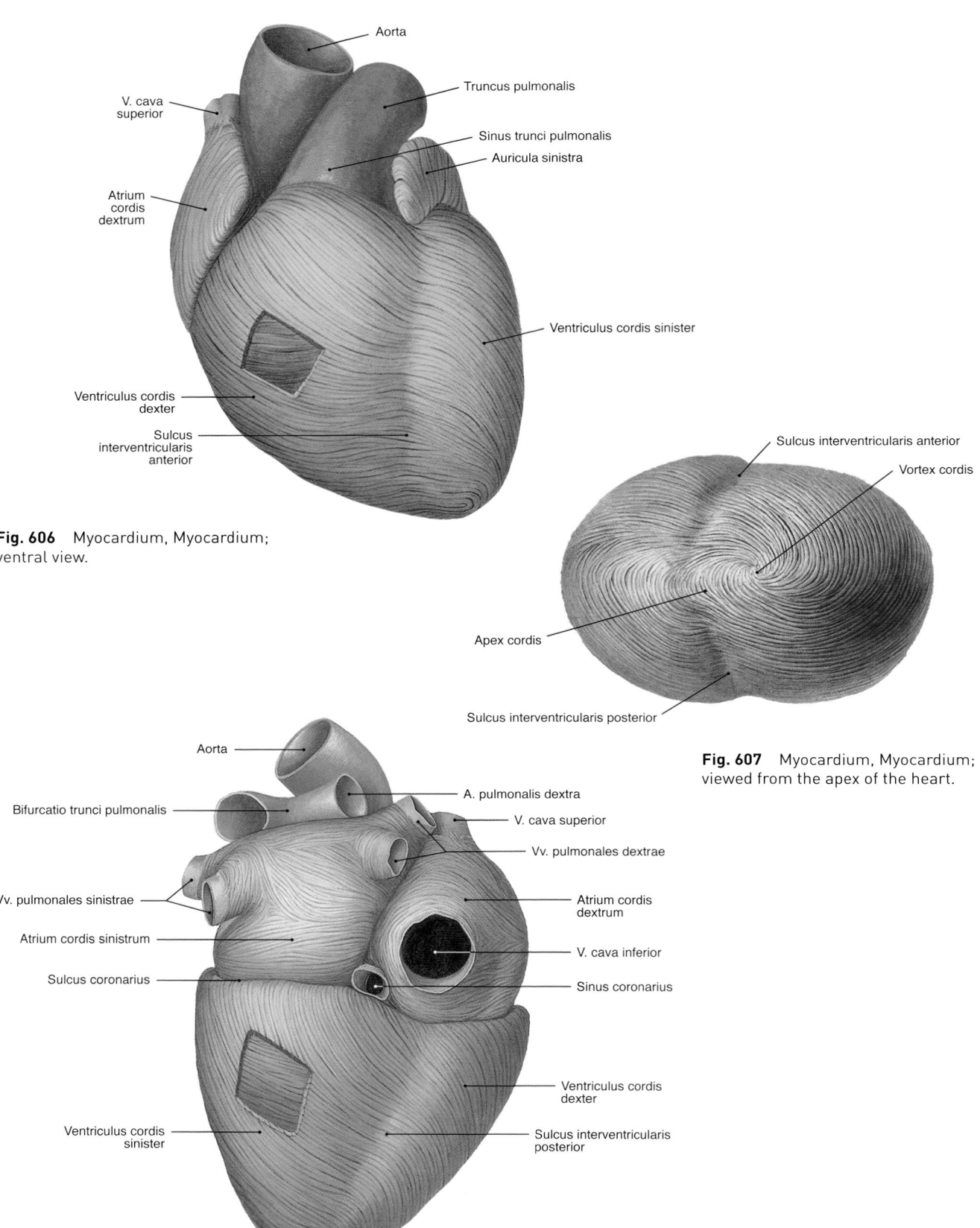

Aorta

Truncus pulmonalis

V. cava
superior

Sinus trunci pulmonalis

Auricula sinistra

Atrium
cordis
dextrum

Ventriculus cordis sinister

Ventriculus cordis
dexter

Sulcus
interventricularis
anterior

Fig. 606 Myocardium, Myocardium;
ventral view.

Sulcus interventricularis anterior

Vortex cordis

Apex cordis

Sulcus interventricularis posterior

Fig. 607 Myocardium, Myocardium;
viewed from the apex of the heart.

Aorta

A. pulmonalis dextra

Bifurcatio trunci pulmonalis

V. cava superior

Vv. pulmonales dextrae

Vv. pulmonales sinistrae

Atrium cordis
dextrum

Atrium cordis sinistrum

V. cava inferior

Sulcus coronarius

Sinus coronarius

Ventriculus cordis
dexter

Ventriculus cordis
sinister

Sulcus interventricularis
posterior

Fig. 608 Myocardium, Myocardium;
dorsoinferior view.

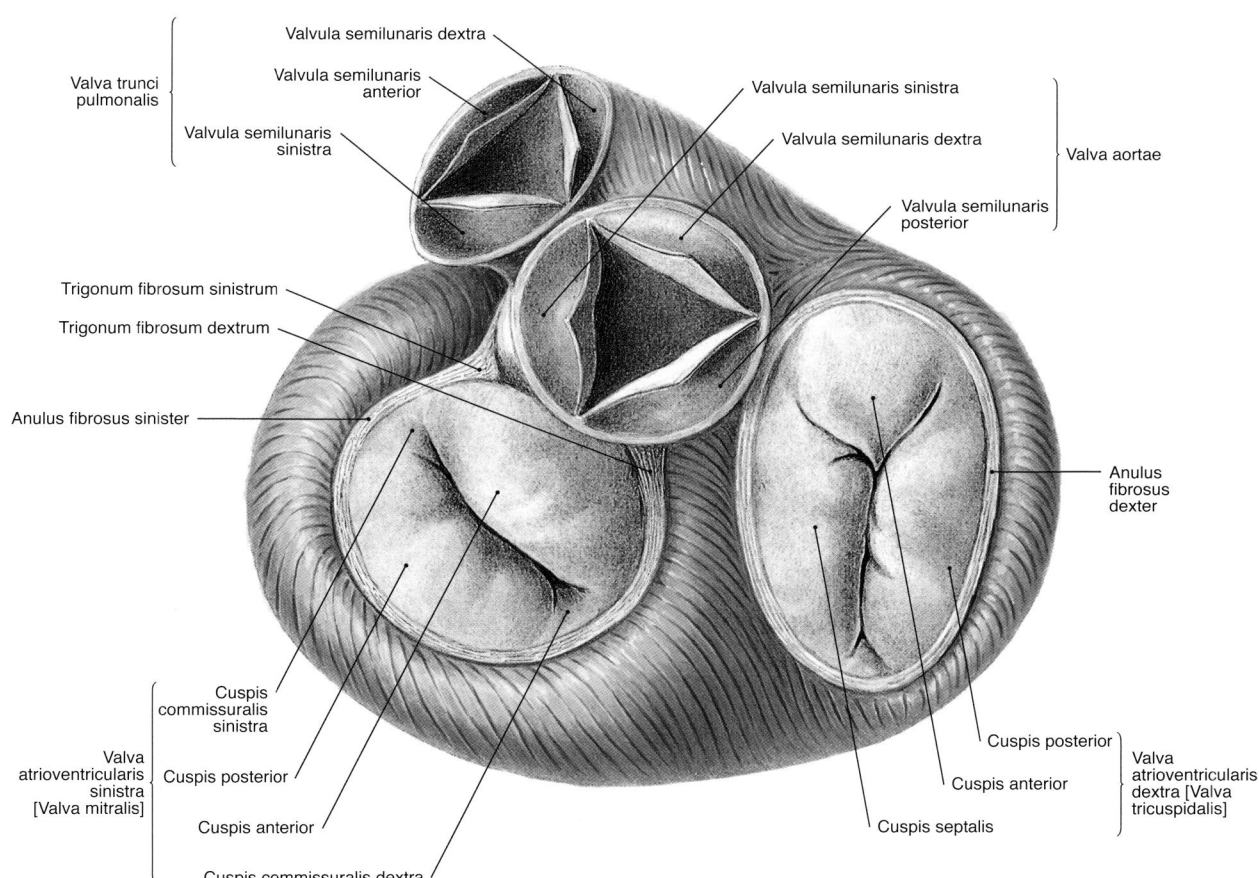

Valva trunci pulmonalis
- Valvula semilunaris dextra
- Valvula semilunaris anterior
- Valvula semilunaris sinistra

Valva aortae
- Valvula semilunaris sinistra
- Valvula semilunaris dextra
- Valvula semilunaris posterior

Trigonum fibrosum sinistrum

Trigonum fibrosum dextrum

Anulus fibrosus sinister

Anulus fibrosus dexter

Valva atrioventricularis sinistra [Valva mitralis]
- Cuspis commissuralis sinistra
- Cuspis posterior
- Cuspis anterior
- Cuspis commissuralis dextra

Valva atrioventricularis dextra [Valva tricuspidalis]
- Cuspis posterior
- Cuspis anterior
- Cuspis septalis

Fig. 609 Valves of the heart, Valvae cordis; superior view.

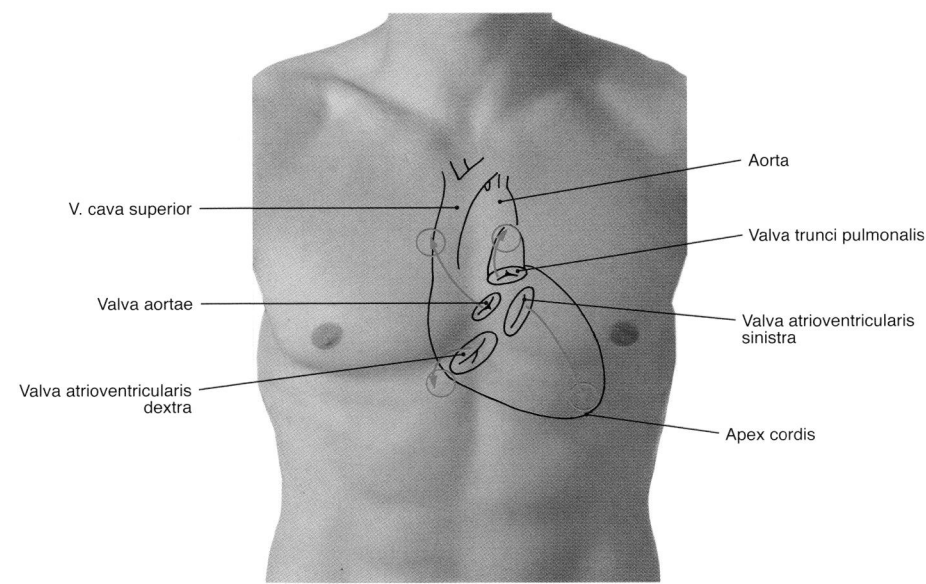

V. cava superior

Aorta

Valva trunci pulmonalis

Valva aortae

Valva atrioventricularis sinistra

Valva atrioventricularis dextra

Apex cordis

Fig. 610 Contour of the heart, valves of the heart, and points of auscultation projected onto the anterior thoracic wall (circles).

The heart sounds and (where applicable) the heart murmurs are spreading in the direction of the arrows.

Internal spaces of the heart

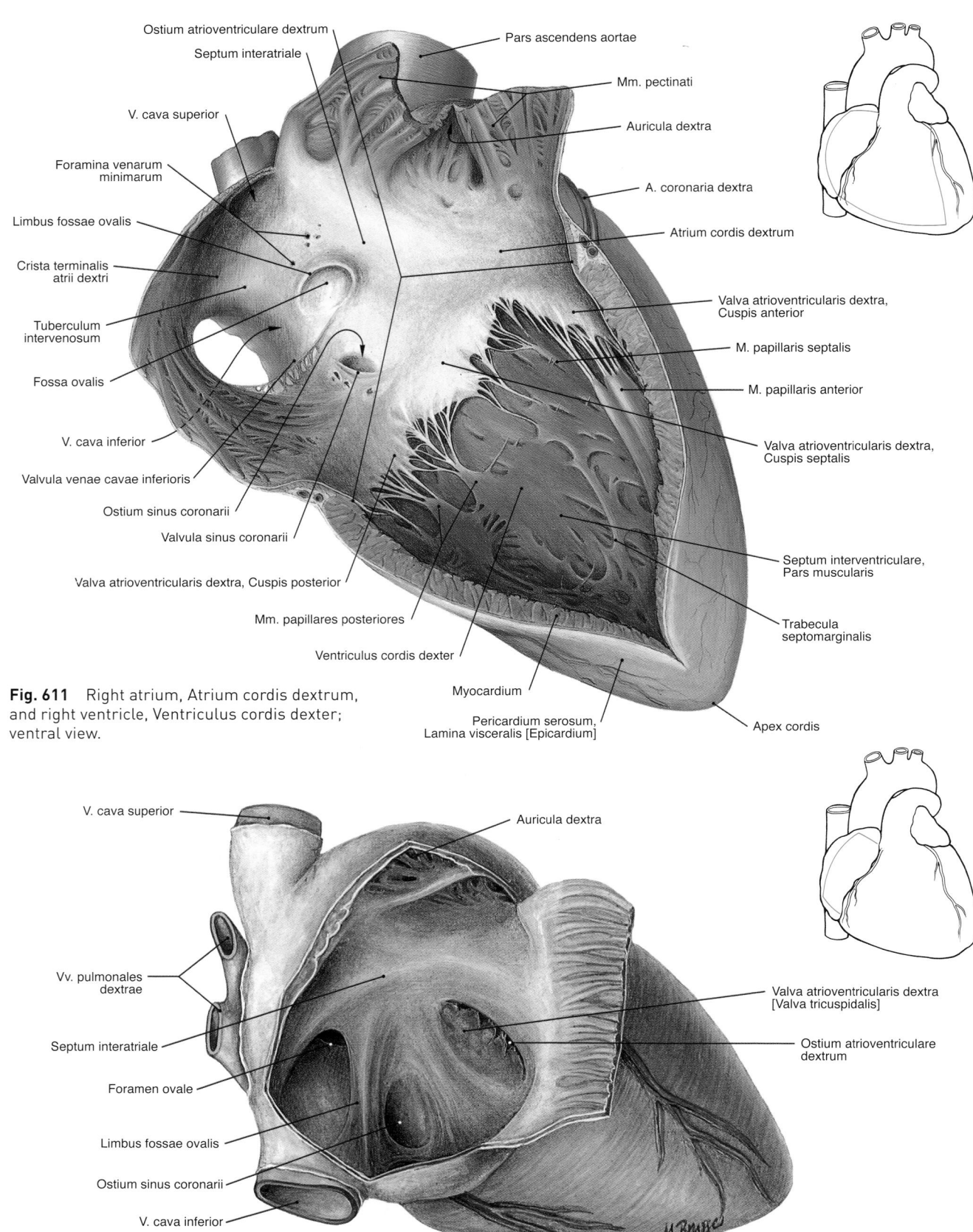

Ostium atrioventriculare dextrum
Septum interatriale
V. cava superior
Foramina venarum minimarum
Limbus fossae ovalis
Crista terminalis atrii dextri
Tuberculum intervenosum
Fossa ovalis
V. cava inferior
Valvula venae cavae inferioris
Ostium sinus coronarii
Valvula sinus coronarii
Valva atrioventricularis dextra, Cuspis posterior
Mm. papillares posteriores
Ventriculus cordis dexter

Pars ascendens aortae
Mm. pectinati
Auricula dextra
A. coronaria dextra
Atrium cordis dextrum
Valva atrioventricularis dextra, Cuspis anterior
M. papillaris septalis
M. papillaris anterior
Valva atrioventricularis dextra, Cuspis septalis
Septum interventriculare, Pars muscularis
Trabecula septomarginalis
Myocardium
Pericardium serosum, Lamina visceralis [Epicardium]
Apex cordis

Fig. 611 Right atrium, Atrium cordis dextrum, and right ventricle, Ventriculus cordis dexter; ventral view.

V. cava superior
Vv. pulmonales dextrae
Septum interatriale
Foramen ovale
Limbus fossae ovalis
Ostium sinus coronarii
V. cava inferior

Auricula dextra
Valva atrioventricularis dextra [Valva tricuspidalis]
Ostium atrioventriculare dextrum

Fig. 612 Right atrium, Atrium cordis dextrum, of a neonate; ventral view from the right.

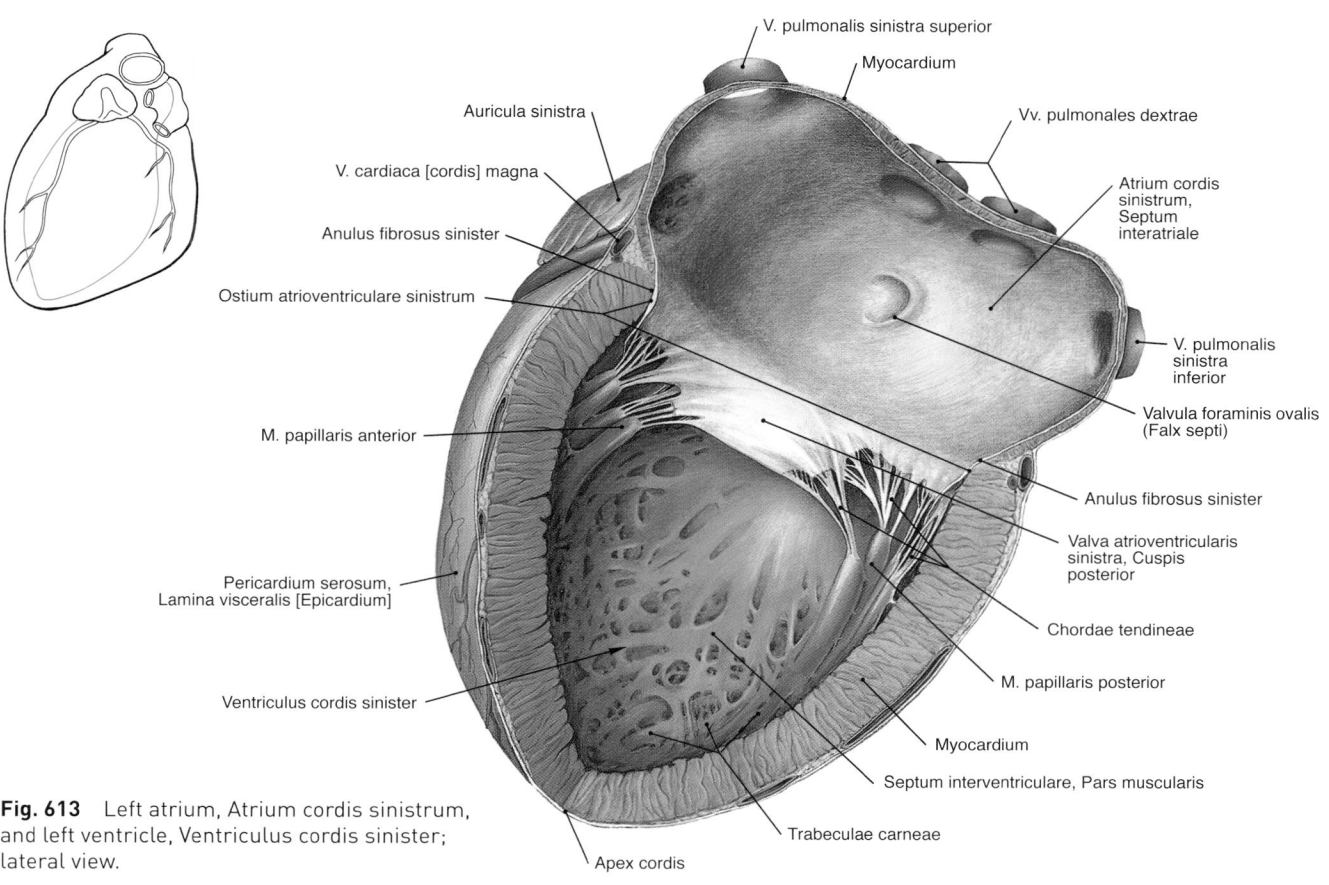

V. pulmonalis sinistra superior

Myocardium

Auricula sinistra

V. cardiaca [cordis] magna

Vv. pulmonales dextrae

Anulus fibrosus sinister

Atrium cordis sinistrum, Septum interatriale

Ostium atrioventriculare sinistrum

V. pulmonalis sinistra inferior

Valvula foraminis ovalis (Falx septi)

M. papillaris anterior

Anulus fibrosus sinister

Valva atrioventricularis sinistra, Cuspis posterior

Pericardium serosum, Lamina visceralis [Epicardium]

Chordae tendineae

M. papillaris posterior

Ventriculus cordis sinister

Myocardium

Septum interventriculare, Pars muscularis

Trabeculae carneae

Fig. 613 Left atrium, Atrium cordis sinistrum, and left ventricle, Ventriculus cordis sinister; lateral view.

Apex cordis

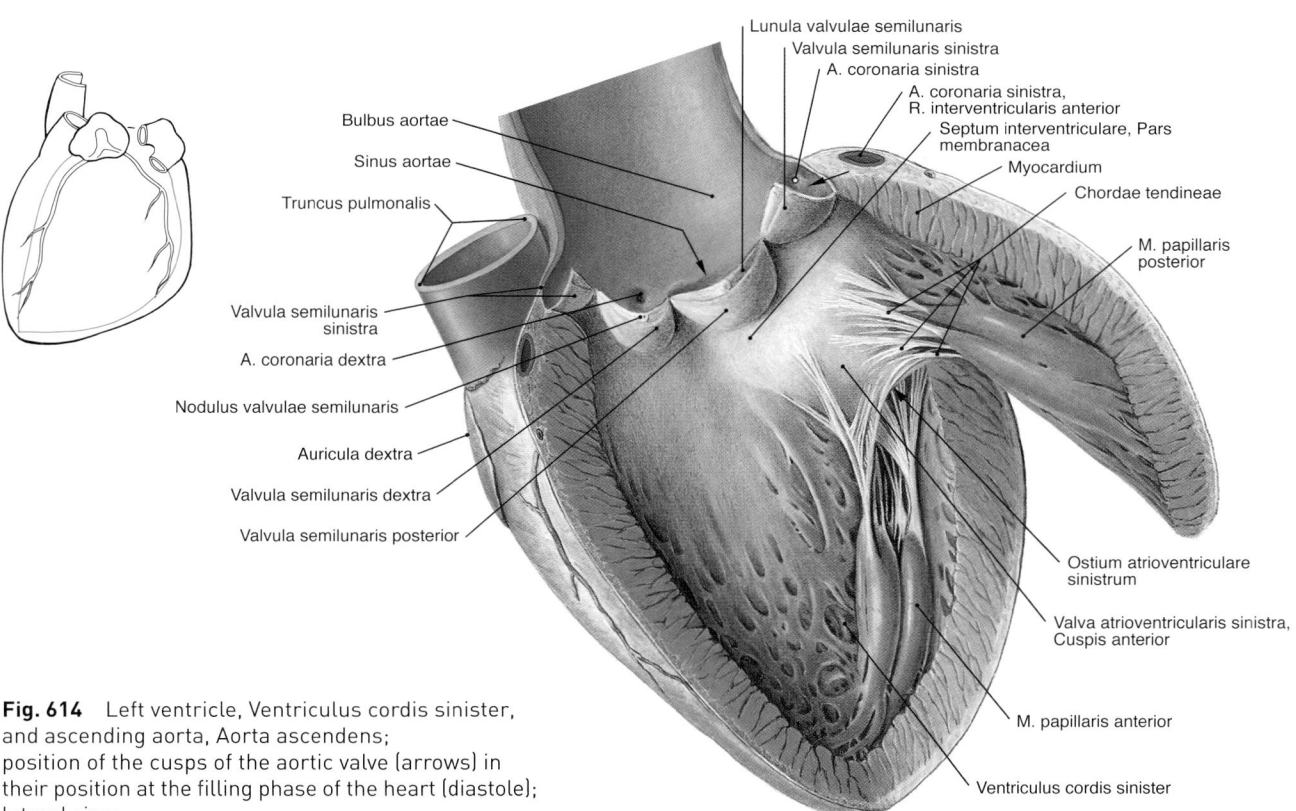

Lunula valvulae semilunaris

Valvula semilunaris sinistra

A. coronaria sinistra

A. coronaria sinistra, R. interventricularis anterior

Bulbus aortae

Septum interventriculare, Pars membranacea

Sinus aortae

Myocardium

Truncus pulmonalis

Chordae tendineae

M. papillaris posterior

Valvula semilunaris sinistra

A. coronaria dextra

Nodulus valvulae semilunaris

Auricula dextra

Valvula semilunaris dextra

Valvula semilunaris posterior

Ostium atrioventriculare sinistrum

Valva atrioventricularis sinistra, Cuspis anterior

M. papillaris anterior

Fig. 614 Left ventricle, Ventriculus cordis sinister, and ascending aorta, Aorta ascendens; position of the cusps of the aortic valve (arrows) in their position at the filling phase of the heart (diastole); lateral view.

Ventriculus cordis sinister

Internal spaces of the heart

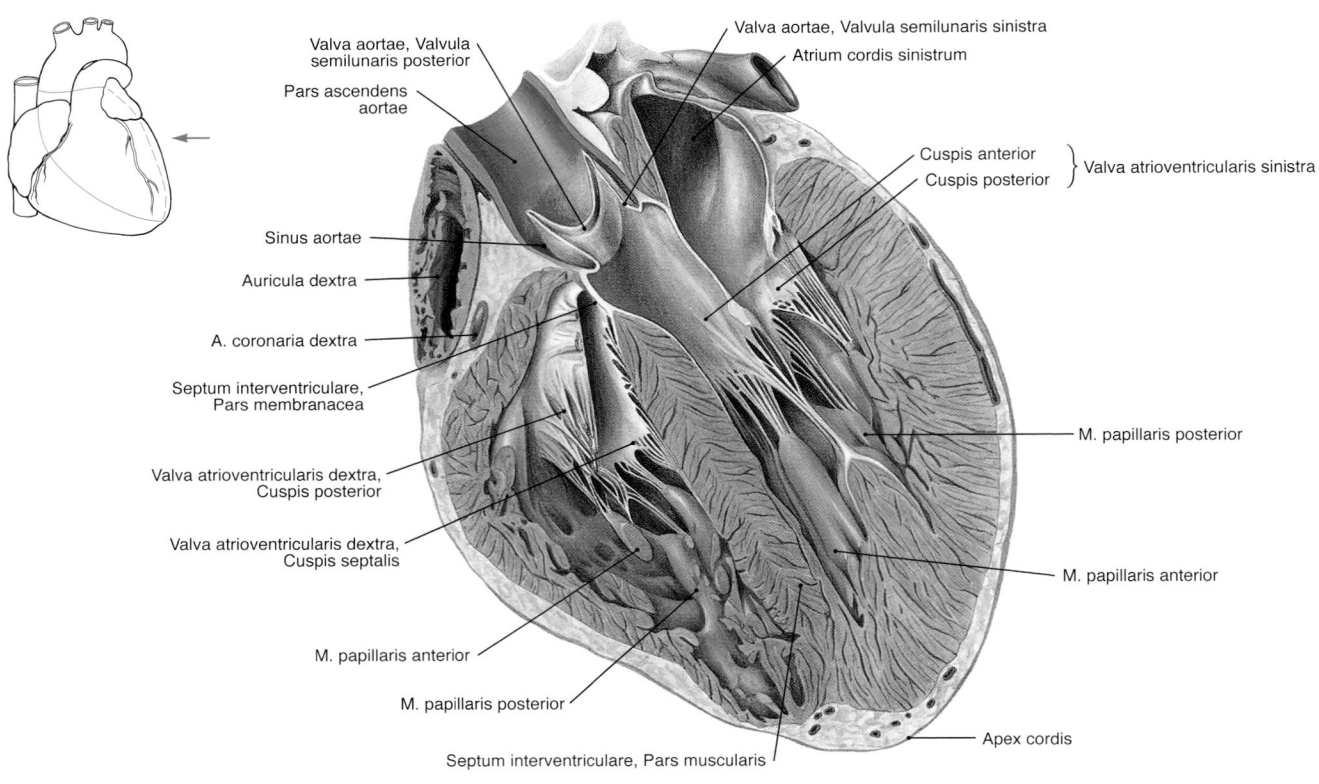

Valva aortae, Valvula semilunaris posterior
Pars ascendens aortae
Valva aortae, Valvula semilunaris sinistra
Atrium cordis sinistrum
Cuspis anterior
Cuspis posterior } Valva atrioventricularis sinistra
Sinus aortae
Auricula dextra
A. coronaria dextra
Septum interventriculare, Pars membranacea
Valva atrioventricularis dextra, Cuspis posterior
Valva atrioventricularis dextra, Cuspis septalis
M. papillaris posterior
M. papillaris anterior
M. papillaris anterior
M. papillaris posterior
Apex cordis
Septum interventriculare, Pars muscularis

Fig. 615 Left and right ventricle, Ventriculus cordis sinister et dexter.

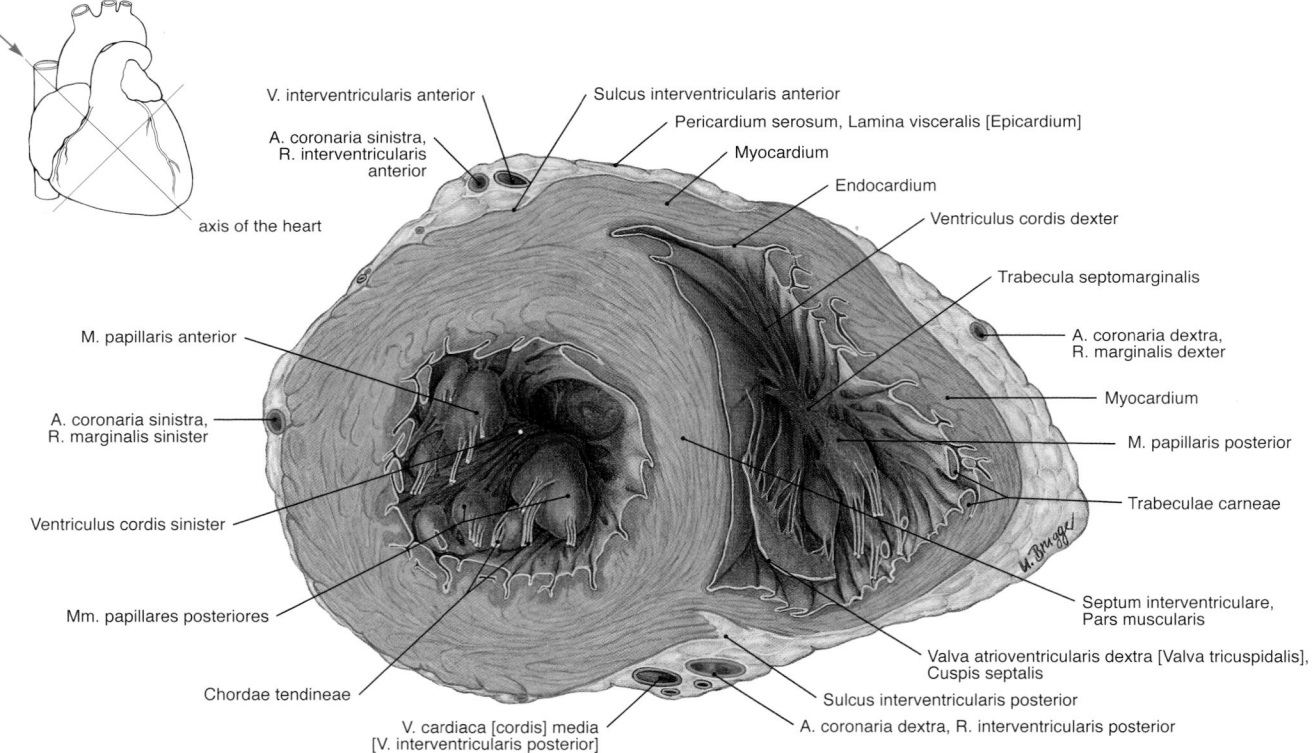

V. interventricularis anterior
A. coronaria sinistra, R. interventricularis anterior
axis of the heart
Sulcus interventricularis anterior
Pericardium serosum, Lamina visceralis [Epicardium]
Myocardium
Endocardium
Ventriculus cordis dexter
Trabecula septomarginalis
A. coronaria dextra, R. marginalis dexter
Myocardium
M. papillaris anterior
A. coronaria sinistra, R. marginalis sinister
Ventriculus cordis sinister
M. papillaris posterior
Trabeculae carneae
Mm. papillares posteriores
Chordae tendineae
Septum interventriculare, Pars muscularis
Valva atrioventricularis dextra [Valva tricuspidalis], Cuspis septalis
Sulcus interventricularis posterior
A. coronaria dextra, R. interventricularis posterior
V. cardiaca [cordis] media [V. interventricularis posterior]

Fig. 616 Left and right ventricle, Ventriculus cordis sinister et dexter; superior view.

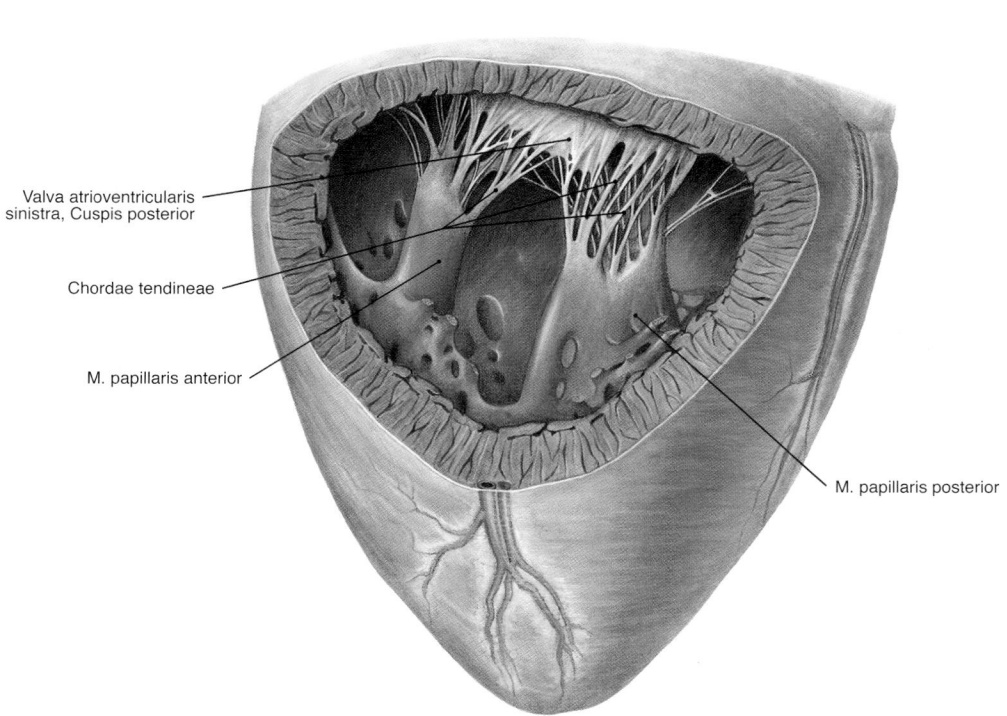
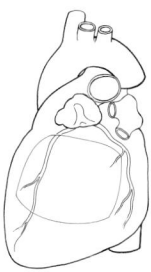

Valva atrioventricularis
sinistra, Cuspis posterior

Chordae tendineae

M. papillaris anterior

M. papillaris posterior

Fig. 617 Left ventricle, Ventriculus cordis sinister;
ventrosuperior view from the left.

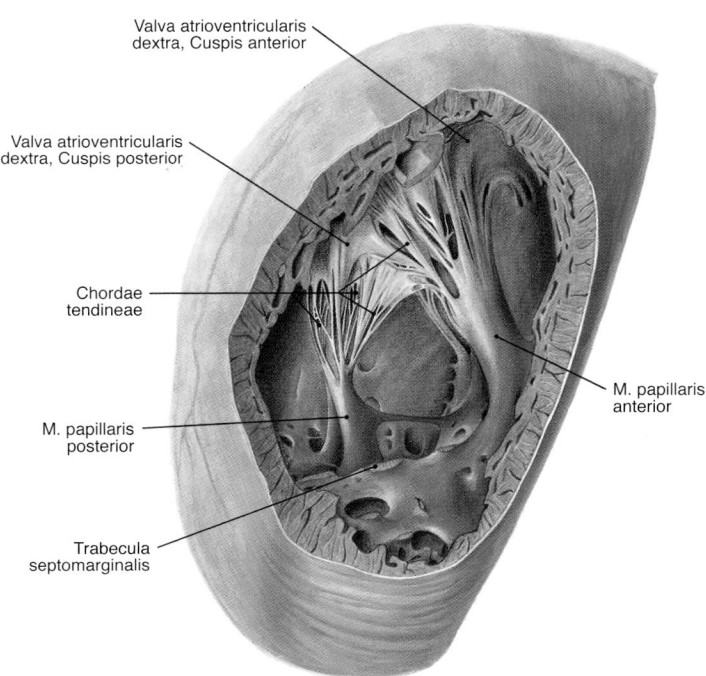

Valva atrioventricularis
dextra, Cuspis anterior

Valva atrioventricularis
dextra, Cuspis posterior

Chordae
tendineae

M. papillaris
anterior

M. papillaris
posterior

Trabecula
septomarginalis

Fig. 618 Right ventricle, Ventriculus cordis dexter;
dorsal view.

Conducting system

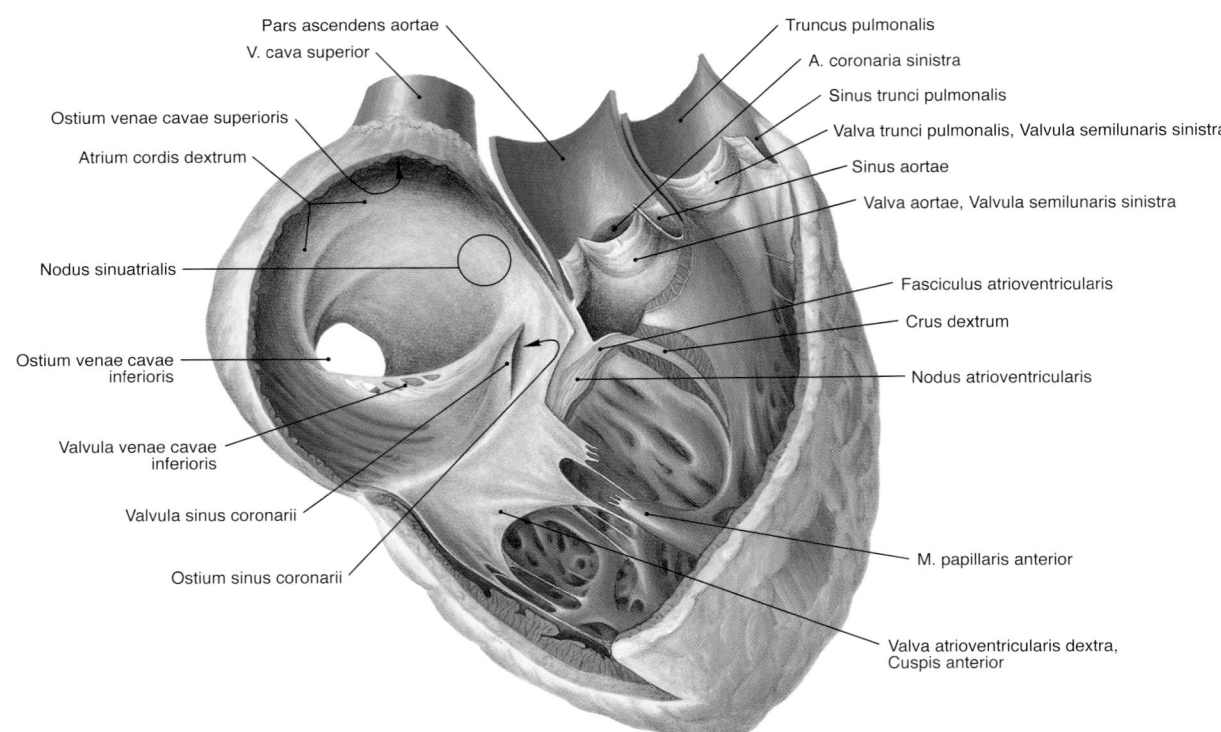

Fig. 619 Right atrium, Atrium cordis dextrum, and right ventricle, Ventriculus cordis dexter; conducting system, Complexus stimulans cordis [Systema conducente cordis], highlighted in yellow; ventral view.

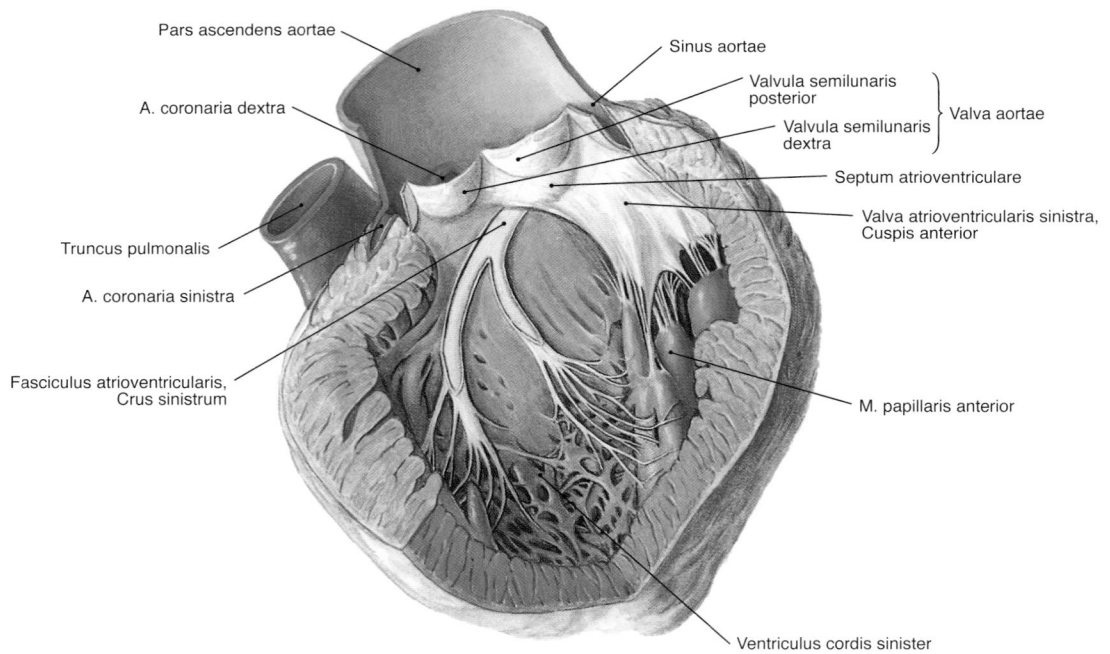

Fig. 620 Left ventricle, Ventriculus cordis sinister; conducting system, Complexus stimulans cordis [Systema conducente cordis], highlighted in yellow; ventral view from the left.

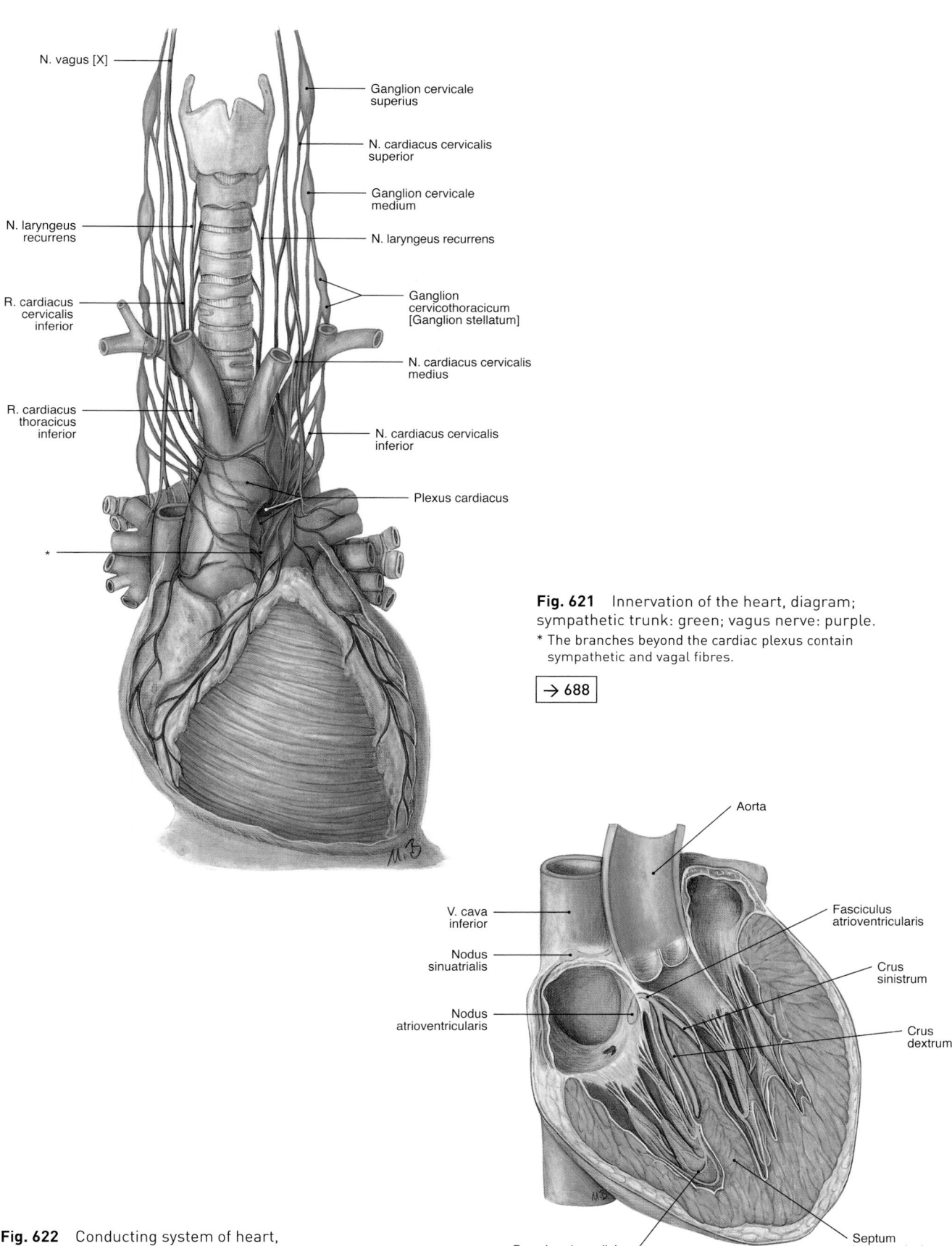

N. vagus [X]

Ganglion cervicale
superius

N. cardiacus cervicalis
superior

Ganglion cervicale
medium

N. laryngeus
recurrens

N. laryngeus recurrens

Ganglion
cervicothoracicum
[Ganglion stellatum]

R. cardiacus
cervicalis
inferior

N. cardiacus cervicalis
medius

R. cardiacus
thoracicus
inferior

N. cardiacus cervicalis
inferior

Plexus cardiacus

*

Fig. 621 Innervation of the heart, diagram;
sympathetic trunk: green; vagus nerve: purple.
* The branches beyond the cardiac plexus contain
sympathetic and vagal fibres.

→ 688

Fig. 622 Conducting system of heart,
Complexus stimulans cordis [Systema conducente cordis];
section at the plane of the axis of the heart.

Aorta

V. cava
inferior

Fasciculus
atrioventricularis

Nodus
sinuatrialis

Crus
sinistrum

Nodus
atrioventricularis

Crus
dextrum

Rr. subendocardiales

Septum
interventriculare

Coronary arteries

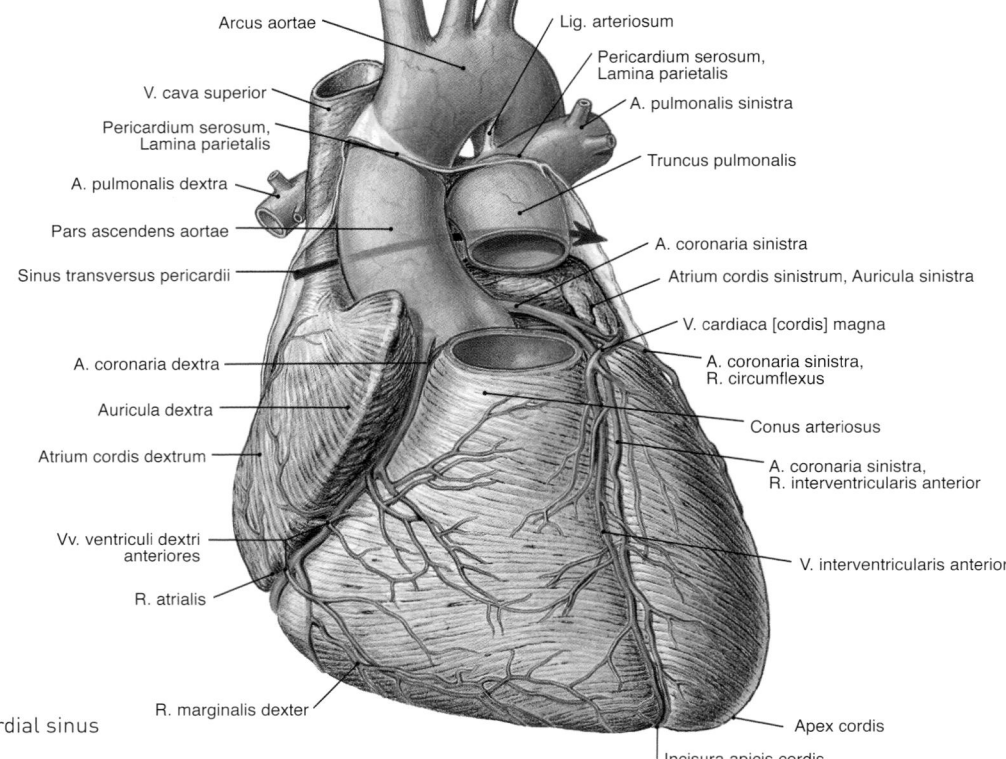

Arcus aortae
Lig. arteriosum
V. cava superior
Pericardium serosum, Lamina parietalis
Pericardium serosum, Lamina parietalis
A. pulmonalis sinistra
A. pulmonalis dextra
Truncus pulmonalis
Pars ascendens aortae
A. coronaria sinistra
Sinus transversus pericardii
Atrium cordis sinistrum, Auricula sinistra
V. cardiaca [cordis] magna
A. coronaria dextra
A. coronaria sinistra, R. circumflexus
Auricula dextra
Conus arteriosus
Atrium cordis dextrum
A. coronaria sinistra, R. interventricularis anterior
Vv. ventriculi dextri anteriores
V. interventricularis anterior
R. atrialis
R. marginalis dexter
Apex cordis
Incisura apicis cordis

Fig. 623 Coronary arteries, Aa. coronariae; ventral view.
Arrow in the transverse pericardial sinus

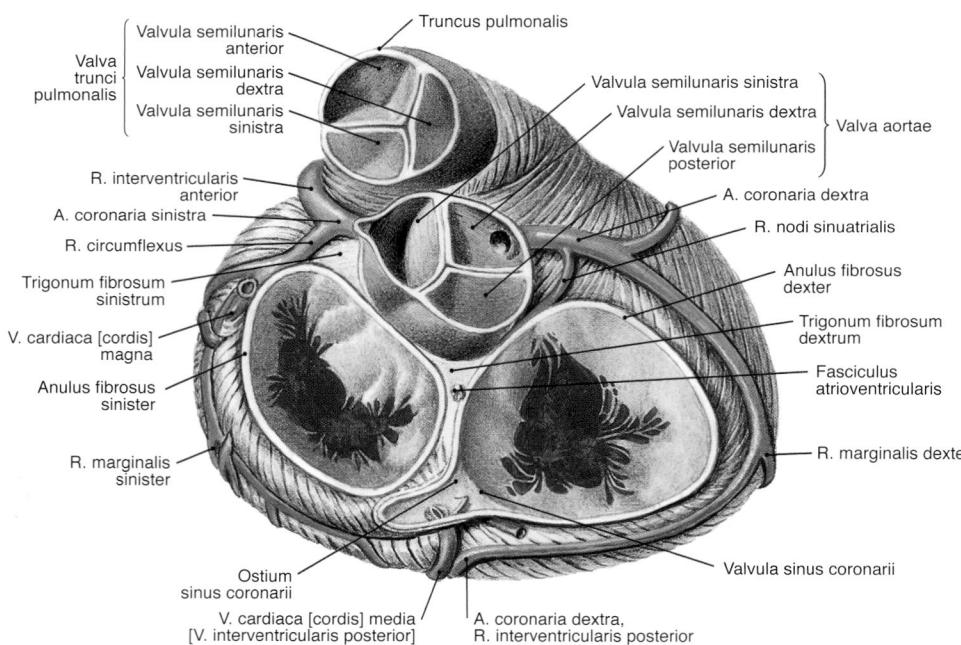

Valvula semilunaris anterior
Truncus pulmonalis
Valva trunci pulmonalis
Valvula semilunaris dextra
Valvula semilunaris sinistra
Valvula semilunaris sinistra
Valvula semilunaris dextra
Valva aortae
Valvula semilunaris posterior
R. interventricularis anterior
A. coronaria sinistra
A. coronaria dextra
R. circumflexus
R. nodi sinuatrialis
Trigonum fibrosum sinistrum
Anulus fibrosus dexter
V. cardiaca [cordis] magna
Trigonum fibrosum dextrum
Anulus fibrosus sinister
Fasciculus atrioventricularis
R. marginalis sinister
R. marginalis dexter
Valvula sinus coronarii
Ostium sinus coronarii
V. cardiaca [cordis] media [V. interventricularis posterior]
A. coronaria dextra, R. interventricularis posterior

Fig. 624 Coronary arteries, Aa. coronariae; superior view.

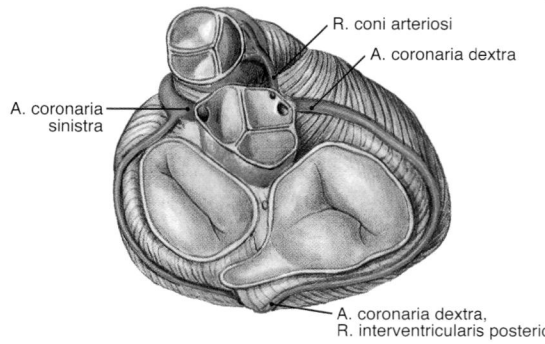

R. coni arteriosi
A. coronaria dextra
A. coronaria sinistra
A. coronaria dextra, R. interventricularis posterior

Fig. 625 Variability of the coronary arteries. The conus arteriosus branch arises from the aorta as an independent artery (~37%).

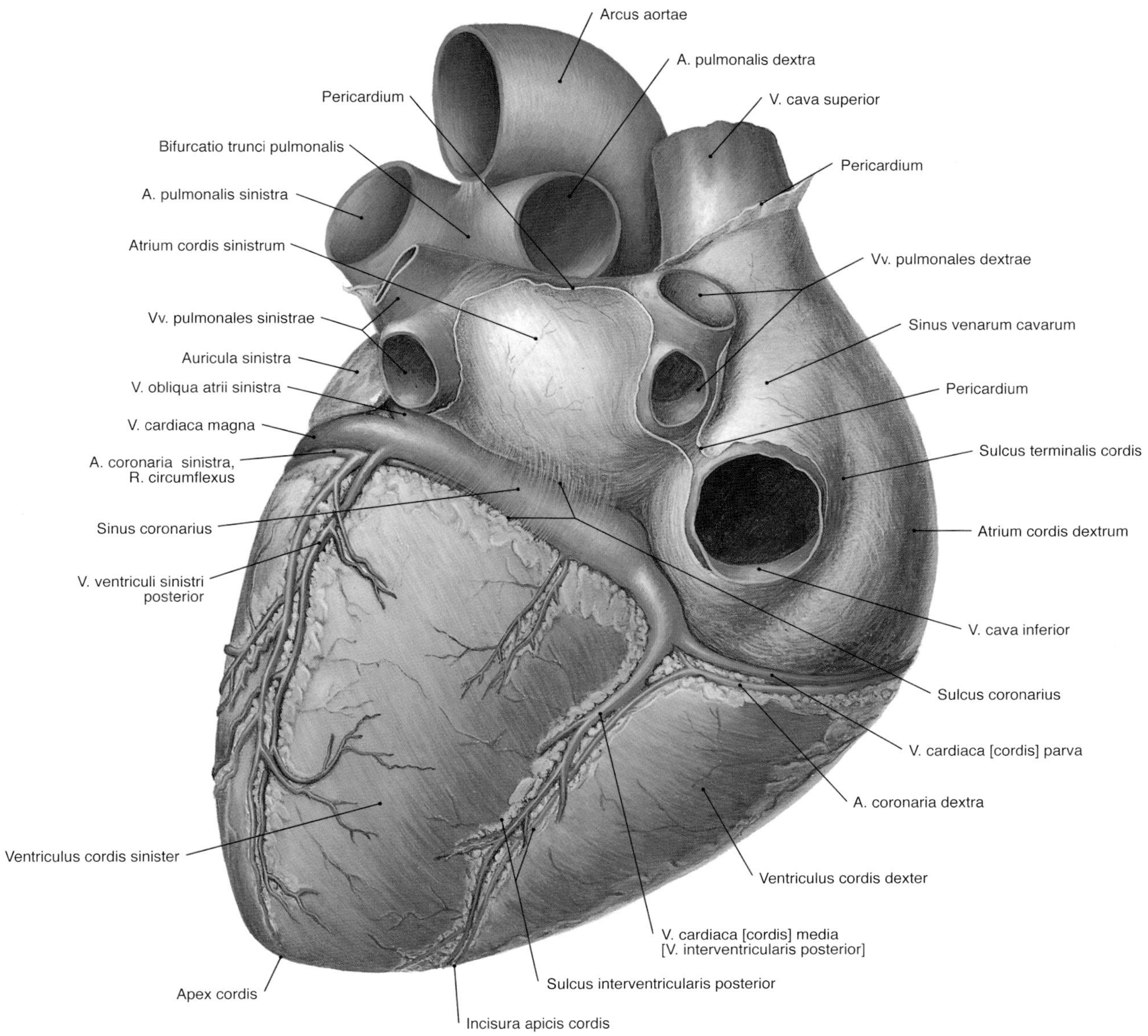

Arcus aortae

A. pulmonalis dextra

V. cava superior

Pericardium

Pericardium

Bifurcatio trunci pulmonalis

A. pulmonalis sinistra

Atrium cordis sinistrum

Vv. pulmonales dextrae

Vv. pulmonales sinistrae

Auricula sinistra

V. obliqua atrii sinistra

V. cardiaca magna

Sinus venarum cavarum

Pericardium

Sulcus terminalis cordis

A. coronaria sinistra, R. circumflexus

Sinus coronarius

Atrium cordis dextrum

V. ventriculi sinistri posterior

V. cava inferior

Sulcus coronarius

V. cardiaca [cordis] parva

A. coronaria dextra

Ventriculus cordis sinister

Ventriculus cordis dexter

V. cardiaca [cordis] media [V. interventricularis posterior]

Apex cordis

Sulcus interventricularis posterior

Incisura apicis cordis

Fig. 626   Veins of the heart, Vv. cordis.

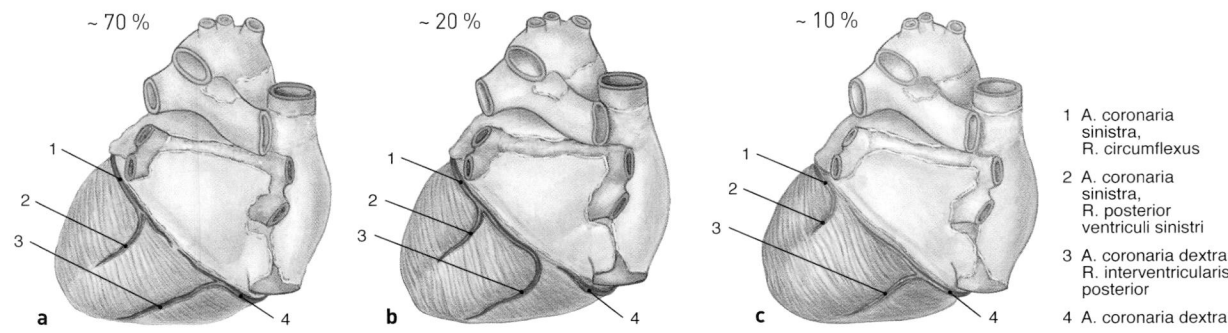

~ 70 %

~ 20 %

~ 10 %

1
2
3
a   4

1
2
3
b   4

1
2
3
c   4

1 A. coronaria sinistra, R. circumflexus

2 A. coronaria sinistra, R. posterior ventriculi sinistri

3 A. coronaria dextra, R. interventricularis posterior

4 A. coronaria dextra

Fig. 627 a–c   Variations in the arterial supply of the posterior aspect of the heart; dorsal view.

a Balanced coronary artery supply
b Dominant left coronary artery supply
c Dominant right coronary artery supply

Coronary arteries, variability of supply

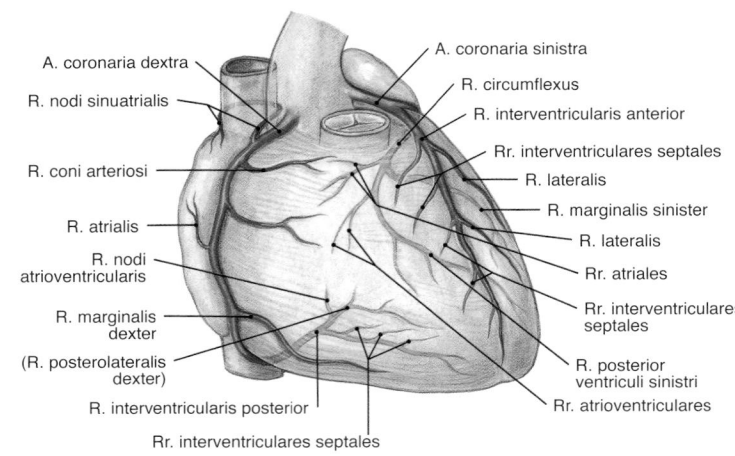

Fig. 628 Coronary arteries, Aa. coronariae; posterior arterial branches are shown in a lighter colour; the posterior interventricular branch arises from the right coronary artery (balanced coronary artery supply); ventral view.

A. coronaria dextra
R. nodi sinuatrialis
R. coni arteriosi
R. atrialis
R. nodi atrioventricularis
R. marginalis dexter
(R. posterolateralis dexter)
R. interventricularis posterior
Rr. interventriculares septales
A. coronaria sinistra
R. circumflexus
R. interventricularis anterior
Rr. interventriculares septales
R. lateralis
R. marginalis sinister
R. lateralis
Rr. atriales
Rr. interventriculares septales
R. posterior ventriculi sinistri
Rr. atrioventriculares

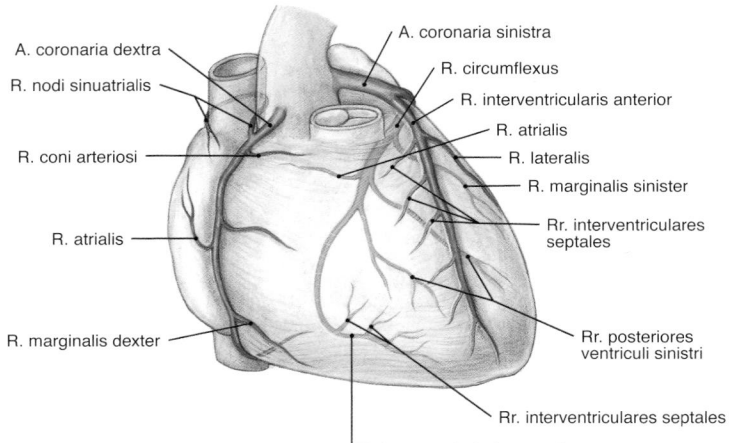

Fig. 629 Coronary arteries, Aa. coronariae; the posterior interventricular branch arises from the left coronary artery (dominant left coronary artery supply); ventral view.

A. coronaria dextra
R. nodi sinuatrialis
R. coni arteriosi
R. atrialis
R. marginalis dexter
A. coronaria sinistra
R. circumflexus
R. interventricularis anterior
R. atrialis
R. lateralis
R. marginalis sinister
Rr. interventriculares septales
Rr. posteriores ventriculi sinistri
Rr. interventriculares septales
R. interventricularis posterior

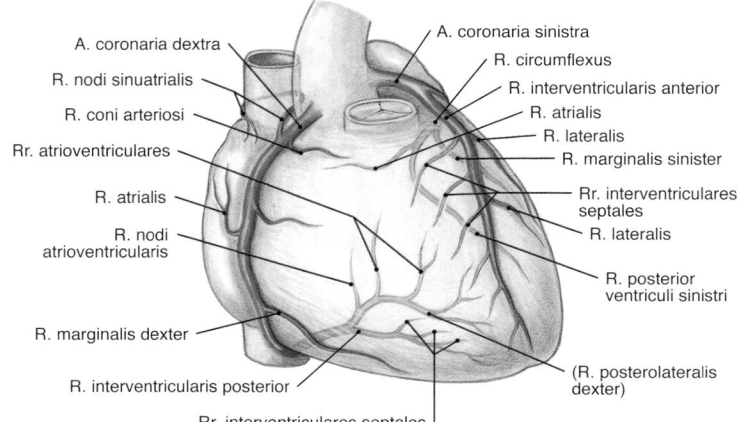

Fig. 630 Coronary arteries, Aa. coronariae; the posterior wall of the ventricles is mainly supplied by branches of the right coronary artery (dominant right coronary artery supply); ventral view.

A. coronaria dextra
R. nodi sinuatrialis
R. coni arteriosi
Rr. atrioventriculares
R. atrialis
R. nodi atrioventricularis
R. marginalis dexter
R. interventricularis posterior
Rr. interventriculares septales
A. coronaria sinistra
R. circumflexus
R. interventricularis anterior
R. atrialis
R. lateralis
R. marginalis sinister
Rr. interventriculares septales
R. lateralis
R. posterior ventriculi sinistri
(R. posterolateralis dexter)

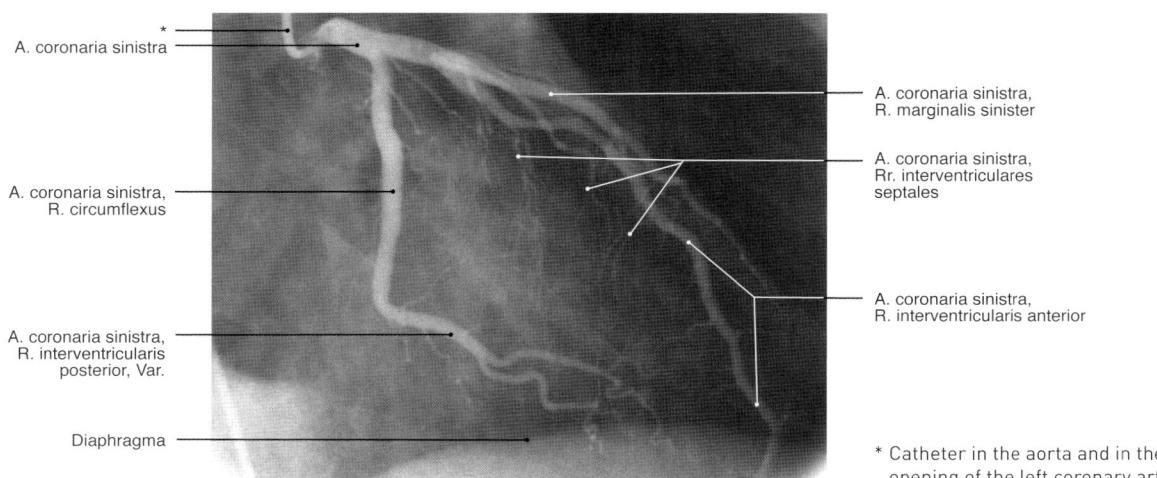

A. coronaria sinistra *

A. coronaria sinistra, R. circumflexus

A. coronaria sinistra, R. interventricularis posterior, Var.

Diaphragma

A. coronaria sinistra, R. marginalis sinister

A. coronaria sinistra, Rr. interventriculares septales

A. coronaria sinistra, R. interventricularis anterior

* Catheter in the aorta and in the opening of the left coronary artery

Fig. 631 Left coronary artery, A. coronaria sinistra; coronary angiography; the beam is directed obliquely from right anterior to left posterior (RAO).

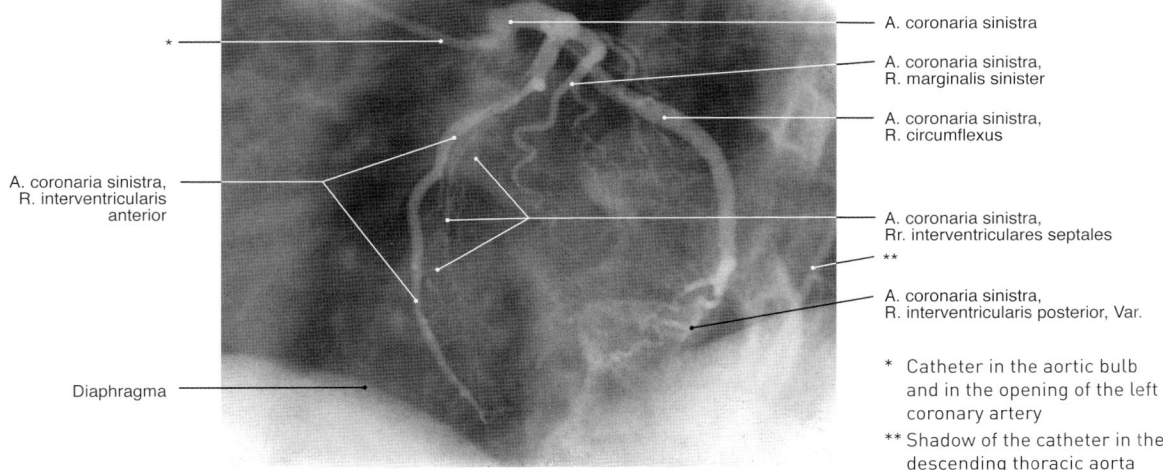

*

A. coronaria sinistra, R. interventricularis anterior

Diaphragma

A. coronaria sinistra

A. coronaria sinistra, R. marginalis sinister

A. coronaria sinistra, R. circumflexus

A. coronaria sinistra, Rr. interventriculares septales

**

A. coronaria sinistra, R. interventricularis posterior, Var.

* Catheter in the aortic bulb and in the opening of the left coronary artery

** Shadow of the catheter in the descending thoracic aorta

Fig. 632 Left coronary artery, A. coronaria sinistra; coronary angiography; the beam is directed obliquely from left anterior to right posterior (LAO).

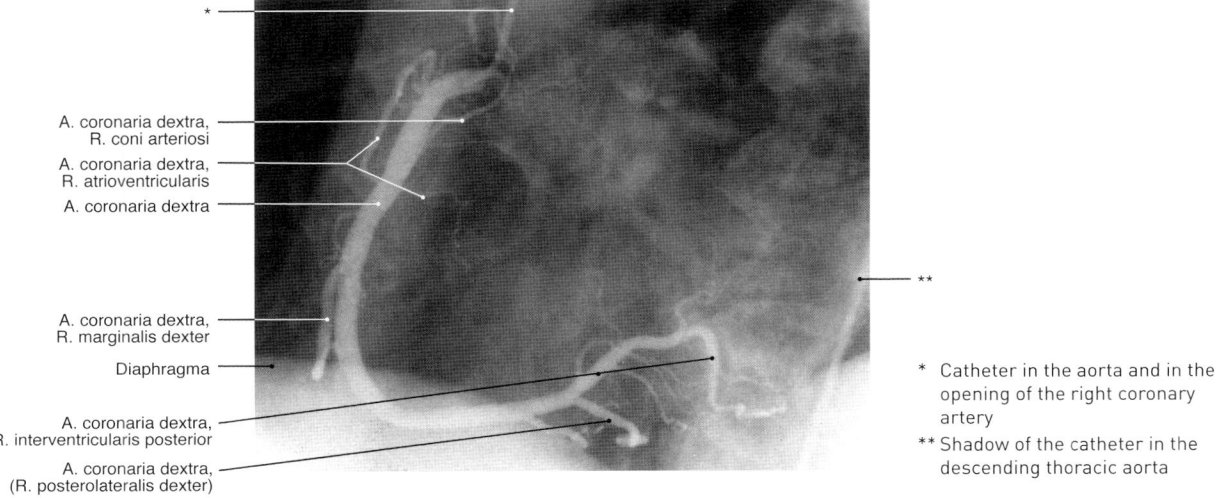

*

A. coronaria dextra, R. coni arteriosi

A. coronaria dextra, R. atrioventricularis

A. coronaria dextra

A. coronaria dextra, R. marginalis dexter

Diaphragma

A. coronaria dextra, R. interventricularis posterior

A. coronaria dextra, (R. posterolateralis dexter)

**

* Catheter in the aorta and in the opening of the right coronary artery

** Shadow of the catheter in the descending thoracic aorta

Fig. 633 Right coronary artery, A. coronaria dextra; coronary angiography; the beam is directed obliquely from left anterior to right posterior (LAO).

Heart situs

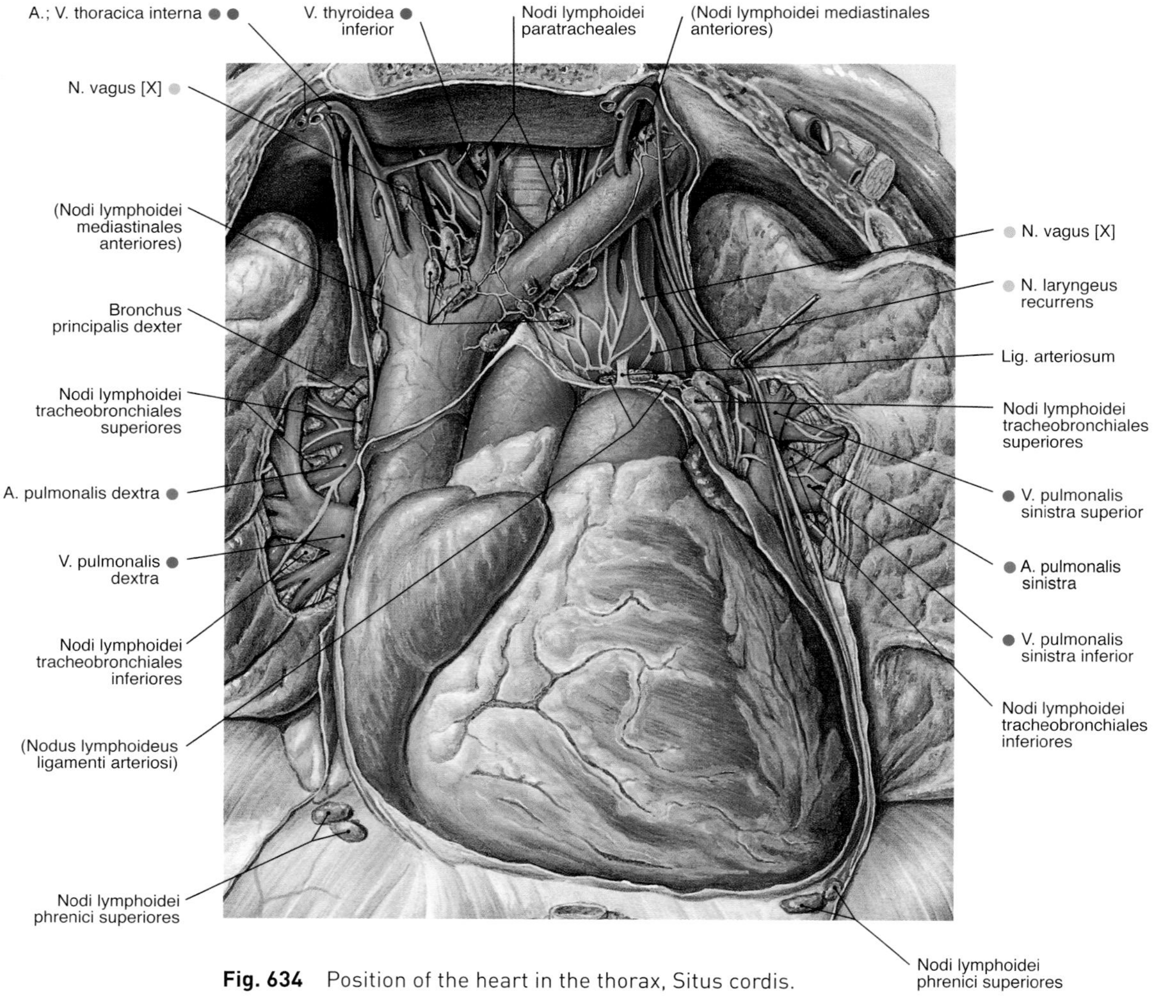

A.; V. thoracica interna ● ●
V. thyroidea ●
inferior
Nodi lymphoidei
paratracheales
(Nodi lymphoidei mediastinales
anteriores)

N. vagus [X] ●

(Nodi lymphoidei
mediastinales
anteriores)

Bronchus
principalis dexter

Nodi lymphoidei
tracheobronchiales
superiores

A. pulmonalis dextra ●

V. pulmonalis ●
dextra

Nodi lymphoidei
tracheobronchiales
inferiores

(Nodus lymphoideus
ligamenti arteriosi)

Nodi lymphoidei
phrenici superiores

● N. vagus [X]

● N. laryngeus
recurrens

Lig. arteriosum

Nodi lymphoidei
tracheobronchiales
superiores

● V. pulmonalis
sinistra superior

● A. pulmonalis
sinistra

● V. pulmonalis
sinistra inferior

Nodi lymphoidei
tracheobronchiales
inferiores

Nodi lymphoidei
phrenici superiores

Fig. 634   Position of the heart in the thorax, Situs cordis.

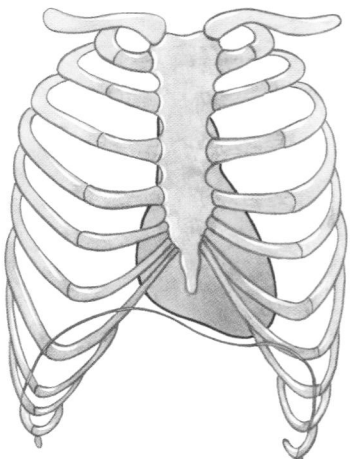

Fig. 635   Position of the heart;
inspiration.

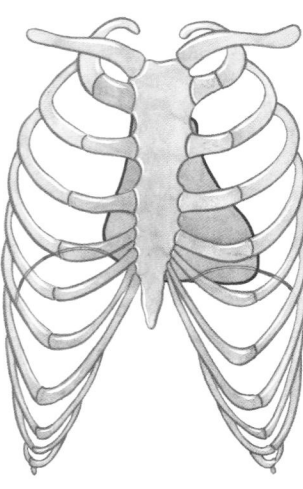

Fig. 636   Position of the heart;
expiration.

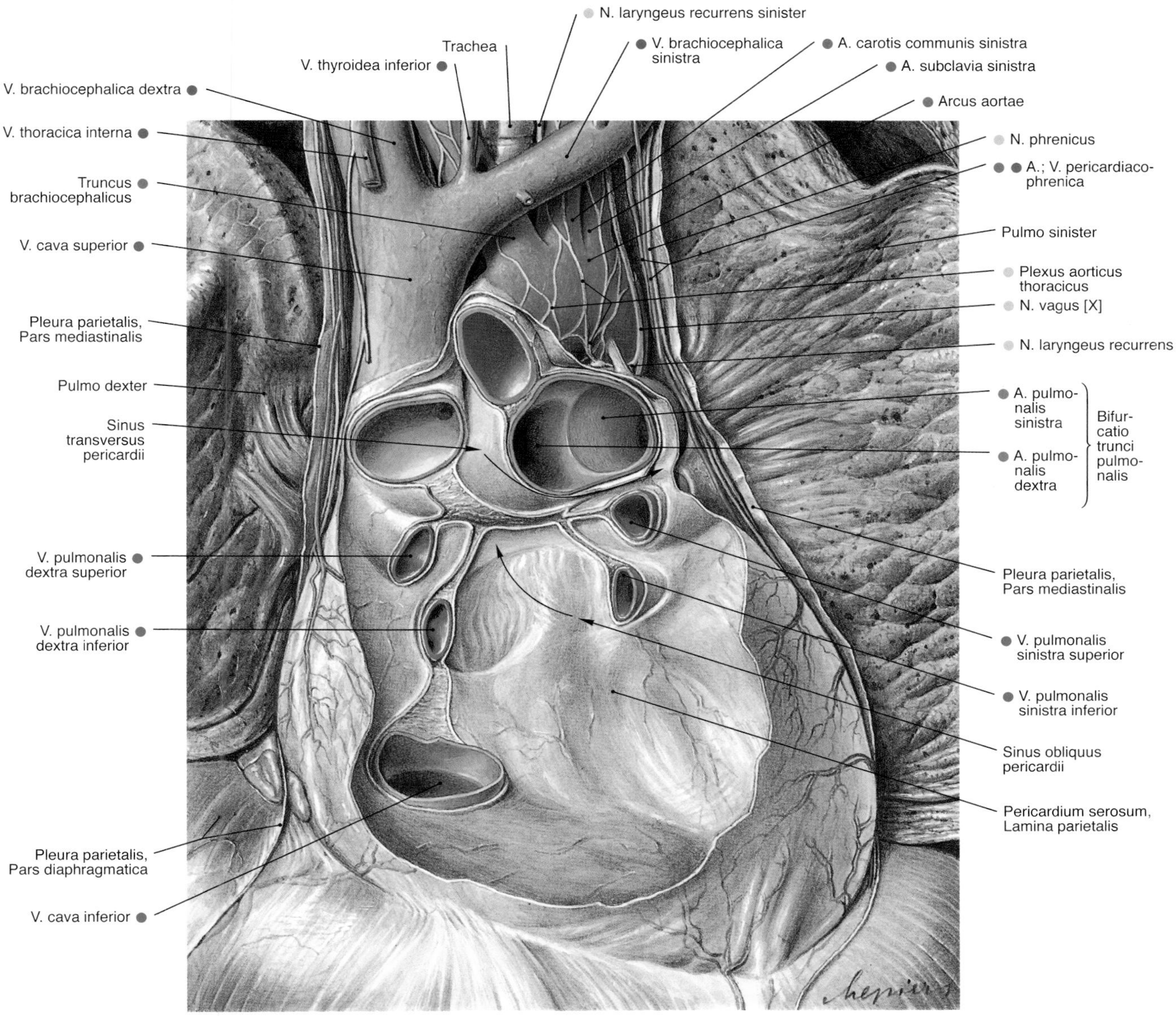

N. laryngeus recurrens sinister

Trachea

V. thyroidea inferior ●

● V. brachiocephalica sinistra

● A. carotis communis sinistra

● A. subclavia sinistra

● Arcus aortae

V. brachiocephalica dextra ●

V. thoracica interna ●

Truncus brachiocephalicus ●

V. cava superior ●

Pleura parietalis, Pars mediastinalis

Pulmo dexter

Sinus transversus pericardii

V. pulmonalis ● dextra superior

V. pulmonalis ● dextra inferior

Pleura parietalis, Pars diaphragmatica

V. cava inferior ●

● N. phrenicus

● ● A.; V. pericardiaco-phrenica

Pulmo sinister

● Plexus aorticus thoracicus

● N. vagus [X]

● N. laryngeus recurrens

● A. pulmonalis sinistra ⎫
● A. pulmonalis dextra ⎬ Bifurcatio trunci pulmonalis

Pleura parietalis, Pars mediastinalis

● V. pulmonalis sinistra superior

● V. pulmonalis sinistra inferior

Sinus obliquus pericardii

Pericardium serosum, Lamina parietalis

Fig. 637 Pericardium, Pericardium.

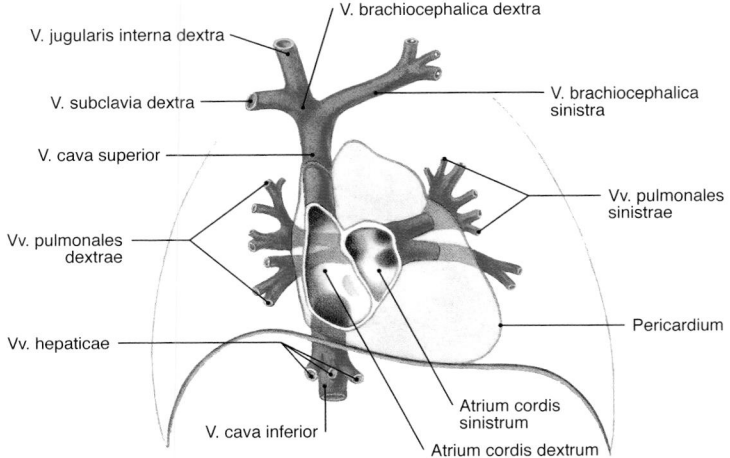

V. jugularis interna dextra

V. brachiocephalica dextra

V. subclavia dextra

V. cava superior

Vv. pulmonales dextrae

Vv. hepaticae

V. cava inferior

Atrium cordis sinistrum

Atrium cordis dextrum

V. brachiocephalica sinistra

Vv. pulmonales sinistrae

Pericardium

Fig. 638 Openings of the large veins into the heart; ventral view.

Trachea and bronchi

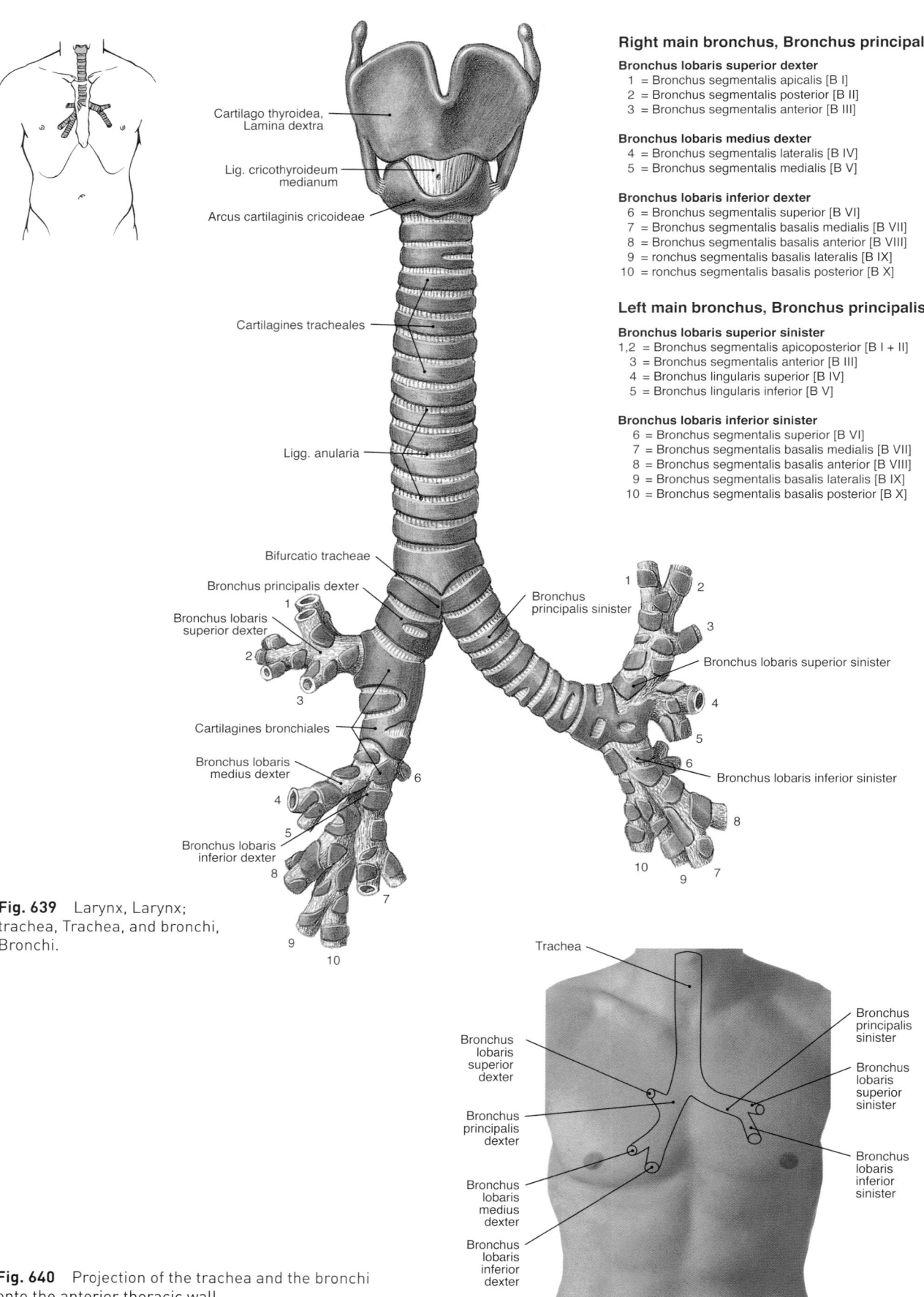

Right main bronchus, Bronchus principalis dexter

Bronchus lobaris superior dexter
1 = Bronchus segmentalis apicalis [B I]
2 = Bronchus segmentalis posterior [B II]
3 = Bronchus segmentalis anterior [B III]

Bronchus lobaris medius dexter
4 = Bronchus segmentalis lateralis [B IV]
5 = Bronchus segmentalis medialis [B V]

Bronchus lobaris inferior dexter
6 = Bronchus segmentalis superior [B VI]
7 = Bronchus segmentalis basalis medialis [B VII]
8 = Bronchus segmentalis basalis anterior [B VIII]
9 = ronchus segmentalis basalis lateralis [B IX]
10 = ronchus segmentalis basalis posterior [B X]

Left main bronchus, Bronchus principalis sinister

Bronchus lobaris superior sinister
1,2 = Bronchus segmentalis apicoposterior [B I + II]
3 = Bronchus segmentalis anterior [B III]
4 = Bronchus lingularis superior [B IV]
5 = Bronchus lingularis inferior [B V]

Bronchus lobaris inferior sinister
6 = Bronchus segmentalis superior [B VI]
7 = Bronchus segmentalis basalis medialis [B VII]
8 = Bronchus segmentalis basalis anterior [B VIII]
9 = Bronchus segmentalis basalis lateralis [B IX]
10 = Bronchus segmentalis basalis posterior [B X]

Cartilago thyroidea, Lamina dextra

Lig. cricothyroideum medianum

Arcus cartilaginis cricoideae

Cartilagines tracheales

Ligg. anularia

Bifurcatio tracheae

Bronchus principalis dexter

Bronchus lobaris superior dexter

Cartilagines bronchiales

Bronchus lobaris medius dexter

Bronchus lobaris inferior dexter

Bronchus principalis sinister

Bronchus lobaris superior sinister

Bronchus lobaris inferior sinister

Fig. 639 Larynx, Larynx; trachea, Trachea, and bronchi, Bronchi.

Trachea

Bronchus lobaris superior dexter

Bronchus principalis dexter

Bronchus lobaris medius dexter

Bronchus lobaris inferior dexter

Bronchus principalis sinister

Bronchus lobaris superior sinister

Bronchus lobaris inferior sinister

Fig. 640 Projection of the trachea and the bronchi onto the anterior thoracic wall.

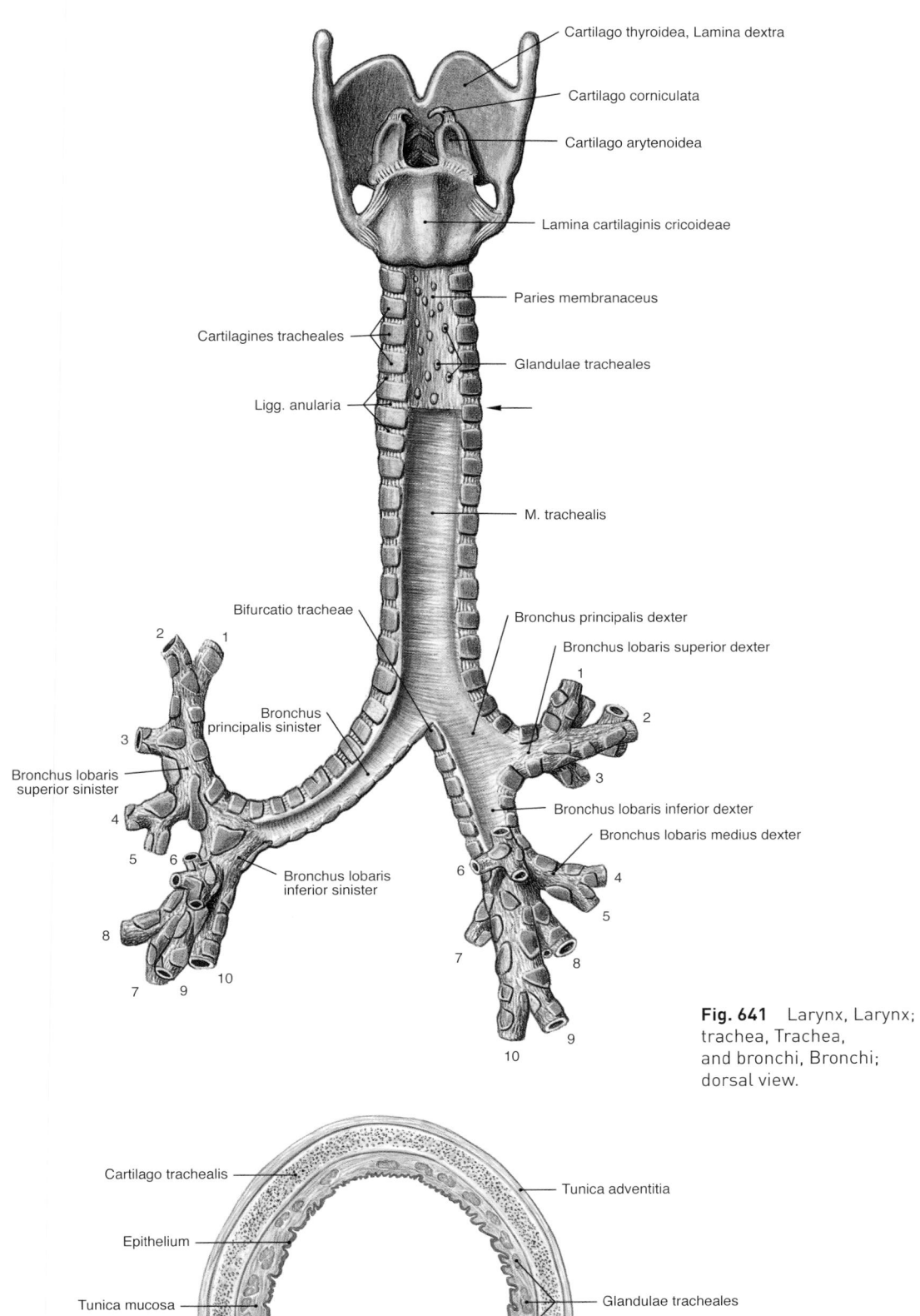

Cartilago thyroidea, Lamina dextra

Cartilago corniculata

Cartilago arytenoidea

Lamina cartilaginis cricoideae

Paries membranaceus

Cartilagines tracheales

Glandulae tracheales

Ligg. anularia

M. trachealis

Bifurcatio tracheae

Bronchus principalis dexter

Bronchus lobaris superior dexter

Bronchus principalis sinister

Bronchus lobaris superior sinister

Bronchus lobaris inferior dexter

Bronchus lobaris medius dexter

Bronchus lobaris inferior sinister

Fig. 641 Larynx, Larynx; trachea, Trachea, and bronchi, Bronchi; dorsal view.

Cartilago trachealis

Tunica adventitia

Epithelium

Tunica mucosa

Glandulae tracheales

Paries membranaceus

M. trachealis

Fig. 642 Trachea, Trachea; cross-section; microscopic enlargement at low magnification.

Segmental bronchi

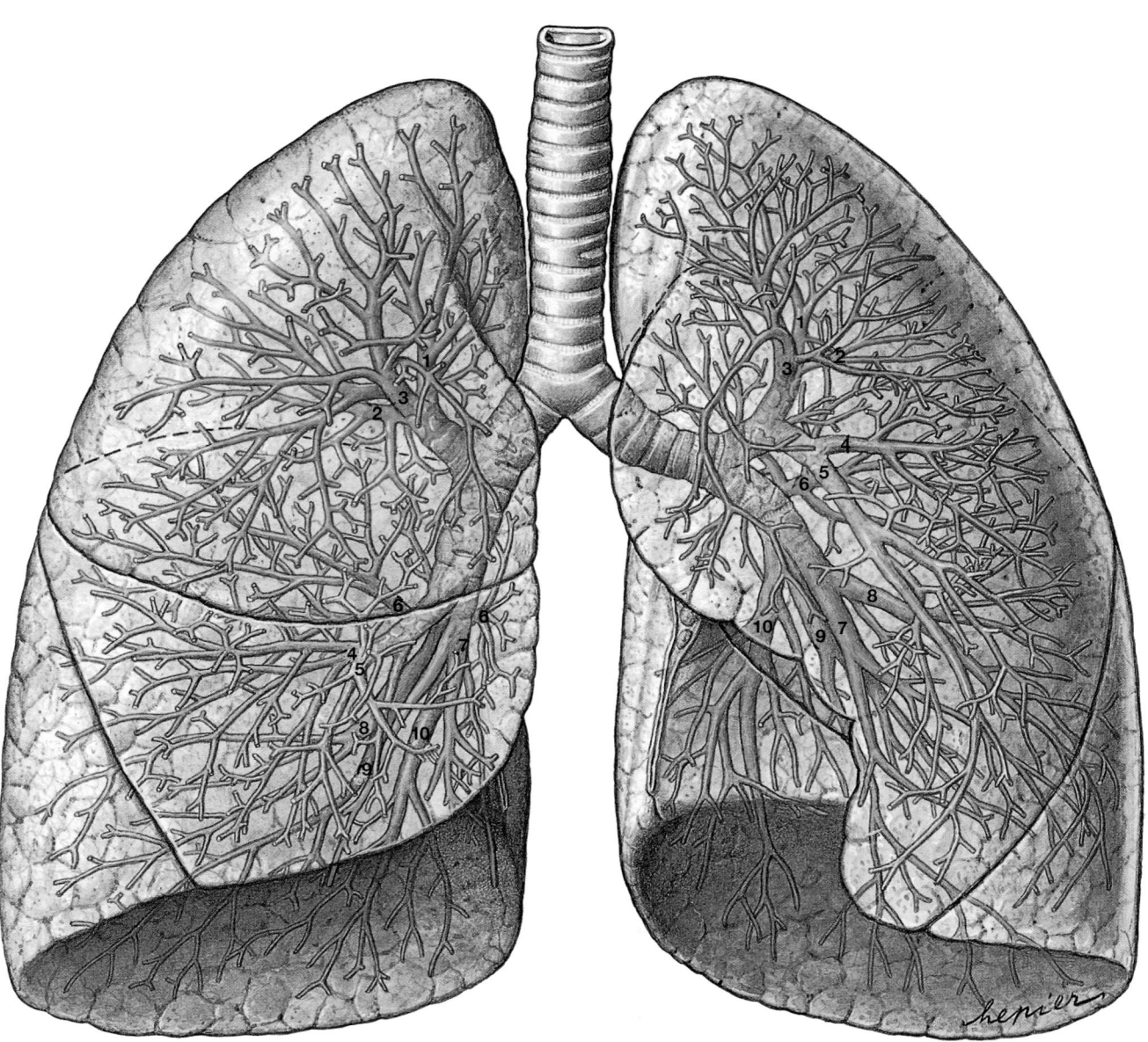

Fig. 643 Bronchi, Bronchi;
the lobar and the segmental bronchi have been projected
onto the lungs and are illustrated with different colours;
ventral view.
Numbers indicate the segmental bronchi (see p. 348).

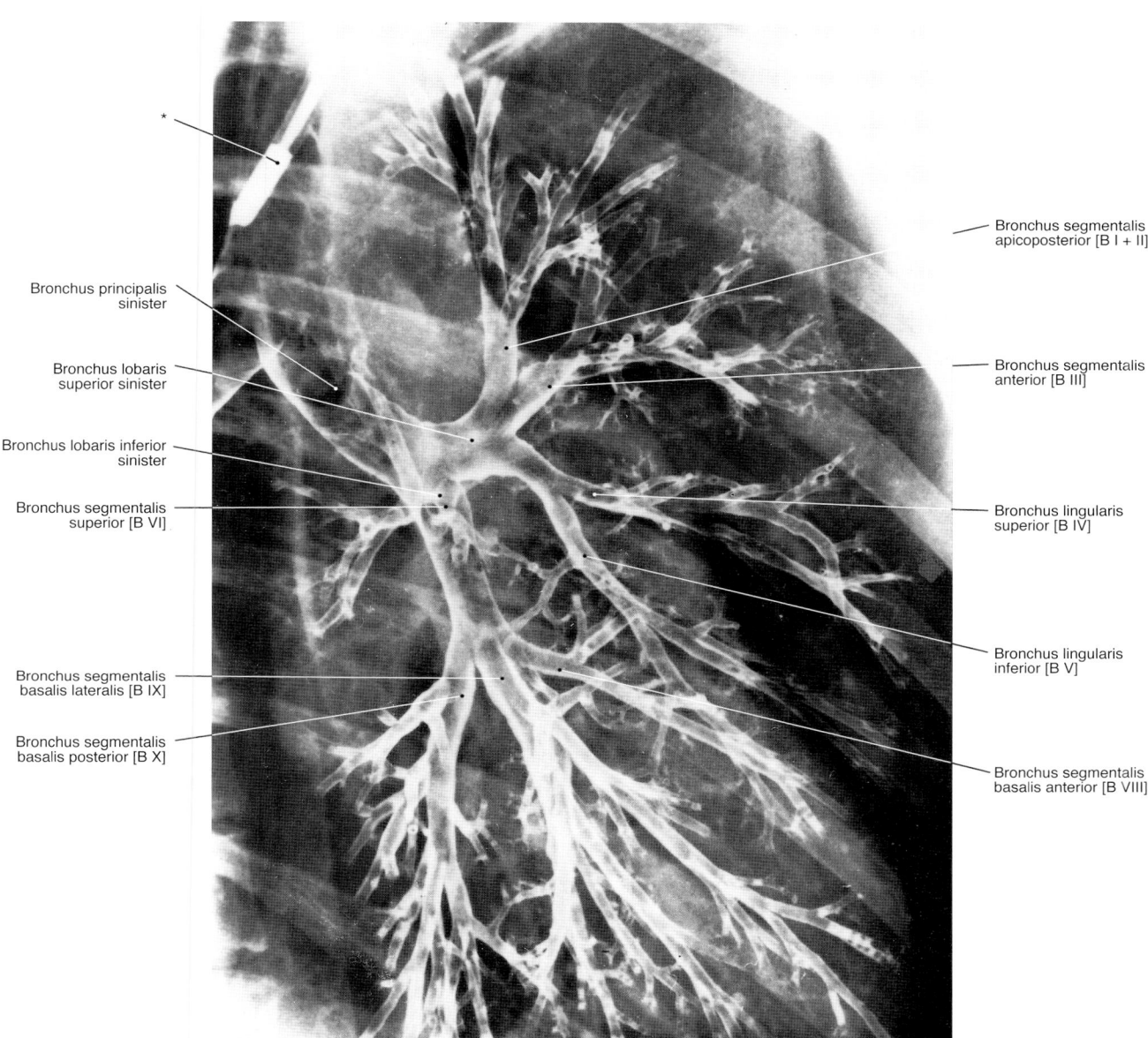

Bronchus segmentalis
apicoposterior [B I + II]

Bronchus principalis
sinister

Bronchus segmentalis
anterior [B III]

Bronchus lobaris
superior sinister

Bronchus lobaris inferior
sinister

Bronchus segmentalis
superior [B VI]

Bronchus lingularis
superior [B IV]

Bronchus lingularis
inferior [B V]

Bronchus segmentalis
basalis lateralis [B IX]

Bronchus segmentalis
basalis posterior [B X]

Bronchus segmentalis
basalis anterior [B VIII]

Fig. 644 Bronchi, Bronchi;
AP-radiograph; bronchography of the left lung.
* Bronchography catheter in the trachea

Lungs

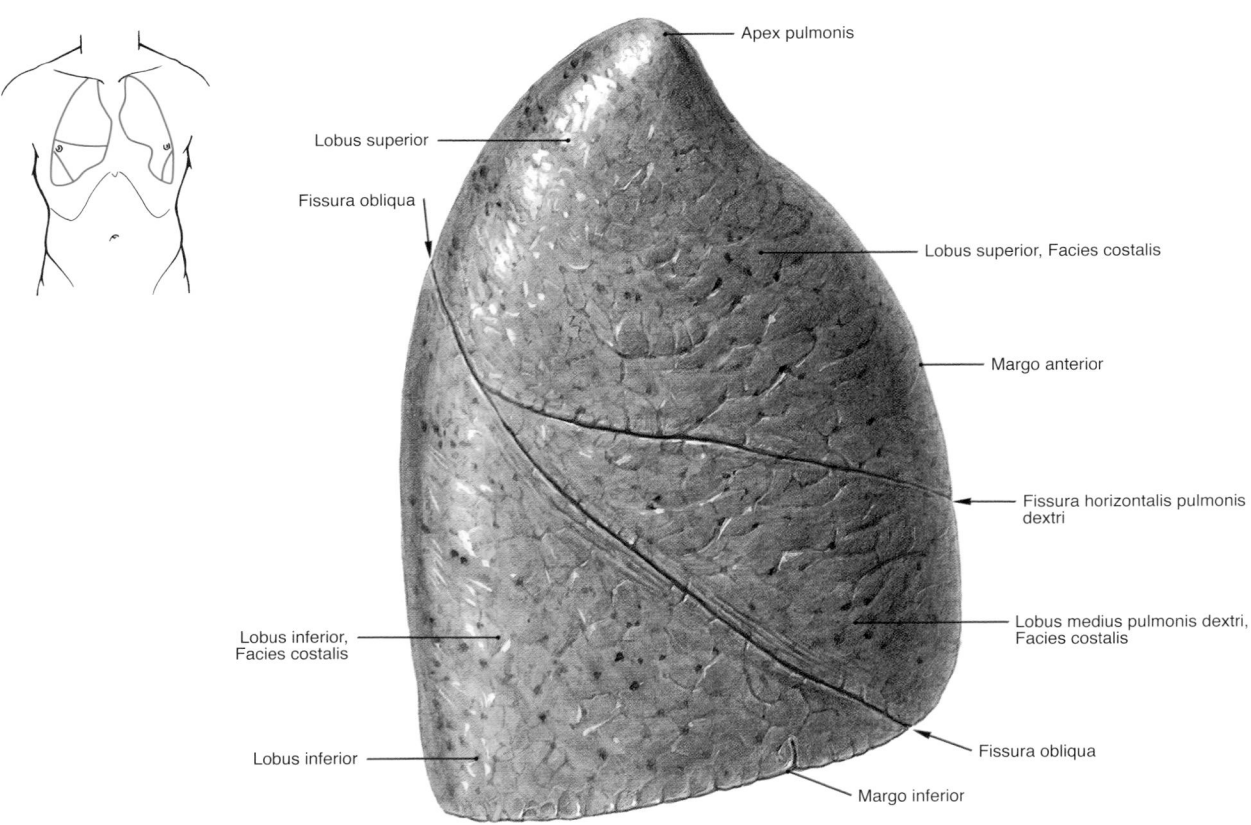

Apex pulmonis

Lobus superior

Fissura obliqua

Lobus superior, Facies costalis

Margo anterior

Fissura horizontalis pulmonis dextri

Lobus inferior, Facies costalis

Lobus medius pulmonis dextri, Facies costalis

Lobus inferior

Fissura obliqua

Margo inferior

Fig. 645   Right lung, Pulmo dexter; lateral view.

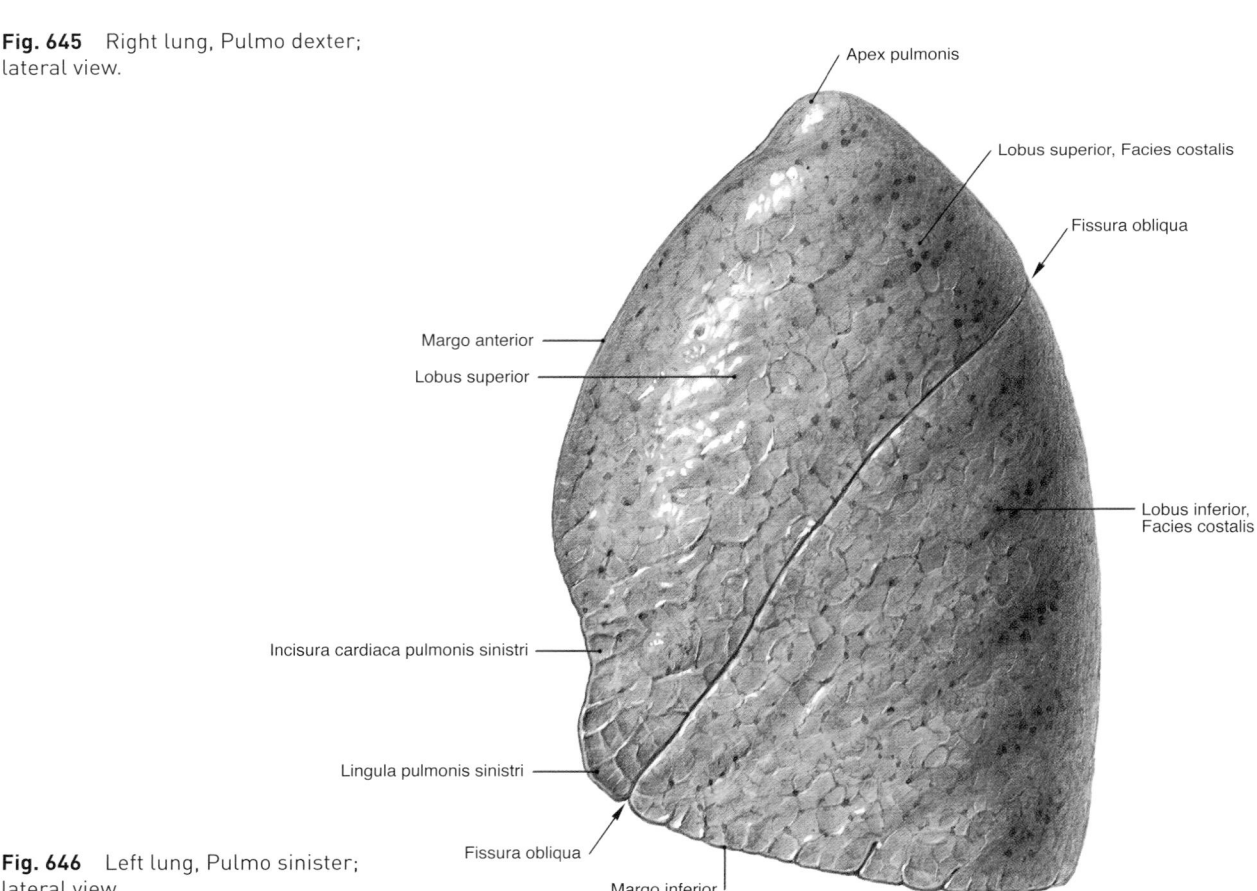

Apex pulmonis

Lobus superior, Facies costalis

Fissura obliqua

Margo anterior

Lobus superior

Lobus inferior, Facies costalis

Incisura cardiaca pulmonis sinistri

Lingula pulmonis sinistri

Fissura obliqua

Margo inferior

Fig. 646   Left lung, Pulmo sinister; lateral view.

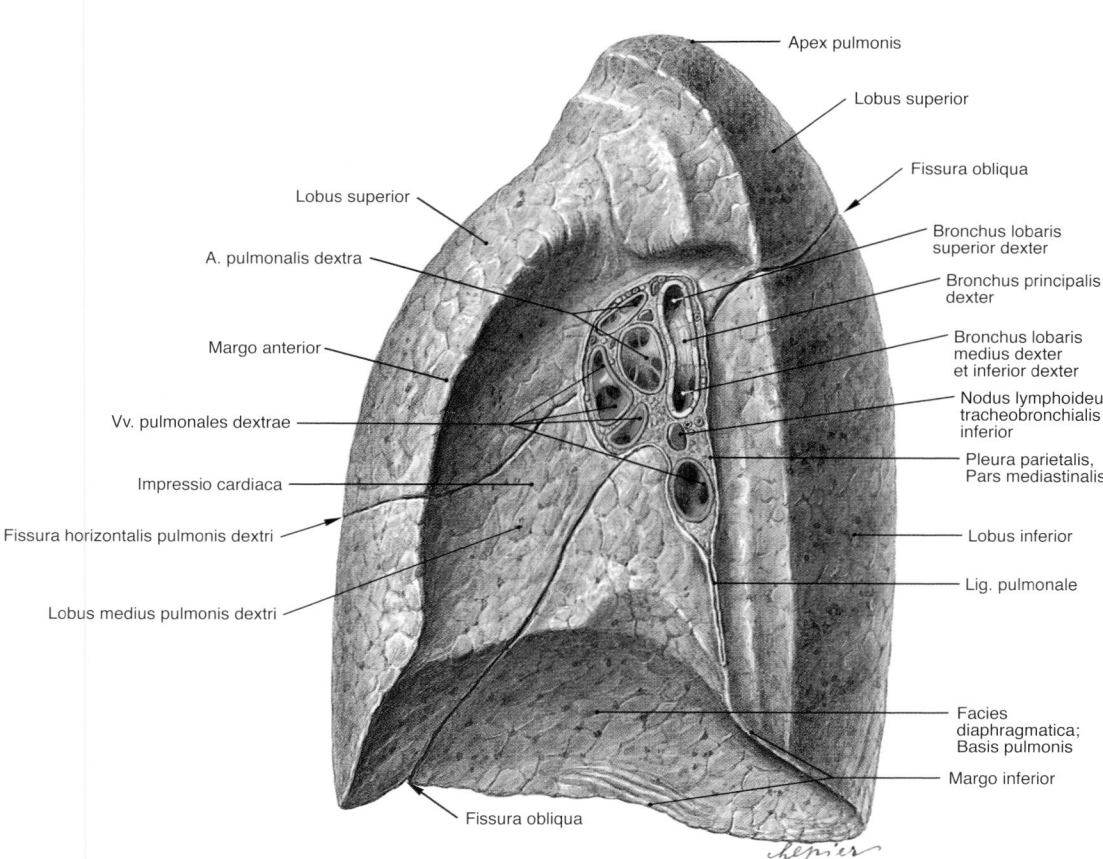

Apex pulmonis

Lobus superior

Lobus superior

Fissura obliqua

A. pulmonalis dextra

Bronchus lobaris superior dexter

Margo anterior

Bronchus principalis dexter

Bronchus lobaris medius dexter et inferior dexter

Vv. pulmonales dextrae

Nodus lymphoideus tracheobronchialis inferior

Impressio cardiaca

Pleura parietalis, Pars mediastinalis

Fissura horizontalis pulmonis dextri

Lobus inferior

Lig. pulmonale

Lobus medius pulmonis dextri

Facies diaphragmatica; Basis pulmonis

Margo inferior

Fissura obliqua

Fig. 647 Right lung, Pulmo dexter; sagittal section at the plane of the hilum of the lung; medial view.

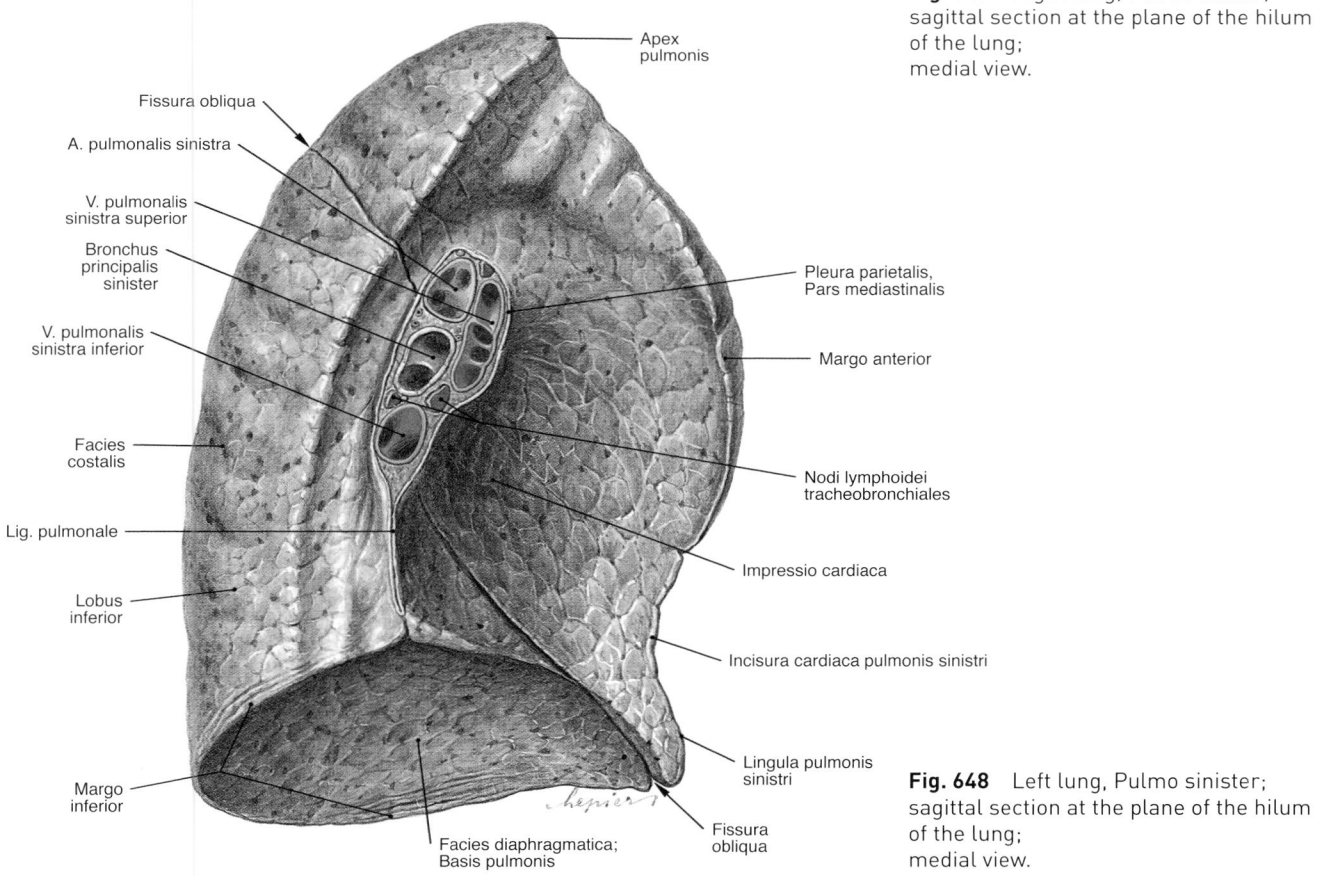

Apex pulmonis

Fissura obliqua

A. pulmonalis sinistra

V. pulmonalis sinistra superior

Bronchus principalis sinister

Pleura parietalis, Pars mediastinalis

V. pulmonalis sinistra inferior

Margo anterior

Facies costalis

Lig. pulmonale

Nodi lymphoidei tracheobronchiales

Lobus inferior

Impressio cardiaca

Incisura cardiaca pulmonis sinistri

Lingula pulmonis sinistri

Margo inferior

Facies diaphragmatica; Basis pulmonis

Fissura obliqua

Fig. 648 Left lung, Pulmo sinister; sagittal section at the plane of the hilum of the lung; medial view.

Bronchopulmonary segments

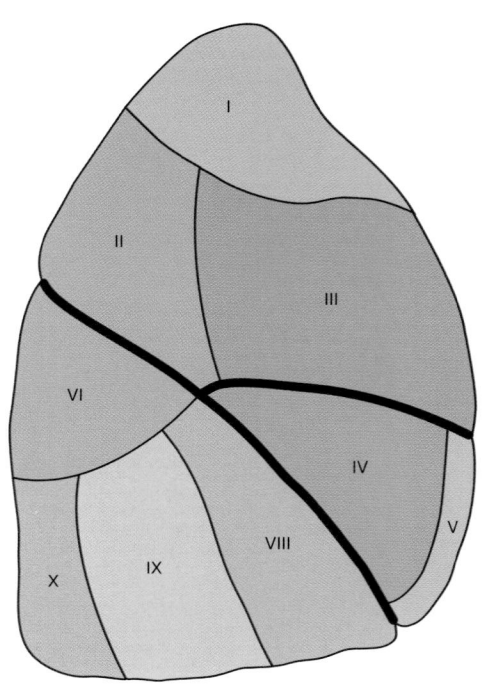

Pulmo dexter

Pulmo dexter, Lobus superior

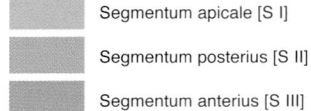

Segmentum apicale [S I]

Segmentum posterius [S II]

Segmentum anterius [S III]

Pulmo dexter, Lobus medius

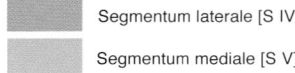

Segmentum laterale [S IV]

Segmentum mediale [S V]

Pulmo dexter, Lobus inferior

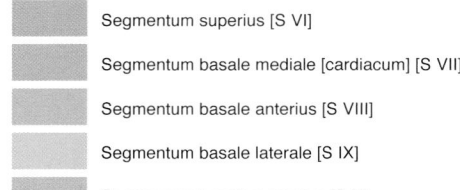

Segmentum superius [S VI]

Segmentum basale mediale [cardiacum] [S VII]*

Segmentum basale anterius [S VIII]

Segmentum basale laterale [S IX]

Segmentum basale posterius [S X]

* This segment is generally not an independent segment,
but rather fused with the anterior basal segment [S VIII].

Fig. 649 Right lung, Pulmo dexter;
bronchopulmonary segments,
Segmenta bronchopulmonalia;
lateral view.

Pulmo sinister

Pulmo sinister, Lobus superior

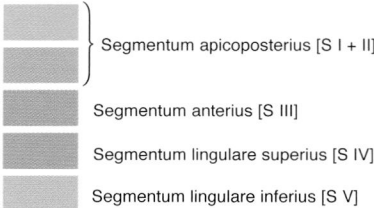

} Segmentum apicoposterius [S I + II]

Segmentum anterius [S III]

Segmentum lingulare superius [S IV]

Segmentum lingulare inferius [S V]

Pulmo sinister, Lobus inferior

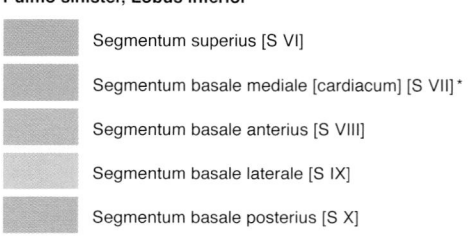

Segmentum superius [S VI]

Segmentum basale mediale [cardiacum] [S VII]*

Segmentum basale anterius [S VIII]

Segmentum basale laterale [S IX]

Segmentum basale posterius [S X]

* This segment is generally not an independent segment,
but rather fused with the anterior basal segment [S VIII].

Fig. 650 Left lung, Pulmo sinister;
bronchopulmonary segments,
Segmenta bronchopulmonalia;
lateral view.

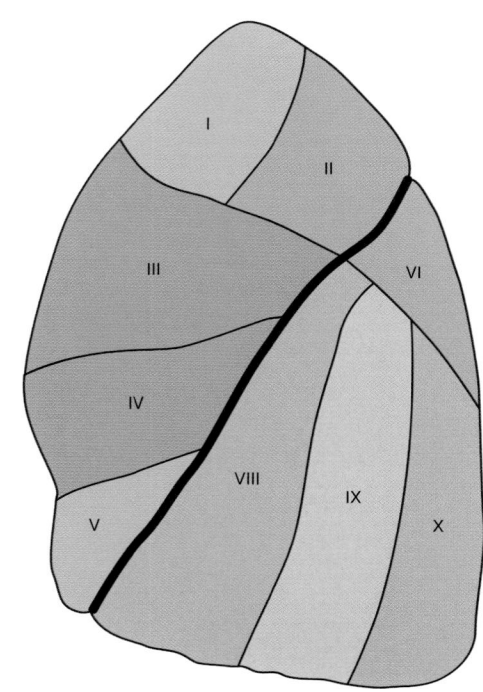

Bronchopulmonary segments

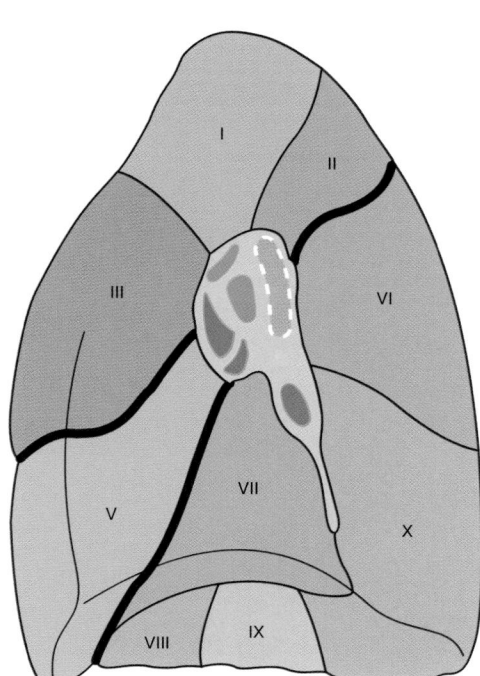

Fig. 651   Right lung, Pulmo dexter;
bronchopulmonary segments,
Segmenta bronchopulmonalia;
medial view.

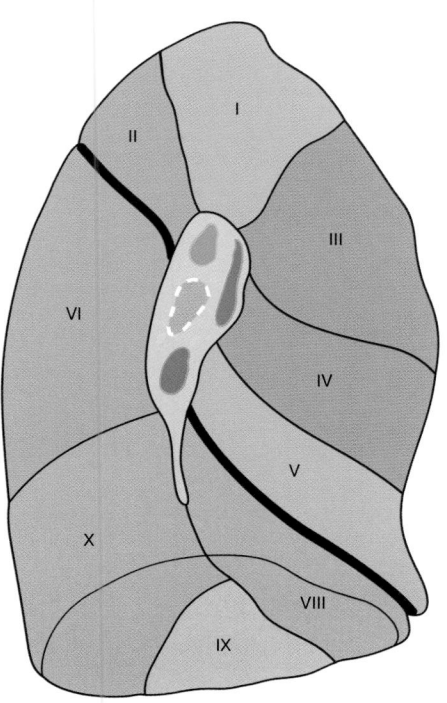

Fig. 652   Left lung, Pulmo sinister;
bronchopulmonary segments,
Segmenta bronchopulmonalia;
medial view.

Lungs, structure

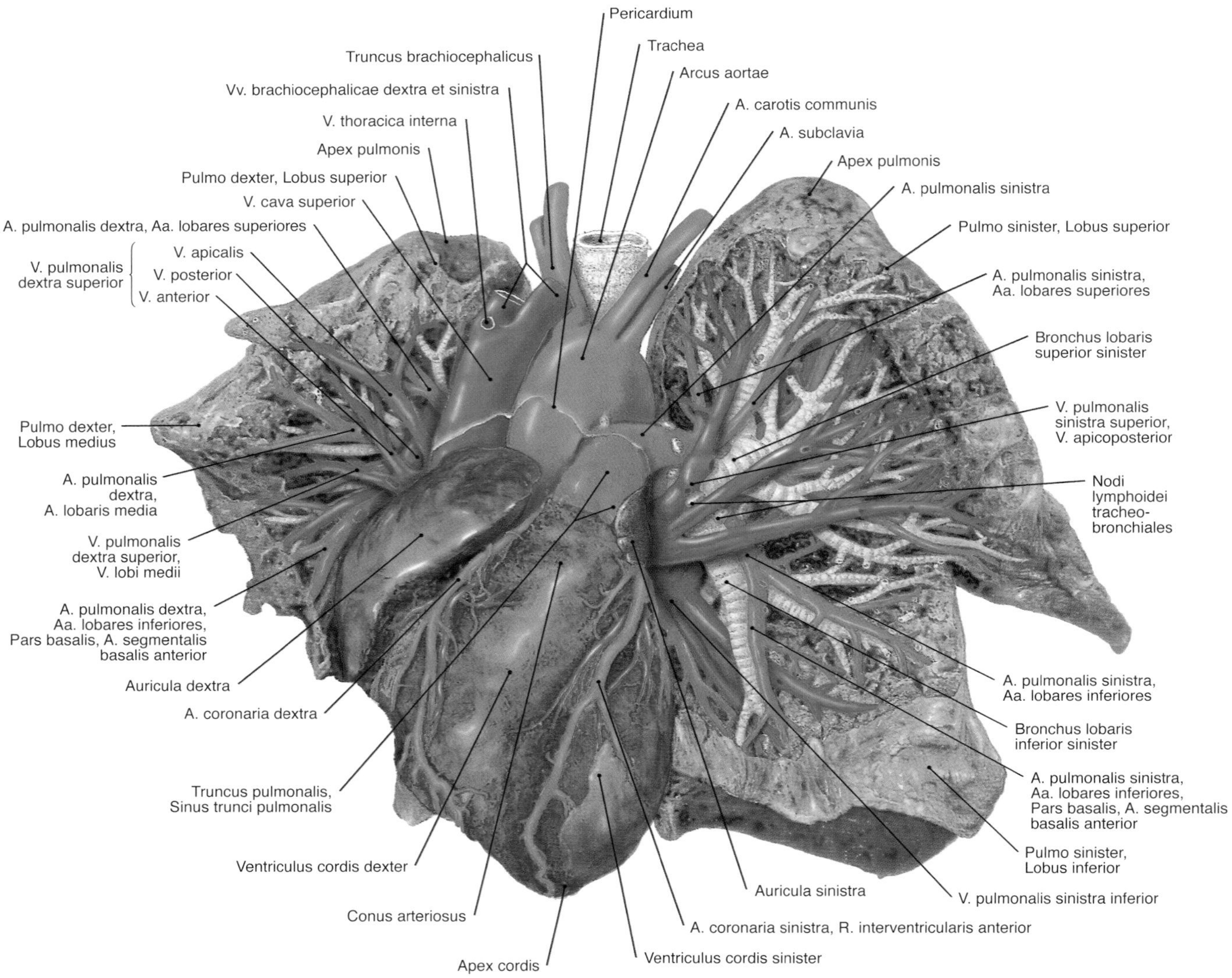

Pericardium

Truncus brachiocephalicus

Trachea

Vv. brachiocephalicae dextra et sinistra

Arcus aortae

V. thoracica interna

A. carotis communis

Apex pulmonis

A. subclavia

Pulmo dexter, Lobus superior

Apex pulmonis

V. cava superior

A. pulmonalis sinistra

A. pulmonalis dextra, Aa. lobares superiores

Pulmo sinister, Lobus superior

V. apicalis

V. pulmonalis dextra superior

V. posterior

A. pulmonalis sinistra, Aa. lobares superiores

V. anterior

Bronchus lobaris superior sinister

V. pulmonalis sinistra superior, V. apicoposterior

Pulmo dexter, Lobus medius

Nodi lymphoidei tracheobronchiales

A. pulmonalis dextra, A. lobaris media

V. pulmonalis dextra superior, V. lobi medii

A. pulmonalis dextra, Aa. lobares inferiores, Pars basalis, A. segmentalis basalis anterior

A. pulmonalis sinistra, Aa. lobares inferiores

Auricula dextra

Bronchus lobaris inferior sinister

A. coronaria dextra

A. pulmonalis sinistra, Aa. lobares inferiores, Pars basalis, A. segmentalis basalis anterior

Pulmo sinister, Lobus inferior

Truncus pulmonalis, Sinus trunci pulmonalis

Ventriculus cordis dexter

Auricula sinistra

V. pulmonalis sinistra inferior

Conus arteriosus

A. coronaria sinistra, R. interventricularis anterior

Apex cordis

Ventriculus cordis sinister

Fig. 653 Lungs, Pulmones, and heart, Cor; the arteries, the veins and the bronchi have been dissected up to the external surface of the lungs.

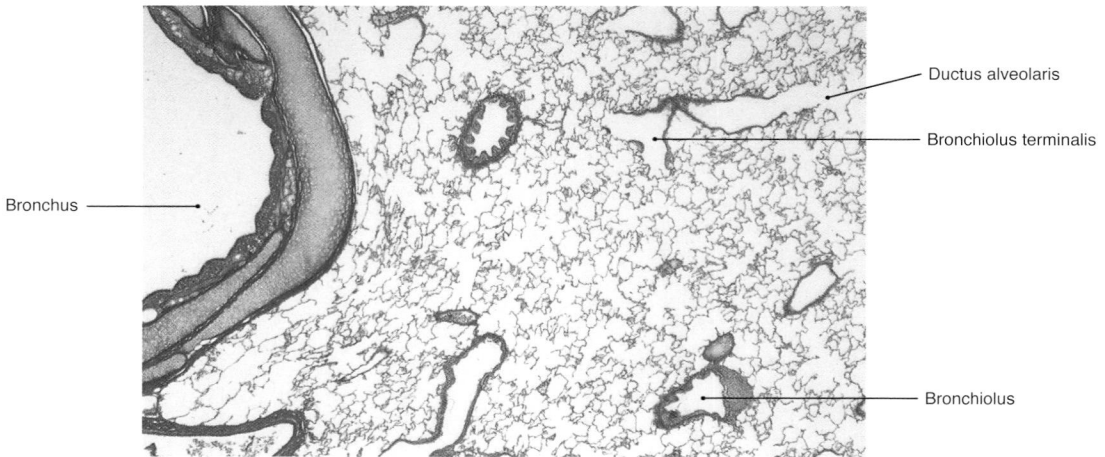

Bronchus

Ductus alveolaris

Bronchiolus terminalis

Bronchiolus

Fig. 654 Lung, Pulmo; overview of the lung structure; microscopic enlargement at low magnification.

Vessels of the lungs and bronchi

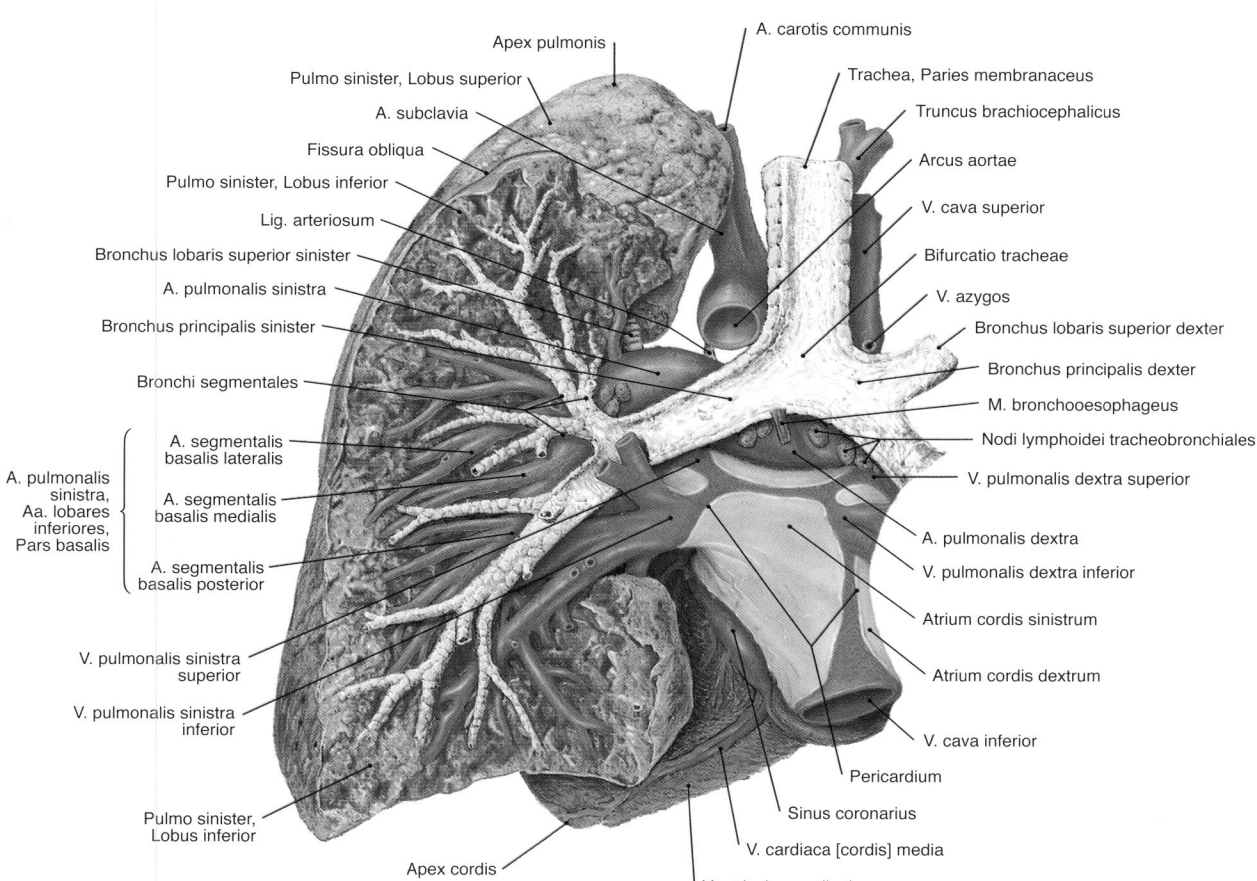

Apex pulmonis
Pulmo sinister, Lobus superior
A. subclavia
Fissura obliqua
Pulmo sinister, Lobus inferior
Lig. arteriosum
Bronchus lobaris superior sinister
A. pulmonalis sinistra
Bronchus principalis sinister
Bronchi segmentales
A. segmentalis basalis lateralis
A. pulmonalis sinistra, Aa. lobares inferiores, Pars basalis
A. segmentalis basalis medialis
A. segmentalis basalis posterior
V. pulmonalis sinistra superior
V. pulmonalis sinistra inferior
Pulmo sinister, Lobus inferior
Apex cordis

A. carotis communis
Trachea, Paries membranaceus
Truncus brachiocephalicus
Arcus aortae
V. cava superior
Bifurcatio tracheae
V. azygos
Bronchus lobaris superior dexter
Bronchus principalis dexter
M. bronchooesophageus
Nodi lymphoidei tracheobronchiales
V. pulmonalis dextra superior
A. pulmonalis dextra
V. pulmonalis dextra inferior
Atrium cordis sinistrum
Atrium cordis dextrum
V. cava inferior
Pericardium
Sinus coronarius
V. cardiaca [cordis] media
Ventriculus cordis dexter

Fig. 655   Vessels of the left lung, Pulmo sinister; dorsal view.

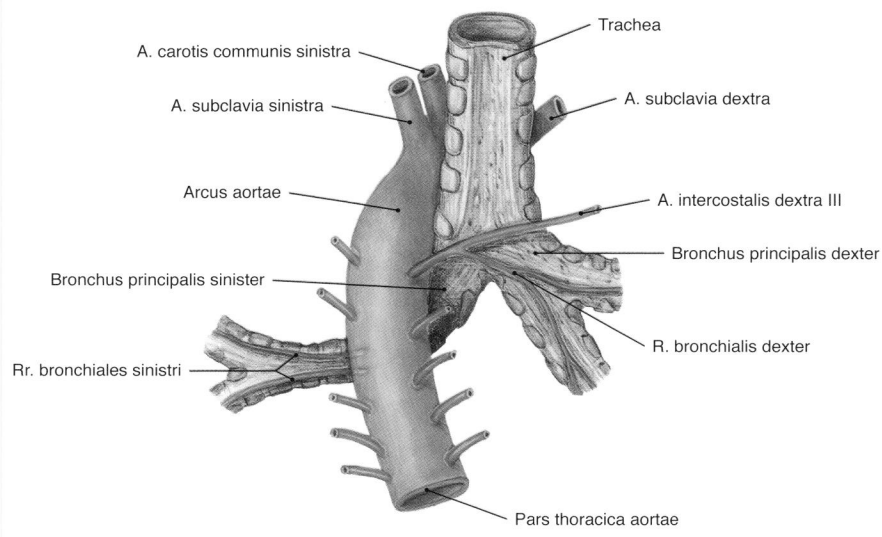

A. carotis communis sinistra
A. subclavia sinistra
Arcus aortae
Bronchus principalis sinister
Rr. bronchiales sinistri

Trachea
A. subclavia dextra
A. intercostalis dextra III
Bronchus principalis dexter
R. bronchialis dexter
Pars thoracica aortae

Fig. 656   Bronchi, Bronchi; arterial supply.

Vessels of the lung, radiography

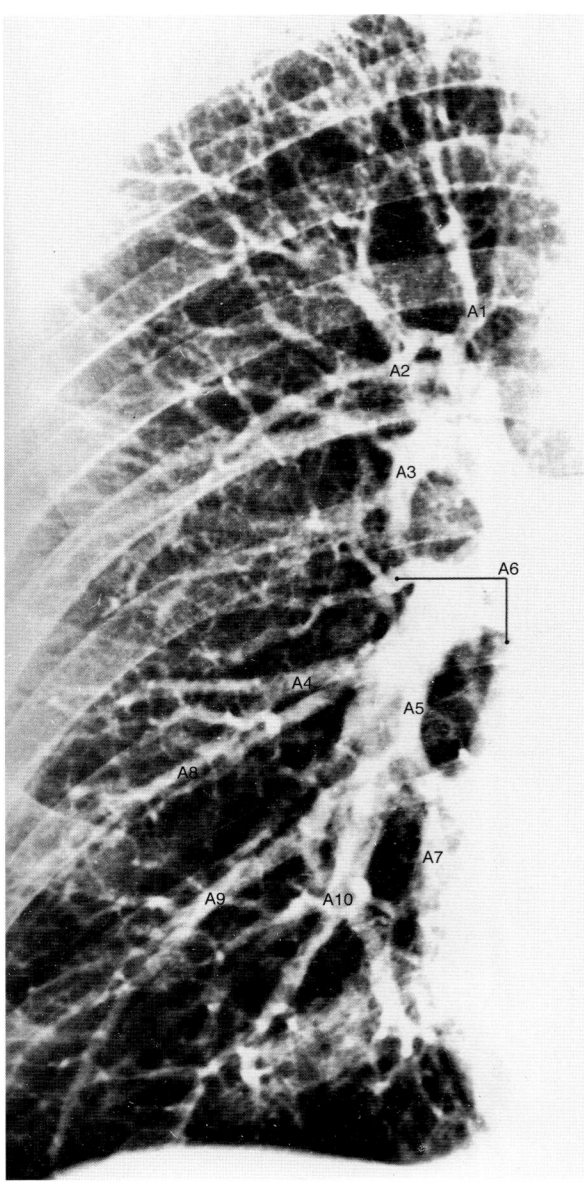

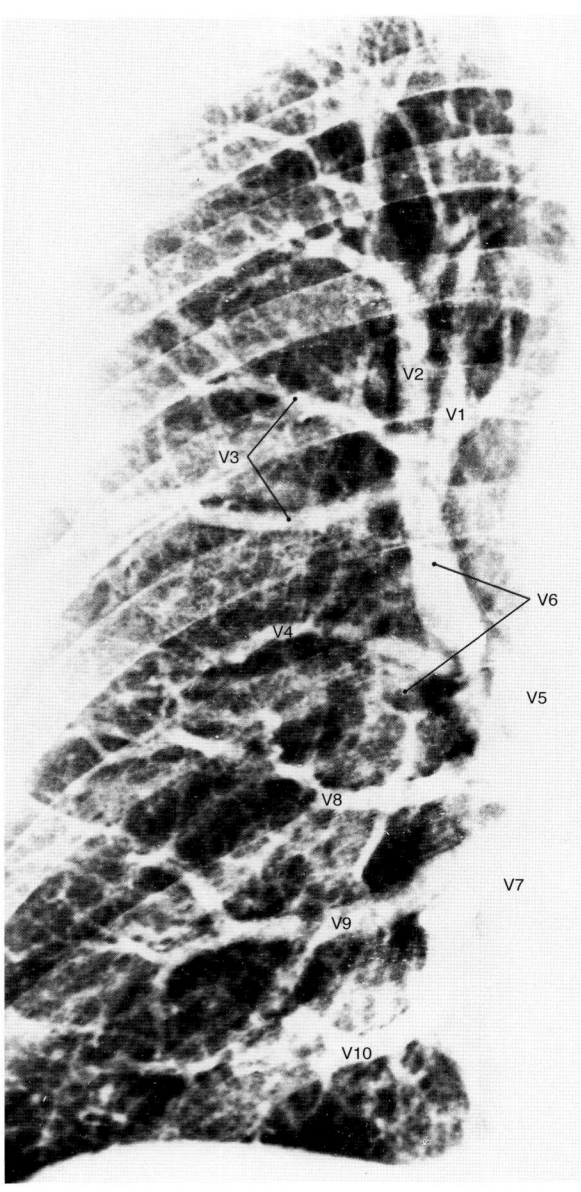

Fig. 657 Arteries of the right lung,
Aa. pulmonales dextrae;
AP-radiograph (pulmonary angiography); after
injection of a contrast medium into the right ventricle;
ventral view.
The numbers designate the segmental arteries
(compare p. 354).

Fig. 658 Veins of the right lung,
Vv. pulmonales dextrae;
AP-radiograph (return via pulmonary veins of the contrast
medium injected into the right ventricle);
ventral view.
Numbers indicate the segmental veins (compare p. 354).

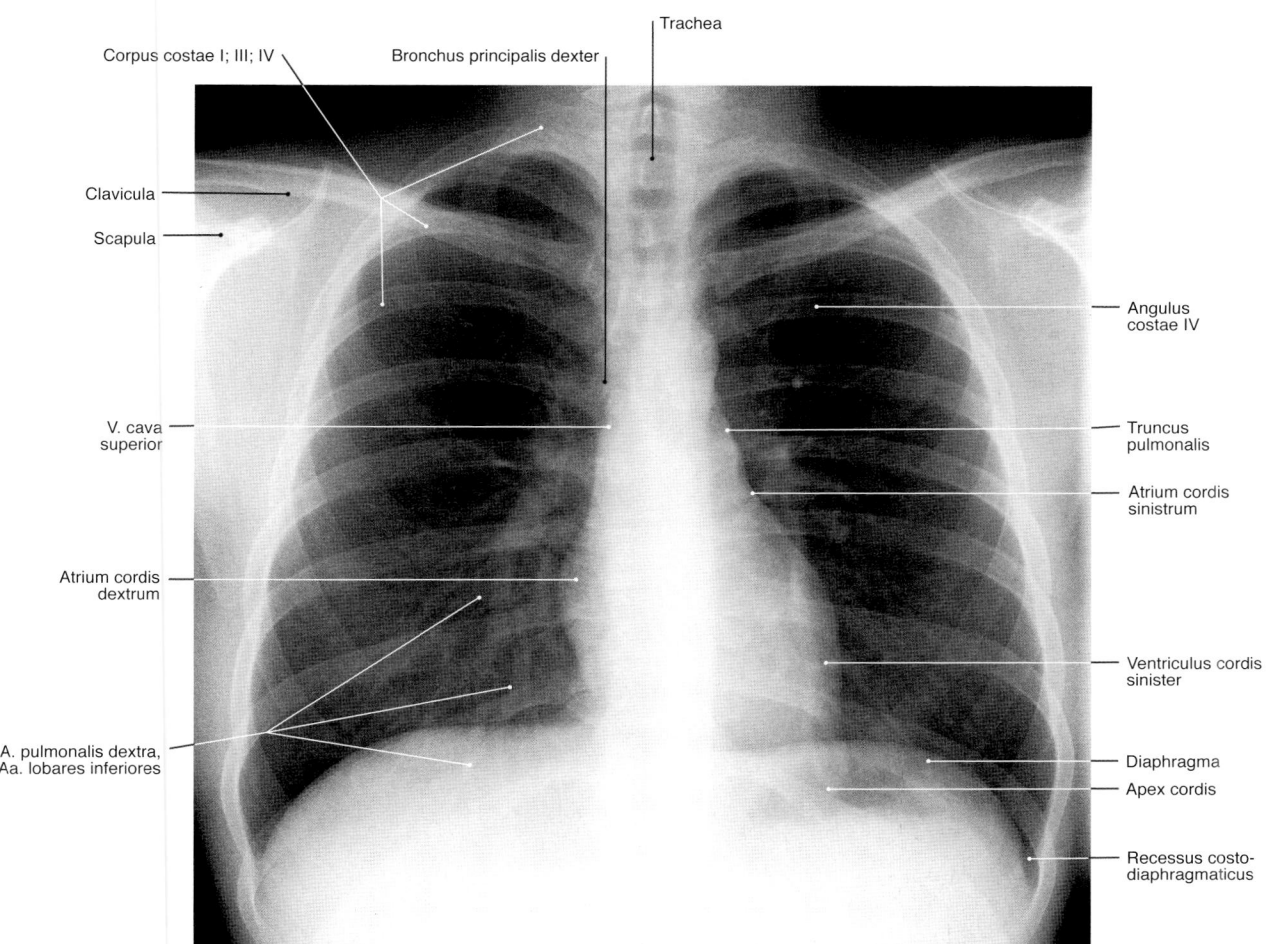

Corpus costae I; III; IV
Bronchus principalis dexter
Trachea
Clavicula
Scapula
Angulus costae IV
V. cava superior
Truncus pulmonalis
Atrium cordis sinistrum
Atrium cordis dextrum
Ventriculus cordis sinister
A. pulmonalis dextra, Aa. lobares inferiores
Diaphragma
Apex cordis
Recessus costo-diaphragmaticus

Fig. 659 Thoracic cage, Cavea thoracis, and thoracic viscera; PA-radiograph of a 27-year-old male (thorax radiograph).

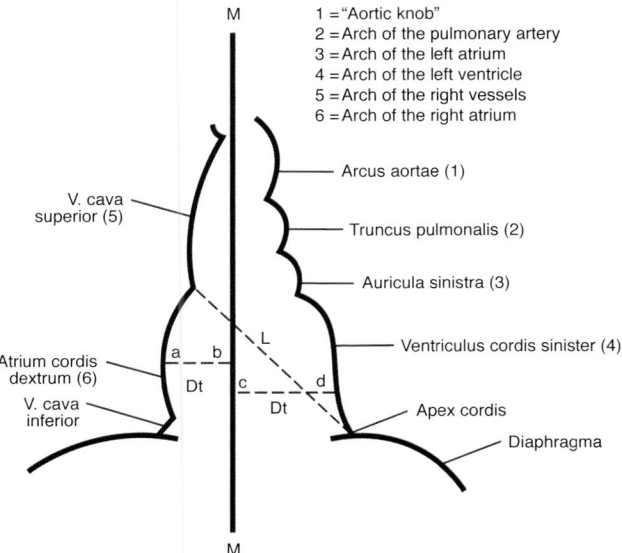

M

1 = "Aortic knob"
2 = Arch of the pulmonary artery
3 = Arch of the left atrium
4 = Arch of the left ventricle
5 = Arch of the right vessels
6 = Arch of the right atrium

Arcus aortae (1)
Truncus pulmonalis (2)
Auricula sinistra (3)
Ventriculus cordis sinister (4)

V. cava superior (5)
Atrium cordis dextrum (6)
V. cava inferior
Apex cordis
Diaphragma

Fig. 660 Outline of the heart shadow in the radiograph;
Dt = Transverse diameter,
    ab + cd = 13–14 cm
L = Longitudinal axis of the heart (from the superior border of the right atrial contour to the apex of the heart) = 15–16 cm
M = Median plane of the body

Bronchoscopy

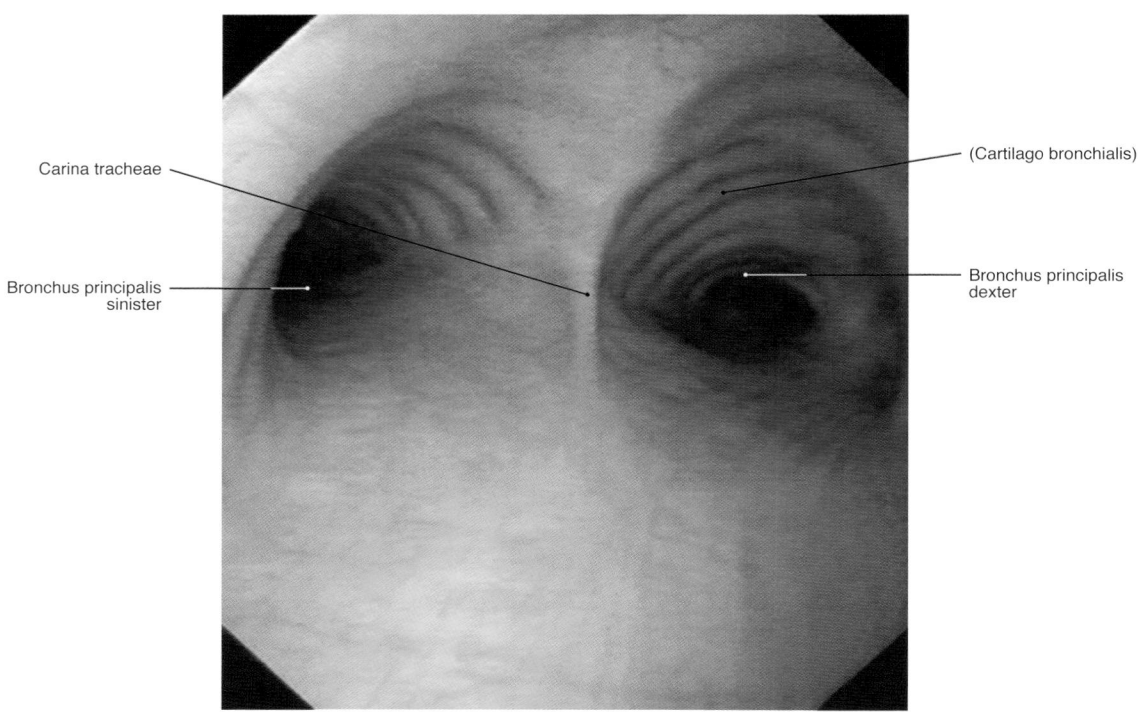

Carina tracheae

(Cartilago bronchialis)

Bronchus principalis
sinister

Bronchus principalis
dexter

Fig. 661 Bronchi, Bronchi;
bronchoscopy of a healthy individual displaying the tracheal
bifurcation and the carina of trachea.

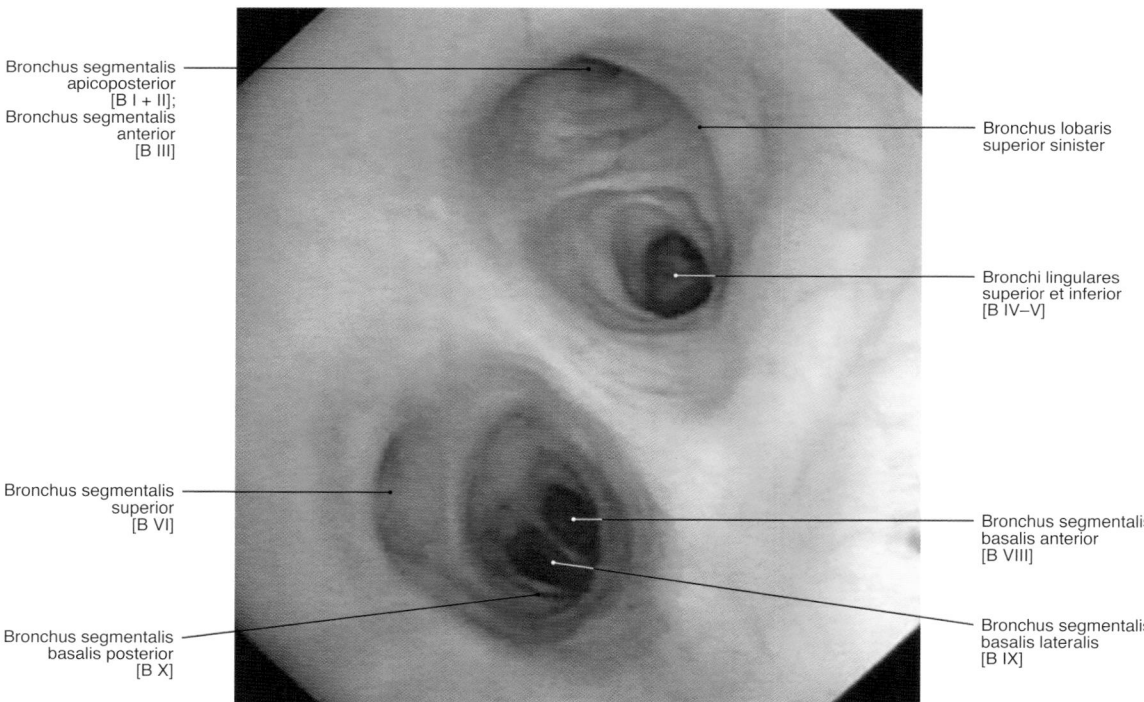

Bronchus segmentalis
apicoposterior
[B I + II];
Bronchus segmentalis
anterior
[B III]

Bronchus lobaris
superior sinister

Bronchi lingulares
superior et inferior
[B IV–V]

Bronchus segmentalis
superior
[B VI]

Bronchus segmentalis
basalis anterior
[B VIII]

Bronchus segmentalis
basalis posterior
[B X]

Bronchus segmentalis
basalis lateralis
[B IX]

Fig. 662 Bronchi, Bronchi;
bronchoscopic view of the left segmental bronchi.

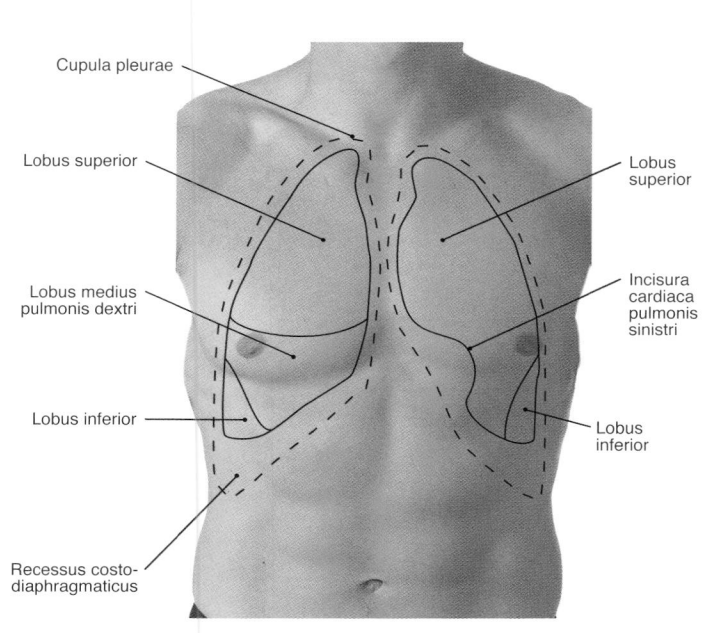

Cupula pleurae

Lobus superior

Lobus medius pulmonis dextri

Lobus inferior

Recessus costo-diaphragmaticus

Lobus superior

Incisura cardiaca pulmonis sinistri

Lobus inferior

Fig. 663 Projection of the pulmonary and the pleural borders onto the anterior thoracic wall.

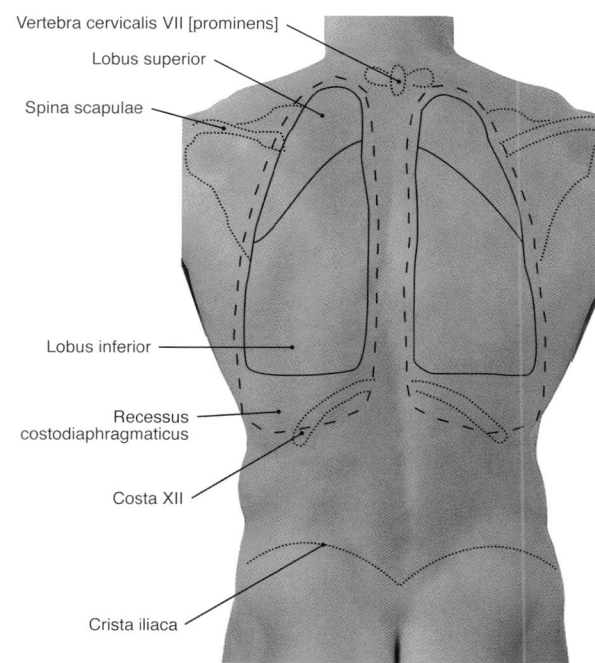

Vertebra cervicalis VII [prominens]

Lobus superior

Spina scapulae

Lobus inferior

Recessus costodiaphragmaticus

Costa XII

Crista iliaca

Fig. 664 Projection of the pulmonary and the pleural borders onto the posterior thoracic wall.

Borders of the lungs – line
Borders of the pleura – dashed line

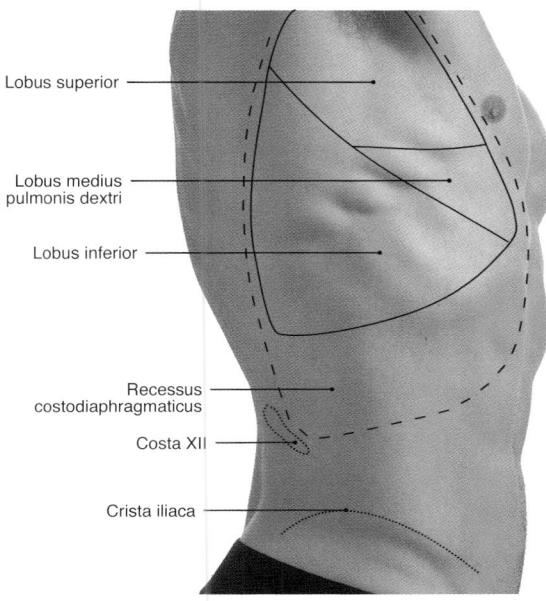

Lobus superior

Lobus medius pulmonis dextri

Lobus inferior

Recessus costodiaphragmaticus

Costa XII

Crista iliaca

Fig. 665 Projection of the pulmonary and the pleural borders onto the lateral thoracic wall.

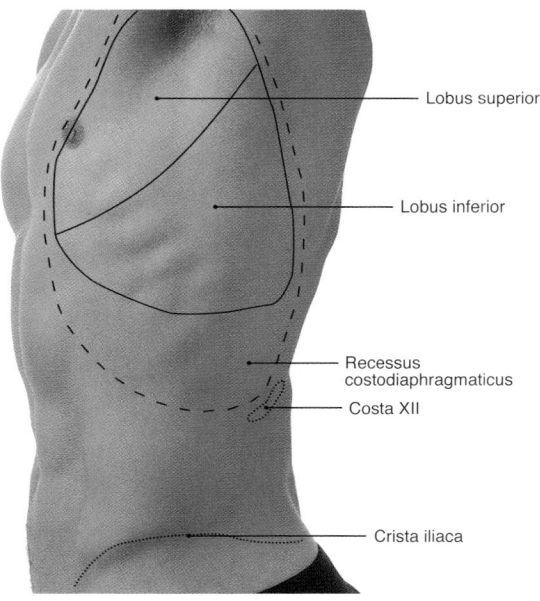

Lobus superior

Lobus inferior

Recessus costodiaphragmaticus

Costa XII

Crista iliaca

Fig. 666 Projection of the pulmonary and the pleural borders onto the lateral thoracic wall.

Oesophagus

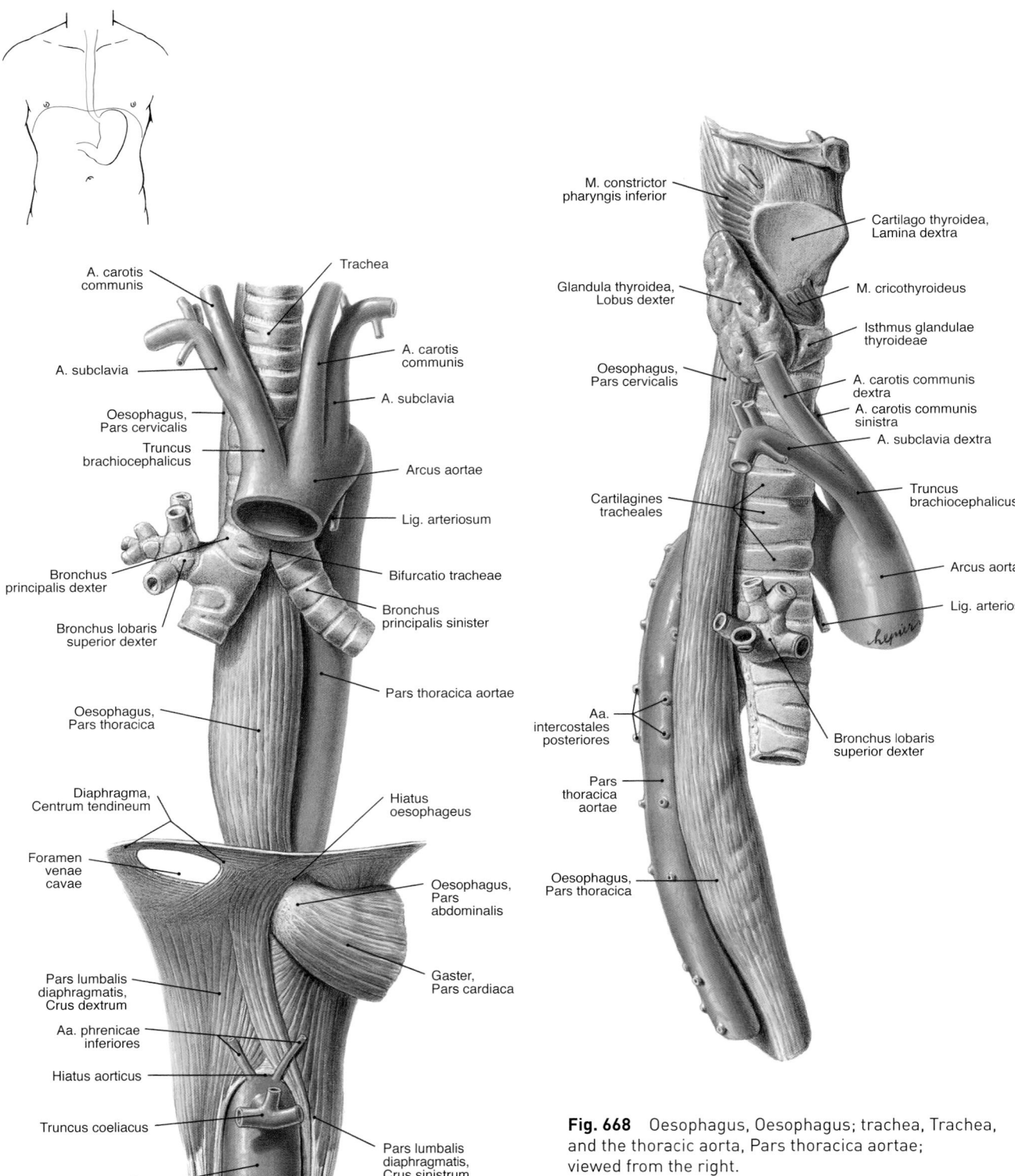

A. carotis communis

Trachea

A. subclavia

A. carotis communis

Oesophagus, Pars cervicalis

A. subclavia

Truncus brachiocephalicus

Arcus aortae

Lig. arteriosum

Bronchus principalis dexter

Bifurcatio tracheae

Bronchus lobaris superior dexter

Bronchus principalis sinister

Oesophagus, Pars thoracica

Pars thoracica aortae

Diaphragma, Centrum tendineum

Hiatus oesophageus

Foramen venae cavae

Oesophagus, Pars abdominalis

Pars lumbalis diaphragmatis, Crus dextrum

Gaster, Pars cardiaca

Aa. phrenicae inferiores

Hiatus aorticus

Truncus coeliacus

Pars lumbalis diaphragmatis, Crus sinistrum

Pars abdominalis aortae

M. constrictor pharyngis inferior

Cartilago thyroidea, Lamina dextra

Glandula thyroidea, Lobus dexter

M. cricothyroideus

Isthmus glandulae thyroideae

Oesophagus, Pars cervicalis

A. carotis communis dextra

A. carotis communis sinistra

A. subclavia dextra

Cartilagines tracheales

Truncus brachiocephalicus

Arcus aortae

Lig. arteriosum

Aa. intercostales posteriores

Bronchus lobaris superior dexter

Pars thoracica aortae

Oesophagus, Pars thoracica

Fig. 668 Oesophagus, Oesophagus; trachea, Trachea, and the thoracic aorta, Pars thoracica aortae; viewed from the right.

Fig. 667 Oesophagus, Oesophagus; trachea, Trachea, and the thoracic aorta, Pars thoracica aortae; ventral view.

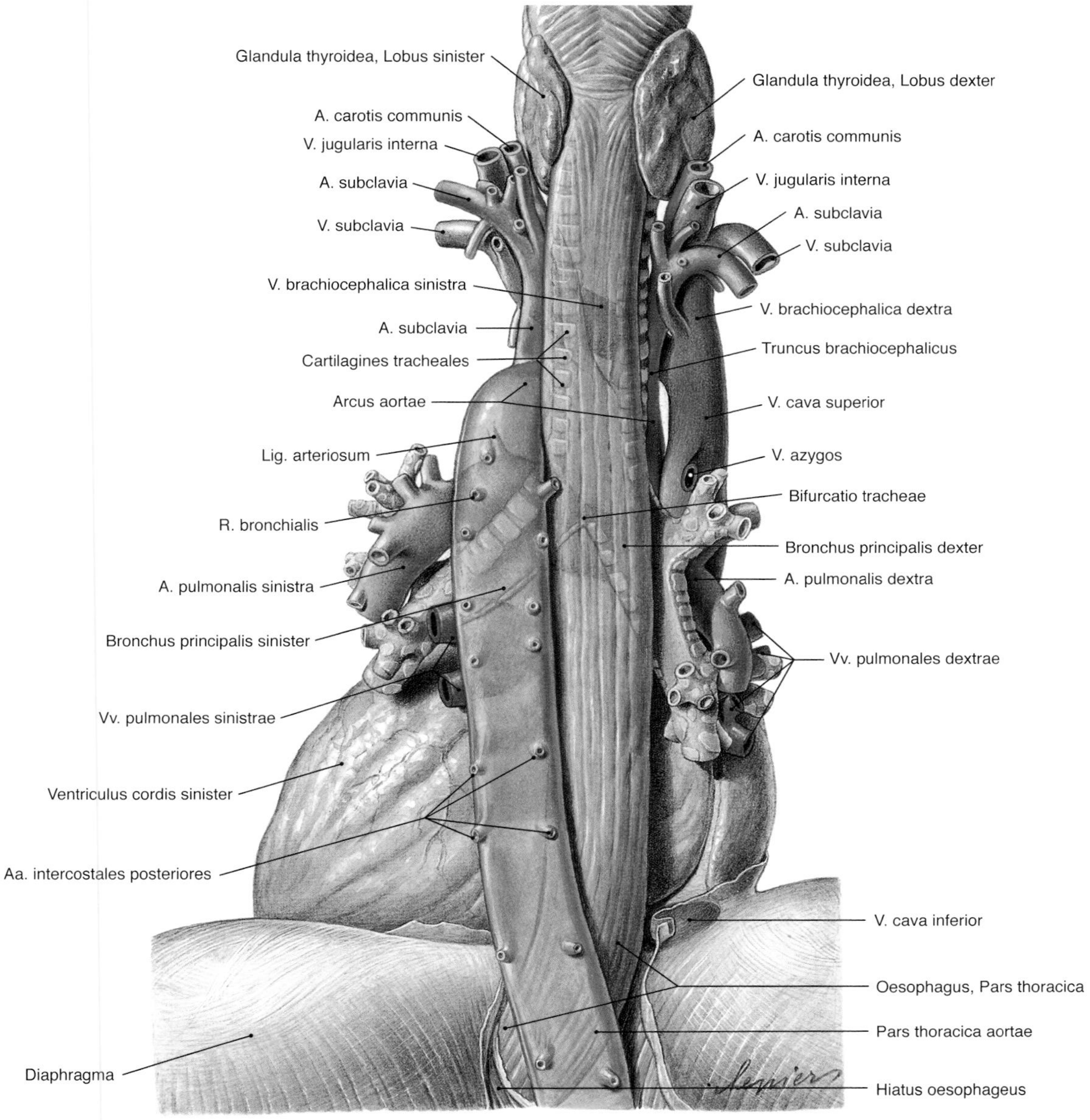

Glandula thyroidea, Lobus sinister
A. carotis communis
V. jugularis interna
A. subclavia
V. subclavia
V. brachiocephalica sinistra
A. subclavia
Cartilagines tracheales
Arcus aortae
Lig. arteriosum
R. bronchialis
A. pulmonalis sinistra
Bronchus principalis sinister
Vv. pulmonales sinistrae
Ventriculus cordis sinister
Aa. intercostales posteriores
Diaphragma

Glandula thyroidea, Lobus dexter
A. carotis communis
V. jugularis interna
A. subclavia
V. subclavia
V. brachiocephalica dextra
Truncus brachiocephalicus
V. cava superior
V. azygos
Bifurcatio tracheae
Bronchus principalis dexter
A. pulmonalis dextra
Vv. pulmonales dextrae
V. cava inferior
Oesophagus, Pars thoracica
Pars thoracica aortae
Hiatus oesophageus

Fig. 669   Oesophagus, Oesophagus, and the thoracic aorta,
Pars thoracica aortae;
dorsal view.

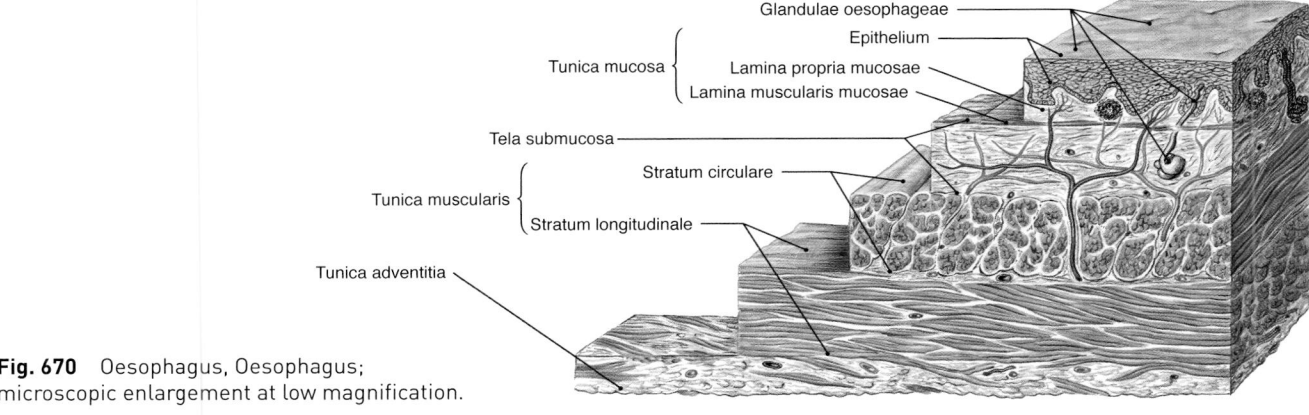

Glandulae oesophageae
Epithelium
Tunica mucosa
Lamina propria mucosae
Lamina muscularis mucosae
Tela submucosa
Stratum circulare
Tunica muscularis
Stratum longitudinale
Tunica adventitia

Fig. 670   Oesophagus, Oesophagus;
microscopic enlargement at low magnification.

Vessels of the oesophagus

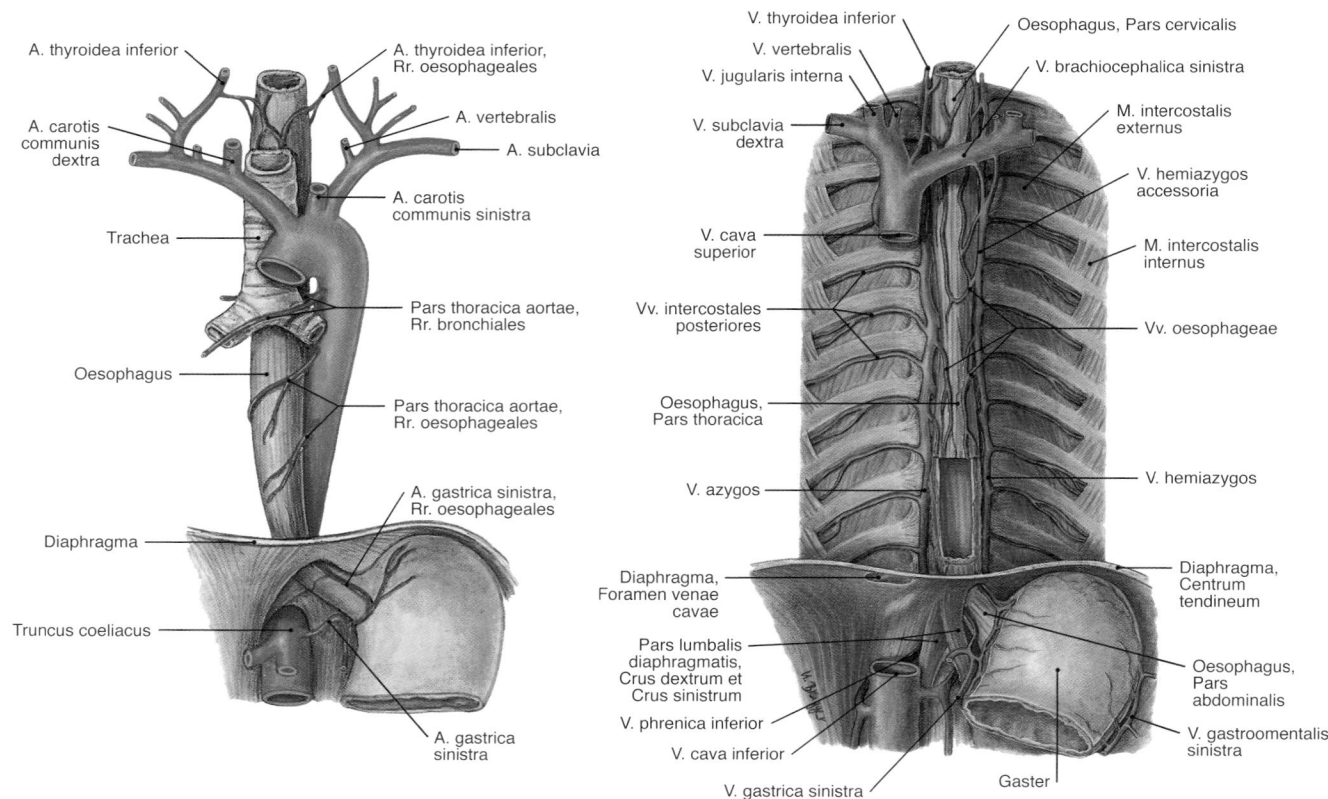

Fig. 671   Oesophagus, Oesophagus; supplying arteries; ventral view.

Fig. 672   Veins of the oesophagus, Vv. oesophageae.

→ 809, 810

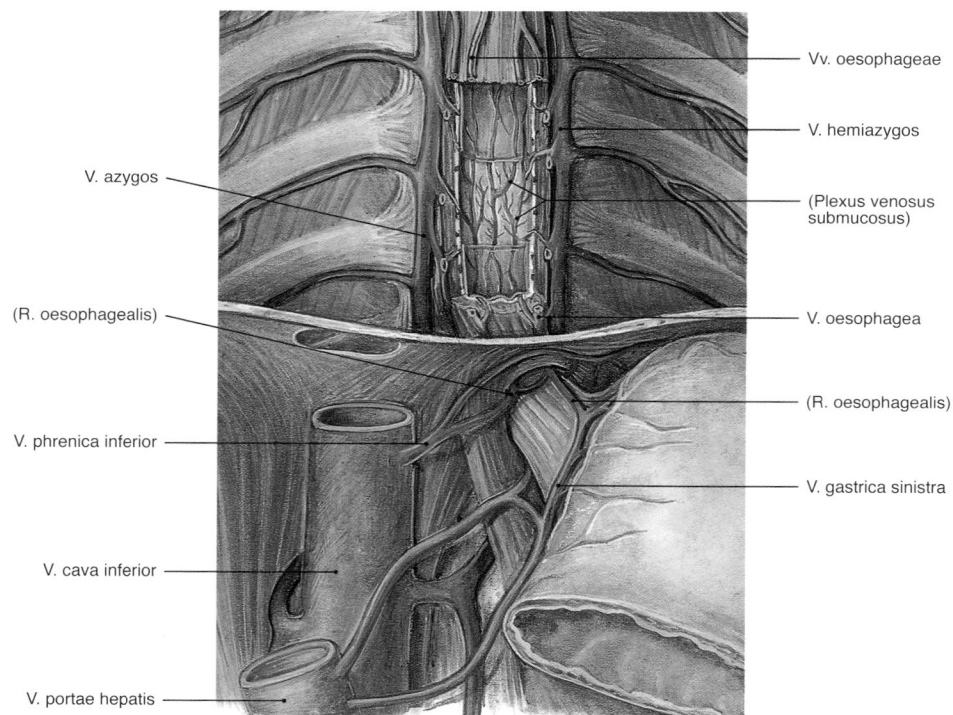

→ 810

Fig. 673   Veins of the oesophagus, Vv. oesophageae; magnification of Fig. 672; demonstration of anastomoses between branches of the hepatic portal vein and the superior vena cava.

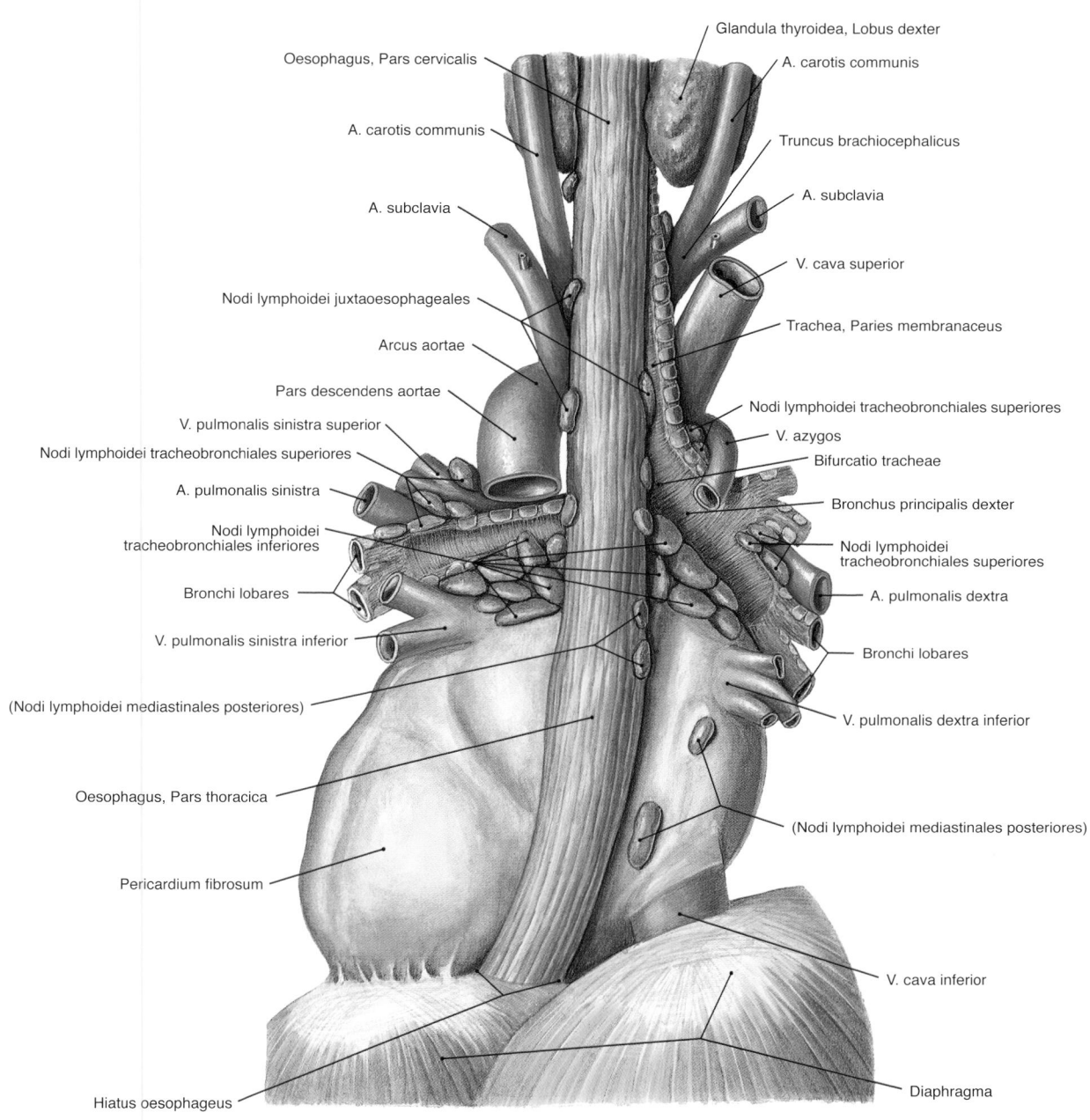

Glandula thyroidea, Lobus dexter

Oesophagus, Pars cervicalis

A. carotis communis

A. carotis communis

Truncus brachiocephalicus

A. subclavia

A. subclavia

V. cava superior

Nodi lymphoidei juxtaoesophageales

Trachea, Paries membranaceus

Arcus aortae

Pars descendens aortae

Nodi lymphoidei tracheobronchiales superiores

V. pulmonalis sinistra superior

V. azygos

Nodi lymphoidei tracheobronchiales superiores

Bifurcatio tracheae

A. pulmonalis sinistra

Bronchus principalis dexter

Nodi lymphoidei
tracheobronchiales inferiores

Nodi lymphoidei
tracheobronchiales superiores

Bronchi lobares

A. pulmonalis dextra

V. pulmonalis sinistra inferior

Bronchi lobares

(Nodi lymphoidei mediastinales posteriores)

V. pulmonalis dextra inferior

Oesophagus, Pars thoracica

(Nodi lymphoidei mediastinales posteriores)

Pericardium fibrosum

V. cava inferior

Diaphragma

Hiatus oesophageus

Fig. 674 Thoracic lymph nodes;
Nodi lymphoidei thoracis;
dorsal view.

Oesophagus, radiography and oesophagoscopy

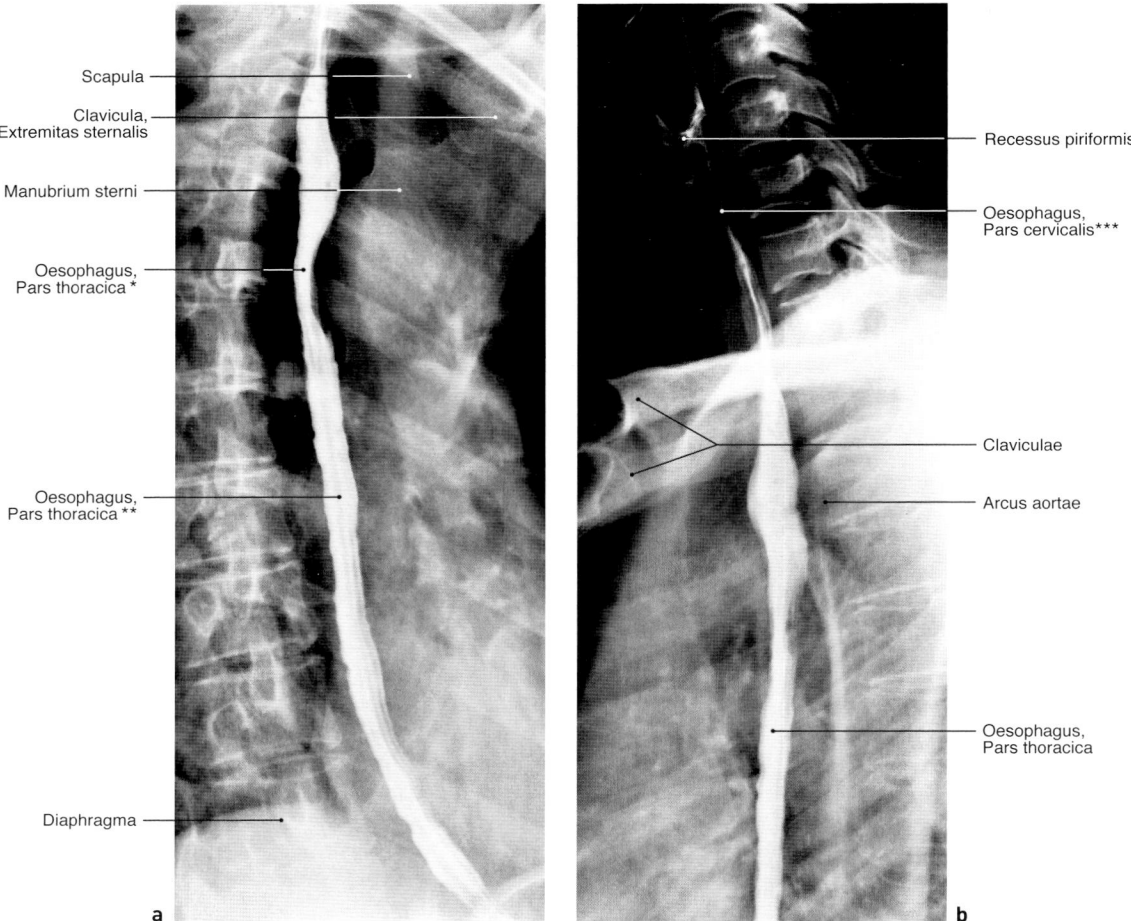

Scapula

Clavicula,
Extremitas sternalis

Manubrium sterni

Oesophagus,
Pars thoracica *

Oesophagus,
Pars thoracica **

Diaphragma

a

Recessus piriformis

Oesophagus,
Pars cervicalis***

Claviculae

Arcus aortae

Oesophagus,
Pars thoracica

b

Fig. 675 a, b Oesophagus, Oesophagus;
radiograph after swallowing of a contrast medium.
a Right anterior oblique position, oblique diameter I (beam
directed from left anterior to right posterior)
b Left anterior oblique position, oblique diameter II (beam
directed from right anterior to left posterior)

* Oesophageal constriction caused by the aortic arch
** Retrocardial portion of the oesophagus
*** Oesophageal constriction at the junction of the pharynx with the
oesophagus

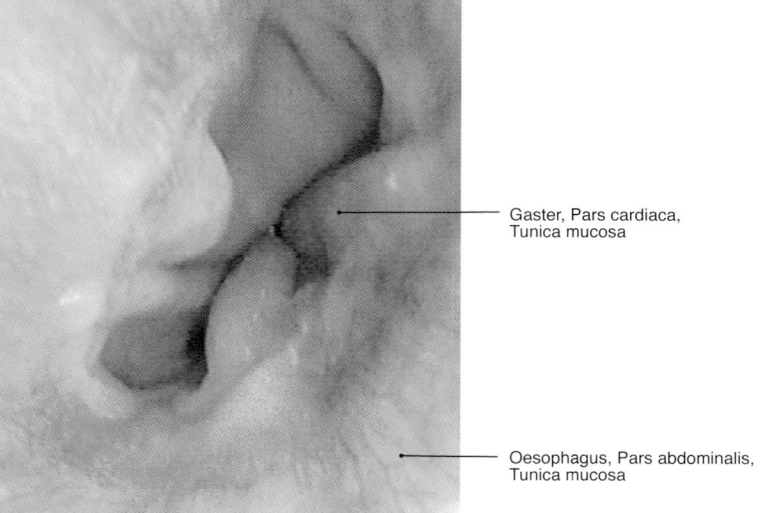

Gaster, Pars cardiaca,
Tunica mucosa

Oesophagus, Pars abdominalis,
Tunica mucosa

Fig. 676 Oesophagus, Oesophagus;
oesophagoscopy (technical details see Fig. 718);
superior view.

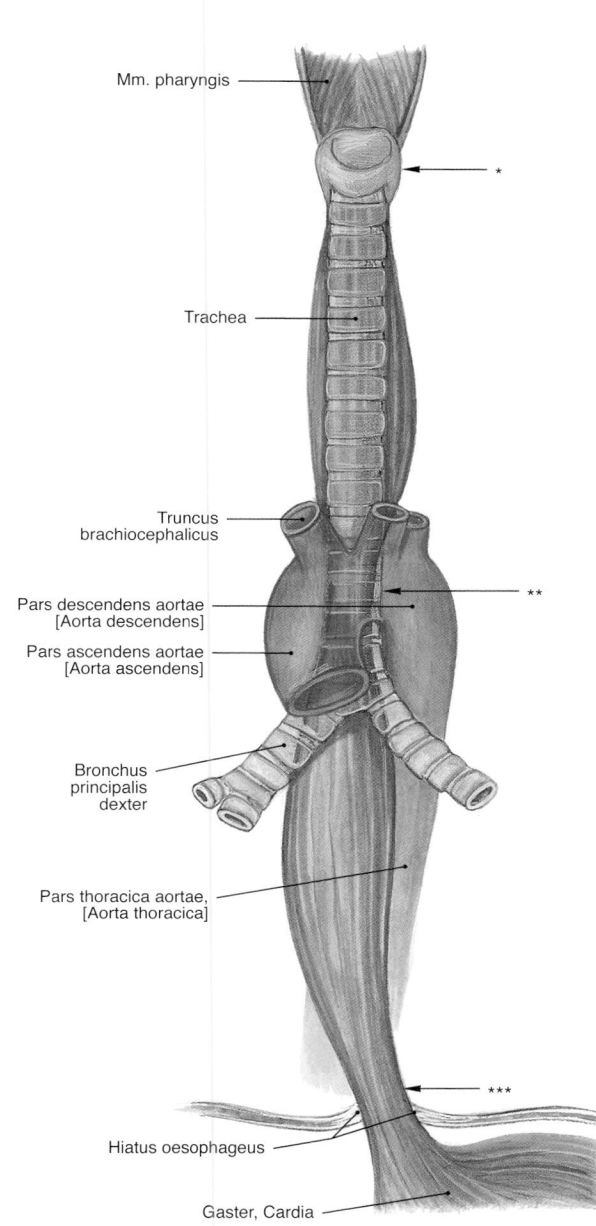

Fig. 677 Oesophagus, Oesophagus;
constrictions.

* Upper oesophageal sphincter
** Narrowing caused by the aortic arch
*** Diaphragmatic constriction

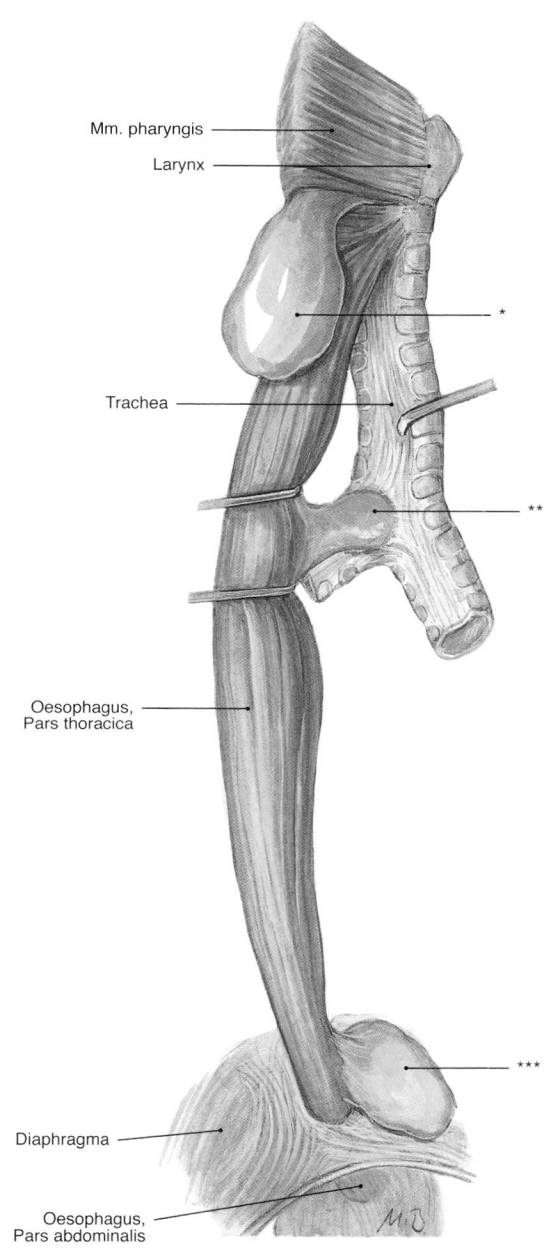

Fig. 678 Oesophagus, Oesophagus;
typical location and frequency of diverticula.

* Cervical diverticulum
  (ZENKER's diverticulum), (~70%)
** Mid-oesophageal diverticulum (~22%)
*** Epiphrenic diverticulum (~8%)

Thymus

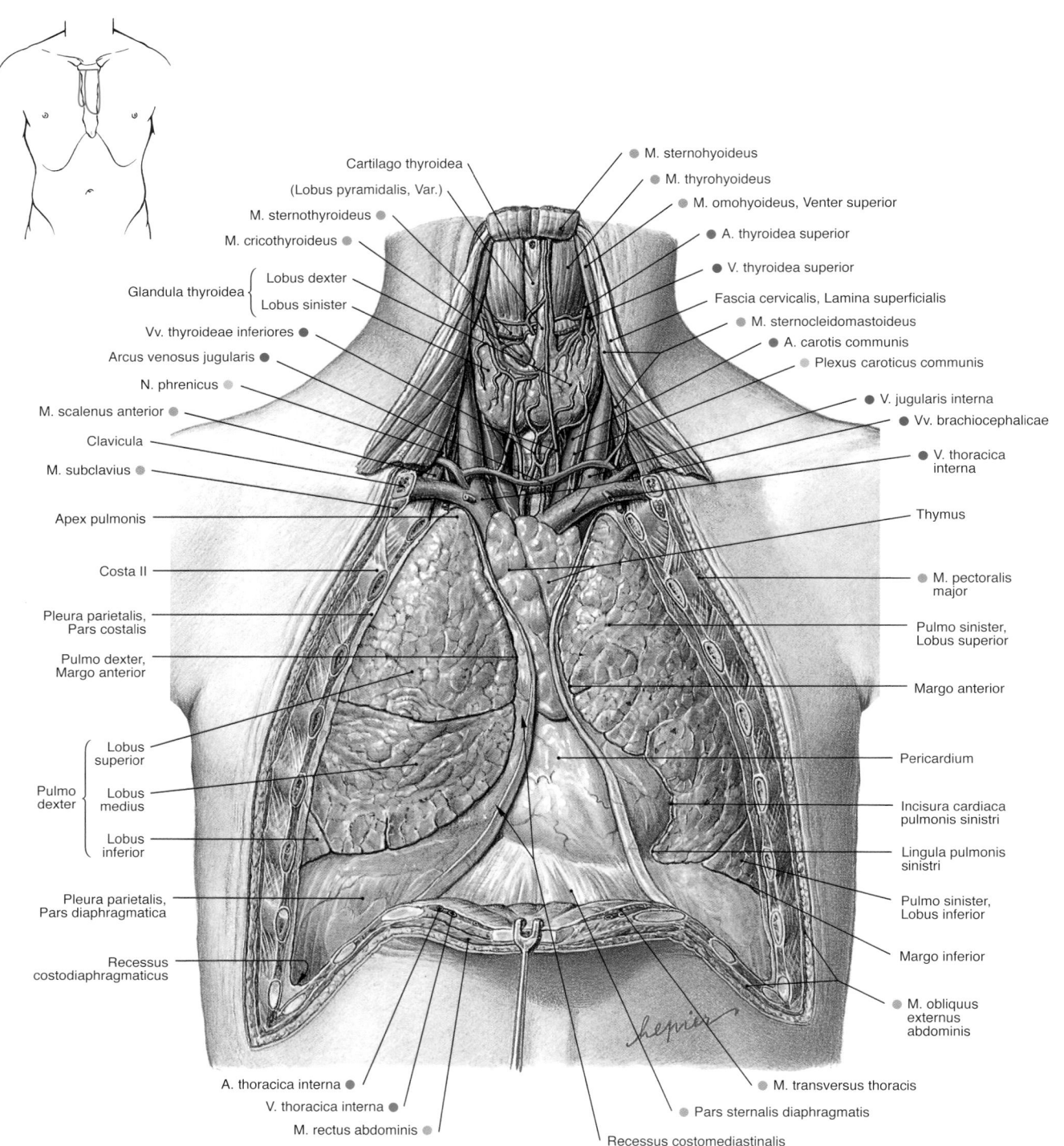

Cartilago thyroidea
(Lobus pyramidalis, Var.)
M. sternothyroideus ●
M. cricothyroideus ●
Glandula thyroidea { Lobus dexter
Lobus sinister
Vv. thyroideae inferiores ●
Arcus venosus jugularis ●
N. phrenicus ●
M. scalenus anterior ●
Clavicula
M. subclavius ●
Apex pulmonis
Costa II
Pleura parietalis, Pars costalis
Pulmo dexter, Margo anterior
Pulmo dexter { Lobus superior
Lobus medius
Lobus inferior
Pleura parietalis, Pars diaphragmatica
Recessus costodiaphragmaticus
A. thoracica interna ●
V. thoracica interna ●
M. rectus abdominis ●

● M. sternohyoideus
● M. thyrohyoideus
● M. omohyoideus, Venter superior
● A. thyroidea superior
● V. thyroidea superior
Fascia cervicalis, Lamina superficialis
● M. sternocleidomastoideus
● A. carotis communis
● Plexus caroticus communis
● V. jugularis interna
● Vv. brachiocephalicae
● V. thoracica interna
Thymus
● M. pectoralis major
Pulmo sinister, Lobus superior
Margo anterior
Pericardium
Incisura cardiaca pulmonis sinistri
Lingula pulmonis sinistri
Pulmo sinister, Lobus inferior
Margo inferior
● M. obliquus externus abdominis
● M. transversus thoracis
● Pars sternalis diaphragmatis
Recessus costomediastinalis

→ 781

Fig. 679 Thymus, Thymus; pericardium, Pericardium, and lungs, Pulmones, of an adolescent.
Note the size of the adolescent thymus. In older individuals, the thymic tissue is almost entirely replaced by adipose tissue.

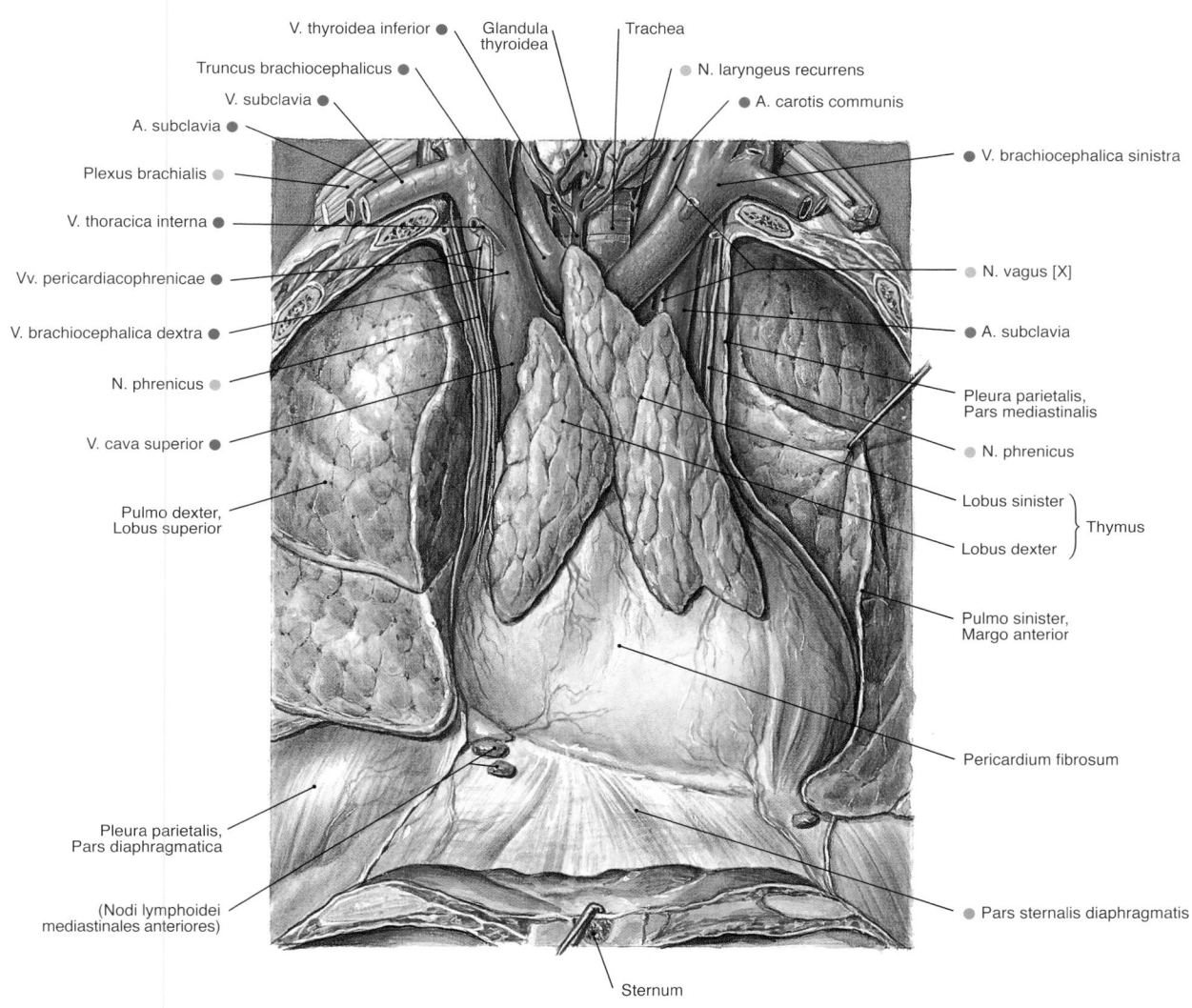

V. thyroidea inferior ●   Glandula thyroidea   Trachea

Truncus brachiocephalicus ●   ● N. laryngeus recurrens

V. subclavia ●   ● A. carotis communis

A. subclavia ●   ● V. brachiocephalica sinistra

Plexus brachialis ●

V. thoracica interna ●   ● N. vagus [X]

Vv. pericardiacophrenicae ●   ● A. subclavia

V. brachiocephalica dextra ●   Pleura parietalis, Pars mediastinalis

N. phrenicus ●   ● N. phrenicus

V. cava superior ●   Lobus sinister ⎫
   Lobus dexter ⎭ Thymus

Pulmo dexter, Lobus superior   Pulmo sinister, Margo anterior

Pericardium fibrosum

Pleura parietalis, Pars diaphragmatica

(Nodi lymphoidei mediastinales anteriores)   ● Pars sternalis diaphragmatis

Sternum

Fig. 680   Thymus, Thymus, of an adolescent.

→ 781

Plexus brachialis, Pars infraclavicularis ●

Truncus sympathicus, Ganglion thoracicum II ●

N. vagus [X], N. laryngeus recurrens ●

N. vagus [X], Rr. cardiaci thoracici ●

N. vagus [X], Plexus pulmonalis ●

V. azygos ●

Bronchus principalis dexter

R. bronchialis (Aorta); ● ●
V. bronchialis

N. vagus [X], ●
Rr. cardiaci thoracici

V. intercostalis posterior ●

N. thoracicus [T 7], ●
N. intercostalis

Truncus sympathicus, ●
Rr. communicantes

N. splanchnicus ●
major

Aa. intercostales ●
posteriores

Pleura parietalis,
Pars costalis

Diaphragma, Centrum tendineum ●

● A. subclavia

Clavicula

● M. subclavius

● M. scalenus anterior

● V. subclavia

● A. thoracica interna

○ N. phrenicus

● V. brachiocephalica dextra

Thymus

● V. cava superior

● Aa. pulmonales

○ ● ● N. phrenicus; A.; V.
pericardiacophrenica

● Vv. pulmonales

Pericardium
fibrosum;
Pleura parietalis,
Pars mediastinalis

Lig. pulmonale

● N. vagus [X],
Plexus
oesophageus

Pleura parietalis,
Pars costalis

Oesophagus

● Diaphragma; Pleura parietalis, Pars diaphragmatica

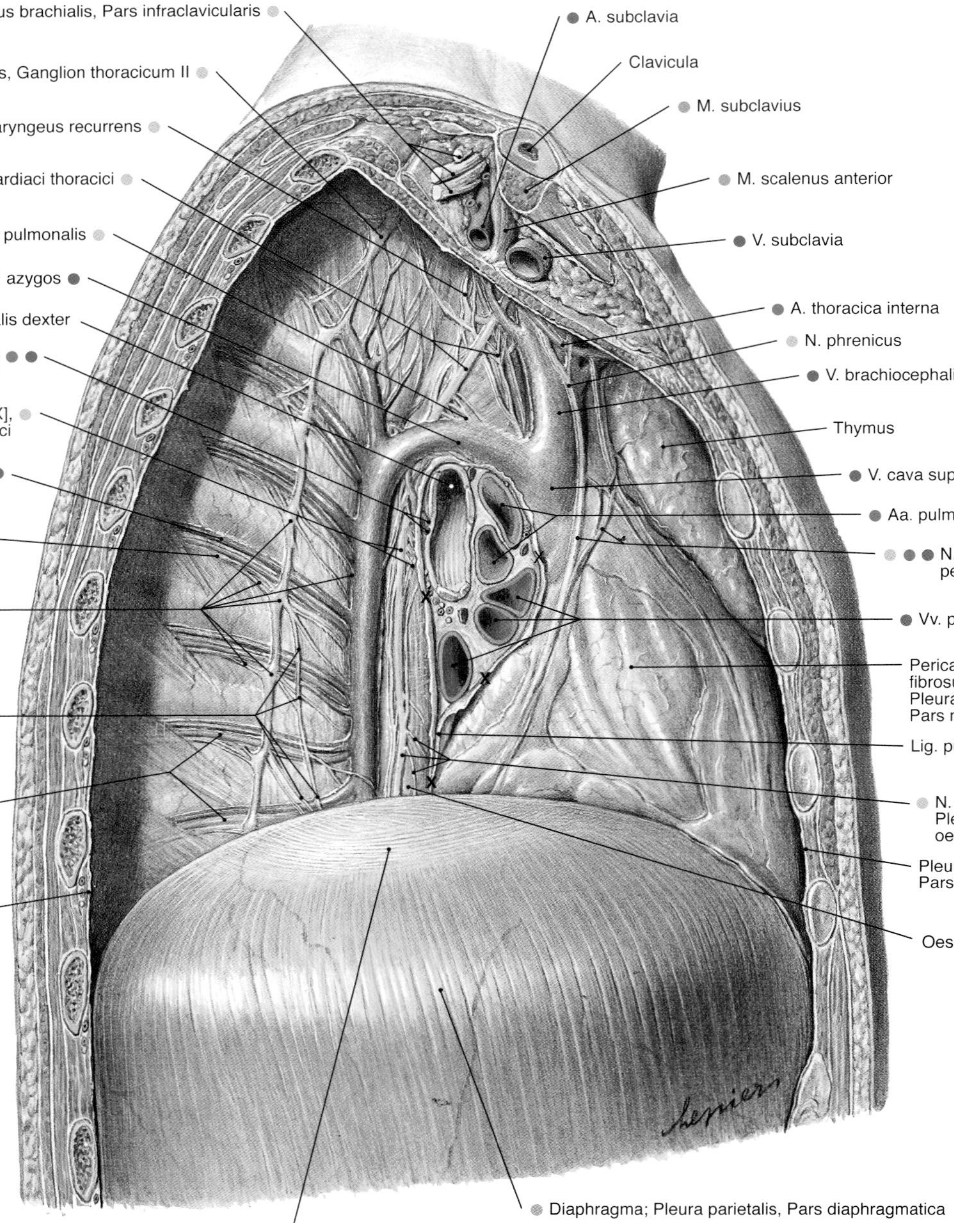

Fig. 681 Pleural cavity, Cavitas pleuralis, and mediastinum,
Mediastinum, of an adolescent;
lateral thoracic wall and right lung have been removed;
viewed from the right.
The x indicate the areas at the root of the lung and the
pulmonary ligament, respectively, where the visceral pleura
folds back into the parietal pleura.

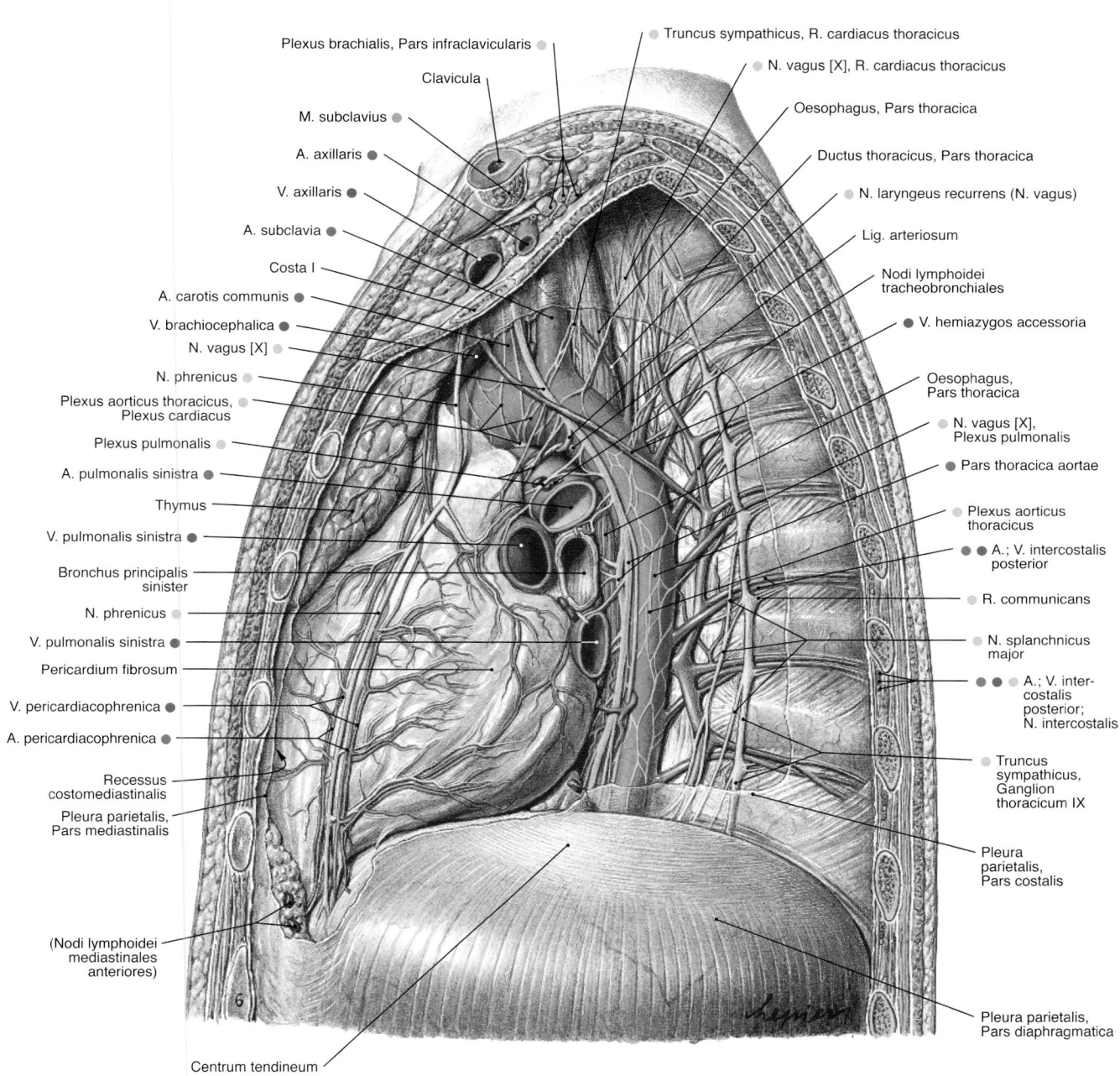

Plexus brachialis, Pars infraclavicularis
Clavicula
M. subclavius
A. axillaris
V. axillaris
A. subclavia
Costa I
A. carotis communis
V. brachiocephalica
N. vagus [X]
N. phrenicus
Plexus aorticus thoracicus, Plexus cardiacus
Plexus pulmonalis
A. pulmonalis sinistra
Thymus
V. pulmonalis sinistra
Bronchus principalis sinister
N. phrenicus
V. pulmonalis sinistra
Pericardium fibrosum
V. pericardiacophrenica
A. pericardiacophrenica
Recessus costomediastinalis
Pleura parietalis, Pars mediastinalis
(Nodi lymphoidei mediastinales anteriores)
Centrum tendineum

Truncus sympathicus, R. cardiacus thoracicus
N. vagus [X], R. cardiacus thoracicus
Oesophagus, Pars thoracica
Ductus thoracicus, Pars thoracica
N. laryngeus recurrens (N. vagus)
Lig. arteriosum
Nodi lymphoidei tracheobronchiales
V. hemiazygos accessoria
Oesophagus, Pars thoracica
N. vagus [X], Plexus pulmonalis
Pars thoracica aortae
Plexus aorticus thoracicus
A.; V. intercostalis posterior
R. communicans
N. splanchnicus major
A.; V. intercostalis posterior; N. intercostalis
Truncus sympathicus, Ganglion thoracicum IX
Pleura parietalis, Pars costalis
Pleura parietalis, Pars diaphragmatica

6

Fig. 682   Pleural cavity, Cavitas pleuralis, and mediastinum,
Mediastinum, of an adolescent;
viewed from the left.
In older individuals, the thymic tissue is almost entirely
replaced by adipose tissue.

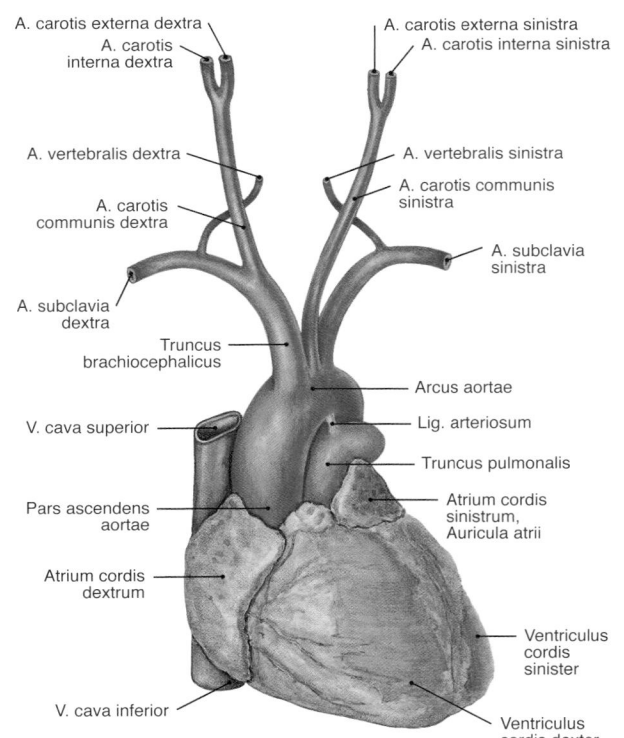

Fig. 683   Heart, Cor, and aortic arch, Arcus aortae, with the origins of the major arteries; ventral view.

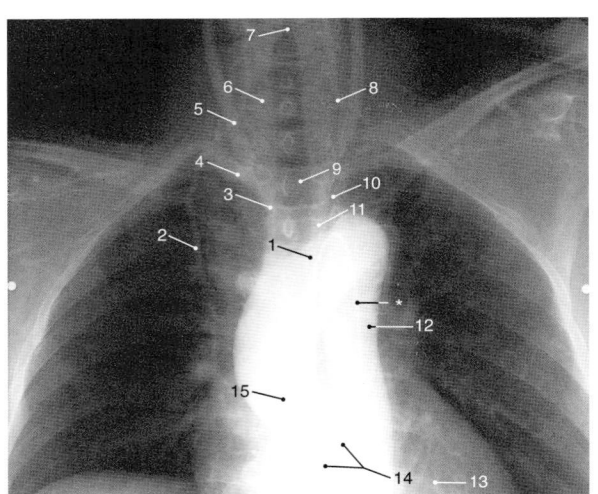

1	Arcus aortae	9	Trachea
2	A. thoracica interna	10	A. subclavia sinistra
3	Truncus brachiocephalicus	11	A. carotis communis sinistra
4	A. subclavia dextra	12	Pars descendens aortae
5	A. carotis communis dextra	13	Cor
6	A. vertebralis dextra	14	Valva aortae
7	Rima glottidis	15	Pars ascendens aortae
8	A. vertebralis sinistra		

Fig. 684   Aortic arch, Arcus aortae, and branches; AP-radiograph after injection of a contrast medium into the aortic bulb; ventral view.
* Catheter

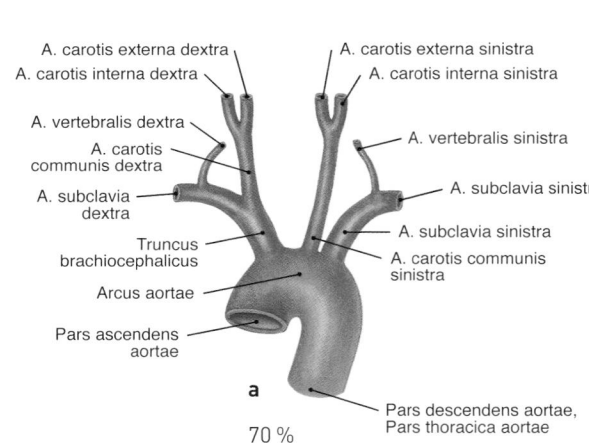

Fig. 685 a–e   Variability of the origin of the major arteries from the aortic arch, Arcus aortae.
a   "Textbook case"
b   Common origin of the brachiocephalic trunk and the left common carotid artery
c   Common trunk for the brachiocephalic trunk and the left common carotid artery

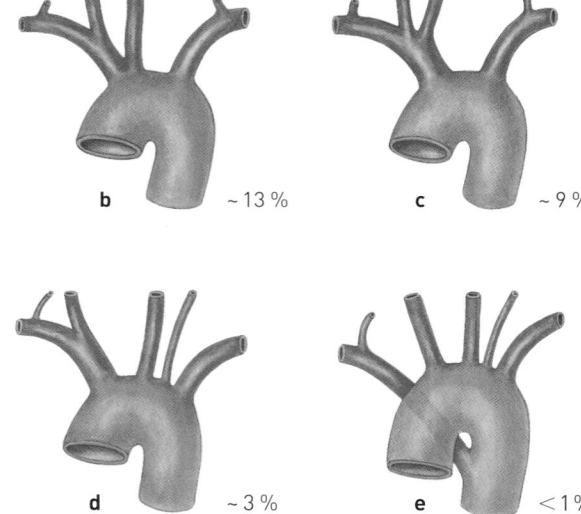

d   Left vertebral artery branching off the aortic arch independently
e   Right subclavian artery as the ultimate branch of the aortic arch
     This abnormal artery frequently passes behind the oesophagus to the right, which can result in swallowing difficulties (Dysphagia lusoria).

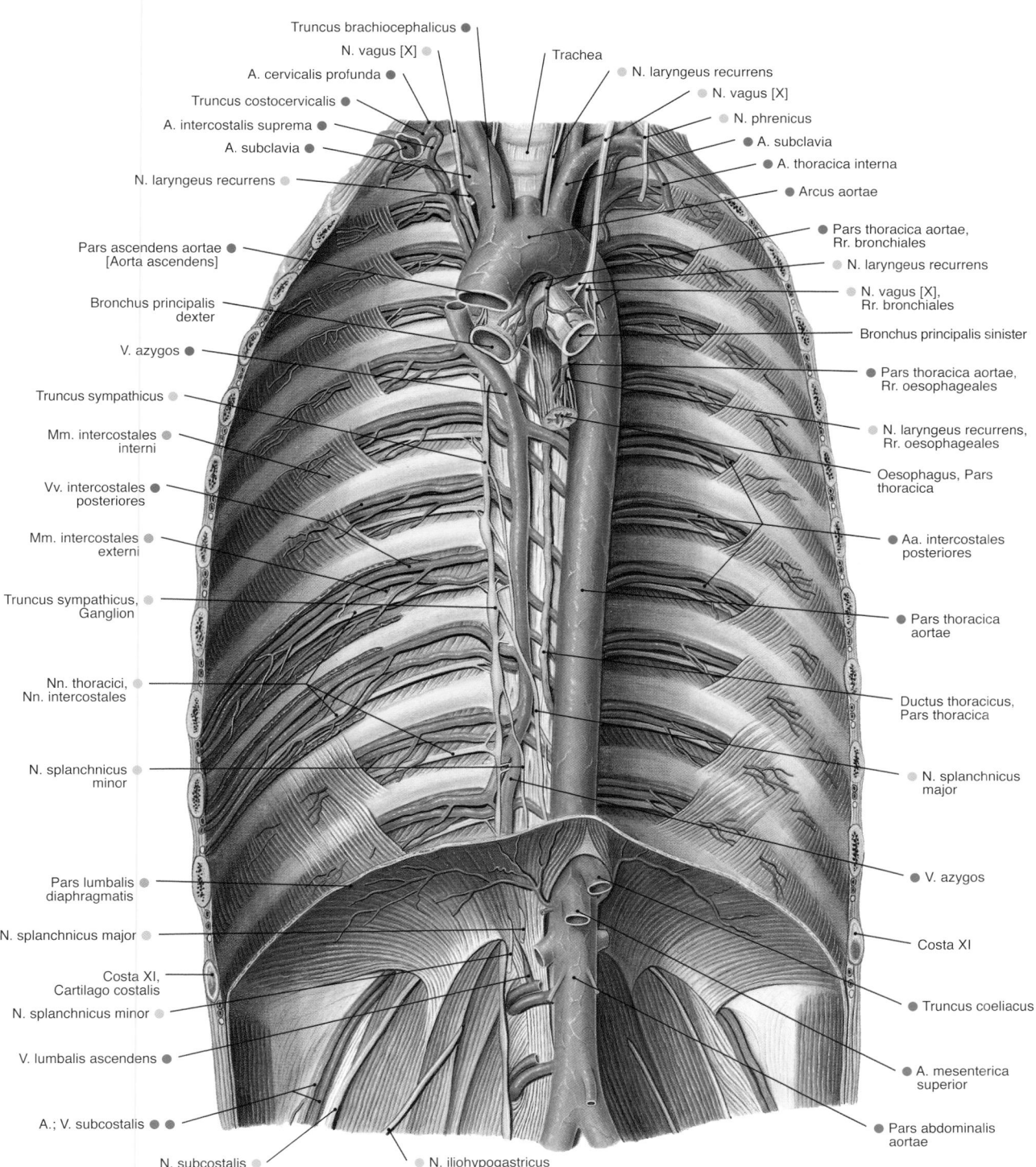

Truncus brachiocephalicus ●
N. vagus [X] ●
A. cervicalis profunda ●
Truncus costocervicalis ●
A. intercostalis suprema ●
A. subclavia ●
N. laryngeus recurrens ●

Trachea
● N. laryngeus recurrens
● N. vagus [X]
● N. phrenicus
● A. subclavia
● A. thoracica interna
● Arcus aortae

Pars ascendens aortae ●
[Aorta ascendens]

Bronchus principalis
dexter

V. azygos ●

Truncus sympathicus ●

Mm. intercostales ●
interni

Vv. intercostales ●
posteriores

Mm. intercostales ●
externi

Truncus sympathicus, ●
Ganglion

Nn. thoracici, ●
Nn. intercostales

N. splanchnicus ●
minor

Pars lumbalis ●
diaphragmatis

N. splanchnicus major ●

Costa XI, ●
Cartilago costalis

N. splanchnicus minor ●

V. lumbalis ascendens ●

A.; V. subcostalis ● ●

N. subcostalis ●

● Pars thoracica aortae,
Rr. bronchiales
● N. laryngeus recurrens
● N. vagus [X],
Rr. bronchiales

Bronchus principalis sinister

● Pars thoracica aortae,
Rr. oesophageales

● N. laryngeus recurrens,
Rr. oesophageales

Oesophagus, Pars
thoracica

● Aa. intercostales
posteriores

● Pars thoracica
aortae

Ductus thoracicus,
Pars thoracica

● N. splanchnicus
major

● V. azygos

● Costa XI

● Truncus coeliacus

● A. mesenterica
superior

● Pars abdominalis
aortae

N. iliohypogastricus ●

Fig. 686 Thoracic and abdominal aorta, Pars thoracica
aortae et Pars abdominalis aortae.

Posterior mediastinum

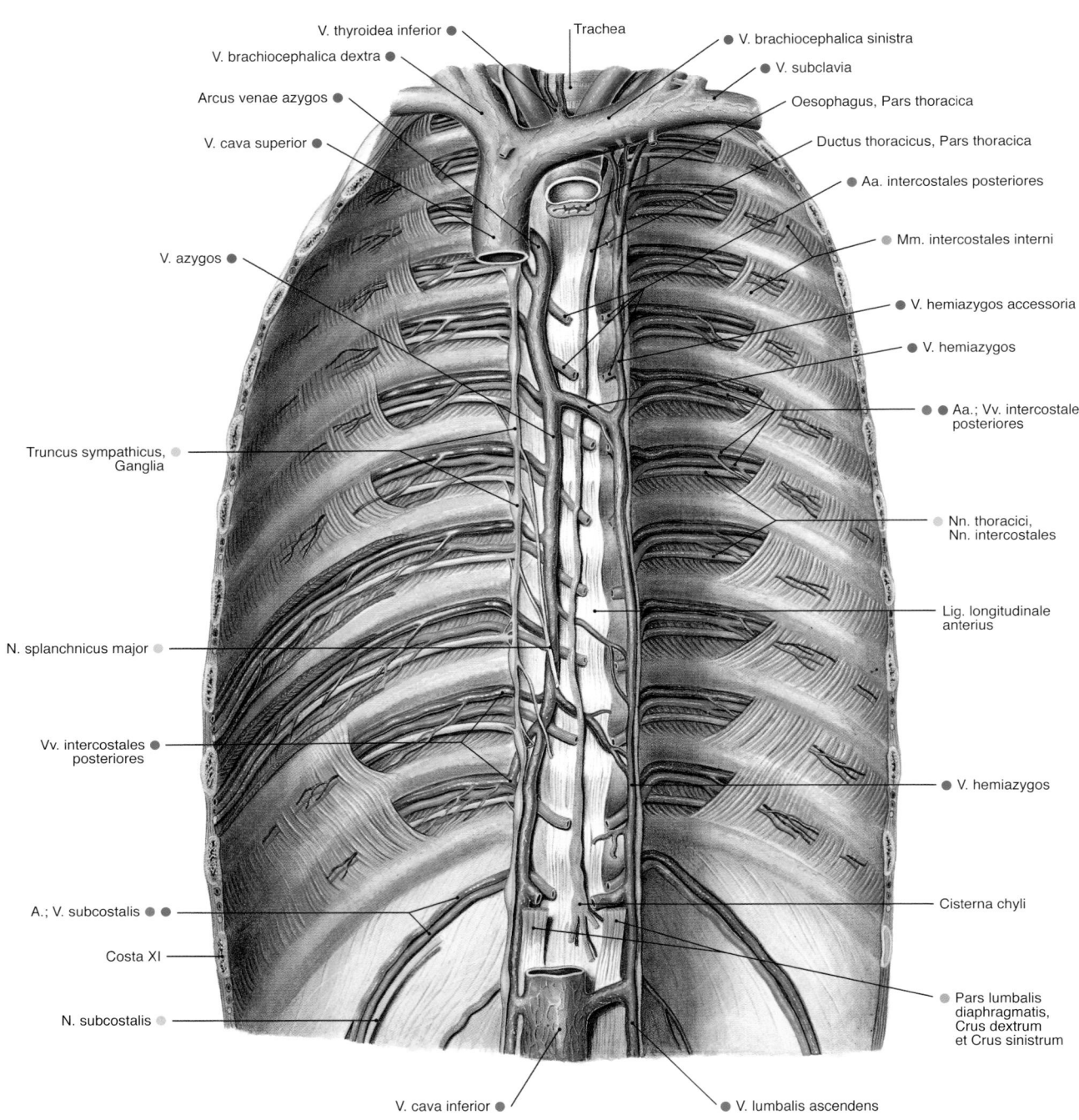

V. thyroidea inferior ●
Trachea
● V. brachiocephalica sinistra
V. brachiocephalica dextra ●
● V. subclavia
Arcus venae azygos ●
Oesophagus, Pars thoracica
V. cava superior ●
Ductus thoracicus, Pars thoracica
● Aa. intercostales posteriores
● Mm. intercostales interni
V. azygos ●
● V. hemiazygos accessoria
● V. hemiazygos
● ● Aa.; Vv. intercostales posteriores
Truncus sympathicus, ● Ganglia
● Nn. thoracici, Nn. intercostales
Lig. longitudinale anterius
N. splanchnicus major ●
Vv. intercostales ● posteriores
● V. hemiazygos
A.; V. subcostalis ● ●
Cisterna chyli
Costa XI
● Pars lumbalis diaphragmatis, Crus dextrum et Crus sinistrum
N. subcostalis ●
V. cava inferior ●
● V. lumbalis ascendens

Fig. 687   Vessels and nerves of the posterior mediastinum, Mediastinum posterius.

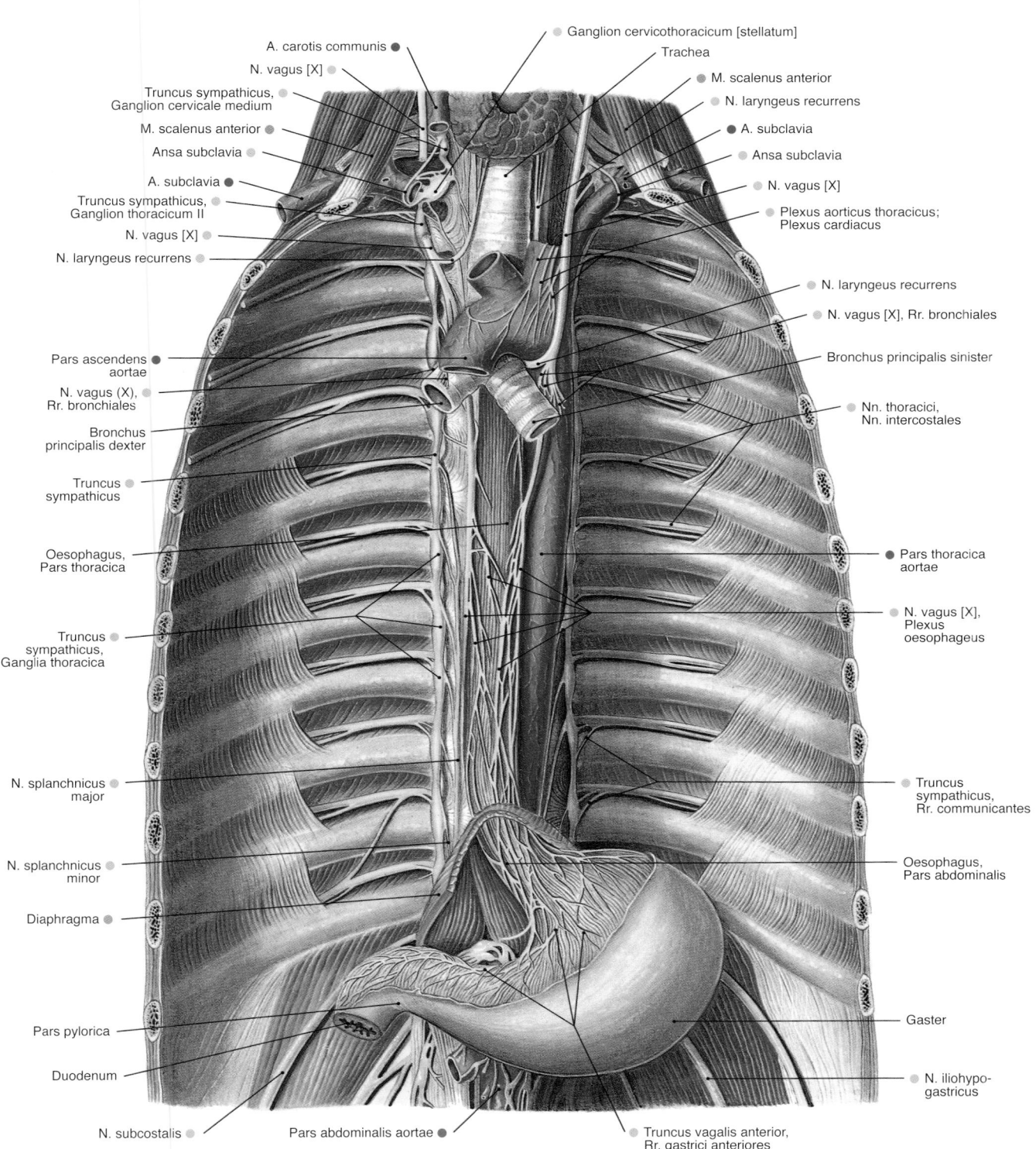

A. carotis communis ●
N. vagus [X] ●
Truncus sympathicus, ●
Ganglion cervicale medium
M. scalenus anterior ●
Ansa subclavia ●
A. subclavia ●
Truncus sympathicus, ●
Ganglion thoracicum II
N. vagus [X] ●
N. laryngeus recurrens ●

Ganglion cervicothoracicum [stellatum] ●
Trachea
● M. scalenus anterior
● N. laryngeus recurrens
● A. subclavia
● Ansa subclavia
● N. vagus [X]
● Plexus aorticus thoracicus; Plexus cardiacus

Pars ascendens ● aortae
N. vagus (X), ● Rr. bronchiales
Bronchus principalis dexter
Truncus ● sympathicus
Oesophagus, Pars thoracica
Truncus ● sympathicus, Ganglia thoracica

● N. laryngeus recurrens
● N. vagus [X], Rr. bronchiales
Bronchus principalis sinister
● Nn. thoracici, Nn. intercostales
● Pars thoracica aortae
● N. vagus [X], Plexus oesophageus

N. splanchnicus ● major
N. splanchnicus ● minor
Diaphragma ●
Pars pylorica
Duodenum

● Truncus sympathicus, Rr. communicantes
Oesophagus, Pars abdominalis
Gaster
● N. iliohypo-gastricus

N. subcostalis ●   Pars abdominalis aortae ●   ● Truncus vagalis anterior, Rr. gastrici anteriores

Fig. 688 Autonomous nervous system of the thoracic cavity, Pars thoracica autonomica.

→ 49, 50

Phrenic nerve

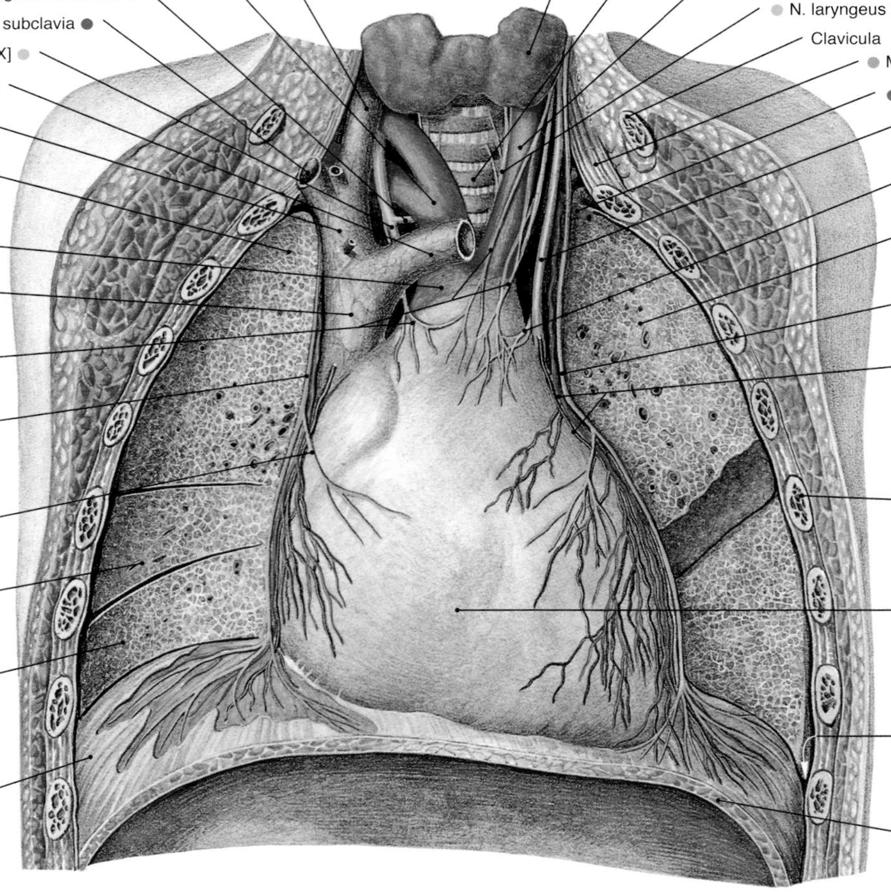

V. jugularis interna ●
Truncus brachiocephalicus ●
N. laryngeus recurrens ○
V. subclavia ●
N. vagus [X] ○
V. brachiocephalica sinistra ●
V. brachiocephalica ● dextra
Pulmo dexter, Lobus superior
Arcus aortae ●
V. cava ● superior
Plexus ○ cardiacus
N. phrenicus ○
N. phrenicus, ○ R. pericardiacus
Pulmo dexter, Lobus medius
Pulmo dexter, Lobus inferior
Pleura parietalis, Pars diaphragmatica

Glandula thyroidea
Trachea
● A. carotis communis
○ N. laryngeus recurrens
Clavicula
● M. scalenus anterior
● A. thoracica interna
○ N. vagus [X]
○ N. vagus [X], Rr. cardiaci thoracici
Pulmo sinister, Lobus superior
○ N. phrenicus
● ● A.; V. pericardiacophrenica
Costa V
Pericardium
Recessus costodiaphragmaticus
● Diaphragma

Fig. 689   Thoracic viscera of an adult; the anterior thoracic wall has been removed, and the right and the left lung have been sectioned in the frontal plane; ventral view.

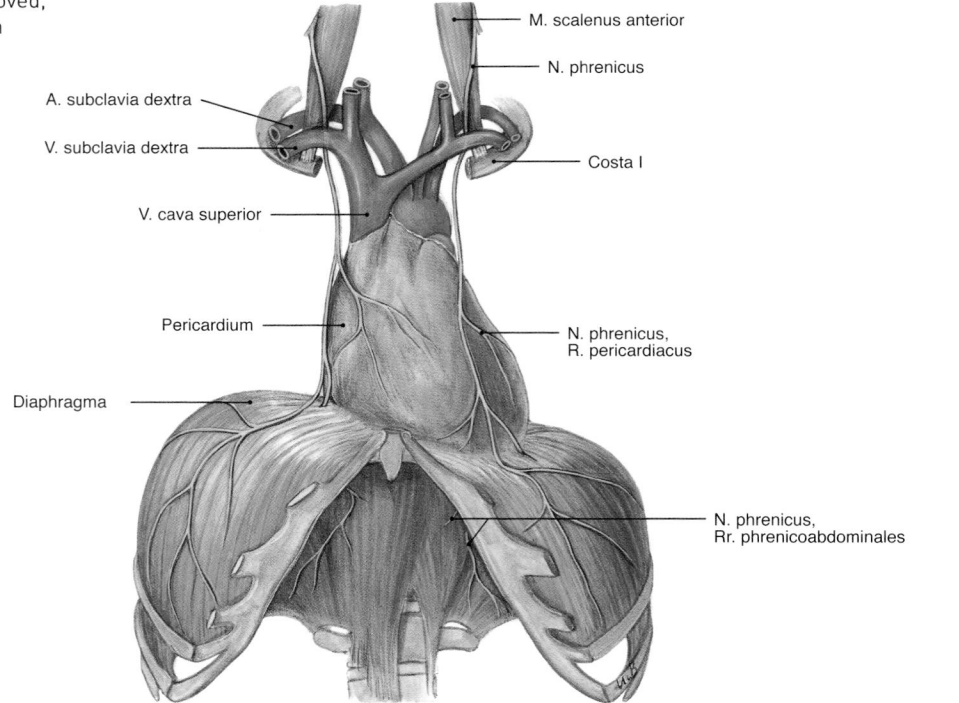

M. scalenus anterior
N. phrenicus
A. subclavia dextra
V. subclavia dextra
Costa I
V. cava superior
Pericardium
N. phrenicus, R. pericardiacus
Diaphragma
N. phrenicus, Rr. phrenicoabdominales

Fig. 690   Course of the phrenic nerve, N. phrenicus.

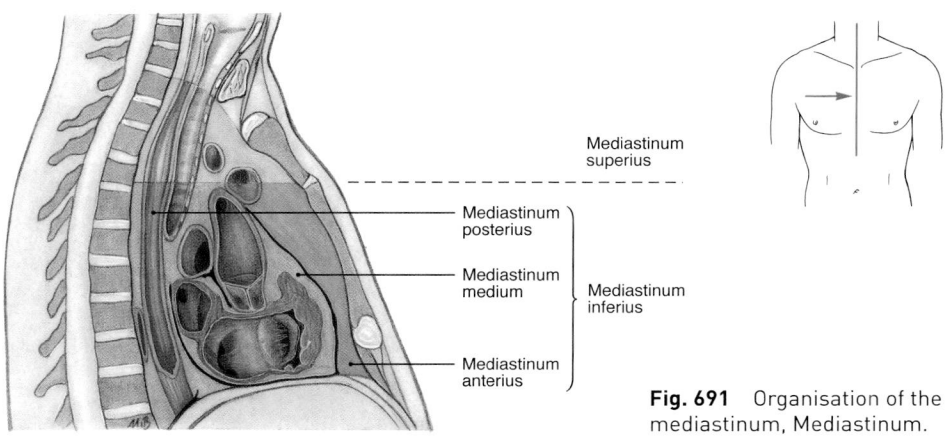

Mediastinum superius

Mediastinum posterius
Mediastinum medium
Mediastinum anterius

Mediastinum inferius

Fig. 691 Organisation of the mediastinum, Mediastinum.

M. arytenoideus transversus ●
Oesophagus, Pars cervicalis
Cartilago cricoidea, Lamina
Cavitas infraglottica
Lig. vocale
Trachea, Paries membranaceus
Cartilago thyroidea
Vertebra cervicalis VII [prominens]
● M. sternothyroideus
Bronchus principalis sinister
Fascia cervicalis, Lamina superficialis
● V. jugularis anterior
Nodi lymphoidei tracheobronchiales superiores
Glandula thyroidea
Cartilagines tracheales
Vertebra cervicalis VII [prominens], Proc. spinosus
● M. sternocleidomastoideus
Articulatio sternoclavicularis
Ligg. interspinalia
Manubrium sterni
● Truncus brachiocephalicus
Bifurcatio tracheae, Carina tracheae
● M. pectoralis major
Vv. basivertebrales ●
● V. brachiocephalica sinistra
Bronchus principalis dexter
● Arcus aortae
Nodus lymphoideus tracheobronchialis inferior
Corpus sterni
● Pars ascendens aortae
Thymus
Plexus venosus ● vertebralis internus posterior
Valva aortae, Valvulae semilunares sinistra, posterior et dextra
M. interspinalis ●
● A. coronaria sinistra
A. pulmonalis dextra ●
Myocardium
Oesophagus, Pars thoracica
V. pulmonalis sinistra ●
Valva atrioventricularis dextra [Valva tricuspidalis]
Sinus transversus pericardii
V. hemiazygos ●
Costae VI; VII
Atrium cordis sinistrum
Septum interatriale
Cavitas pericardiaca
A. coronaria dextra; ● ●
V. cardiaca media
Sternum, Proc. xiphoideus
Medulla spinalis
● M. rectus abdominis
Dura mater spinalis
● Pars sternalis diaphragmatis
Spatium subarachnoideum

Oesophagus, Tunica muscularis
Hepar
Lamina visceralis [Epicardium]
Pericardium serosum
Pars lumbalis diaphragmatis ●
Hepar, Area nuda
Lamina parietalis
Nodus lymphoideus phrenicus superior
Atrium cordis dextrum

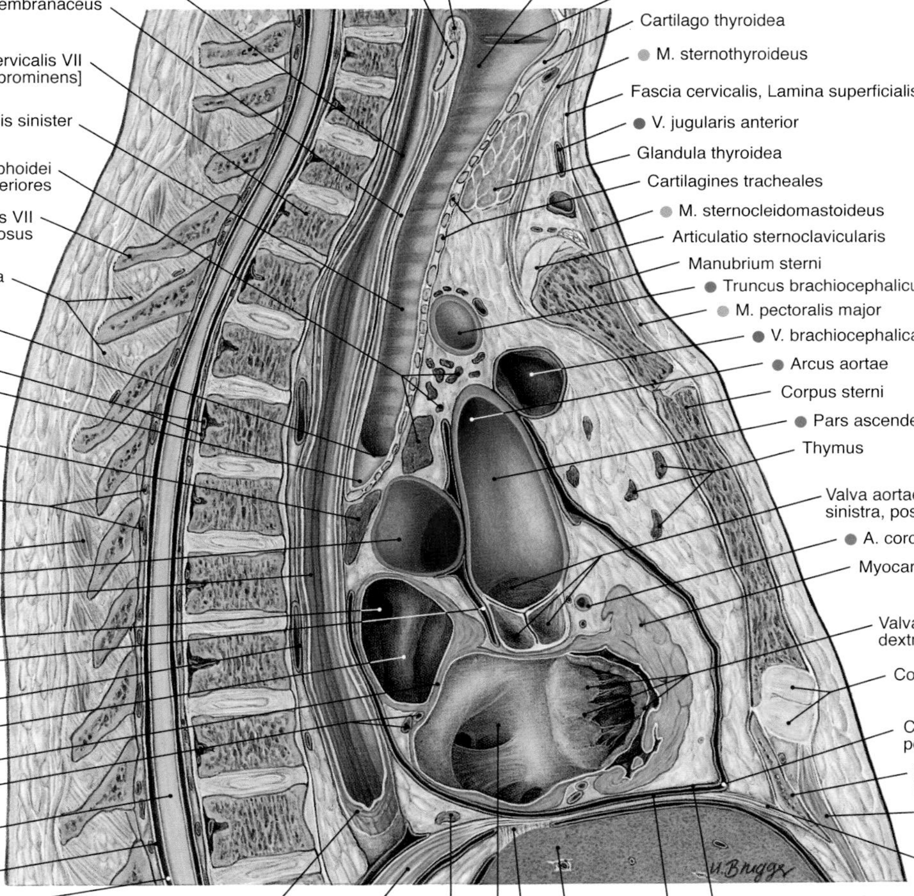

Fig. 692 Thoracic cavity, Cavitas thoracis, and mediastinum, Mediastinum; median sagittal section through the neck and the thorax; lateral view from the right.

Thorax, frontal sections

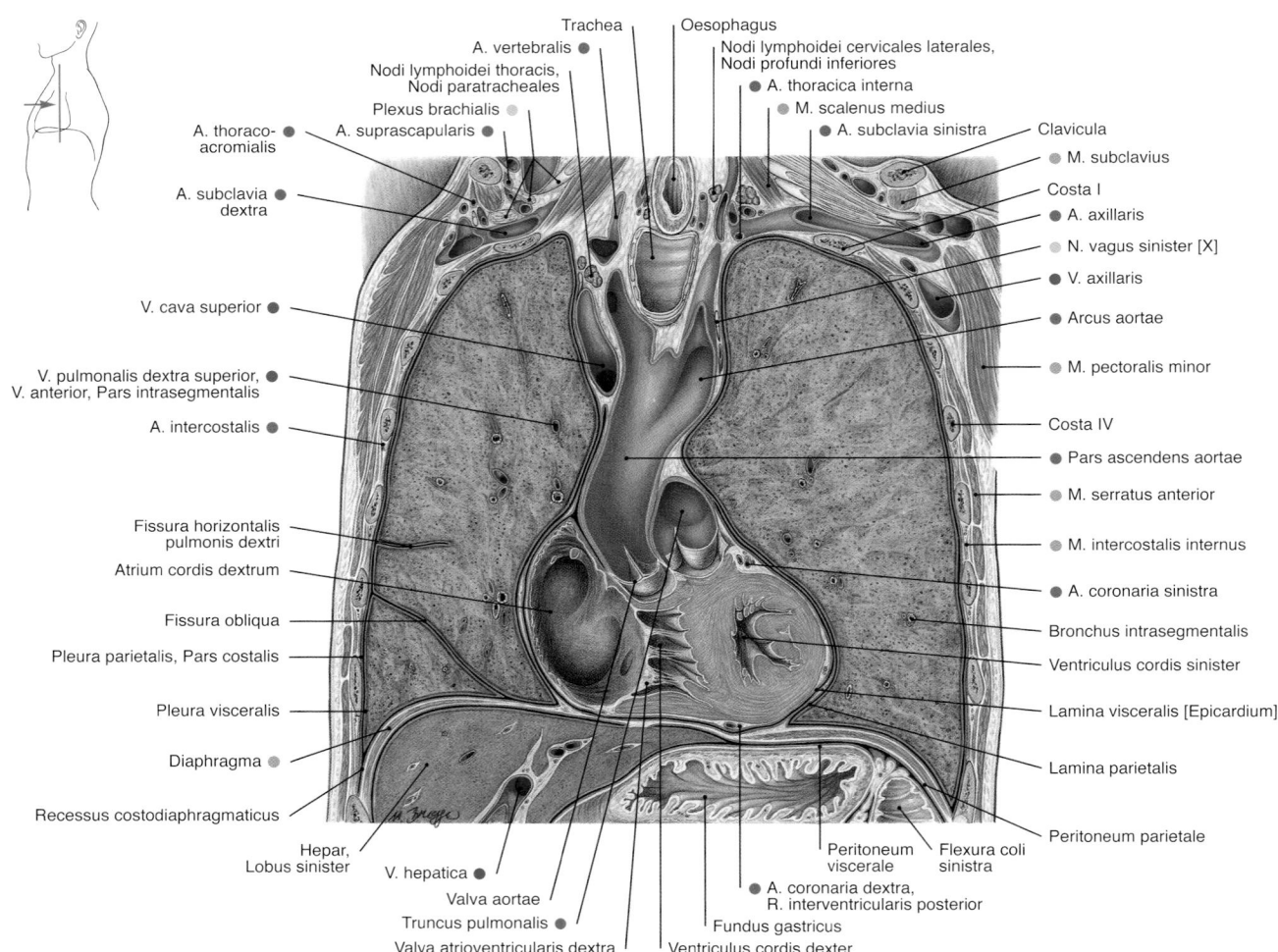

Trachea
Oesophagus
A. vertebralis ●
Nodi lymphoidei cervicales laterales,
Nodi profundi inferiores
Nodi lymphoidei thoracis,
Nodi paratracheales
● A. thoracica interna
Plexus brachialis ●
● M. scalenus medius
A. thoraco-
acromialis ●
A. suprascapularis ●
● A. subclavia sinistra
Clavicula
● M. subclavius
A. subclavia
dextra ●
Costa I
● A. axillaris
● N. vagus sinister [X]
V. cava superior ●
● V. axillaris
● Arcus aortae
V. pulmonalis dextra superior, ●
V. anterior, Pars intrasegmentalis
● M. pectoralis minor
A. intercostalis ●
Costa IV
● Pars ascendens aortae
● M. serratus anterior
Fissura horizontalis
pulmonis dextri
● M. intercostalis internus
Atrium cordis dextrum
● A. coronaria sinistra
Fissura obliqua
Bronchus intrasegmentalis
Pleura parietalis, Pars costalis
Ventriculus cordis sinister
Pleura visceralis
Lamina visceralis [Epicardium]
Diaphragma ●
Lamina parietalis
Recessus costodiaphragmaticus
Peritoneum parietale
Hepar,
Lobus sinister
Peritoneum
viscerale
Flexura coli
sinistra
V. hepatica ●
Valva aortae
● A. coronaria dextra,
R. interventricularis posterior
Truncus pulmonalis ●
Fundus gastricus
Valva atrioventricularis dextra
Ventriculus cordis dexter

Fig. 693   Thoracic cavity, Cavitas thoracis.

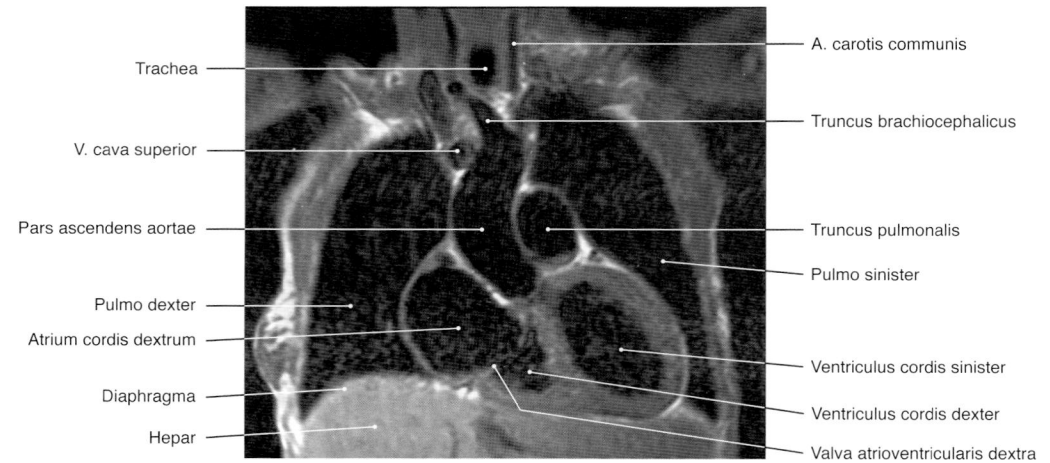

Trachea
A. carotis communis
V. cava superior
Truncus brachiocephalicus
Pars ascendens aortae
Truncus pulmonalis
Pulmo dexter
Pulmo sinister
Atrium cordis dextrum
Diaphragma
Ventriculus cordis sinister
Hepar
Ventriculus cordis dexter
Valva atrioventricularis dextra

Fig. 694   Thoracic cavity, Cavitas thoracis;
magnetic resonance tomographic image (MRI);
frontal section at the level of the superior vena cava;
ventral view.

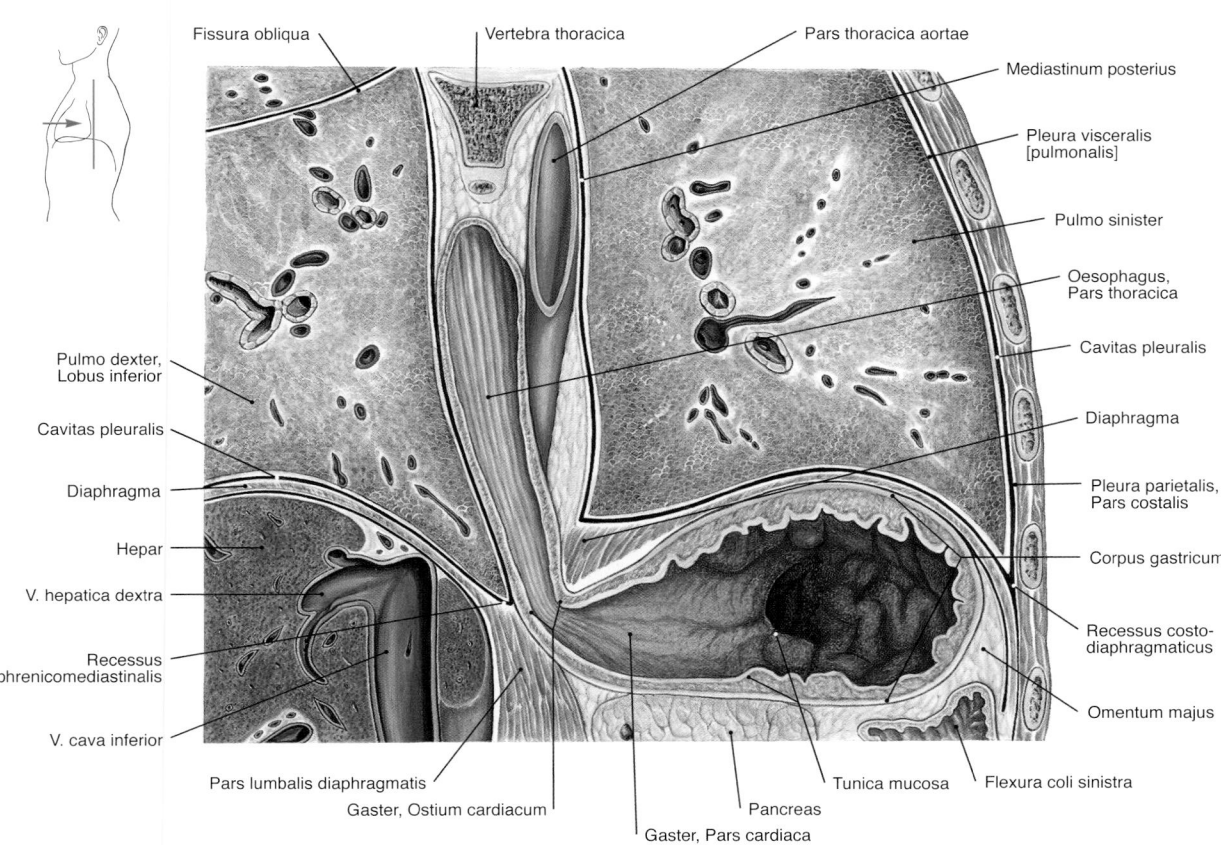

Fissura obliqua
Vertebra thoracica
Pars thoracica aortae
Mediastinum posterius
Pleura visceralis [pulmonalis]
Pulmo sinister
Oesophagus, Pars thoracica
Cavitas pleuralis
Diaphragma
Pleura parietalis, Pars costalis
Corpus gastricum
Recessus costo-diaphragmaticus
Omentum majus
Flexura coli sinistra
Tunica mucosa
Pancreas
Gaster, Pars cardiaca
Gaster, Ostium cardiacum
Pars lumbalis diaphragmatis
V. cava inferior
Recessus phrenicomediastinalis
V. hepatica dextra
Hepar
Diaphragma
Cavitas pleuralis
Pulmo dexter, Lobus inferior

Fig. 695 Diaphragm, Diaphragma, and oesophagus, Oesophagus, with its transition into the stomach, Gaster; frontal section through the lower part of the thoracic cavity and the upper part of the abdominal cavity.

→ 919

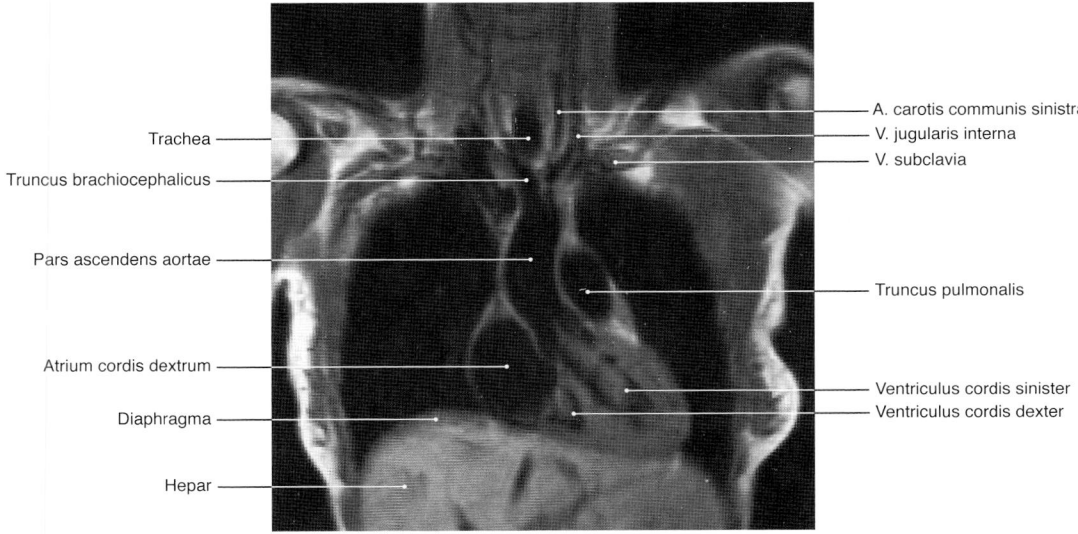

Trachea
Truncus brachiocephalicus
Pars ascendens aortae
Atrium cordis dextrum
Diaphragma
Hepar
A. carotis communis sinistra
V. jugularis interna
V. subclavia
Truncus pulmonalis
Ventriculus cordis sinister
Ventriculus cordis dexter

Fig. 696 Thoracic cavity, Cavitas thoracis; magnetic resonance tomographic image (MRI); frontal section at the level of the aortic valve; ventral view.

Thorax, frontal sections

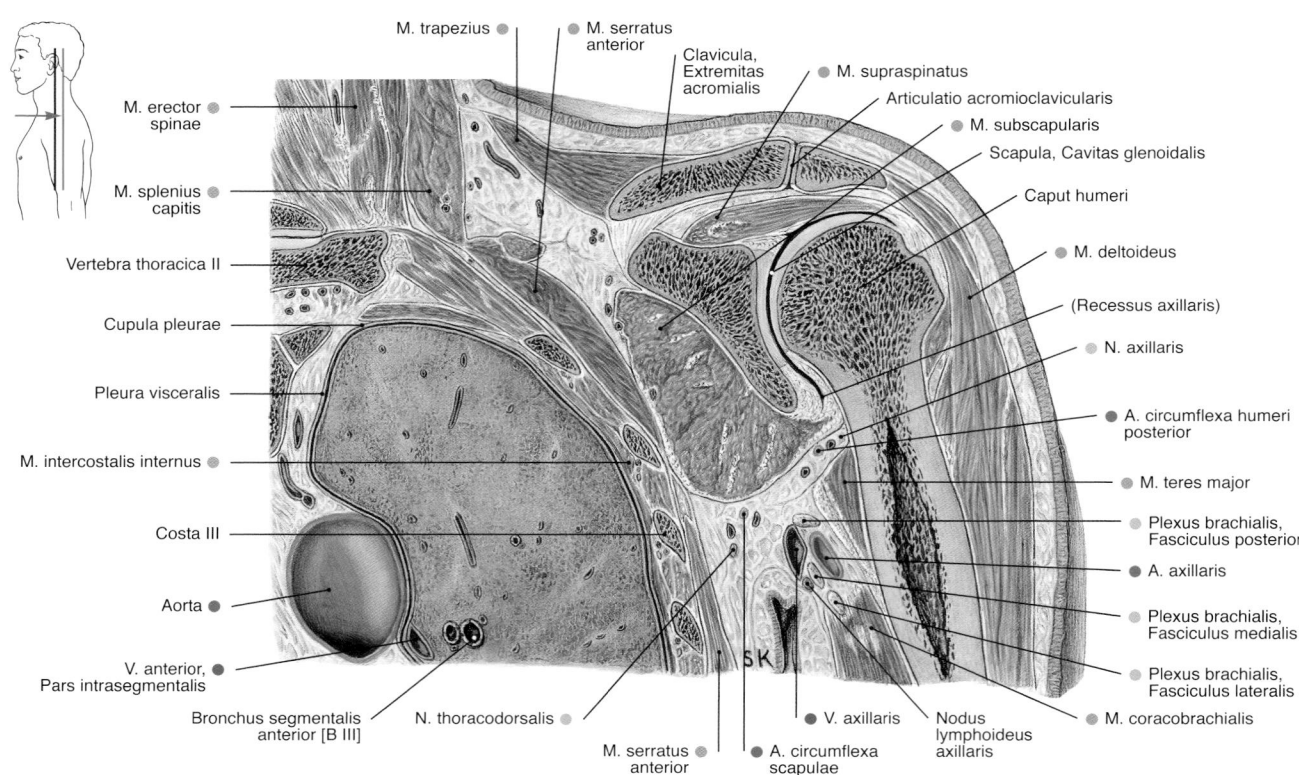

M. trapezius

M. serratus anterior

Clavicula, Extremitas acromialis

M. supraspinatus

Articulatio acromioclavicularis

M. subscapularis

Scapula, Cavitas glenoidalis

Caput humeri

M. deltoideus

(Recessus axillaris)

N. axillaris

A. circumflexa humeri posterior

M. teres major

Plexus brachialis, Fasciculus posterior

A. axillaris

Plexus brachialis, Fasciculus medialis

Plexus brachialis, Fasciculus lateralis

M. coracobrachialis

M. erector spinae

M. splenius capitis

Vertebra thoracica II

Cupula pleurae

Pleura visceralis

M. intercostalis internus

Costa III

Aorta

V. anterior, Pars intrasegmentalis

Bronchus segmentalis anterior [B III]

N. thoracodorsalis

M. serratus anterior

A. circumflexa scapulae

V. axillaris

Nodus lymphoideus axillaris

Fig. 697 Thoracic cavity, Cavitas thoracis; axilla, Axilla, and shoulder joint, Articulatio humeri.

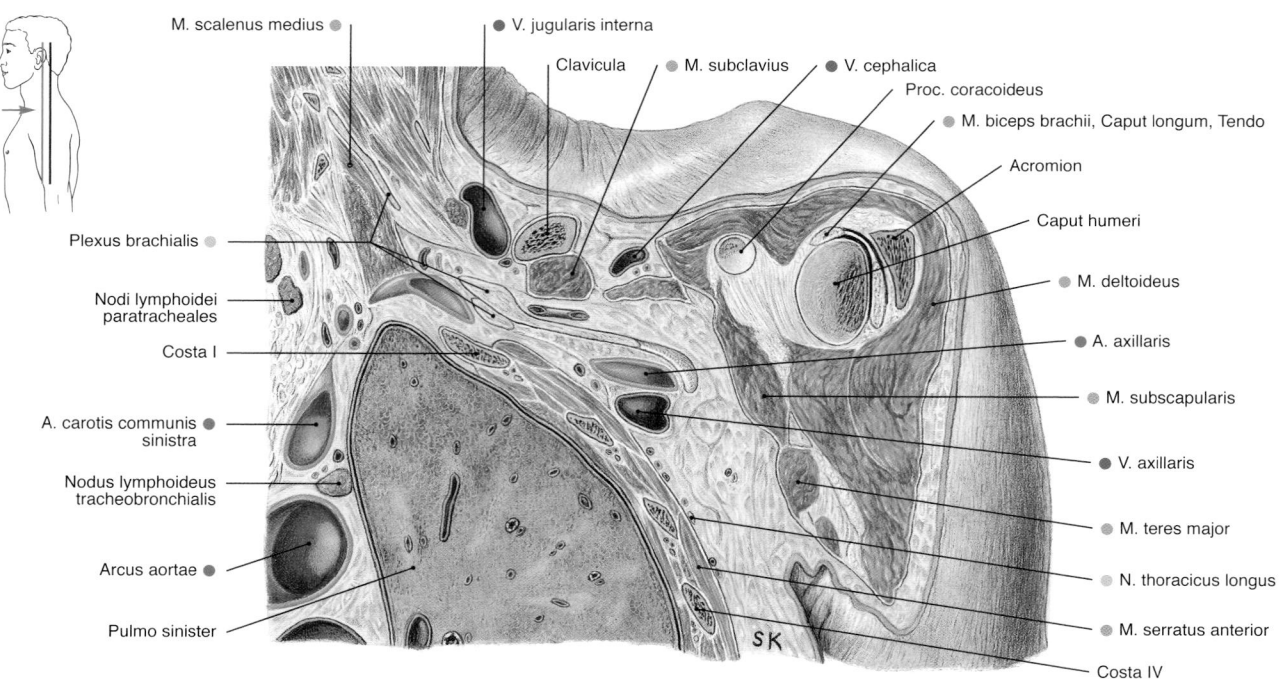

M. scalenus medius

V. jugularis interna

Clavicula

M. subclavius

V. cephalica

Proc. coracoideus

M. biceps brachii, Caput longum, Tendo

Acromion

Caput humeri

M. deltoideus

A. axillaris

M. subscapularis

V. axillaris

M. teres major

N. thoracicus longus

M. serratus anterior

Costa IV

Plexus brachialis

Nodi lymphoidei paratracheales

Costa I

A. carotis communis sinistra

Nodus lymphoideus tracheobronchialis

Arcus aortae

Pulmo sinister

Fig. 698 Thoracic cavity, Cavitas thoracis; axilla, Axilla, and shoulder joint, Articulatio humeri.

Thorax, transverse section

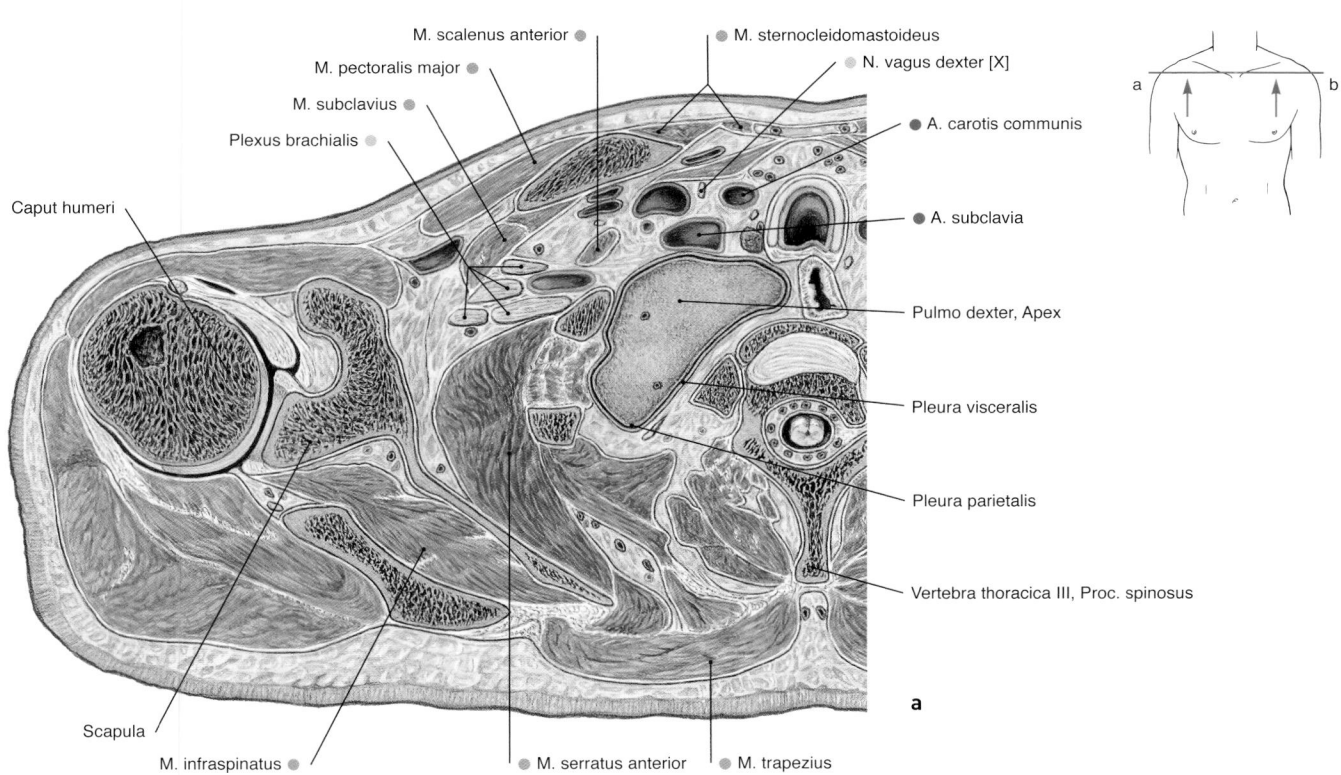

M. scalenus anterior ●
M. pectoralis major ●
M. subclavius ●
Plexus brachialis ●
● M. sternocleidomastoideus
● N. vagus dexter [X]
● A. carotis communis
● A. subclavia
Caput humeri
Pulmo dexter, Apex
Pleura visceralis
Pleura parietalis
Vertebra thoracica III, Proc. spinosus
Scapula
M. infraspinatus ●
● M. serratus anterior
● M. trapezius

a

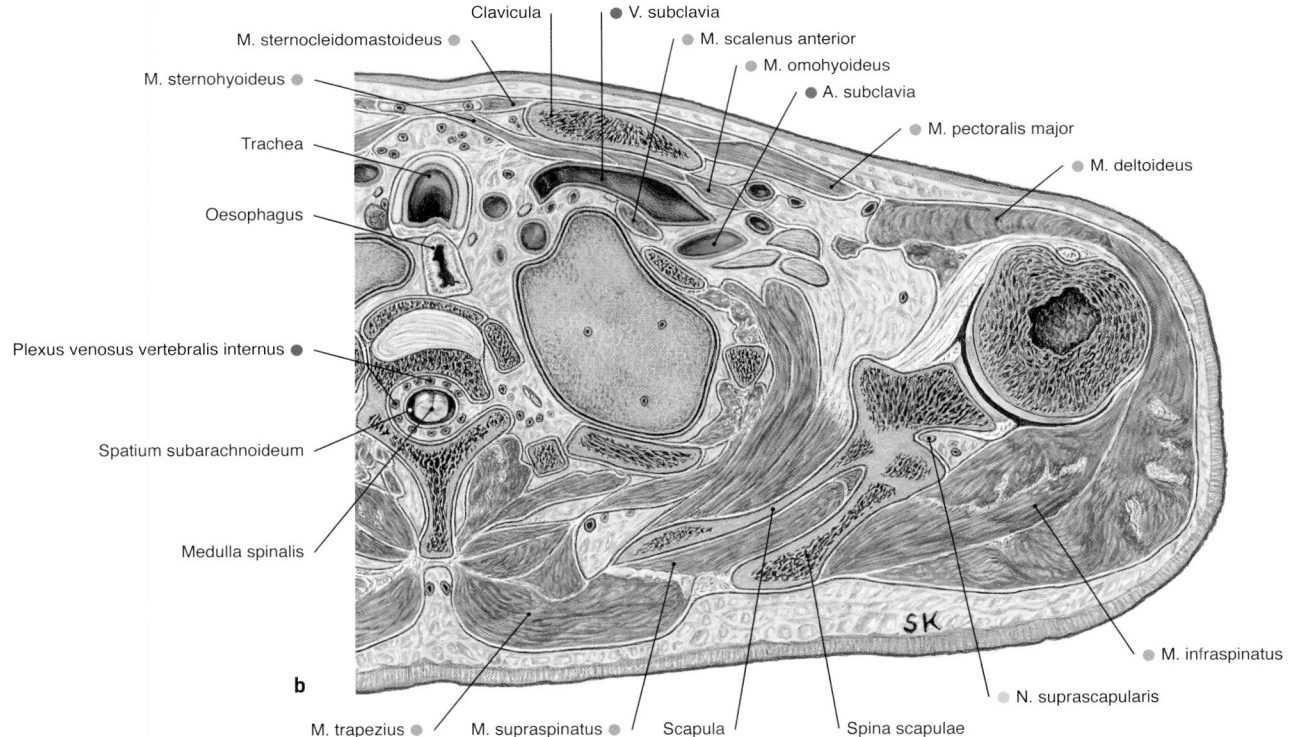

Clavicula
● V. subclavia
M. sternocleidomastoideus ●
● M. scalenus anterior
M. sternohyoideus ●
● M. omohyoideus
● A. subclavia
Trachea
● M. pectoralis major
Oesophagus
● M. deltoideus
Plexus venosus vertebralis internus ●
Spatium subarachnoideum
Medulla spinalis
● M. infraspinatus
● N. suprascapularis
SK
b
M. trapezius ●
● M. supraspinatus ●
Scapula
Spina scapulae

Fig. 699 a, b Thoracic cavity, Cavitas thoracis; axilla, Axilla,
and shoulder joint, Articulatio humeri.

a Right part of the body
b Left part of the body

→ 294

Thorax, transverse sections

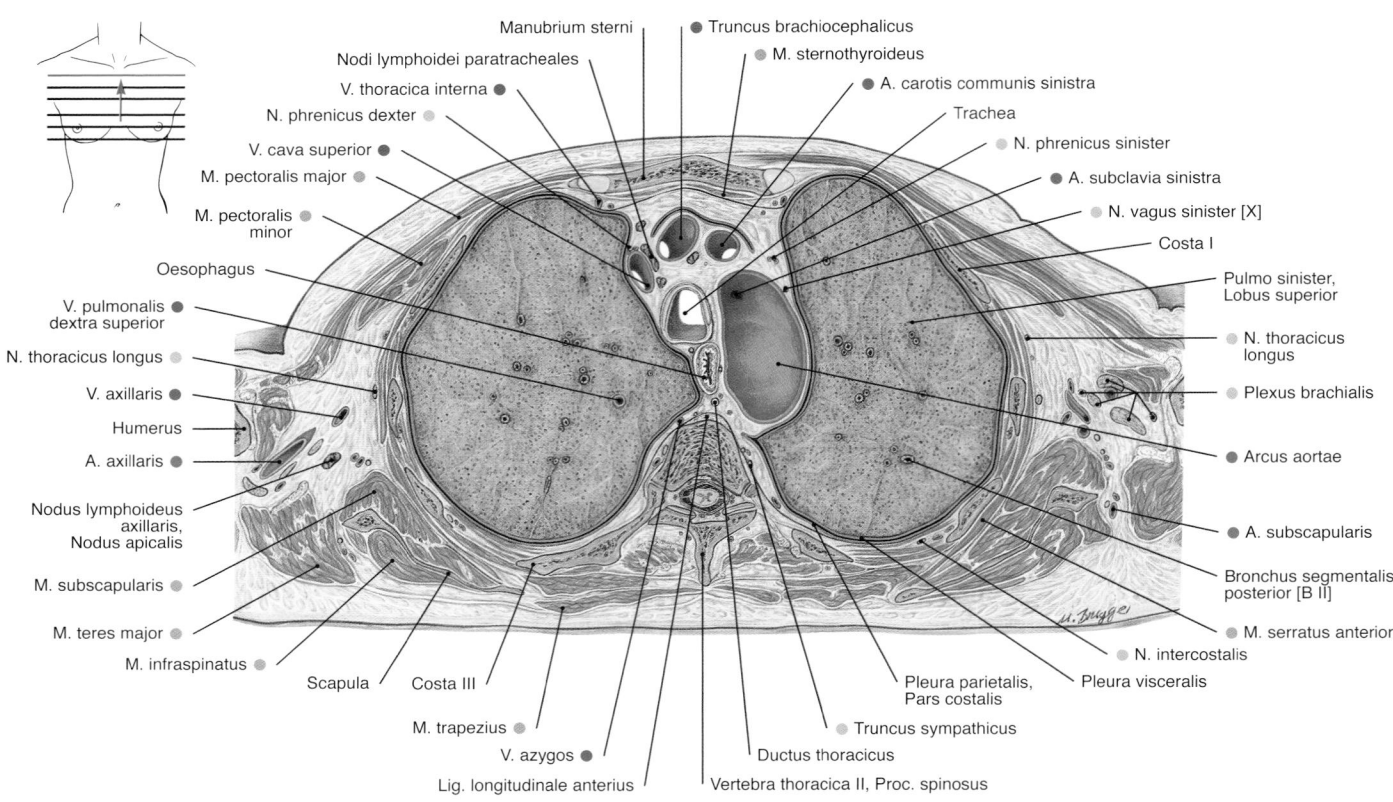

Manubrium sterni
Nodi lymphoidei paratracheales
V. thoracica interna ●
N. phrenicus dexter ●
V. cava superior ●
M. pectoralis major ●
M. pectoralis ● minor
Oesophagus
V. pulmonalis ● dextra superior
N. thoracicus longus ●
V. axillaris ●
Humerus
A. axillaris ●
Nodus lymphoideus axillaris, Nodus apicalis
M. subscapularis ●
M. teres major ●
M. infraspinatus ●
Scapula
Costa III
M. trapezius ●
V. azygos ●
Lig. longitudinale anterius

● Truncus brachiocephalicus
● M. sternothyroideus
● A. carotis communis sinistra
Trachea
● N. phrenicus sinister
● A. subclavia sinistra
● N. vagus sinister [X]
Costa I
Pulmo sinister, Lobus superior
● N. thoracicus longus
● Plexus brachialis
● Arcus aortae
● A. subscapularis
Bronchus segmentalis posterior [B II]
● M. serratus anterior
● N. intercostalis
Pleura visceralis
Pleura parietalis, Pars costalis
● Truncus sympathicus
Ductus thoracicus
Vertebra thoracica II, Proc. spinosus

Fig. 700 Thoracic cavity, Cavitas thoracis.

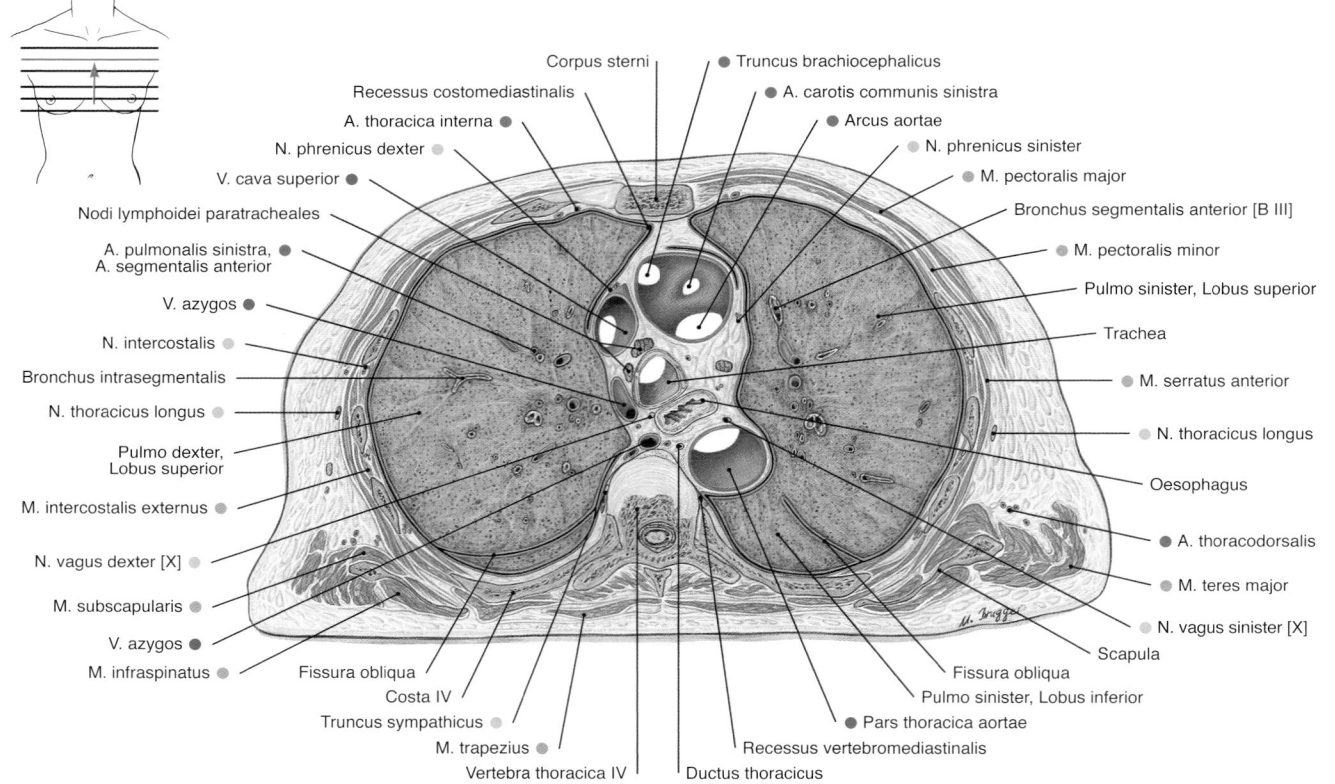

Corpus sterni
Recessus costomediastinalis
A. thoracica interna ●
N. phrenicus dexter ●
V. cava superior ●
Nodi lymphoidei paratracheales
A. pulmonalis sinistra, ● A. segmentalis anterior
V. azygos ●
N. intercostalis ●
Bronchus intrasegmentalis
N. thoracicus longus ●
Pulmo dexter, Lobus superior
M. intercostalis externus ●
N. vagus dexter [X] ●
M. subscapularis ●
V. azygos ●
M. infraspinatus ●
Fissura obliqua
Costa IV
Truncus sympathicus ●
M. trapezius ●
Vertebra thoracica IV

● Truncus brachiocephalicus
● A. carotis communis sinistra
● Arcus aortae
● N. phrenicus sinister
● M. pectoralis major
Bronchus segmentalis anterior [B III]
● M. pectoralis minor
Pulmo sinister, Lobus superior
Trachea
● M. serratus anterior
● N. thoracicus longus
Oesophagus
● A. thoracodorsalis
● M. teres major
● N. vagus sinister [X]
Scapula
Fissura obliqua
Pulmo sinister, Lobus inferior
● Pars thoracica aortae
Recessus vertebromediastinalis
Ductus thoracicus

Fig. 701 Thoracic cavity, Cavitas thoracis.

Thorax, transverse sections

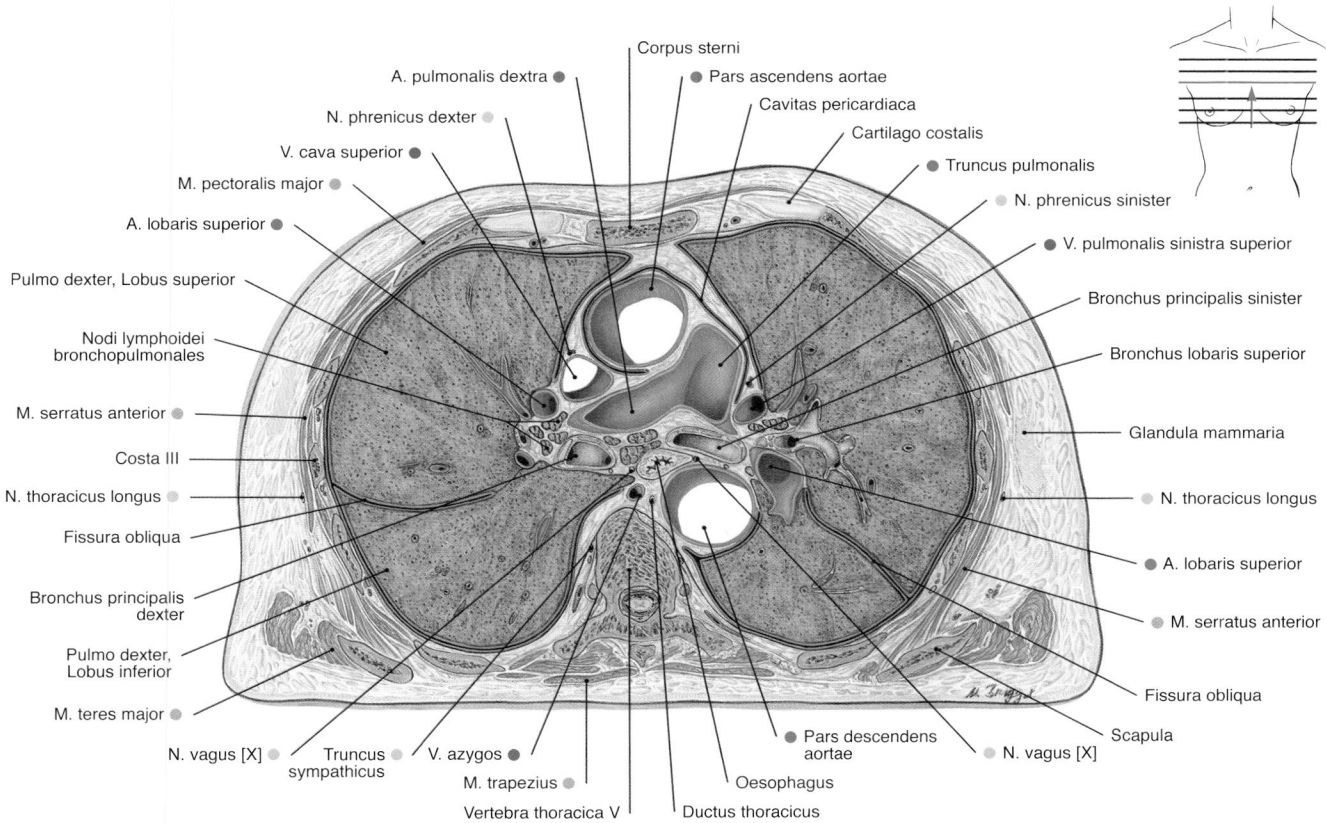

Corpus sterni
A. pulmonalis dextra ●
Pars ascendens aortae ●
N. phrenicus dexter ●
Cavitas pericardiaca
V. cava superior ●
Cartilago costalis
M. pectoralis major ●
Truncus pulmonalis ●
A. lobaris superior ●
N. phrenicus sinister ○
Pulmo dexter, Lobus superior
V. pulmonalis sinistra superior ●
Nodi lymphoidei bronchopulmonales
Bronchus principalis sinister
M. serratus anterior ○
Bronchus lobaris superior
Costa III
Glandula mammaria
N. thoracicus longus ○
N. thoracicus longus ○
Fissura obliqua
A. lobaris superior ●
Bronchus principalis dexter
M. serratus anterior ○
Pulmo dexter, Lobus inferior
Fissura obliqua
M. teres major ●
Scapula
N. vagus [X] ●   Truncus sympathicus ●   V. azygos ●
Pars descendens aortae ●
N. vagus [X] ●
M. trapezius ●
Oesophagus
Vertebra thoracica V
Ductus thoracicus

Fig. 702   Thoracic cavity, Cavitas thoracis.

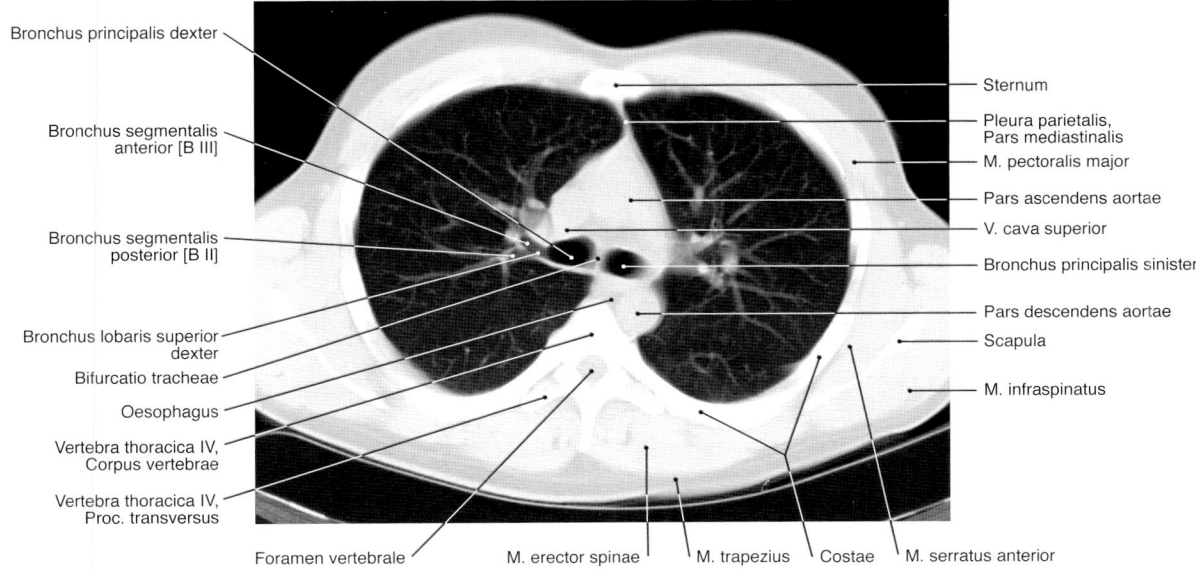

Bronchus principalis dexter
Sternum
Pleura parietalis, Pars mediastinalis
Bronchus segmentalis anterior [B III]
M. pectoralis major
Pars ascendens aortae
Bronchus segmentalis posterior [B II]
V. cava superior
Bronchus principalis sinister
Bronchus lobaris superior dexter
Pars descendens aortae
Bifurcatio tracheae
Scapula
Oesophagus
M. infraspinatus
Vertebra thoracica IV, Corpus vertebrae
Vertebra thoracica IV, Proc. transversus
Foramen vertebrale   M. erector spinae   M. trapezius   Costae   M. serratus anterior

Fig. 703   Thoracic cavity, Cavitas thoracis; computed tomographic cross-section (CT).

Thorax, transverse sections

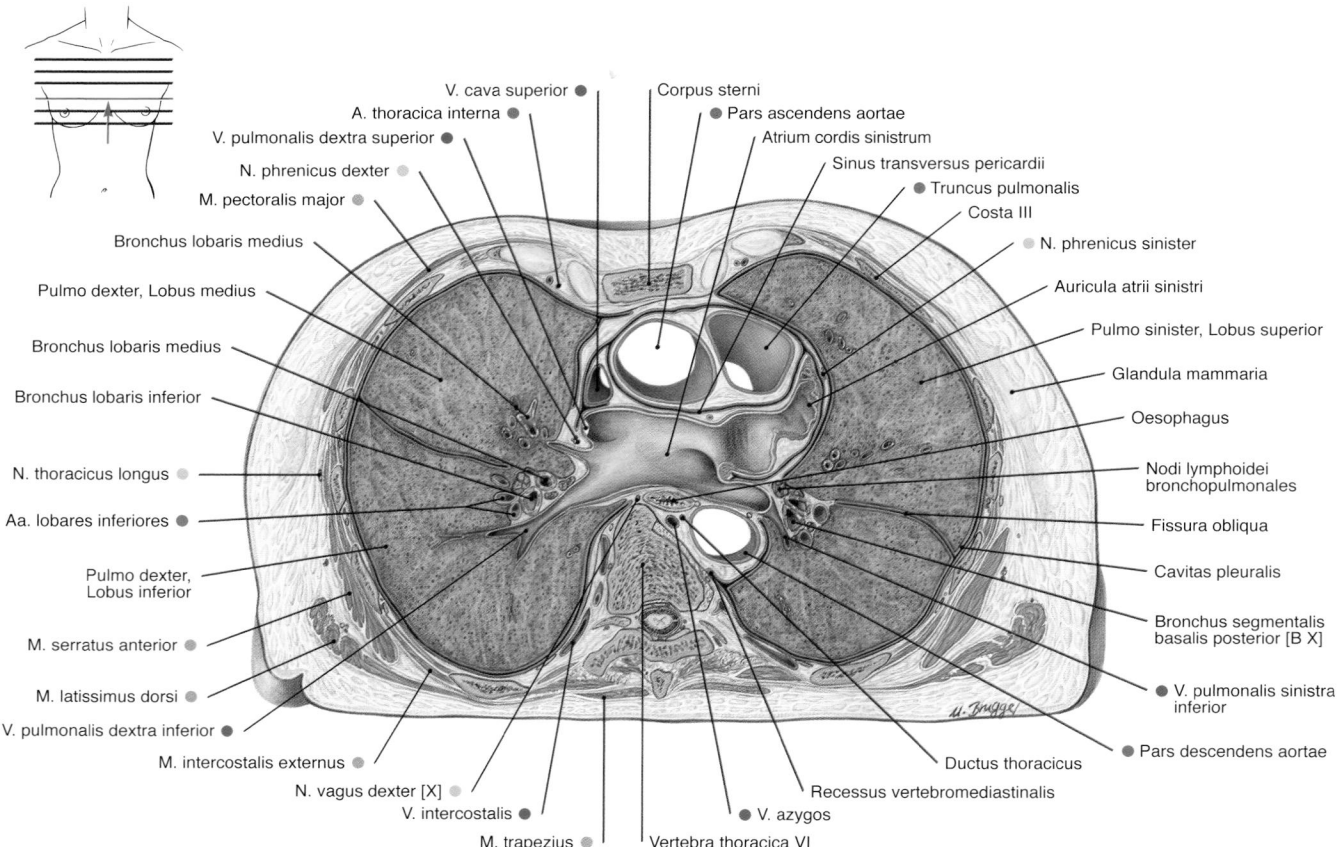

V. cava superior ●
A. thoracica interna ●
V. pulmonalis dextra superior ●
N. phrenicus dexter ●
M. pectoralis major ●
Bronchus lobaris medius
Pulmo dexter, Lobus medius
Bronchus lobaris medius
Bronchus lobaris inferior
N. thoracicus longus ●
Aa. lobares inferiores ●
Pulmo dexter, Lobus inferior
M. serratus anterior ●
M. latissimus dorsi ●
V. pulmonalis dextra inferior ●
M. intercostalis externus ●
N. vagus dexter [X] ●
V. intercostalis ●
M. trapezius ●

Corpus sterni
● Pars ascendens aortae
Atrium cordis sinistrum
Sinus transversus pericardii
● Truncus pulmonalis
Costa III
● N. phrenicus sinister
Auricula atrii sinistri
Pulmo sinister, Lobus superior
Glandula mammaria
Oesophagus
Nodi lymphoidei bronchopulmonales
Fissura obliqua
Cavitas pleuralis
Bronchus segmentalis basalis posterior [B X]
● V. pulmonalis sinistra inferior
● Pars descendens aortae
Ductus thoracicus
Recessus vertebromediastinalis
● V. azygos
Vertebra thoracica VI

Fig. 704   Thoracic cavity, Cavitas thoracis.

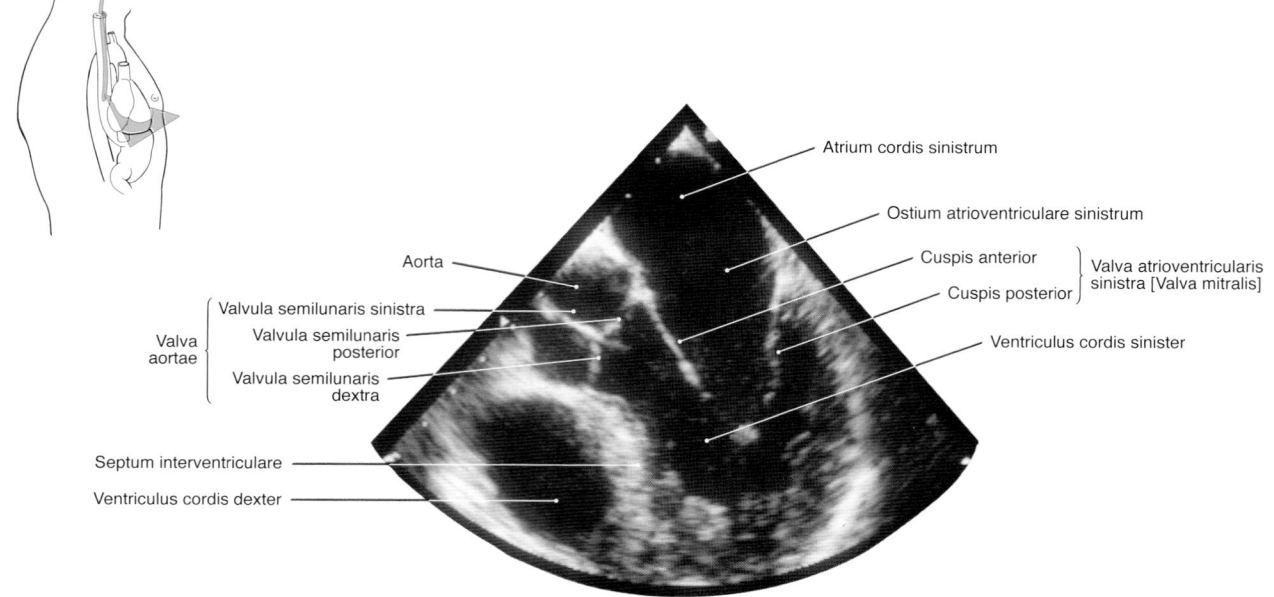

Aorta
Valvula semilunaris sinistra
Valva aortae
Valvula semilunaris posterior
Valvula semilunaris dextra
Septum interventriculare
Ventriculus cordis dexter

Atrium cordis sinistrum
Ostium atrioventriculare sinistrum
Cuspis anterior
Valva atrioventricularis sinistra [Valva mitralis]
Cuspis posterior
Ventriculus cordis sinister

Fig. 705   Heart, Cor;
ultrasound image viewed from the oesophagus
(transoesophageal echocardiography).

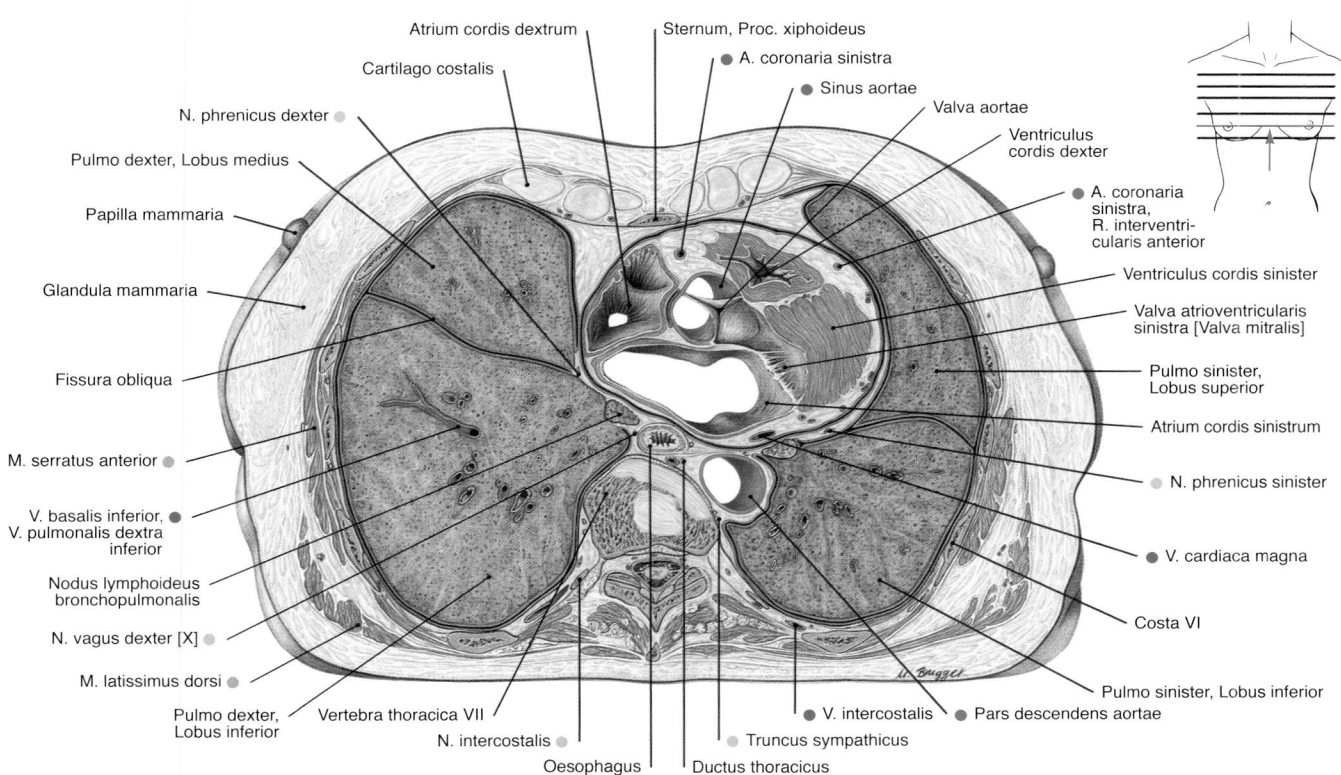

Atrium cordis dextrum
Cartilago costalis
N. phrenicus dexter
Pulmo dexter, Lobus medius
Papilla mammaria
Glandula mammaria
Fissura obliqua
M. serratus anterior
V. basalis inferior,
V. pulmonalis dextra inferior
Nodus lymphoideus bronchopulmonalis
N. vagus dexter [X]
M. latissimus dorsi
Pulmo dexter, Lobus inferior
Vertebra thoracica VII
N. intercostalis
Oesophagus
Sternum, Proc. xiphoideus
A. coronaria sinistra
Sinus aortae
Valva aortae
Ventriculus cordis dexter
A. coronaria sinistra, R. interventricularis anterior
Ventriculus cordis sinister
Valva atrioventricularis sinistra [Valva mitralis]
Pulmo sinister, Lobus superior
Atrium cordis sinistrum
N. phrenicus sinister
V. cardiaca magna
Costa VI
Pulmo sinister, Lobus inferior
Pars descendens aortae
V. intercostalis
Truncus sympathicus
Ductus thoracicus

Fig. 706 Thoracic cavity, Cavitas thoracis.

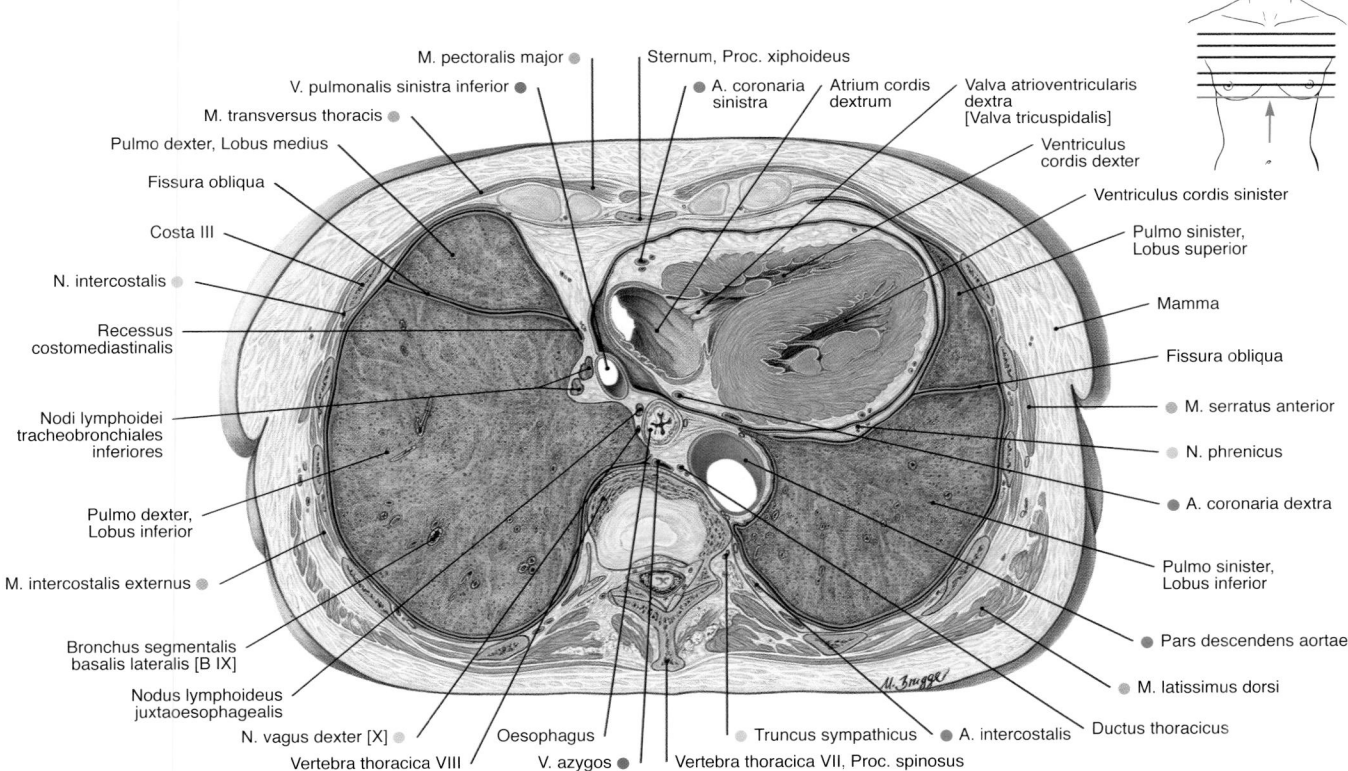

M. pectoralis major
V. pulmonalis sinistra inferior
M. transversus thoracis
Pulmo dexter, Lobus medius
Fissura obliqua
Costa III
N. intercostalis
Recessus costomediastinalis
Nodi lymphoidei tracheobronchiales inferiores
Pulmo dexter, Lobus inferior
M. intercostalis externus
Bronchus segmentalis basalis lateralis [B IX]
Nodus lymphoideus juxtaoesophagealis
N. vagus dexter [X]
Vertebra thoracica VIII
Oesophagus
V. azygos
Sternum, Proc. xiphoideus
A. coronaria sinistra
Atrium cordis dextrum
Valva atrioventricularis dextra [Valva tricuspidalis]
Ventriculus cordis dexter
Ventriculus cordis sinister
Pulmo sinister, Lobus superior
Mamma
Fissura obliqua
M. serratus anterior
N. phrenicus
A. coronaria dextra
Pulmo sinister, Lobus inferior
Pars descendens aortae
M. latissimus dorsi
Ductus thoracicus
A. intercostalis
Truncus sympathicus
Vertebra thoracica VII, Proc. spinosus

Fig. 707 Thoracic cavity, Cavitas thoracis.

Stomach

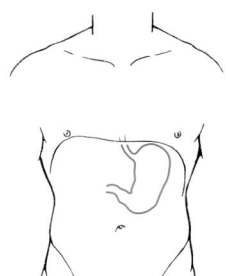

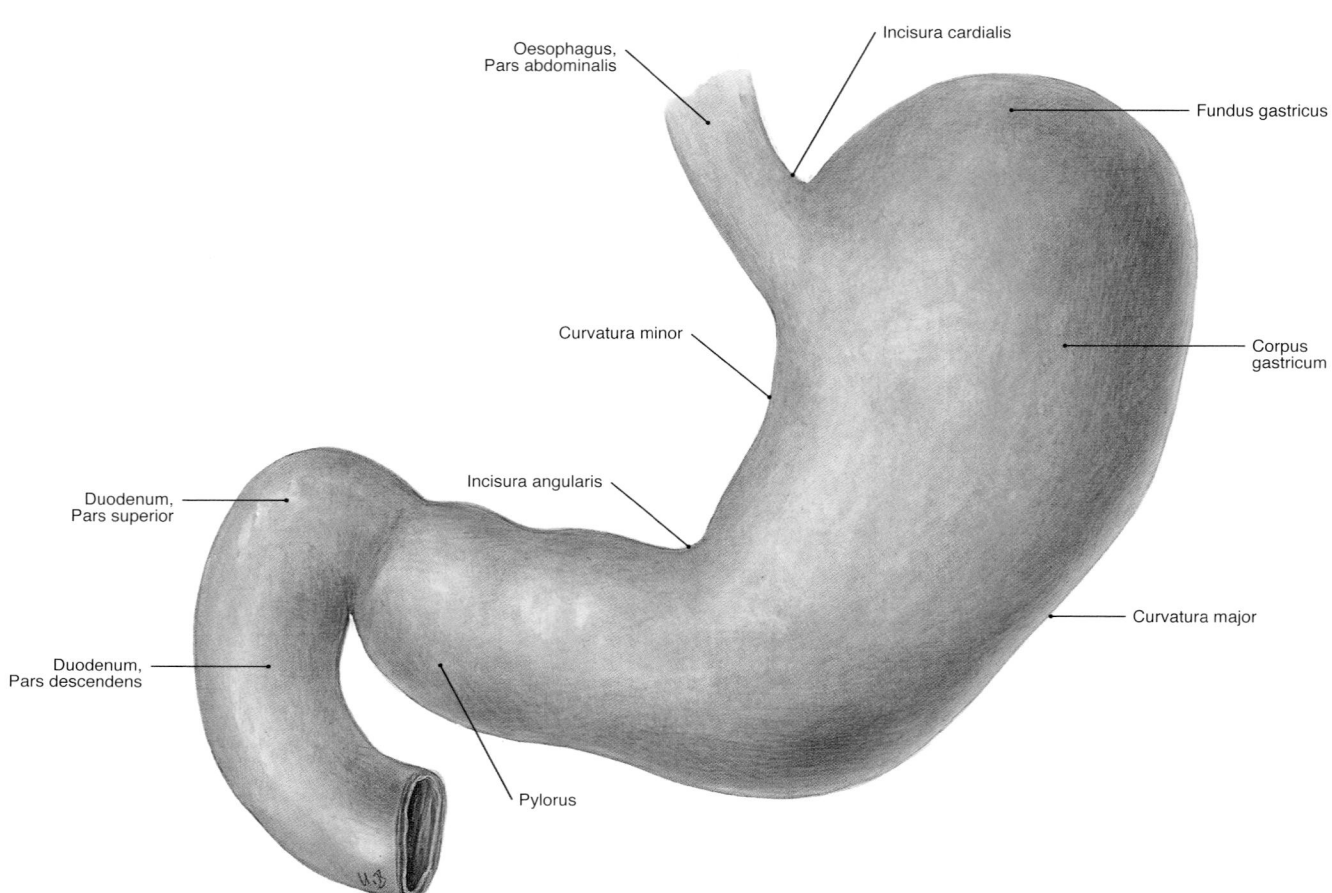

Oesophagus,
Pars abdominalis

Incisura cardialis

Fundus gastricus

Curvatura minor

Corpus
gastricum

Duodenum,
Pars superior

Incisura angularis

Duodenum,
Pars descendens

Curvatura major

Pylorus

Fig. 708   Stomach, Gaster;
ventral view.

Muscles of the stomach

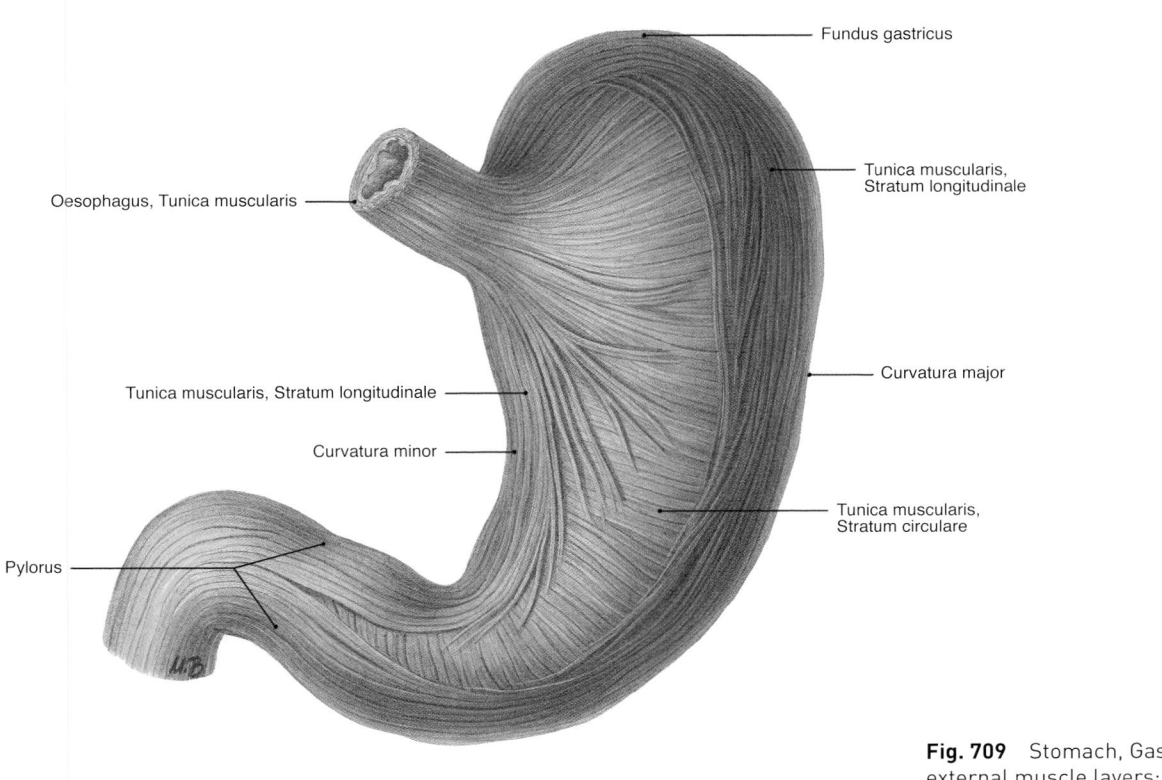

Fundus gastricus

Oesophagus, Tunica muscularis

Tunica muscularis, Stratum longitudinale

Tunica muscularis, Stratum longitudinale

Curvatura major

Curvatura minor

Tunica muscularis, Stratum circulare

Pylorus

Fig. 709 Stomach, Gaster; external muscle layers; ventral view.

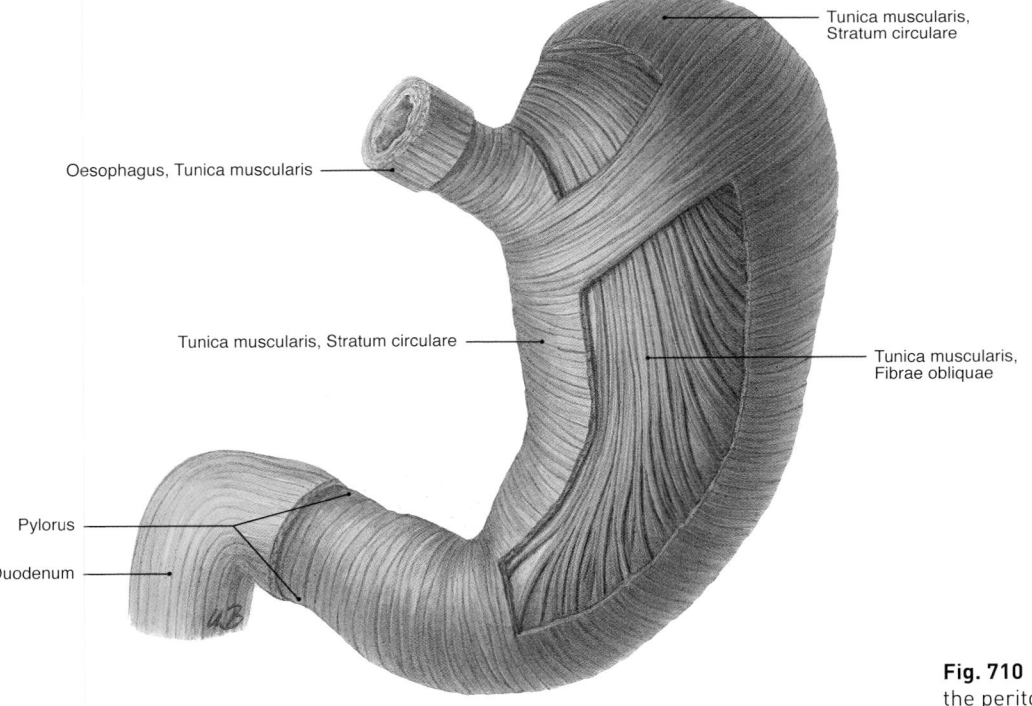

Tunica muscularis, Stratum circulare

Oesophagus, Tunica muscularis

Tunica muscularis, Stratum circulare

Tunica muscularis, Fibrae obliquae

Pylorus

Duodenum

Fig. 710 Stomach, Gaster; the peritoneum has been removed to demonstrate the internal muscle layers; ventral view.

Stomach, structure

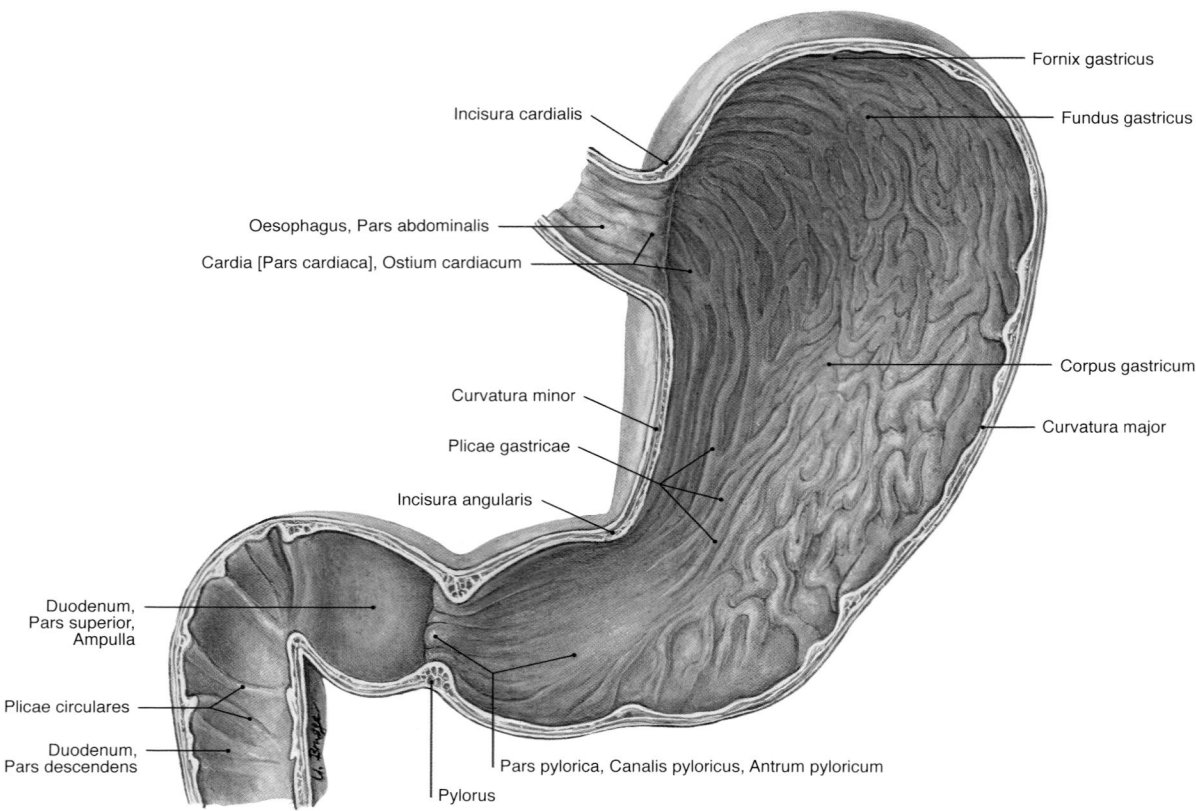

Incisura cardialis

Oesophagus, Pars abdominalis

Cardia [Pars cardiaca], Ostium cardiacum

Curvatura minor

Plicae gastricae

Incisura angularis

Duodenum, Pars superior, Ampulla

Plicae circulares

Duodenum, Pars descendens

Pars pylorica, Canalis pyloricus, Antrum pyloricum

Pylorus

Fornix gastricus

Fundus gastricus

Corpus gastricum

Curvatura major

Fig. 711 Stomach, Gaster, and duodenum, Duodenum; ventral view.

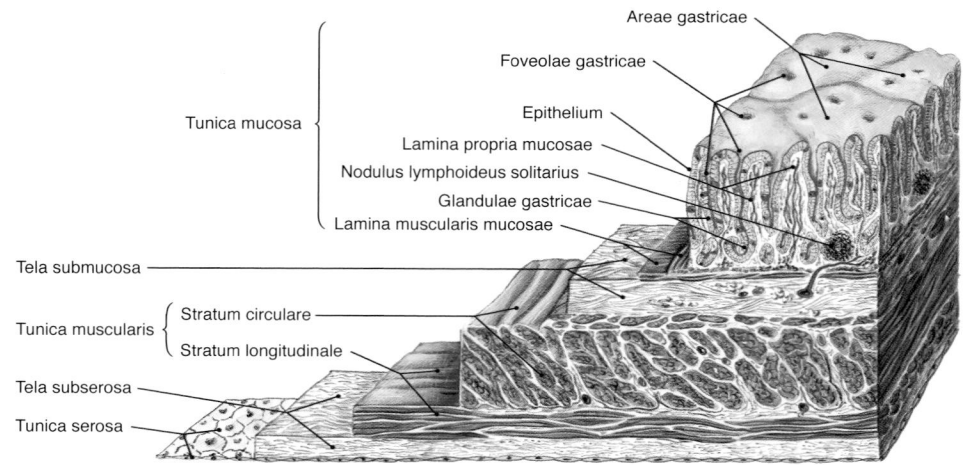

Areae gastricae

Foveolae gastricae

Epithelium

Lamina propria mucosae

Nodulus lymphoideus solitarius

Glandulae gastricae

Lamina muscularis mucosae

Tunica mucosa

Tela submucosa

Tunica muscularis {
Stratum circulare
Stratum longitudinale
}

Tela subserosa

Tunica serosa

Fig. 712 Diagram of the stomach wall; the layers of the wall have been removed stepwise; microscopic enlargement at low magnification.

Vessels of the stomach

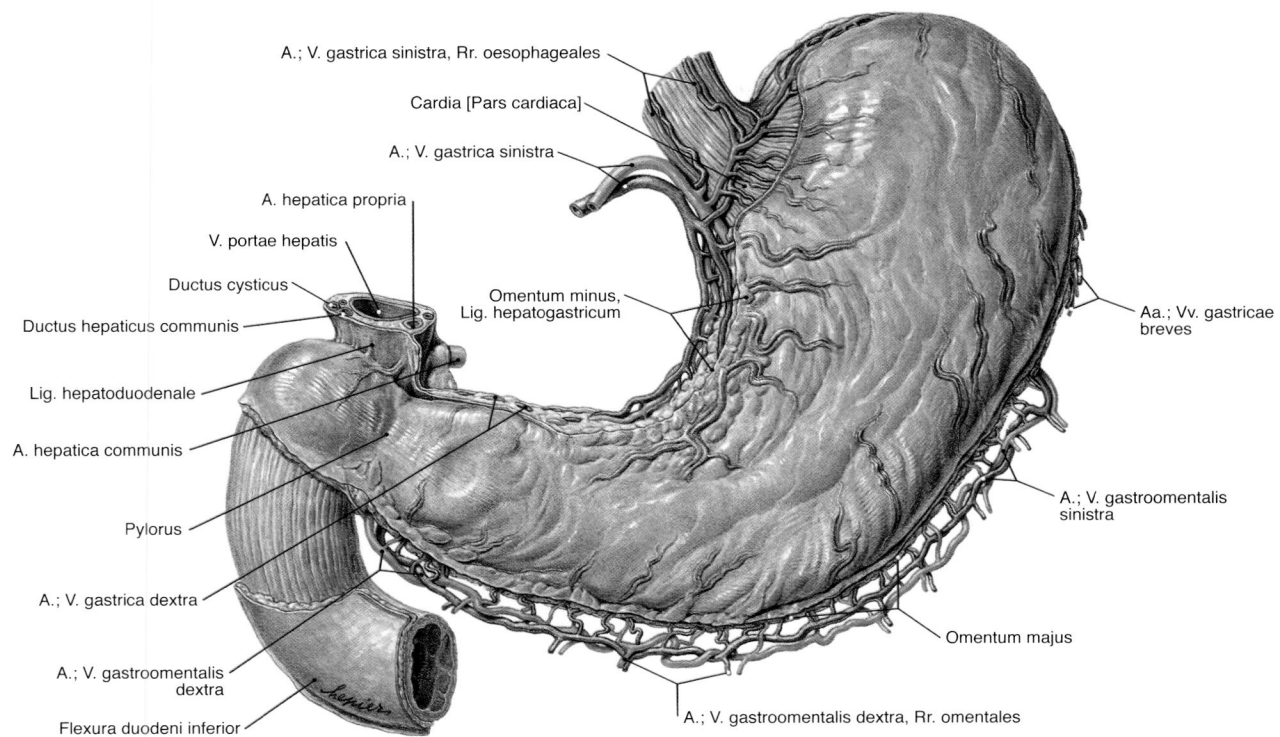

Fig. 713 Blood vessels of the stomach, Gaster; ventral view.

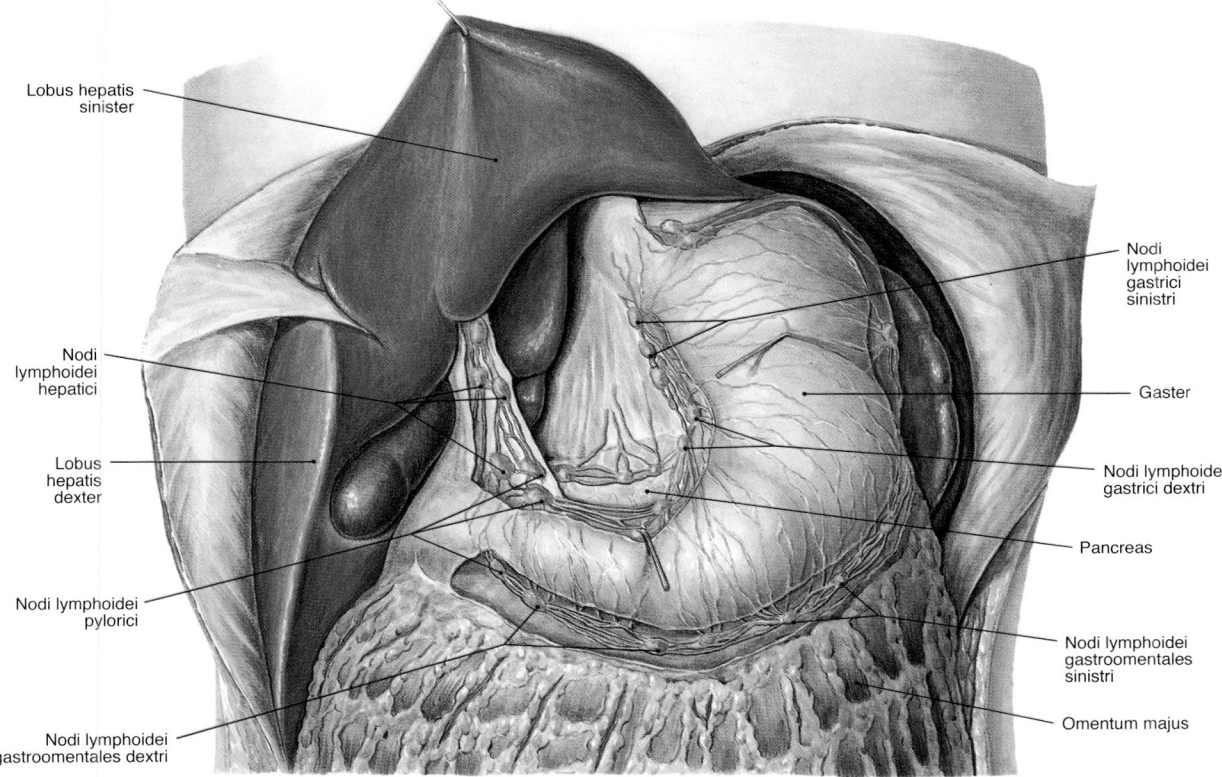

Fig. 714 Stomach, Gaster, and liver, Hepar, with lymph nodes, Nodi lymphoidei; ventral view.

Stomach, radiography

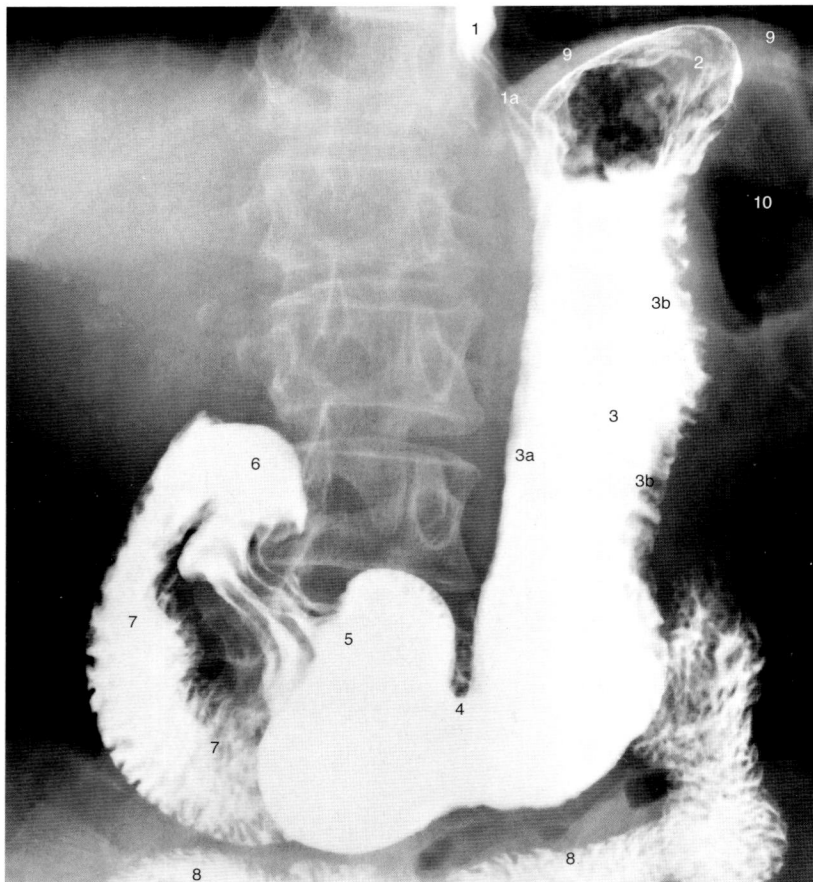

1 = Oesophagus with contrast medium.
  At the transition (1a) into the fundus
  of stomach, the grooves between
  the folds appear as dark striations.
2 = Fundus of stomach with air bubble
3 = Body of stomach
3a = Lesser curvature
3b = Greater curvature.
  In the linings of the latter, notches
  corresponding to the contour
  of the mucous are visible.
4 = Peristaltic constriction at
  the angular notch
5 = Pyloric part prior to the progression of
  a portion of the stomach's content
6 = Ampulla of duodenum
7 = Descending part of the duodenum
  with circular folds
8 = Jejunum
9 = Left "dome" of diaphragm
10 = Left colic flexure (filled with air)

Fig. 715 Stomach, Gaster, and
duodenum, Duodenum;
AP-radiograph after oral
administration of a contrast medium;
upright position;
ventral view.

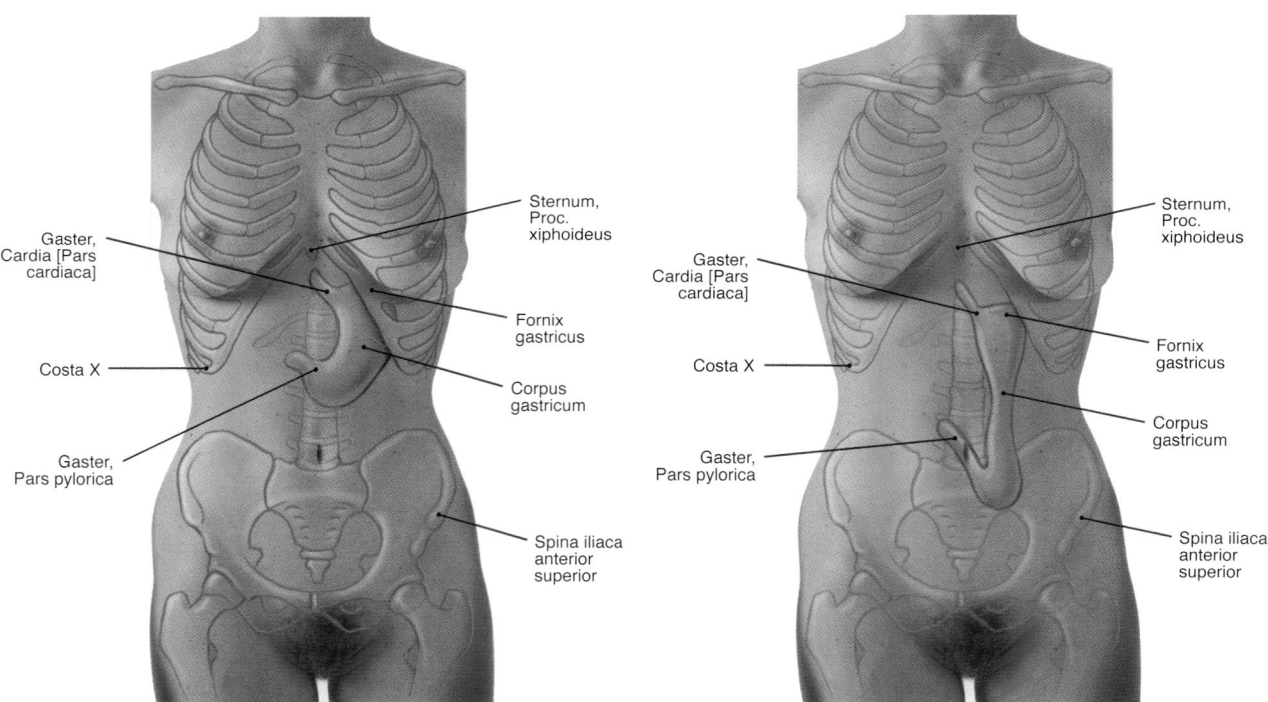

Fig. 716 Stomach, Gaster;
projection of a "normal" stomach onto the anterior abdominal
wall;
upright position.

Fig. 717 Stomach, Gaster;
projection of a "long" stomach onto the anterior abdominal
wall;
upright position.

Gastroscopy

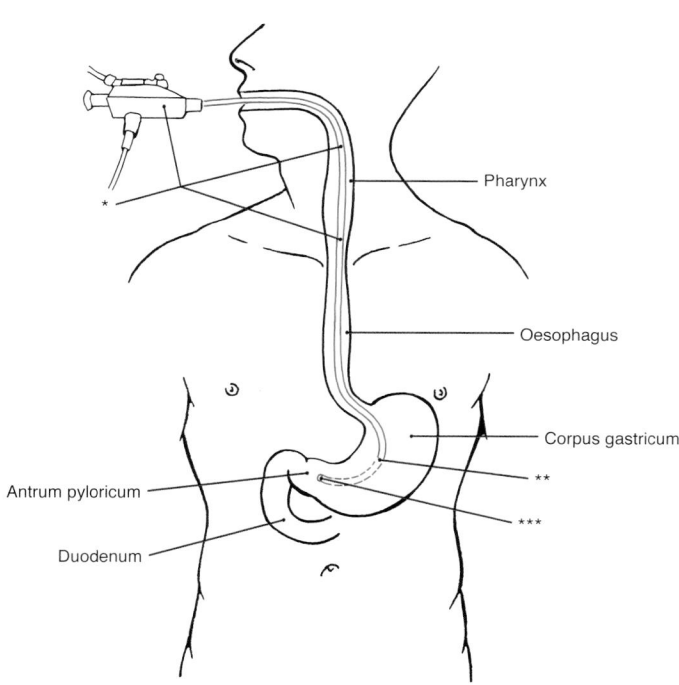

Pharynx

Oesophagus

Corpus gastricum

**

***

Antrum pyloricum

Duodenum

Fig. 718   Technical procedure of oesophagoscopy
and gastroscopy.

*   Gastroscope
**   The gastroscope's tip located in the body of stomach (compare Fig. 719 a)
***The gastroscope's tip located in the pyloric antrum (compare Fig. 719 b)

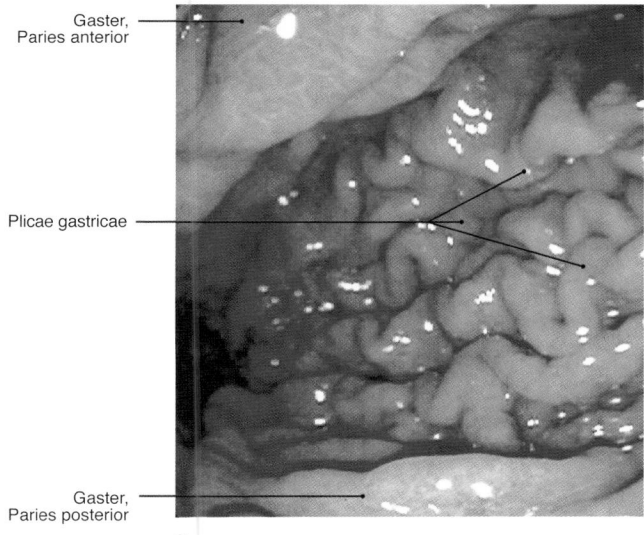

Gaster,
Paries anterior

Plicae gastricae

Gaster,
Paries posterior

a

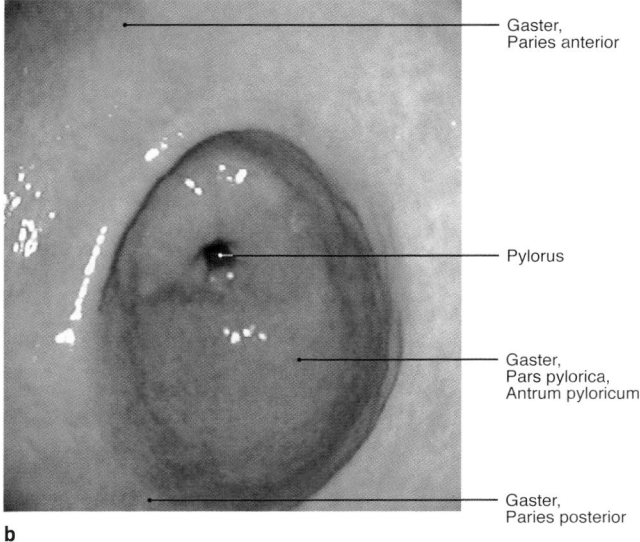

Gaster,
Paries anterior

Pylorus

Gaster,
Pars pylorica,
Antrum pyloricum

Gaster,
Paries posterior

b

Fig. 719 a, b   Stomach, Gaster;
endoscopic image of the stomach (gastroscopy);
superior view.

a View of the body of stomach, Corpus gastricum, with distinct
longitudinal folds of the mucosa (Plica gastricae)
b View of the pyloric antrum, Antrum pyloricum, predominantly
covered with smooth mucosa

Duodenum

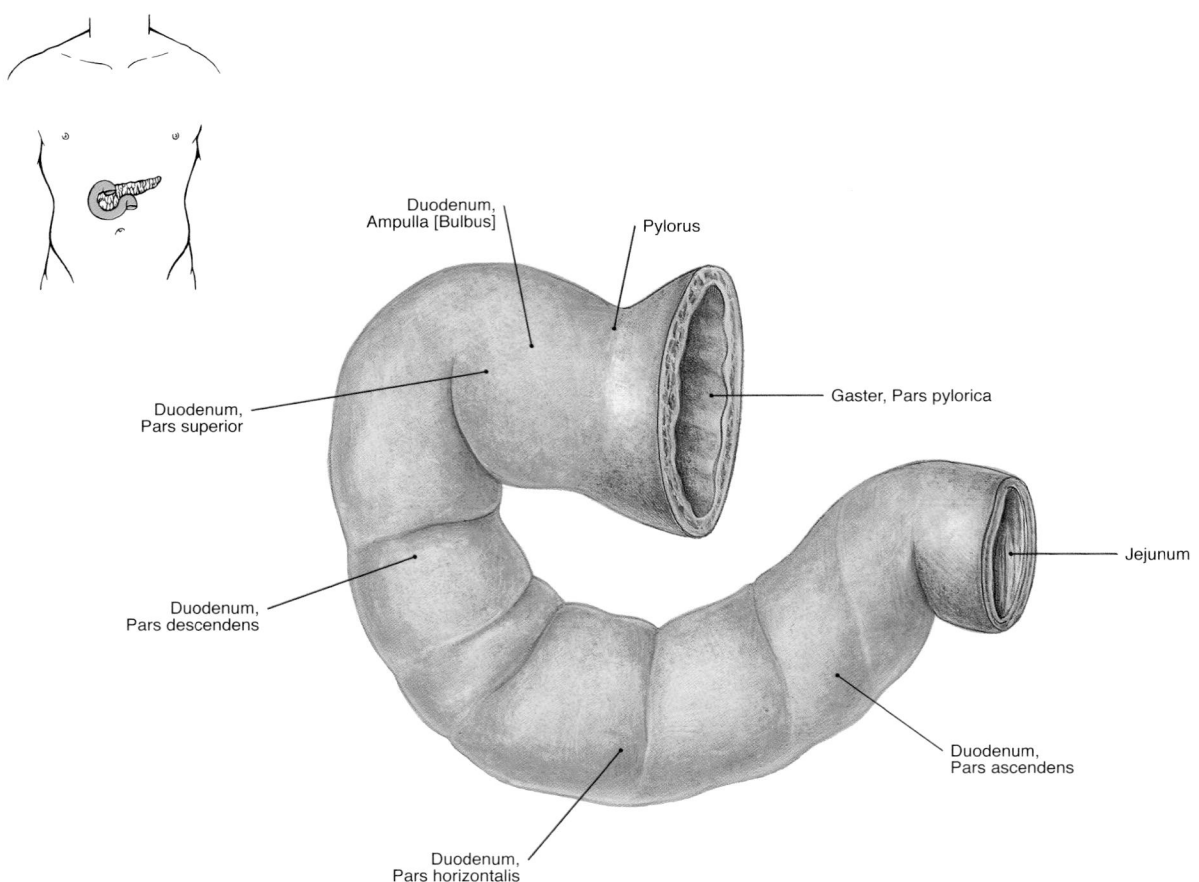

Duodenum,
Ampulla [Bulbus]

Pylorus

Duodenum,
Pars superior

Gaster, Pars pylorica

Duodenum,
Pars descendens

Jejunum

Duodenum,
Pars ascendens

Duodenum,
Pars horizontalis

Fig. 720   Duodenum, Duodenum.

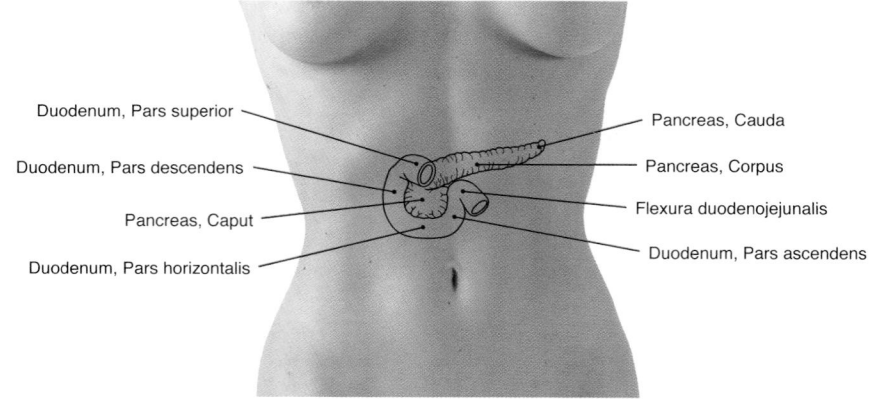

Duodenum, Pars superior

Pancreas, Cauda

Duodenum, Pars descendens

Pancreas, Corpus

Pancreas, Caput

Flexura duodenojejunalis

Duodenum, Pars horizontalis

Duodenum, Pars ascendens

Fig. 721   Duodenum, Duodenum, and
pancreas, Pancreas;
projected onto the anterior abdominal wall.

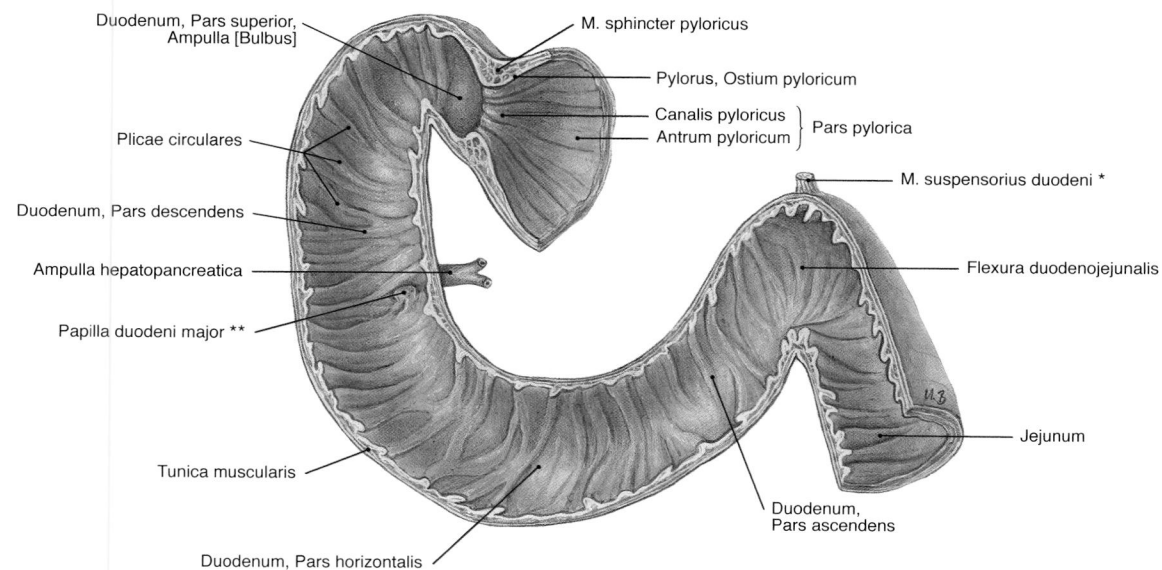

Duodenum, Pars superior, Ampulla [Bulbus]

M. sphincter pyloricus

Pylorus, Ostium pyloricum

Canalis pyloricus

Antrum pyloricum } Pars pylorica

Plicae circulares

Duodenum, Pars descendens

M. suspensorius duodeni *

Flexura duodenojejunalis

Ampulla hepatopancreatica

Papilla duodeni major **

Jejunum

Tunica muscularis

Duodenum, Pars ascendens

Duodenum, Pars horizontalis

Fig. 722 Duodenum, Duodenum; ventral view.
* Clinical term: muscle of TREITZ
** Clinical term: papilla of VATER

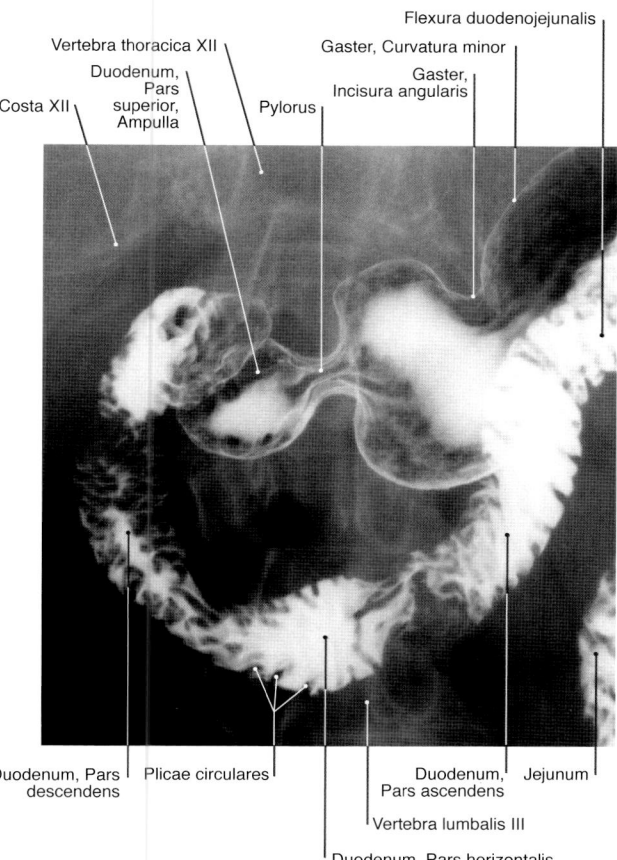

Vertebra thoracica XII

Flexura duodenojejunalis

Gaster, Curvatura minor

Duodenum, Pars superior, Ampulla

Gaster, Incisura angularis

Costa XII

Pylorus

Duodenum, Pars descendens

Plicae circulares

Duodenum, Pars ascendens

Jejunum

Vertebra lumbalis III

Duodenum, Pars horizontalis

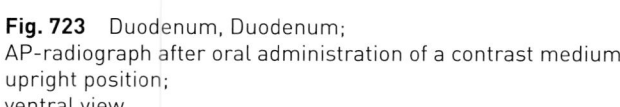

Fig. 723 Duodenum, Duodenum;
AP-radiograph after oral administration of a contrast medium; upright position; ventral view.

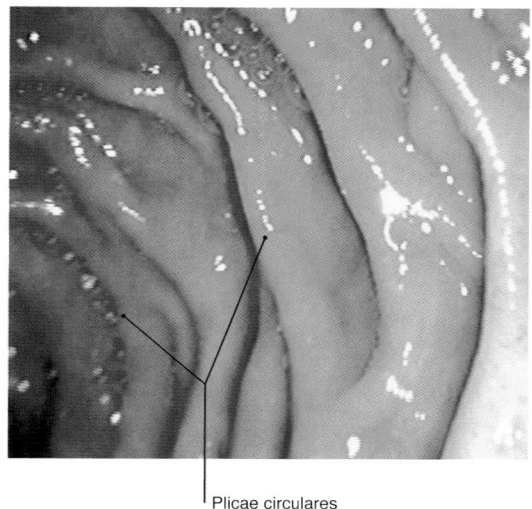

Plicae circulares

Fig. 724 Duodenum, Duodenum; endoscopic image.

Small intestine, structure

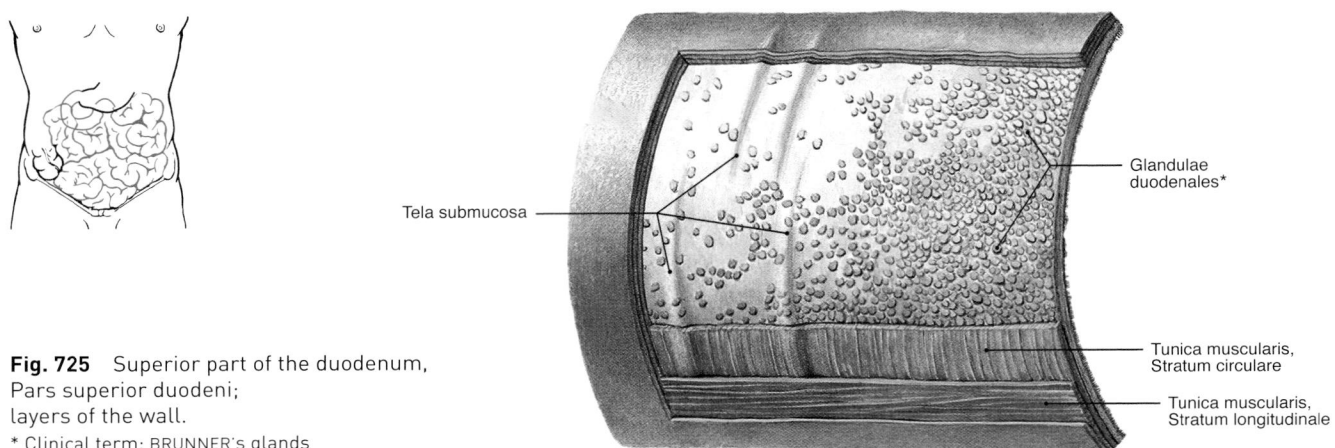

Fig. 725 Superior part of the duodenum,
Pars superior duodeni;
layers of the wall.
* Clinical term: BRUNNER's glands

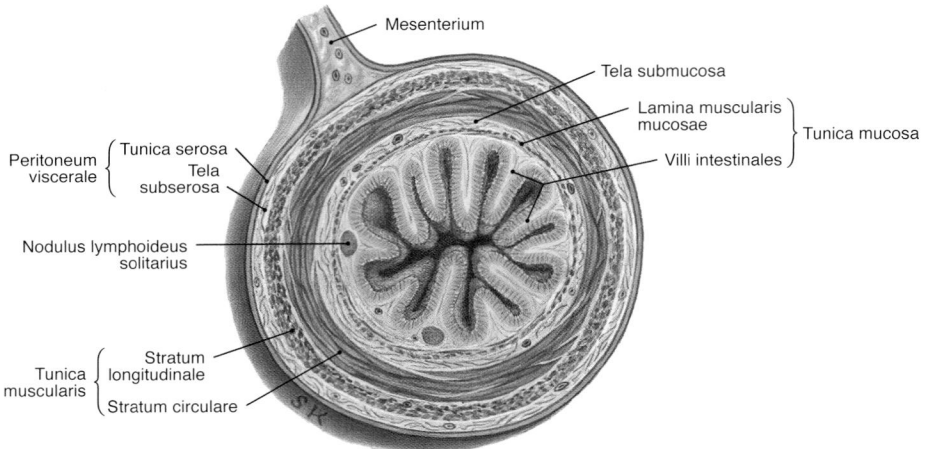

Fig. 726 Small intestine, Intestinum tenue;
cross-section through the upper small intestine.

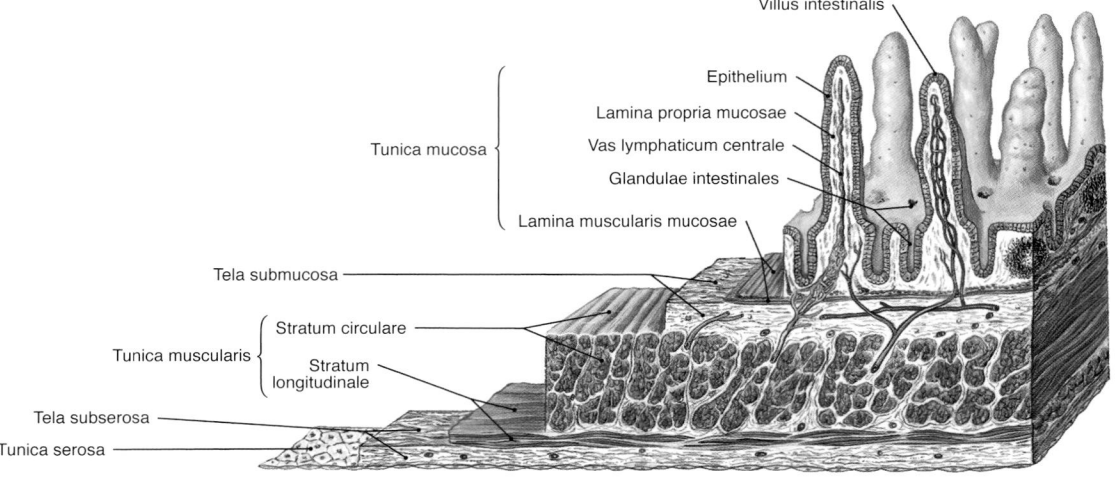

Fig. 727 Small intestine, Intestinum tenue;
layers of the wall;
microscopic enlargement at low magnification.

Mucosa of the small intestine

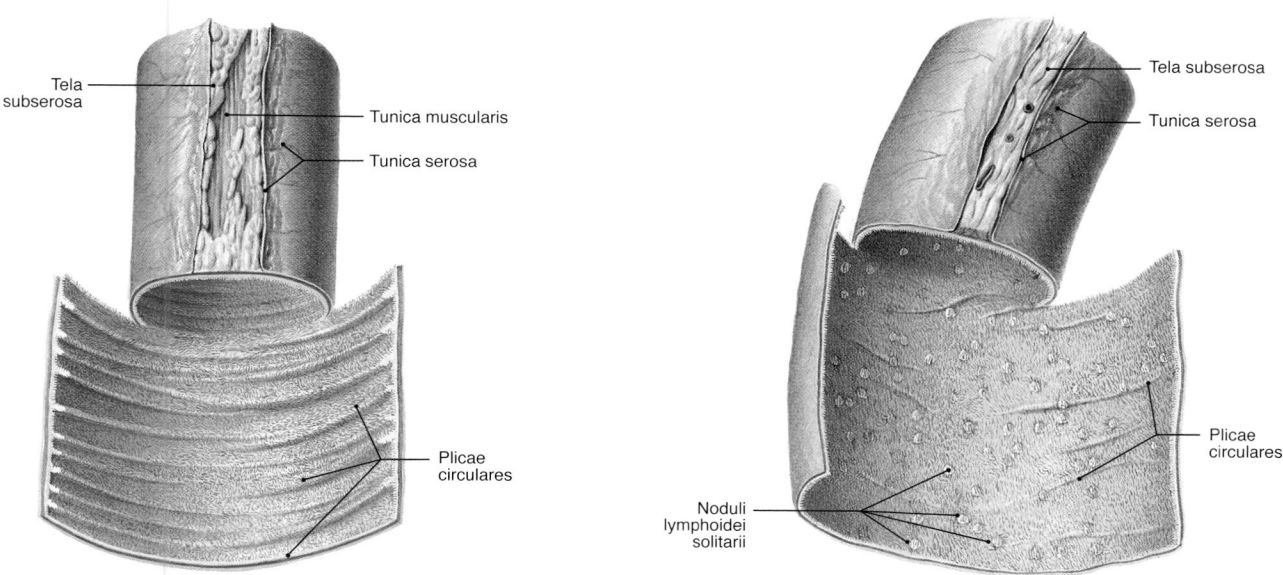

Fig. 728 Jejunum, Jejunum.

Fig. 729 Ileum, Ileum.

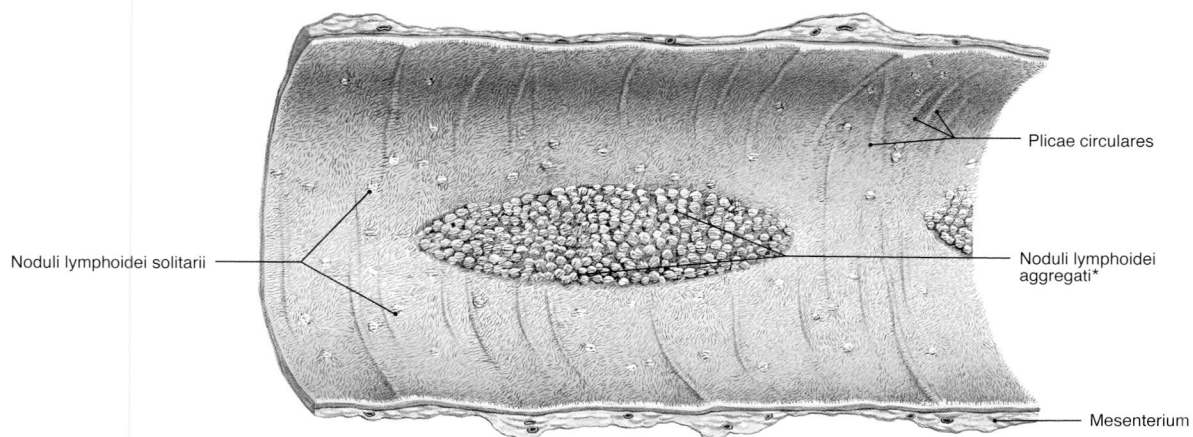

Fig. 730 Terminal ileum,
Pars terminalis ilei.
* Clinical term: PEYER's patches

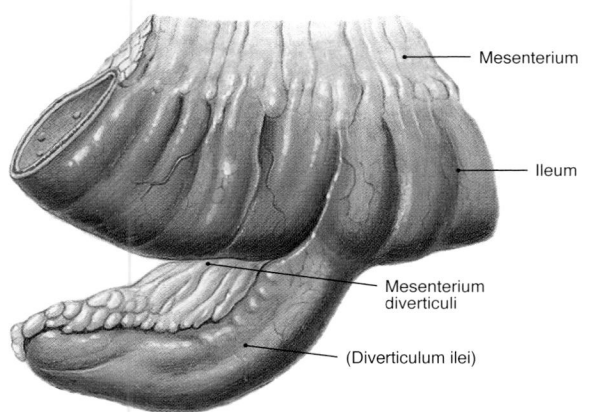

Fig. 731 MECKEL's diverticulum (Diverticulum ilei).
This vestige of the yolk stalk (Ductus omphaloentericus)
occurs in 1–3% of cases. It is located 30–70 cm oral to
the ileocaecal junction opposite to the attachment of the
mesentery.

Large intestine

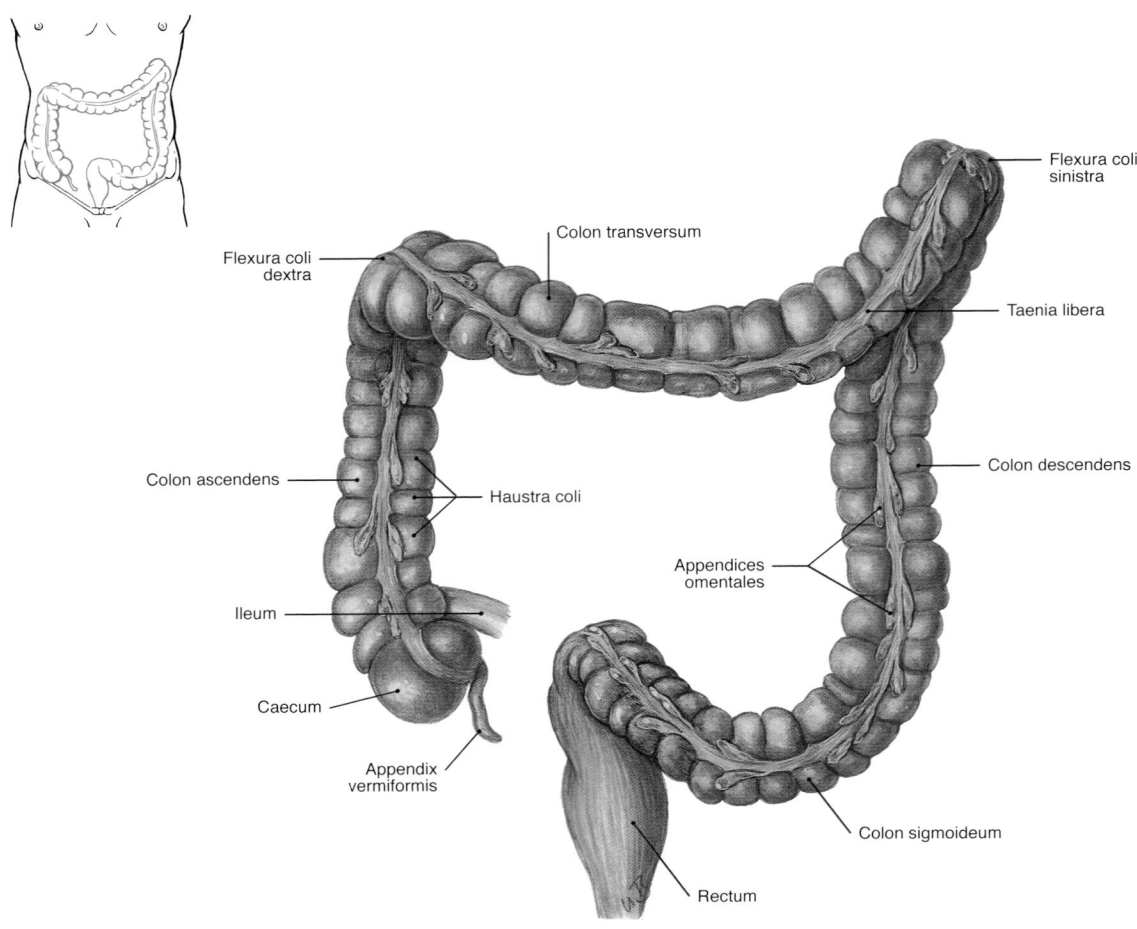

Fig. 732   Large intestine, Intestinum crassum;
ventral view.

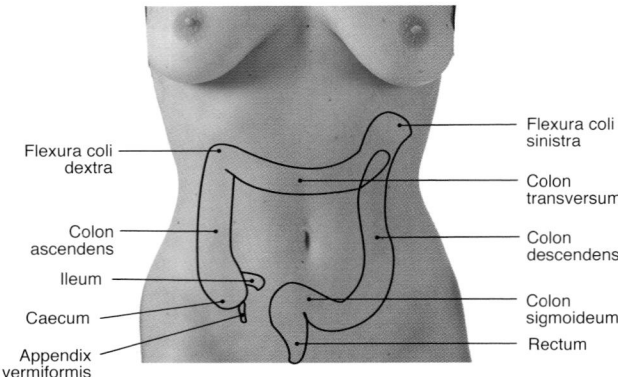

Fig. 733   Large intestine, Intestinum crassum;
projected onto the anterior abdominal wall.
The positions of the transverse colon and of the sigmoid
colon are highly variable (compare Fig. 742).

Large intestine, structure

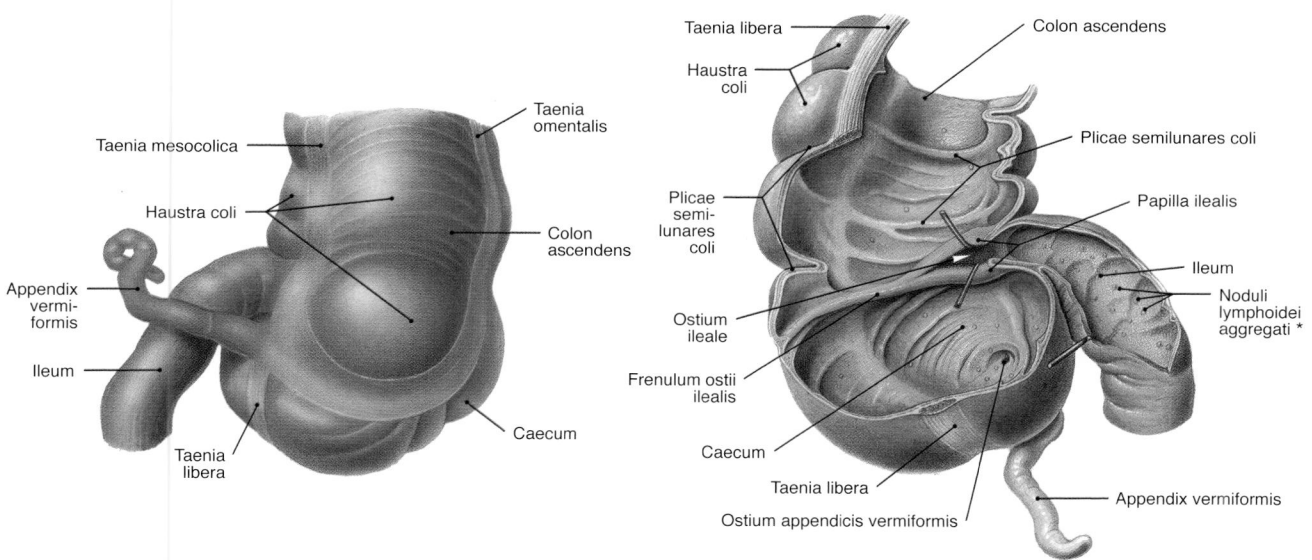

Fig. 734   Caecum, Caecum; vermiform appendix,
Appendix vermiformis, and terminal ileum,
Pars terminalis ilei;
dorsal view.

Fig. 735   Ascending colon, Colon ascendens;
caecum, Caecum, and vermiform appendix, Appendix vermiformis;
ventral view.
* Clinical term: PEYER's patches

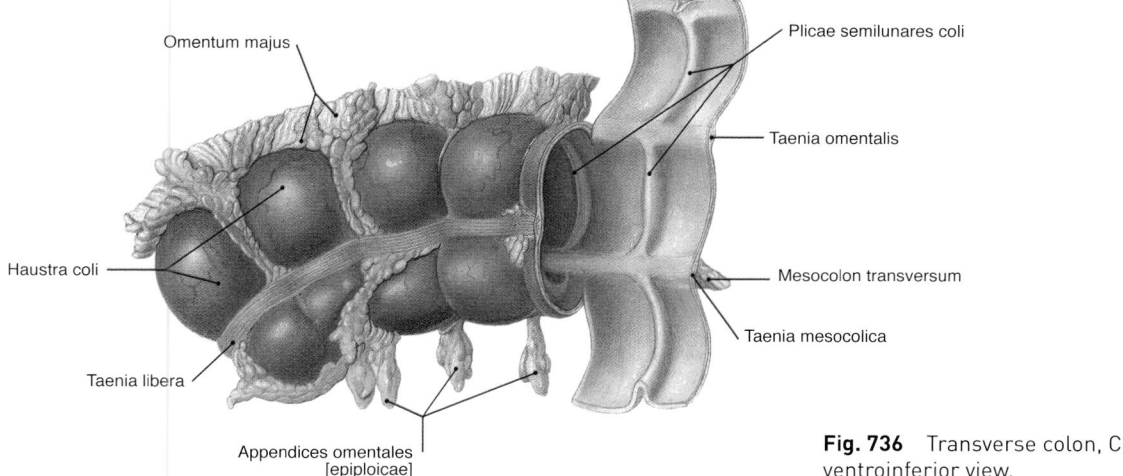

Fig. 736   Transverse colon, Colon transversum;
ventroinferior view.

Fig. 737   Colon, Colon;
layers of the wall;
microscopic enlargement
at low magnification.

Vermiform appendix

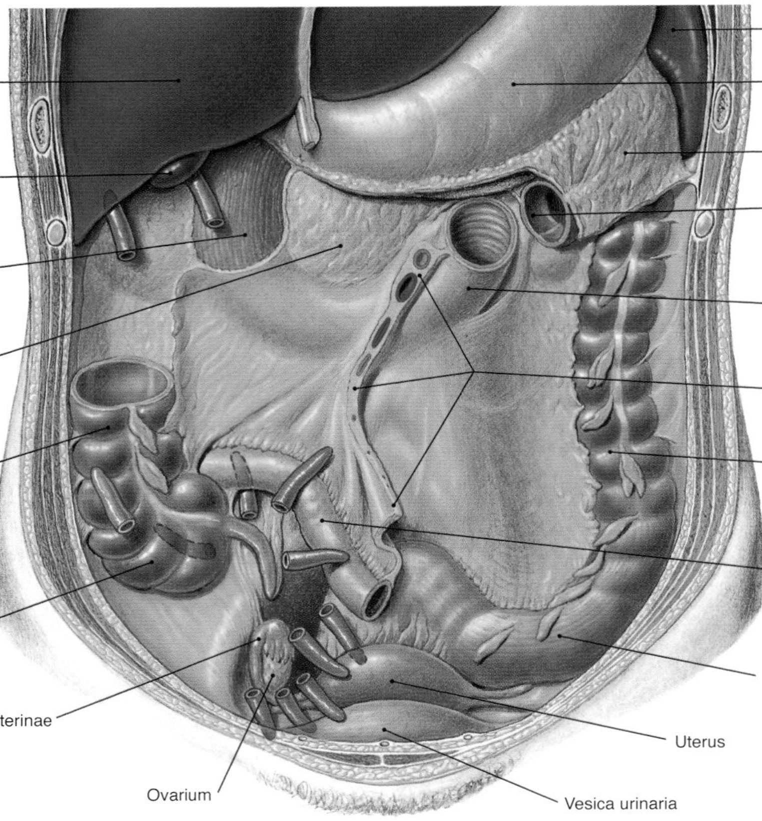

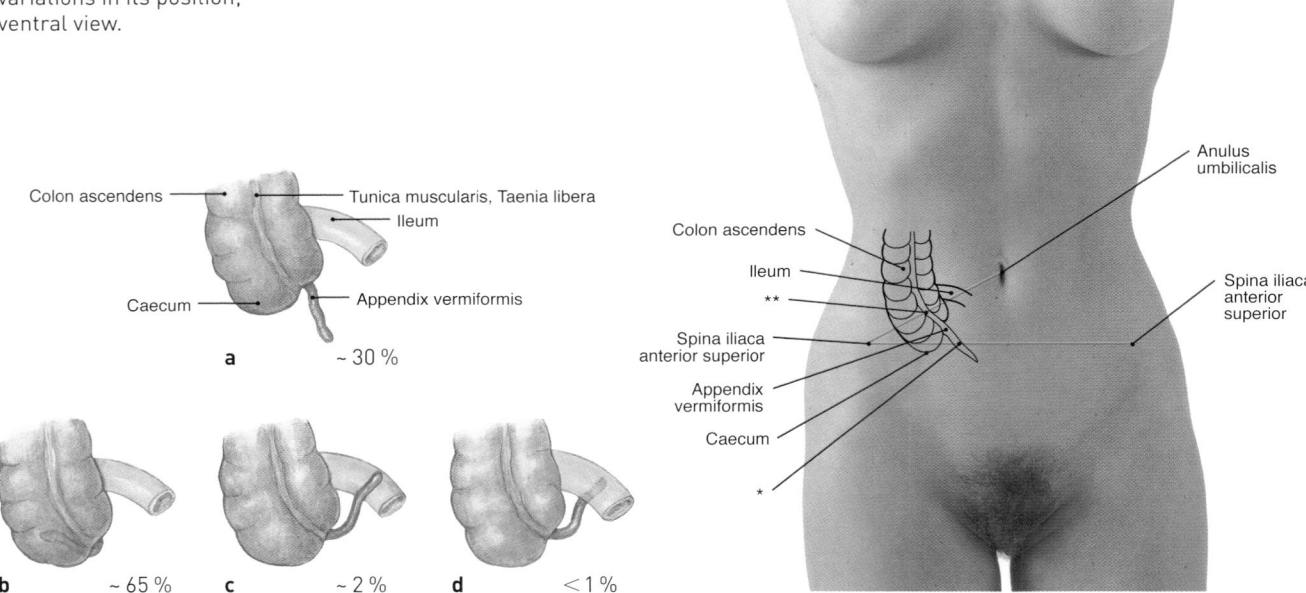

Lobus hepatis dexter

Vesica biliaris

Duodenum,
Pars descendens

Caput pancreatis

Colon ascendens

Caecum

Ampulla tubae uterinae

Ovarium

Splen [Lien]

Gaster

Omentum majus

Colon transversum

Duodenum, Pars ascendens

Radix mesenterii

Colon descendens

Ileum

Colon sigmoideum

Uterus

Vesica urinaria

Fig. 738 Vermiform appendix, Appendix vermiformis;
variations in its position;
ventral view.

Colon ascendens

Caecum

Tunica muscularis, Taenia libera
Ileum

Appendix vermiformis

a ~ 30 %

b ~ 65 %   **c** ~ 2 %   **d** < 1 %

Fig. 739 a–d Vermiform appendix, Appendix vermiformis;
variations in its position.
a Descending into the lesser pelvis
b Behind the caecum
c In front of the ileum
d Behind the ileum

Anulus
umbilicalis

Colon ascendens

Ileum

**

Spina iliaca
anterior superior

Appendix
vermiformis

Caecum

*

Spina iliaca
anterior
superior

Fig. 740 Caecum, Caecum, and vermiform appendix,
Appendix vermiformis;
projection onto the anterior abdominal wall.

* Clinical term: v. LANZ's point, at the right third of a line
  connecting the anterior superior iliac spines, locates the tip
  of the vermiform appendix
** Clinical term: McBURNEY's point, at the outer third of a line
  connecting the right anterior superior iliac spine and the
  umbilicus, locates the base of the vermiform appendix

Large intestine, imaging

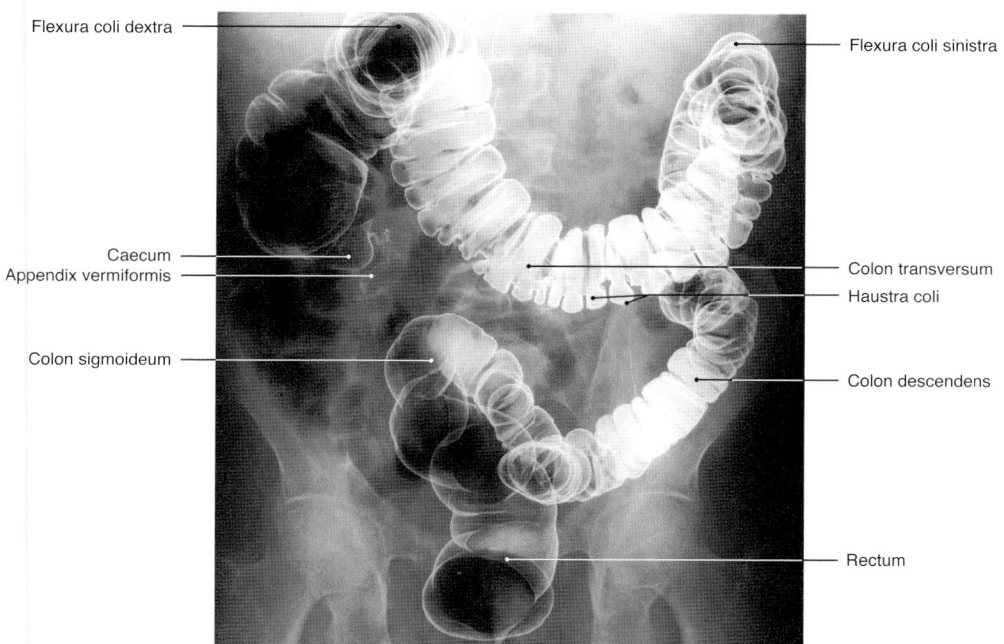

Flexura coli dextra

Flexura coli sinistra

Caecum

Appendix vermiformis

Colon transversum

Haustra coli

Colon sigmoideum

Colon descendens

Rectum

Fig. 741 Colon, Colon, and rectum, Rectum;
AP-radiograph after filling with a contrast medium
and air (double contrast method).

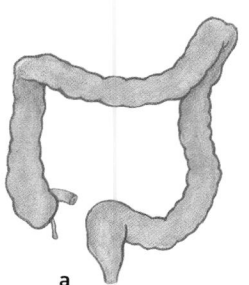
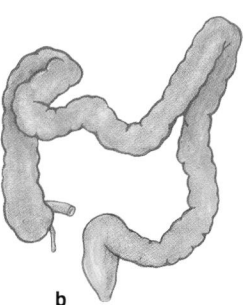
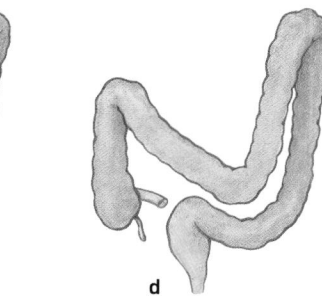

a

b

c

d

Fig. 742 a–d Transverse colon, Colon transversum;
common variations in its position;
ventral view.

a Normal position
b Twisted

c U-shaped
d V-shaped

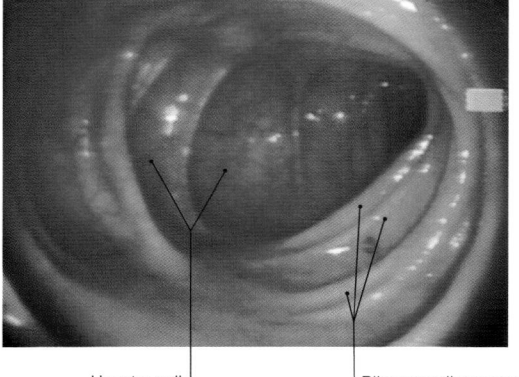

Haustra coli

Plicae semilunares coli

Fig. 743 Ascending colon, Colon ascendens;
endoscopic image after passage of the rectum,
the sigmoid colon, the descending colon
and the transverse colon (colonoscopy).

Liver

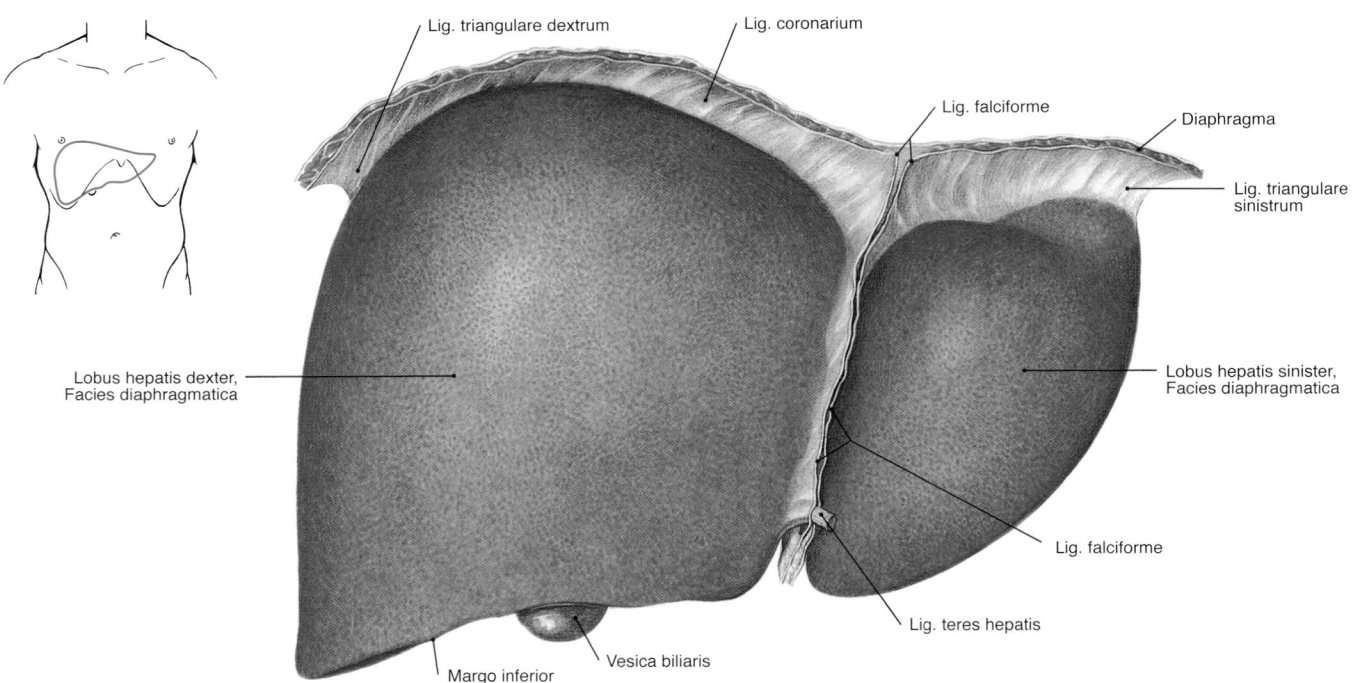

Lig. triangulare dextrum
Lig. coronarium
Lig. falciforme
Diaphragma
Lig. triangulare sinistrum
Lobus hepatis dexter, Facies diaphragmatica
Lobus hepatis sinister, Facies diaphragmatica
Lig. falciforme
Lig. teres hepatis
Vesica biliaris
Margo inferior

Fig. 744 Liver, Hepar; ventral view.

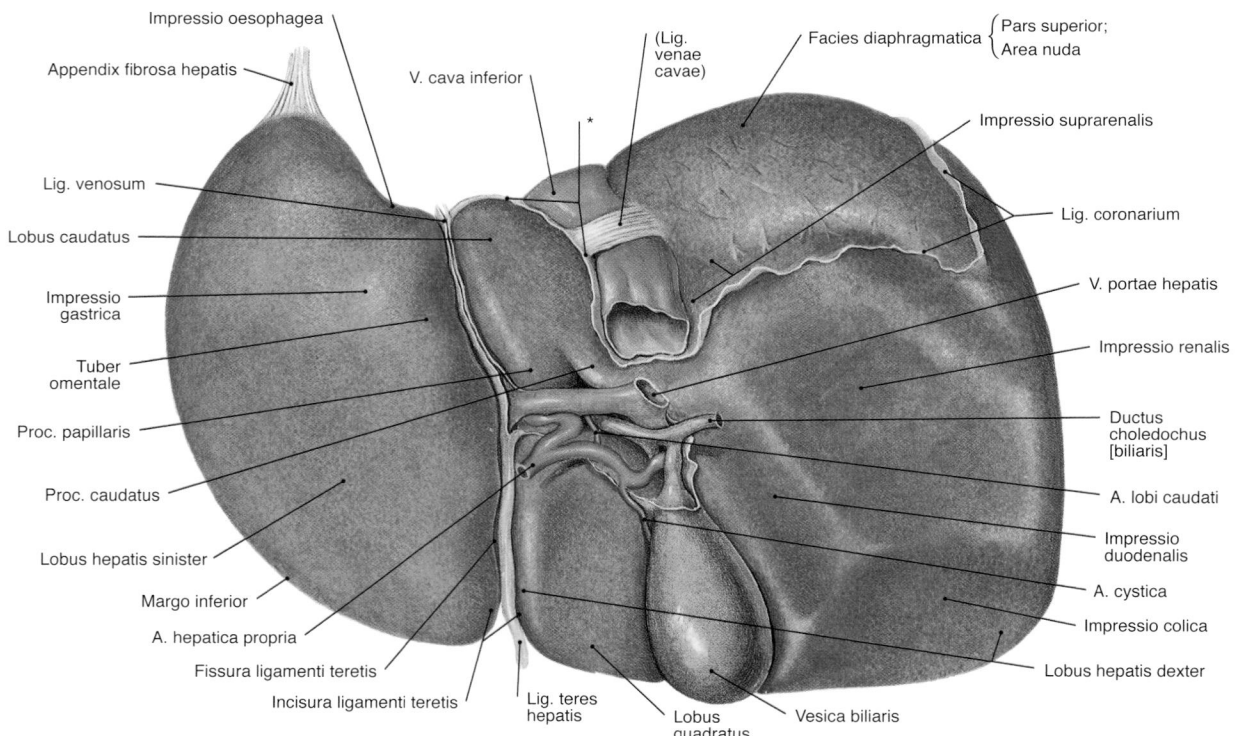

Impressio oesophagea
Appendix fibrosa hepatis
V. cava inferior
(Lig. venae cavae)
Facies diaphragmatica { Pars superior; Area nuda
Impressio suprarenalis
Lig. venosum
Lobus caudatus
Lig. coronarium
Impressio gastrica
V. portae hepatis
Tuber omentale
Impressio renalis
Proc. papillaris
Ductus choledochus [biliaris]
Proc. caudatus
A. lobi caudati
Lobus hepatis sinister
Impressio duodenalis
Margo inferior
A. cystica
A. hepatica propria
Impressio colica
Fissura ligamenti teretis
Lobus hepatis dexter
Incisura ligamenti teretis
Lig. teres hepatis
Lobus quadratus
Vesica biliaris

Fig. 745 Liver, Hepar, and porta hepatis, Porta hepatis; dorsal view.

* Borders of the superior recess of the omental bursa

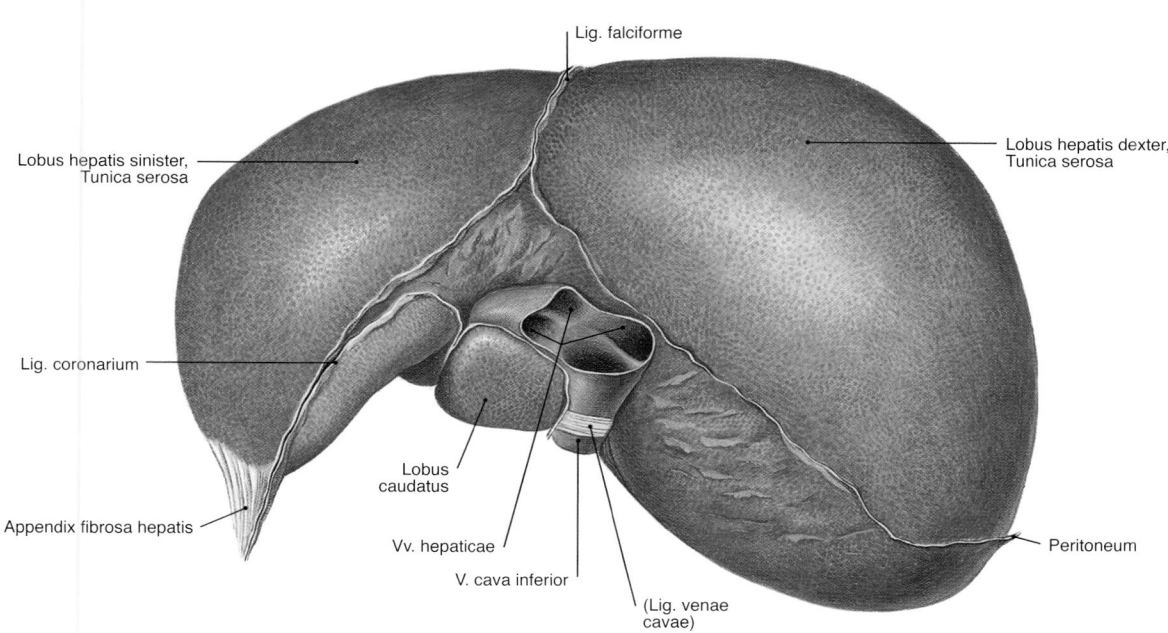

Lig. falciforme

Lobus hepatis sinister,
Tunica serosa

Lobus hepatis dexter,
Tunica serosa

Lig. coronarium

Appendix fibrosa hepatis

Lobus
caudatus

Vv. hepaticae

V. cava inferior

(Lig. venae
cavae)

Peritoneum

Fig. 746 Liver, Hepar;
superior view.

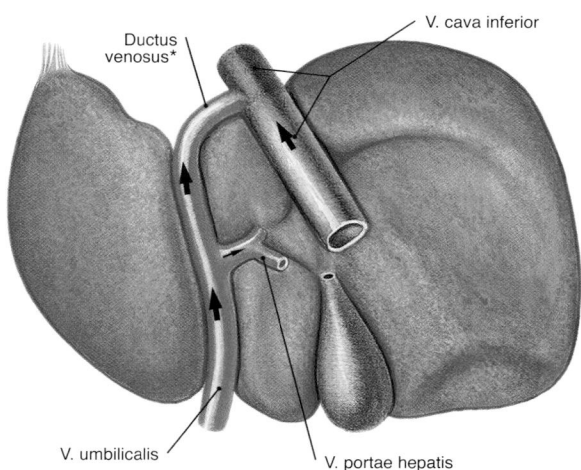

Ductus
venosus*

V. cava inferior

V. umbilicalis

V. portae hepatis

Fig. 747 Liver, Hepar, of a foetus;
oxygen content of the blood is shown
by different colours and the direction
of flow by arrows;
dorsal view.
* Also: Ductus ARANTII

Liver puncture

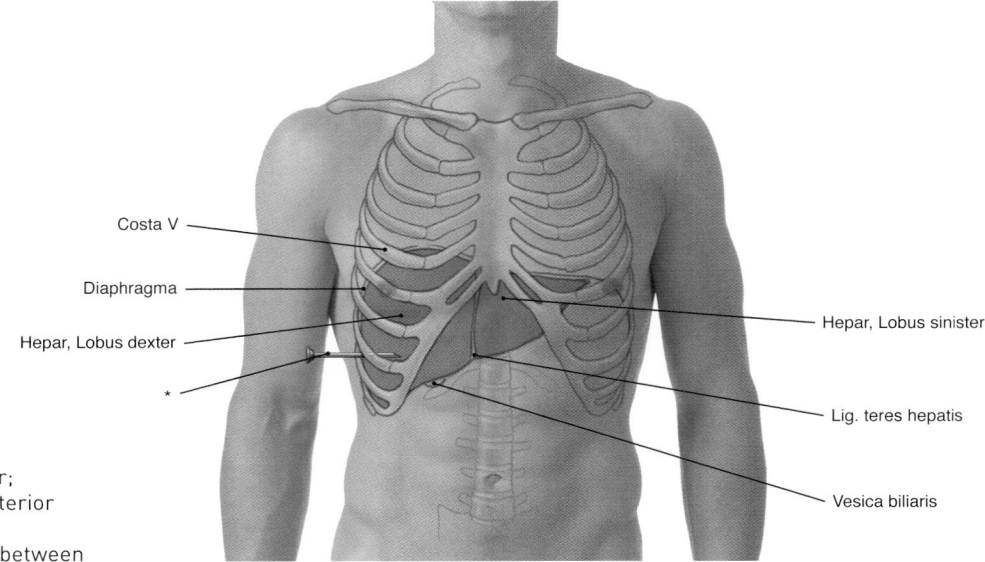

Fig. 748   Liver, Hepar;
projection onto the anterior
abdominal wall;
intermediate position between
inspiration and expiration.
* Position of the needle for liver puncture

Costa V
Diaphragma
Hepar, Lobus dexter
*
Hepar, Lobus sinister
Lig. teres hepatis
Vesica biliaris

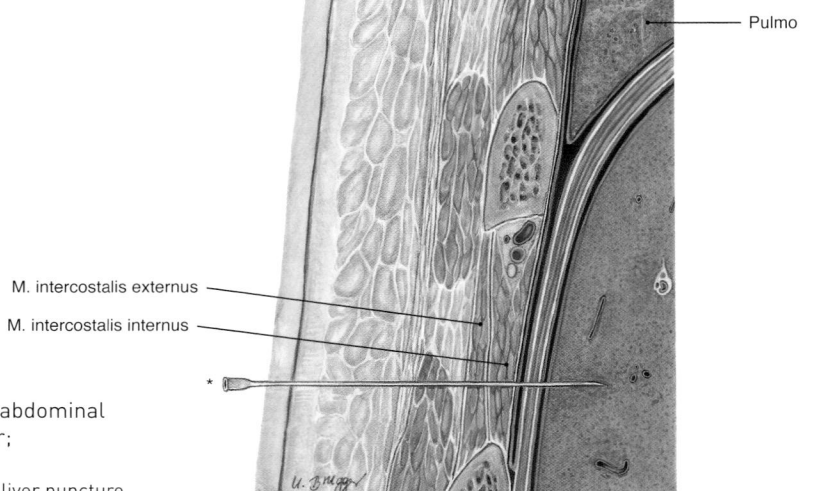

Pulmo
M. intercostalis externus
M. intercostalis internus
*

Fig. 749   Layers of the abdominal
wall and the liver, Hepar;
frontal section.
* Position of the needle for liver puncture

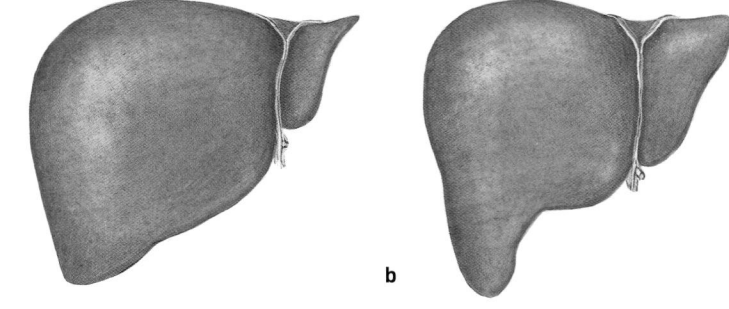

a   b

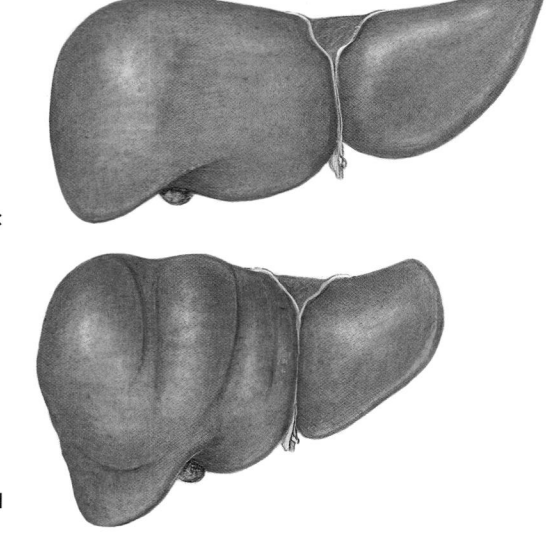

c

d

Fig. 750 a–d   Liver, Hepar;
variations in shape.
a Small left lobe of liver, Lobus hepatis sinister
b Tongue-shaped process of the right lobe of liver,
    Lobus hepatis dexter
c Bridged flat shape
d Diaphragmatic furrows

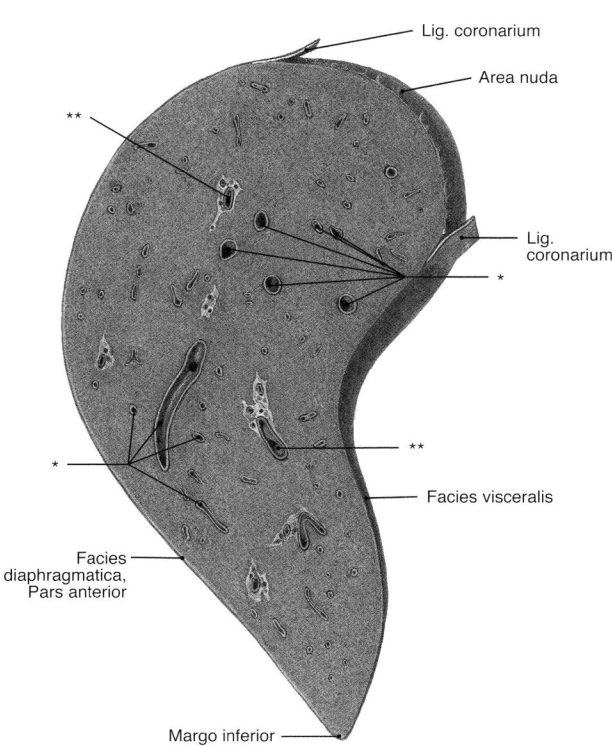

Fig. 751 Liver, Hepar;
sagittal section through the right lobe of liver to demonstrate
the branches of the hepatic veins and the hepatic portal vein.
* Intrahepatic branches of the hepatic veins
** Intrahepatic branches of the hepatic portal vein and the hepatic artery

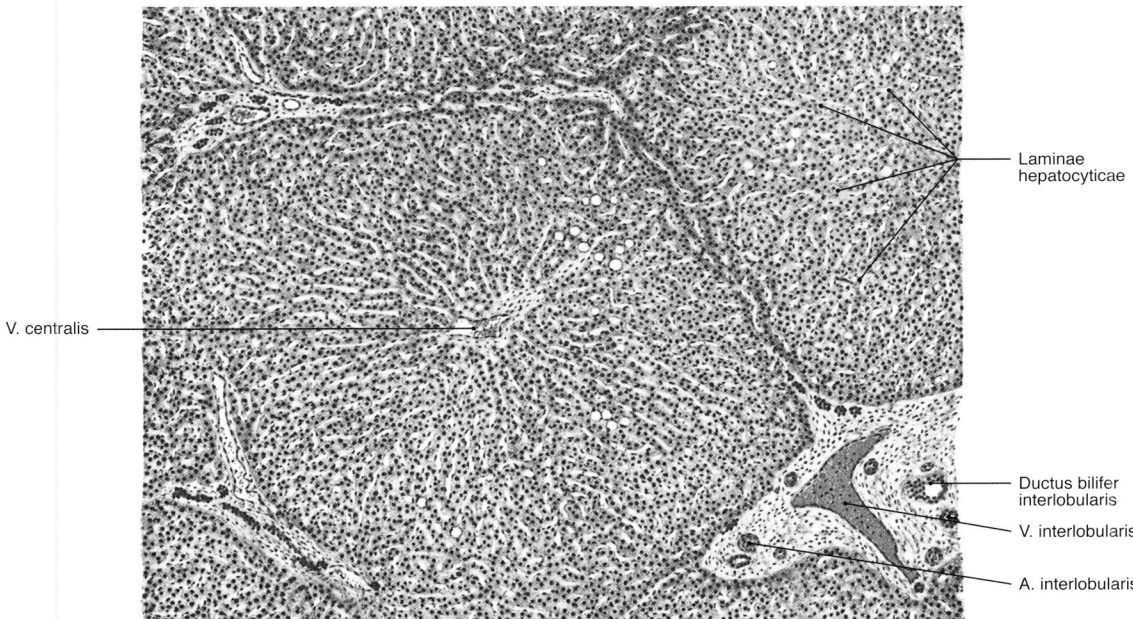

Fig. 752 Liver, Hepar;
microscopic structure (microscopic enlargement at low
magnification);

trias of GLISSON (consists of a branch of the hepatic portal
vein, a branch of the hepatic artery proper and a small bile duct),
and a small liver lobule surrounding a central vein.

Blood vessels of the liver

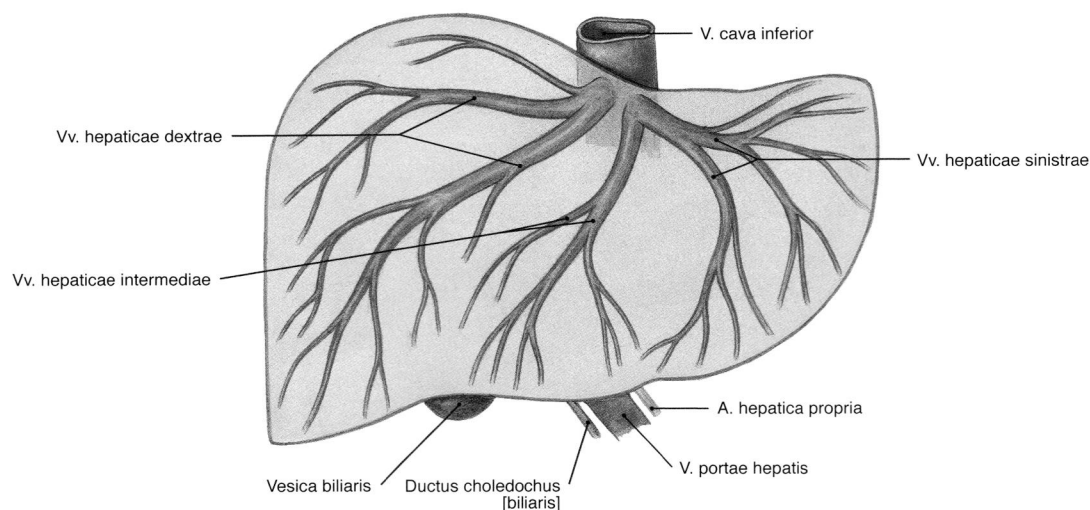

Fig. 753   Liver, Hepar, and hepatic veins, Vv. hepaticae; ventral view.

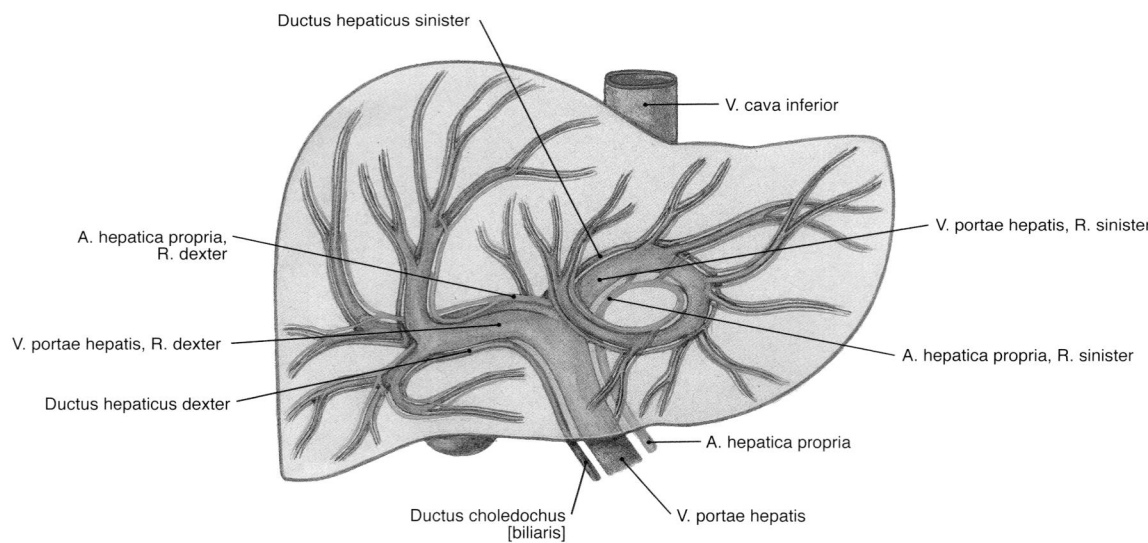

Fig. 754   Liver, Hepar, and the hepatic portal vein, V. portae hepatis; ventral view.

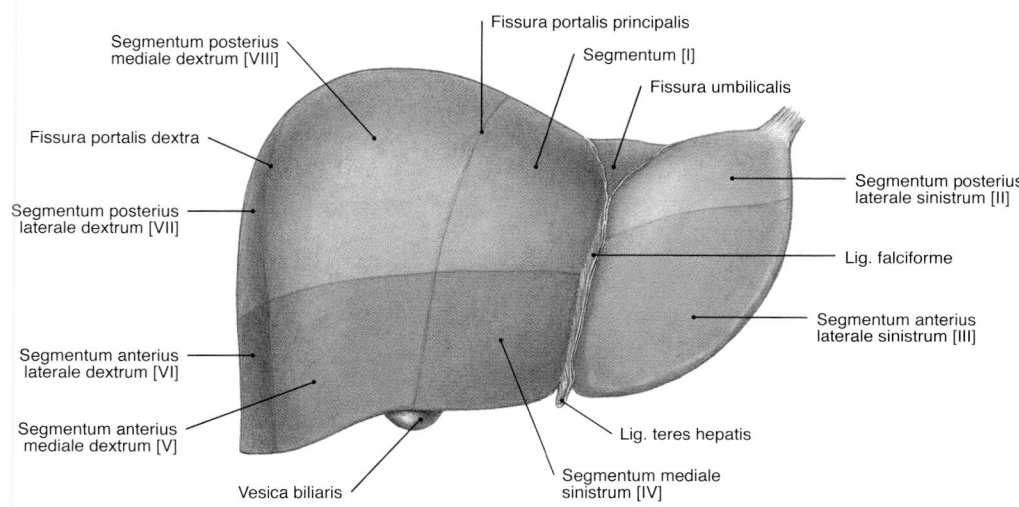

Segmentum posterius mediale dextrum [VIII]

Fissura portalis principalis

Segmentum [I]

Fissura umbilicalis

Fissura portalis dextra

Segmentum posterius laterale sinistrum [II]

Segmentum posterius laterale dextrum [VII]

Lig. falciforme

Segmentum anterius laterale sinistrum [III]

Segmentum anterius laterale dextrum [VI]

Segmentum anterius mediale dextrum [V]

Lig. teres hepatis

Vesica biliaris

Segmentum mediale sinistrum [IV]

Fig. 755 Liver, Hepar;
the segments of the lobes are shown in different colours;
ventral view.

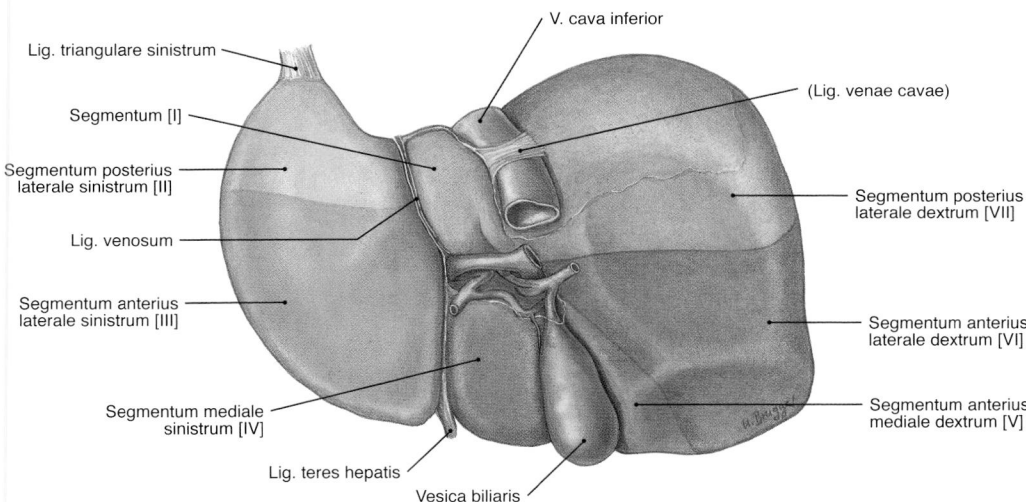

V. cava inferior

Lig. triangulare sinistrum

(Lig. venae cavae)

Segmentum [I]

Segmentum posterius laterale sinistrum [II]

Segmentum posterius laterale dextrum [VII]

Lig. venosum

Segmentum anterius laterale sinistrum [III]

Segmentum anterius laterale dextrum [VI]

Segmentum mediale sinistrum [IV]

Segmentum anterius mediale dextrum [V]

Lig. teres hepatis

Vesica biliaris

Fig. 756 Liver, Hepar;
the segments of the lobes are shown in different colours;
dorsal view.

Liver, ultrasound

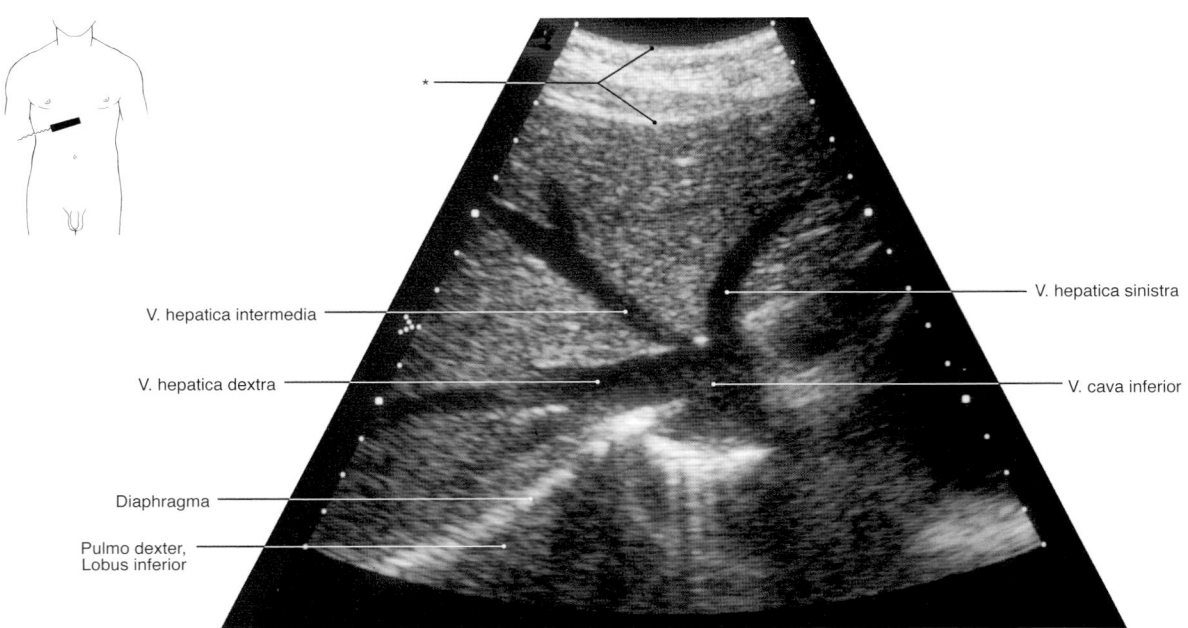

V. hepatica intermedia

V. hepatica dextra

Diaphragma

Pulmo dexter,
Lobus inferior

V. hepatica sinistra

V. cava inferior

→ 753

Fig. 757 Hepatic veins, Vv. hepaticae;
ultrasound image showing the opening of the hepatic veins
into the inferior vena cava;
inferior view.
* Abdominal wall

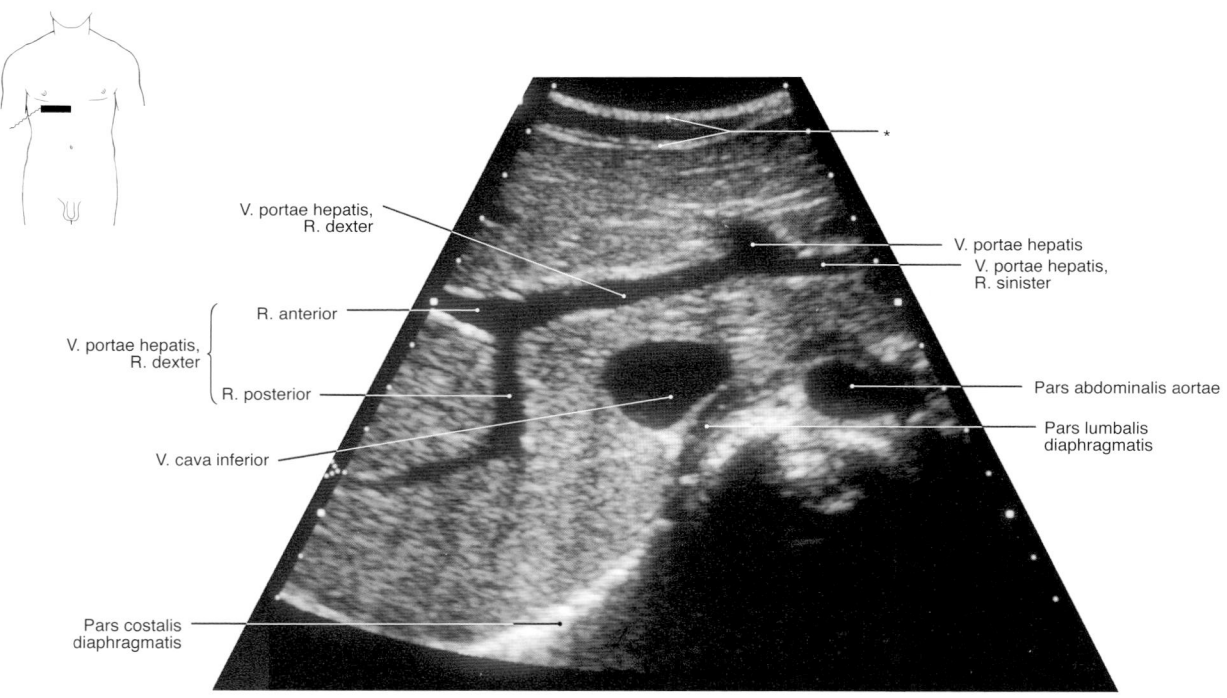

V. portae hepatis,
R. dexter

R. anterior

V. portae hepatis,
R. dexter

R. posterior

V. cava inferior

Pars costalis
diaphragmatis

V. portae hepatis

V. portae hepatis,
R. sinister

Pars abdominalis aortae

Pars lumbalis
diaphragmatis

→ 754

Fig. 758 Hepatic portal vein, V. portae hepatis;
ultrasound image showing the division of the hepatic portal vein
into the main branches;
inferior view.
* Abdominal wall

Liver, laparoscopy

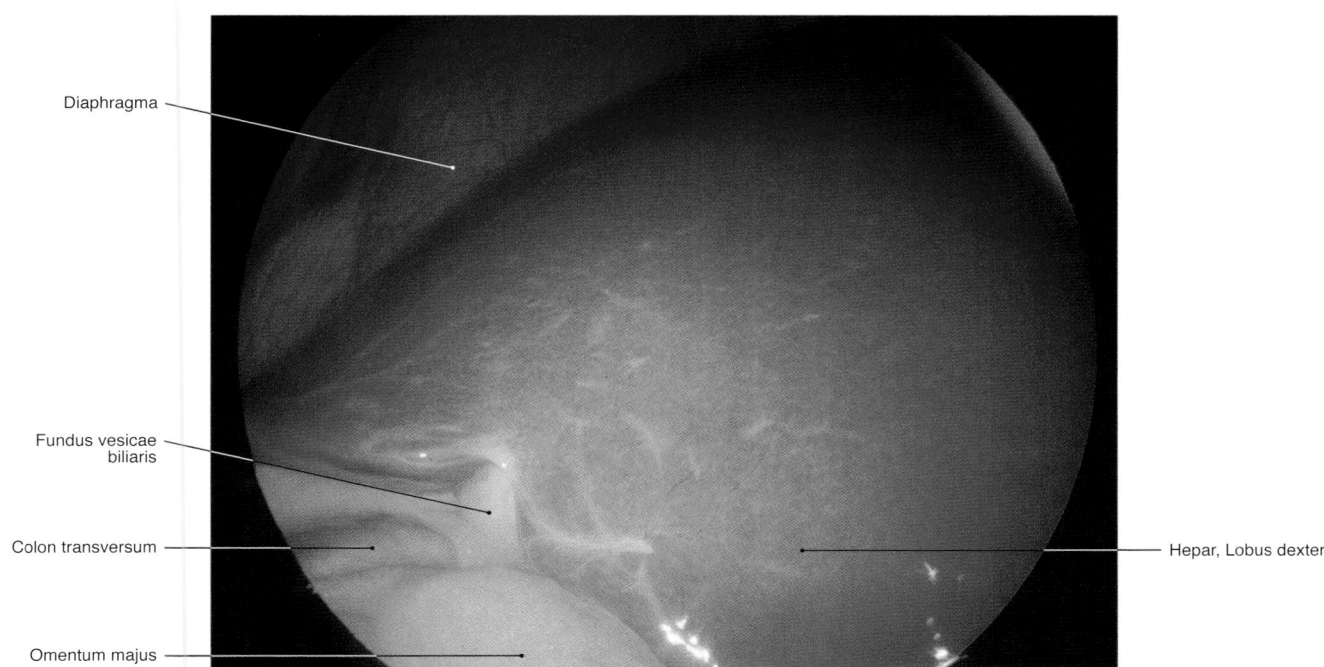

Diaphragma

Fundus vesicae biliaris

Colon transversum

Omentum majus

Hepar, Lobus dexter

Fig. 759   Liver, Hepar, and gallbladder, Vesica biliaris [fellea];
laparoscopy;
oblique inferior view from the left.

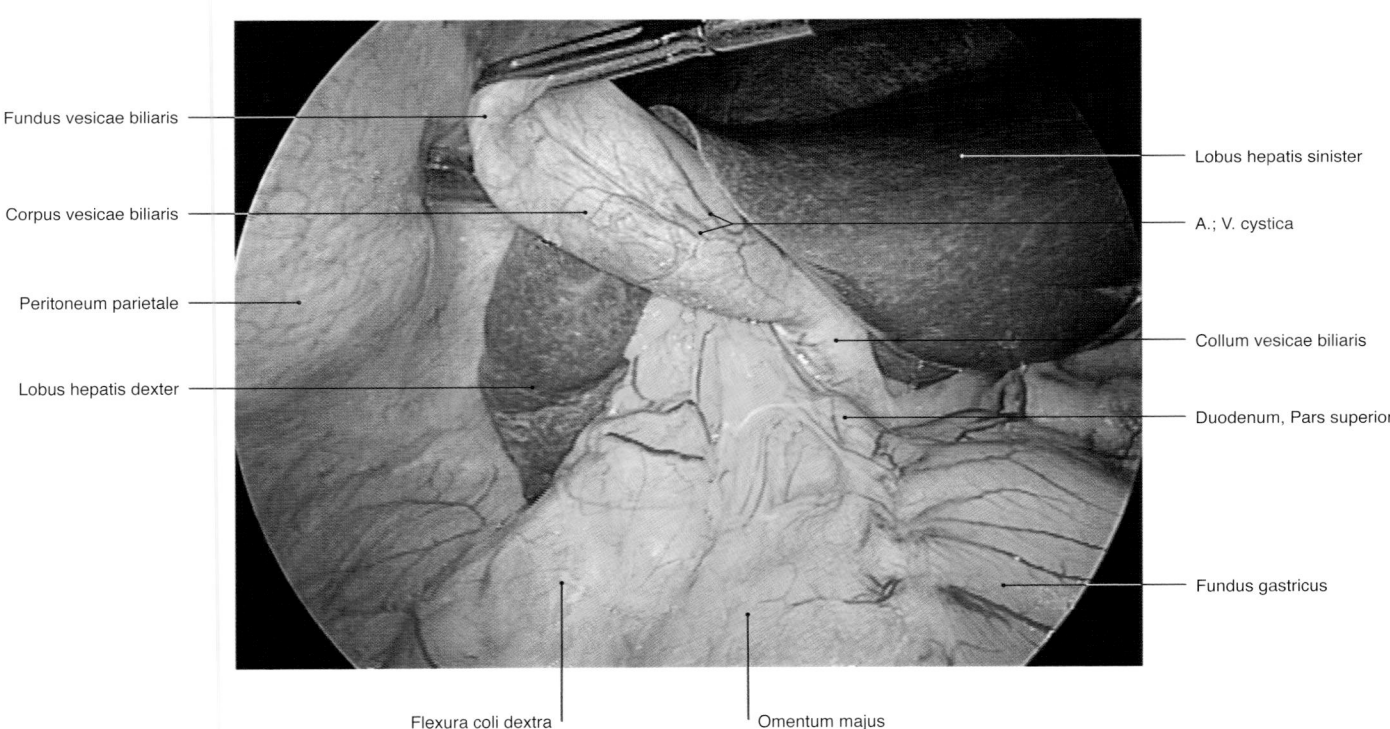

Fundus vesicae biliaris

Corpus vesicae biliaris

Peritoneum parietale

Lobus hepatis dexter

Lobus hepatis sinister

A.; V. cystica

Collum vesicae biliaris

Duodenum, Pars superior

Fundus gastricus

Flexura coli dextra

Omentum majus

Fig. 760   Gallbladder, Vesica biliaris [fellea], and liver, Hepar;
laparoscopy;
ventral view.

Gallbladder and bile duct system

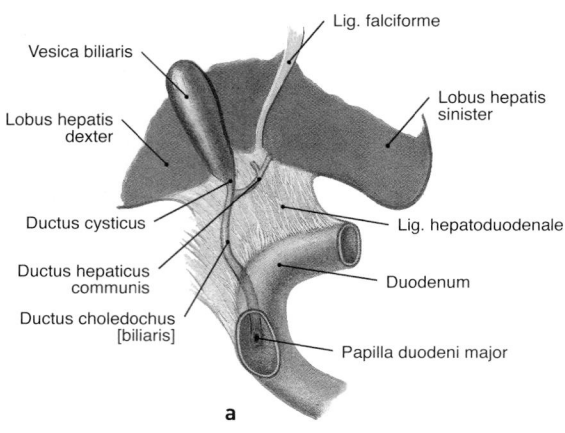

Vesica biliaris

Lobus hepatis dexter

Ductus cysticus

Ductus hepaticus communis

Ductus choledochus [biliaris]

Lig. falciforme

Lobus hepatis sinister

Lig. hepatoduodenale

Duodenum

Papilla duodeni major

a

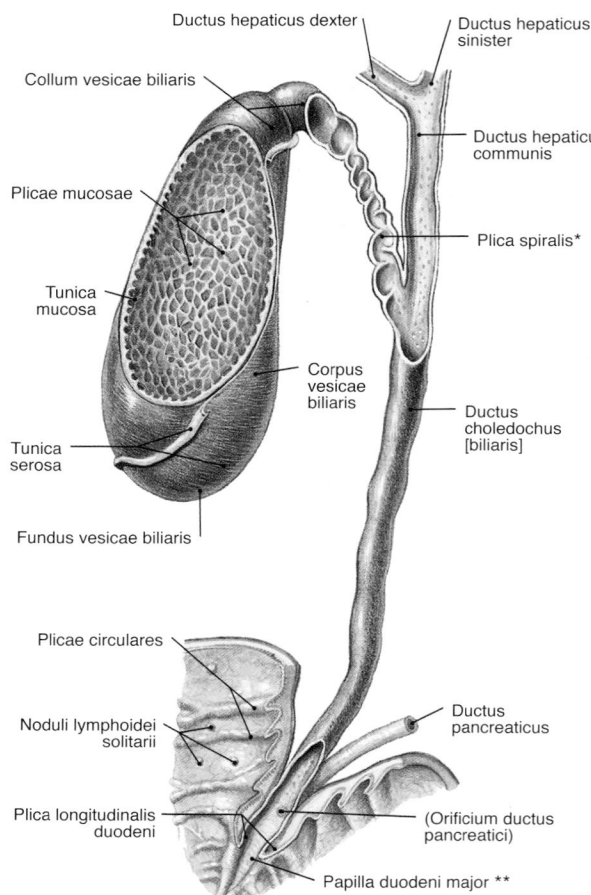

Ductus hepaticus dexter

Collum vesicae biliaris

Plicae mucosae

Tunica mucosa

Tunica serosa

Fundus vesicae biliaris

Plicae circulares

Noduli lymphoidei solitarii

Plica longitudinalis duodeni

Ductus hepaticus sinister

Ductus hepaticus communis

Plica spiralis*

Corpus vesicae biliaris

Ductus choledochus [biliaris]

Ductus pancreaticus

(Orificium ductus pancreatici)

Papilla duodeni major **

Fig. 761 Gallbladder, Vesica biliaris [fellea], and bile duct system; ventral view.
* Clinical term: HEISTER's valve
** Clinical term: tubercle of VATER

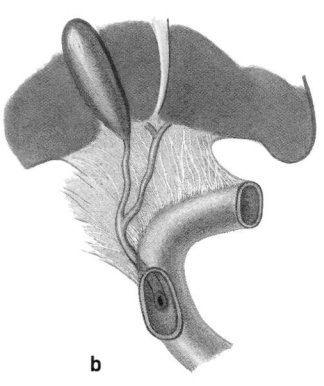

b

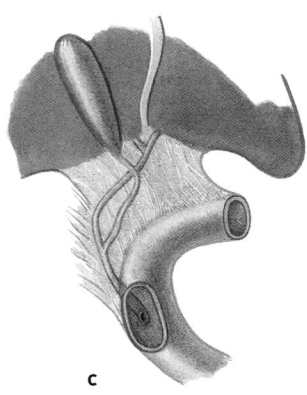

c

Fig. 762 a–c Variations in the bile duct system: common hepatic duct, Ductus hepaticus communis, and bile duct, Ductus choledochus.
a High union of the common hepatic duct, Ductus hepaticus communis, and the cystic duct, Ductus cysticus
b Low union of the common hepatic duct, Ductus hepaticus communis, and the cystic duct, Ductus cysticus
c Low union after the cystic duct, Ductus cysticus, crosses over the common hepatic duct, Ductus hepaticus communis

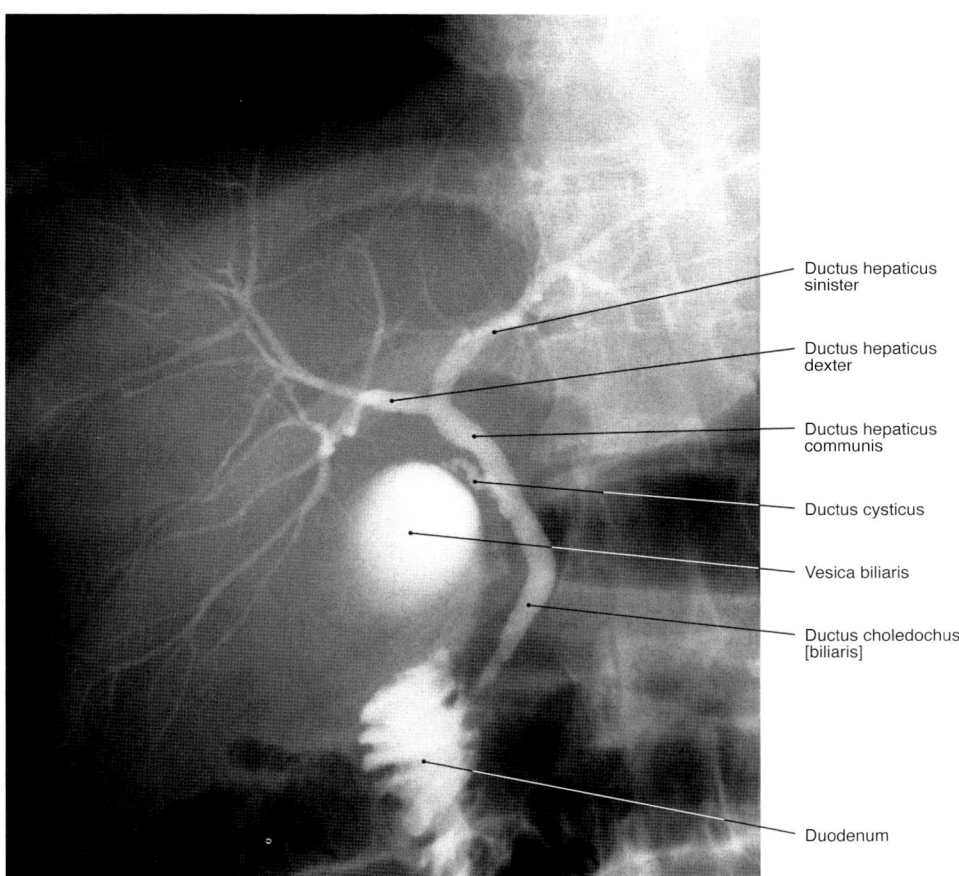

Ductus hepaticus sinister

Ductus hepaticus dexter

Ductus hepaticus communis

Ductus cysticus

Vesica biliaris

Ductus choledochus [biliaris]

Duodenum

Fig. 763 Bile duct system;
AP-radiograph after administration of a contrast medium;
upright position;
ventral view.

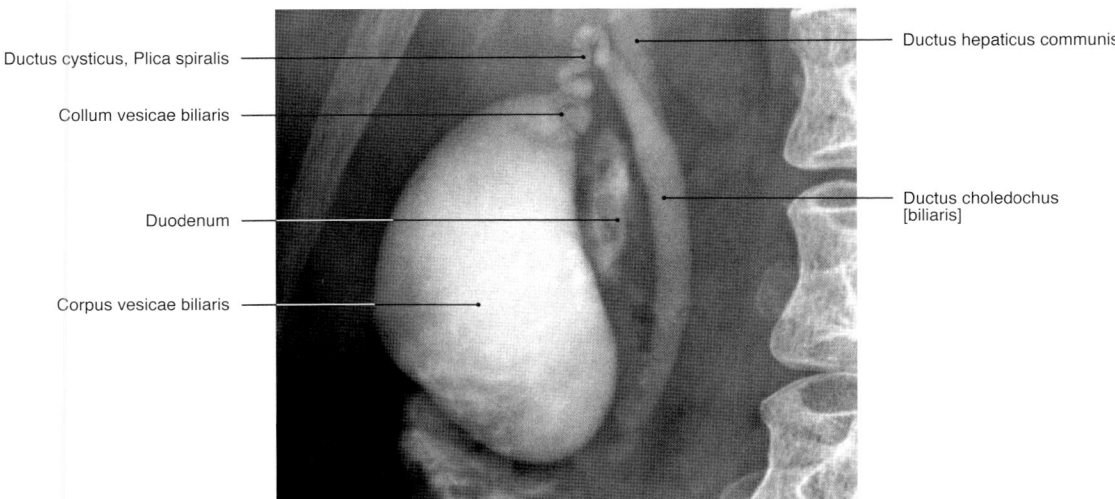

Ductus cysticus, Plica spiralis

Collum vesicae biliaris

Duodenum

Corpus vesicae biliaris

Ductus hepaticus communis

Ductus choledochus [biliaris]

Fig. 764 Gallbladder, Vesica biliaris [fellea],
and bile duct system;
AP-radiograph after administration of a contrast medium;
upright position;
ventral view.

Pancreas

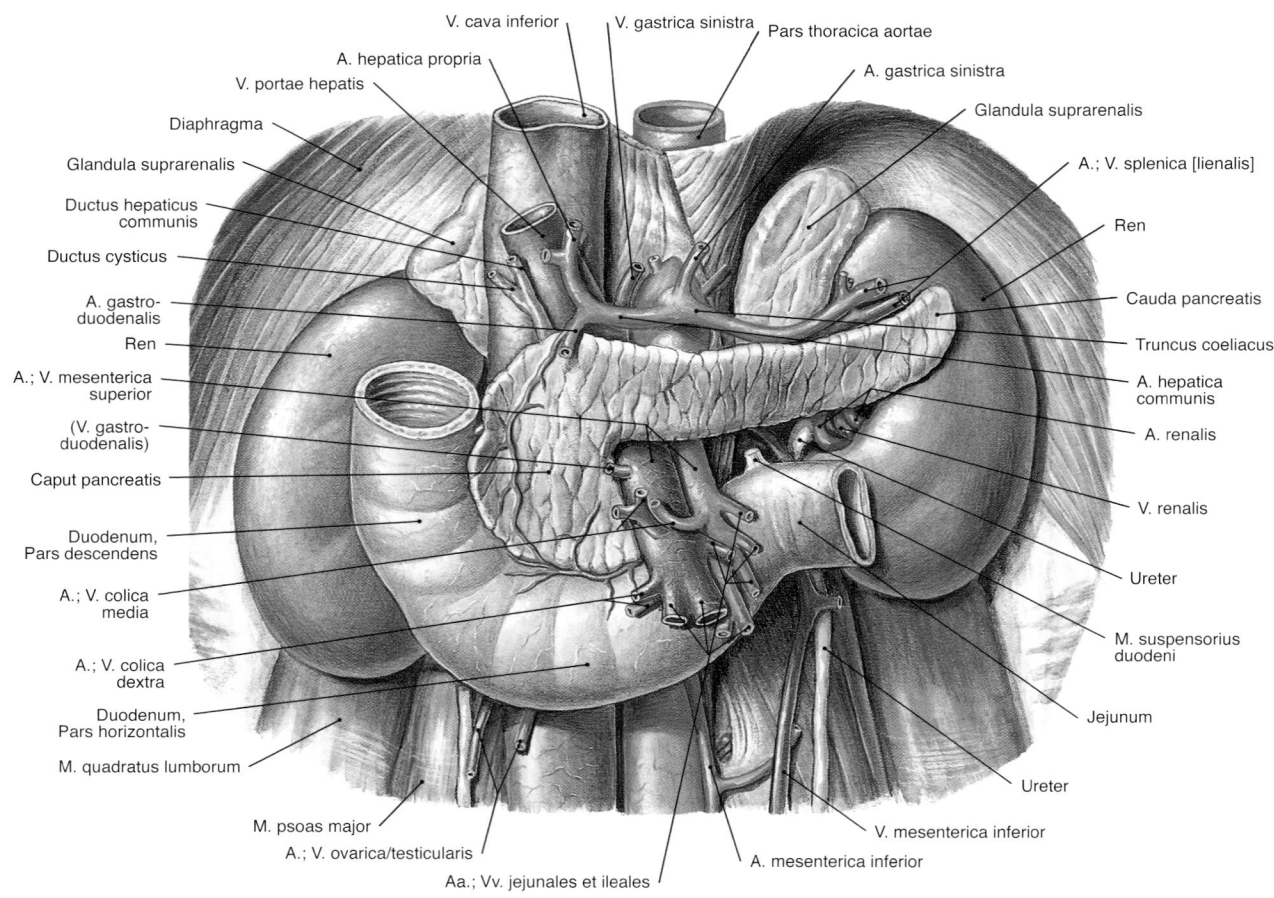

V. cava inferior
V. gastrica sinistra
Pars thoracica aortae
A. hepatica propria
A. gastrica sinistra
V. portae hepatis
Glandula suprarenalis
Diaphragma
Glandula suprarenalis
A.; V. splenica [lienalis]
Ductus hepaticus communis
Ren
Ductus cysticus
Cauda pancreatis
A. gastro-duodenalis
Truncus coeliacus
Ren
A. hepatica communis
A.; V. mesenterica superior
A. renalis
(V. gastro-duodenalis)
V. renalis
Caput pancreatis
Ureter
Duodenum, Pars descendens
M. suspensorius duodeni
A.; V. colica media
Jejunum
A.; V. colica dextra
Ureter
Duodenum, Pars horizontalis
M. quadratus lumborum
M. psoas major
V. mesenterica inferior
A.; V. ovarica/testicularis
A. mesenterica inferior
Aa.; Vv. jejunales et ileales

Fig. 765 Retroperitoneal organs and vessels of the upper abdomen; ventral view.

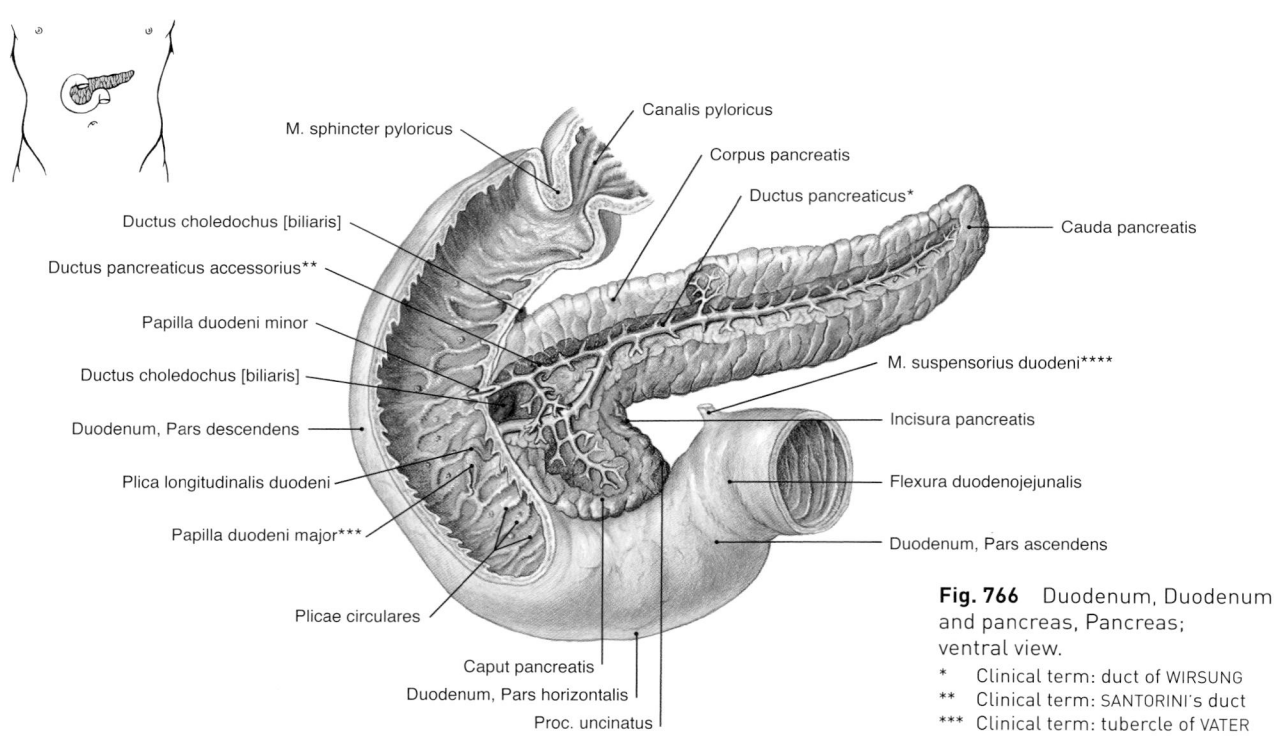

M. sphincter pyloricus
Canalis pyloricus
Corpus pancreatis
Ductus choledochus [biliaris]
Ductus pancreaticus*
Ductus pancreaticus accessorius**
Cauda pancreatis
Papilla duodeni minor
Ductus choledochus [biliaris]
M. suspensorius duodeni****
Duodenum, Pars descendens
Incisura pancreatis
Plica longitudinalis duodeni
Flexura duodenojejunalis
Papilla duodeni major***
Duodenum, Pars ascendens
Plicae circulares
Caput pancreatis
Duodenum, Pars horizontalis
Proc. uncinatus

Fig. 766 Duodenum, Duodenum, and pancreas, Pancreas; ventral view.
*   Clinical term: duct of WIRSUNG
**   Clinical term: SANTORINI's duct
***   Clinical term: tubercle of VATER
**** Clinical term: muscle of TREITZ

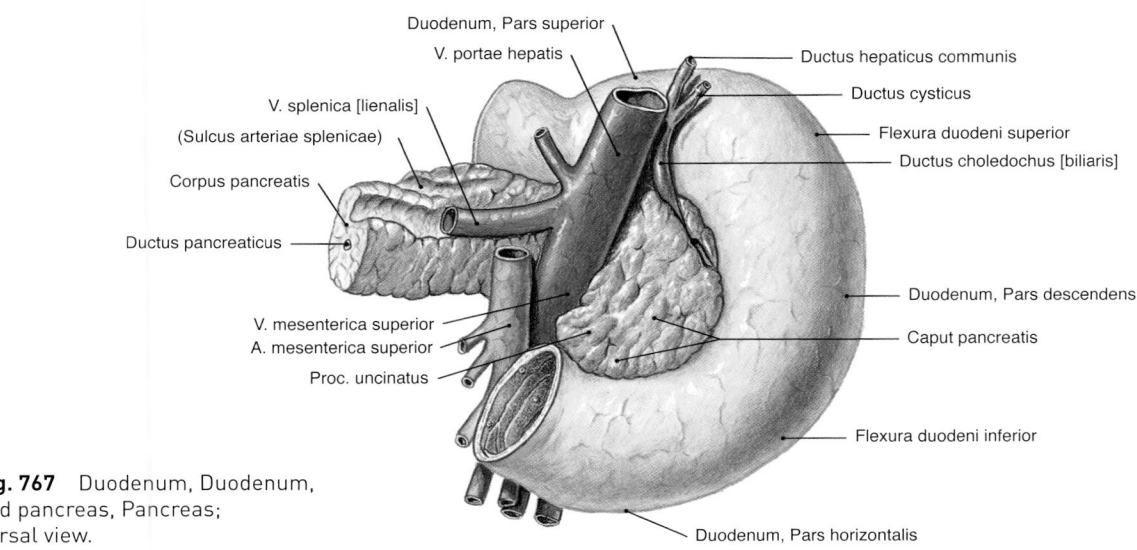

Fig. 767 Duodenum, Duodenum, and pancreas, Pancreas; dorsal view.

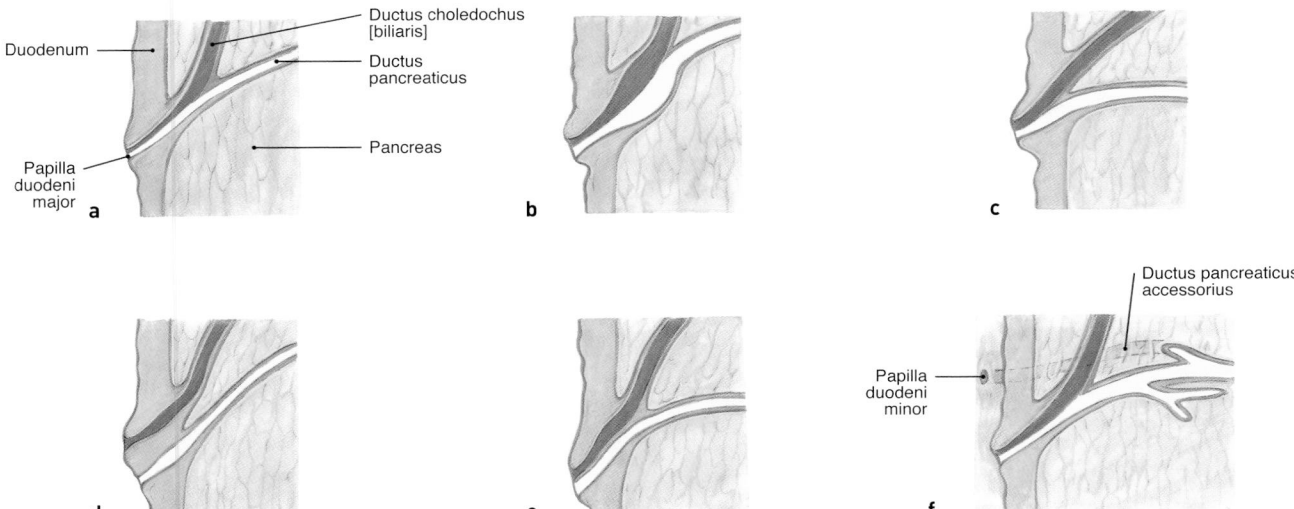

Fig. 768 a–f Variations in the opening of the bile duct, Ductus choledochus, and the pancreatic duct, Ductus pancreaticus.
a Long common part
b Ampullary enlargement at the terminal part

c Short common part
d Separate opening
e Single opening with a septum dividing the common duct
f Accessory duct, Ductus pancreaticus accessorius

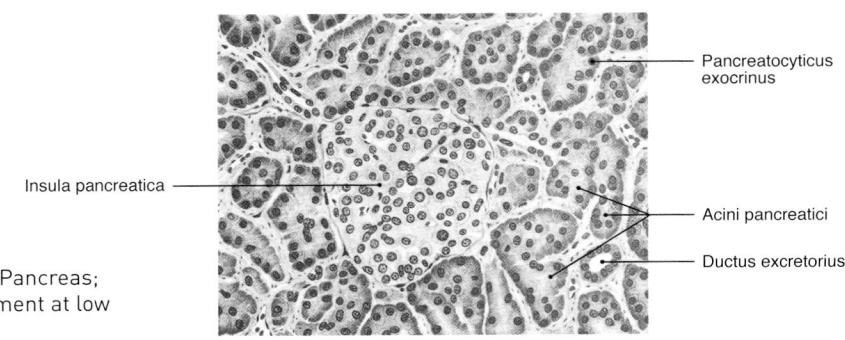

Fig. 769 Pancreas, Pancreas; microscopic enlargement at low magnification.

Pancreas, imaging

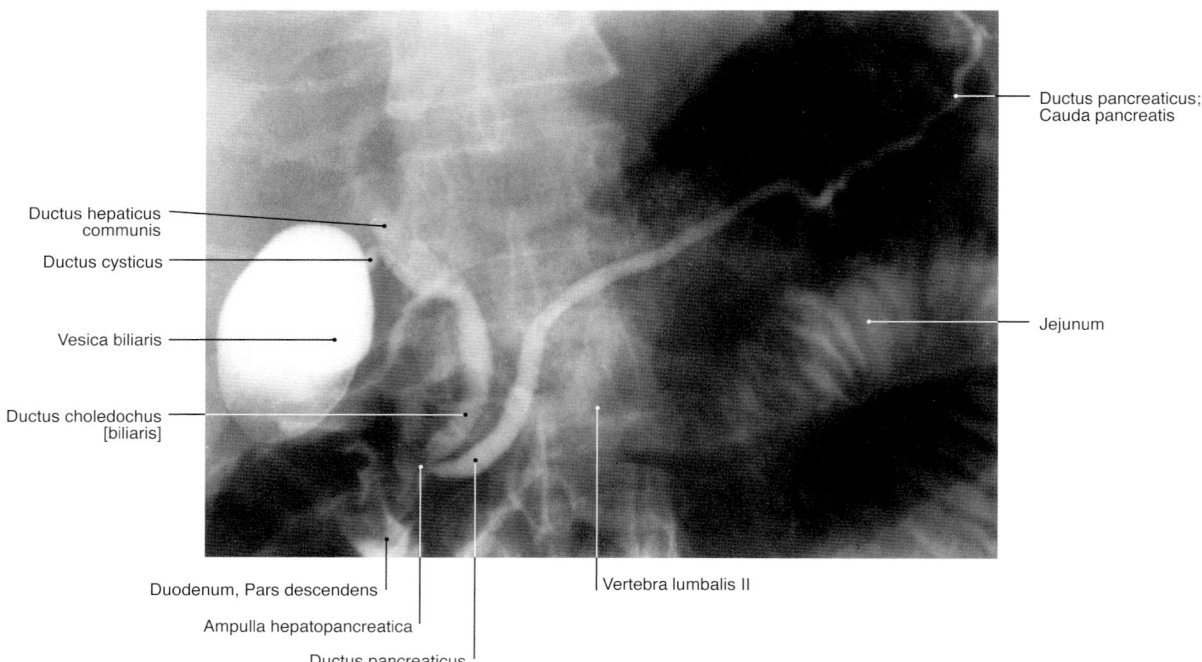

Ductus hepaticus communis

Ductus cysticus

Vesica biliaris

Ductus choledochus [biliaris]

Duodenum, Pars descendens

Ampulla hepatopancreatica

Ductus pancreaticus

Ductus pancreaticus; Cauda pancreatis

Jejunum

Vertebra lumbalis II

Fig. 770 Pancreatic duct, Ductus pancreaticus; bile duct, Ductus choledochus, and gallbladder, Vesica biliaris [fellea]; AP-radiograph; supine position; after endoscopic intubation of the common excretory duct of the liver and the pancreas, as well as injection of a contrast medium; ventral view.
Clinical term: ERCP (endoscopic retrograde cholangio-pancreaticography).

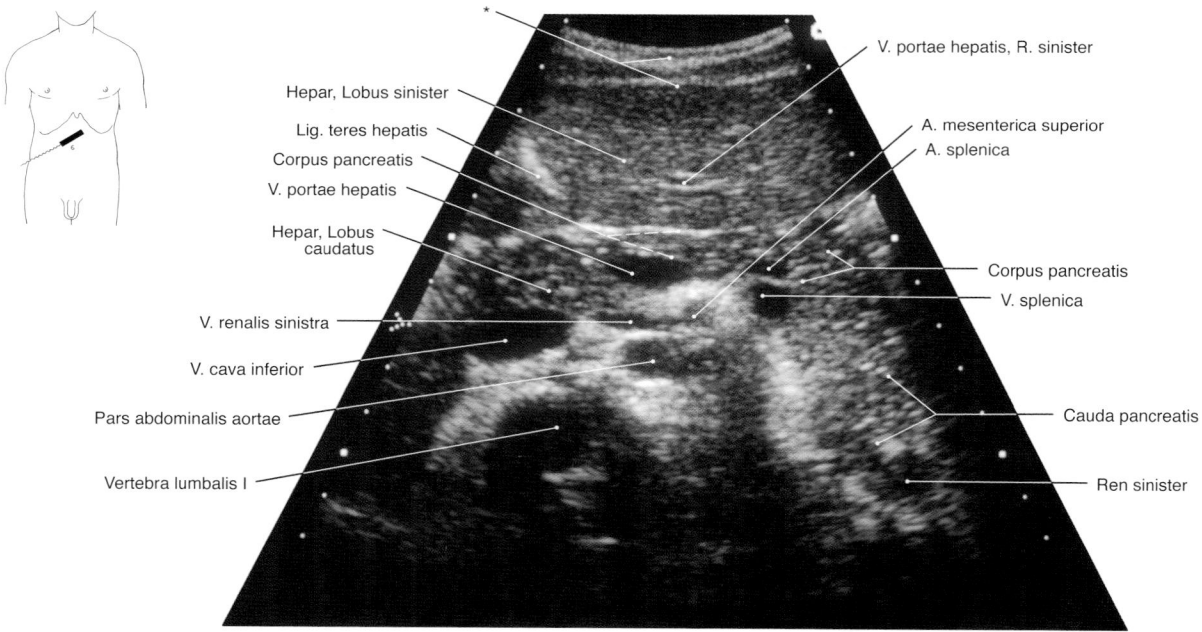

Hepar, Lobus sinister

Lig. teres hepatis

Corpus pancreatis

V. portae hepatis

Hepar, Lobus caudatus

V. renalis sinistra

V. cava inferior

Pars abdominalis aortae

Vertebra lumbalis I

*

V. portae hepatis, R. sinister

A. mesenterica superior

A. splenica

Corpus pancreatis

V. splenica

Cauda pancreatis

Ren sinister

Fig. 771 Pancreas, Pancreas; ultrasound image showing the pancreas and adjacent large vessels in deep inspiration; oblique inferior view.
* Abdominal wall

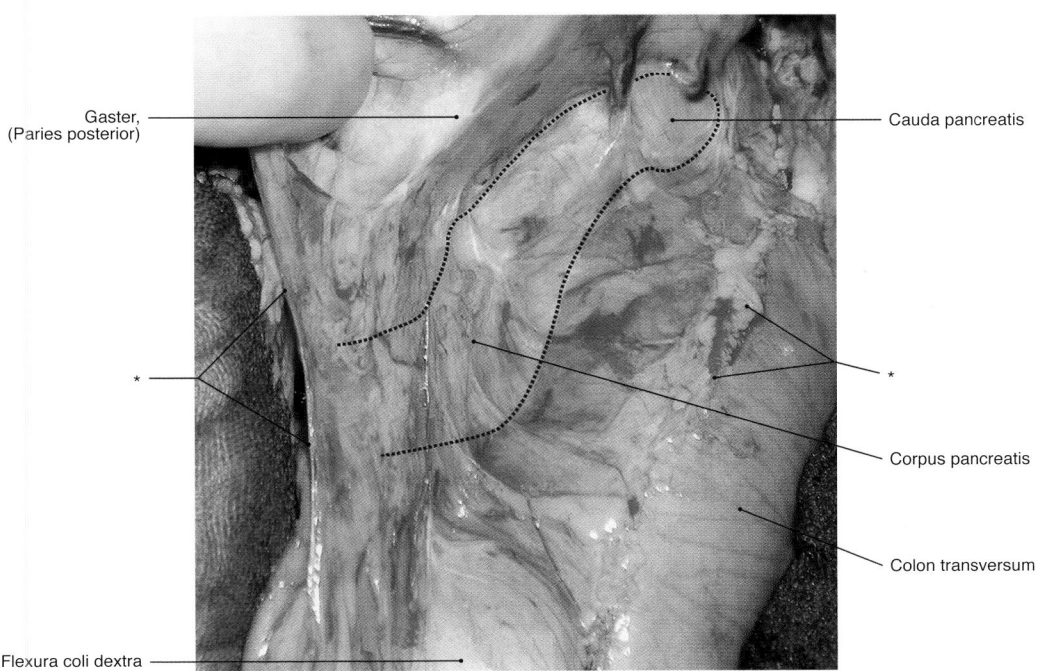

Gaster, (Paries posterior)
Cauda pancreatis
*
Corpus pancreatis
Colon transversum
Flexura coli dextra

Fig. 772 Pancreas, Pancreas;
the gastrocolic ligament of the greater omentum has been
dissected to expose the omental bursa;
photograph taken during surgery.
* Dissection line at the greater omentum

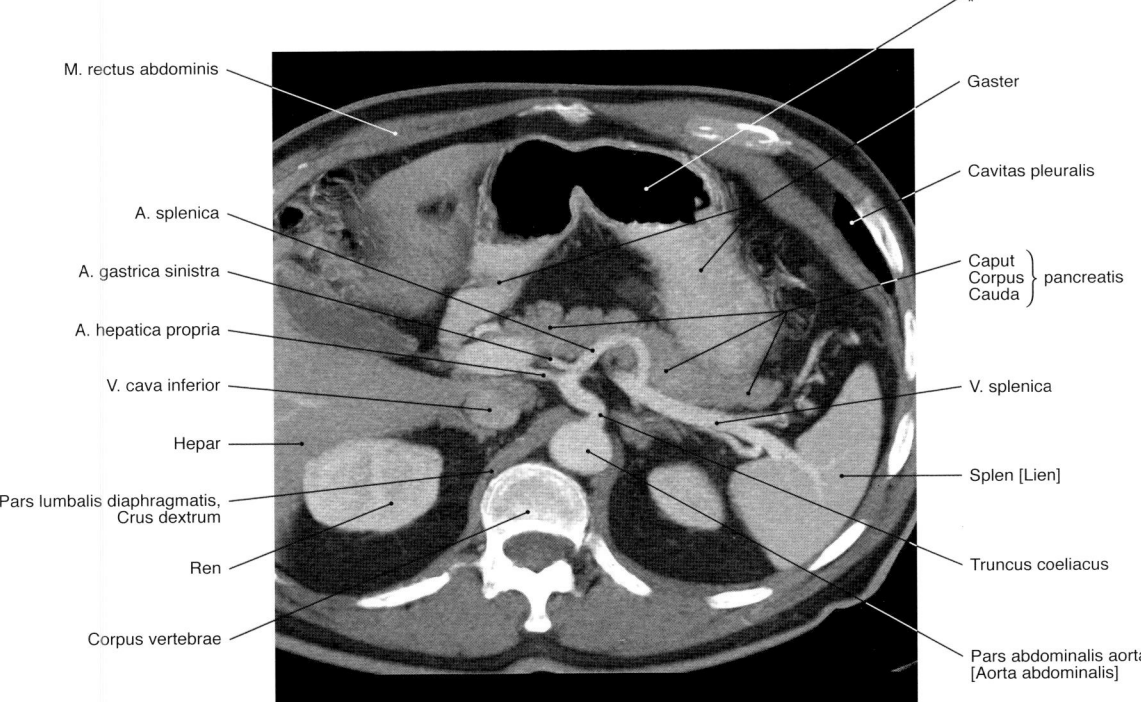

M. rectus abdominis
A. splenica
A. gastrica sinistra
A. hepatica propria
V. cava inferior
Hepar
Pars lumbalis diaphragmatis, Crus dextrum
Ren
Corpus vertebrae

*
Gaster
Cavitas pleuralis
Caput
Corpus } pancreatis
Cauda
V. splenica
Splen [Lien]
Truncus coeliacus
Pars abdominalis aortae [Aorta abdominalis]

Fig. 773 Pancreas, Pancreas;
computed tomographic horizontal section (CT);
inferior view.
In this subject, the coeliac trunk is located remarkably low.
* Air bubble in the stomach

Spleen

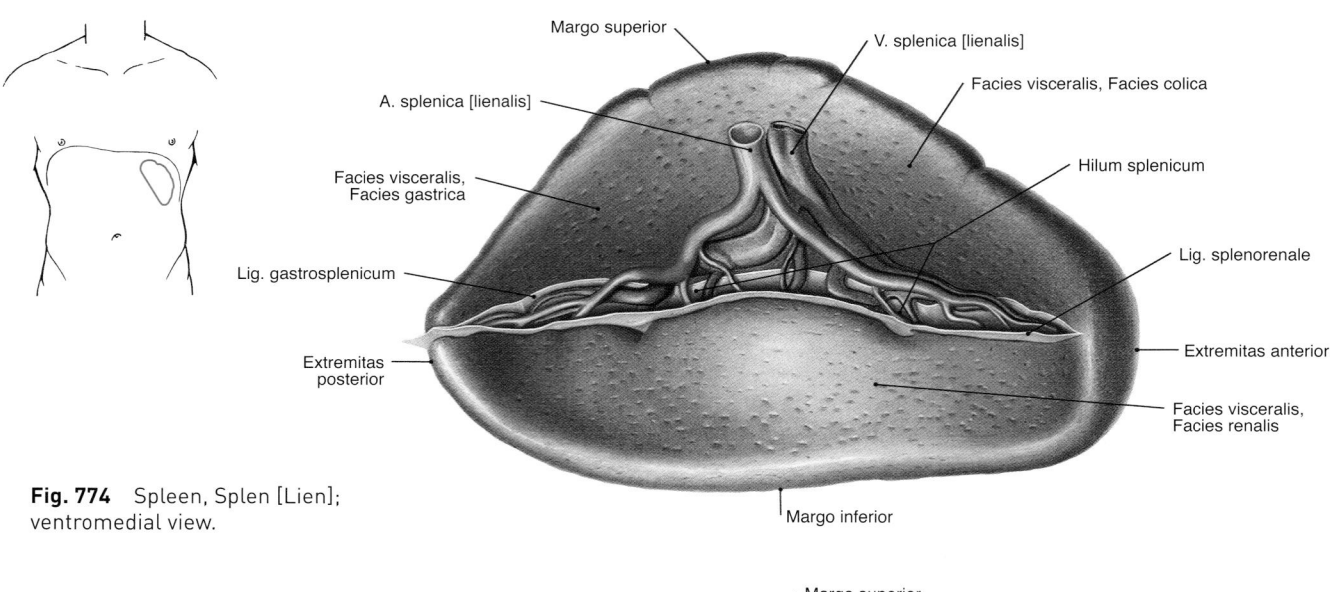

Fig. 774 Spleen, Splen [Lien];
ventromedial view.

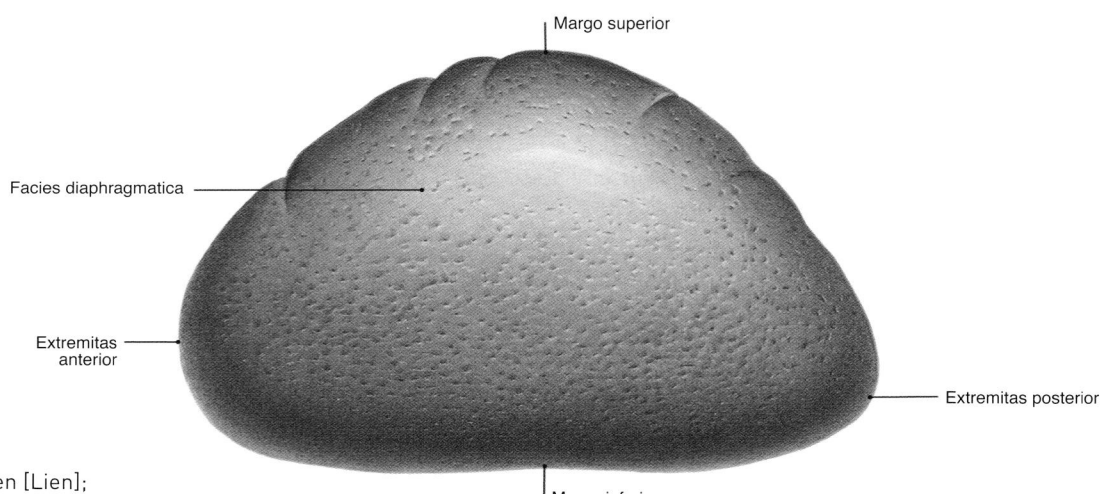

Fig. 775 Spleen, Splen [Lien];
superolateral view.

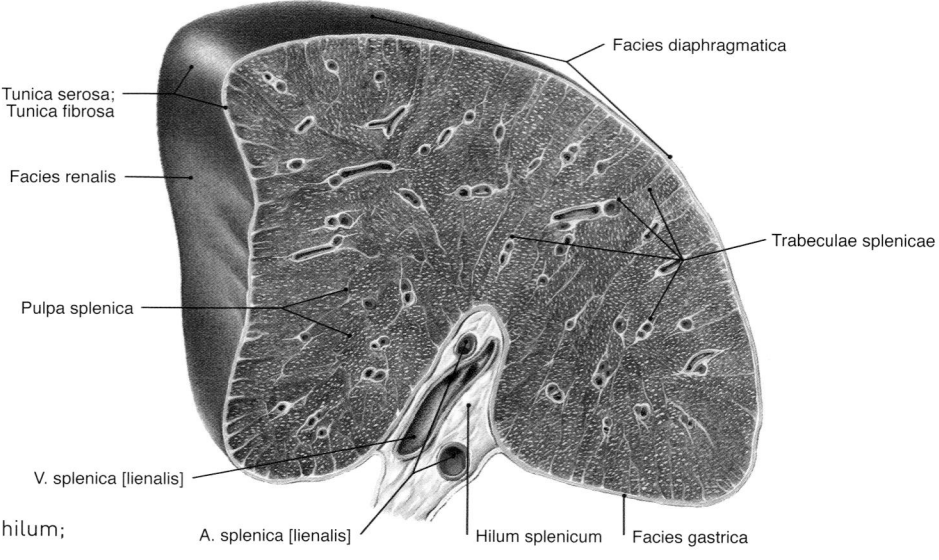

Fig. 776 Spleen, Splen [Lien];
cross-section through the splenic hilum;
superomedial view.

Development of the intestines

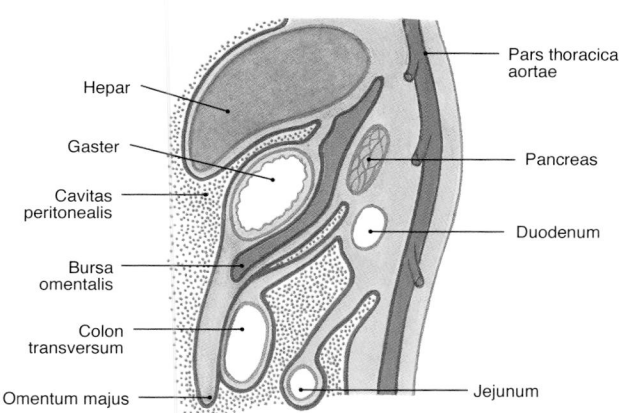

Fig. 777 Development of the peritoneal cavity, Cavitas peritonealis, and the visceral relationships; schematic median section; lateral view.

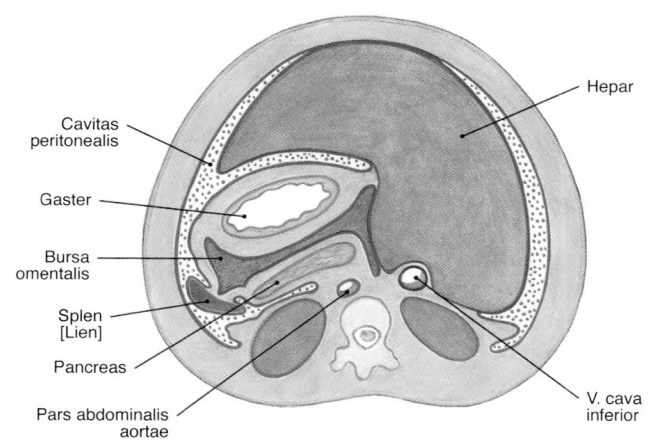

Fig. 778 Development of the peritoneal cavity, Cavitas peritonealis; schematic horizontal section; superior view.

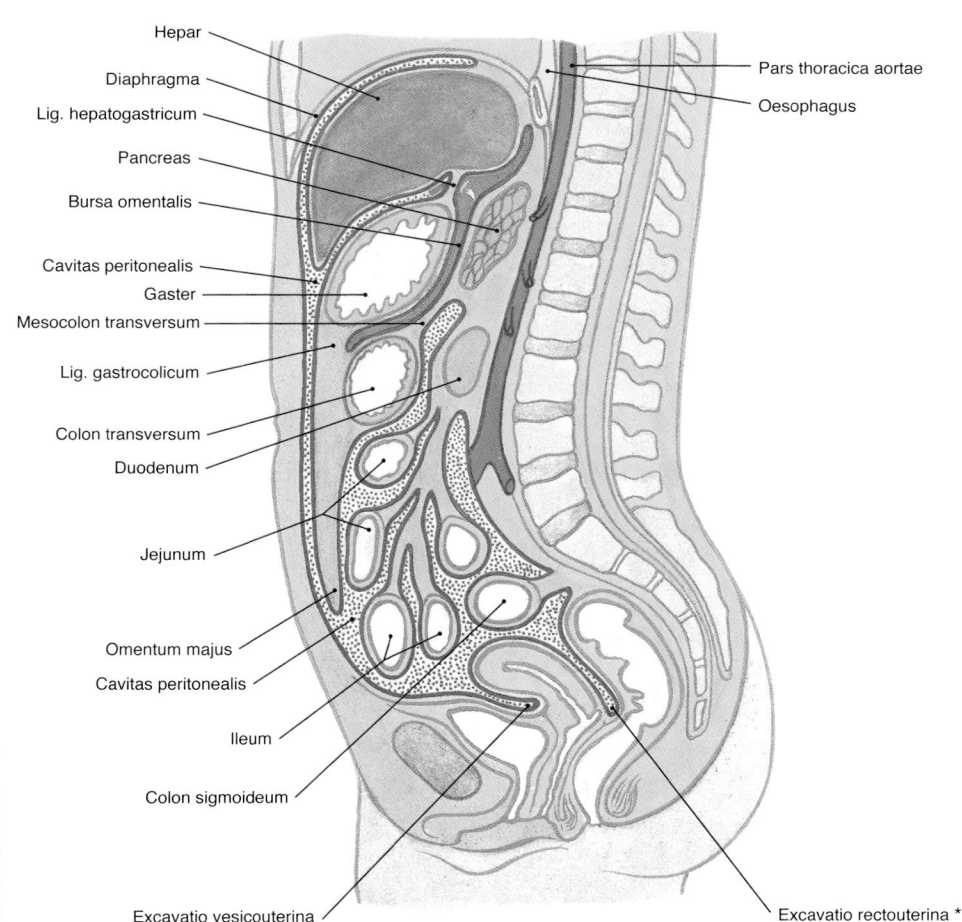

Fig. 779 Development of the peritoneal cavity, Cavitas peritonealis, and the visceral relationships of the female; final state of the peritoneal cavity with adhesion of the greater omentum to the transverse colon; schematic median section; lateral view.

The omental bursa corresponds with the peritoneal cavity via the omental foramen.

* Clinical term: pouch of DOUGLAS

Greater omentum

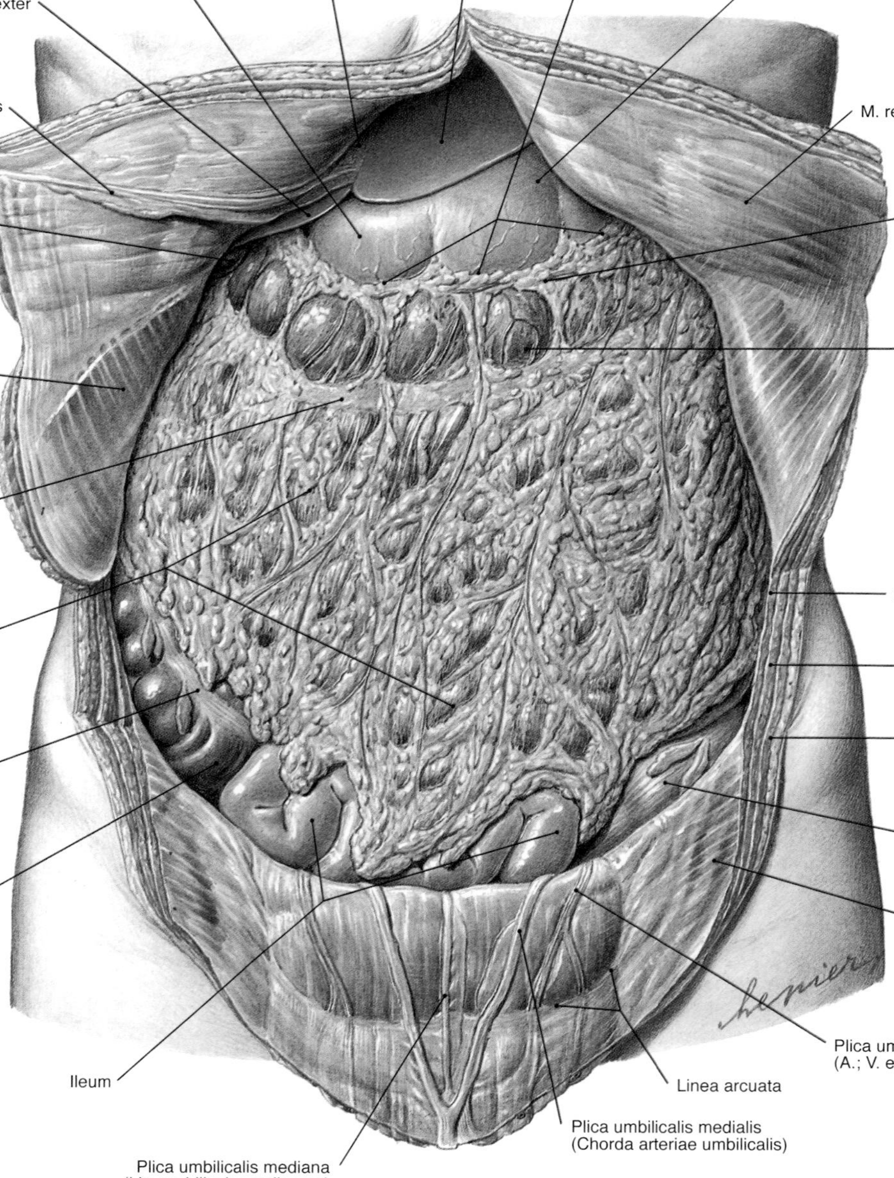

Fig. 780 Position of the abdominal viscera, Situs viscerum, and greater omentum, Omentum majus.

→ 578

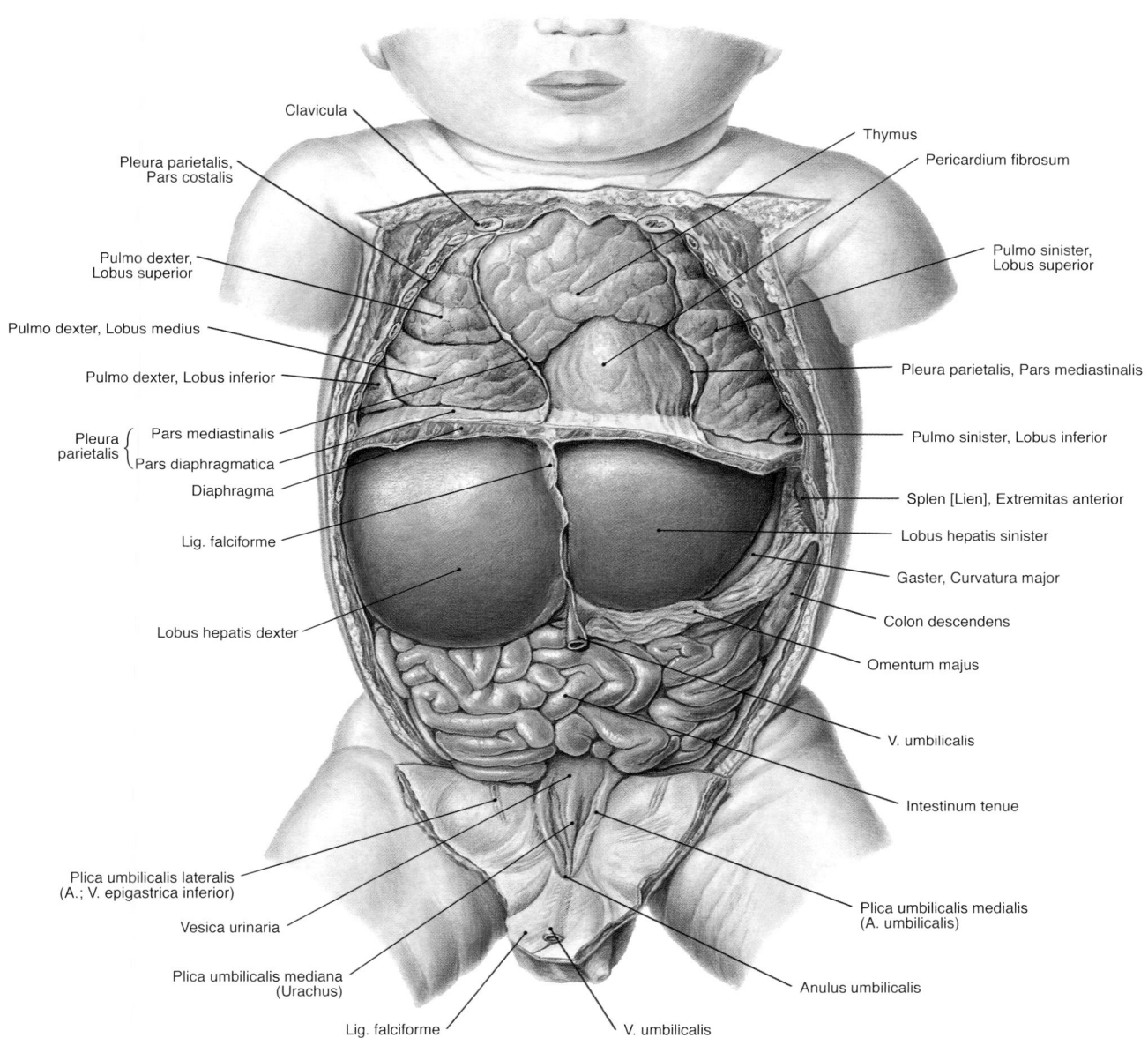

Clavicula

Pleura parietalis,
Pars costalis

Pulmo dexter,
Lobus superior

Pulmo dexter, Lobus medius

Pulmo dexter, Lobus inferior

Pleura   Pars mediastinalis
parietalis {
             Pars diaphragmatica

Diaphragma

Lig. falciforme

Lobus hepatis dexter

Plica umbilicalis lateralis
(A.; V. epigastrica inferior)

Vesica urinaria

Plica umbilicalis mediana
(Urachus)

Lig. falciforme

Thymus

Pericardium fibrosum

Pulmo sinister,
Lobus superior

Pleura parietalis, Pars mediastinalis

Pulmo sinister, Lobus inferior

Splen [Lien], Extremitas anterior

Lobus hepatis sinister

Gaster, Curvatura major

Colon descendens

Omentum majus

V. umbilicalis

Intestinum tenue

Plica umbilicalis medialis
(A. umbilicalis)

Anulus umbilicalis

V. umbilicalis

Fig. 781 Position of the abdominal viscera of the neonate.

Abdominal viscera in the upper abdomen

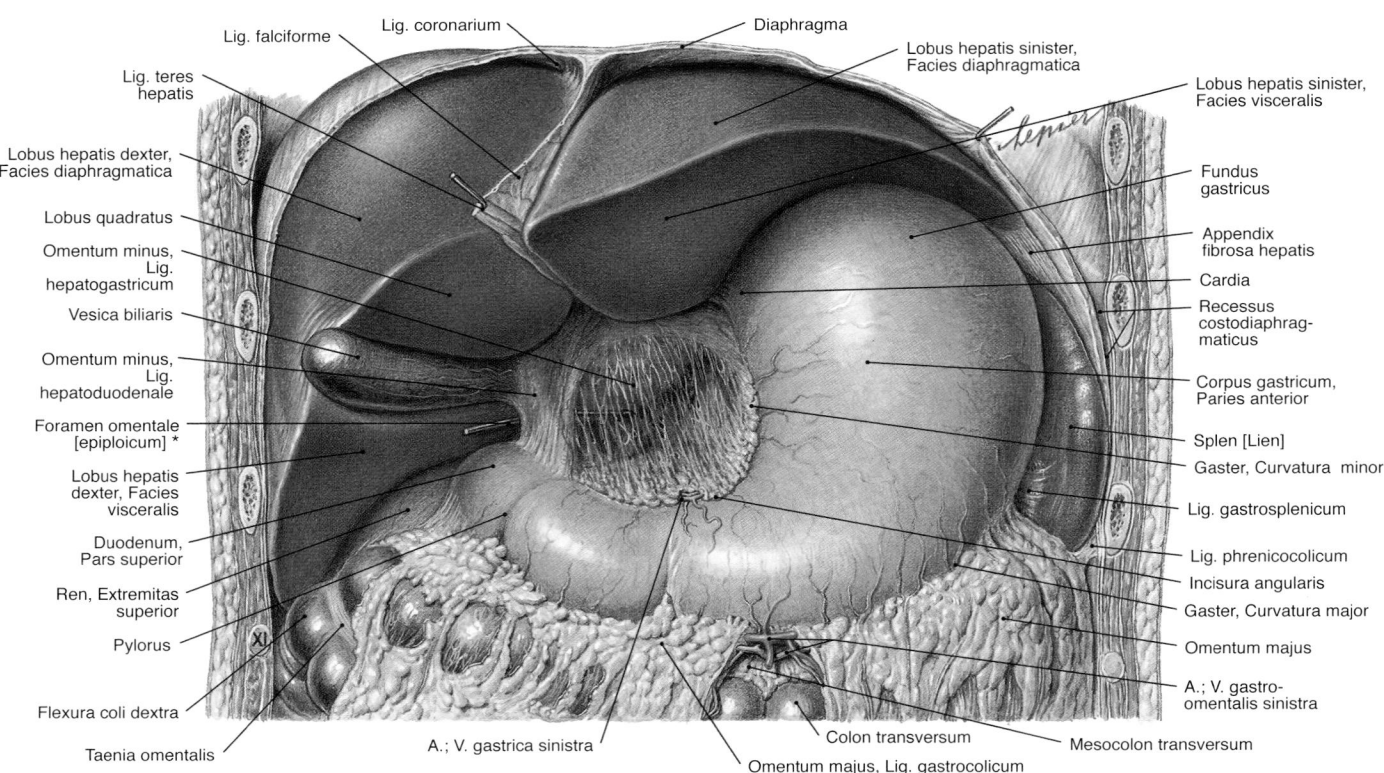

Fig. 782 Position of the abdominal viscera in the upper abdomen; ventral view.

* Also: foramen of WINSLOW

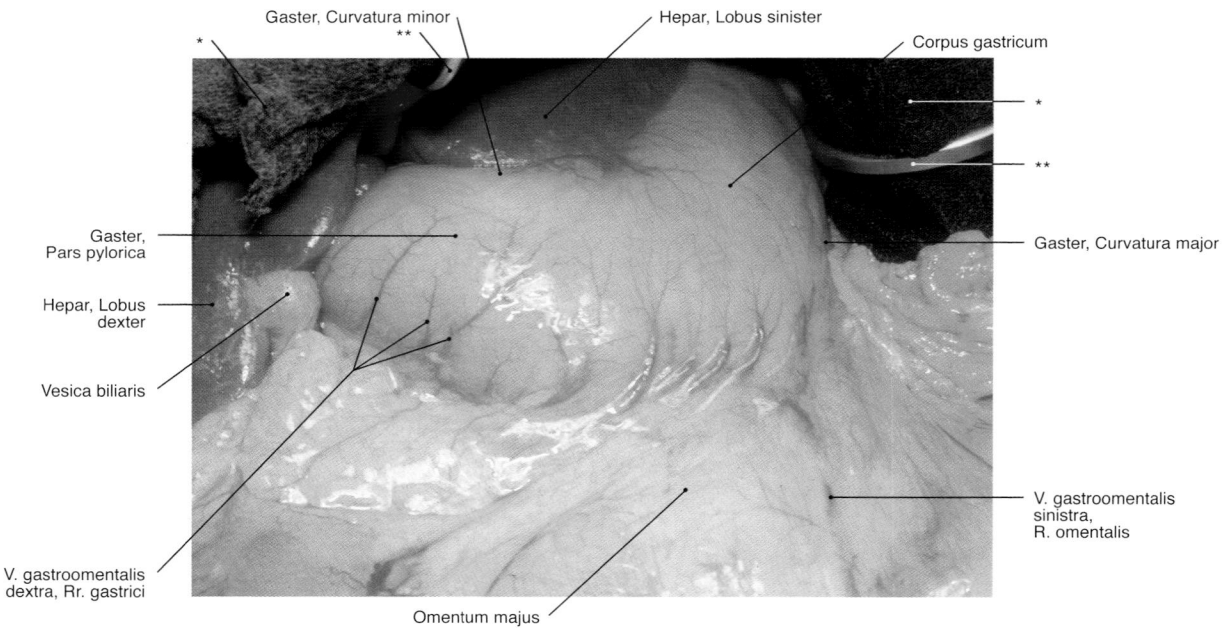

Fig. 783 Stomach, Gaster, and greater omentum, Omentum majus; photograph taken during surgery; ventral view.

* Surgical drape
** Surgical retractor

Abdominal viscera in the upper abdomen

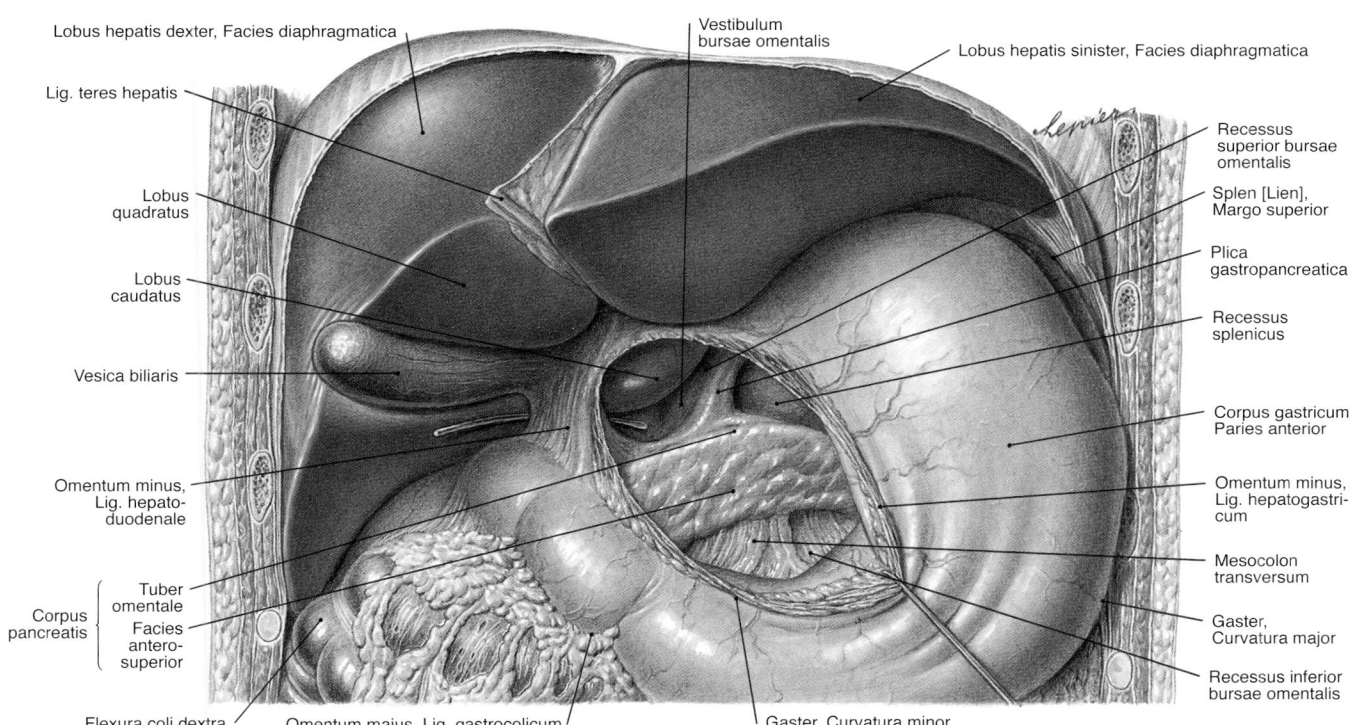

Lobus hepatis dexter, Facies diaphragmatica
Vestibulum bursae omentalis
Lobus hepatis sinister, Facies diaphragmatica
Lig. teres hepatis
Recessus superior bursae omentalis
Lobus quadratus
Splen [Lien], Margo superior
Lobus caudatus
Plica gastropancreatica
Recessus splenicus
Vesica biliaris
Corpus gastricum, Paries anterior
Omentum minus, Lig. hepato-duodenale
Omentum minus, Lig. hepatogastri-cum
Mesocolon transversum
Corpus pancreatis
Tuber omentale
Facies antero-superior
Gaster, Curvatura major
Recessus inferior bursae omentalis
Flexura coli dextra
Omentum majus, Lig. gastrocolicum
Gaster, Curvatura minor

Fig. 784 Abdominal viscera in the upper abdomen; parts of the lesser omentum have been removed to expose the omental bursa and the pancreas; oblique view from superior.

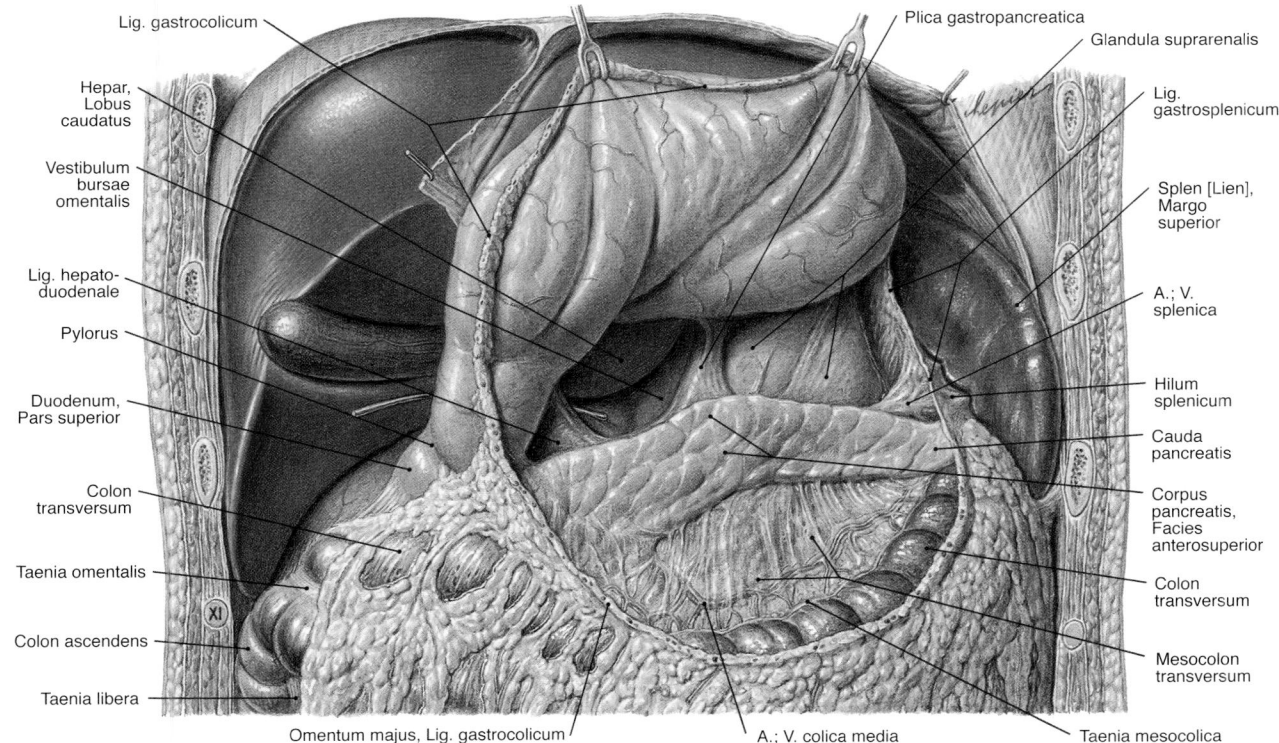

Lig. gastrocolicum
Plica gastropancreatica
Glandula suprarenalis
Hepar, Lobus caudatus
Lig. gastrosplenicum
Vestibulum bursae omentalis
Splen [Lien], Margo superior
Lig. hepato-duodenale
A.; V. splenica
Pylorus
Hilum splenicum
Duodenum, Pars superior
Cauda pancreatis
Colon transversum
Corpus pancreatis, Facies anterosuperior
Taenia omentalis
Colon transversum
Colon ascendens
Mesocolon transversum
Taenia libera
Omentum majus, Lig. gastrocolicum
A.; V. colica media
Taenia mesocolica

Fig. 785 Omental bursa, Bursa omentalis; after dissection of the gastrocolic ligament; oblique view from inferior.

Abdominal viscera in the lower abdomen

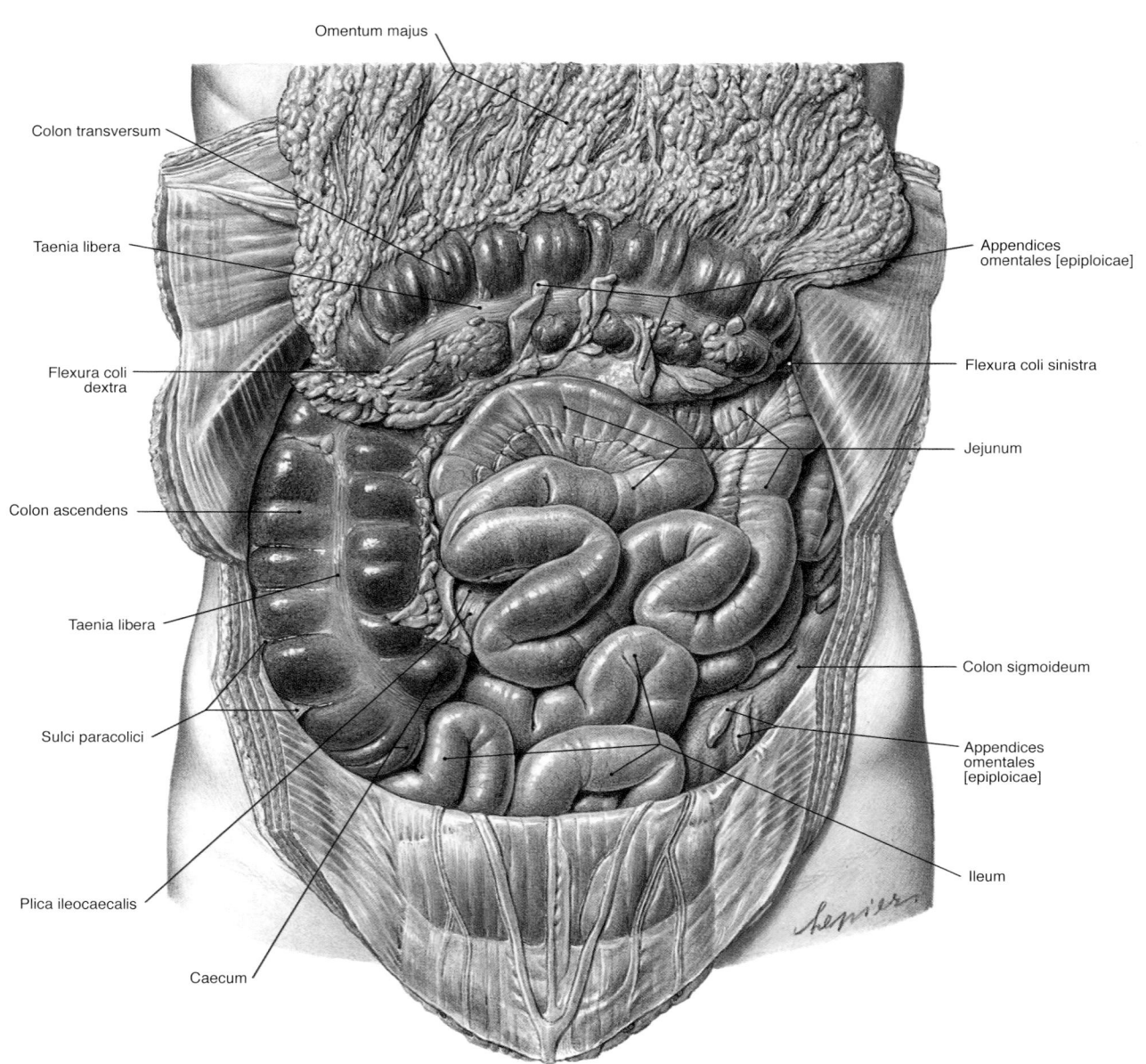

Omentum majus

Colon transversum

Taenia libera

Flexura coli dextra

Colon ascendens

Taenia libera

Sulci paracolici

Plica ileocaecalis

Caecum

Appendices omentales [epiploicae]

Flexura coli sinistra

Jejunum

Colon sigmoideum

Appendices omentales [epiploicae]

Ileum

Fig. 786   Position of the abdominal viscera, Situs viscerum.

Abdominal viscera in the lower abdomen

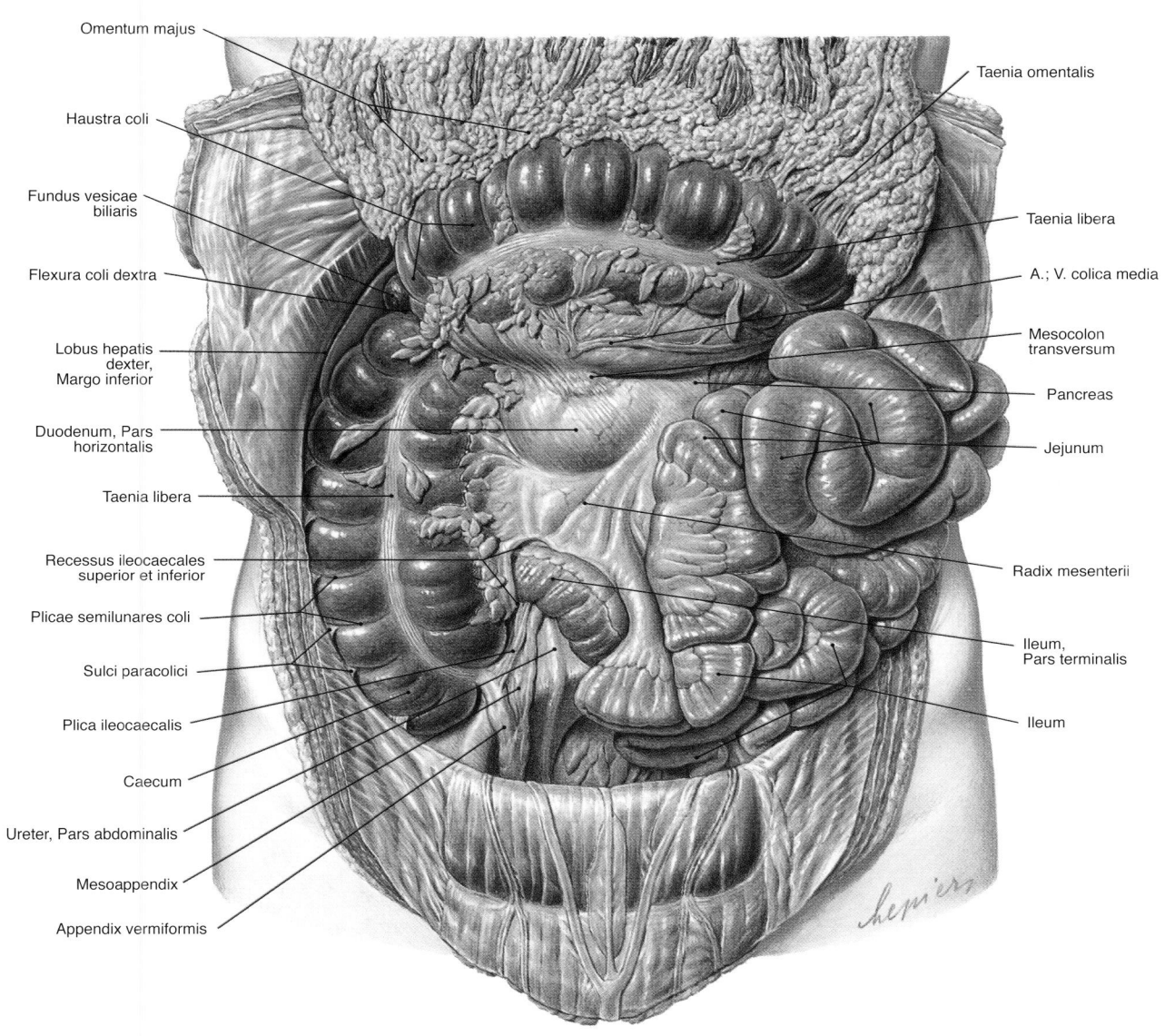

Omentum majus

Haustra coli

Fundus vesicae biliaris

Flexura coli dextra

Lobus hepatis dexter, Margo inferior

Duodenum, Pars horizontalis

Taenia libera

Recessus ileocaecales superior et inferior

Plicae semilunares coli

Sulci paracolici

Plica ileocaecalis

Caecum

Ureter, Pars abdominalis

Mesoappendix

Appendix vermiformis

Taenia omentalis

Taenia libera

A.; V. colica media

Mesocolon transversum

Pancreas

Jejunum

Radix mesenterii

Ileum, Pars terminalis

Ileum

Fig. 787 Small intestine, Intestinum tenue, and large intestine, Intestinum crassum.

Abdominal viscera in the lower abdomen

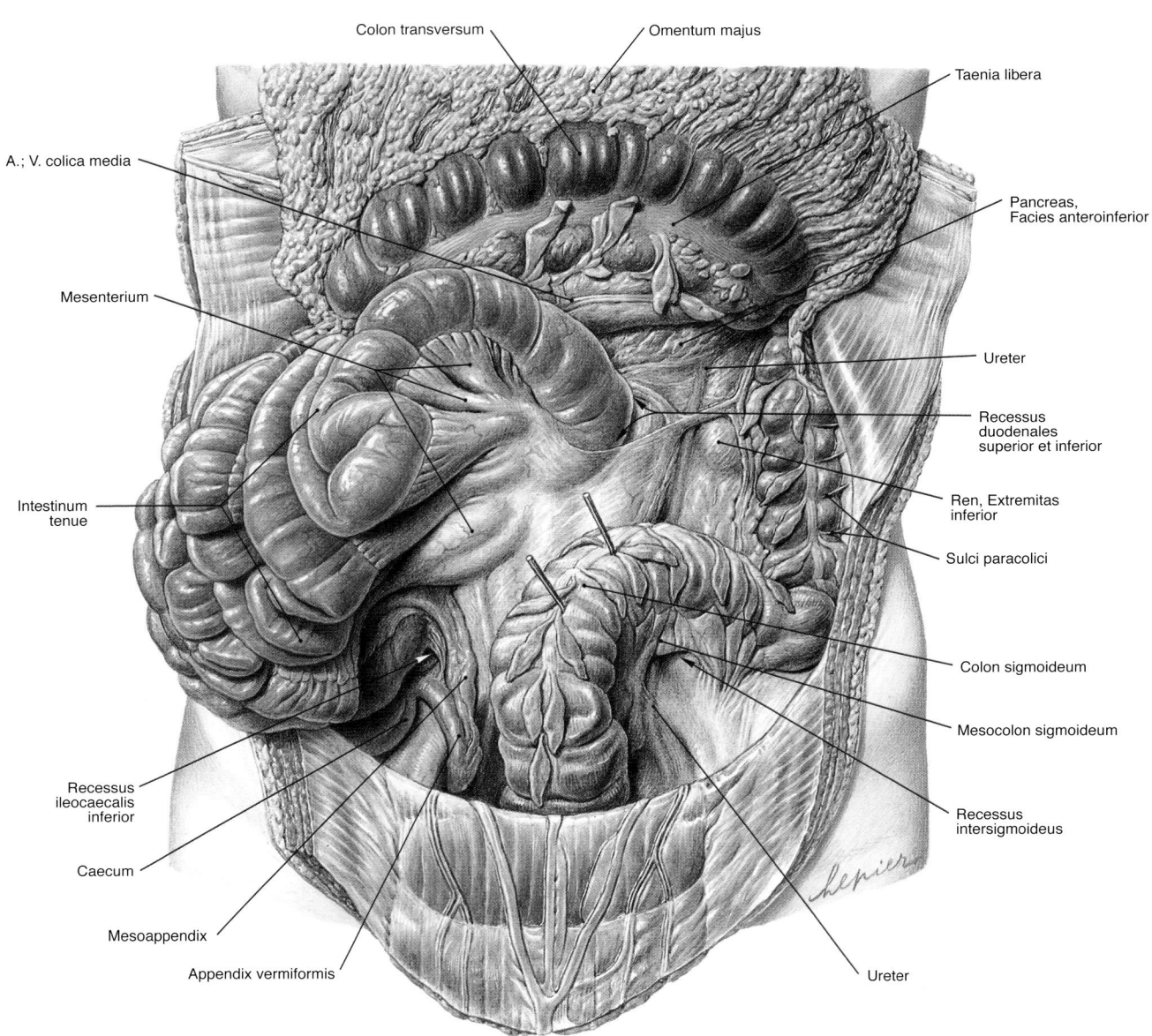

Fig. 788 Small intestine, Intestinum tenue, and large intestine, Intestinum crassum.

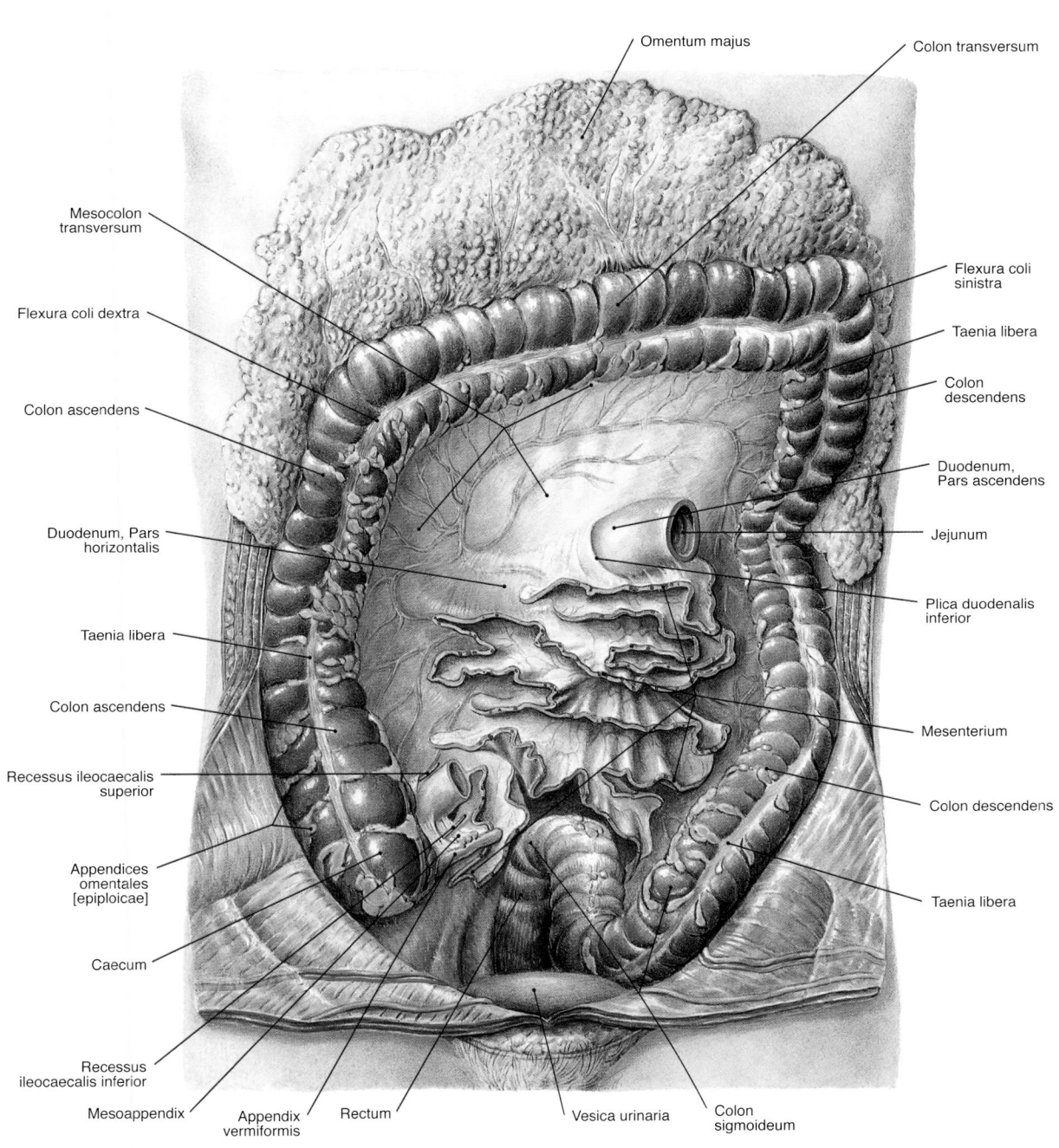

Omentum majus

Colon transversum

Mesocolon transversum

Flexura coli sinistra

Flexura coli dextra

Taenia libera

Colon ascendens

Colon descendens

Duodenum, Pars ascendens

Duodenum, Pars horizontalis

Jejunum

Taenia libera

Plica duodenalis inferior

Colon ascendens

Mesenterium

Recessus ileocaecalis superior

Colon descendens

Appendices omentales [epiploicae]

Taenia libera

Caecum

Recessus ileocaecalis inferior

Mesoappendix

Appendix vermiformis

Rectum

Vesica urinaria

Colon sigmoideum

Fig. 789 Mesentery, Mesenterium, and large intestine, Intestinum crassum.

Mesenteric root and retroperitoneal space

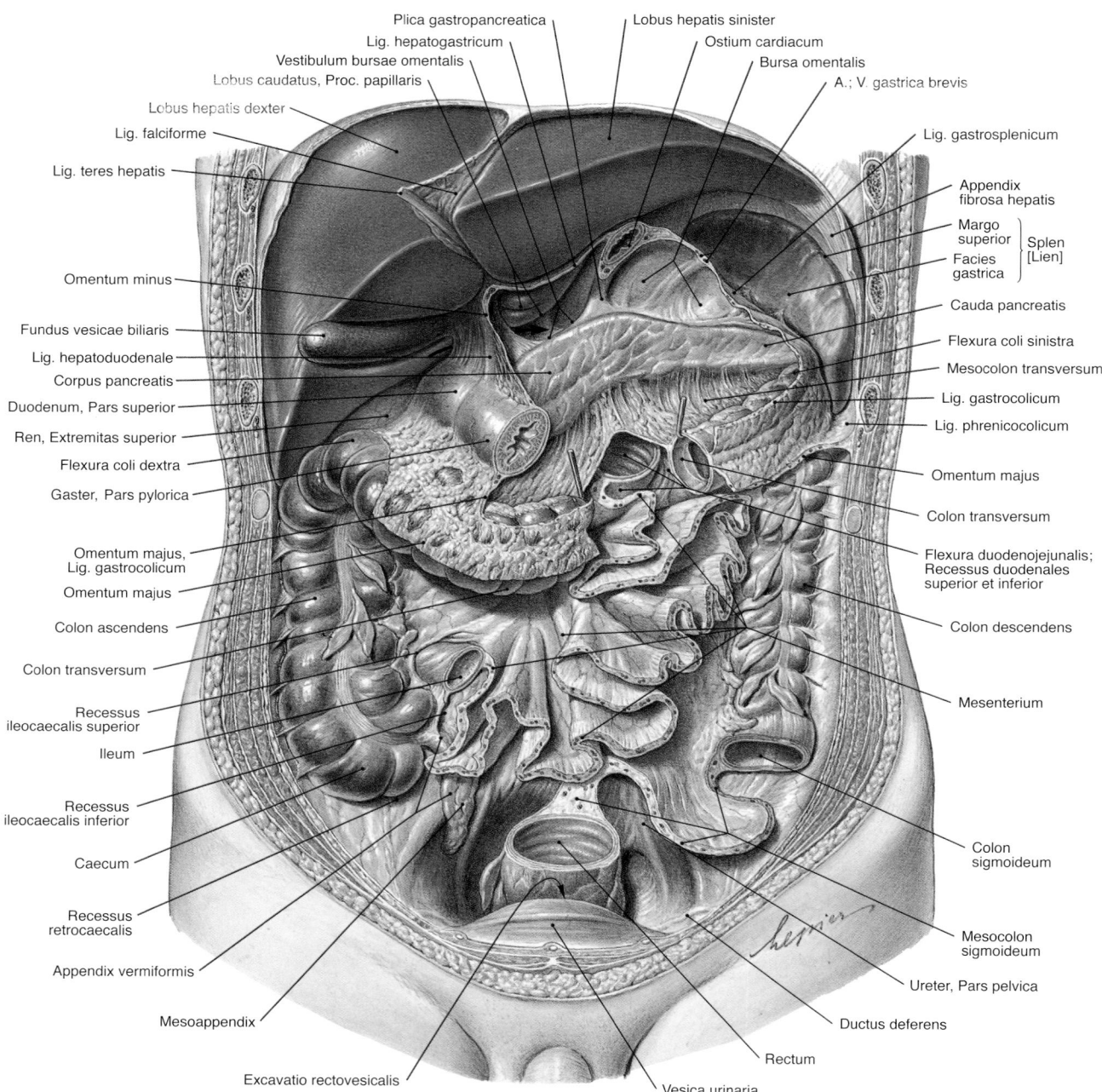

Plica gastropancreatica
Lig. hepatogastricum
Vestibulum bursae omentalis
Lobus caudatus, Proc. papillaris
Lobus hepatis dexter
Lig. falciforme
Lig. teres hepatis
Omentum minus
Fundus vesicae biliaris
Lig. hepatoduodenale
Corpus pancreatis
Duodenum, Pars superior
Ren, Extremitas superior
Flexura coli dextra
Gaster, Pars pylorica
Omentum majus, Lig. gastrocolicum
Omentum majus
Colon ascendens
Colon transversum
Recessus ileocaecalis superior
Ileum
Recessus ileocaecalis inferior
Caecum
Recessus retrocaecalis
Appendix vermiformis
Mesoappendix
Excavatio rectovesicalis

Lobus hepatis sinister
Ostium cardiacum
Bursa omentalis
A.; V. gastrica brevis
Lig. gastrosplenicum
Appendix fibrosa hepatis
Margo superior
Facies gastrica
Splen [Lien]
Cauda pancreatis
Flexura coli sinistra
Mesocolon transversum
Lig. gastrocolicum
Lig. phrenicocolicum
Omentum majus
Colon transversum
Flexura duodenojejunalis; Recessus duodenales superior et inferior
Colon descendens
Mesenterium
Colon sigmoideum
Mesocolon sigmoideum
Ureter, Pars pelvica
Ductus deferens
Rectum
Vesica urinaria

Fig. 790 Position of the abdominal viscera, Situs viscerum, and the omental bursa, Bursa omentalis. An arrow indicates the omental [epiploic] foramen.

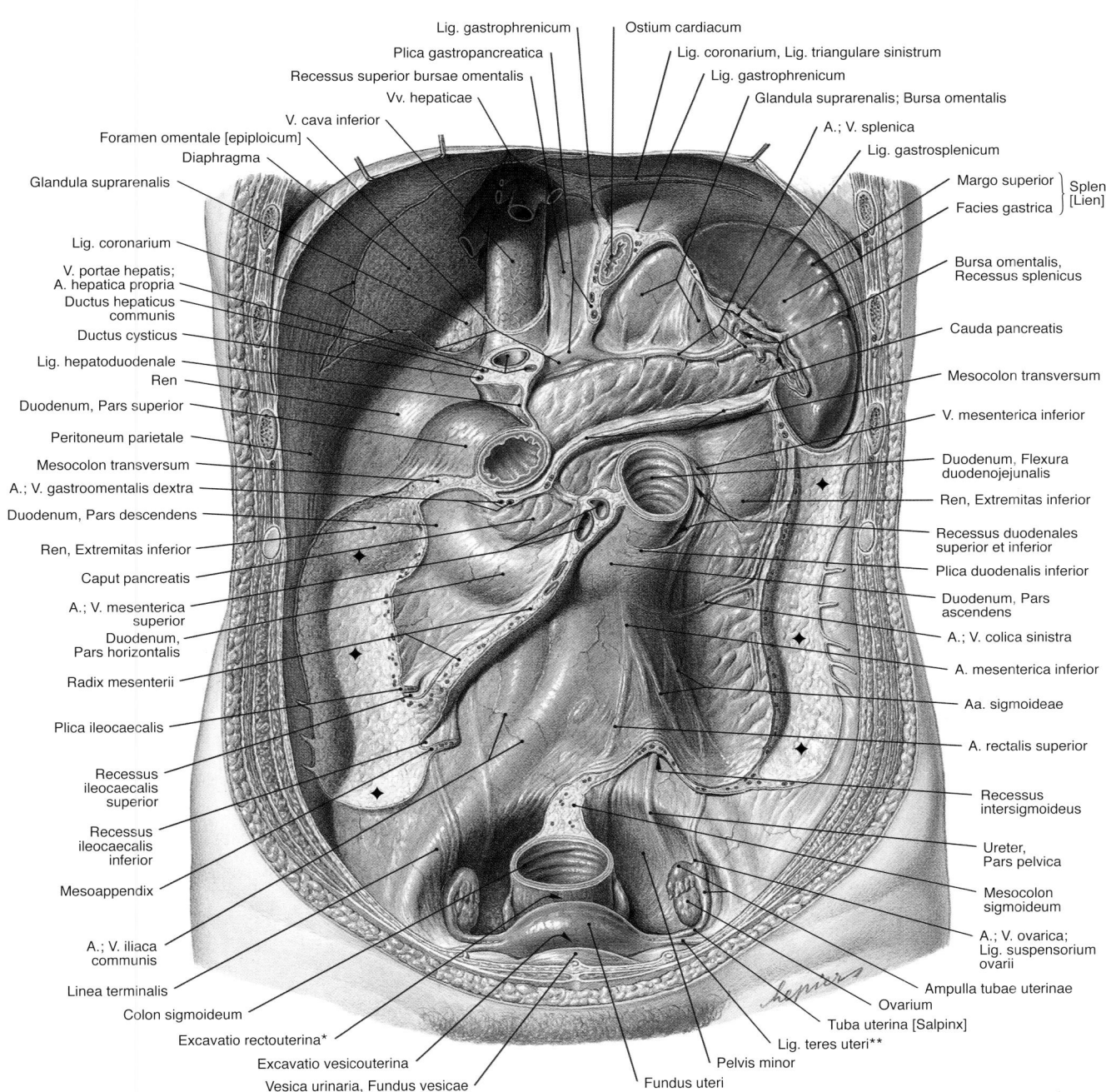

Lig. gastrophrenicum
Plica gastropancreatica
Recessus superior bursae omentalis
Vv. hepaticae
V. cava inferior
Foramen omentale [epiploicum]
Diaphragma
Glandula suprarenalis
Lig. coronarium
V. portae hepatis;
A. hepatica propria
Ductus hepaticus
communis
Ductus cysticus
Lig. hepatoduodenale
Ren
Duodenum, Pars superior
Peritoneum parietale
Mesocolon transversum
A.; V. gastroomentalis dextra
Duodenum, Pars descendens
Ren, Extremitas inferior
Caput pancreatis
A.; V. mesenterica
superior
Duodenum,
Pars horizontalis
Radix mesenterii
Plica ileocaecalis
Recessus
ileocaecalis
superior
Recessus
ileocaecalis
inferior
Mesoappendix
A.; V. iliaca
communis
Linea terminalis
Colon sigmoideum
Excavatio rectouterina*
Excavatio vesicouterina
Vesica urinaria, Fundus vesicae

Ostium cardiacum
Lig. coronarium, Lig. triangulare sinistrum
Lig. gastrophrenicum
Glandula suprarenalis; Bursa omentalis
A.; V. splenica
Lig. gastrosplenicum
Margo superior ⎫ Splen
Facies gastrica ⎭ [Lien]
Bursa omentalis,
Recessus splenicus
Cauda pancreatis
Mesocolon transversum
V. mesenterica inferior
Duodenum, Flexura
duodenojejunalis
Ren, Extremitas inferior
Recessus duodenales
superior et inferior
Plica duodenalis inferior
Duodenum, Pars
ascendens
A.; V. colica sinistra
A. mesenterica inferior
Aa. sigmoideae
A. rectalis superior
Recessus
intersigmoideus
Ureter,
Pars pelvica
Mesocolon
sigmoideum
A.; V. ovarica;
Lig. suspensorium
ovarii
Ampulla tubae uterinae
Ovarium
Tuba uterina [Salpinx]
Lig. teres uteri**
Pelvis minor
Fundus uteri

Fig. 791 Posterior wall of the peritoneal cavity, Cavitas
peritonealis, and spleen, Splen [Lien], of the female.
Sites of attachment of the ascending and descending colon
are indicated (◆).
* Clinical term: pouch of DOUGLAS
** Clinical term: round ligament

Abdominal arteries, overview

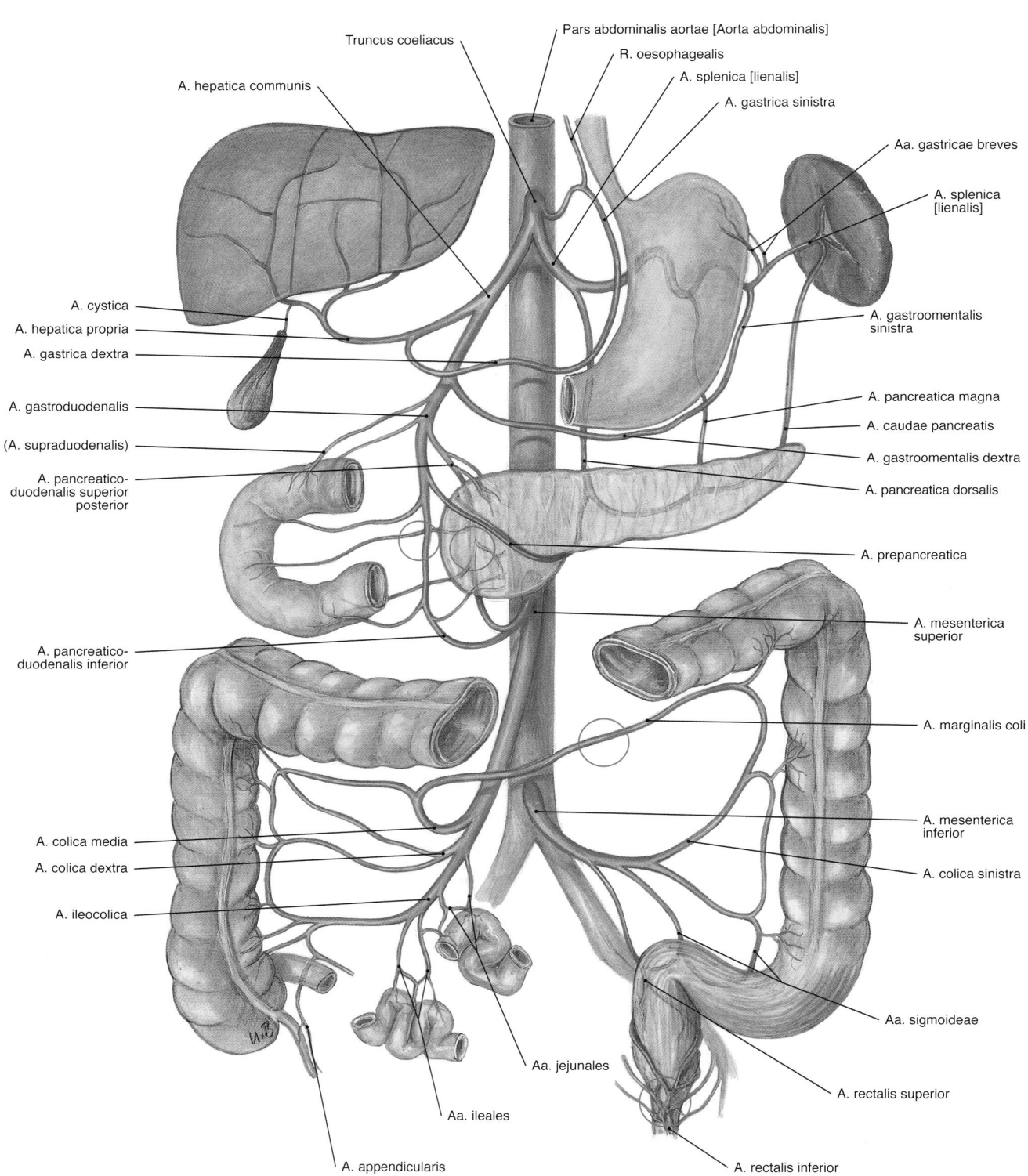

Truncus coeliacus

Pars abdominalis aortae [Aorta abdominalis]

R. oesophagealis

A. hepatica communis

A. splenica [lienalis]

A. gastrica sinistra

Aa. gastricae breves

A. splenica [lienalis]

A. cystica

A. hepatica propria

A. gastrica dextra

A. gastroomentalis sinistra

A. gastroduodenalis

(A. supraduodenalis)

A. pancreatico-duodenalis superior posterior

A. pancreatica magna

A. caudae pancreatis

A. gastroomentalis dextra

A. pancreatica dorsalis

A. prepancreatica

A. mesenterica superior

A. pancreatico-duodenalis inferior

A. marginalis coli

A. colica media

A. colica dextra

A. ileocolica

A. mesenterica inferior

A. colica sinistra

Aa. sigmoideae

A. rectalis superior

Aa. jejunales

Aa. ileales

A. appendicularis

A. rectalis inferior

Fig. 792 Arteries of the abdominal viscera;
semi-schematic;
possible anastomoses are indicated (O).

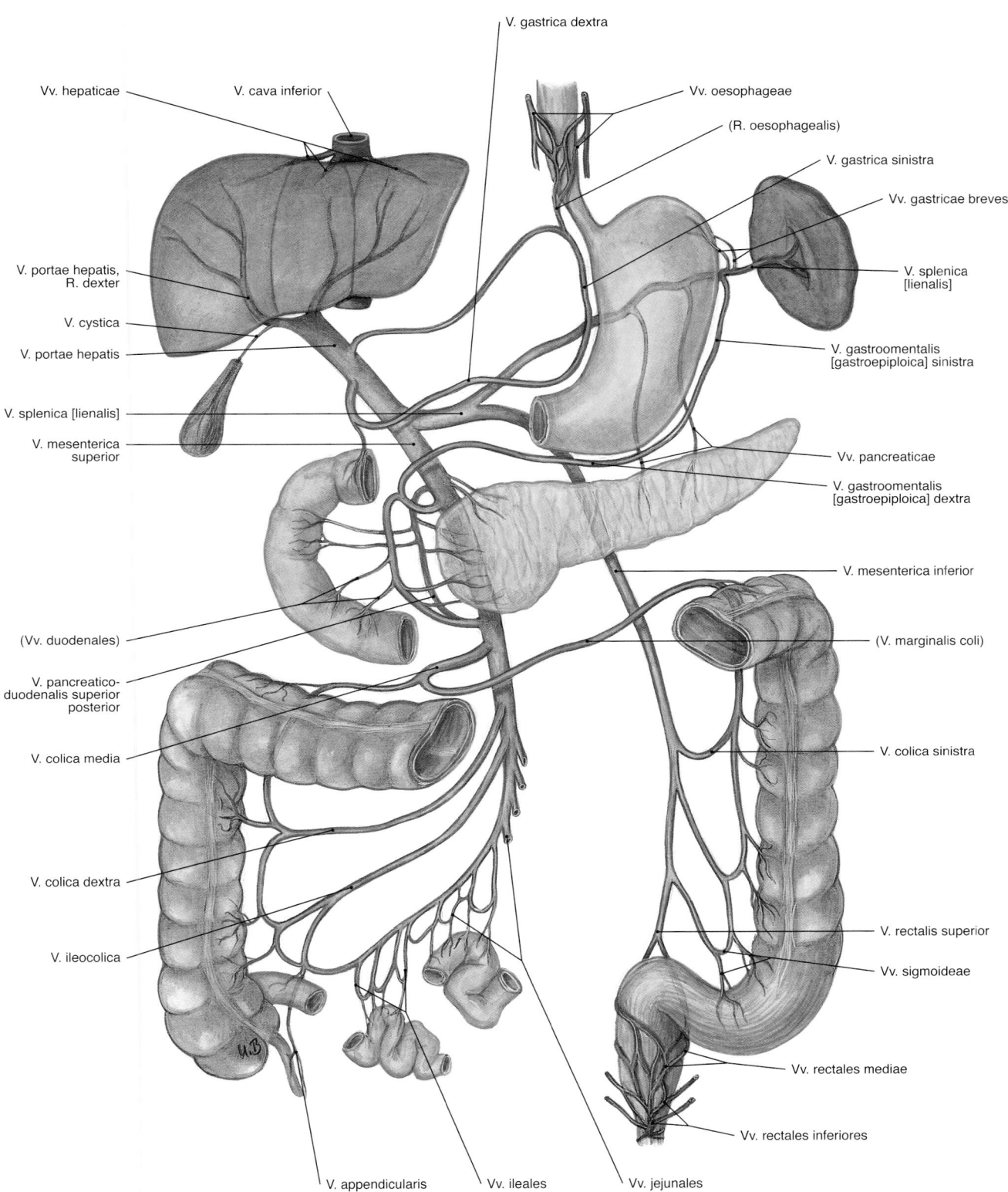

V. gastrica dextra

Vv. hepaticae

V. cava inferior

Vv. oesophageae

(R. oesophagealis)

V. gastrica sinistra

Vv. gastricae breves

V. portae hepatis, R. dexter

V. splenica [lienalis]

V. cystica

V. portae hepatis

V. gastroomentalis [gastroepiploica] sinistra

V. splenica [lienalis]

V. mesenterica superior

Vv. pancreaticae

V. gastroomentalis [gastroepiploica] dextra

V. mesenterica inferior

(Vv. duodenales)

(V. marginalis coli)

V. pancreatico-duodenalis superior posterior

V. colica media

V. colica sinistra

V. colica dextra

V. rectalis superior

V. ileocolica

Vv. sigmoideae

Vv. rectales mediae

Vv. rectales inferiores

V. appendicularis

Vv. ileales

Vv. jejunales

Fig. 793 Hepatic portal vein, V. portae hepatis, with tributaries; semi-schematic.

Coeliac trunk

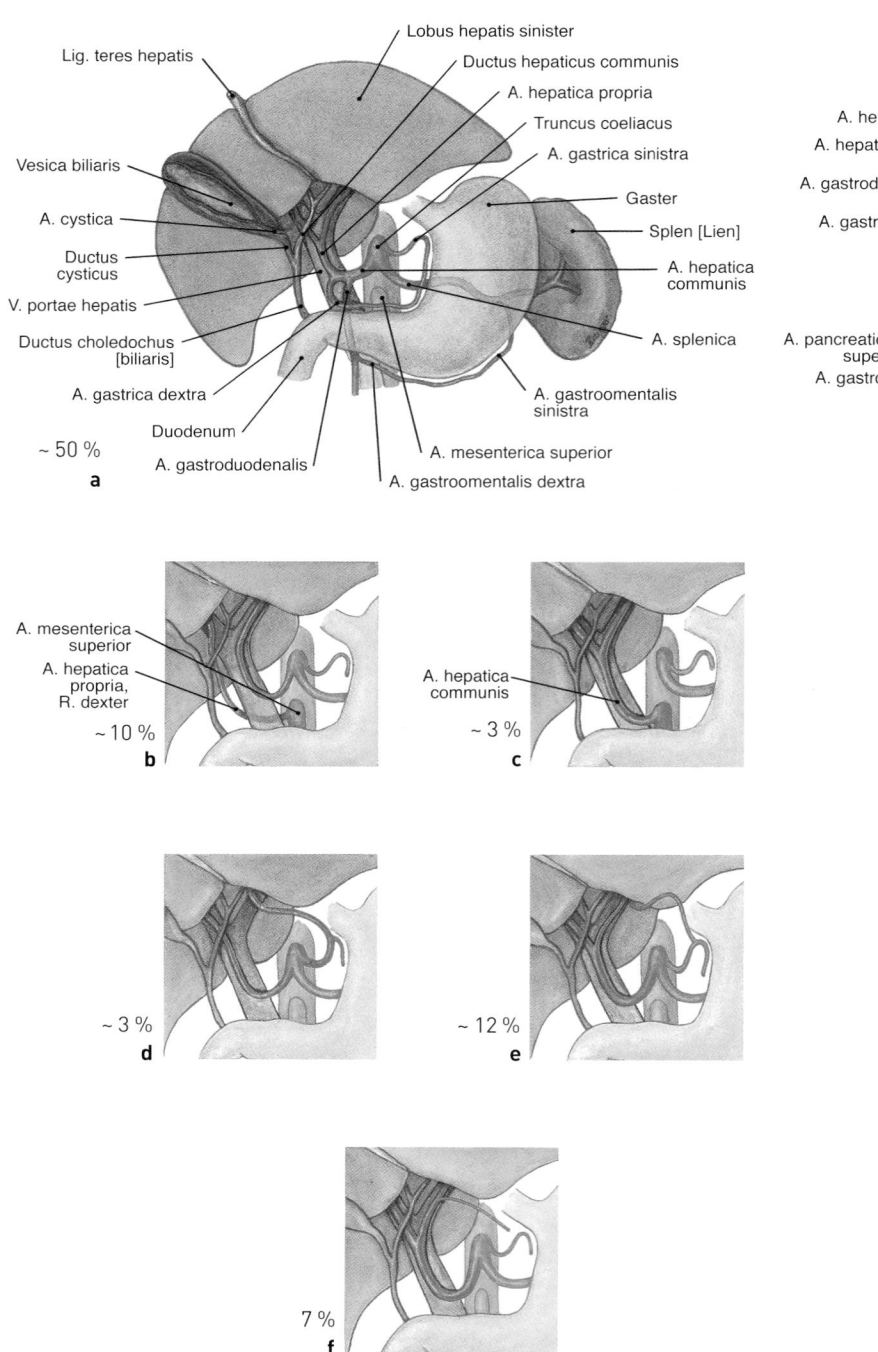

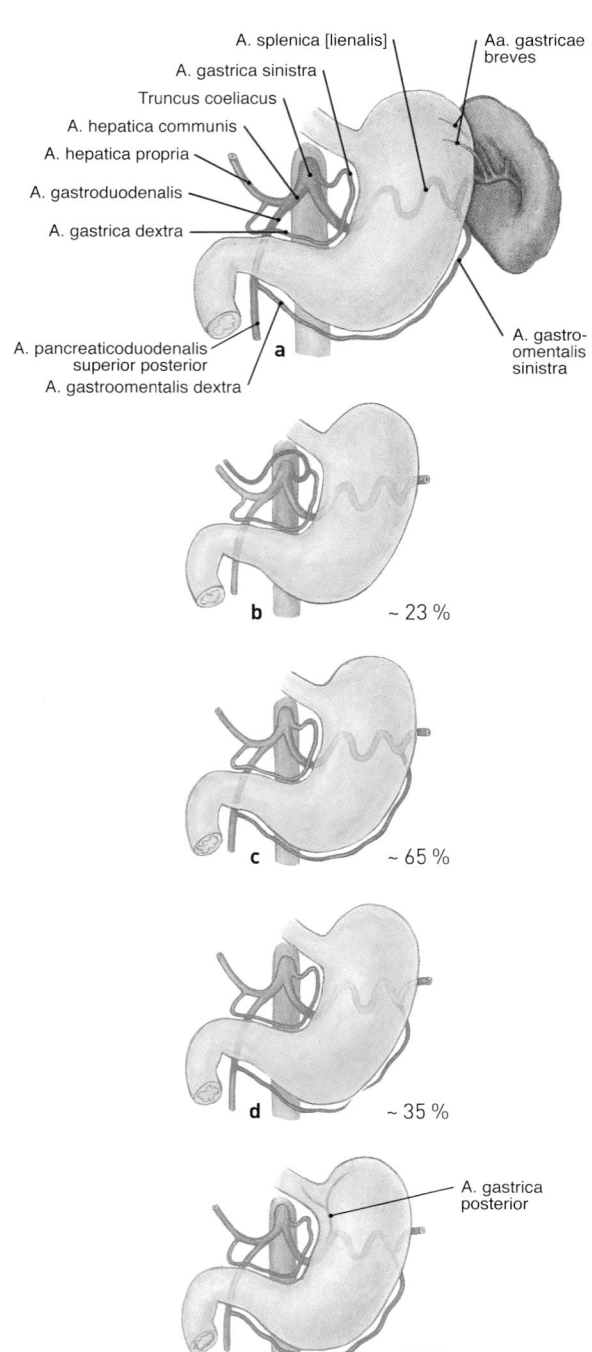

Fig. 794 a–f Variability of the arterial blood supply of the liver.
a "Textbook case"
b The superior mesenteric artery, A. mesenterica superior, participates in the supply of the right lobe of the liver.
c The common hepatic artery, A. hepatica communis, arises from the superior mesenteric artery, A. mesenterica superior.
d The left lobe of the liver is supplied by the left gastric artery, A. gastrica sinistra.
e A branch of the left gastric artery, A. gastrica sinistra, supplies the left lobe of the liver along with the left branch of the hepatic artery proper, A. hepatica propria.
f An accessory branch of the hepatic artery proper, A. hepatica propria, supplies the lesser curvature of the stomach.

Fig. 795 a–e Variability of the arterial blood supply of the stomach.
a "Textbook case", closed arterial arcade supplying both the lesser and the greater curvature
b The left gastric artery, A. gastrica sinistra, participates in the supply of the left lobe of the liver.
c Anastomosis between the right and left gastro-omental arteries, Aa. gastromentales dextra et sinistra, at the greater curvature
d Absence of an anastomosis between the right and left gastro-omental arteries, Aa. gastromentales dextra et sinistra, at the greater curvature
e An accessory posterior gastric artery, A. gastrica posterior, arising from the splenic artery, A. splenica, supplies the posterior wall of the stomach.

Arteries of the upper abdomen, radiography

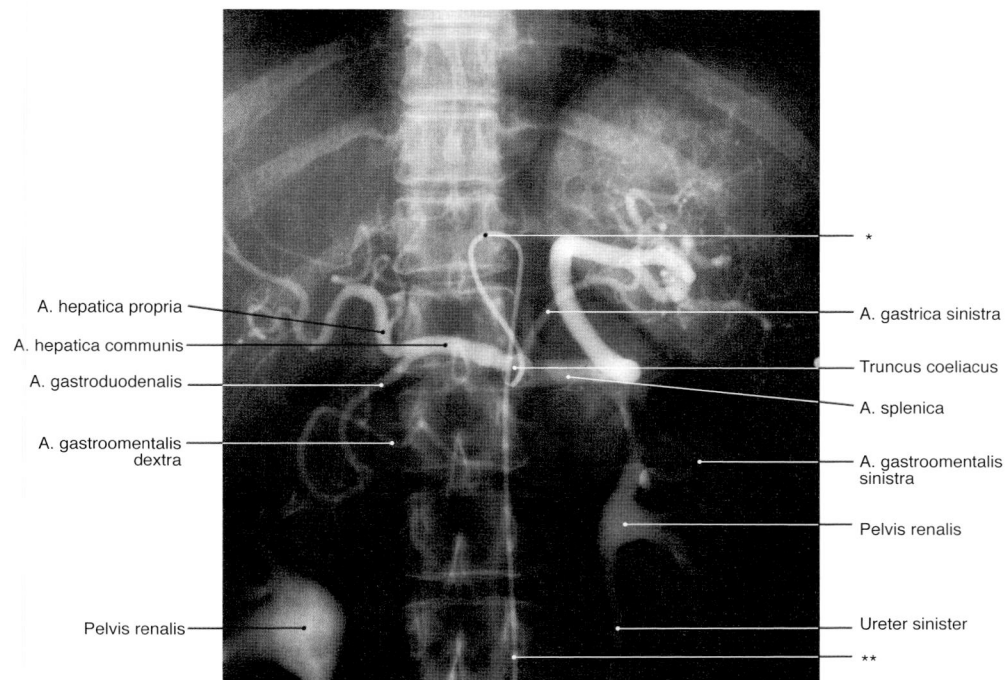

A. hepatica propria
A. hepatica communis
A. gastroduodenalis

A. gastroomentalis dextra

Pelvis renalis

*
A. gastrica sinistra
Truncus coeliacus
A. splenica
A. gastroomentalis sinistra
Pelvis renalis
Ureter sinister
**

Fig. 796 Arteries of the stomach, Gaster; the spleen, Splen [Lien], and the liver, Hepar;
AP-radiograph after selective injection of a contrast medium into the coeliac trunk (coeliacography) with concomitant visualization of the renal pelvis due to the renal excretion of the medium; ventral view.
* Catheter loop in the aorta
** Catheter in the aorta

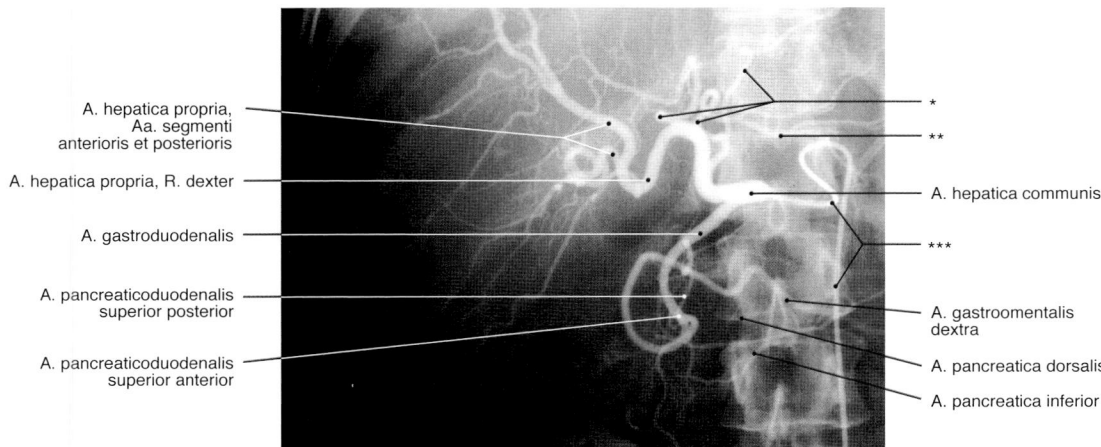

A. hepatica propria, Aa. segmenti anterioris et posterioris
A. hepatica propria, R. dexter
A. gastroduodenalis
A. pancreaticoduodenalis superior posterior
A. pancreaticoduodenalis superior anterior

*
**
A. hepatica communis
***
A. gastroomentalis dextra
A. pancreatica dorsalis
A. pancreatica inferior

Fig. 797 Common hepatic artery, A. hepatica communis;
AP-radiograph after selective injection of a contrast medium into the common hepatic artery;
ventral view.

* Branches to the left lobe of the liver replacing a single left branch of the hepatic artery proper
** An accessory branch of the hepatic artery to the lesser curvature of the stomach
*** Catheter in the aorta

Vessels of the upper abdomen

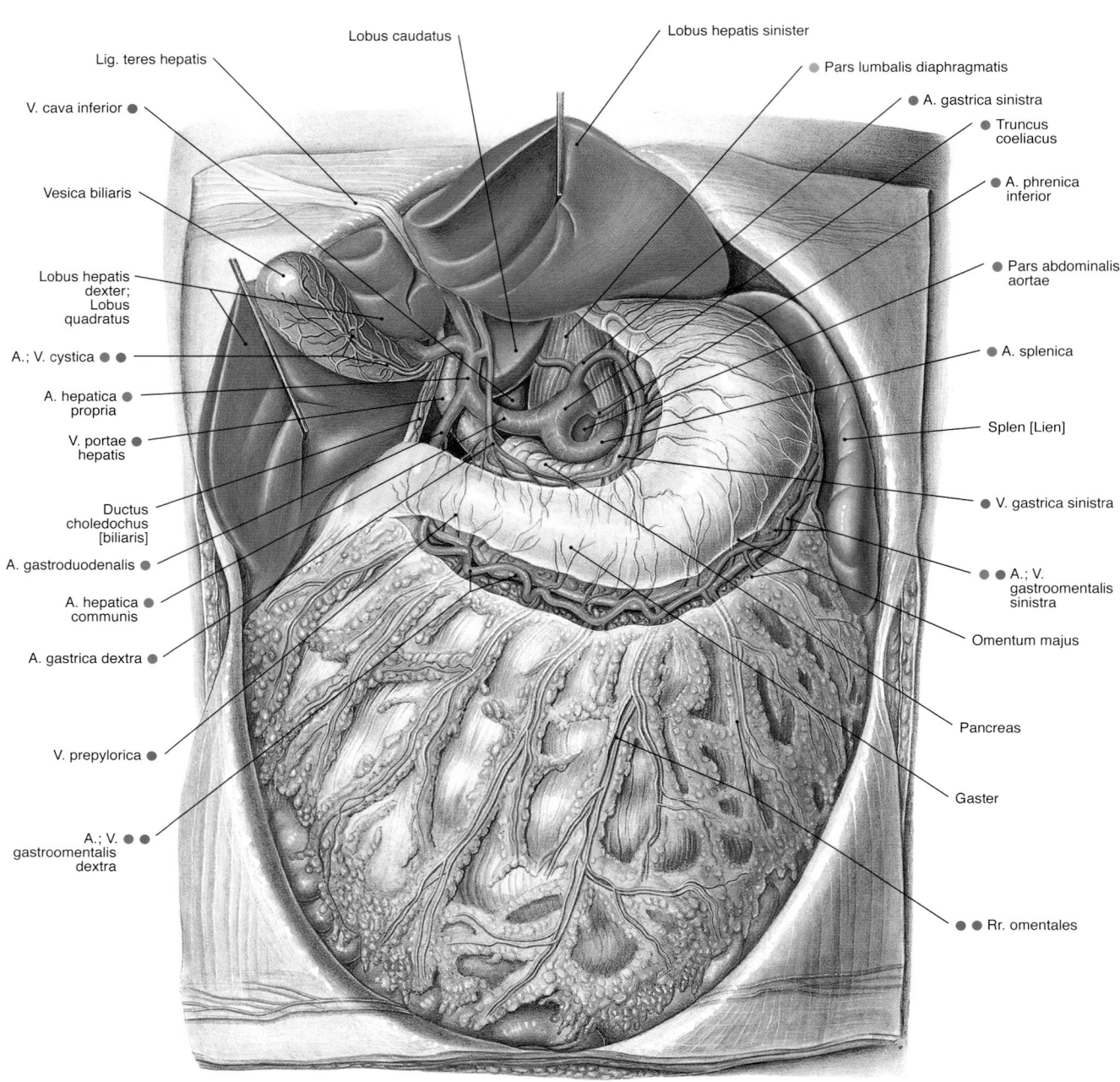

Lobus caudatus
Lobus hepatis sinister
Lig. teres hepatis
Pars lumbalis diaphragmatis
V. cava inferior ●
A. gastrica sinistra
Truncus coeliacus
Vesica biliaris
A. phrenica inferior
Lobus hepatis dexter; Lobus quadratus
Pars abdominalis aortae
A.; V. cystica ● ●
A. splenica
A. hepatica propria ●
Splen [Lien]
V. portae hepatis ●
V. gastrica sinistra
Ductus choledochus [biliaris]
A.; V. gastroomentalis sinistra
A. gastroduodenalis ●
Omentum majus
A. hepatica communis ●
A. gastrica dextra ●
Pancreas
V. prepylorica ●
Gaster
A.; V. ● ● gastroomentalis dextra
Rr. omentales

Fig. 798   Vessels of the upper abdomen.

Vessels of the upper abdomen

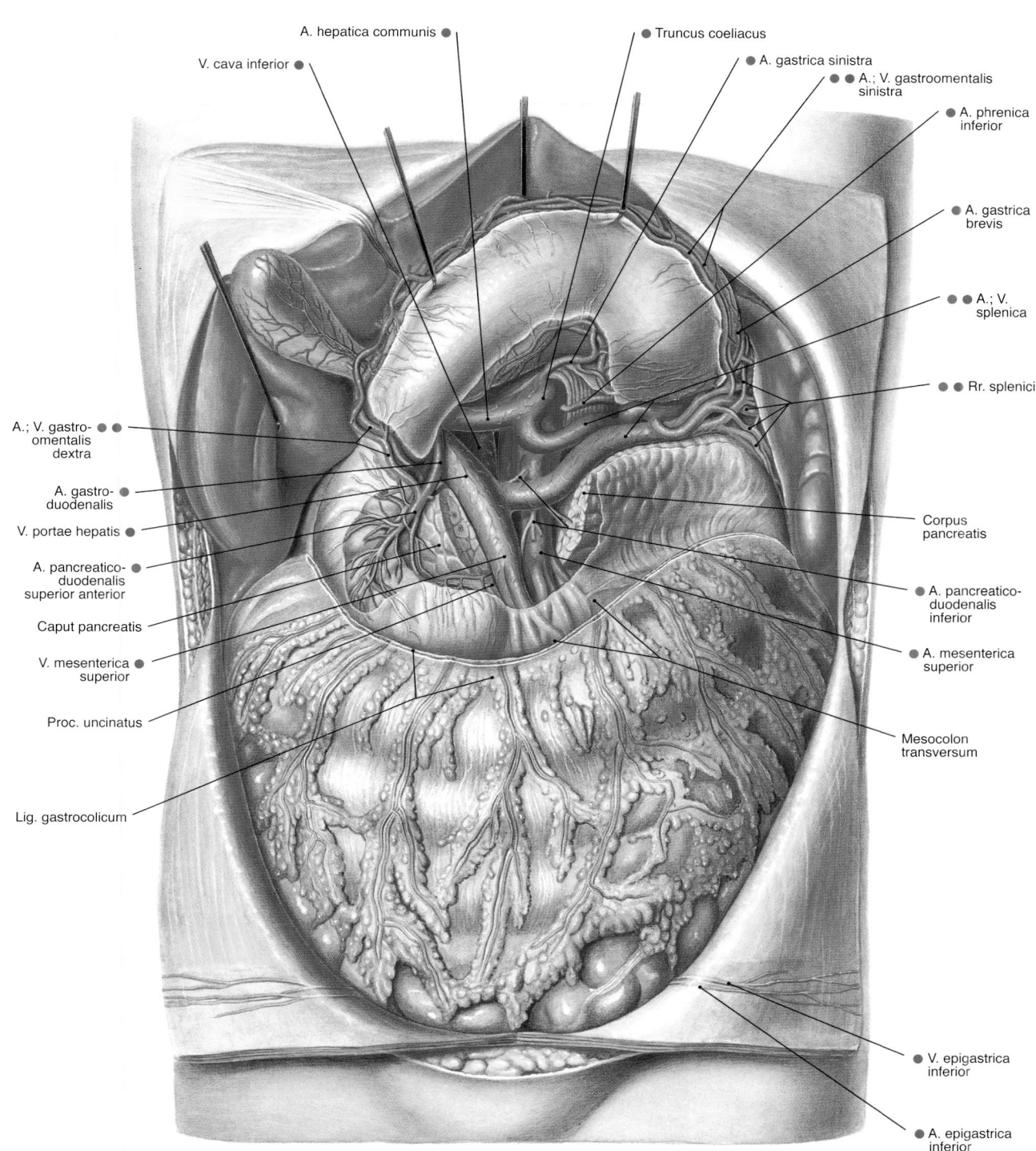

A. hepatica communis ●

V. cava inferior ●

● Truncus coeliacus

● A. gastrica sinistra

● ● A.; V. gastroomentalis sinistra

● A. phrenica inferior

● A. gastrica brevis

● ● A.; V. splenica

● ● Rr. splenici

A.; V. gastro- ● ●
omentalis
dextra

A. gastro- ●
duodenalis

V. portae hepatis ●

A. pancreatico- ●
duodenalis
superior anterior

Caput pancreatis

V. mesenterica ●
superior

Proc. uncinatus

Lig. gastrocolicum

Corpus pancreatis

● A. pancreatico-
duodenalis
inferior

● A. mesenterica
superior

Mesocolon
transversum

● V. epigastrica
inferior

● A. epigastrica
inferior

Fig. 799   Vessels of the upper abdomen.

Superior mesenteric artery

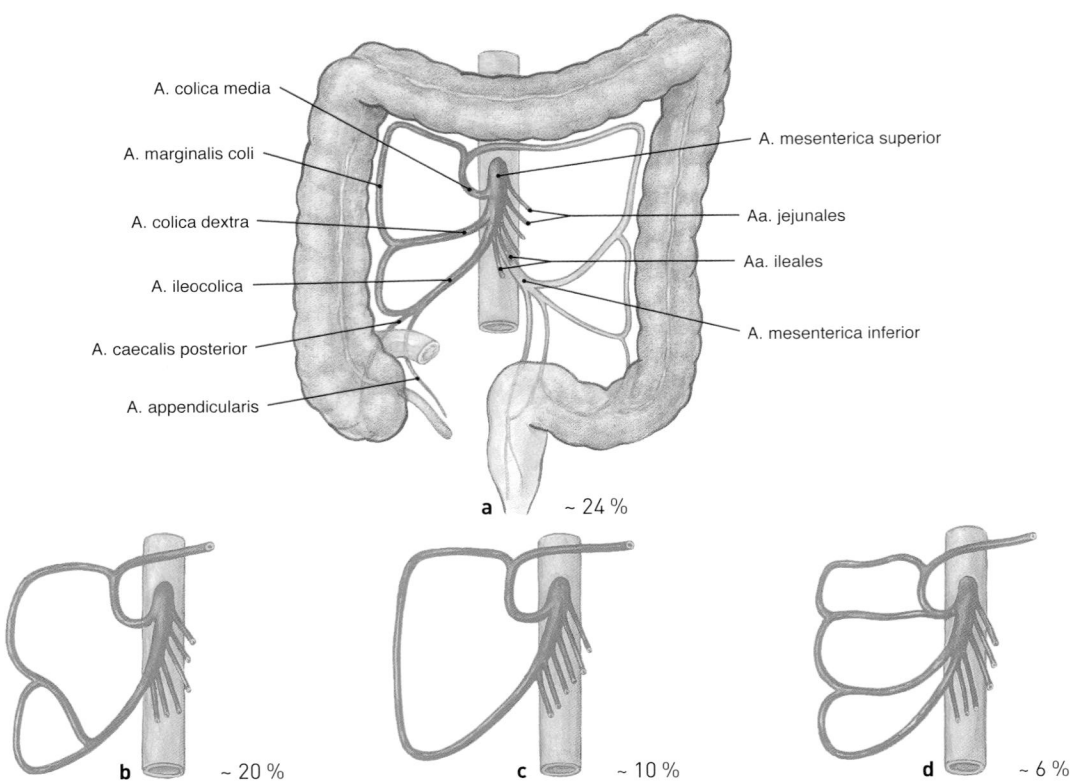

Fig. 800 a–d Variability of the branches of the superior mesenteric artery, A. mesenterica superior, supplying the large intestine.
a "Textbook case", the ascending and the transverse colon, Colon ascendens et transversum, are supplied by three branches.

b The ileocolic artery, A. ileocolica, and the right colic artery, A. colica dextra, form a common trunk.
c Only two branches arise from the mesenteric artery while the right colic artery, A. colica dextra, is absent.
d Duplication of the right colic artery, A. colica dextra

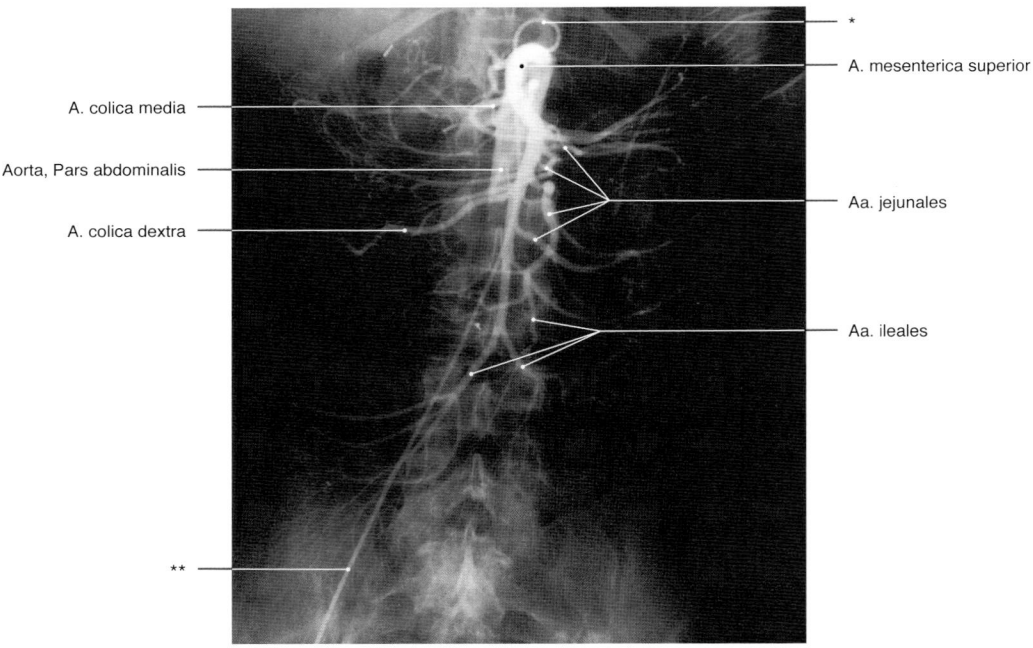

Fig. 801 Superior mesenteric artery, A. mesenterica superior; AP-radiograph after injection of a contrast medium into the origin of the superior mesenteric artery; ventral view.

* Catheter in the aorta
** Catheter in the common iliac artery

Vessels of the lower abdomen

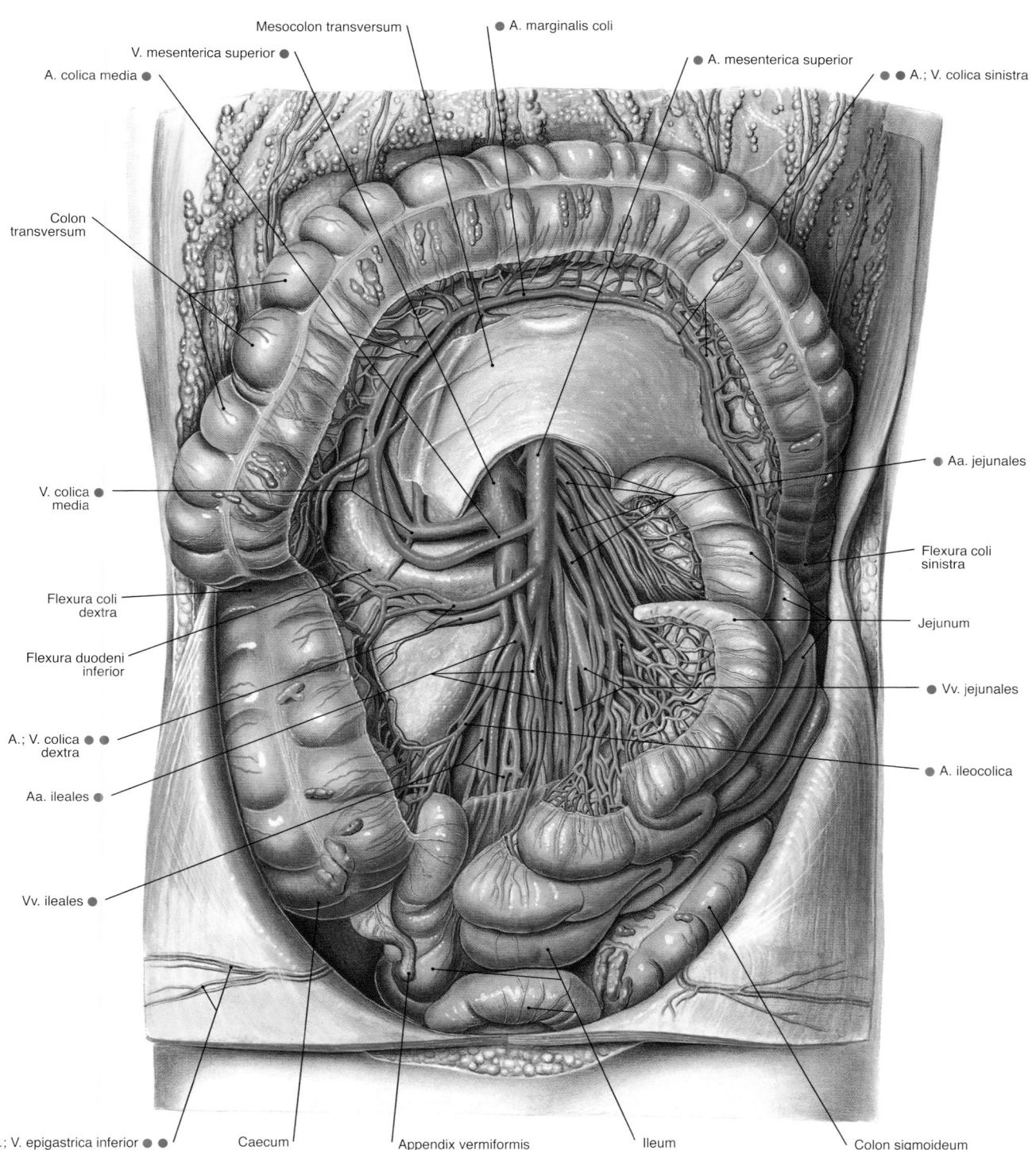

Mesocolon transversum
A. marginalis coli
V. mesenterica superior
A. mesenterica superior
A. colica media
A.; V. colica sinistra
Colon transversum
Aa. jejunales
V. colica media
Flexura coli sinistra
Flexura coli dextra
Jejunum
Flexura duodeni inferior
Vv. jejunales
A.; V. colica dextra
Aa. ileales
A. ileocolica
Vv. ileales
A.; V. epigastrica inferior
Caecum
Appendix vermiformis
Ileum
Colon sigmoideum

Fig. 802 Superior mesenteric artery and vein, A. et V. mesenterica superior.
The arteries supplying the small intestine form a series of arcades.

Inferior mesenteric artery

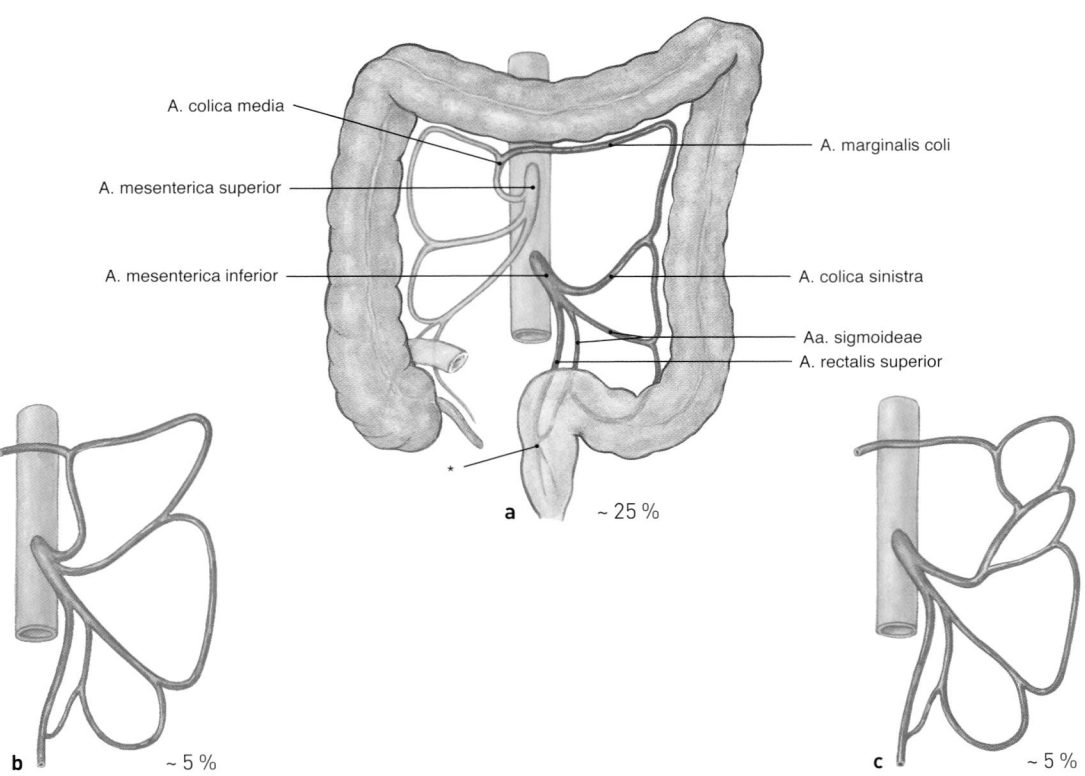

A. colica media

A. mesenterica superior

A. mesenterica inferior

A. marginalis coli

A. colica sinistra

Aa. sigmoideae
A. rectalis superior

*

a ~ 25 %

b ~ 5 %

c ~ 5 %

Fig. 803 a–c Variations in the branches of the inferior mesenteric artery, A. mesenterica inferior.
a The inferior mesenteric artery, A. mesenterica inferior, divides into three parts supplying the descending and sigmoid colon, as well as the rectum.

b An accessory middle colic artery, A. colica media, arises from the inferior mesenteric artery, A. mesenterica inferior.
c An accessory middle colic artery, A. colica media, arises from the left colic artery, A. colica sinistra.
* Clinical term: SUDECK's point

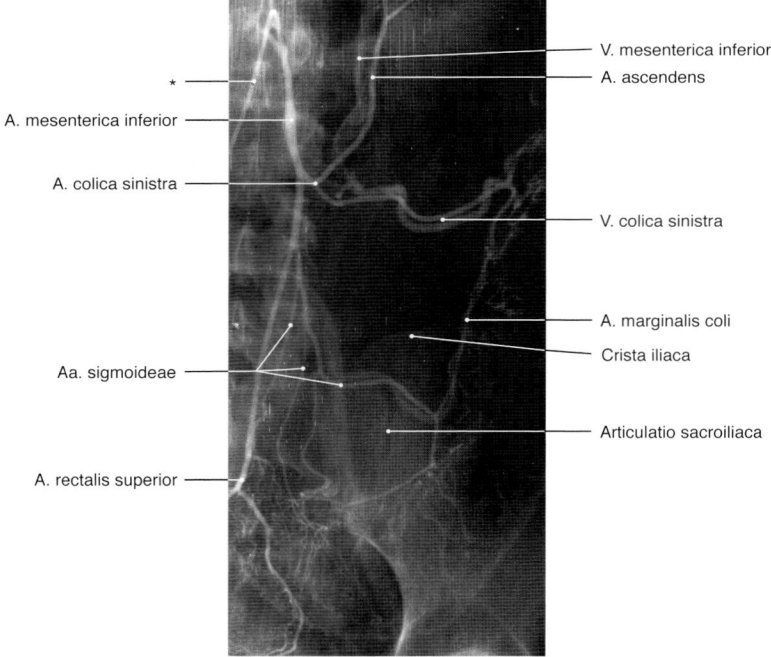

V. mesenterica inferior
A. ascendens

*

A. mesenterica inferior

A. colica sinistra

V. colica sinistra

A. marginalis coli
Crista iliaca

Aa. sigmoideae

Articulatio sacroiliaca

A. rectalis superior

Fig. 804 Inferior mesenteric artery, A. mesenterica inferior; AP-radiograph after selective injection of a contrast medium into the origin of the inferior mesenteric artery; ventral view.
* Catheter in the aorta

Vessels of the lower abdomen

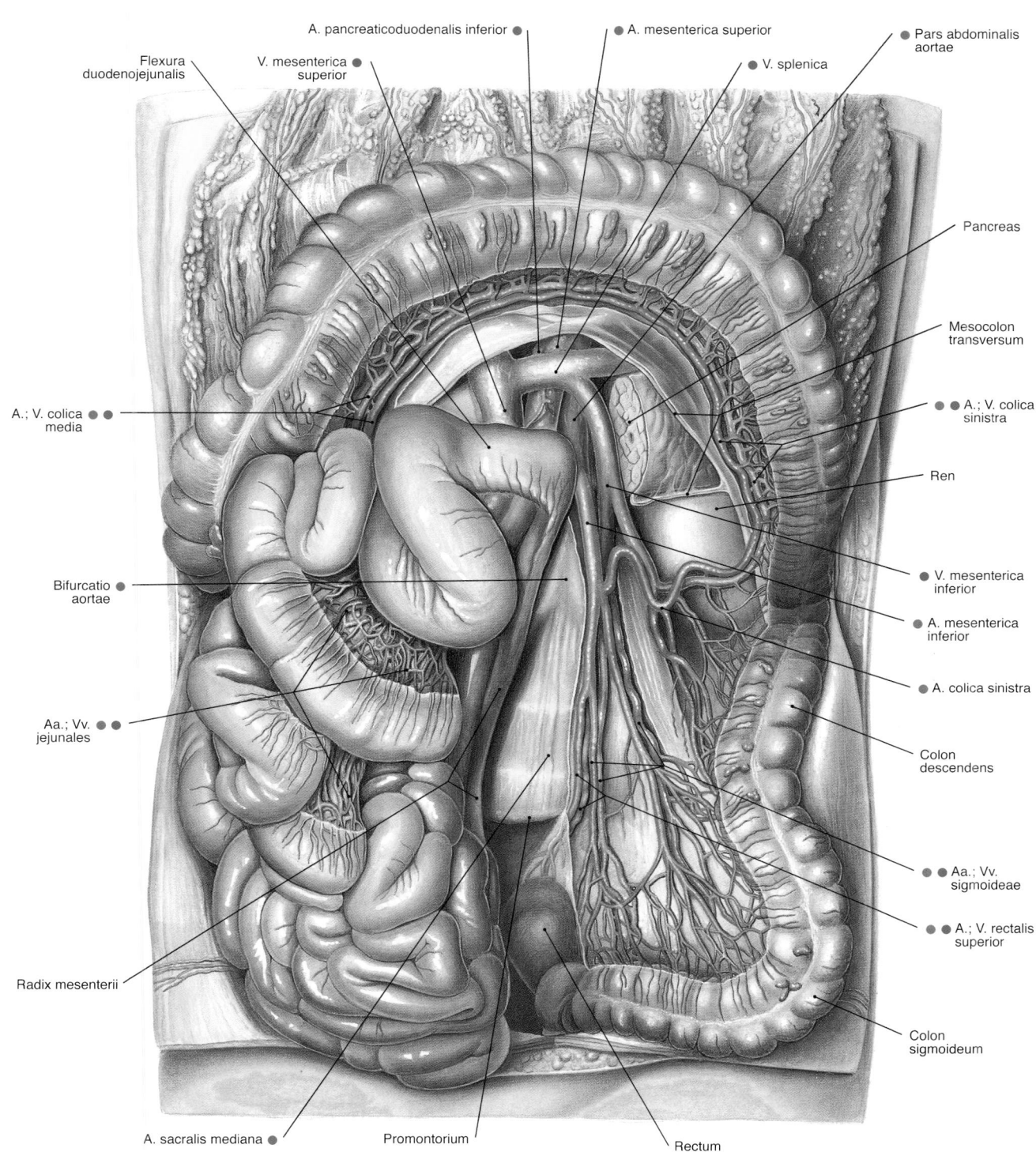

Flexura duodenojejunalis

A. pancreaticoduodenalis inferior ●

V. mesenterica ● superior

● A. mesenterica superior

● V. splenica

● Pars abdominalis aortae

Pancreas

Mesocolon transversum

A.; V. colica ● ● media

● ● A.; V. colica sinistra

Ren

Bifurcatio ● aortae

● V. mesenterica inferior

● A. mesenterica inferior

● A. colica sinistra

Colon descendens

Aa.; Vv. ● ● jejunales

● ● Aa.; Vv. sigmoideae

● ● A.; V. rectalis superior

Radix mesenterii

Colon sigmoideum

A. sacralis mediana ●

Promontorium

Rectum

Fig. 805   Inferior mesenteric artery and vein, A. et V. mesenterica inferior.

Coeliac trunk

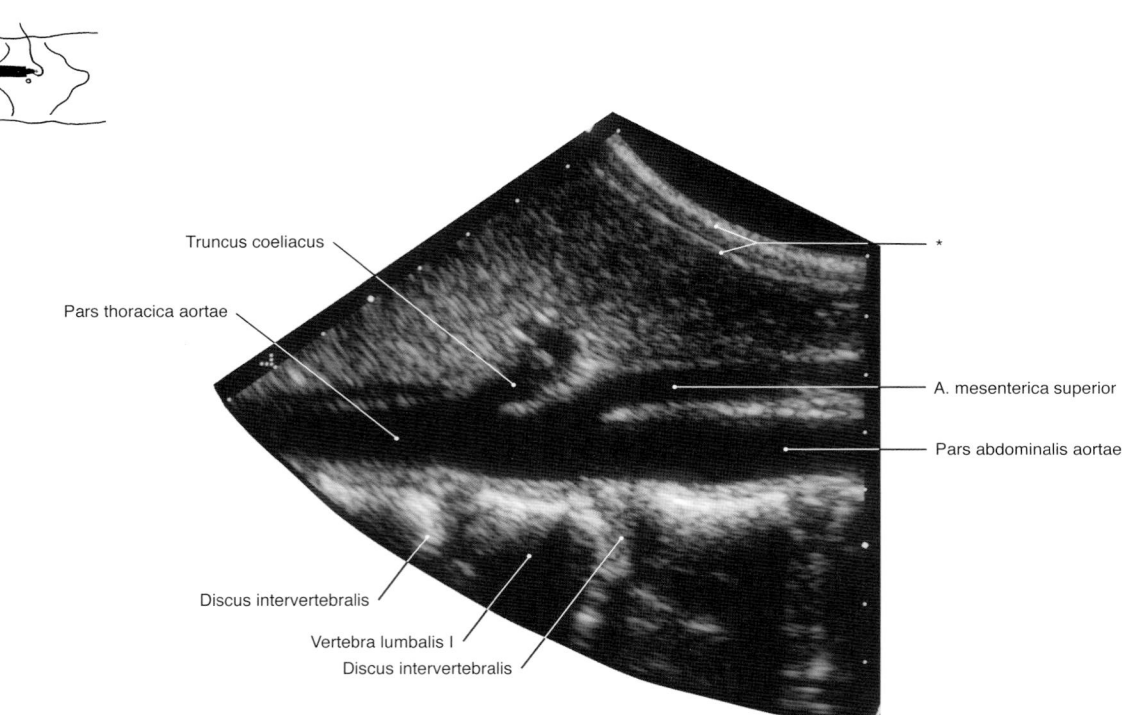

Fig. 806 Abdominal aorta, Pars abdominalis aortae, with the coeliac trunk, Truncus coeliacus, and the superior mesenteric artery, A. mesenterica superior; ultrasound image; almost in the sagittal plane.
* Abdominal wall

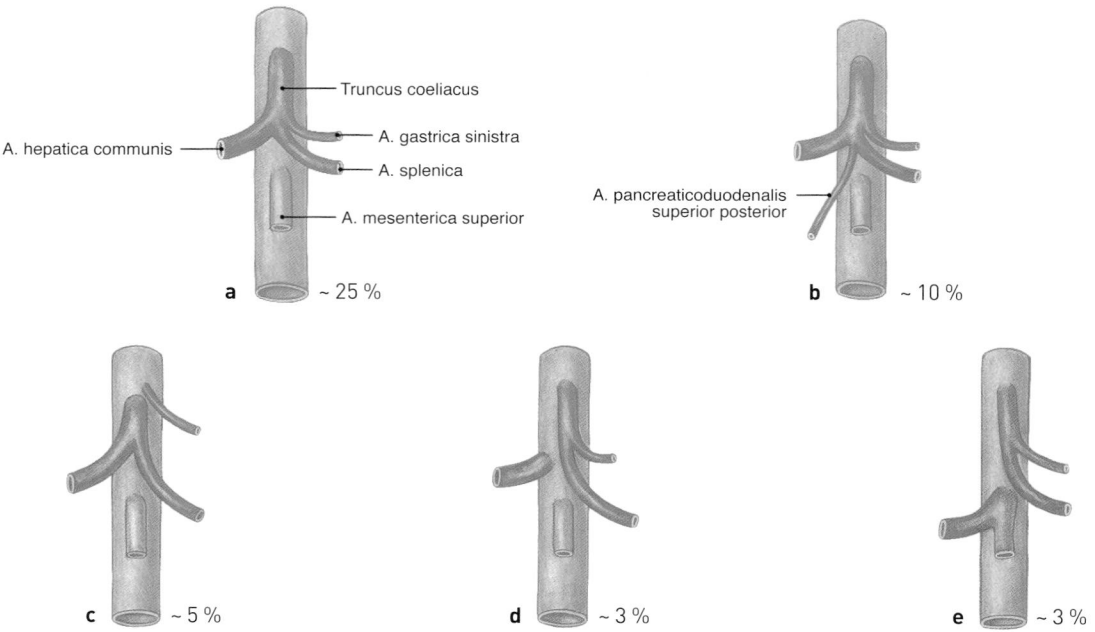

Fig. 807 a–e Variability of the coeliac trunk, Truncus coeliacus.
a "Textbook case", division of the trunk into three branches
b Division of the trunk into four branches
c Development of a hepatosplenic trunk, Truncus hepatosplenicus

d Development of a gastrosplenic trunk, Truncus gastrosplenicus
e Development of a gastrosplenic trunk, Truncus gastrosplenicus, and a hepatomesenteric trunk, Truncus hepatomesentericus

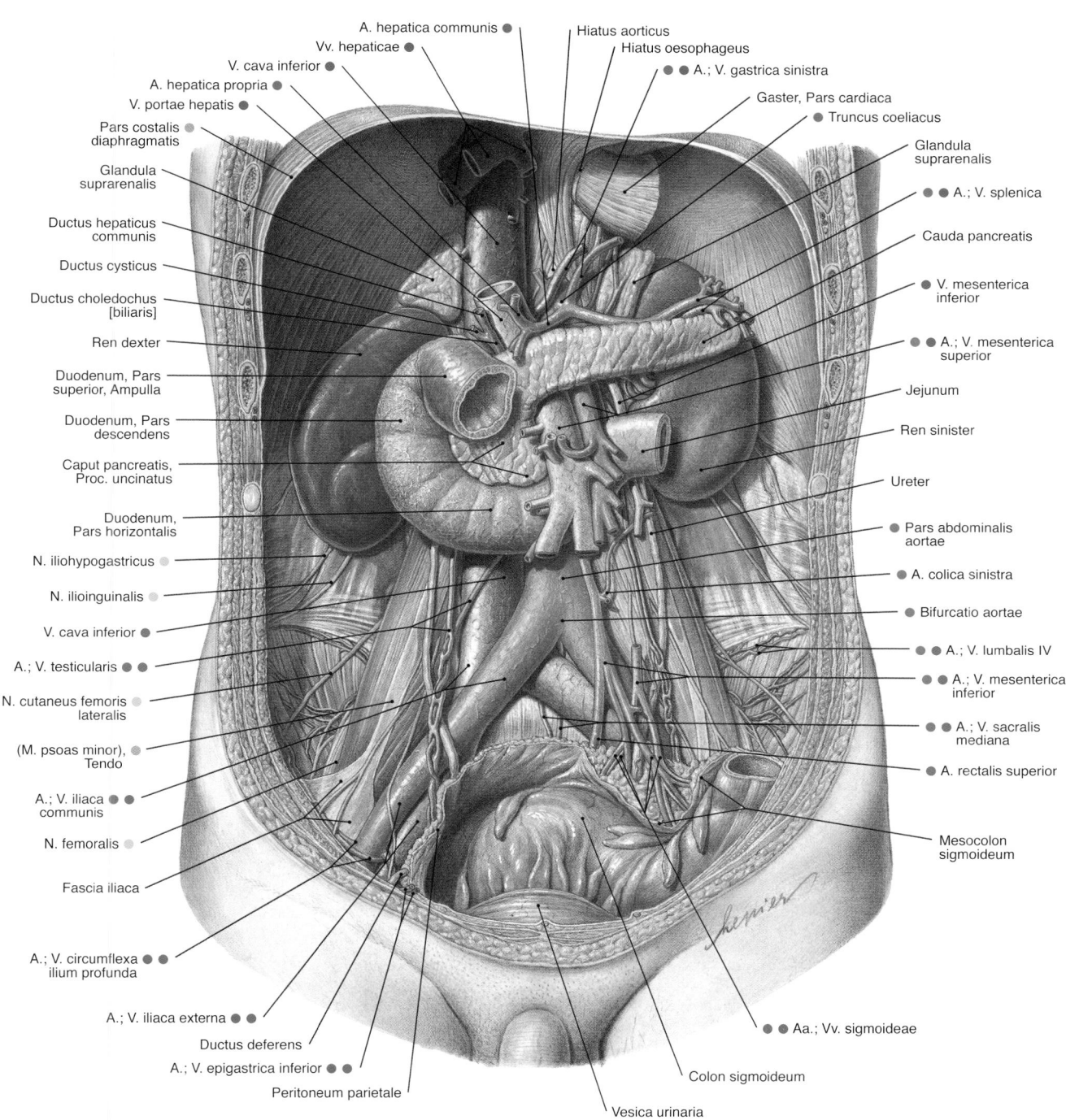

A. hepatica communis
Vv. hepaticae
V. cava inferior
A. hepatica propria
V. portae hepatis
Pars costalis diaphragmatis
Glandula suprarenalis
Ductus hepaticus communis
Ductus cysticus
Ductus choledochus [biliaris]
Ren dexter
Duodenum, Pars superior, Ampulla
Duodenum, Pars descendens
Caput pancreatis, Proc. uncinatus
Duodenum, Pars horizontalis
N. iliohypogastricus
N. ilioinguinalis
V. cava inferior
A.; V. testicularis
N. cutaneus femoris lateralis
(M. psoas minor), Tendo
A.; V. iliaca communis
N. femoralis
Fascia iliaca
A.; V. circumflexa ilium profunda
A.; V. iliaca externa
Ductus deferens
A.; V. epigastrica inferior
Peritoneum parietale

Hiatus aorticus
Hiatus oesophageus
A.; V. gastrica sinistra
Gaster, Pars cardiaca
Truncus coeliacus
Glandula suprarenalis
A.; V. splenica
Cauda pancreatis
V. mesenterica inferior
A.; V. mesenterica superior
Jejunum
Ren sinister
Ureter
Pars abdominalis aortae
A. colica sinistra
Bifurcatio aortae
A.; V. lumbalis IV
A.; V. mesenterica inferior
A.; V. sacralis mediana
A. rectalis superior
Mesocolon sigmoideum
Aa.; Vv. sigmoideae
Colon sigmoideum
Vesica urinaria

Fig. 808   Vessels of the retroperitoneal space,
Situs retroperitonealis, of the male.

Hepatic portal vein, overview

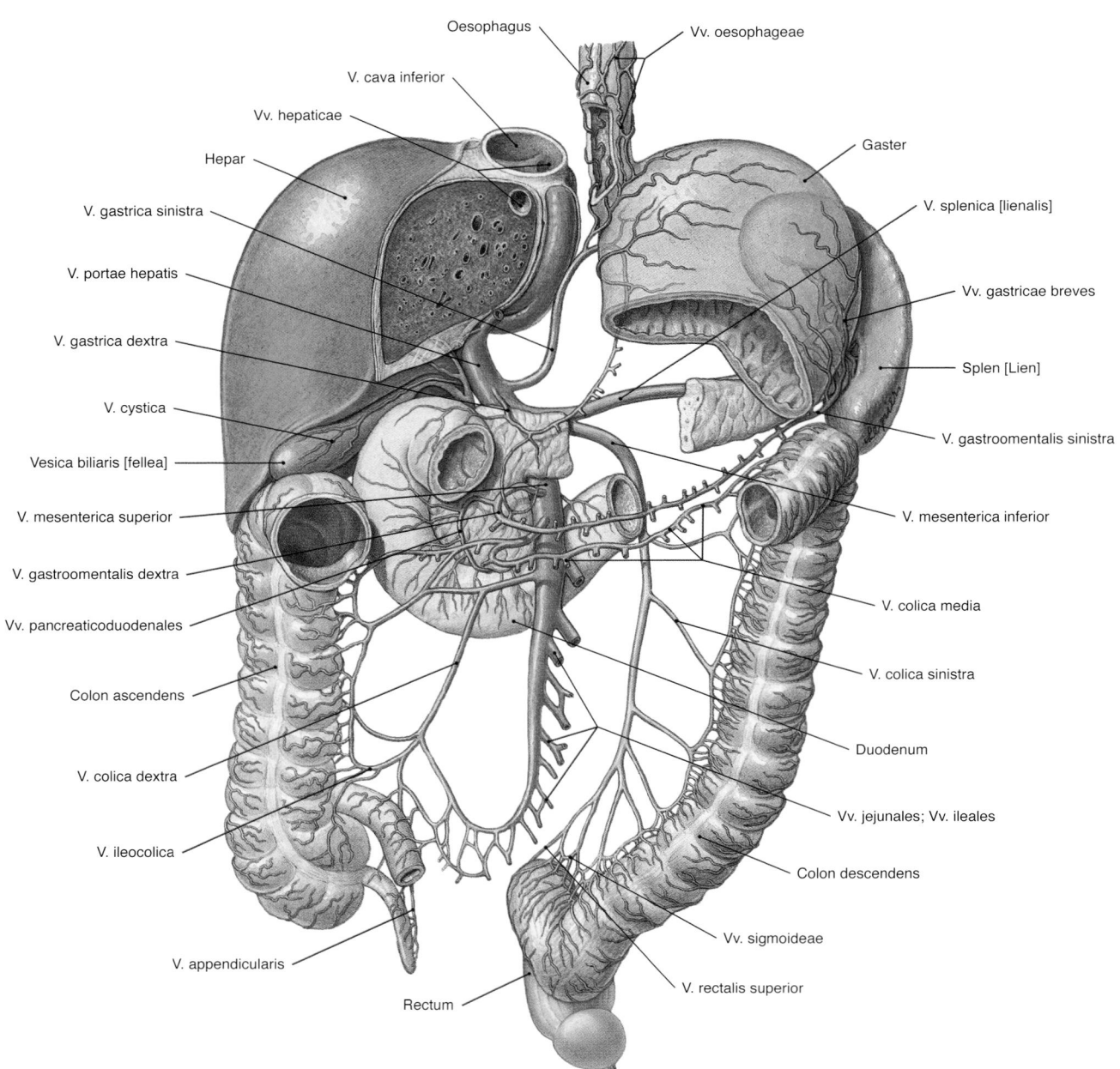

Oesophagus

Vv. oesophageae

V. cava inferior

Vv. hepaticae

Gaster

Hepar

V. splenica [lienalis]

V. gastrica sinistra

V. portae hepatis

Vv. gastricae breves

V. gastrica dextra

Splen [Lien]

V. cystica

V. gastroomentalis sinistra

Vesica biliaris [fellea]

V. mesenterica superior

V. mesenterica inferior

V. gastroomentalis dextra

V. colica media

Vv. pancreaticoduodenales

V. colica sinistra

Colon ascendens

Duodenum

V. colica dextra

Vv. jejunales; Vv. ileales

V. ileocolica

Colon descendens

Vv. sigmoideae

V. appendicularis

V. rectalis superior

Rectum

Fig. 809   Hepatic portal vein, V. portae hepatis;
ventral view.

Portocaval anastomoses

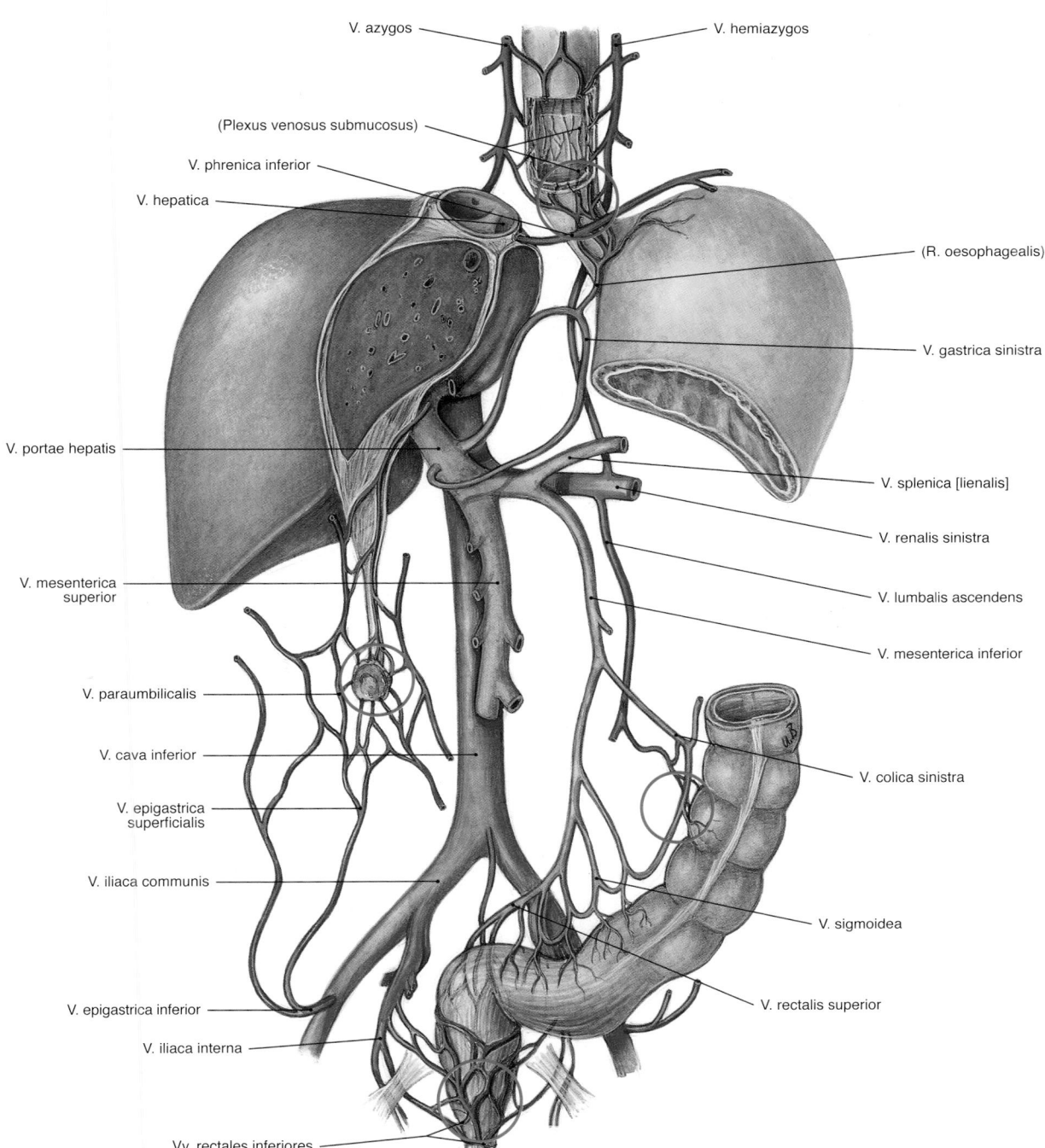

V. azygos

V. hemiazygos

(Plexus venosus submucosus)

V. phrenica inferior

V. hepatica

(R. oesophagealis)

V. gastrica sinistra

V. portae hepatis

V. splenica [lienalis]

V. renalis sinistra

V. mesenterica superior

V. lumbalis ascendens

V. mesenterica inferior

V. paraumbilicalis

V. cava inferior

V. colica sinistra

V. epigastrica superficialis

V. iliaca communis

V. sigmoidea

V. epigastrica inferior

V. rectalis superior

V. iliaca interna

Vv. rectales inferiores

Fig. 810 Hepatic portal vein, V. portae hepatis,
and inferior vena cava, V. cava inferior;
semi-schematic;
tributaries of the inferior vena cava in blue;
tributaries of the hepatic portal vein in purple;
potential portocaval anastomoses are indicated
by circles.

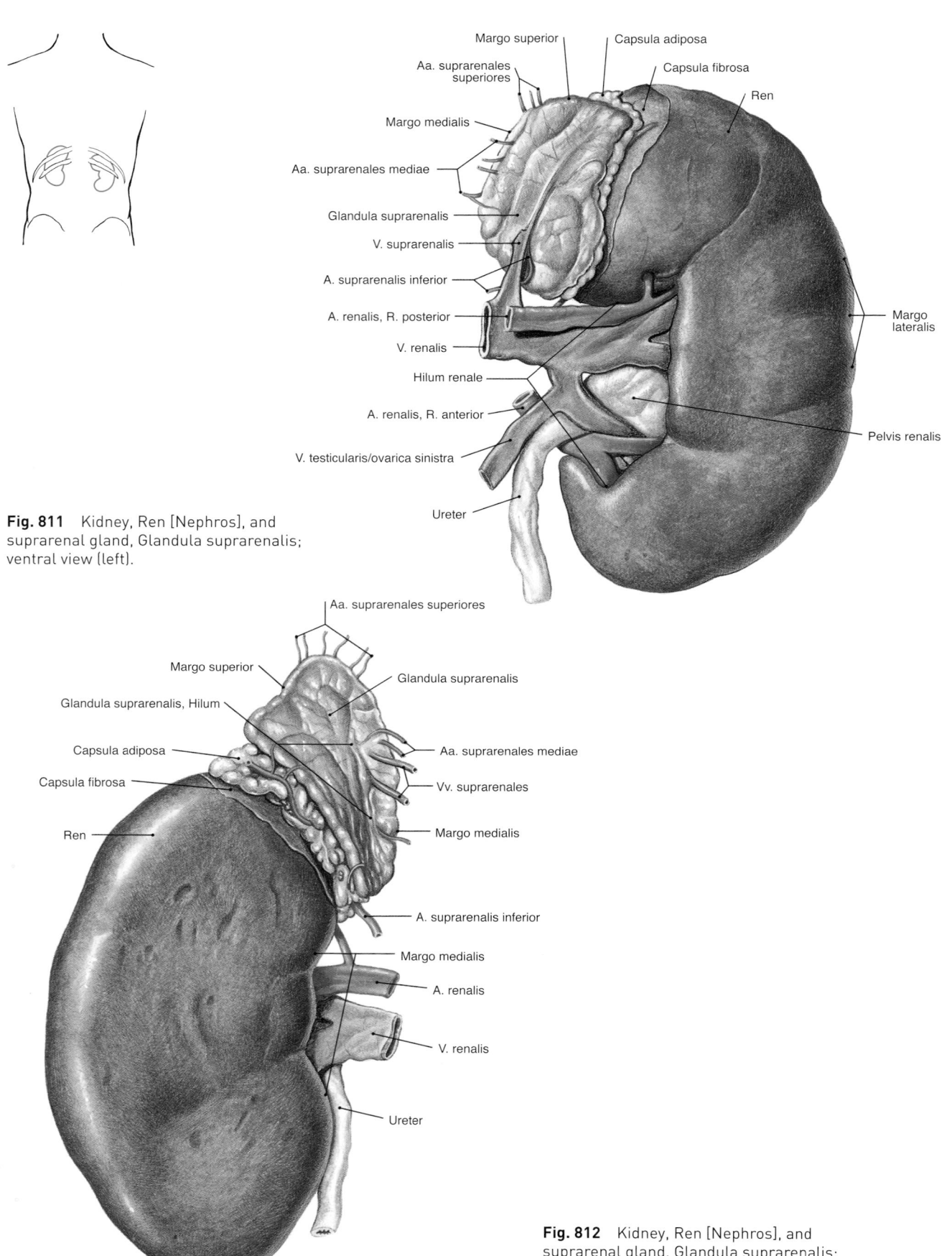

Margo superior

Capsula adiposa

Aa. suprarenales superiores

Capsula fibrosa

Ren

Margo medialis

Aa. suprarenales mediae

Glandula suprarenalis

V. suprarenalis

A. suprarenalis inferior

A. renalis, R. posterior

V. renalis

Margo lateralis

Hilum renale

A. renalis, R. anterior

V. testicularis/ovarica sinistra

Pelvis renalis

Ureter

Fig. 811 Kidney, Ren [Nephros], and suprarenal gland, Glandula suprarenalis; ventral view (left).

Aa. suprarenales superiores

Margo superior

Glandula suprarenalis

Glandula suprarenalis, Hilum

Capsula adiposa

Aa. suprarenales mediae

Capsula fibrosa

Vv. suprarenales

Ren

Margo medialis

A. suprarenalis inferior

Margo medialis

A. renalis

V. renalis

Ureter

Fig. 812 Kidney, Ren [Nephros], and suprarenal gland, Glandula suprarenalis; ventral view (right).

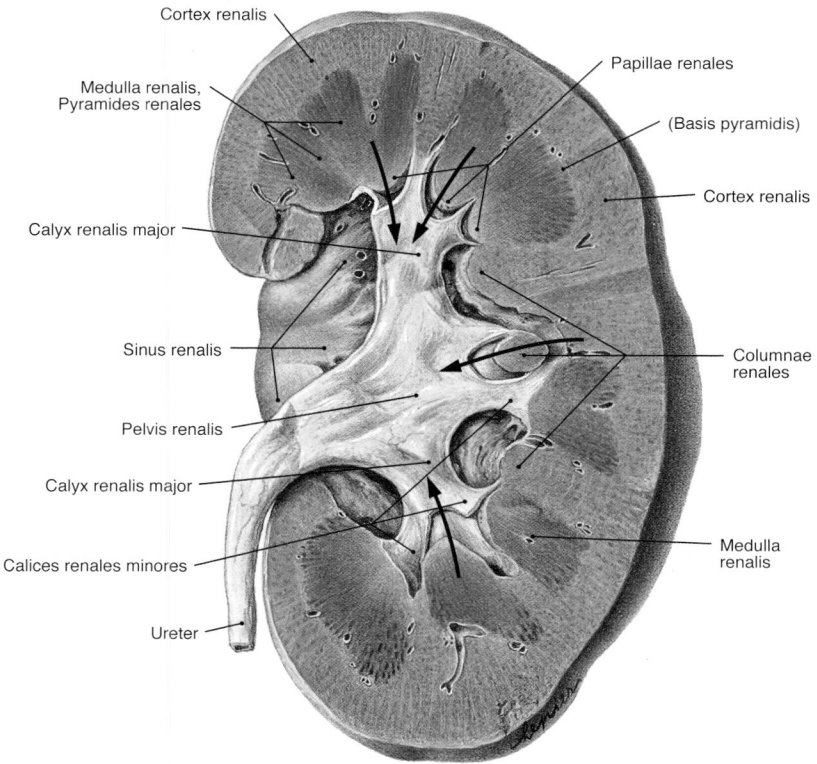

Cortex renalis

Medulla renalis,
Pyramides renales

Calyx renalis major

Sinus renalis

Pelvis renalis

Calyx renalis major

Calices renales minores

Ureter

Papillae renales

(Basis pyramidis)

Cortex renalis

Columnae
renales

Medulla
renalis

Fig. 813 Kidney, Ren [Nephros];
oblique and vertical hemisection
displaying the renal cortex, the medulla
and the pelvis;
ventral view (left).
Arrows point from the pyramids to the
calyces.

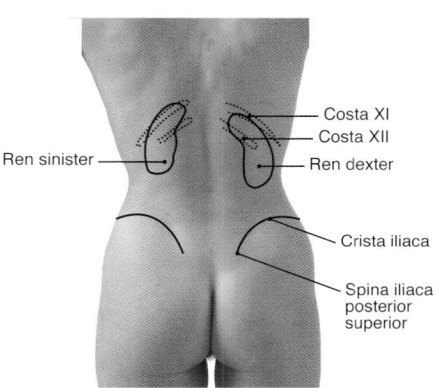

Ren sinister

Costa XI
Costa XII
Ren dexter

Crista iliaca

Spina iliaca
posterior
superior

Fig. 814 Projection of the kidneys
onto the back.

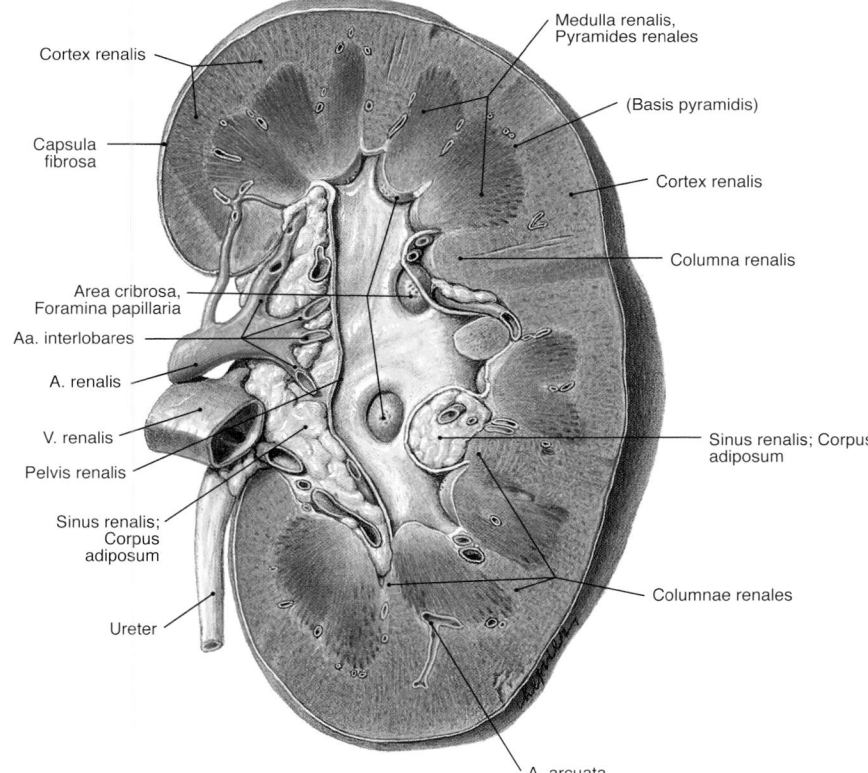

Cortex renalis

Capsula
fibrosa

Area cribrosa,
Foramina papillaria

Aa. interlobares

A. renalis

V. renalis

Pelvis renalis

Sinus renalis;
Corpus
adiposum

Ureter

Medulla renalis,
Pyramides renales

(Basis pyramidis)

Cortex renalis

Columna renalis

Sinus renalis; Corpus
adiposum

Columnae renales

A. arcuata

Fig. 815 Kidney, Ren [Nephros];
oblique and vertical hemisection;
ventral view (left).

Kidney, structure

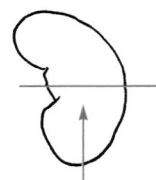

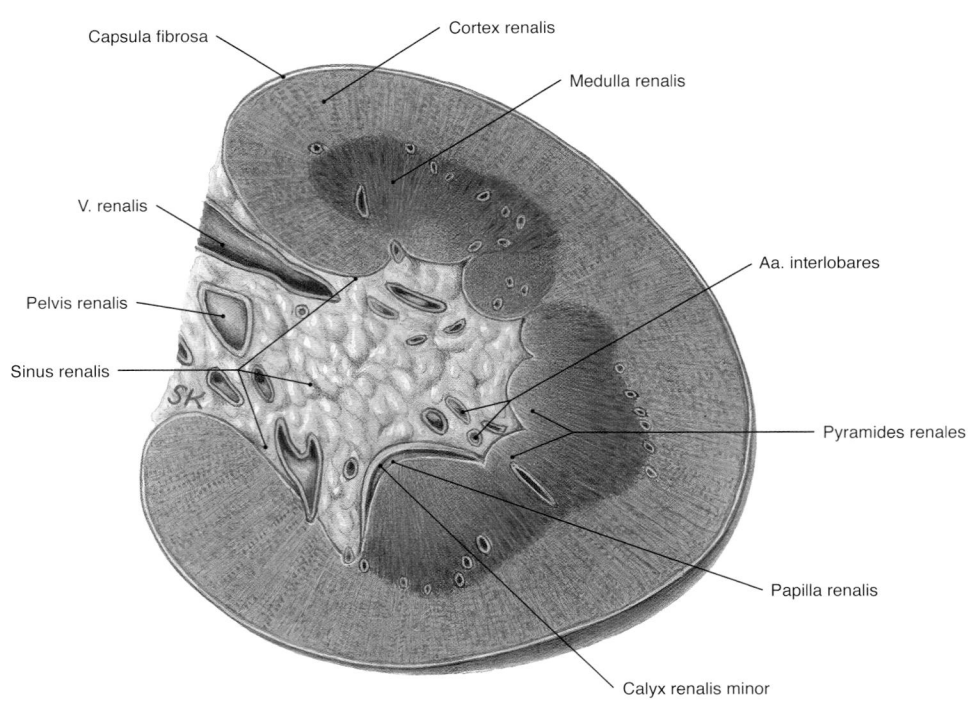

Capsula fibrosa

Cortex renalis

Medulla renalis

V. renalis

Pelvis renalis

Sinus renalis

Aa. interlobares

Pyramides renales

Papilla renalis

Calyx renalis minor

Fig. 816   Kidney, Ren [Nephros];
transverse section through the renal sinus;
inferior view (left).

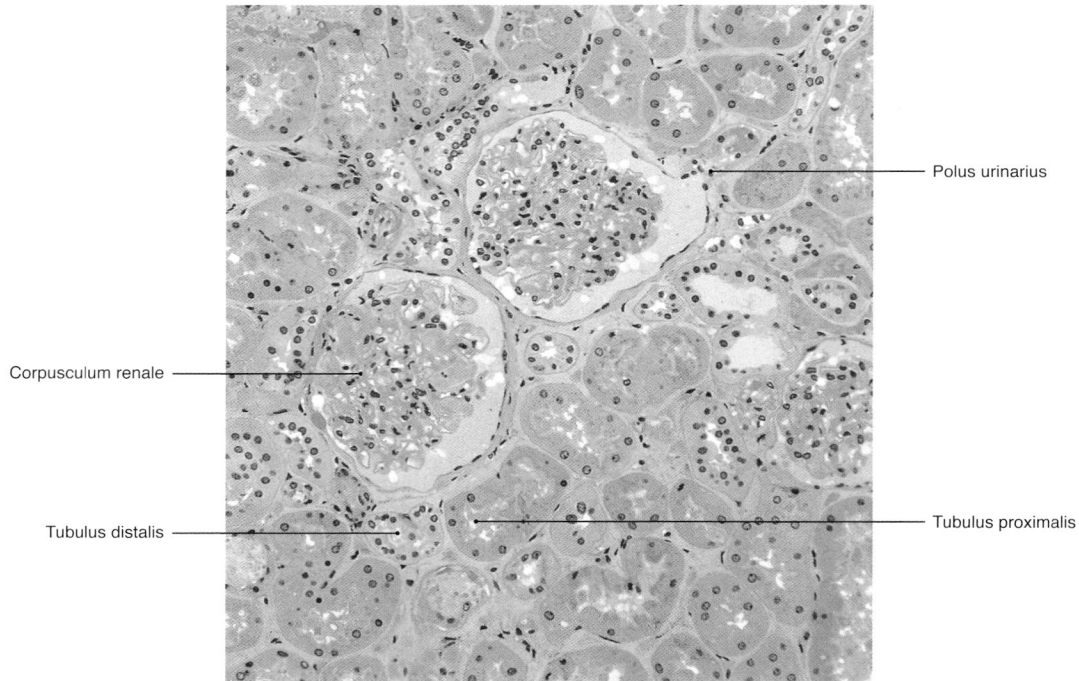

Polus urinarius

Corpusculum renale

Tubulus distalis

Tubulus proximalis

Fig. 817   Kidney, Ren [Nephros];
microscopic section of the cortex (100×).

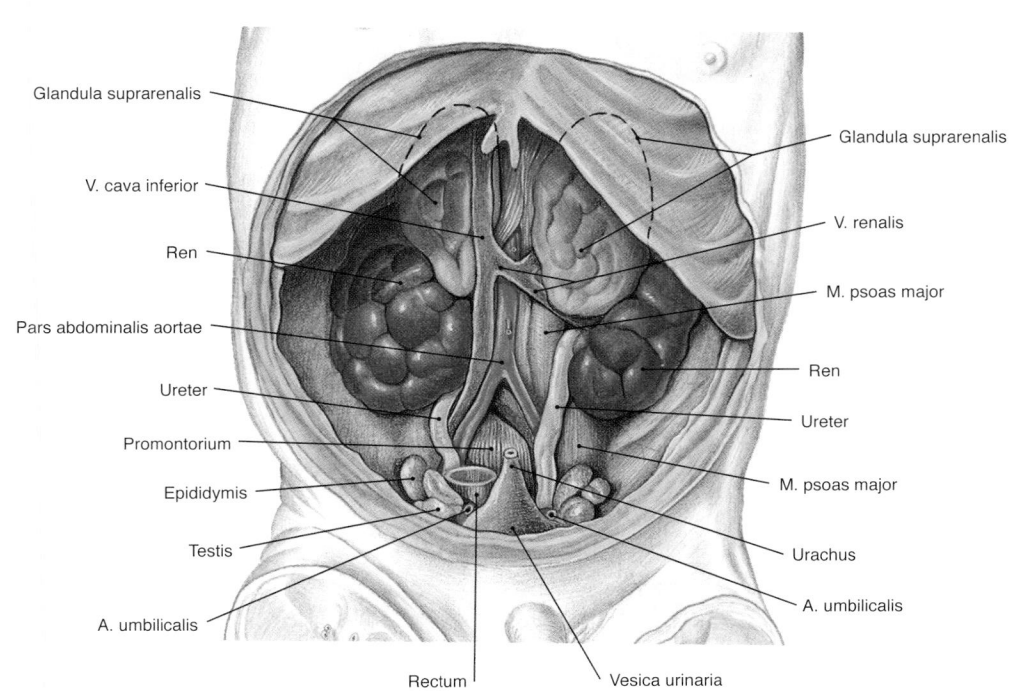

Glandula suprarenalis

V. cava inferior

Ren

Pars abdominalis aortae

Ureter

Promontorium

Epididymis

Testis

A. umbilicalis

Glandula suprarenalis

V. renalis

M. psoas major

Ren

Ureter

M. psoas major

Urachus

A. umbilicalis

Rectum

Vesica urinaria

Fig. 818 Kidney, Ren [Nephros], and
the suprarenal gland, Glandula suprarenalis,
of a ~ 5-month-old foetus.

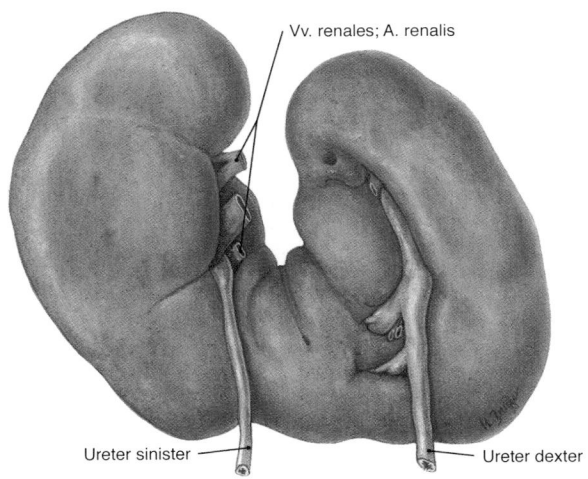

Vv. renales; A. renalis

Ureter sinister

Ureter dexter

Fig. 819 Kidney, Ren [Nephros];
dorsal view.
The lower poles of both kidneys are fused
(= horseshoe kidney).

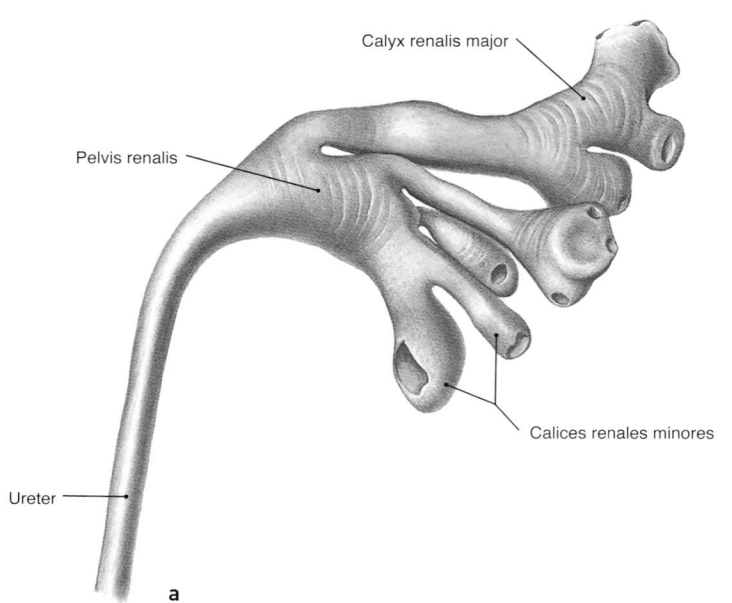

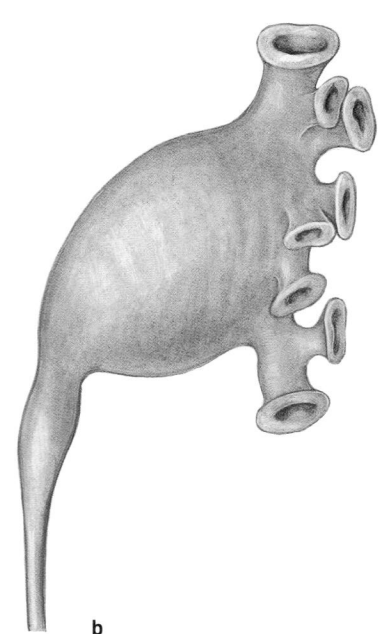

Fig. 820 a, b   Renal pelvis, Pelvis renalis;
corrosion casts;
ventral view (left).
a Dendritic type
b Ampullar type

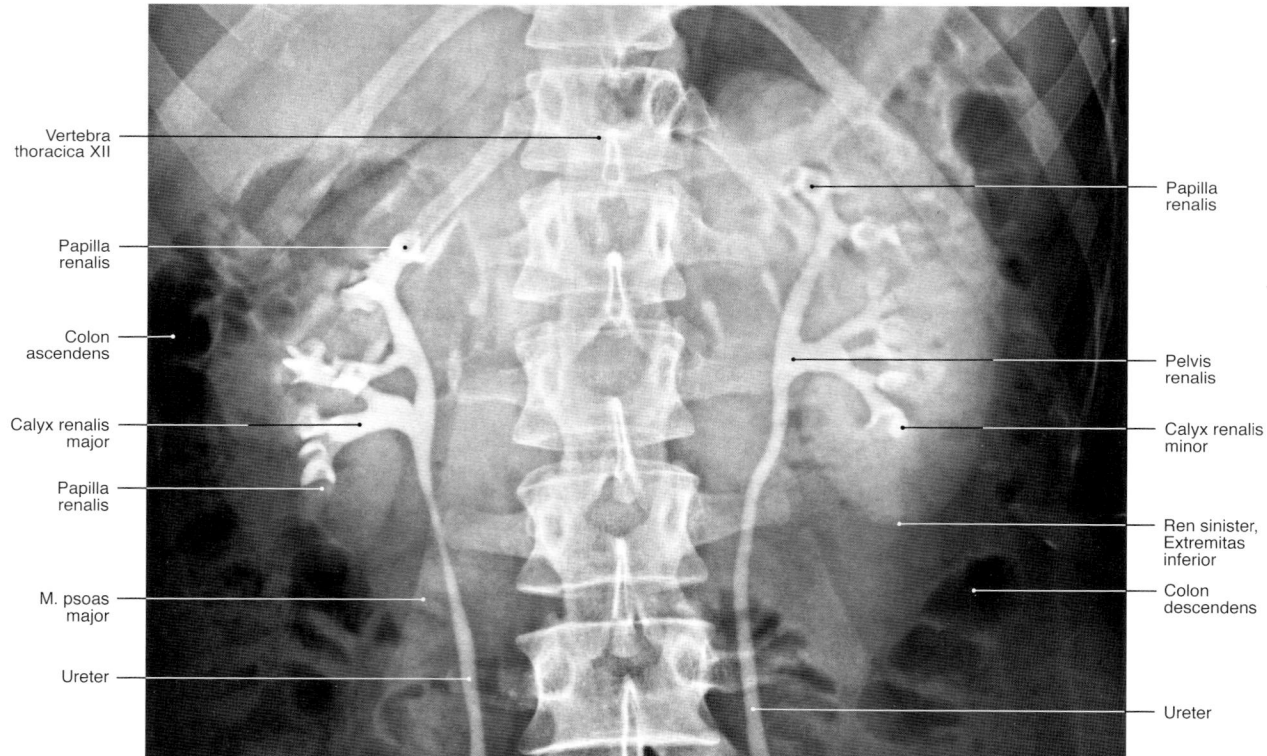

Fig. 821   Kidney, Ren [Nephros];
renal pelvis, Pelvis renalis, and ureter, Ureter;
AP-radiograph after retrograde injection of a
contrast medium via both ureters.

Areas of contact and renal segments

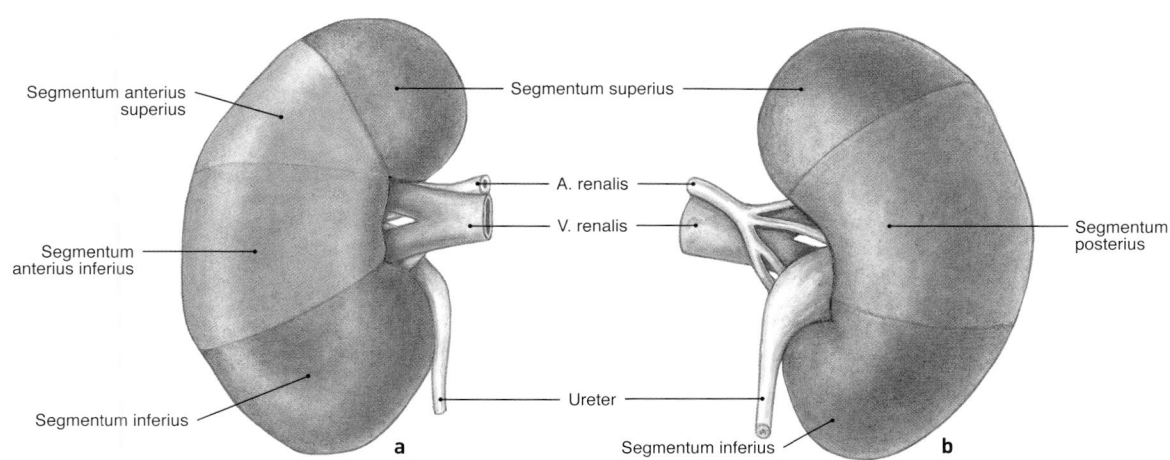

Segmentum anterius superius
Segmentum superius
A. renalis
V. renalis
Segmentum posterius
Segmentum anterius inferius
Segmentum inferius
Ureter
Segmentum inferius
a
b

Fig. 822 a, b Renal segments, Segmenta renalia.

a Ventral view (right)
b Dorsal view (right)

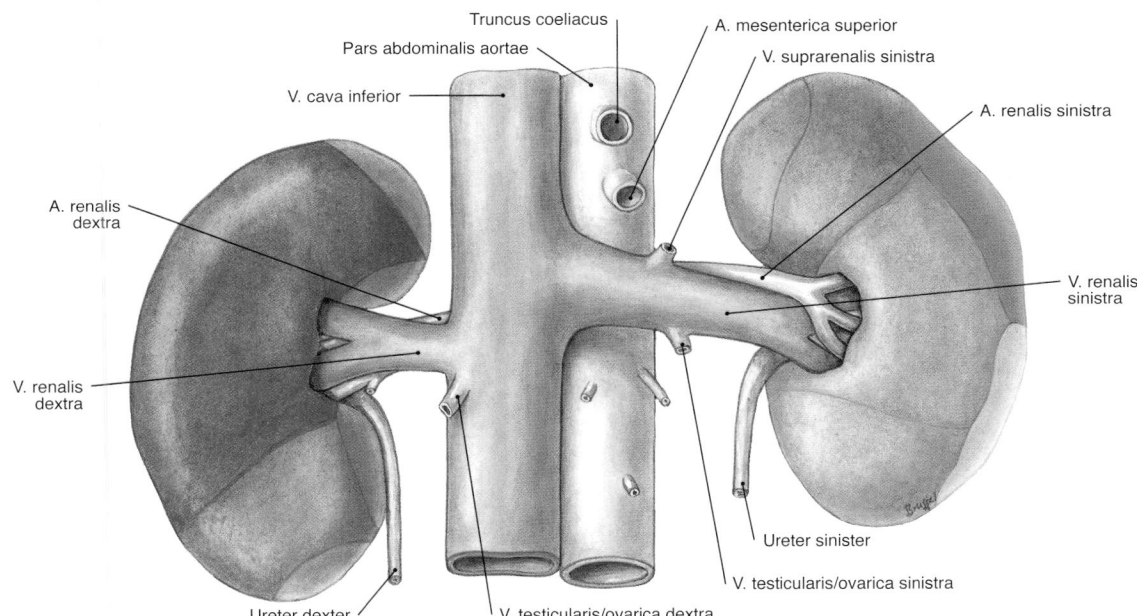

Truncus coeliacus
Pars abdominalis aortae
A. mesenterica superior
V. suprarenalis sinistra
V. cava inferior
A. renalis sinistra
A. renalis dextra
V. renalis sinistra
V. renalis dextra
Ureter sinister
V. testicularis/ovarica sinistra
Ureter dexter
V. testicularis/ovarica dextra

Fig. 823 Kidney, Ren; areas of contact with adjacent organs; ventral view.

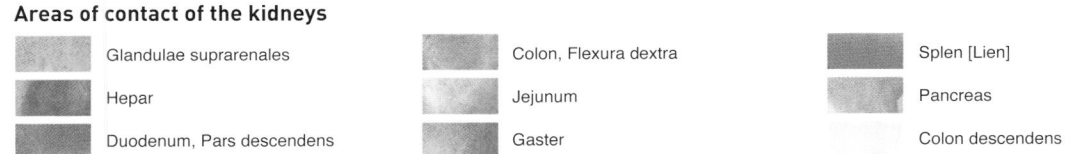

Areas of contact of the kidneys

Glandulae suprarenales
Colon, Flexura dextra
Splen [Lien]

Hepar
Jejunum
Pancreas

Duodenum, Pars descendens
Gaster
Colon descendens

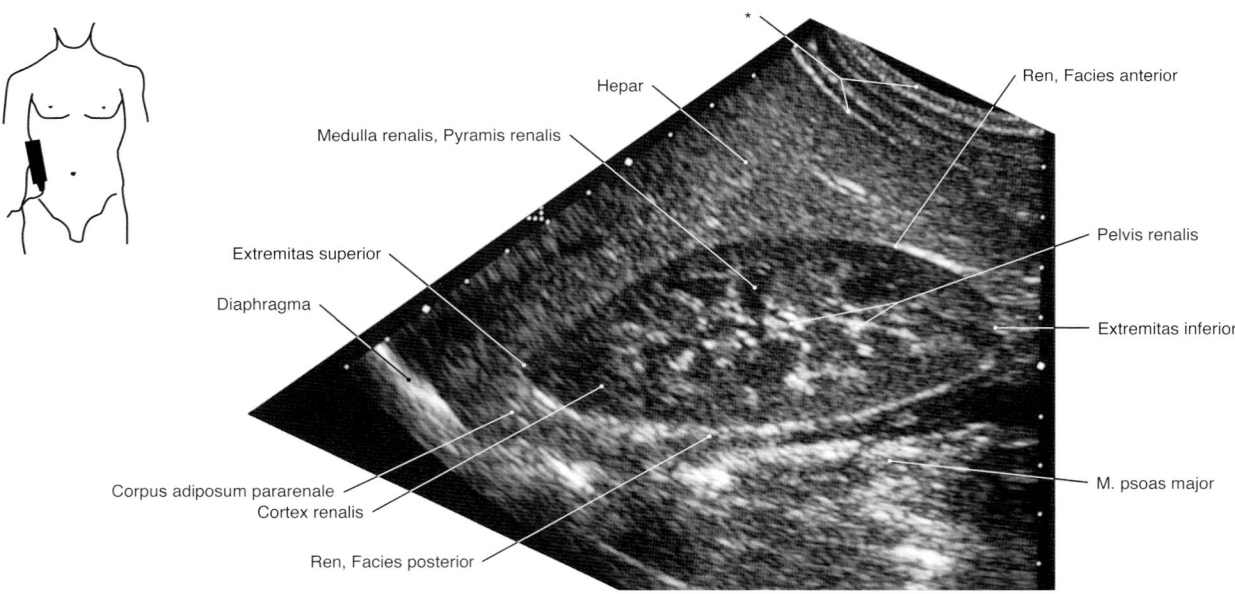

Fig. 824 Kidney, Ren [Nephros];
ultrasound image;
the transducer is directed from ventroinferior to dorsosuperior;
lateral view (right).
* Abdominal wall

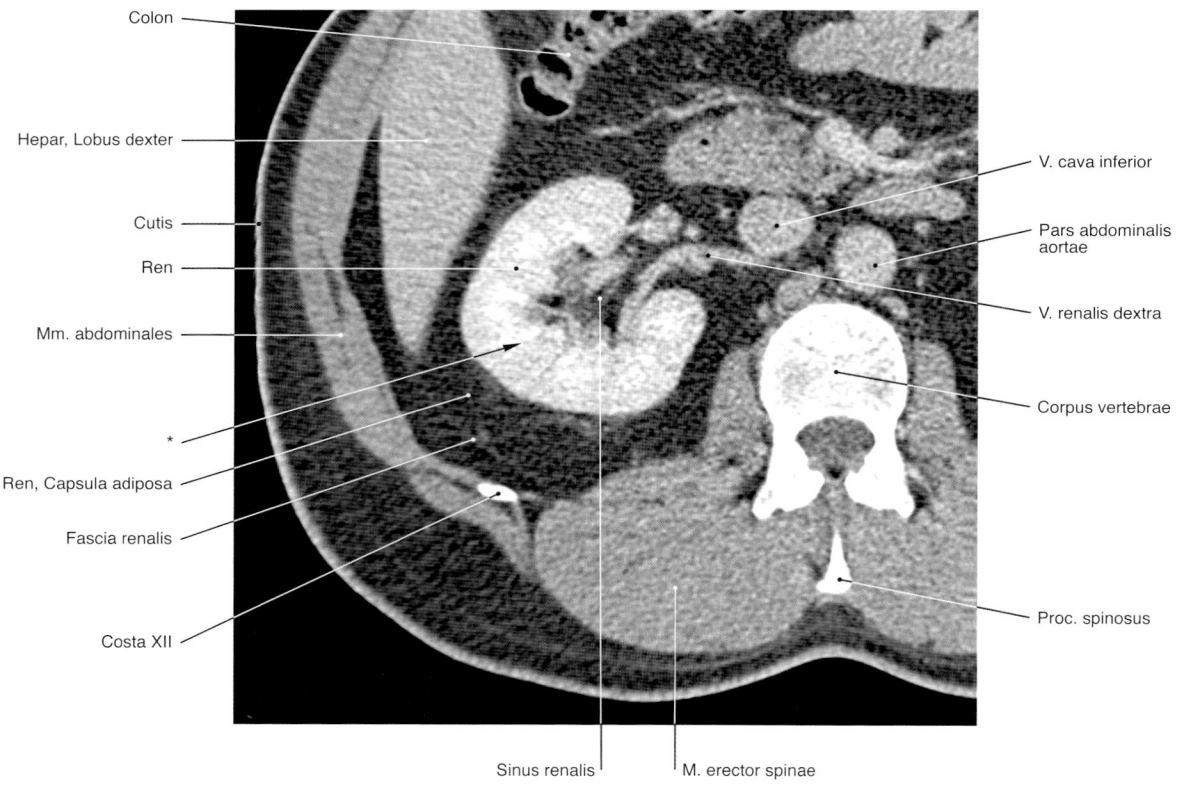

→ 928

Fig. 825 Kidney, Ren [Nephros];
puncture of the right kidney;
computed tomographic cross-section (CT);
inferior view.
* Guidance of a needle for kidney biopsy

Suprarenal gland

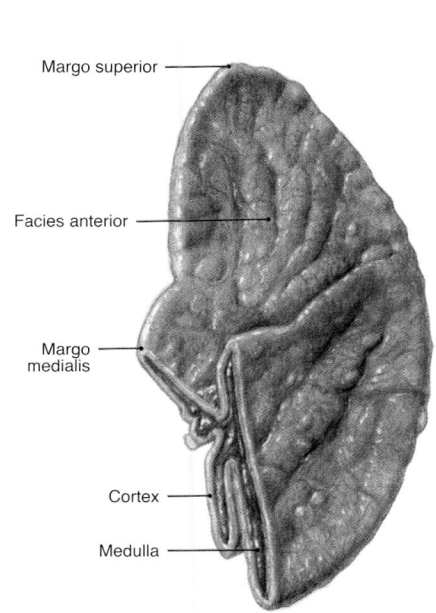

Fig. 826   Suprarenal gland, Glandula suprarenalis; ventral view (right).

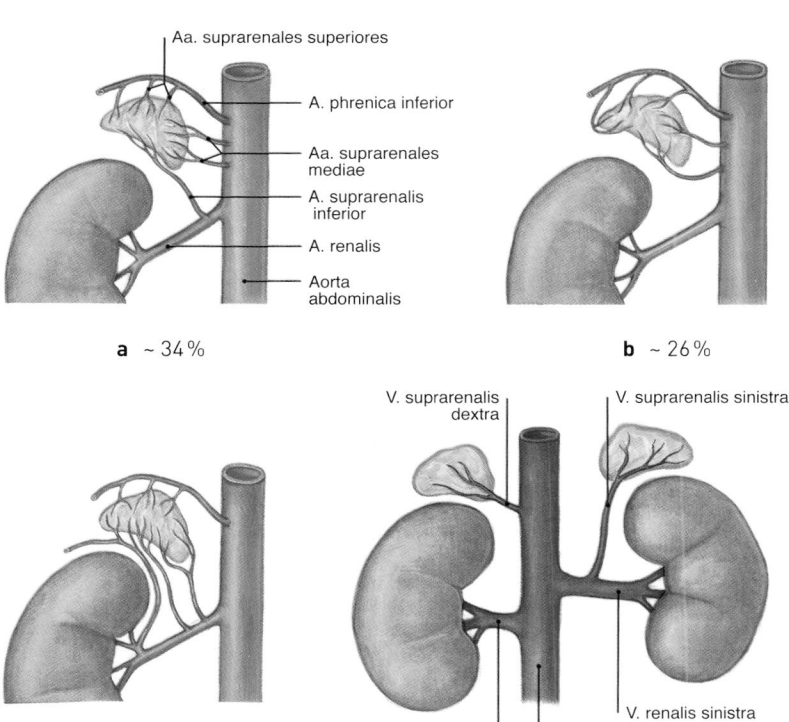

a ~ 34%

b ~ 26%

c ~ 33%

d V. renalis dextra   V. cava inferior

Fig. 827 a–d   Variability of the suprarenal arteries, Aa. suprarenales, and course of the suprarenal veins, Vv. suprarenales.
a   Arterial supply by three arteries ("textbook case")
b   Arterial supply without a branch from the renal artery, A. renalis
c   Arterial supply without a direct branch from the aorta, Aorta
d   Course of the suprarenal veins, Vv. suprarenales

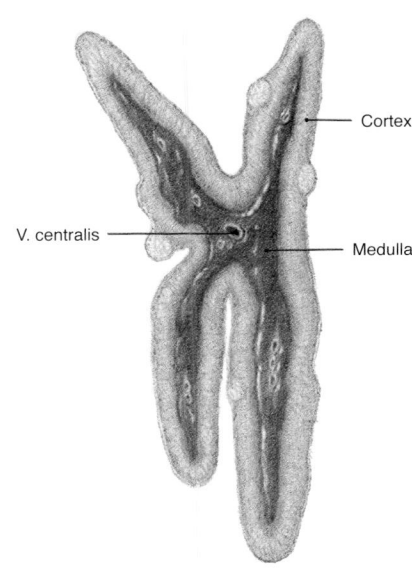

Fig. 828   Suprarenal gland, Glandula suprarenalis; sagittal section; lateral view (right).

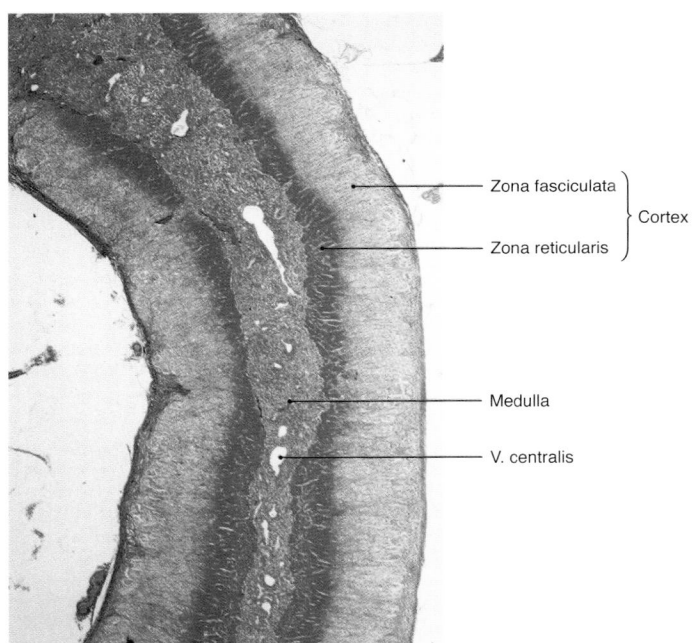

Fig. 829   Suprarenal gland, Glandula suprarenalis; microscopic enlargement at low magnification.

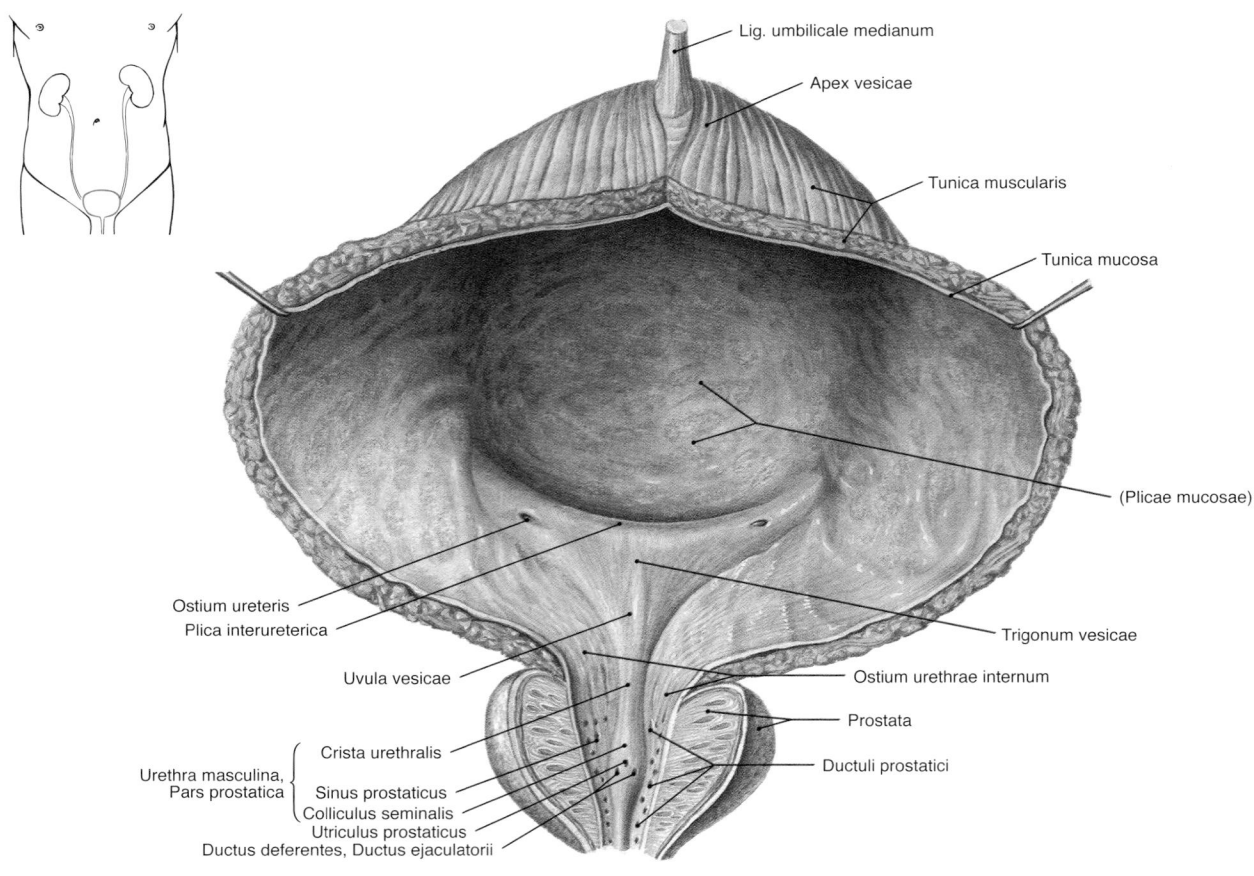

Lig. umbilicale medianum

Apex vesicae

Tunica muscularis

Tunica mucosa

(Plicae mucosae)

Ostium ureteris

Plica interureterica

Uvula vesicae

Trigonum vesicae

Ostium urethrae internum

Prostata

Ductuli prostatici

Crista urethralis

Urethra masculina, Pars prostatica

Sinus prostaticus

Colliculus seminalis

Utriculus prostaticus

Ductus deferentes, Ductus ejaculatorii

Fig. 830   Urinary bladder, Vesica urinaria; prostate, Prostata, and urethra, Urethra; ventral view.

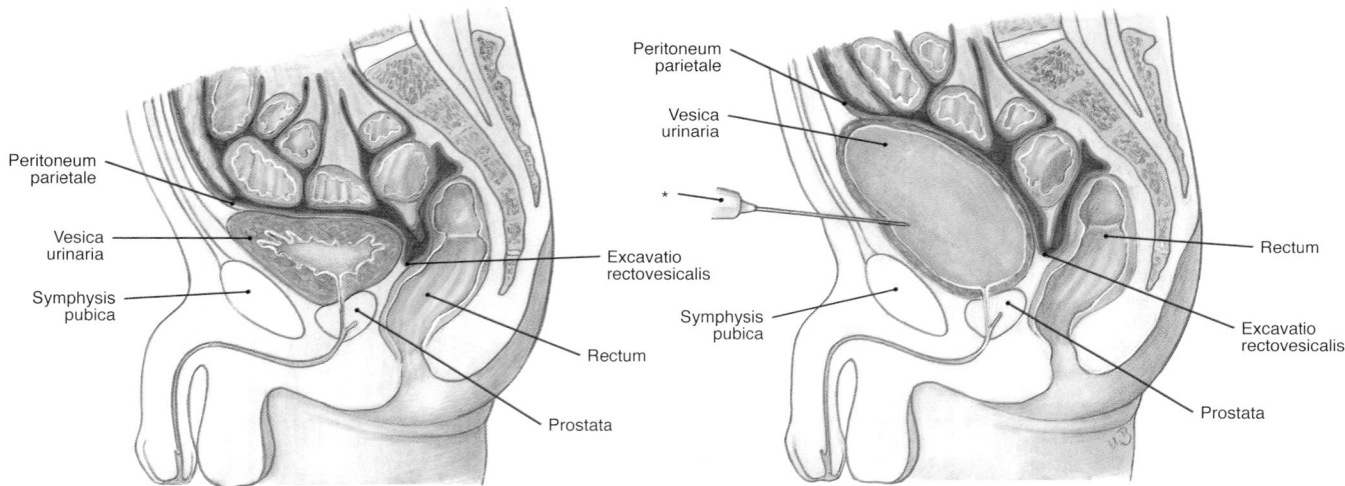

Peritoneum parietale

Vesica urinaria

Symphysis pubica

Excavatio rectovesicalis

Rectum

Prostata

Peritoneum parietale

Vesica urinaria

*

Symphysis pubica

Rectum

Excavatio rectovesicalis

Prostata

Fig. 831   Urinary bladder, Vesica urinaria, almost completely voided.

Fig. 832   Urinary bladder, Vesica urinaria, filled. In this situation, the bladder can be punctured from just above the pubic bone without passing through the peritoneal cavity.

* Puncture needle

Urinary bladder, ductus deferens and seminal vesicle

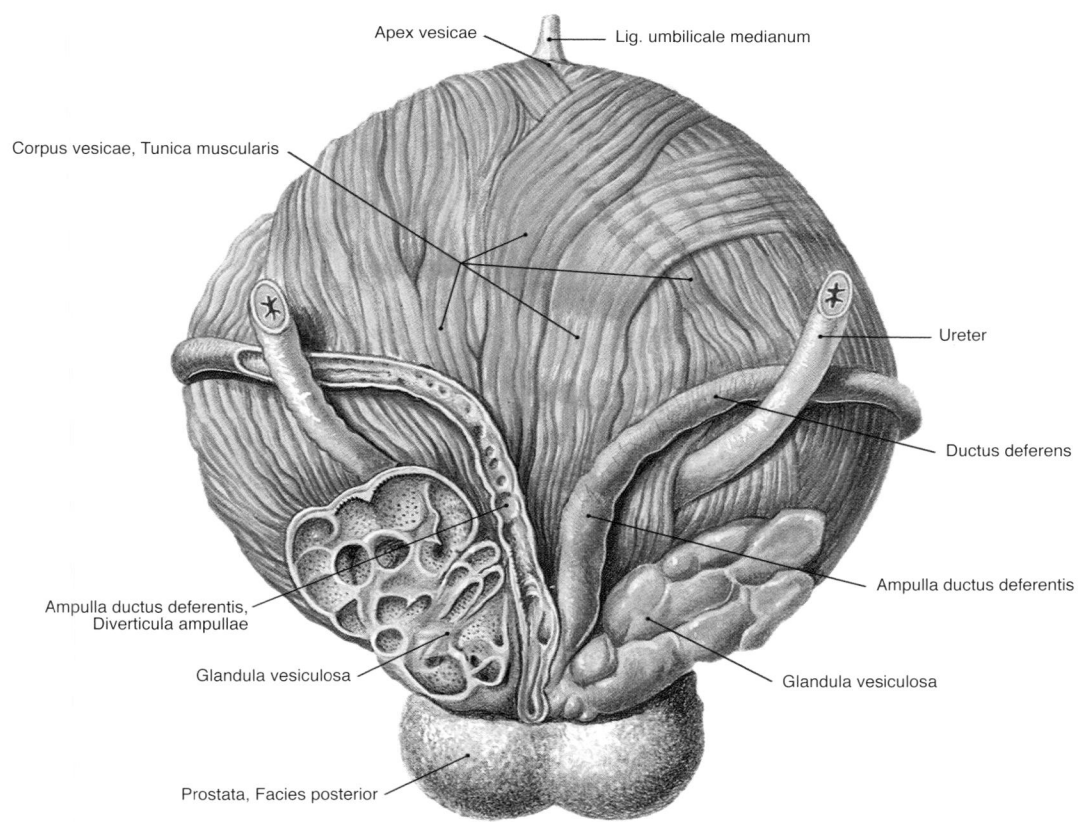

Apex vesicae — Lig. umbilicale medianum

Corpus vesicae, Tunica muscularis

Ureter

Ductus deferens

Ampulla ductus deferentis

Ampulla ductus deferentis,
Diverticula ampullae

Glandula vesiculosa

Glandula vesiculosa

Prostata, Facies posterior

Fig. 833 Urinary bladder, Vesica urinaria; ductus deferentes,
Ductus deferentes; seminal vesicles, Glandulae vesiculosae,
and prostate, Prostata;
dorsal view.

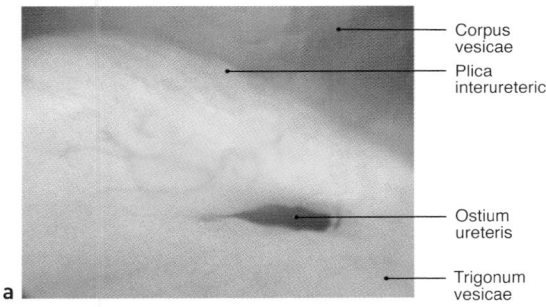

Corpus
vesicae

Plica
interureterica

Ostium
ureteris

Trigonum
vesicae

a

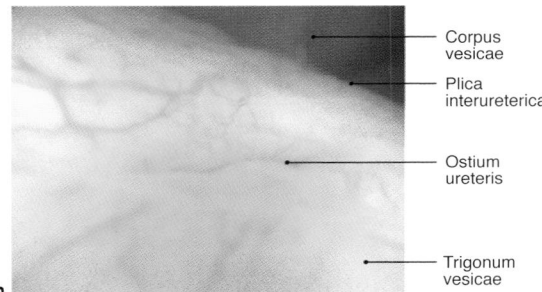

Corpus
vesicae

Plica
interureterica

Ostium
ureteris

Trigonum
vesicae

b

Fig. 834 a, b Urinary bladder, Vesica urinaria;
endoscopic view of the opening of the ureter
(cystoscopy).
a Open ostium of the ureter with a peristaltic
wave transporting urine into the bladder
b Closed ostium of the ureter

Fig. 835 Urinary bladder, Vesica urinaria;
endoscopic view of the mucosa in the body of
the bladder (cystoscopy);
inferior view.

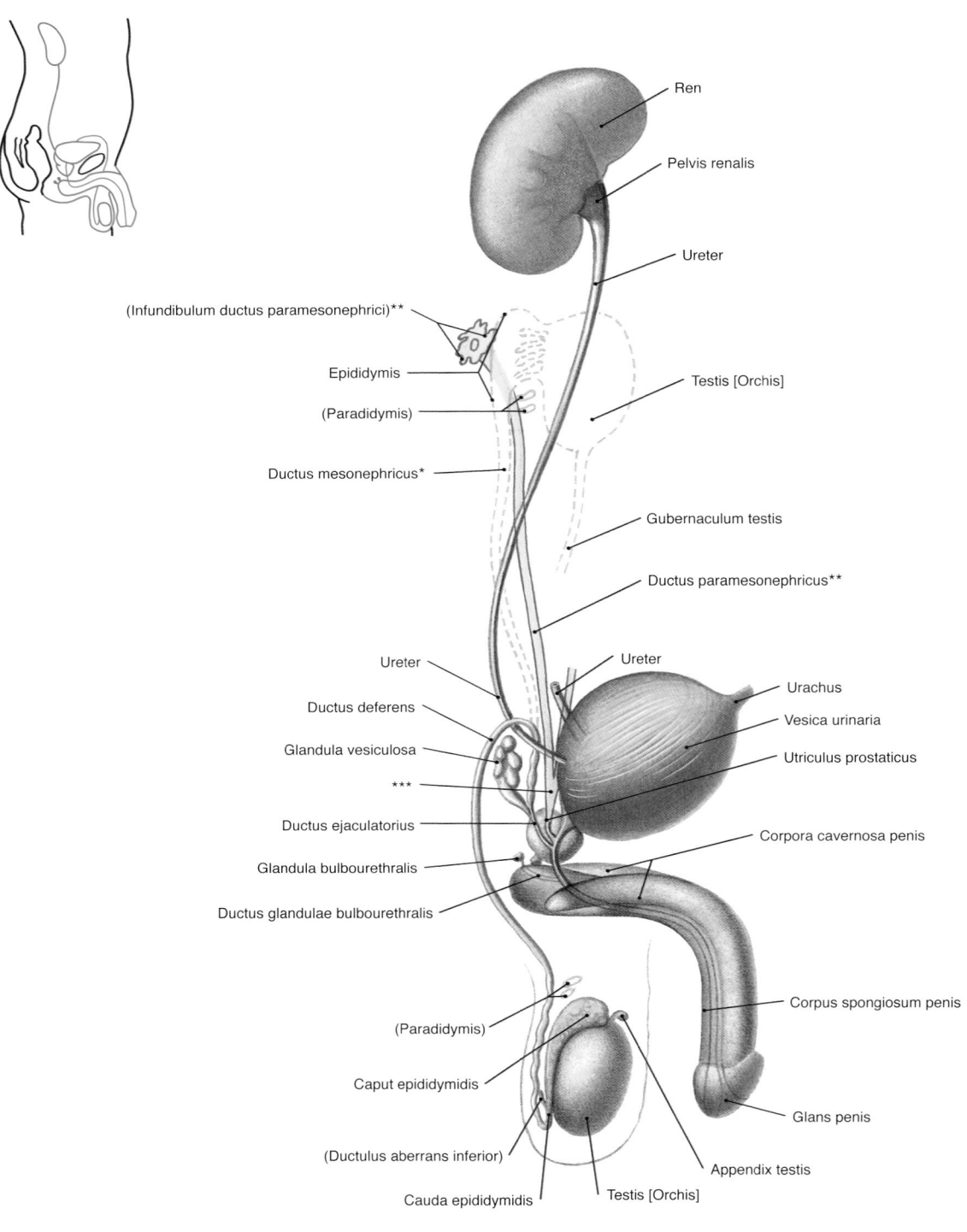

→ 851

Fig. 836   Male urinary and genital organs;
Organa urogenitalia masculina;
diagram of the development: the parts that degenerate are
displayed in pale pink, and the position of the testis prior to its
descent is indicated by the dashed line;
viewed from the right.

Epididymis   = genital part of the mesonephros;
Paradidymis = remnants of tubules of the mesonephros

*   WOLFFian duct
**   MÜLLERian duct
***   Junction of the MÜLLERian ducts,
       Ductus paramesonephrici

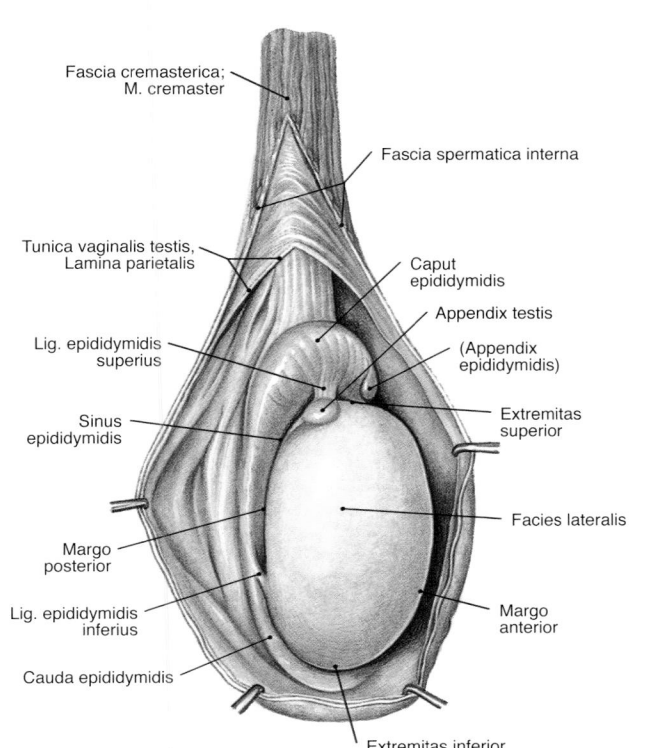

Fascia cremasterica;
M. cremaster

Fascia spermatica interna

Tunica vaginalis testis,
Lamina parietalis

Caput
epididymidis

Lig. epididymidis
superius

Appendix testis

(Appendix
epididymidis)

Sinus
epididymidis

Extremitas
superior

Margo
posterior

Facies lateralis

Lig. epididymidis
inferius

Margo
anterior

Cauda epididymidis

Extremitas inferior

Fig. 837   Testis, Testis [Orchis], and
epididymis, Epididymis;
viewed from the right.

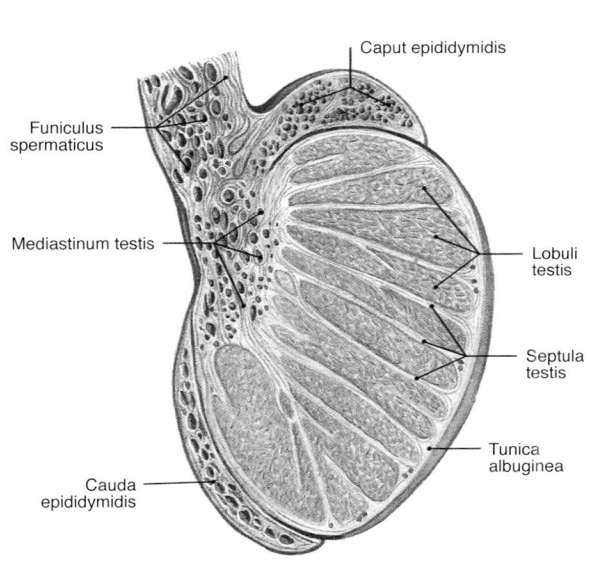

Caput epididymidis

Funiculus
spermaticus

Mediastinum testis

Lobuli
testis

Septula
testis

Cauda
epididymidis

Tunica
albuginea

Fig. 838   Testis, Testis [Orchis], and
epididymis, Epididymis;
viewed from the right.

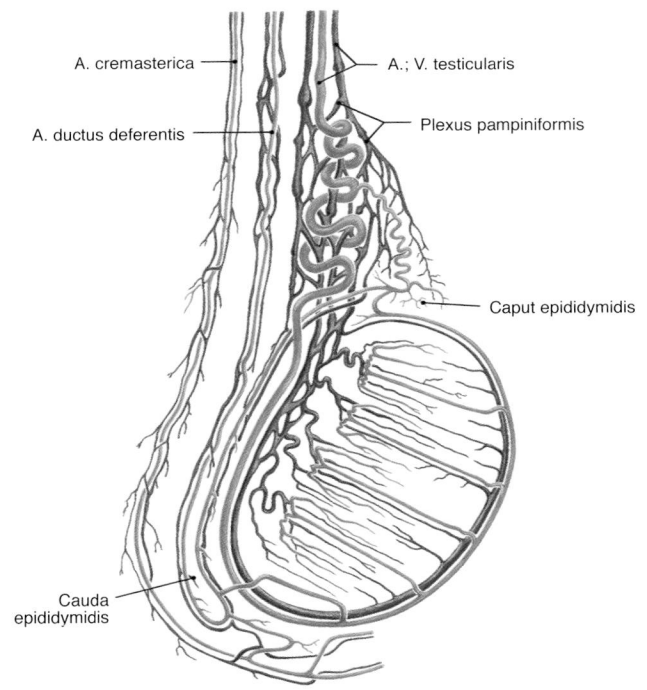

A. cremasterica

A.; V. testicularis

A. ductus deferentis

Plexus pampiniformis

Caput epididymidis

Cauda
epididymidis

Fig. 839   Blood vessels of the testis, Testis,
the epididymis, Epididymis, and the spermatic cord,
Funiculus spermaticus;
viewed from the right.

452

▶ **Pelvic viscera
and retroperitoneal space**

Testis and epididymis

▶▶ | Kidney | Suprarenal gland | Urinary blad� |

▶▶▶ **Male genit◀**

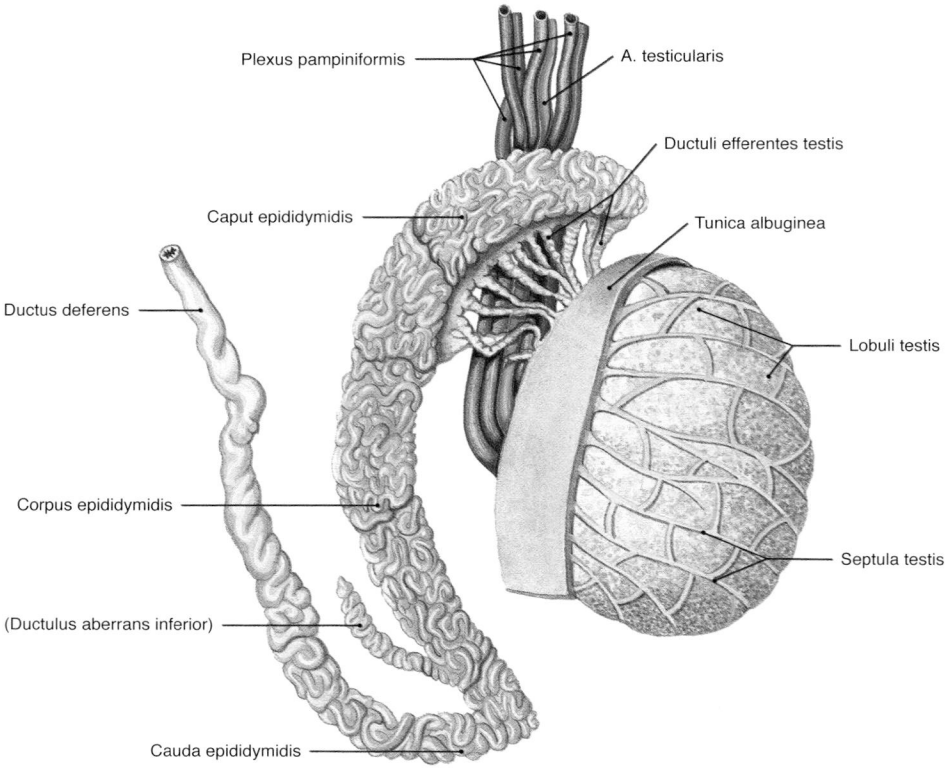

Fig. 840 Testis, Testis; epididymis, Epididymis,
and ductus deferens (vas deferens), Ductus deferens;
lateral view.

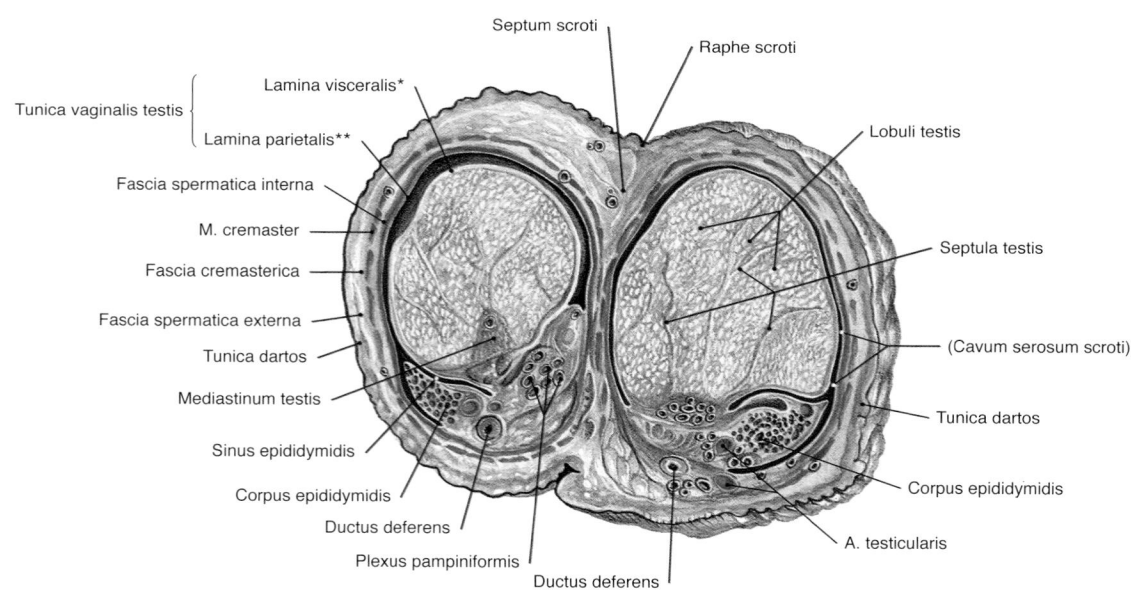

Fig. 841 Testis, Testis; epididymis, Epididymis,
and scrotum, Scrotum;
superior view.
* Also: Epiorchium
** Also: Periorchium

Ductus deferens and seminal vesicle

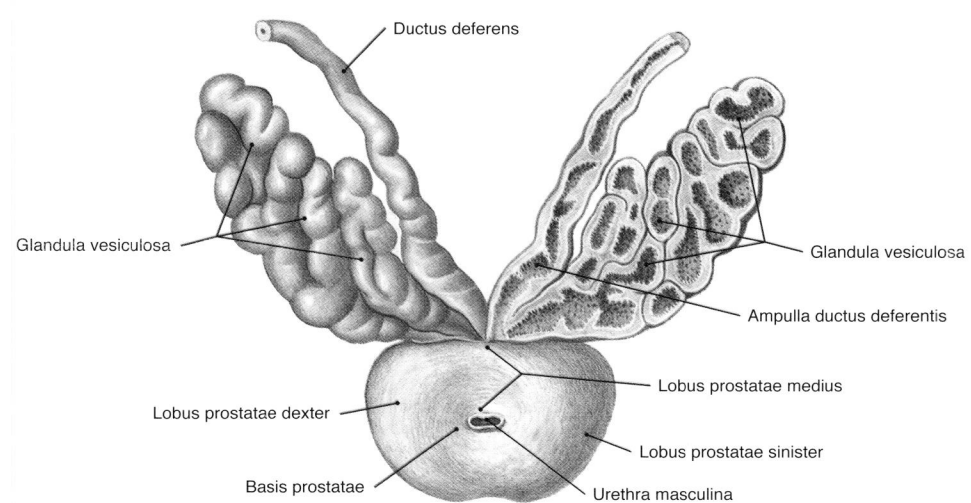

Ductus deferens

Glandula vesiculosa

Glandula vesiculosa

Ampulla ductus deferentis

Lobus prostatae medius

Lobus prostatae dexter

Lobus prostatae sinister

Basis prostatae

Urethra masculina

Fig. 842 Ductus deferentes, Ductus deferentes, seminal vesicles, Glandulae vesiculosae, and prostate, Prostata; superior view.

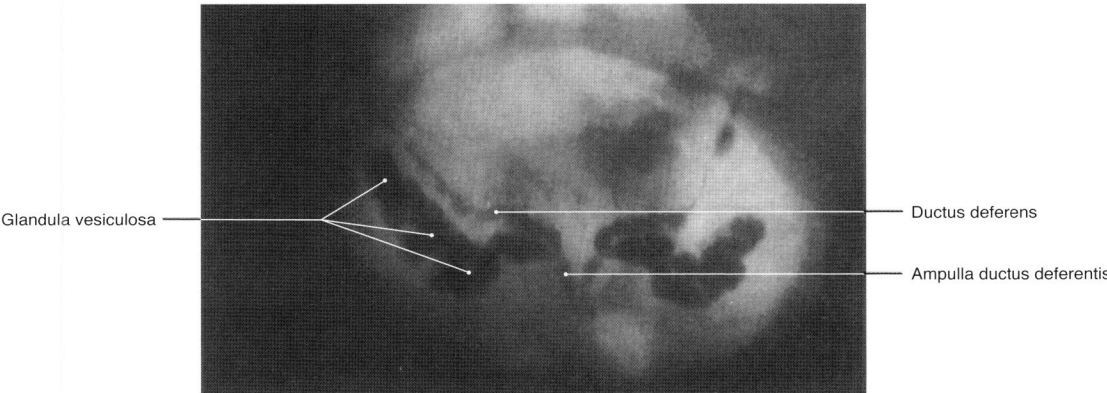

Glandula vesiculosa

Ductus deferens

Ampulla ductus deferentis

Fig. 843 Ductus deferentes, Ductus deferentes, and seminal vesicles, Glandulae vesiculosae; AP-radiograph after injection of a contrast medium via the ejaculatory ducts; ventral view.

Though this technique demonstrates size and position of the seminal vesicles, it is no more applied under clinical circumstances.

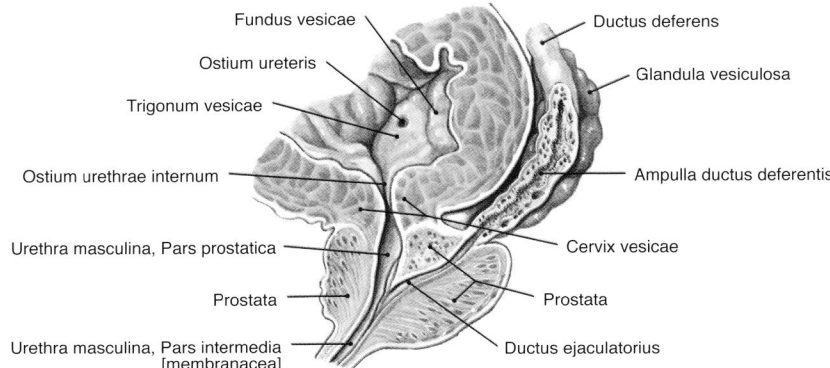

Fundus vesicae

Ductus deferens

Ostium ureteris

Glandula vesiculosa

Trigonum vesicae

Ostium urethrae internum

Ampulla ductus deferentis

Urethra masculina, Pars prostatica

Cervix vesicae

Prostata

Prostata

Urethra masculina, Pars intermedia [membranacea]

Ductus ejaculatorius

Fig. 844 Urinary bladder, Vesica urinaria; prostate, Prostata; ductus deferens (vas deferens), Ductus deferens, and seminal vesicle, Glandula vesiculosa; viewed from the right.

454

► **Pelvic viscera
and retroperitoneal space**

Urinary bladder and male genitalia

►► | Kidney | Suprarenal gland | Urinary blad

►►► **Male genit**

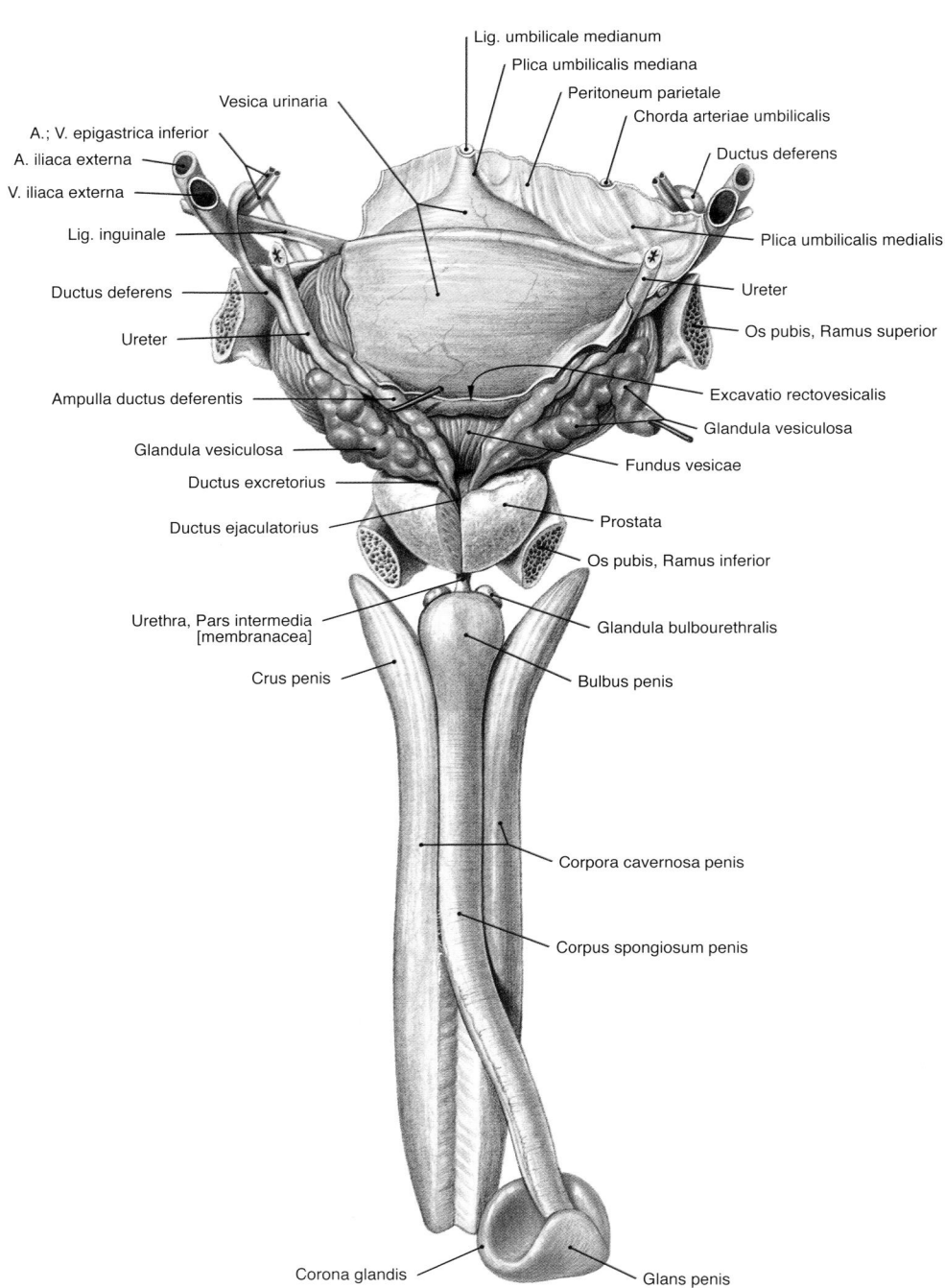

Lig. umbilicale medianum
Plica umbilicalis mediana
Peritoneum parietale
Chorda arteriae umbilicalis
Vesica urinaria
A.; V. epigastrica inferior
Ductus deferens
A. iliaca externa
V. iliaca externa
Plica umbilicalis medialis
Lig. inguinale
Ureter
Ductus deferens
Os pubis, Ramus superior
Ureter
Excavatio rectovesicalis
Ampulla ductus deferentis
Glandula vesiculosa
Glandula vesiculosa
Fundus vesicae
Ductus excretorius
Prostata
Ductus ejaculatorius
Os pubis, Ramus inferior
Urethra, Pars intermedia
[membranacea]
Glandula bulbourethralis
Crus penis
Bulbus penis
Corpora cavernosa penis
Corpus spongiosum penis
Corona glandis
Glans penis

Fig. 845   Urinary bladder, Vesica urinaria; ductus deferentes,
Ductus deferentes; seminal vesicles, Glandulae vesiculosae;
prostate, Prostata, and male urethra, Urethra masculina;
dorsal view.

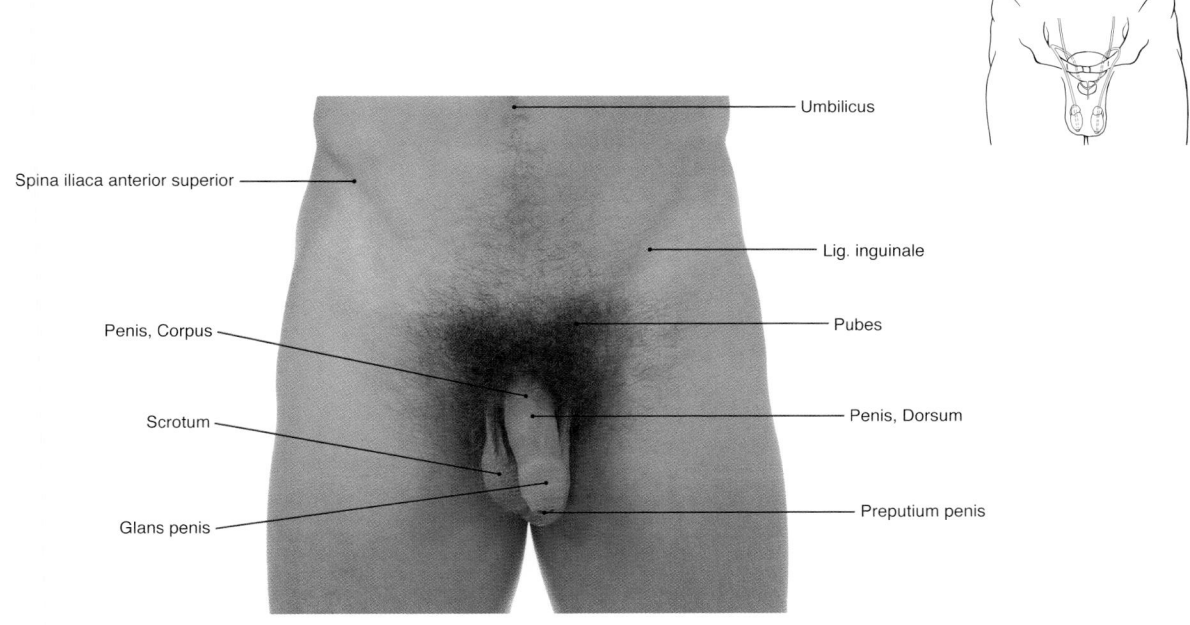

Fig. 846 Male external genitalia, Organa genitalia masculina externa.

Umbilicus

Spina iliaca anterior superior

Lig. inguinale

Penis, Corpus

Pubes

Scrotum

Penis, Dorsum

Glans penis

Preputium penis

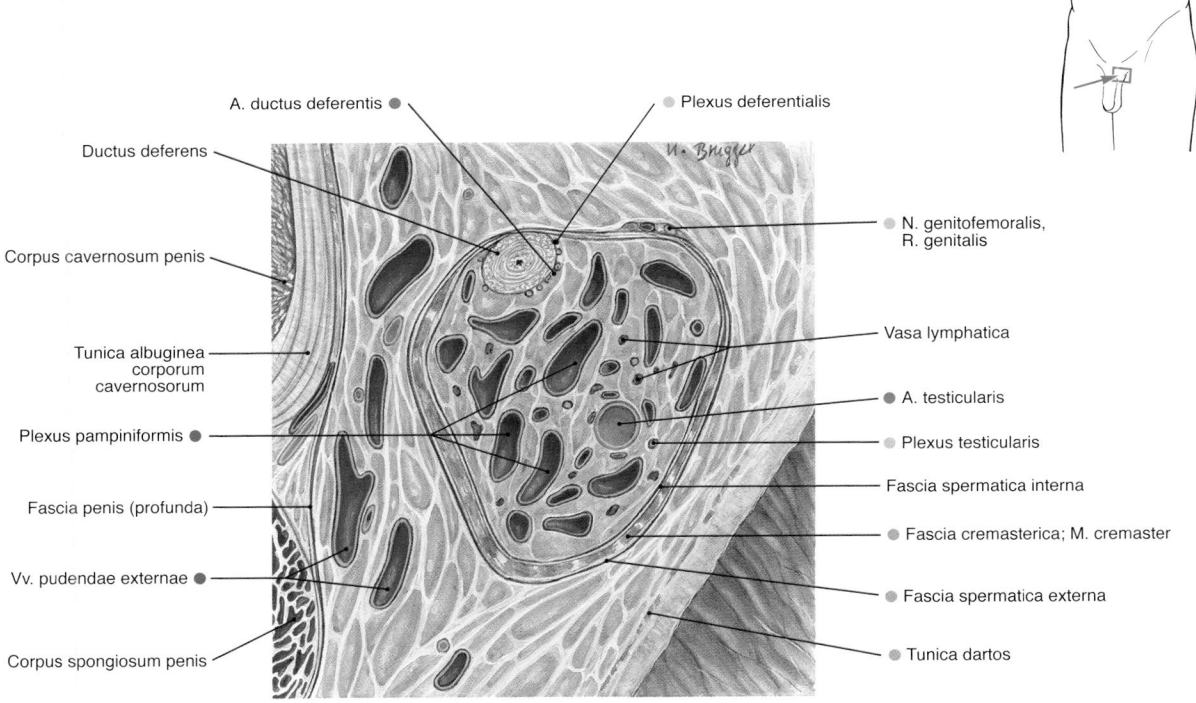

Fig. 847 Spermatic cord, Funiculus spermaticus; frontal section; ventral view (left, 250 %).

A. ductus deferentis

Plexus deferentialis

Ductus deferens

N. genitofemoralis, R. genitalis

Corpus cavernosum penis

Tunica albuginea corporum cavernosorum

Vasa lymphatica

A. testicularis

Plexus pampiniformis

Plexus testicularis

Fascia penis (profunda)

Fascia spermatica interna

Fascia cremasterica; M. cremaster

Vv. pudendae externae

Fascia spermatica externa

Corpus spongiosum penis

Tunica dartos

456

► **Pelvic viscera
and retroperitoneal space**

Male urethra

►► | Kidney | Suprarenal gland | Urinary blad◌

►►► **Male genita**

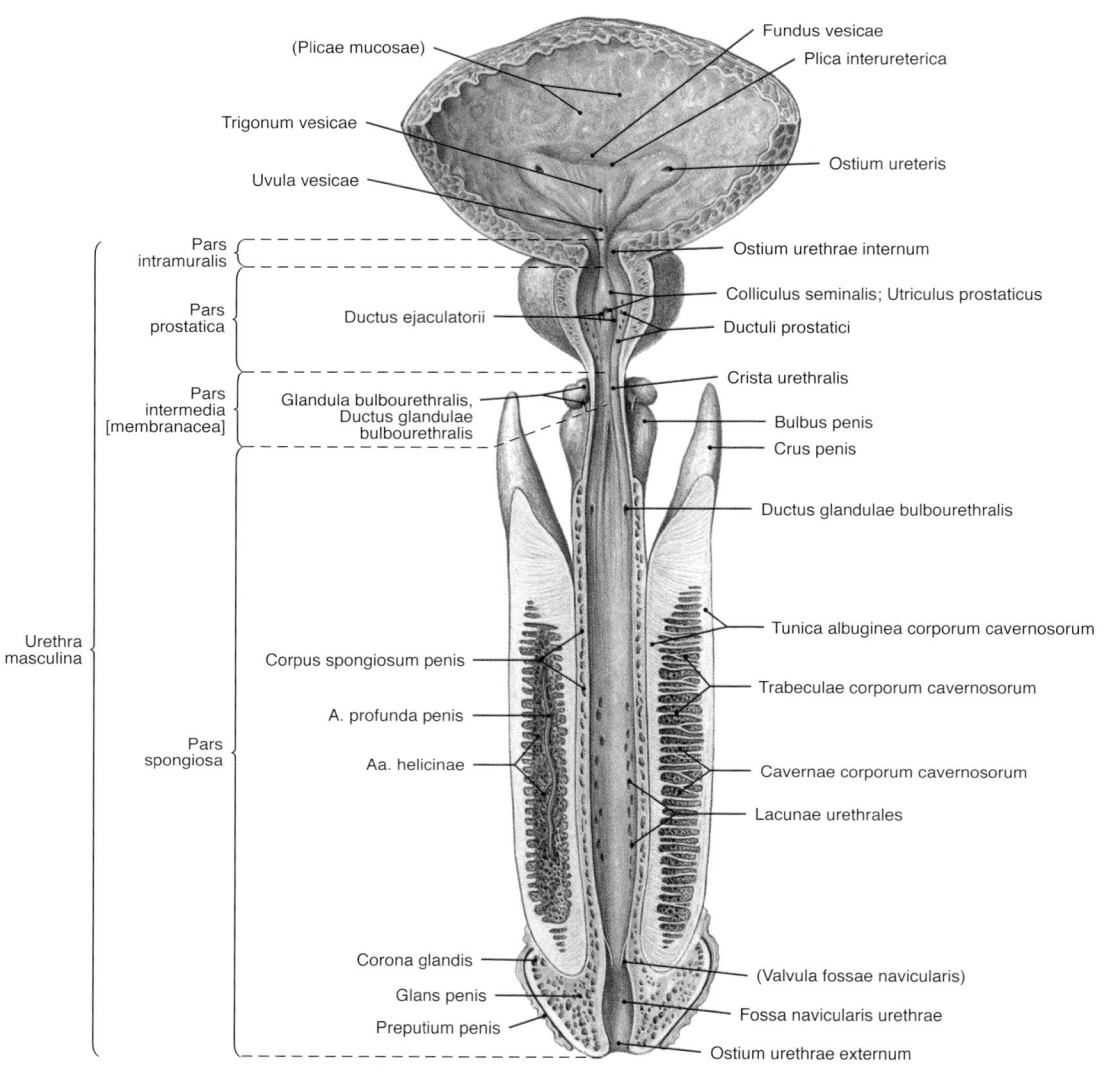

(Plicae mucosae)

Trigonum vesicae

Uvula vesicae

Fundus vesicae

Plica interureterica

Ostium ureteris

Pars
intramuralis

Pars
prostatica

Ductus ejaculatorii

Pars
intermedia
[membranacea]

Glandula bulbourethralis,
Ductus glandulae
bulbourethralis

Urethra
masculina

Corpus spongiosum penis

A. profunda penis

Aa. helicinae

Pars
spongiosa

Corona glandis

Glans penis

Preputium penis

Ostium urethrae internum

Colliculus seminalis; Utriculus prostaticus

Ductuli prostatici

Crista urethralis

Bulbus penis

Crus penis

Ductus glandulae bulbourethralis

Tunica albuginea corporum cavernosorum

Trabeculae corporum cavernosorum

Cavernae corporum cavernosorum

Lacunae urethrales

(Valvula fossae navicularis)

Fossa navicularis urethrae

Ostium urethrae externum

→ 931

Fig. 848 Urinary bladder, Vesica urinaria;
prostate, Prostata, and male urethra, Urethra masculina;
ventral view.

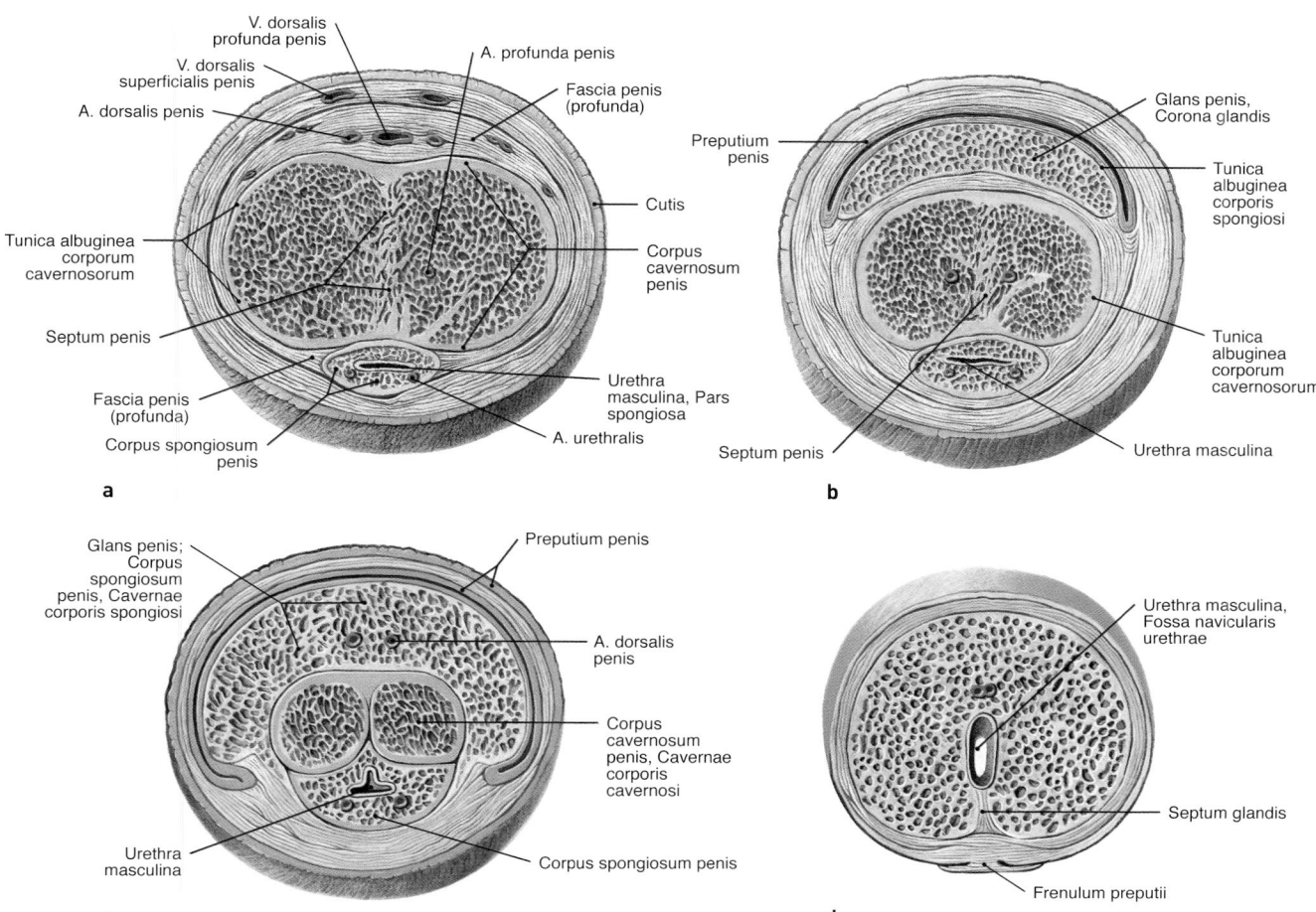

Fig. 849 a–d   Penis, Penis;
cross-sections; planes indicated in Fig. 850;
ventral view.

a   Cross-section through the middle of the shaft
b   Cross-section at the level of the proximal part of the glans penis
c   Cross-section through the middle of the glans penis
d   Cross-section at the level of the distal part of the glans penis

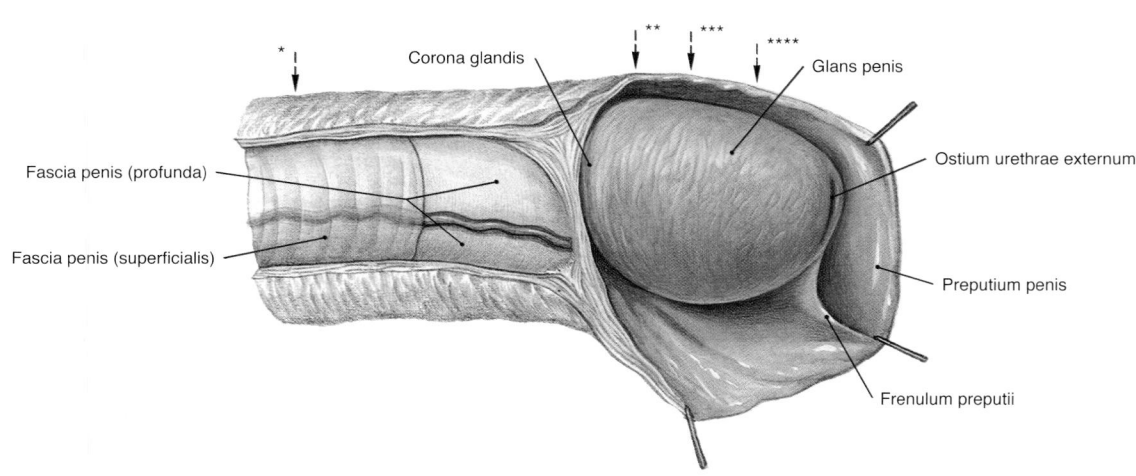

Fig. 850   Penis, Penis, with glans penis, Glans penis,
and prepuce, Preputium penis.

*   Level of section of Fig. 849a
**   Level of section of Fig. 849b
***   Level of section of Fig. 849c
****   Level of section of Fig. 849d

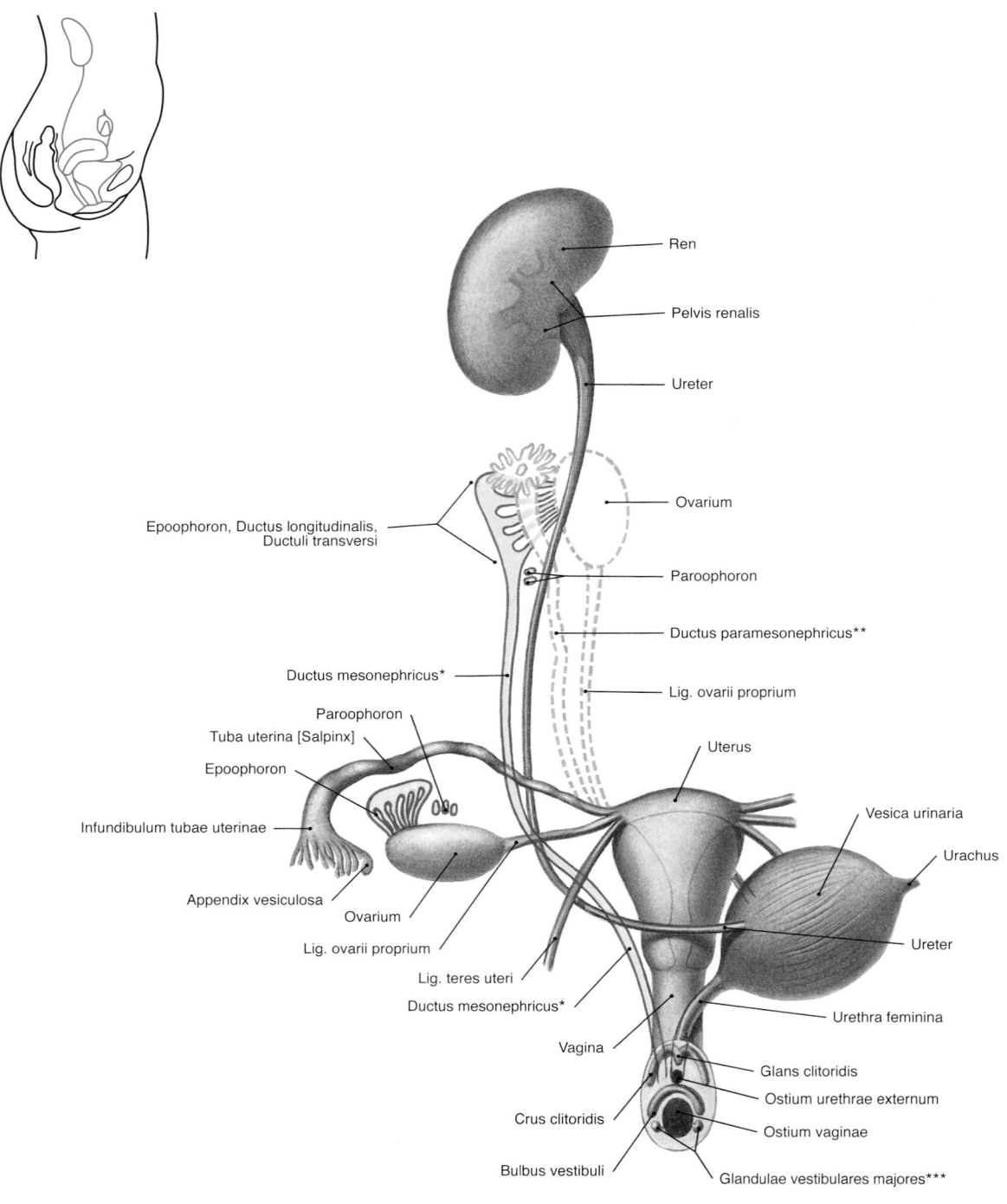

Ren

Pelvis renalis

Ureter

Ovarium

Epoophoron, Ductus longitudinalis,
Ductuli transversi

Paroophoron

Ductus paramesonephricus**

Ductus mesonephricus*

Lig. ovarii proprium

Paroophoron

Tuba uterina [Salpinx]

Uterus

Epoophoron

Vesica urinaria

Infundibulum tubae uterinae

Urachus

Appendix vesiculosa

Ovarium

Ureter

Lig. ovarii proprium

Lig. teres uteri

Urethra feminina

Ductus mesonephricus*

Glans clitoridis

Vagina

Ostium urethrae externum

Crus clitoridis

Ostium vaginae

Bulbus vestibuli

Glandulae vestibulares majores***

→ 836

Fig. 851   Female urinary and genital organs,
Organa urogenitalia feminina;
diagram of the development: the parts that degenerate are
displayed in pale pink, and the position of the ovary prior to its
descent is indicated by the dashed line;
ventral view.

Epoophoron = genital part of the mesonephros;
Paroophoron = remnants of the tubules of the mesonephros

*   WOLFFian duct
**   MÜLLERian duct
*** BARTHOLIN's glands

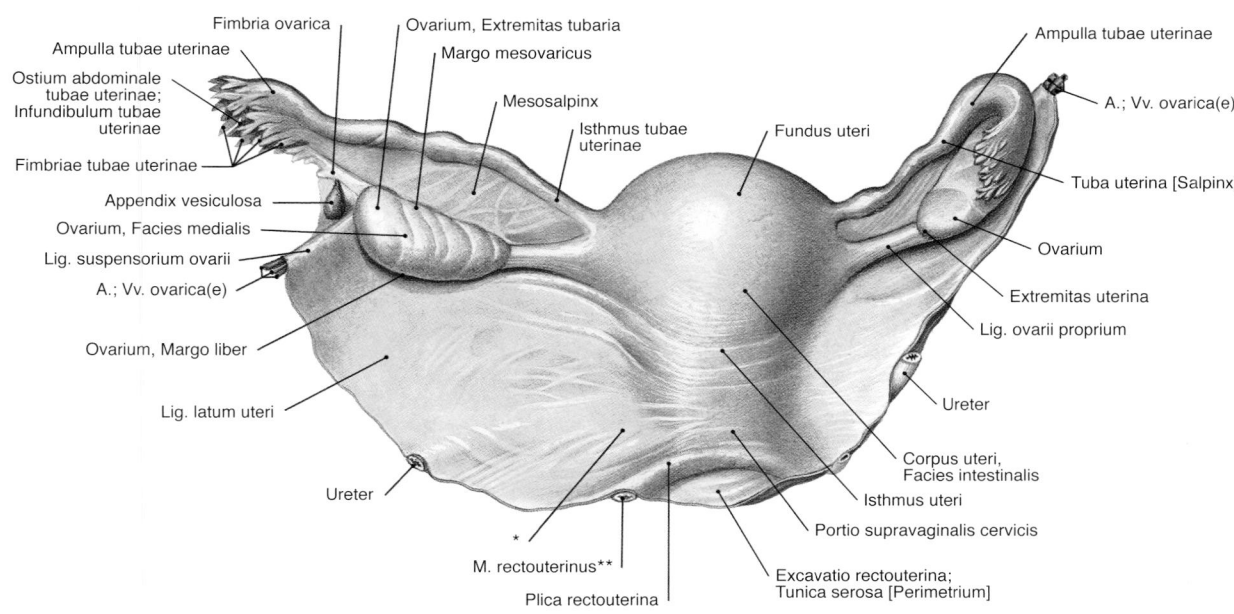

Fimbria ovarica
Ampulla tubae uterinae
Ostium abdominale tubae uterinae; Infundibulum tubae uterinae
Fimbriae tubae uterinae
Appendix vesiculosa
Ovarium, Facies medialis
Lig. suspensorium ovarii
A.; Vv. ovarica(e)
Ovarium, Margo liber
Lig. latum uteri
Ureter

Ovarium, Extremitas tubaria
Margo mesovaricus
Mesosalpinx
Isthmus tubae uterinae
Fundus uteri

Ampulla tubae uterinae
A.; Vv. ovarica(e)
Tuba uterina [Salpinx]
Ovarium
Extremitas uterina
Lig. ovarii proprium
Ureter
Corpus uteri, Facies intestinalis
Isthmus uteri
Portio supravaginalis cervicis

*
M. rectouterinus**
Plica rectouterina
Excavatio rectouterina; Tunica serosa [Perimetrium]

Fig. 852   Uterus, Uterus;
ovary, Ovar, and uterine tube, Tuba uterina;
dorsal view.

*   Clinical term: cardinal ligament
** Clinical term: sacrouterine ligament

Lig. ovarii proprium
Stroma ovarii
Isthmus tubae uterinae
Fundus uteri
Mesosalpinx
Ductus longitudinalis
Ampulla tubae uterinae
Ductuli transversi
Plicae tubariae

Tuba uterina [Salpinx]
Lig. teres uteri***
Lig. ovarii proprium
Tunica serosa [Perimetrium]
Cavitas uteri; Tunica mucosa [Endometrium]
Tunica muscularis [Myometrium]
Canalis cervicis uteri, Plicae palmatae
Portio vaginalis cervicis
Ostium uteri
Rugae vaginales
Vagina

Infundibulum tubae uterinae; Fimbriae tubae uterinae
Appendix vesiculosa
Fimbria ovarica
Corpus albicans
Vv. ovaricae; A. ovarica
Appendix vesiculosa**
Folliculi ovarici vesiculosi*
Corpus luteum
Lig. latum uteri
Pars uterina; Ostium uterinum } Tuba uterina
Corpus uteri
Isthmus uteri
Portio supravaginalis cervicis

Fig. 853   Uterus, Uterus;
ovary, Ovar, and uterine tube, Tuba uterina;
dorsal view.

*   Clinical term: GRAAFian follicle
** Stalked hydatid
*** Clinical term: round ligament

Ovaries and uterus

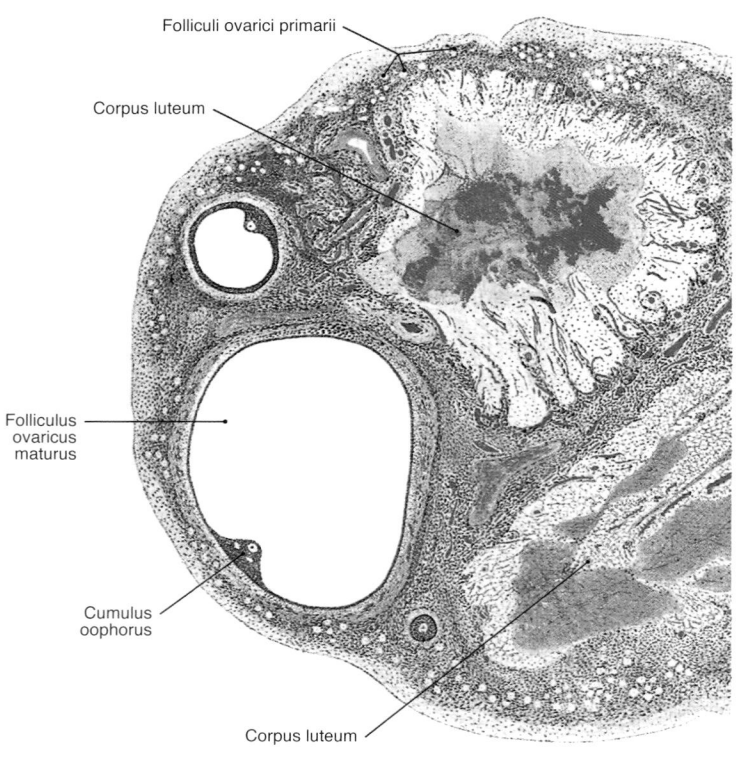
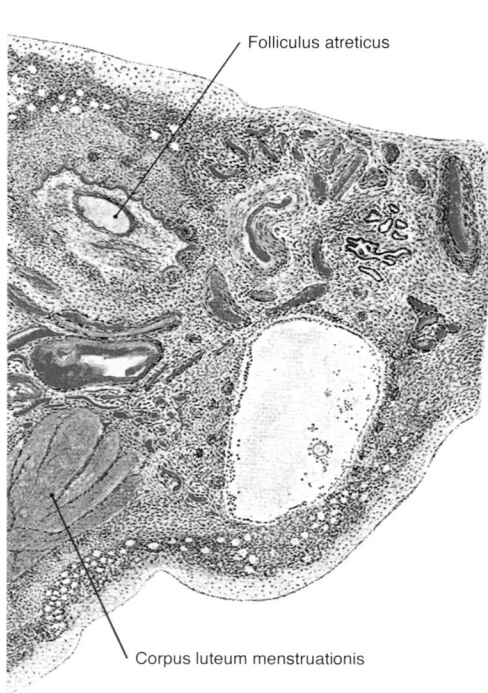

Folliculi ovarici primarii

Corpus luteum

Folliculus ovaricus maturus

Cumulus oophorus

Corpus luteum

Folliculus atreticus

Corpus luteum menstruationis

Fig. 854   Ovary, Ovar;
microscopic enlargement at low magnification.

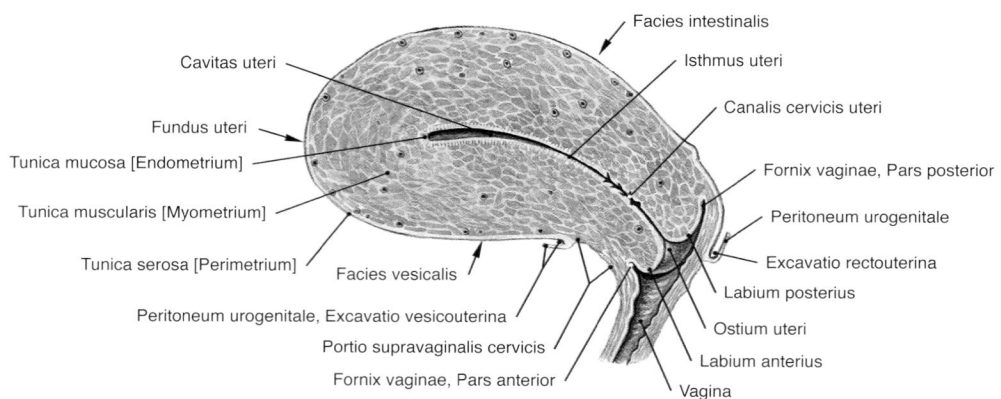

Cavitas uteri

Fundus uteri

Tunica mucosa [Endometrium]

Tunica muscularis [Myometrium]

Tunica serosa [Perimetrium]

Facies vesicalis

Peritoneum urogenitale, Excavatio vesicouterina

Portio supravaginalis cervicis

Fornix vaginae, Pars anterior

Facies intestinalis

Isthmus uteri

Canalis cervicis uteri

Fornix vaginae, Pars posterior

Peritoneum urogenitale

Excavatio rectouterina

Labium posterius

Ostium uteri

Labium anterius

Vagina

Fig. 855   Uterus, Uterus, and vagina, Vagina;
viewed from the right.

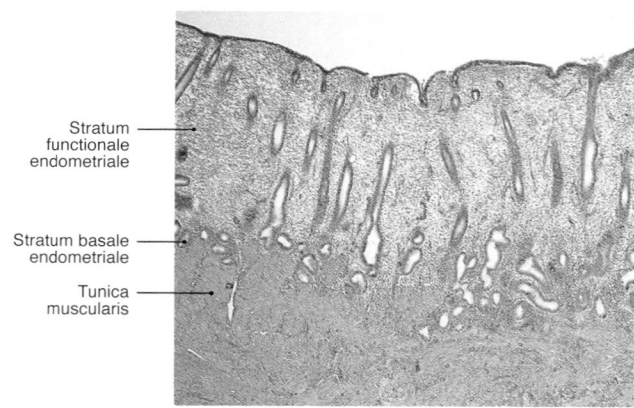
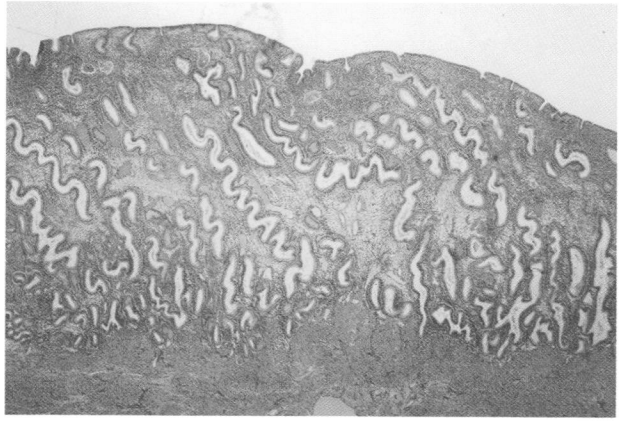

Stratum functionale endometriale

Stratum basale endometriale

Tunica muscularis

Fig. 856   Mucosa of the uterus, Uterus;
early phase of proliferation.

Fig. 857   Mucosa of the uterus, Uterus;
late phase of proliferation with excretory glands.

Uterus

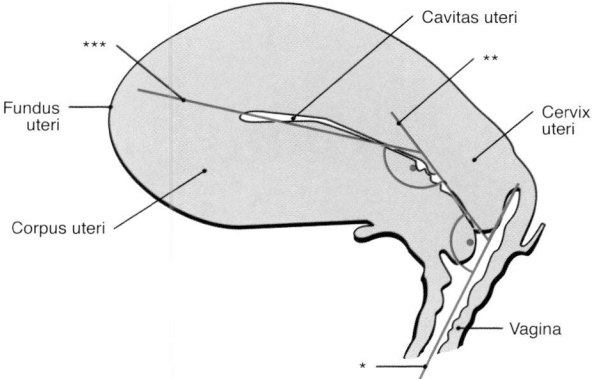

Fundus uteri

Cavitas uteri

Cervix uteri

Corpus uteri

Vagina

Fig. 858 Uterus, Uterus, and vagina, Vagina;
normal angles between the vagina, the cervix, and the
body of uterus;
viewed from the right.
* Longitudinal axis of the vagina
** Longitudinal axis of the cervix of uterus
*** Longitudinal axis of the body of uterus
Angle between vagina and cervix of uterus = version
Angle between cervix and body of uterus = flexion
Normal topographical situation of the uterus:
anteversion, anteflexion
Relation to the median plane = position

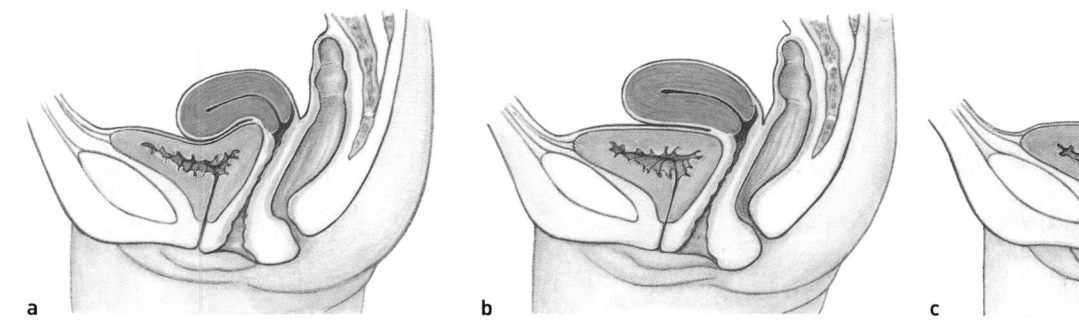
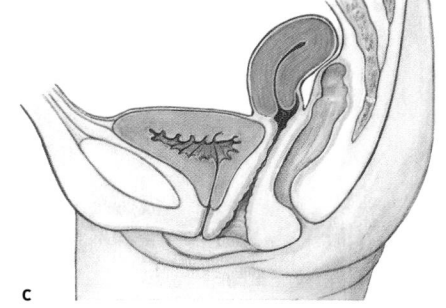

a b c

Fig. 859 a–c Uterus, Uterus, and vagina, Vagina.
a Anteversion, anteflexion = normal position
b Anteversion, but no anteflexion
c Retroversion, retroflexion

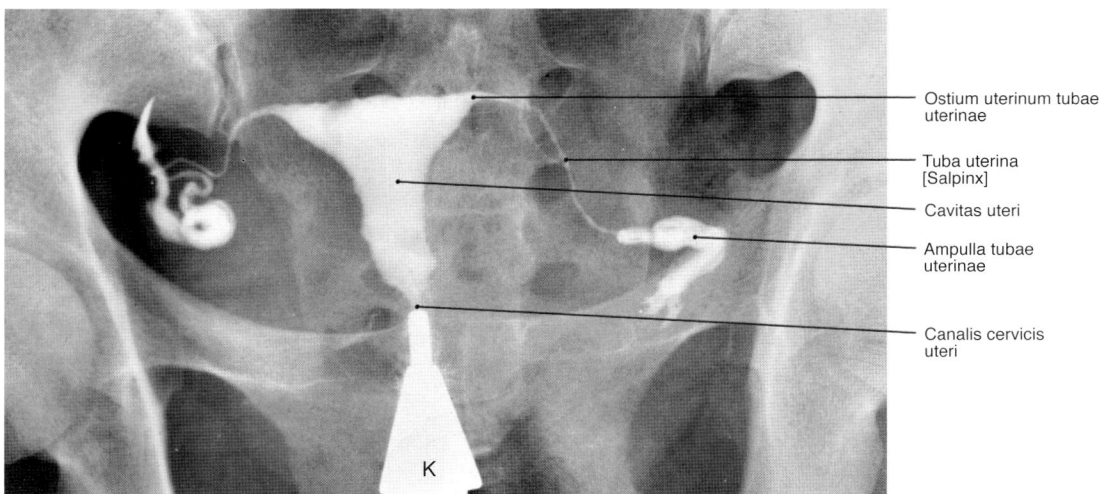

Ostium uterinum tubae uterinae

Tuba uterina [Salpinx]

Cavitas uteri

Ampulla tubae uterinae

Canalis cervicis uteri

Fig. 860 Uterus, Uterus, and uterine tube, Tuba uterina;
AP-radiograph after injection of to contrast medium into the
cervix of uterus (hysterosalpingography);
uterus in dextroposition;
ventral view.

This formerly clinically applied technique allows to determine
the position of the organs and the patency of the tubes.
K = tube adaptor for injection of the contrast medium

462

▶ **Pelvic viscera
and retroperitoneal space**

Arteries of the female internal genitalia

▶▶ | Kidney | Suprarenal gland | Urinary bladd

▶▶▶ Male geni

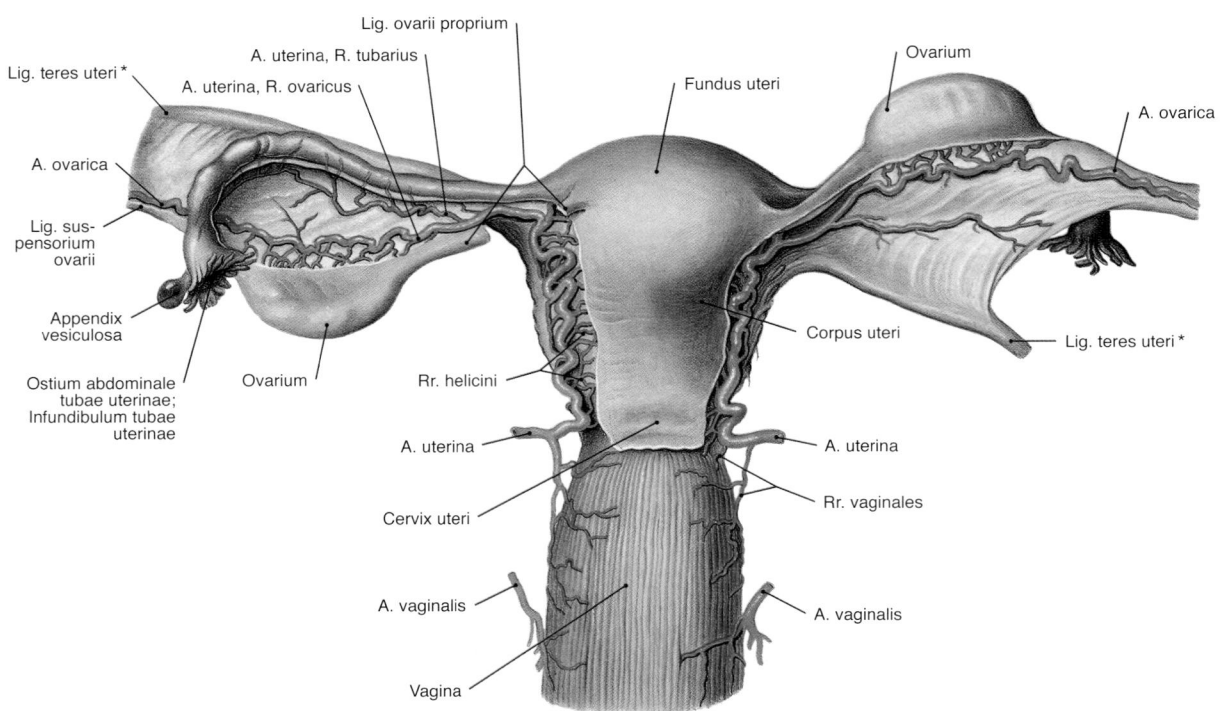

Fig. 861 Arteries of the female internal genitalia,
Organa genitalia feminina interna;
dorsal view.
* Clinical term: round ligament

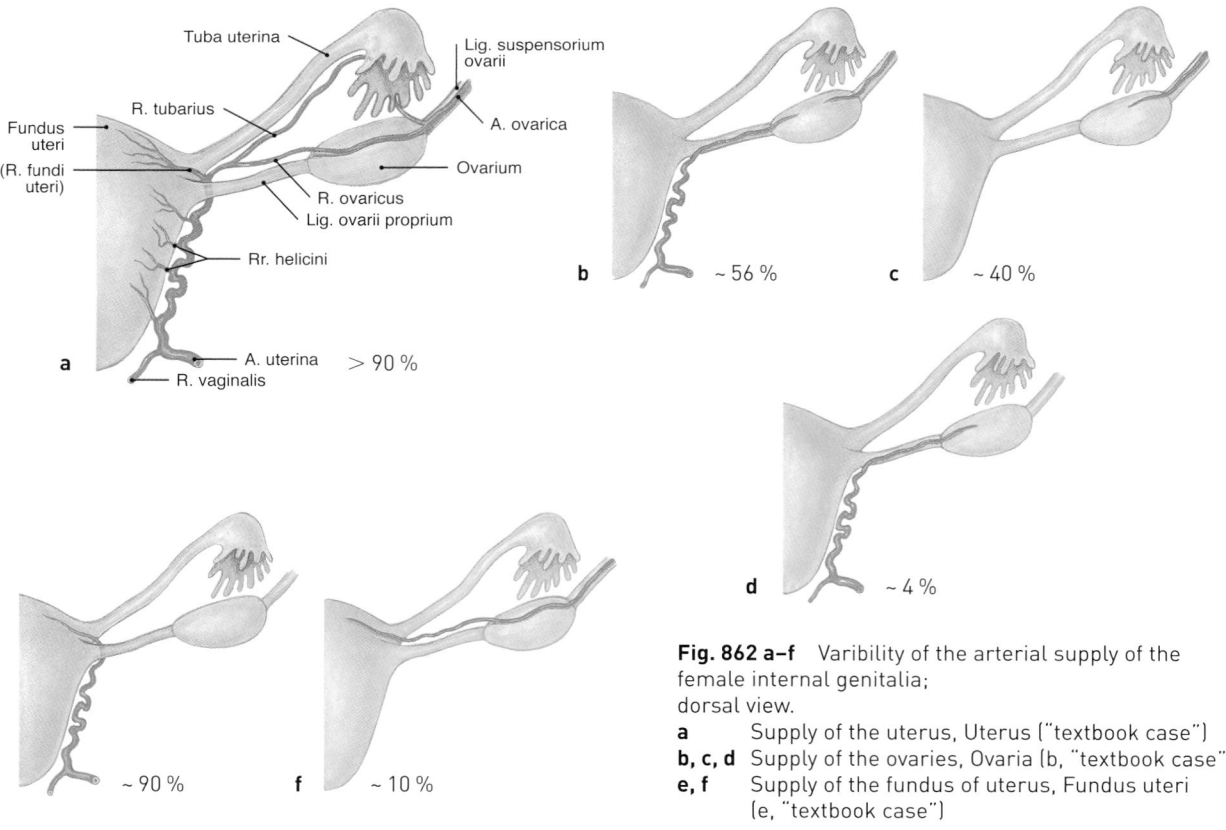

Fig. 862 a–f Varibility of the arterial supply of the
female internal genitalia;
dorsal view.
a Supply of the uterus, Uterus ("textbook case")
b, c, d Supply of the ovaries, Ovaria (b, "textbook case")
e, f Supply of the fundus of uterus, Fundus uteri
(e, "textbook case")

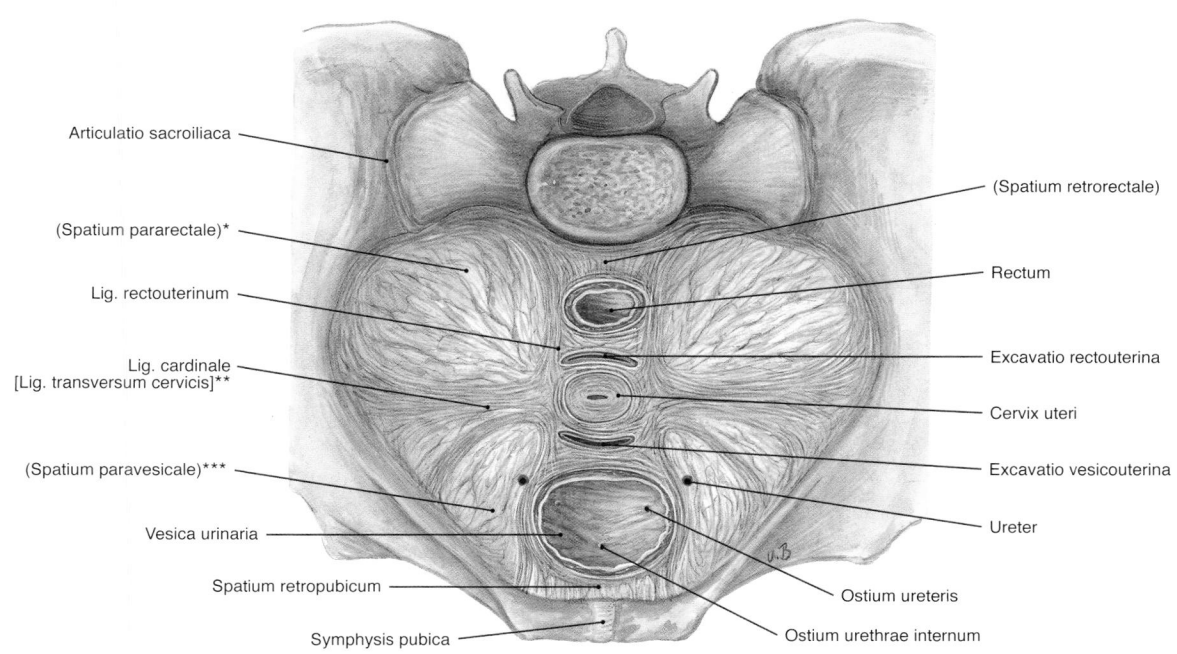

Articulatio sacroiliaca

(Spatium pararectale)*

Lig. rectouterinum

Lig. cardinale
[Lig. transversum cervicis]**

(Spatium paravesicale)***

Vesica urinaria

Spatium retropubicum

Symphysis pubica

(Spatium retrorectale)

Rectum

Excavatio rectouterina

Cervix uteri

Excavatio vesicouterina

Ureter

Ostium ureteris

Ostium urethrae internum

Fig. 863 Uterus, Uterus;
uterine ligaments and connective tissue spaces;
semi-schematic transverse section at the
level of the cervix of uterus;
superior view.

*   Clinical term: Paraproctium
**   Clinical term: Parametrium
      (existence of this structure is controversial)
*** Clinical term: Paracystium

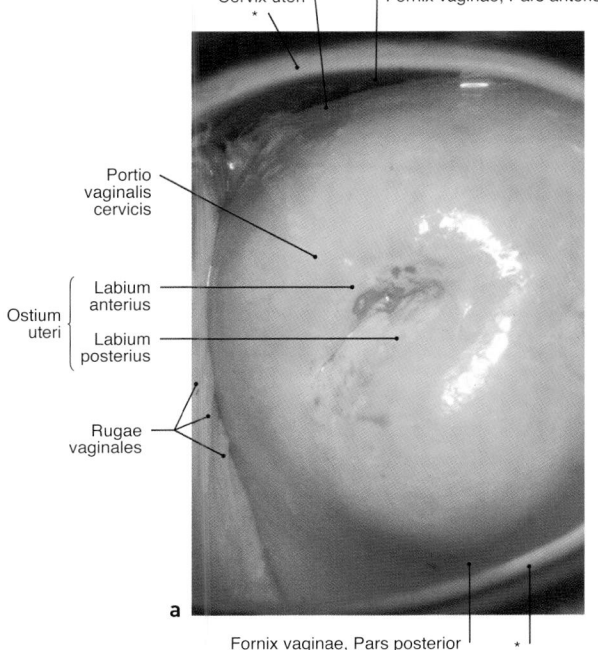

Cervix uteri

Fornix vaginae, Pars anterior

Portio
vaginalis
cervicis

Ostium
uteri

Labium
anterius

Labium
posterius

Rugae
vaginales

a

Fornix vaginae, Pars posterior *

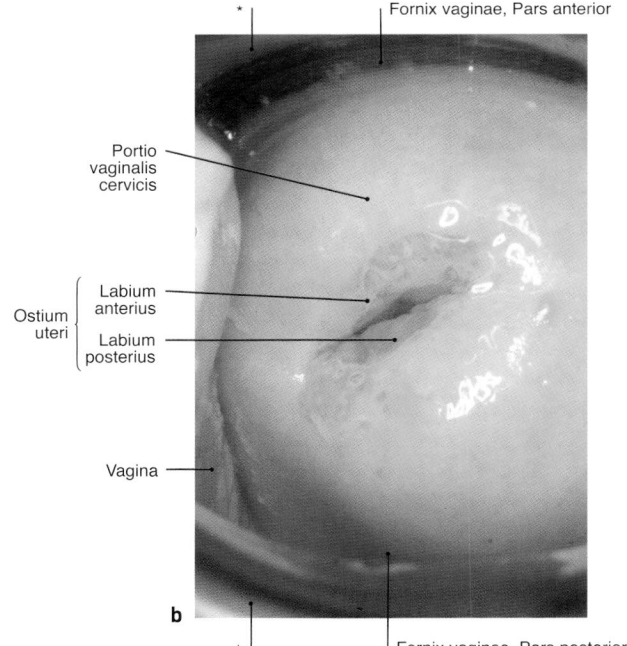

*

Fornix vaginae, Pars anterior

Portio
vaginalis
cervicis

Ostium
uteri

Labium
anterius

Labium
posterius

Vagina

b

*

Fornix vaginae, Pars posterior

Fig. 864 a, b Vaginal portion of the cervix of uterus, Portio
vaginalis cervicis.
a Photograph of the cervix of a young nulliparous woman
b Photograph of the cervix of a young woman who has given
birth to two children

For the inspection of the vaginal portion of the cervix the
normally slit-like vagina is spreaded by means of a bivalve
speculum (*);
inferior view.

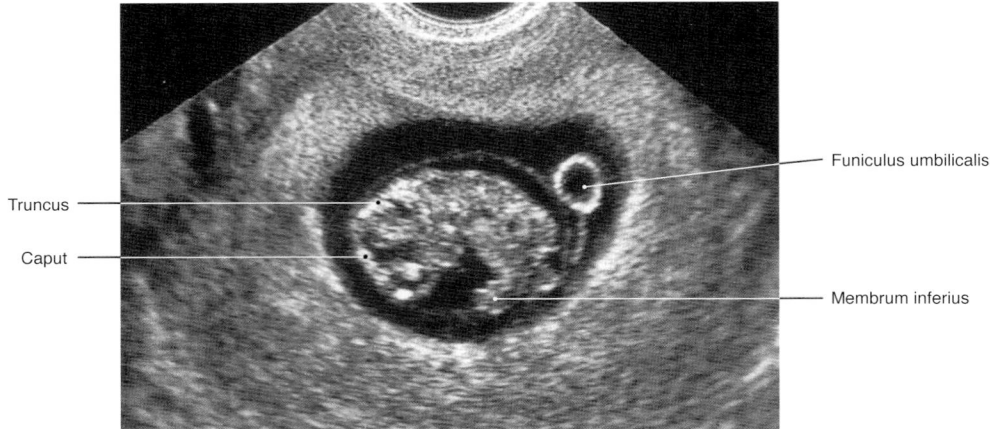

Truncus

Caput

Funiculus umbilicalis

Membrum inferius

Fig. 865 Uterus, Uterus, with an embryo; ultrasound image taken in the eighth week of pregnancy; lateral view (right).

The embryo is immersed in the amniotic fluid of the chorionic cavity.

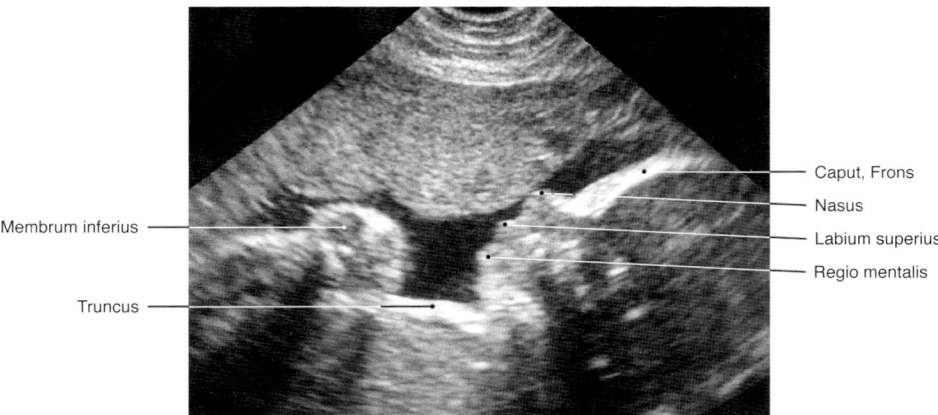

Membrum inferius

Truncus

Caput, Frons

Nasus

Labium superius

Regio mentalis

Fig. 866 Uterus, Uterus, with a foetus; ultrasound image taken in the 28th week of pregnancy; lateral view (left).

Ultrasound examination allows the visualization of movements of the extremities and the opening of the mouth.

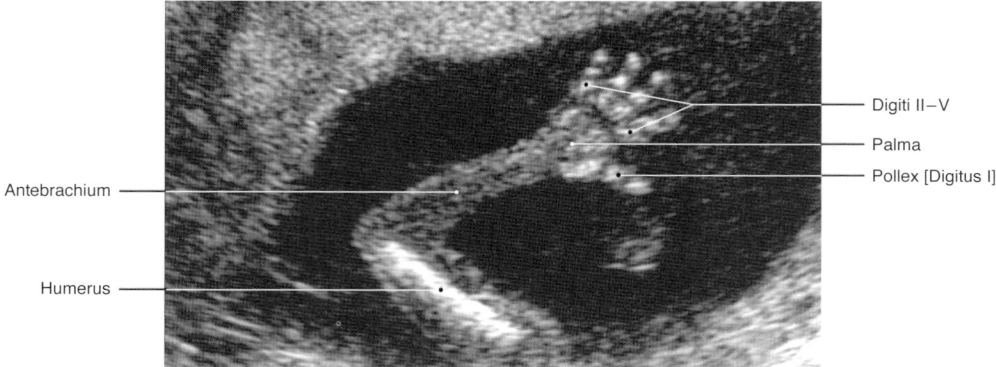

Antebrachium

Humerus

Digiti II–V

Palma

Pollex [Digitus I]

Fig. 867 Hand, Manus, of a foetus; ultrasound image taken in the 18th week of pregnancy; lateral view.

Details such as fingers can be observed.

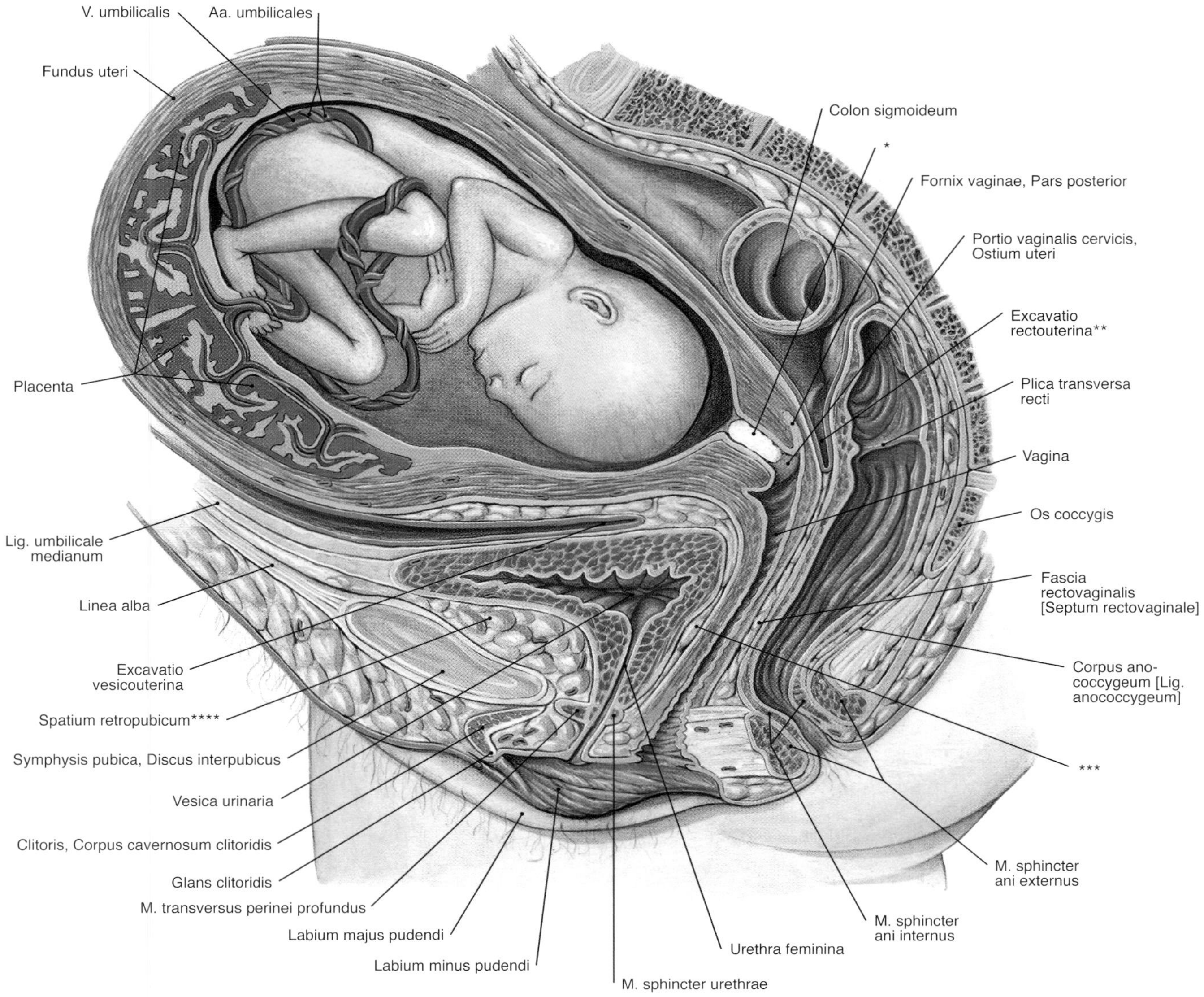

male genitalia

Pregnancy

V. umbilicalis   Aa. umbilicales

Fundus uteri

Colon sigmoideum

*

Fornix vaginae, Pars posterior

Portio vaginalis cervicis, Ostium uteri

Excavatio rectouterina**

Plica transversa recti

Placenta

Vagina

Os coccygis

Lig. umbilicale medianum

Linea alba

Fascia rectovaginalis [Septum rectovaginale]

Excavatio vesicouterina

Corpus ano-coccygeum [Lig. anococcygeum]

Spatium retropubicum****

***

Symphysis pubica, Discus interpubicus

Vesica urinaria

M. sphincter ani externus

Clitoris, Corpus cavernosum clitoridis

Glans clitoridis

M. sphincter ani internus

M. transversus perinei profundus

Labium majus pudendi

M. sphincter ani internus

Labium minus pudendi

Urethra feminina

M. sphincter urethrae

Fig. 868 Uterus, Uterus, with a foetus;
the pelvis has been sectioned in the median plane.

*   Mucous plug (of KRISTELLER) in the cervical canal of the uterus
**   Clinical term: pouch of DOUGLAS
***   Clinical term: vesicovaginal septum
****   Clinical term: cave of RETZIUS

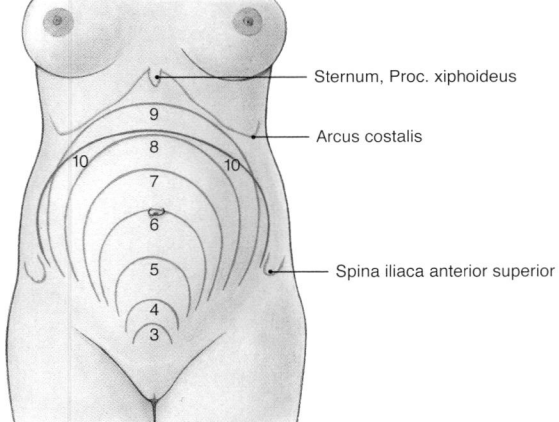

Sternum, Proc. xiphoideus

Arcus costalis

Spina iliaca anterior superior

Fig. 869 Uterus, Uterus;
position of the fundus of uterus during pregnancy.
Numbers refer to the end of the respective
month of pregnancy (= 28 days).

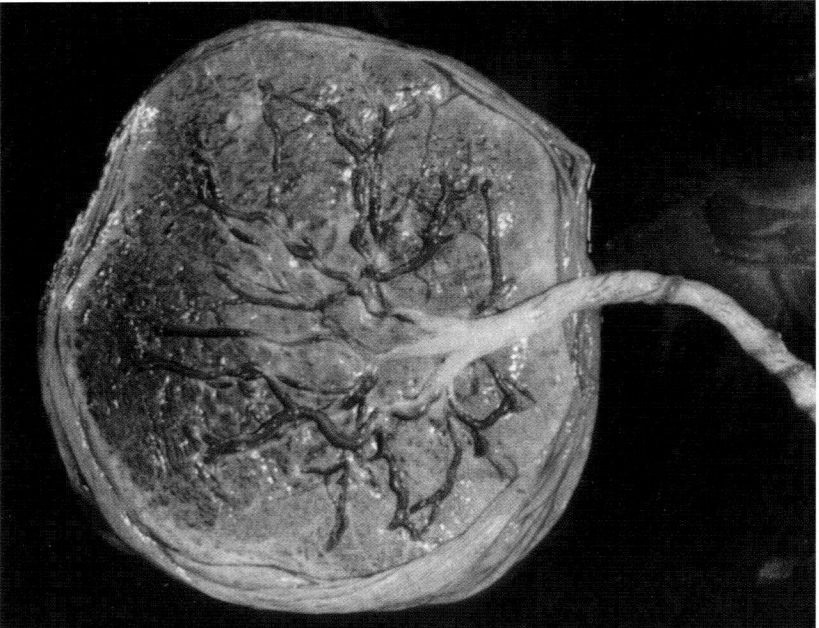

a

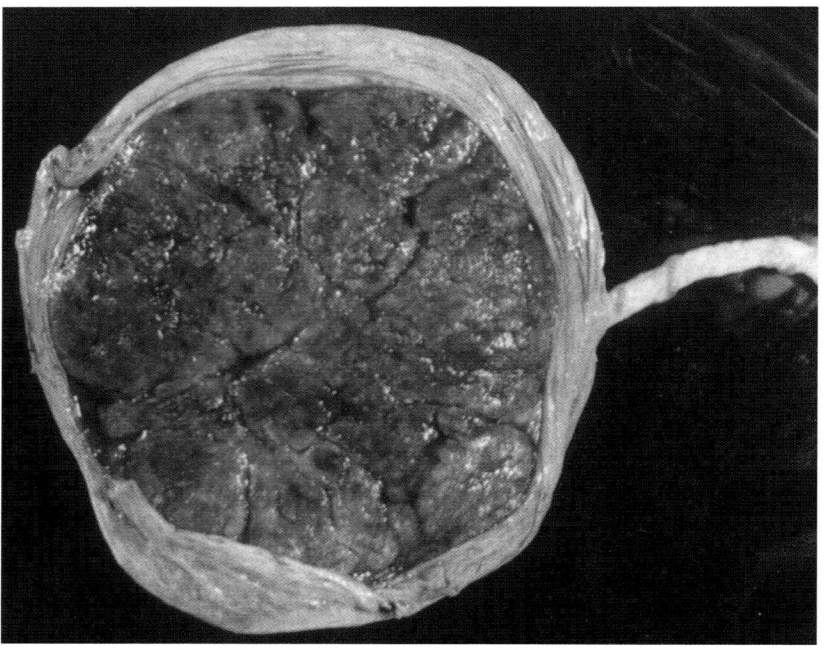

b

Fig. 870 a, b Placenta, Placenta, and
umbilical cord, Funiculus umbilicalis.
a View of the foetal surface
b View of the maternal surface of a
parturient placenta

Ovaries and uterine tubes

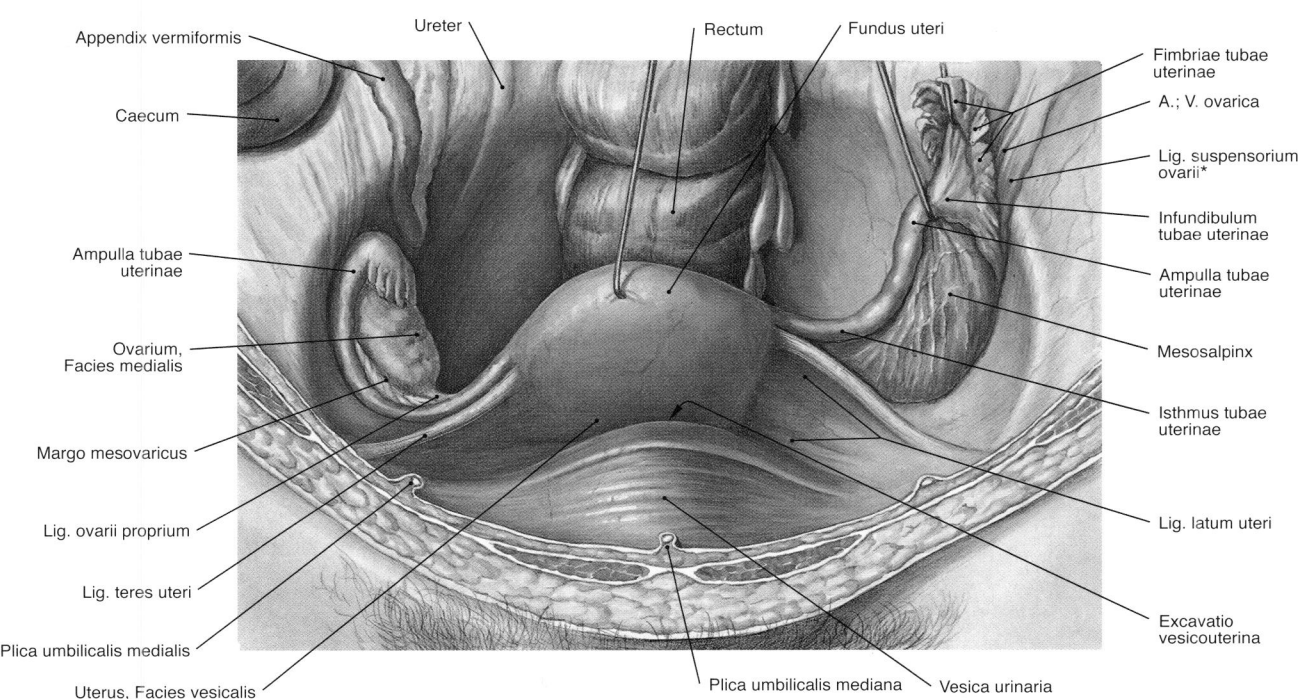

Appendix vermiformis

Caecum

Ampulla tubae uterinae

Ovarium, Facies medialis

Margo mesovaricus

Lig. ovarii proprium

Lig. teres uteri

Plica umbilicalis medialis

Uterus, Facies vesicalis

Ureter

Rectum

Fundus uteri

Fimbriae tubae uterinae

A.; V. ovarica

Lig. suspensorium ovarii*

Infundibulum tubae uterinae

Ampulla tubae uterinae

Mesosalpinx

Isthmus tubae uterinae

Lig. latum uteri

Excavatio vesicouterina

Plica umbilicalis mediana

Vesica urinaria

Fig. 871   Female internal genitalia,
Organa genitalia feminina interna;
ventral view.
* Clinical term: infundibulopelvic ligament

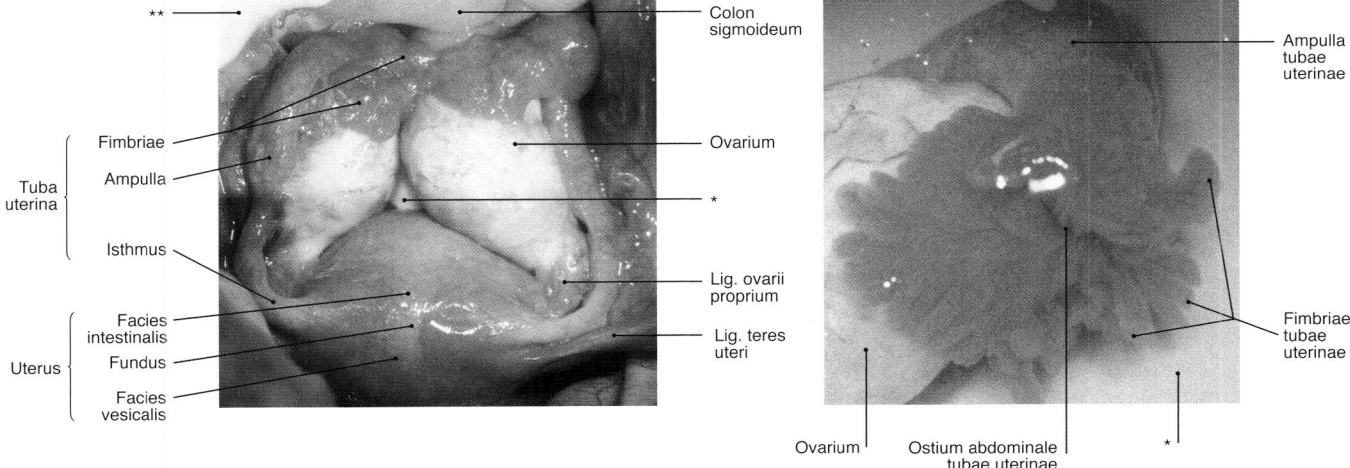

Fig. 872   Female internal genitalia,
Organa genitalia feminina interna;
surgical exposure in a young woman;
ovaries displaced both medially and superiorly by
compresses (*) in the pouch of DOUGLAS;
ventrosuperior view.
** Swab

Colon sigmoideum

Ovarium

*

Lig. ovarii proprium

Lig. teres uteri

**

Fimbriae

Ampulla

Tuba uterina

Isthmus

Facies intestinalis

Fundus

Facies vesicalis

Uterus

Fig. 873   Abdominal ostium of the uterine tube,
Ostium abdominale tubae uterinae;
surgical exposure in a young woman;
the pelvic cavity is filled with saline to demonstrate
the fimbria;
dorsosuperior view.
* Plastic tray to support the uterine tube

Ampulla tubae uterinae

Fimbriae tubae uterinae

Ovarium

Ostium abdominale tubae uterinae

*

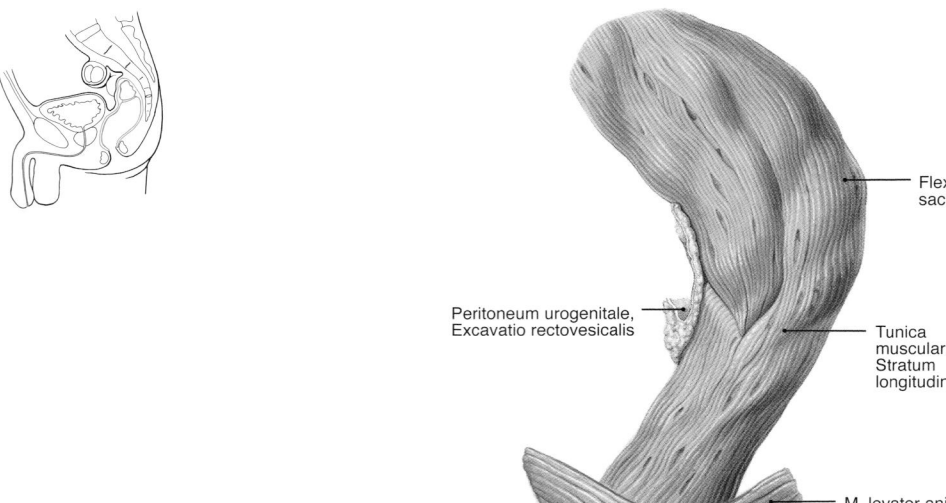

Flexura sacralis

Peritoneum urogenitale, Excavatio rectovesicalis

Tunica muscularis, Stratum longitudinale

M. levator ani

Flexura anorectalis [perinealis]

M. sphincter ani externus

Tela subcutanea, Panniculus adiposus

Anus

Fig. 874 Rectum, Rectum; viewed from the left.

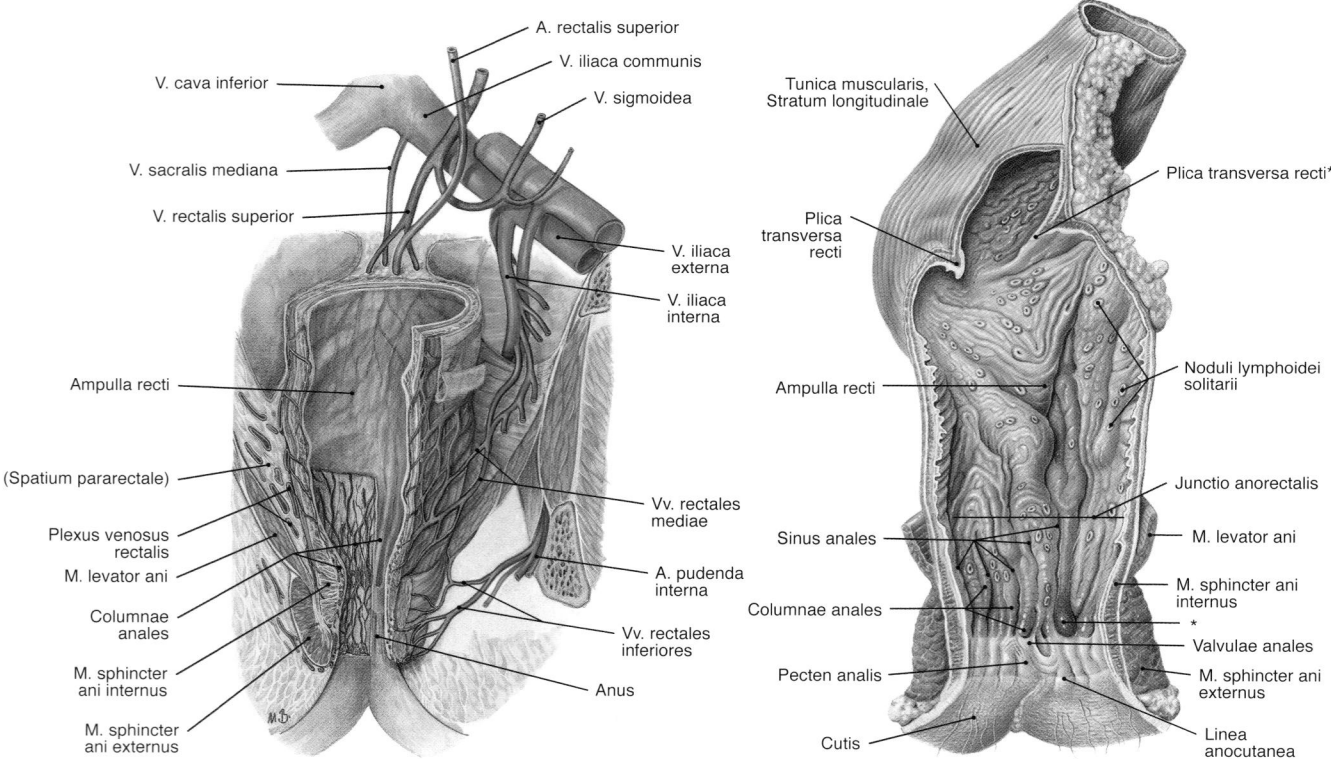

A. rectalis superior

V. iliaca communis

V. cava inferior

V. sigmoidea

V. sacralis mediana

V. rectalis superior

V. iliaca externa

V. iliaca interna

Ampulla recti

(Spatium pararectale)

Plexus venosus rectalis

M. levator ani

Columnae anales

Vv. rectales mediae

A. pudenda interna

Vv. rectales inferiores

M. sphincter ani internus

Anus

M. sphincter ani externus

Tunica muscularis, Stratum longitudinale

Plica transversa recti**

Plica transversa recti

Noduli lymphoidei solitarii

Ampulla recti

Junctio anorectalis

Sinus anales

M. levator ani

M. sphincter ani internus

Columnae anales

*

Valvulae anales

Pecten analis

M. sphincter ani externus

Cutis

Linea anocutanea

Fig. 875 Rectum, Rectum; blood supply; the mucosa and the pararectal adipose tissues have been partly removed; openings into the hepatic portal vein in purple.

Fig. 876 Rectum, Rectum, and anus, Anus; ventral view.

* Haemorrhoidal node
** KOHLRAUSCH's fold

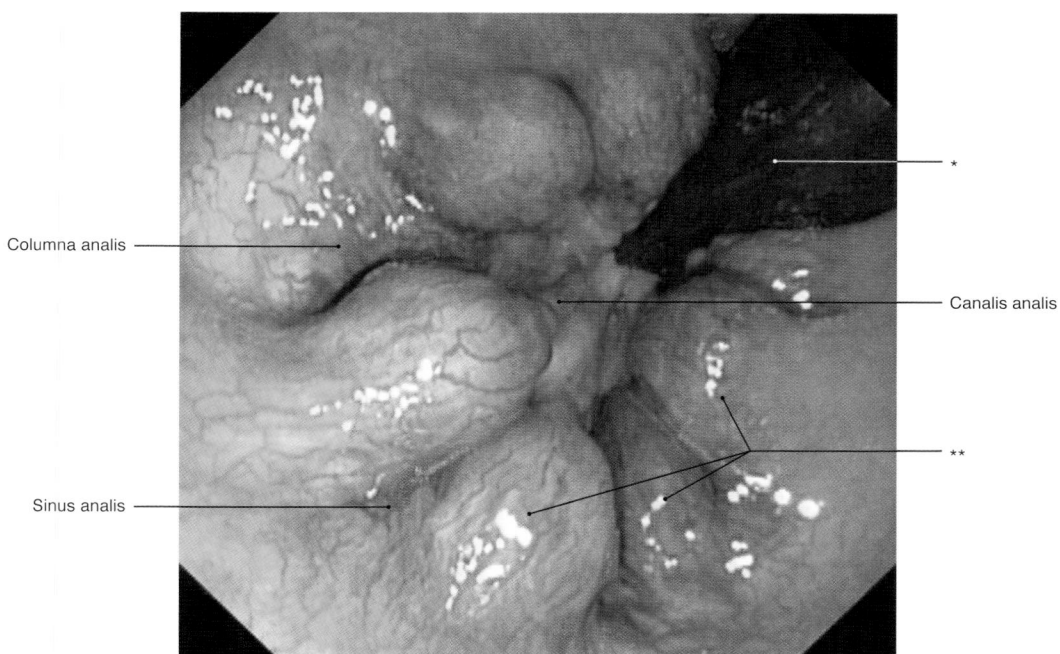

Columna analis

Sinus analis

Canalis analis

*

**

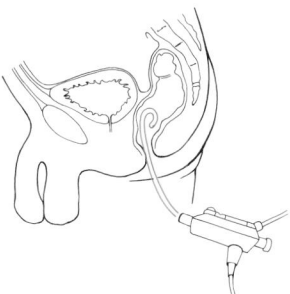

Fig. 877 Rectum, Rectum;
endoscopic image of the anal canal with six enlarged
nodes of the cavernous rectal body, haemorrhoids;
superior view.
* Colonoscope
** Three haemorrhoidal nodes

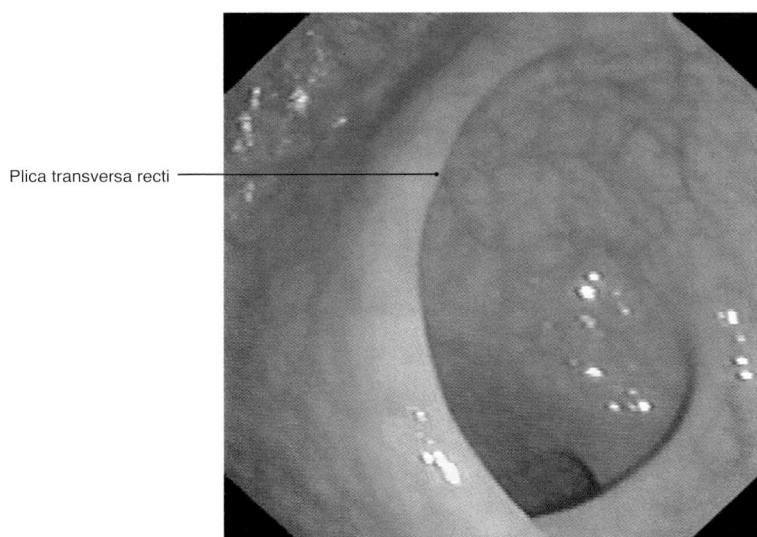

Plica transversa recti

Fig. 878 Rectum, Rectum;
endoscopic image of the rectal ampulla (rectoscopy);
inferior view.

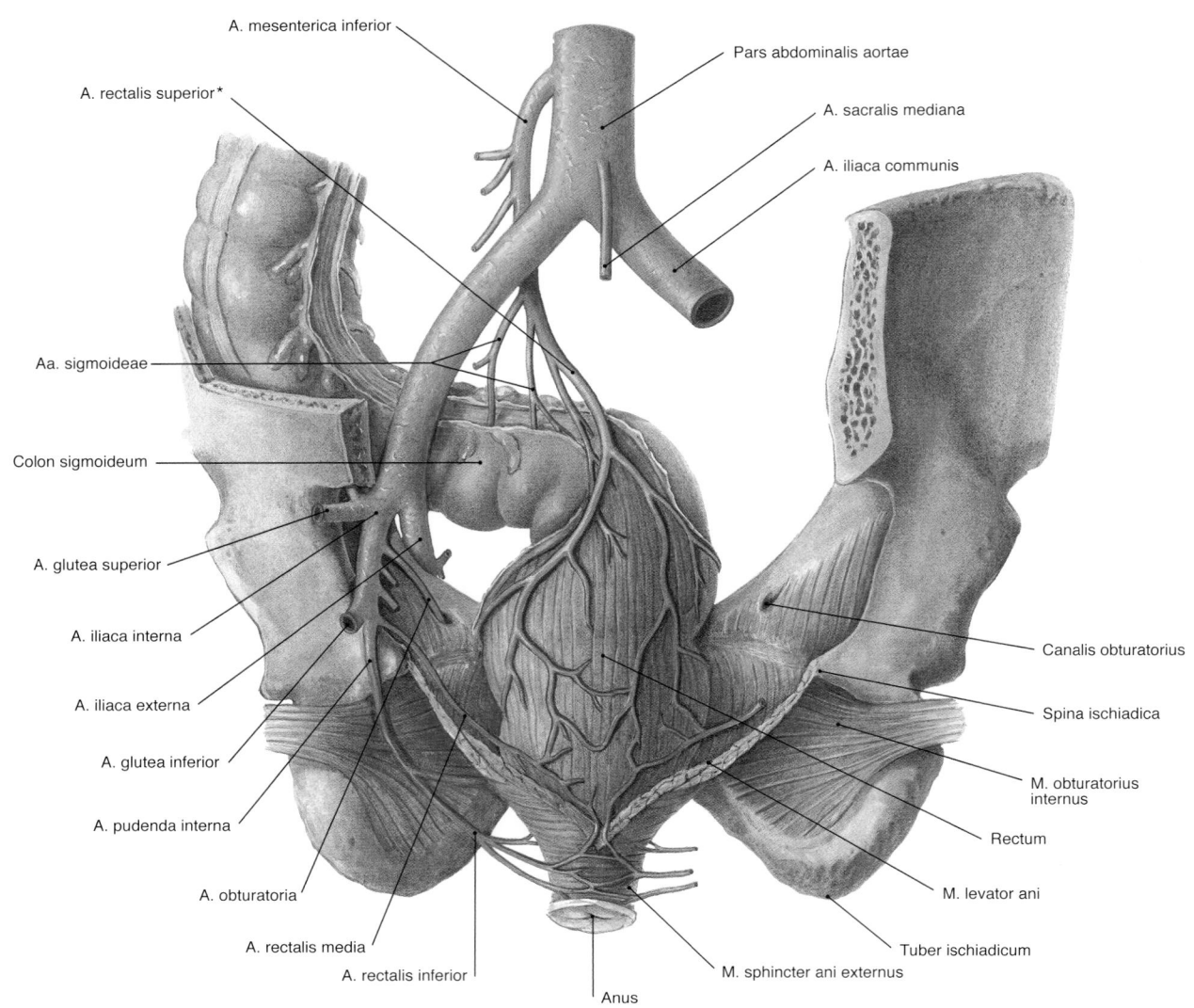

A. mesenterica inferior

Pars abdominalis aortae

A. rectalis superior*

A. sacralis mediana

A. iliaca communis

Aa. sigmoideae

Colon sigmoideum

A. glutea superior

A. iliaca interna

Canalis obturatorius

A. iliaca externa

Spina ischiadica

A. glutea inferior

M. obturatorius internus

A. pudenda interna

Rectum

A. obturatoria

M. levator ani

A. rectalis media

Tuber ischiadicum

A. rectalis inferior

M. sphincter ani externus

Anus

Fig. 879 Rectal arteries, Aa. rectales; dorsal view.

* Clinical term: SUDECK's point (from this point on there are no further anastomoses with the sigmoid arteries)

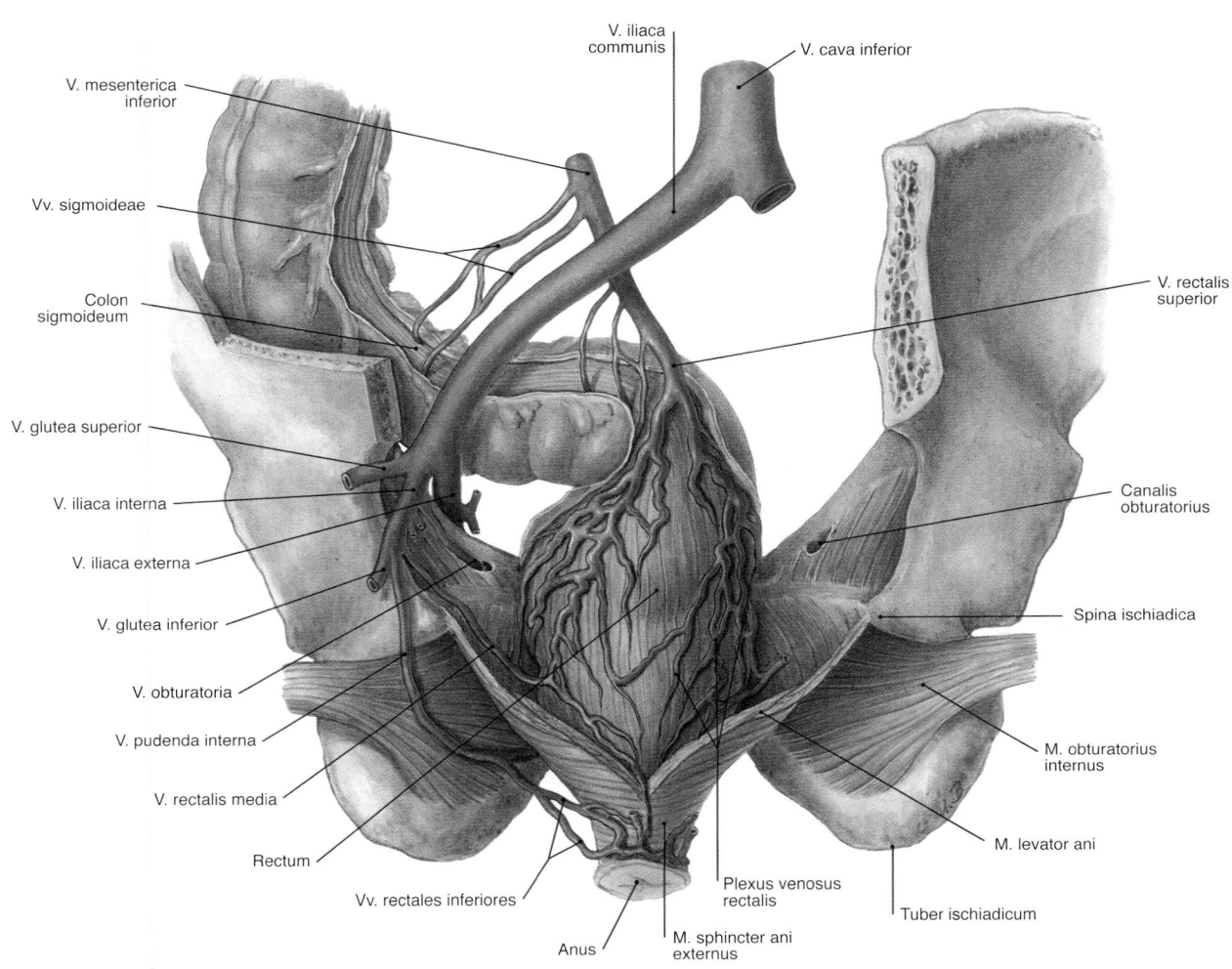

V. iliaca communis

V. cava inferior

V. mesenterica inferior

Vv. sigmoideae

Colon sigmoideum

V. rectalis superior

V. glutea superior

V. iliaca interna

V. iliaca externa

Canalis obturatorius

V. glutea inferior

Spina ischiadica

V. obturatoria

V. pudenda interna

M. obturatorius internus

V. rectalis media

Rectum

M. levator ani

Vv. rectales inferiores

Plexus venosus rectalis

Tuber ischiadicum

Anus

M. sphincter ani externus

Fig. 880 Rectal veins, Vv. rectales;
diagram with parts of the pelvis and the pelvic
diaphragm;
dorsal view.
There are numerous connections between the veins
draining into the hepatic portal vein (superior
rectal vein) and those draining into the inferior vena
cava (middle and inferior rectal veins). They form
the portocaval anastomoses, which are of particular
clinical importance.

→ 809, 810

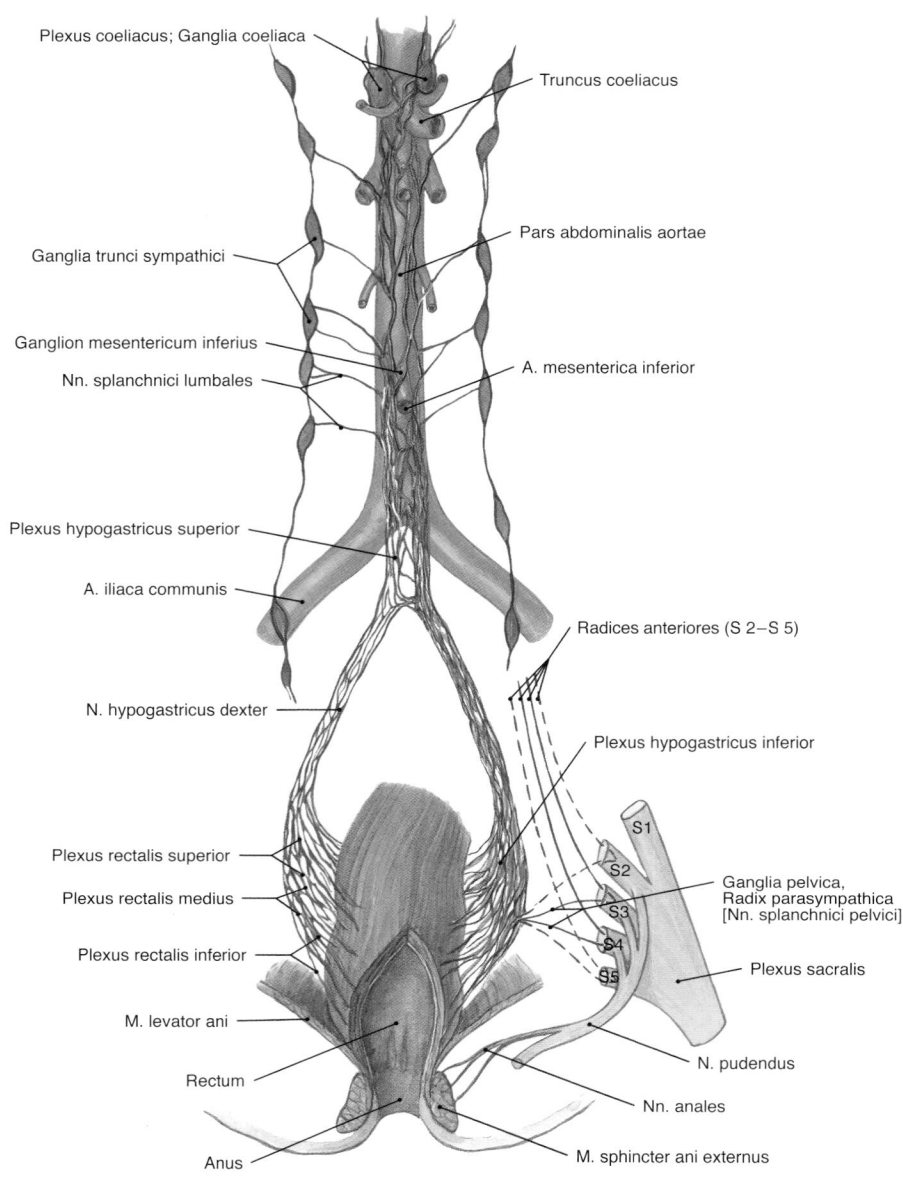

Plexus coeliacus; Ganglia coeliaca

Truncus coeliacus

Ganglia trunci sympathici

Pars abdominalis aortae

Ganglion mesentericum inferius

Nn. splanchnici lumbales

A. mesenterica inferior

Plexus hypogastricus superior

A. iliaca communis

Radices anteriores (S 2–S 5)

N. hypogastricus dexter

Plexus hypogastricus inferior

S1
S2
S3
S4
S5

Plexus rectalis superior

Plexus rectalis medius

Ganglia pelvica, Radix parasympathica [Nn. splanchnici pelvici]

Plexus rectalis inferior

Plexus sacralis

M. levator ani

Rectum

N. pudendus

Nn. anales

Anus

M. sphincter ani externus

Fig. 881   Rectum, Rectum;
schematic overview of the innervation;
ventral view.
Green = sympathetic nervous system
Purple = parasympathetic nervous system

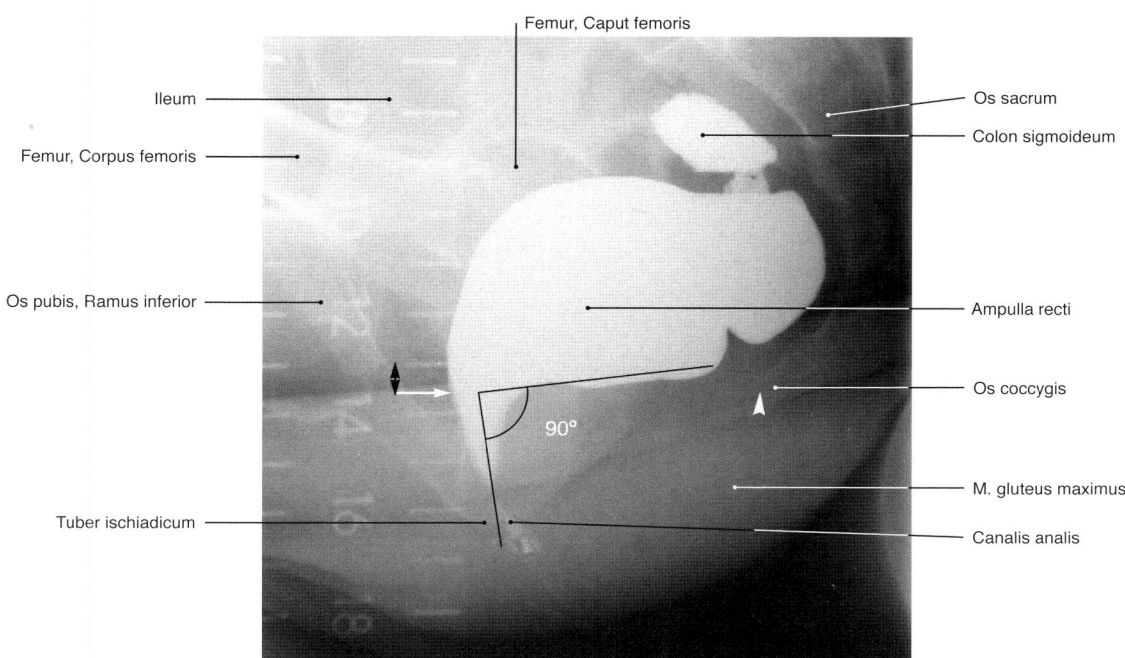

Fig. 882 Rectum, Rectum;
lateral radiograph in voluntary closure of the anus after filling with a contrast medium (defaecography).

The transitional zone between the anus and the rectum (arrow) is located at the level of the tip of the coccyx (triangle). The angle between the axes of the anus and the rectum (∡) is approximately 90° and depends upon the curvature of the levator ani muscle (puborectal muscle). Scale in cm.

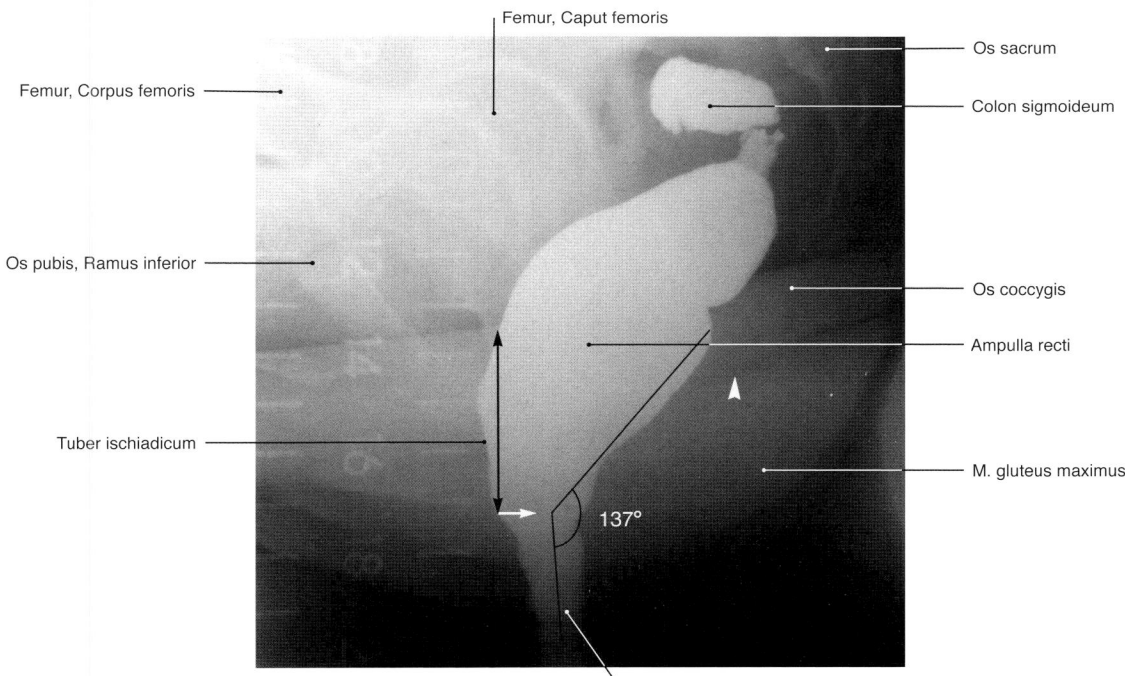

Fig. 883 Rectum, Rectum;
lateral radiograph of the defaecation after filling with a contrast medium (defaecography).

In comparison to Fig. 882, the anorectal transitional zone has descended and the angle (∡) increased to 137° due to the relaxation of the curvature of the levator ani muscle. As the bending acts like a valve, the elongation results in an unimpeded pressure of the faeces on the anal canal leading to defaecation.

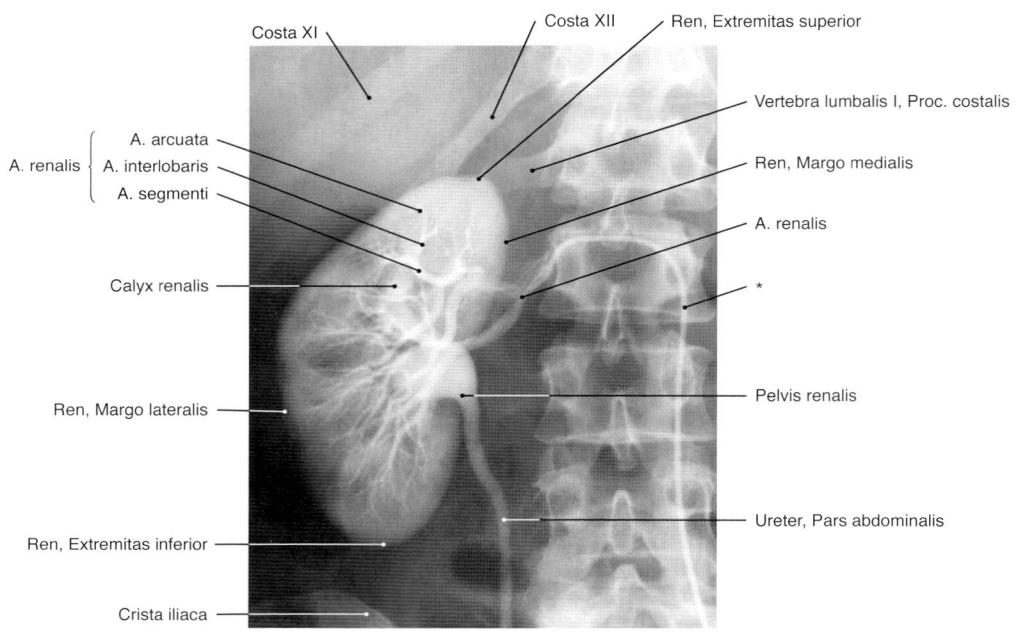

Fig. 884 Kidney, Ren;
AP-radiograph after intravenous injection of a contrast medium which is excreted via the kidneys to demonstrate the renal pelvis and the ureters (intravenous pyelography);

concomitant visualization of the arteries by injection of a contrast medium into the renal artery through a catheter* introduced into the aorta (arteriography).

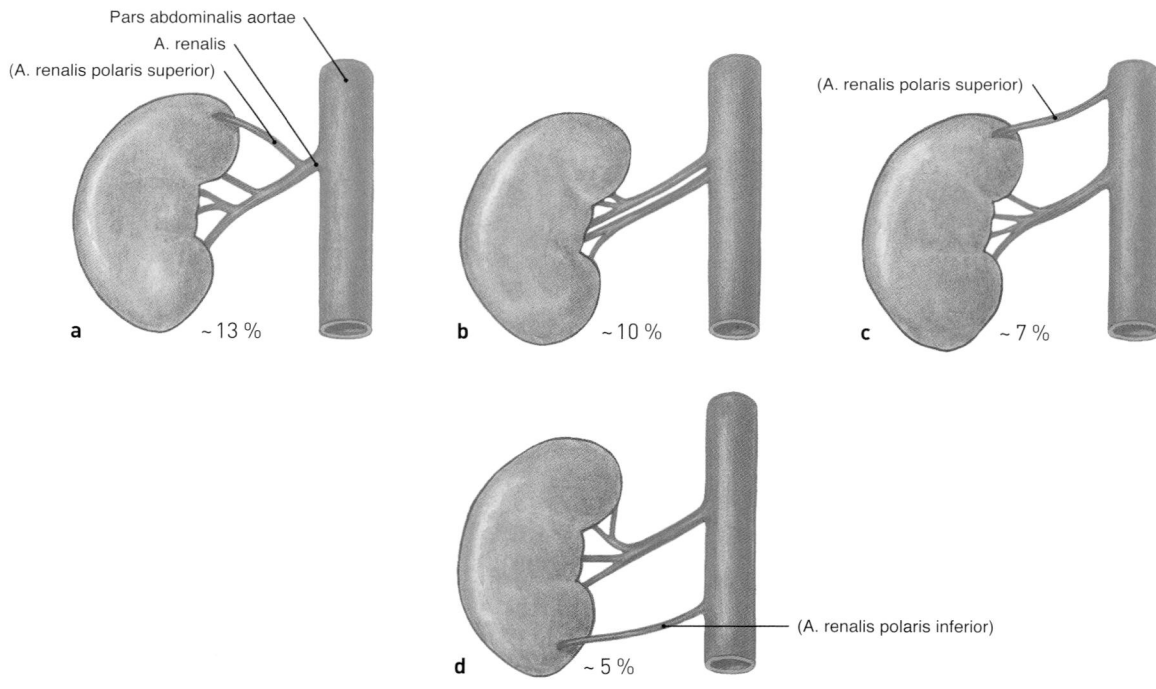

Fig. 885 a–d Variations in the arterial supply of the kidney.
  a One renal artery, A. renalis, with a branch to the superior pole
  b Two renal arteries to the renal hilum
  c Two renal arteries, one of which supplies the superior pole
  d Two renal arteries, one of which supplies the inferior pole

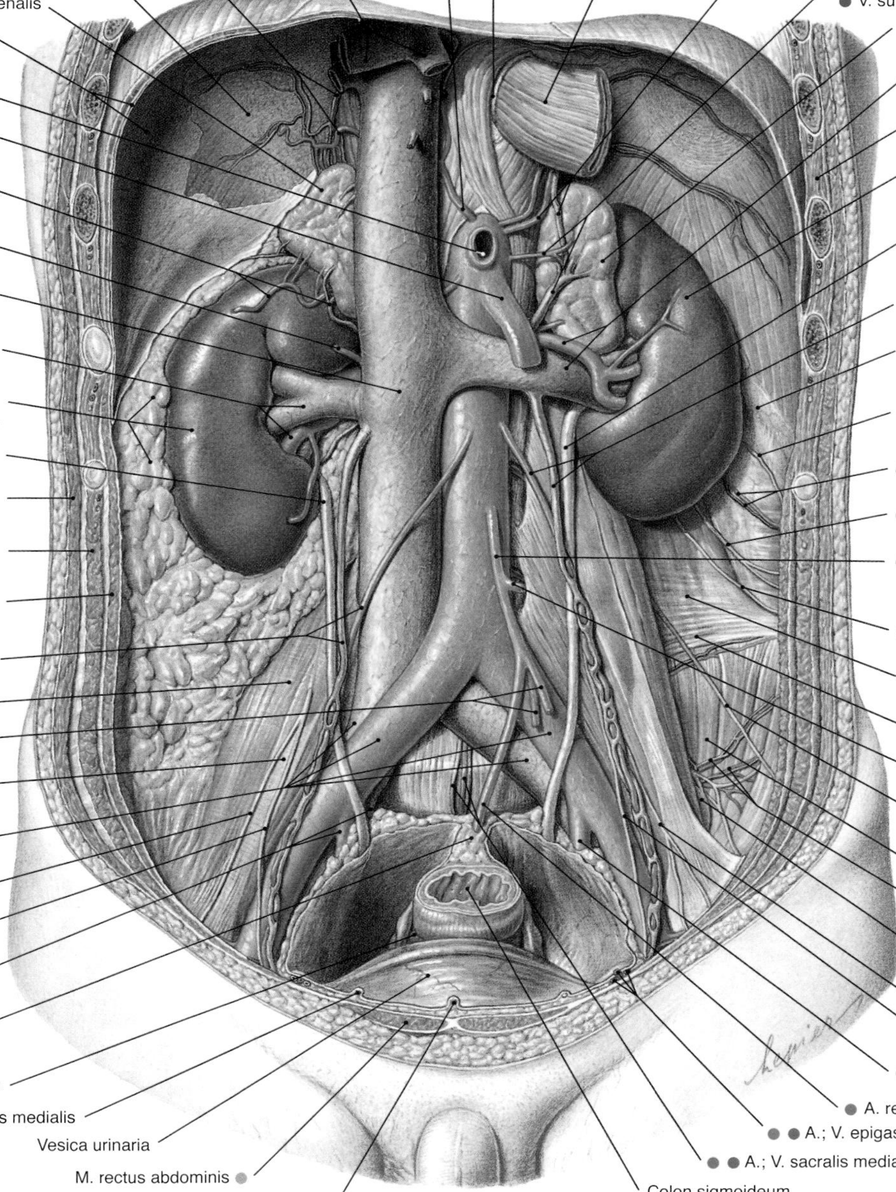

Retroperitoneal space, overview

A.; V. phrenica inferior
(Facies contacta hepatis)
Glandula suprarenalis
Peritoneum parietale
Truncus coeliacus
A. mesenterica superior
A. suprarenalis inferior; V. suprarenalis dextra
(A. renalis accessoria)
V. cava inferior
A.; V. renalis
Ren, Capsula adiposa
Ureter
M. obliquus externus abdominis
M. obliquus internus abdominis
M. transversus abdominis
V.; A. testicularis
M. psoas major
Aa. sigmoideae
(M. psoas minor)
Aa.; Vv. iliacae communes
N. genito-femoralis { R. femoralis / R. genitalis
A.; V. iliaca interna
Mesocolon sigmoideum
Excavatio rectovesicalis
Plica umbilicalis medialis
Vesica urinaria
M. rectus abdominis
Plica umbilicalis mediana

Vv. hepaticae
A. phrenica inferior
Hiatus oesophageus
Gaster, Pars cardiaca
A.; V. phrenica inferior
A. suprarenalis media; V. suprarenalis sinistra
Glandula suprarenalis
A.; V. renalis
Mm. intercostales
Ren
Ureter
A.; V. testicularis
Costa XI
N. subcostalis
A.; V. lumbalis I
N. iliohypogastricus
A. mesenterica inferior
N. ilioinguinalis
M. quadratus lumborum
Lig. iliolumbale
A. colica sinistra
N. cutaneus femoris lateralis
M. iliacus
A.; V. iliolumbalis, Rr. iliaci
N. femoralis
R. femoralis } N. genito-femoralis
R. genitalis }
A. iliaca interna
A. rectalis superior
A.; V. epigastrica inferior
A.; V. sacralis mediana
Colon sigmoideum

Fig. 886 Position of the retroperitoneal structures, Situs retroperitonealis, of the male.
Whereas the left testicular vein opens into the left renal vein, the right testicular vein drains directly into the inferior vena cava. The same applies to the ovarian veins.

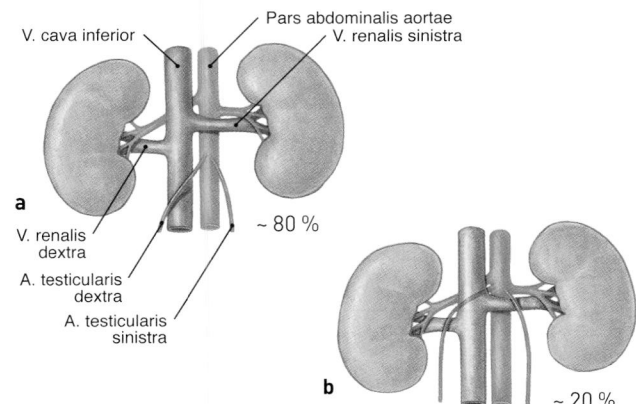

V. cava inferior
Pars abdominalis aortae
V. renalis sinistra
V. renalis dextra
A. testicularis dextra
A. testicularis sinistra
a ~ 80 %
b ~ 20 %

Fig. 887 a, b Variability of the course of the testicular arteries, Aa. testiculares.
a "Textbook case"
b Both testicular arteries, Aa. testiculares, branch off cranially to the renal veins, Vv. renales; the right artery passes posterior to the inferior vena cava, V. cava inferior, and the left artery passes anterior to the left renal vein, V. renalis sinistra.

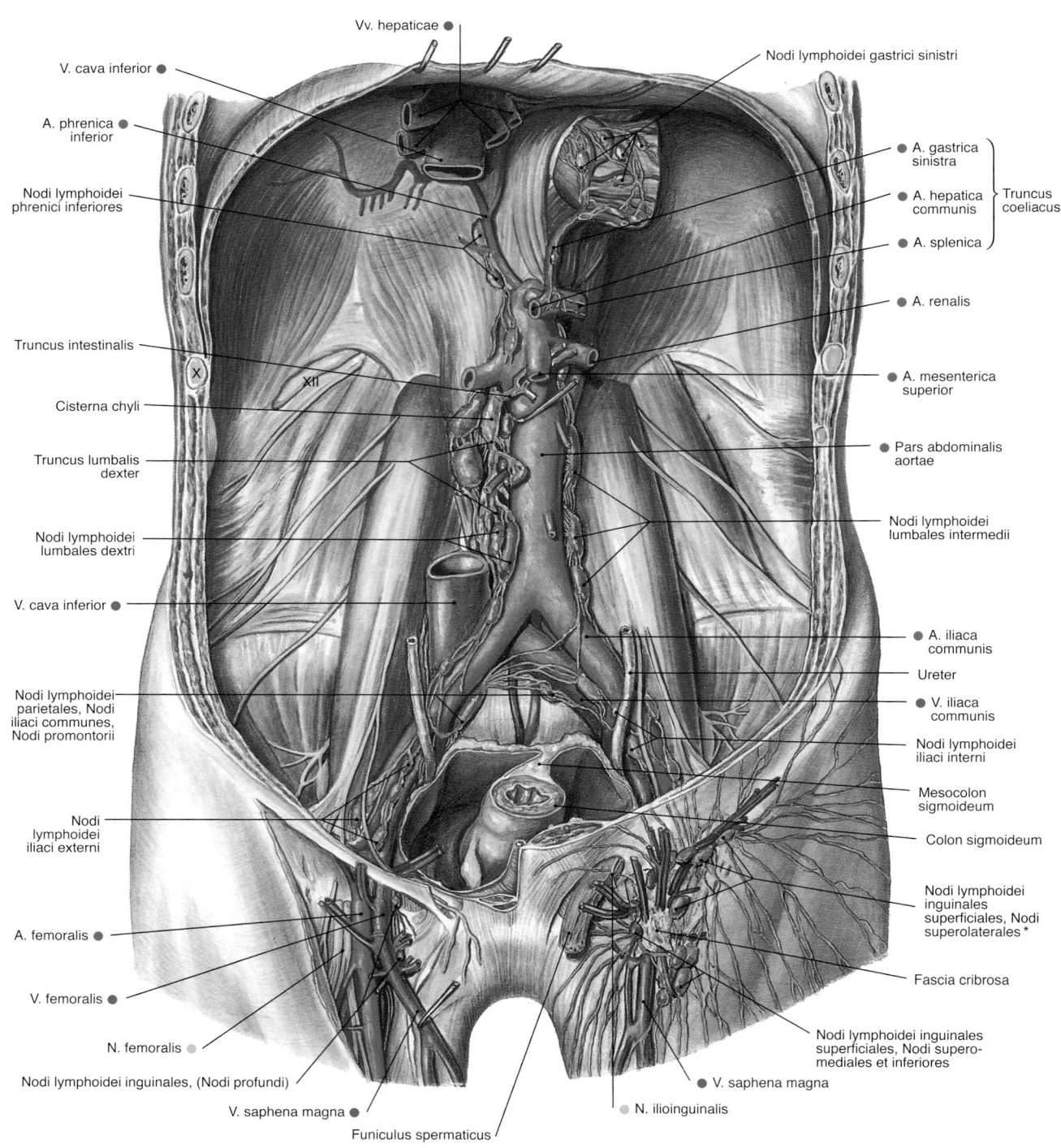

Vv. hepaticae ●

Nodi lymphoidei gastrici sinistri

V. cava inferior ●

A. phrenica ●
inferior

A. gastrica
sinistra ●

A. hepatica
communis ●   } Truncus
coeliacus

A. splenica ●

Nodi lymphoidei
phrenici inferiores

A. renalis ●

Truncus intestinalis

A. mesenterica ●
superior

X

XII

Cisterna chyli

Pars abdominalis ●
aortae

Truncus lumbalis
dexter

Nodi lymphoidei
lumbales intermedii

Nodi lymphoidei
lumbales dextri

V. cava inferior ●

A. iliaca ●
communis

Ureter

V. iliaca ●
communis

Nodi lymphoidei
parietales, Nodi
iliaci communes,
Nodi promontorii

Nodi lymphoidei
iliaci interni

Mesocolon
sigmoideum

Nodi
lymphoidei
iliaci externi

Colon sigmoideum

Nodi lymphoidei
inguinales
superficiales, Nodi
superolaterales *

A. femoralis ●

Fascia cribrosa

V. femoralis ●

Nodi lymphoidei inguinales
superficiales, Nodi superomediales et inferiores

N. femoralis ●

V. saphena magna ●

Nodi lymphoidei inguinales, (Nodi profundi)

N. ilioinguinalis ●

V. saphena magna ●

Funiculus spermaticus

→ 1121

Fig. 888 Lymph nodes, Nodi lymphoidei, and lymphatics,
Vasa lymphatica, of the posterior abdominal wall and the
inguinal region;
ventral view.

The numbers X and XII indicate the respective ribs.
* Clinical term: "horizontal chain", draining the lower abdominal wall,
the gluteal region, the perineum and the external genital

Lymphatics of the retroperitoneal space, radiography

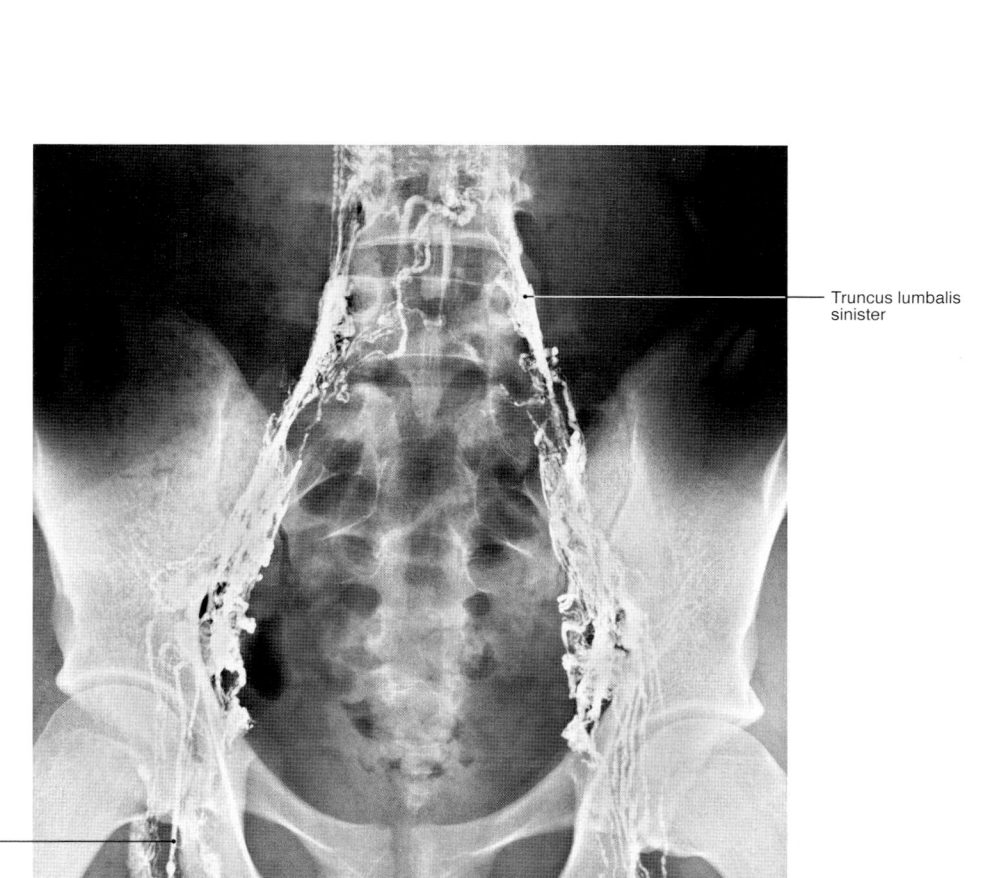

Truncus lumbalis sinister

Vas lymphaticum efferens

Vasa lymphatica afferentia

Nodus lymphoideus inguinalis superficialis

Fig. 889 Lymphatics, Vasa lymphatica, and lymph nodes, Nodi lymphoidei, of the inguinal, the pelvic and the lumbar region;
AP-radiograph after bilateral injection of a contrast medium into lymphatics of the foot (lymphography).
This formerly applied technique visualizes the position and size of lymphatics and lymph nodes.

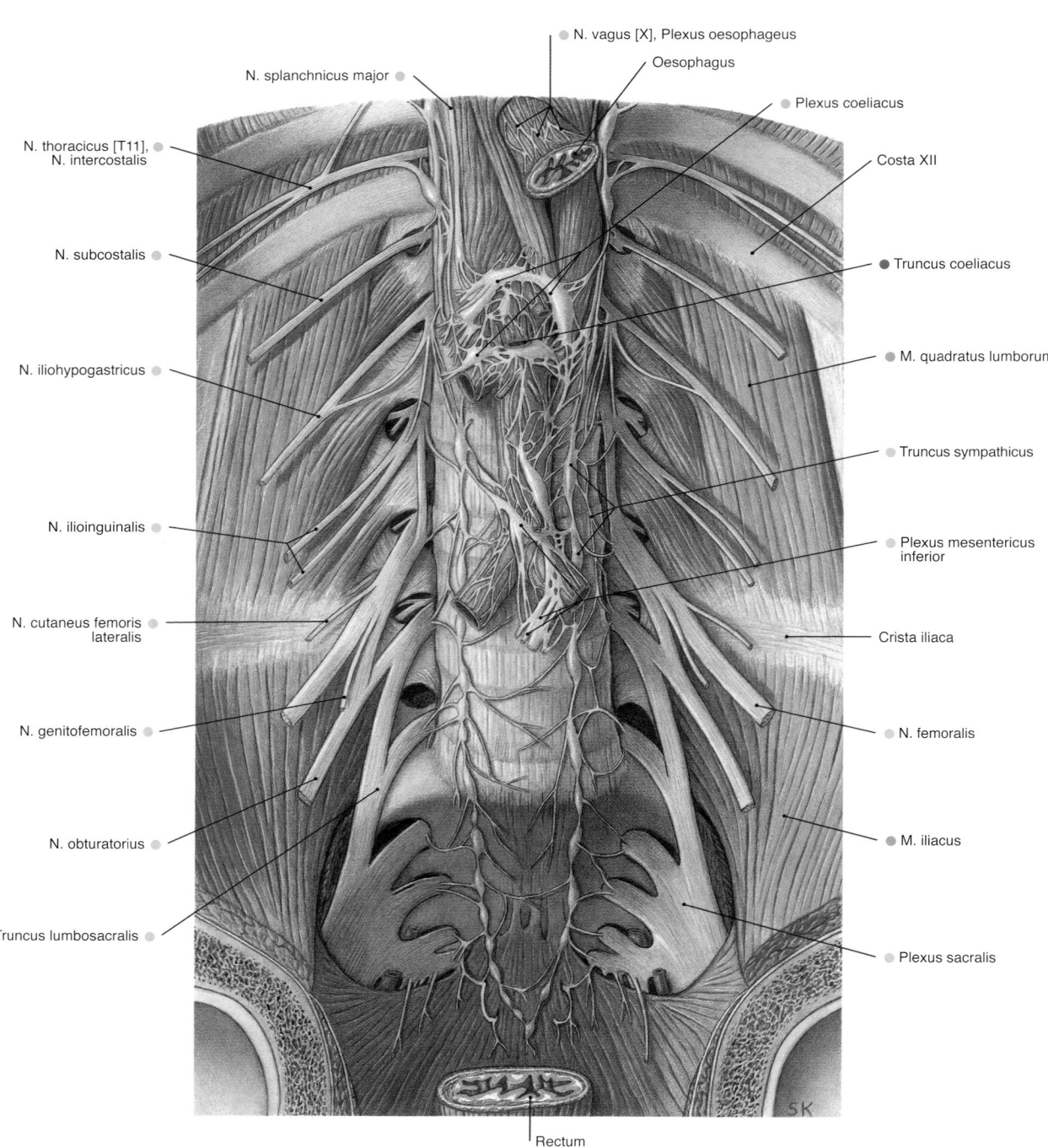

N. vagus [X], Plexus oesophageus

Oesophagus

N. splanchnicus major

Plexus coeliacus

N. thoracicus [T11], N. intercostalis

Costa XII

N. subcostalis

Truncus coeliacus

N. iliohypogastricus

M. quadratus lumborum

Truncus sympathicus

N. ilioinguinalis

Plexus mesentericus inferior

N. cutaneus femoris lateralis

Crista iliaca

N. genitofemoralis

N. femoralis

N. obturatorius

M. iliacus

Truncus lumbosacralis

Plexus sacralis

Rectum

→ 47, 49, 50

Fig. 890 Nerves of the posterior abdominal wall, the lumbosacral plexus, Plexus lumbosacralis, and the abdominal part of the autonomous nervous system, Pars abdominalis autonomica; ventral view.

Vessels and nerves of the retroperitoneal space

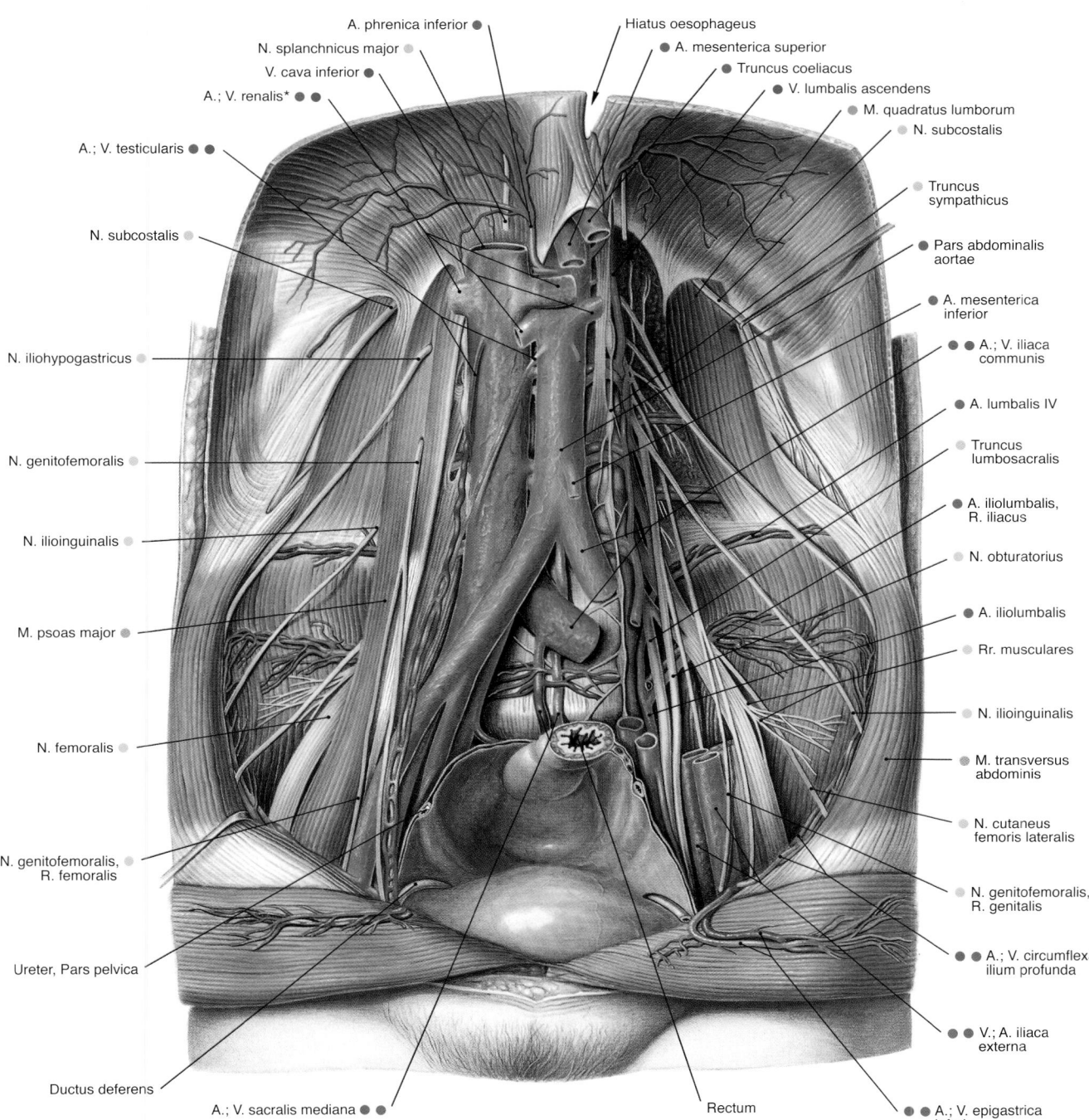

A. phrenica inferior

N. splanchnicus major

V. cava inferior

A.; V. renalis*

A.; V. testicularis

N. subcostalis

N. iliohypogastricus

N. genitofemoralis

N. ilioinguinalis

M. psoas major

N. femoralis

N. genitofemoralis, R. femoralis

Ureter, Pars pelvica

Ductus deferens

A.; V. sacralis mediana

Hiatus oesophageus

A. mesenterica superior

Truncus coeliacus

V. lumbalis ascendens

M. quadratus lumborum

N. subcostalis

Truncus sympathicus

Pars abdominalis aortae

A. mesenterica inferior

A.; V. iliaca communis

A. lumbalis IV

Truncus lumbosacralis

A. iliolumbalis, R. iliacus

N. obturatorius

A. iliolumbalis

Rr. musculares

N. ilioinguinalis

M. transversus abdominis

N. cutaneus femoris lateralis

N. genitofemoralis, R. genitalis

A.; V. circumflexa ilium profunda

V.; A. iliaca externa

Rectum

A.; V. epigastrica inferior

Fig. 891 Vessels and nerves of the posterior abdominal
wall of the male.
* In ~10% the left renal vein passes posterior to the aorta.

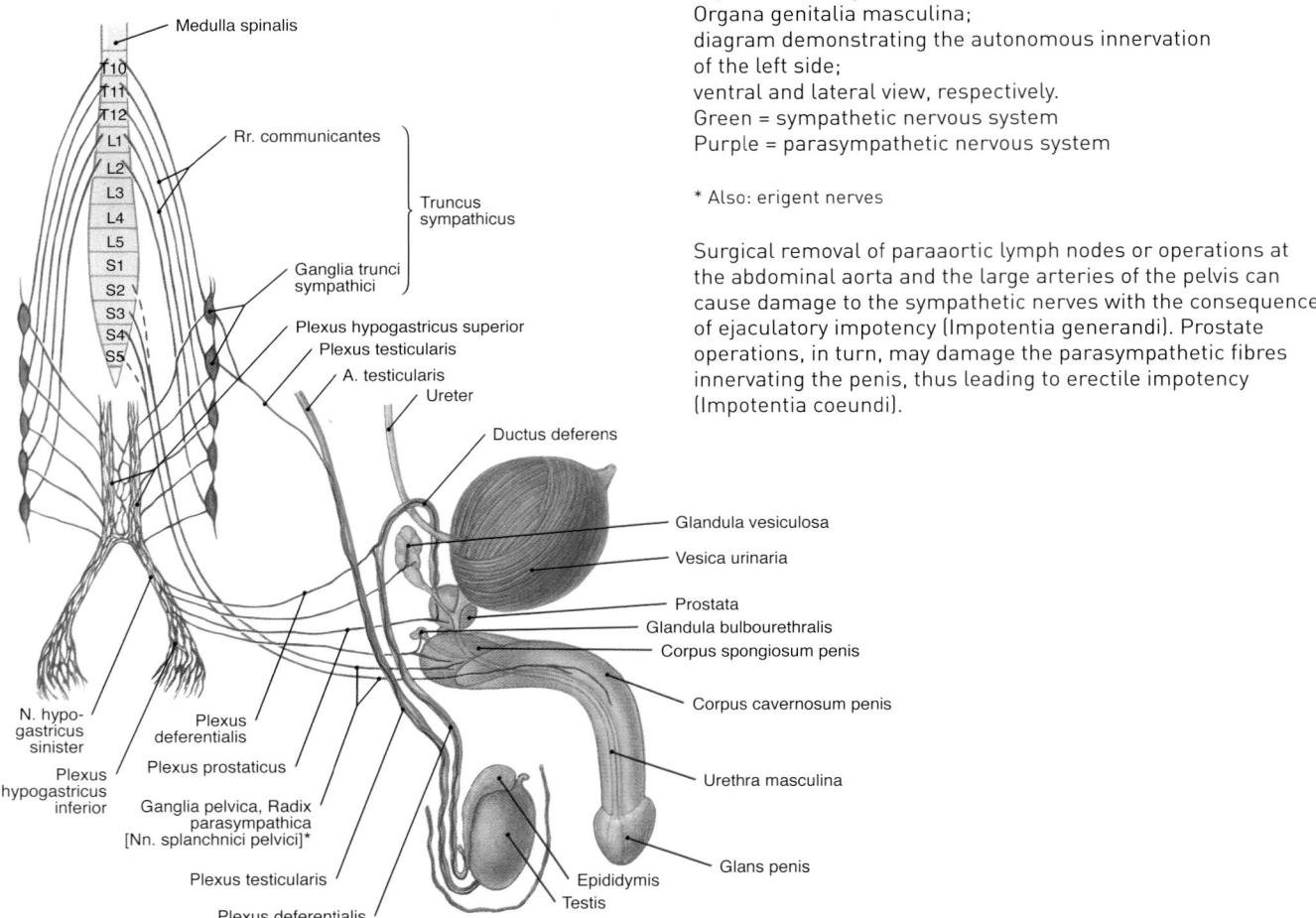

Fig. 892 Male genitalia,
Organa genitalia masculina;
diagram demonstrating the autonomous innervation
of the left side;
ventral and lateral view, respectively.
Green = sympathetic nervous system
Purple = parasympathetic nervous system

* Also: erigent nerves

Surgical removal of paraaortic lymph nodes or operations at
the abdominal aorta and the large arteries of the pelvis can
cause damage to the sympathetic nerves with the consequence
of ejaculatory impotency (Impotentia generandi). Prostate
operations, in turn, may damage the parasympathetic fibres
innervating the penis, thus leading to erectile impotency
(Impotentia coeundi).

Innervation of the male genitalia

	Origin	Course	Organ	Function
Parasympathetic	Sacral part of the spinal cord (S2 – S4)	Ganglia pelvica, Radix parasympathica [Nn. splanchnici pelvici]	Penis Corpus cavernosum	Vasodilatation Erection
Sympathetic	Thoracic part of the spinal cord (T10 – T12)	Plexus mesenterici superior et inferior ↓ Truncus sympathicus ↓ Plexus testicularis ↓	Testis	Regulation of blood flow
	Lumbar part of the spinal cord (L1 – L2)	Plexus hypogastricus superior ↓ N. hypogastricus ↓		
		Plexus hypogastricus inferior	Glandula bulbo-urethralis	Expulsion of its fluid
			Ductus (vas) deferens	Contraction, transport of the sperms into the urethra
			Glandula vesiculosa Prostata	Expulsion of its content into the urethra
Somatomotor, somatosensory	Sacral part of the spinal cord (S2 – S4)	N. pudendus	(M. sphincter vesicae)	Closure of the urinary bladder to prevent retrograde ejaculation
			M. ischiocavernosus M. bulbospongiosus	Expulsion of the ejaculate out of the urethra
		Nn. scrotales posteriores N. dorsalis penis	Scrotal skin Penile skin	

Innervation of the female genitalia

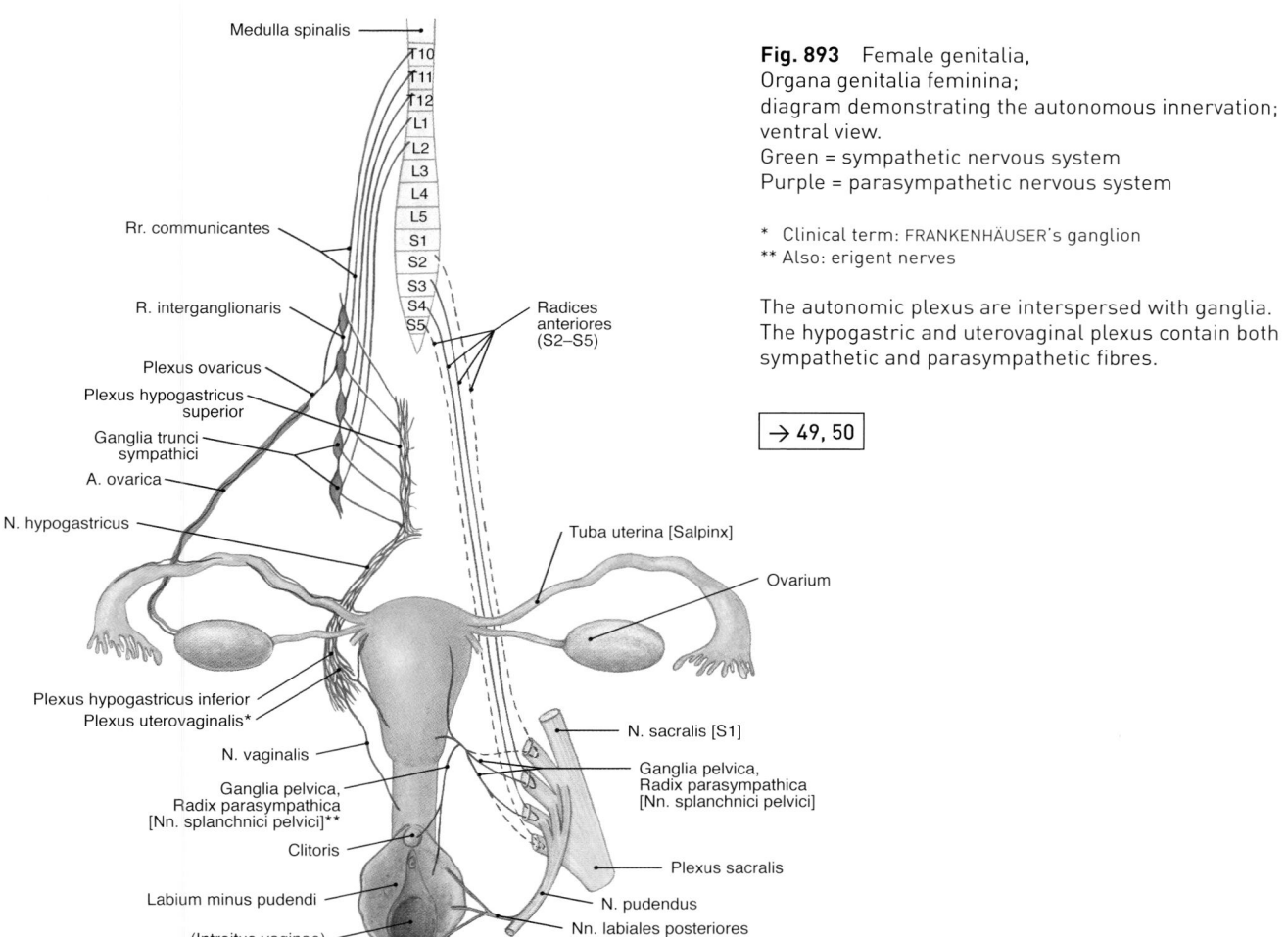

Fig. 893 Female genitalia,
Organa genitalia feminina;
diagram demonstrating the autonomous innervation;
ventral view.
Green = sympathetic nervous system
Purple = parasympathetic nervous system

* Clinical term: FRANKENHÄUSER's ganglion
** Also: erigent nerves

The autonomic plexus are interspersed with ganglia.
The hypogastric and uterovaginal plexus contain both
sympathetic and parasympathetic fibres.

→ 49, 50

Innervation of the female genitalia

	Origin	Course	Organ	Function
Parasympathetic	Sacral part of the spinal cord (S2 – S4)	Ganglia pelvica, Radix parasympathica [Nn. splanchnici pelvici] ↓ Nn. cavernosi clitoridis	Tuba uterina Uterus Vagina Clitoris	Vasodilatation Vasodilatation Transsudation Erection
Sympathetic	Thoracic part of the spinal cord (T10 – T12)	Plexus mesentericus superior ↘ Plexus ovaricus ↗ Plexus renalis Truncus sympathicus ↓	Ovar	Vasoconstriction
	Lumbar part of the spinal cord (L1 – L2)	Plexus hypogastricus superior ↓ N. hypogastricus Plexus hypogastricus inferior ↓ Plexus uterovaginalis (FRANKENHÄUSER's ganglion)	- Tuba uterina Uterus Vagina	Contraction
Somatomotor, somatosensory	Sacral part of the spinal cord (S2 – S4)	N. pudendus ↗ N. dorsalis clitoridis ↘ Nn. labiales posteriores	Clitoris Labia majora M. ischiocavernosus M. bulbospongiosus	Contraction

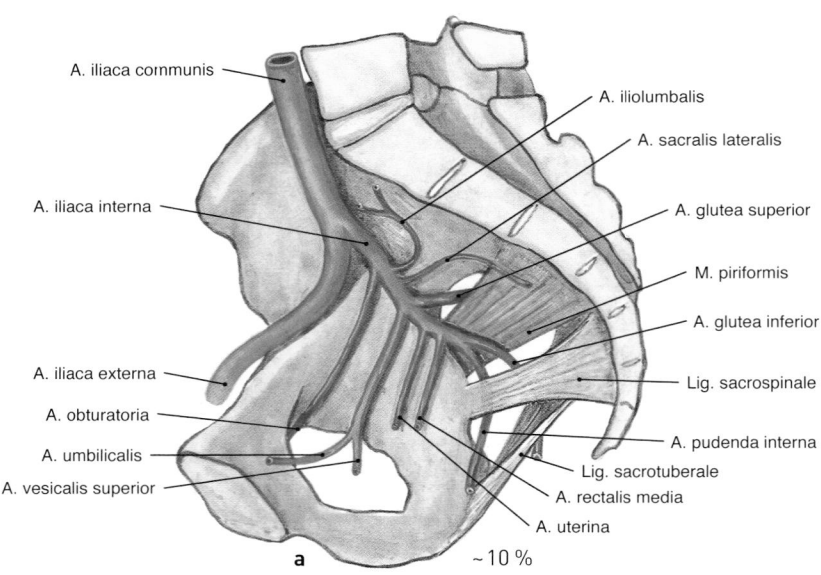

A. iliaca communis

A. iliolumbalis

A. sacralis lateralis

A. iliaca interna

A. glutea superior

M. piriformis

A. glutea inferior

Lig. sacrospinale

A. iliaca externa

A. obturatoria

A. umbilicalis

A. vesicalis superior

A. pudenda interna

Lig. sacrotuberale

A. rectalis media

A. uterina

a　　　　～10 %

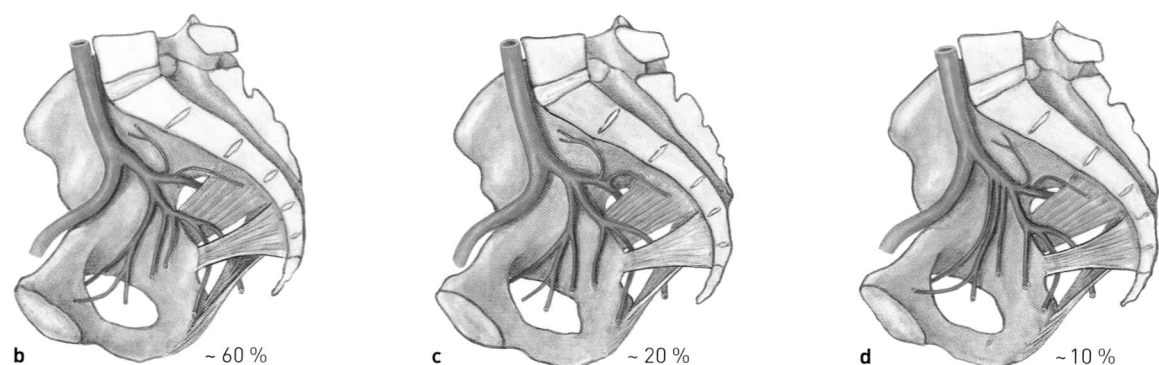

b　　　～60 %　　　**c**　　　～20 %　　　**d**　　　～10 %

Fig. 894 a–d　Variability of the branching pattern of the internal iliac artery, A. iliaca interna; viewed from the left.
a　All branches arise from the same stem.
b　The internal iliac artery, A. iliaca interna, divides into two major branches ("textbook case").
c　The internal iliac artery, A. iliaca interna, divides into three major branches.
d　The internal iliac artery, A. iliaca interna, divides into more than three major branches.

Vessels and nerves of the pelvic wall

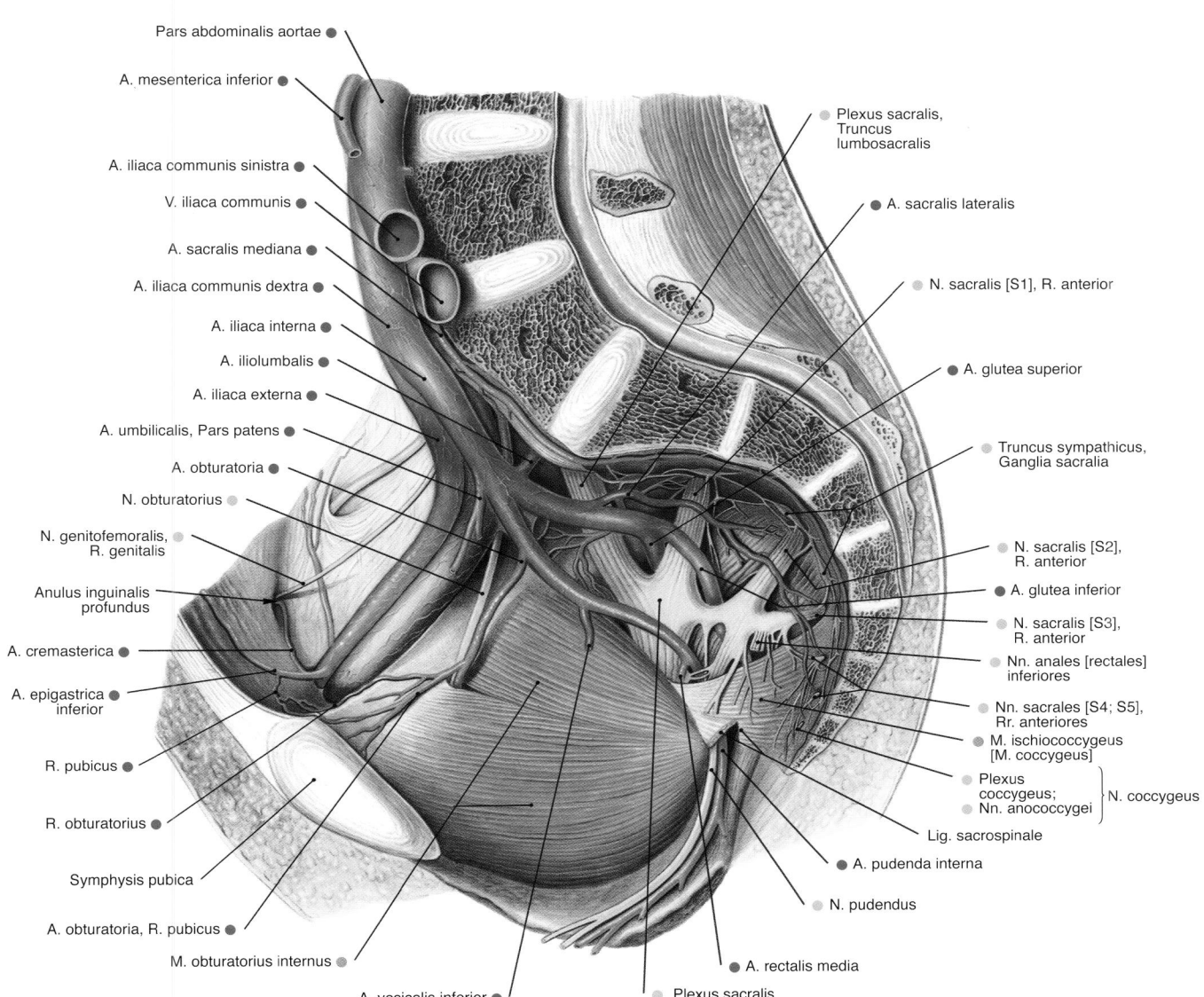

Pars abdominalis aortae ●

A. mesenterica inferior ●

A. iliaca communis sinistra ●

V. iliaca communis ●

A. sacralis mediana ●

A. iliaca communis dextra ●

A. iliaca interna ●

A. iliolumbalis ●

A. iliaca externa ●

A. umbilicalis, Pars patens ●

A. obturatoria ●

N. obturatorius ●

N. genitofemoralis, ●
R. genitalis

Anulus inguinalis
profundus

A. cremasterica ●

A. epigastrica ●
inferior

R. pubicus ●

R. obturatorius ●

Symphysis pubica

A. obturatoria, R. pubicus ●

M. obturatorius internus ●

A. vesicalis inferior ●

A. rectalis media ●

Plexus sacralis ●

N. pudendus ●

A. pudenda interna ●

Lig. sacrospinale

Plexus
coccygeus; ●
Nn. anococcygei ●   } N. coccygeus

M. ischiococcygeus ●
[M. coccygeus]

Nn. sacrales [S4; S5], ●
Rr. anteriores

Nn. anales [rectales]
inferiores

N. sacralis [S3], ●
R. anterior

A. glutea inferior ●

N. sacralis [S2], ●
R. anterior

Truncus sympathicus, ●
Ganglia sacralia

A. glutea superior ●

N. sacralis [S1], R. anterior ●

A. sacralis lateralis ●

Plexus sacralis, ●
Truncus
lumbosacralis

Fig. 895 Internal iliac artery, A. iliaca interna,
and sacral plexus, Plexus sacralis;
viewed from the left.

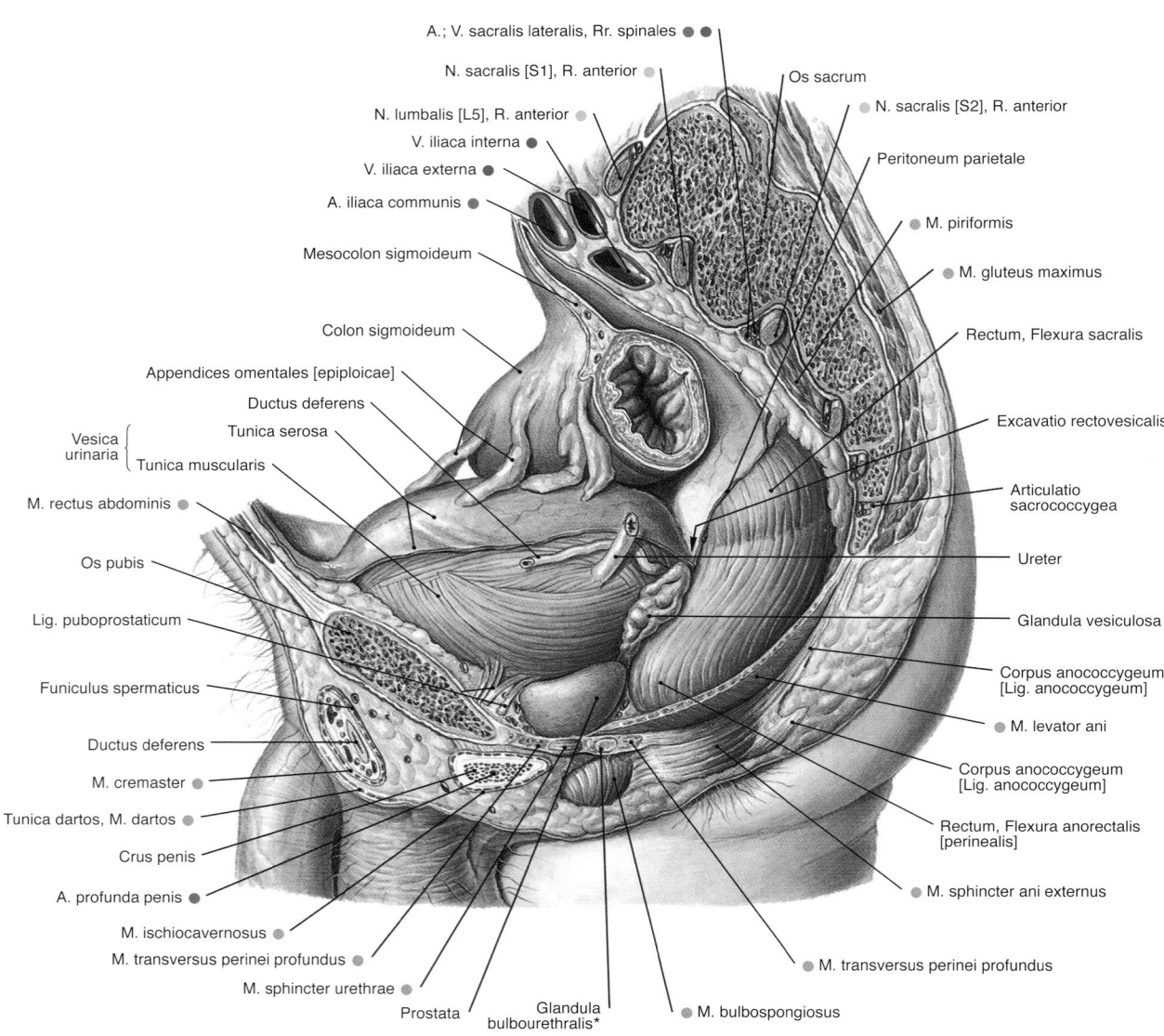

A.; V. sacralis lateralis, Rr. spinales
N. sacralis [S1], R. anterior
N. lumbalis [L5], R. anterior
V. iliaca interna
V. iliaca externa
A. iliaca communis
Mesocolon sigmoideum
Colon sigmoideum
Appendices omentales [epiploicae]
Ductus deferens
Tunica serosa
Vesica urinaria
Tunica muscularis
M. rectus abdominis
Os pubis
Lig. puboprostaticum
Funiculus spermaticus
Ductus deferens
M. cremaster
Tunica dartos, M. dartos
Crus penis
A. profunda penis
M. ischiocavernosus
M. transversus perinei profundus
M. sphincter urethrae
Prostata
Glandula bulbourethralis*

Os sacrum
N. sacralis [S2], R. anterior
Peritoneum parietale
M. piriformis
M. gluteus maximus
Rectum, Flexura sacralis
Excavatio rectovesicalis
Articulatio sacrococcygea
Ureter
Glandula vesiculosa
Corpus anococcygeum [Lig. anococcygeum]
M. levator ani
Corpus anococcygeum [Lig. anococcygeum]
Rectum, Flexura anorectalis [perinealis]
M. sphincter ani externus
M. transversus perinei profundus
M. bulbospongiosus

Fig. 896 Organs of the male pelvis.
* Clinical term: COWPER's gland

Vessels of the male pelvis

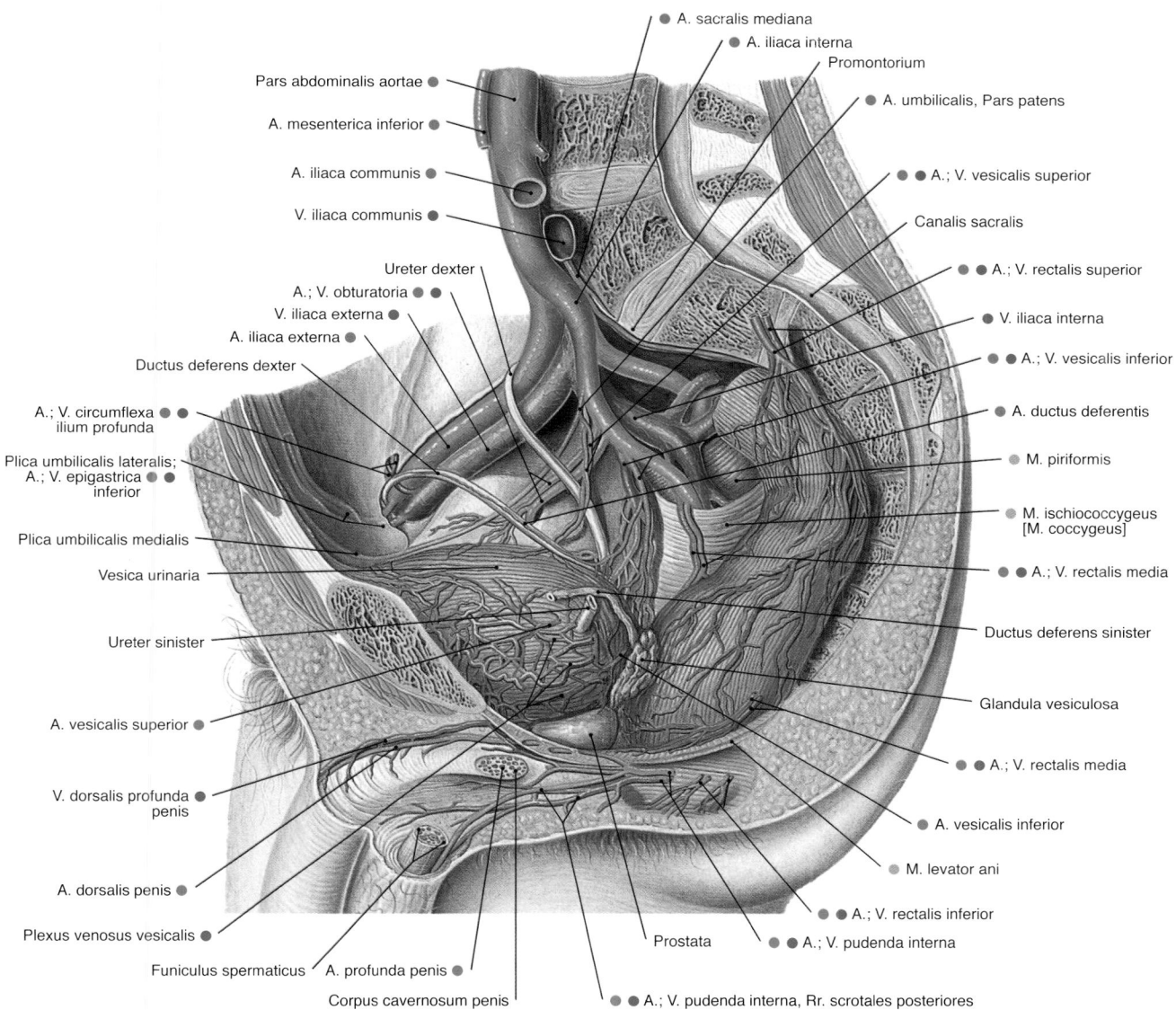

A. sacralis mediana
A. iliaca interna
Promontorium
Pars abdominalis aortae
A. umbilicalis, Pars patens
A. mesenterica inferior
A.; V. vesicalis superior
A. iliaca communis
Canalis sacralis
V. iliaca communis
A.; V. rectalis superior
Ureter dexter
A.; V. obturatoria
V. iliaca interna
V. iliaca externa
A.; V. vesicalis inferior
A. iliaca externa
Ductus deferens dexter
A. ductus deferentis
A.; V. circumflexa
ilium profunda
M. piriformis
Plica umbilicalis lateralis;
A.; V. epigastrica
inferior
M. ischiococcygeus
[M. coccygeus]
Plica umbilicalis medialis
A.; V. rectalis media
Vesica urinaria
Ductus deferens sinister
Ureter sinister
Glandula vesiculosa
A. vesicalis superior
A.; V. rectalis media
V. dorsalis profunda
penis
A. vesicalis inferior
M. levator ani
A. dorsalis penis
A.; V. rectalis inferior
Plexus venosus vesicalis
Prostata
A.; V. pudenda interna
Funiculus spermaticus   A. profunda penis
Corpus cavernosum penis
A.; V. pudenda interna, Rr. scrotales posteriores

Fig. 897 Blood supply of the male pelvis.

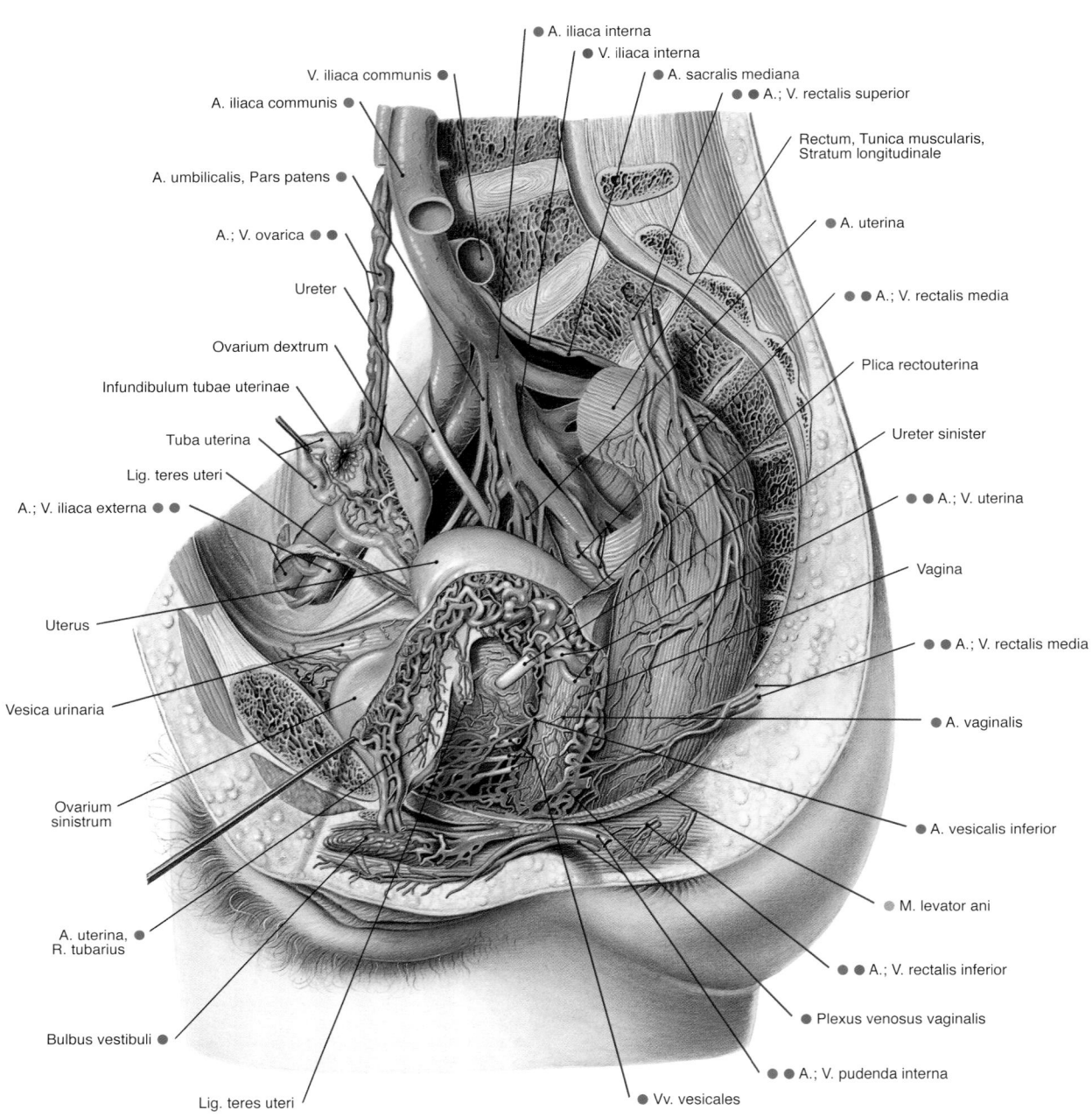

A. iliaca interna

V. iliaca interna

V. iliaca communis

A. iliaca communis

A. sacralis mediana

A.; V. rectalis superior

A. umbilicalis, Pars patens

Rectum, Tunica muscularis, Stratum longitudinale

A.; V. ovarica

A. uterina

Ureter

A.; V. rectalis media

Ovarium dextrum

Infundibulum tubae uterinae

Plica rectouterina

Tuba uterina

Ureter sinister

Lig. teres uteri

A.; V. iliaca externa

A.; V. uterina

Vagina

Uterus

A.; V. rectalis media

Vesica urinaria

A. vaginalis

Ovarium sinistrum

A. vesicalis inferior

M. levator ani

A. uterina, R. tubarius

A.; V. rectalis inferior

Plexus venosus vaginalis

Bulbus vestibuli

A.; V. pudenda interna

Lig. teres uteri

Vv. vesicales

Fig. 898 Blood supply of the female pelvis.

Vessels of the female pelvis

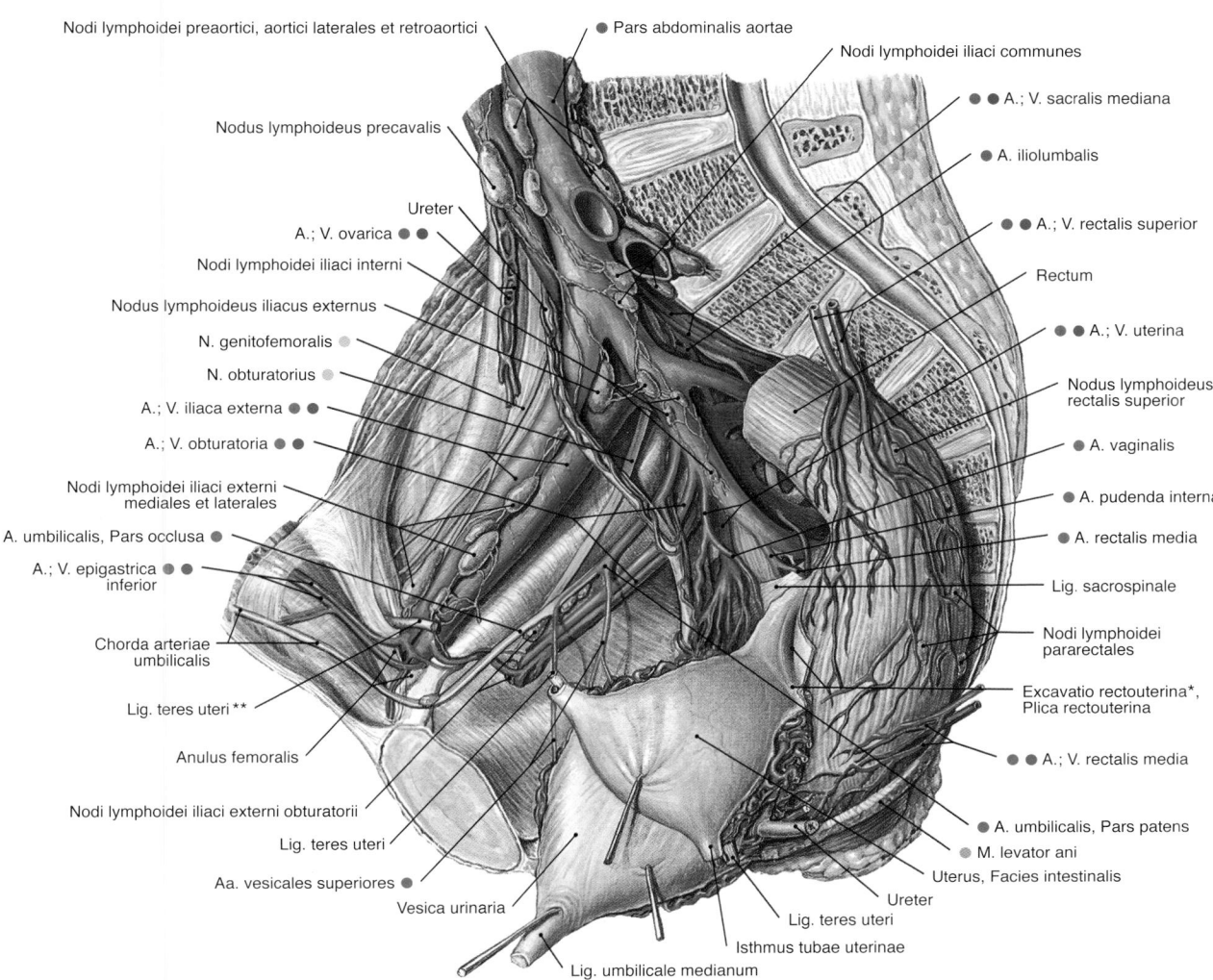

Nodi lymphoidei preaortici, aortici laterales et retroaortici
Pars abdominalis aortae
Nodi lymphoidei iliaci communes
Nodus lymphoideus precavalis
A.; V. sacralis mediana
A. iliolumbalis
Ureter
A.; V. ovarica
A.; V. rectalis superior
Nodi lymphoidei iliaci interni
Rectum
Nodus lymphoideus iliacus externus
A.; V. uterina
N. genitofemoralis
Nodus lymphoideus rectalis superior
N. obturatorius
A.; V. iliaca externa
A. vaginalis
A.; V. obturatoria
A. pudenda interna
Nodi lymphoidei iliaci externi mediales et laterales
A. rectalis media
A. umbilicalis, Pars occlusa
Lig. sacrospinale
A.; V. epigastrica inferior
Nodi lymphoidei pararectales
Chorda arteriae umbilicalis
Excavatio rectouterina*, Plica rectouterina
Lig. teres uteri**
A.; V. rectalis media
Anulus femoralis
A. umbilicalis, Pars patens
Nodi lymphoidei iliaci externi obturatorii
M. levator ani
Lig. teres uteri
Uterus, Facies intestinalis
Aa. vesicales superiores
Ureter
Vesica urinaria
Lig. teres uteri
Isthmus tubae uterinae
Lig. umbilicale medianum

Fig. 899 Lymphatics, Vasa lymphatica, and lymph nodes, Nodi lymphoidei, of the pelvic wall of the female.

The lymph nodes are frequently much smaller than illustrated but they are always present. Tumour cells from the uterus can reach the superficial inguinal lymph nodes via lymphatics of the round ligament of uterus.

* Clinical term: pouch of DOUGLAS
** Clinical term: round ligament

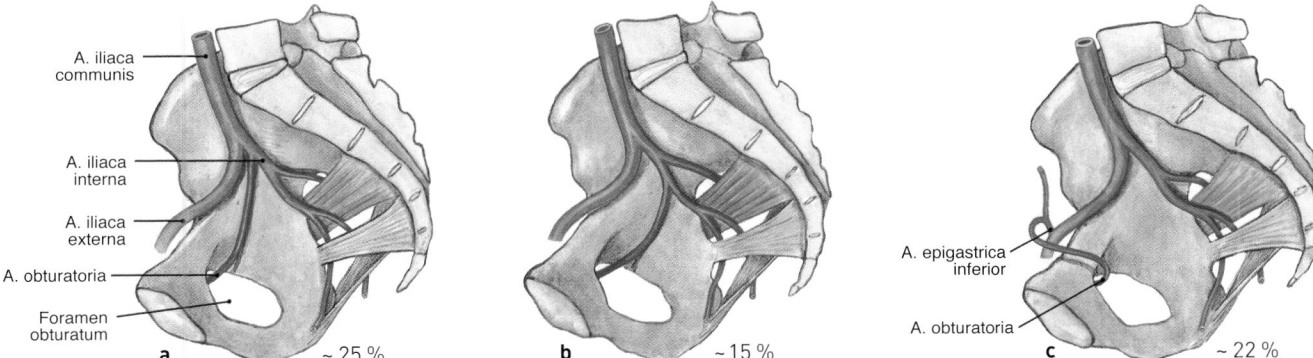

A. iliaca communis
A. iliaca interna
A. iliaca externa
A. obturatoria
Foramen obturatum

a ~ 25 %
b ~ 15 %
c ~ 22 %

A. epigastrica inferior
A. obturatoria

Fig. 900 a–c Variability of the origin of the obturator artery, A. obturatoria; medial view.
a Origin from the anterior branch of the internal iliac artery, A. iliaca interna ("textbook case")

b Origin as an independent branch from the internal iliac artery, A. iliaca interna
c Origin from the external iliac artery, A. iliaca externa
Only in 75% of the cases, the obturator artery originates from the trunk of the internal iliac artery.

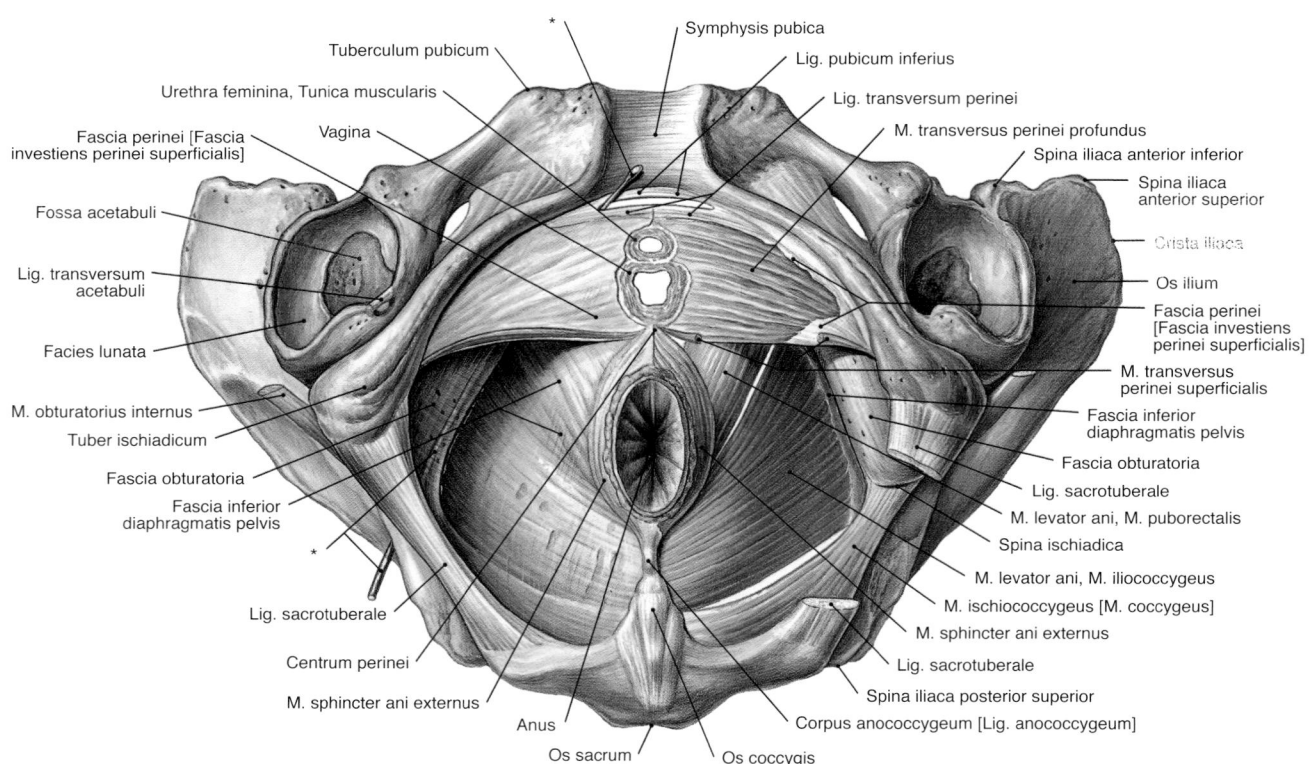

Fig. 901   Perineal muscles, Mm. perinei, and the pelvic diaphragm, Diaphragma pelvis, of the female; inferior view.

* Probe in the pudendal canal (ALCOCK's canal)

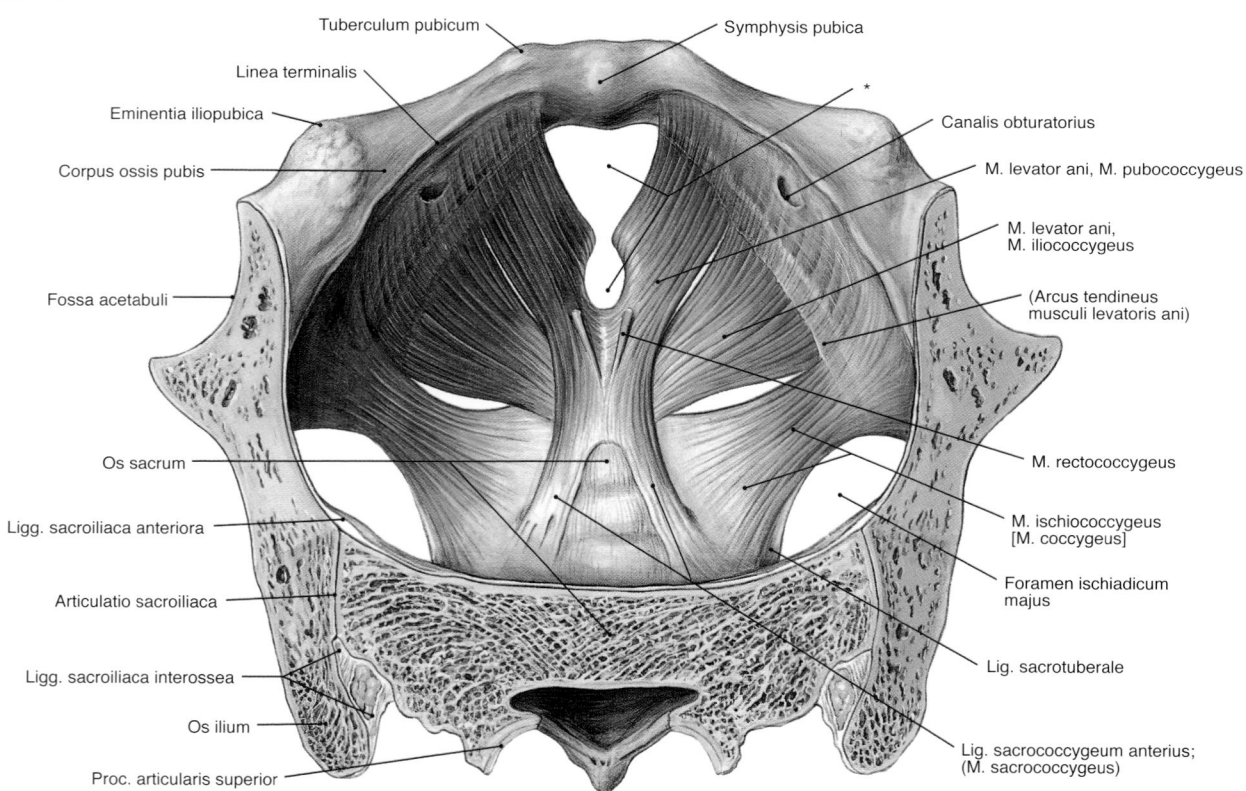

Fig. 902   Pelvic diaphragm, Diaphragma pelvis, of the female; superior view.

* Clinical term: levator hiatus (Hiatus urogenitalis et ani)

Female pelvic diaphragm

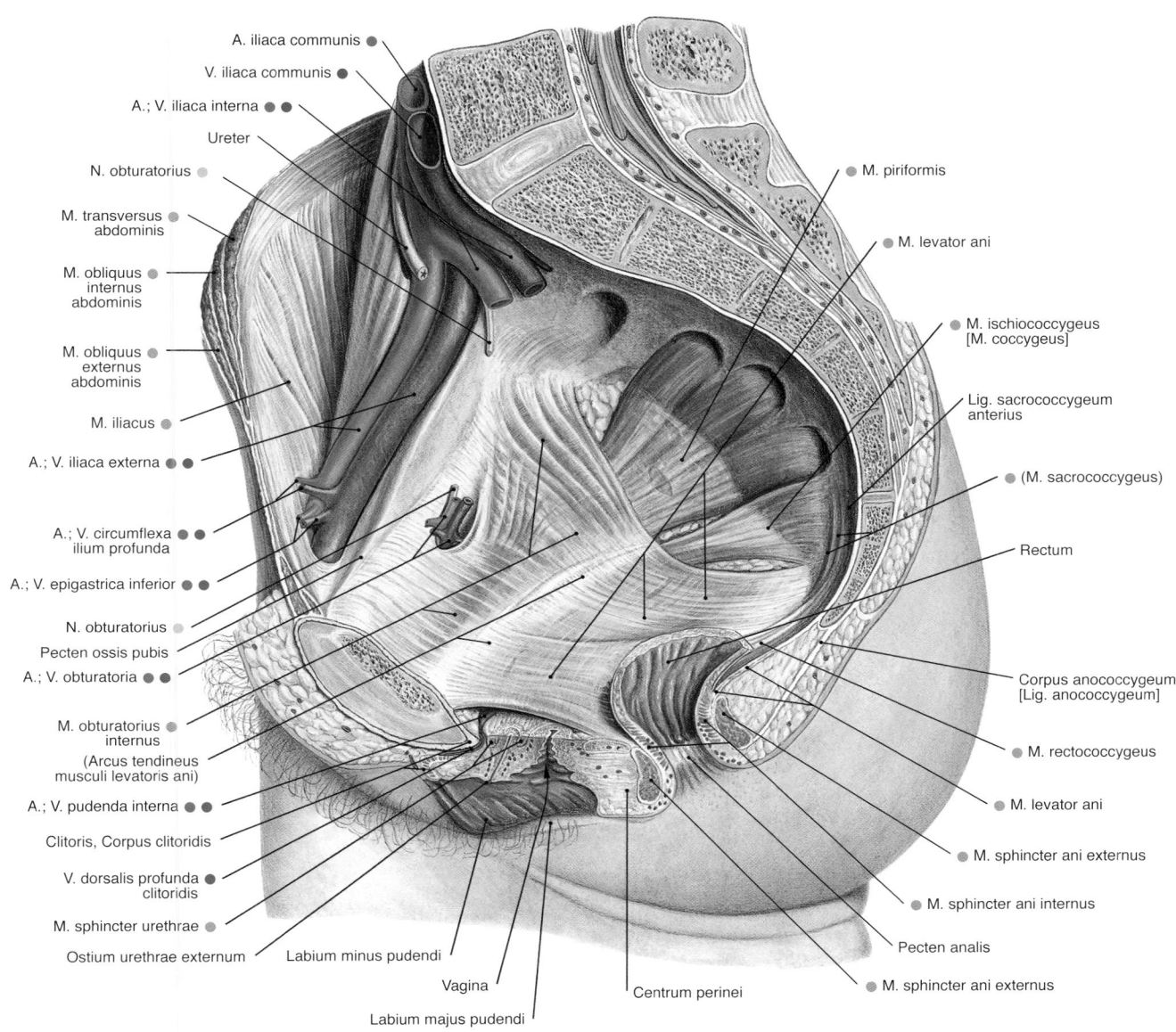

A. iliaca communis ●
V. iliaca communis ●
A.; V. iliaca interna ● ●
Ureter
N. obturatorius ●
M. transversus ● abdominis
M. obliquus ● internus abdominis
M. obliquus ● externus abdominis
M. iliacus ●
A.; V. iliaca externa ● ●
A.; V. circumflexa ● ● ilium profunda
A.; V. epigastrica inferior ● ●
N. obturatorius ●
Pecten ossis pubis
A.; V. obturatoria ● ●
M. obturatorius ● internus
(Arcus tendineus musculi levatoris ani)
A.; V. pudenda interna ● ●
Clitoris, Corpus clitoridis
V. dorsalis profunda ● clitoridis
M. sphincter urethrae ●
Ostium urethrae externum
Labium minus pudendi
Vagina
Labium majus pudendi

● M. piriformis
● M. levator ani
● M. ischiococcygeus [M. coccygeus]
Lig. sacrococcygeum anterius
● (M. sacrococcygeus)
Rectum
Corpus anococcygeum [Lig. anococcygeum]
● M. rectococcygeus
● M. levator ani
● M. sphincter ani externus
● M. sphincter ani internus
Pecten analis
● M. sphincter ani externus
Centrum perinei

Fig. 903 Muscles of the pelvic diaphragm, Diaphragma pelvis, of the female.

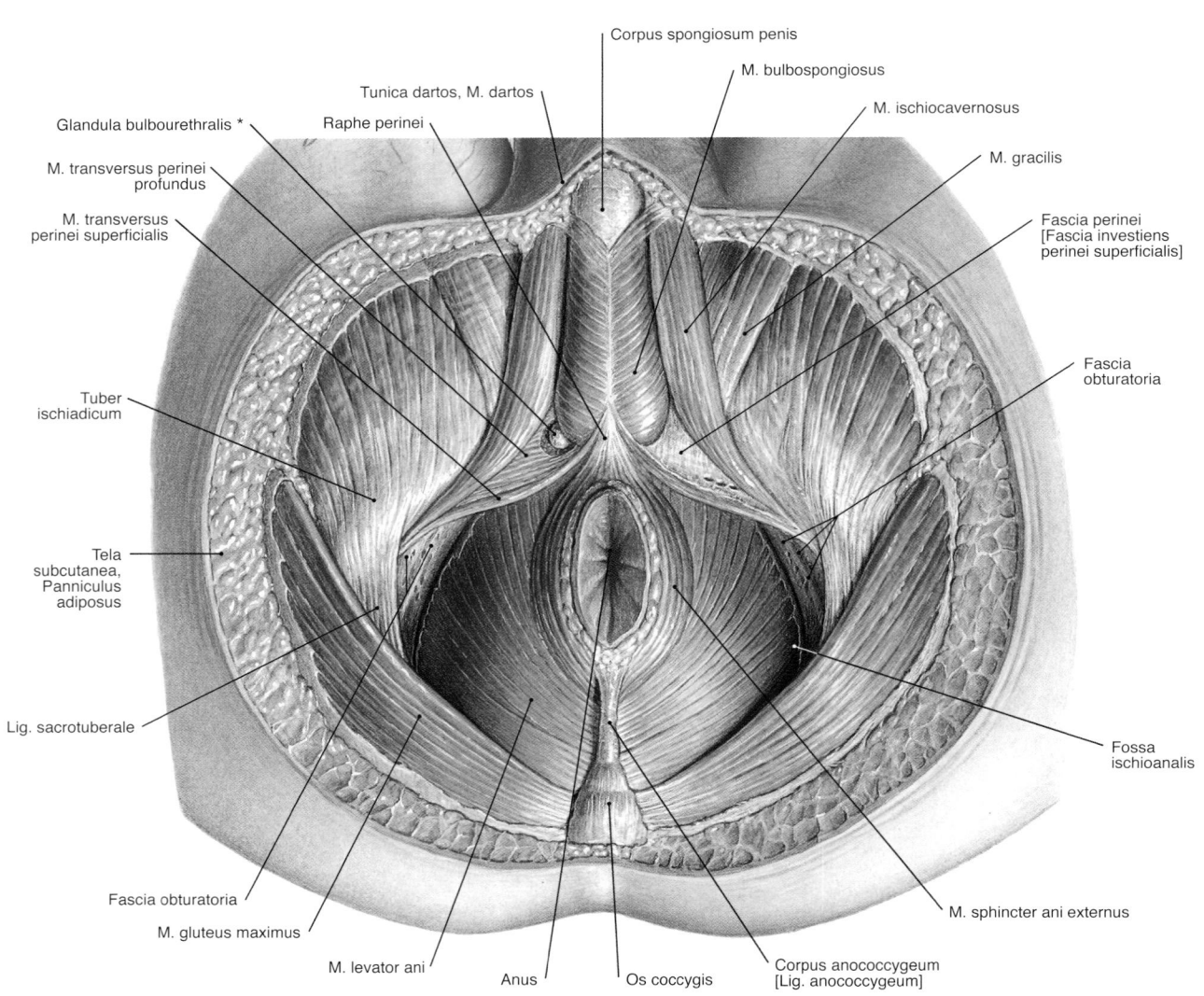

Glandula bulbourethralis *

M. transversus perinei profundus

M. transversus perinei superficialis

Tunica dartos, M. dartos

Raphe perinei

Corpus spongiosum penis

M. bulbospongiosus

M. ischiocavernosus

M. gracilis

Fascia perinei [Fascia investiens perinei superficialis]

Fascia obturatoria

Tuber ischiadicum

Tela subcutanea, Panniculus adiposus

Lig. sacrotuberale

Fascia obturatoria

M. gluteus maximus

M. levator ani

Anus

Os coccygis

Corpus anococcygeum [Lig. anococcygeum]

M. sphincter ani externus

Fossa ischioanalis

→ T 22

Fig. 904 Perineum, Perineum, and pelvic diaphragm, Diaphragma pelvis, of the male; inferior view.
* Clinical term: COWPER's gland

Female pelvic diaphragm

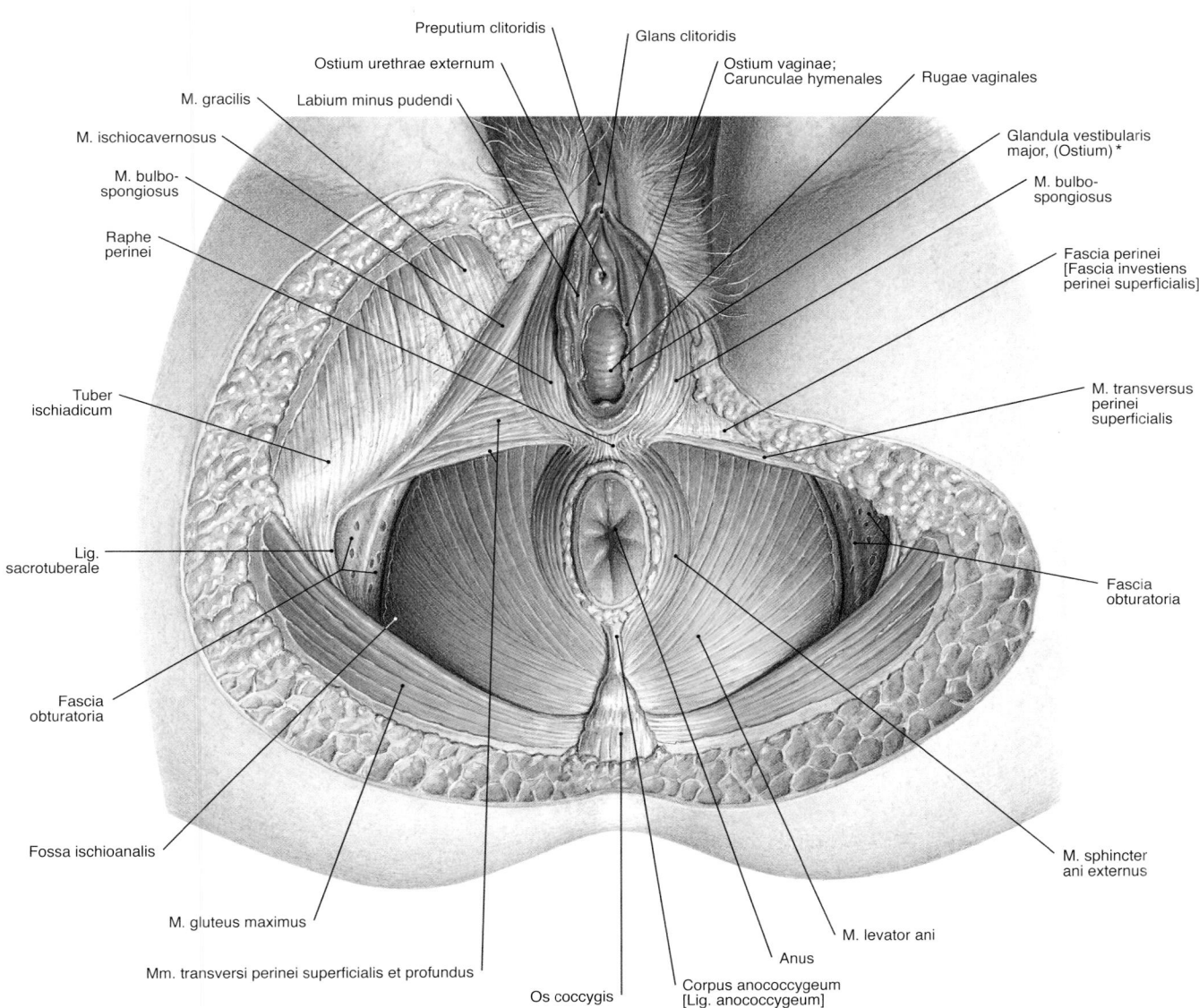

Preputium clitoridis
Glans clitoridis
Ostium urethrae externum
Ostium vaginae;
Carunculae hymenales
Rugae vaginales
M. gracilis
Labium minus pudendi
M. ischiocavernosus
Glandula vestibularis
major, (Ostium) *
M. bulbo-
spongiosus
M. bulbo-
spongiosus
Raphe
perinei
Fascia perinei
[Fascia investiens
perinei superficialis]
Tuber
ischiadicum
M. transversus
perinei
superficialis
Lig.
sacrotuberale
Fascia
obturatoria
Fascia
obturatoria
M. sphincter
ani externus
Fossa ischioanalis
M. gluteus maximus
M. levator ani
Mm. transversi perinei superficialis et profundus
Anus
Os coccygis
Corpus anococcygeum
[Lig. anococcygeum]

Fig. 905 Perineum, Perineum; pelvic diaphragm,
Diaphragma pelvis, and female external genitalia,
Organa genitalia feminina externa;
inferior view.
* Clinical term: BARTHOLIN's gland

→ T 22

The vaginal and the anal orifices are located in close proximity.
During delivery the skin and muscles of the perineum can
rupture up to the sphincter muscles of the anus (I. – III. degree
perineal lacerations). These can be prevented by surgical
incisions directed either laterally or in the median plane
(perineal incision = lateral or medial episiotomy).

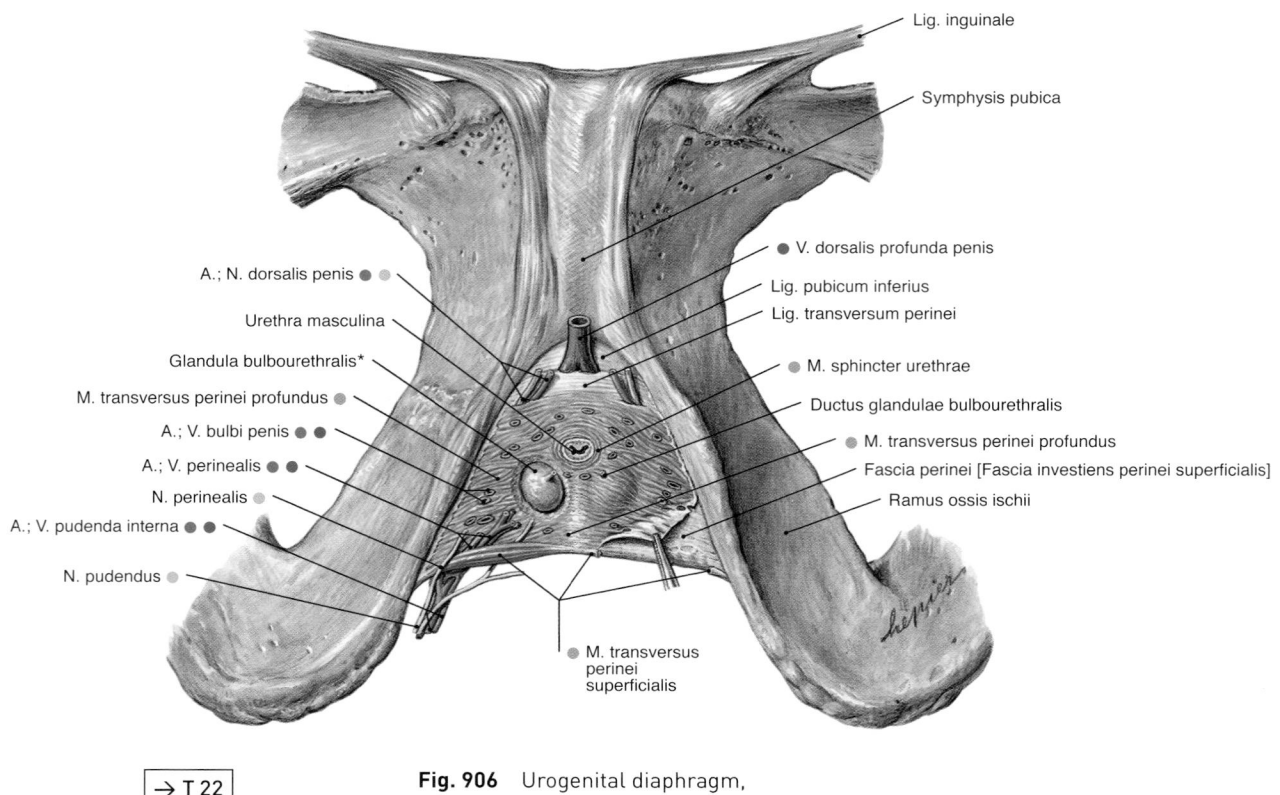

A.; N. dorsalis penis ● ●
Urethra masculina
Glandula bulbourethralis*
M. transversus perinei profundus ●
A.; V. bulbi penis ● ●
A.; V. perinealis ● ●
N. perinealis ●
A.; V. pudenda interna ● ●
N. pudendus ●

V. dorsalis profunda penis ●
Lig. pubicum inferius
Lig. transversum perinei
M. sphincter urethrae ●
Ductus glandulae bulbourethralis
M. transversus perinei profundus ●
Fascia perinei [Fascia investiens perinei superficialis]
Ramus ossis ischii

Lig. inguinale
Symphysis pubica

M. transversus
perinei
superficialis ●

→ T 22

Fig. 906 Urogenital diaphragm,
Diaphragma urogenitale, of the male;
inferior view.
* Clinical term: COWPER's gland

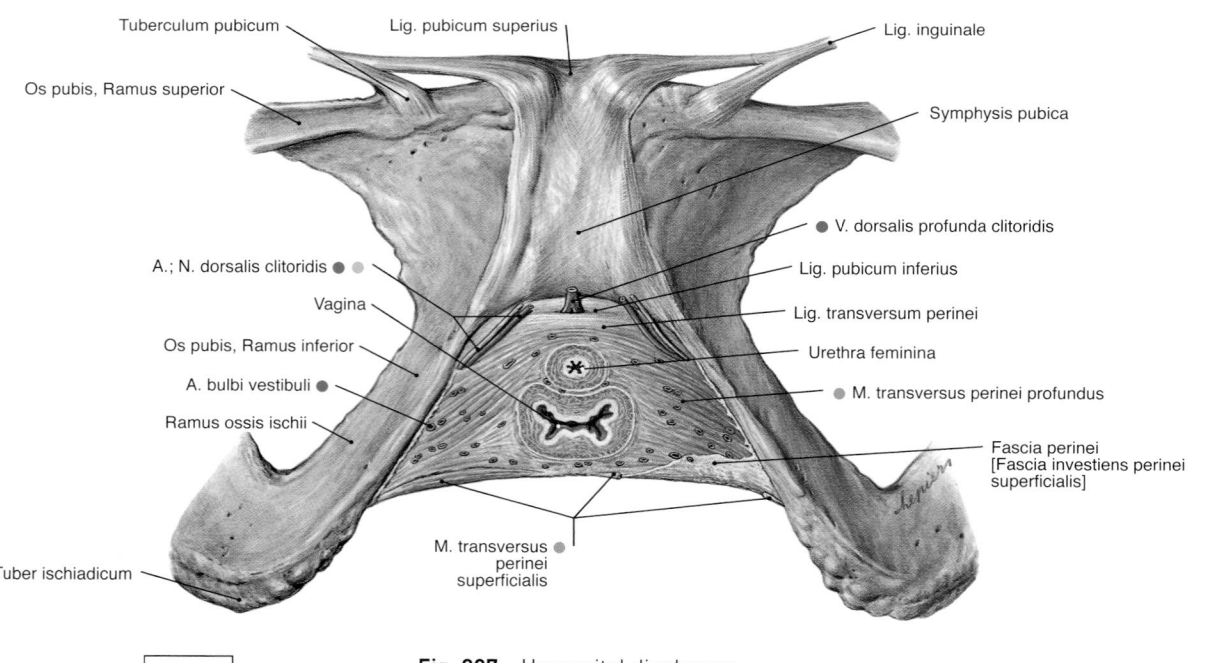

Tuberculum pubicum
Os pubis, Ramus superior

A.; N. dorsalis clitoridis ● ●
Vagina
Os pubis, Ramus inferior
A. bulbi vestibuli ●
Ramus ossis ischii

Tuber ischiadicum

M. transversus ●
perinei
superficialis

Lig. pubicum superius
Lig. inguinale
Symphysis pubica

V. dorsalis profunda clitoridis ●
Lig. pubicum inferius
Lig. transversum perinei
Urethra feminina
M. transversus perinei profundus ●
Fascia perinei
[Fascia investiens perinei
superficialis]

→ T 22

Fig. 907 Urogenital diaphragm,
Diaphragma urogenitale, of the female;
inferior view.

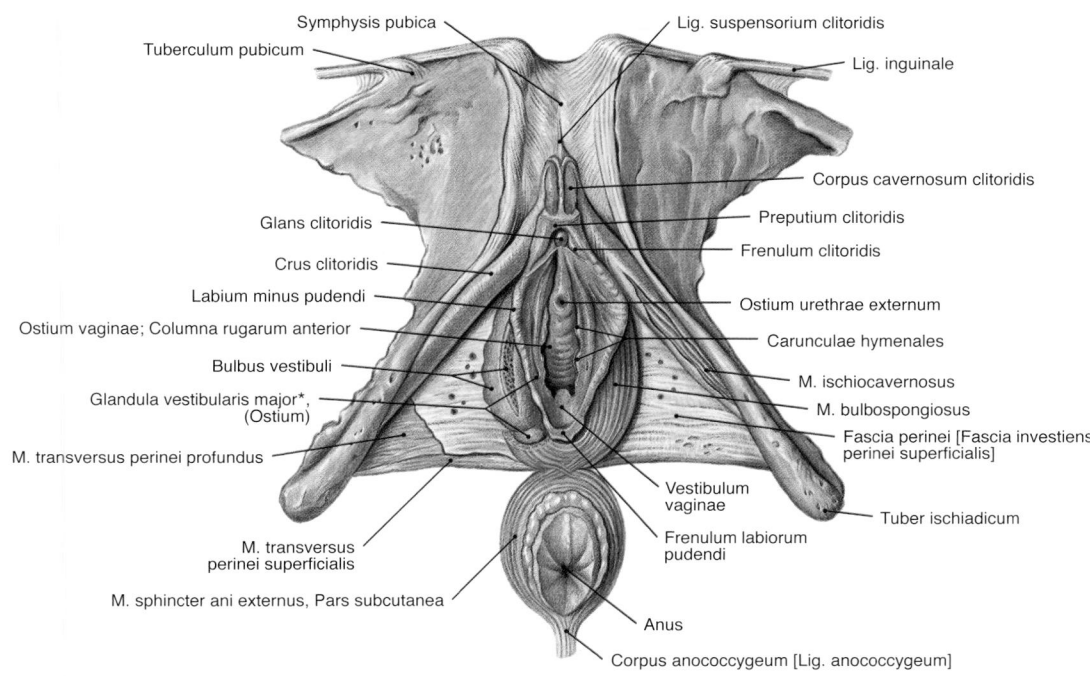

Symphysis pubica

Tuberculum pubicum

Lig. suspensorium clitoridis

Lig. inguinale

Corpus cavernosum clitoridis

Glans clitoridis

Preputium clitoridis

Crus clitoridis

Frenulum clitoridis

Labium minus pudendi

Ostium urethrae externum

Ostium vaginae; Columna rugarum anterior

Carunculae hymenales

Bulbus vestibuli

M. ischiocavernosus

Glandula vestibularis major*, (Ostium)

M. bulbospongiosus

M. transversus perinei profundus

Fascia perinei [Fascia investiens perinei superficialis]

Vestibulum vaginae

Tuber ischiadicum

M. transversus perinei superficialis

Frenulum labiorum pudendi

M. sphincter ani externus, Pars subcutanea

Anus

Corpus anococcygeum [Lig. anococcygeum]

Fig. 908 Female external genitalia, Organa genitalia feminina externa; ventroinferior view.

* Clinical term: BARTHOLIN's gland

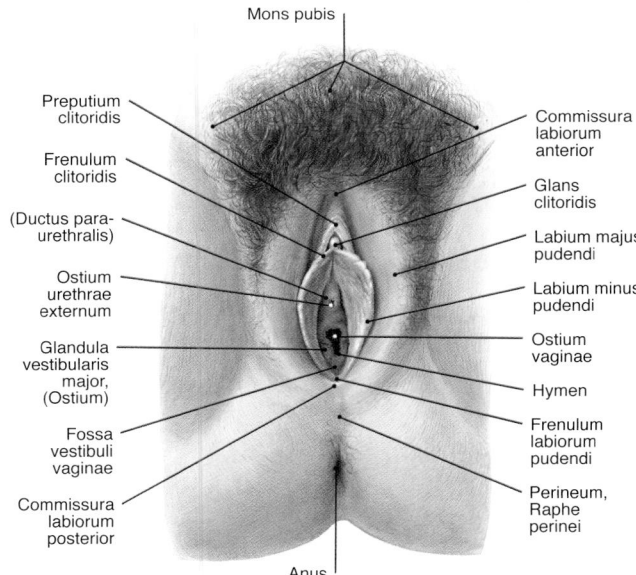

Mons pubis

Preputium clitoridis

Frenulum clitoridis

(Ductus para-urethralis)

Ostium urethrae externum

Glandula vestibularis major, (Ostium)

Fossa vestibuli vaginae

Commissura labiorum posterior

Anus

Commissura labiorum anterior

Glans clitoridis

Labium majus pudendi

Labium minus pudendi

Ostium vaginae

Hymen

Frenulum labiorum pudendi

Perineum, Raphe perinei

Fig. 909 Female external genitalia, Organa genitalia feminina externa; inferior view.

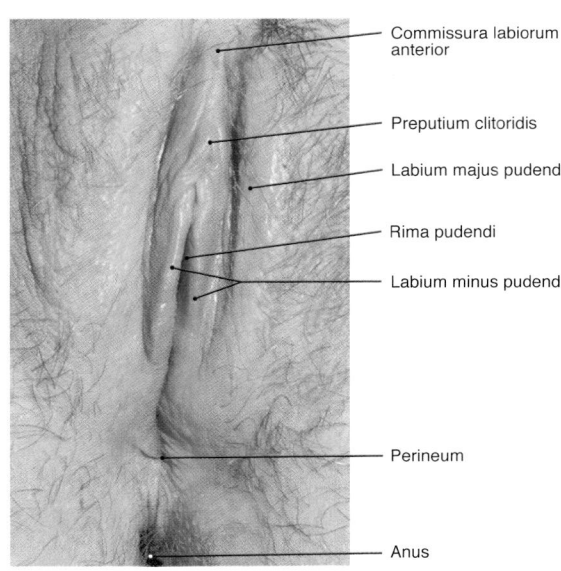

Commissura labiorum anterior

Preputium clitoridis

Labium majus pudendi

Rima pudendi

Labium minus pudendi

Perineum

Anus

Fig. 910 Female external genitalia, Organa genitalia feminina externa; inferior view.

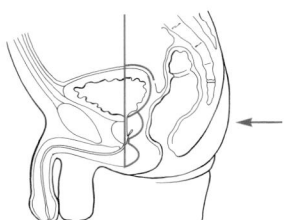

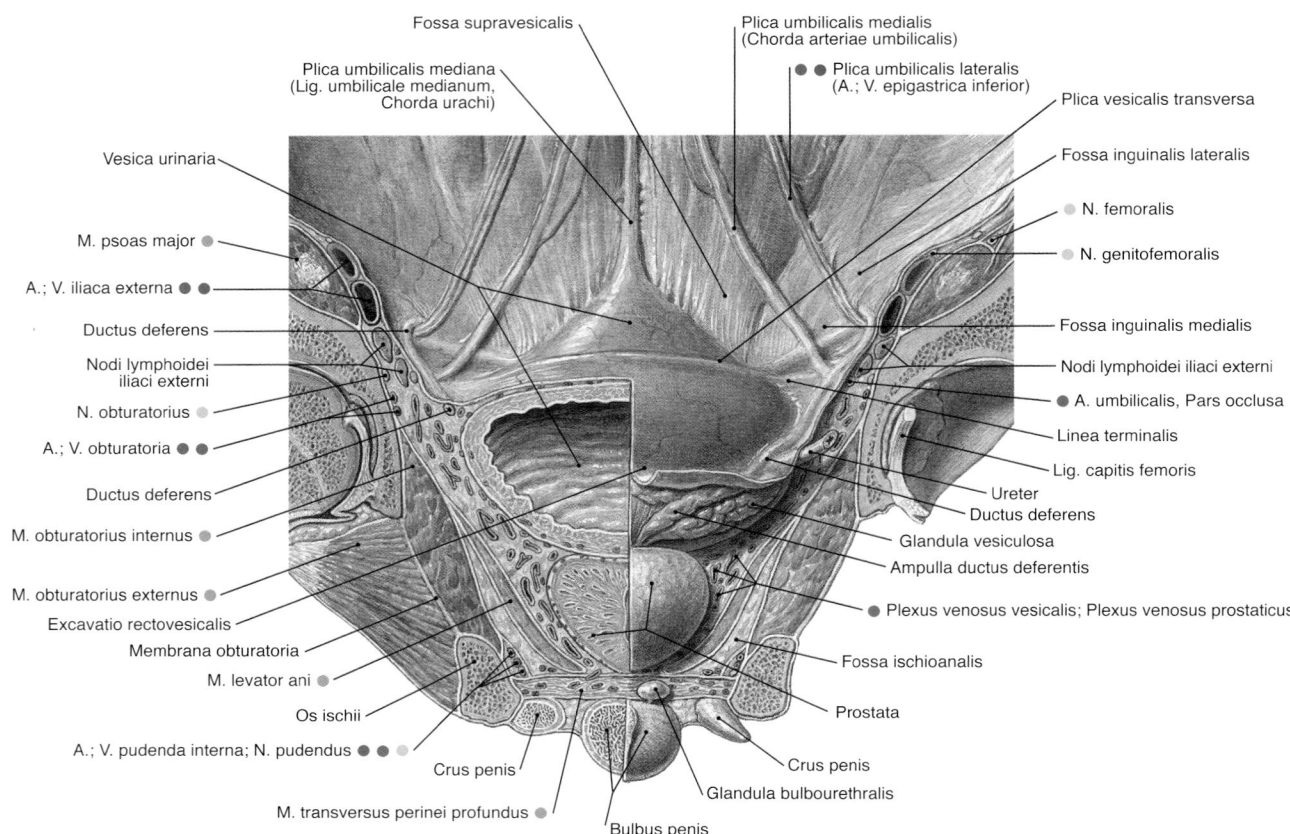

Fossa supravesicalis

Plica umbilicalis mediana
(Lig. umbilicale medianum,
Chorda urachi)

Vesica urinaria

M. psoas major ●

A.; V. iliaca externa ● ●

Ductus deferens

Nodi lymphoidei
iliaci externi

N. obturatorius ●

A.; V. obturatoria ● ●

Ductus deferens

M. obturatorius internus ●

M. obturatorius externus ●

Excavatio rectovesicalis

Membrana obturatoria

M. levator ani ●

Os ischii

A.; V. pudenda interna; N. pudendus ● ● ●

M. transversus perinei profundus ●

Crus penis

Bulbus penis

Plica umbilicalis medialis
(Chorda arteriae umbilicalis)

● ● Plica umbilicalis lateralis
(A.; V. epigastrica inferior)

Plica vesicalis transversa

Fossa inguinalis lateralis

● N. femoralis

● N. genitofemoralis

Fossa inguinalis medialis

Nodi lymphoidei iliaci externi

● A. umbilicalis, Pars occlusa

Linea terminalis

Lig. capitis femoris

Ureter

Ductus deferens

Glandula vesiculosa

Ampulla ductus deferentis

● Plexus venosus vesicalis; Plexus venosus prostaticus

Fossa ischioanalis

Prostata

Crus penis

Glandula bulbourethralis

Fig. 911   Pelvic diaphragm, Diaphragma pelvis;
pelvic organs and anterior abdominal wall,
Organa abdominis et pelvis, of the male;
frontal section through the head of the femur
and the urinary bladder on the left;
dorsal view.

Female pelvic organs and retroperitoneal space

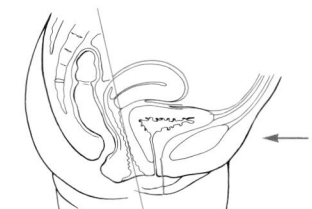

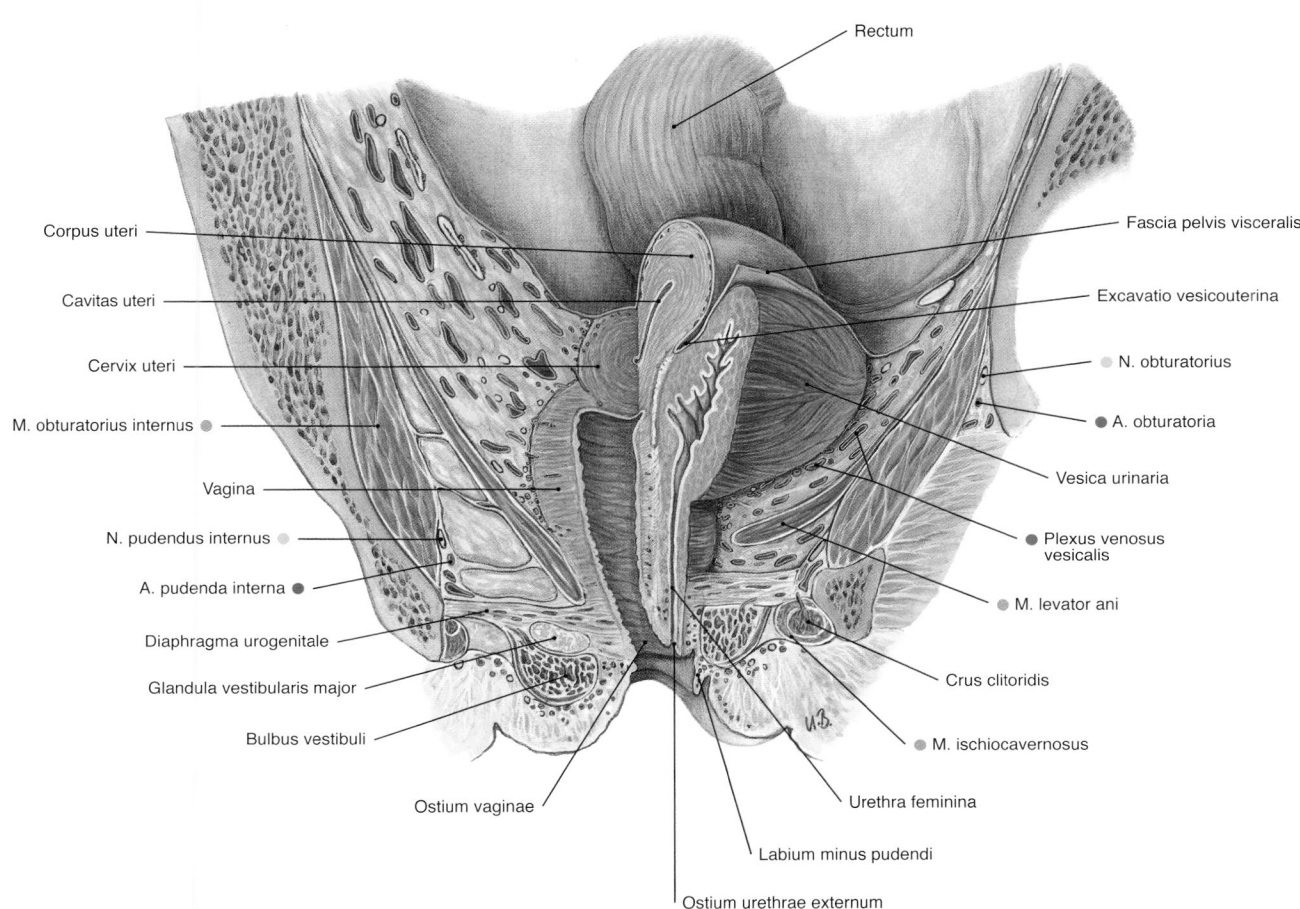

Rectum

Corpus uteri

Cavitas uteri

Cervix uteri

M. obturatorius internus ●

Vagina

N. pudendus internus ●

A. pudenda interna ●

Diaphragma urogenitale

Glandula vestibularis major

Bulbus vestibuli

Ostium vaginae

Fascia pelvis visceralis

Excavatio vesicouterina

● N. obturatorius

● A. obturatoria

Vesica urinaria

● Plexus venosus vesicalis

● M. levator ani

Crus clitoridis

● M. ischiocavernosus

Urethra feminina

Labium minus pudendi

Ostium urethrae externum

Fig. 912   Pelvic diaphragm, Diaphragma pelvis, and
pelvic organs, Organa pelvis, of the female;
frontal section (on the right) combined with a median section;
ventral view.

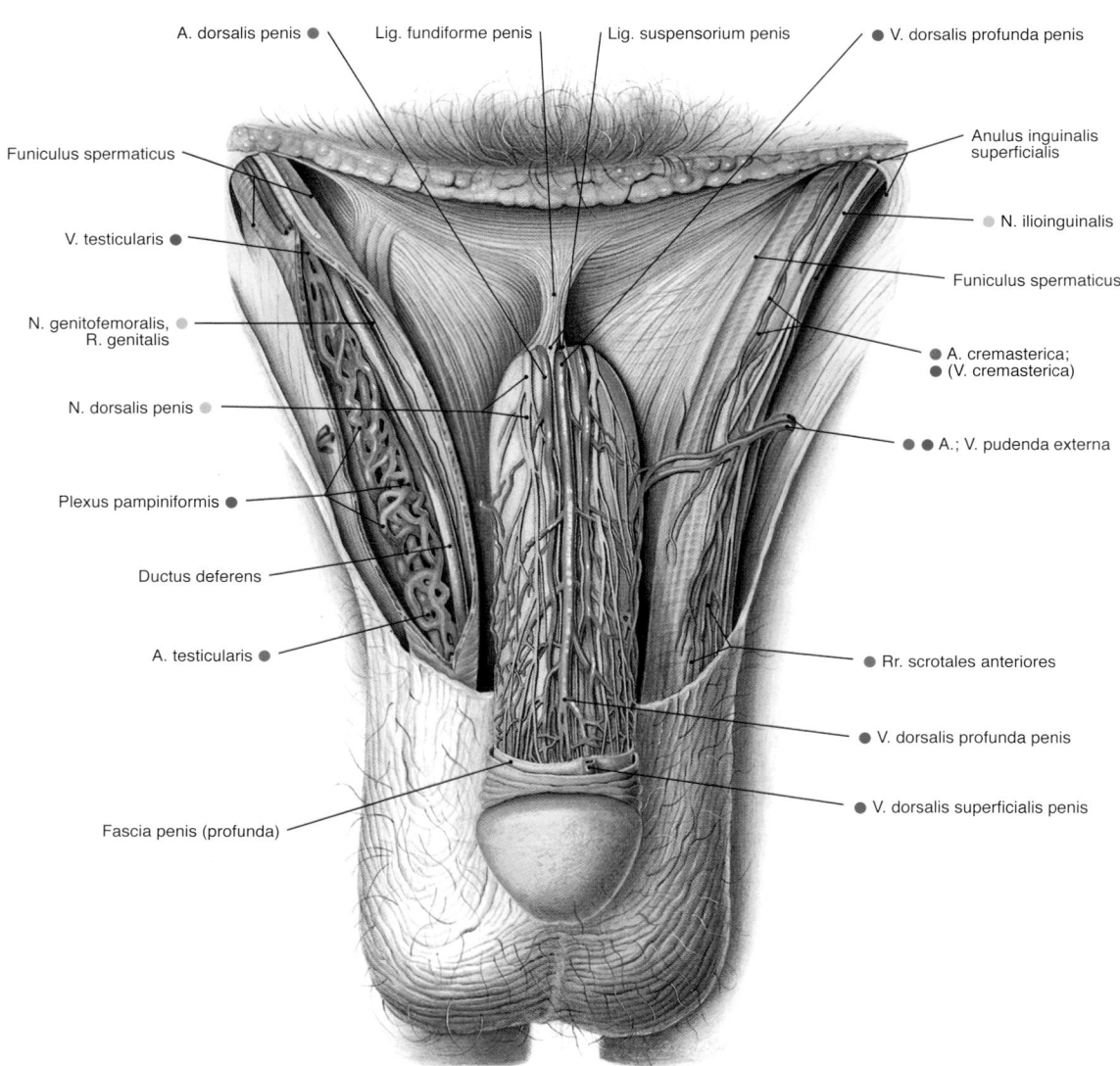

A. dorsalis penis ●
Lig. fundiforme penis
Lig. suspensorium penis
● V. dorsalis profunda penis

Funiculus spermaticus

Anulus inguinalis
superficialis

V. testicularis ●

● N. ilioinguinalis

Funiculus spermaticus

N. genitofemoralis, ●
R. genitalis

● A. cremasterica;
● (V. cremasterica)

N. dorsalis penis ●

● ● A.; V. pudenda externa

Plexus pampiniformis ●

Ductus deferens

A. testicularis ●

● Rr. scrotales anteriores

● V. dorsalis profunda penis

● V. dorsalis superficialis penis

Fascia penis (profunda)

Fig. 913   Male external genitalia,
Organa genitalia masculina externa.

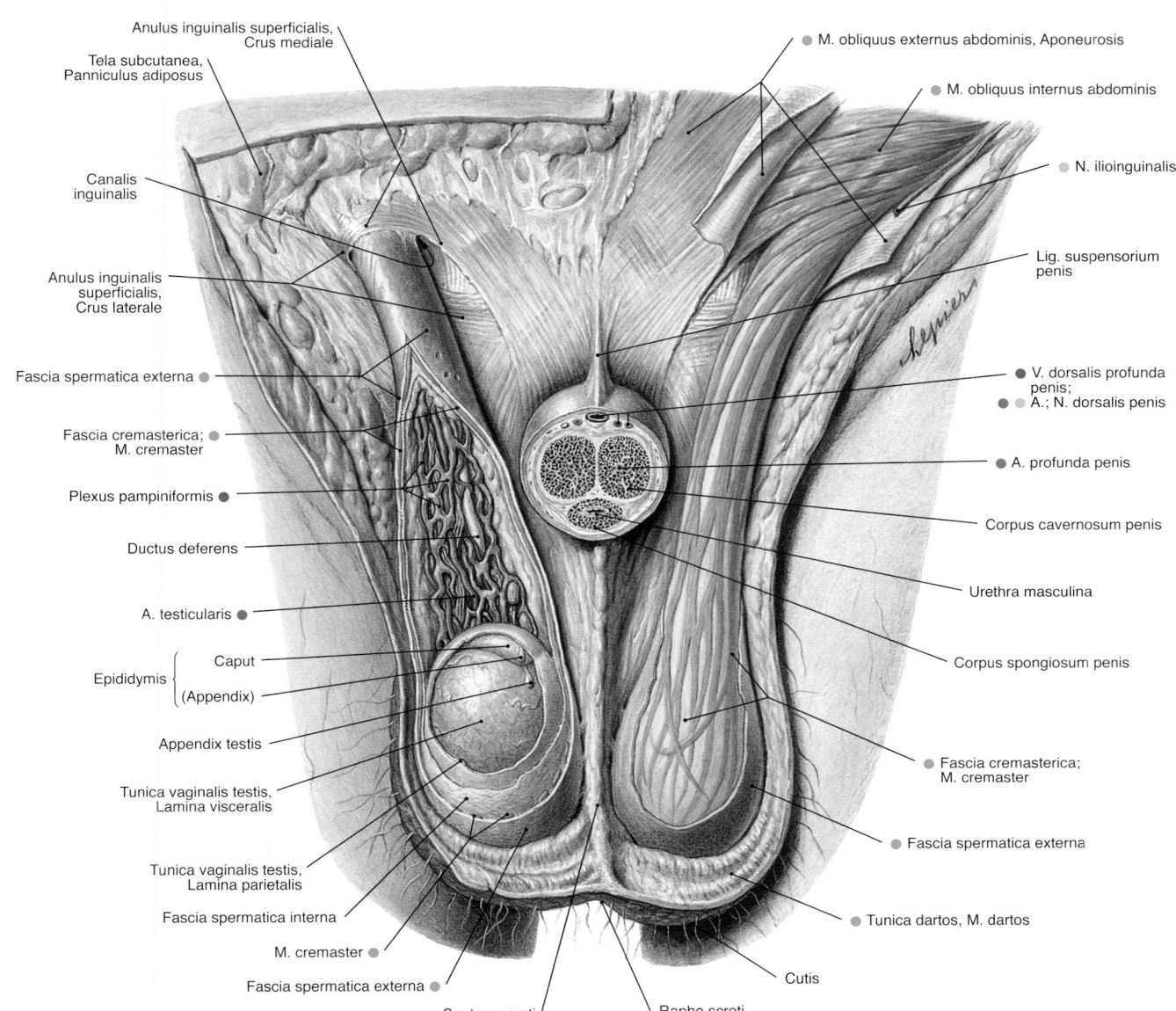

Anulus inguinalis superficialis, Crus mediale

Tela subcutanea, Panniculus adiposus

Canalis inguinalis

Anulus inguinalis superficialis, Crus laterale

Fascia spermatica externa ●

Fascia cremasterica; M. cremaster ●

Plexus pampiniformis ●

Ductus deferens

A. testicularis ●

Epididymis { Caput
(Appendix) }

Appendix testis

Tunica vaginalis testis, Lamina visceralis

Tunica vaginalis testis, Lamina parietalis

Fascia spermatica interna

M. cremaster ●

Fascia spermatica externa ●

Septum scroti

M. obliquus externus abdominis, Aponeurosis ●

M. obliquus internus abdominis ●

N. ilioinguinalis ●

Lig. suspensorium penis

V. dorsalis profunda penis; ●
A.; N. dorsalis penis ● ●

A. profunda penis ●

Corpus cavernosum penis

Urethra masculina

Corpus spongiosum penis

Fascia cremasterica; M. cremaster ●

Fascia spermatica externa ●

Tunica dartos, M. dartos ●

Cutis

Raphe scroti

Fig. 914 Male genitalia, Organa genitalia masculina.

→ 837, 849

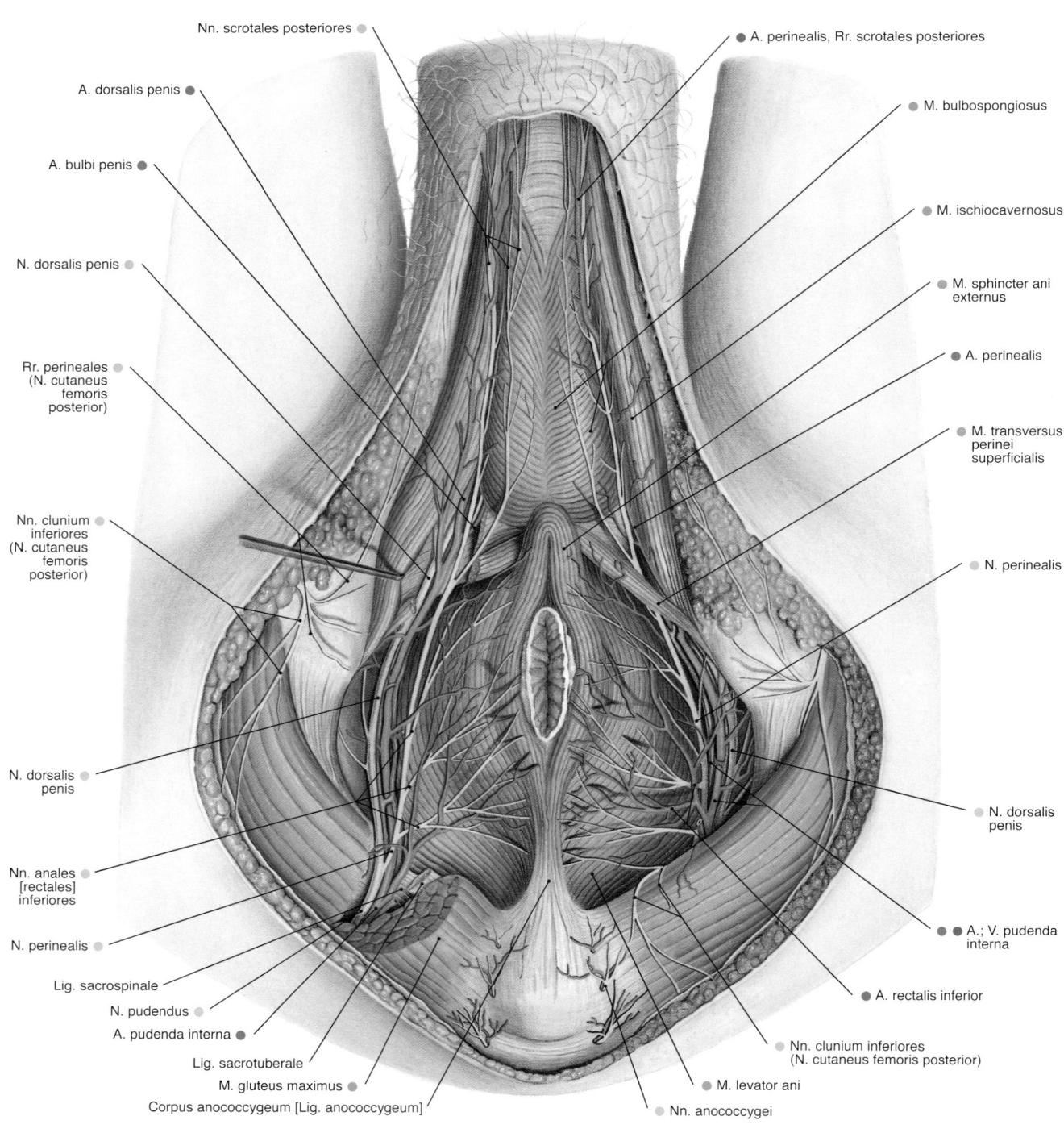

Nn. scrotales posteriores

A. dorsalis penis

A. bulbi penis

N. dorsalis penis

Rr. perineales
(N. cutaneus
femoris
posterior)

Nn. clunium
inferiores
(N. cutaneus
femoris
posterior)

N. dorsalis
penis

Nn. anales
[rectales]
inferiores

N. perinealis

Lig. sacrospinale

N. pudendus

A. pudenda interna

Lig. sacrotuberale

M. gluteus maximus

Corpus anococcygeum [Lig. anococcygeum]

A. perinealis, Rr. scrotales posteriores

M. bulbospongiosus

M. ischiocavernosus

M. sphincter ani
externus

A. perinealis

M. transversus
perinei
superficialis

N. perinealis

N. dorsalis
penis

A.; V. pudenda
interna

A. rectalis inferior

Nn. clunium inferiores
(N. cutaneus femoris posterior)

M. levator ani

Nn. anococcygei

Fig. 915   Vessels and nerves of the perineum,
Regio perinealis, and the male external genitalia,
Organa genitalia masculina externa.

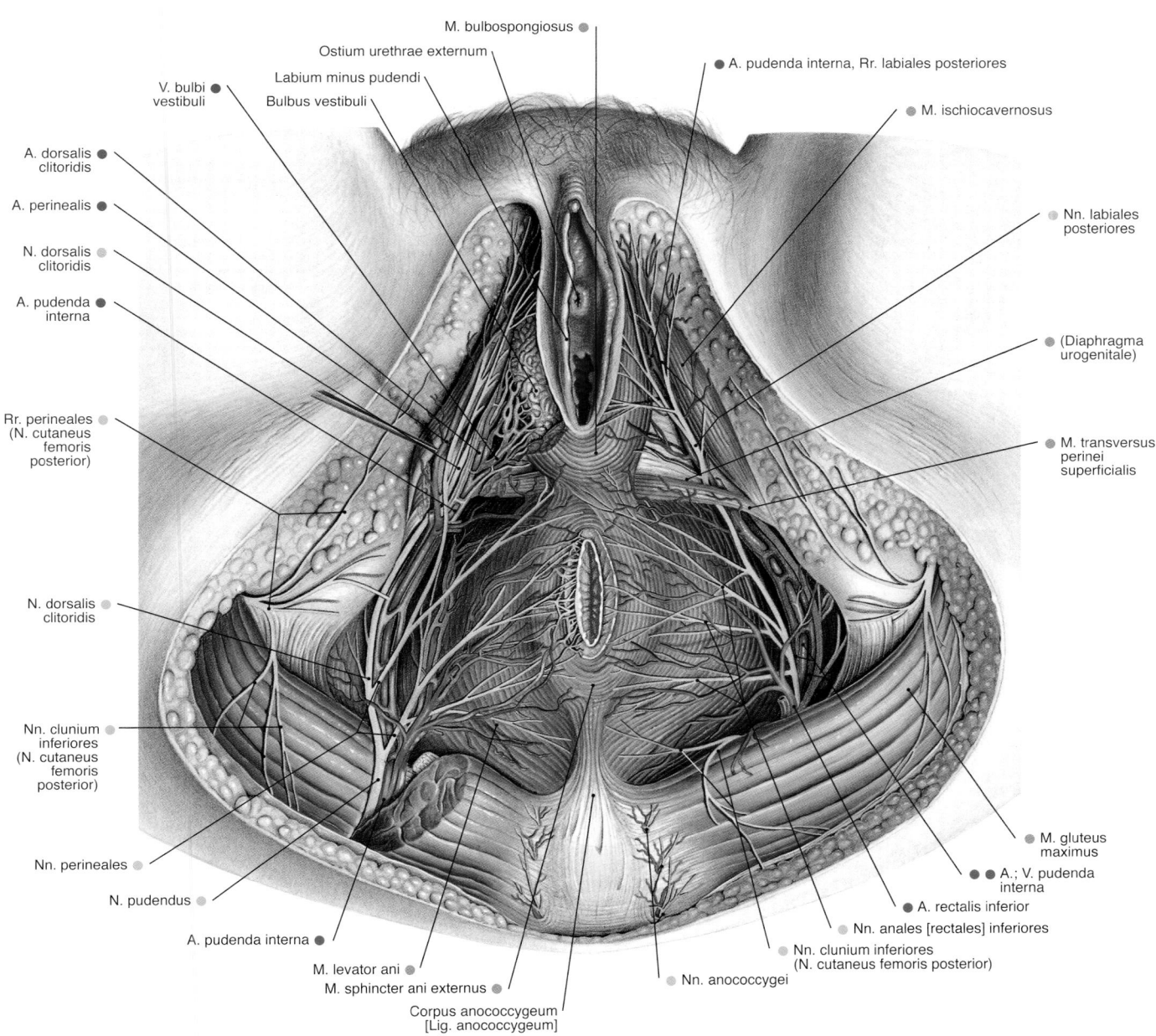

M. bulbospongiosus ●

Ostium urethrae externum

V. bulbi ● vestibuli

Labium minus pudendi

Bulbus vestibuli

● A. pudenda interna, Rr. labiales posteriores

● M. ischiocavernosus

A. dorsalis ● clitoridis

A. perinealis ●

N. dorsalis ● clitoridis

A. pudenda ● interna

● Nn. labiales posteriores

● (Diaphragma urogenitale)

Rr. perineales ● (N. cutaneus femoris posterior)

● M. transversus perinei superficialis

N. dorsalis ● clitoridis

Nn. clunium ● inferiores (N. cutaneus femoris posterior)

● M. gluteus maximus

Nn. perineales ●

● ● A.; V. pudenda interna

N. pudendus ●

● A. rectalis inferior

A. pudenda interna ●

● Nn. anales [rectales] inferiores

M. levator ani ●

● Nn. clunium inferiores (N. cutaneus femoris posterior)

M. sphincter ani externus ●

● Nn. anococcygei

Corpus anococcygeum [Lig. anococcygeum]

Fig. 916 Vessels and nerves of the perineum,
Regio perinealis, and the female external genitalia,
Organa genitalia feminina externa.

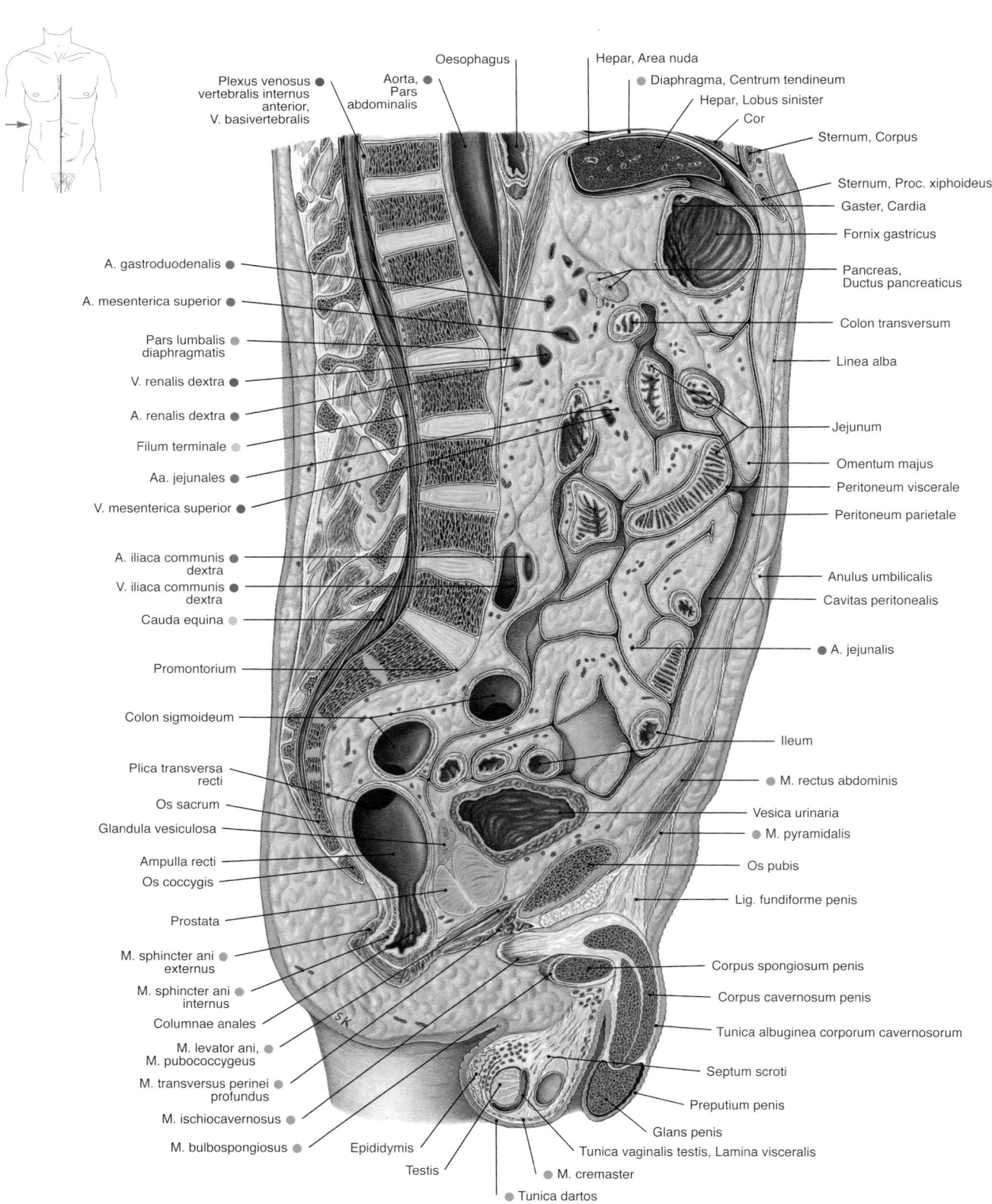

Plexus venosus vertebralis internus anterior, V. basivertebralis

Oesophagus

Aorta, Pars abdominalis

Hepar, Area nuda

Diaphragma, Centrum tendineum

Hepar, Lobus sinister

Cor

Sternum, Corpus

Sternum, Proc. xiphoideus

Gaster, Cardia

Fornix gastricus

A. gastroduodenalis

A. mesenterica superior

Pars lumbalis diaphragmatis

V. renalis dextra

A. renalis dextra

Filum terminale

Aa. jejunales

V. mesenterica superior

A. iliaca communis dextra

V. iliaca communis dextra

Cauda equina

Promontorium

Colon sigmoideum

Plica transversa recti

Os sacrum

Glandula vesiculosa

Ampulla recti

Os coccygis

Prostata

M. sphincter ani externus

M. sphincter ani internus

Columnae anales

M. levator ani, M. pubococcygeus

M. transversus perinei profundus

M. ischiocavernosus

M. bulbospongiosus

Epididymis

Testis

Pancreas, Ductus pancreaticus

Colon transversum

Linea alba

Jejunum

Omentum majus

Peritoneum viscerale

Peritoneum parietale

Anulus umbilicalis

Cavitas peritonealis

A. jejunalis

Ileum

M. rectus abdominis

Vesica urinaria

M. pyramidalis

Os pubis

Lig. fundiforme penis

Corpus spongiosum penis

Corpus cavernosum penis

Tunica albuginea corporum cavernosorum

Septum scroti

Preputium penis

Glans penis

Tunica vaginalis testis, Lamina visceralis

M. cremaster

Tunica dartos

Fig. 917 Abdomen, Abdomen, and pelvis, Pelvis, of the male; median section.

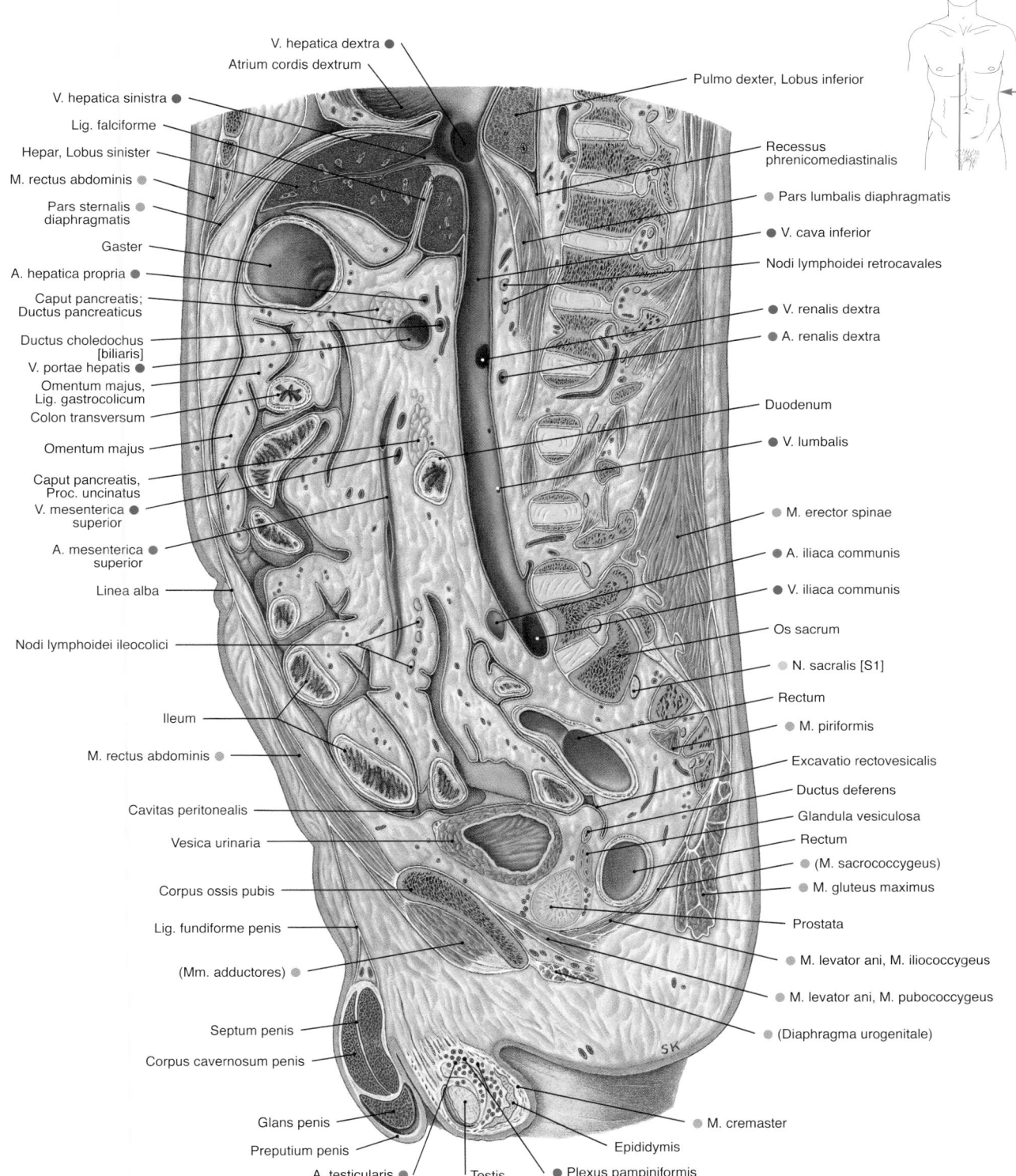

V. hepatica dextra ●
Atrium cordis dextrum
V. hepatica sinistra ●
Lig. falciforme
Hepar, Lobus sinister
M. rectus abdominis ●
Pars sternalis diaphragmatis ●
Gaster
A. hepatica propria ●
Caput pancreatis; Ductus pancreaticus
Ductus choledochus [biliaris]
V. portae hepatis ●
Omentum majus, Lig. gastrocolicum
Colon transversum
Omentum majus
Caput pancreatis, Proc. uncinatus
V. mesenterica ● superior
A. mesenterica ● superior
Linea alba
Nodi lymphoidei ileocolici
Ileum
M. rectus abdominis ●
Cavitas peritonealis
Vesica urinaria
Corpus ossis pubis
Lig. fundiforme penis
(Mm. adductores) ●
Septum penis
Corpus cavernosum penis
Glans penis
Preputium penis
A. testicularis ●
Testis

Pulmo dexter, Lobus inferior
Recessus phrenicomediastinalis
● Pars lumbalis diaphragmatis
● V. cava inferior
Nodi lymphoidei retrocavales
● V. renalis dextra
● A. renalis dextra
Duodenum
● V. lumbalis
● M. erector spinae
● A. iliaca communis
● V. iliaca communis
Os sacrum
● N. sacralis [S1]
Rectum
● M. piriformis
Excavatio rectovesicalis
Ductus deferens
Glandula vesiculosa
Rectum
● (M. sacrococcygeus)
● M. gluteus maximus
Prostata
● M. levator ani, M. iliococcygeus
● M. levator ani, M. pubococcygeus
● (Diaphragma urogenitale)
● M. cremaster
Epididymis
● Plexus pampiniformis

SK

Fig. 918 Abdomen, Abdomen, and pelvis, Pelvis, of the male;
sagittal section to the right of the median plane.

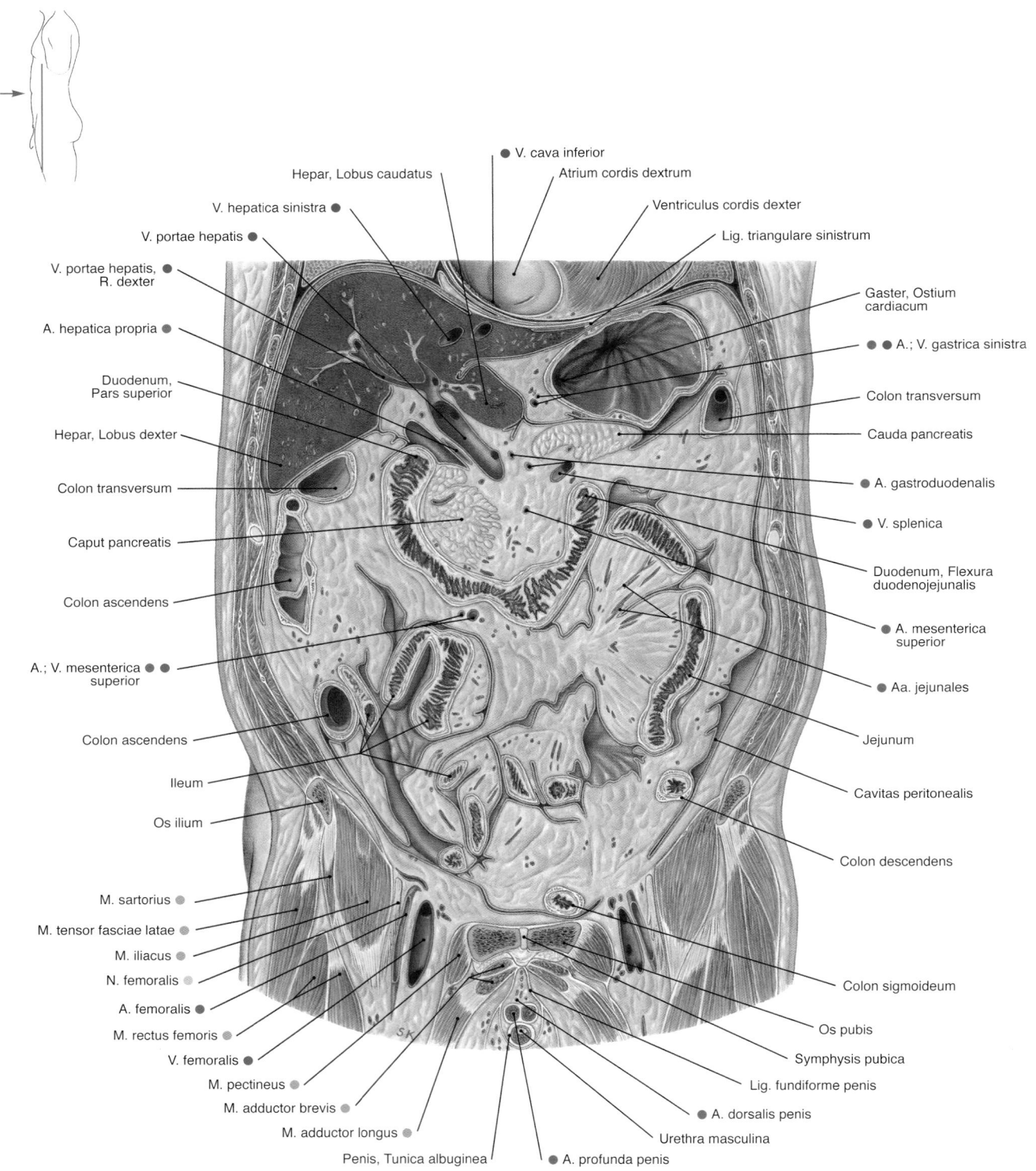

● V. cava inferior

Hepar, Lobus caudatus

Atrium cordis dextrum

V. hepatica sinistra ●

Ventriculus cordis dexter

V. portae hepatis ●

Lig. triangulare sinistrum

V. portae hepatis, ●
R. dexter

Gaster, Ostium
cardiacum

A. hepatica propria ●

● ● A.; V. gastrica sinistra

Duodenum,
Pars superior

Colon transversum

Hepar, Lobus dexter

Cauda pancreatis

Colon transversum

● A. gastroduodenalis

Caput pancreatis

● V. splenica

Colon ascendens

Duodenum, Flexura
duodenojejunalis

A.; V. mesenterica ● ● ●
superior

● A. mesenterica
superior

Colon ascendens

● Aa. jejunales

Ileum

Jejunum

Os ilium

Cavitas peritonealis

M. sartorius ●

Colon descendens

M. tensor fasciae latae ●

M. iliacus ●

N. femoralis ●

A. femoralis ●

Colon sigmoideum

M. rectus femoris ●

Os pubis

V. femoralis ●

Symphysis pubica

M. pectineus ●

Lig. fundiforme penis

M. adductor brevis ●

● A. dorsalis penis

M. adductor longus ●

Urethra masculina

Penis, Tunica albuginea

● A. profunda penis

→ 602

Fig. 919 Abdomen, Abdomen;
frontal section through the most anterior part of the abdominal cavity.

Upper abdomen, frontal section

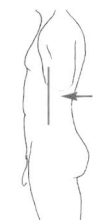

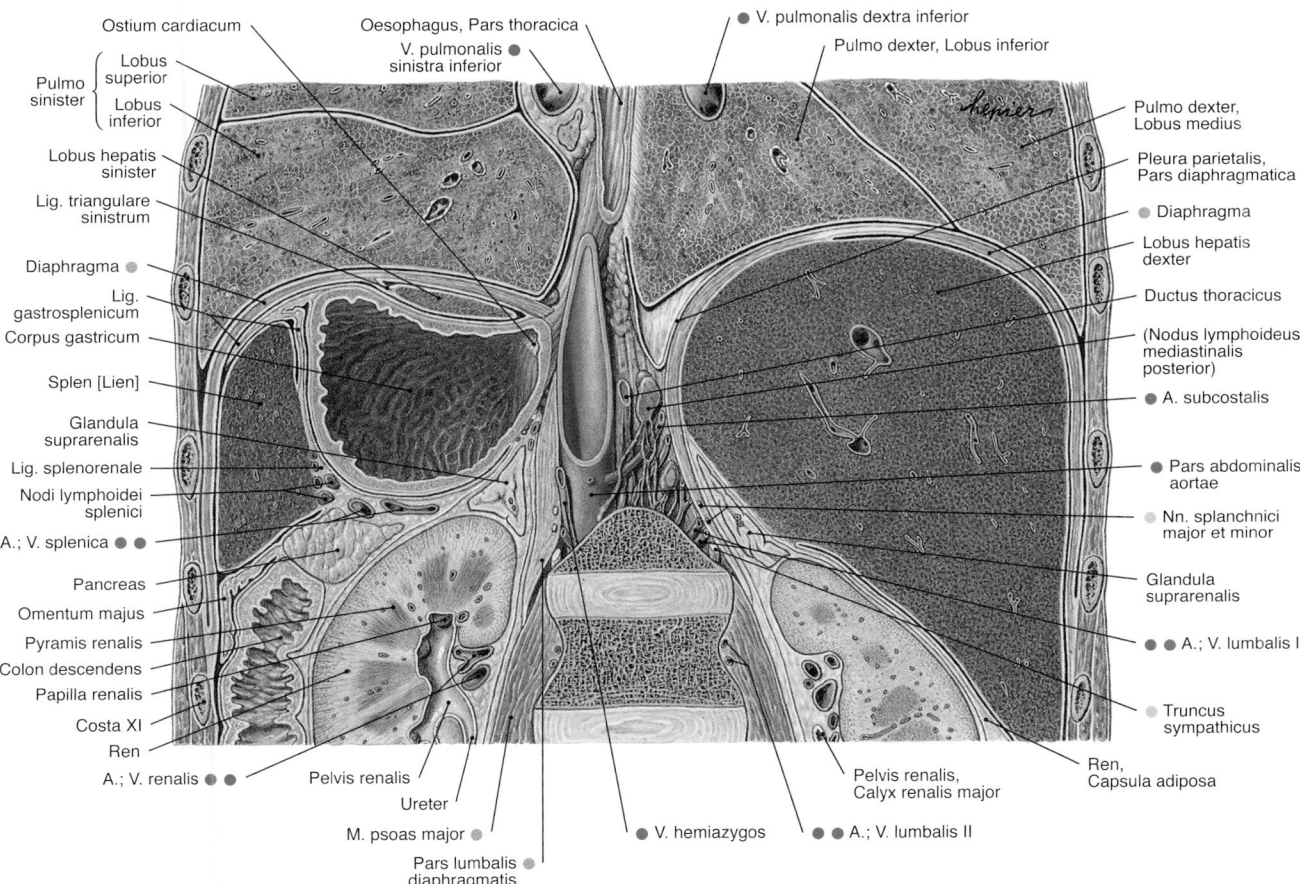

Ostium cardiacum

Oesophagus, Pars thoracica

● V. pulmonalis dextra inferior

V. pulmonalis ●
sinistra inferior

Pulmo dexter, Lobus inferior

Pulmo
sinister { Lobus
superior
Lobus
inferior

Lobus hepatis
sinister

Lig. triangulare
sinistrum

Diaphragma ●

Lig.
gastrosplenicum

Corpus gastricum

Splen [Lien]

Glandula
suprarenalis

Lig. splenorenale

Nodi lymphoidei
splenici

A.; V. splenica ● ●

Pancreas

Omentum majus

Pyramis renalis

Colon descendens

Papilla renalis

Costa XI

Ren

A.; V. renalis ● ●

Pelvis renalis

Ureter

M. psoas major ●

Pars lumbalis
diaphragmatis

V. hemiazygos ●

A.; V. lumbalis II ● ●

Pelvis renalis,
Calyx renalis major

Ren,
Capsula adiposa

Pulmo dexter,
Lobus medius

Pleura parietalis,
Pars diaphragmatica

● Diaphragma

Lobus hepatis
dexter

Ductus thoracicus

(Nodus lymphoideus
mediastinalis
posterior)

● A. subcostalis

● Pars abdominalis
aortae

● Nn. splanchnici
major et minor

Glandula
suprarenalis

● ● A.; V. lumbalis I

● Truncus
sympathicus

Fig. 920 Abdomen, Abdomen;
frontal section demonstrating the diaphragm,
the organs of the upper abdomen and the kidneys;
dorsal view.

Upper abdomen, sagittal section

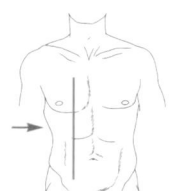

Diaphragma, Centrum tendineum
Hepar, Lobus dexter
Pulmo dexter, Lobus inferior
Costa V
Pleura visceralis [pulmonalis]
Pleura parietalis, Pars costalis
Pars costalis diaphragmatis
V. hepatica dextra
Costa XI
Pars costalis diaphragmatis
Recessus costodiaphragmaticus
M. erector spinae
Columna renalis
V. renalis
A. renalis
Pelvis renalis
Medulla renalis
Calyx renalis minor
M. quadratus lumborum
Cortex renalis
Ren, Capsula adiposa
Ren, Capsula fibrosa
M. psoas major
Fascia renalis
V. portae hepatis, R. dexter, R. anterior
M. rectus abdominis
Peritoneum viscerale
Gaster
Omentum majus
Colon transversum
SK

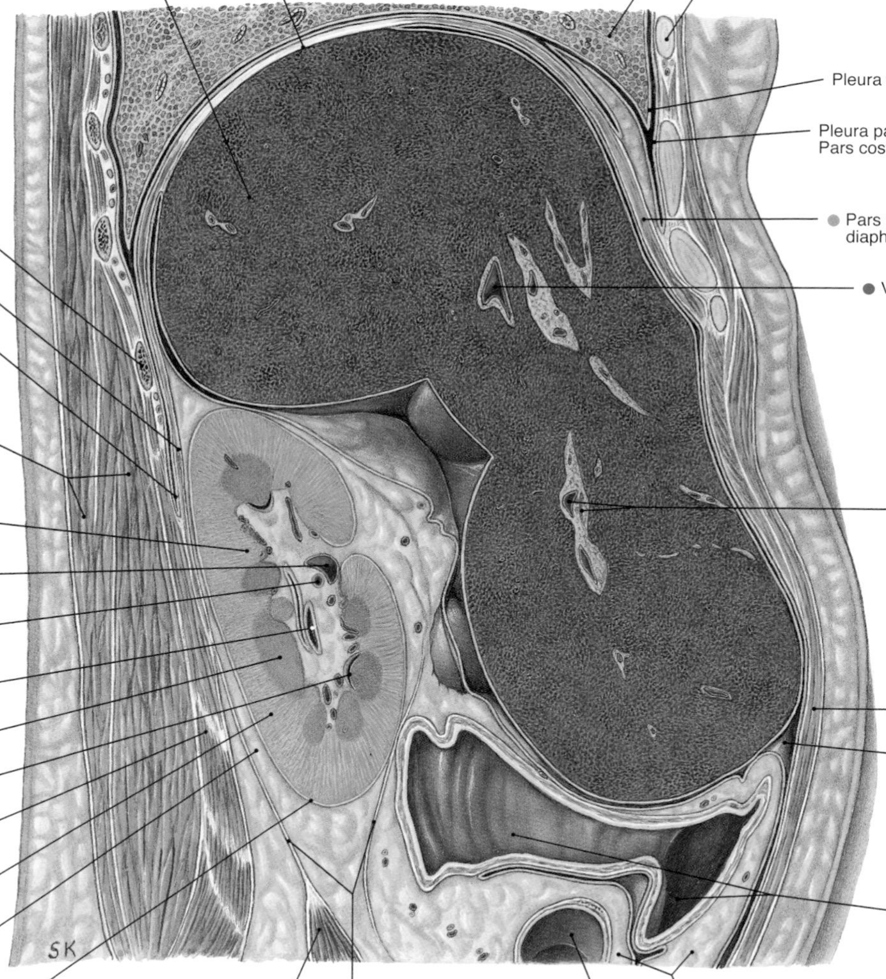

Fig. 921 Abdomen, Abdomen;
sagittal section through the upper abdomen
at the level of the right kidney;
viewed from the right.

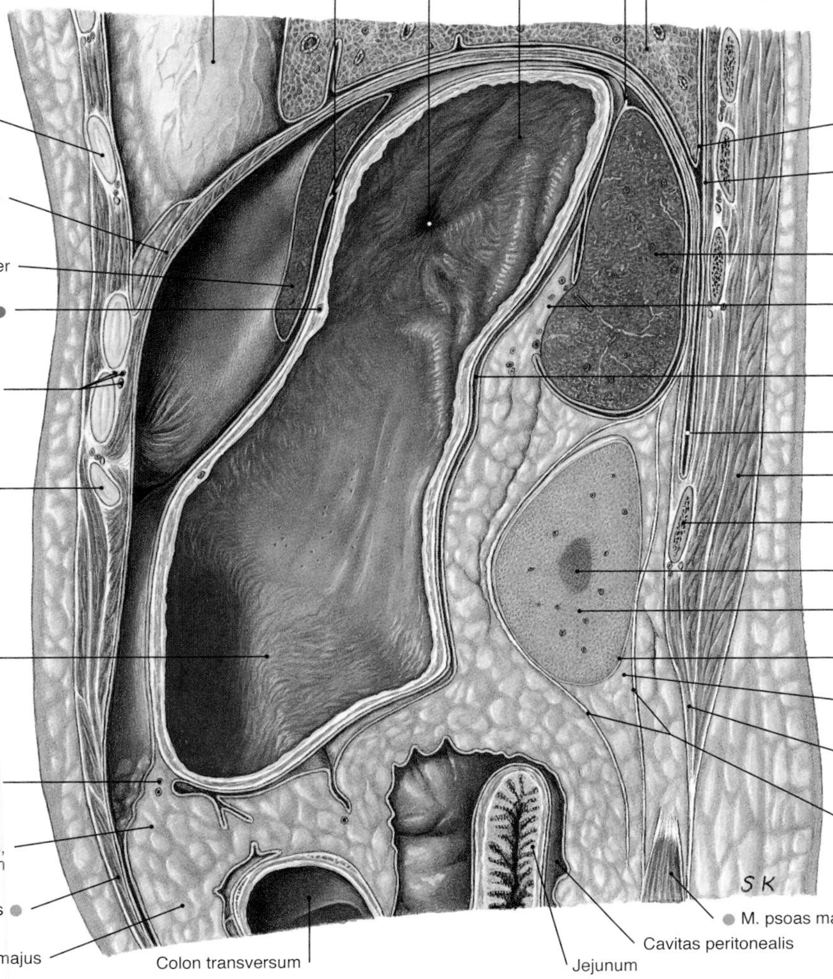

Upper abdomen, sagittal section

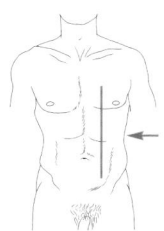

Gaster, Cardia, Ostium cardiacum

Gaster, Fornix gastricus

Lig. phrenicosplenicum

Omentum minus, Lig. hepatogastricum

Pericardium

Pulmo sinister, Lobus inferior

Costa VI

Pleura visceralis [pulmonalis]

Pars costalis diaphragmatis

Pleura parietalis, Pars costalis

Hepar, Lobus sinister

A. gastrica sinistra ●

Splen [Lien]

Lig. gastrosplenicum

R. intercostalis anterior; ●
V. intercostalis anterior; ●
N. intercostalis ●

Bursa omentalis

Recessus costodiaphragmaticus

● M. erector spinae

Costa IX

Costa XII

Medulla renalis

Cortex renalis

Ren

Gaster, Pars pylorica, Antrum pyloricum

Capsula fibrosa

Capsula adiposa

● M. quadratus lumborum

A. gastroomentalis ●
sinistra

Fascia renalis

Omentum majus, Lig. gastrocolicum

M. rectus abdominis ●

● M. psoas major

Cavitas peritonealis

Omentum majus

Colon transversum

Jejunum

S K

Fig. 922 Abdomen, Abdomen;
sagittal section through the upper abdomen at the level of the spleen;
viewed from the left.

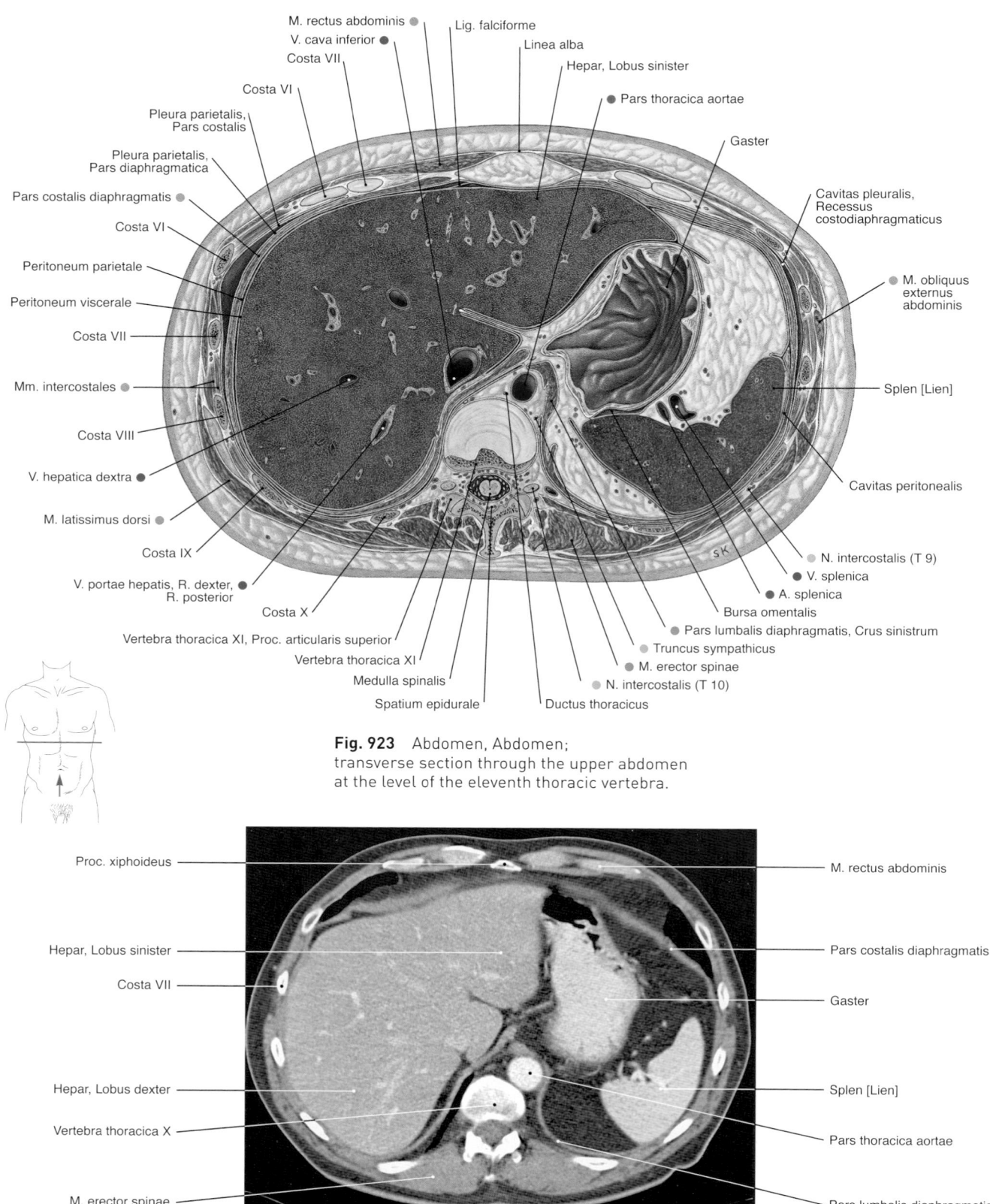

M. rectus abdominis ●
V. cava inferior ●
Costa VII
Costa VI
Pleura parietalis,
Pars costalis
Pleura parietalis,
Pars diaphragmatica
Pars costalis diaphragmatis ●
Costa VI
Peritoneum parietale
Peritoneum viscerale
Costa VII
Mm. intercostales ●
Costa VIII
V. hepatica dextra ●
M. latissimus dorsi ●
Costa IX
V. portae hepatis, R. dexter, ●
R. posterior
Costa X
Vertebra thoracica XI, Proc. articularis superior
Vertebra thoracica XI
Medulla spinalis
Spatium epidurale

Lig. falciforme
Linea alba
Hepar, Lobus sinister
● Pars thoracica aortae
Gaster

Cavitas pleuralis,
Recessus
costodiaphragmaticus

● M. obliquus
externus
abdominis

Splen [Lien]

Cavitas peritonealis

● N. intercostalis (T 9)
● V. splenica
● A. splenica
Bursa omentalis
● Pars lumbalis diaphragmatis, Crus sinistrum
● Truncus sympathicus
● M. erector spinae
● N. intercostalis (T 10)
Ductus thoracicus

Fig. 923 Abdomen, Abdomen;
transverse section through the upper abdomen
at the level of the eleventh thoracic vertebra.

Proc. xiphoideus
Hepar, Lobus sinister
Costa VII
Hepar, Lobus dexter
Vertebra thoracica X
M. erector spinae

M. rectus abdominis
Pars costalis diaphragmatis
Gaster
Splen [Lien]
Pars thoracica aortae
Pars lumbalis diaphragmatis

Fig. 924 Abdomen, Abdomen;
computed tomographic cross-section (CT)
at the level of the tenth thoracic vertebra;
inferior view.

Upper abdomen, transverse sections

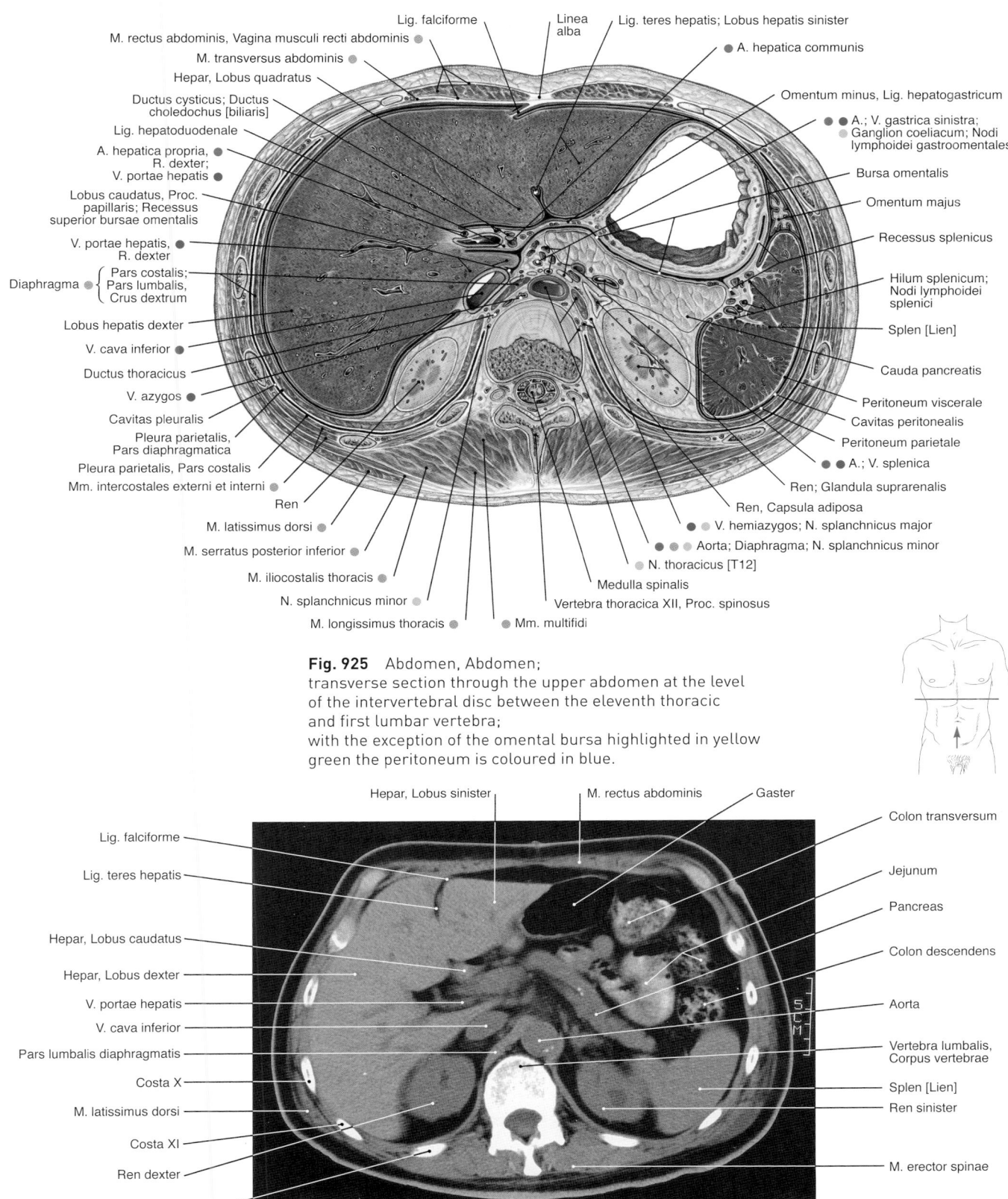

Lig. falciforme
Linea alba
Lig. teres hepatis; Lobus hepatis sinister
M. rectus abdominis, Vagina musculi recti abdominis ●
M. transversus abdominis ●
Hepar, Lobus quadratus
Ductus cysticus; Ductus choledochus [biliaris]
Lig. hepatoduodenale
A. hepatica propria, R. dexter; V. portae hepatis ●
Lobus caudatus, Proc. papillaris; Recessus superior bursae omentalis
V. portae hepatis, ● R. dexter
Diaphragma ● { Pars costalis; Pars lumbalis, Crus dextrum
Lobus hepatis dexter
V. cava inferior ●
Ductus thoracicus
V. azygos ●
Cavitas pleuralis
Pleura parietalis, Pars diaphragmatica
Pleura parietalis, Pars costalis
Mm. intercostales externi et interni ●
Ren
M. latissimus dorsi ●
M. serratus posterior inferior ●
M. iliocostalis thoracis ●
N. splanchnicus minor ●
M. longissimus thoracis ●

● A. hepatica communis
Omentum minus, Lig. hepatogastricum
● ● A.; V. gastrica sinistra; Ganglion coeliacum; Nodi lymphoidei gastroomentales
Bursa omentalis
Omentum majus
Recessus splenicus
Hilum splenicum; Nodi lymphoidei splenici
Splen [Lien]
Cauda pancreatis
Peritoneum viscerale
Cavitas peritonealis
Peritoneum parietale
● ● A.; V. splenica
Ren; Glandula suprarenalis
Ren, Capsula adiposa
● ● V. hemiazygos; N. splanchnicus major
● ● ● Aorta; Diaphragma; N. splanchnicus minor
● N. thoracicus [T12]
Medulla spinalis
Vertebra thoracica XII, Proc. spinosus
● Mm. multifidi

Fig. 925 Abdomen, Abdomen;
transverse section through the upper abdomen at the level of the intervertebral disc between the eleventh thoracic and first lumbar vertebra;
with the exception of the omental bursa highlighted in yellow green the peritoneum is coloured in blue.

Hepar, Lobus sinister
M. rectus abdominis
Gaster
Colon transversum
Lig. falciforme
Jejunum
Lig. teres hepatis
Pancreas
Hepar, Lobus caudatus
Colon descendens
Hepar, Lobus dexter
V. portae hepatis
Aorta
V. cava inferior
Pars lumbalis diaphragmatis
Vertebra lumbalis, Corpus vertebrae
Costa X
Splen [Lien]
M. latissimus dorsi
Ren sinister
Costa XI
Ren dexter
M. erector spinae
Costa XII

Fig. 926 Abdomen, Abdomen;
computed tomographic section (CT)
at the level of the first lumbar vertebra.
The intestine is partially filled with a contrast medium.

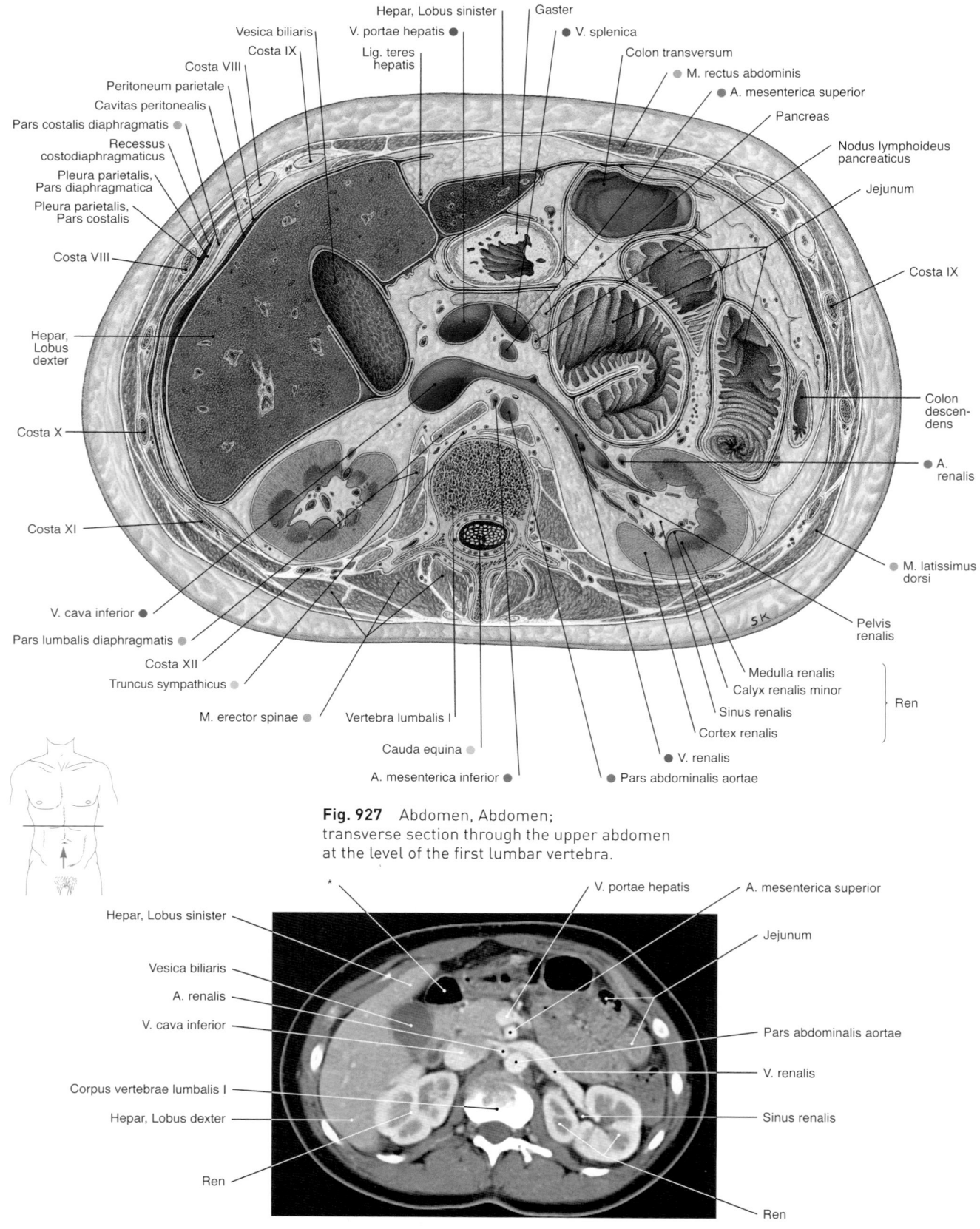

Hepar, Lobus sinister
V. portae hepatis ●
Gaster
● V. splenica
Vesica biliaris
Costa IX
Lig. teres hepatis
Colon transversum
● M. rectus abdominis
Costa VIII
● A. mesenterica superior
Peritoneum parietale
Pancreas
Cavitas peritonealis
Nodus lymphoideus pancreaticus
Pars costalis diaphragmatis ●
Recessus costodiaphragmaticus
Jejunum
Pleura parietalis, Pars diaphragmatica
Pleura parietalis, Pars costalis
Costa VIII
Costa IX
Hepar, Lobus dexter
Colon descendens
Costa X
● A. renalis
Costa XI
● M. latissimus dorsi
V. cava inferior ●
Pelvis renalis
Pars lumbalis diaphragmatis ●
Medulla renalis
Costa XII
Calyx renalis minor
Ren
Truncus sympathicus ●
Sinus renalis
Cortex renalis
M. erector spinae ●
Vertebra lumbalis I
Cauda equina ●
● V. renalis
A. mesenterica inferior ●
● Pars abdominalis aortae

Fig. 927 Abdomen, Abdomen; transverse section through the upper abdomen at the level of the first lumbar vertebra.

*
V. portae hepatis
A. mesenterica superior
Hepar, Lobus sinister
Jejunum
Vesica biliaris
A. renalis
V. cava inferior
Pars abdominalis aortae
V. renalis
Corpus vertebrae lumbalis I
Hepar, Lobus dexter
Sinus renalis
Ren
Ren

Fig. 928 Abdomen, Abdomen; computed tomographic section (CT) at the level of the first lumbar vertebra; inferior view.
* Intestinal gas

Lower abdomen, transverse sections

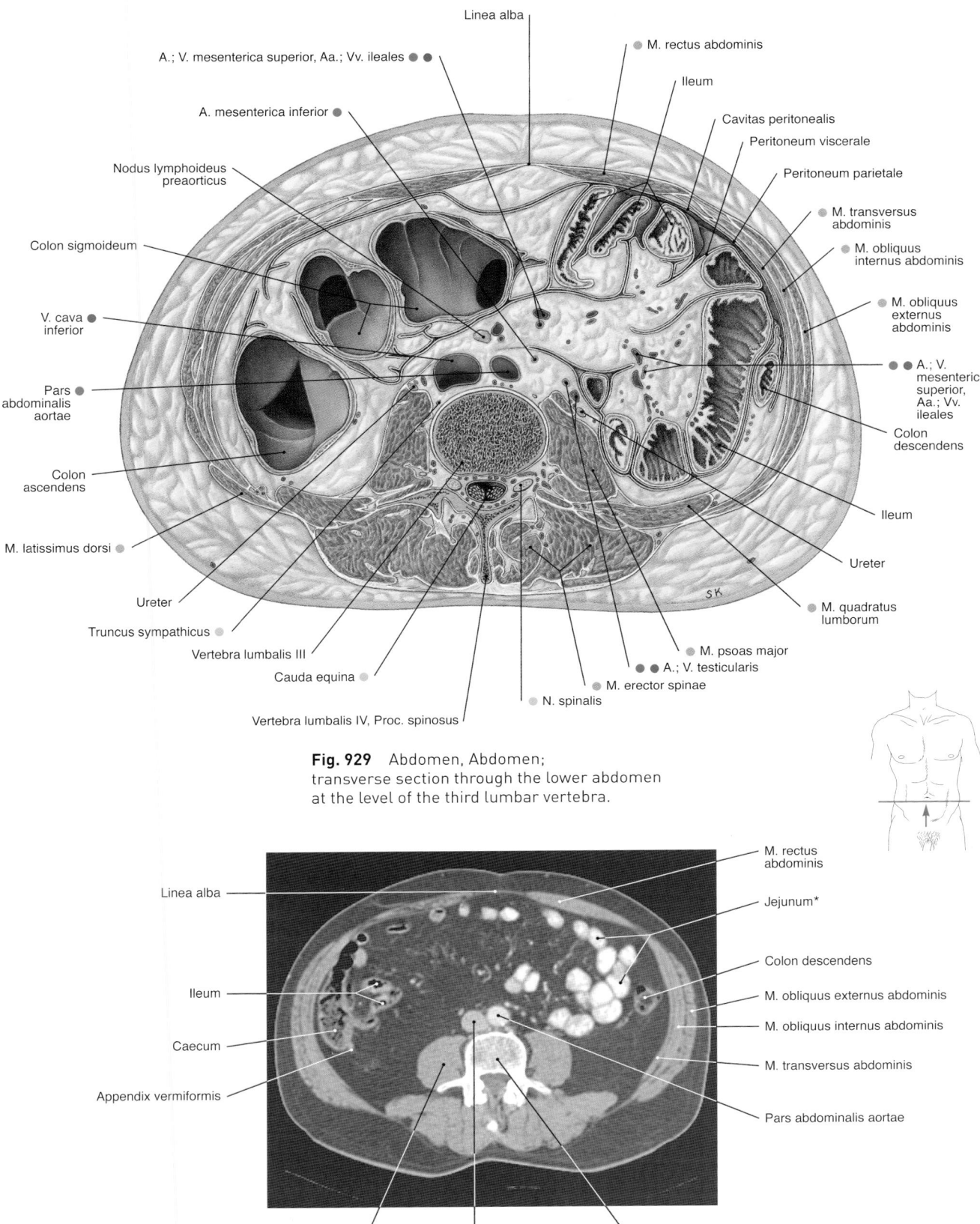

Linea alba

A.; V. mesenterica superior, Aa.; Vv. ileales ● ●

A. mesenterica inferior ●

Nodus lymphoideus preaorticus

Colon sigmoideum

V. cava ● inferior

Pars ● abdominalis aortae

Colon ascendens

M. latissimus dorsi ●

Ureter

Truncus sympathicus ●

Vertebra lumbalis III

Cauda equina ●

Vertebra lumbalis IV, Proc. spinosus

● M. rectus abdominis

Ileum

Cavitas peritonealis

Peritoneum viscerale

Peritoneum parietale

● M. transversus abdominis

● M. obliquus internus abdominis

● M. obliquus externus abdominis

● ● A.; V. mesenterica superior, Aa.; Vv. ileales

Colon descendens

Ileum

Ureter

● M. quadratus lumborum

● M. psoas major

● ● A.; V. testicularis

● M. erector spinae

● N. spinalis

Fig. 929 Abdomen, Abdomen;
transverse section through the lower abdomen
at the level of the third lumbar vertebra.

Linea alba

Ileum

Caecum

Appendix vermiformis

M. rectus abdominis

Jejunum*

Colon descendens

M. obliquus externus abdominis

M. obliquus internus abdominis

M. transversus abdominis

Pars abdominalis aortae

M. psoas major

V. cava inferior

Corpus vertebrae lumbalis III

Fig. 930 Abdomen, Abdomen;
computed tomographic section (CT)
at the level of the third lumbar vertebra;
inferior view.
* Jejunum filled with a contrast medium

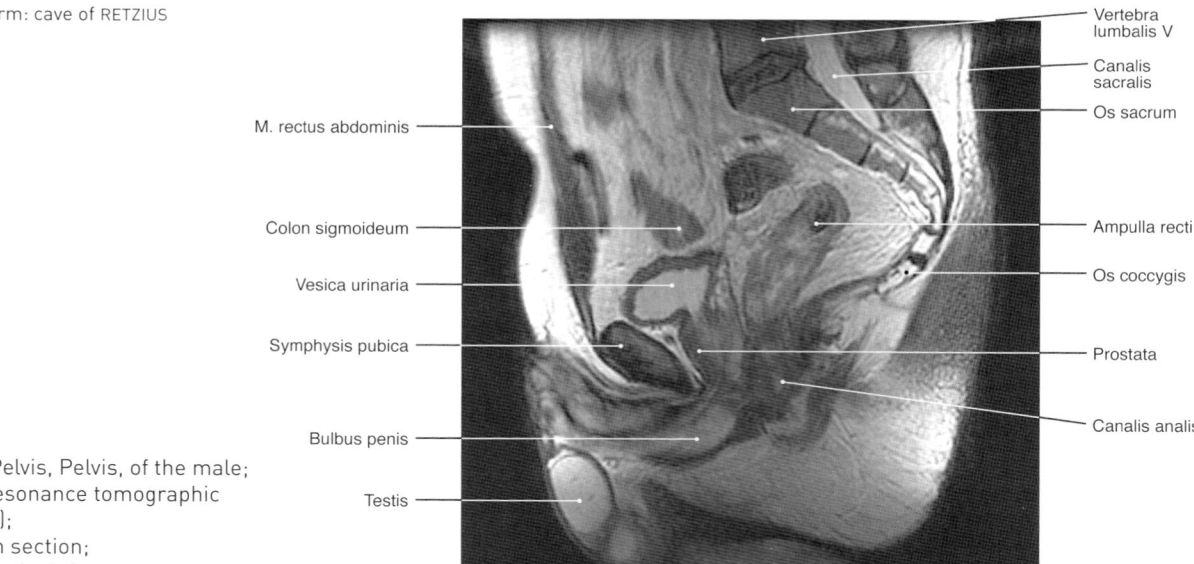

Mesenterium

Ostium urethrae internum

Intestinum tenue

Omentum majus

Apex vesicae

Plica umbilicalis mediana
(Lig. umbilicale medianum)

Spatium
retropubicum**

Linea alba

Symphysis pubica

Lig. fundiforme penis

V. dorsalis profunda penis ●

V. dorsalis superficialis penis ●

Urethra, Pars spongiosa

Ductus deferens

Caput epididymidis

Tunica albuginea
corporum cavernosorum

Corpus cavernosum penis

Corpus spongiosum penis

Septula testis

Corona glandis

Glans penis

Fossa navicularis urethrae

Preputium penis

Ostium urethrae externum

M. cremaster; Fascia cremasterica ●

Lobuli testis

Colon sigmoideum

Filum terminale

Ostium ureteris

Plica transversa recti*

Lig. sacrococcygeum
posterius superficiale

Excavatio rectovesicalis

Articulatio
sacrococcygea

Ampulla recti

Fascia rectoprostatica

Prostata

Fascia pelvis visceralis

Corpus anococcygeum
[Lig. anococcygeum]

● M. sphincter ani
externus

● M. sphincter ani
internus

Columnae anales; Sinus anales

(Pecten analis)

● M. sphincter ani externus

● M. transversus perinei profundus

Membrana perinei

Urethra, Pars intermedia [membranacea]

Lig. puboprostaticum

Bulbus penis, Corpus spongiosum penis

Ductuli efferentes testis

Mediastinum testis

Ductus deferens; Cauda epididymidis

● Scrotum, Tunica dartos, M. dartos

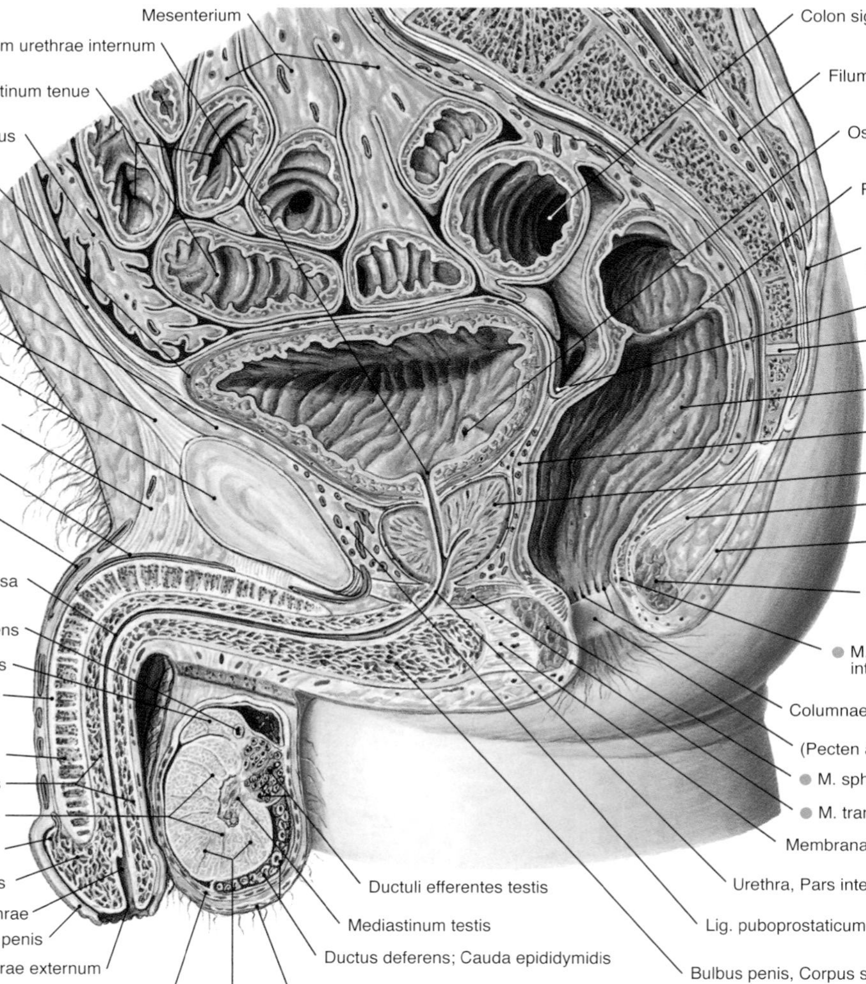

Fig. 931 Pelvis, Pelvis, of the male;
median section;
viewed from the left.
* Clinical term: KOHLRAUSCH's fold
** Clinical term: cave of RETZIUS

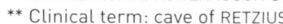

M. rectus abdominis

Colon sigmoideum

Vesica urinaria

Symphysis pubica

Bulbus penis

Testis

Vertebra
lumbalis V

Canalis
sacralis

Os sacrum

Ampulla recti

Os coccygis

Prostata

Canalis analis

Fig. 932 Pelvis, Pelvis, of the male;
magnetic resonance tomographic
image (MRI);
paramedian section;
viewed from the left.

Female pelvis, median sections

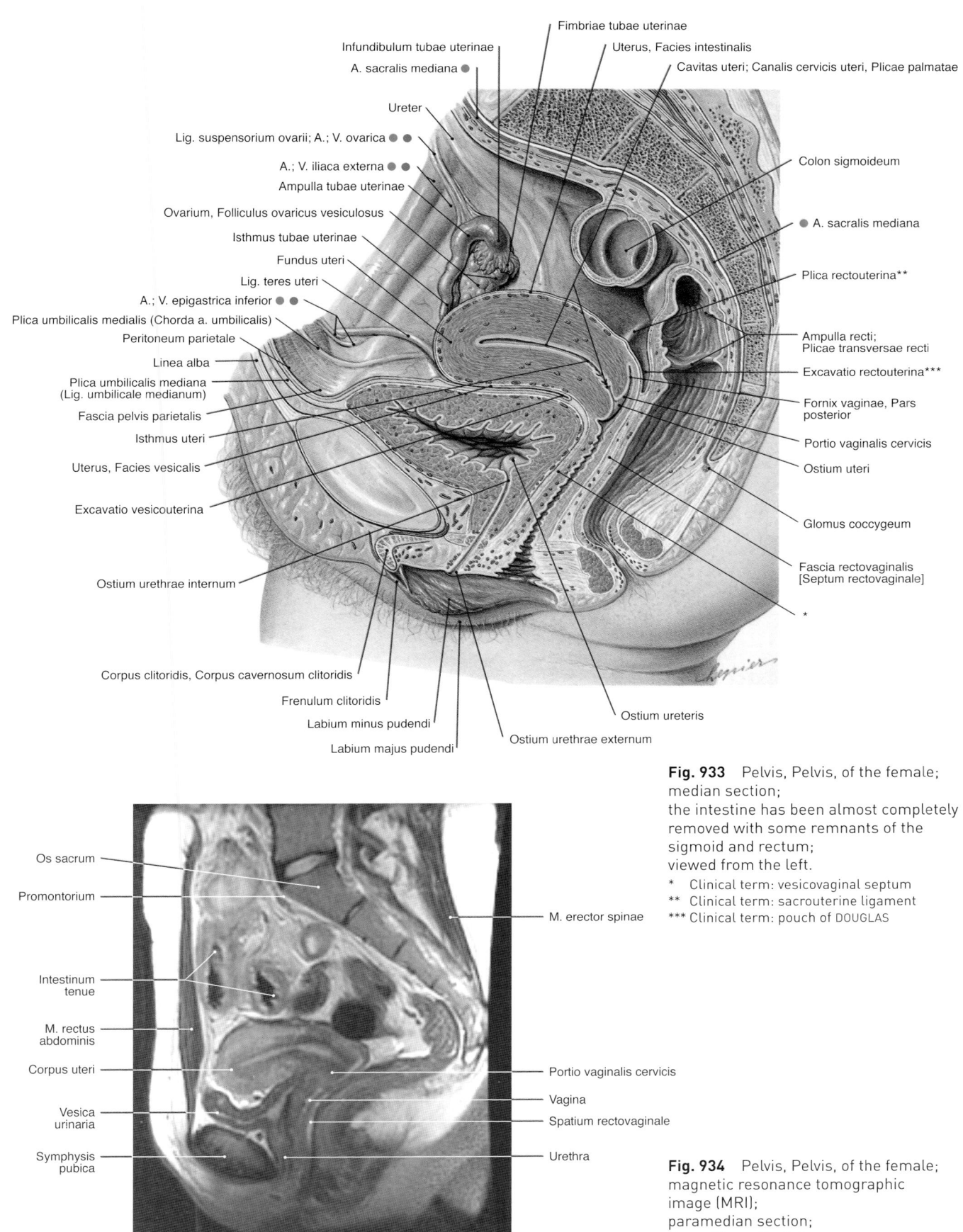

Fimbriae tubae uterinae
Infundibulum tubae uterinae
Uterus, Facies intestinalis
A. sacralis mediana ●
Cavitas uteri; Canalis cervicis uteri, Plicae palmatae
Ureter
Lig. suspensorium ovarii; A.; V. ovarica ● ●
Colon sigmoideum
A.; V. iliaca externa ● ●
Ampulla tubae uterinae
Ovarium, Folliculus ovaricus vesiculosus
● A. sacralis mediana
Isthmus tubae uterinae
Fundus uteri
Plica rectouterina**
Lig. teres uteri
A.; V. epigastrica inferior ● ●
Ampulla recti;
Plica umbilicalis medialis (Chorda a. umbilicalis)
Plicae transversae recti
Peritoneum parietale
Excavatio rectouterina***
Linea alba
Plica umbilicalis mediana
(Lig. umbilicale medianum)
Fornix vaginae, Pars posterior
Fascia pelvis parietalis
Portio vaginalis cervicis
Isthmus uteri
Ostium uteri
Uterus, Facies vesicalis
Excavatio vesicouterina
Glomus coccygeum
Fascia rectovaginalis
[Septum rectovaginale]
Ostium urethrae internum
*
Corpus clitoridis, Corpus cavernosum clitoridis
Frenulum clitoridis
Labium minus pudendi
Ostium ureteris
Labium majus pudendi
Ostium urethrae externum

Fig. 933 Pelvis, Pelvis, of the female;
median section;
the intestine has been almost completely
removed with some remnants of the
sigmoid and rectum;
viewed from the left.
* Clinical term: vesicovaginal septum
** Clinical term: sacrouterine ligament
*** Clinical term: pouch of DOUGLAS

Os sacrum
Promontorium
M. erector spinae
Intestinum
tenue
M. rectus
abdominis
Corpus uteri
Portio vaginalis cervicis
Vesica
urinaria
Vagina
Spatium rectovaginale
Symphysis
pubica
Urethra

Fig. 934 Pelvis, Pelvis, of the female;
magnetic resonance tomographic
image (MRI);
paramedian section;
viewed from the left.

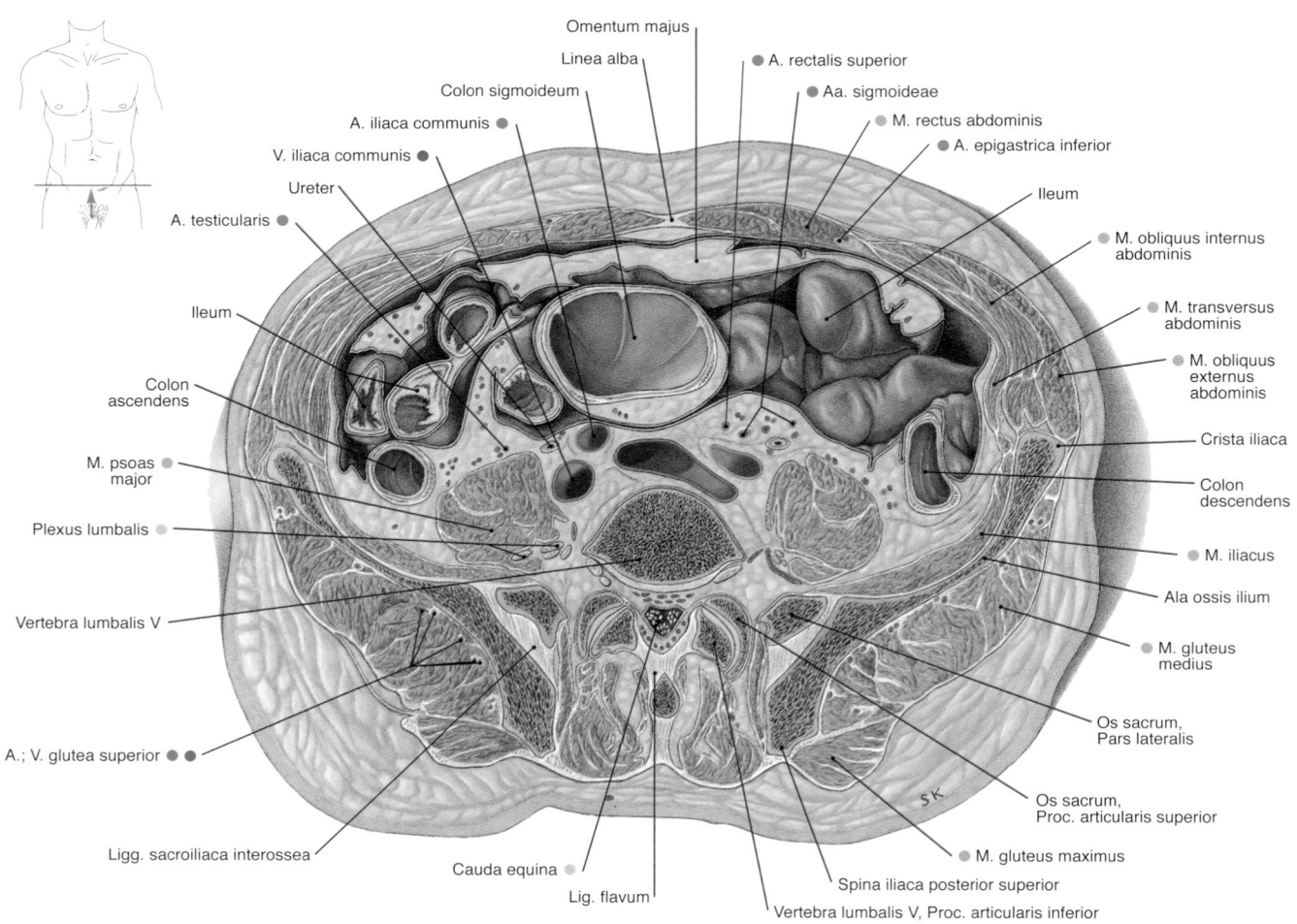

Omentum majus
Linea alba
Colon sigmoideum
A. iliaca communis ●
V. iliaca communis ●
Ureter
A. testicularis ●
Ileum
Colon ascendens
M. psoas major ●
Plexus lumbalis ●
Vertebra lumbalis V
A.; V. glutea superior ● ●
Ligg. sacroiliaca interossea
Cauda equina ●
Lig. flavum

● A. rectalis superior
● Aa. sigmoideae
● M. rectus abdominis
● A. epigastrica inferior
Ileum
● M. obliquus internus abdominis
● M. transversus abdominis
● M. obliquus externus abdominis
Crista iliaca
Colon descendens
● M. iliacus
Ala ossis ilium
● M. gluteus medius
Os sacrum, Pars lateralis
Os sacrum, Proc. articularis superior
● M. gluteus maximus
Spina iliaca posterior superior
Vertebra lumbalis V, Proc. articularis inferior

Fig. 935 Pelvis, Pelvis;
transverse section at the level of the fifth lumbar vertebra. This male specimen is different from Fig. 923, 925, 927 and 929.

As the sigmoid reaches far into the upper abdomen the figure also displays the dome of colonic flexure. The thickness of the adipose tissue layer on the gluteus medius muscle must be taken into consideration when injecting intramuscularly.

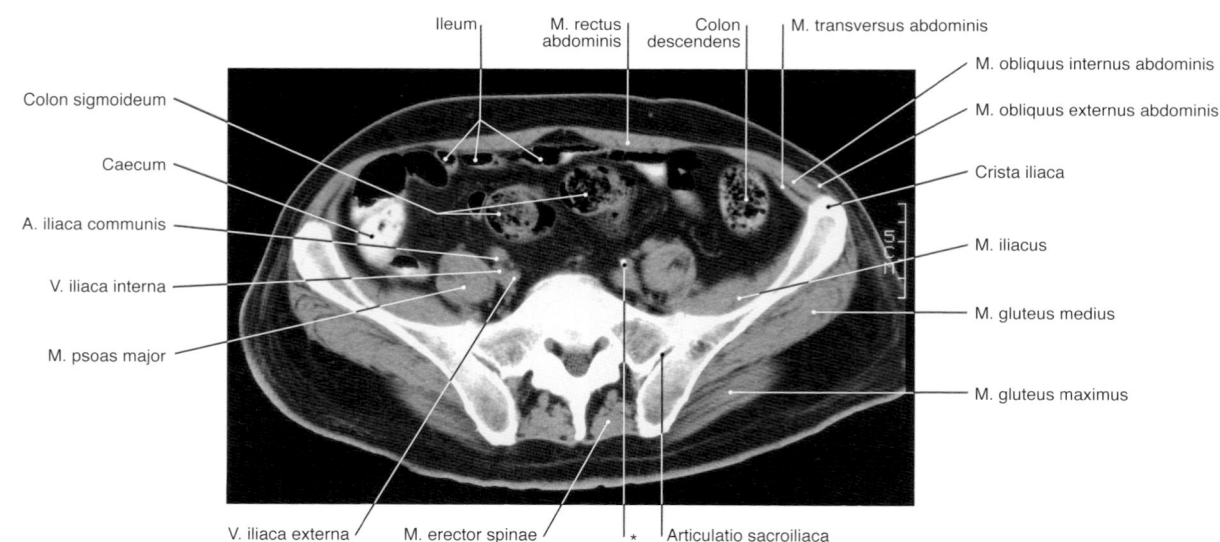

Ileum
M. rectus abdominis
Colon descendens
M. transversus abdominis
M. obliquus internus abdominis
M. obliquus externus abdominis
Crista iliaca
M. iliacus
M. gluteus medius
M. gluteus maximus

Colon sigmoideum
Caecum
A. iliaca communis
V. iliaca interna
M. psoas major
V. iliaca externa
M. erector spinae
*
Articulatio sacroiliaca

Fig. 936 Pelvis, Pelvis;
computed tomographic cross-section (CT) at the level of the first sacral vertebra after administration

of a contrast medium into the colon; supine position; inferior view.
* Calcification in the wall of the iliac artery.

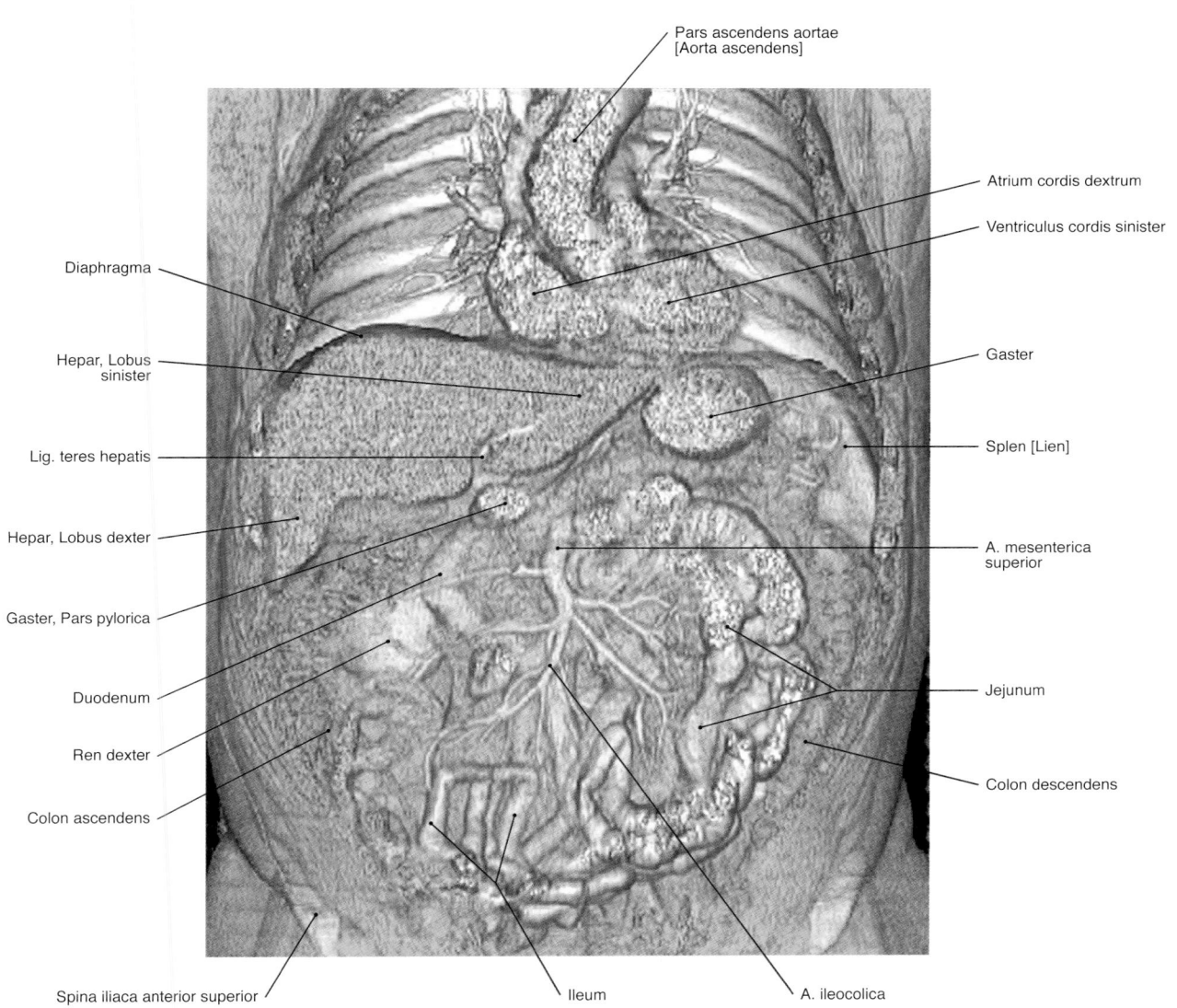

Pars ascendens aortae
[Aorta ascendens]

Atrium cordis dextrum

Ventriculus cordis sinister

Diaphragma

Hepar, Lobus sinister

Gaster

Lig. teres hepatis

Splen [Lien]

Hepar, Lobus dexter

A. mesenterica superior

Gaster, Pars pylorica

Duodenum

Jejunum

Ren dexter

Colon ascendens

Colon descendens

Spina iliaca anterior superior

Ileum

A. ileocolica

Fig. 937 Abdomen, Abdomen;
volume-guided reconstruction in the frontal plane
based on horizontal computed tomographic sections (CT).
The section planes of organs such as the heart,
the stomach, the liver and parts of the small intestine,
appear granulated.

→ 802, 919

Male pelvis, transverse sections

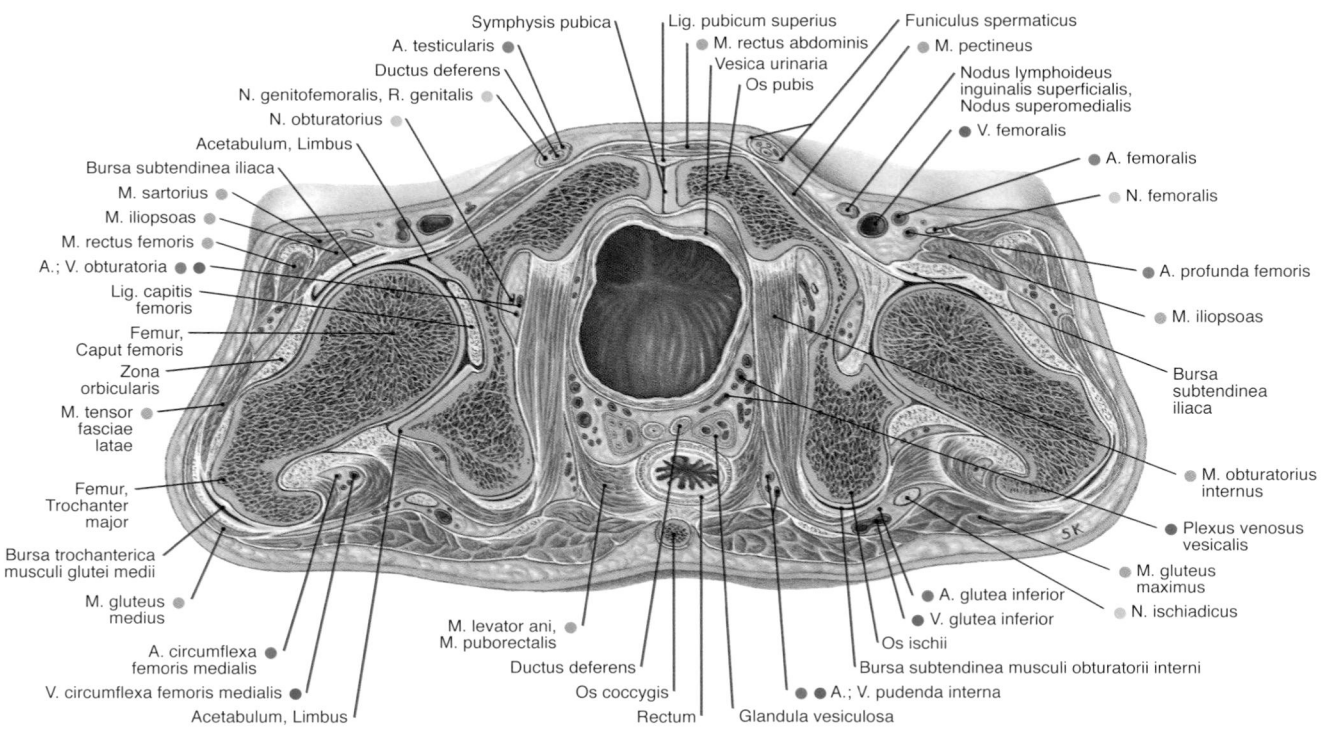

Fig. 938 Pelvis, Pelvis, of the male;
transverse section through the lesser pelvis.

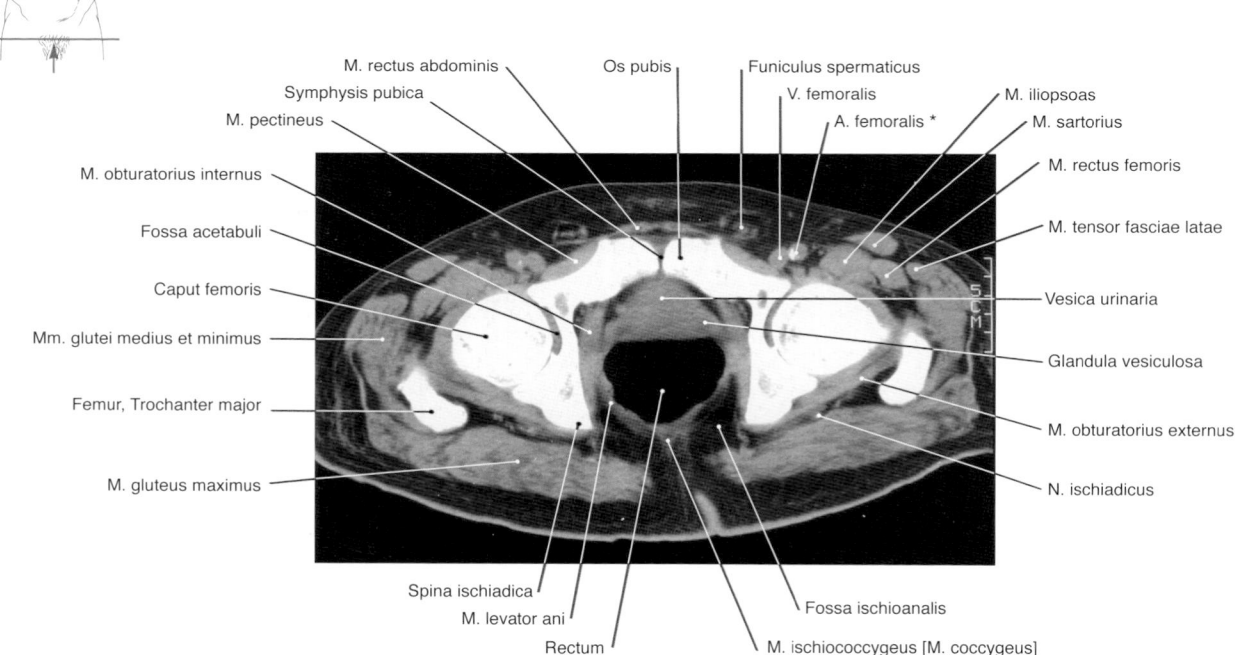

Fig. 939 Pelvis, Pelvis, of the male;
computed tomographic cross-section (CT) through
the lesser pelvis with the subject in supine position.
* Calcification in the medial part of the femoral artery

Female pelvis, transverse sections

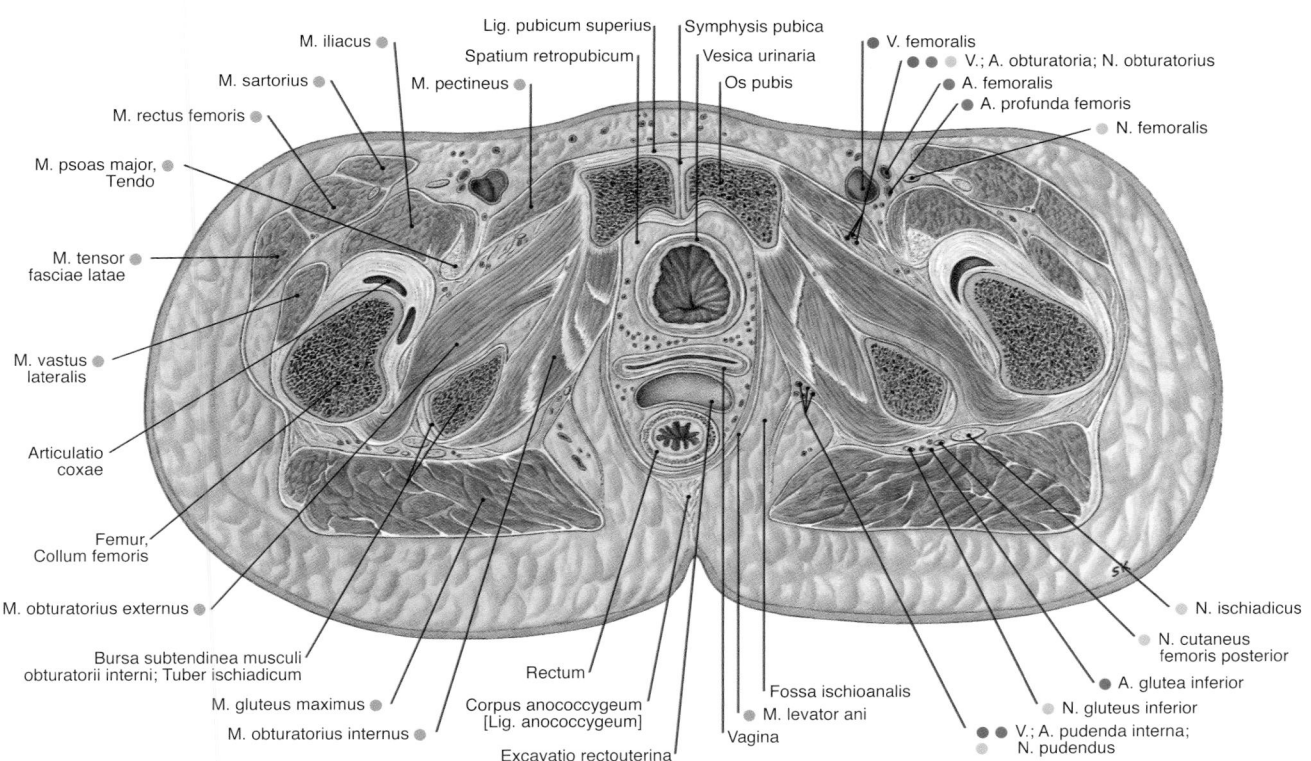

M. iliacus
Lig. pubicum superius
Symphysis pubica
V. femoralis
M. sartorius
Spatium retropubicum
Vesica urinaria
V.; A. obturatoria; N. obturatorius
M. pectineus
Os pubis
A. femoralis
M. rectus femoris
A. profunda femoris
N. femoralis
M. psoas major, Tendo
M. tensor fasciae latae
M. vastus lateralis
Articulatio coxae
Femur, Collum femoris
M. obturatorius externus
N. ischiadicus
N. cutaneus femoris posterior
Bursa subtendinea musculi obturatorii interni; Tuber ischiadicum
A. glutea inferior
M. gluteus maximus
Rectum
Fossa ischioanalis
N. gluteus inferior
Corpus anococcygeum [Lig. anococcygeum]
M. levator ani
V.; A. pudenda interna; N. pudendus
M. obturatorius internus
Vagina
Excavatio rectouterina

Fig. 940   Pelvis, Pelvis, of the female;
transverse section through the lesser pelvis
at the level of the symphysis.

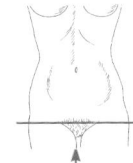

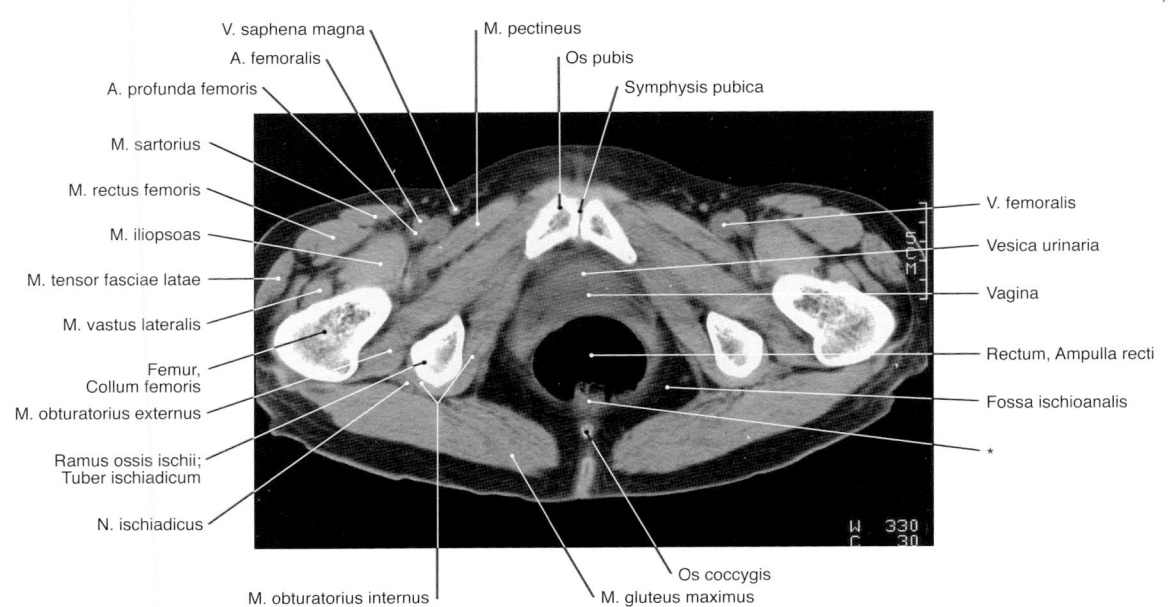

V. saphena magna
M. pectineus
A. femoralis
Os pubis
A. profunda femoris
Symphysis pubica
M. sartorius
M. rectus femoris
V. femoralis
M. iliopsoas
Vesica urinaria
M. tensor fasciae latae
Vagina
M. vastus lateralis
Femur, Collum femoris
Rectum, Ampulla recti
M. obturatorius externus
Fossa ischioanalis
Ramus ossis ischii; Tuber ischiadicum
*
N. ischiadicus
Os coccygis
M. obturatorius internus
M. gluteus maximus

Fig. 941   Pelvis, Pelvis, of the female;
computed tomographic cross-section (CT) through
the lesser pelvis with the subject in supine position.
* Remnants of contrasting intestinal contents

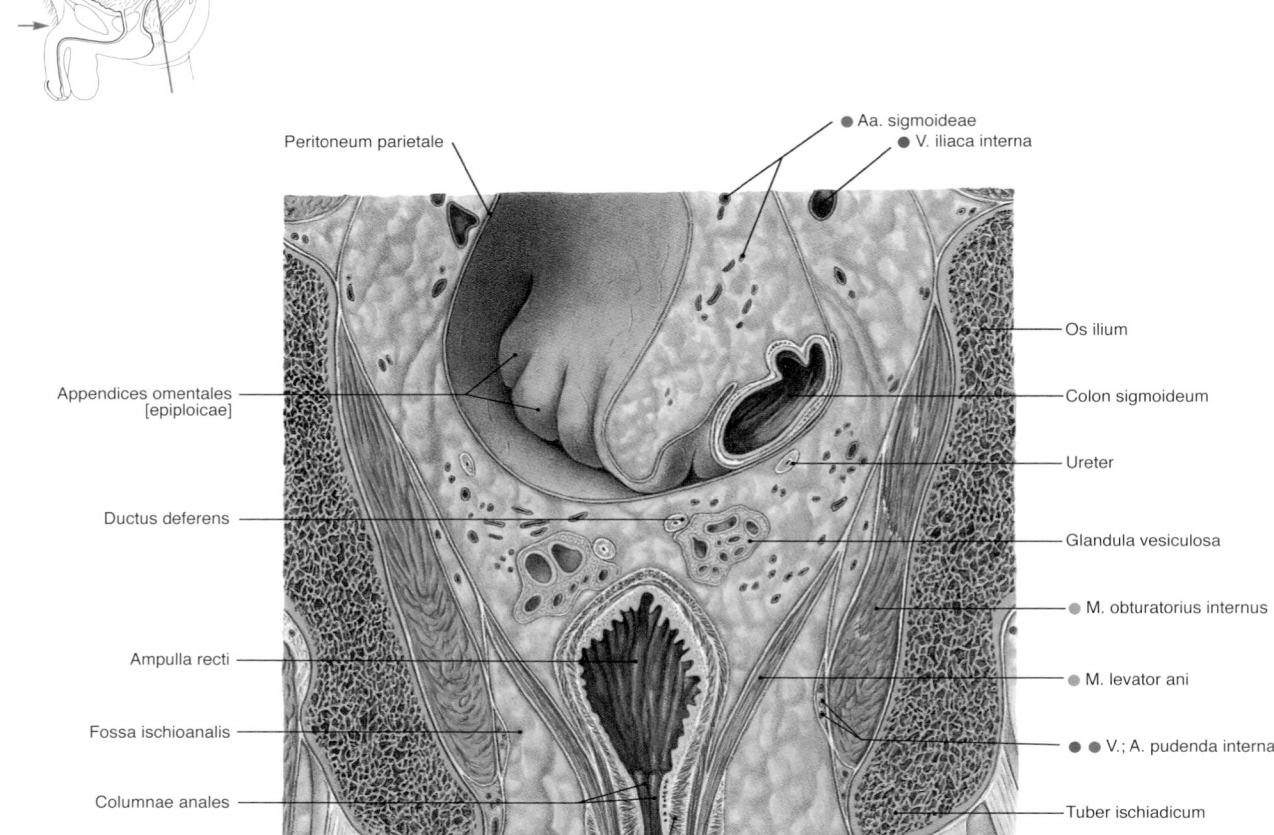

Peritoneum parietale

● Aa. sigmoideae
● V. iliaca interna

Appendices omentales
[epiploicae]

Ductus deferens

Ampulla recti

Fossa ischioanalis

Columnae anales

Os ilium

Colon sigmoideum

Ureter

Glandula vesiculosa

● M. obturatorius internus

● M. levator ani

● ● V.; A. pudenda interna*

Tuber ischiadicum

● M. biceps femoris;
M. semitendinosus;
M. semimembranosus

Cutis

M. sphincter ani internus ●

● M. levator ani, M. puborectalis

● M. sphincter ani externus

Fig. 942   Pelvis, Pelvis, of the male;
oblique frontal section through the lesser pelvis.
* Clinical term: ALCOCK's canal

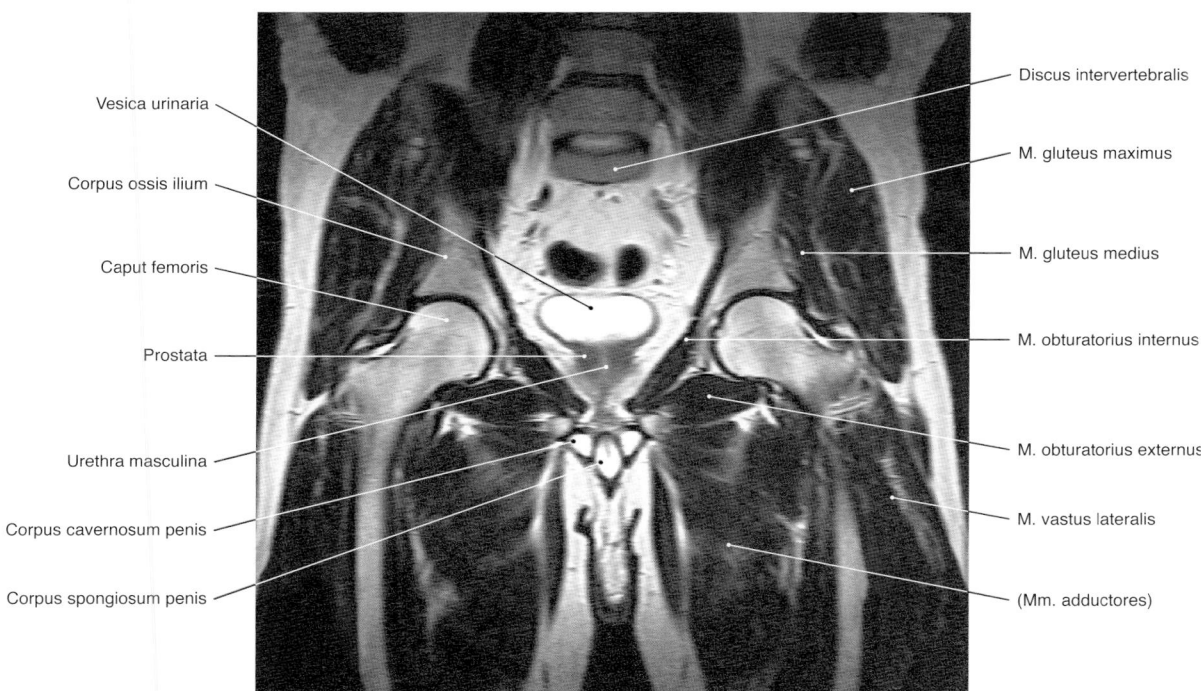

Vesica urinaria

Corpus ossis ilium

Caput femoris

Prostata

Urethra masculina

Corpus cavernosum penis

Corpus spongiosum penis

Discus intervertebralis

M. gluteus maximus

M. gluteus medius

M. obturatorius internus

M. obturatorius externus

M. vastus lateralis

(Mm. adductores)

Fig. 943   Pelvis, Pelvis, of the male;
magnetic resonance tomographic image (MRI);
frontal section at the level of the hip joints;
ventral view.

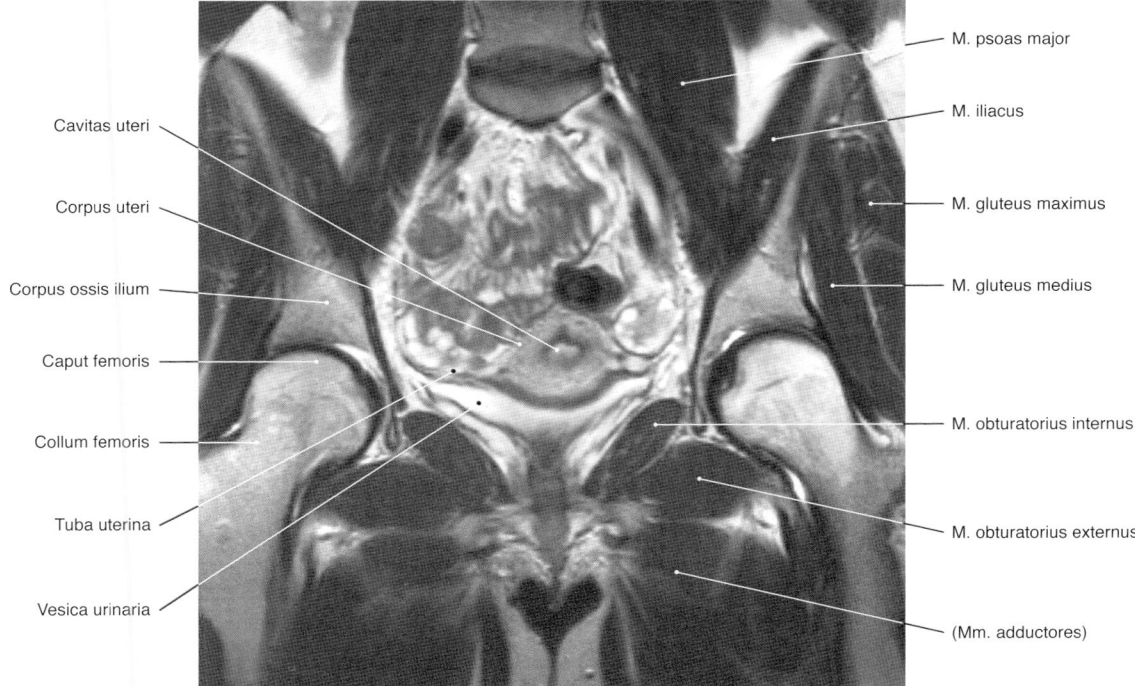

Cavitas uteri

Corpus uteri

Corpus ossis ilium

Caput femoris

Collum femoris

Tuba uterina

Vesica urinaria

M. psoas major

M. iliacus

M. gluteus maximus

M. gluteus medius

M. obturatorius internus

M. obturatorius externus

(Mm. adductores)

Fig. 944   Pelvis, Pelvis, of the female;
magnetic resonance tomographic image (MRI);
frontal section at the level of the hip joints;
ventral view.

When the urinary bladder is empty, the uterus lies on the apex
of the bladder due to its anteflexion.

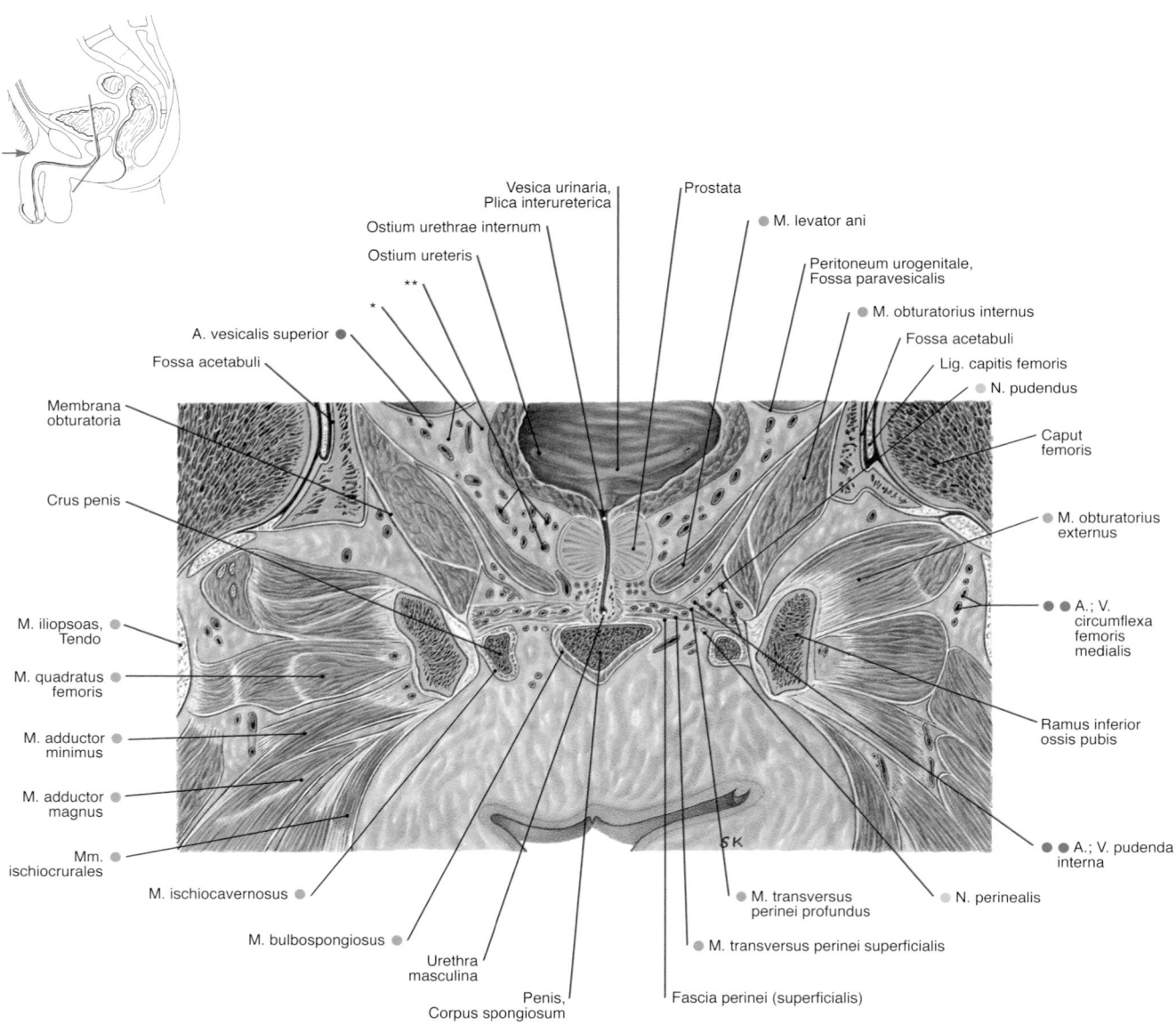

Vesica urinaria,
Plica interureterica

Prostata

Ostium urethrae internum

● M. levator ani

Ostium ureteris

Peritoneum urogenitale,
Fossa paravesicalis

**

*

● M. obturatorius internus

A. vesicalis superior ●

Fossa acetabuli

Fossa acetabuli

Lig. capitis femoris

● N. pudendus

Membrana
obturatoria

Caput
femoris

Crus penis

● M. obturatorius
externus

M. iliopsoas,
Tendo ●

● ● A.; V.
circumflexa
femoris
medialis

M. quadratus ●
femoris

M. adductor ●
minimus

M. adductor ●
magnus

Ramus inferior
ossis pubis

Mm. ●
ischiocrurales

● ● A.; V. pudenda
interna

M. ischiocavernosus ●

● M. transversus
perinei profundus

● N. perinealis

M. bulbospongiosus ●

● M. transversus perinei superficialis

Urethra
masculina

Penis,
Corpus spongiosum

Fascia perinei (superficialis)

Fig. 945 Pelvis, Pelvis, of the male;
angled-frontal section through the urinary bladder.
*   Clinical term: paracystium
** Clinical term: prostatic venous plexus

Female pelvic diaphragm, angled-frontal section

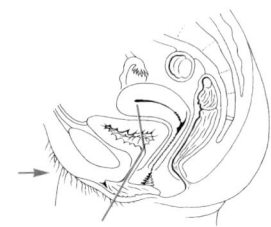

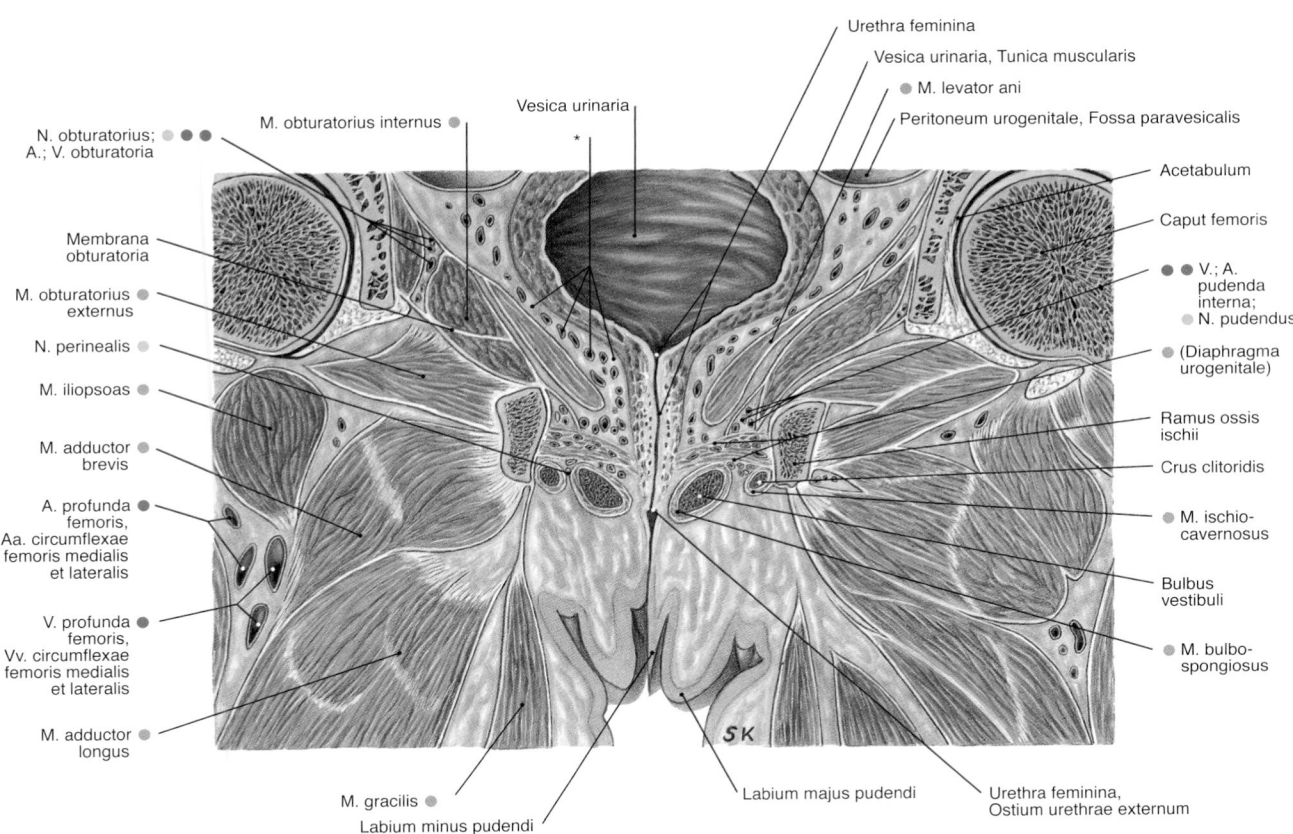

N. obturatorius;
A.; V. obturatoria

M. obturatorius internus

Vesica urinaria

*

Urethra feminina

Vesica urinaria, Tunica muscularis

M. levator ani

Peritoneum urogenitale, Fossa paravesicalis

Acetabulum

Caput femoris

V.; A. pudenda interna;
N. pudendus

(Diaphragma urogenitale)

Ramus ossis ischii

Crus clitoridis

M. ischio-cavernosus

Bulbus vestibuli

M. bulbo-spongiosus

Membrana obturatoria

M. obturatorius externus

N. perinealis

M. iliopsoas

M. adductor brevis

A. profunda femoris,
Aa. circumflexae femoris medialis et lateralis

V. profunda femoris,
Vv. circumflexae femoris medialis et lateralis

M. adductor longus

M. gracilis

Labium minus pudendi

Labium majus pudendi

Urethra feminina,
Ostium urethrae externum

SK

Fig. 946 Pelvis, Pelvis, of the female;
angled-frontal section through the urinary bladder.
* Paracystium with venous plexus

Surface anatomy

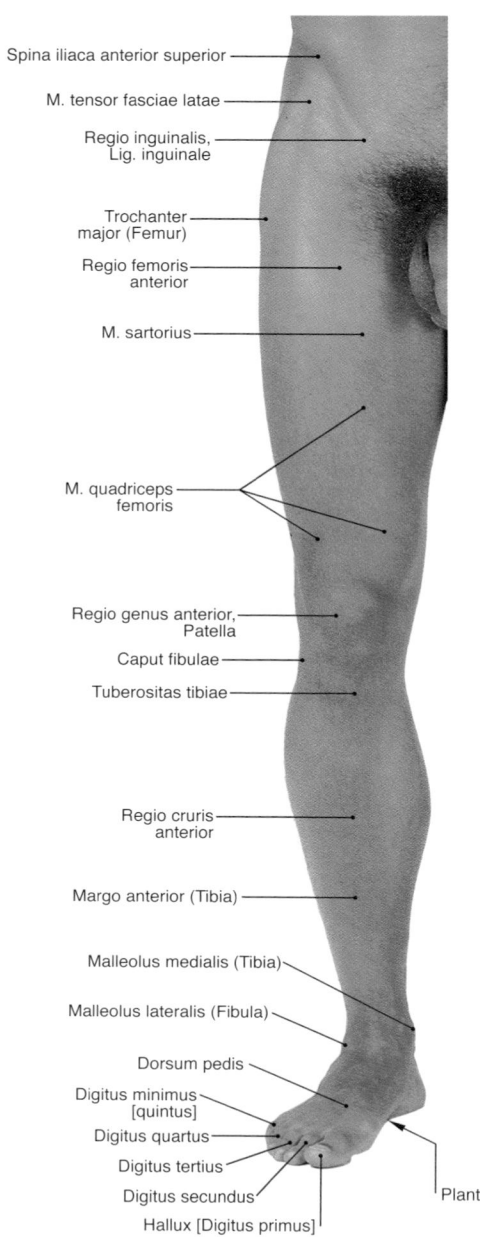

Spina iliaca anterior superior

M. tensor fasciae latae

Regio inguinalis, Lig. inguinale

Trochanter major (Femur)

Regio femoris anterior

M. sartorius

M. quadriceps femoris

Regio genus anterior, Patella

Caput fibulae

Tuberositas tibiae

Regio cruris anterior

Margo anterior (Tibia)

Malleolus medialis (Tibia)

Malleolus lateralis (Fibula)

Dorsum pedis

Digitus minimus [quintus]

Digitus quartus

Digitus tertius

Digitus secundus

Hallux [Digitus primus]

Planta

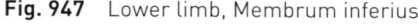

Fig. 947   Lower limb, Membrum inferius.

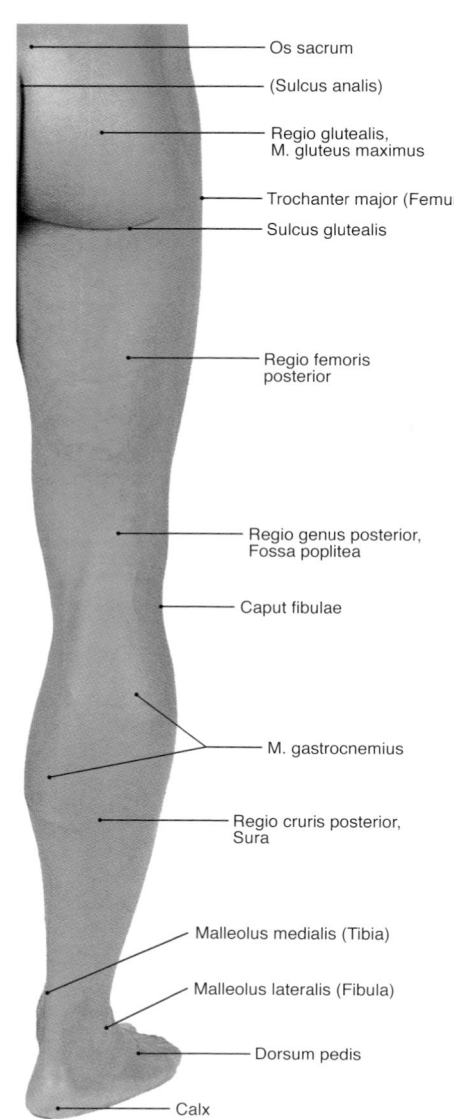

Os sacrum

(Sulcus analis)

Regio glutealis, M. gluteus maximus

Trochanter major (Femur)

Sulcus glutealis

Regio femoris posterior

Regio genus posterior, Fossa poplitea

Caput fibulae

M. gastrocnemius

Regio cruris posterior, Sura

Malleolus medialis (Tibia)

Malleolus lateralis (Fibula)

Dorsum pedis

Calx

Fig. 948   Lower limb, Membrum inferius.

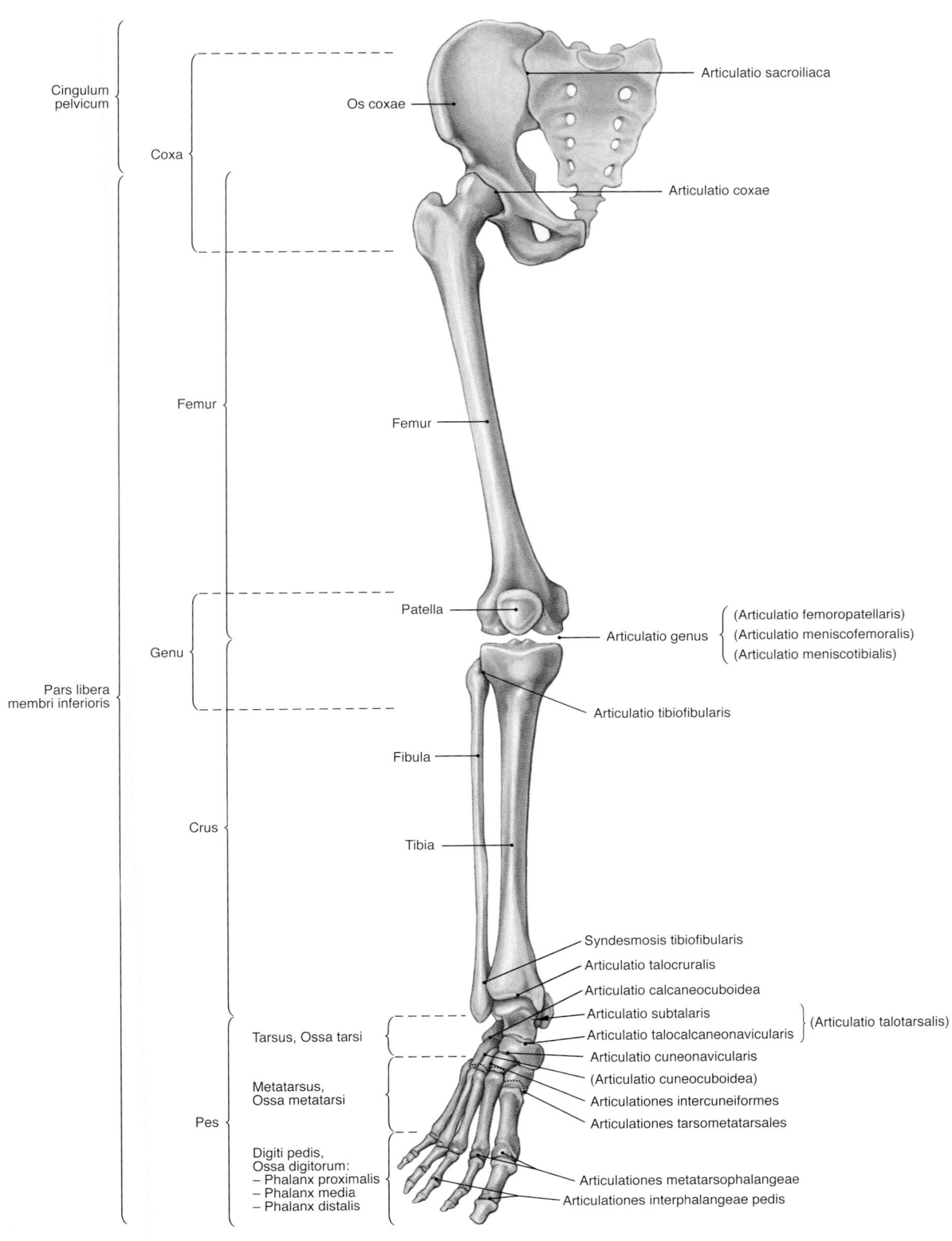

Cingulum
pelvicum

Coxa

Os coxae

Articulatio sacroiliaca

Articulatio coxae

Femur

Femur

Pars libera
membri inferioris

Genu

Patella

Articulatio genus

(Articulatio femoropatellaris)
(Articulatio meniscofemoralis)
(Articulatio meniscotibialis)

Articulatio tibiofibularis

Fibula

Crus

Tibia

Syndesmosis tibiofibularis
Articulatio talocruralis
Articulatio calcaneocuboidea
Articulatio subtalaris
Articulatio talocalcaneonavicularis

(Articulatio talotarsalis)

Tarsus, Ossa tarsi

Articulatio cuneonavicularis
(Articulatio cuneocuboidea)
Articulationes intercuneiformes
Articulationes tarsometatarsales

Metatarsus,
Ossa metatarsi

Pes

Digiti pedis,
Ossa digitorum:
– Phalanx proximalis
– Phalanx media
– Phalanx distalis

Articulationes metatarsophalangeae
Articulationes interphalangeae pedis

Fig. 949 Lower limb, Membrum inferius;
skeleton and joints.

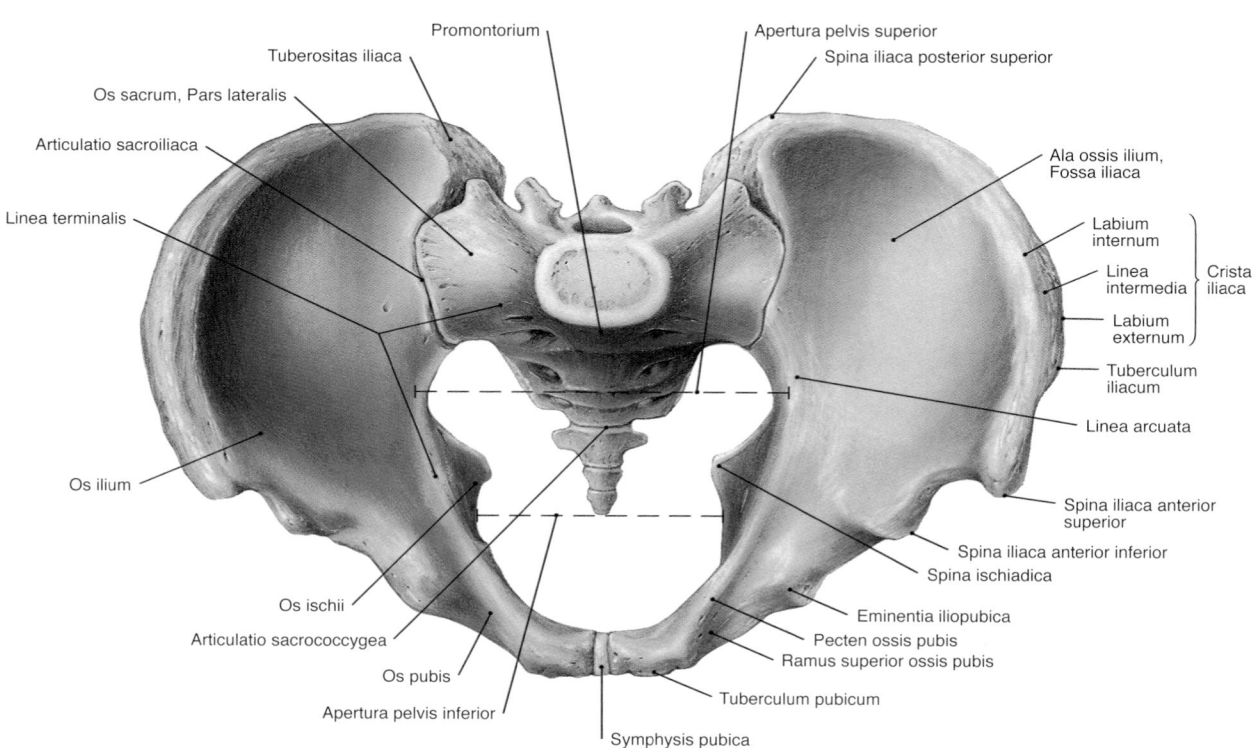

Fig. 950   Sacrum, Os sacrum, and pelvic girdle,
Cingulum pelvicum.
The region cranial to the linea terminalis is referred
to as the greater pelvis, Pelvis major, and the region
caudal to it is known as lesser pelvis, Pelvis minor.

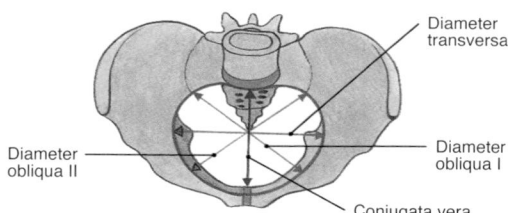

Fig. 951   Pelvis, Pelvis;
shape and dimensions of the pelvic inlet
of the female.

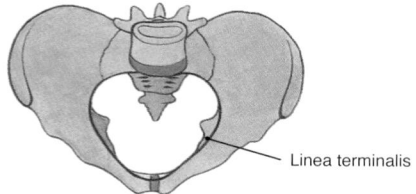

Fig. 952   Pelvis, Pelvis;
shape of the pelvic inlet
of the male.

k–k = Pelvic axis
a–b = Anatomical conjugate
a–e = Diagonal conjugate
         12.5–13 cm
a–c = True conjugate
         10.4–11 cm

h–d = Sagittal diameter of the
         pelvic brim 12–12.5 cm
e–g = Sagittal diameter of the
         pelvic constriction
         11–11.5 cm
e–f = Sagittal diameter of the
         pelvic outlet (= Distantia
         pubococcygea)
         9–10 cm

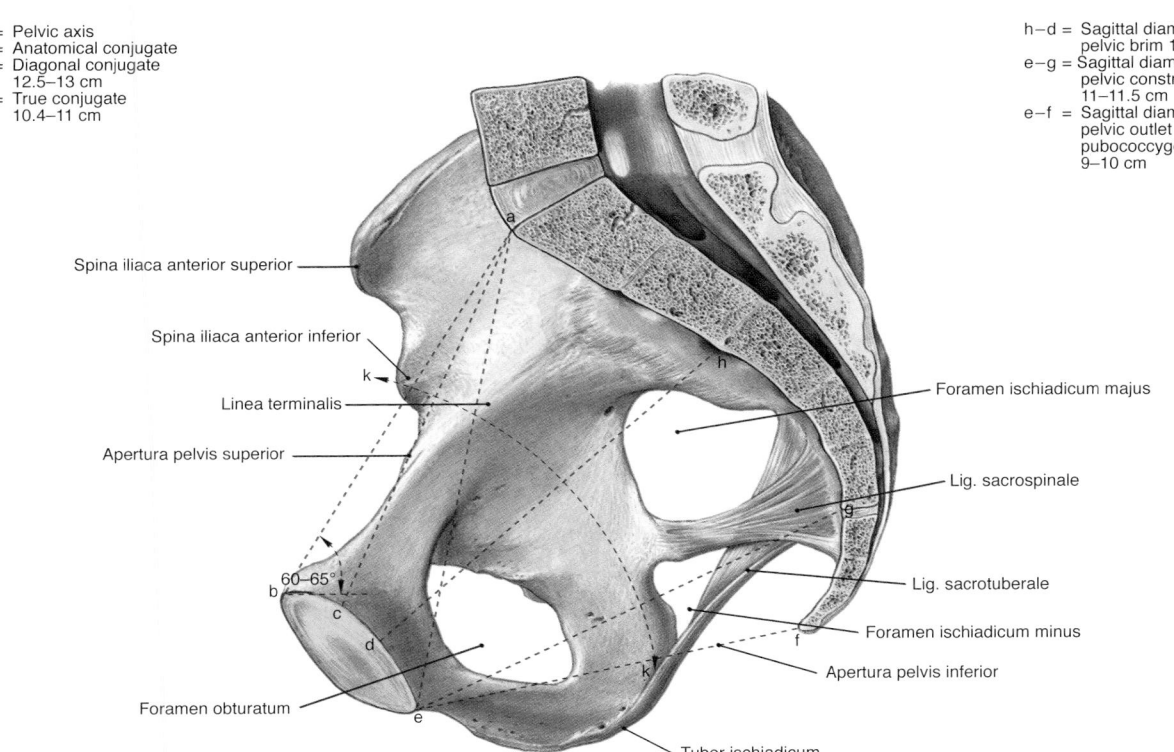

Spina iliaca anterior superior
Spina iliaca anterior inferior
Linea terminalis
Apertura pelvis superior
60–65°
Foramen obturatum

Foramen ischiadicum majus
Lig. sacrospinale
Lig. sacrotuberale
Foramen ischiadicum minus
Apertura pelvis inferior
Tuber ischiadicum

Fig. 953   Pelvis, Pelvis;
dimensions in the female;
median section.

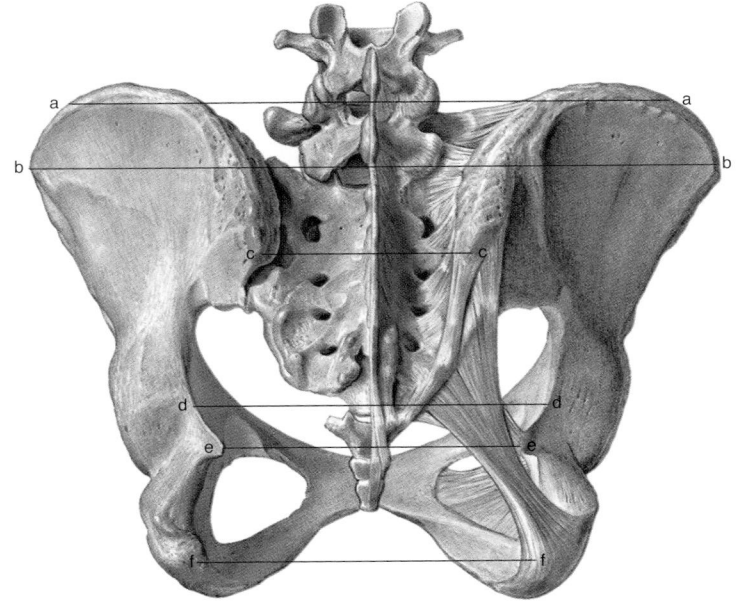

a–a = Crestal distance
         28–29 cm*
b–b = Anterior spinal distance
         25–26 cm*
c–c = Posterior spinal distance
         (width of the sacrum)
         10 cm
         * In this perspective, the crestal
         distance appears shorter than
         the anterior spinal distance.

d–d = Transverse diameter
         of the pelvic brim
         (= interacetabular line)
         12–12.5 cm
e–e = Transverse diameter of
         the pelvic constriction
         (= interspinal line)
         10.5 cm
f–f = Transverse diameter of
         the pelvic outlet
         (= tuberal diameter)
         11–12 cm)

Fig. 954   Pelvis, Pelvis,
dimensions in the female.

Hip bone

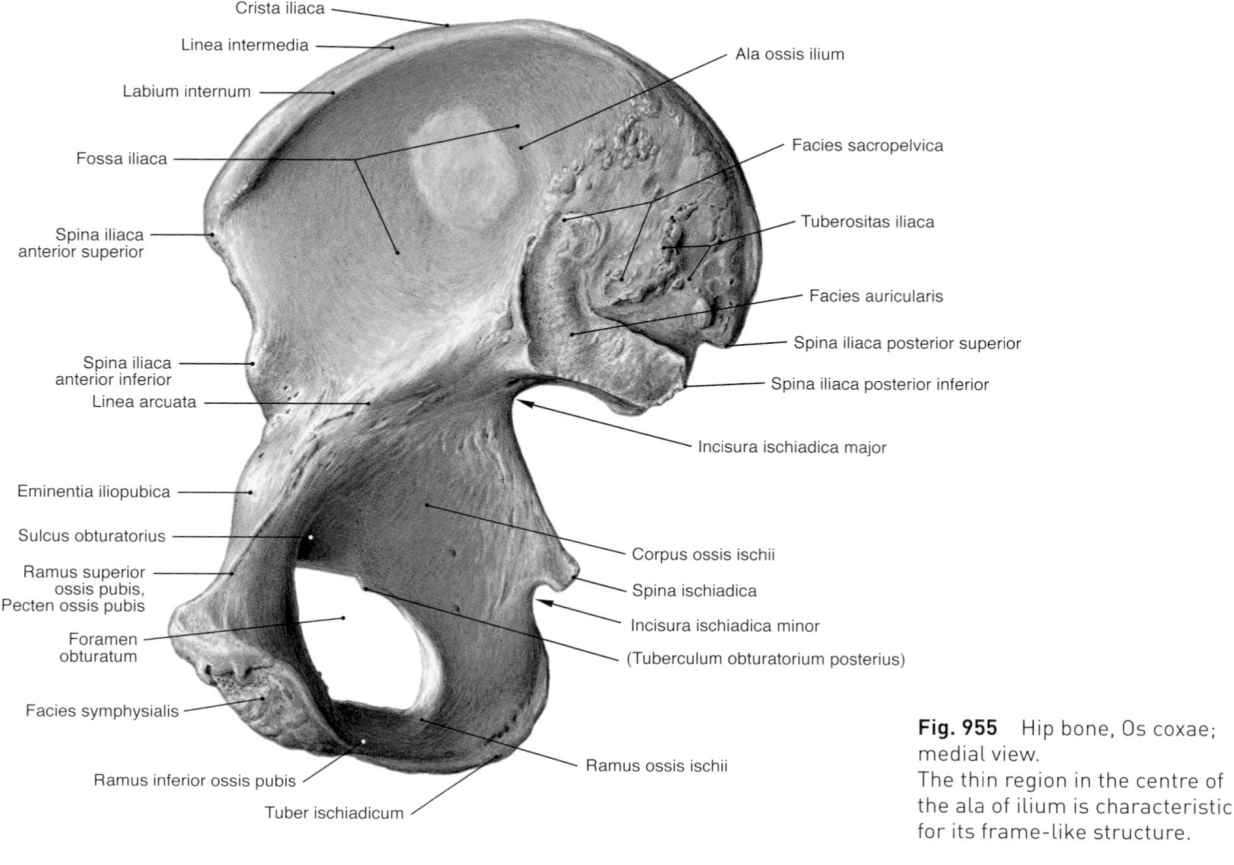

Crista iliaca
Linea intermedia
Labium internum
Fossa iliaca
Spina iliaca anterior superior
Spina iliaca anterior inferior
Linea arcuata
Eminentia iliopubica
Sulcus obturatorius
Ramus superior ossis pubis, Pecten ossis pubis
Foramen obturatum
Facies symphysialis
Ramus inferior ossis pubis
Tuber ischiadicum

Ala ossis ilium
Facies sacropelvica
Tuberositas iliaca
Facies auricularis
Spina iliaca posterior superior
Spina iliaca posterior inferior
Incisura ischiadica major
Corpus ossis ischii
Spina ischiadica
Incisura ischiadica minor
(Tuberculum obturatorium posterius)
Ramus ossis ischii

Fig. 955 Hip bone, Os coxae; medial view.
The thin region in the centre of the ala of ilium is characteristic for its frame-like structure.

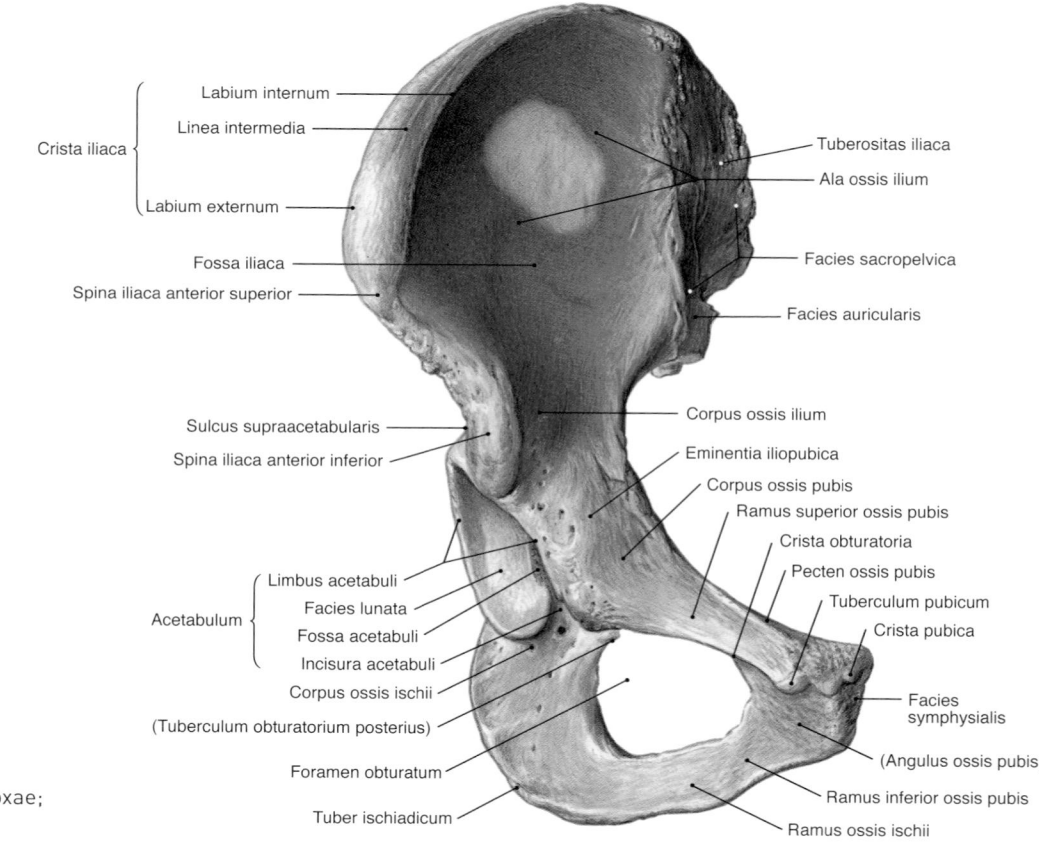

Crista iliaca
Labium internum
Linea intermedia
Labium externum
Fossa iliaca
Spina iliaca anterior superior
Sulcus supraacetabularis
Spina iliaca anterior inferior
Acetabulum
Limbus acetabuli
Facies lunata
Fossa acetabuli
Incisura acetabuli
Corpus ossis ischii
(Tuberculum obturatorium posterius)
Foramen obturatum
Tuber ischiadicum

Tuberositas iliaca
Ala ossis ilium
Facies sacropelvica
Facies auricularis
Corpus ossis ilium
Eminentia iliopubica
Corpus ossis pubis
Ramus superior ossis pubis
Crista obturatoria
Pecten ossis pubis
Tuberculum pubicum
Crista pubica
Facies symphysialis
(Angulus ossis pubis)
Ramus inferior ossis pubis
Ramus ossis ischii

Fig. 956 Hip bone, Os coxae; ventral view.

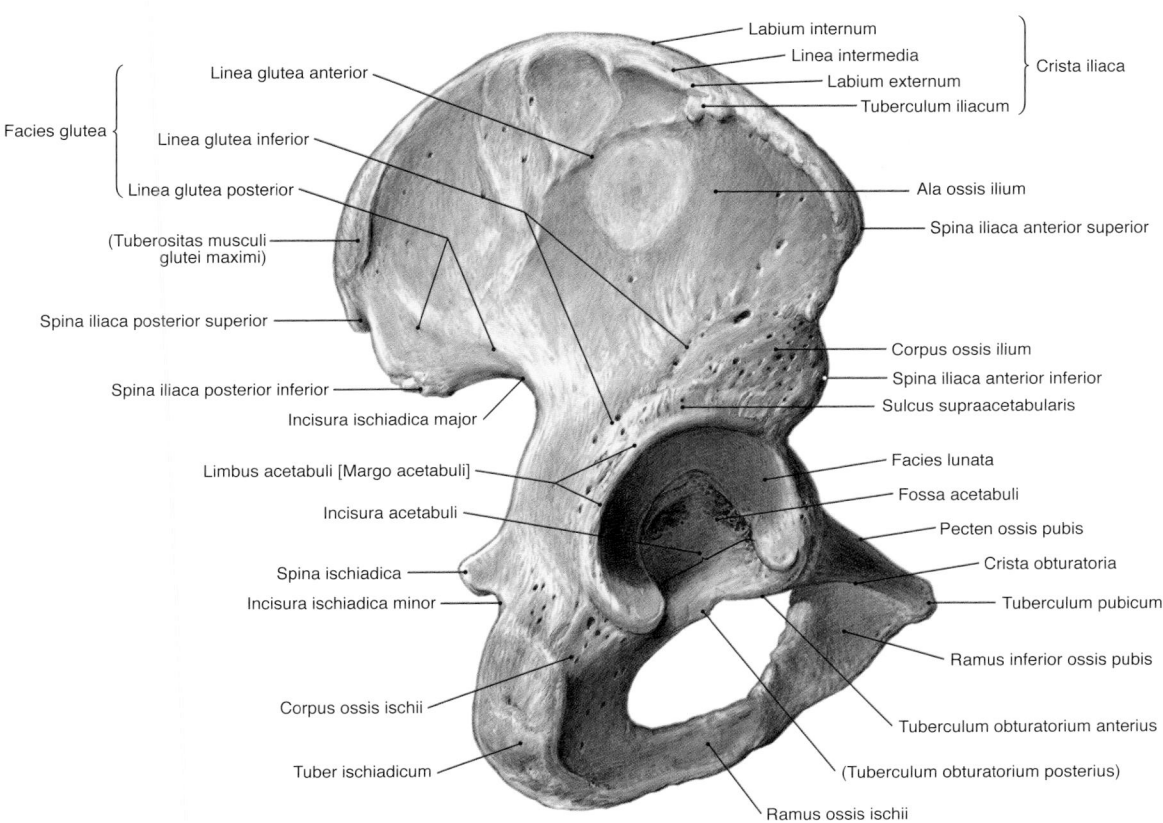

Facies glutea
- Linea glutea anterior
- Linea glutea inferior
- Linea glutea posterior

(Tuberositas musculi glutei maximi)

Spina iliaca posterior superior

Spina iliaca posterior inferior

Incisura ischiadica major

Limbus acetabuli [Margo acetabuli]

Incisura acetabuli

Spina ischiadica

Incisura ischiadica minor

Corpus ossis ischii

Tuber ischiadicum

Labium internum
Linea intermedia
Labium externum
Tuberculum iliacum
} Crista iliaca

Ala ossis ilium

Spina iliaca anterior superior

Corpus ossis ilium
Spina iliaca anterior inferior
Sulcus supraacetabularis

Facies lunata
Fossa acetabuli
Pecten ossis pubis
Crista obturatoria
Tuberculum pubicum

Ramus inferior ossis pubis

Tuberculum obturatorium anterius
(Tuberculum obturatorium posterius)

Ramus ossis ischii

Fig. 957   Hip bone, Os coxae; dorsolateral view.

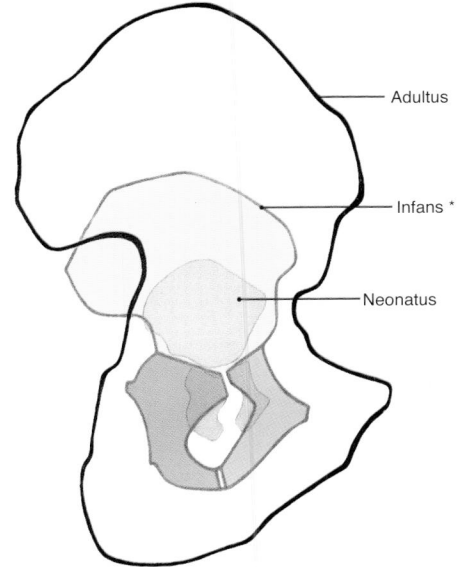

Adultus

Infans *

Neonatus

Fig. 958   Hip bone, Os coxae; development.
* Approximately sixth year of life

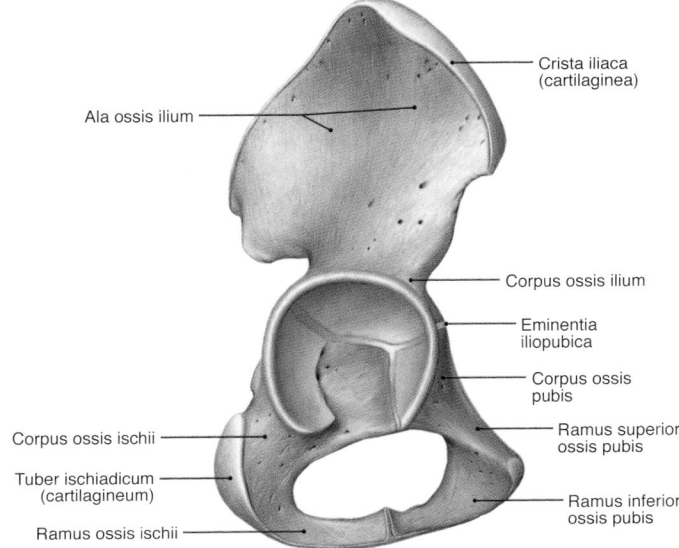

Ala ossis ilium

Crista iliaca (cartilaginea)

Corpus ossis ilium

Eminentia iliopubica

Corpus ossis pubis

Ramus superior ossis pubis

Ramus inferior ossis pubis

Corpus ossis ischii

Tuber ischiadicum (cartilagineum)

Ramus ossis ischii

Fig. 959   Hip bone, Os coxae;
stage of development in a 6-year-old child.
In the acetabulum, the three parts of the hip bone are fused to a Y-shaped cartilaginous junction. This junction ossifies at the age of 13–18 years.

Joints of the pelvic girdle

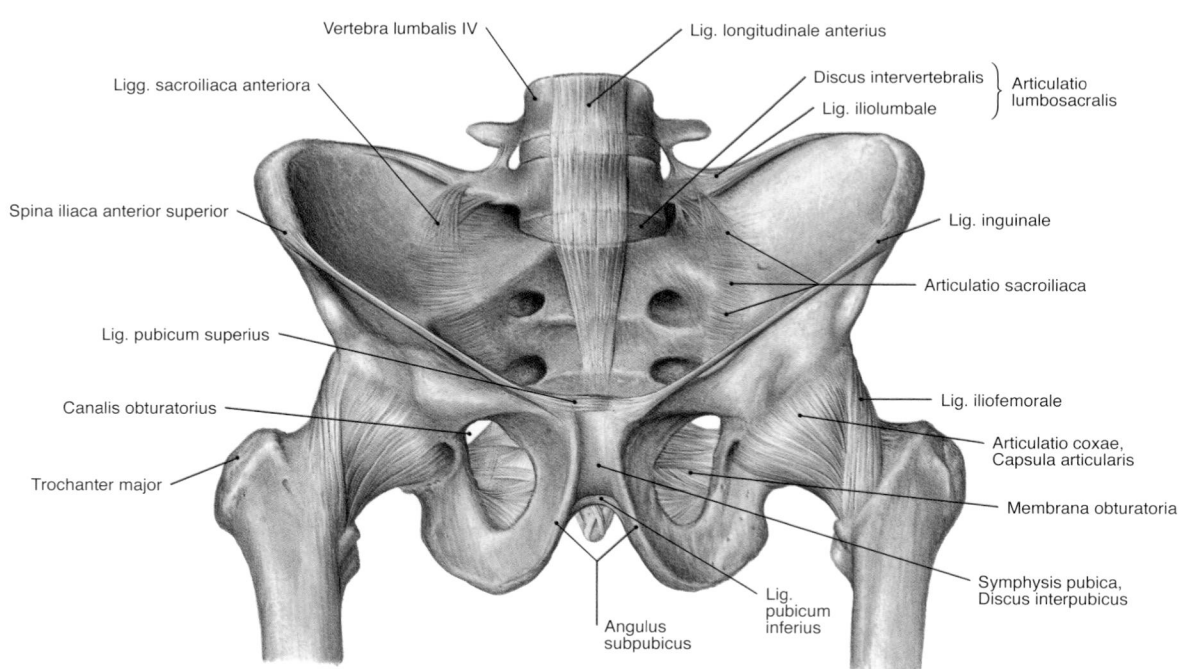

Vertebra lumbalis IV

Lig. longitudinale anterius

Ligg. sacroiliaca anteriora

Discus intervertebralis
Lig. iliolumbale } Articulatio lumbosacralis

Spina iliaca anterior superior

Lig. inguinale

Articulatio sacroiliaca

Lig. pubicum superius

Canalis obturatorius

Lig. iliofemorale

Trochanter major

Articulatio coxae, Capsula articularis

Membrana obturatoria

Symphysis pubica, Discus interpubicus

Angulus subpubicus

Lig. pubicum inferius

Fig. 960   Joints of the pelvic girdle,
Juncturae cinguli pelvici, and the lumbosacral joint,
Articulatio lumbosacralis, of the male.

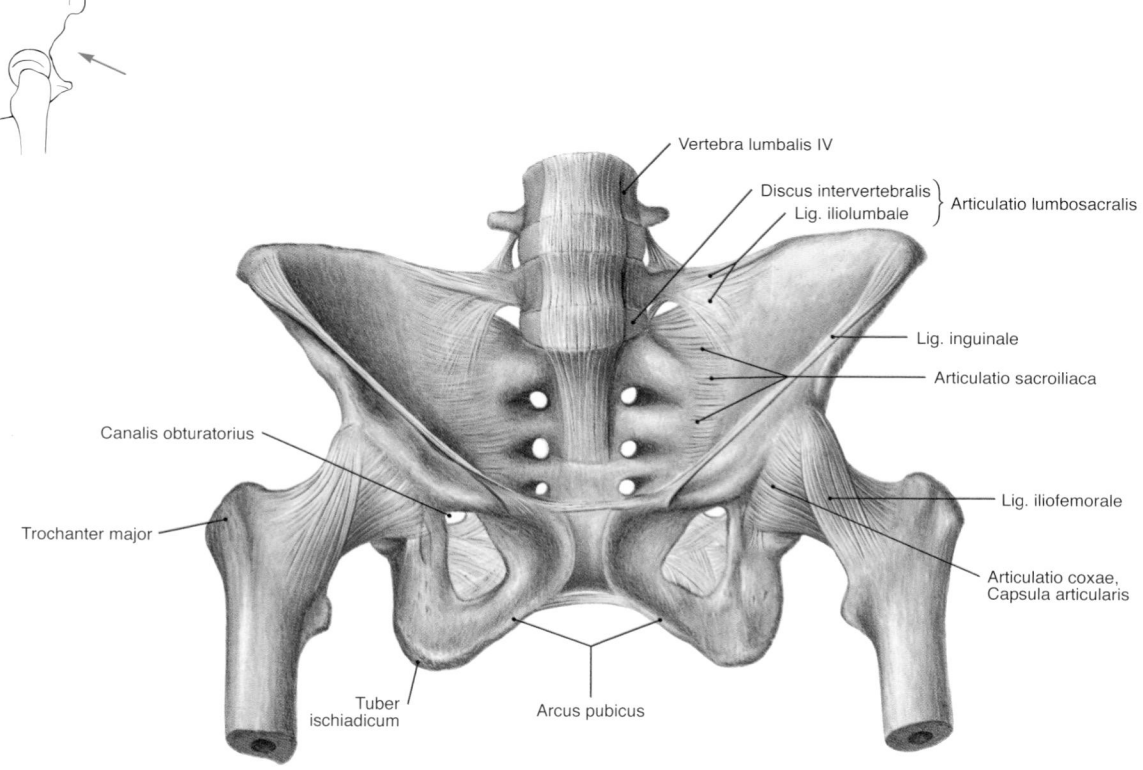

Vertebra lumbalis IV

Discus intervertebralis
Lig. iliolumbale } Articulatio lumbosacralis

Lig. inguinale

Articulatio sacroiliaca

Canalis obturatorius

Trochanter major

Lig. iliofemorale

Articulatio coxae, Capsula articularis

Tuber ischiadicum

Arcus pubicus

Fig. 961   Joints of the pelvic girdle,
Juncturae cinguli pelvici, and the lumbosacral joint,
Articulatio lumbosacralis, of the female.

Joints of the pelvic girdle

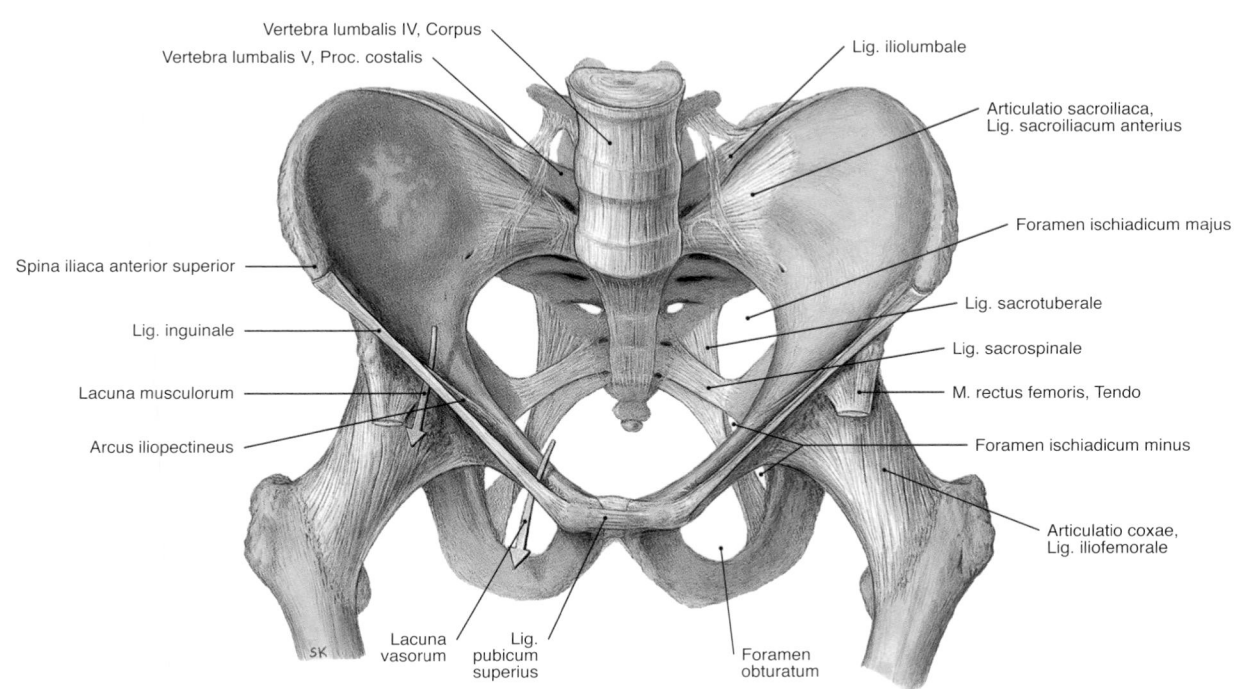

Vertebra lumbalis IV, Corpus
Vertebra lumbalis V, Proc. costalis
Lig. iliolumbale
Articulatio sacroiliaca, Lig. sacroiliacum anterius
Foramen ischiadicum majus
Spina iliaca anterior superior
Lig. sacrotuberale
Lig. inguinale
Lig. sacrospinale
Lacuna musculorum
M. rectus femoris, Tendo
Arcus iliopectineus
Foramen ischiadicum minus
Articulatio coxae, Lig. iliofemorale
Lacuna vasorum
Lig. pubicum superius
Foramen obturatum

Fig. 962 Joints of the pelvic girdle,
Juncturae cinguli pelvici, and the lumbosacral joint,
Articulatio lumbosacralis, of the male.

Vertebra lumbalis IV, Corpus
Vertebra lumbalis V, Proc. costalis
Lig. iliolumbale
Articulatio sacroiliaca, Lig. sacroiliacum anterius
Foramen ischiadicum majus
Spina iliaca anterior superior
Lig. sacrospinale
Lig. inguinale
Lig. sacrotuberale
Lacuna musculorum
Foramen ischiadicum minus
Arcus iliopectineus
M. rectus femoris, Tendo
Lacuna vasorum
Articulatio coxae, Lig. iliofemorale
Lig. pubicum superius
Foramen obturatum

Fig. 963 Joints of the pelvic girdle,
Juncturae cinguli pelvici, and the lumbosacral joint,
Articulatio lumbosacralis, of the female.

Joints of the pelvic girdle

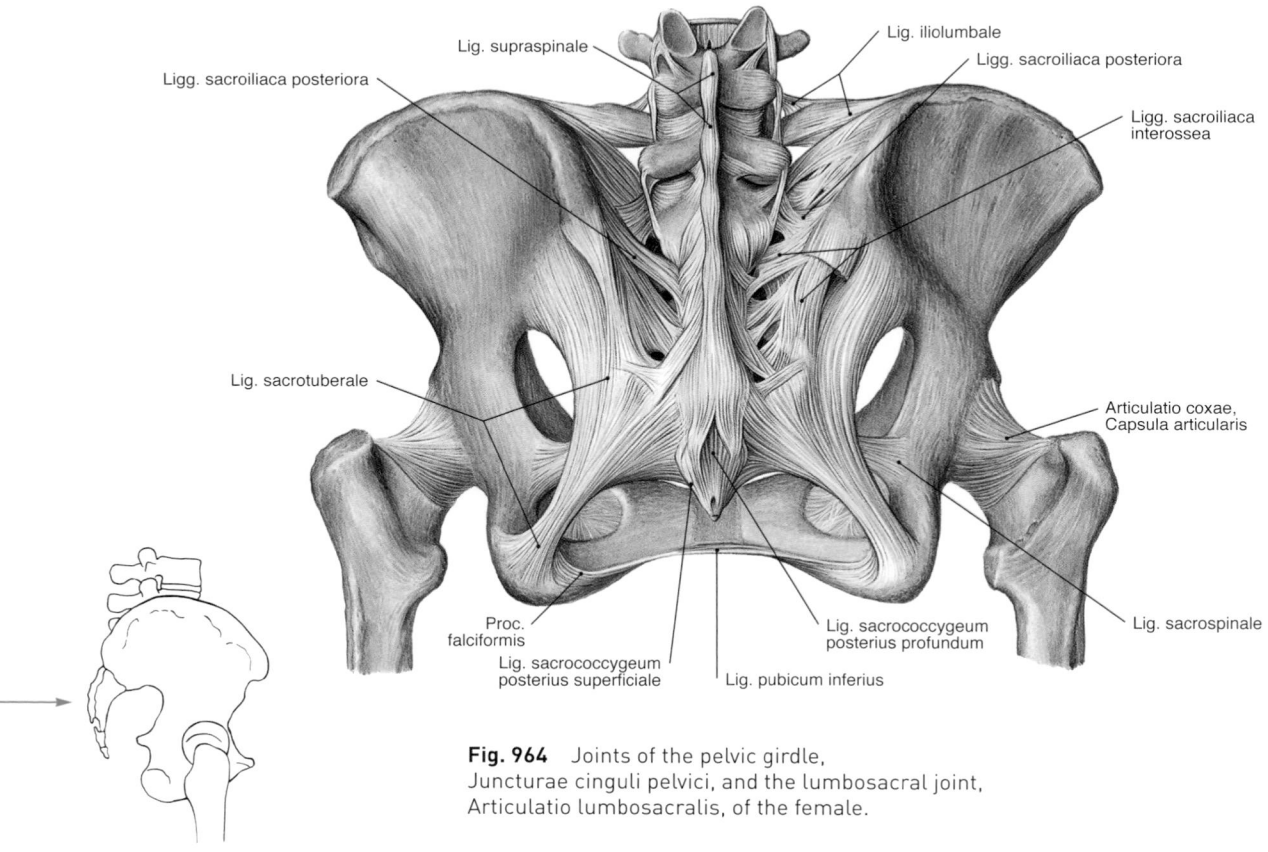

Ligg. sacroiliaca posteriora

Lig. supraspinale

Lig. iliolumbale

Ligg. sacroiliaca posteriora

Ligg. sacroiliaca interossea

Lig. sacrotuberale

Articulatio coxae, Capsula articularis

Proc. falciformis

Lig. sacrococcygeum posterius superficiale

Lig. sacrococcygeum posterius profundum

Lig. pubicum inferius

Lig. sacrospinale

Fig. 964 Joints of the pelvic girdle,
Juncturae cinguli pelvici, and the lumbosacral joint,
Articulatio lumbosacralis, of the female.

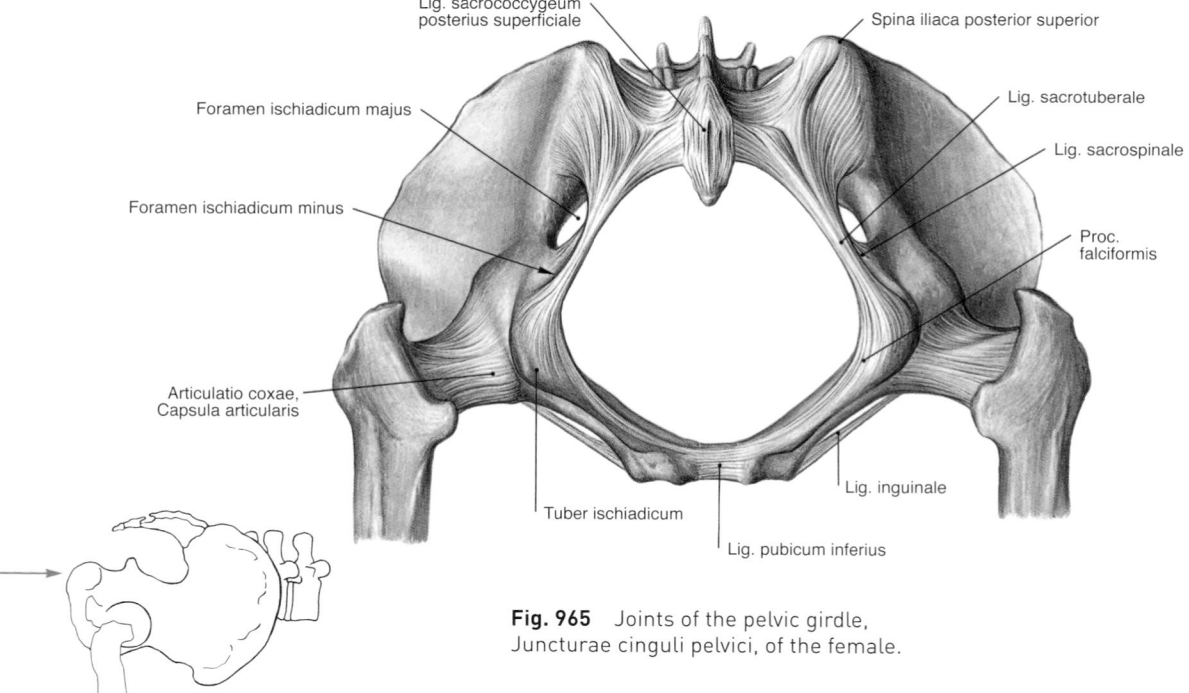

Lig. sacrococcygeum posterius superficiale

Spina iliaca posterior superior

Foramen ischiadicum majus

Lig. sacrotuberale

Lig. sacrospinale

Foramen ischiadicum minus

Proc. falciformis

Articulatio coxae, Capsula articularis

Lig. inguinale

Tuber ischiadicum

Lig. pubicum inferius

Fig. 965 Joints of the pelvic girdle,
Juncturae cinguli pelvici, of the female.

Joints of the pelvic girdle

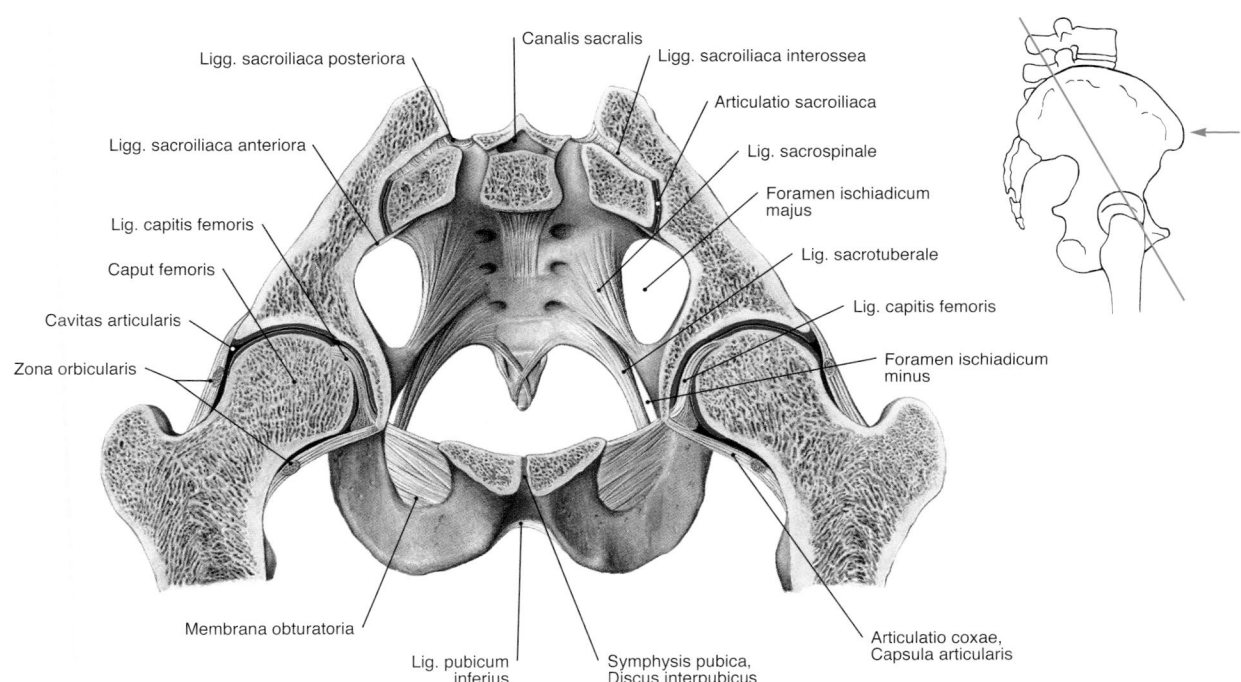

Ligg. sacroiliaca posteriora

Canalis sacralis

Ligg. sacroiliaca interossea

Articulatio sacroiliaca

Lig. sacrospinale

Ligg. sacroiliaca anteriora

Lig. capitis femoris

Foramen ischiadicum majus

Caput femoris

Lig. sacrotuberale

Cavitas articularis

Lig. capitis femoris

Zona orbicularis

Foramen ischiadicum minus

Membrana obturatoria

Articulatio coxae, Capsula articularis

Lig. pubicum inferius

Symphysis pubica, Discus interpubicus

Fig. 966   Joints of the pelvic girdle,
Juncturae cinguli pelvici, of the female.

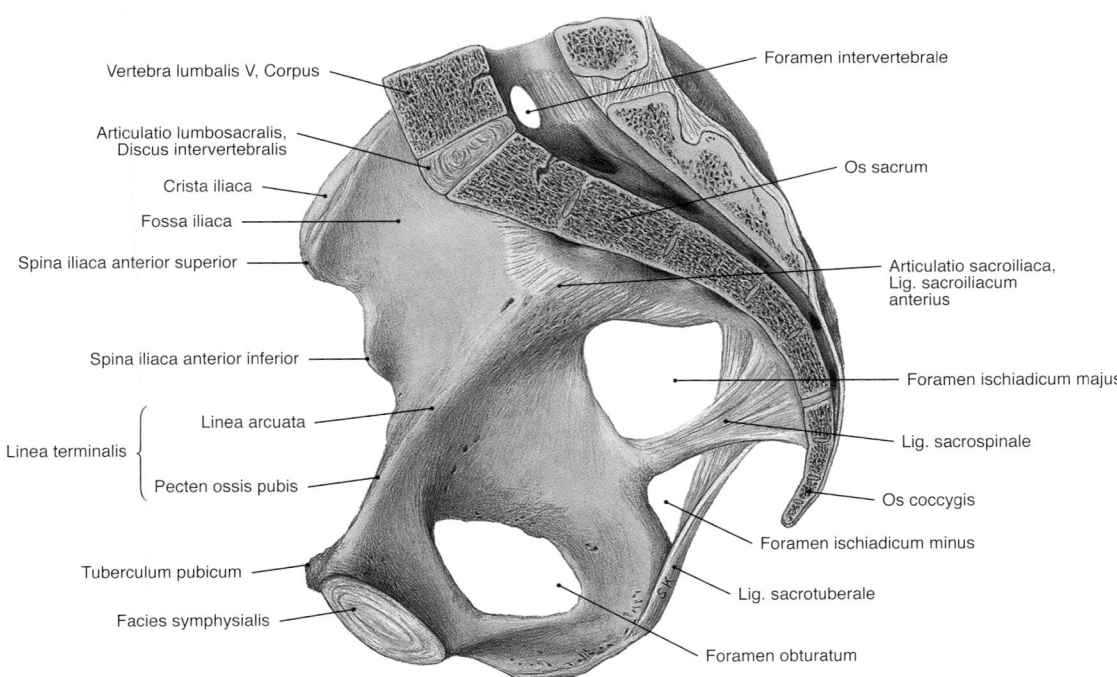

Vertebra lumbalis V, Corpus

Foramen intervertebrale

Articulatio lumbosacralis, Discus intervertebralis

Os sacrum

Crista iliaca

Fossa iliaca

Spina iliaca anterior superior

Articulatio sacroiliaca, Lig. sacroiliacum anterius

Spina iliaca anterior inferior

Foramen ischiadicum majus

Linea arcuata

Lig. sacrospinale

Linea terminalis

Pecten ossis pubis

Os coccygis

Foramen ischiadicum minus

Tuberculum pubicum

Lig. sacrotuberale

Facies symphysialis

Foramen obturatum

Fig. 967   Joints of the pelvic girdle,
Juncturae cinguli pelvici, and the lumbosacral joint,
Articulatio lumbosacralis, of the female;
median section.

Normally, the anterior border of the lowest intervertebral disc
forms the furthest projecting point of the posterior circumference
of the pelvic inlet. Radiographically, the most anterior part of the
sacrum is referred to as promontory.

Joints of the pelvic girdle

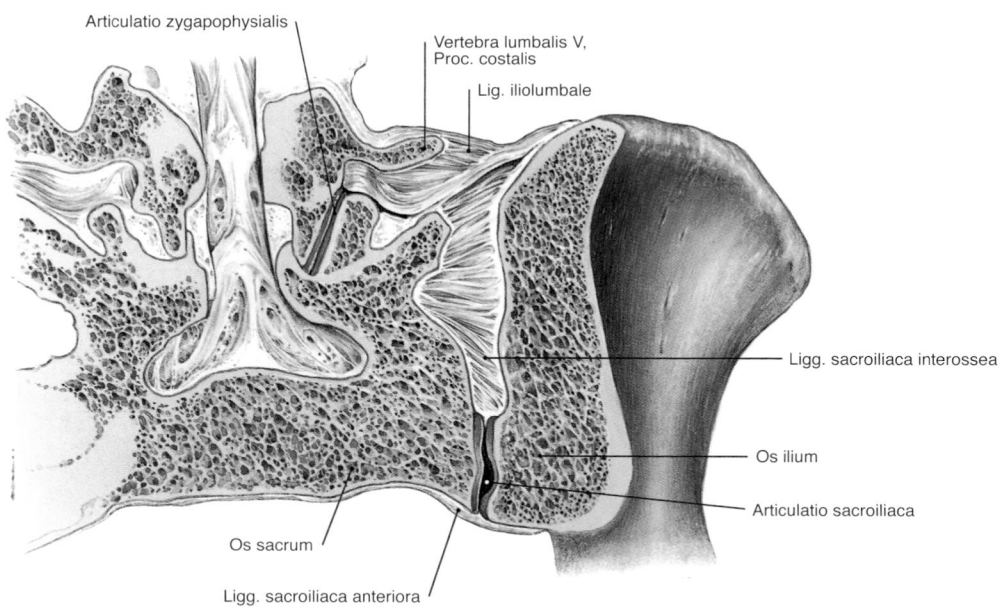

Fig. 968   Sacroiliac joint, Articulatio sacroiliaca; frontal section.

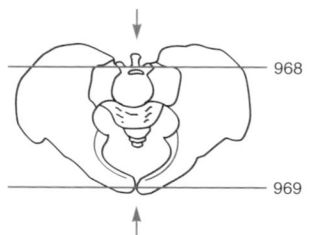

Fig. 969   Pubic symphysis, Symphysis pubica; oblique section in the direction of the longitudinal axis of the symphysis.
The interpubic disc consists of fibrous cartilage, with the exception of the articular symphysial surfaces of both pubic bones that are covered with hyaline cartilage. A longitudinal flat cleft occurs after the first decade of life (*).

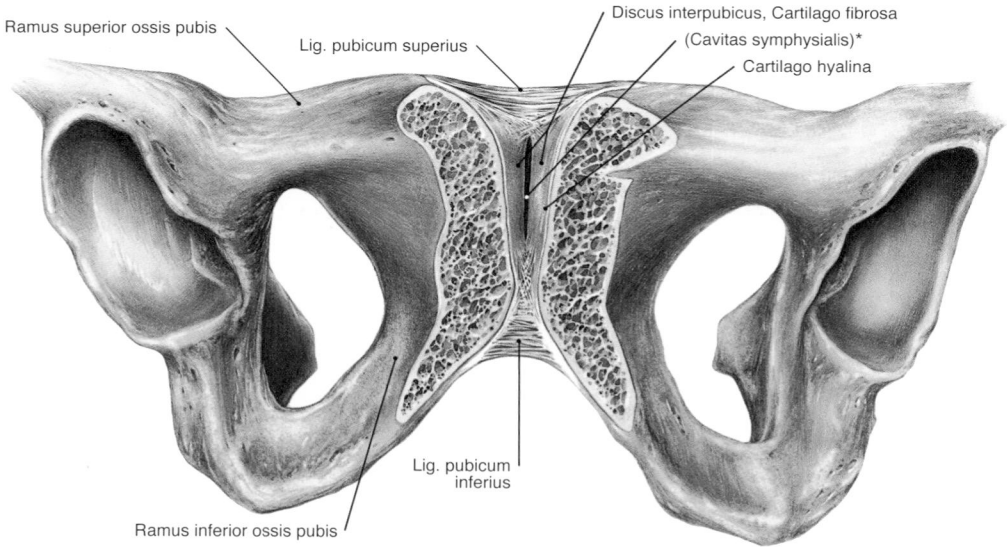

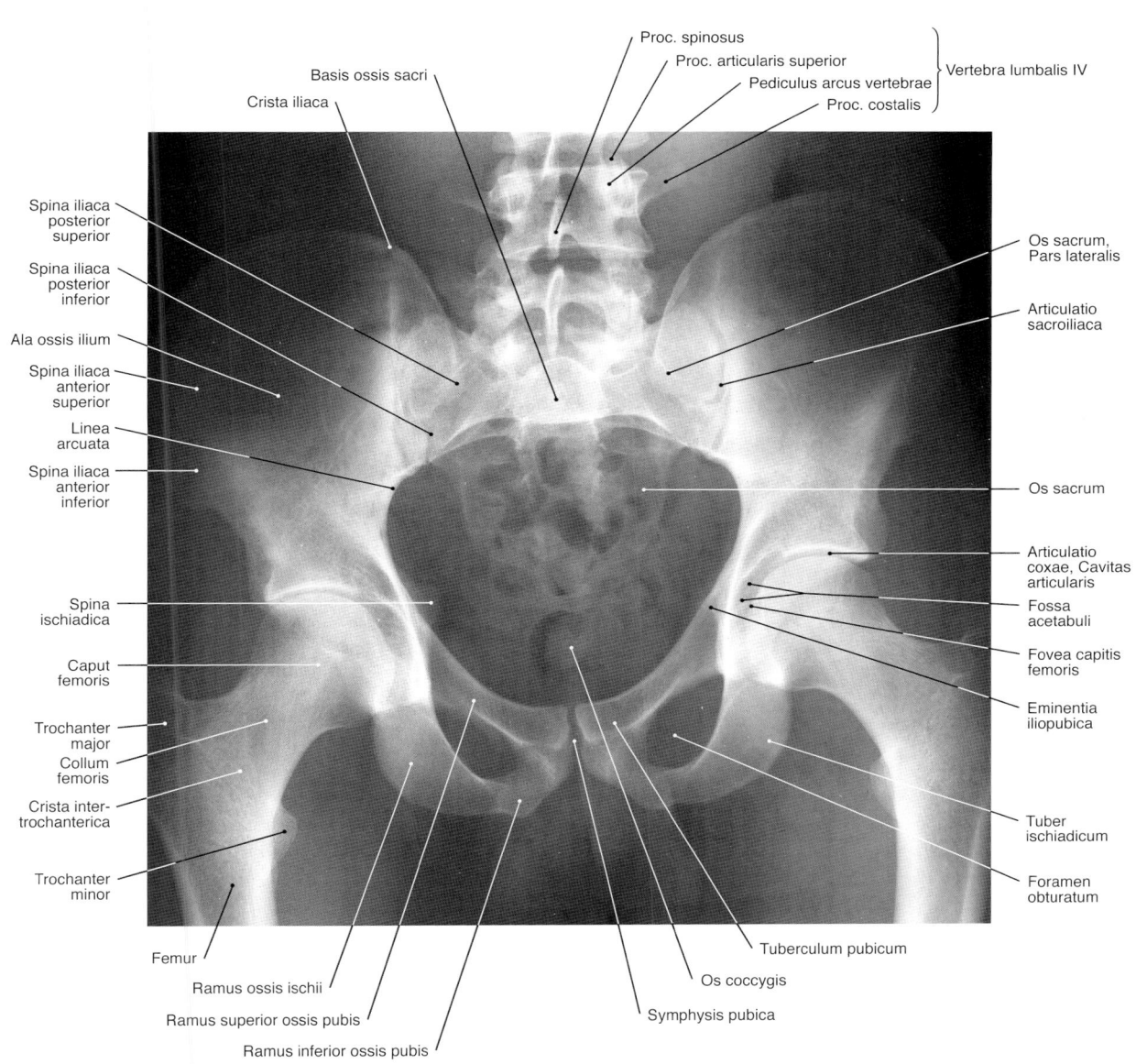

Proc. spinosus
Proc. articularis superior
Basis ossis sacri
Pediculus arcus vertebrae
Crista iliaca
Proc. costalis
Vertebra lumbalis IV

Spina iliaca posterior superior
Spina iliaca posterior inferior
Ala ossis ilium
Spina iliaca anterior superior
Linea arcuata
Spina iliaca anterior inferior

Spina ischiadica
Caput femoris
Trochanter major
Collum femoris
Crista inter-trochanterica
Trochanter minor

Femur
Ramus ossis ischii
Ramus superior ossis pubis
Ramus inferior ossis pubis

Os sacrum, Pars lateralis
Articulatio sacroiliaca
Os sacrum
Articulatio coxae, Cavitas articularis
Fossa acetabuli
Fovea capitis femoris
Eminentia iliopubica
Tuber ischiadicum
Foramen obturatum

Tuberculum pubicum
Os coccygis
Symphysis pubica

Fig. 970   Pelvis, Pelvis, of the male;
AP-radiograph with the central beam directed
onto the third sacral segment; upright position.

Pelvis, development

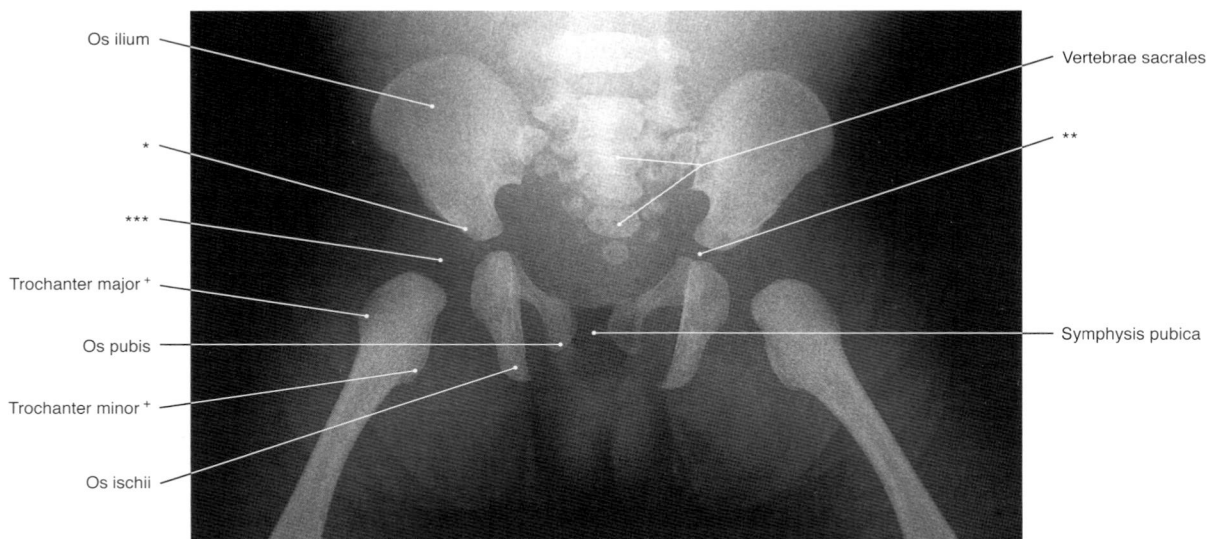

Os ilium

Vertebrae sacrales

*

**

***

Trochanter major⁺

Os pubis

Symphysis pubica

Trochanter minor⁺

Os ischii

Fig. 971 Pelvis, Pelvis, and femur, Femur; AP-radiograph of a female, premature baby (eighth month of pregnancy).

* Osseous roof of the acetabulum
** Y-shaped junction in the acetabular fossa
*** The ossification centre in the head of the femur does not appear before the third to fifth month of life.
\+ At this age, both greater trochanters only become apparent as small protuberances of the bone of the diaphysis.

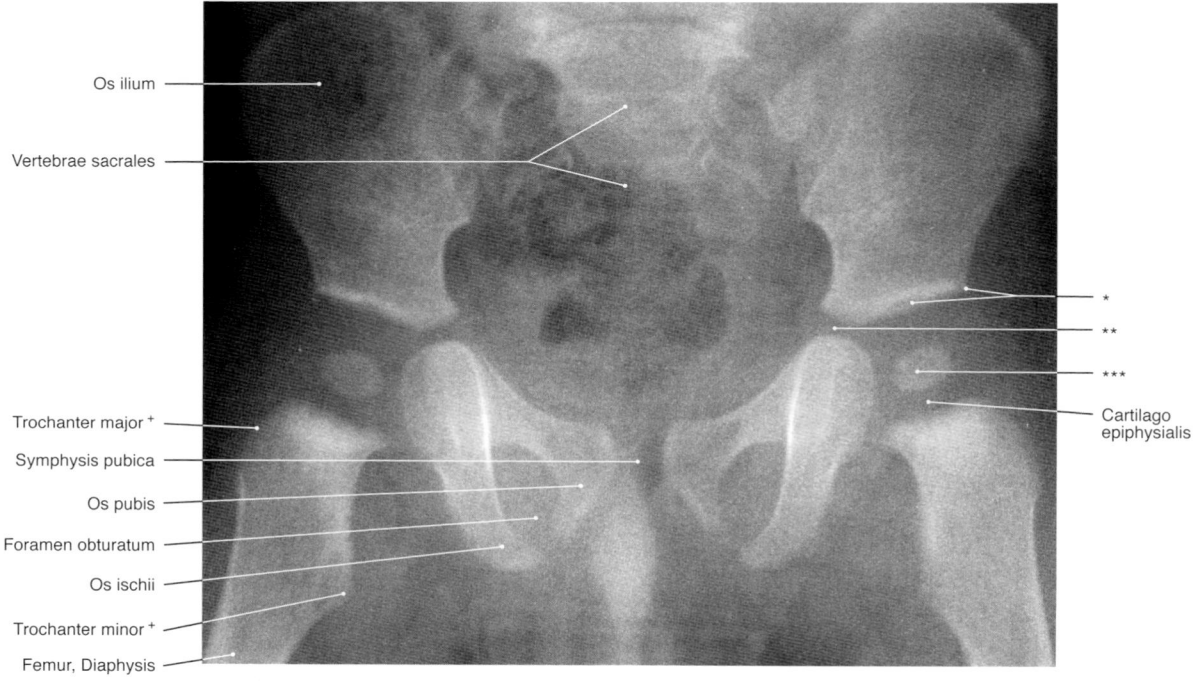

Os ilium

Vertebrae sacrales

Trochanter major⁺

Symphysis pubica

Os pubis

Foramen obturatum

Os ischii

Trochanter minor⁺

Femur, Diaphysis

*

**

***

Cartilago epiphysialis

Fig. 972 Pelvis, Pelvis, and femur, Femur; AP-radiograph of a 12-month-old boy.

* Osseous roof of the acetabulum
** Y-shaped junction in the acetabular fossa
*** Ossification centre in the epiphysis of the head of the femur
\+ At this age, both greater trochanters only become apparent as small protuberances of the bone of the diaphysis.

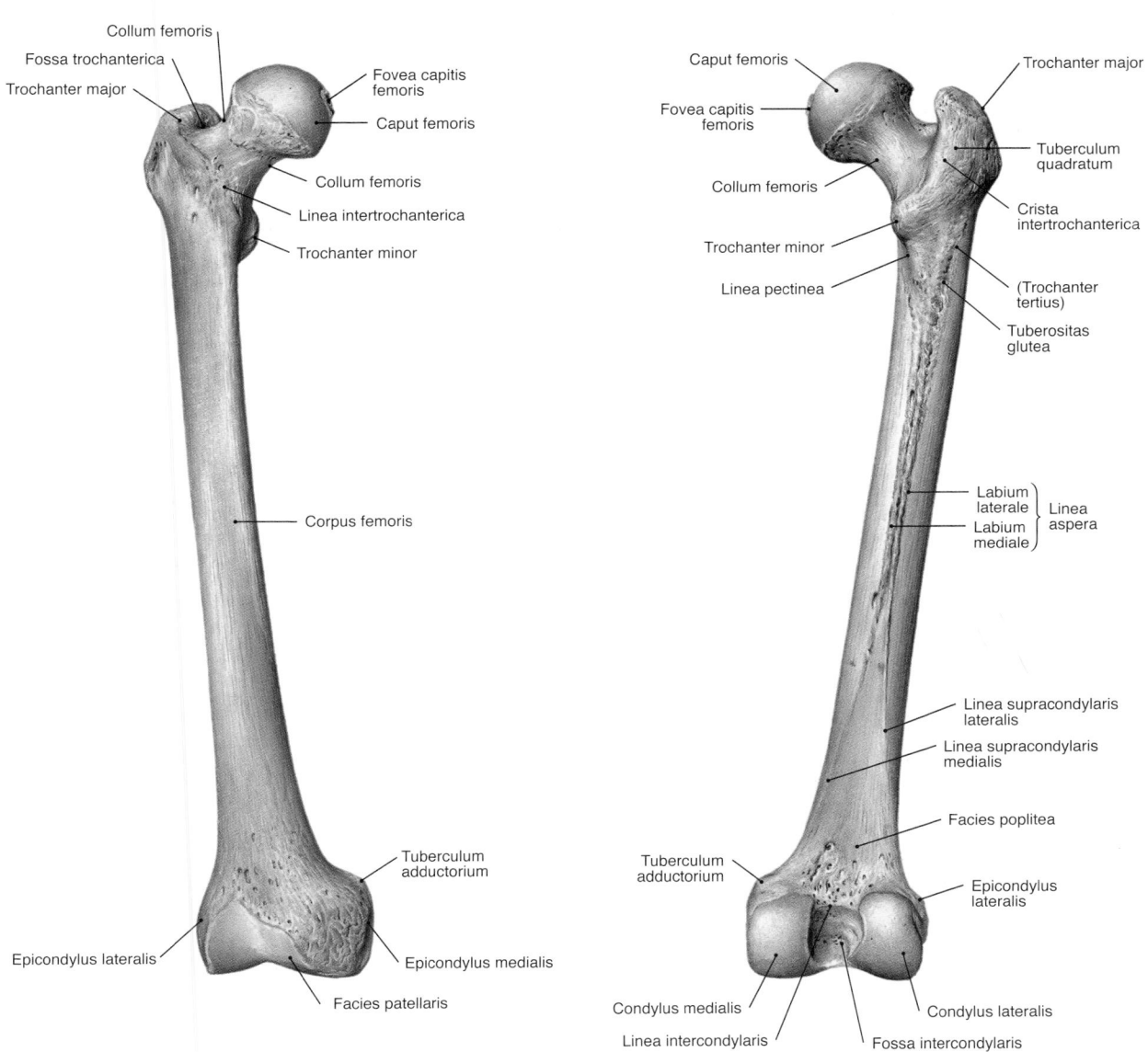

Collum femoris
Fossa trochanterica
Trochanter major
Fovea capitis femoris
Caput femoris
Collum femoris
Linea intertrochanterica
Trochanter minor
Corpus femoris
Tuberculum adductorium
Epicondylus lateralis
Epicondylus medialis
Facies patellaris

Caput femoris
Trochanter major
Fovea capitis femoris
Collum femoris
Tuberculum quadratum
Crista intertrochanterica
Trochanter minor
Linea pectinea
(Trochanter tertius)
Tuberositas glutea
Labium laterale
Labium mediale
Linea aspera
Linea supracondylaris lateralis
Linea supracondylaris medialis
Facies poplitea
Tuberculum adductorium
Epicondylus lateralis
Condylus medialis
Linea intercondylaris
Fossa intercondylaris
Condylus lateralis

Fig. 973   Femur, Femur; ventral view.

Fig. 974   Femur, Femur; dorsal view.

Femur

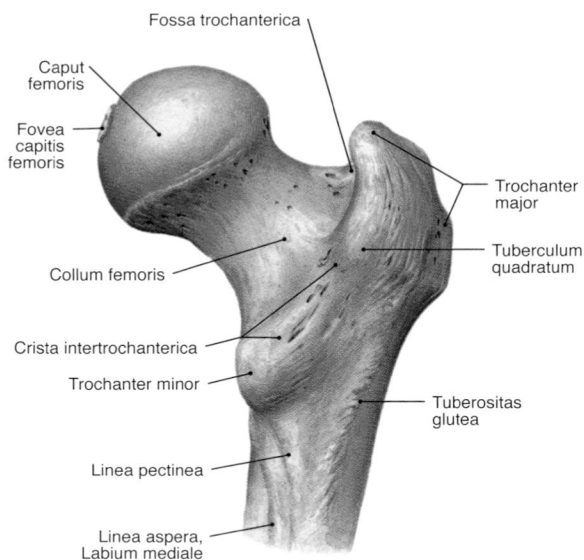

Fig. 975 Femur, Femur;
proximal extremity;
dorsal view.

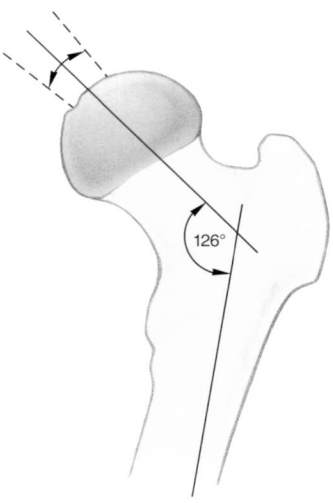

Fig. 976 Femur, Femur;
variability of the angle of the neck of the femur;
dorsal view.
The angle between the neck and the shaft of the femur is
referred to as neck-shaft angle. It is 150° in infants and about
126° in the adult.

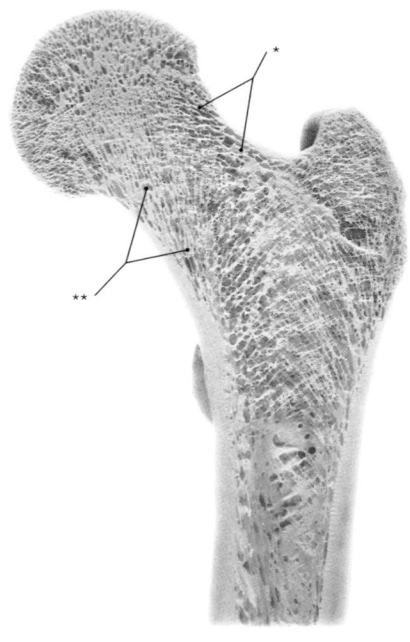

Fig. 977 Femur, Femur;
trabecular structure of the femoral bone with a large
neck-shaft angle (Coxa valga); section in the plane of the
angle of anterior torsion (60%).
The lateral plates of the trabecular bone* ("tensile system")
are only poorly developed, whereas the medial plates**
("compressive system") are much stronger.

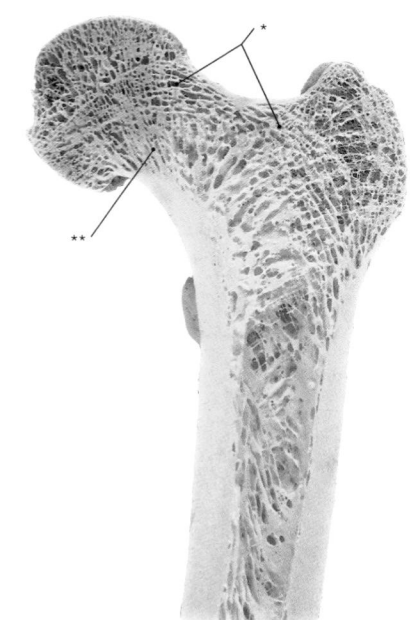

Fig. 978 Femur, Femur;
trabecular structure of the femoral bone with a small
neck-shaft angle (Coxa vara); section in the plane of the
angle of anterior torsion (60%).
The lateral plates of the trabecular bone * ("tensile system")
are well developed, while the medial plates **
("compressive system") are developed less strong. As a
result of the high demand of flexion, the cortex on the inner
side of the femoral neck is particularly thick.

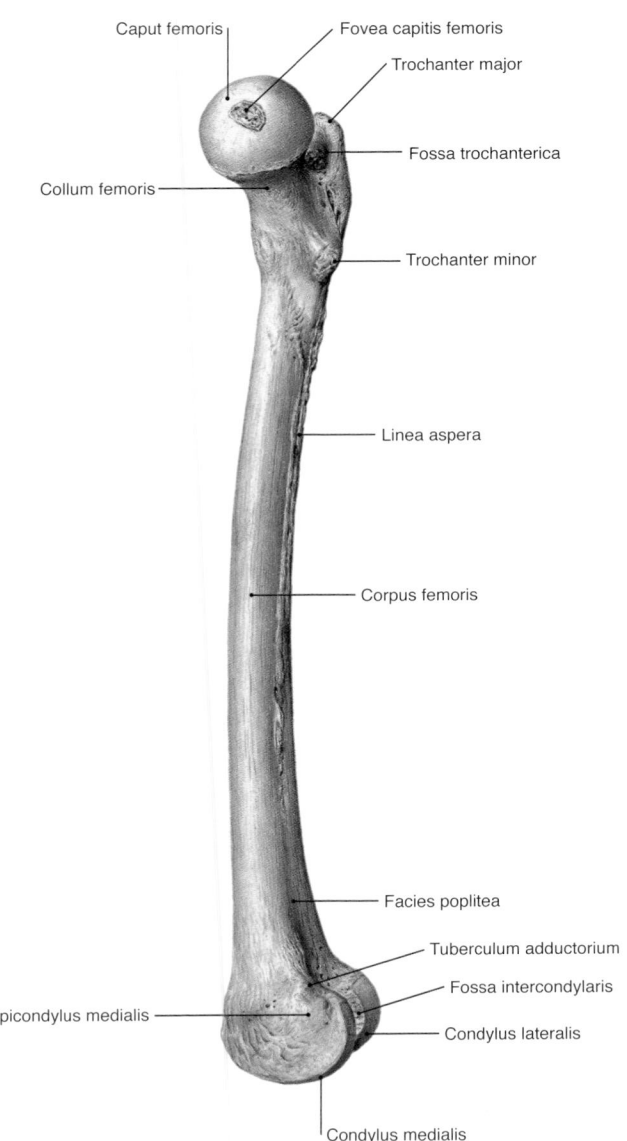

Caput femoris

Fovea capitis femoris

Trochanter major

Fossa trochanterica

Collum femoris

Trochanter minor

Linea aspera

Corpus femoris

Facies poplitea

Tuberculum adductorium

Fossa intercondylaris

Epicondylus medialis

Condylus lateralis

Condylus medialis

Fig. 979   Femur, Femur;
medial view.

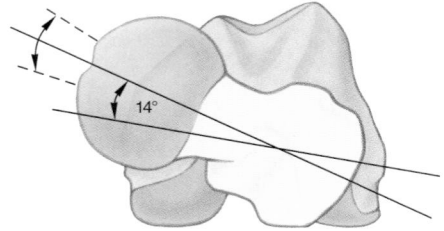

14°

Fig. 980   Femur, Femur;
variability of the angle of anterior torsion; the proximal
end of the femur has been projected over the distal end;
proximal view.
The angle of anterior torsion is about 30° in infants
and about 14° in adults.

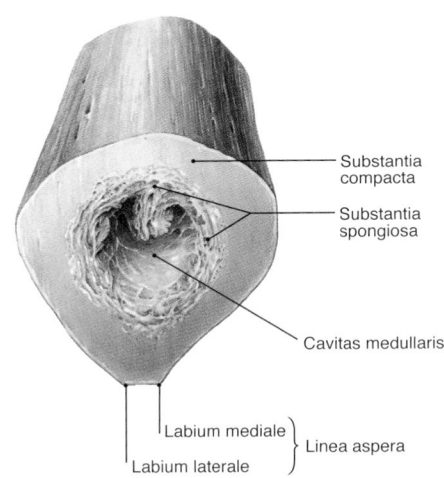

Substantia
compacta

Substantia
spongiosa

Cavitas medullaris

Labium mediale
Labium laterale   } Linea aspera

Fig. 981   Femur, Femur;
cross-section through the middle of the shaft;
distal view.

Hip joint

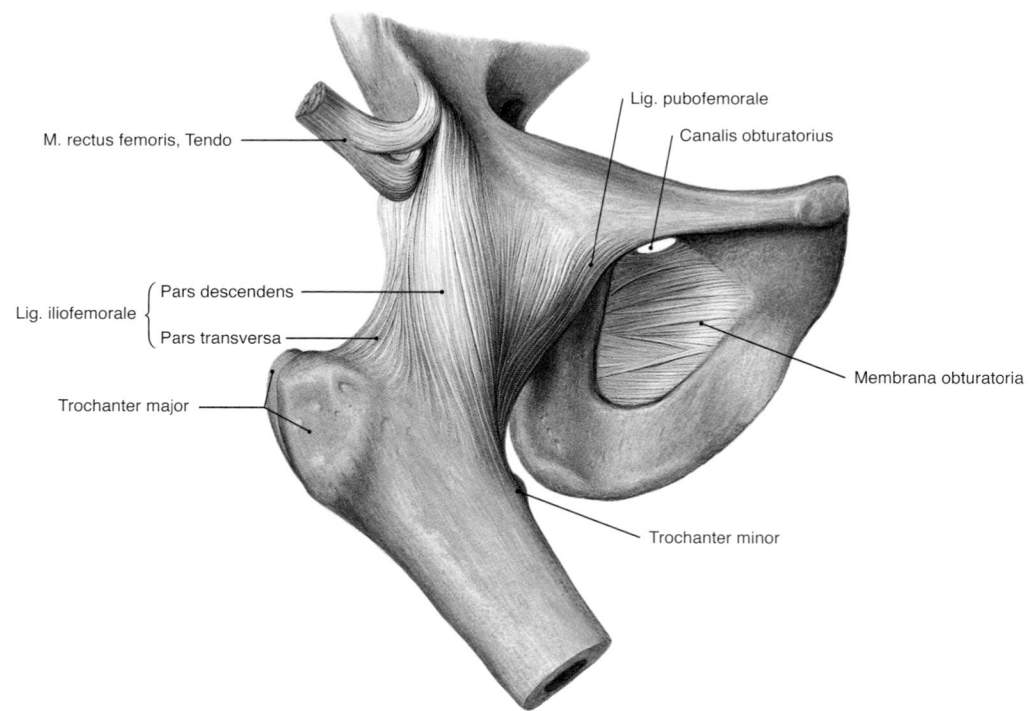

M. rectus femoris, Tendo

Lig. iliofemorale { Pars descendens
Pars transversa

Trochanter major

Lig. pubofemorale

Canalis obturatorius

Membrana obturatoria

Trochanter minor

Fig. 982   Hip joint, Articulatio coxae;
ventrodistal view.

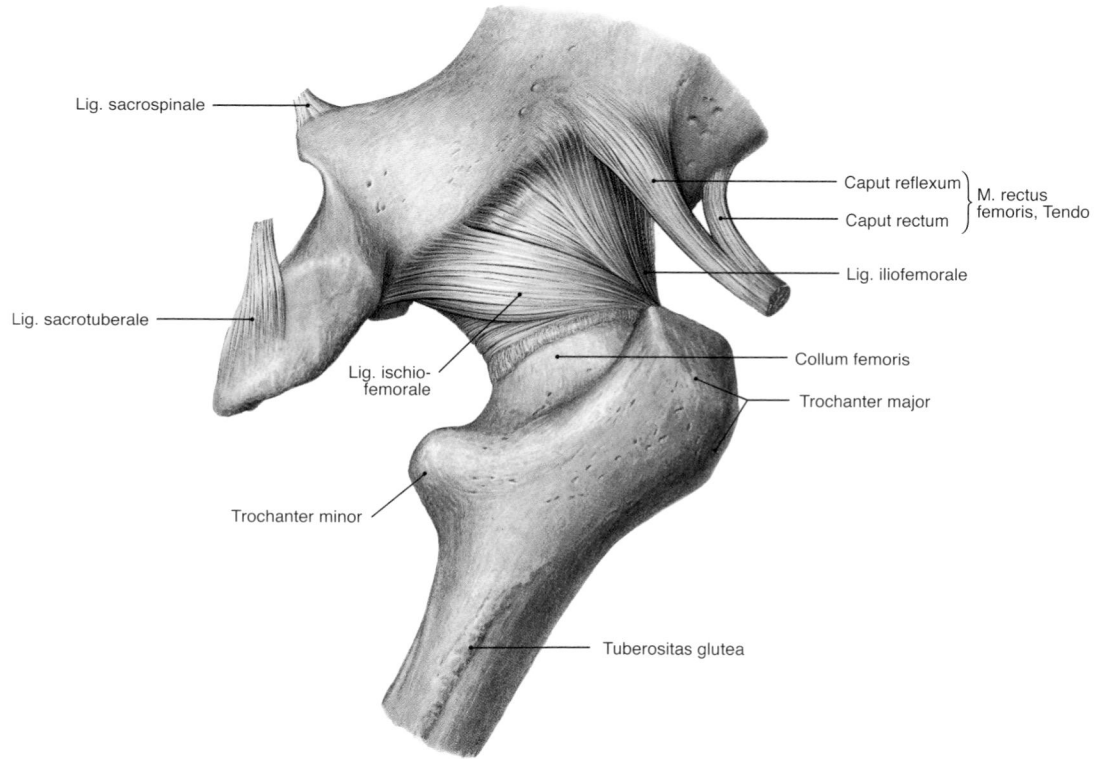

Lig. sacrospinale

Lig. sacrotuberale

Lig. ischio-femorale

Trochanter minor

Caput reflexum } M. rectus
Caput rectum } femoris, Tendo

Lig. iliofemorale

Collum femoris

Trochanter major

Tuberositas glutea

Fig. 983   Hip joint, Articulatio coxae;
dorsal view.

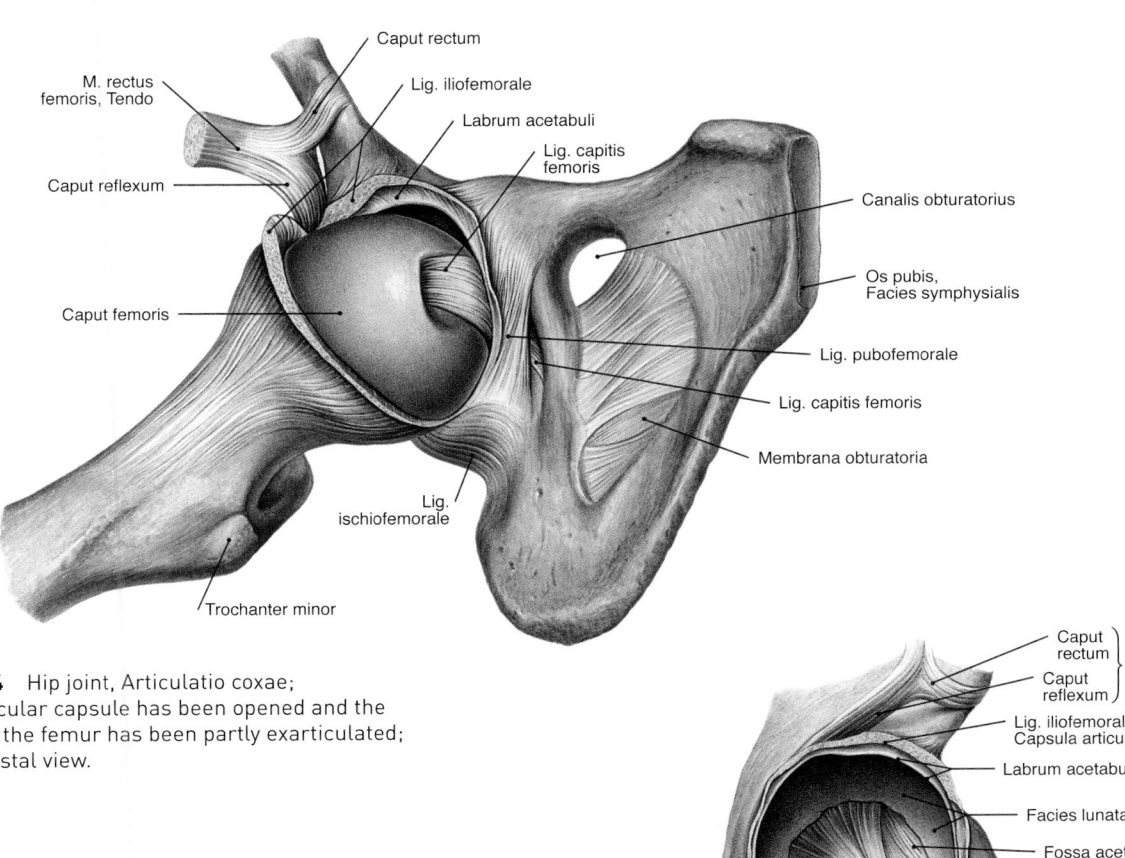

Caput rectum
M. rectus femoris, Tendo
Lig. iliofemorale
Labrum acetabuli
Lig. capitis femoris
Caput reflexum
Canalis obturatorius
Caput femoris
Os pubis, Facies symphysialis
Lig. pubofemorale
Caput femoris
Lig. capitis femoris
Membrana obturatoria
Lig. ischiofemorale
Trochanter minor

Fig. 984 Hip joint, Articulatio coxae;
the articular capsule has been opened and the
head of the femur has been partly exarticulated;
laterodistal view.

Caput rectum ⎱ M. rectus
Caput reflexum ⎰ femoris, Tendo
Lig. iliofemorale; Capsula articularis
Labrum acetabuli
Facies lunata
Fossa acetabuli
Lig. capitis femoris
Canalis obturatorius
Lig. transversum acetabuli
Lig. ischiofemorale; Capsula articularis

Fig. 985 Hip joint, Articulatio coxae;
aspect of the acetabulum after removal of the articular
capsule and exarticulation of the head of the femur;
laterodistal view.

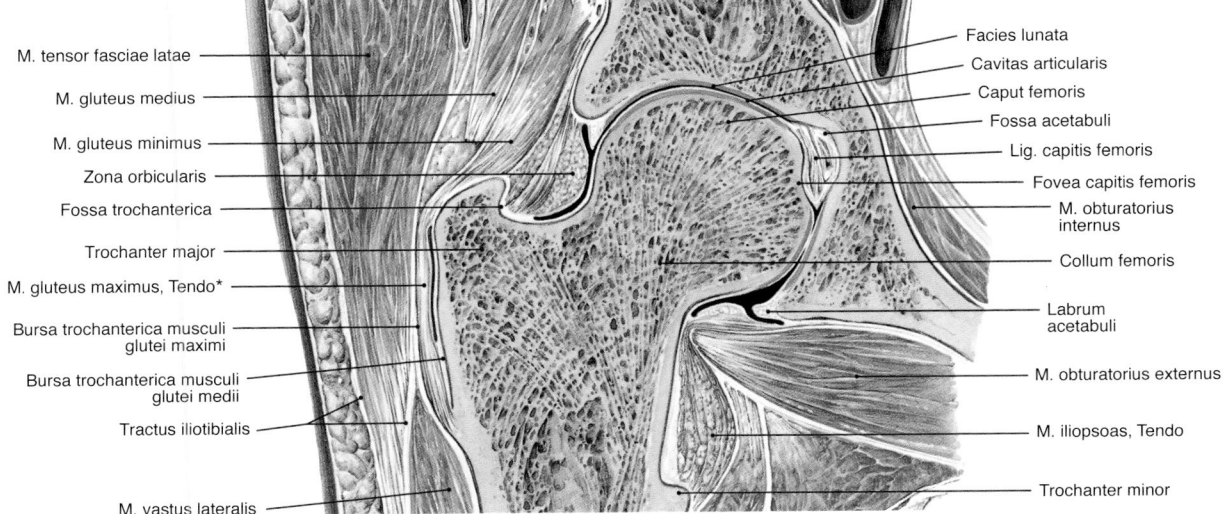

M. tensor fasciae latae
M. gluteus medius
M. gluteus minimus
Zona orbicularis
Fossa trochanterica
Trochanter major
M. gluteus maximus, Tendo*
Bursa trochanterica musculi glutei maximi
Bursa trochanterica musculi glutei medii
Tractus iliotibialis
M. vastus lateralis

Facies lunata
Cavitas articularis
Caput femoris
Fossa acetabuli
Lig. capitis femoris
Fovea capitis femoris
M. obturatorius internus
Collum femoris
Labrum acetabuli
M. obturatorius externus
M. iliopsoas, Tendo
Trochanter minor

Fig. 986 Hip joint, Articulatio coxae;
vertical section at the plane of the angle of antetorsion.
* Radiations into the iliotibial tract

Hip joint, radiography

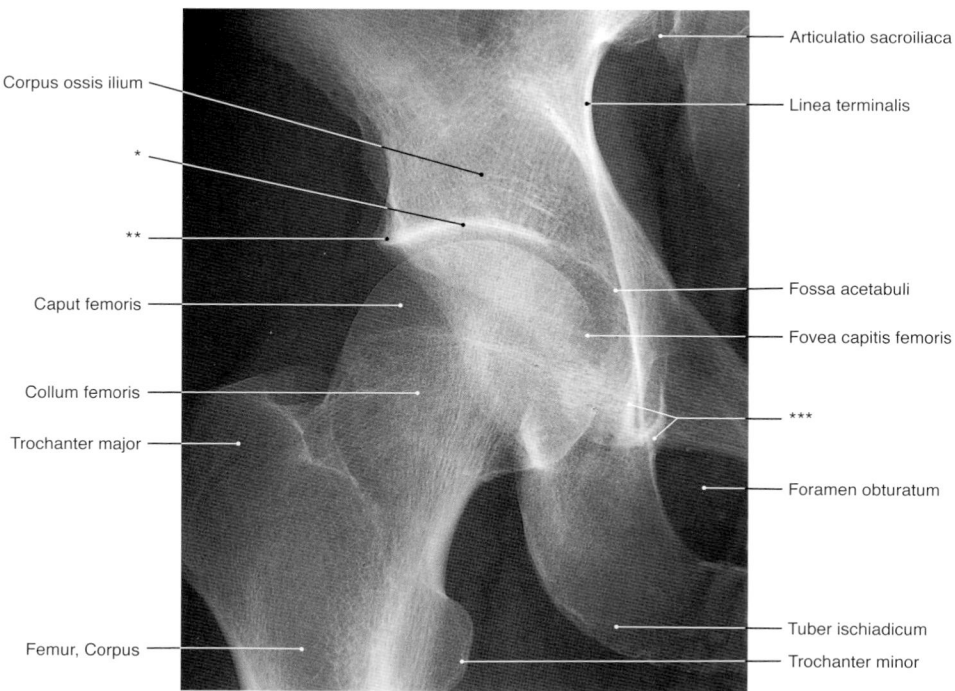

Corpus ossis ilium

Articulatio sacroiliaca

Linea terminalis

*

**

Caput femoris

Fossa acetabuli

Fovea capitis femoris

Collum femoris

***

Trochanter major

Foramen obturatum

Tuber ischiadicum

Femur, Corpus

Trochanter minor

Fig. 987   Hip joint, Articulatio coxae;
AP-radiograph; upright position on both legs.

*   Clinical term: acetabular roof = tangential projection of the lunate surface
**   Clinical term: edge of the acetabular roof = the most lateral projection
    of the acetabulum
*** Clinical term: KÖHLER's teardrop = projection of the acetabular fossa

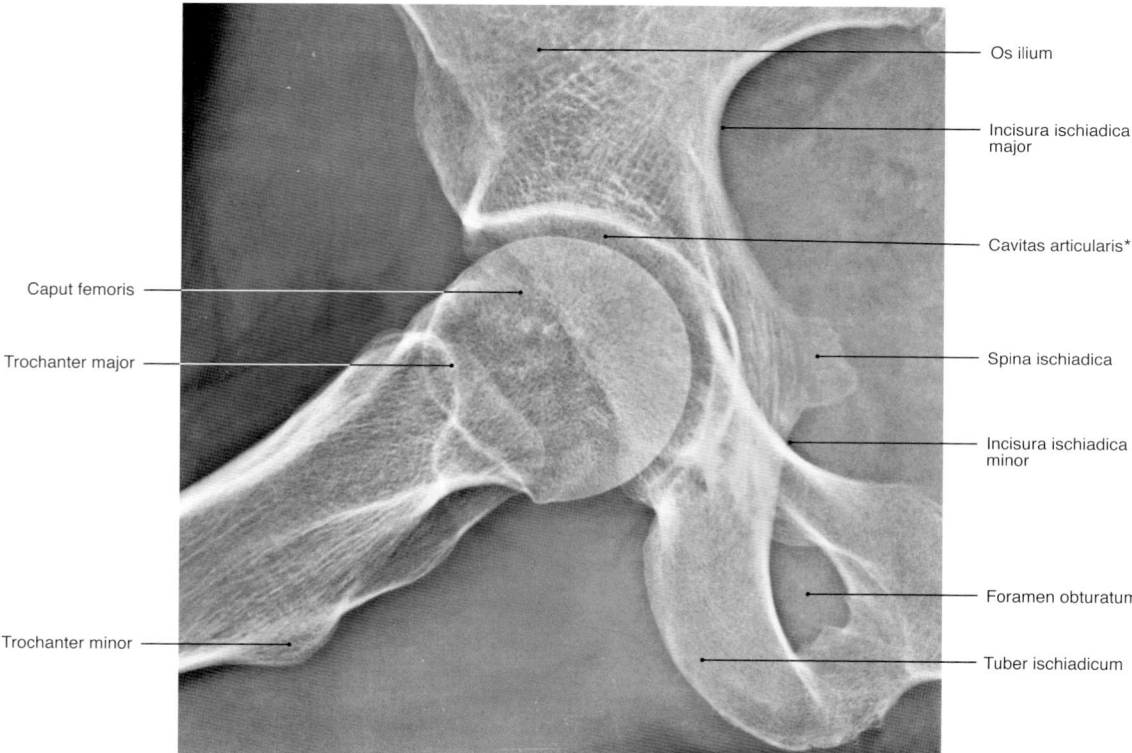

Os ilium

Incisura ischiadica
major

Cavitas articularis*

Caput femoris

Trochanter major

Spina ischiadica

Incisura ischiadica
minor

Foramen obturatum

Trochanter minor

Tuber ischiadicum

Fig. 988   Hip joint, Articulatio coxae;
AP-radiograph; supine position with the thigh abducted
and flexed (so-called LAUENSTEIN projection).

* Due to minimal absorption of X-rays by cartilage, the articular cleft
appears abnormally broad.

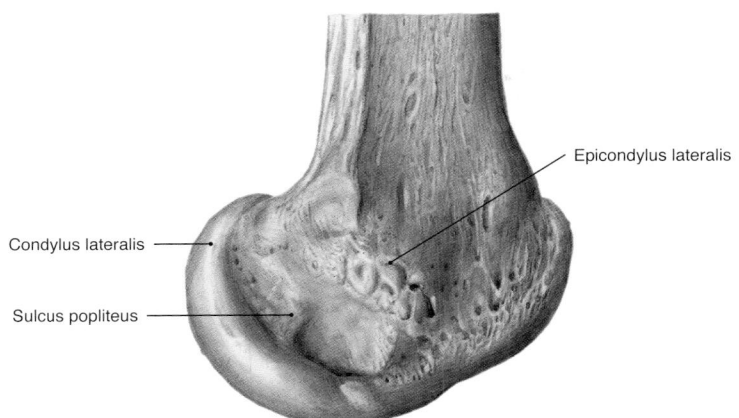

Fig. 989   Femur, Femur;
distal extremity;
lateral view.

Epicondylus lateralis

Condylus lateralis

Sulcus popliteus

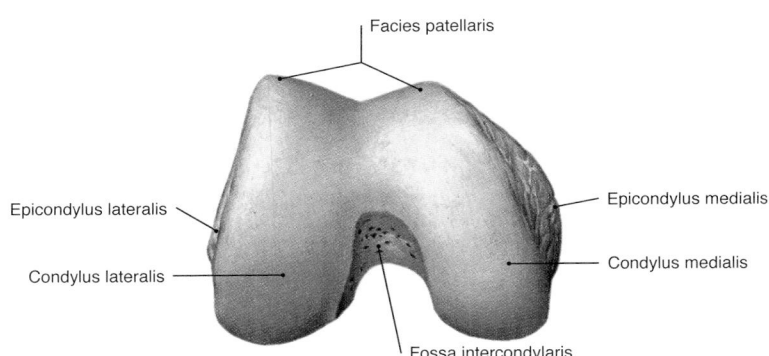

Facies patellaris

Epicondylus lateralis

Condylus lateralis

Epicondylus medialis

Condylus medialis

Fossa intercondylaris

Fig. 990   Femur, Femur;
distal extremity;
distal view.

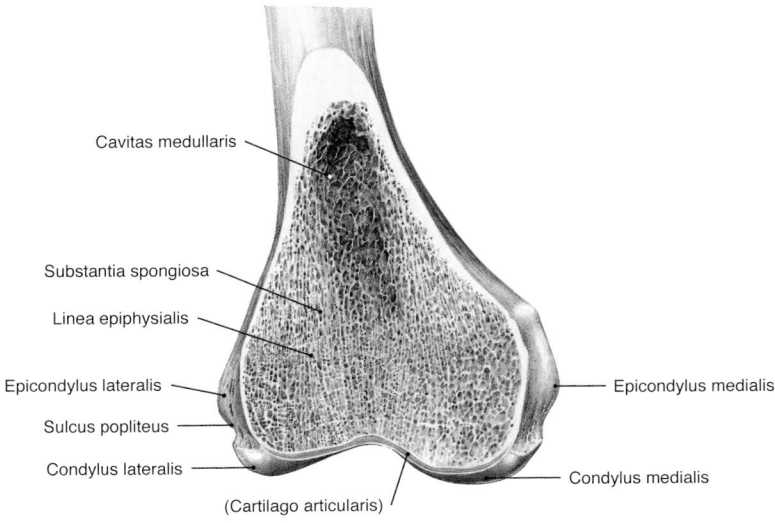

Cavitas medullaris

Substantia spongiosa

Linea epiphysialis

Epicondylus lateralis

Sulcus popliteus

Condylus lateralis

(Cartilago articularis)

Epicondylus medialis

Condylus medialis

Fig. 991   Femur, Femur;
frontal section through the distal part;
ventral view.

Tibia

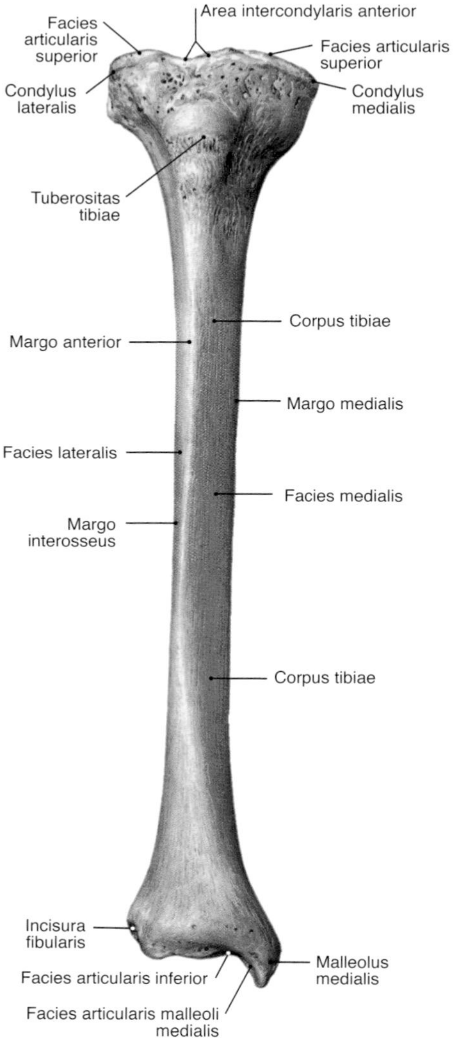

Facies articularis superior
Area intercondylaris anterior
Facies articularis superior
Condylus lateralis
Condylus medialis
Tuberositas tibiae
Margo anterior
Corpus tibiae
Margo medialis
Facies lateralis
Facies medialis
Margo interosseus
Corpus tibiae
Incisura fibularis
Malleolus medialis
Facies articularis inferior
Facies articularis malleoli medialis

Fig. 992　Tibia, Tibia; ventral view.

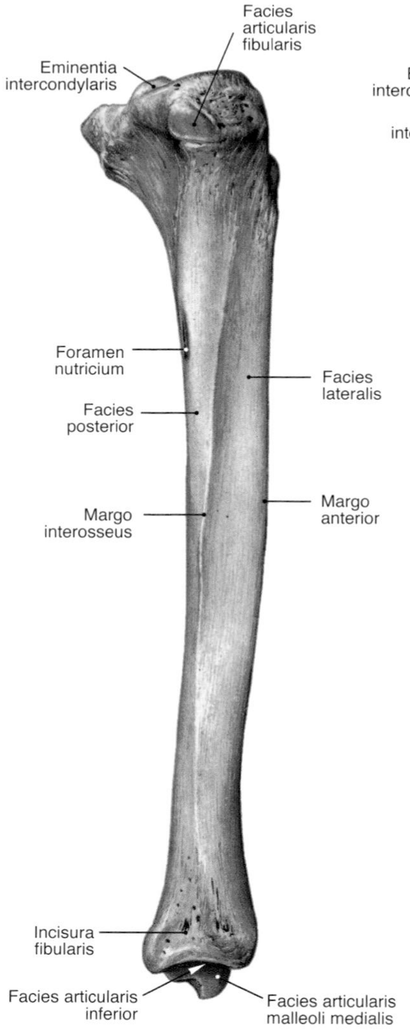

Facies articularis fibularis
Eminentia intercondylaris
Foramen nutricium
Facies posterior
Margo interosseus
Facies lateralis
Margo anterior
Incisura fibularis
Facies articularis inferior
Facies articularis malleoli medialis

Fig. 993　Tibia, Tibia; lateral view.

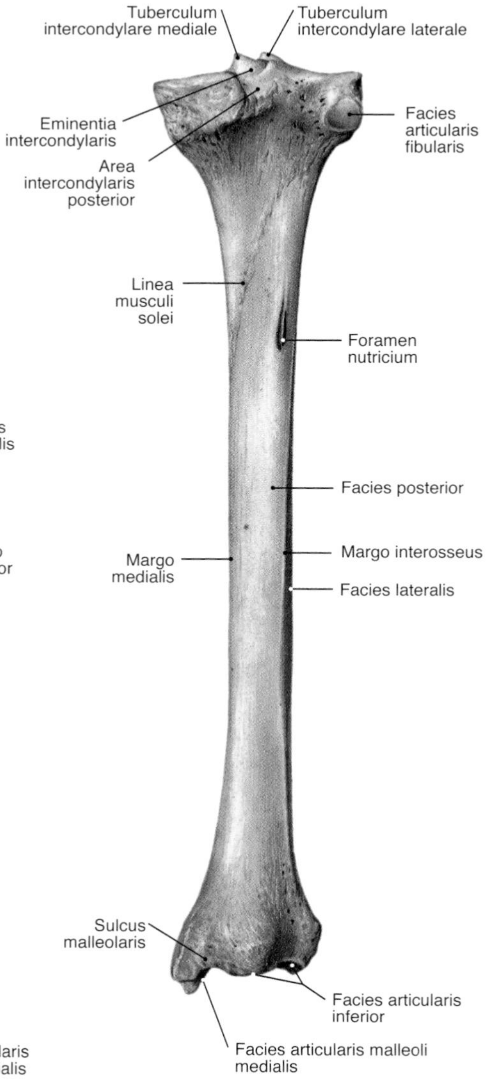

Tuberculum intercondylare mediale
Tuberculum intercondylare laterale
Eminentia intercondylaris
Area intercondylaris posterior
Facies articularis fibularis
Linea musculi solei
Foramen nutricium
Facies posterior
Margo medialis
Margo interosseus
Facies lateralis
Sulcus malleolaris
Facies articularis inferior
Facies articularis malleoli medialis

Fig. 994　Tibia, Tibia; dorsal view.

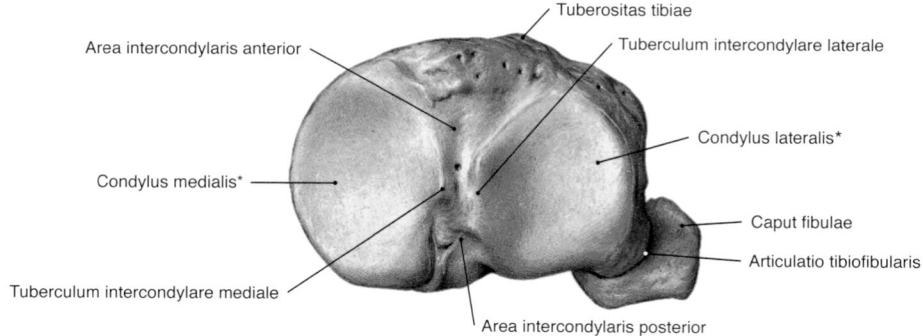

Tuberositas tibiae
Area intercondylaris anterior
Tuberculum intercondylare laterale
Condylus medialis*
Condylus lateralis*
Caput fibulae
Articulatio tibiofibularis
Tuberculum intercondylare mediale
Area intercondylaris posterior

Fig. 995　Tibia, Tibia, and fibula, Fibula; proximal view.

* The articular surfaces of the condyles together are referred to as superior articular surface.

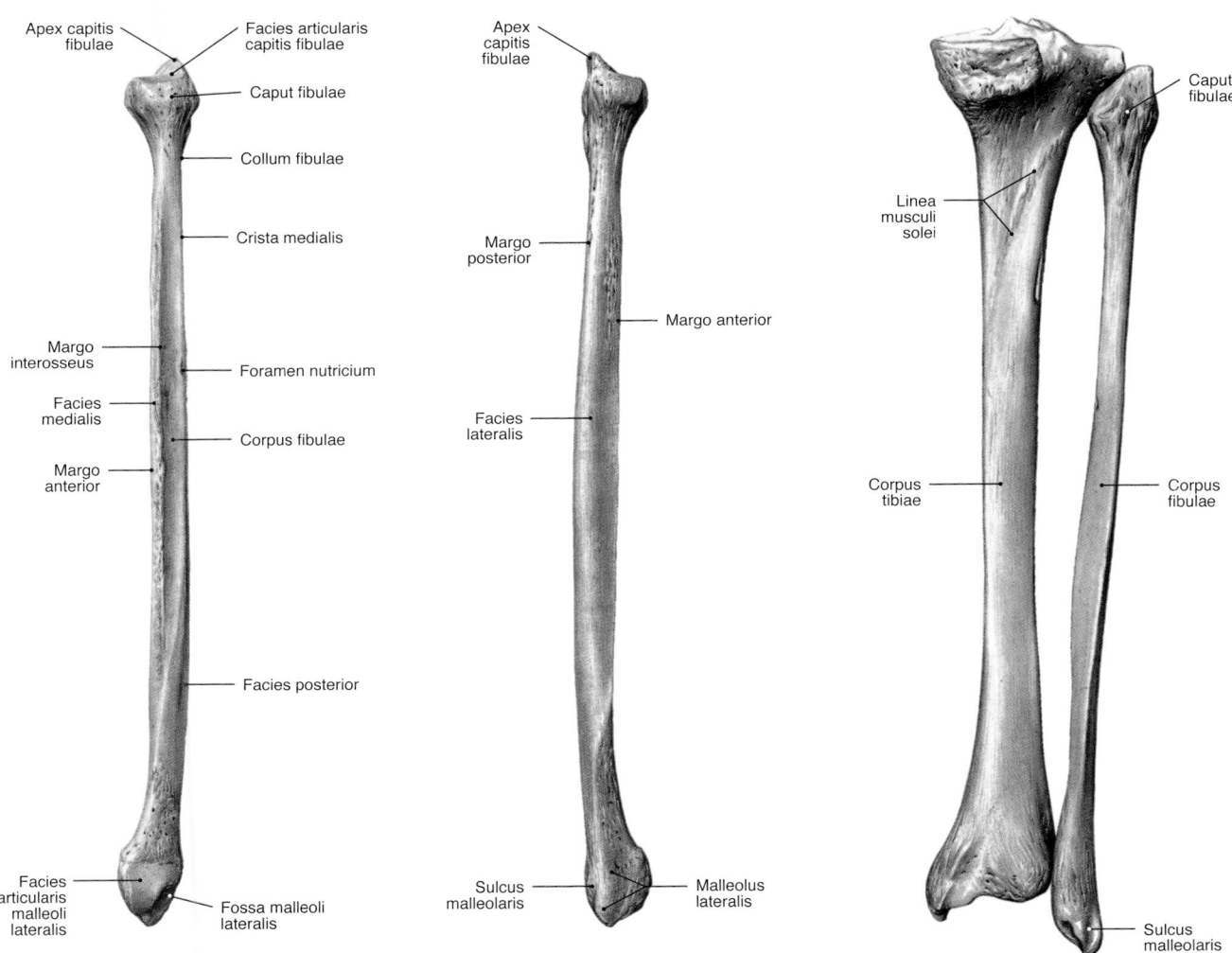

Apex capitis fibulae
Facies articularis capitis fibulae
Caput fibulae
Collum fibulae
Crista medialis
Margo interosseus
Facies medialis
Margo anterior
Foramen nutricium
Corpus fibulae
Facies posterior
Facies articularis malleoli lateralis
Fossa malleoli lateralis

Fig. 996 Fibula, Fibula; medial view.

Apex capitis fibulae
Margo posterior
Margo anterior
Facies lateralis
Sulcus malleolaris
Malleolus lateralis

Fig. 997 Fibula, Fibula; lateral view.

Caput fibulae
Linea musculi solei
Corpus tibiae
Corpus fibulae
Sulcus malleolaris

Fig. 998 Tibia, Tibia, and fibula, Fibula; dorsal view.

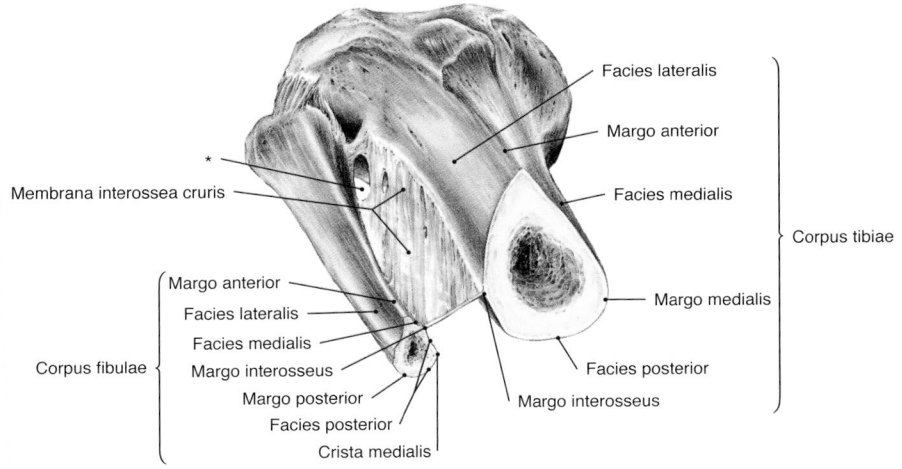

Facies lateralis
Margo anterior
Facies medialis
*
Membrana interossea cruris
Corpus tibiae
Margo anterior
Facies lateralis
Facies medialis
Margo medialis
Margo interosseus
Facies posterior
Corpus fibulae
Margo posterior
Margo interosseus
Facies posterior
Crista medialis

Fig. 999 Tibia, Tibia, and fibula, Fibula; cross-section with the interosseous membrane of leg; distal view.
* Opening for the anterior tibial artery

Patella and knee joint

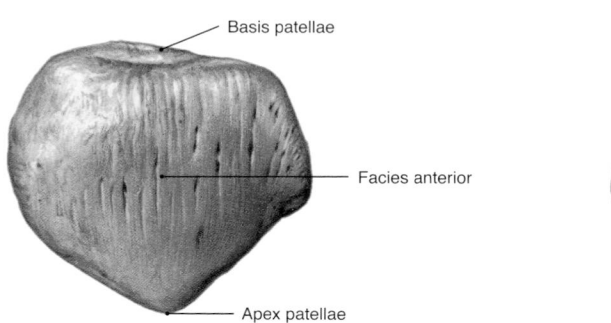

Fig. 1000 Patella, Patella; ventral view.

Fig. 1001 Patella, Patella; dorsal view.

Basis patellae

Facies anterior

Apex patellae

Basis patellae

Facies articularis

Apex patellae

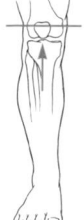

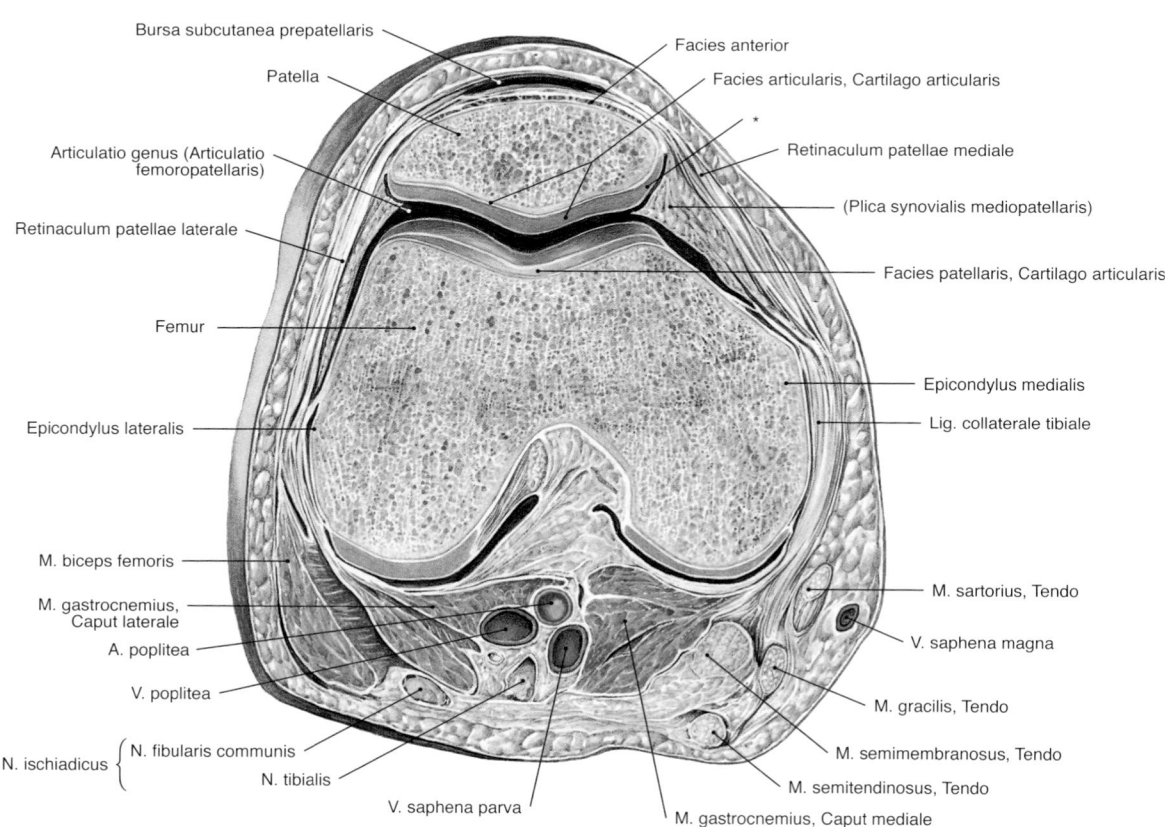

Bursa subcutanea prepatellaris

Patella

Articulatio genus (Articulatio femoropatellaris)

Retinaculum patellae laterale

Femur

Epicondylus lateralis

M. biceps femoris

M. gastrocnemius, Caput laterale

A. poplitea

V. poplitea

N. ischiadicus { N. fibularis communis

N. tibialis

V. saphena parva

Facies anterior

Facies articularis, Cartilago articularis

*

Retinaculum patellae mediale

(Plica synovialis mediopatellaris)

Facies patellaris, Cartilago articularis

Epicondylus medialis

Lig. collaterale tibiale

M. sartorius, Tendo

V. saphena magna

M. gracilis, Tendo

M. semimembranosus, Tendo

M. semitendinosus, Tendo

M. gastrocnemius, Caput mediale

Fig. 1002 Knee joint, Articulatio genus; cross-section.
* Medial border facet

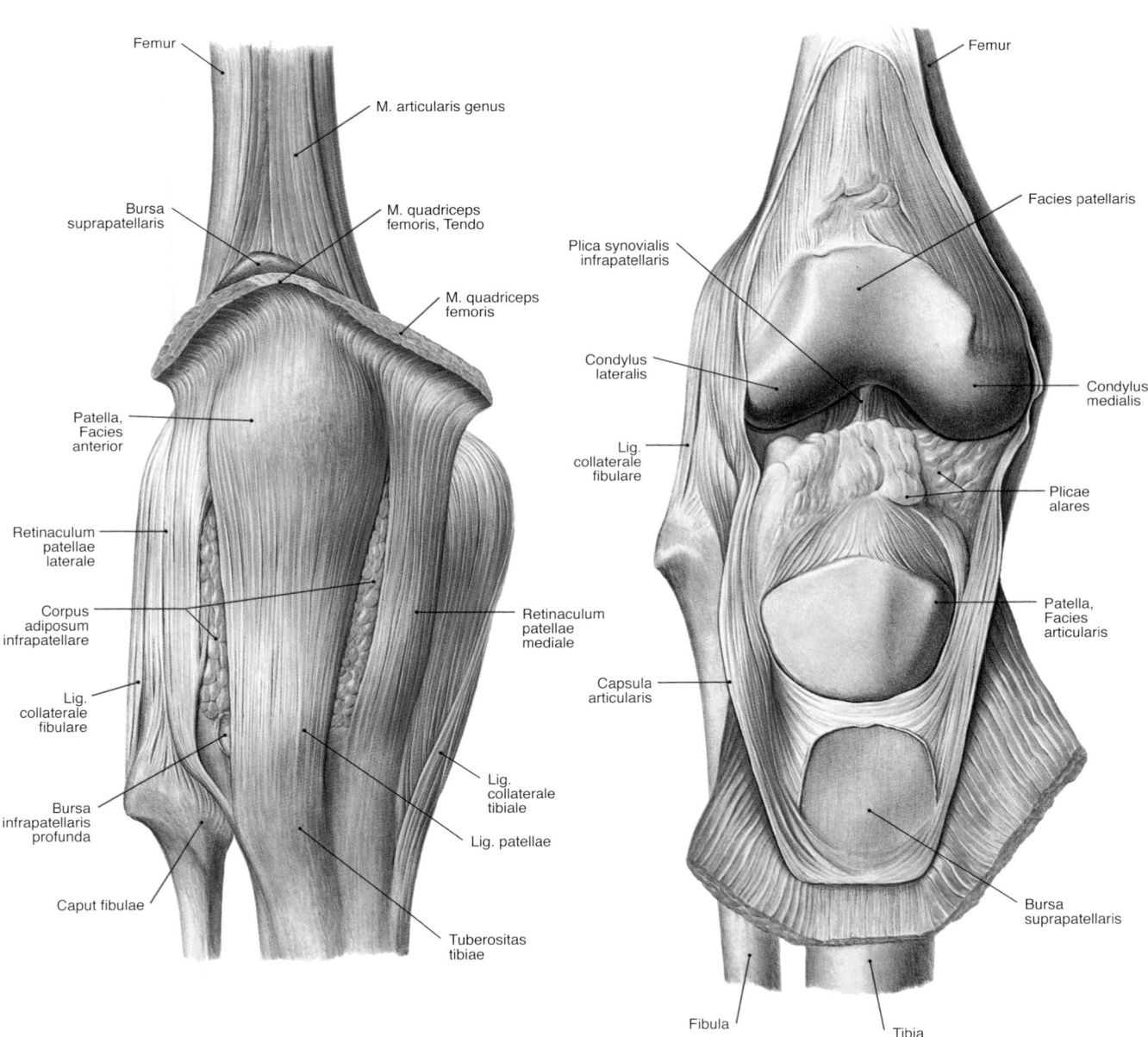

Fig. 1003 Knee joint, Articulatio genus;
intact articular capsule;
ventral view.

Fig. 1004 Knee joint, Articulatio genus;
the anterior part of the articular capsule has
been reflected downwards after dissection of
the quadriceps muscle;
the suprapatellar bursa has been opened;
ventral view.

Knee joint

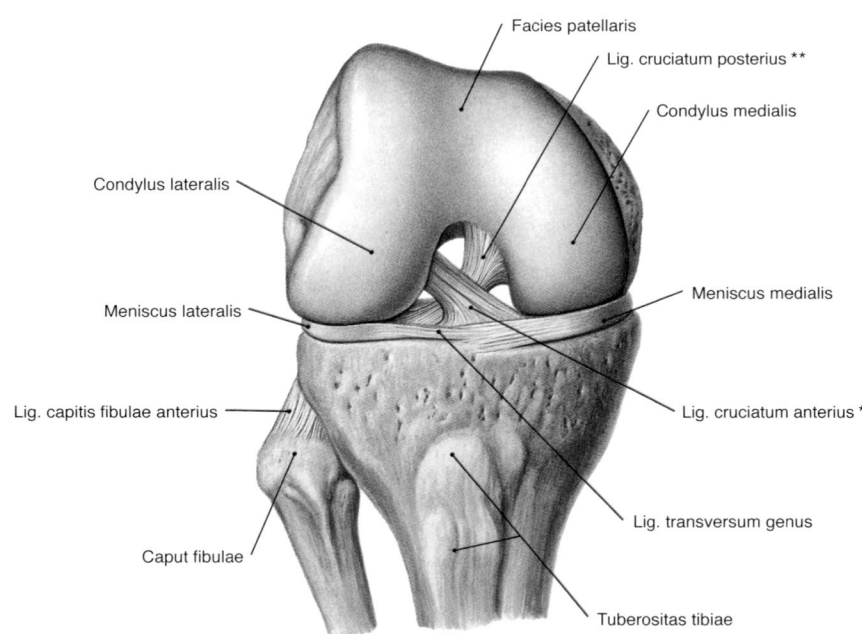

Facies patellaris
Lig. cruciatum posterius **
Condylus medialis
Condylus lateralis
Meniscus medialis
Meniscus lateralis
Lig. capitis fibulae anterius
Lig. cruciatum anterius *
Lig. transversum genus
Caput fibulae
Tuberositas tibiae

Fig. 1005   Knee joint, Articulatio genus;
in 90° flexion; the articular capsule and the lateral
ligaments have been removed;
ventral view.

   * Clinical term: ACL (= anterior cruciate ligament)
** Clinical term: PCL (= posterior cruciate ligament)

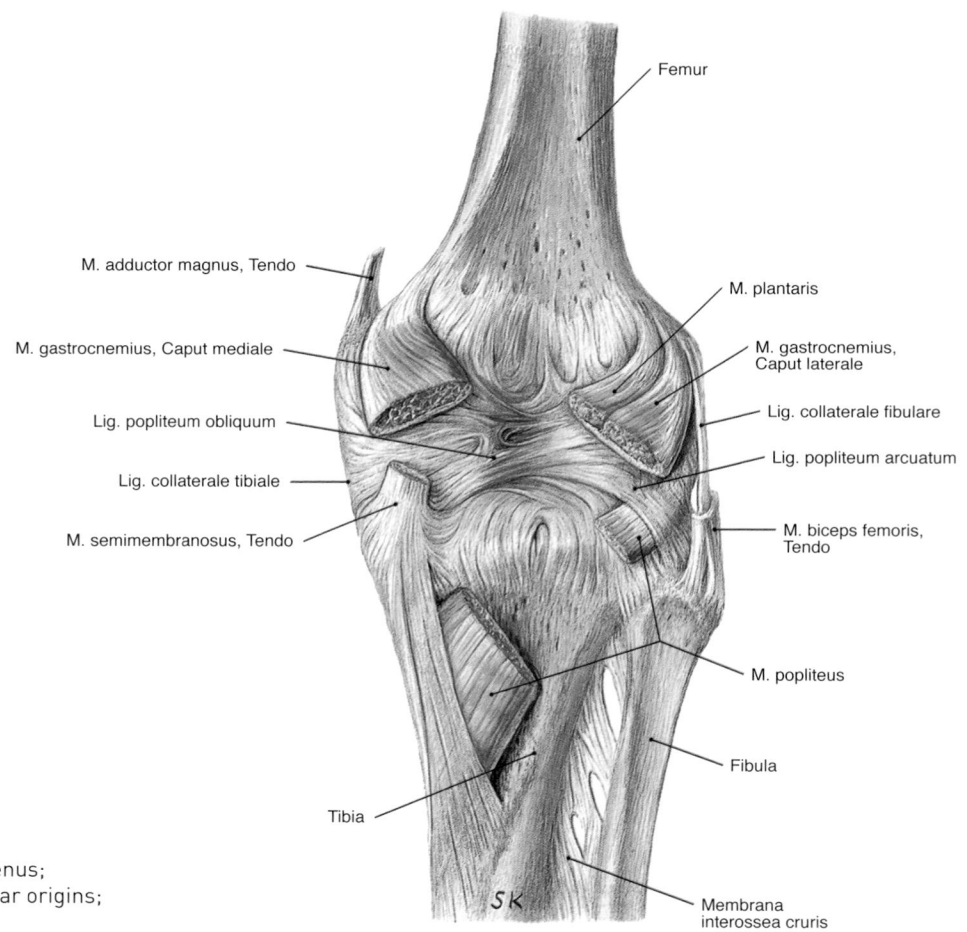

Femur
M. adductor magnus, Tendo
M. plantaris
M. gastrocnemius, Caput mediale
M. gastrocnemius, Caput laterale
Lig. popliteum obliquum
Lig. collaterale fibulare
Lig. collaterale tibiale
Lig. popliteum arcuatum
M. semimembranosus, Tendo
M. biceps femoris, Tendo
M. popliteus
Fibula
Tibia
SK
Membrana interossea cruris

Fig. 1006   Knee joint, Articulatio genus;
intact articular capsule with muscular origins;
dorsal view.

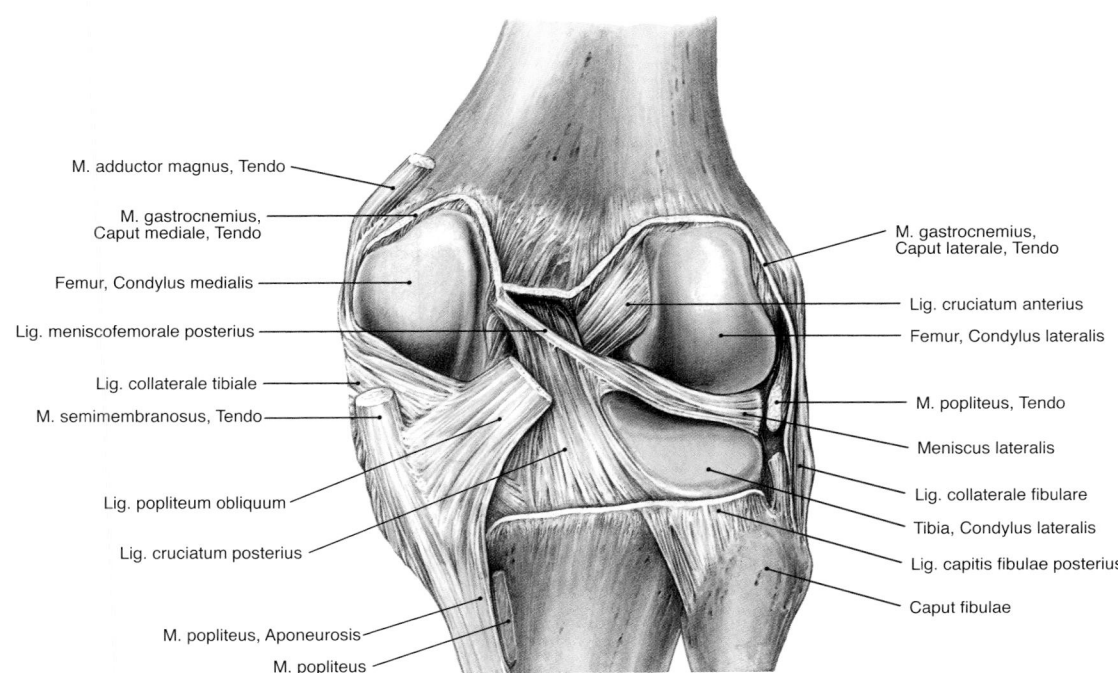

M. adductor magnus, Tendo

M. gastrocnemius, Caput mediale, Tendo

Femur, Condylus medialis

Lig. meniscofemorale posterius

Lig. collaterale tibiale

M. semimembranosus, Tendo

Lig. popliteum obliquum

Lig. cruciatum posterius

M. popliteus, Aponeurosis

M. popliteus

M. gastrocnemius, Caput laterale, Tendo

Lig. cruciatum anterius

Femur, Condylus lateralis

M. popliteus, Tendo

Meniscus lateralis

Lig. collaterale fibulare

Tibia, Condylus lateralis

Lig. capitis fibulae posterius

Caput fibulae

Fig. 1007 Knee joint, Articulatio genus; exposure of the cruciate ligaments and the menisci; dorsal view.

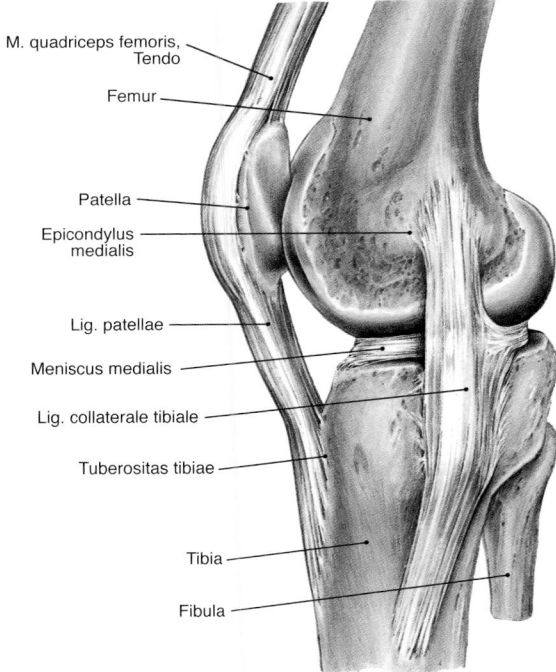

M. quadriceps femoris, Tendo

Femur

Patella

Epicondylus medialis

Lig. patellae

Meniscus medialis

Lig. collaterale tibiale

Tuberositas tibiae

Tibia

Fibula

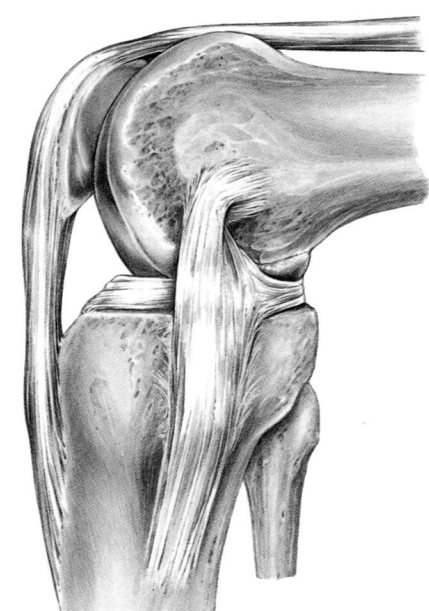

Fig. 1008 Tibial collateral ligament, Lig. collaterale tibiale; knee in extended position; medial view.
Only the posterior fibres of the tibial collateral ligament are attached to the medial meniscus.

Fig. 1009 Tibial collateral ligament, Lig. collaterale tibiale; knee in flexed position (90°); medial view.
In the course of flexion, the posterior and proximal fibres of the tibial collateral ligament become twisted, thereby stabilizing the medial meniscus.

Knee joint

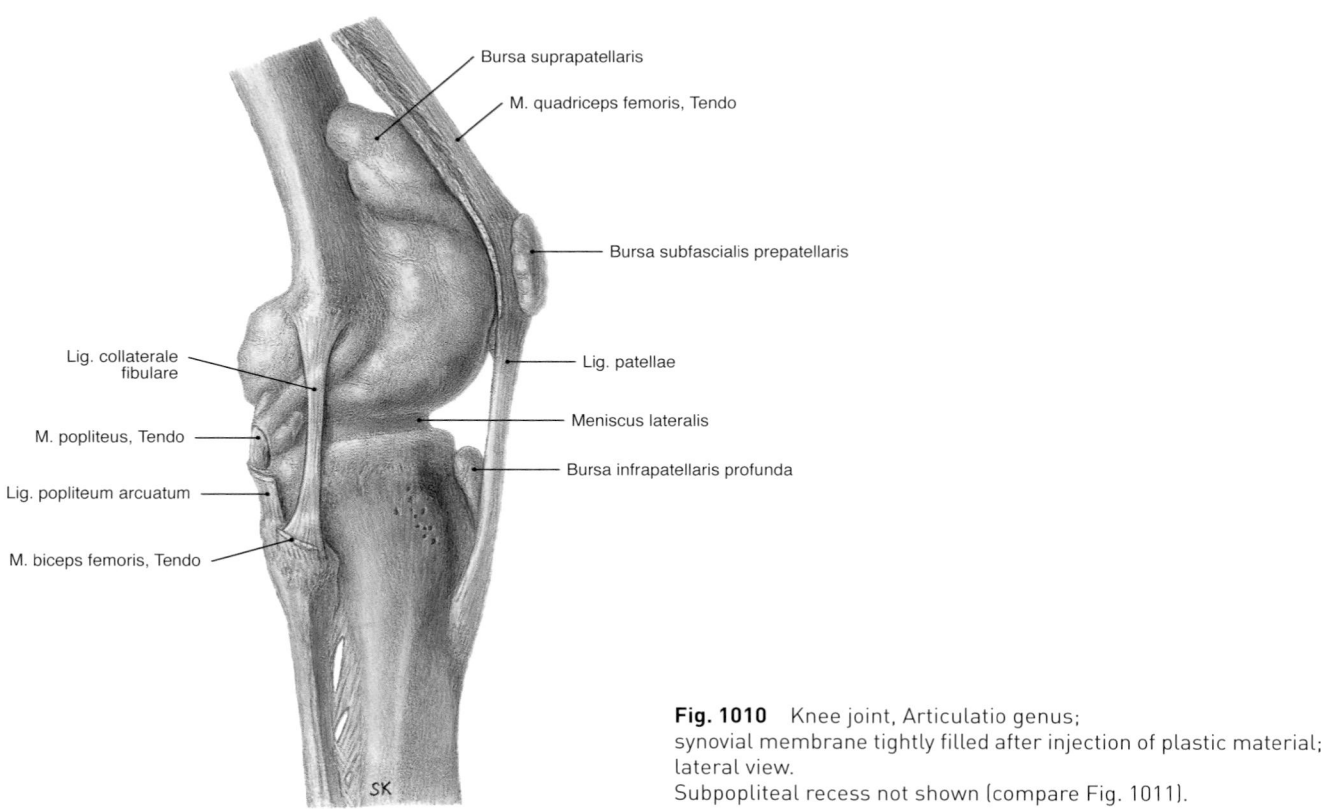

Fig. 1010 Knee joint, Articulatio genus;
synovial membrane tightly filled after injection of plastic material;
lateral view.
Subpopliteal recess not shown (compare Fig. 1011).

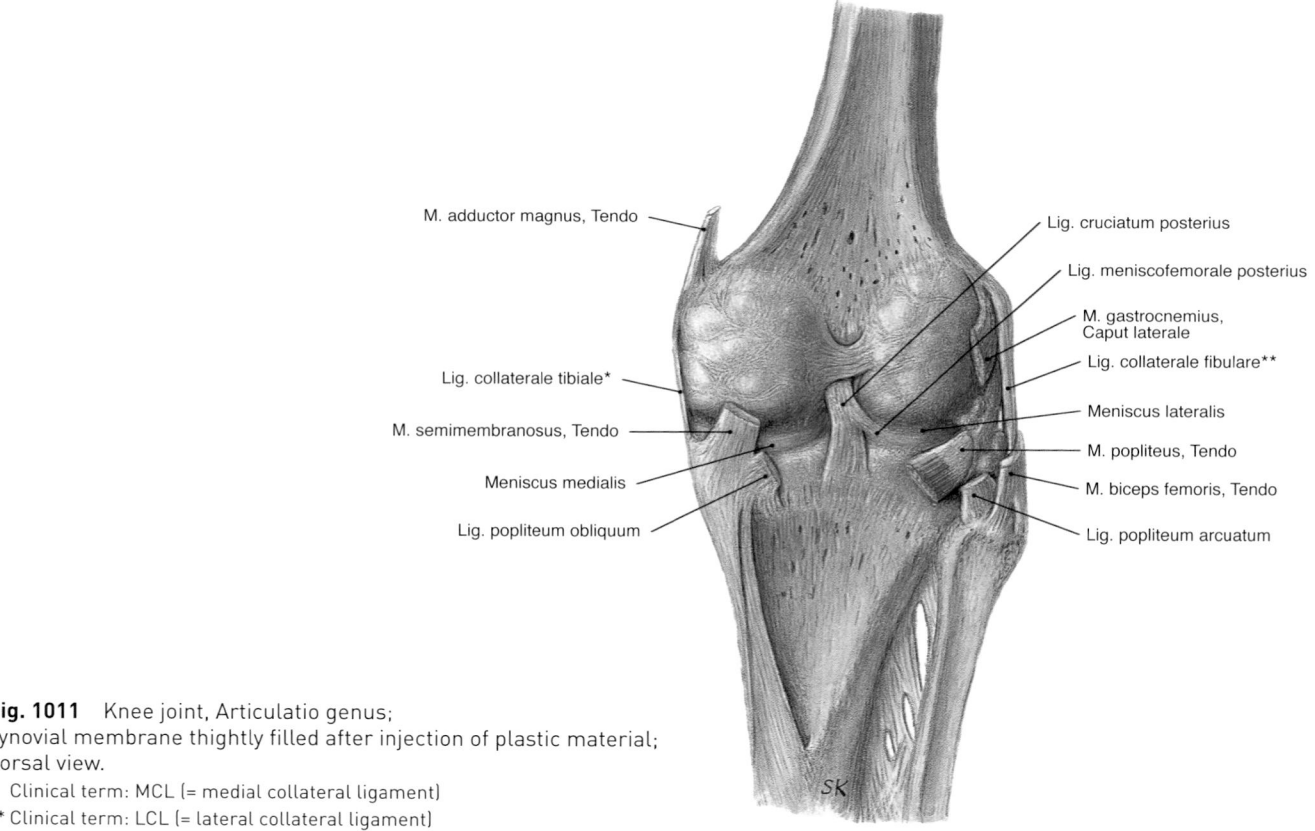

Fig. 1011 Knee joint, Articulatio genus;
synovial membrane thightly filled after injection of plastic material;
dorsal view.
* Clinical term: MCL (= medial collateral ligament)
** Clinical term: LCL (= lateral collateral ligament)

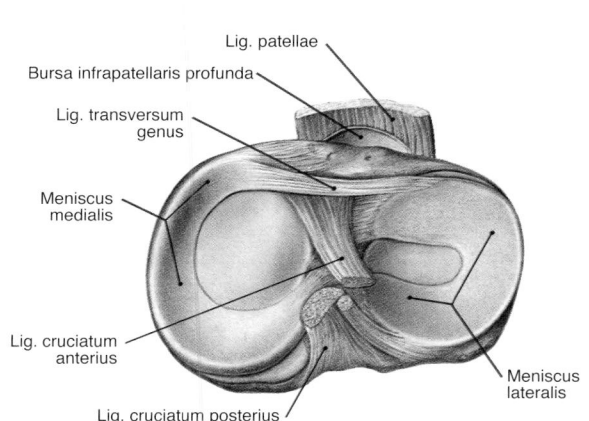

Fig. 1012 Menisci of the knee joint, Articulatio genus, and cruciate ligaments, Ligg. cruciata; proximal view.

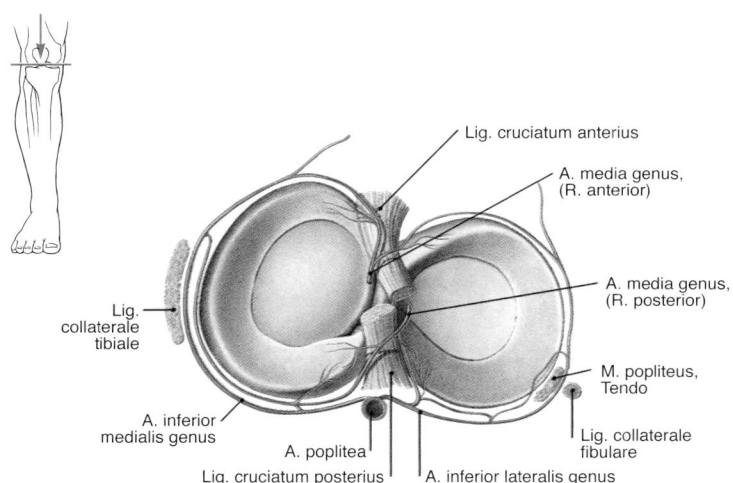

Fig. 1013 Menisci of the knee joint, Articulatio genus; arterial supply; proximal view.

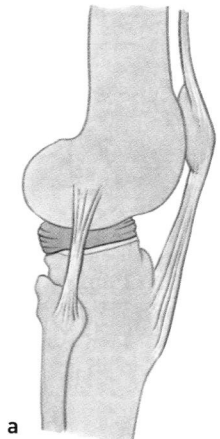

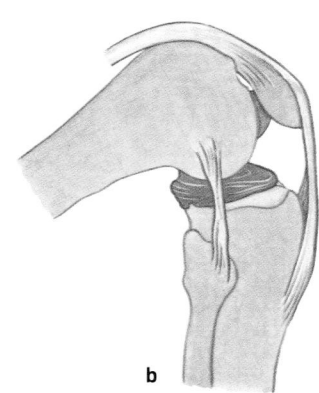

Fig. 1014 a, b Displacement of the menisci during flexion; lateral view.

a Extended position
b Flexed position

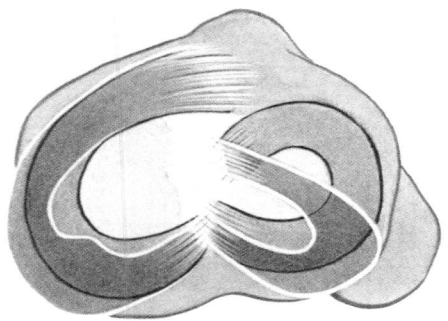

Fig. 1015 Displacement of the menisci during flexion; proximal view.
In flexion, both menisci are displaced posteriorly over the edges of the tibial condyles. The greater mobility of the lateral meniscus accounts for its lesser risk of damage.

Knee joint, sections

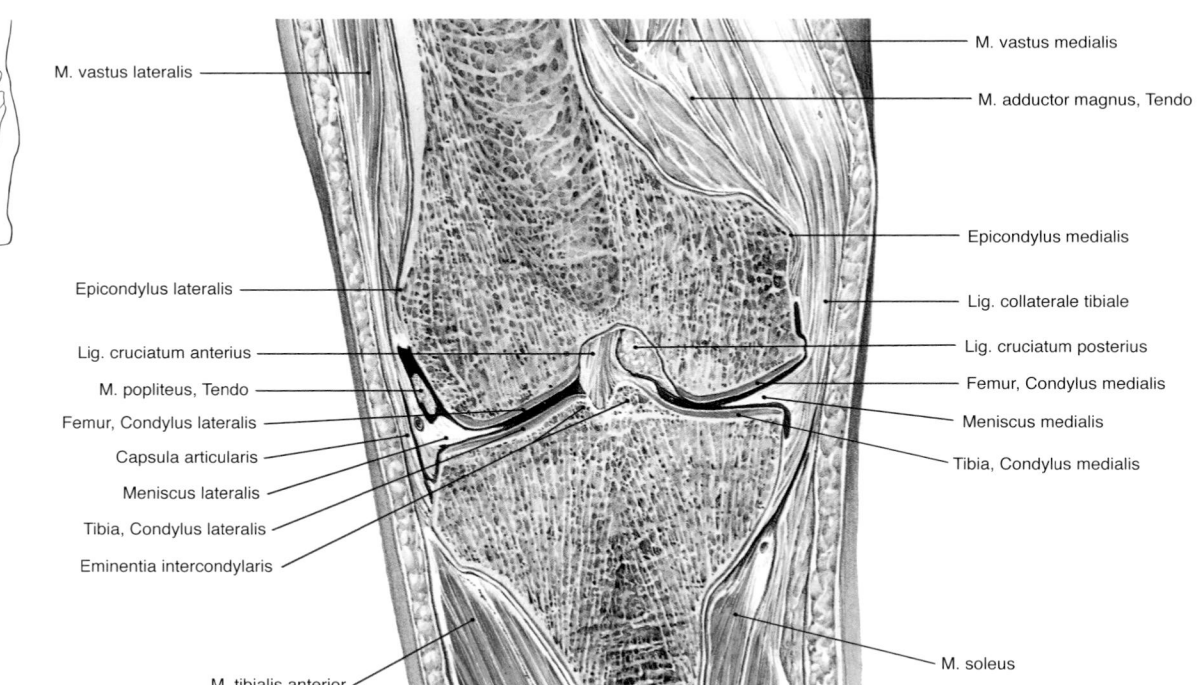

M. vastus lateralis

M. vastus medialis

M. adductor magnus, Tendo

Epicondylus medialis

Epicondylus lateralis

Lig. collaterale tibiale

Lig. cruciatum anterius

Lig. cruciatum posterius

M. popliteus, Tendo

Femur, Condylus medialis

Femur, Condylus lateralis

Meniscus medialis

Capsula articularis

Tibia, Condylus medialis

Meniscus lateralis

Tibia, Condylus lateralis

Eminentia intercondylaris

M. soleus

M. tibialis anterior

Fig. 1016 Knee joint, Articulatio genus; frontal section.

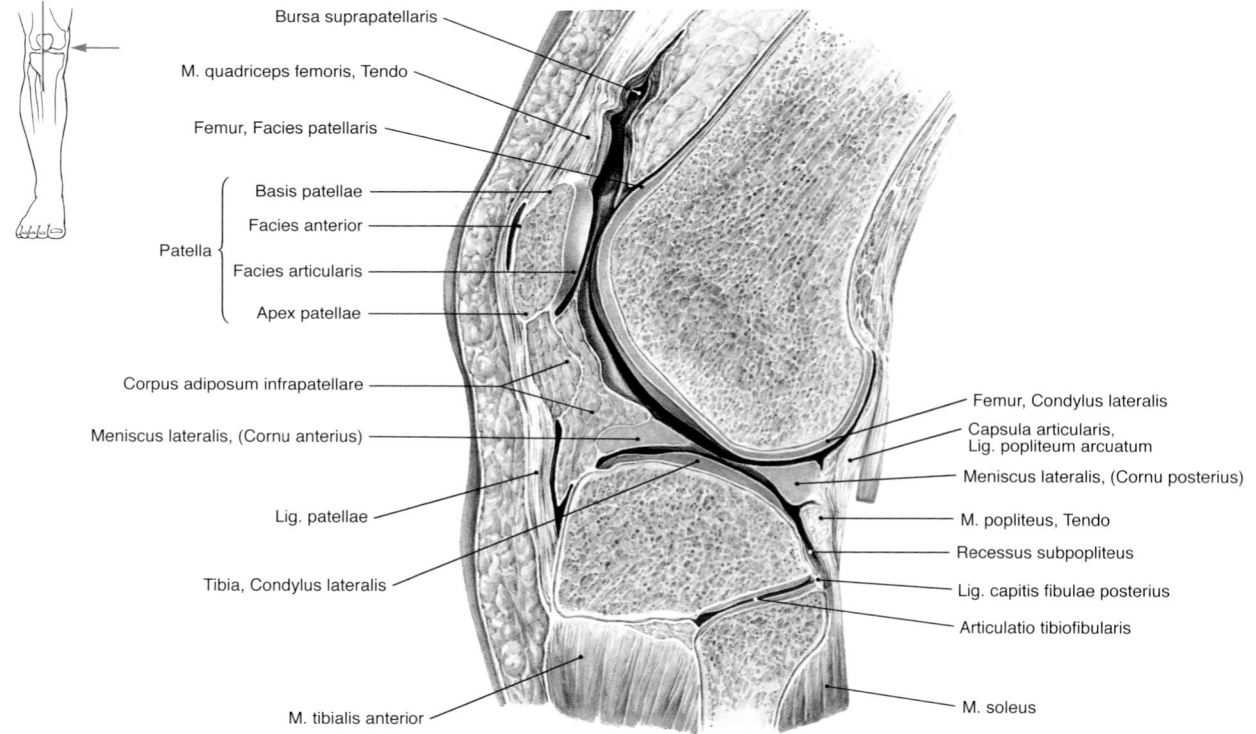

Bursa suprapatellaris

M. quadriceps femoris, Tendo

Femur, Facies patellaris

Basis patellae

Facies anterior

Patella

Facies articularis

Apex patellae

Corpus adiposum infrapatellare

Femur, Condylus lateralis

Meniscus lateralis, (Cornu anterius)

Capsula articularis, Lig. popliteum arcuatum

Meniscus lateralis, (Cornu posterius)

Lig. patellae

M. popliteus, Tendo

Recessus subpopliteus

Tibia, Condylus lateralis

Lig. capitis fibulae posterius

Articulatio tibiofibularis

M. tibialis anterior

M. soleus

Fig. 1017 Knee joint, Articulatio genus; sagittal section through the lateral part of the joint.

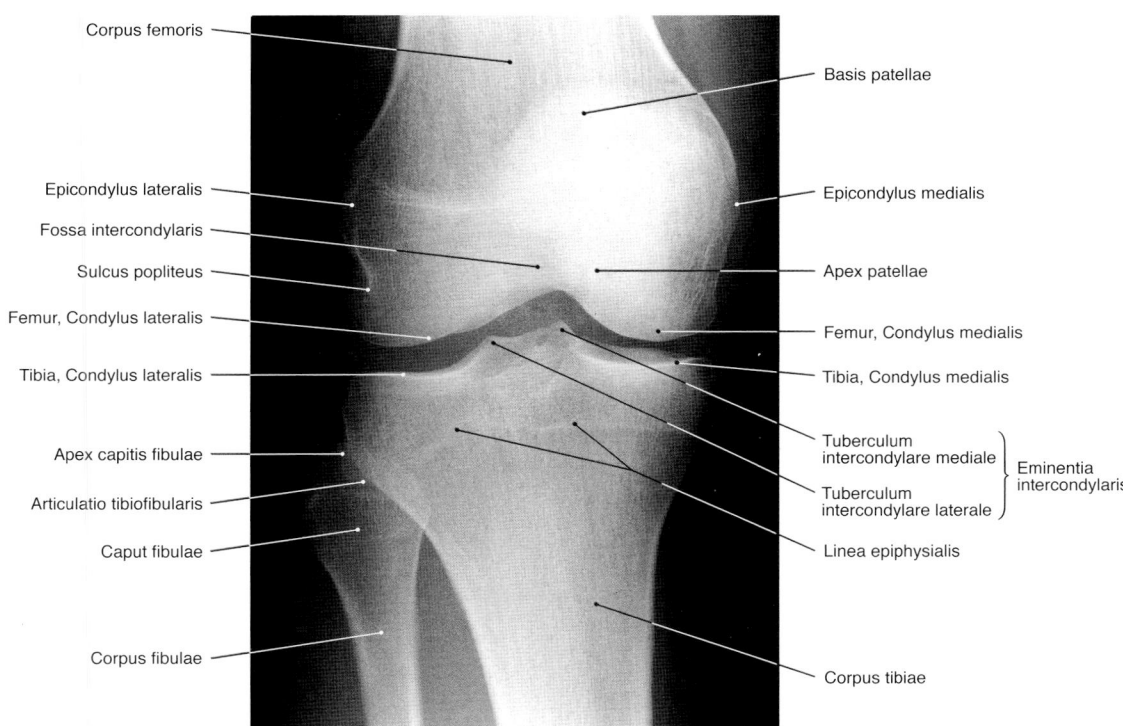

Corpus femoris

Basis patellae

Epicondylus lateralis

Epicondylus medialis

Fossa intercondylaris

Sulcus popliteus

Apex patellae

Femur, Condylus lateralis

Femur, Condylus medialis

Tibia, Condylus lateralis

Tibia, Condylus medialis

Apex capitis fibulae

Tuberculum intercondylare mediale ⎫
Tuberculum intercondylare laterale ⎬ Eminentia intercondylaris

Articulatio tibiofibularis

Caput fibulae

Linea epiphysialis

Corpus fibulae

Corpus tibiae

Fig. 1018 Knee joint, Articulatio genus;
AP-radiograph with the central beam directed onto
the middle of the joint; subject reclined.

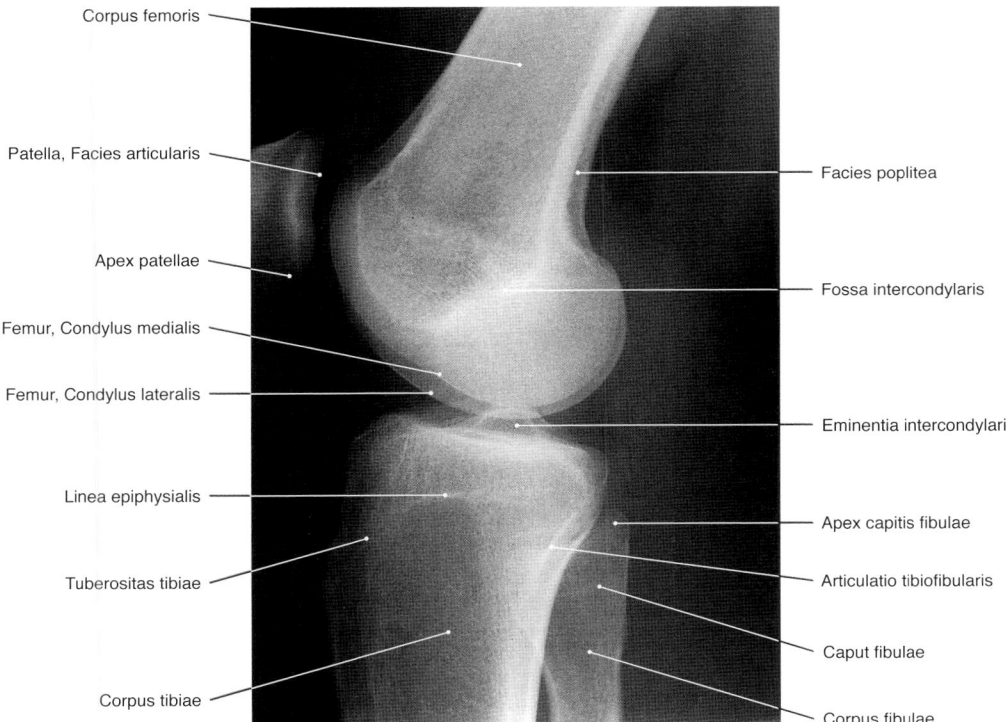

Corpus femoris

Patella, Facies articularis

Facies poplitea

Apex patellae

Fossa intercondylaris

Femur, Condylus medialis

Femur, Condylus lateralis

Eminentia intercondylaris

Linea epiphysialis

Apex capitis fibulae

Tuberositas tibiae

Articulatio tibiofibularis

Caput fibulae

Corpus tibiae

Corpus fibulae

Fig. 1019 Knee joint, Articulatio genus;
lateral radiograph with the central beam directed onto
the middle of the joint; subject reclined.

Knee joint, arthroscopy

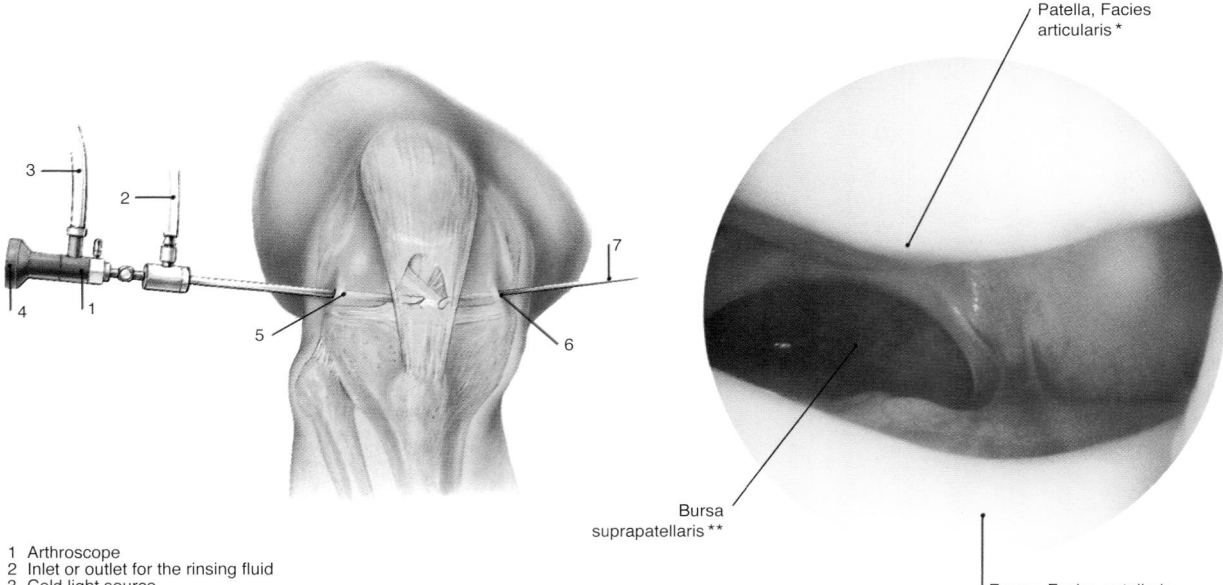

1 Arthroscope
2 Inlet or outlet for the rinsing fluid
3 Cold light source
4 Ocular or connector for the video system
5 Anterolateral access
6 Anteromedial access
7 Additional instrument

Fig. 1020   Accesses for arthroscopy.

Patella, Facies articularis *

Bursa suprapatellaris **

Femur, Facies patellaris

Fig. 1021 a–c   Knee joint, Articulatio genus; arthroscopy.
a Distal view into the femoropatellar joint
* Patellar roof ridge: ridge between the medial and lateral articular surfaces
** Clinical term: suprapatellar recess

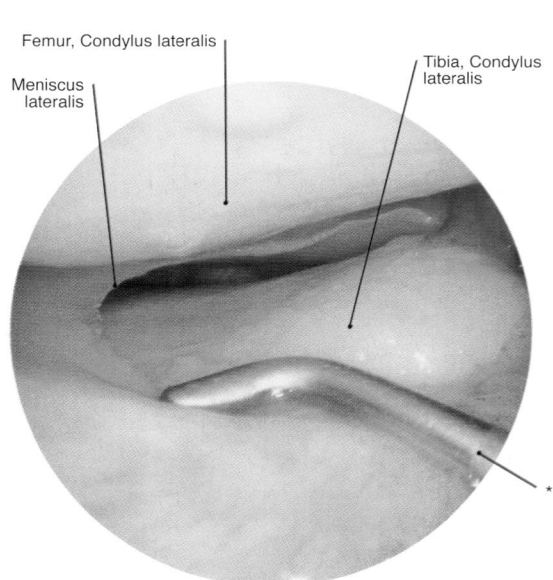

Femur, Condylus lateralis

Meniscus lateralis

Tibia, Condylus lateralis

b Medial view of the free inner edge of the lateral meniscus;
retractor (*) slightly depressing the anterior part of the meniscus

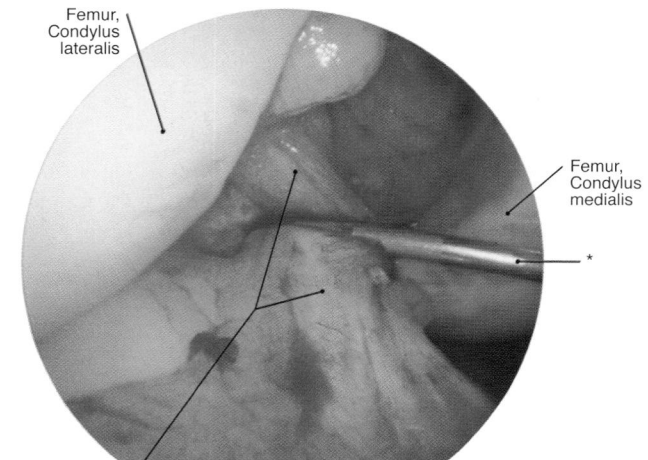

Femur, Condylus lateralis

Femur, Condylus medialis

Lig. cruciatum anterius

c Anterolateral view of the distal part of the anterior cruciate ligament, Lig. cruciatum anterius.
The ligament is covered by a richly vascularized synovial membrane. It is drawn medially by a retractor (*).

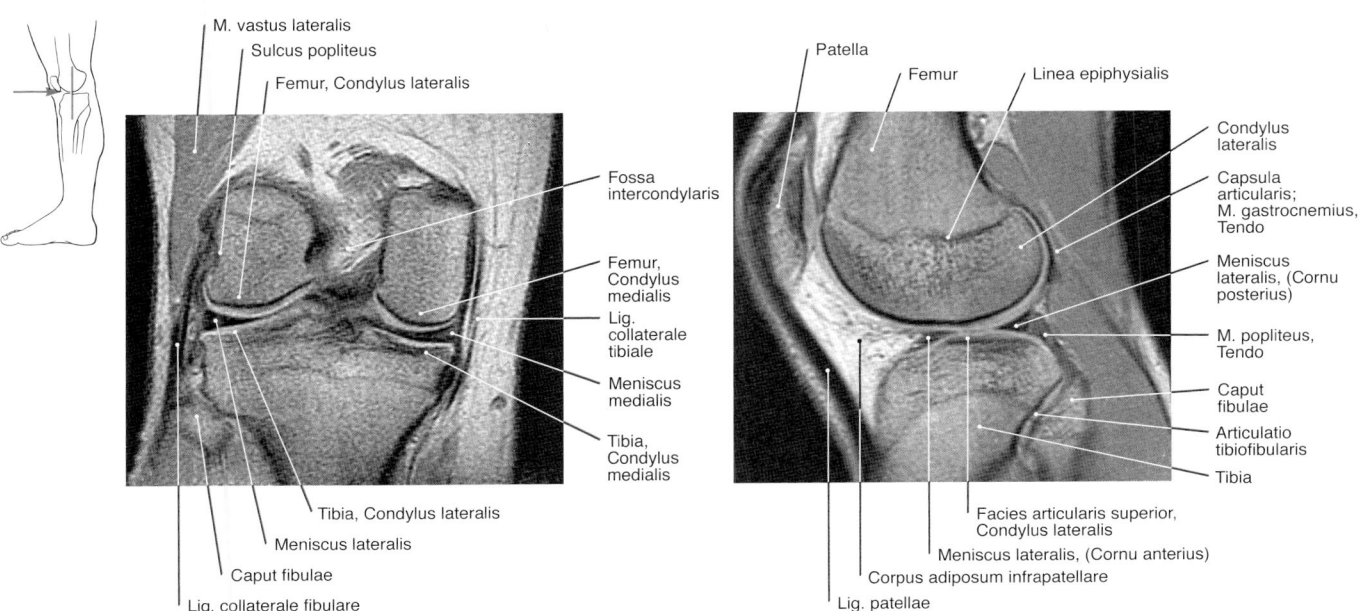

M. vastus lateralis
Sulcus popliteus
Femur, Condylus lateralis

Fossa intercondylaris

Femur, Condylus medialis

Lig. collaterale tibiale

Meniscus medialis

Tibia, Condylus medialis

Tibia, Condylus lateralis
Meniscus lateralis
Caput fibulae
Lig. collaterale fibulare

Patella
Femur
Linea epiphysialis

Condylus lateralis

Capsula articularis; M. gastrocnemius, Tendo

Meniscus lateralis, (Cornu posterius)

M. popliteus, Tendo

Caput fibulae

Articulatio tibiofibularis

Tibia

Facies articularis superior, Condylus lateralis
Meniscus lateralis, (Cornu anterius)
Corpus adiposum infrapatellare
Lig. patellae

Fig. 1022 Knee joint, Articulatio genus;
magnetic resonance tomographic image (MRI);
frontal section;
knee in the extended position.
In this imaging technique, compact bone appears black.

Fig. 1023 Knee joint, Articulatio genus;
magnetic resonance tomographic image (MRI);
sagittal section through the lateral part of the joint;
knee in the extended position.

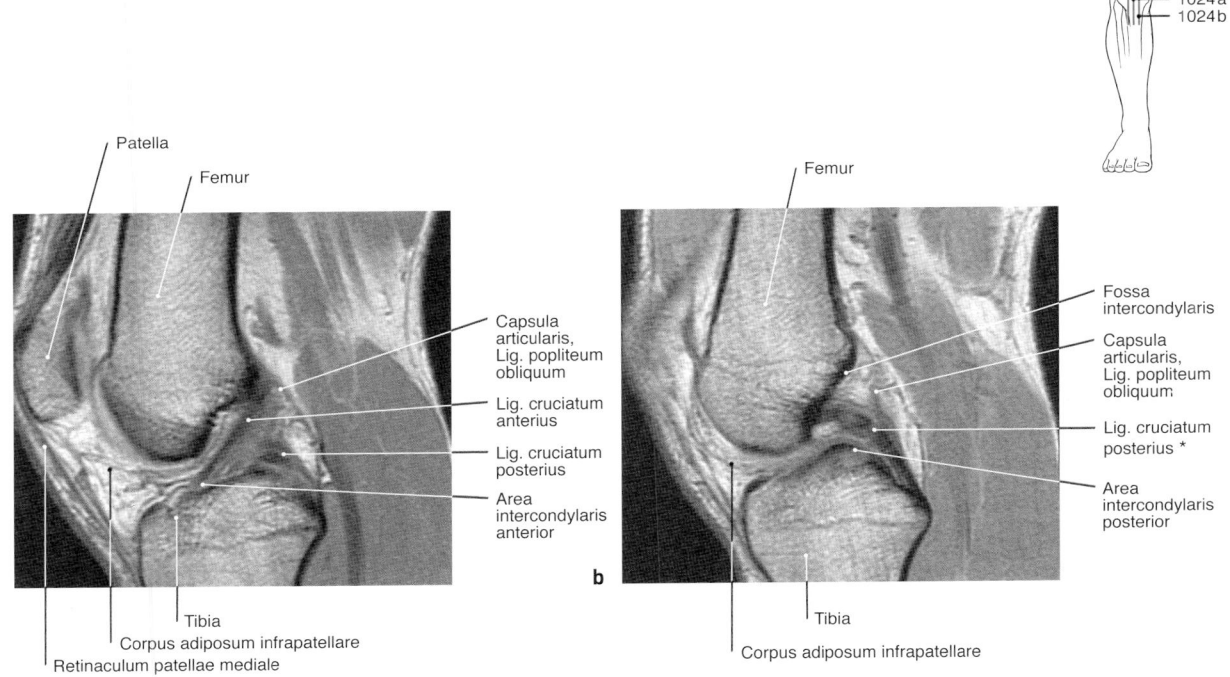

1023
1024a
1024b

Patella
Femur

Capsula articularis, Lig. popliteum obliquum

Lig. cruciatum anterius

Lig. cruciatum posterius

Area intercondylaris anterior

a

Tibia
Corpus adiposum infrapatellare
Retinaculum patellae mediale

Femur

Fossa intercondylaris

Capsula articularis, Lig. popliteum obliquum

Lig. cruciatum posterius *

Area intercondylaris posterior

b

Tibia
Corpus adiposum infrapatellare

Fig. 1024 a, b Knee joint, Articulatio genus;
magnetic resonance tomographic image (MRI);
sagittal sections to demonstrate the cruciate
ligaments;
knee in the extended position.

a Anterior cruciate ligament, Lig. cruciatum anterius, (ACL)
b Posterior cruciate ligament, Lig. cruciatum posterius, (PCL)
* The inhomogeneity is due to oblique sectioning of the fibre bundles.

Joints of the bones of the leg

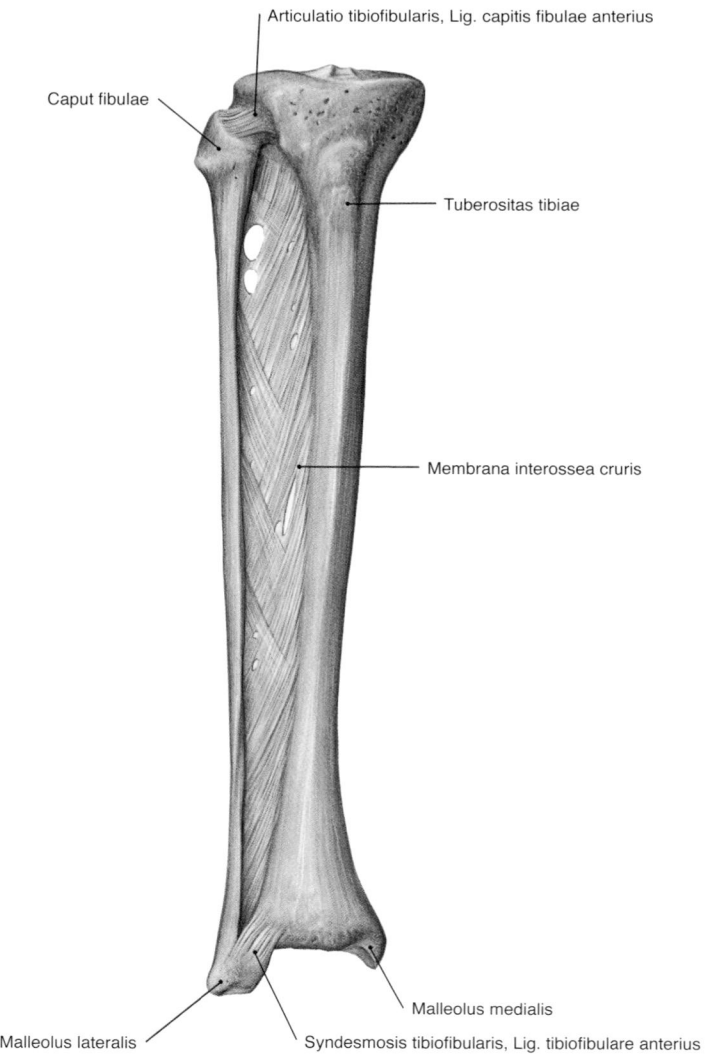

Articulatio tibiofibularis, Lig. capitis fibulae anterius

Caput fibulae

Tuberositas tibiae

Membrana interossea cruris

Malleolus medialis

Malleolus lateralis

Syndesmosis tibiofibularis, Lig. tibiofibulare anterius

Fig. 1025 Joints of the bones of the leg;
ventral view.

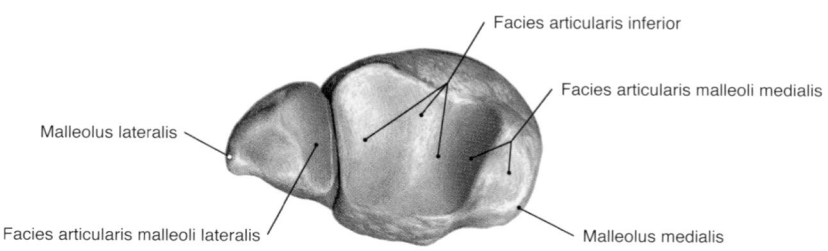

Facies articularis inferior

Facies articularis malleoli medialis

Malleolus lateralis

Facies articularis malleoli lateralis

Malleolus medialis

Fig. 1026 Tibia, Tibia, and fibula, Fibula;
distal view.

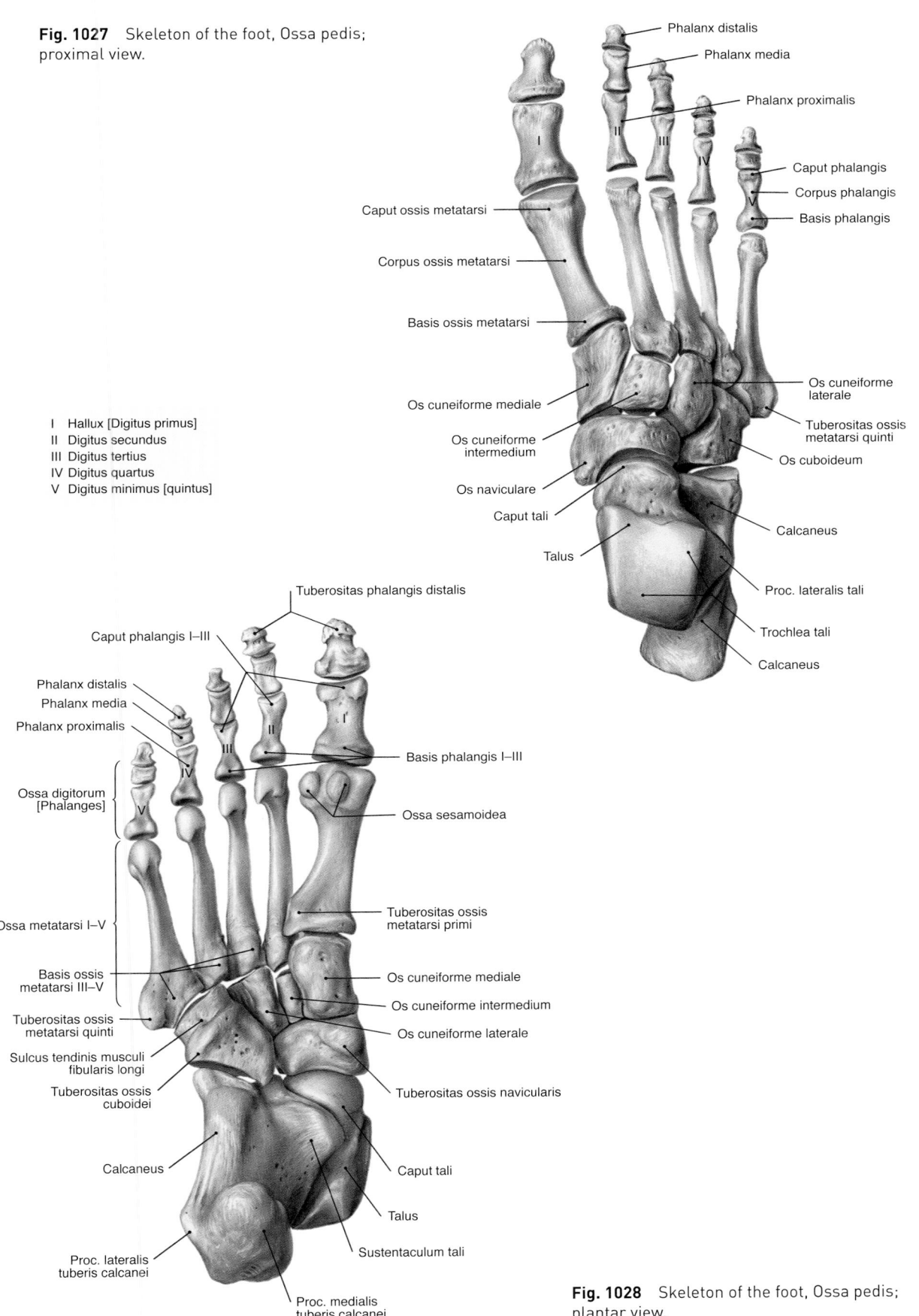

Fig. 1027 Skeleton of the foot, Ossa pedis; proximal view.

Phalanx distalis

Phalanx media

Phalanx proximalis

Caput phalangis

Corpus phalangis

Basis phalangis

Caput ossis metatarsi

Corpus ossis metatarsi

Basis ossis metatarsi

Os cuneiforme laterale

I   Hallux [Digitus primus]
II Digitus secundus
III Digitus tertius
IV Digitus quartus
V Digitus minimus [quintus]

Os cuneiforme mediale

Os cuneiforme intermedium

Tuberositas ossis metatarsi quinti

Os cuboideum

Os naviculare

Caput tali

Calcaneus

Talus

Proc. lateralis tali

Trochlea tali

Calcaneus

Tuberositas phalangis distalis

Caput phalangis I–III

Phalanx distalis
Phalanx media
Phalanx proximalis

Basis phalangis I–III

Ossa digitorum [Phalanges]

Ossa sesamoidea

Tuberositas ossis metatarsi primi

Ossa metatarsi I–V

Os cuneiforme mediale

Os cuneiforme intermedium

Basis ossis metatarsi III–V

Os cuneiforme laterale

Tuberositas ossis metatarsi quinti

Sulcus tendinis musculi fibularis longi

Tuberositas ossis navicularis

Tuberositas ossis cuboidei

Calcaneus

Caput tali

Talus

Proc. lateralis tuberis calcanei

Sustentaculum tali

Proc. medialis tuberis calcanei

Fig. 1028 Skeleton of the foot, Ossa pedis; plantar view.

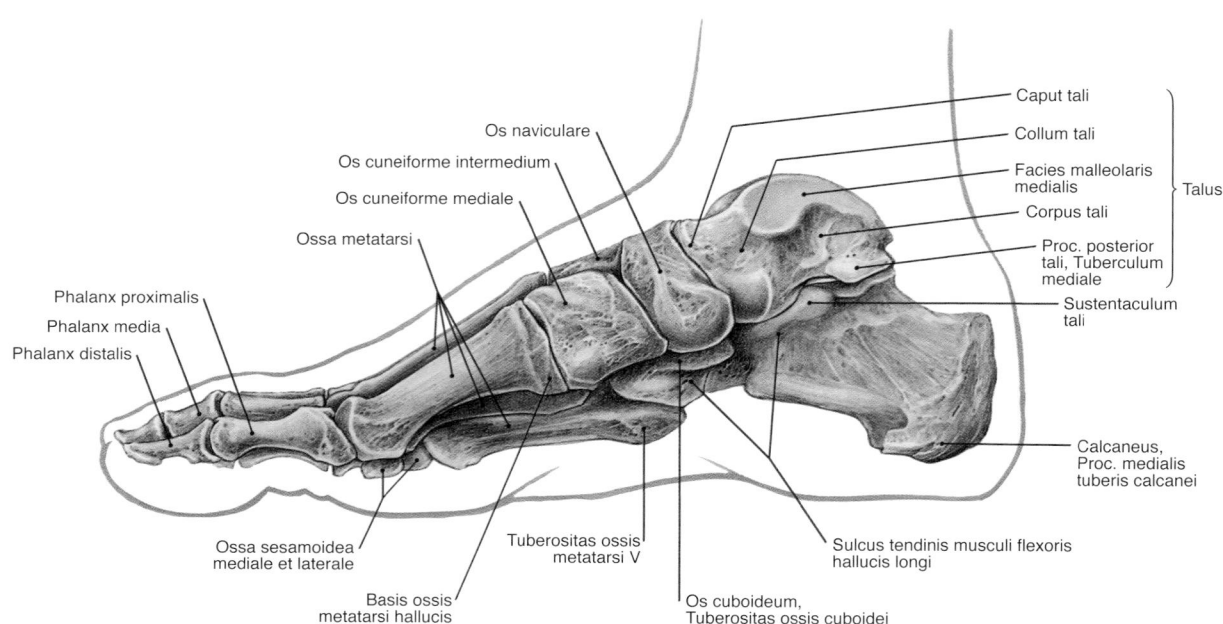

Caput tali
Collum tali
Facies malleolaris medialis
Corpus tali ⎱ Talus
Proc. posterior tali, Tuberculum mediale
Os naviculare
Os cuneiforme intermedium
Os cuneiforme mediale
Ossa metatarsi
Sustentaculum tali
Phalanx proximalis
Phalanx media
Phalanx distalis
Calcaneus, Proc. medialis tuberis calcanei
Ossa sesamoidea mediale et laterale
Tuberositas ossis metatarsi V
Sulcus tendinis musculi flexoris hallucis longi
Basis ossis metatarsi hallucis
Os cuboideum, Tuberositas ossis cuboidei

Fig. 1029 Skeleton of the foot, Ossa pedis; medial view.

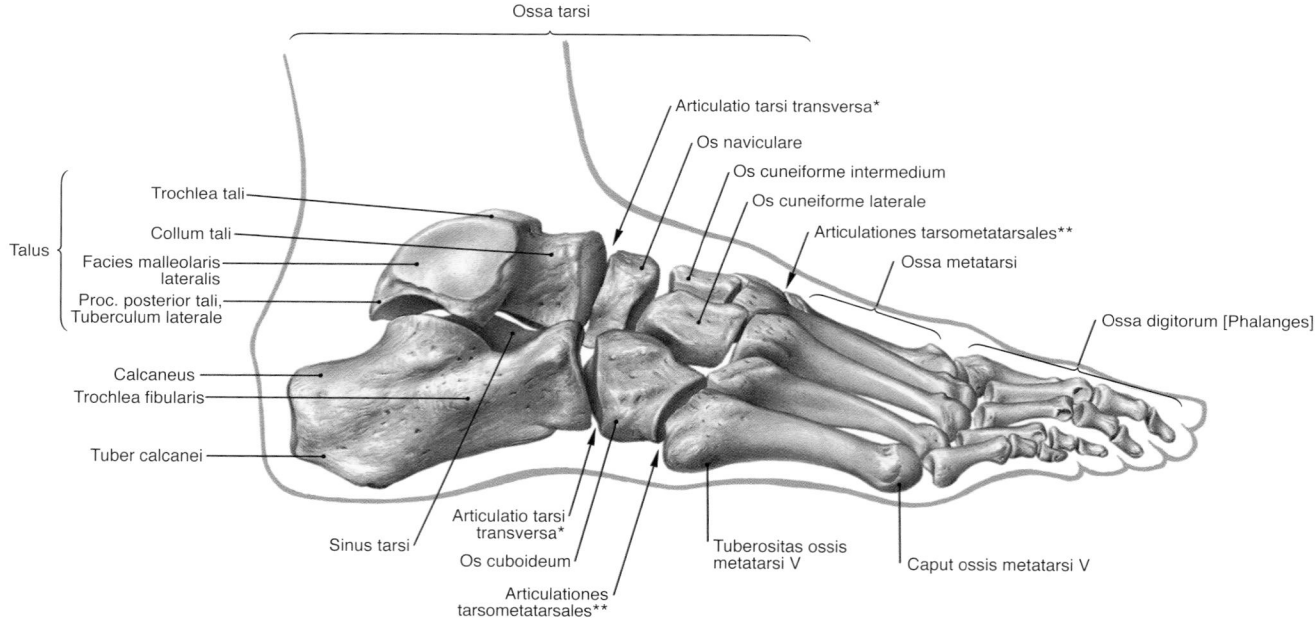

Ossa tarsi

Articulatio tarsi transversa*
Os naviculare
Os cuneiforme intermedium
Os cuneiforme laterale
Articulationes tarsometatarsales**
Ossa metatarsi
Trochlea tali
Collum tali
Talus {
Facies malleolaris lateralis
Proc. posterior tali, Tuberculum laterale
Ossa digitorum [Phalanges]
Calcaneus
Trochlea fibularis
Tuber calcanei
Sinus tarsi
Articulatio tarsi transversa*
Os cuboideum
Articulationes tarsometatarsales**
Tuberositas ossis metatarsi V
Caput ossis metatarsi V

Fig. 1030 Skeleton of the foot, Ossa pedis; lateral view.
* Also: CHOPART's joint
** Also: LISFRANC's joint

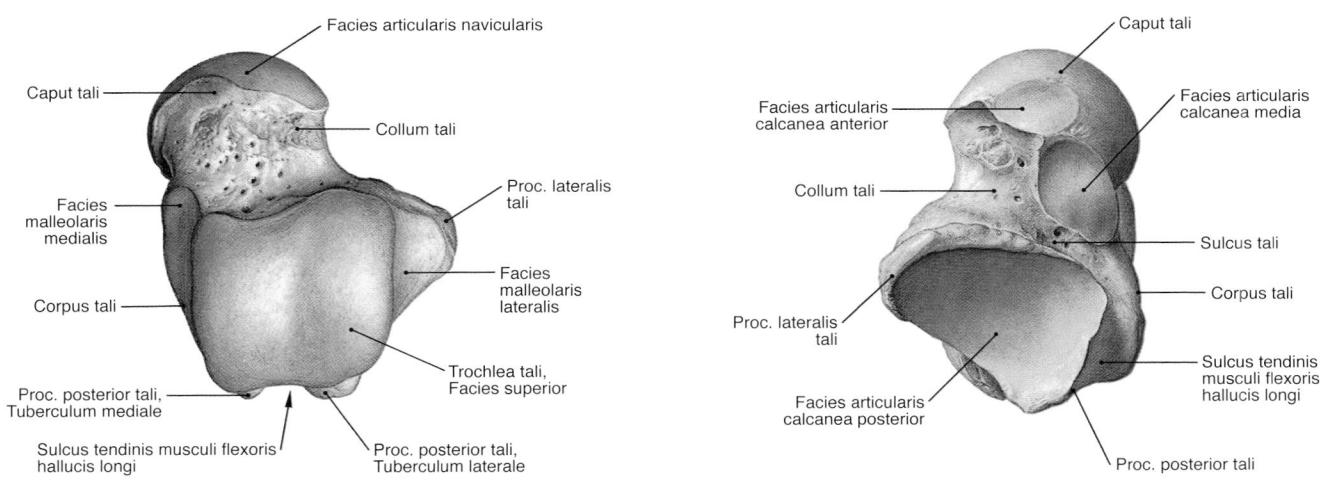

Facies articularis navicularis

Caput tali

Collum tali

Proc. lateralis tali

Facies malleolaris medialis

Facies malleolaris lateralis

Corpus tali

Facies malleolaris lateralis

Trochlea tali, Facies superior

Proc. posterior tali, Tuberculum mediale

Sulcus tendinis musculi flexoris hallucis longi

Proc. posterior tali, Tuberculum laterale

Fig. 1031 Talus, Talus; proximal view.

Caput tali

Facies articularis calcanea anterior

Facies articularis calcanea media

Collum tali

Sulcus tali

Corpus tali

Proc. lateralis tali

Sulcus tendinis musculi flexoris hallucis longi

Facies articularis calcanea posterior

Proc. posterior tali

Fig. 1032 Talus, Talus; plantar view.

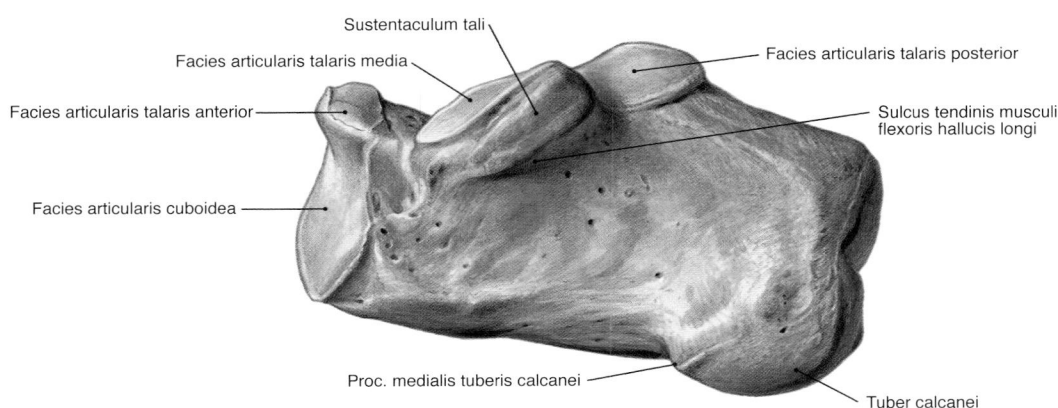

Sustentaculum tali

Facies articularis talaris media

Facies articularis talaris posterior

Facies articularis talaris anterior

Sulcus tendinis musculi flexoris hallucis longi

Facies articularis cuboidea

Proc. medialis tuberis calcanei

Tuber calcanei

Fig. 1033 Calcaneus, Calcaneus; medial view.

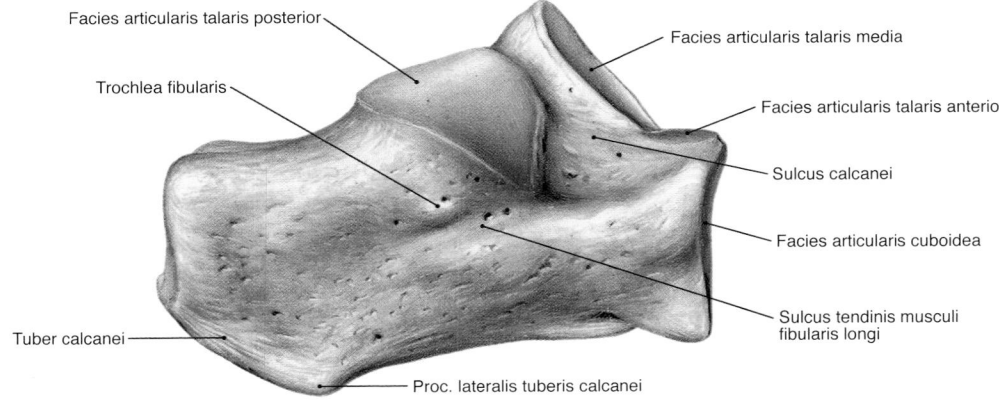

Facies articularis talaris posterior

Facies articularis talaris media

Trochlea fibularis

Facies articularis talaris anterior

Sulcus calcanei

Facies articularis cuboidea

Sulcus tendinis musculi fibularis longi

Tuber calcanei

Proc. lateralis tuberis calcanei

Fig. 1034 Calcaneus, Calcaneus; lateral view.

Tarsal bones

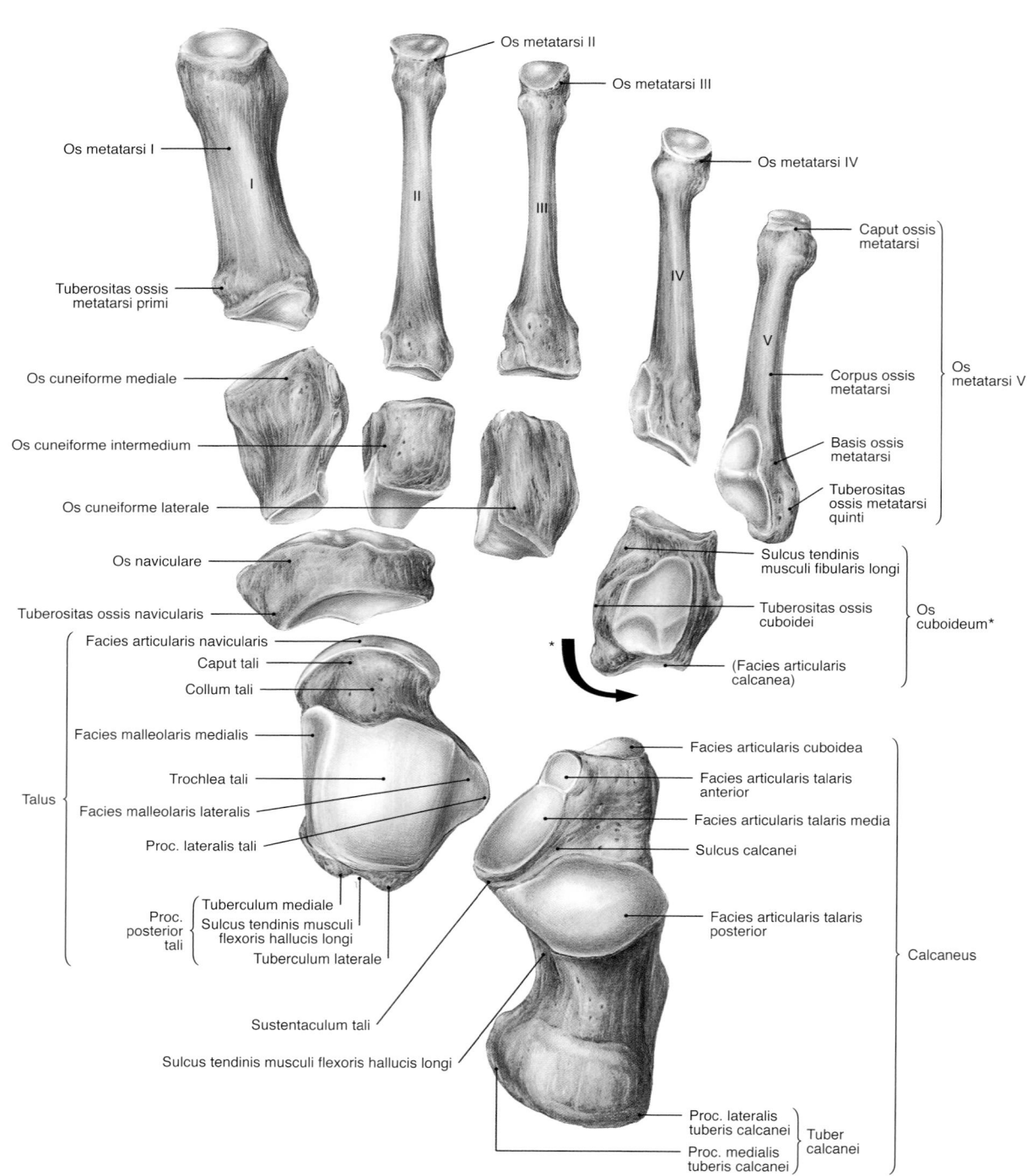

Os metatarsi I

Tuberositas ossis metatarsi primi

Os cuneiforme mediale

Os cuneiforme intermedium

Os cuneiforme laterale

Os naviculare

Tuberositas ossis navicularis

Talus
- Facies articularis navicularis
- Caput tali
- Collum tali
- Facies malleolaris medialis
- Trochlea tali
- Facies malleolaris lateralis
- Proc. lateralis tali
- Proc. posterior tali
  - Tuberculum mediale
  - Sulcus tendinis musculi flexoris hallucis longi
  - Tuberculum laterale

Sustentaculum tali

Sulcus tendinis musculi flexoris hallucis longi

Os metatarsi II

Os metatarsi III

Os metatarsi IV

Caput ossis metatarsi

Corpus ossis metatarsi

Basis ossis metatarsi

Tuberositas ossis metatarsi quinti

Os metatarsi V

Sulcus tendinis musculi fibularis longi

Tuberositas ossis cuboidei

(Facies articularis calcanea)

Os cuboideum*

Facies articularis cuboidea

Facies articularis talaris anterior

Facies articularis talaris media

Sulcus calcanei

Facies articularis talaris posterior

Calcaneus

Proc. lateralis tuberis calcanei

Proc. medialis tuberis calcanei

Tuber calcanei

Fig. 1035   Tarsal bones, Ossa tarsi, and metatarsal bones, Ossa metatarsi; proximal view.

* The cuboid bone is shown in a medial view.

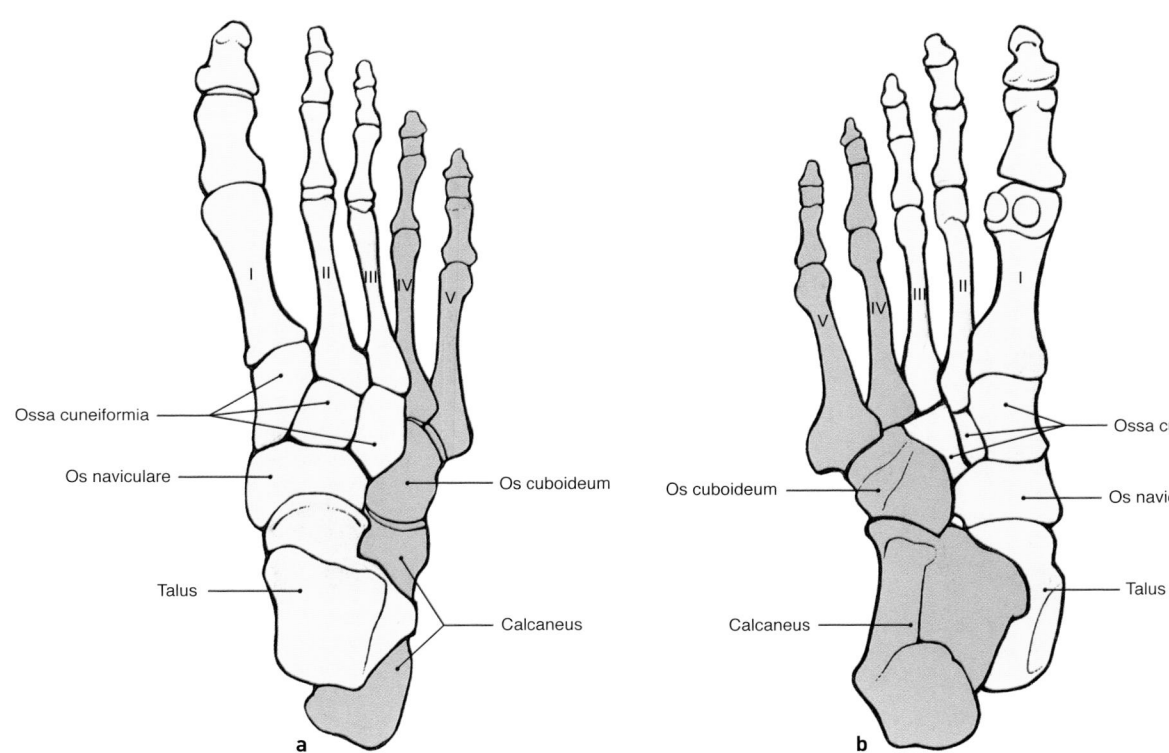

Fig. 1036 a, b   Skeleton of the foot, Ossa pedis;
structural organisation.
a Proximal view
b Plantar view

The heads of all metatarsal bones lie in the plantar plane. The
cuneiform bones, the navicular bone and the talus rest upon the
lateral parts of the skeleton, especially in the posterior part of
the foot. The talus is therefore situated above the calcaneus and
the longitudinal arch is formed.
The wedge-shaped cross-section of the cuneiform bones and
the bases of the metatarsal bones contribute to the formation
of the transverse vault.

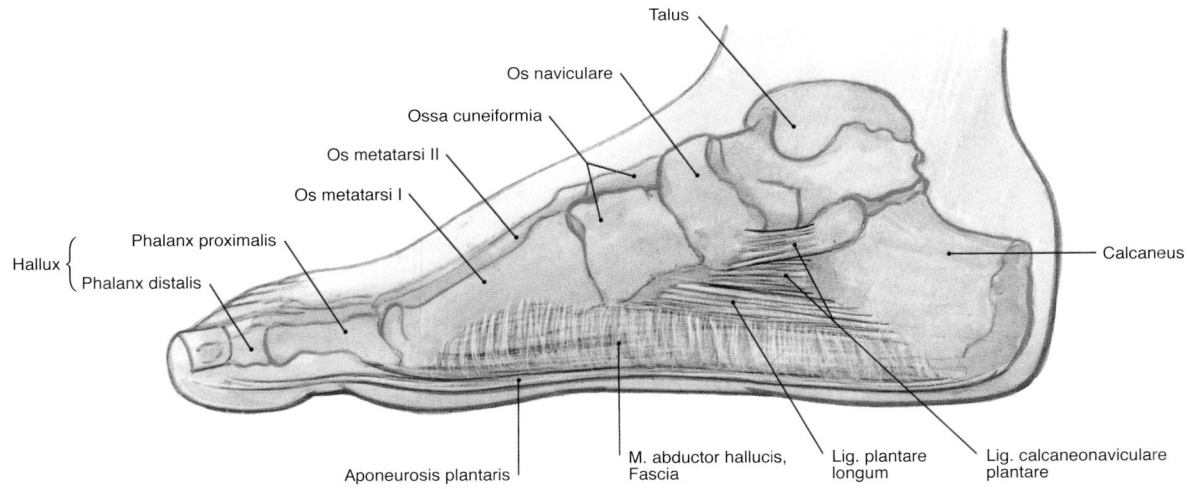

Fig. 1037   Supporting structures of the medial arch of the
longitudinal vault of the foot;
medial view.

The ligaments shown in this illustration are mostly directed in
the longitudinal axis of the foot and support passively the
longitudinal vault of the foot. The short muscles of the foot
primarily support this construction.

Joints of the foot

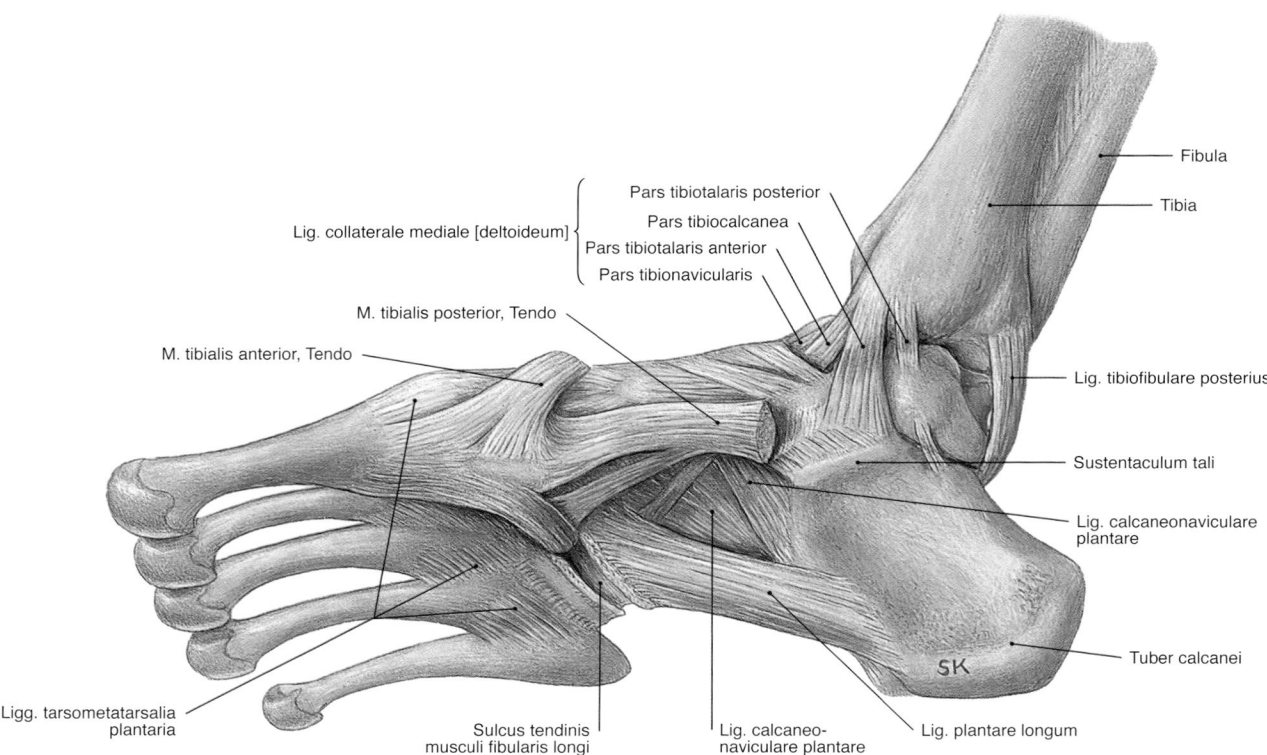

Fibula

Tibia

Pars tibiotalaris posterior
Pars tibiocalcanea
Pars tibiotalaris anterior
Pars tibionavicularis

Lig. collaterale mediale [deltoideum]

M. tibialis posterior, Tendo

M. tibialis anterior, Tendo

Lig. tibiofibulare posterius

Sustentaculum tali

Lig. calcaneonaviculare plantare

Tuber calcanei

Ligg. tarsometatarsalia plantaria

Sulcus tendinis musculi fibularis longi

Lig. calcaneo-naviculare plantare

Lig. plantare longum

SK

Fig. 1038 Joints of the foot, Articulationes pedis; ligaments and tendons; medial view.

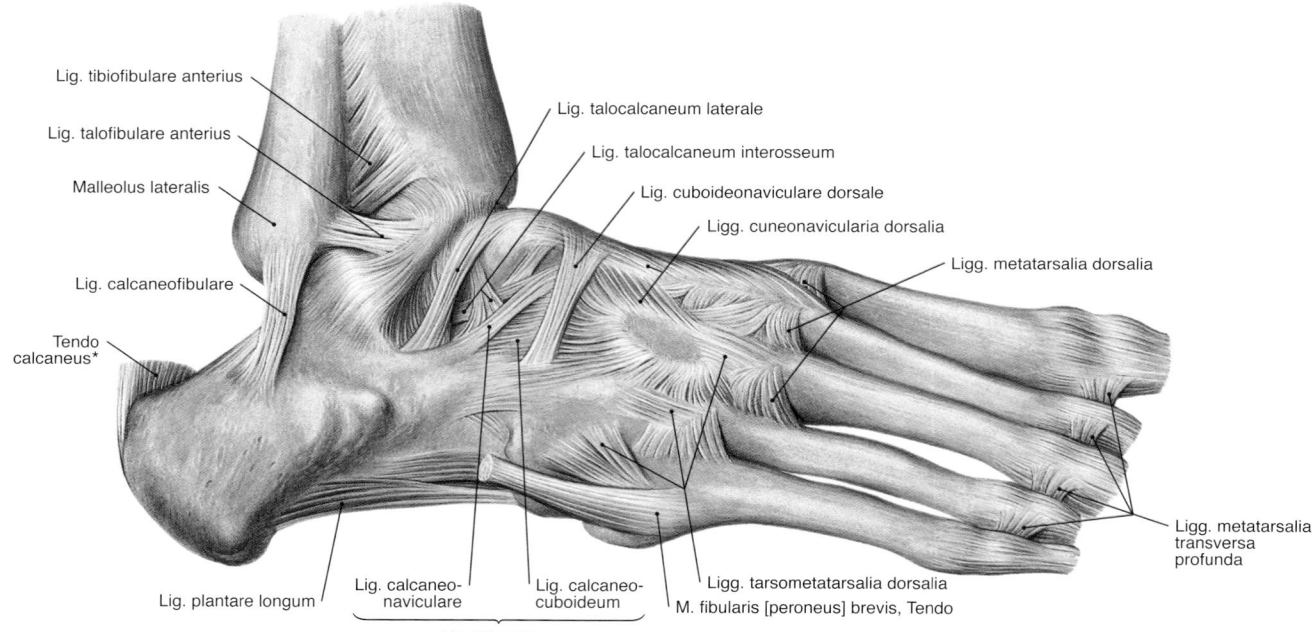

Lig. tibiofibulare anterius

Lig. talofibulare anterius

Malleolus lateralis

Lig. calcaneofibulare

Tendo calcaneus*

Lig. talocalcaneum laterale

Lig. talocalcaneum interosseum

Lig. cuboideonaviculare dorsale

Ligg. cuneonavicularia dorsalia

Ligg. metatarsalia dorsalia

Ligg. metatarsalia transversa profunda

Lig. plantare longum

Lig. calcaneo-naviculare

Lig. calcaneo-cuboideum

Ligg. tarsometatarsalia dorsalia

M. fibularis [peroneus] brevis, Tendo

Lig. bifurcatum

Fig. 1039 Joints of the foot, Articulationes pedis; ligaments and tendons; lateral view.

* Also: Achilles tendon

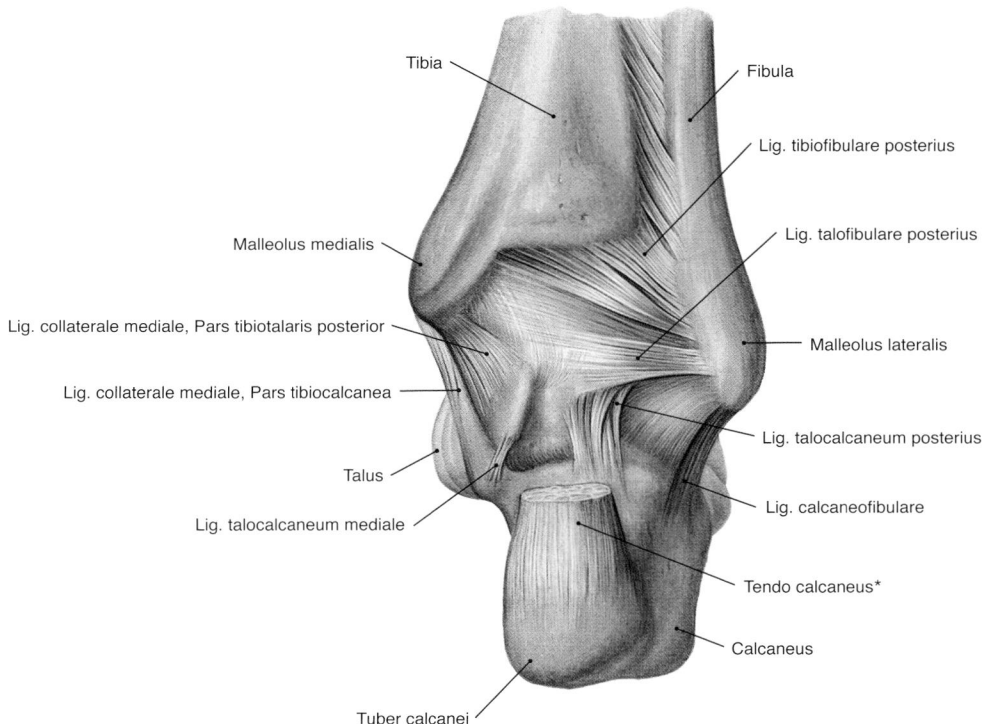

Tibia

Fibula

Lig. tibiofibulare posterius

Lig. talofibulare posterius

Malleolus medialis

Lig. collaterale mediale, Pars tibiotalaris posterior

Malleolus lateralis

Lig. collaterale mediale, Pars tibiocalcanea

Lig. talocalcaneum posterius

Talus

Lig. calcaneofibulare

Lig. talocalcaneum mediale

Tendo calcaneus*

Calcaneus

Tuber calcanei

Fig. 1040   Joints of the foot, Articulationes pedis;
ligaments and tendons of the posterior part of the foot.
* Also: Achilles tendon

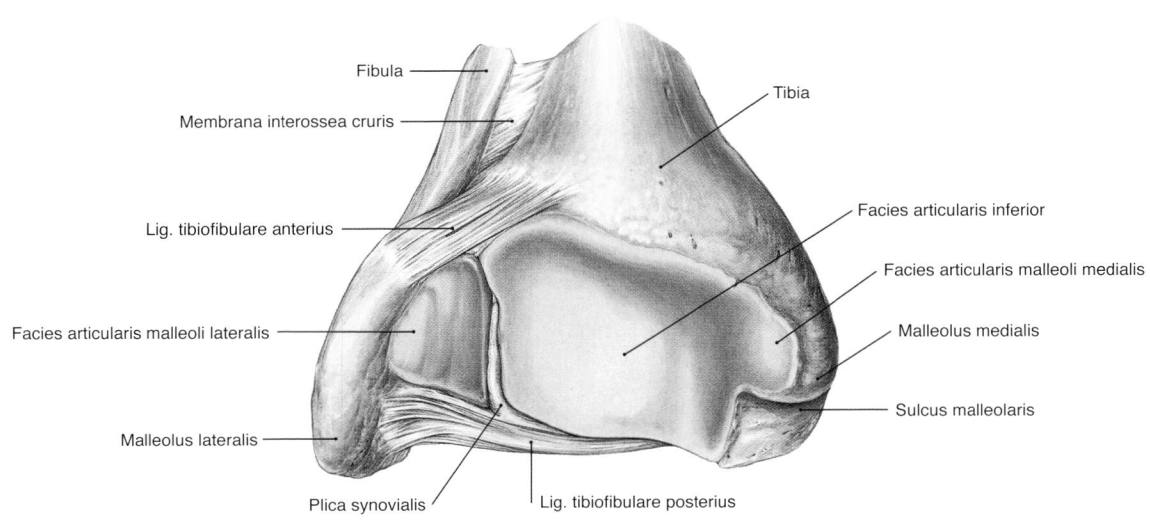

Fibula

Tibia

Membrana interossea cruris

Lig. tibiofibulare anterius

Facies articularis inferior

Facies articularis malleoli medialis

Facies articularis malleoli lateralis

Malleolus medialis

Malleolus lateralis

Sulcus malleolaris

Plica synovialis

Lig. tibiofibulare posterius

Fig. 1041   Ankle joint, Articulatio talocruralis;
proximal articular surfaces;
distal view.

Joints of the foot

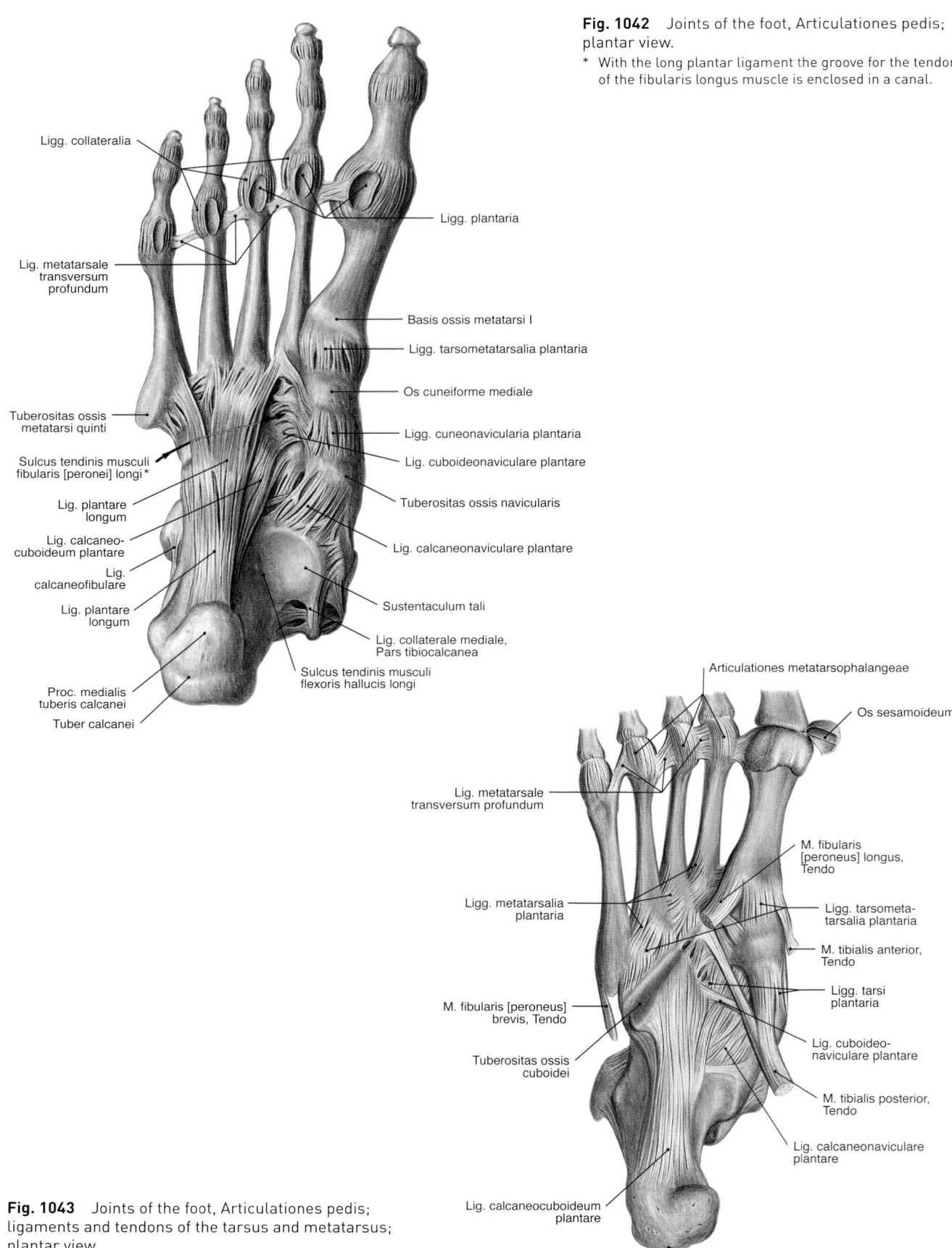

Fig. 1042   Joints of the foot, Articulationes pedis; plantar view.
* With the long plantar ligament the groove for the tendon of the fibularis longus muscle is enclosed in a canal.

Ligg. collateralia

Ligg. plantaria

Lig. metatarsale transversum profundum

Basis ossis metatarsi I

Ligg. tarsometatarsalia plantaria

Os cuneiforme mediale

Tuberositas ossis metatarsi quinti

Ligg. cuneonavicularia plantaria

Lig. cuboideonaviculare plantare

Sulcus tendinis musculi fibularis [peronei] longi*

Tuberositas ossis navicularis

Lig. plantare longum

Lig. calcaneo-cuboideum plantare

Lig. calcaneonaviculare plantare

Lig. calcaneofibulare

Lig. plantare longum

Sustentaculum tali

Lig. collaterale mediale, Pars tibiocalcanea

Proc. medialis tuberis calcanei

Sulcus tendinis musculi flexoris hallucis longi

Tuber calcanei

Articulationes metatarsophalangeae

Os sesamoideum

Lig. metatarsale transversum profundum

M. fibularis [peroneus] longus, Tendo

Ligg. metatarsalia plantaria

Ligg. tarsometa-tarsalia plantaria

M. tibialis anterior, Tendo

Ligg. tarsi plantaria

M. fibularis [peroneus] brevis, Tendo

Lig. cuboideo-naviculare plantare

Tuberositas ossis cuboidei

M. tibialis posterior, Tendo

Lig. calcaneonaviculare plantare

Lig. calcaneocuboideum plantare

Tuber calcanei

Fig. 1043   Joints of the foot, Articulationes pedis; ligaments and tendons of the tarsus and metatarsus; plantar view.

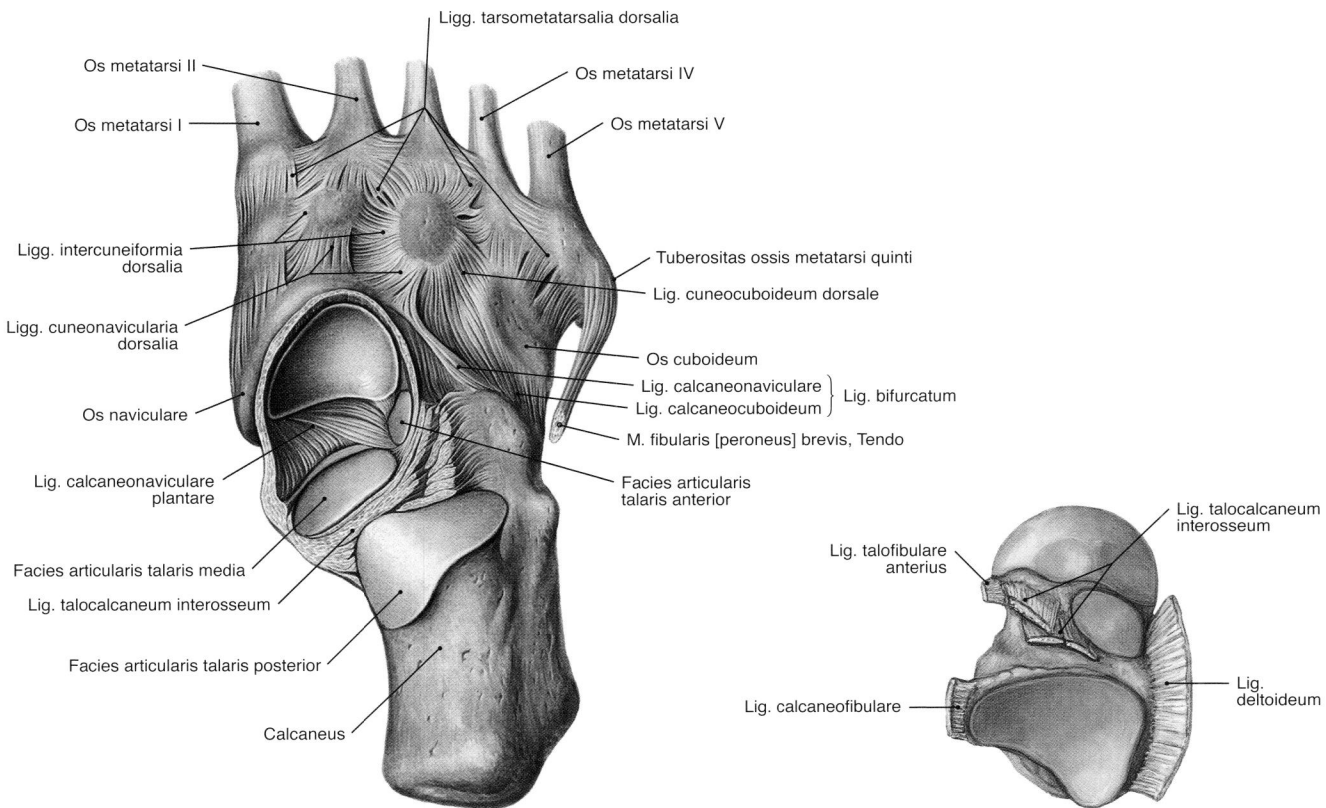

Ligg. tarsometatarsalia dorsalia

Os metatarsi II

Os metatarsi I

Ligg. intercuneiformia dorsalia

Ligg. cuneonavicularia dorsalia

Os naviculare

Lig. calcaneonaviculare plantare

Facies articularis talaris media

Lig. talocalcaneum interosseum

Facies articularis talaris posterior

Calcaneus

Os metatarsi IV

Os metatarsi V

Tuberositas ossis metatarsi quinti

Lig. cuneocuboideum dorsale

Os cuboideum

Lig. calcaneonaviculare
Lig. calcaneocuboideum } Lig. bifurcatum

M. fibularis [peroneus] brevis, Tendo

Facies articularis talaris anterior

Fig. 1044   Talotarsal joint,
Articulatio talotarsalis;
distal articular surfaces;
proximal view.

Lig. talofibulare anterius

Lig. calcaneofibulare

Lig. talocalcaneum interosseum

Lig. deltoideum

Fig. 1045   Talotarsal joint,
Articulatio talotarsalis;
proximal articular surfaces;
distal view.

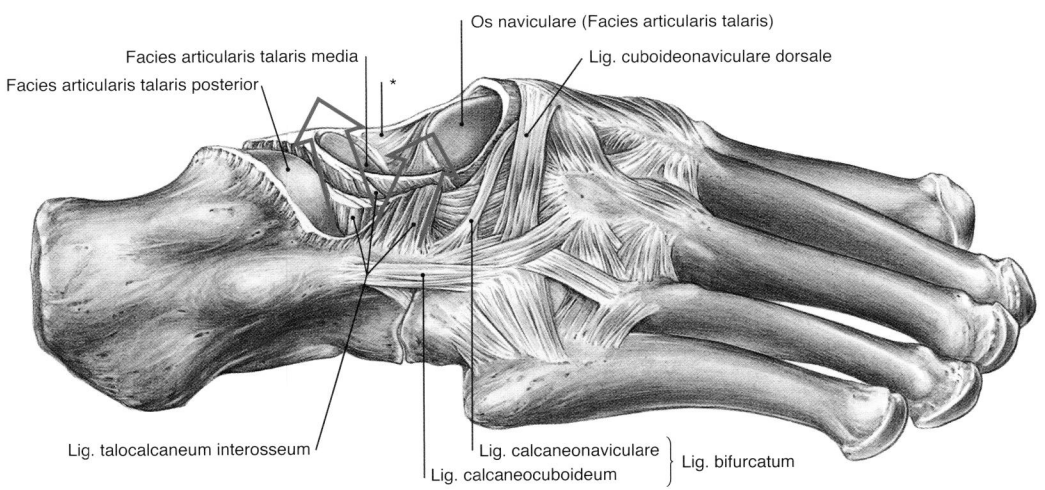

Facies articularis talaris media

Facies articularis talaris posterior

Os naviculare (Facies articularis talaris)

Lig. cuboideonaviculare dorsale

*

Lig. talocalcaneum interosseum

Lig. calcaneonaviculare
Lig. calcaneocuboideum } Lig. bifurcatum

Fig. 1046   Talotarsal joint, Articulatio talotarsalis;
the talus and the lateral ligaments have been removed;
lateral view.
The two arrows point out the helical distorsion of the
talocalcaneal interosseous ligament.

* Tight connective tissue layer between the plantar calcaneonavicular
ligament and the tibionavicular part of the deltoid ligament limiting
a medially directed gliding of the head of the talus; slackening of this
layer results in flattening of the longitudinal vault (flat-foot, pes valgus)

Ankle and talotarsal joint, sections

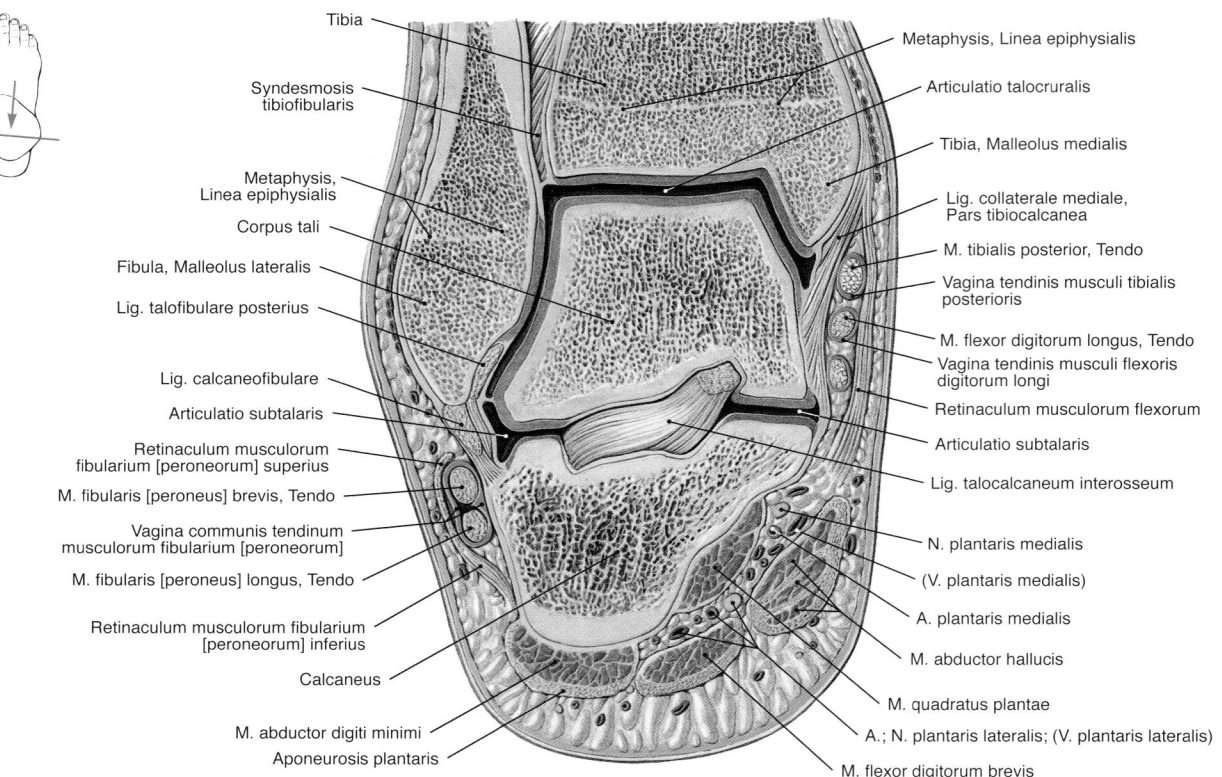

Tibia

Syndesmosis tibiofibularis

Metaphysis, Linea epiphysialis

Corpus tali

Fibula, Malleolus lateralis

Lig. talofibulare posterius

Lig. calcaneofibulare

Articulatio subtalaris

Retinaculum musculorum fibularium [peroneorum] superius

M. fibularis [peroneus] brevis, Tendo

Vagina communis tendinum musculorum fibularium [peroneorum]

M. fibularis [peroneus] longus, Tendo

Retinaculum musculorum fibularium [peroneorum] inferius

Calcaneus

M. abductor digiti minimi

Aponeurosis plantaris

Metaphysis, Linea epiphysialis

Articulatio talocruralis

Tibia, Malleolus medialis

Lig. collaterale mediale, Pars tibiocalcanea

M. tibialis posterior, Tendo

Vagina tendinis musculi tibialis posterioris

M. flexor digitorum longus, Tendo

Vagina tendinis musculi flexoris digitorum longi

Retinaculum musculorum flexorum

Articulatio subtalaris

Lig. talocalcaneum interosseum

N. plantaris medialis

(V. plantaris medialis)

A. plantaris medialis

M. abductor hallucis

M. quadratus plantae

A.; N. plantaris lateralis; (V. plantaris lateralis)

M. flexor digitorum brevis

Fig. 1047   Ankle and talotarsal joint, Articulationes talocruralis et talotarsalis; frontal section.

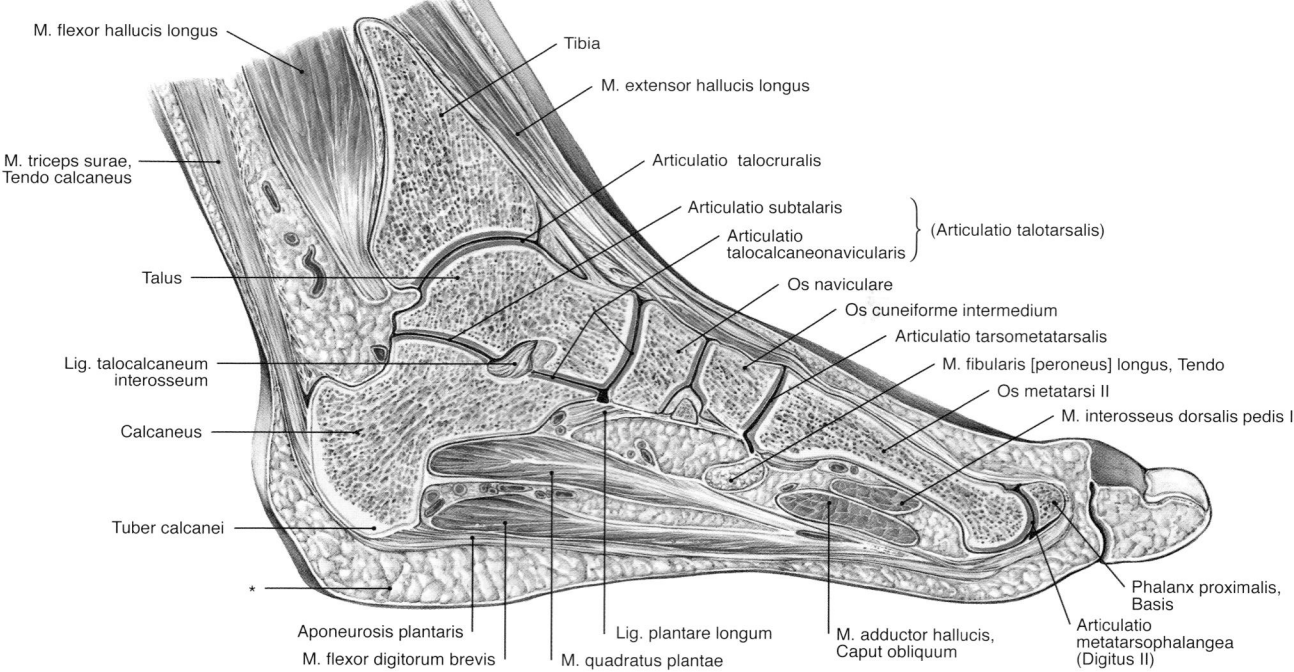

M. flexor hallucis longus

M. triceps surae, Tendo calcaneus

Talus

Lig. talocalcaneum interosseum

Calcaneus

Tuber calcanei

*

Aponeurosis plantaris

M. flexor digitorum brevis

Tibia

M. extensor hallucis longus

Articulatio talocruralis

Articulatio subtalaris

Articulatio talocalcaneonavicularis

} (Articulatio talotarsalis)

Os naviculare

Os cuneiforme intermedium

Articulatio tarsometatarsalis

M. fibularis [peroneus] longus, Tendo

Os metatarsi II

M. interosseus dorsalis pedis I

Lig. plantare longum

M. quadratus plantae

M. adductor hallucis, Caput obliquum

Phalanx proximalis, Basis

Articulatio metatarsophalangea (Digitus II)

Fig. 1048   Ankle and talotarsal joint, Articulationes talocruralis et talotarsalis; sagittal section.
* Fat pad of the heel

Ankle and talotarsal joint, radiography

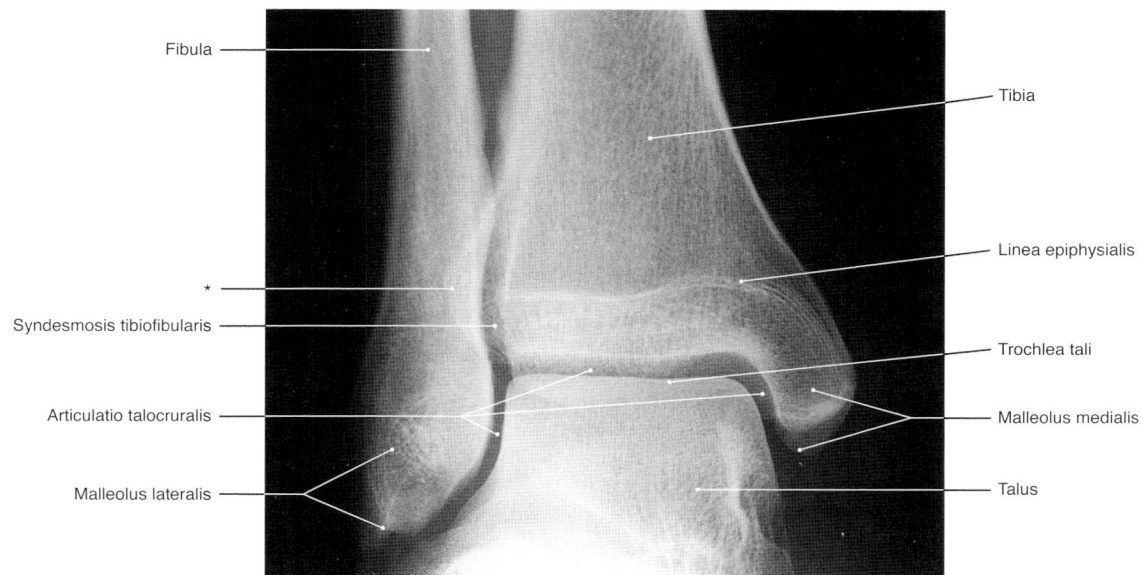

Fibula

Tibia

Linea epiphysialis

*

Syndesmosis tibiofibularis

Trochlea tali

Articulatio talocruralis

Malleolus medialis

Malleolus lateralis

Talus

Fig. 1049 Ankle joint, Articulatio talocruralis;
AP-radiograph with the subject reclined and the central beam
directed tangentially onto the trochlea of talus.

* Clinically, the posterior border of the fibular notch is also referred to
  as the third malleolus.

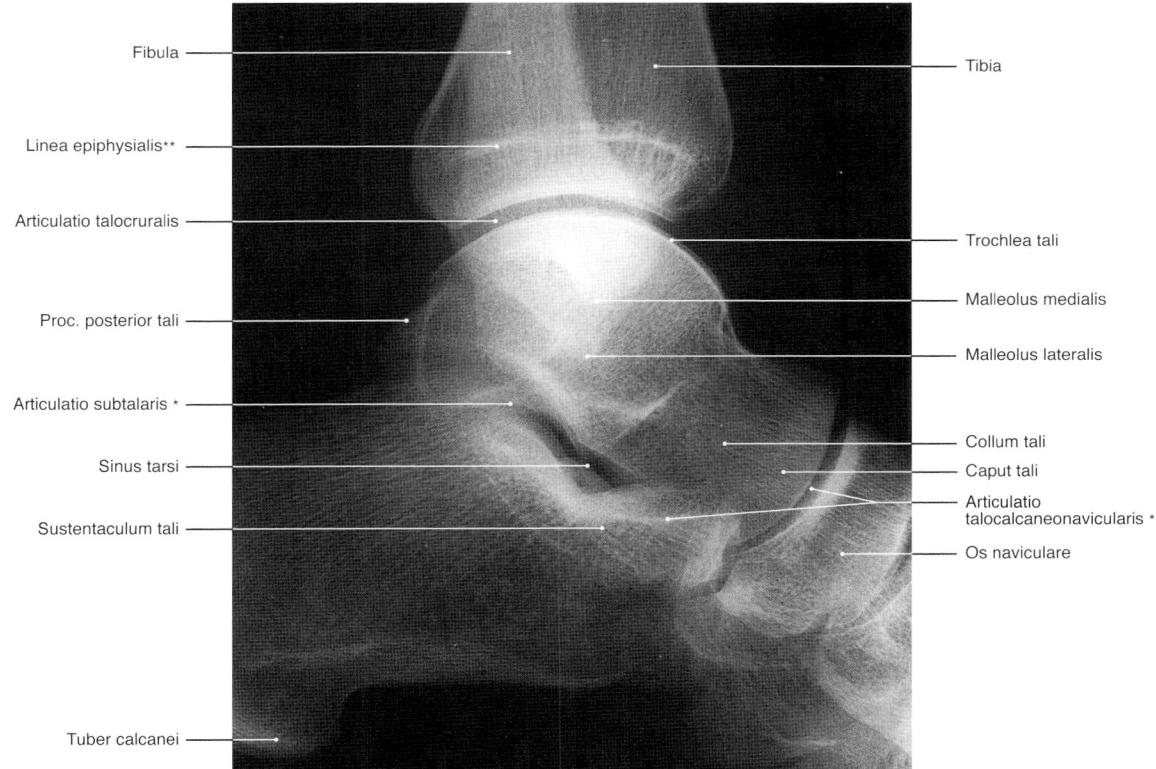

Fibula

Tibia

Linea epiphysialis**

Articulatio talocruralis

Trochlea tali

Malleolus medialis

Proc. posterior tali

Malleolus lateralis

Articulatio subtalaris *

Collum tali

Sinus tarsi

Caput tali

Articulatio
talocalcaneonavicularis *

Sustentaculum tali

Os naviculare

Tuber calcanei

Fig. 1050 Ankle and talotarsal joint,
Articulationes talocruralis et talotarsalis;
AP-radiograph with the subject reclined and the central beam
directed tangentially onto the apex of the trochlea of talus.

* Due to their helical distorsion, the joint clefts are not displayed
  orthogonally.
** Overlapping epiphyseal lines of the tibia and fibula

→ 1160, 1162

Fasciae of the lower limb

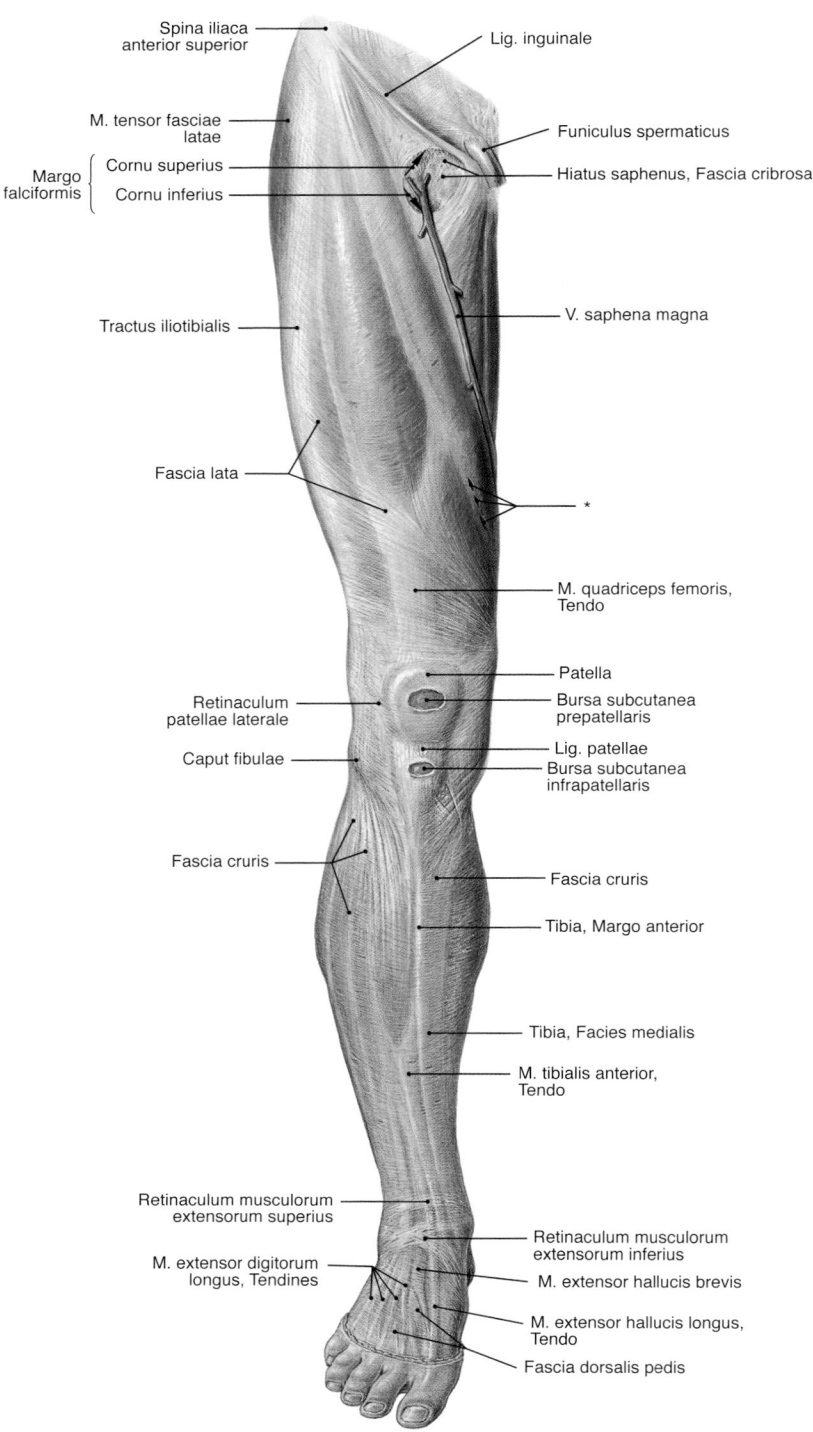

Spina iliaca anterior superior
Lig. inguinale
M. tensor fasciae latae
Funiculus spermaticus
Margo falciformis — Cornu superius / Cornu inferius
Hiatus saphenus, Fascia cribrosa
Tractus iliotibialis
V. saphena magna
Fascia lata
*
M. quadriceps femoris, Tendo
Patella
Retinaculum patellae laterale
Bursa subcutanea prepatellaris
Caput fibulae
Lig. patellae
Bursa subcutanea infrapatellaris
Fascia cruris
Fascia cruris
Tibia, Margo anterior
Tibia, Facies medialis
M. tibialis anterior, Tendo
Retinaculum musculorum extensorum superius
Retinaculum musculorum extensorum inferius
M. extensor digitorum longus, Tendines
M. extensor hallucis brevis
M. extensor hallucis longus, Tendo
Fascia dorsalis pedis

Fig. 1051   Fascia lata, Fascia lata, and deep fascia of leg, Fascia cruris.
The transition zone between the aponeurosis of the external oblique abdominal muscle and the fascia lata is known as inguinal ligament. This ligament extends laterally from the anterior superior iliac spine to its attachment on the pubic tubercle medially.
* Openings in the fascia for the perforator veins (DODD's veins)

Fasciae of the lower limb

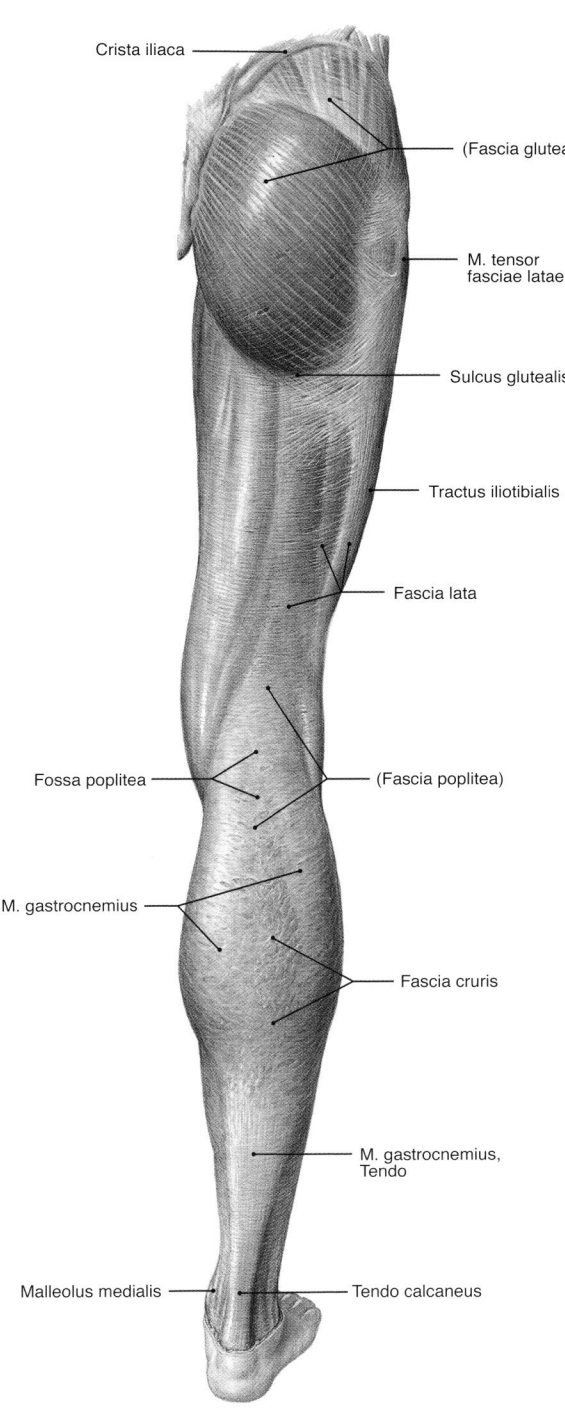

Crista iliaca

(Fascia glutea)

M. tensor
fasciae latae

Sulcus glutealis

Tractus iliotibialis

Fascia lata

Fossa poplitea

(Fascia poplitea)

M. gastrocnemius

Fascia cruris

M. gastrocnemius,
Tendo

Malleolus medialis

Tendo calcaneus

Fig. 1052   Fascia lata, Fascia lata,
and deep fascia of leg, Fascia cruris.

Muscles of the lower limb, overview

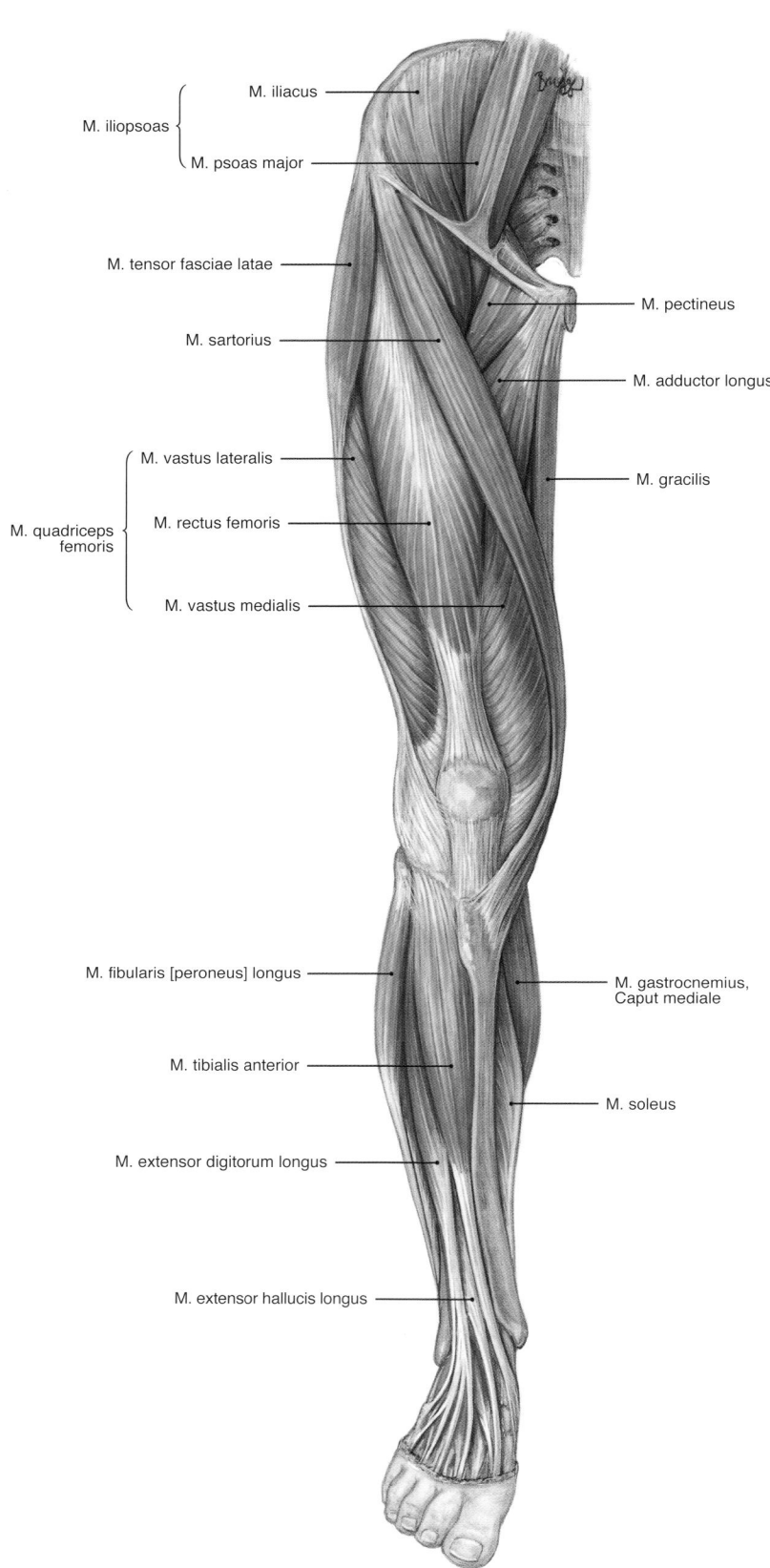

M. iliacus

M. iliopsoas

M. psoas major

M. tensor fasciae latae

M. pectineus

M. sartorius

M. adductor longus

M. vastus lateralis

M. gracilis

M. quadriceps
femoris

M. rectus femoris

M. vastus medialis

M. fibularis [peroneus] longus

M. gastrocnemius,
Caput mediale

M. tibialis anterior

M. soleus

M. extensor digitorum longus

M. extensor hallucis longus

→ T 42, T 44, T 45,
T 47, T 48

Fig. 1053 Muscles of the lower limb, Mm. extremitatis inferioris;
overview.

Muscles of the lower limb, overview

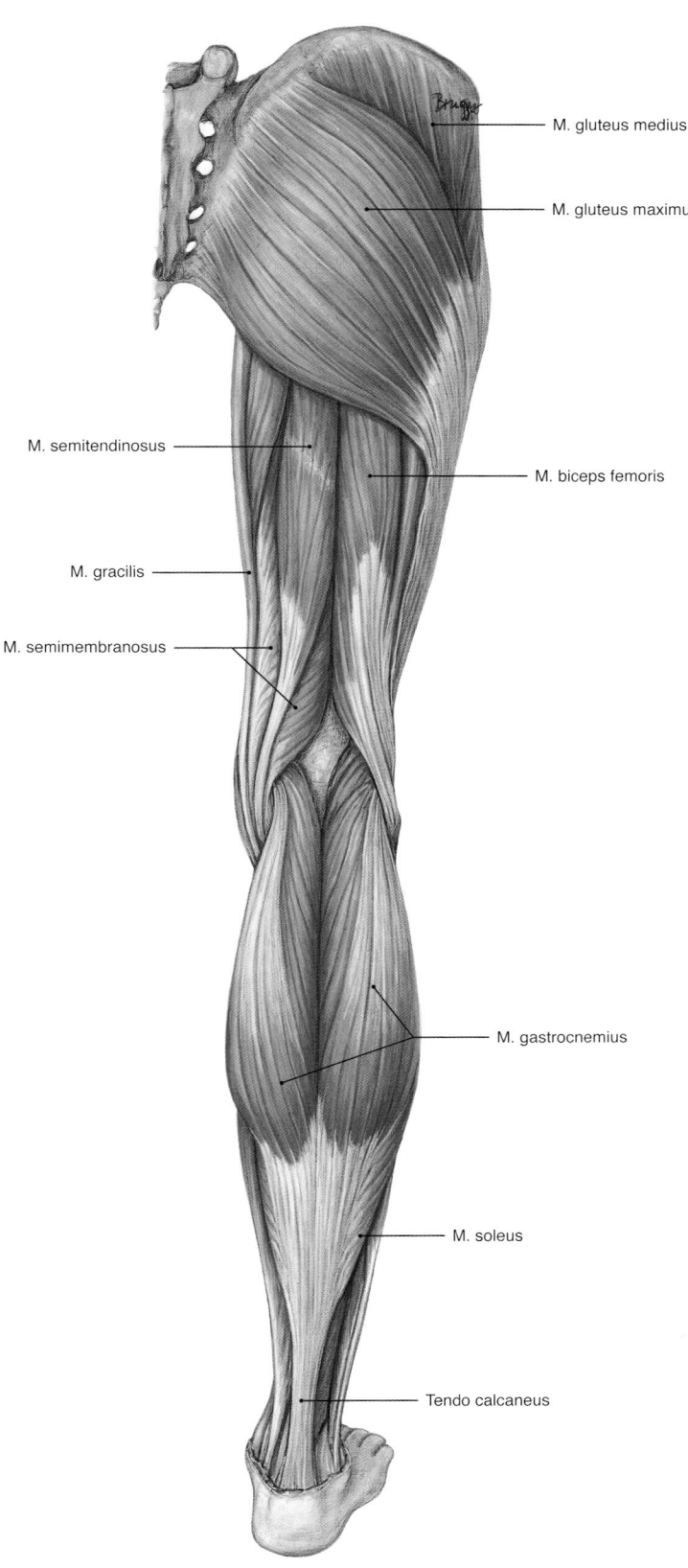

M. gluteus medius

M. gluteus maximus

M. semitendinosus

M. biceps femoris

M. gracilis

M. semimembranosus

M. gastrocnemius

M. soleus

Tendo calcaneus

Fig. 1054   Muscles of the lower limb, Mm. extremitatis inferioris; overview.

→ T 43, T 46, T 49

Origins and insertions of the muscles of the hip, the thigh and the leg

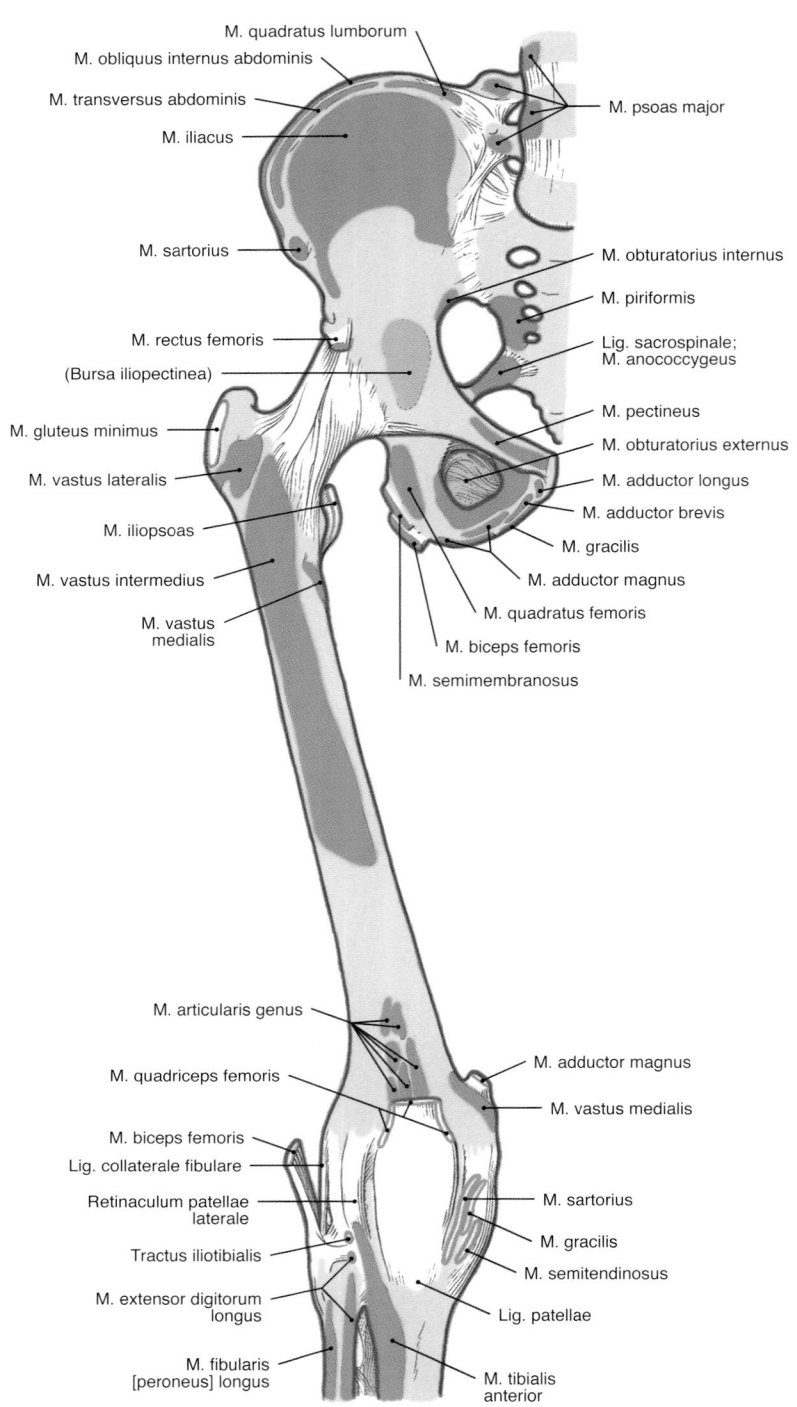

- M. quadratus lumborum
- M. obliquus internus abdominis
- M. transversus abdominis
- M. iliacus
- M. psoas major
- M. sartorius
- M. obturatorius internus
- M. piriformis
- M. rectus femoris
- (Bursa iliopectinea)
- Lig. sacrospinale; M. anococcygeus
- M. gluteus minimus
- M. pectineus
- M. obturatorius externus
- M. vastus lateralis
- M. adductor longus
- M. iliopsoas
- M. adductor brevis
- M. gracilis
- M. vastus intermedius
- M. adductor magnus
- M. vastus medialis
- M. quadratus femoris
- M. biceps femoris
- M. semimembranosus
- M. articularis genus
- M. adductor magnus
- M. vastus medialis
- M. quadriceps femoris
- M. biceps femoris
- M. sartorius
- Lig. collaterale fibulare
- Retinaculum patellae laterale
- M. gracilis
- Tractus iliotibialis
- M. semitendinosus
- M. extensor digitorum longus
- Lig. patellae
- M. fibularis [peroneus] longus
- M. tibialis anterior

→ T 42–T 48

Fig. 1055 Origins and insertions of the muscles at the lower lumbar vertebrae, the pelvic bones, the femur and the proximal extremities of the bones of the leg; ventral view.

Origins and insertions of the muscles of the hip, the thigh and the leg

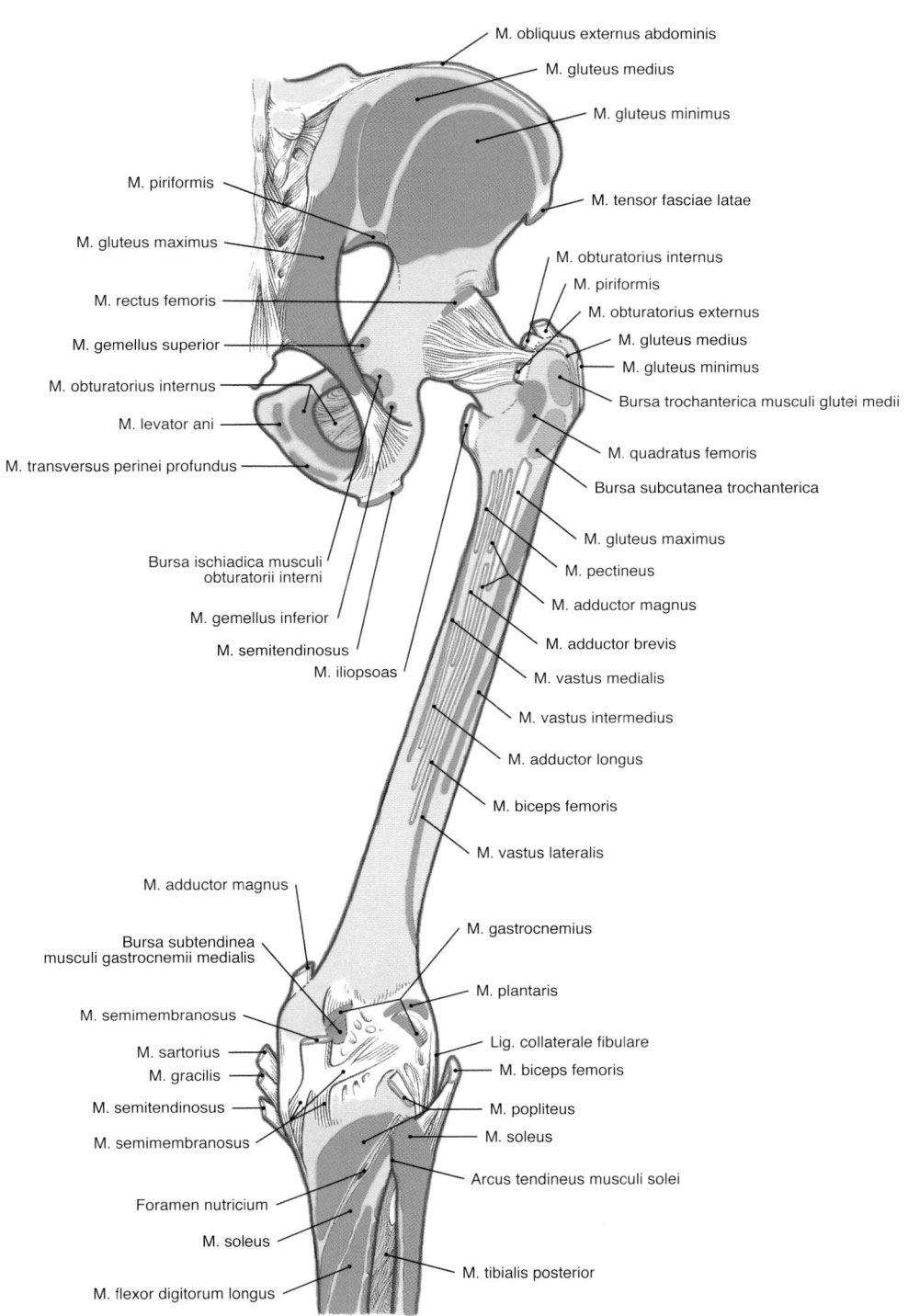

M. obliquus externus abdominis
M. gluteus medius
M. gluteus minimus
M. tensor fasciae latae
M. piriformis
M. gluteus maximus
M. rectus femoris
M. gemellus superior
M. obturatorius internus
M. levator ani
M. transversus perinei profundus

M. obturatorius internus
M. piriformis
M. obturatorius externus
M. gluteus medius
M. gluteus minimus
Bursa trochanterica musculi glutei medii
M. quadratus femoris
Bursa subcutanea trochanterica
M. gluteus maximus
M. pectineus
M. adductor magnus
M. adductor brevis
M. vastus medialis
M. vastus intermedius
M. adductor longus
M. biceps femoris
M. vastus lateralis

Bursa ischiadica musculi obturatorii interni
M. gemellus inferior
M. semitendinosus
M. iliopsoas

M. adductor magnus
Bursa subtendinea musculi gastrocnemii medialis
M. semimembranosus
M. sartorius
M. gracilis
M. semitendinosus
M. semimembranosus
Foramen nutricium
M. soleus
M. flexor digitorum longus

M. gastrocnemius
M. plantaris
Lig. collaterale fibulare
M. biceps femoris
M. popliteus
M. soleus
Arcus tendineus musculi solei
M. tibialis posterior

Fig. 1056 Origins and insertions of the muscles at the pelvic bones, the femur and the proximal extremities of the bones of the leg; dorsal view.

→ T 43–T 46, T 49, T 50

Muscles of the thigh

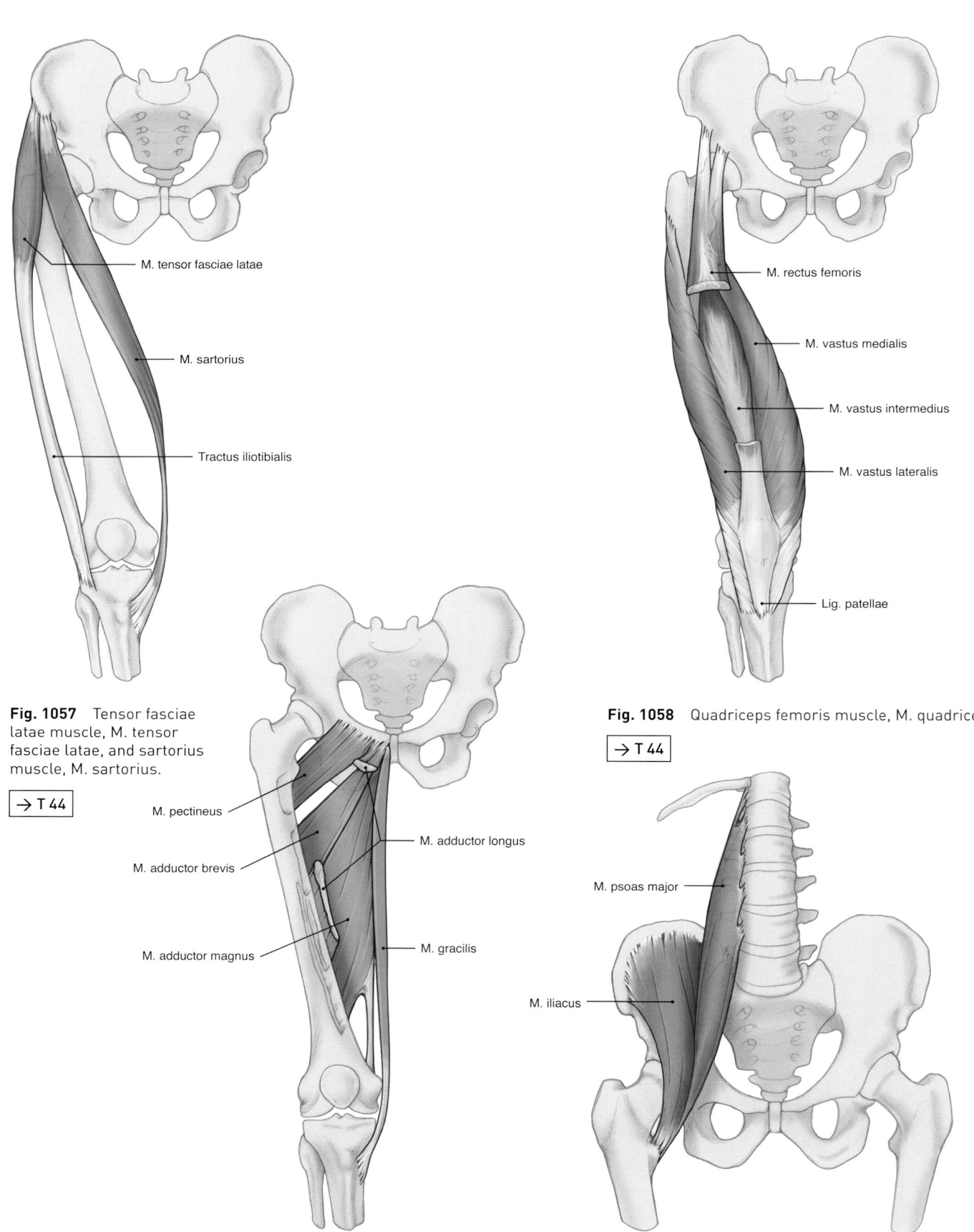

Fig. 1057   Tensor fasciae latae muscle, M. tensor fasciae latae, and sartorius muscle, M. sartorius.

→ T 44

Fig. 1058   Quadriceps femoris muscle, M. quadriceps femoris.

→ T 44

Fig. 1059   Adductor muscles, Mm. adductores.

→ T 45

Fig. 1060   Iliopsoas muscle, M. iliopsoas.

→ T 42

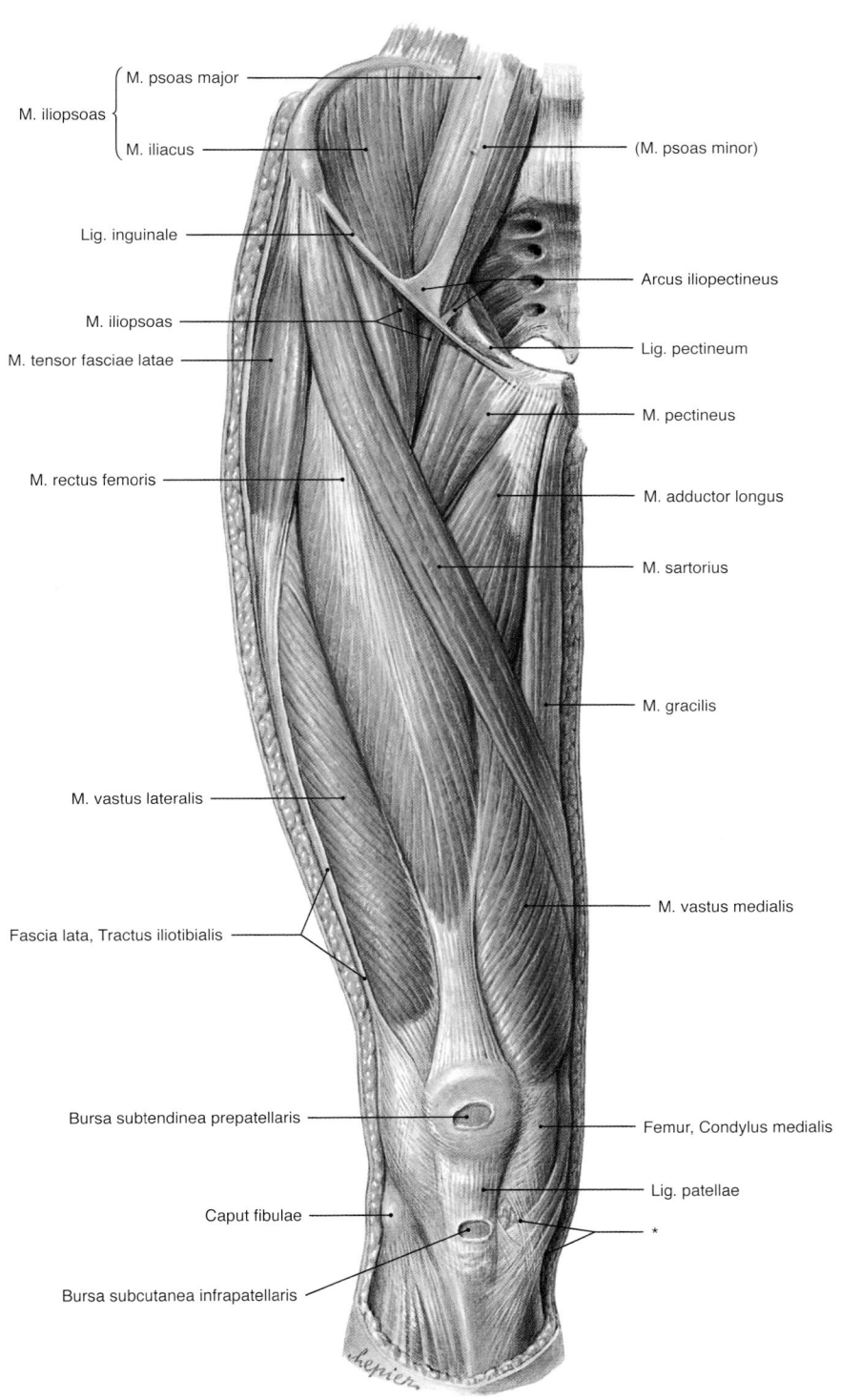

M. psoas major

M. iliopsoas {

M. iliacus

(M. psoas minor)

Lig. inguinale

Arcus iliopectineus

M. iliopsoas

Lig. pectineum

M. tensor fasciae latae

M. pectineus

M. rectus femoris

M. adductor longus

M. sartorius

M. gracilis

M. vastus lateralis

M. vastus medialis

Fascia lata, Tractus iliotibialis

Bursa subtendinea prepatellaris

Femur, Condylus medialis

Lig. patellae

Caput fibulae

*

Bursa subcutanea infrapatellaris

Fig. 1061 Muscles of the thigh and the hip;
after removal of the fascia lata except for the iliotibial tract.
* Common insertion of the sartorius, gracilis and semitendinosus
muscles just below the medial condyle of the tibia (formerly known
as the superficial pes anserinus, Pes anserinus superficialis)

→ T 42, T 44, T 45

Muscles of the thigh

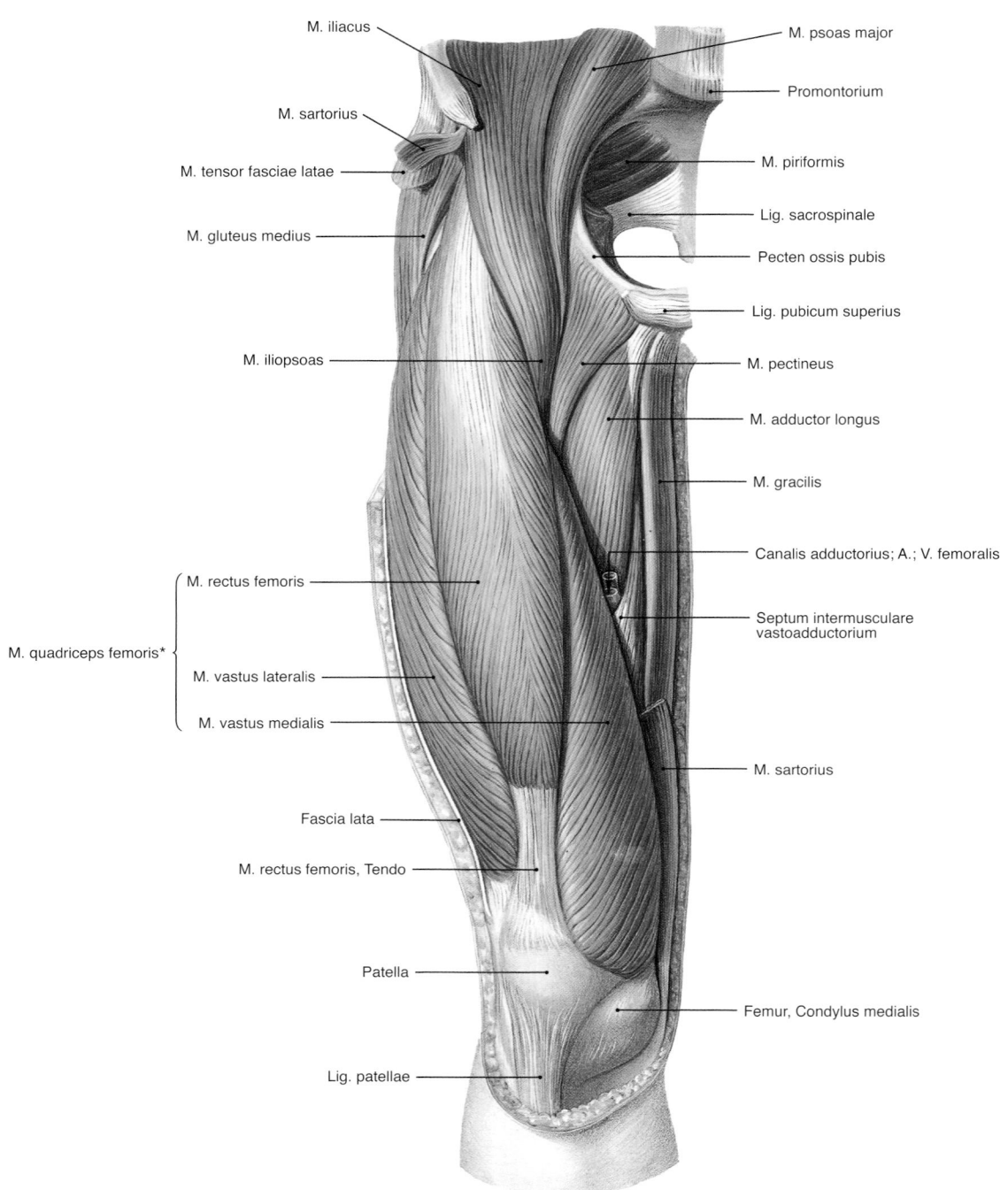

M. iliacus

M. sartorius

M. tensor fasciae latae

M. gluteus medius

M. iliopsoas

M. quadriceps femoris*

M. rectus femoris

M. vastus lateralis

M. vastus medialis

Fascia lata

M. rectus femoris, Tendo

Patella

Lig. patellae

M. psoas major

Promontorium

M. piriformis

Lig. sacrospinale

Pecten ossis pubis

Lig. pubicum superius

M. pectineus

M. adductor longus

M. gracilis

Canalis adductorius; A.; V. femoralis

Septum intermusculare vastoadductorium

M. sartorius

Femur, Condylus medialis

→ T 42, T 44, T 45

Fig. 1062 Muscles of the thigh and the hip; after removal of the fascia lata, the tensor fasciae latae muscle and the sartorius muscle.

* The fourth head of the quadriceps muscle, the vastus intermedius muscle, is covered by the rectus femoris muscle.

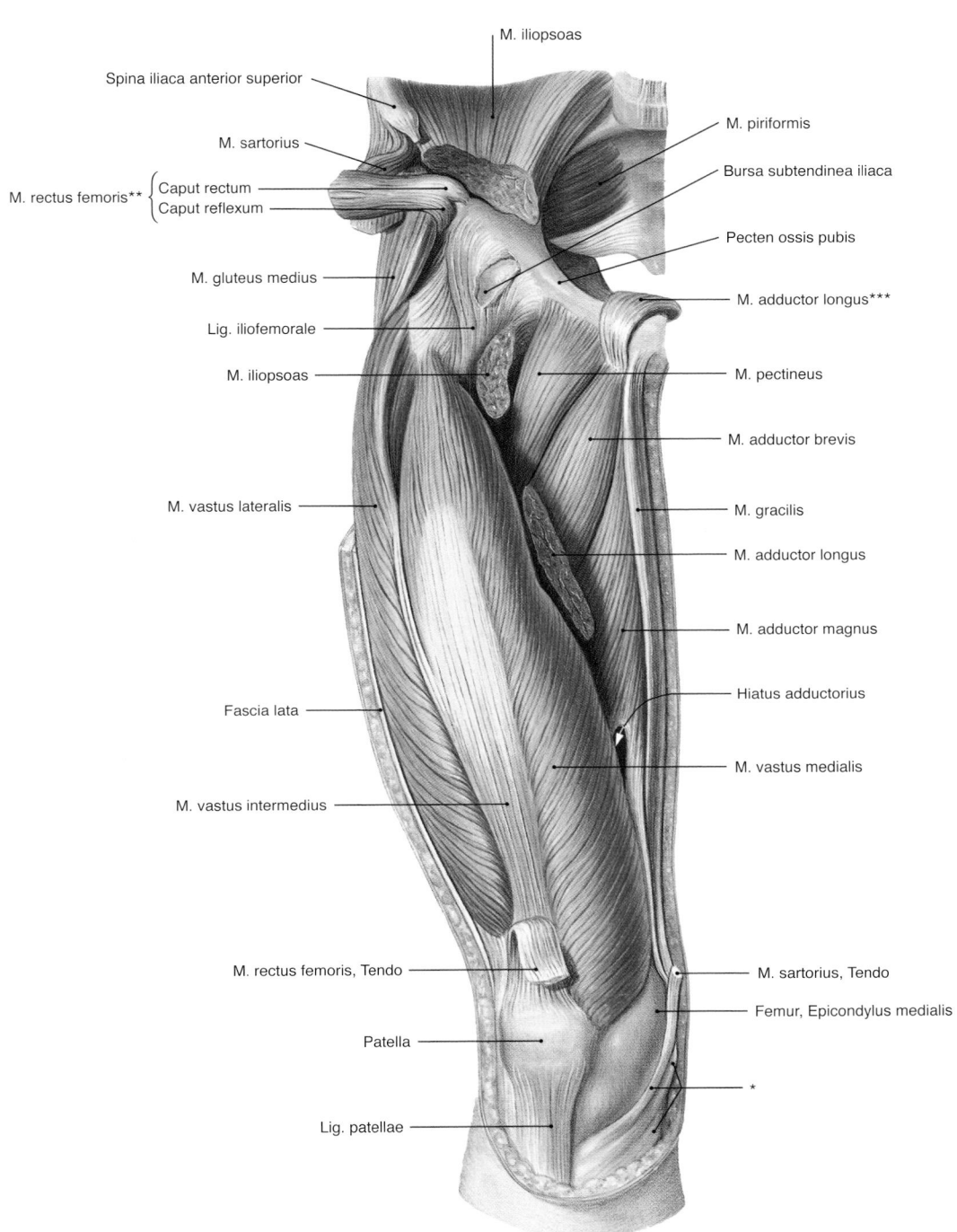

M. iliopsoas

Spina iliaca anterior superior

M. sartorius

M. rectus femoris** { Caput rectum / Caput reflexum

M. gluteus medius

Lig. iliofemorale

M. iliopsoas

M. vastus lateralis

Fascia lata

M. vastus intermedius

M. rectus femoris, Tendo

Patella

Lig. patellae

M. piriformis

Bursa subtendinea iliaca

Pecten ossis pubis

M. adductor longus***

M. pectineus

M. adductor brevis

M. gracilis

M. adductor longus

M. adductor magnus

Hiatus adductorius

M. vastus medialis

M. sartorius, Tendo

Femur, Epicondylus medialis

*

Fig. 1063 Muscles of the thigh and the hip;
deep layer after removal of the sartorius, the rectus femoris
and the adductor longus muscles as well as parts of the
iliopsoas muscle in the joint region.

* Common insertion of the sartorius, gracilis and semitendinosus
muscles just below the medial condyle of the tibia
** The origin of the rectus femoris muscle has been flapped laterally
upwards.
*** A part of the adductor longus muscle has been flapped upwards.

→ T 42, T 44, T 45

Muscles of the thigh

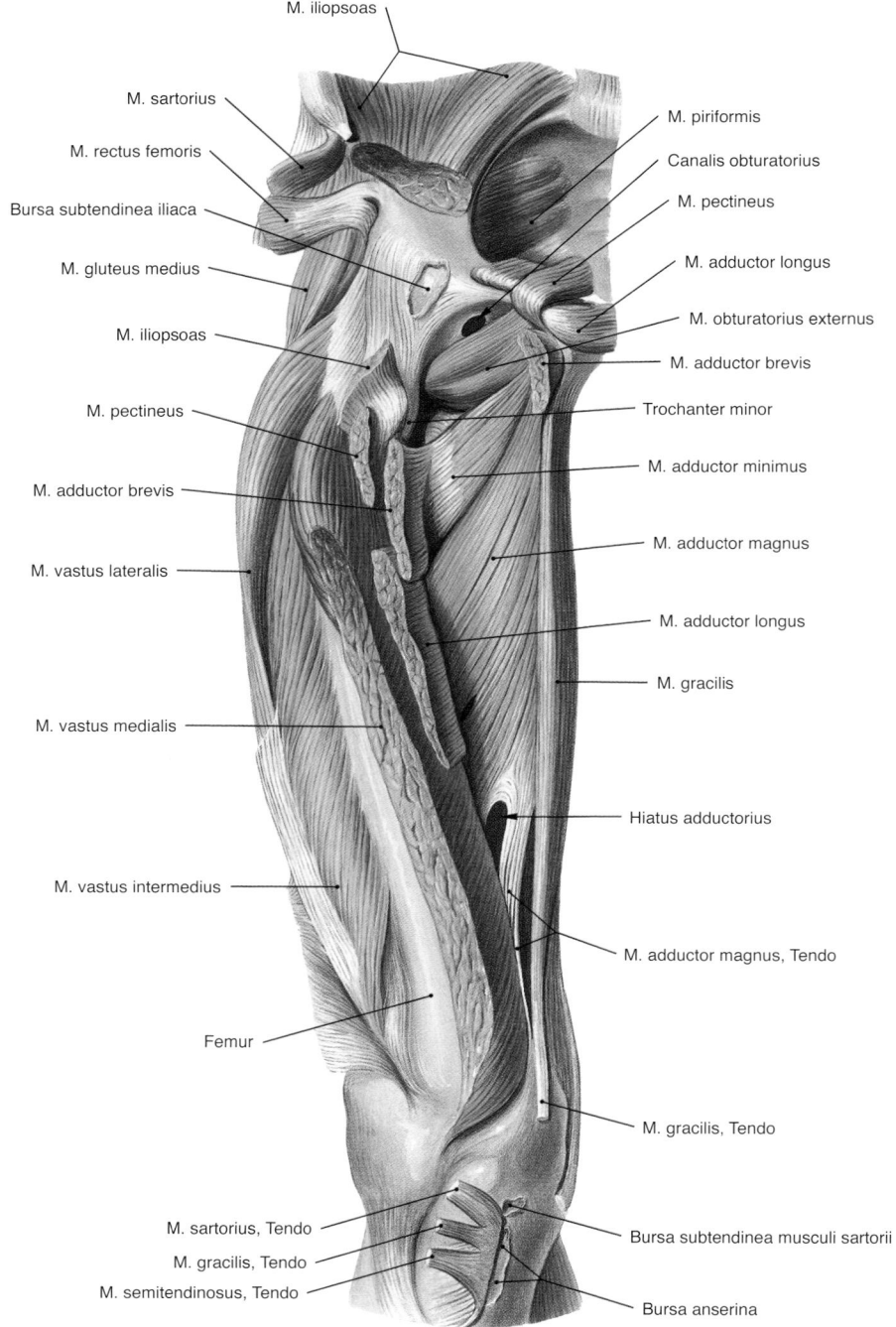

M. iliopsoas

M. sartorius

M. rectus femoris

Bursa subtendinea iliaca

M. gluteus medius

M. iliopsoas

M. pectineus

M. adductor brevis

M. vastus lateralis

M. vastus medialis

M. vastus intermedius

Femur

M. sartorius, Tendo

M. gracilis, Tendo

M. semitendinosus, Tendo

M. piriformis

Canalis obturatorius

M. pectineus

M. adductor longus

M. obturatorius externus

M. adductor brevis

Trochanter minor

M. adductor minimus

M. adductor magnus

M. adductor longus

M. gracilis

Hiatus adductorius

M. adductor magnus, Tendo

M. gracilis, Tendo

Bursa subtendinea musculi sartorii

Bursa anserina

→ T 42, T 44, T 45

Fig. 1064   Muscles of the thigh and the hip;
after almost complete removal of superficial and
several deeper muscles;
ventral view.

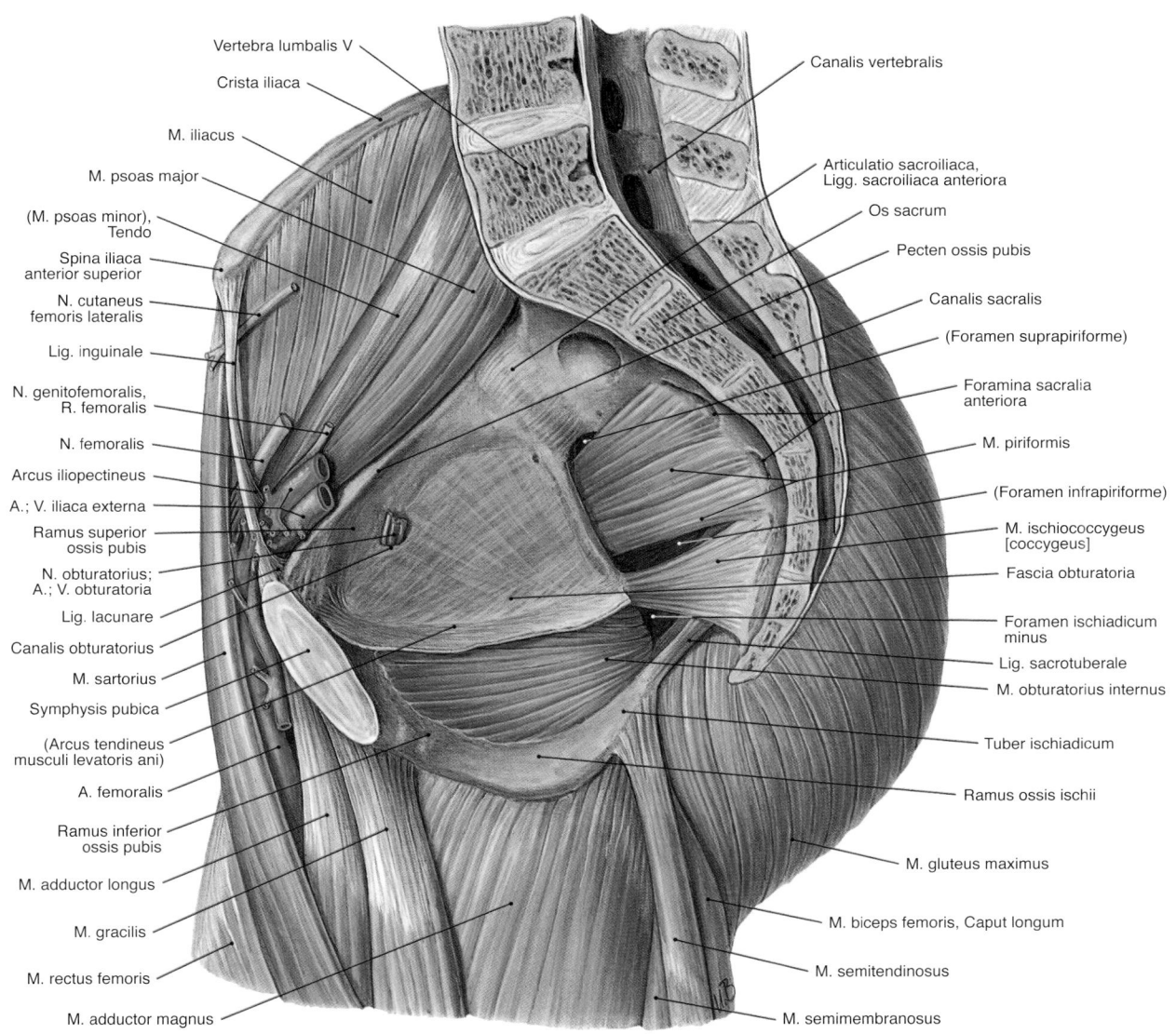

Vertebra lumbalis V

Crista iliaca

M. iliacus

M. psoas major

(M. psoas minor),
Tendo

Spina iliaca
anterior superior

N. cutaneus
femoris lateralis

Lig. inguinale

N. genitofemoralis,
R. femoralis

N. femoralis

Arcus iliopectineus

A.; V. iliaca externa

Ramus superior
ossis pubis

N. obturatorius;
A.; V. obturatoria

Lig. lacunare

Canalis obturatorius

M. sartorius

Symphysis pubica

(Arcus tendineus
musculi levatoris ani)

A. femoralis

Ramus inferior
ossis pubis

M. adductor longus

M. gracilis

M. rectus femoris

M. adductor magnus

Canalis vertebralis

Articulatio sacroiliaca,
Ligg. sacroiliaca anteriora

Os sacrum

Pecten ossis pubis

Canalis sacralis

(Foramen suprapiriforme)

Foramina sacralia
anteriora

M. piriformis

(Foramen infrapiriforme)

M. ischiococcygeus
[coccygeus]

Fascia obturatoria

Foramen ischiadicum
minus

Lig. sacrotuberale

M. obturatorius internus

Tuber ischiadicum

Ramus ossis ischii

M. gluteus maximus

M. biceps femoris, Caput longum

M. semitendinosus

M. semimembranosus

Fig. 1065   Muscles of the thigh and the hip;
medial view.

→ T 22a, T 42–T 46

Muscles of the thigh and the hip

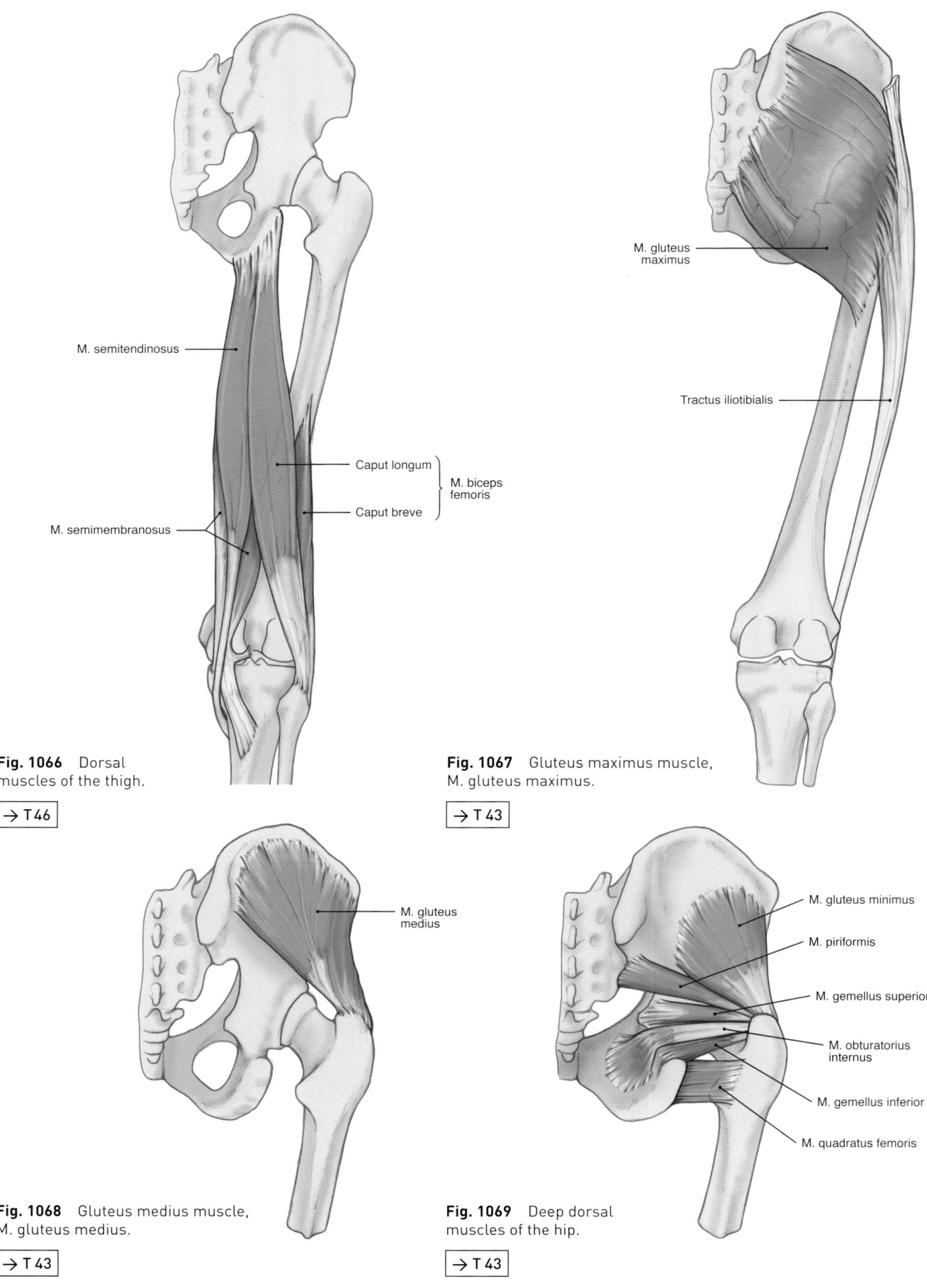

M. semitendinosus

Caput longum ⎫
                ⎬ M. biceps
Caput breve ⎭ femoris

M. semimembranosus

M. gluteus maximus

Tractus iliotibialis

Fig. 1066 Dorsal muscles of the thigh.

→ T 46

Fig. 1067 Gluteus maximus muscle, M. gluteus maximus.

→ T 43

M. gluteus medius

M. gluteus minimus

M. piriformis

M. gemellus superior

M. obturatorius internus

M. gemellus inferior

M. quadratus femoris

Fig. 1068 Gluteus medius muscle, M. gluteus medius.

→ T 43

Fig. 1069 Deep dorsal muscles of the hip.

→ T 43

Muscles of the thigh and the hip

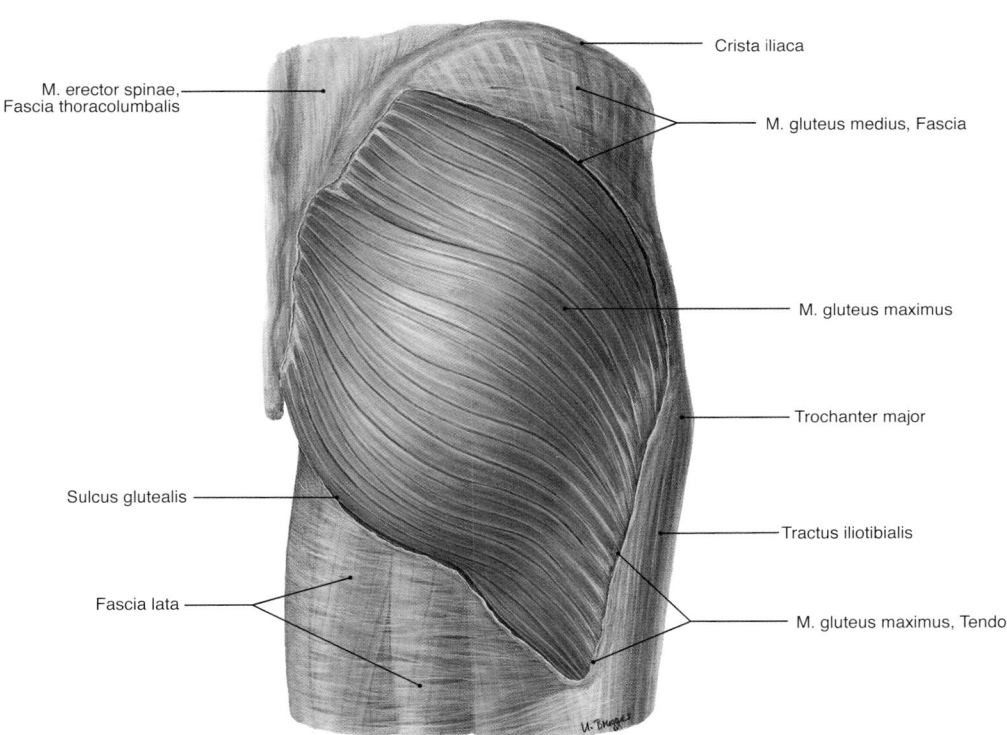

M. erector spinae,
Fascia thoracolumbalis

Crista iliaca

M. gluteus medius, Fascia

M. gluteus maximus

Trochanter major

Sulcus glutealis

Tractus iliotibialis

Fascia lata

M. gluteus maximus, Tendo

Fig. 1070 Muscles of the thigh and the hip.

→ T 43

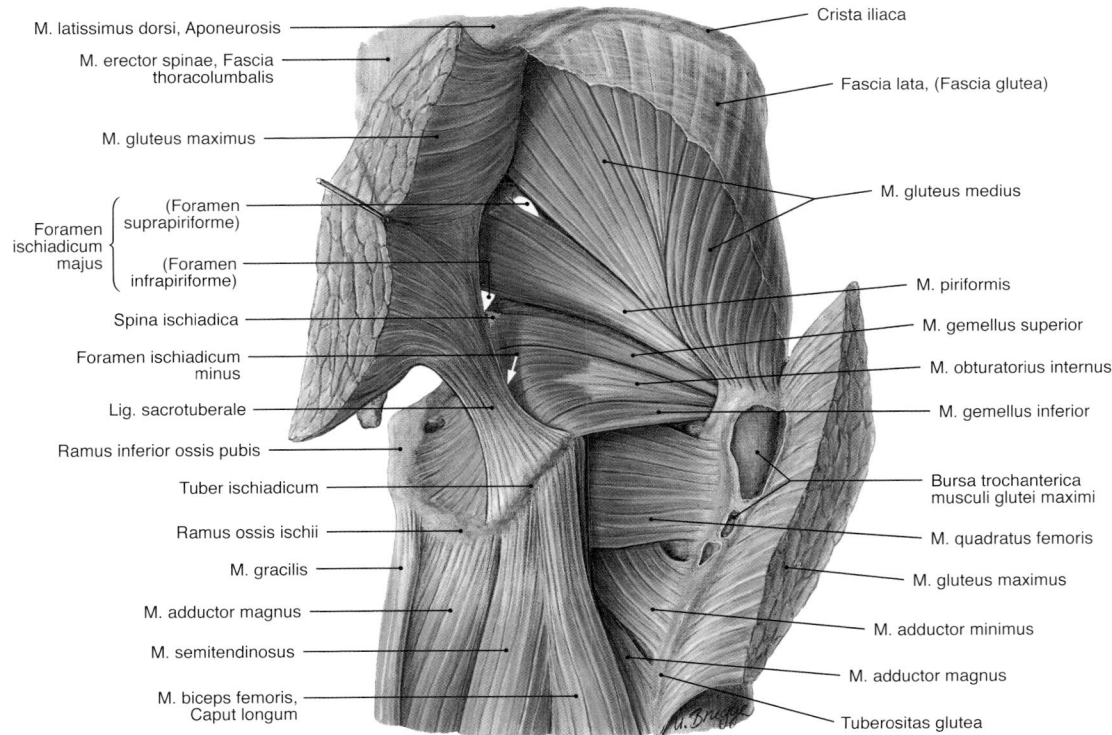

M. latissimus dorsi, Aponeurosis

M. erector spinae, Fascia
thoracolumbalis

M. gluteus maximus

Foramen
ischiadicum
majus
{ (Foramen
suprapiriforme)
(Foramen
infrapiriforme) }

Spina ischiadica

Foramen ischiadicum
minus

Lig. sacrotuberale

Ramus inferior ossis pubis

Tuber ischiadicum

Ramus ossis ischii

M. gracilis

M. adductor magnus

M. semitendinosus

M. biceps femoris,
Caput longum

Crista iliaca

Fascia lata, (Fascia glutea)

M. gluteus medius

M. piriformis

M. gemellus superior

M. obturatorius internus*

M. gemellus inferior

Bursa trochanterica
musculi glutei maximi

M. quadratus femoris

M. gluteus maximus

M. adductor minimus

M. adductor magnus

Tuberositas glutea

Fig. 1071 Muscles of the thigh and the hip;
the gluteus maximus muscle has been sectioned;
dorsal view.

* The part of the obturator internus muscle between the curved edge
of the lesser sciatic notch and the insertion in the trochanteric fossa
frequently consists of tendinous bands.

→ T 43, T 45, T 46

Muscles of the thigh and the hip

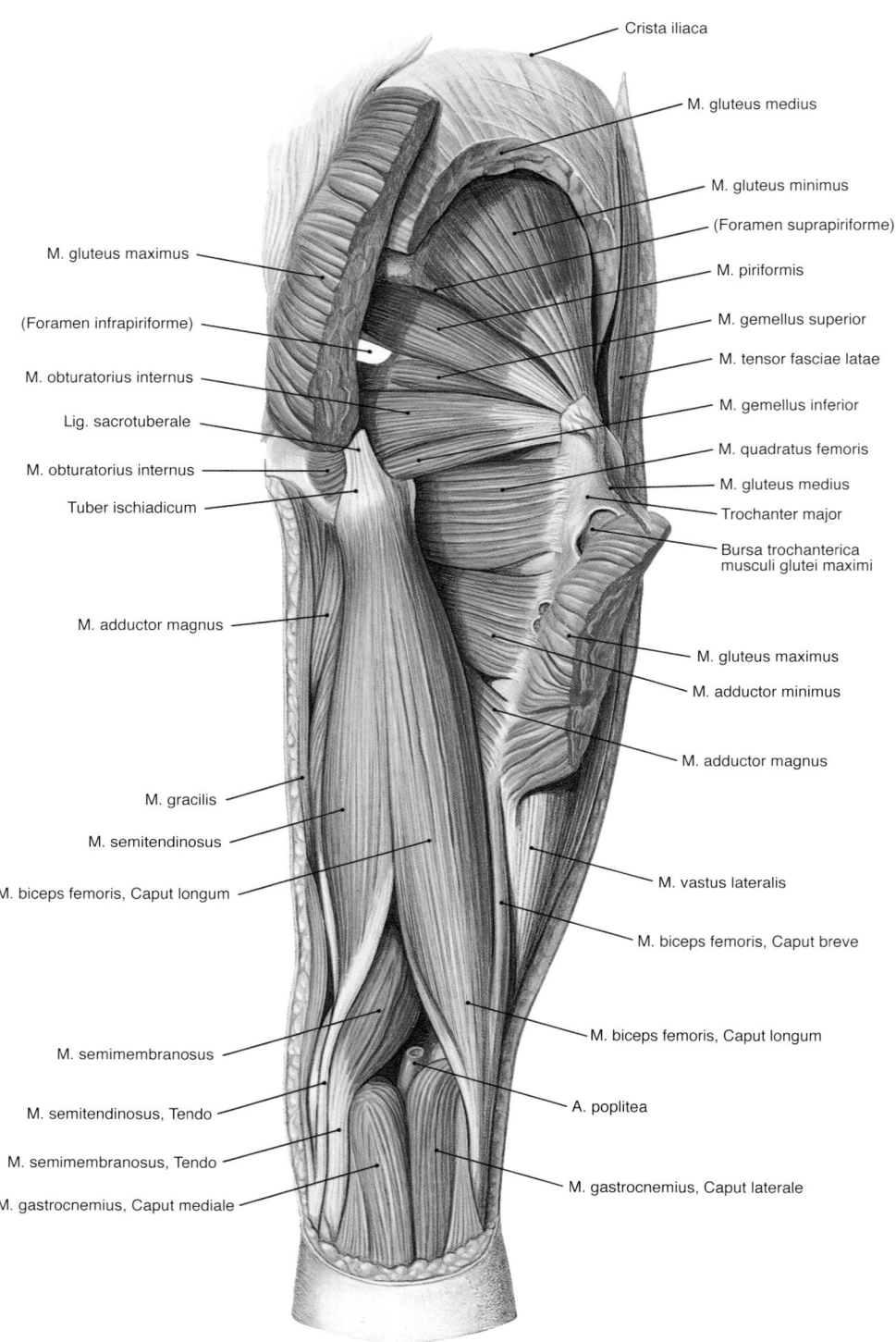

Crista iliaca

M. gluteus medius

M. gluteus minimus

(Foramen suprapiriforme)

M. piriformis

M. gemellus superior

M. tensor fasciae latae

M. gemellus inferior

M. quadratus femoris

M. gluteus medius

Trochanter major

Bursa trochanterica musculi glutei maximi

M. gluteus maximus

M. adductor minimus

M. adductor magnus

M. vastus lateralis

M. biceps femoris, Caput breve

M. biceps femoris, Caput longum

A. poplitea

M. gastrocnemius, Caput laterale

M. gluteus maximus

(Foramen infrapiriforme)

M. obturatorius internus

Lig. sacrotuberale

M. obturatorius internus

Tuber ischiadicum

M. adductor magnus

M. gracilis

M. semitendinosus

M. biceps femoris, Caput longum

M. semimembranosus

M. semitendinosus, Tendo

M. semimembranosus, Tendo

M. gastrocnemius, Caput mediale

→ T 43, T 45, T 46

Fig. 1072 Muscles of the thigh and the hip;
the gluteus maximus and medius muscles have
been partially removed;
dorsal view.

Muscles of the thigh and the hip

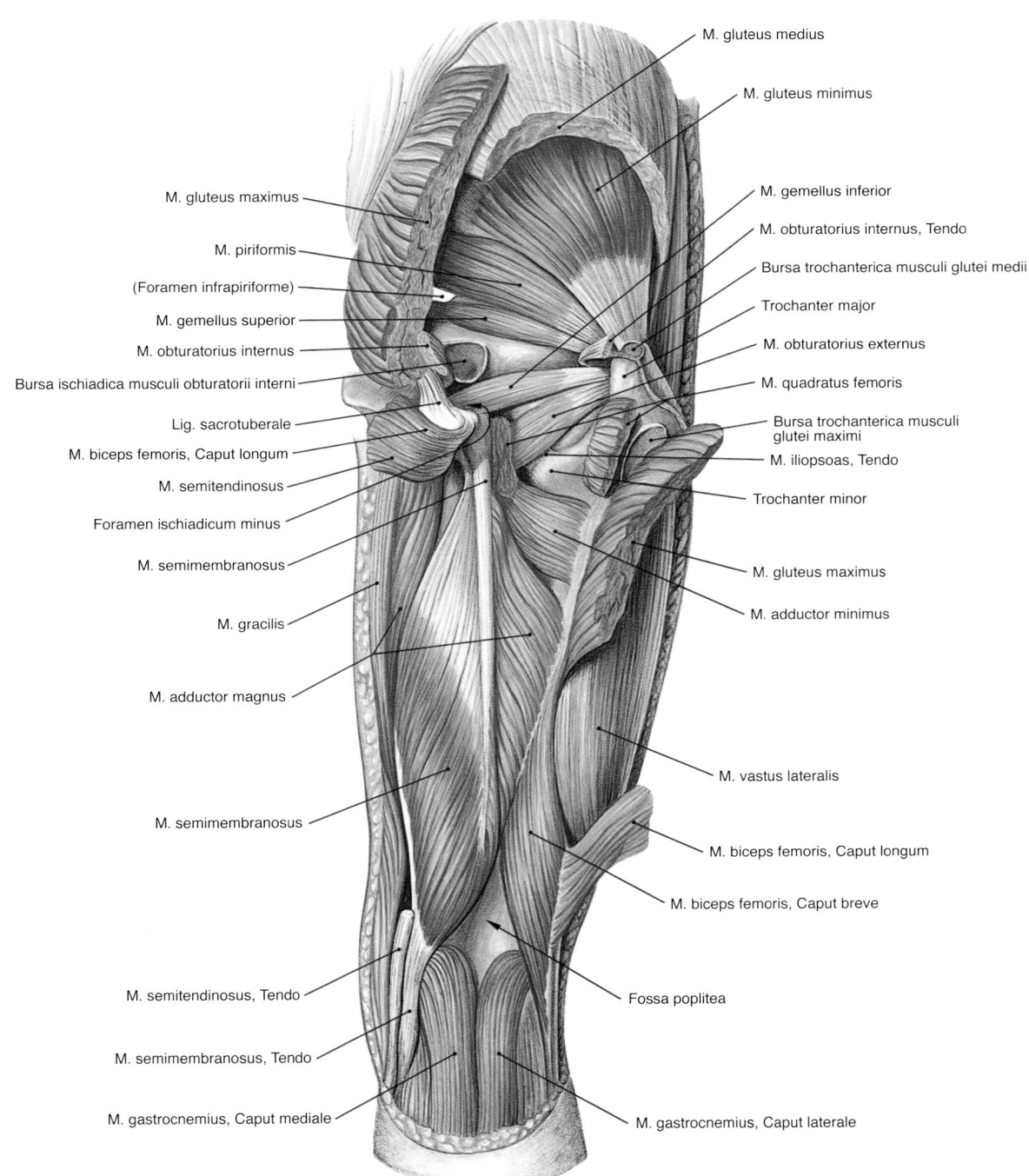

M. gluteus medius

M. gluteus minimus

M. gluteus maximus

M. piriformis

(Foramen infrapiriforme)

M. gemellus superior

M. obturatorius internus

Bursa ischiadica musculi obturatorii interni

Lig. sacrotuberale

M. biceps femoris, Caput longum

M. semitendinosus

Foramen ischiadicum minus

M. semimembranosus

M. gracilis

M. adductor magnus

M. semimembranosus

M. semitendinosus, Tendo

M. semimembranosus, Tendo

M. gastrocnemius, Caput mediale

M. gemellus inferior

M. obturatorius internus, Tendo

Bursa trochanterica musculi glutei medii

Trochanter major

M. obturatorius externus

M. quadratus femoris

Bursa trochanterica musculi glutei maximi

M. iliopsoas, Tendo

Trochanter minor

M. gluteus maximus

M. adductor minimus

M. vastus lateralis

M. biceps femoris, Caput longum

M. biceps femoris, Caput breve

Fossa poplitea

M. gastrocnemius, Caput laterale

Fig. 1073 Muscles of the thigh and the hip; deep layer after almost complete removal of the superficial gluteal and the ischiocrural muscles; dorsal view.

→ T 43, T 45, T 46

Muscles of the thigh and the hip

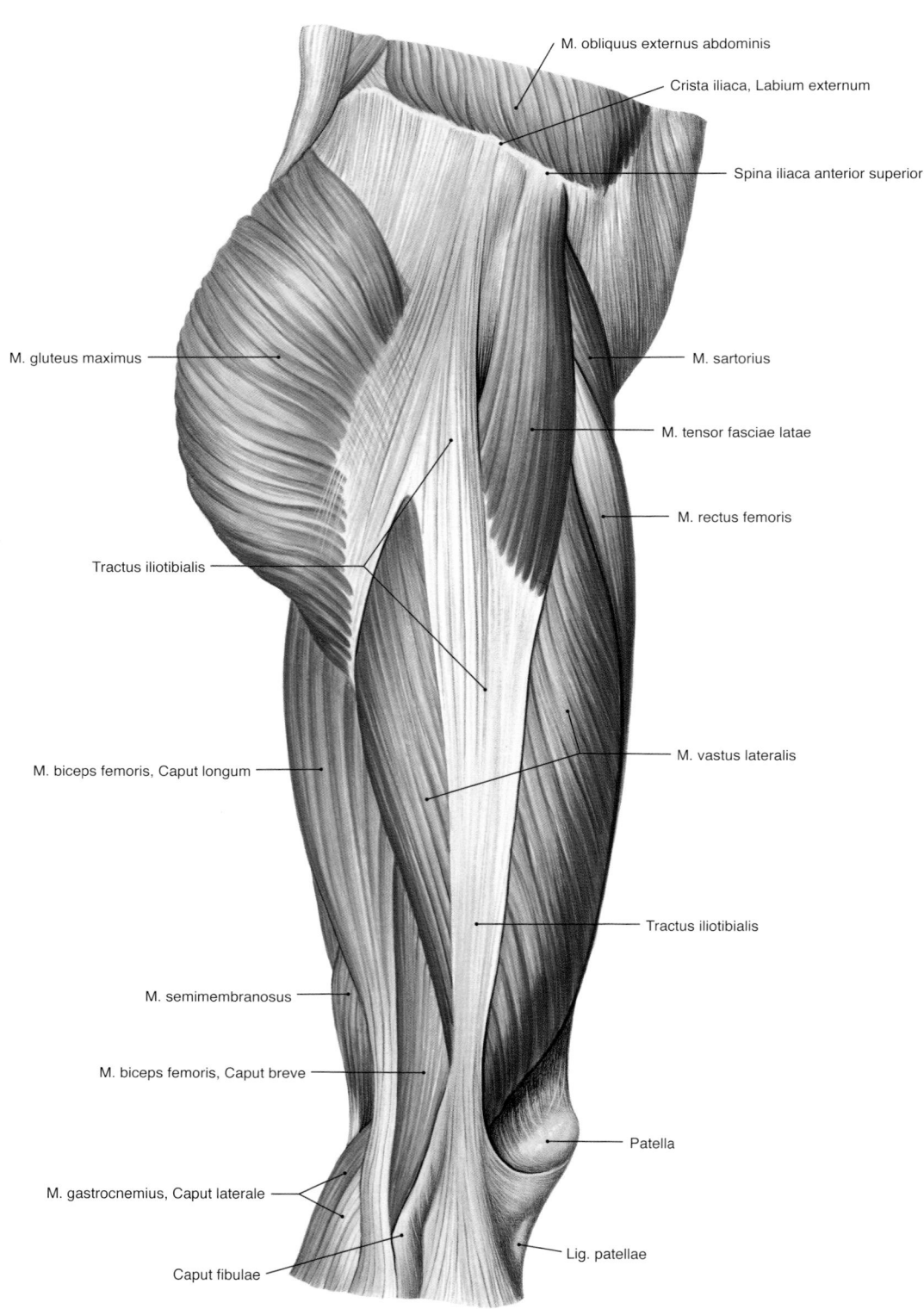

M. obliquus externus abdominis

Crista iliaca, Labium externum

Spina iliaca anterior superior

M. gluteus maximus

M. sartorius

M. tensor fasciae latae

M. rectus femoris

Tractus iliotibialis

M. vastus lateralis

M. biceps femoris, Caput longum

Tractus iliotibialis

M. semimembranosus

M. biceps femoris, Caput breve

Patella

M. gastrocnemius, Caput laterale

Lig. patellae

Caput fibulae

→ T 43, T 44, T 46

Fig. 1074   Muscles of the thigh and the hip;
after removal of the fascia lata except for the iliotibial tract.

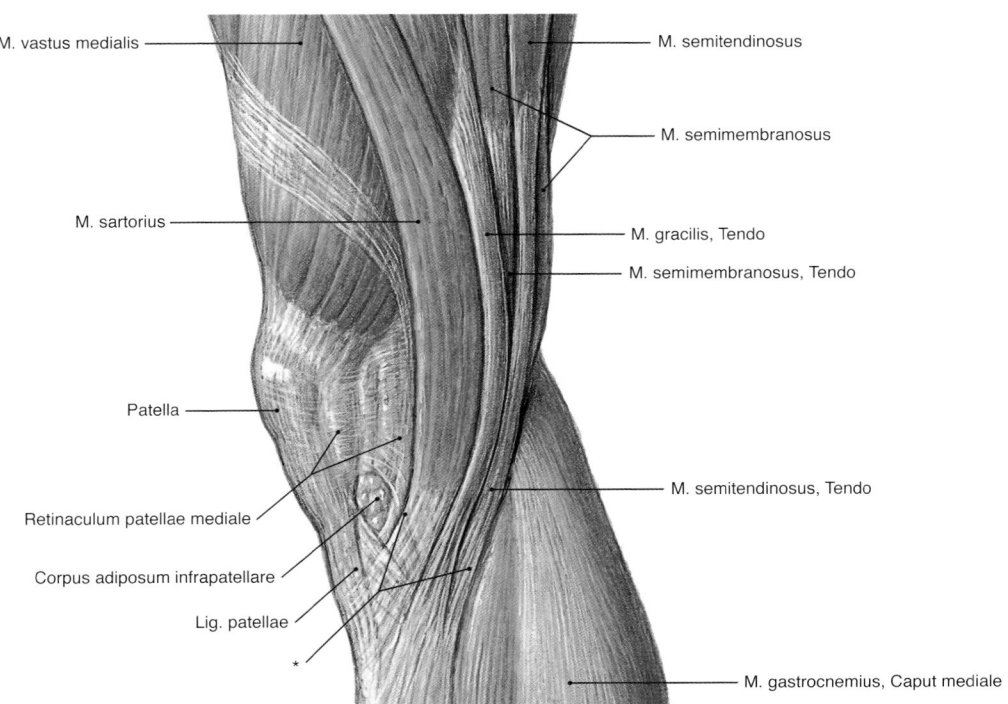

M. vastus medialis

M. semitendinosus

M. semimembranosus

M. sartorius

M. gracilis, Tendo

M. semimembranosus, Tendo

Patella

Retinaculum patellae mediale

M. semitendinosus, Tendo

Corpus adiposum infrapatellare

Lig. patellae

*

M. gastrocnemius, Caput mediale

Fig. 1075   Muscles in the region of the knee joint;
medial view.
* Common insertion just below the medial condyle of the tibia
(formerly known as superficial pes anserinus, Pes anserinus superficialis)

→ T 44–T 46, T 49

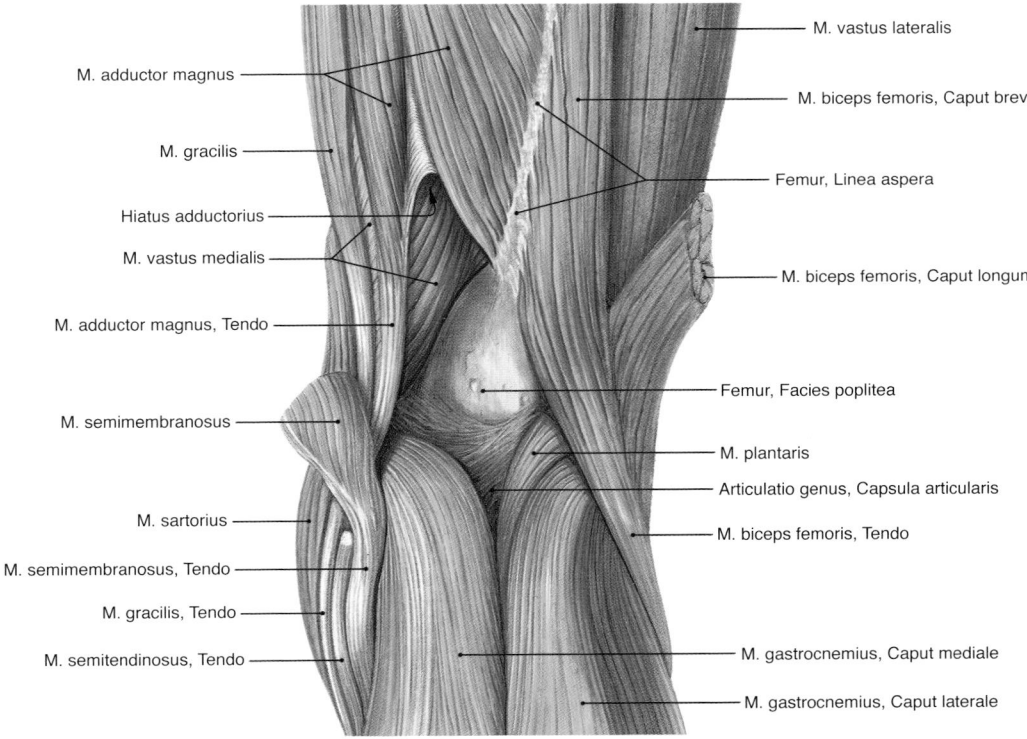

M. vastus lateralis

M. adductor magnus

M. biceps femoris, Caput breve

M. gracilis

Femur, Linea aspera

Hiatus adductorius

M. vastus medialis

M. adductor magnus, Tendo

M. biceps femoris, Caput longum

M. semimembranosus

Femur, Facies poplitea

M. plantaris

Articulatio genus, Capsula articularis

M. sartorius

M. biceps femoris, Tendo

M. semimembranosus, Tendo

M. gracilis, Tendo

M. semitendinosus, Tendo

M. gastrocnemius, Caput mediale

M. gastrocnemius, Caput laterale

Fig. 1076   Muscles in the region of the knee joint;
after almost complete removal of the ischiocrural muscles;
dorsal view.

→ T 44–T 46, T 49

Origins and insertions of the muscles of the thigh and the ventral part of the leg

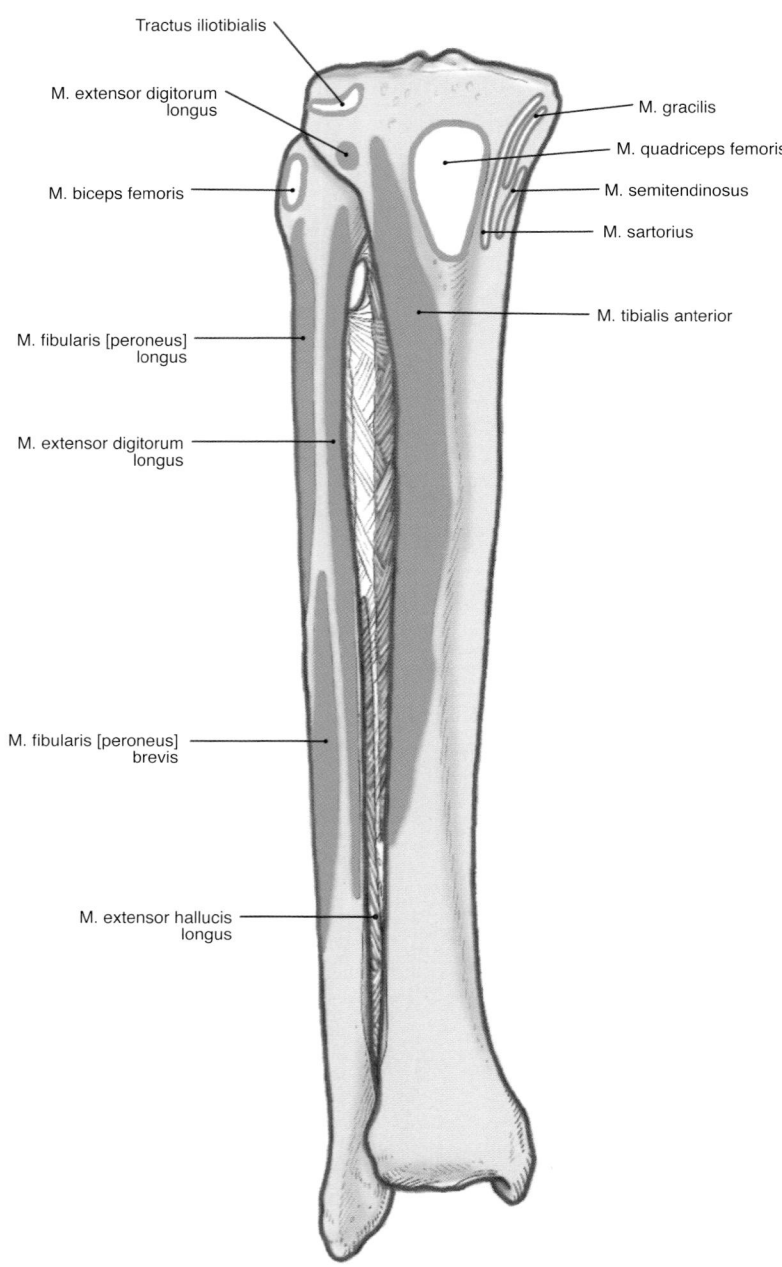

Tractus iliotibialis

M. extensor digitorum
longus

M. biceps femoris

M. fibularis [peroneus]
longus

M. extensor digitorum
longus

M. fibularis [peroneus]
brevis

M. extensor hallucis
longus

M. gracilis

M. quadriceps femoris

M. semitendinosus

M. sartorius

M. tibialis anterior

→ T 44–T 47

Fig. 1077　Origins and insertions of the muscles
at the bones of the leg;
ventral view.

Origins and insertions of the muscles of the thigh and the dorsal part of the leg

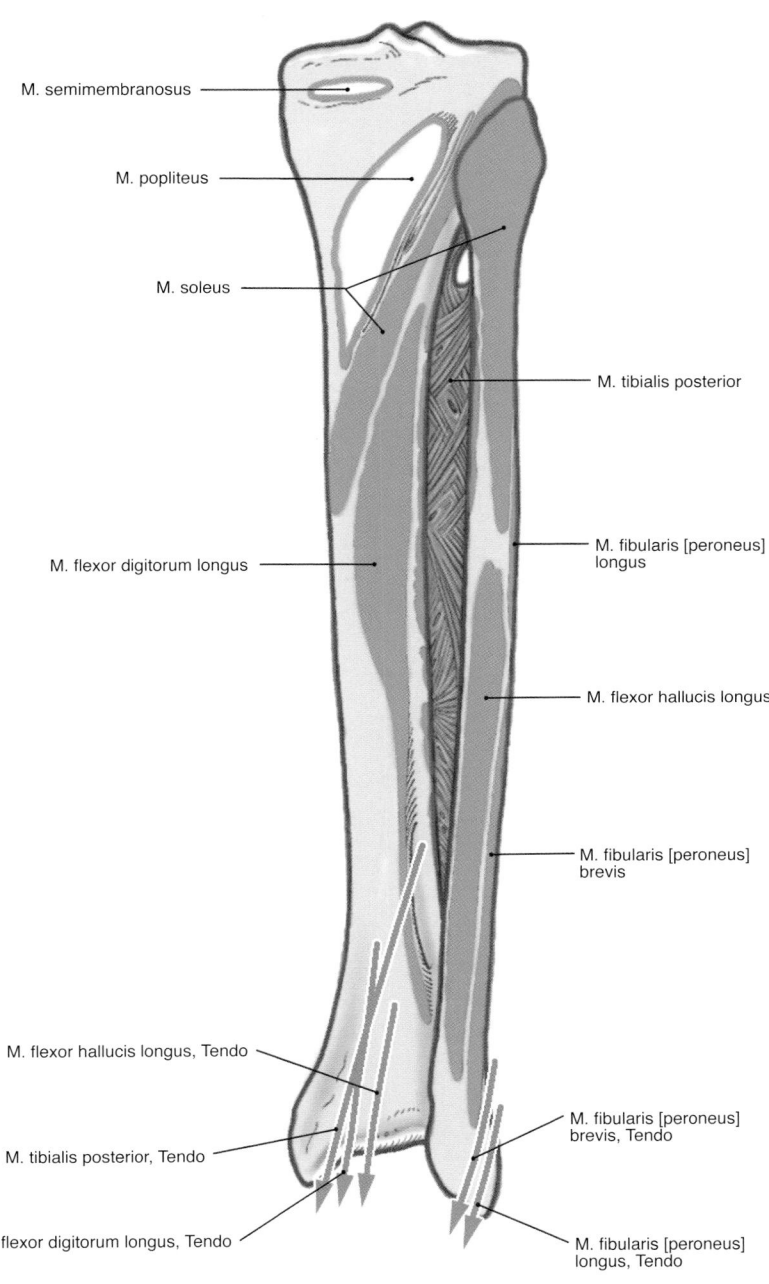

M. semimembranosus

M. popliteus

M. soleus

M. tibialis posterior

M. flexor digitorum longus

M. fibularis [peroneus] longus

M. flexor hallucis longus

M. fibularis [peroneus] brevis

M. flexor hallucis longus, Tendo

M. tibialis posterior, Tendo

M. fibularis [peroneus] brevis, Tendo

M. flexor digitorum longus, Tendo

M. fibularis [peroneus] longus, Tendo

Fig. 1078 Origins and insertions of the muscles at the bones of the leg; dorsal view.

→ T 46, T 48–T 50

Muscles of the leg

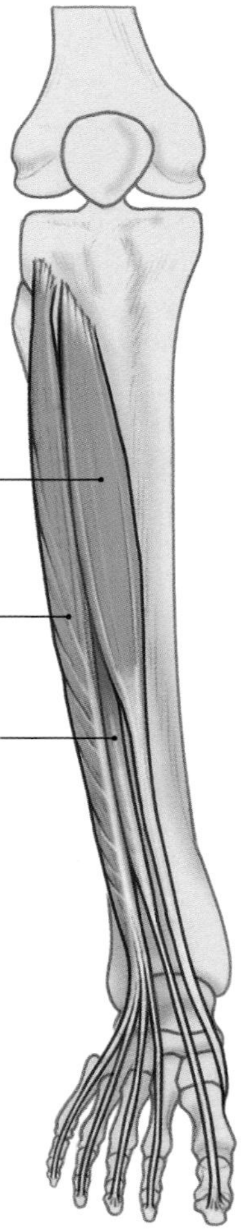

Fig. 1079 Extensor muscles of the leg.
→ T 47

M. tibialis anterior

M. extensor digitorum longus

M. extensor hallucis longus

Caput laterale ⎫
Caput mediale ⎬ M. gastrocnemius

M. soleus

Tendo calcaneus

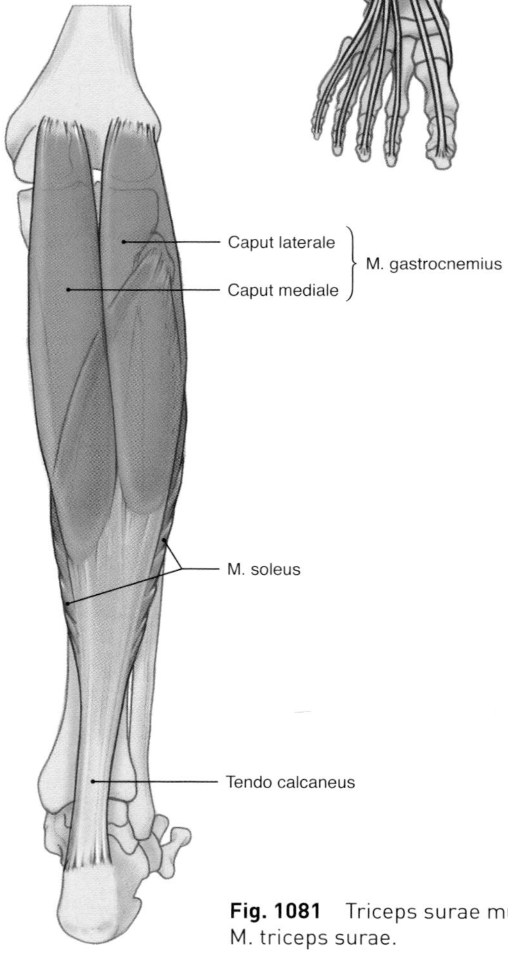

Fig. 1081 Triceps surae muscle, M. triceps surae.
→ T 49

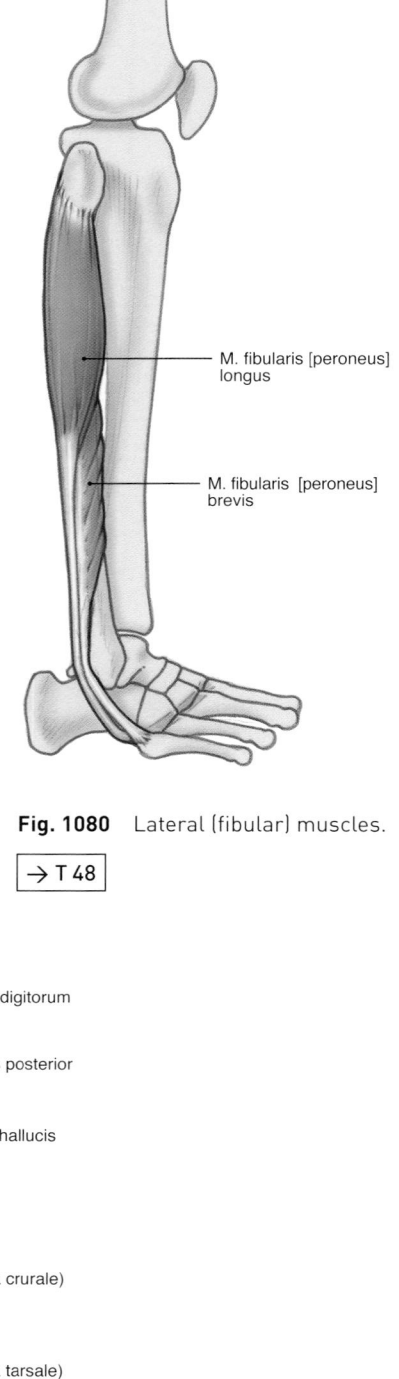

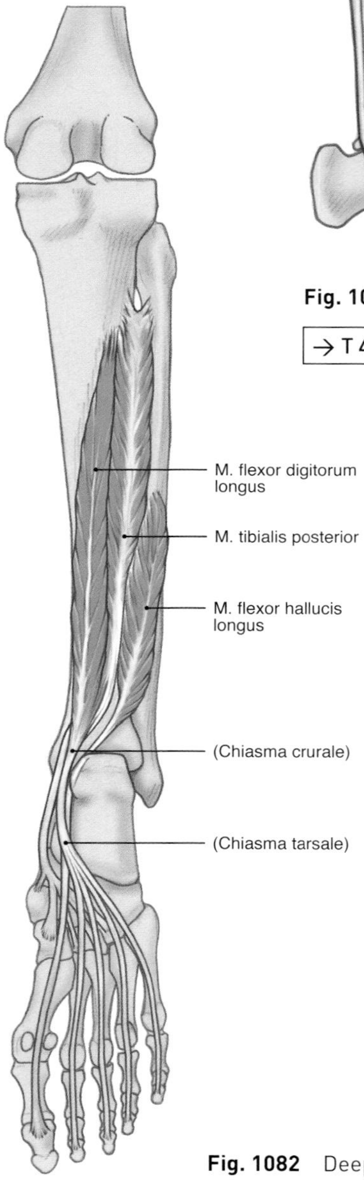

M. fibularis [peroneus] longus

M. fibularis [peroneus] brevis

Fig. 1080 Lateral (fibular) muscles.
→ T 48

M. flexor digitorum longus

M. tibialis posterior

M. flexor hallucis longus

(Chiasma crurale)

(Chiasma tarsale)

Fig. 1082 Deep flexor muscles of the leg.
→ T 50

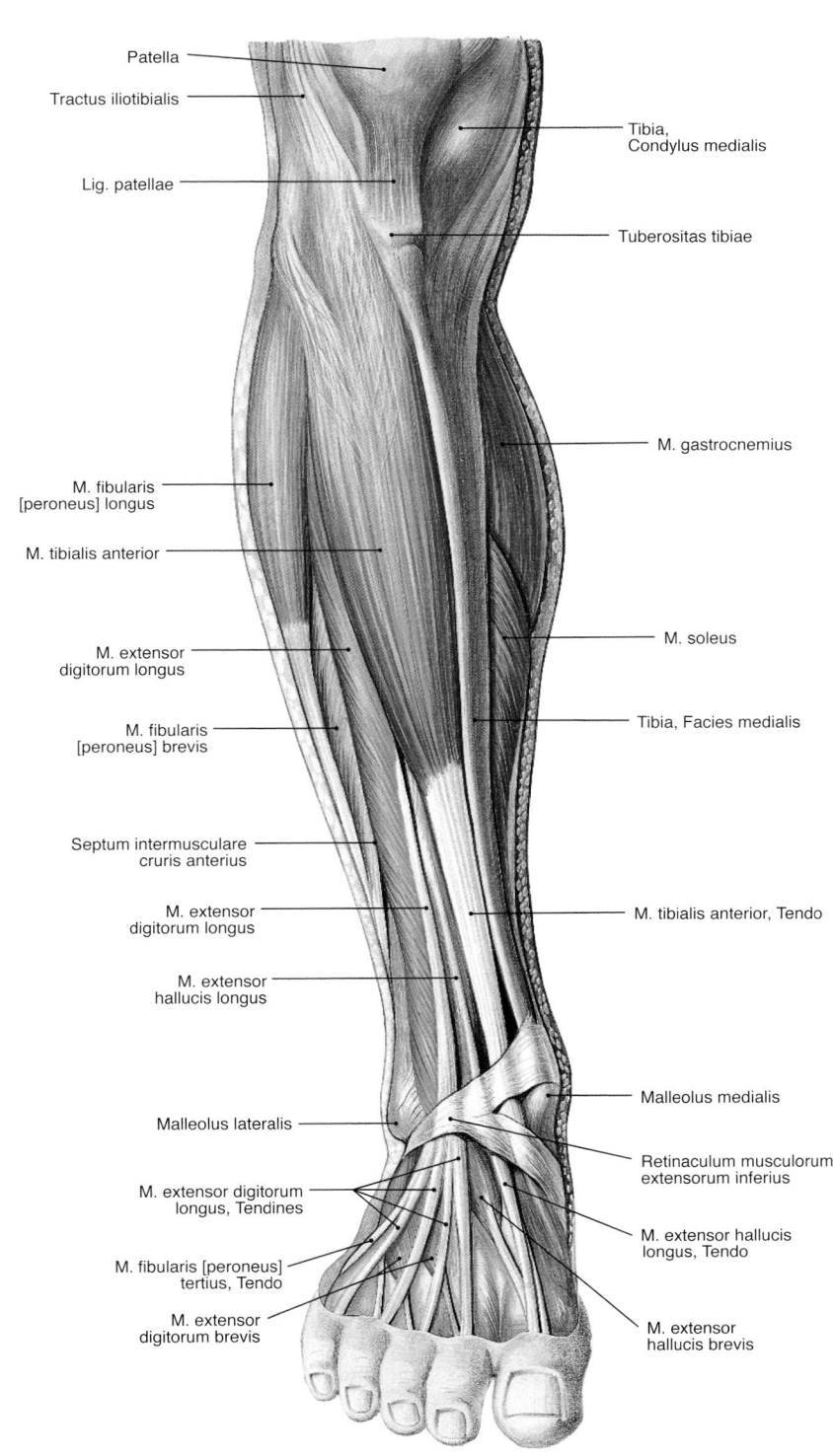

Patella

Tractus iliotibialis

Lig. patellae

Tibia, Condylus medialis

Tuberositas tibiae

M. gastrocnemius

M. fibularis [peroneus] longus

M. tibialis anterior

M. soleus

M. extensor digitorum longus

Tibia, Facies medialis

M. fibularis [peroneus] brevis

Septum intermusculare cruris anterius

M. extensor digitorum longus

M. tibialis anterior, Tendo

M. extensor hallucis longus

Malleolus medialis

Malleolus lateralis

Retinaculum musculorum extensorum inferius

M. extensor digitorum longus, Tendines

M. extensor hallucis longus, Tendo

M. fibularis [peroneus] tertius, Tendo

M. extensor digitorum brevis

M. extensor hallucis brevis

Fig. 1083 Muscles of the leg and the foot.

→ T 47, T 48

Muscles of the leg

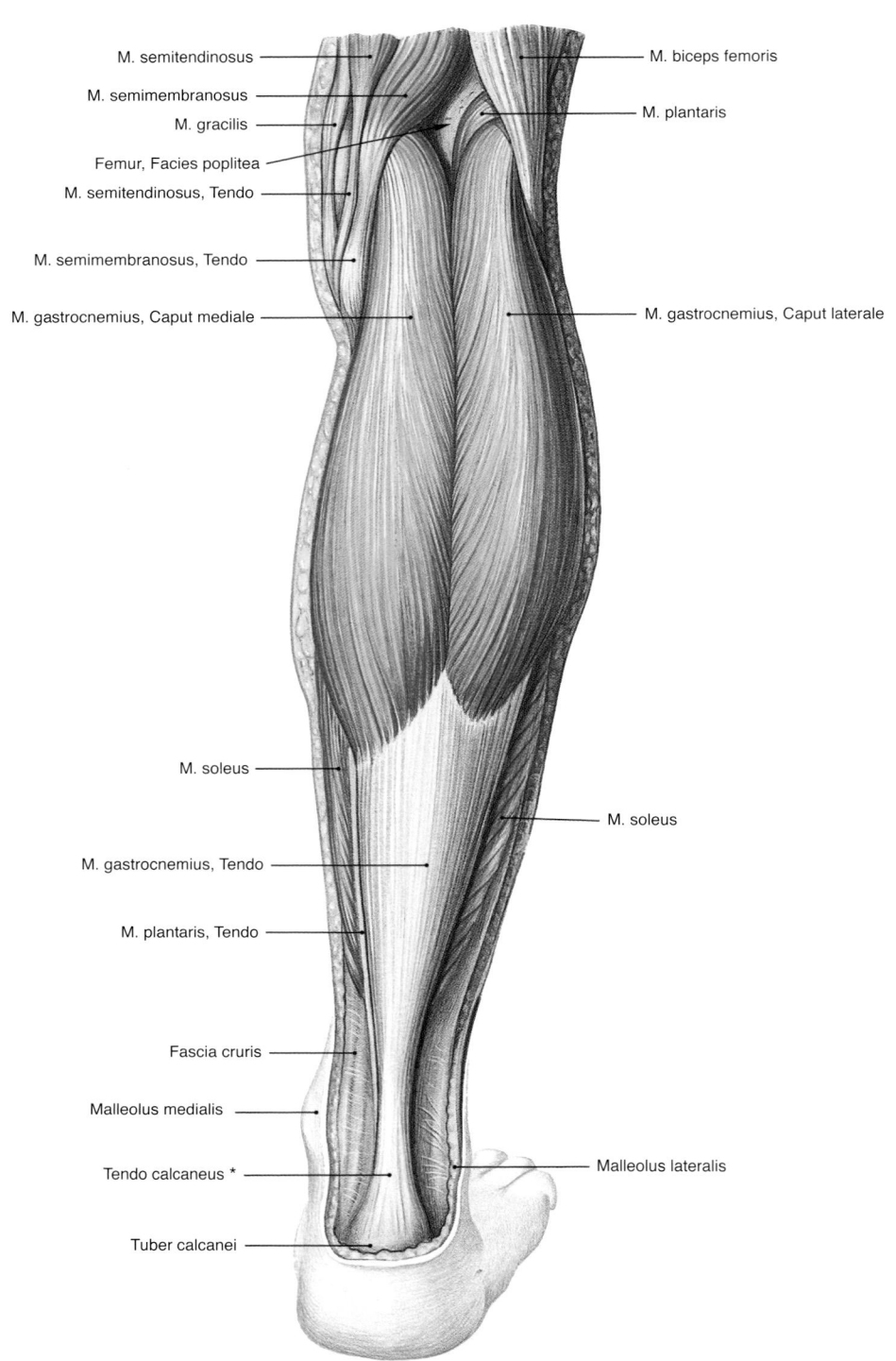

M. semitendinosus

M. semimembranosus

M. gracilis

Femur, Facies poplitea

M. semitendinosus, Tendo

M. semimembranosus, Tendo

M. gastrocnemius, Caput mediale

M. biceps femoris

M. plantaris

M. gastrocnemius, Caput laterale

M. soleus

M. gastrocnemius, Tendo

M. plantaris, Tendo

M. soleus

Fascia cruris

Malleolus medialis

Tendo calcaneus *

Tuber calcanei

Malleolus lateralis

→ T 49

Fig. 1084 Muscles of the leg;
superficial layer.
* Also: Achilles tendon

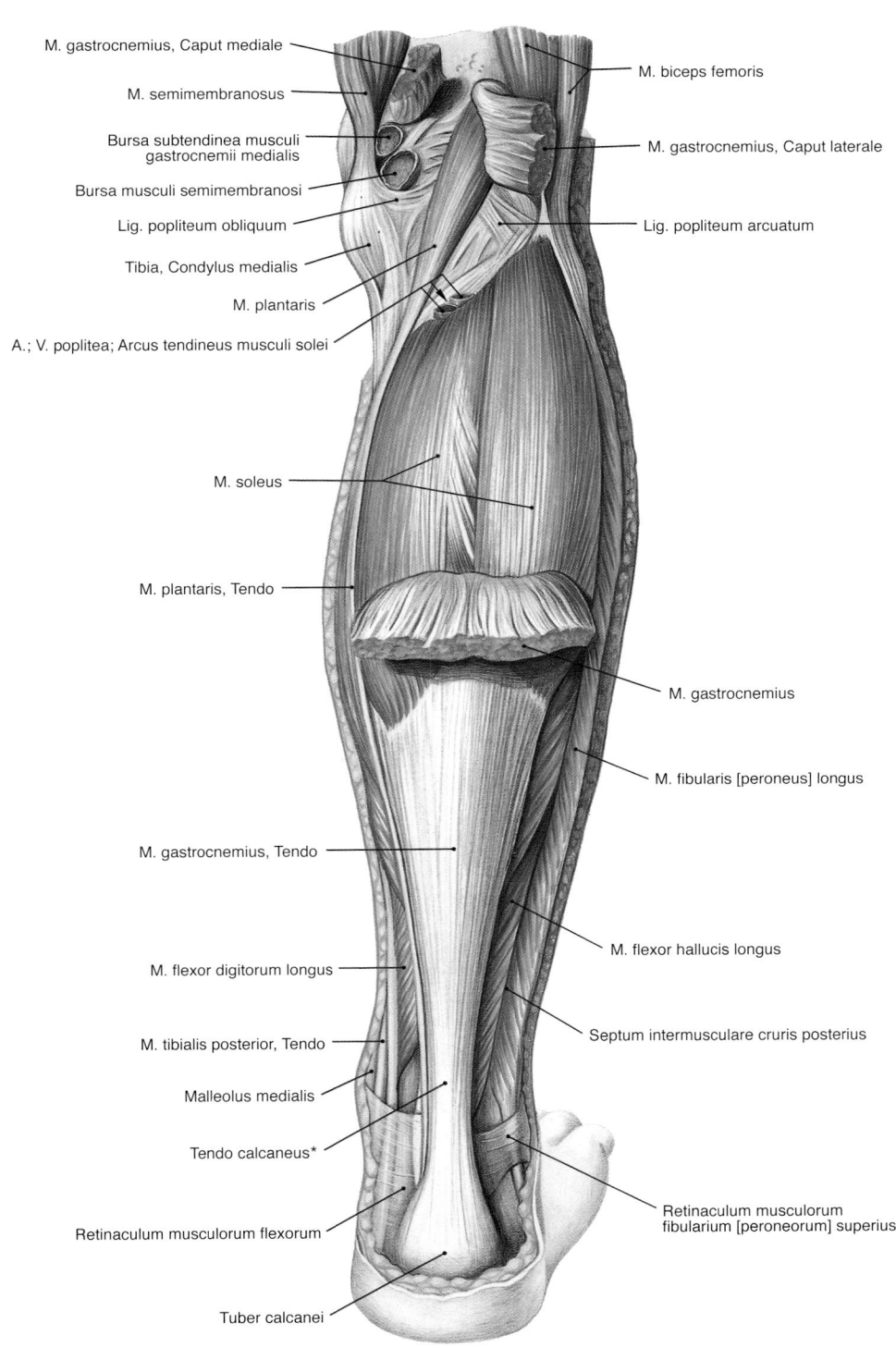

M. gastrocnemius, Caput mediale

M. semimembranosus

Bursa subtendinea musculi gastrocnemii medialis

Bursa musculi semimembranosi

Lig. popliteum obliquum

Tibia, Condylus medialis

M. plantaris

A.; V. poplitea; Arcus tendineus musculi solei

M. soleus

M. plantaris, Tendo

M. gastrocnemius, Tendo

M. flexor digitorum longus

M. tibialis posterior, Tendo

Malleolus medialis

Tendo calcaneus*

Retinaculum musculorum flexorum

Tuber calcanei

M. biceps femoris

M. gastrocnemius, Caput laterale

Lig. popliteum arcuatum

M. gastrocnemius

M. fibularis [peroneus] longus

M. flexor hallucis longus

Septum intermusculare cruris posterius

Retinaculum musculorum fibularium [peroneorum] superius

Fig. 1085 Muscles of the leg; superficial layer after partial removal of the gastrocnemius muscle.
* Also: Achilles tendon

→ T 49

Muscles of the leg

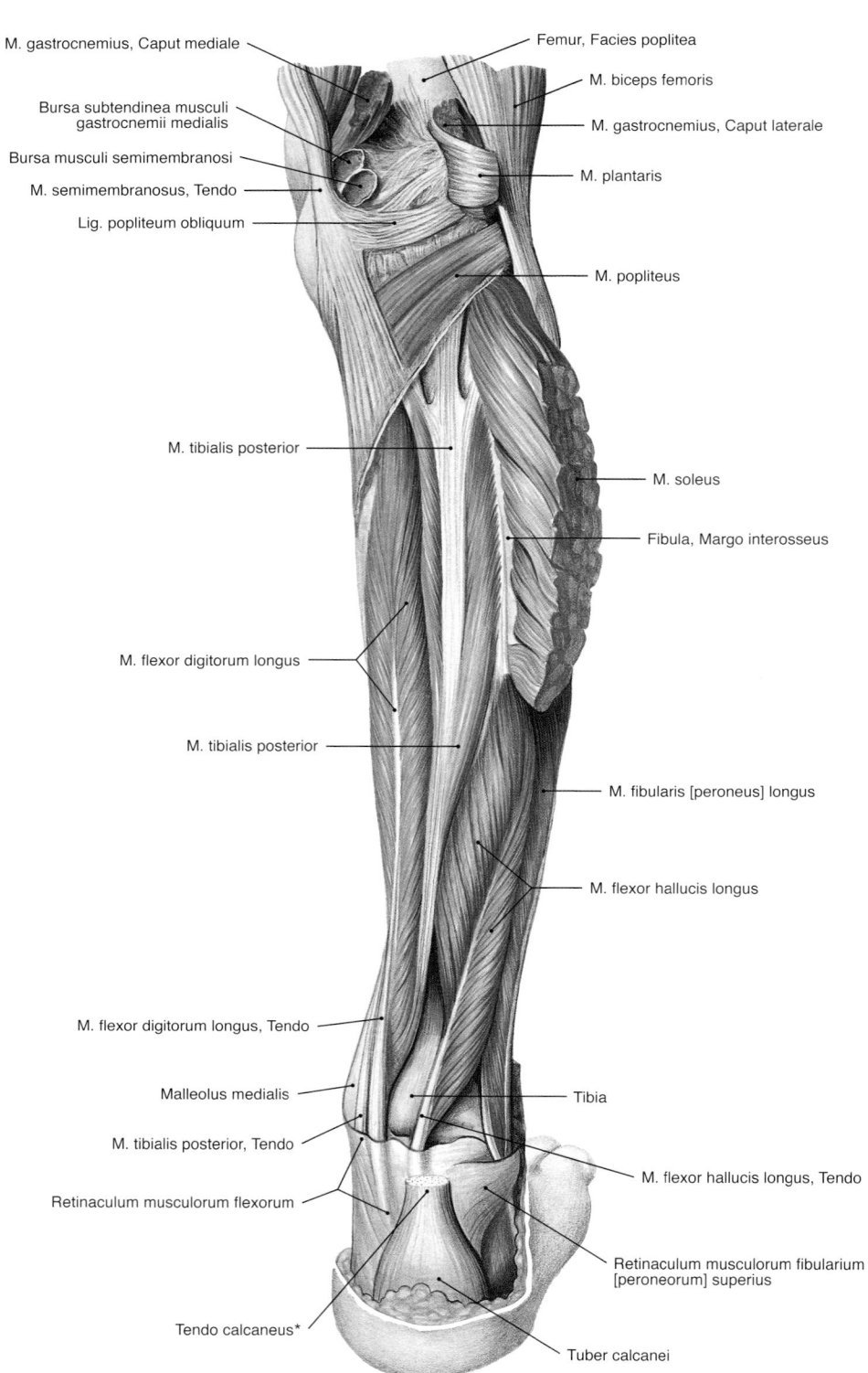

M. gastrocnemius, Caput mediale

Bursa subtendinea musculi gastrocnemii medialis

Bursa musculi semimembranosi

M. semimembranosus, Tendo

Lig. popliteum obliquum

M. tibialis posterior

M. flexor digitorum longus

M. tibialis posterior

M. flexor digitorum longus, Tendo

Malleolus medialis

M. tibialis posterior, Tendo

Retinaculum musculorum flexorum

Tendo calcaneus*

Femur, Facies poplitea

M. biceps femoris

M. gastrocnemius, Caput laterale

M. plantaris

M. popliteus

M. soleus

Fibula, Margo interosseus

M. fibularis [peroneus] longus

M. flexor hallucis longus

Tibia

M. flexor hallucis longus, Tendo

Retinaculum musculorum fibularium [peroneorum] superius

Tuber calcanei

→ T 50

Fig. 1086   Muscles of the leg; deep layer.
* Also: Achilles tendon

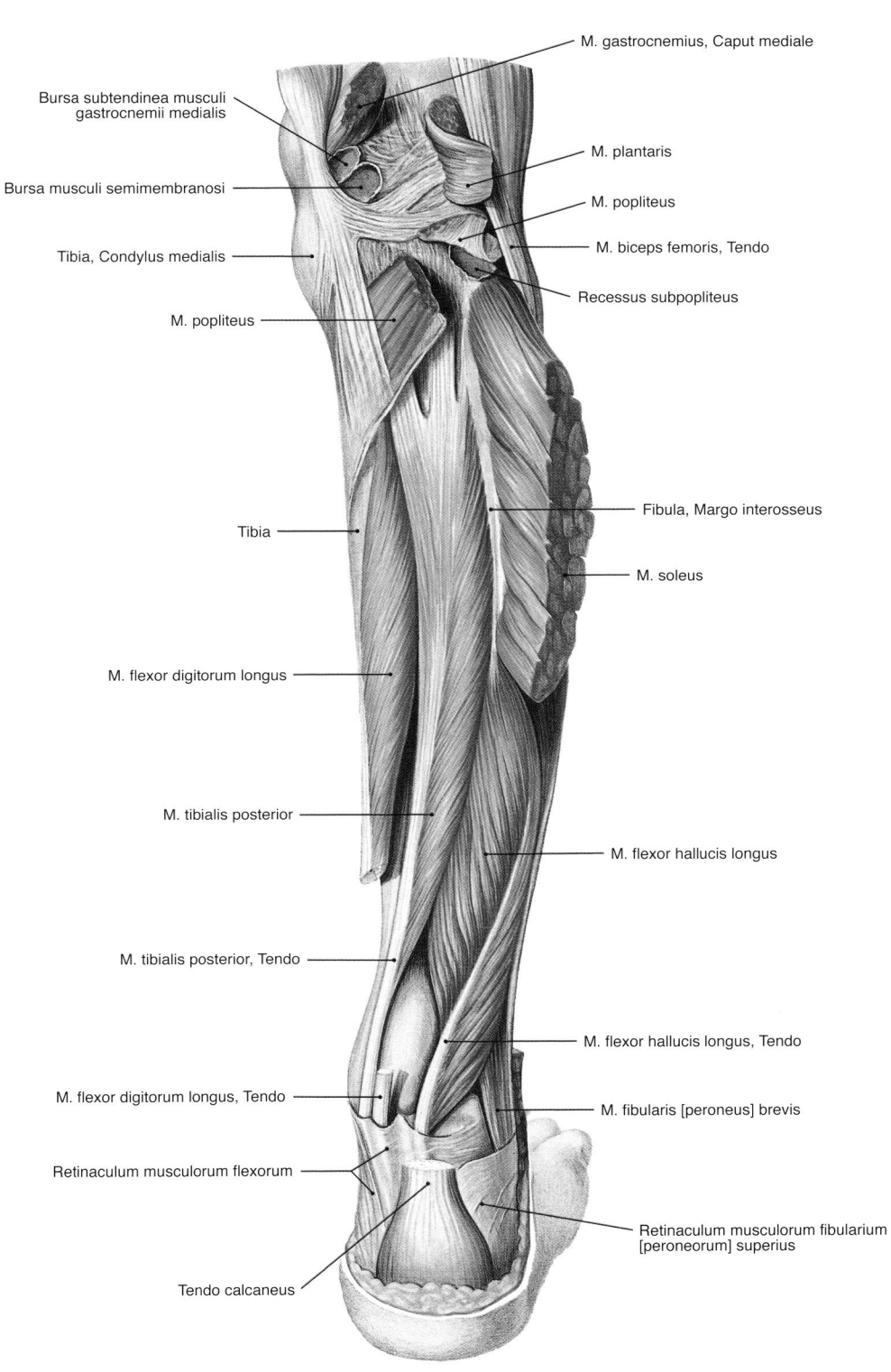

M. gastrocnemius, Caput mediale

Bursa subtendinea musculi gastrocnemii medialis

Bursa musculi semimembranosi

Tibia, Condylus medialis

M. popliteus

Tibia

M. flexor digitorum longus

M. tibialis posterior

M. tibialis posterior, Tendo

M. flexor digitorum longus, Tendo

Retinaculum musculorum flexorum

Tendo calcaneus

M. plantaris

M. popliteus

M. biceps femoris, Tendo

Recessus subpopliteus

Fibula, Margo interosseus

M. soleus

M. flexor hallucis longus

M. flexor hallucis longus, Tendo

M. fibularis [peroneus] brevis

Retinaculum musculorum fibularium [peroneorum] superius

Fig. 1087 Muscles of the leg; deepest layer.

→ T 50

Muscles of the leg

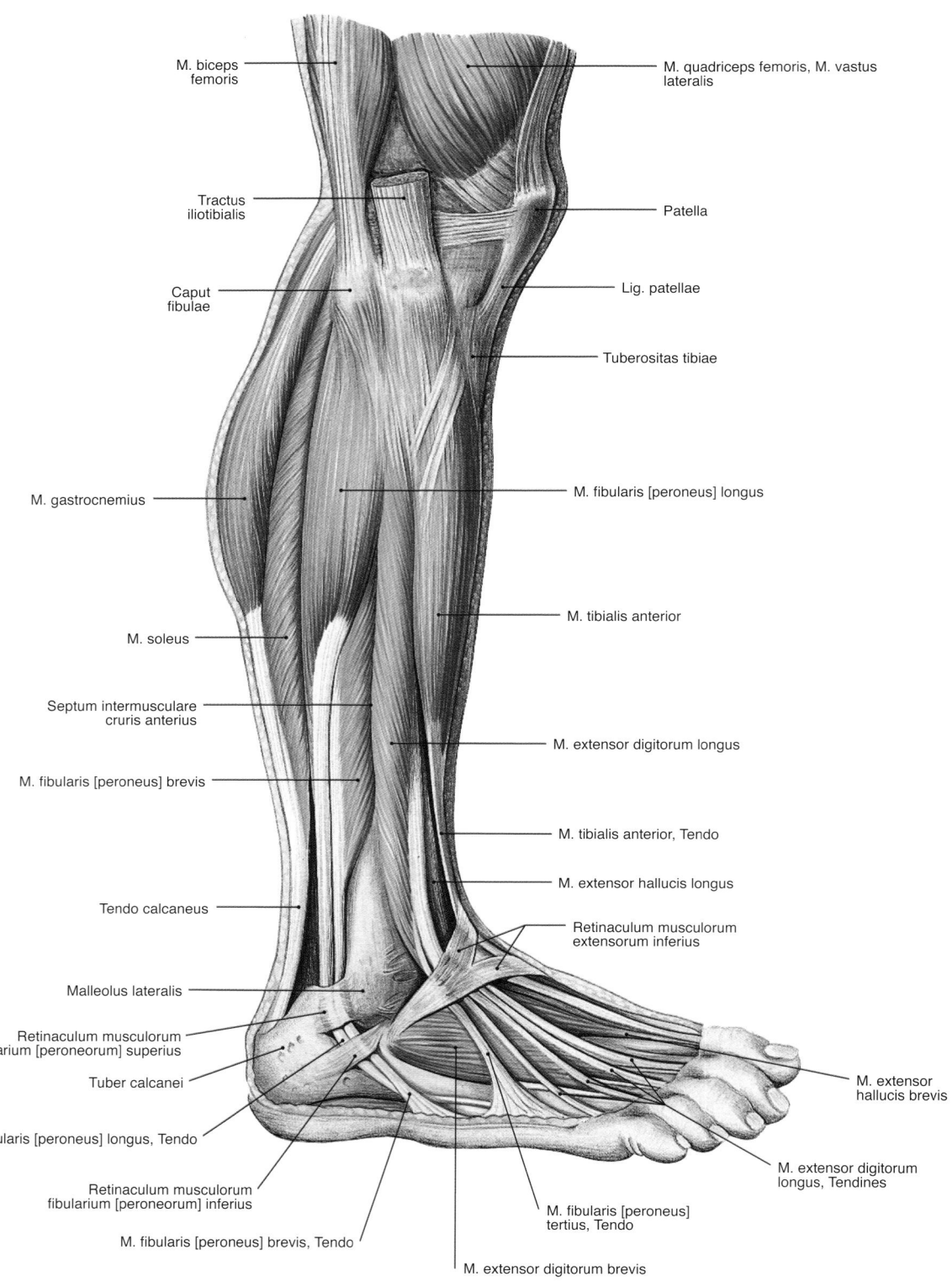

M. biceps femoris

Tractus iliotibialis

Caput fibulae

M. gastrocnemius

M. soleus

Septum intermusculare cruris anterius

M. fibularis [peroneus] brevis

Tendo calcaneus

Malleolus lateralis

Retinaculum musculorum fibularium [peroneorum] superius

Tuber calcanei

M. fibularis [peroneus] longus, Tendo

Retinaculum musculorum fibularium [peroneorum] inferius

M. fibularis [peroneus] brevis, Tendo

M. quadriceps femoris, M. vastus lateralis

Patella

Lig. patellae

Tuberositas tibiae

M. fibularis [peroneus] longus

M. tibialis anterior

M. extensor digitorum longus

M. tibialis anterior, Tendo

M. extensor hallucis longus

Retinaculum musculorum extensorum inferius

M. extensor hallucis brevis

M. extensor digitorum longus, Tendines

M. fibularis [peroneus] tertius, Tendo

M. extensor digitorum brevis

→ T 47 – T 49, T 51

Fig. 1088   Muscles of the leg and the foot.

Origins and insertions of the muscles of the the foot and the leg

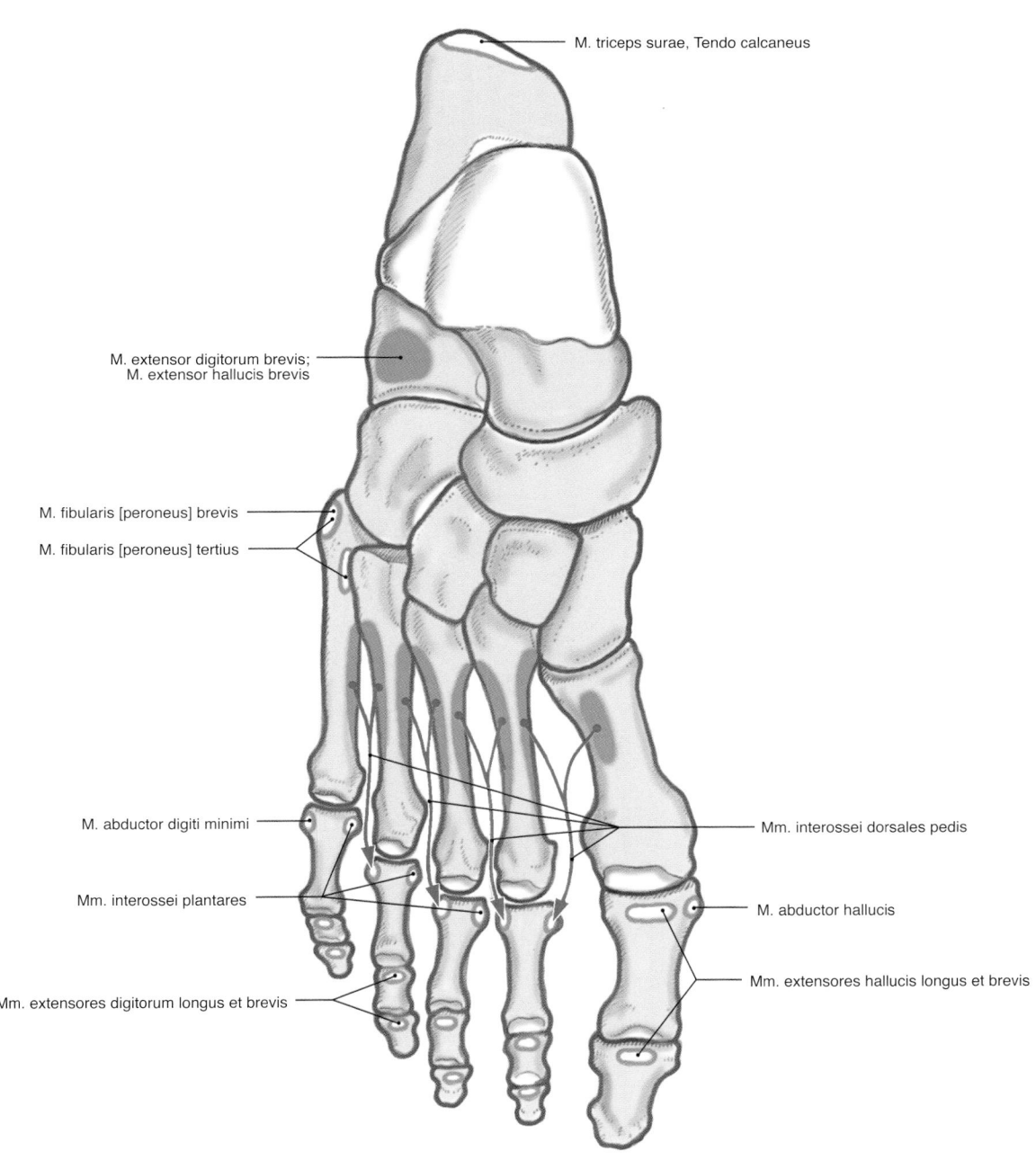

M. triceps surae, Tendo calcaneus

M. extensor digitorum brevis;
M. extensor hallucis brevis

M. fibularis [peroneus] brevis

M. fibularis [peroneus] tertius

M. abductor digiti minimi

Mm. interossei plantares

Mm. extensores digitorum longus et brevis

Mm. interossei dorsales pedis

M. abductor hallucis

Mm. extensores hallucis longus et brevis

Fig. 1089 Origins and insertions of the muscles
at the bones of the foot;
dorsal view.

→ T 47, T 48, T 51,
T 53, T 54

Tendon sheaths of the foot

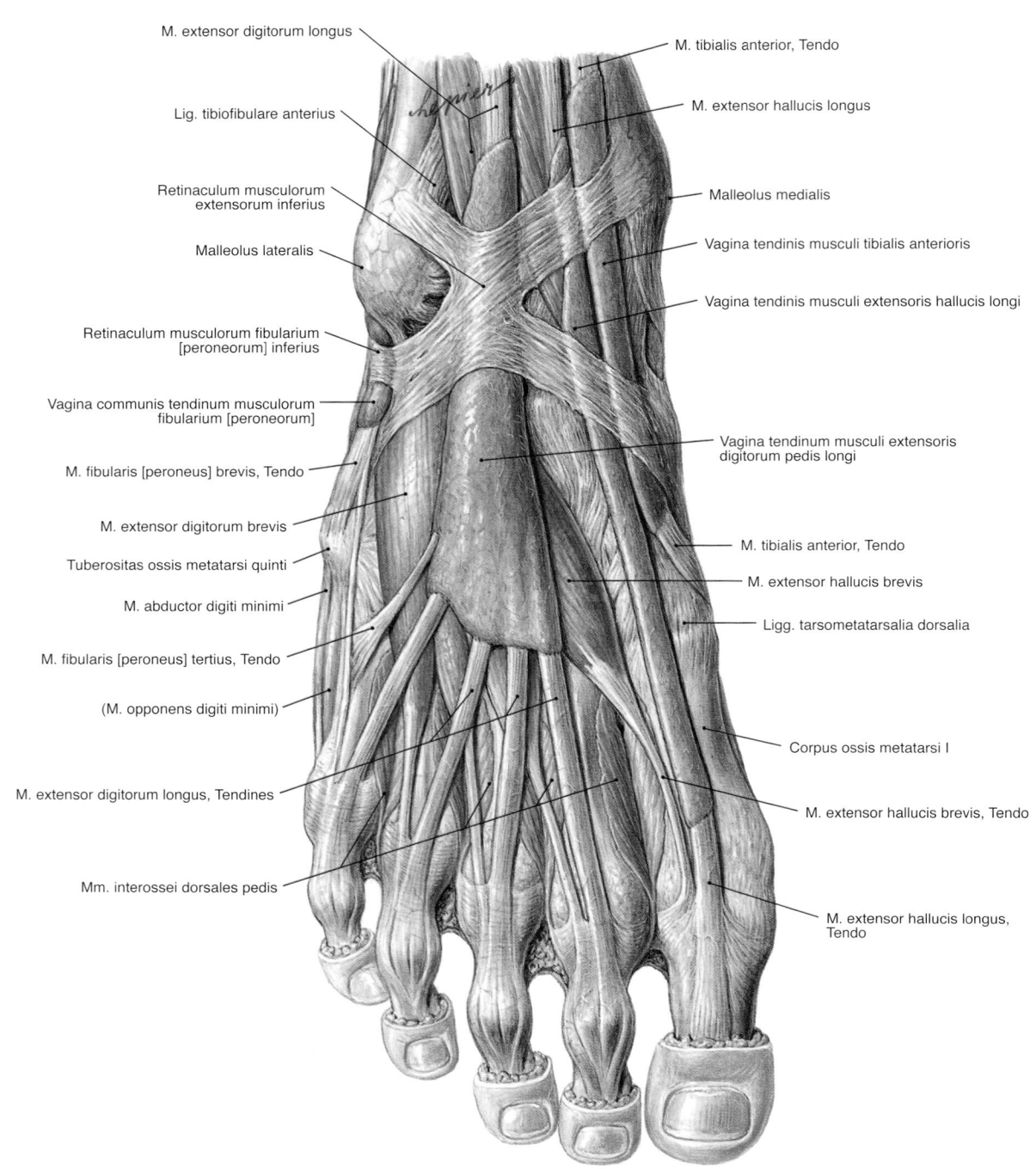

M. extensor digitorum longus

Lig. tibiofibulare anterius

Retinaculum musculorum
extensorum inferius

Malleolus lateralis

Retinaculum musculorum fibularium
[peroneorum] inferius

Vagina communis tendinum musculorum
fibularium [peroneorum]

M. fibularis [peroneus] brevis, Tendo

M. extensor digitorum brevis

Tuberositas ossis metatarsi quinti

M. abductor digiti minimi

M. fibularis [peroneus] tertius, Tendo

(M. opponens digiti minimi)

M. extensor digitorum longus, Tendines

Mm. interossei dorsales pedis

M. tibialis anterior, Tendo

M. extensor hallucis longus

Malleolus medialis

Vagina tendinis musculi tibialis anterioris

Vagina tendinis musculi extensoris hallucis longi

Vagina tendinum musculi extensoris
digitorum pedis longi

M. tibialis anterior, Tendo

M. extensor hallucis brevis

Ligg. tarsometatarsalia dorsalia

Corpus ossis metatarsi I

M. extensor hallucis brevis, Tendo

M. extensor hallucis longus,
Tendo

Fig. 1090   Tendon sheaths, Vaginae tendinum,
of the foot.

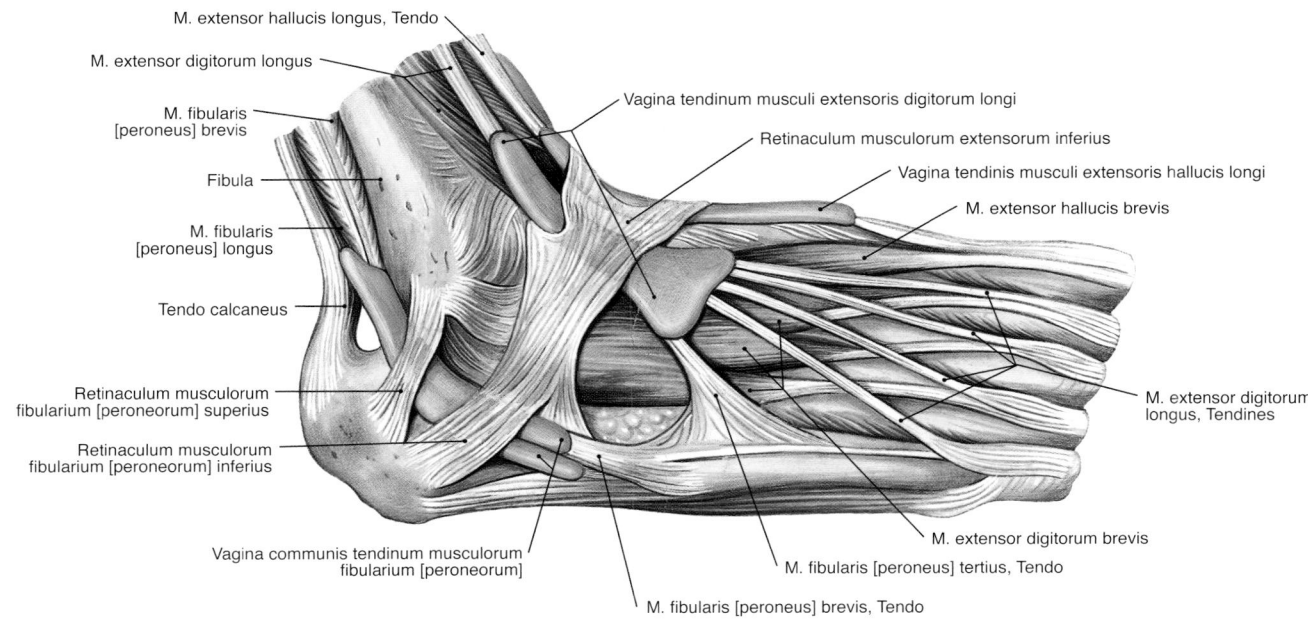

M. extensor hallucis longus, Tendo

M. extensor digitorum longus

M. fibularis [peroneus] brevis

Fibula

M. fibularis [peroneus] longus

Tendo calcaneus

Retinaculum musculorum fibularium [peroneorum] superius

Retinaculum musculorum fibularium [peroneorum] inferius

Vagina tendinum musculi extensoris digitorum longi

Retinaculum musculorum extensorum inferius

Vagina tendinis musculi extensoris hallucis longi

M. extensor hallucis brevis

M. extensor digitorum longus, Tendines

M. extensor digitorum brevis

Vagina communis tendinum musculorum fibularium [peroneorum]

M. fibularis [peroneus] tertius, Tendo

M. fibularis [peroneus] brevis, Tendo

Fig. 1091   Tendon sheaths, Vaginae tendinum, of the foot.

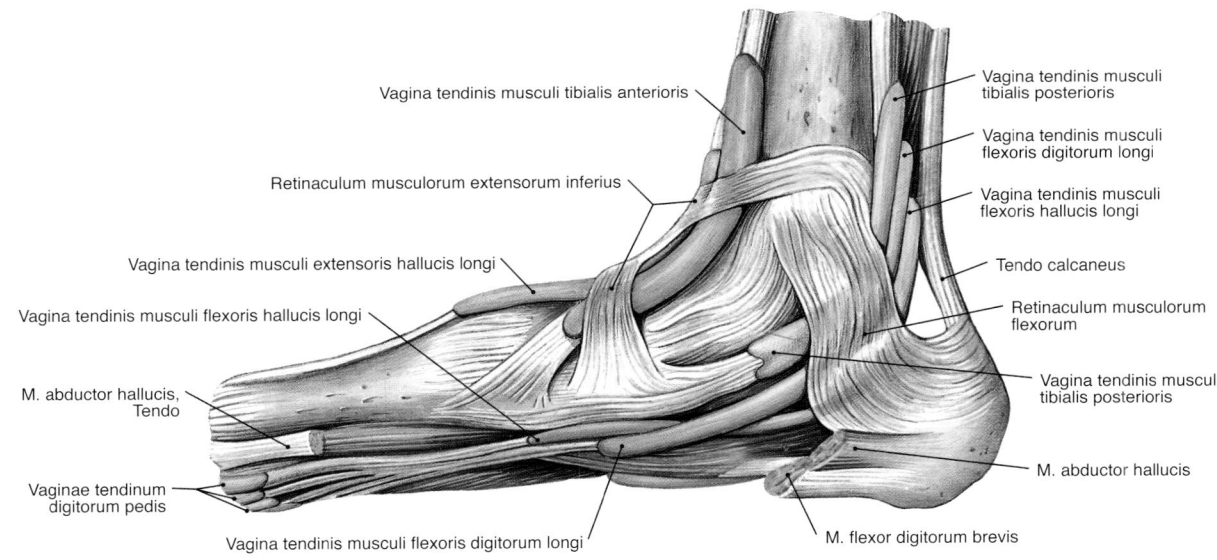

Vagina tendinis musculi tibialis anterioris

Vagina tendinis musculi tibialis posterioris

Vagina tendinis musculi flexoris digitorum longi

Retinaculum musculorum extensorum inferius

Vagina tendinis musculi flexoris hallucis longi

Vagina tendinis musculi extensoris hallucis longi

Tendo calcaneus

Vagina tendinis musculi flexoris hallucis longi

Retinaculum musculorum flexorum

M. abductor hallucis, Tendo

Vagina tendinis musculi tibialis posterioris

Vaginae tendinum digitorum pedis

M. abductor hallucis

Vagina tendinis musculi flexoris digitorum longi

M. flexor digitorum brevis

Fig. 1092   Tendon sheaths, Vaginae tendinum, of the foot.

Muscles of the foot

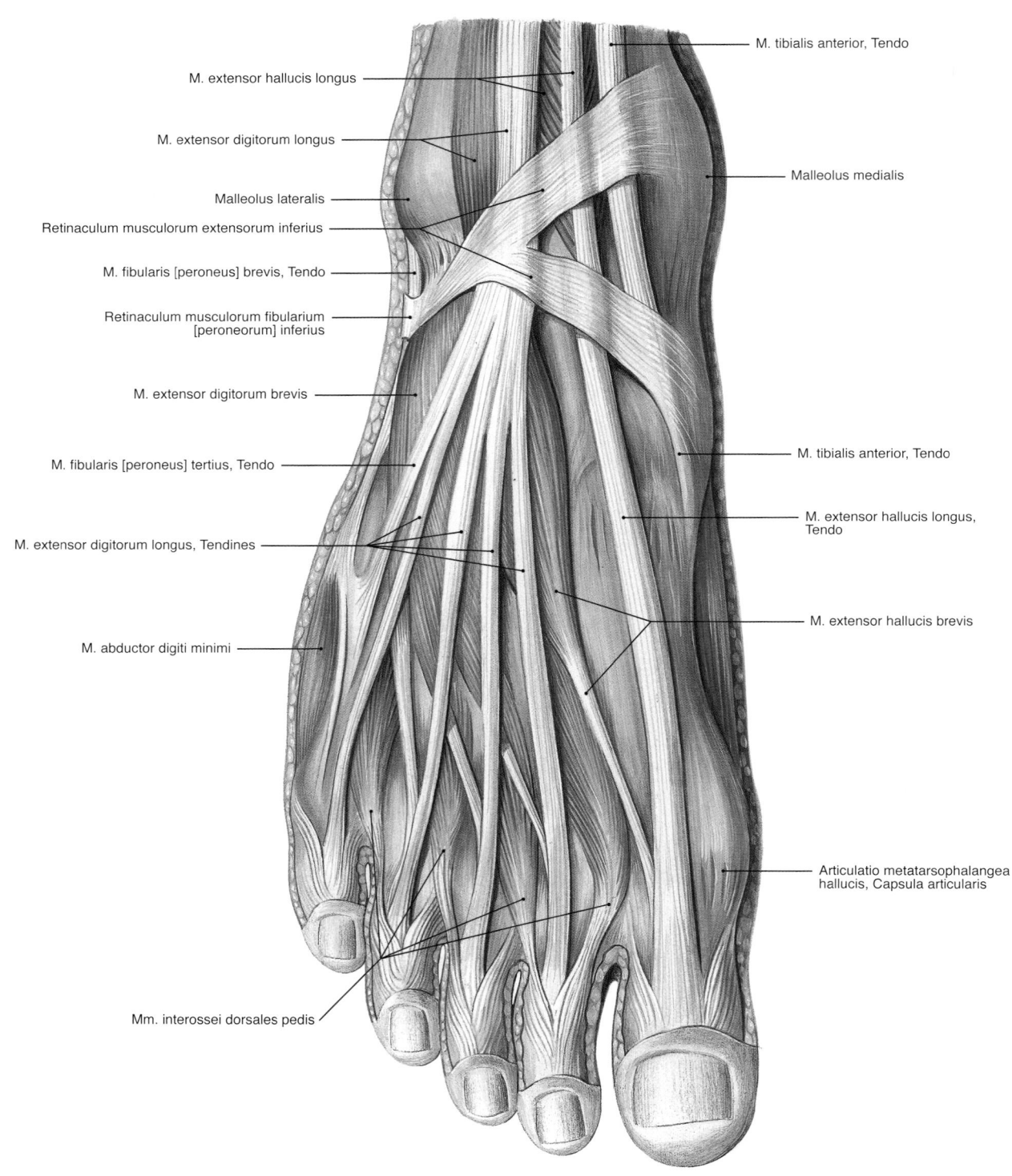

M. tibialis anterior, Tendo

M. extensor hallucis longus

M. extensor digitorum longus

Malleolus lateralis

Retinaculum musculorum extensorum inferius

M. fibularis [peroneus] brevis, Tendo

Retinaculum musculorum fibularium [peroneorum] inferius

M. extensor digitorum brevis

M. fibularis [peroneus] tertius, Tendo

M. extensor digitorum longus, Tendines

M. abductor digiti minimi

Mm. interossei dorsales pedis

Malleolus medialis

M. tibialis anterior, Tendo

M. extensor hallucis longus, Tendo

M. extensor hallucis brevis

Articulatio metatarsophalangea hallucis, Capsula articularis

→ T 47, T 51, T 53

Fig. 1093   Muscles of the foot;
after removal of the tendon sheaths.

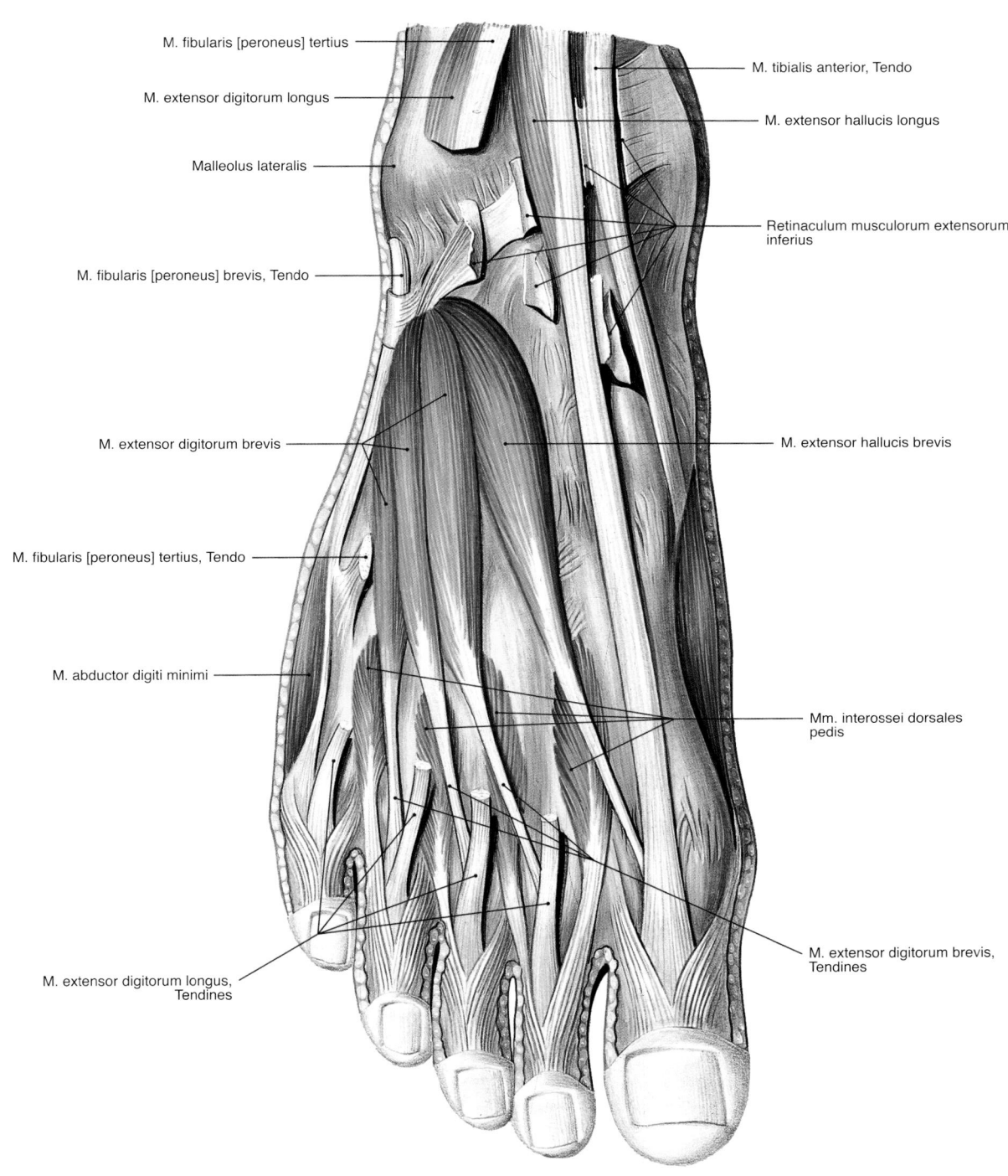

M. fibularis [peroneus] tertius

M. extensor digitorum longus

Malleolus lateralis

M. fibularis [peroneus] brevis, Tendo

M. extensor digitorum brevis

M. fibularis [peroneus] tertius, Tendo

M. abductor digiti minimi

M. extensor digitorum longus, Tendines

M. tibialis anterior, Tendo

M. extensor hallucis longus

Retinaculum musculorum extensorum inferius

M. extensor hallucis brevis

Mm. interossei dorsales pedis

M. extensor digitorum brevis, Tendines

Fig. 1094   Muscles of the foot;
after section of the inferior
extensor retinaculum.

→ T 47, T 51, T 53

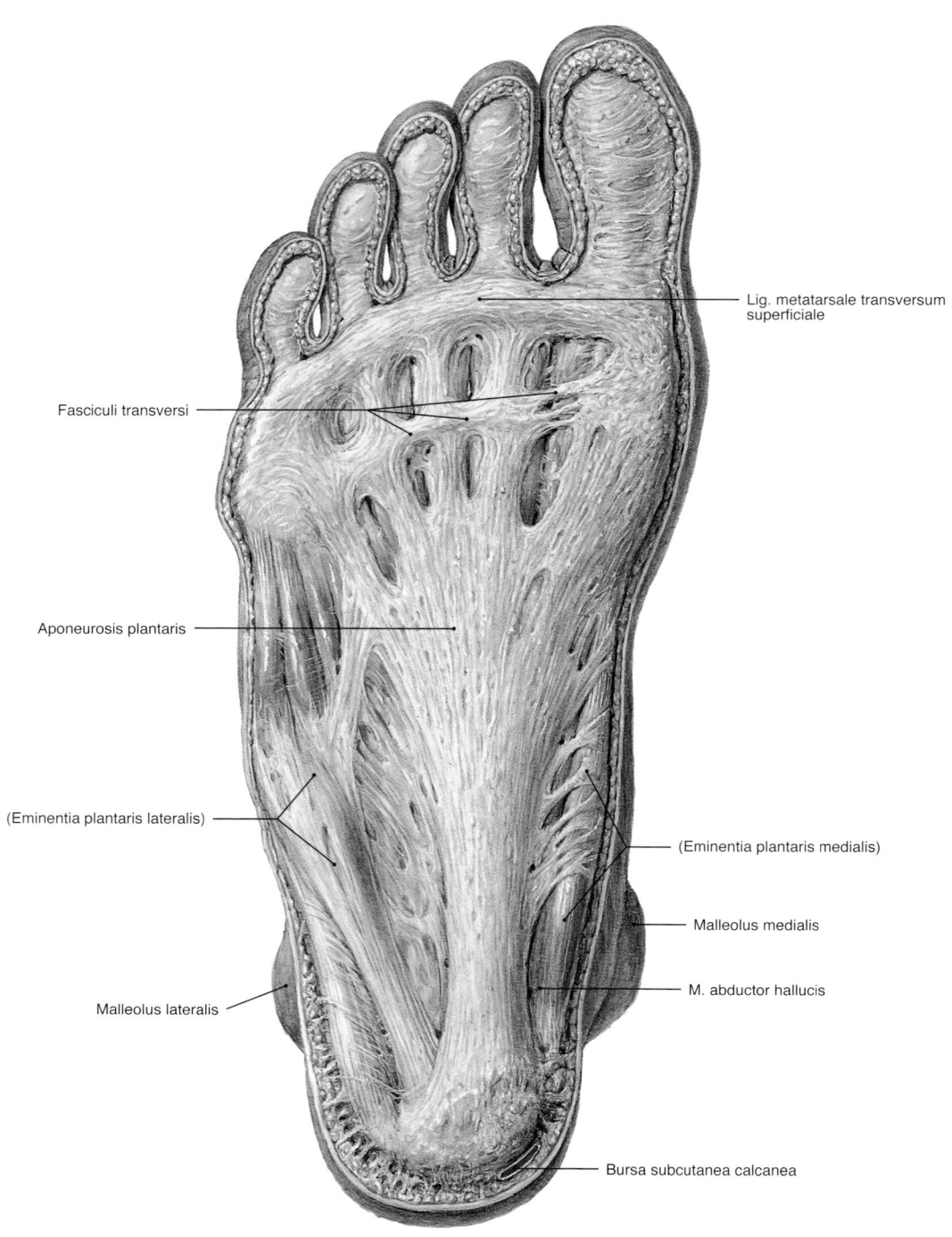

Lig. metatarsale transversum superficiale

Fasciculi transversi

Aponeurosis plantaris

(Eminentia plantaris lateralis)

(Eminentia plantaris medialis)

Malleolus medialis

M. abductor hallucis

Malleolus lateralis

Bursa subcutanea calcanea

Fig. 1095 Muscles of the foot; plantar aponeurosis, Aponeurosis plantaris.

Origins and insertions of the muscles of the foot and the leg

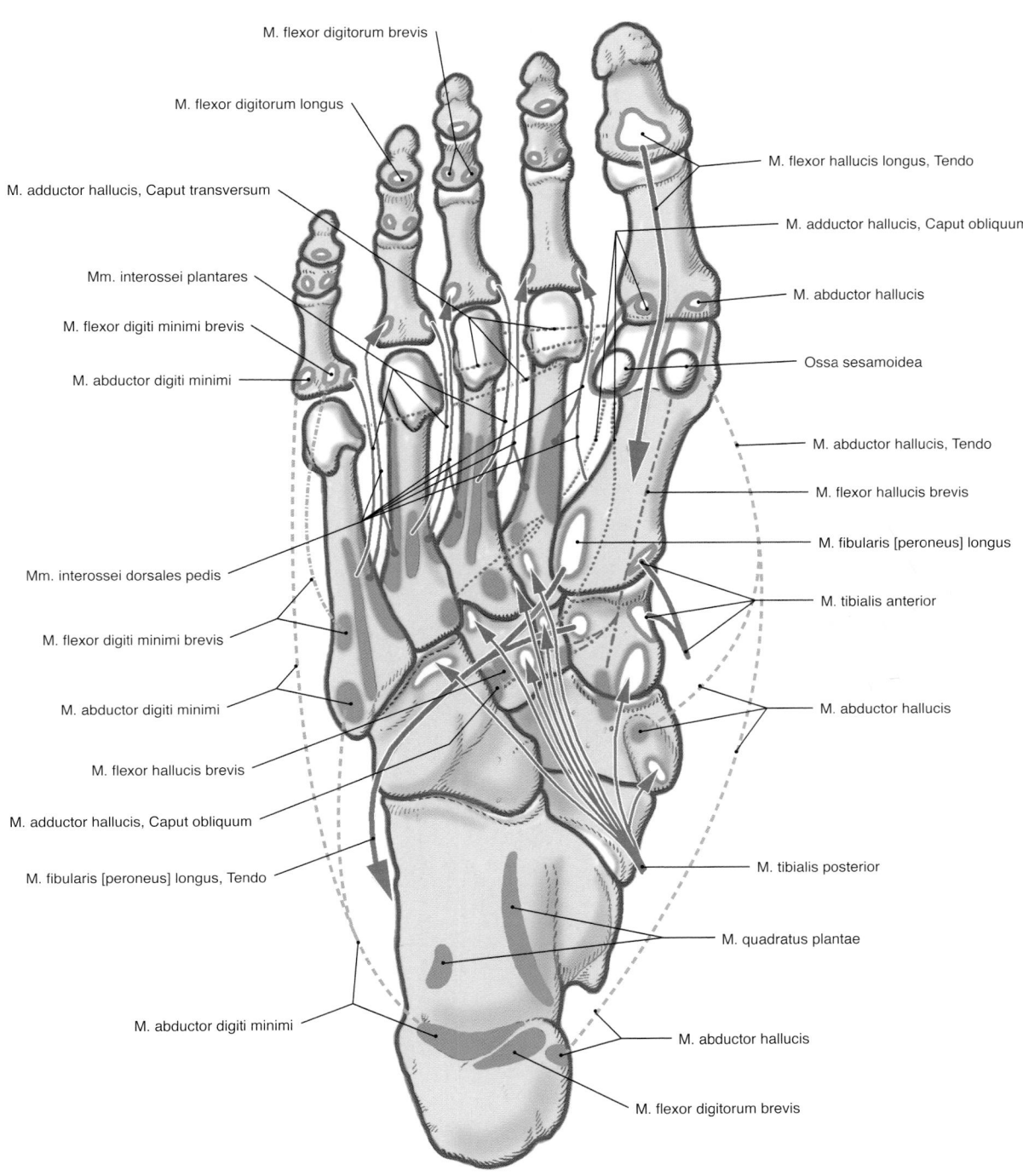

M. flexor digitorum brevis

M. flexor digitorum longus

M. adductor hallucis, Caput transversum

Mm. interossei plantares

M. flexor digiti minimi brevis

M. abductor digiti minimi

Mm. interossei dorsales pedis

M. flexor digiti minimi brevis

M. abductor digiti minimi

M. flexor hallucis brevis

M. adductor hallucis, Caput obliquum

M. fibularis [peroneus] longus, Tendo

M. abductor digiti minimi

M. flexor hallucis longus, Tendo

M. adductor hallucis, Caput obliquum

M. abductor hallucis

Ossa sesamoidea

M. abductor hallucis, Tendo

M. flexor hallucis brevis

M. fibularis [peroneus] longus

M. tibialis anterior

M. abductor hallucis

M. tibialis posterior

M. quadratus plantae

M. abductor hallucis

M. flexor digitorum brevis

Fig. 1096   Origins and insertions of the muscles
at the bones of the foot;
plantar view.

→ T 47, T 48, T 50,
T 52–T 54

Muscles of the foot

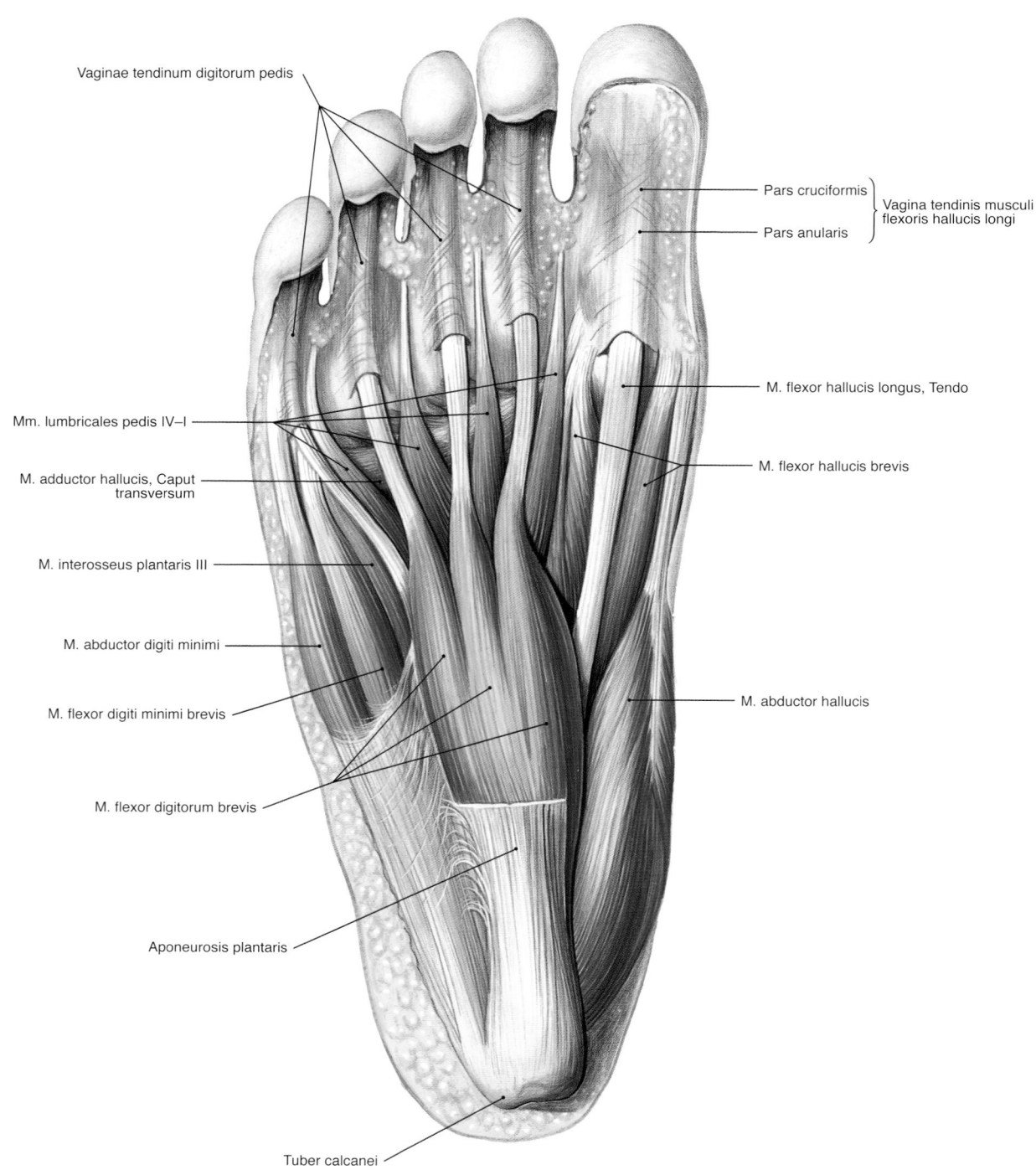

Vaginae tendinum digitorum pedis

Pars cruciformis ⎫ Vagina tendinis musculi flexoris hallucis longi
Pars anularis ⎭

M. flexor hallucis longus, Tendo

Mm. lumbricales pedis IV–I

M. adductor hallucis, Caput transversum

M. flexor hallucis brevis

M. interosseus plantaris III

M. abductor digiti minimi

M. flexor digiti minimi brevis

M. abductor hallucis

M. flexor digitorum brevis

Aponeurosis plantaris

Tuber calcanei

→ T 52 – T 54

Fig. 1097 Muscles of the foot;
the plantar aponeurosis has been removed.

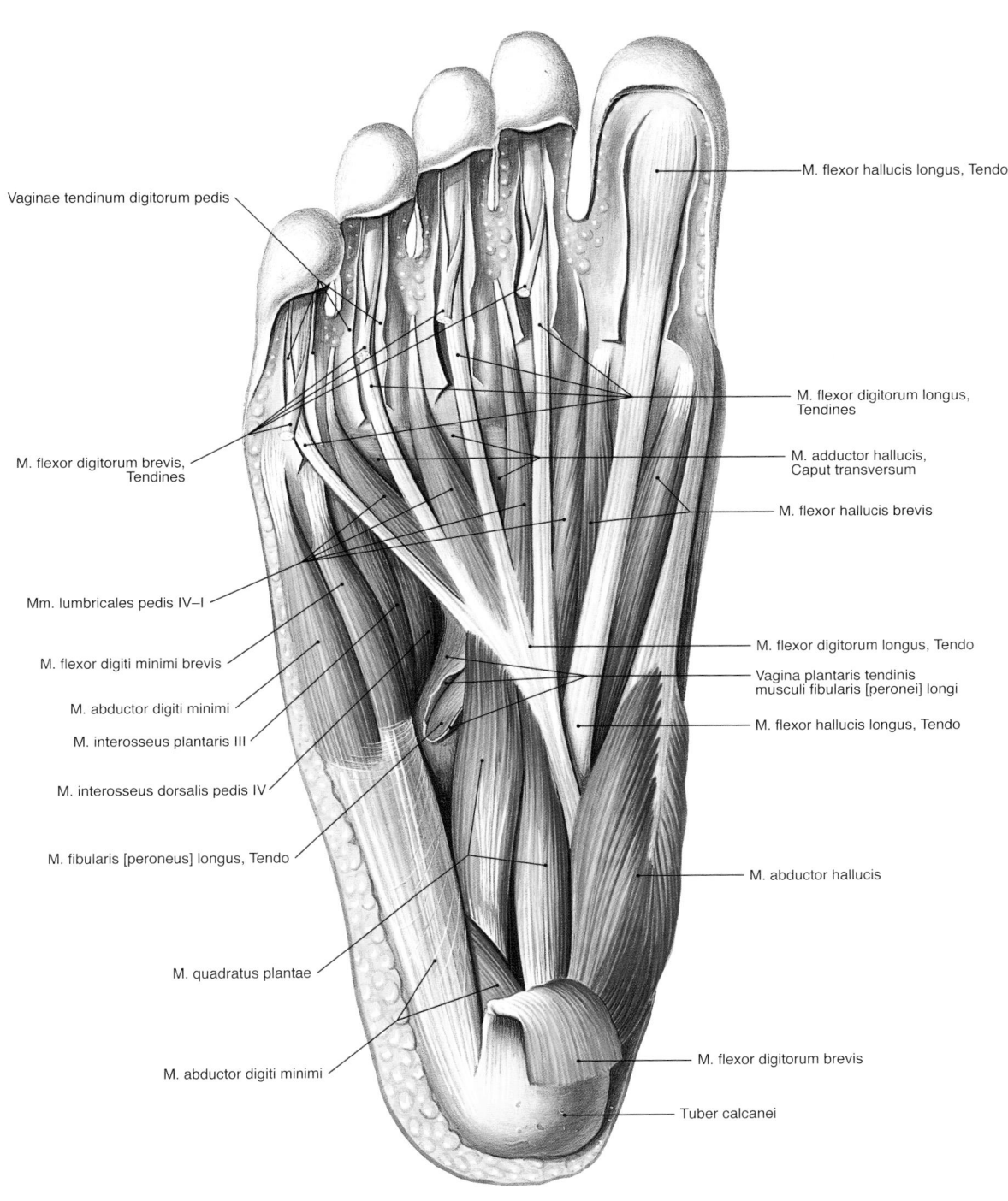

Vaginae tendinum digitorum pedis

M. flexor hallucis longus, Tendo

M. flexor digitorum brevis, Tendines

M. flexor digitorum longus, Tendines

M. adductor hallucis, Caput transversum

M. flexor hallucis brevis

Mm. lumbricales pedis IV–I

M. flexor digiti minimi brevis

M. abductor digiti minimi

M. interosseus plantaris III

M. interosseus dorsalis pedis IV

M. fibularis [peroneus] longus, Tendo

M. flexor digitorum longus, Tendo

Vagina plantaris tendinis musculi fibularis [peronei] longi

M. flexor hallucis longus, Tendo

M. abductor hallucis

M. quadratus plantae

M. flexor digitorum brevis

M. abductor digiti minimi

Tuber calcanei

Fig. 1098 Muscles of the foot;
middle layer after almost complete removal of the
flexor digitorum brevis muscle.

→ T 50, T 52 – T 54

Muscles of the foot

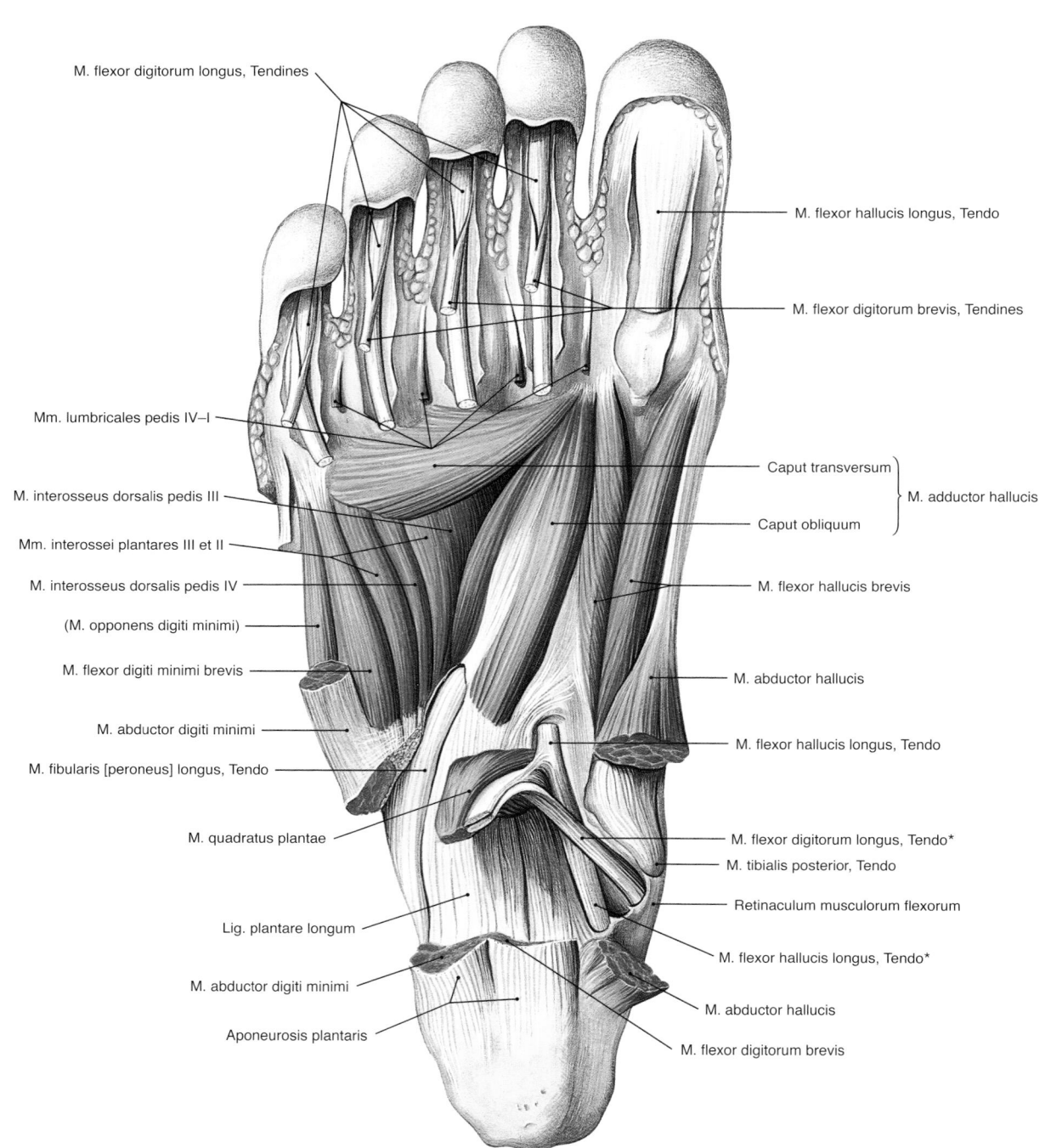

M. flexor digitorum longus, Tendines

M. flexor hallucis longus, Tendo

M. flexor digitorum brevis, Tendines

Mm. lumbricales pedis IV–I

Caput transversum
M. adductor hallucis
Caput obliquum

M. interosseus dorsalis pedis III

Mm. interossei plantares III et II

M. interosseus dorsalis pedis IV

M. flexor hallucis brevis

(M. opponens digiti minimi)

M. flexor digiti minimi brevis

M. abductor hallucis

M. abductor digiti minimi

M. flexor hallucis longus, Tendo

M. fibularis [peroneus] longus, Tendo

M. quadratus plantae

M. flexor digitorum longus, Tendo*

M. tibialis posterior, Tendo

Retinaculum musculorum flexorum

Lig. plantare longum

M. flexor hallucis longus, Tendo*

M. abductor digiti minimi

M. abductor hallucis

Aponeurosis plantaris

M. flexor digitorum brevis

→ T 50, T 52–T 54

Fig. 1099   Muscles of the foot;
deep layer.

* The site where the tendon of the flexor digitorum longus muscle
crosses the tendon of the flexor hallucis longus muscle is
commonly referred to as plantar chiasm, Chiasma plantare.

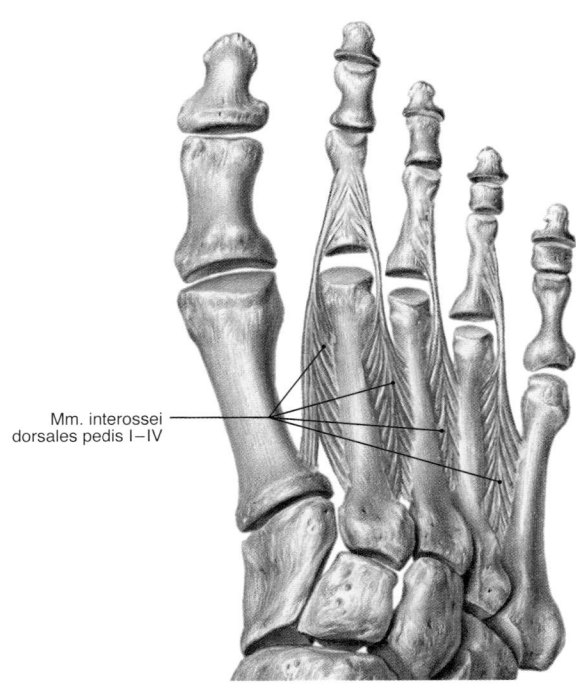

Mm. interossei
dorsales pedis I–IV

Fig. 1100 Dorsal interossei muscles, Mm. interossei dorsales pedis; dorsal view.

→ T 53

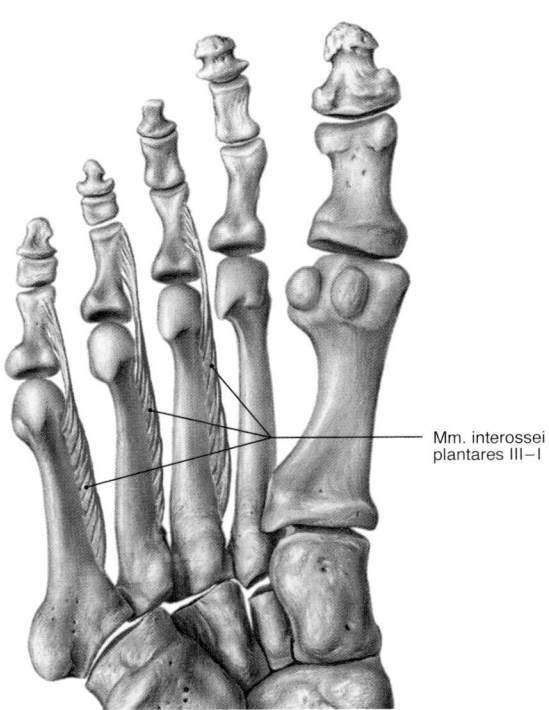

Mm. interossei
plantares III–I

Fig. 1101 Plantar interossei muscles, Mm. interossei plantares; plantar view.

→ T 53

Lumbosacral plexus

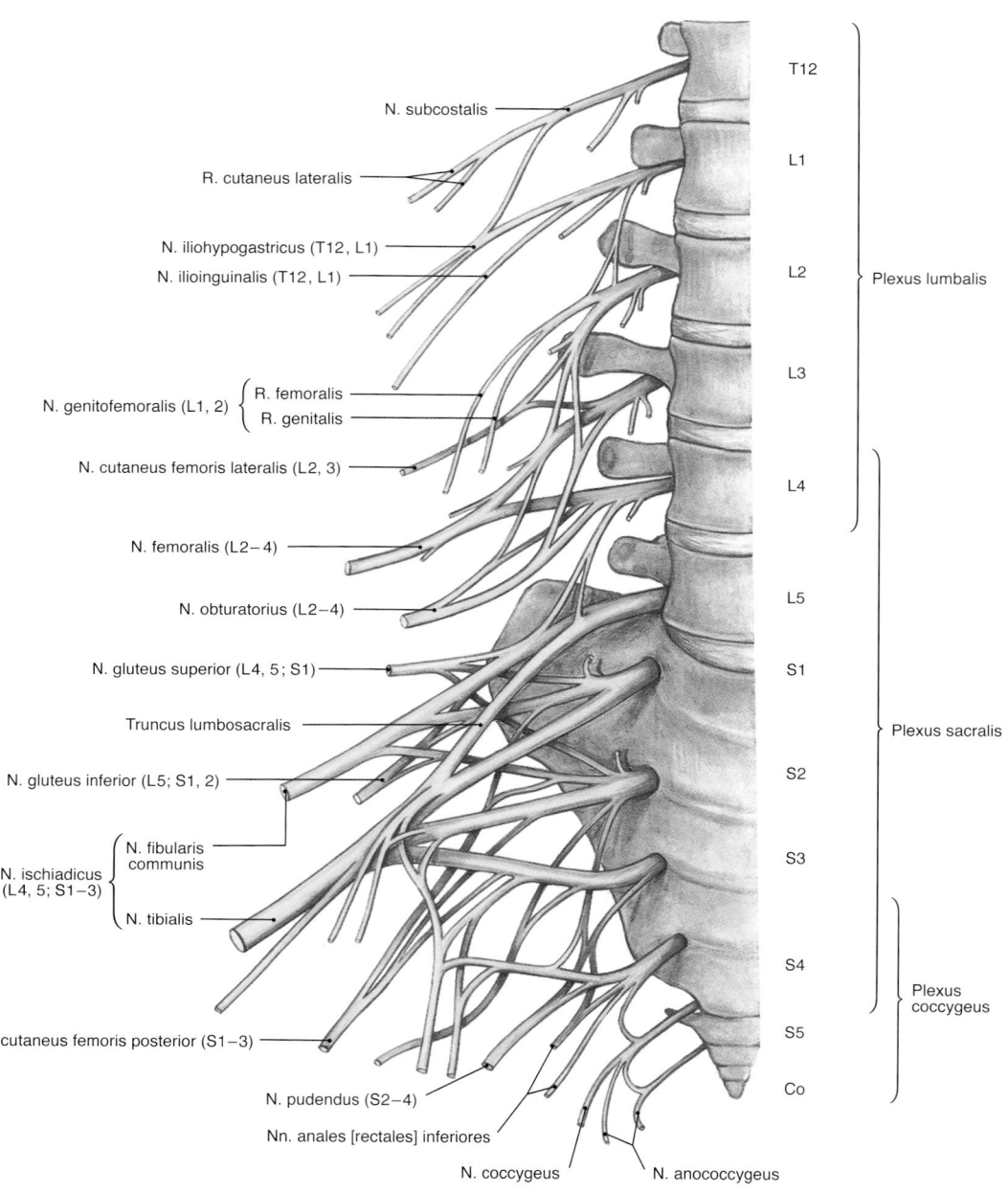

N. subcostalis

R. cutaneus lateralis

N. iliohypogastricus (T12, L1)
N. ilioinguinalis (T12, L1)

N. genitofemoralis (L1, 2) { R. femoralis
R. genitalis

N. cutaneus femoris lateralis (L2, 3)

N. femoralis (L2–4)

N. obturatorius (L2–4)

N. gluteus superior (L4, 5; S1)

Truncus lumbosacralis

N. gluteus inferior (L5; S1, 2)

N. ischiadicus (L4, 5; S1–3) { N. fibularis communis
N. tibialis

N. cutaneus femoris posterior (S1–3)

N. pudendus (S2–4)

Nn. anales [rectales] inferiores

N. coccygeus   N. anococcygeus

T12
L1
L2
L3
L4
L5
S1
S2
S3
S4
S5
Co

Plexus lumbalis

Plexus sacralis

Plexus coccygeus

→ 595

Fig. 1102 Lumbosacral and coccygeal plexus,
Plexus lumbosacralis (Plexus lumbalis et sacralis) et coccygeus;
segmental organisation of nerves.

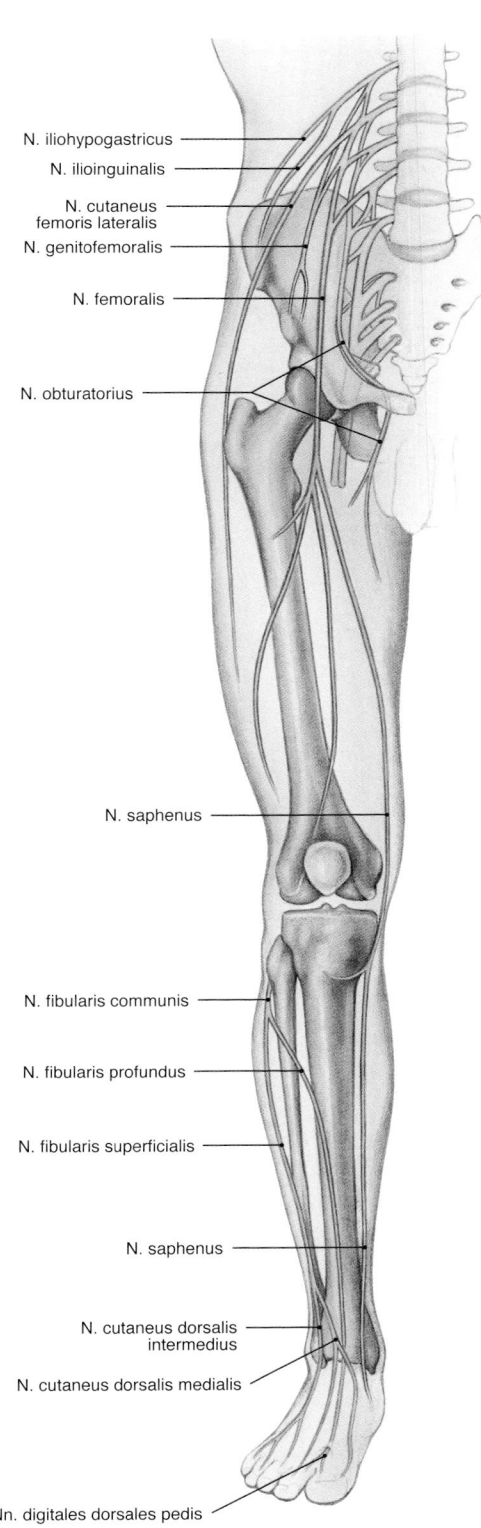

N. iliohypogastricus
N. ilioinguinalis
N. cutaneus femoris lateralis
N. genitofemoralis
N. femoralis
N. obturatorius
N. saphenus
N. fibularis communis
N. fibularis profundus
N. fibularis superficialis
N. saphenus
N. cutaneus dorsalis intermedius
N. cutaneus dorsalis medialis
Nn. digitales dorsales pedis

Fig. 1103   Nerves of the lower limb; overview.

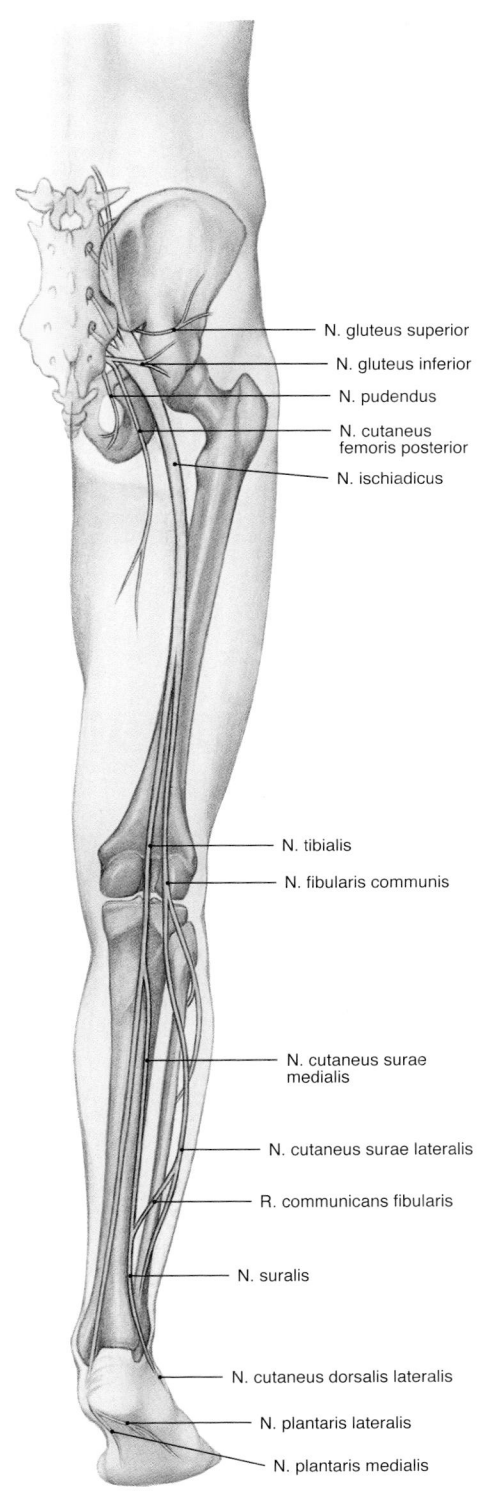

N. gluteus superior
N. gluteus inferior
N. pudendus
N. cutaneus femoris posterior
N. ischiadicus
N. tibialis
N. fibularis communis
N. cutaneus surae medialis
N. cutaneus surae lateralis
R. communicans fibularis
N. suralis
N. cutaneus dorsalis lateralis
N. plantaris lateralis
N. plantaris medialis

Fig. 1104   Nerves of the lower limb; overview.

Cutaneous innervation

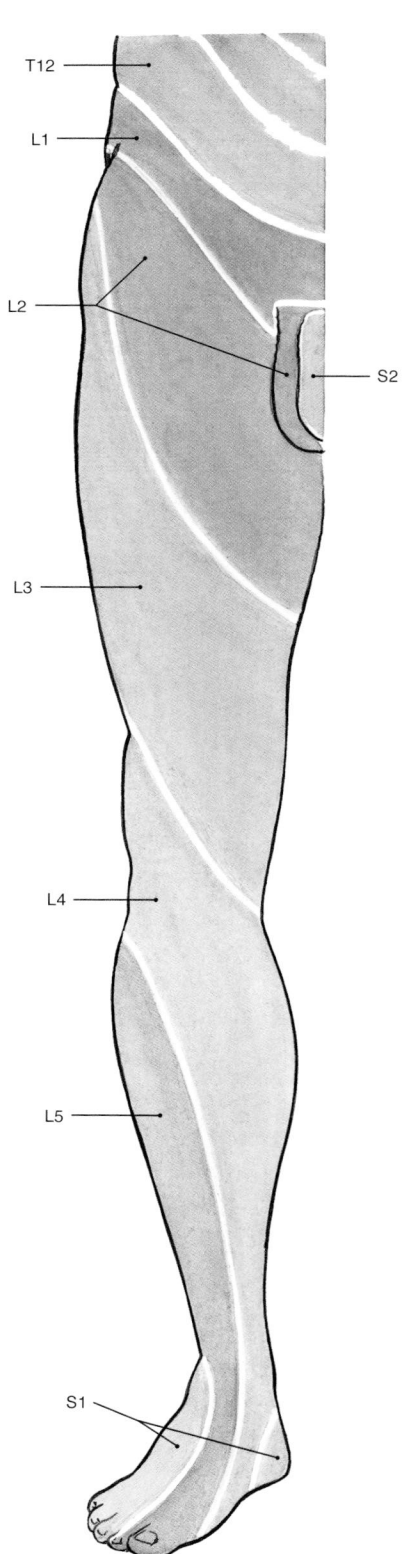

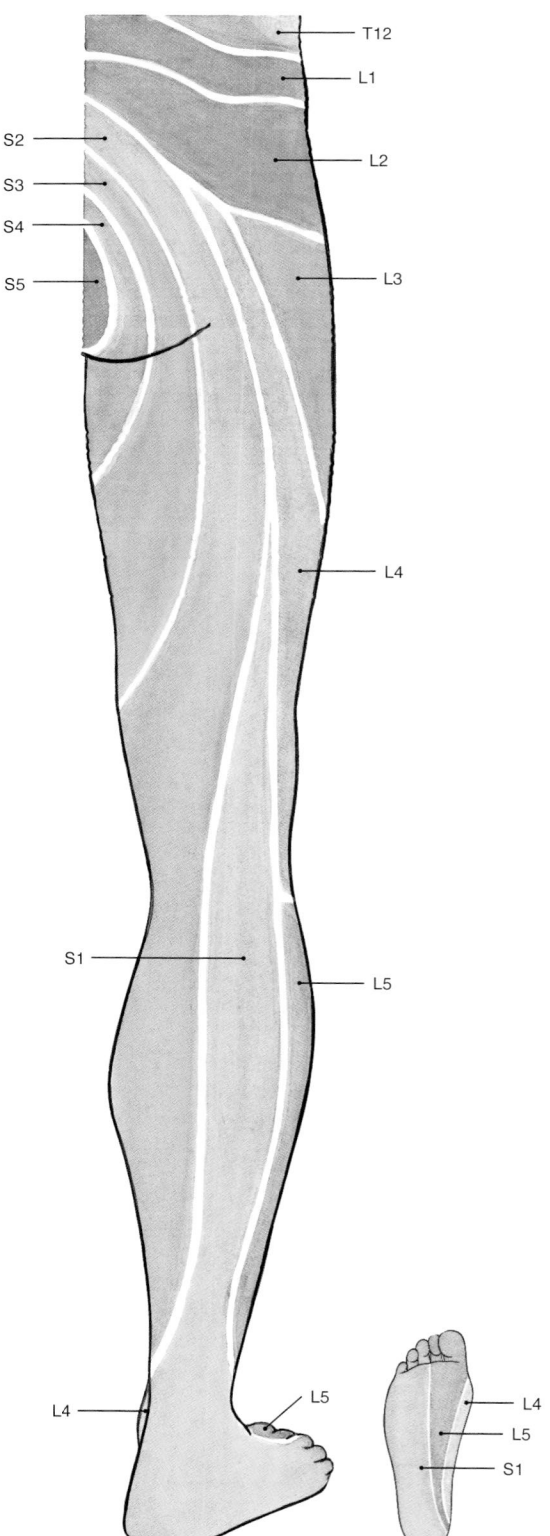

Fig. 1105 Segmental cutaneous innervation (dermatomes) of the lower limb.

Fig. 1106 Segmental cutaneous innervation (dermatomes) of the lower limb.

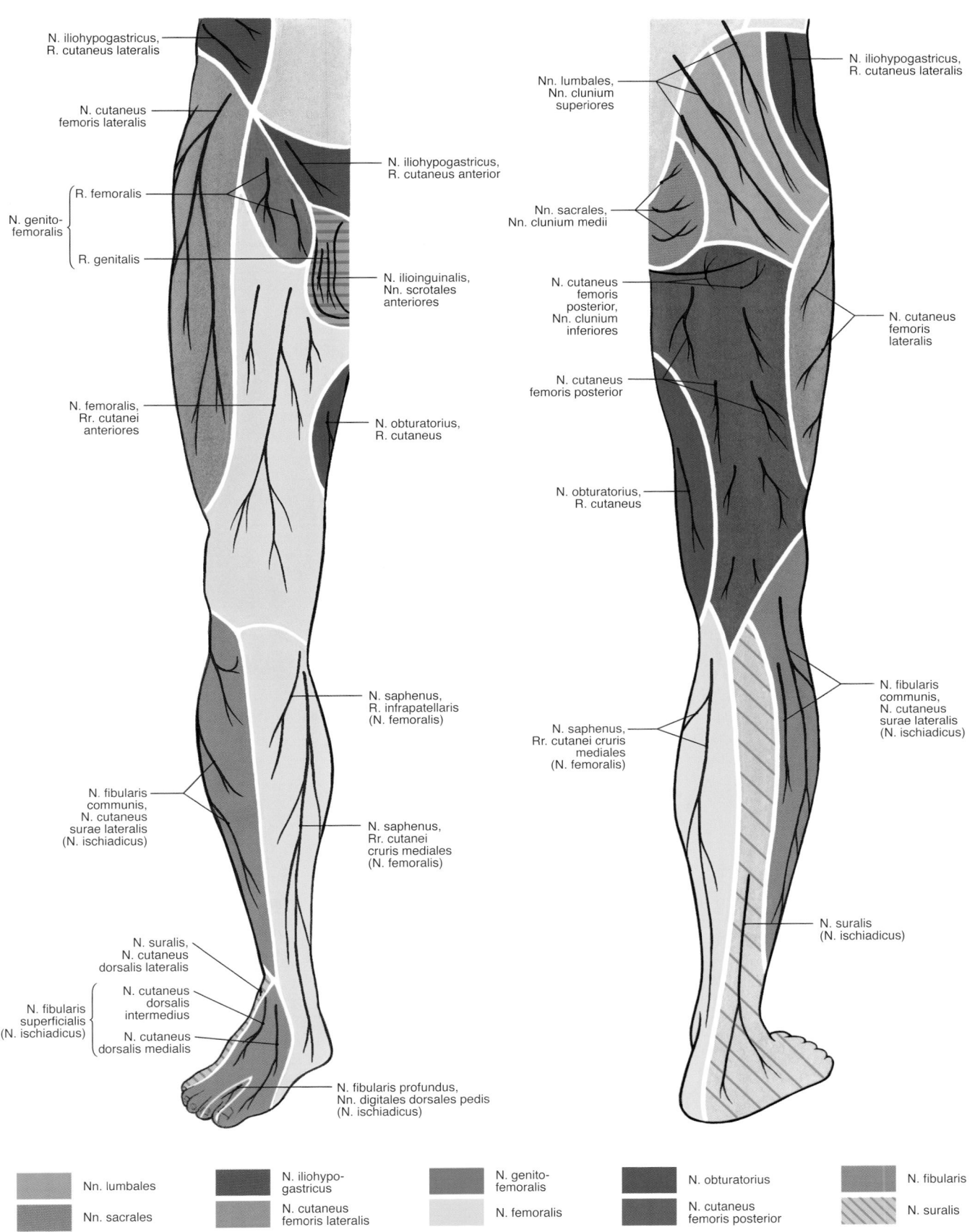

N. iliohypogastricus,
R. cutaneus lateralis

N. cutaneus
femoris lateralis

N. genito-
femoralis { R. femoralis

R. genitalis

N. femoralis,
Rr. cutanei
anteriores

N. fibularis
communis,
N. cutaneus
surae lateralis
(N. ischiadicus)

N. suralis,
N. cutaneus
dorsalis lateralis

N. fibularis
superficialis
(N. ischiadicus) { N. cutaneus
dorsalis
intermedius

N. cutaneus
dorsalis medialis

N. iliohypogastricus,
R. cutaneus anterior

N. ilioinguinalis,
Nn. scrotales
anteriores

N. obturatorius,
R. cutaneus

N. saphenus,
R. infrapatellaris
(N. femoralis)

N. saphenus,
Rr. cutanei
cruris mediales
(N. femoralis)

N. fibularis profundus,
Nn. digitales dorsales pedis
(N. ischiadicus)

Nn. lumbales,
Nn. clunium
superiores

Nn. sacrales,
Nn. clunium medii

N. cutaneus
femoris
posterior,
Nn. clunium
inferiores

N. cutaneus
femoris posterior

N. obturatorius,
R. cutaneus

N. saphenus,
Rr. cutanei cruris
mediales
(N. femoralis)

N. iliohypogastricus,
R. cutaneus lateralis

N. cutaneus
femoris
lateralis

N. fibularis
communis,
N. cutaneus
surae lateralis
(N. ischiadicus)

N. suralis
(N. ischiadicus)

Nn. lumbales

Nn. sacrales

N. iliohypo-
gastricus

N. cutaneus
femoris lateralis

N. genito-
femoralis

N. femoralis

N. obturatorius

N. cutaneus
femoris posterior

N. fibularis

N. suralis

Fig. 1107   Cutaneous nerves of the lower limb.

Fig. 1108   Cutaneous nerves of the lower limb.

Femoral and obturator nerve

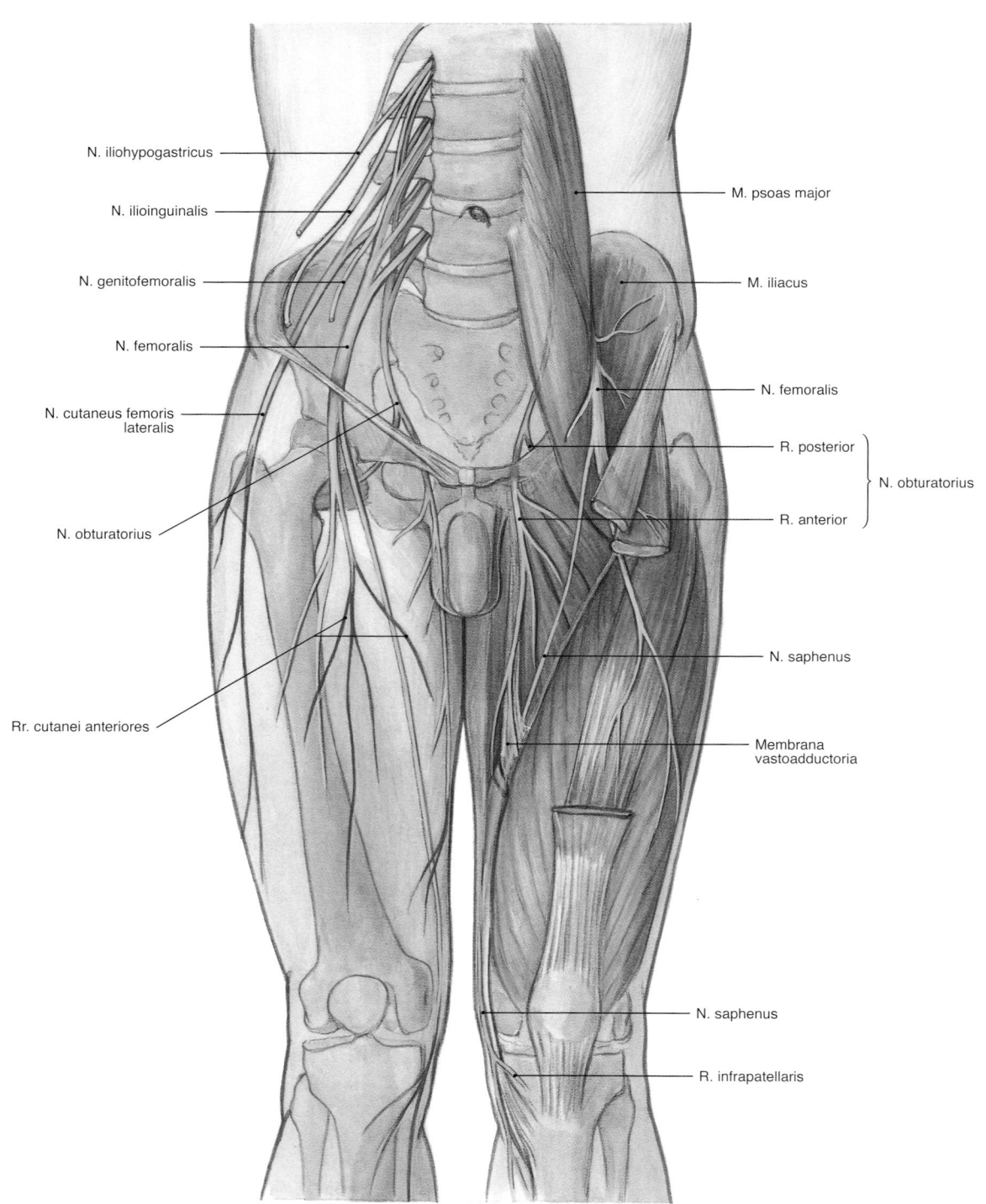

N. iliohypogastricus

N. ilioinguinalis

N. genitofemoralis

N. femoralis

N. cutaneus femoris lateralis

N. obturatorius

Rr. cutanei anteriores

M. psoas major

M. iliacus

N. femoralis

R. posterior ⎫
⎬ N. obturatorius
R. anterior ⎭

N. saphenus

Membrana vastoadductoria

N. saphenus

R. infrapatellaris

Fig. 1109   Femoral and obturator nerve, Nn. femoralis et obturatorius;
overview;
cutaneous innervation illustrated with purple.

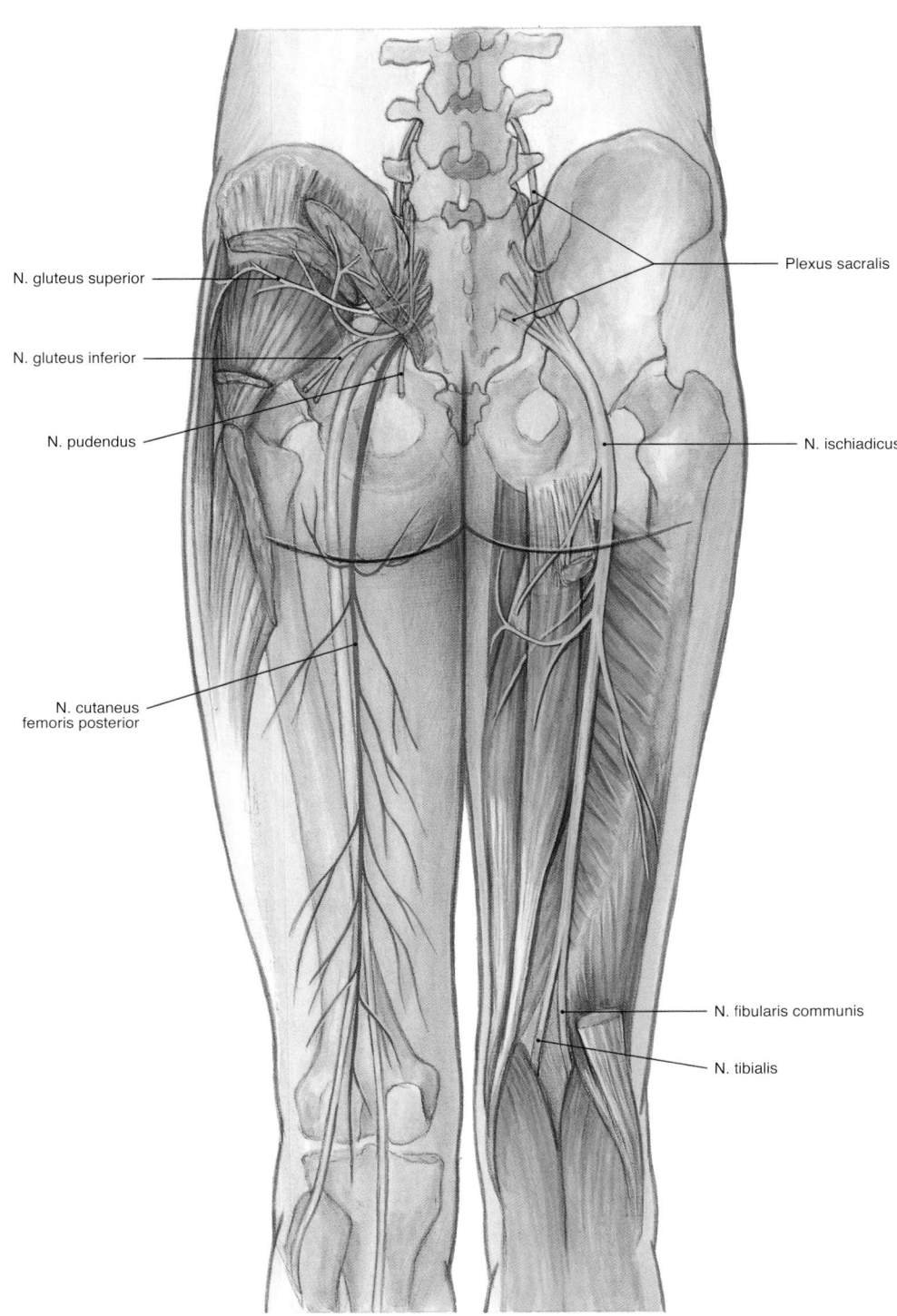

N. gluteus superior

N. gluteus inferior

N. pudendus

N. cutaneus
femoris posterior

Plexus sacralis

N. ischiadicus

N. fibularis communis

N. tibialis

Fig. 1110   Gluteal nerves, Nn. glutei, and sciatic nerve, N. ischiadicus;
overview;
cutaneous innervation illustrated with purple.

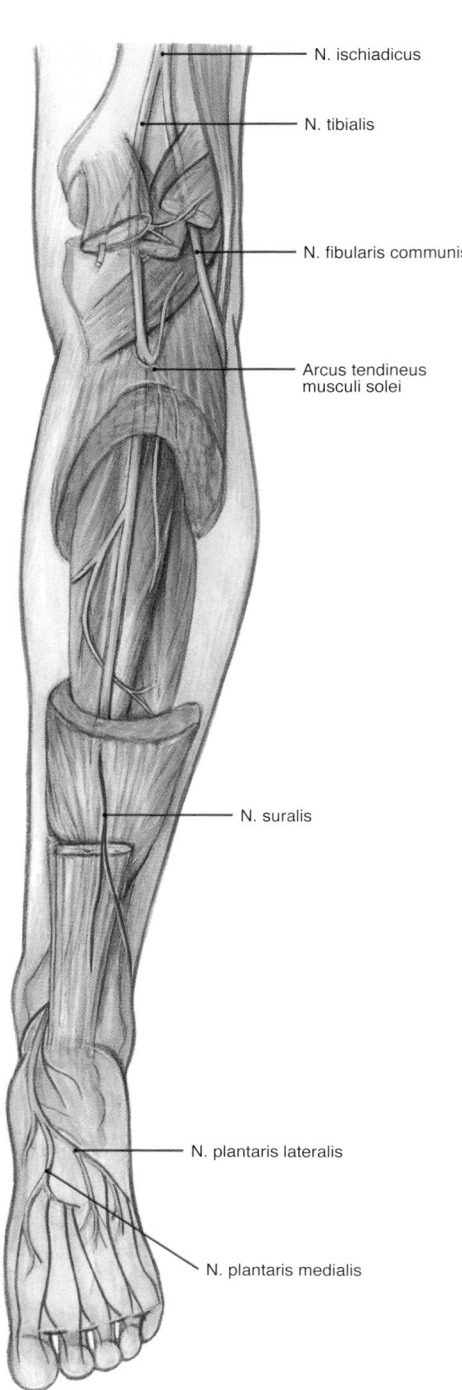

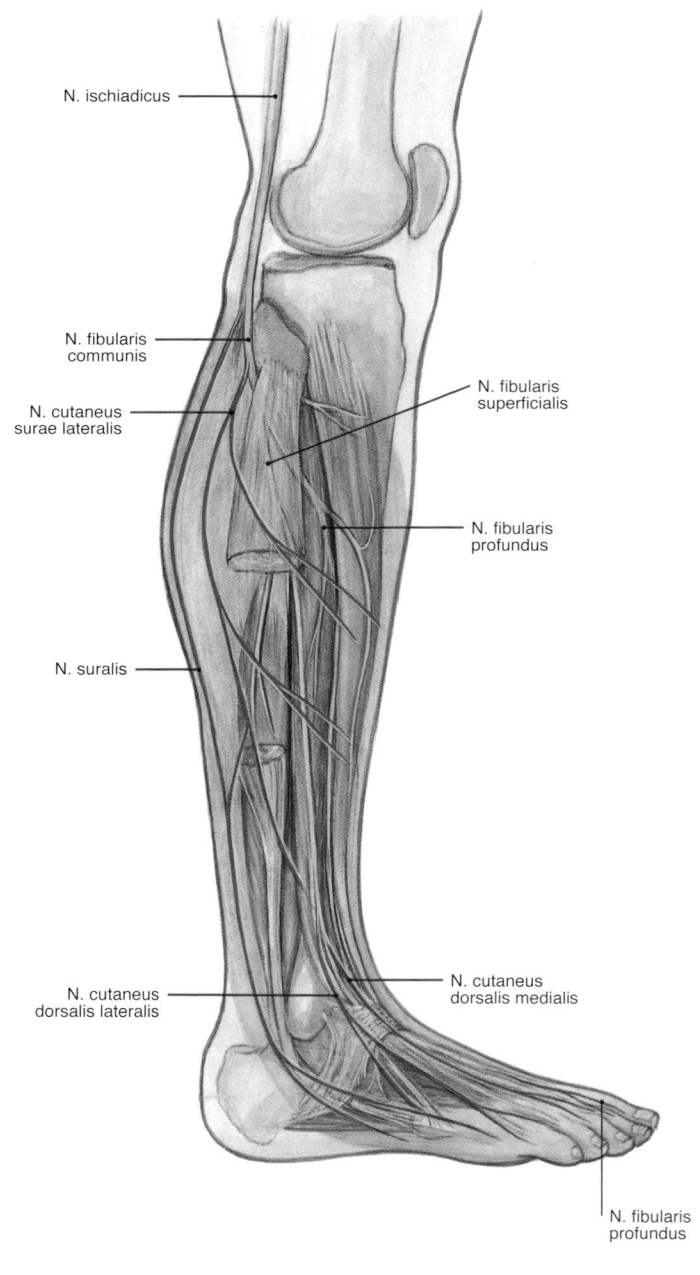

Fig. 1111 Tibial nerve, N. tibialis; overview; cutaneous innervation illustrated with purple.

Fig. 1112 Fibular nerve, N. fibularis; overview; cutaneous innervation illustrated with purple.

Arteries of the lower limb

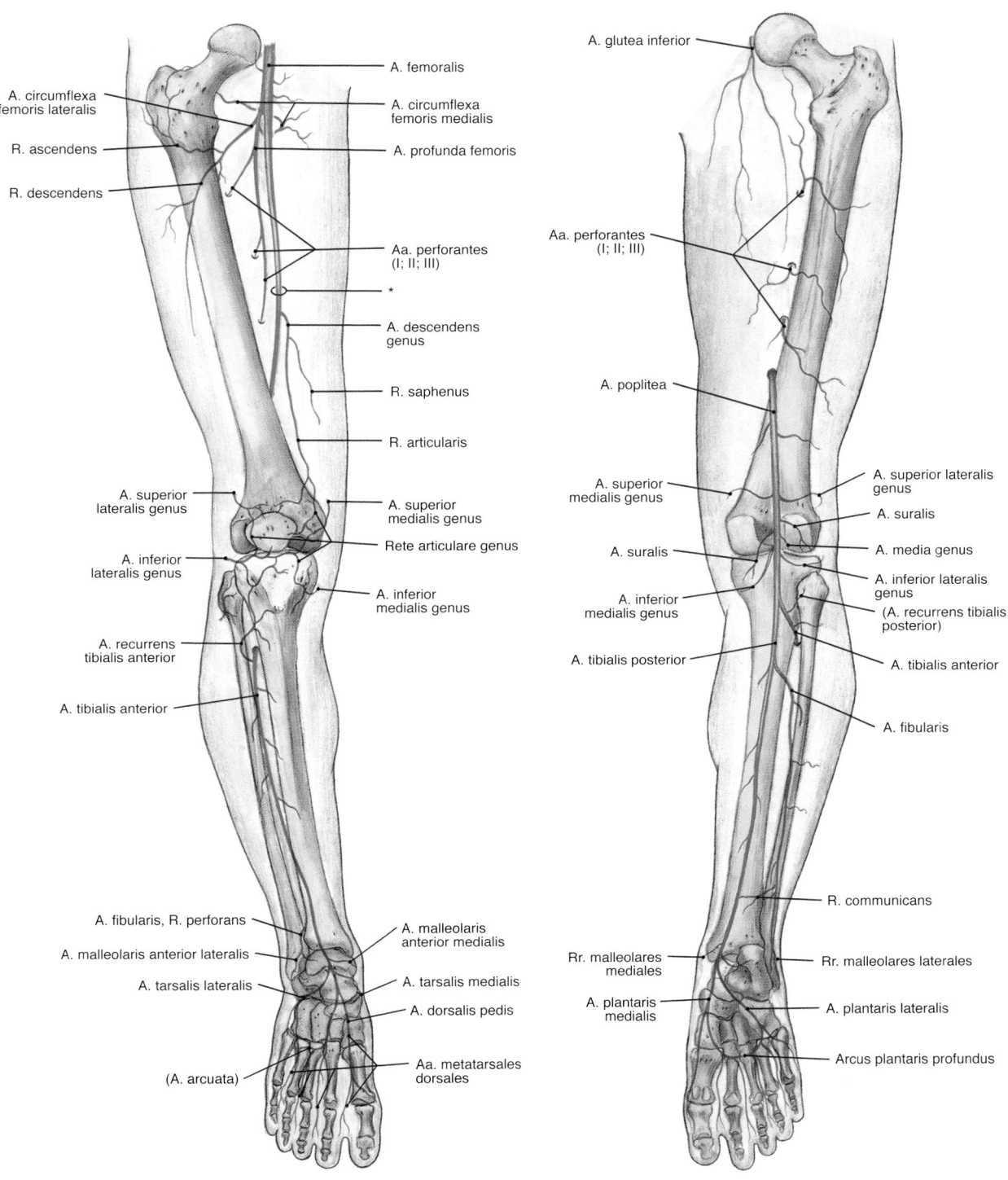

A. circumflexa
femoris lateralis
R. ascendens
R. descendens

A. femoralis
A. circumflexa
femoris medialis
A. profunda femoris

Aa. perforantes
(I; II; III)
*

A. descendens
genus
R. saphenus

R. articularis

A. superior
lateralis genus
A. inferior
lateralis genus

A. superior
medialis genus
Rete articulare genus

A. inferior
medialis genus

A. recurrens
tibialis anterior

A. tibialis anterior

A. fibularis, R. perforans
A. malleolaris anterior lateralis
A. tarsalis lateralis

(A. arcuata)

A. malleolaris
anterior medialis
A. tarsalis medialis
A. dorsalis pedis
Aa. metatarsales
dorsales

A. glutea inferior

Aa. perforantes
(I; II; III)

A. poplitea

A. superior
medialis genus

A. suralis

A. inferior
medialis genus

A. tibialis posterior

A. superior lateralis
genus
A. suralis
A. media genus
A. inferior lateralis
genus
(A. recurrens tibialis
posterior)
A. tibialis anterior

A. fibularis

R. communicans

Rr. malleolares
mediales
A. plantaris
medialis

Rr. malleolares laterales

A. plantaris lateralis

Arcus plantaris profundus

Fig. 1113 Arteries of the lower limb;
overview;
ventral view.
The segment of the femoral artery between the point where
the deep artery of thigh branches off and the point of entry
into the adductor canal (*) is known clinically as superficial
femoral artery.

Fig. 1114 Arteries of the lower limb;
overview;
dorsal view.

Veins and lymphatics of the lower limb

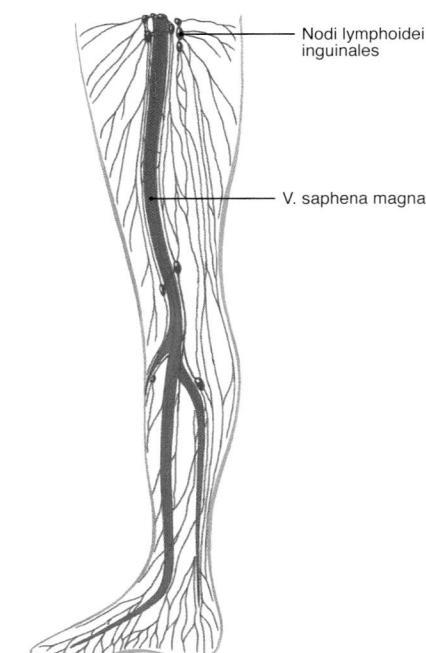

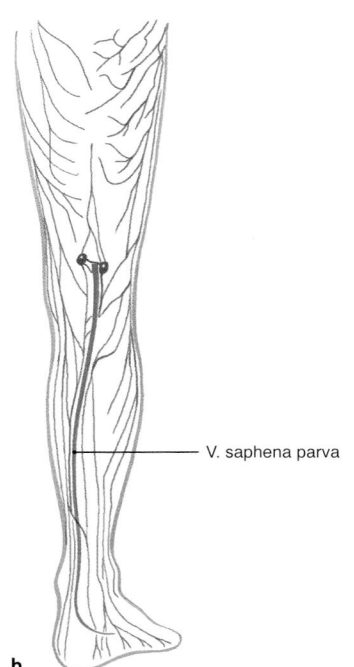

Fig. 1115 a, b Veins and lymphatics of the lower limb; overview.

a Medial view
b Dorsal view

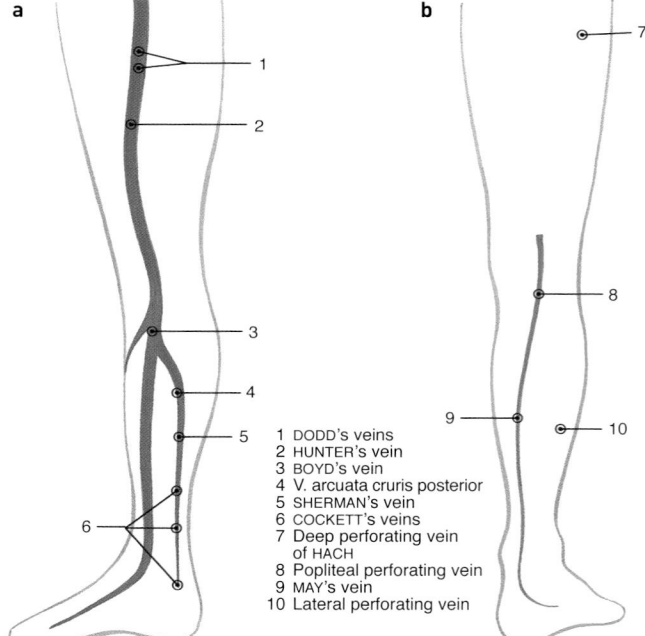

1 DODD's veins
2 HUNTER's vein
3 BOYD's vein
4 V. arcuata cruris posterior
5 SHERMAN's vein
6 COCKETT's veins
7 Deep perforating vein of HACH
8 Popliteal perforating vein
9 MAY's vein
10 Lateral perforating vein

Fig. 1116 a, b Perforating veins, Vv. perforantes; overview (according to HACH, 1986).
a Medial view
b Dorsal view

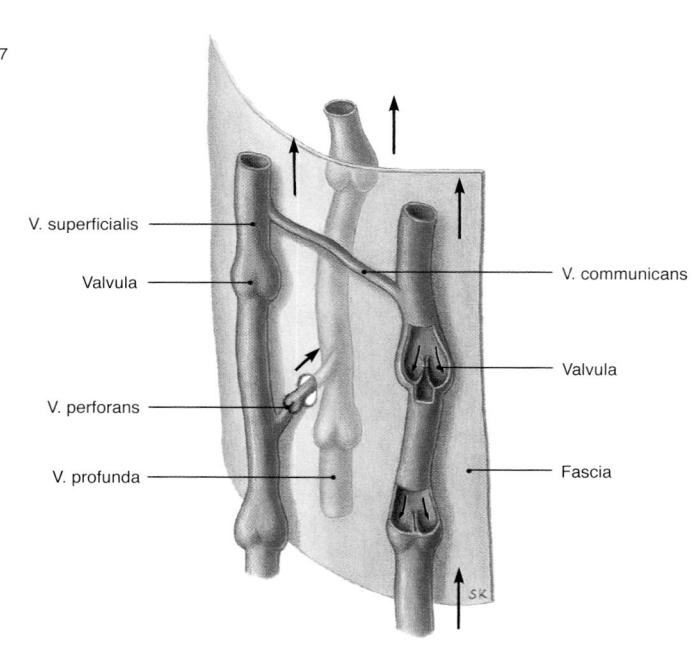

Fig. 1117 Veins of the lower limb; principle of organisation.
Disturbances of the venous flow of the lower limb, especially varicosis, are a common cause of vascular disorders.
If one of the venous systems is entirely occluded, the perforating veins may be of crucial importance to maintain the venous drainage.

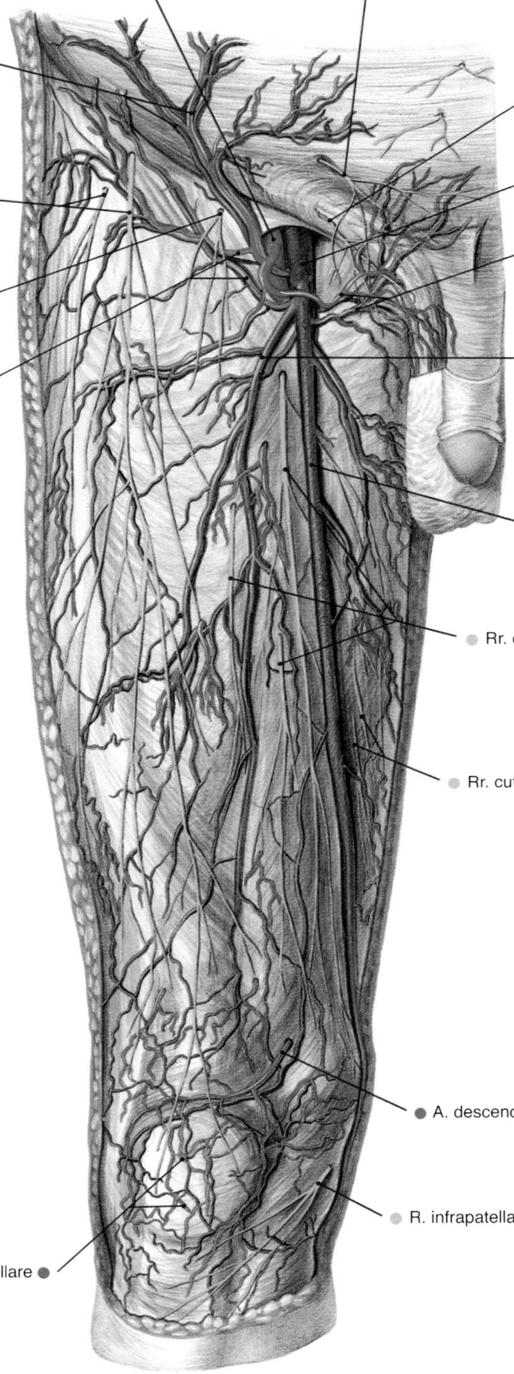

Vessels and nerves of the thigh

A. femoralis

R. cutaneus anterior (N. iliohypogastricus)

A.; V. epigastrica superficialis

N. ilioinguinalis

N. cutaneus femoris lateralis

V. femoralis

R. femoralis (N. genitofemoralis)

Aa.; Vv. pudendae externae

A.; V. circumflexa ilium superficialis

V. saphena accessoria (lateralis)

V. saphena magna

Rr. cutanei anteriores (N. femoralis)

Rr. cutanei (N. obturatorius)

A. descendens genus

R. infrapatellaris (N. saphenus)

Rete patellare

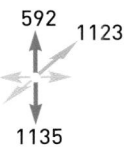

592   1123

1135

Fig. 1118 Epifascial vessels and nerves of the inguinal region, Regio inguinalis, the anterior region of thigh, Regio femoris anterior, and the anterior region of knee, Regio genus anterior.

Lymphatics of the inguinal region

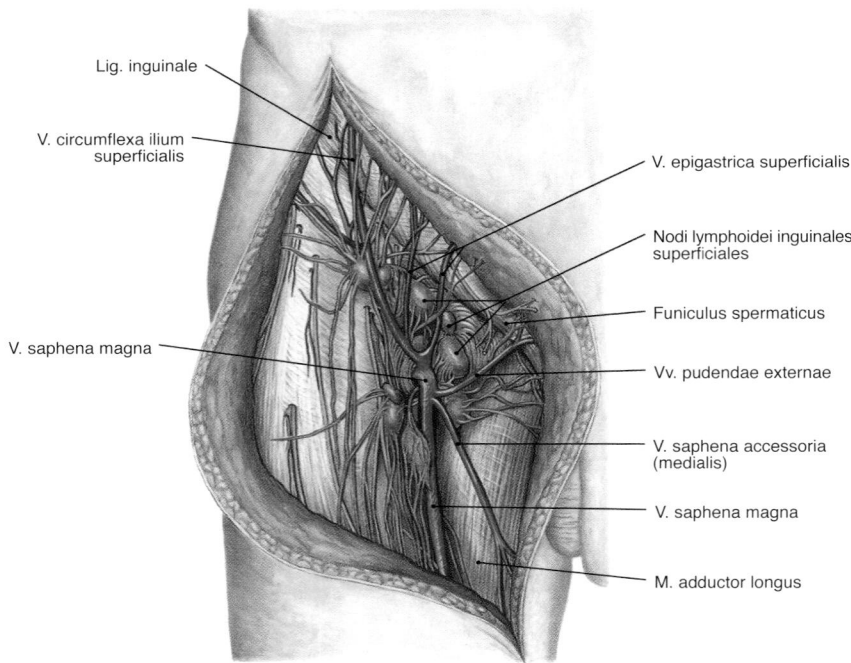

Lig. inguinale

V. circumflexa ilium superficialis

V. saphena magna

V. epigastrica superficialis

Nodi lymphoidei inguinales superficiales

Funiculus spermaticus

Vv. pudendae externae

V. saphena accessoria (medialis)

V. saphena magna

M. adductor longus

Fig. 1119 Superficial lymphatics, lymph nodes and major veins of the inguinal region, Regio inguinalis.

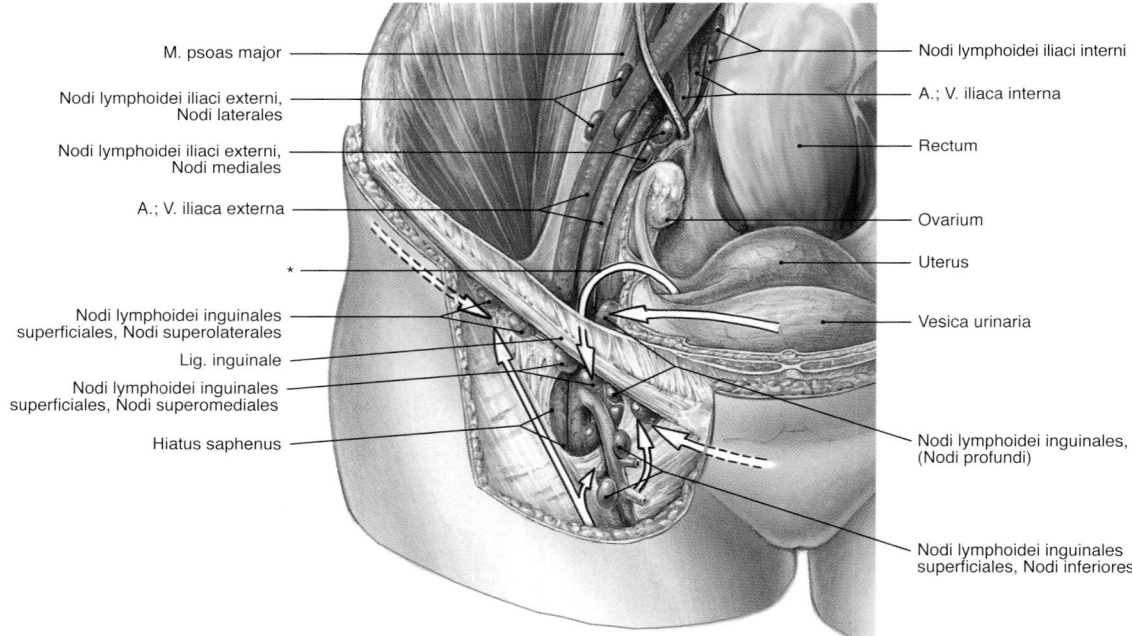

M. psoas major

Nodi lymphoidei iliaci externi, Nodi laterales

Nodi lymphoidei iliaci externi, Nodi mediales

A.; V. iliaca externa

*

Nodi lymphoidei inguinales superficiales, Nodi superolaterales

Lig. inguinale

Nodi lymphoidei inguinales superficiales, Nodi superomediales

Hiatus saphenus

Nodi lymphoidei iliaci interni

A.; V. iliaca interna

Rectum

Ovarium

Uterus

Vesica urinaria

Nodi lymphoidei inguinales, (Nodi profundi)

Nodi lymphoidei inguinales superficiales, Nodi inferiores

Fig. 1120 Draining areas of the lymph nodes in the inguinal region, Regio inguinalis, of the female; overview.
The arrows indicate possible directions of the flow of lymph.

* In some rare cases, the medial parts of the uterine tube and the fundus of the uterus may be drained by superficial lymph nodes in the inguinal region via the round ligament of uterus.

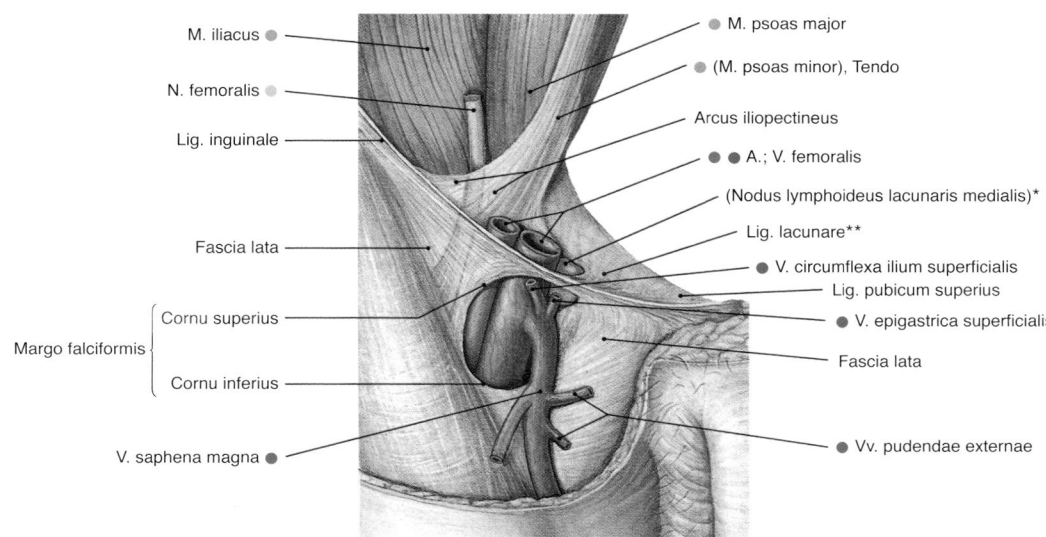

M. iliacus ●
N. femoralis ●
Lig. inguinale
Fascia lata
Margo falciformis { Cornu superius
Cornu inferius
V. saphena magna ●

● M. psoas major
● (M. psoas minor), Tendo
Arcus iliopectineus
● ● A.; V. femoralis
(Nodus lymphoideus lacunaris medialis)*
Lig. lacunare**
● V. circumflexa ilium superficialis
Lig. pubicum superius
● V. epigastrica superficialis
Fascia lata
● Vv. pudendae externae

Fig. 1121   Saphenous opening, Hiatus saphenus,
and vascular space, Lacuna vasorum;
after removal of the anterior abdominal wall and the
contents of the abdomen, as well as dissection of the
iliac fascia and the femoral septum [CLOQUET].
* Also: ROSENMÜLLER's node
** Also: GIMBERNAT's ligament

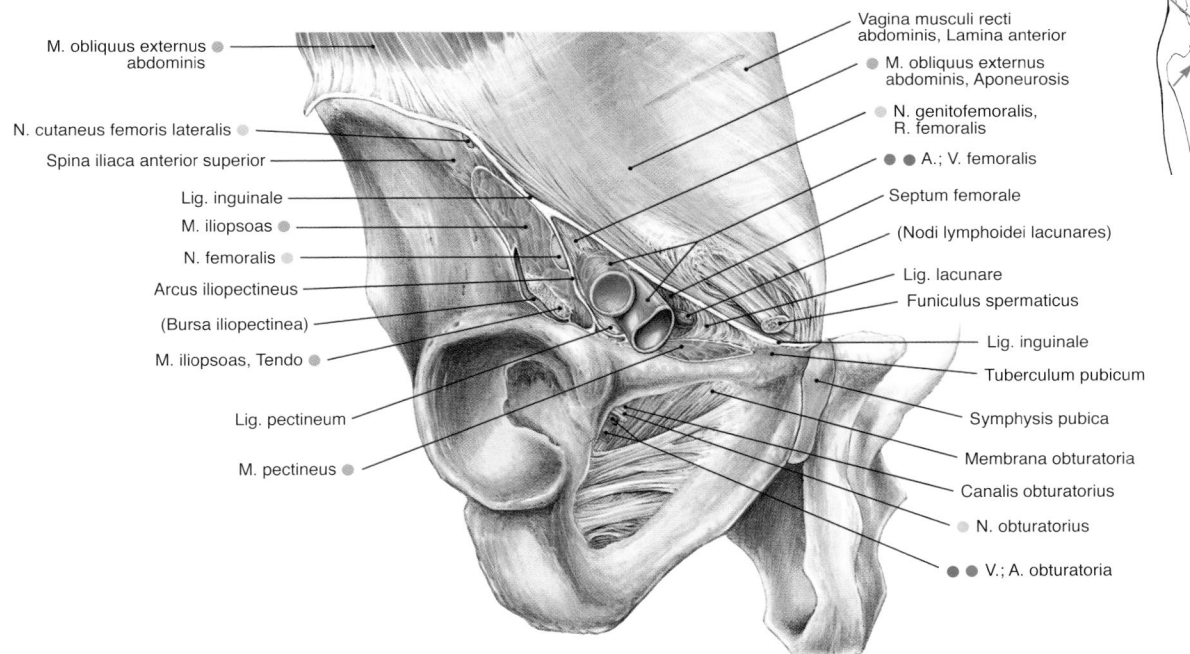

M. obliquus externus ●
abdominis
N. cutaneus femoris lateralis ●
Spina iliaca anterior superior
Lig. inguinale
M. iliopsoas ●
N. femoralis ●
Arcus iliopectineus
(Bursa iliopectinea)
M. iliopsoas, Tendo ●
Lig. pectineum
M. pectineus ●

Vagina musculi recti
abdominis, Lamina anterior
● M. obliquus externus
abdominis, Aponeurosis
● N. genitofemoralis,
R. femoralis
● ● A.; V. femoralis
Septum femorale
(Nodi lymphoidei lacunares)
Lig. lacunare
Funiculus spermaticus
Lig. inguinale
Tuberculum pubicum
Symphysis pubica
Membrana obturatoria
Canalis obturatorius
● N. obturatorius
● ● V.; A. obturatoria

Fig. 1122   Muscular and vascular space,
Lacunae musculorum et vasorum;
oblique section at the level of the inguinal ligament.

Vessels and nerves of the thigh

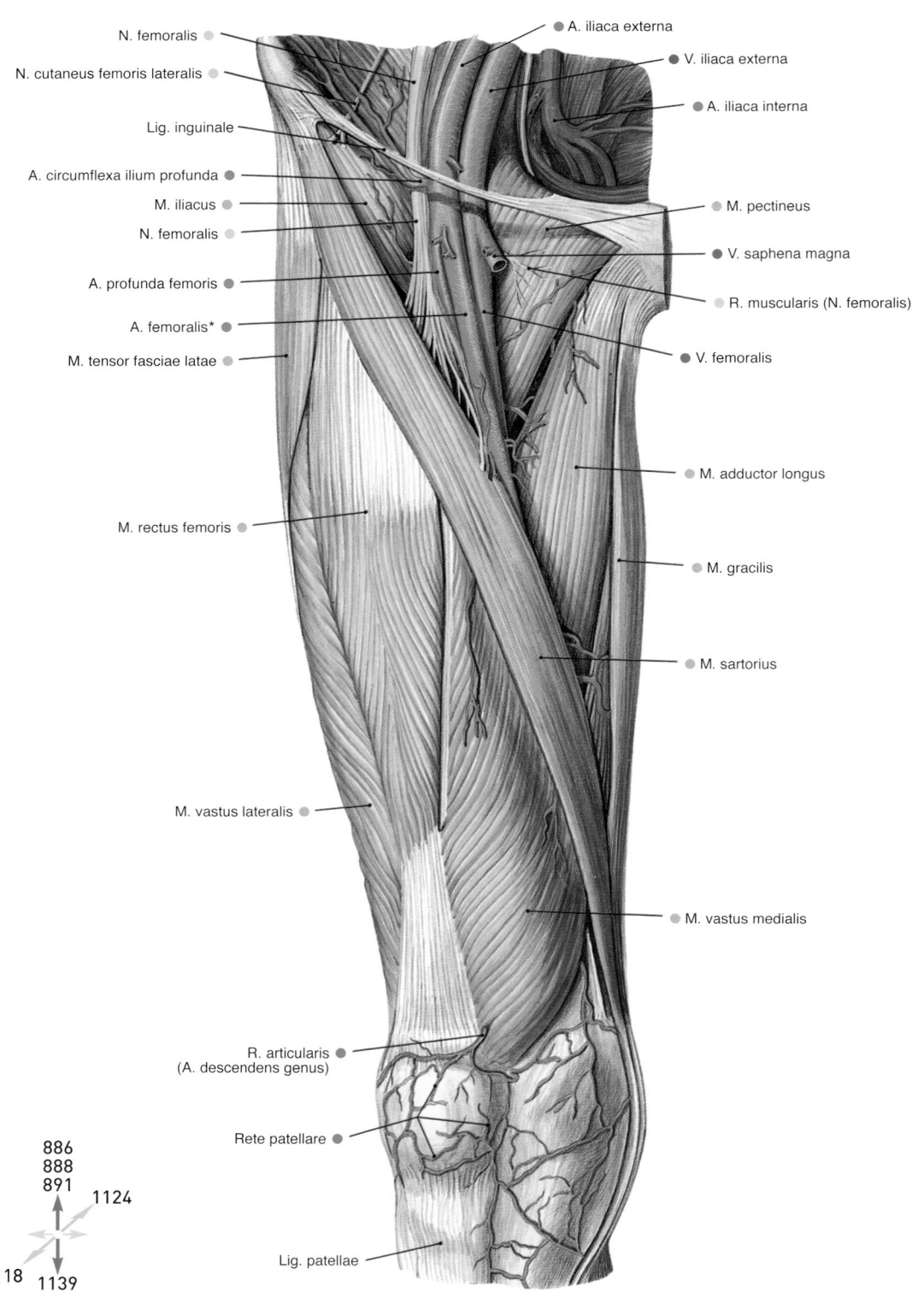

N. femoralis ●
N. cutaneus femoris lateralis ●
Lig. inguinale
A. circumflexa ilium profunda ●
M. iliacus ●
N. femoralis ●
A. profunda femoris ●
A. femoralis* ●
M. tensor fasciae latae ●

M. rectus femoris ●

M. vastus lateralis ●

R. articularis ●
(A. descendens genus)

Rete patellare ●

Lig. patellae

● A. iliaca externa
● V. iliaca externa
● A. iliaca interna

● M. pectineus
● V. saphena magna
● R. muscularis (N. femoralis)
● V. femoralis

● M. adductor longus

● M. gracilis

● M. sartorius

● M. vastus medialis

886
888
891
1124

1118 1139

Fig. 1123 Vessels and nerves of the anterior region of thigh, Regio femoris anterior; after removal of the fascia lata except for the iliotibial tract.

* Clinically the femoral artery is commonly referred to as superficial femoral artery to distinguish it from the deep artery of thigh.

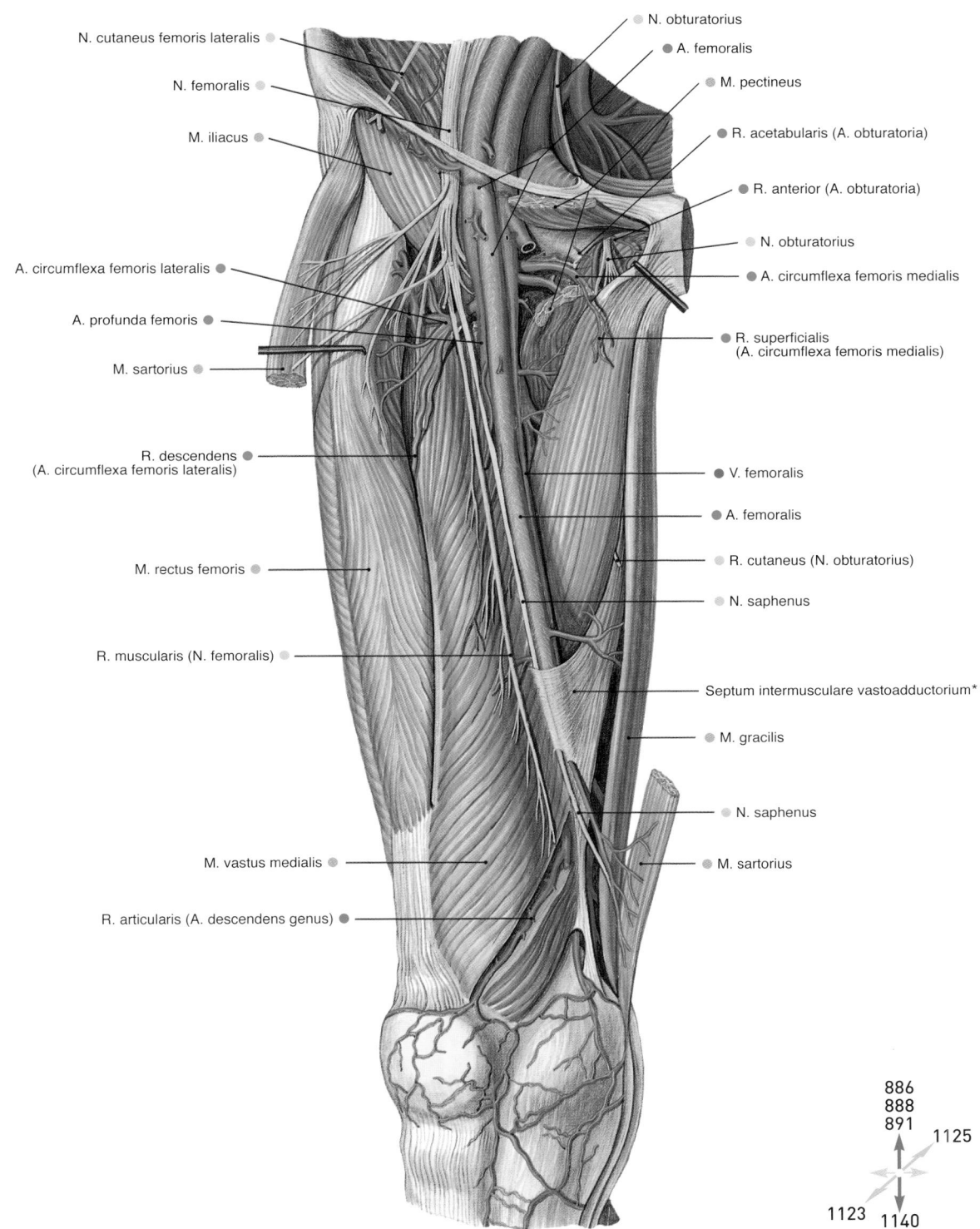

N. cutaneus femoris lateralis

N. femoralis

M. iliacus

A. circumflexa femoris lateralis

A. profunda femoris

M. sartorius

R. descendens
(A. circumflexa femoris lateralis)

M. rectus femoris

R. muscularis (N. femoralis)

M. vastus medialis

R. articularis (A. descendens genus)

N. obturatorius

A. femoralis

M. pectineus

R. acetabularis (A. obturatoria)

R. anterior (A. obturatoria)

N. obturatorius

A. circumflexa femoris medialis

R. superficialis
(A. circumflexa femoris medialis)

V. femoralis

A. femoralis

R. cutaneus (N. obturatorius)

N. saphenus

Septum intermusculare vastoadductorium*

M. gracilis

N. saphenus

M. sartorius

886
888
891
1123   1140   1125

Fig. 1124 Vessels and nerves of the anterior region of thigh,
Regio femoris anterior;
after partial removal of the sartorius muscle and dissection of
the pectineus muscle.

* The entrance into the adductor canal is formed by the vastus medialis
and adductor longus muscles as well as by the anteromedial
intermuscular septum spanning between them.

Vessels and nerves of the thigh

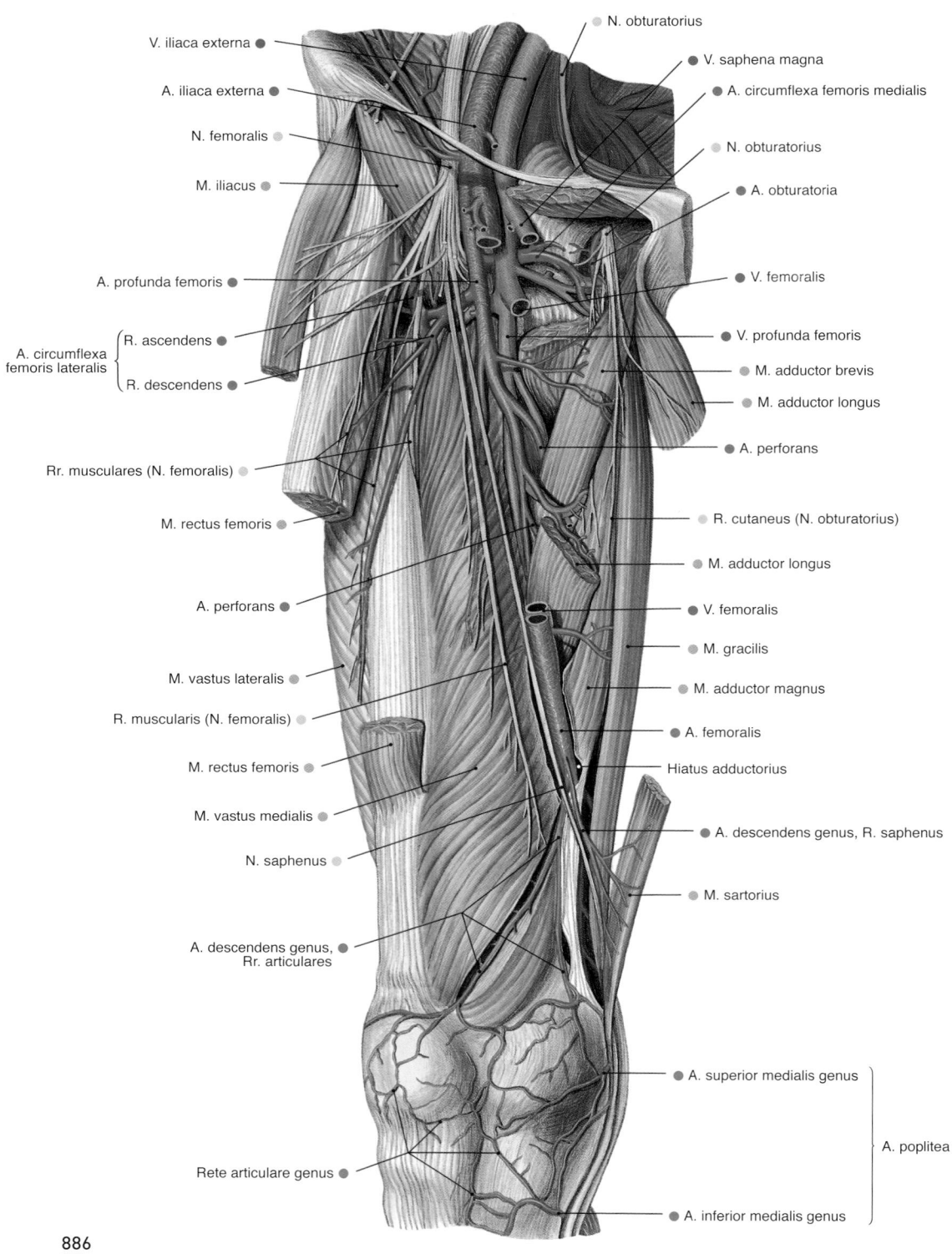

- V. iliaca externa
- A. iliaca externa
- N. femoralis
- M. iliacus

- A. profunda femoris

A. circumflexa femoris lateralis
{ R. ascendens
R. descendens }

- Rr. musculares (N. femoralis)

- M. rectus femoris

- A. perforans

- M. vastus lateralis
- R. muscularis (N. femoralis)

- M. rectus femoris

- M. vastus medialis

- N. saphenus

A. descendens genus, Rr. articulares

Rete articulare genus

- N. obturatorius
- V. saphena magna
- A. circumflexa femoris medialis
- N. obturatorius
- A. obturatoria

- V. femoralis

- V. profunda femoris
- M. adductor brevis
- M. adductor longus

- A. perforans

- R. cutaneus (N. obturatorius)

- M. adductor longus

- V. femoralis

- M. gracilis

- M. adductor magnus

- A. femoralis

Hiatus adductorius

- A. descendens genus, R. saphenus

- M. sartorius

- A. superior medialis genus

A. poplitea

- A. inferior medialis genus

886
888
891

1124 1140

Fig. 1125 Vessels and nerves of the anterior region of thigh,
Regio femoris anterior;
deep layer after partial removal of the sartorius and rectus femoris
muscles, the pectineus and adductor longus muscles have been
dissected; the adductor canal is almost entirely opened.

Arteries of the pelvis and the hip

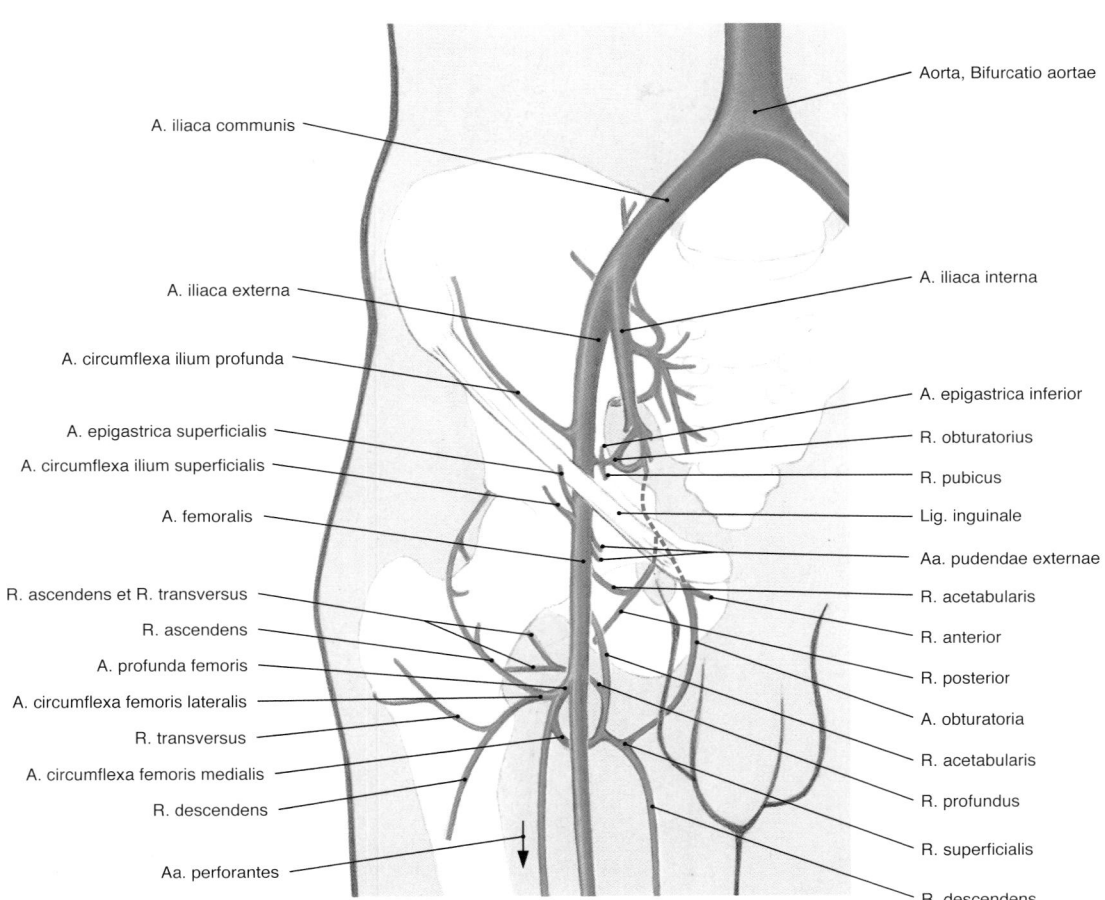

Aorta, Bifurcatio aortae

A. iliaca communis

A. iliaca externa

A. circumflexa ilium profunda

A. epigastrica superficialis

A. circumflexa ilium superficialis

A. femoralis

R. ascendens et R. transversus

R. ascendens

A. profunda femoris

A. circumflexa femoris lateralis

R. transversus

A. circumflexa femoris medialis

R. descendens

Aa. perforantes

A. iliaca interna

A. epigastrica inferior

R. obturatorius

R. pubicus

Lig. inguinale

Aa. pudendae externae

R. acetabularis

R. anterior

R. posterior

A. obturatoria

R. acetabularis

R. profundus

R. superficialis

R. descendens

Fig. 1126   Arteries of the hip and the thigh;
overview.

The branching pattern of these arteries varies considerably.
This type of origin and arborisation of the deep artery of thigh
occurs in approximately 58% of cases.

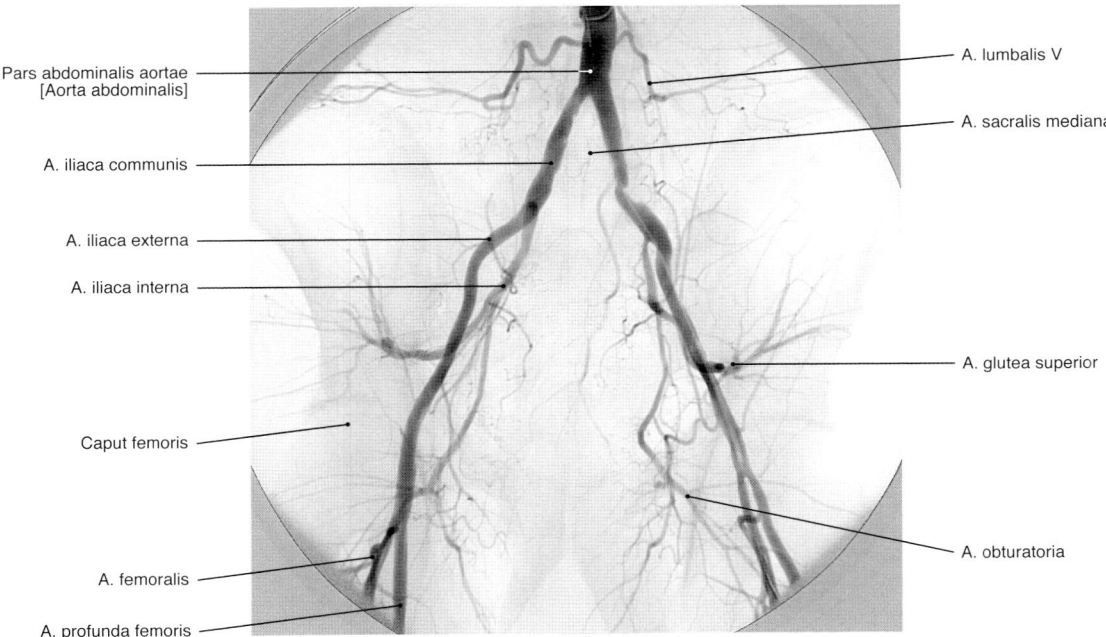

Pars abdominalis aortae
[Aorta abdominalis]

A. iliaca communis

A. iliaca externa

A. iliaca interna

Caput femoris

A. femoralis

A. profunda femoris

A. lumbalis V

A. sacralis mediana

A. glutea superior

A. obturatoria

Fig. 1127   Arteries of the pelvis and the thigh;
digital subtraction angiography (DSA).

Veins and nerves of the thigh

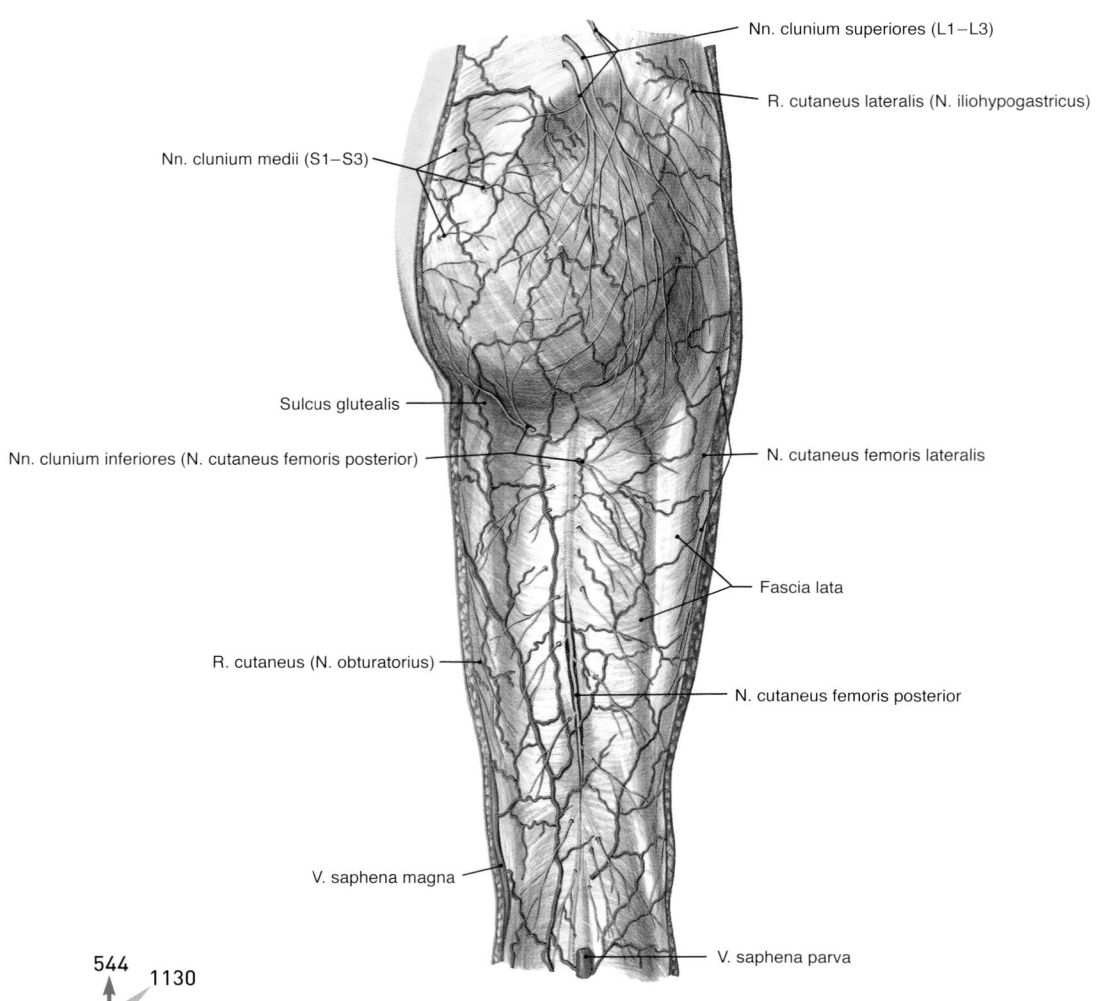

Nn. clunium superiores (L1–L3)

R. cutaneus lateralis (N. iliohypogastricus)

Nn. clunium medii (S1–S3)

Sulcus glutealis

Nn. clunium inferiores (N. cutaneus femoris posterior)

N. cutaneus femoris lateralis

Fascia lata

R. cutaneus (N. obturatorius)

N. cutaneus femoris posterior

V. saphena magna

V. saphena parva

544
1130

1136

Fig. 1128   Epifascial veins and nerves of the posterior region
of thigh, Regio femoris posterior, the gluteal region,
Regio glutealis, and the popliteal fossa, Fossa poplitea.

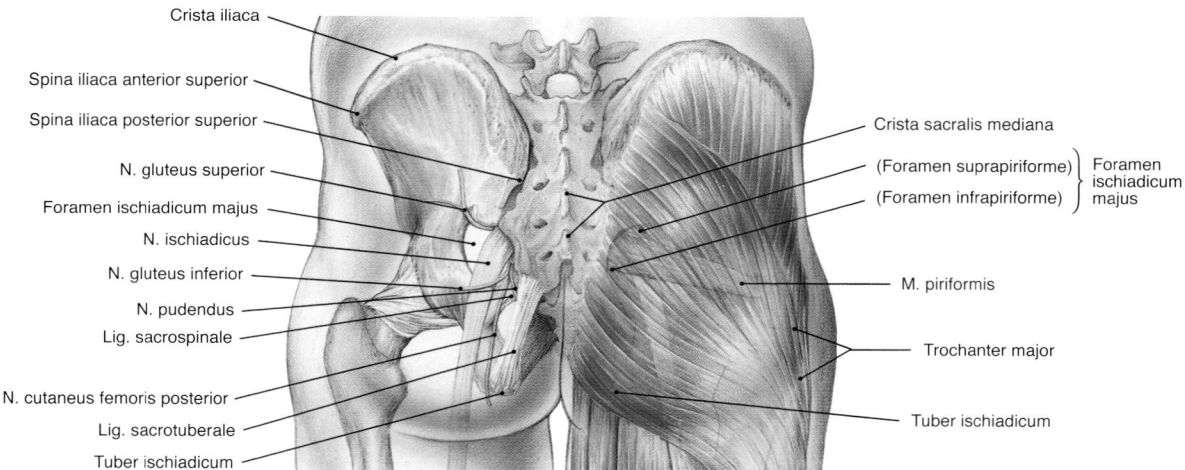

Crista iliaca

Spina iliaca anterior superior

Spina iliaca posterior superior

N. gluteus superior

Foramen ischiadicum majus

N. ischiadicus

N. gluteus inferior

N. pudendus

Lig. sacrospinale

N. cutaneus femoris posterior

Lig. sacrotuberale

Tuber ischiadicum

Crista sacralis mediana

(Foramen suprapiriforme) ⎫ Foramen
                          ⎬ ischiadicum
(Foramen infrapiriforme) ⎭ majus

M. piriformis

Trochanter major

Tuber ischiadicum

Fig. 1129   Skeleton contour and sciatic nerve,
N. ischiadicus, projected onto the surface of the
gluteal region, Regio glutealis.

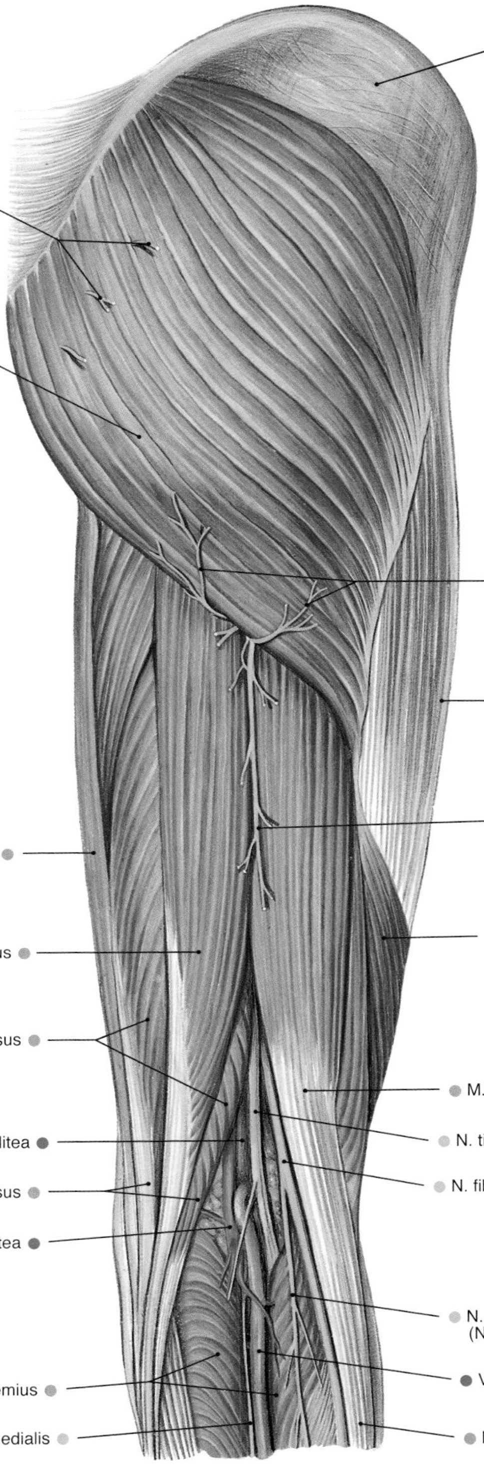

Vessels and nerves of the thigh

M. gluteus medius, Fascia

Nn. clunium medii (S1–S3)

M. gluteus maximus

Nn. clunium inferiores
(N. cutaneus femoris posterior)

Tractus iliotibialis

N. cutaneus femoris posterior

M. gracilis

M. vastus lateralis

M. semitendinosus

M. semimembranosus

M. biceps femoris

V. poplitea

N. tibialis

M. semimembranosus

N. fibularis communis

A. poplitea

N. cutaneus surae lateralis
(N. fibularis communis)

V. saphena parva

M. gastrocnemius

N. cutaneus surae medialis

M. biceps femoris, Tendo

Fig. 1130   Vessels and nerves of the gluteal region,
Regio glutealis, the posterior region of thigh, Regio femoris
posterior, and the popliteal fossa, Fossa poplitea.

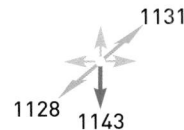

1131

1128   1143

Vessels and nerves of the thigh

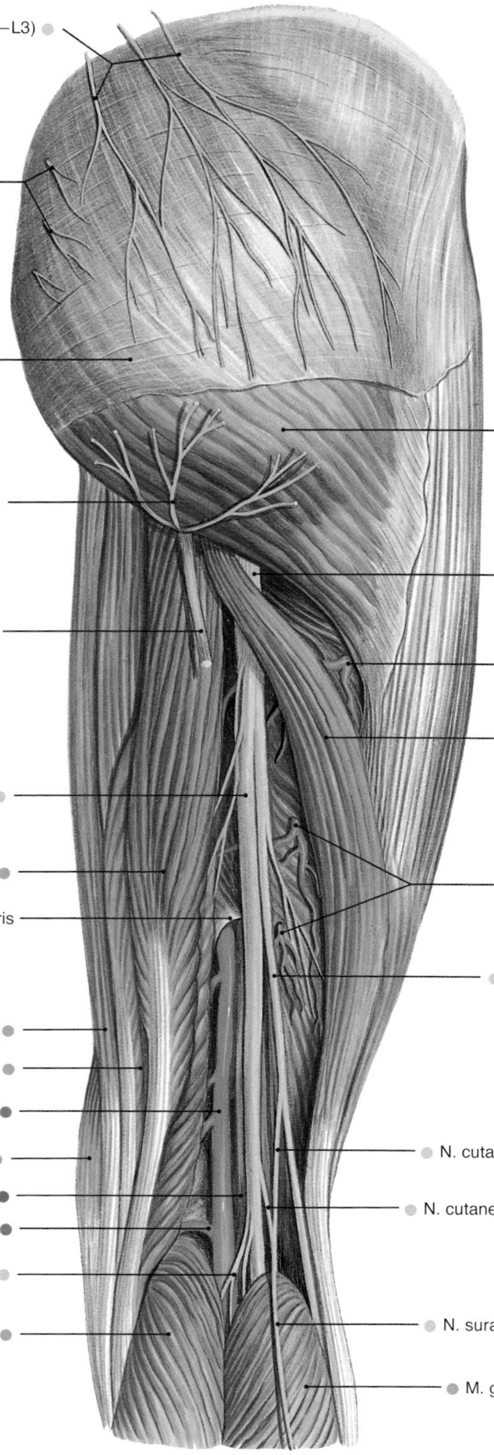

Nn. clunium superiores (L1–L3) ●

Nn. clunium medii (S1–S3) ●

(Fascia glutea)

● M. gluteus maximus

Nn. clunium inferiores ●
(N. cutaneus femoris posterior)

● N. ischiadicus

N. cutaneus femoris posterior ●

● A. perforans

● M. biceps femoris, Caput longum

N. tibialis ●

M. semitendinosus ●

● Aa. perforantes

Hiatus adductoris

● N. fibularis communis

M. gracilis ●

M. semimembranosus ●

A. poplitea ●

● N. cutaneus surae lateralis

M. sartorius ●

V. poplitea ●

● N. cutaneus surae medialis

A. superior medialis genus ●

Rr. musculares (N. tibialis) ●

M. gastrocnemius, ●
Caput mediale

● N. suralis

● M. gastrocnemius, Caput laterale

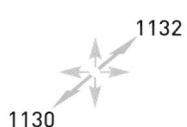

1132

1130

Fig. 1131   Vessels and nerves of the gluteal region, Regio glutealis,
the posterior region of thigh, Regio femoris posterior,
and the popliteal fossa, Fossa poplitea;
the long head of the biceps femoris muscle has been retracted
laterally.
In this specimen, the medial and lateral sural cutaneous nerves branch
off quite far proximally.

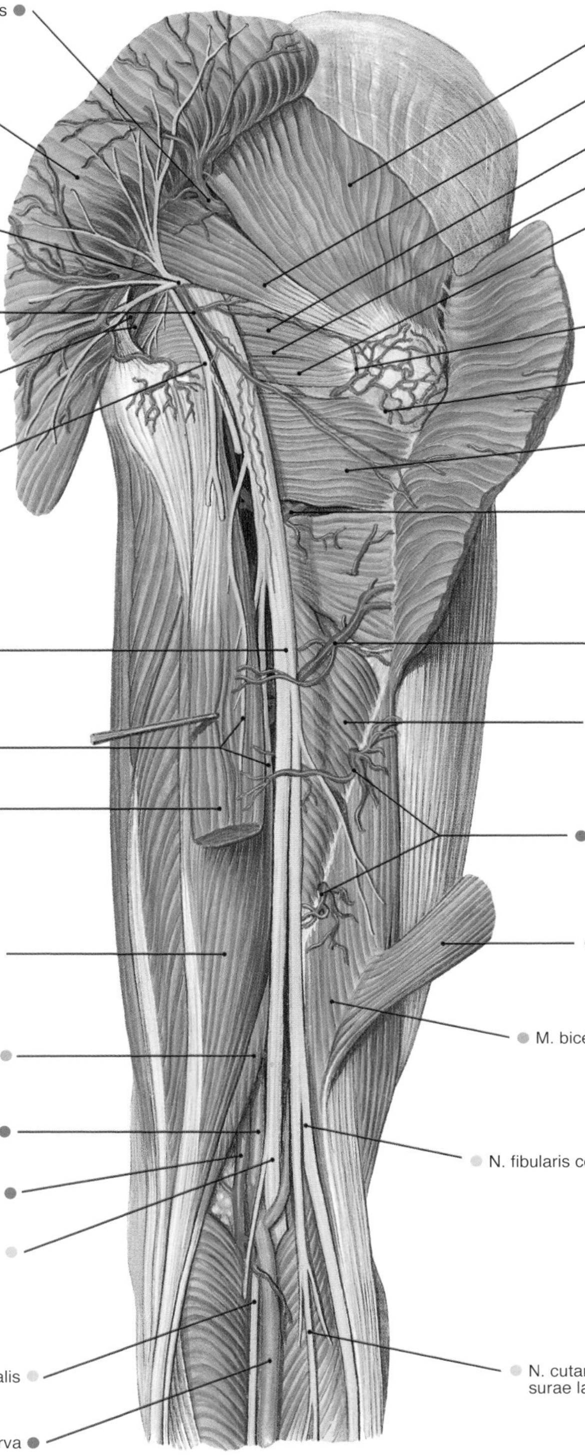

Vessels and nerves of the thigh

A. glutea superior, R. superficialis ●

M. gluteus maximus ●

N. gluteus inferior ●

A. glutea inferior ●

A.; V. pudenda interna ● ●

N. cutaneus femoris posterior ●

N. ischiadicus ●

Rr. musculares (N. tibialis) ●

M. biceps femoris, Caput longum ●

M. semitendinosus ●

M. semimembranosus ●

V. poplitea ●

A. poplitea ●

N. tibialis ●

N. cutaneus surae medialis ●

V. saphena parva ●

● M. gluteus medius

● M. piriformis

● M. gemellus superior

● M. obturatorius internus

● M. gemellus inferior

● R. ascendens (A. circumflexa femoris medialis)

● R. superficialis (A. circumflexa femoris medialis)

● M. quadratus femoris

● R. profundus (A. circumflexa femoris medialis)

● A. perforans

● M. adductor magnus

● Aa. perforantes

● M. biceps femoris, Caput longum

● M. biceps femoris, Caput breve

● N. fibularis communis

● N. cutaneus surae lateralis

Fig. 1132   Vessels and nerves of the gluteal region, Regio glutealis, the posterior region of thigh, Regio femoris posterior, and the popliteal fossa, Fossa poplitea; after dissection of the gluteus maximus muscle and the long head of the biceps femoris muscle.

1131

1143
1145
1146

Vessels and nerves of the gluteal region

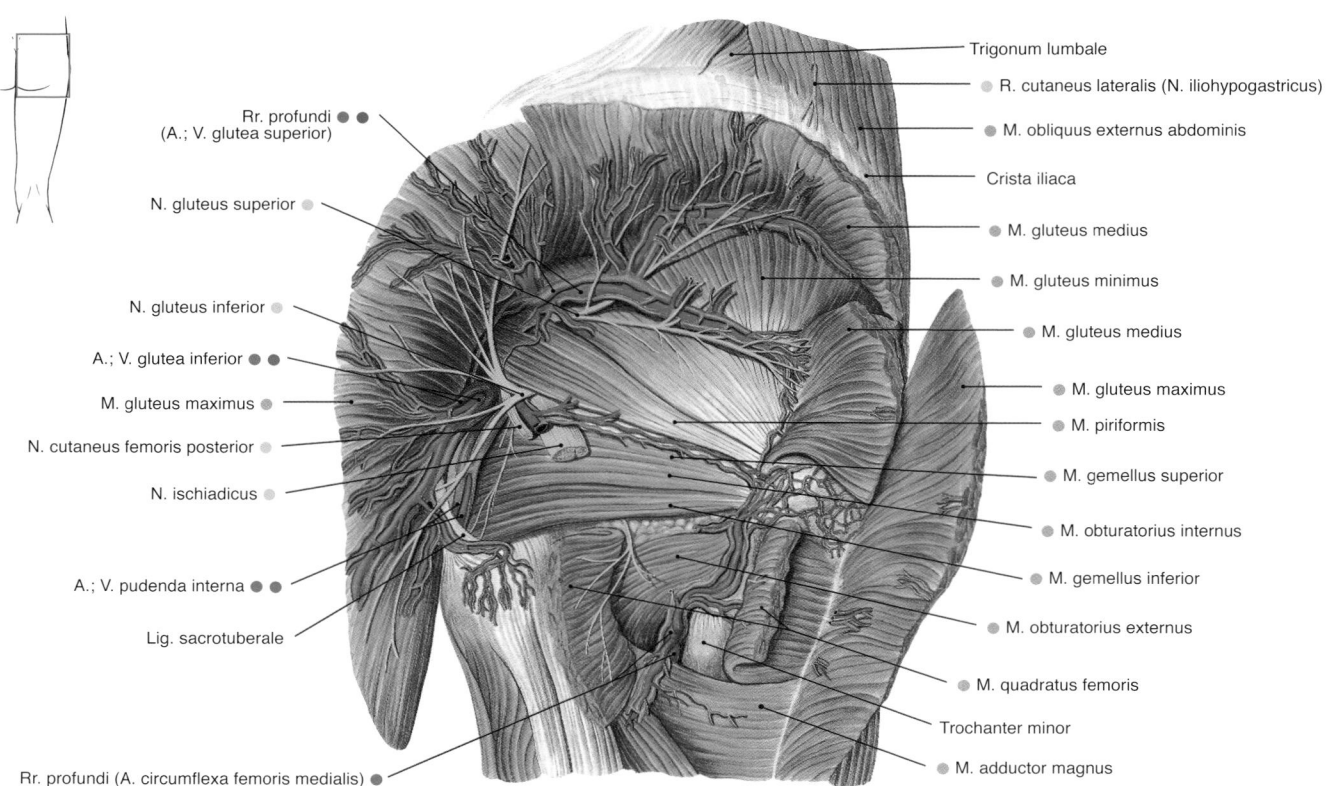

Rr. profundi ●● (A.; V. glutea superior)

N. gluteus superior ○

N. gluteus inferior ○

A.; V. glutea inferior ●●

M. gluteus maximus ○

N. cutaneus femoris posterior ○

N. ischiadicus ○

A.; V. pudenda interna ●●

Lig. sacrotuberale

Rr. profundi (A. circumflexa femoris medialis) ●

Trigonum lumbale

● R. cutaneus lateralis (N. iliohypogastricus)

● M. obliquus externus abdominis

Crista iliaca

● M. gluteus medius

● M. gluteus minimus

● M. gluteus medius

● M. gluteus maximus

● M. piriformis

● M. gemellus superior

● M. obturatorius internus

● M. gemellus inferior

● M. obturatorius externus

● M. quadratus femoris

Trochanter minor

● M. adductor magnus

Fig. 1133   Vessels and nerves of the gluteal region, Regio glutealis;
after dissection and partial removal of the gluteus maximus and medius muscles;
the sciatic nerve has been removed after its passage through the infrapiriform foramen.

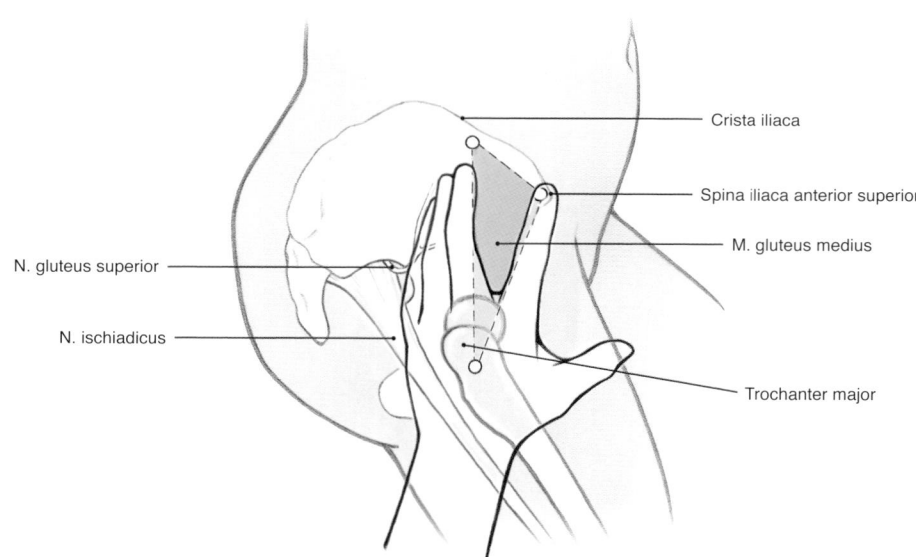

Crista iliaca

Spina iliaca anterior superior

M. gluteus medius

N. gluteus superior

N. ischiadicus

Trochanter major

Fig. 1134   Ventrogluteal injection (according to v. HOCHSTETTER). In order to avoid the superior gluteal nerve and, in particular, the superior gluteal artery the injection is made into the triangular field formed by the two spread fingers and the iliac crest. The index finger – or when using the right hand, the middle finger – is placed on the anterior superior iliac spine and the palm of the hand on the greater trochanter. Since the injected material should be deposited within the belly of the gluteus medius muscle as far away as possible from any vessel, the needle should not cross the lines of the triangle. However, some risk remains for the nerve branch that runs from the superior gluteal nerve to the tensor fasciae latae muscle.

Veins and nerves of the leg

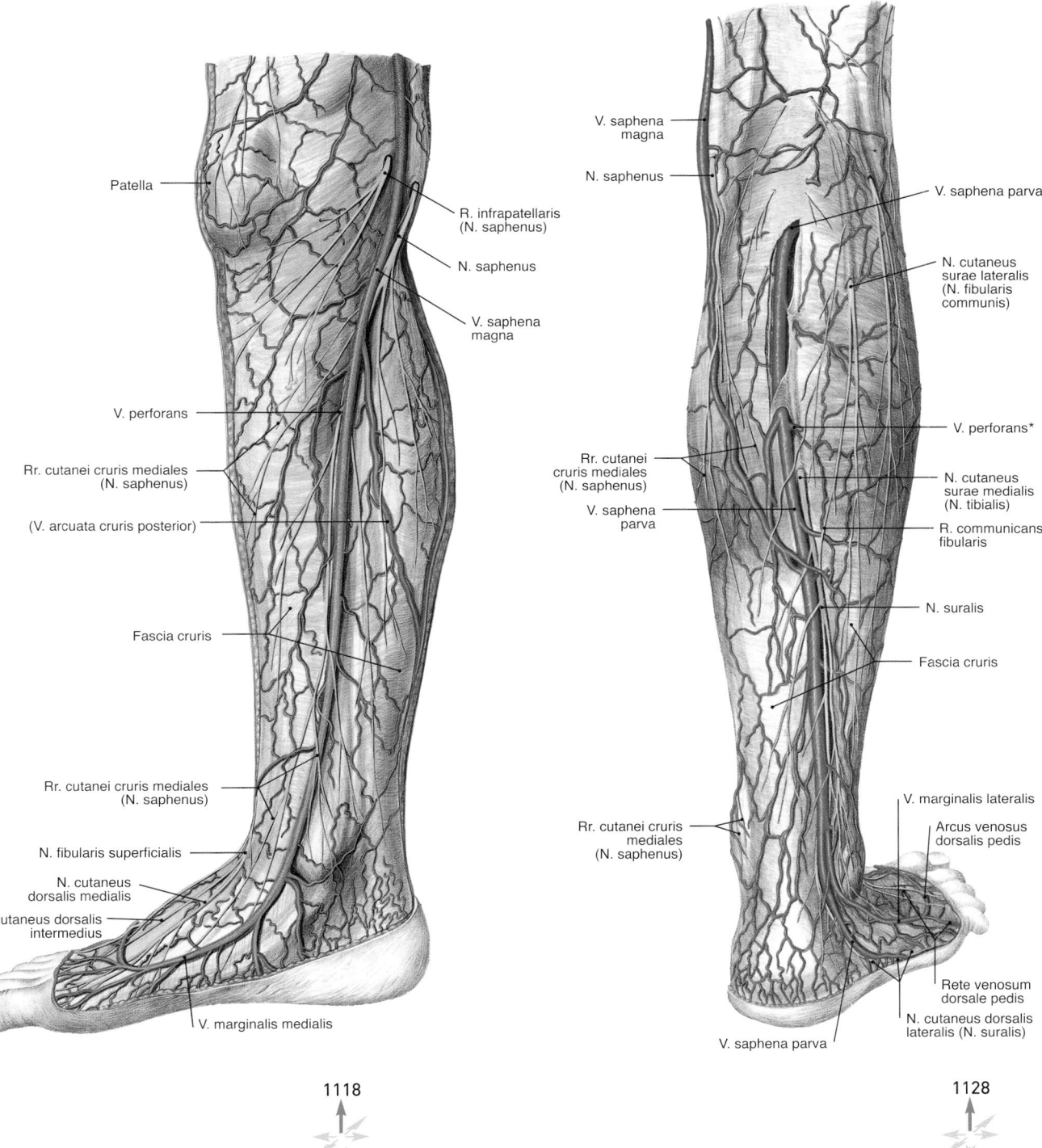

Patella

R. infrapatellaris
(N. saphenus)

N. saphenus

V. saphena
magna

V. perforans

Rr. cutanei cruris mediales
(N. saphenus)

(V. arcuata cruris posterior)

Fascia cruris

Rr. cutanei cruris mediales
(N. saphenus)

N. fibularis superficialis

N. cutaneus
dorsalis medialis

N. cutaneus dorsalis
intermedius

V. marginalis medialis

1118

V. saphena
magna

N. saphenus

V. saphena parva

N. cutaneus
surae lateralis
(N. fibularis
communis)

V. perforans*

Rr. cutanei
cruris mediales
(N. saphenus)

N. cutaneus
surae medialis
(N. tibialis)

V. saphena
parva

R. communicans
fibularis

N. suralis

Fascia cruris

Rr. cutanei cruris
mediales
(N. saphenus)

V. marginalis lateralis

Arcus venosus
dorsalis pedis

Rete venosum
dorsale pedis

N. cutaneus dorsalis
lateralis (N. suralis)

V. saphena parva

1128

Fig. 1135   Epifascial veins and nerves of the leg
and the foot, Regiones cruris et pedis.

Fig. 1136   Epifascial veins and nerves of the leg
and the foot, Regiones cruris et pedis;
the deep fascia of leg has been dissected
proximally.
* Clinical term: MAY's vein

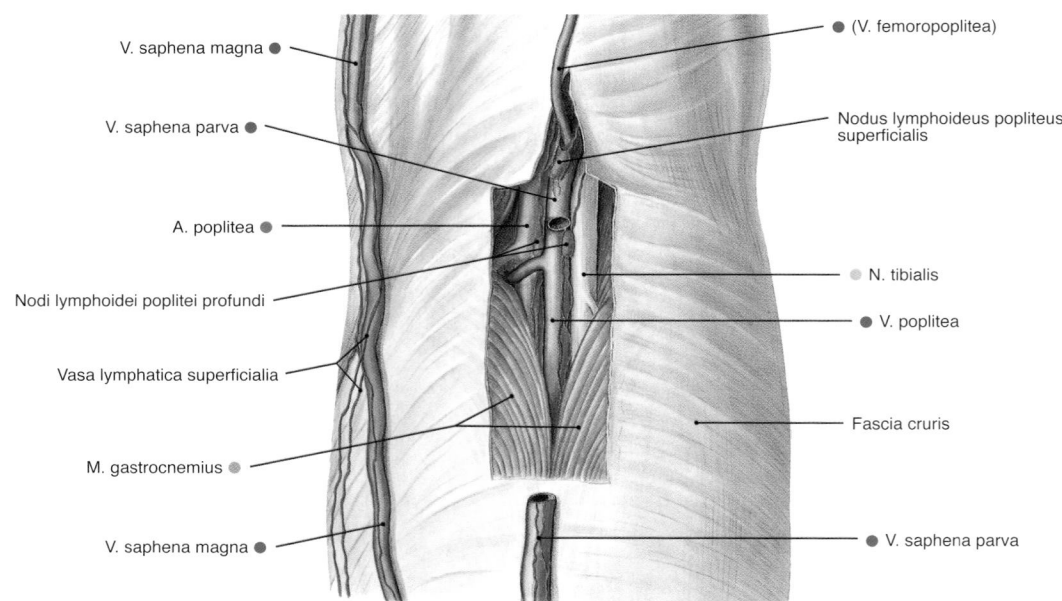

Fig. 1137 Vessels and nerves of the popliteal fossa,
Fossa poplitea;
after dissection of the deep fascia of leg and partial removal
of the small saphenous vein.

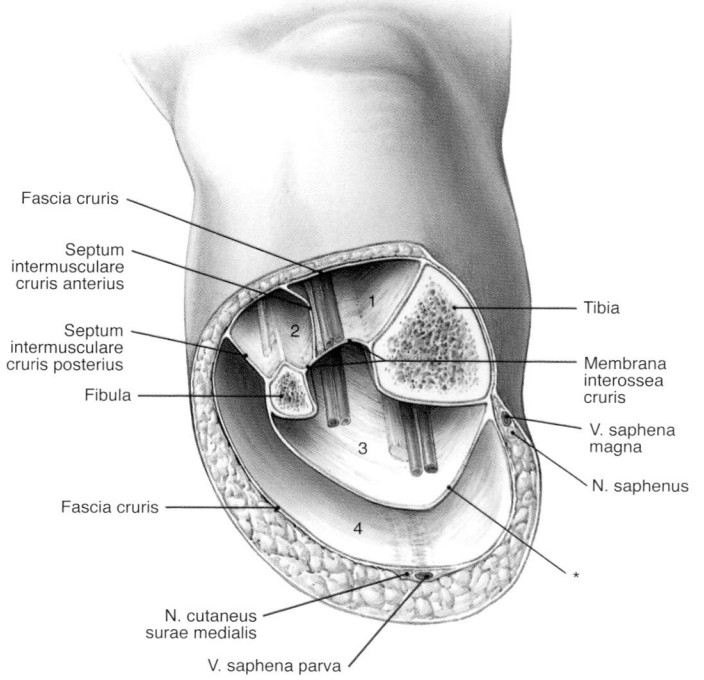

1 **Compartimentum cruris anterius:**
   A.; V. tibialis anterior
   N. fibularis profundus
   M. tibialis anterior
   M. extensor digitorum longus
   M. extensor hallucis longus
   M. fibularis [peroneus] tertius

2 **Compartimentum cruris laterale:**
   N. fibularis superficialis
   M. fibularis [peroneus] longus
   M. fibularis [peroneus] brevis

3 **Compartimentum cruris posterius, Pars profunda:**
   A.; V. tibialis posterior
   A.; V. fibularis
   N. tibialis
   M. flexor digitorum longus
   M. tibialis posterior
   M. flexor hallucis longus

4 **Compartimentum cruris posterius, Pars super-ficialis:**
   M. triceps surae
   M. plantaris

Fig. 1138 Osteofibrous tubes of the leg;
cross-section superior to the middle of the leg.
These osteofibrous tubes together with their contents are
clinically known as compartments.
* Deep part of the deep fascia of leg

→ 1157

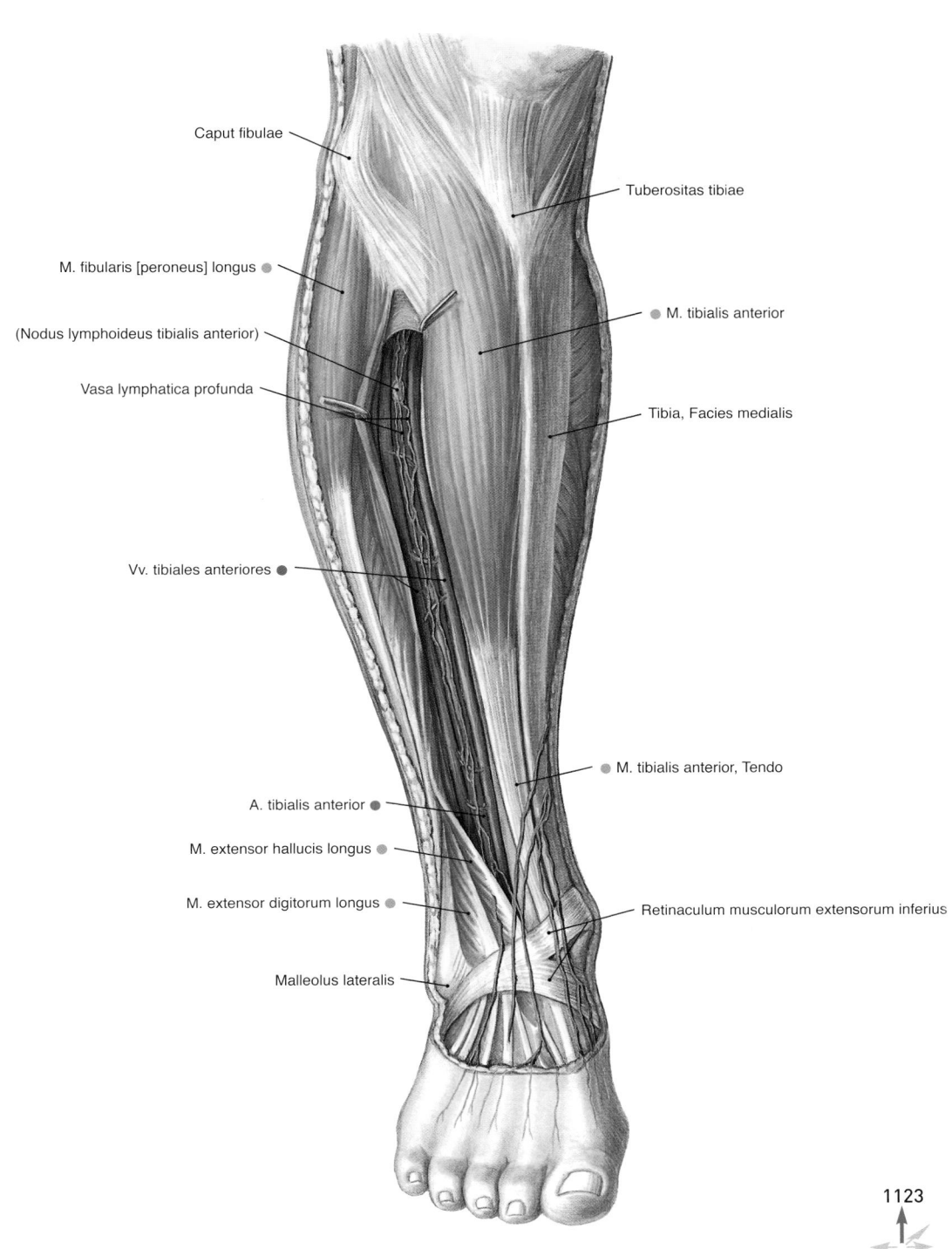

Caput fibulae

Tuberositas tibiae

M. fibularis [peroneus] longus ●

● M. tibialis anterior

(Nodus lymphoideus tibialis anterior)

Vasa lymphatica profunda

Tibia, Facies medialis

Vv. tibiales anteriores ●

M. tibialis anterior, Tendo ●

A. tibialis anterior ●

M. extensor hallucis longus ●

M. extensor digitorum longus ●

Retinaculum musculorum extensorum inferius

Malleolus lateralis

1123

Abb. 1139   Vessels of the anterior region of leg,
Regio cruris anterior;
the extensor muscles spread by retractors.

The superficial lymphatics regularly follow the major epifascial
veins and converge along the great saphenous vein to the
medial side of the leg. The deep lymphatics are found within
the connective tissue sheaths of the deep arteries and veins of
the leg.

Arteries and nerves of the leg

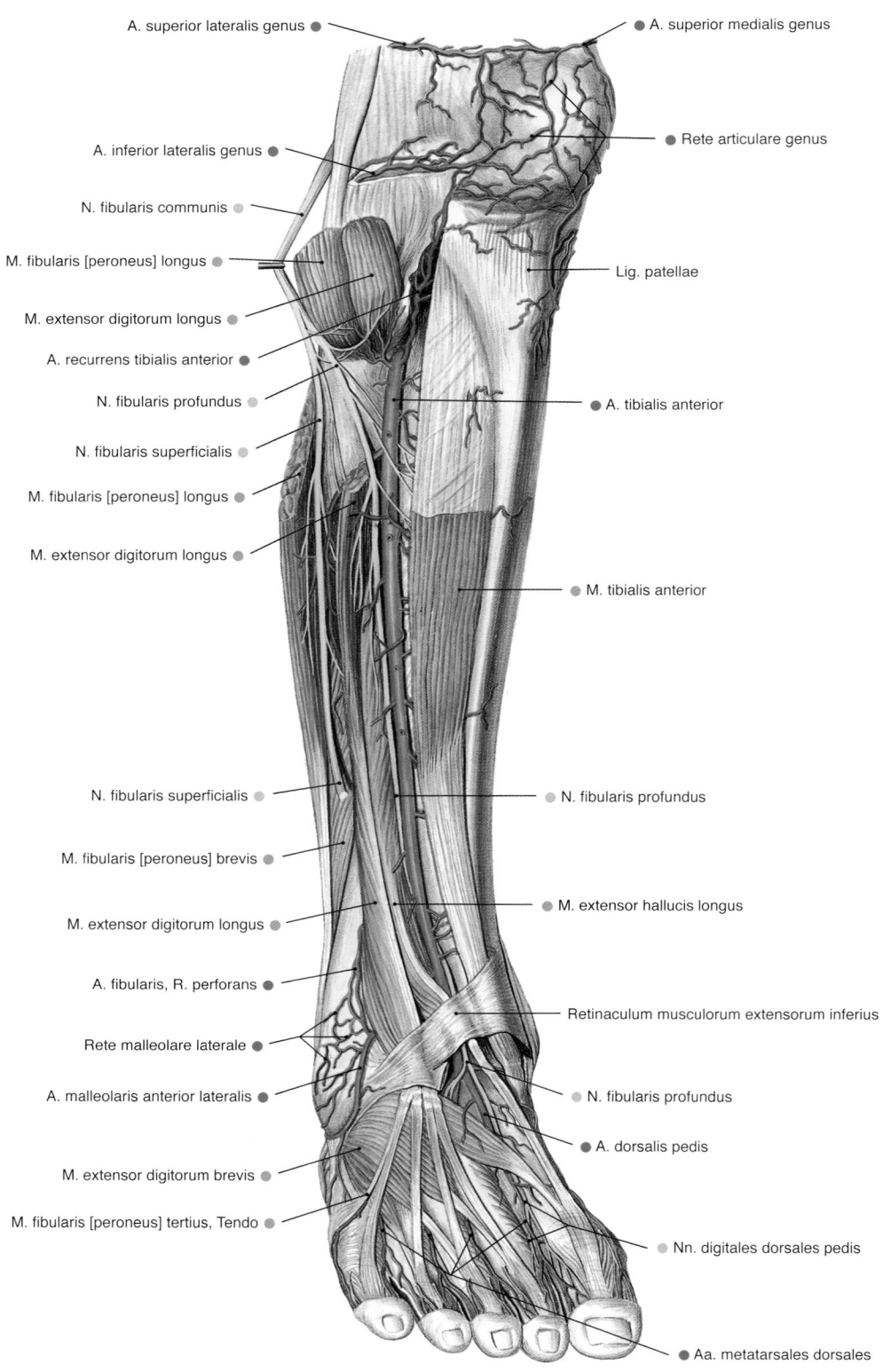

A. superior lateralis genus ●
A. inferior lateralis genus ●
N. fibularis communis ●
M. fibularis [peroneus] longus ●
M. extensor digitorum longus ●
A. recurrens tibialis anterior ●
N. fibularis profundus ●
N. fibularis superficialis ●
M. fibularis [peroneus] longus ●
M. extensor digitorum longus ●

● A. superior medialis genus
● Rete articulare genus
Lig. patellae
● A. tibialis anterior
● M. tibialis anterior

N. fibularis superficialis ●
M. fibularis [peroneus] brevis ●
M. extensor digitorum longus ●
A. fibularis, R. perforans ●
Rete malleolare laterale ●
A. malleolaris anterior lateralis ●
M. extensor digitorum brevis ●
M. fibularis [peroneus] tertius, Tendo ●

● N. fibularis profundus
● M. extensor hallucis longus
Retinaculum musculorum extensorum inferius
● N. fibularis profundus
● A. dorsalis pedis
● Nn. digitales dorsales pedis
● Aa. metatarsales dorsales

1123
1124
1148

1139

Fig. 1140 Arteries and nerves of the anterior region of leg,
Regio cruris anterior, and the dorsum of foot, Dorsum pedis;
after removal of the deep fascia of leg and dissection of the extensor
digitorum longus and fibularis [peroneus] longus muscles.

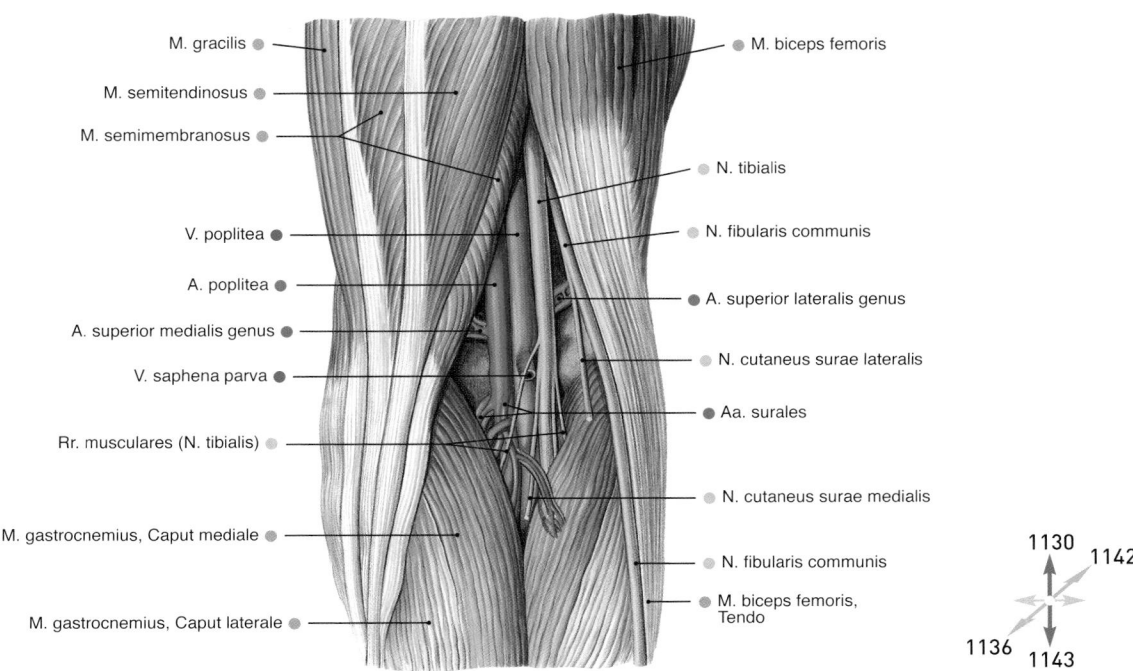

M. gracilis ●
M. semitendinosus ●
M. semimembranosus ●

V. poplitea ●
A. poplitea ●
A. superior medialis genus ●
V. saphena parva ●

Rr. musculares (N. tibialis) ●

M. gastrocnemius, Caput mediale ●

M. gastrocnemius, Caput laterale ●

● M. biceps femoris

● N. tibialis
● N. fibularis communis
● A. superior lateralis genus
● N. cutaneus surae lateralis
● Aa. surales

● N. cutaneus surae medialis

● N. fibularis communis
● M. biceps femoris, Tendo

1130   1142
1136   1143

Fig. 1141   Vessels and nerves of the popliteal fossa, Fossa poplitea; after removal of the fascia lata and the deep fascia of leg.

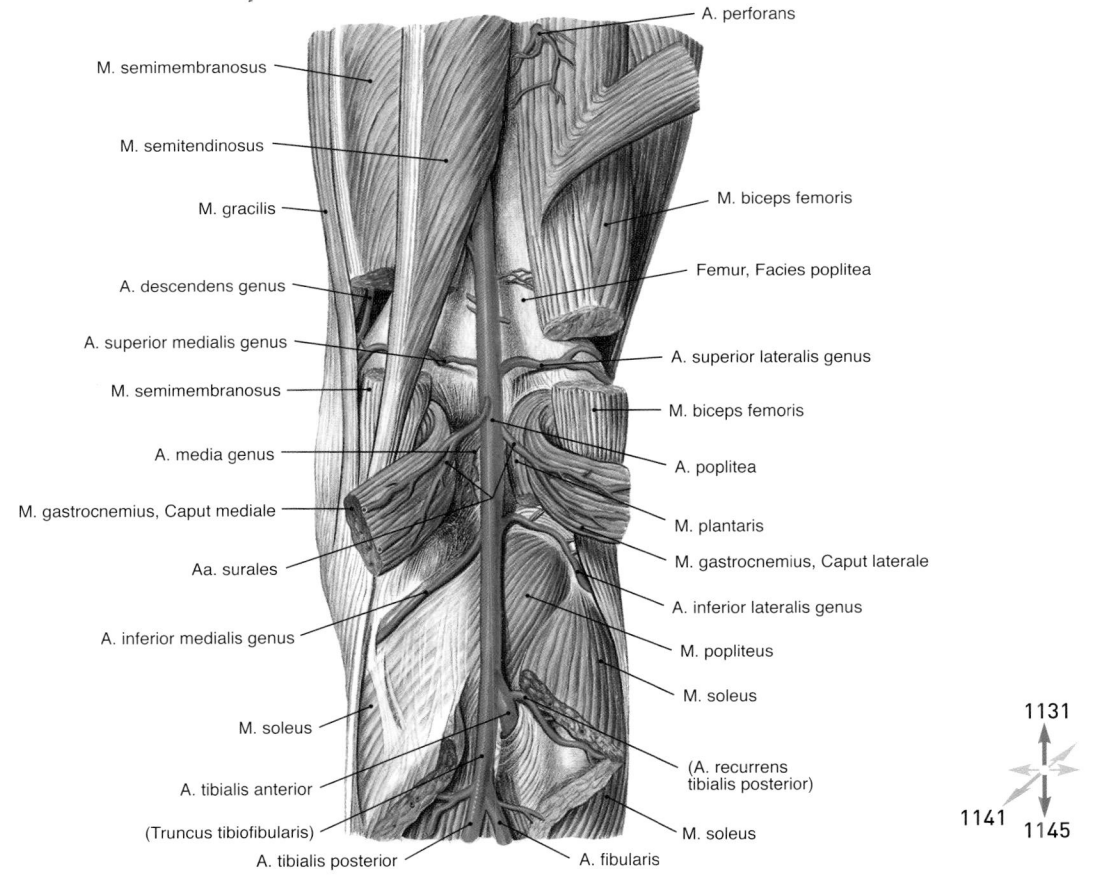

M. semimembranosus
M. semitendinosus
M. gracilis

A. descendens genus
A. superior medialis genus
M. semimembranosus
A. media genus
M. gastrocnemius, Caput mediale
Aa. surales
A. inferior medialis genus

M. soleus

A. tibialis anterior
(Truncus tibiofibularis)
A. tibialis posterior

A. perforans

M. biceps femoris
Femur, Facies poplitea
A. superior lateralis genus
M. biceps femoris
A. poplitea
M. plantaris
M. gastrocnemius, Caput laterale
A. inferior lateralis genus
M. popliteus
M. soleus

(A. recurrens tibialis posterior)
M. soleus
A. fibularis

1131
1141   1145

Fig. 1142   Arteries of the popliteal fossa, Fossa poplitea; demonstration of the arterial supply after partial

removal of the covering muscles.
This branching pattern is found in about 90% of the cases.

Vessels and nerves of the popliteal fossa and the leg

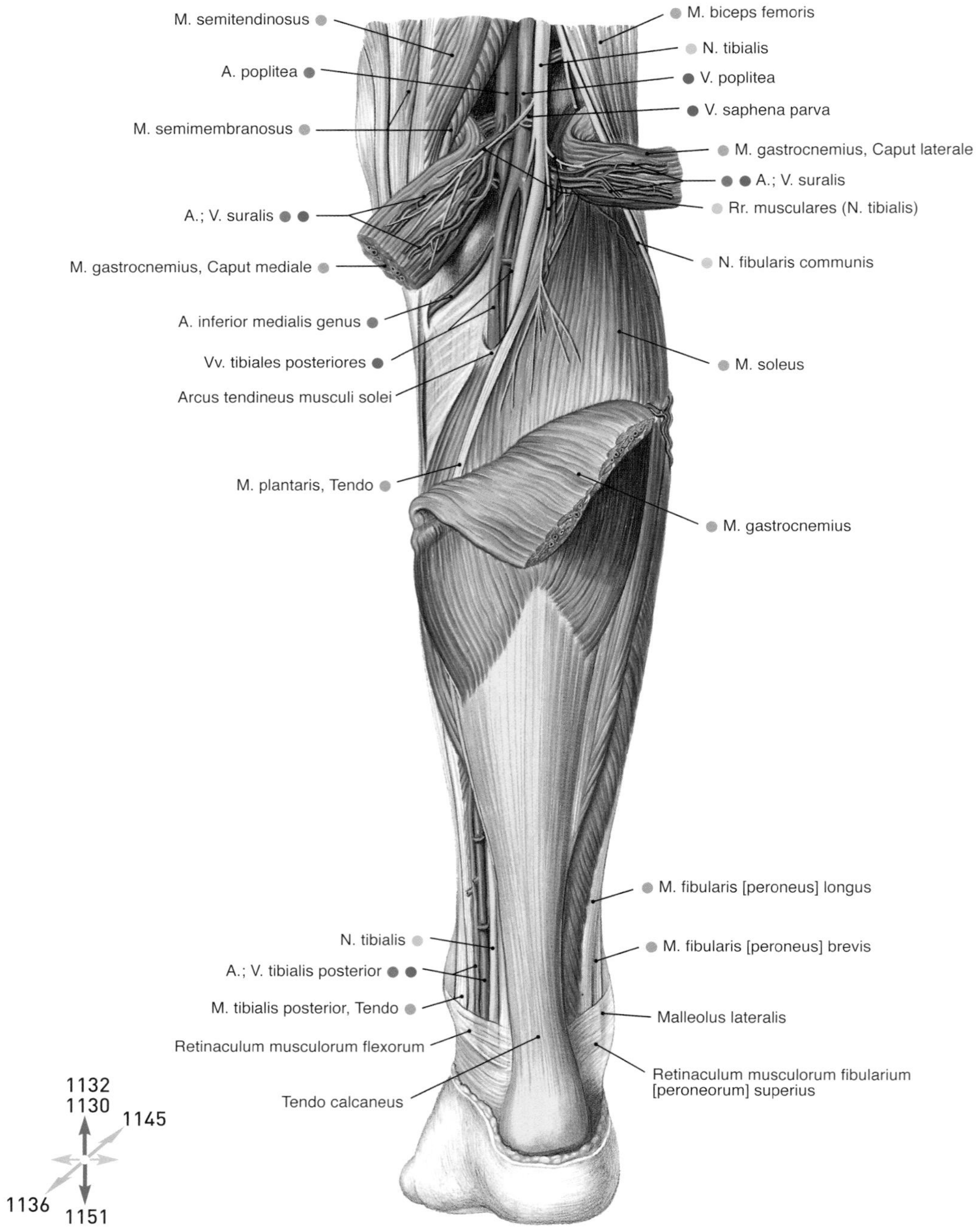

M. semitendinosus ●

A. poplitea ●

M. semimembranosus ●

A.; V. suralis ● ●

M. gastrocnemius, Caput mediale ●

A. inferior medialis genus ●

Vv. tibiales posteriores ●

Arcus tendineus musculi solei

M. plantaris, Tendo ●

M. biceps femoris ●

N. tibialis ●

V. poplitea ●

V. saphena parva ●

M. gastrocnemius, Caput laterale ●

A.; V. suralis ● ●

Rr. musculares (N. tibialis) ●

N. fibularis communis ●

M. soleus ●

M. gastrocnemius ●

N. tibialis ●

A.; V. tibialis posterior ● ●

M. tibialis posterior, Tendo ●

Retinaculum musculorum flexorum

Tendo calcaneus

M. fibularis [peroneus] longus ●

M. fibularis [peroneus] brevis ●

Malleolus lateralis

Retinaculum musculorum fibularium [peroneorum] superius

1132
1130
1145
1136
1151

Fig. 1143 Vessels and nerves of the popliteal fossa, Fossa poplitea, and the posterior region of leg, Regio cruris posterior; after removal of the deep fascia of leg and dissection of the gastrocnemius muscle.

Fig. 1144 a–d Variations in the branching pattern of the popliteal artery, A. poplitea.
a Common trunk of the anterior and posterior tibial artery, Aa. tibiales anterior et posterior, along with the fibular artery, A. fibularis
b The popliteal artery, A. poplitea, branches off proximally to the superior border of the popliteal muscle, M. popliteus.
c Posterior tibial and fibular artery, Aa. tibialis posterior et fibularis, originate from a common proximal trunk.
d The anterior tibial artery, A. tibialis anterior, passes ventrally to the popliteal muscle, M. popliteus.

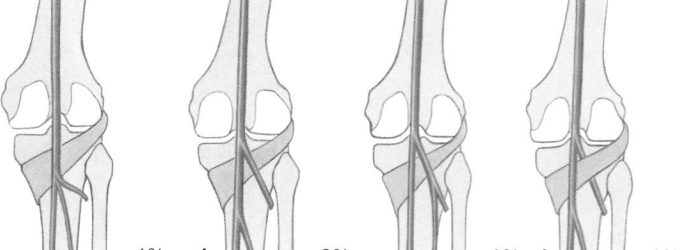

a ~ 4%   **b** ~ 3%   **c** ~ 1%   **d** ~ 1%

Vessels and nerves of the popliteal fossa and the leg

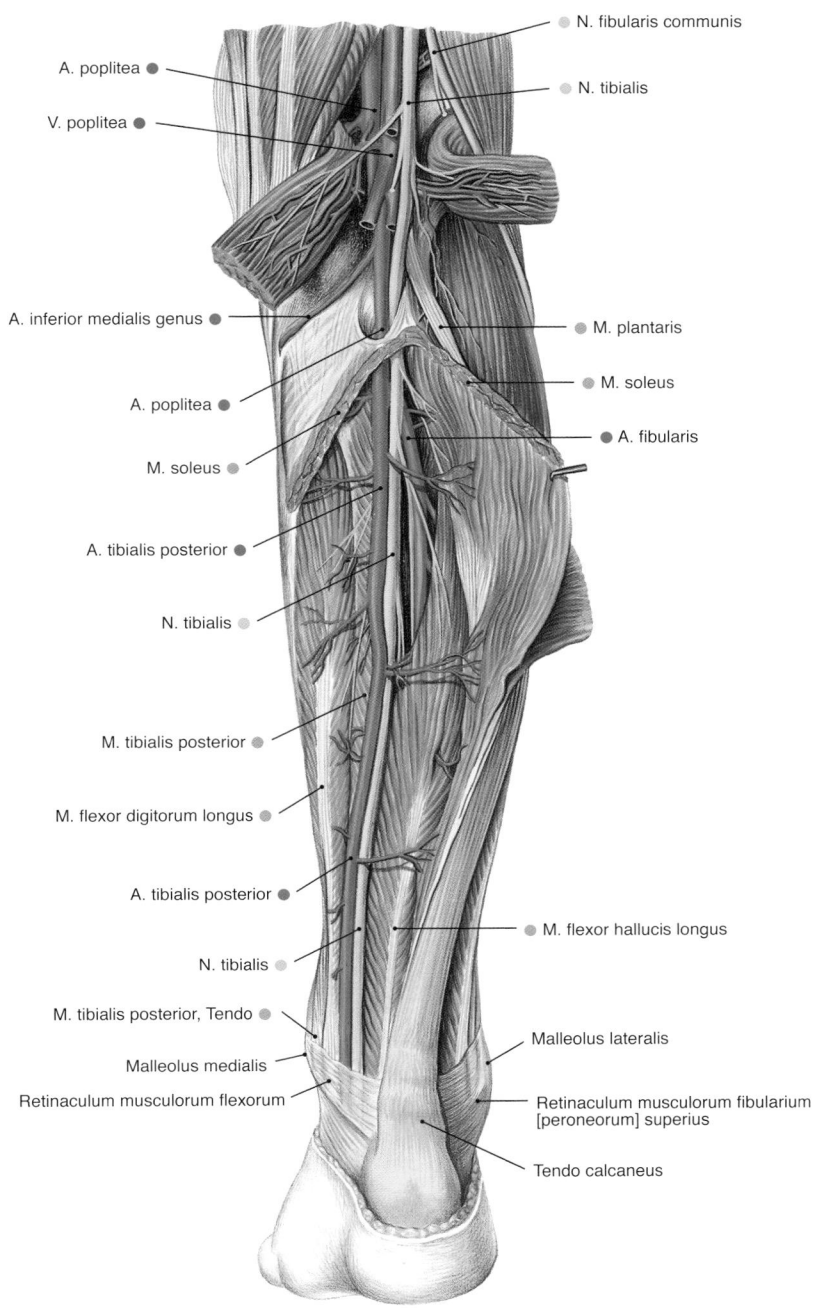

N. fibularis communis

A. poplitea ●

N. tibialis

V. poplitea ●

A. inferior medialis genus ●

M. plantaris

M. soleus

A. poplitea ●

A. fibularis

M. soleus ●

A. tibialis posterior ●

N. tibialis ●

M. tibialis posterior ●

M. flexor digitorum longus ●

A. tibialis posterior ●

M. flexor hallucis longus

N. tibialis ●

M. tibialis posterior, Tendo ●

Malleolus lateralis

Malleolus medialis

Retinaculum musculorum fibularium
[peroneorum] superius

Retinaculum musculorum flexorum

Tendo calcaneus

Fig. 1145 Vessels and nerves of the popliteal fossa, Fossa
poplitea, and the posterior region of leg, Regio cruris posterior;
deep layer.

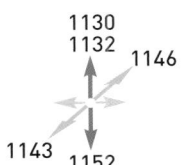

1130
1132
1146
1143
1152

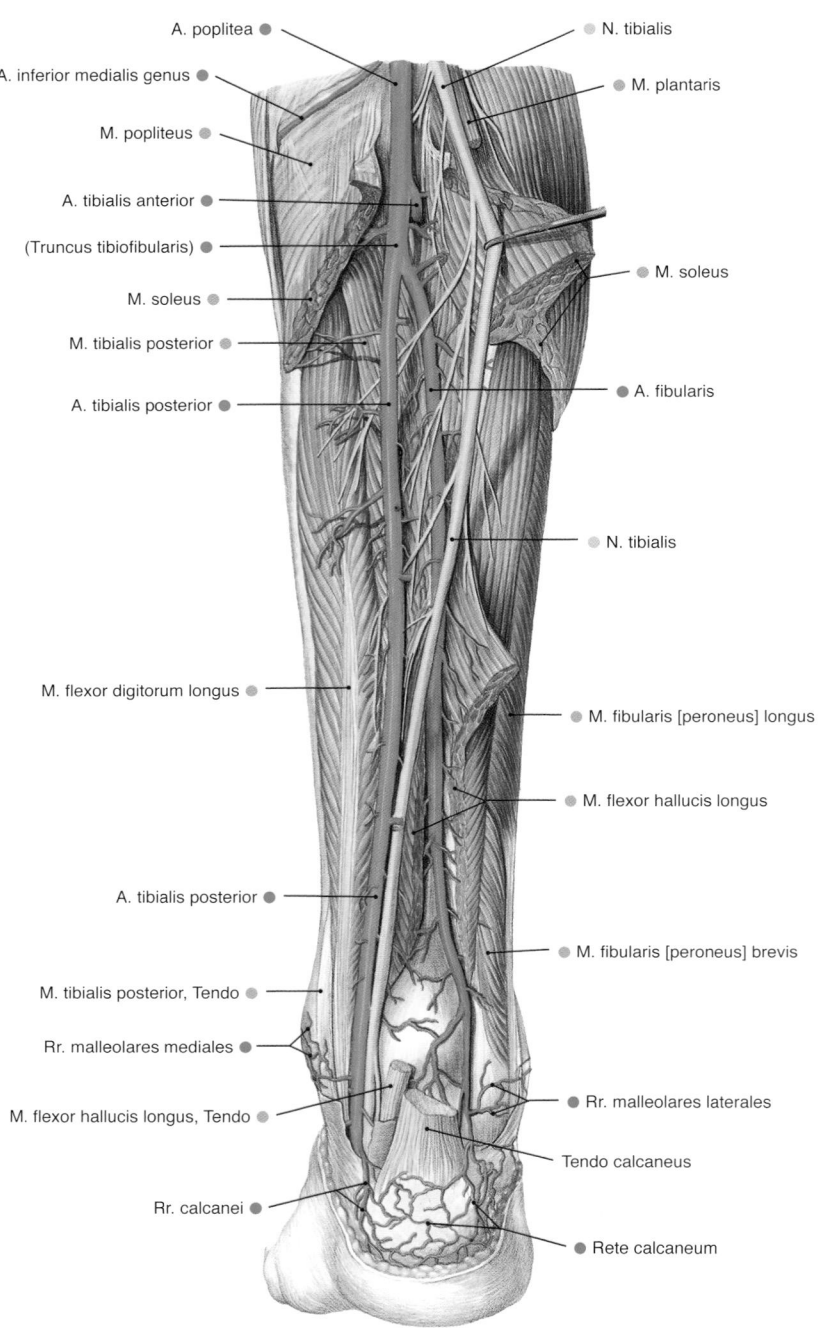

A. poplitea ●
A. inferior medialis genus ●
M. popliteus ●
A. tibialis anterior ●
(Truncus tibiofibularis) ●
M. soleus ●
M. tibialis posterior ●
A. tibialis posterior ●

● N. tibialis
● M. plantaris

● M. soleus

● A. fibularis

● N. tibialis

M. flexor digitorum longus ●

● M. fibularis [peroneus] longus

● M. flexor hallucis longus

A. tibialis posterior ●

● M. fibularis [peroneus] brevis

M. tibialis posterior, Tendo ●
Rr. malleolares mediales ●
M. flexor hallucis longus, Tendo ●

● Rr. malleolares laterales

Tendo calcaneus

Rr. calcanei ●

● Rete calcaneum

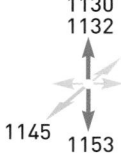

1130
1132

1145 1153

Fig. 1146 Arteries and nerves of the popliteal fossa, Fossa poplitea, and the posterior region of leg, Regio cruris posterior; deepest layer.

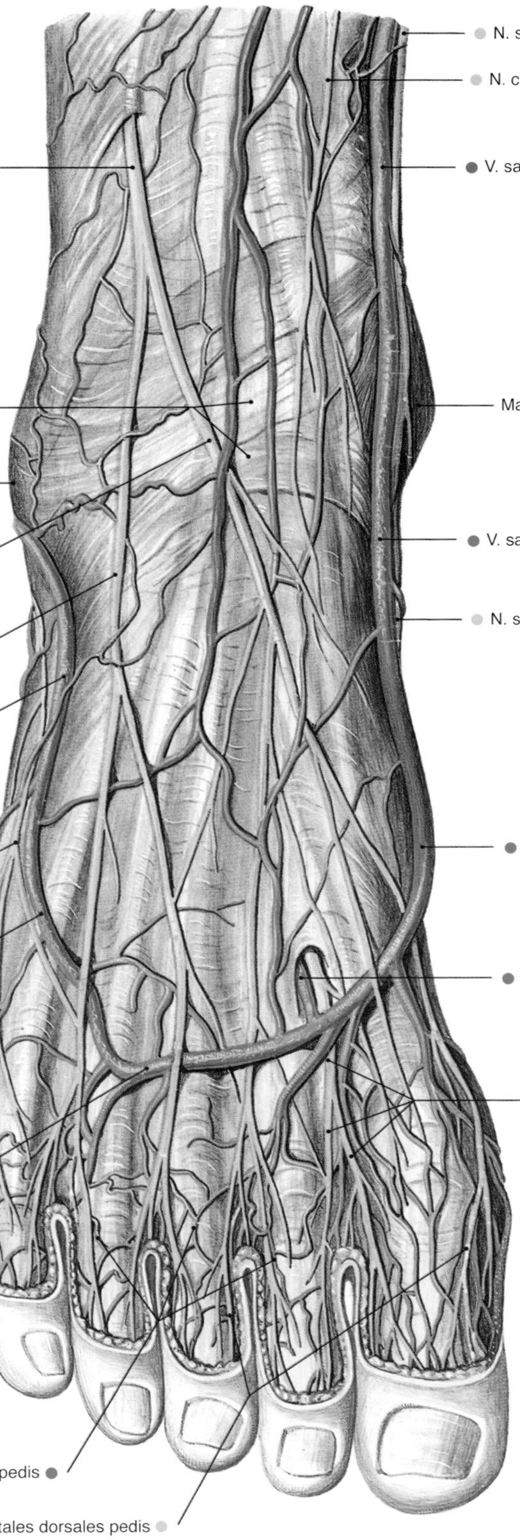

N. fibularis superficialis ●

Retinaculum musculorum extensorum inferius

Malleolus lateralis

N. cutaneus dorsalis medialis ●

N. cutaneus dorsalis intermedius ●

V. saphena parva ●

N. cutaneus dorsalis lateralis ●

V. marginalis lateralis ●

Arcus venosus dorsalis pedis ●

Vv. digitales dorsales pedis ●

Nn. digitales dorsales pedis ●

● N. saphenus

● N. cutaneus surae medialis (N. tibialis)

● V. saphena magna

Malleolus medialis

● V. saphena magna

● N. saphenus

● V. marginalis medialis

● V. perforans

● N. fibularis profundus, Nn. digitales dorsales pedis

1135
1148

Fig. 1147   Epifascial veins and nerves of the dorsum of foot, Dorsum pedis.

Arteries and nerves of the foot

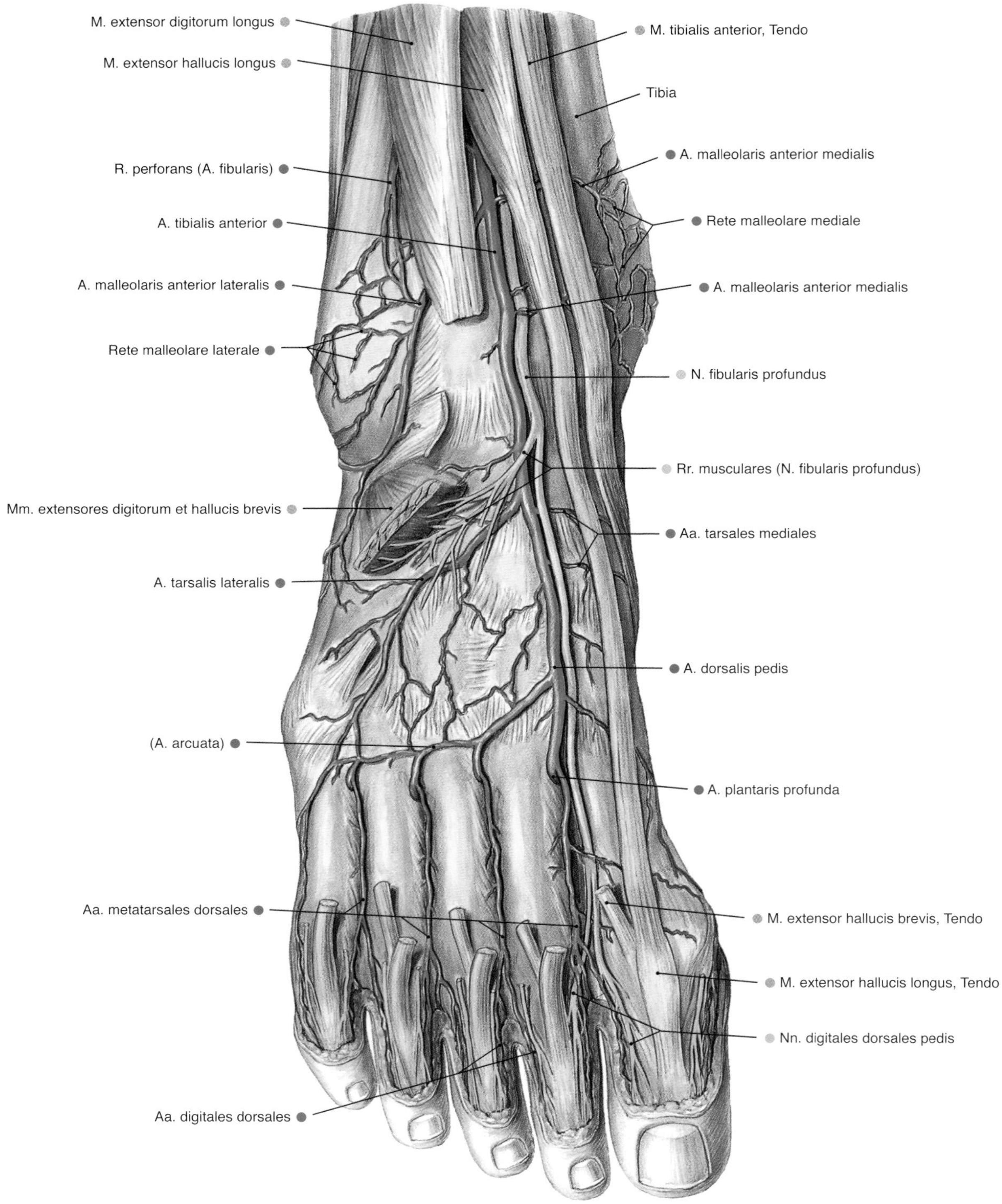

M. extensor digitorum longus ●

M. extensor hallucis longus ●

R. perforans (A. fibularis) ●

A. tibialis anterior ●

A. malleolaris anterior lateralis ●

Rete malleolare laterale ●

Mm. extensores digitorum et hallucis brevis ●

A. tarsalis lateralis ●

(A. arcuata) ●

Aa. metatarsales dorsales ●

Aa. digitales dorsales ●

● M. tibialis anterior, Tendo

Tibia

● A. malleolaris anterior medialis

● Rete malleolare mediale

● A. malleolaris anterior medialis

● N. fibularis profundus

● Rr. musculares (N. fibularis profundus)

● Aa. tarsales mediales

● A. dorsalis pedis

● A. plantaris profunda

● M. extensor hallucis brevis, Tendo

● M. extensor hallucis longus, Tendo

● Nn. digitales dorsales pedis

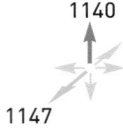

1140

1147

Fig. 1148 Arteries and nerves of the dorsum of foot, Dorsum pedis.

Arteries of the foot

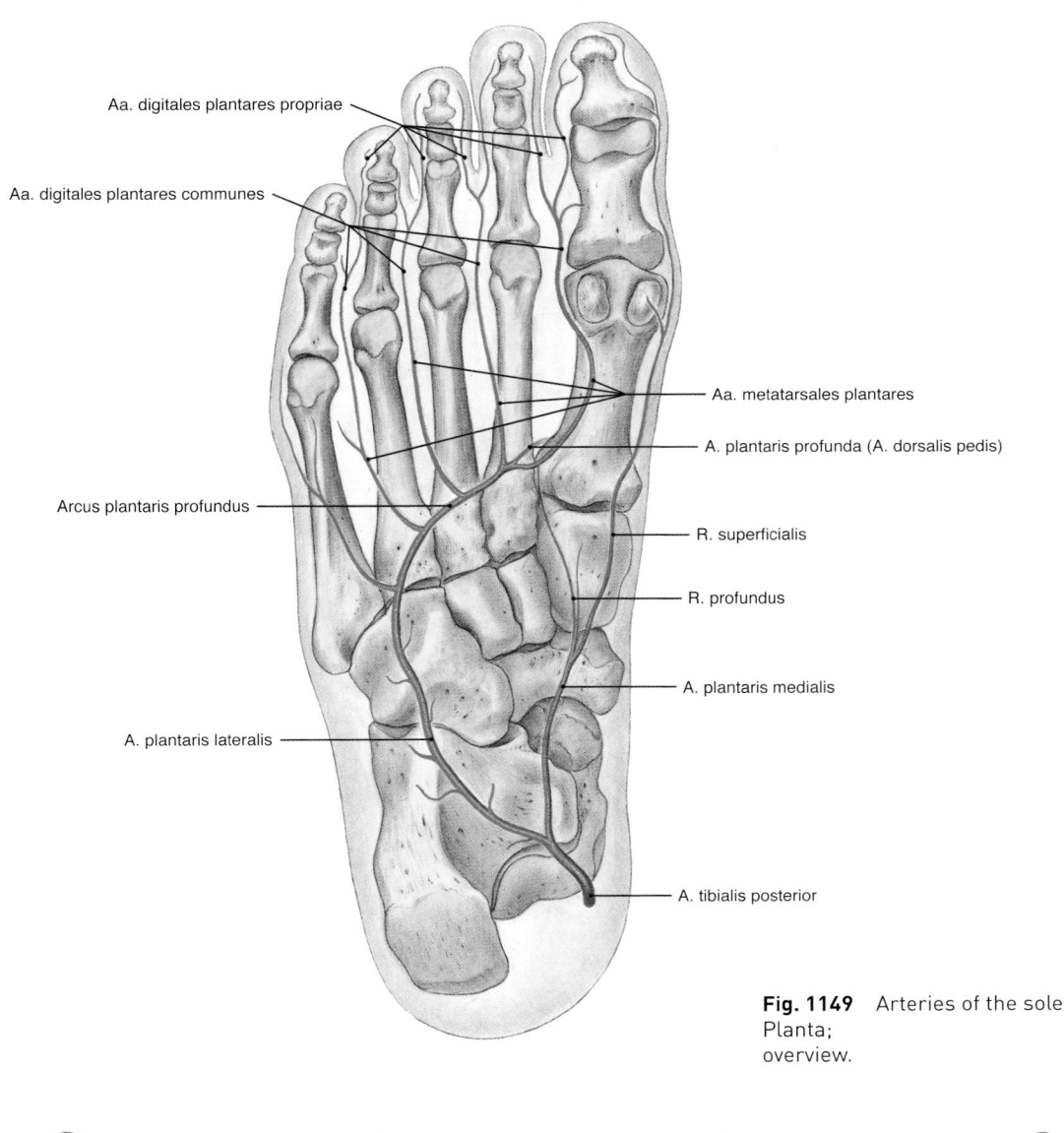

Aa. digitales plantares propriae

Aa. digitales plantares communes

Arcus plantaris profundus

A. plantaris lateralis

Aa. metatarsales plantares

A. plantaris profunda (A. dorsalis pedis)

R. superficialis

R. profundus

A. plantaris medialis

A. tibialis posterior

Fig. 1149 Arteries of the sole of foot, Planta; overview.

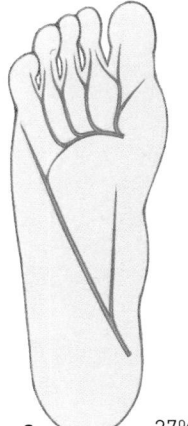

a ~ 27%

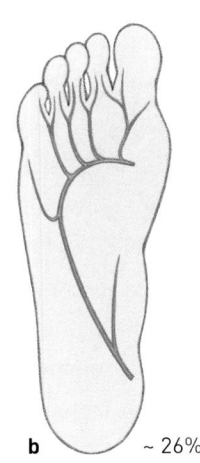

b ~ 26%

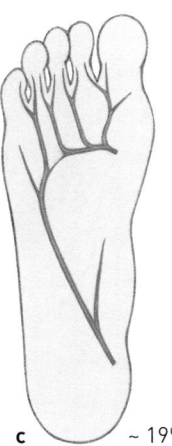

c ~ 19%

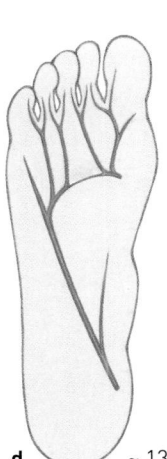

d ~ 13%

Fig. 1150 a–d Variations in the arterial supply of the sole of foot, Planta.
- **a** Dorsalis pedis artery, A. dorsalis pedis, as major supply for the deep plantar arch, Arcus plantaris profundus
- **b** Posterior tibial artery, A. tibialis posterior, as major supply for the deep plantar arch, Arcus plantaris profundus
- **c** The fifth toe and lateral parts of the fourth toe are supplied by the posterior tibial artery, A. tibialis posterior, whereas the

remaining medially located toes receive their arterial supply through the dorsalis pedis artery, A. dorsalis pedis.
- **d** The fifth and fourth toe as well as lateral parts of the third toe are supplied by the posterior tibial artery, A. tibialis posterior, whereas all remaining medially located toes receive their arterial supply through the dorsalis pedis artery, A. dorsalis pedis.

Arteries and nerves of the foot

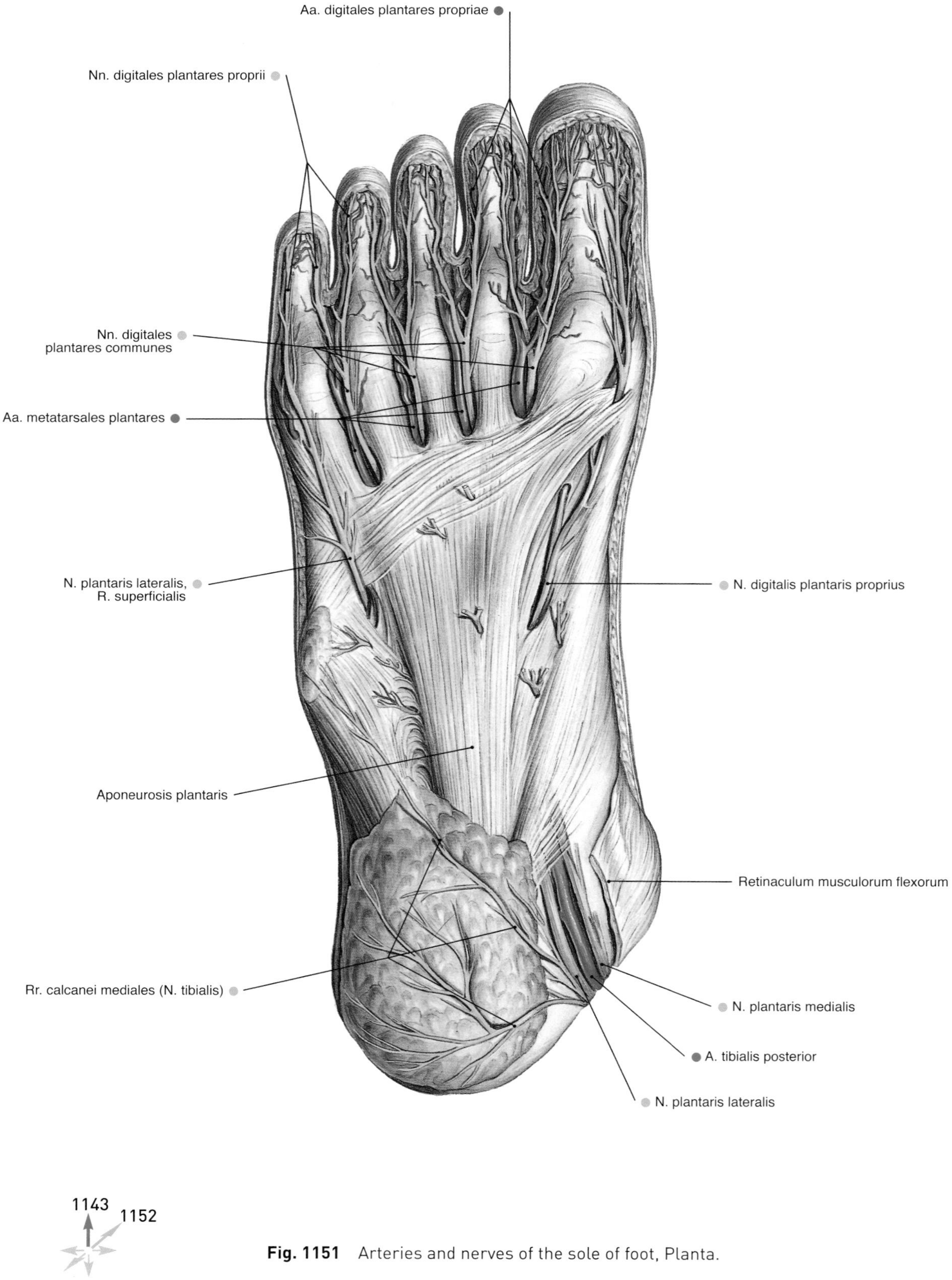

Aa. digitales plantares propriae ●

Nn. digitales plantares proprii ●

Nn. digitales ●
plantares communes

Aa. metatarsales plantares ●

N. plantaris lateralis, ●
R. superficialis

● N. digitalis plantaris proprius

Aponeurosis plantaris

Retinaculum musculorum flexorum

Rr. calcanei mediales (N. tibialis) ●

● N. plantaris medialis

● A. tibialis posterior

● N. plantaris lateralis

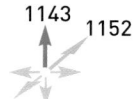
1143
1152

Fig. 1151 Arteries and nerves of the sole of foot, Planta.

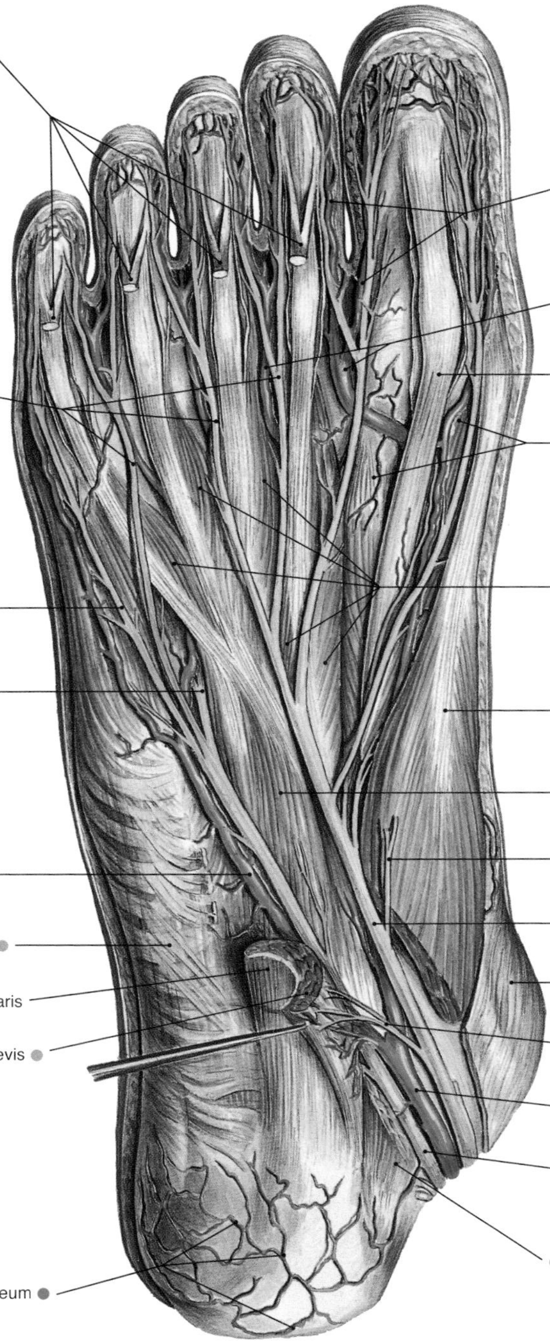

M. flexor digitorum brevis, Tendines ●

Nn. digitales ●
plantares communes

N. plantaris lateralis {
R. superficialis ●

R. profundus ●
}

A. plantaris lateralis ●

M. abductor digiti minimi ●

Aponeurosis plantaris

M. flexor digitorum brevis ●

Rete calcaneum ●

● Aa. digitales plantares propriae

● Aa. digitales plantares communes

● M. flexor hallucis longus, Tendo

● M. flexor hallucis brevis

● M. flexor digitorum longus

● M. abductor hallucis

● M. quadratus plantae

● (R. cutaneus)

● N. plantaris medialis

Retinaculum
musculorum flexorum

● (R. muscularis)

● A. tibialis posterior

● N. plantaris lateralis

● M. abductor hallucis*

Fig. 1152 Arteries and nerves of the sole of foot, Planta;
deep layer.
* The distal extension of the medial retromalleolar space
beneath the abductor hallucis muscle is also known as tarsal
tunnel.

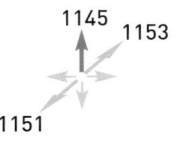

1145
1153

1151

Arteries of the foot

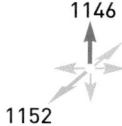

Nn. digitales plantares proprii
M. flexor hallucis longus, Tendo
Nn. digitales plantares communes
Caput transversum
M. adductor hallucis
Aa. metatarsales plantares
Caput obliquum
M. flexor hallucis brevis
Arcus plantaris profundus
R. perforans*
R. superficialis
A. plantaris medialis, R. superficialis
N. plantaris lateralis
R. profundus
M. flexor hallucis longus, Tendo
M. adductor hallucis, Caput obliquum
M. flexor digitorum longus, Tendo
A. plantaris lateralis
M. abductor digiti minimi
M. quadratus plantae
M. abductor hallucis
M. flexor digitorum brevis
N. plantaris medialis
Aponeurosis plantaris
Retinaculum musculorum flexorum
A. tibialis posterior
N. plantaris lateralis
M. abductor hallucis
Rete calcaneum

1146
1152

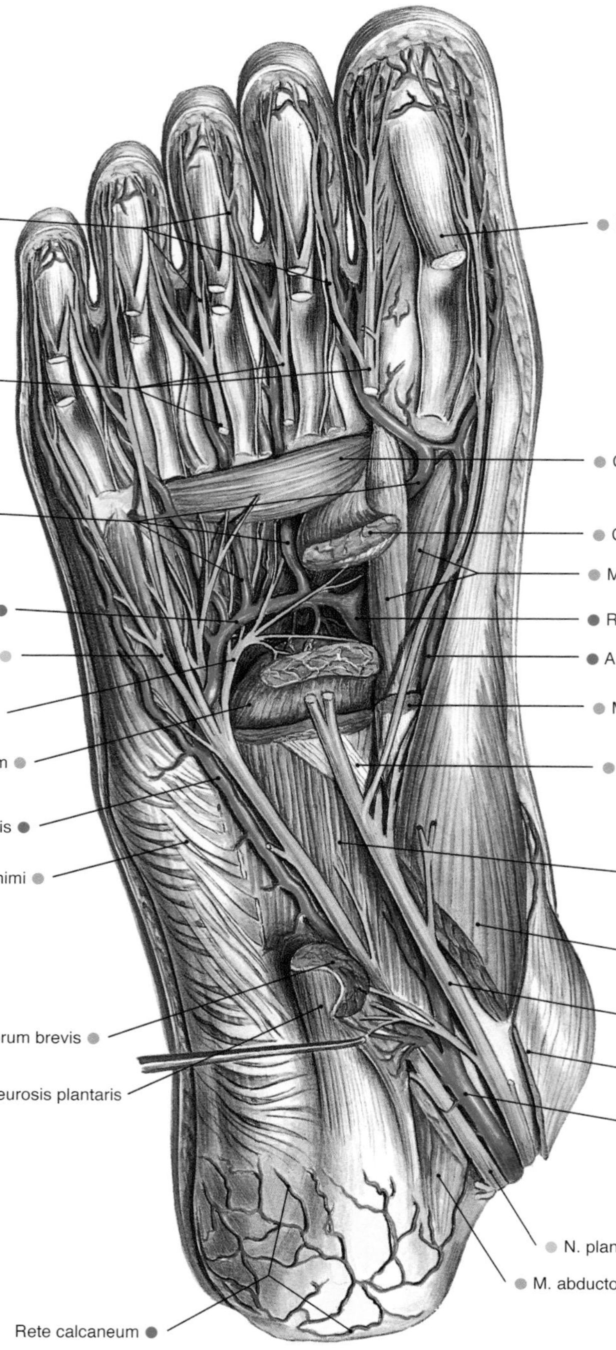

Fig. 1153 Arteries and nerves of the sole of foot, Planta; deepest layer.
* Anastomosis with the dorsalis pedis artery

Compartments of the foot

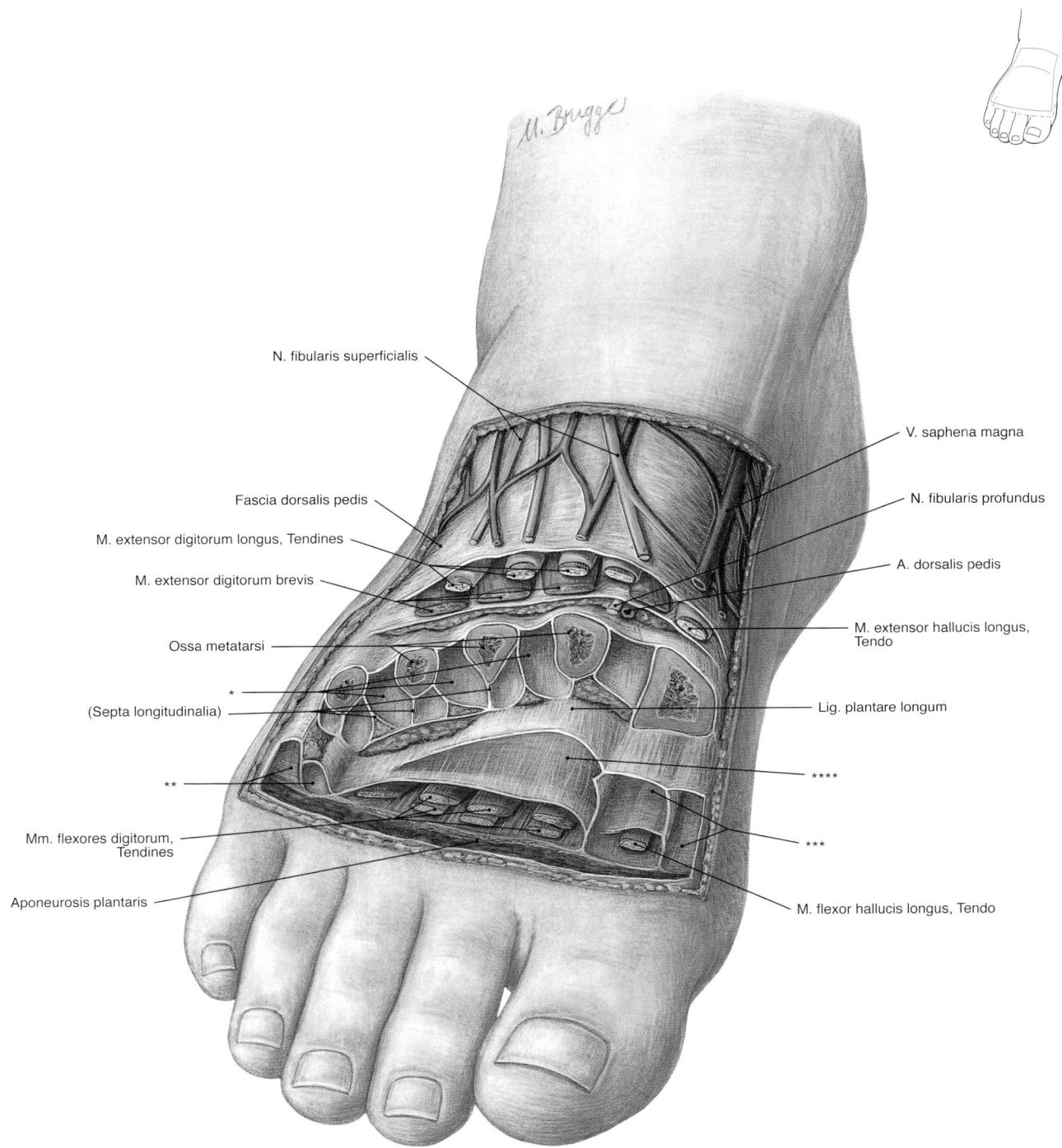

N. fibularis superficialis

Fascia dorsalis pedis

M. extensor digitorum longus, Tendines

M. extensor digitorum brevis

Ossa metatarsi

*

(Septa longitudinalia)

**

Mm. flexores digitorum, Tendines

Aponeurosis plantaris

V. saphena magna

N. fibularis profundus

A. dorsalis pedis

M. extensor hallucis longus, Tendo

Lig. plantare longum

****

***

M. flexor hallucis longus, Tendo

Fig. 1154 Compartments of the foot;
stepwise section.
*   Space of the interossei muscles
**   Lateral compartment
***   Medial compartment
****   Intermediate compartment

Thigh, oblique section

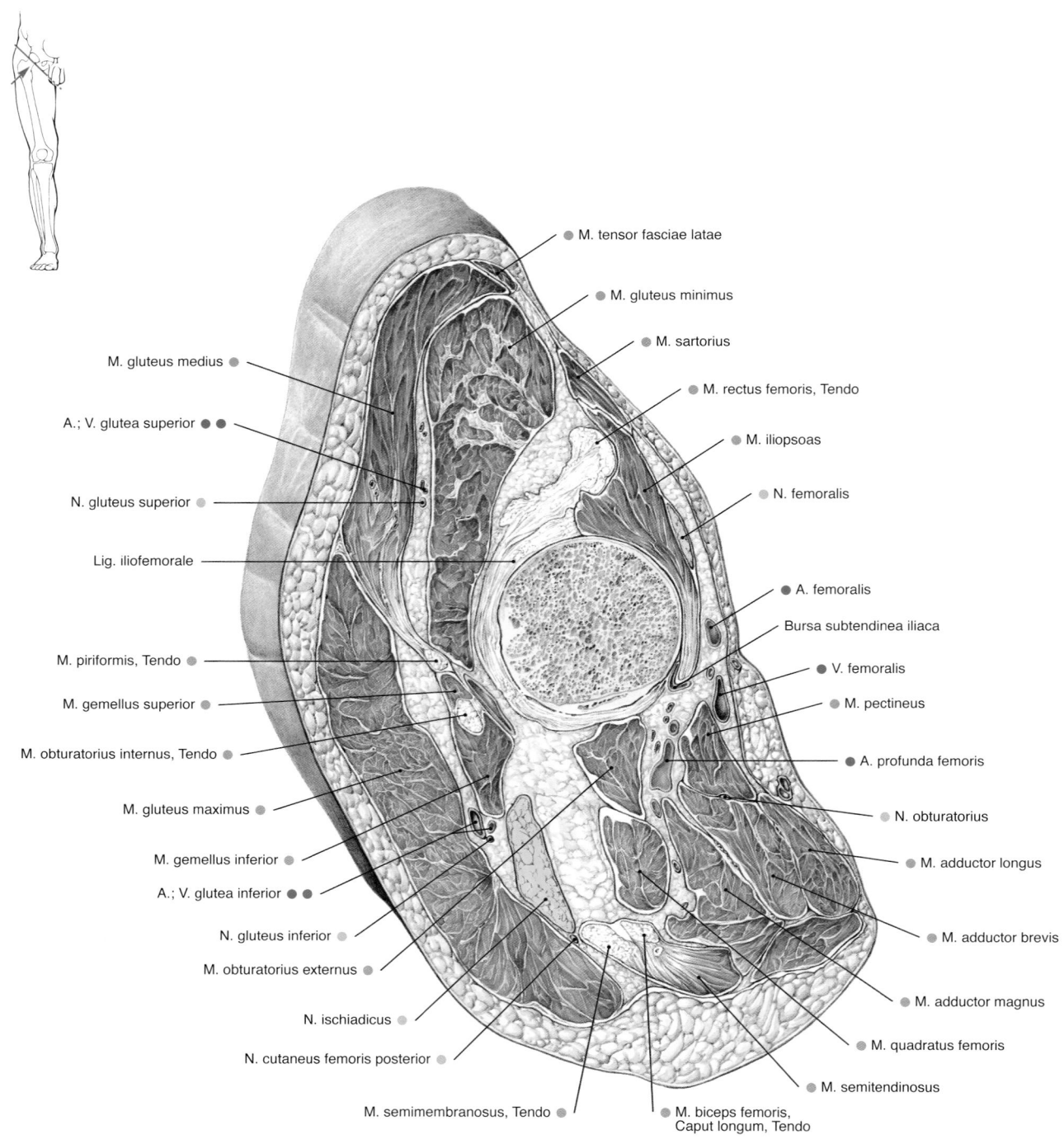

M. gluteus medius

A.; V. glutea superior

N. gluteus superior

Lig. iliofemorale

M. piriformis, Tendo

M. gemellus superior

M. obturatorius internus, Tendo

M. gluteus maximus

M. gemellus inferior

A.; V. glutea inferior

N. gluteus inferior

M. obturatorius externus

N. ischiadicus

N. cutaneus femoris posterior

M. semimembranosus, Tendo

M. tensor fasciae latae

M. gluteus minimus

M. sartorius

M. rectus femoris, Tendo

M. iliopsoas

N. femoralis

A. femoralis

Bursa subtendinea iliaca

V. femoralis

M. pectineus

A. profunda femoris

N. obturatorius

M. adductor longus

M. adductor brevis

M. adductor magnus

M. quadratus femoris

M. semitendinosus

M. biceps femoris, Caput longum, Tendo

Fig. 1155 Thigh, Femur; oblique section through the hip joint.

Thigh, cross-section

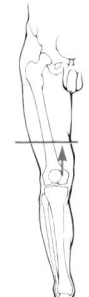

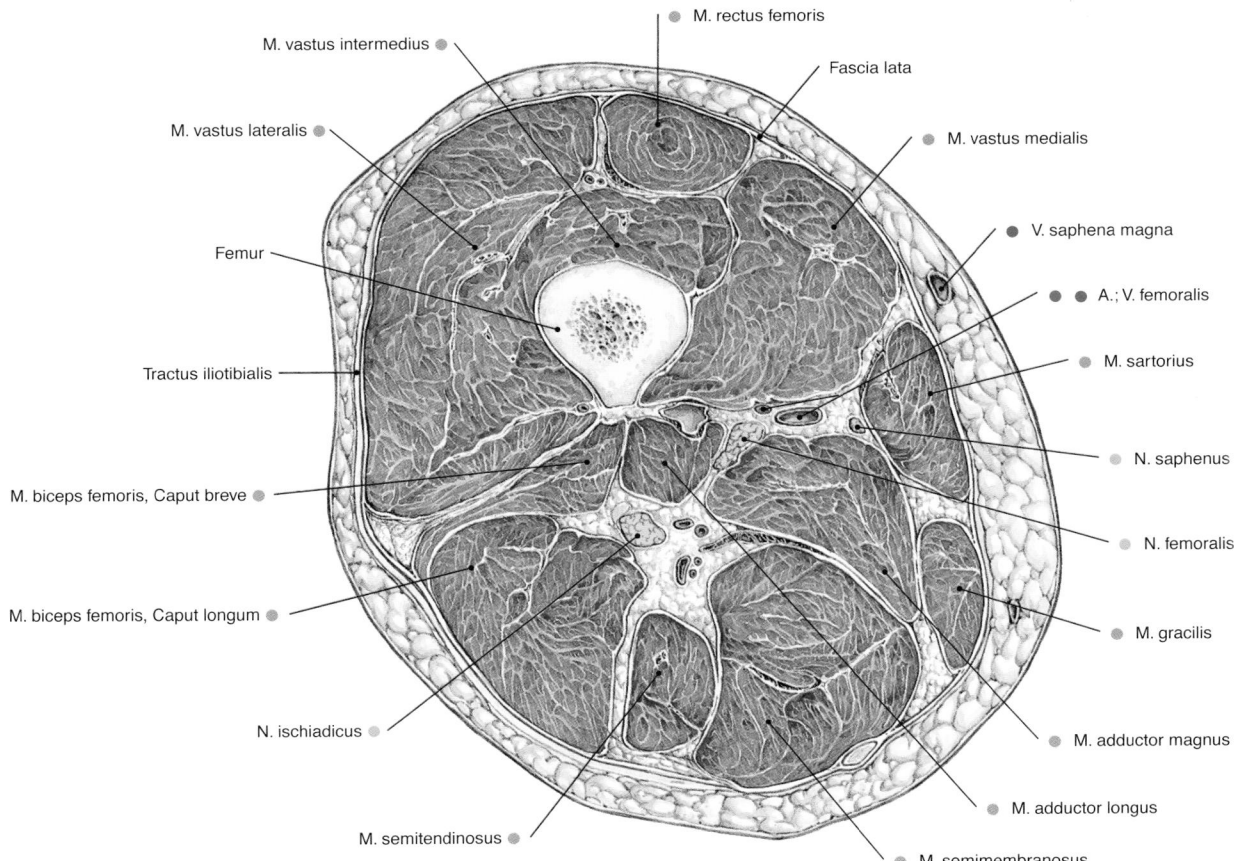

M. rectus femoris

M. vastus intermedius

Fascia lata

M. vastus lateralis

M. vastus medialis

Femur

V. saphena magna

A.; V. femoralis

Tractus iliotibialis

M. sartorius

N. saphenus

M. biceps femoris, Caput breve

N. femoralis

M. biceps femoris, Caput longum

M. gracilis

N. ischiadicus

M. adductor magnus

M. semitendinosus

M. adductor longus

M. semimembranosus

Fig. 1156 Thigh, Femur;
cross-section through the middle of the thigh.

Leg, cross-section

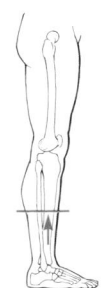

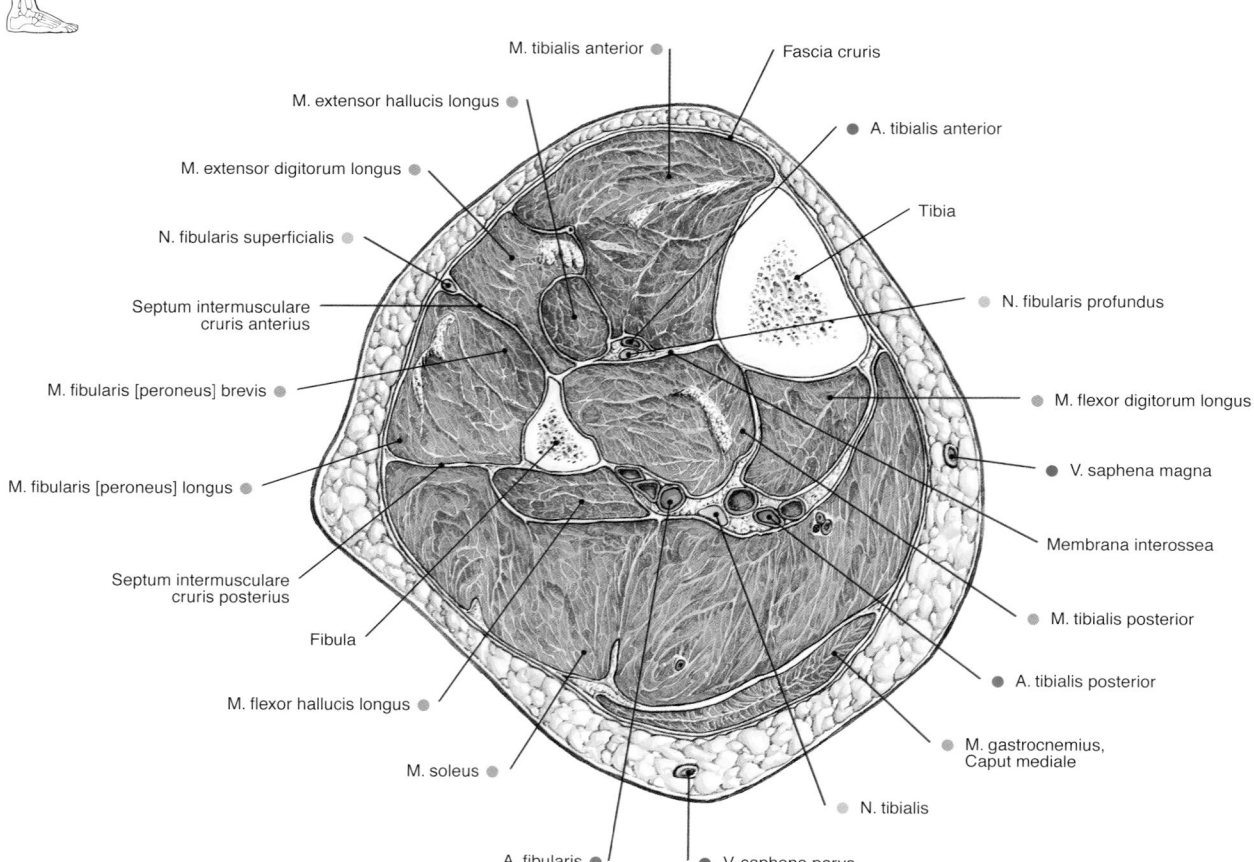

M. tibialis anterior ●

M. extensor hallucis longus ●

M. extensor digitorum longus ●

N. fibularis superficialis ●

Septum intermusculare
cruris anterius

M. fibularis [peroneus] brevis ●

M. fibularis [peroneus] longus ●

Septum intermusculare
cruris posterius

Fibula

M. flexor hallucis longus ●

M. soleus ●

A. fibularis ●

V. saphena parva ●

Fascia cruris

● A. tibialis anterior

Tibia

● N. fibularis profundus

● M. flexor digitorum longus

● V. saphena magna

Membrana interossea

● M. tibialis posterior

● A. tibialis posterior

● M. gastrocnemius,
Caput mediale

● N. tibialis

→ 1138

Fig. 1157 Leg, Crus;
cross-section through the middle of the leg.

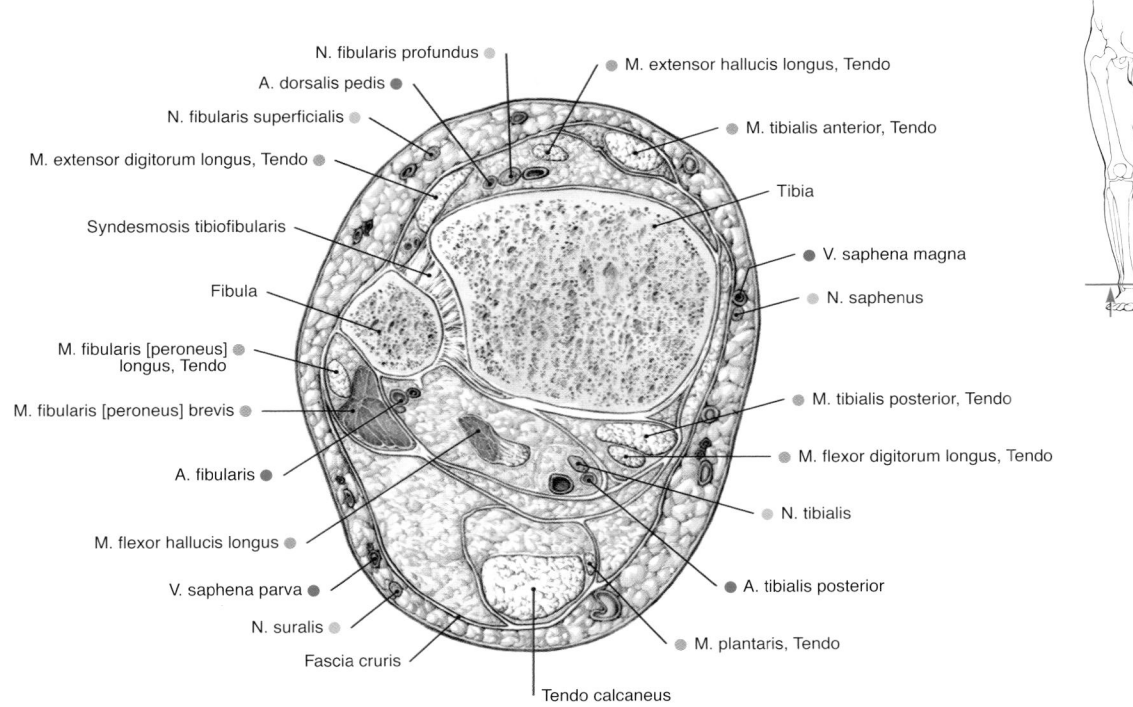

N. fibularis profundus ⬤

A. dorsalis pedis ⬤

N. fibularis superficialis ⬤

M. extensor digitorum longus, Tendo ⬤

Syndesmosis tibiofibularis

Fibula

M. fibularis [peroneus] ⬤
longus, Tendo

M. fibularis [peroneus] brevis ⬤

A. fibularis ⬤

M. flexor hallucis longus ⬤

V. saphena parva ⬤

N. suralis ⬤

Fascia cruris

Tendo calcaneus

⬤ M. extensor hallucis longus, Tendo

⬤ M. tibialis anterior, Tendo

Tibia

⬤ V. saphena magna

⬤ N. saphenus

⬤ M. tibialis posterior, Tendo

⬤ M. flexor digitorum longus, Tendo

⬤ N. tibialis

⬤ A. tibialis posterior

⬤ M. plantaris, Tendo

Fig. 1158   Leg, Crus;
cross-section just above the ankle joint.

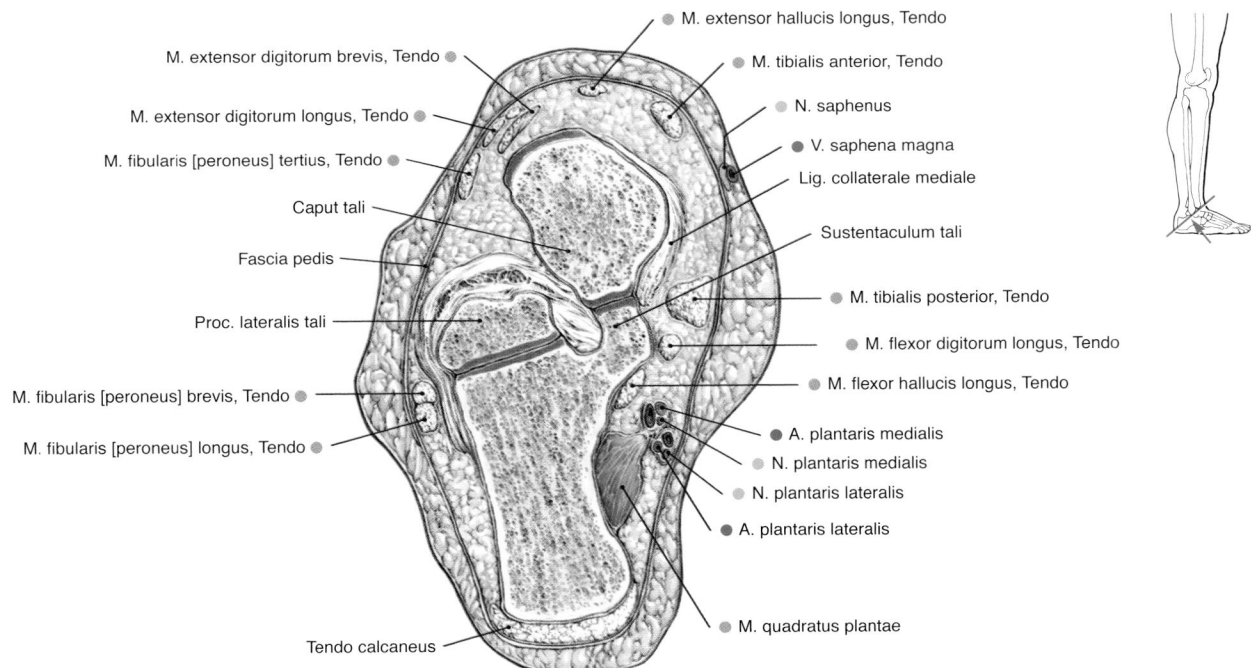

M. extensor digitorum brevis, Tendo ⬤

M. extensor digitorum longus, Tendo ⬤

M. fibularis [peroneus] tertius, Tendo ⬤

Caput tali

Fascia pedis

Proc. lateralis tali

M. fibularis [peroneus] brevis, Tendo ⬤

M. fibularis [peroneus] longus, Tendo ⬤

Tendo calcaneus

⬤ M. extensor hallucis longus, Tendo

⬤ M. tibialis anterior, Tendo

⬤ N. saphenus

⬤ V. saphena magna

Lig. collaterale mediale

Sustentaculum tali

⬤ M. tibialis posterior, Tendo

⬤ M. flexor digitorum longus, Tendo

⬤ M. flexor hallucis longus, Tendo

⬤ A. plantaris medialis

⬤ N. plantaris medialis

⬤ N. plantaris lateralis

⬤ A. plantaris lateralis

⬤ M. quadratus plantae

Fig. 1159   Foot, Pes;
oblique section through the calcaneus and the head of the talus.

Foot, sagittal sections

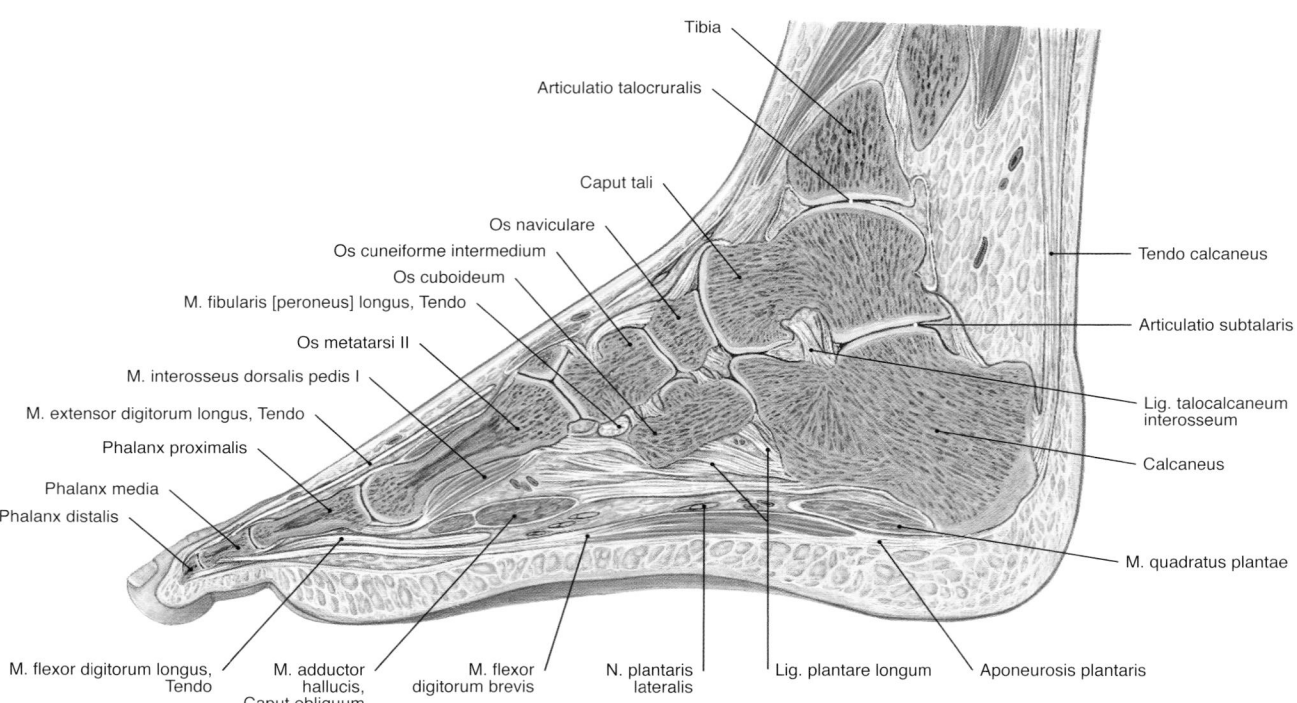

Tibia

Articulatio talocruralis

Caput tali

Os naviculare

Os cuneiforme intermedium

Os cuboideum

M. fibularis [peroneus] longus, Tendo

Os metatarsi II

M. interosseus dorsalis pedis I

M. extensor digitorum longus, Tendo

Phalanx proximalis

Phalanx media

Phalanx distalis

Tendo calcaneus

Articulatio subtalaris

Lig. talocalcaneum interosseum

Calcaneus

M. quadratus plantae

M. flexor digitorum longus, Tendo

M. adductor hallucis, Caput obliquum

M. flexor digitorum brevis

N. plantaris lateralis

Lig. plantare longum

Aponeurosis plantaris

→ 1047, 1048

Fig. 1160 Foot, Pes;
sagittal section through the second toe.

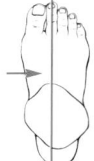

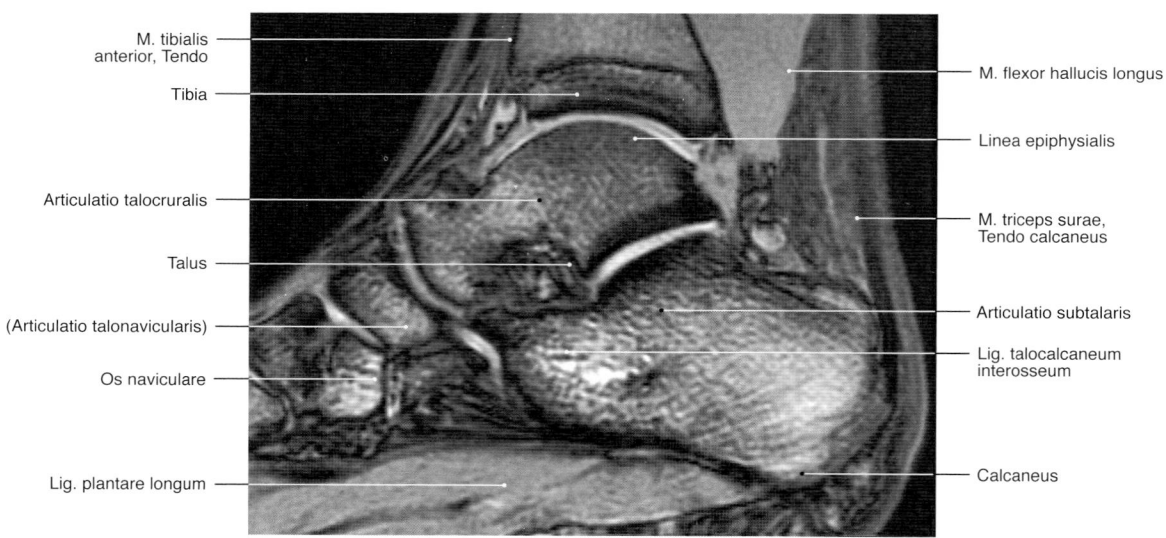

M. tibialis anterior, Tendo

Tibia

Articulatio talocruralis

Talus

(Articulatio talonavicularis)

Os naviculare

Lig. plantare longum

M. flexor hallucis longus

Linea epiphysialis

M. triceps surae, Tendo calcaneus

Articulatio subtalaris

Lig. talocalcaneum interosseum

Calcaneus

→ 1049, 1050

Fig. 1161 Foot, Pes;
magnetic resonance tomography image (MRI); sagittal section.

Foot, cross-section and pedograms

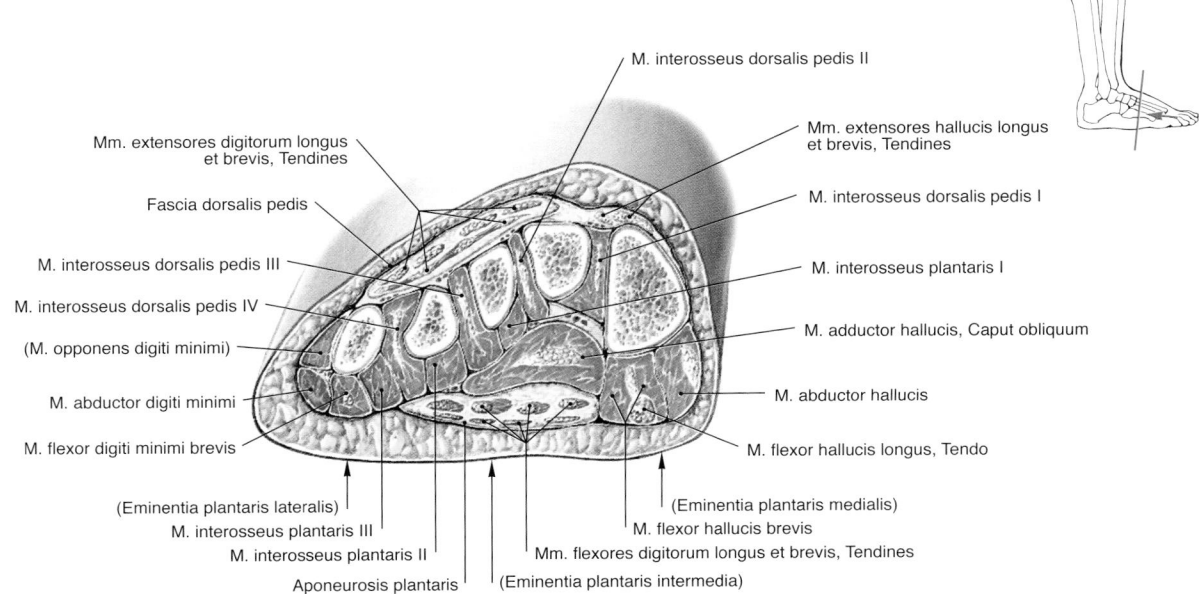

M. interosseus dorsalis pedis II

Mm. extensores digitorum longus et brevis, Tendines

Fascia dorsalis pedis

M. interosseus dorsalis pedis III

M. interosseus dorsalis pedis IV

(M. opponens digiti minimi)

M. abductor digiti minimi

M. flexor digiti minimi brevis

Mm. extensores hallucis longus et brevis, Tendines

M. interosseus dorsalis pedis I

M. interosseus plantaris I

M. adductor hallucis, Caput obliquum

M. abductor hallucis

M. flexor hallucis longus, Tendo

(Eminentia plantaris lateralis)

M. interosseus plantaris III

M. interosseus plantaris II

Aponeurosis plantaris

(Eminentia plantaris medialis)

M. flexor hallucis brevis

Mm. flexores digitorum longus et brevis, Tendines

(Eminentia plantaris intermedia)

Fig. 1162 Osteofibrous tubes of the foot; frontal section through the metatarsus.

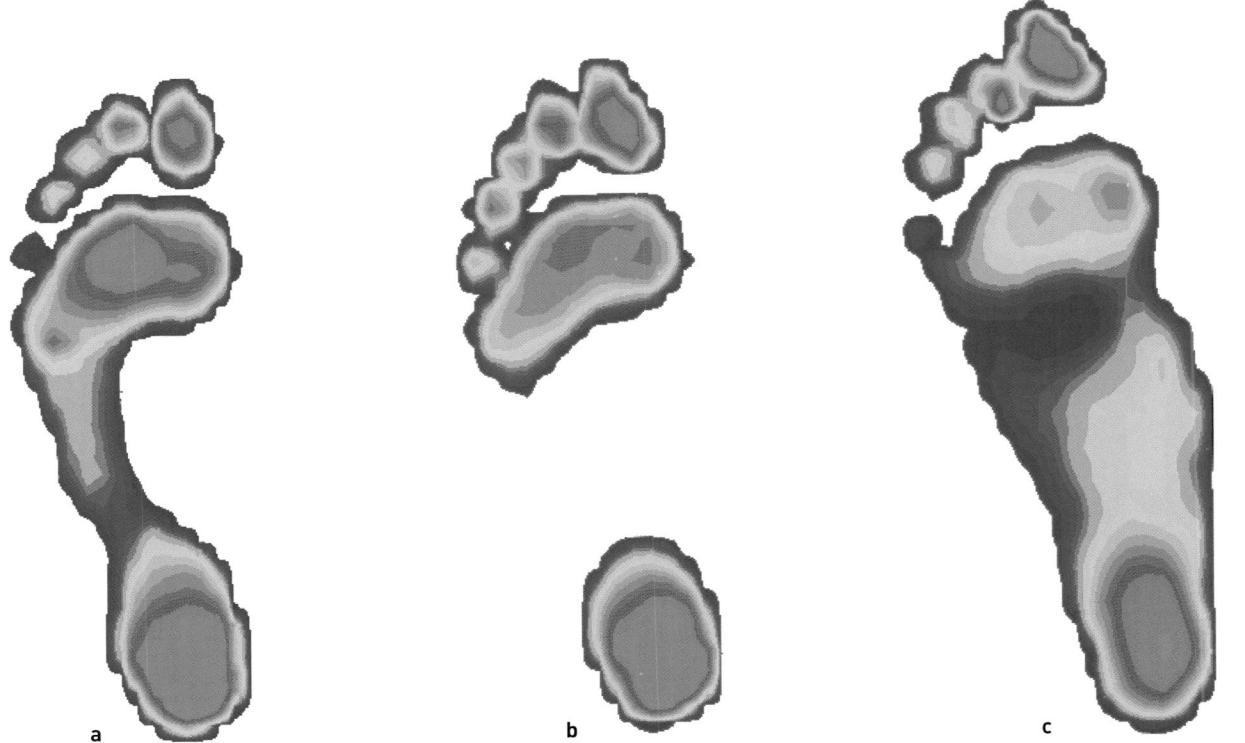

a

b

c

Fig. 1163 a–c Foot prints, pedograms.
a Normal foot
b Pes cavus
c Flat foot

Arteries of the head

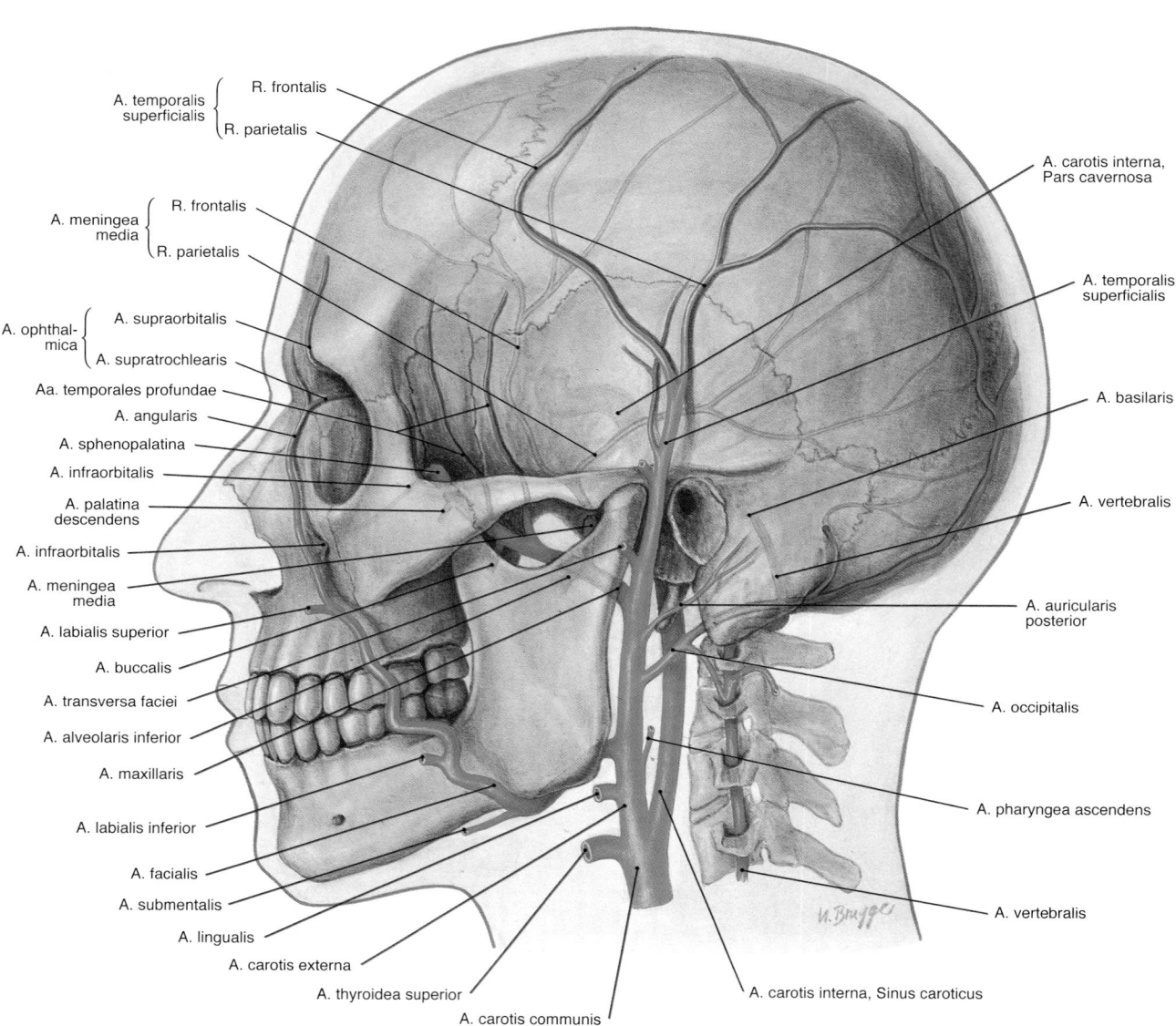

A. temporalis superficialis
  R. frontalis
  R. parietalis

A. meningea media
  R. frontalis
  R. parietalis

A. ophthalmica
  A. supraorbitalis
  A. supratrochlearis

Aa. temporales profundae

A. angularis

A. sphenopalatina

A. infraorbitalis

A. palatina descendens

A. infraorbitalis

A. meningea media

A. labialis superior

A. buccalis

A. transversa faciei

A. alveolaris inferior

A. maxillaris

A. labialis inferior

A. facialis

A. submentalis

A. lingualis

A. carotis externa

A. thyroidea superior

A. carotis communis

A. carotis interna, Pars cavernosa

A. temporalis superficialis

A. basilaris

A. vertebralis

A. auricularis posterior

A. occipitalis

A. pharyngea ascendens

A. vertebralis

A. carotis interna, Sinus caroticus

Fig. 1164   External arteries of the head.

Arteries of the head

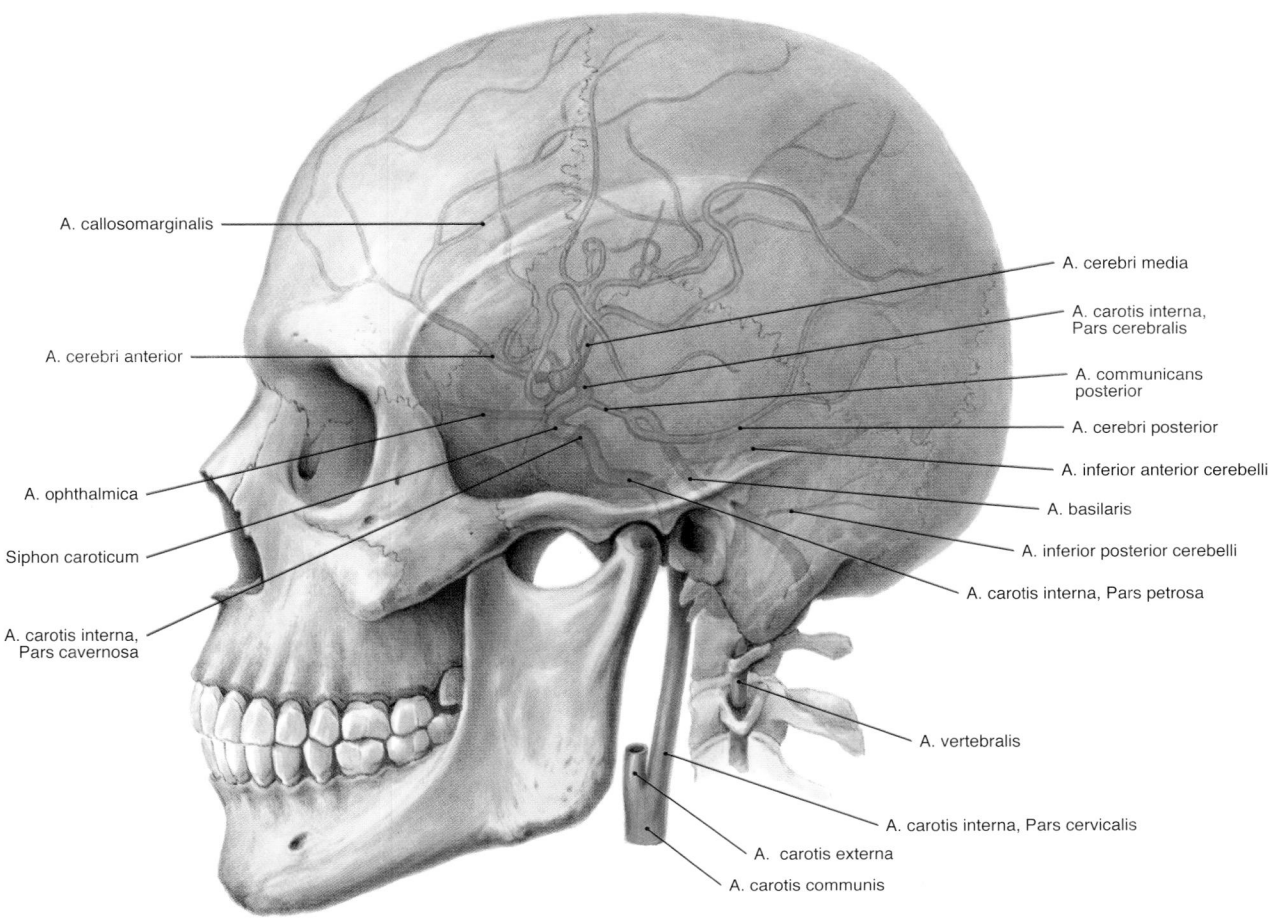

A. callosomarginalis

A. cerebri anterior

A. ophthalmica

Siphon caroticum

A. carotis interna,
Pars cavernosa

A. cerebri media

A. carotis interna,
Pars cerebralis

A. communicans
posterior

A. cerebri posterior

A. inferior anterior cerebelli

A. basilaris

A. inferior posterior cerebelli

A. carotis interna, Pars petrosa

A. vertebralis

A. carotis interna, Pars cervicalis

A. carotis externa

A. carotis communis

Fig. 1165   Internal arteries of the head.

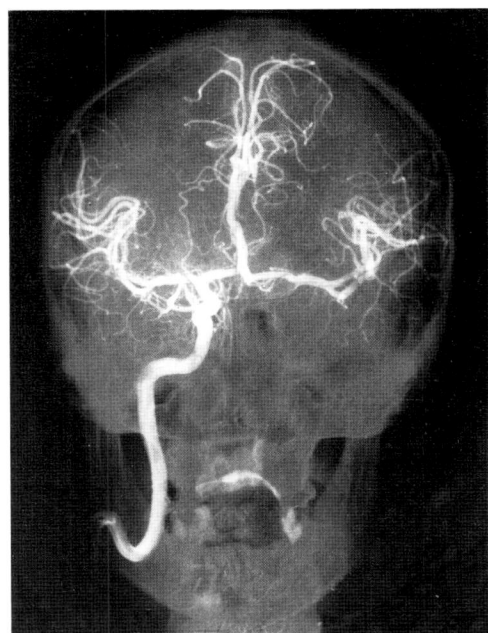

a

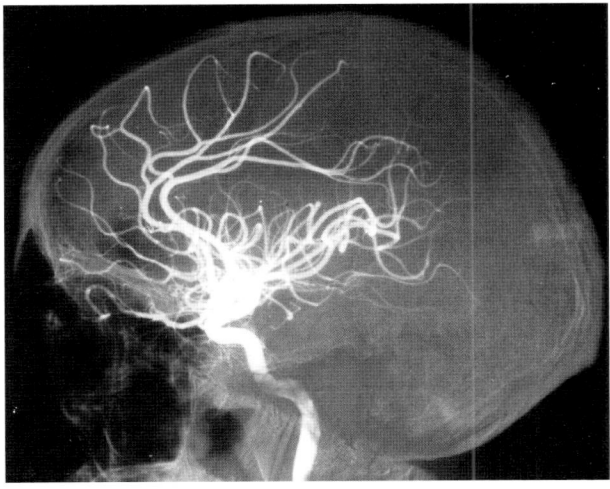

b

Fig. 1166 a, b   Internal carotid artery, A. carotis interna;
radiographs after unilateral injection of a contrast medium
(angiograms).

The contrast medium also distributes to the vessels of the
contralateral side via the arterial circle.
a AP-radiograph, digital subtraction angiography (DSA)
b Lateral radiograph, digital subtraction angiography (DSA)

Veins of the head

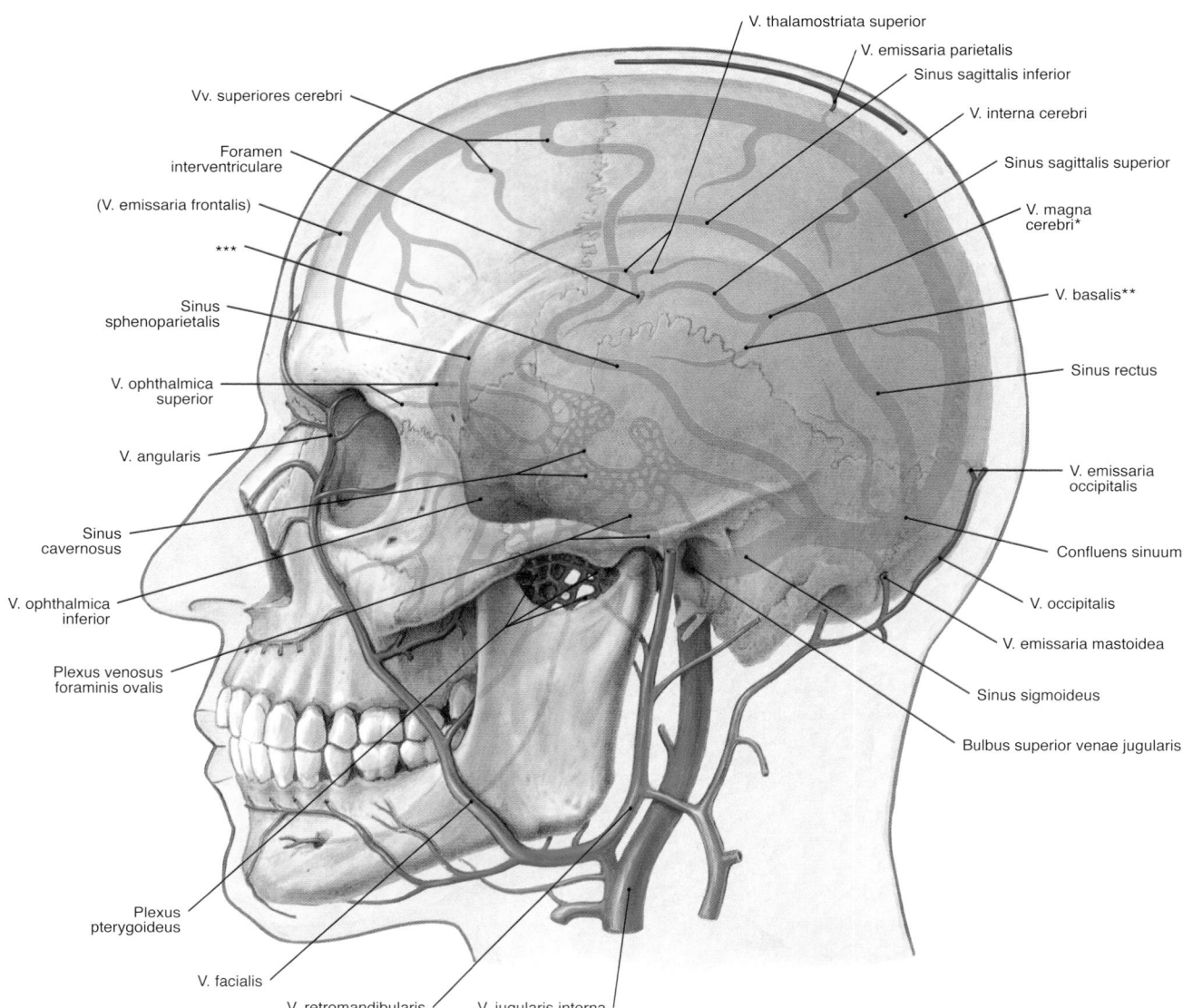

Fig. 1167 Internal and external veins of the head.
*   Vein of GALEN
** ROSENTHAL's vein
***Vein of LABBÉ

Emissary veins, Vv. emissariae – Passages through the skull

V. emissaria parietalis – Foramen parietale
V. emissaria mastoidea – Foramen mastoideum
V. emissaria occipitalis – Passage in the region of the
   Protuberantia occipitalis externa
V. emissaria condylaris – Canalis condylaris

Plexus venosus canalis nervi hypoglossi – Canalis nervi
   hypoglossi
Plexus venosus foraminis ovalis – Foramen ovale
Plexus venosus caroticus internus – Canalis caroticus

Veins of the head

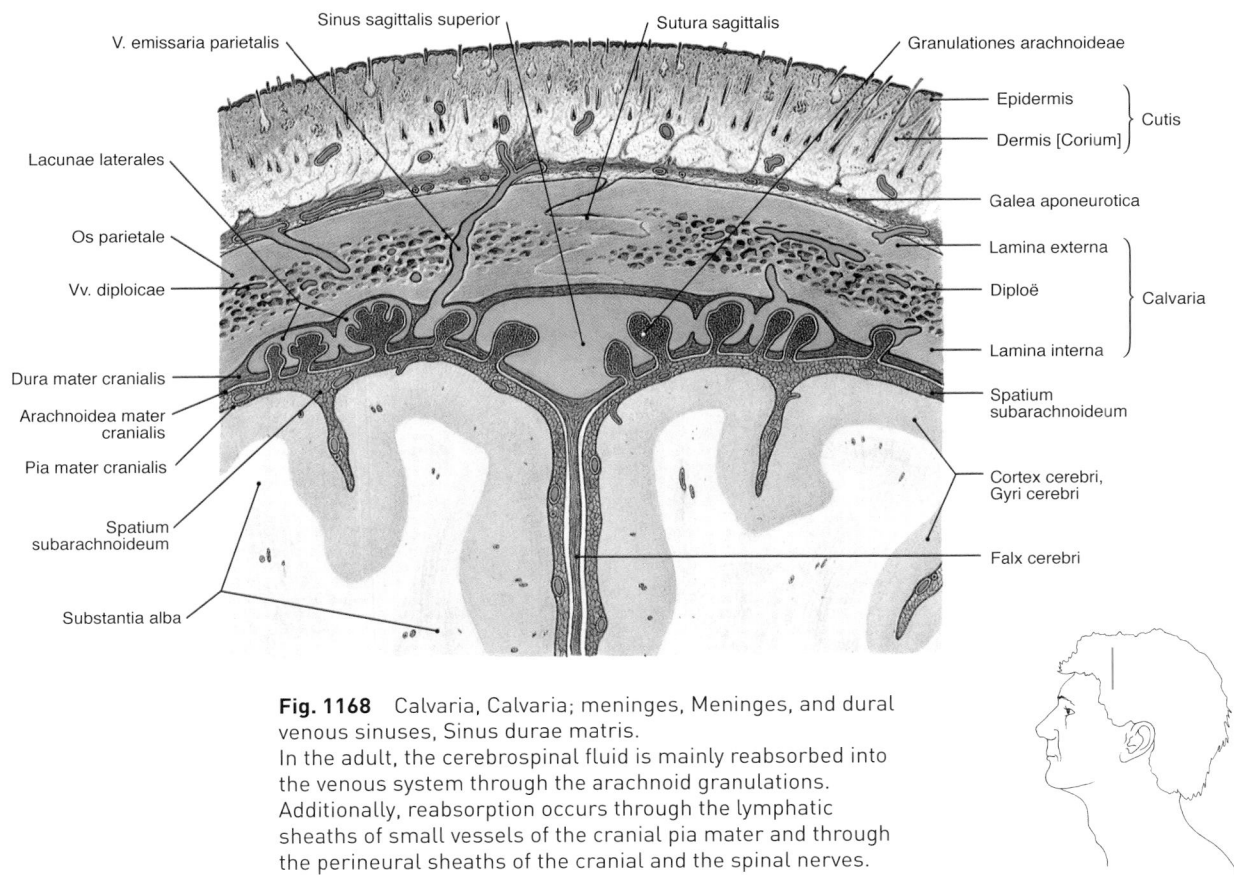

Fig. 1168 Calvaria, Calvaria; meninges, Meninges, and dural venous sinuses, Sinus durae matris.
In the adult, the cerebrospinal fluid is mainly reabsorbed into the venous system through the arachnoid granulations. Additionally, reabsorption occurs through the lymphatic sheaths of small vessels of the cranial pia mater and through the perineural sheaths of the cranial and the spinal nerves.

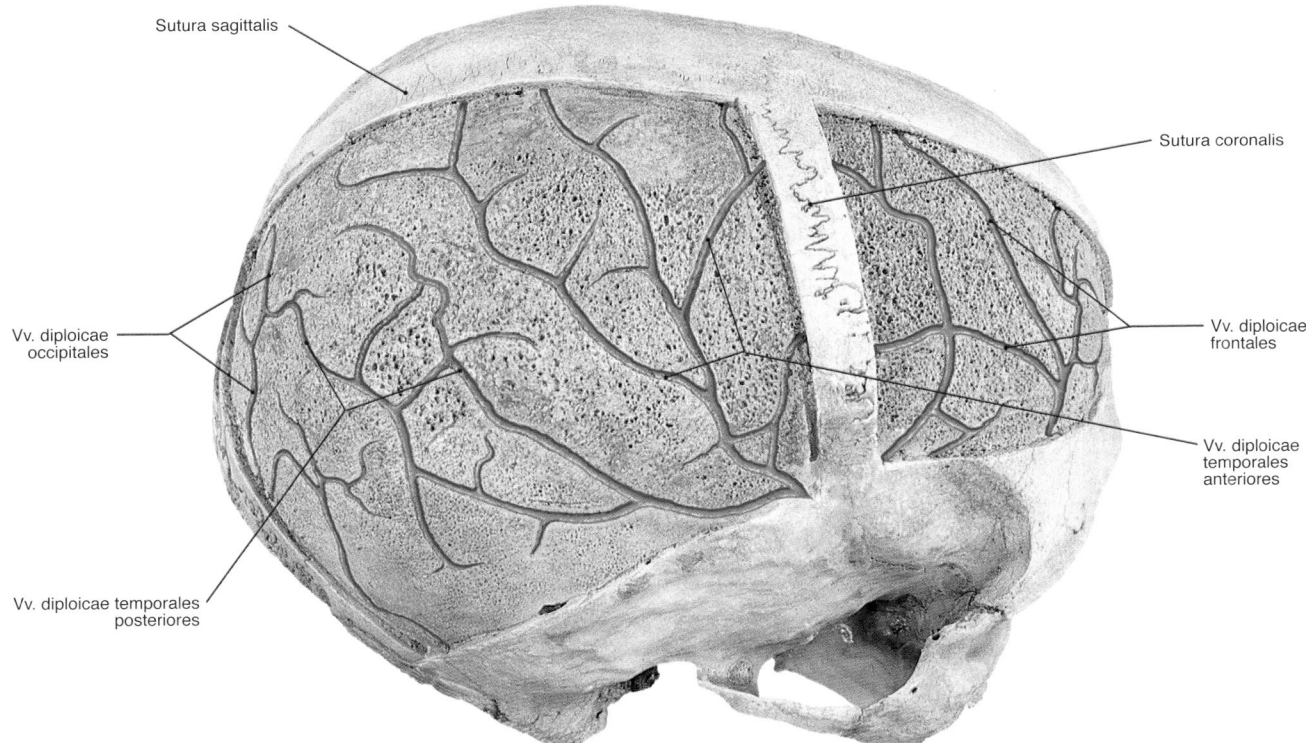

Fig. 1169 Diploic canals, Canales diploici, and diploic veins, Vv. diploicae, of the calvaria;

the external table of compact bone has been removed from the calvaria.

Dural venous sinuses

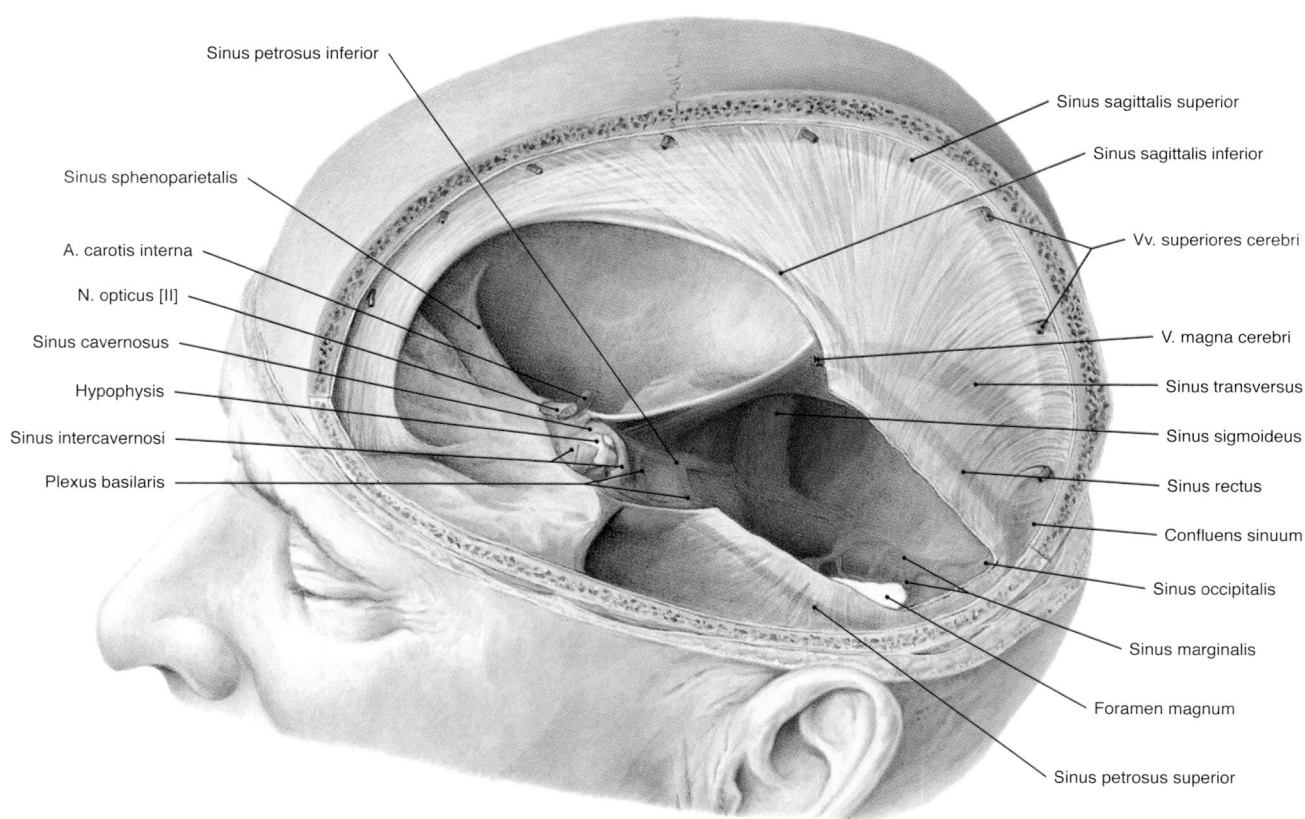

Sinus petrosus inferior

Sinus sphenoparietalis

A. carotis interna

N. opticus [II]

Sinus cavernosus

Hypophysis

Sinus intercavernosi

Plexus basilaris

Sinus sagittalis superior

Sinus sagittalis inferior

Vv. superiores cerebri

V. magna cerebri

Sinus transversus

Sinus sigmoideus

Sinus rectus

Confluens sinuum

Sinus occipitalis

Sinus marginalis

Foramen magnum

Sinus petrosus superior

Fig. 1170 Cranial dura mater, Dura mater cranialis,
and dural venous sinuses, Sinus durae matris;
after partial removal of the tentorium cerebelli.

Cranial dura mater, Dura mater cranialis

The cranial dura mater lines the cranial cavity completely
and tightly adheres to the skull bone. The cerebral falx
protrudes in the sagittal plane in a sickle-like shape and
stretches from the crista galli to the ridge of the tentorium
cerebelli, which, in turn, overstretches the posterior cranial
fossa and is attached along the transverse sinus and the
pyramidal edge. The margins of the tentorial notch envelop
the midbrain and taper off into the anterior and posterior
clinoid process. The cerebral falx and the tentorium
cerebelli divide the cranial cavity into three spaces that are
incompletely separated from one another, containing
the two cerebral hemispheres and the cerebellum.

Dural venous sinuses

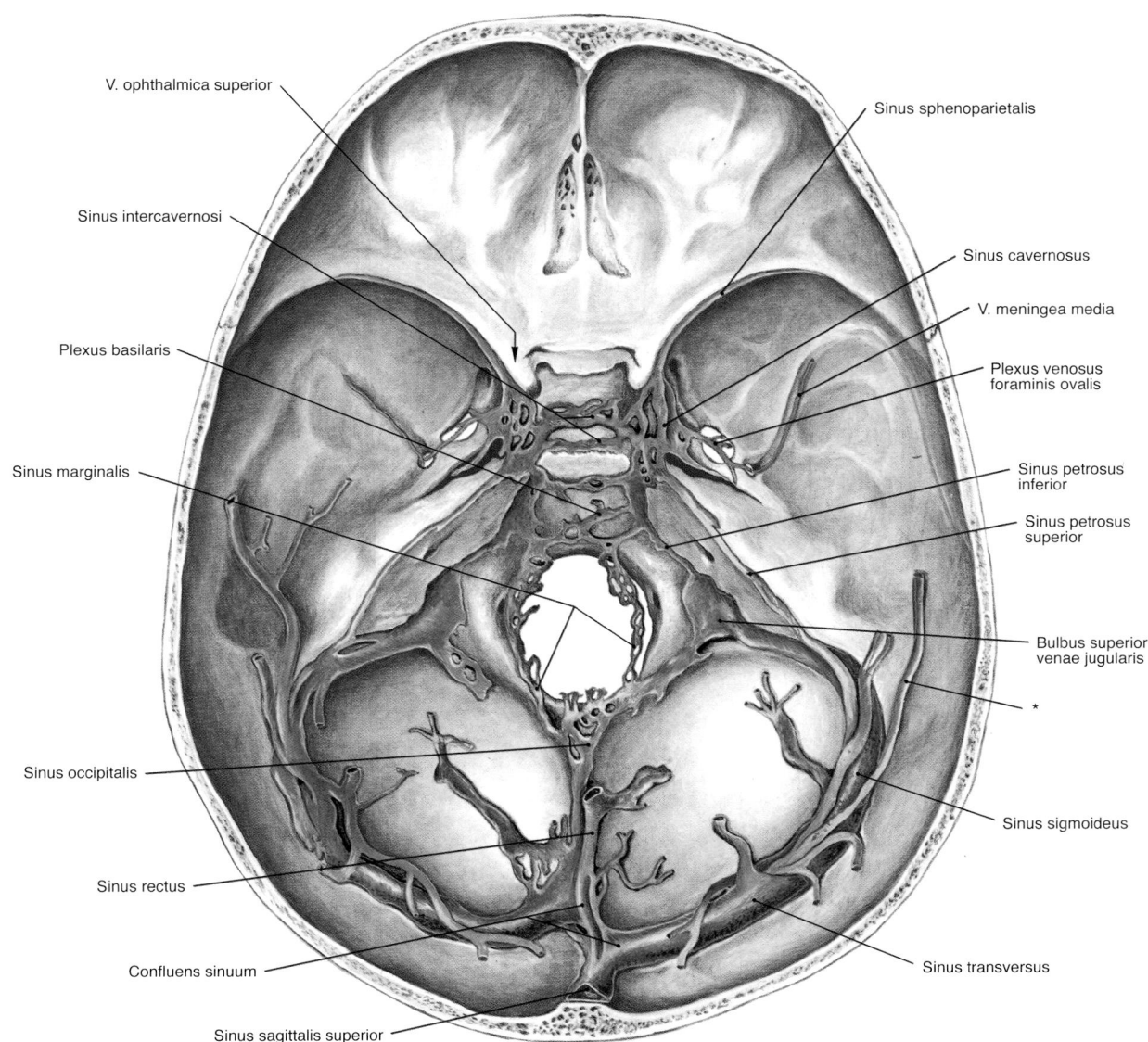

V. ophthalmica superior

Sinus sphenoparietalis

Sinus intercavernosi

Sinus cavernosus

V. meningea media

Plexus basilaris

Plexus venosus
foraminis ovalis

Sinus marginalis

Sinus petrosus
inferior

Sinus petrosus
superior

Bulbus superior
venae jugularis

*

Sinus occipitalis

Sinus sigmoideus

Sinus rectus

Confluens sinuum

Sinus transversus

Sinus sagittalis superior

Fig. 1171 Dural venous sinuses, Sinus durae matris;
corrosion cast.
The sinuses contain no valves and feature rigid walls.
* Vein of LABBÉ to the superficial middle cerebral veins

Dural venous sinuses, Sinus durae matris

The dural venous sinuses are rigid venous channels
without valves draining the venous blood from the brain via
so-called bridging veins.
The main drainage from within the skull occurs via the
sigmoid sinuses into the internal jugular veins. Additionally,
the superior ophthalmic veins and the highly variable emiss-
ary veins form a series of smaller, likewise valveless, venous
connections between the intra- and extracranial regions.

The two cavernous sinuses assume a central position by
being situated in the middle cranial fossa to the right
and the left of the sella turcica. They communicate with
each other through the intercavernous sinuses and either
directly or indirectly with most other sinuses and with the
veins of the orbit and the infratemporal fossa.

External surface of the cranial base

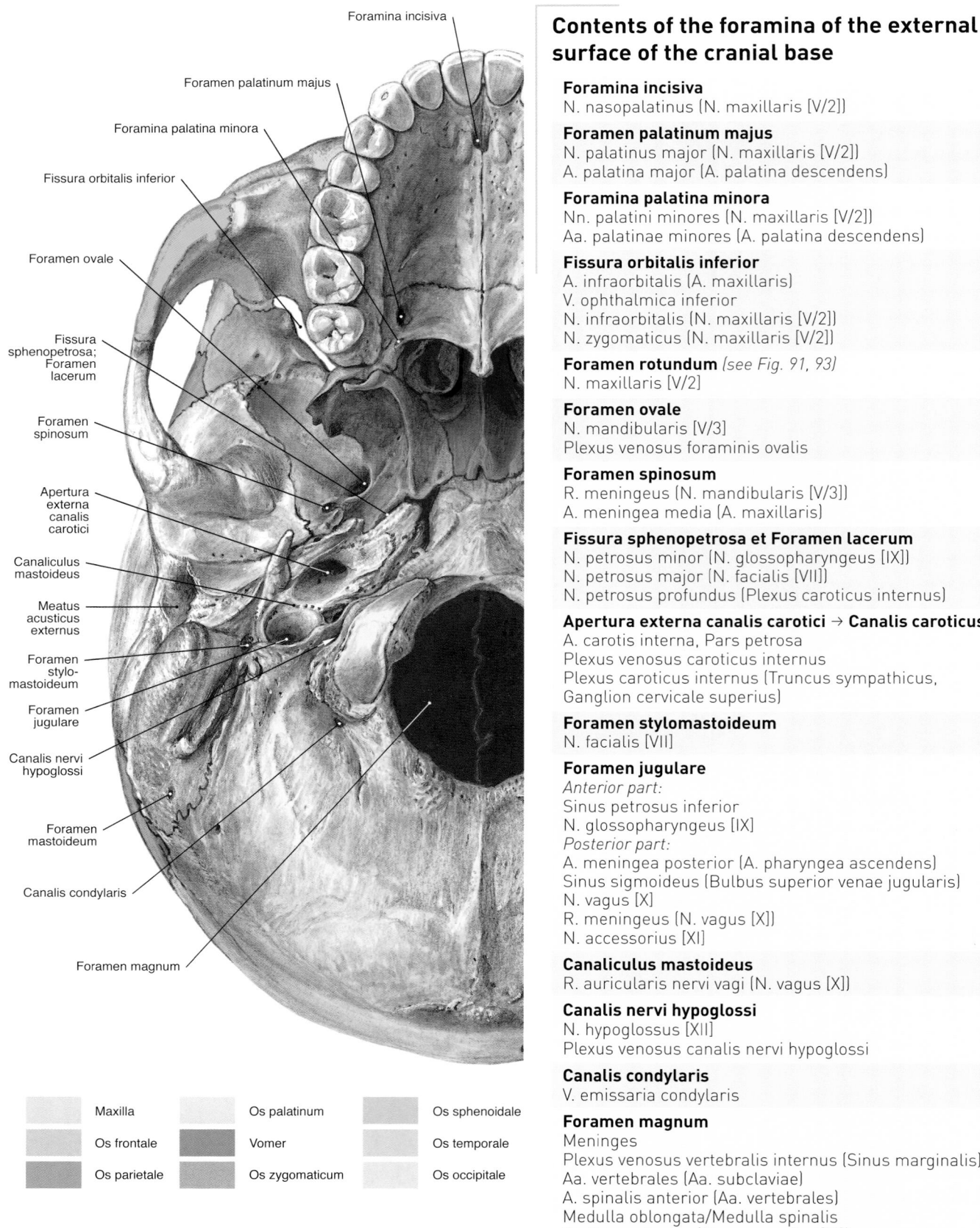

Foramina incisiva

Foramen palatinum majus

Foramina palatina minora

Fissura orbitalis inferior

Foramen ovale

Fissura sphenopetrosa; Foramen lacerum

Foramen spinosum

Apertura externa canalis carotici

Canaliculus mastoideus

Meatus acusticus externus

Foramen stylo-mastoideum

Foramen jugulare

Canalis nervi hypoglossi

Foramen mastoideum

Canalis condylaris

Foramen magnum

Maxilla	Os palatinum	Os sphenoidale
Os frontale	Vomer	Os temporale
Os parietale	Os zygomaticum	Os occipitale

Fig. 1172 External surface of the cranial base, Basis cranii externa, and foramina.

Contents of the foramina of the external surface of the cranial base

Foramina incisiva
N. nasopalatinus (N. maxillaris [V/2])

Foramen palatinum majus
N. palatinus major (N. maxillaris [V/2])
A. palatina major (A. palatina descendens)

Foramina palatina minora
Nn. palatini minores (N. maxillaris [V/2])
Aa. palatinae minores (A. palatina descendens)

Fissura orbitalis inferior
A. infraorbitalis (A. maxillaris)
V. ophthalmica inferior
N. infraorbitalis (N. maxillaris [V/2])
N. zygomaticus (N. maxillaris [V/2])

Foramen rotundum *(see Fig. 91, 93)*
N. maxillaris [V/2]

Foramen ovale
N. mandibularis [V/3]
Plexus venosus foraminis ovalis

Foramen spinosum
R. meningeus (N. mandibularis [V/3])
A. meningea media (A. maxillaris)

Fissura sphenopetrosa et Foramen lacerum
N. petrosus minor (N. glossopharyngeus [IX])
N. petrosus major (N. facialis [VII])
N. petrosus profundus (Plexus caroticus internus)

Apertura externa canalis carotici → Canalis caroticus
A. carotis interna, Pars petrosa
Plexus venosus caroticus internus
Plexus caroticus internus (Truncus sympathicus, Ganglion cervicale superius)

Foramen stylomastoideum
N. facialis [VII]

Foramen jugulare
Anterior part:
Sinus petrosus inferior
N. glossopharyngeus [IX]
Posterior part:
A. meningea posterior (A. pharyngea ascendens)
Sinus sigmoideus (Bulbus superior venae jugularis)
N. vagus [X]
R. meningeus (N. vagus [X])
N. accessorius [XI]

Canaliculus mastoideus
R. auricularis nervi vagi (N. vagus [X])

Canalis nervi hypoglossi
N. hypoglossus [XII]
Plexus venosus canalis nervi hypoglossi

Canalis condylaris
V. emissaria condylaris

Foramen magnum
Meninges
Plexus venosus vertebralis internus (Sinus marginalis)
Aa. vertebrales (Aa. subclaviae)
A. spinalis anterior (Aa. vertebrales)
Medulla oblongata/Medulla spinalis
Radices spinales (N. accessorius [XI])

Internal surface of the cranial base

Contents of the foramina of the internal surface of the cranial base

Lamina cribrosa
Nn. olfactorii [I]
A. ethmoidalis anterior (A. ophthalmica)

Canalis opticus
N. opticus [II]
A. ophthalmica (A. carotis interna)
Meninges; Vaginae nervi optici

Fissura orbitalis superior
Medial part:
N. nasociliaris (N. ophthalmicus [V/1])
N. oculomotorius [III]
N. abducens [VI]
Lateral part:
N. trochlearis [IV]
Common trunk of the:
– N. frontalis (N. ophthalmicus [V/1]
– N. lacrimalis (N. ophthalmicus [V/1]
R. orbitalis (A. meningea media)
V. ophthalmica superior

Foramen rotundum
N. maxillaris [V/2]

Foramen ovale
N. mandibularis [V/3]
Plexus venosus foraminis ovalis

Foramen spinosum
R. meningeus (N. mandibularis [V/3])
A. meningea media (A. maxillaris)

Fissura sphenopetrosa et Foramen lacerum
N. petrosus minor (N. glossopharyngeus [IX])
N. petrosus major (N. facialis [VII])
N. petrosus profundus (Plexus caroticus internus)

Apertura interna canalis carotici → Canalis caroticus
A. carotis interna, Pars petrosa
Plexus venosus caroticus internus
Plexus caroticus internus (Truncus sympathicus,
Ganglion cervicale superius)

Porus → Meatus acusticus internus
N. facialis [VII]
N. vestibulocochlearis [VIII]
A. labyrinthi (A. basilaris)
Vv. labyrinthi

Foramen jugulare
Anterior part:
Sinus petrosus inferior
N. glossopharyngeus [IX]
Posterior part:
A. meningea posterior (A. pharyngea ascendens)
Sinus sigmoideus (Bulbus superior venae jugularis)
N. vagus [X]
N. accessorius [XI]
R. meningeus (N. vagus [X])

Canalis nervi hypoglossi
N. hypoglossus [XII]
Plexus venosus canalis nervi hypoglossi

Canalis condylaris
V. emissaria condylaris

Foramen magnum
Meninges
Plexus venosus vertebralis internus (Sinus marginalis)
Aa. vertebrales (Aa. subclaviae)
A. spinalis anterior (Aa. vertebrales)
Medulla oblongata/Medulla spinalis
Radices spinales (N. accessorius [XI])

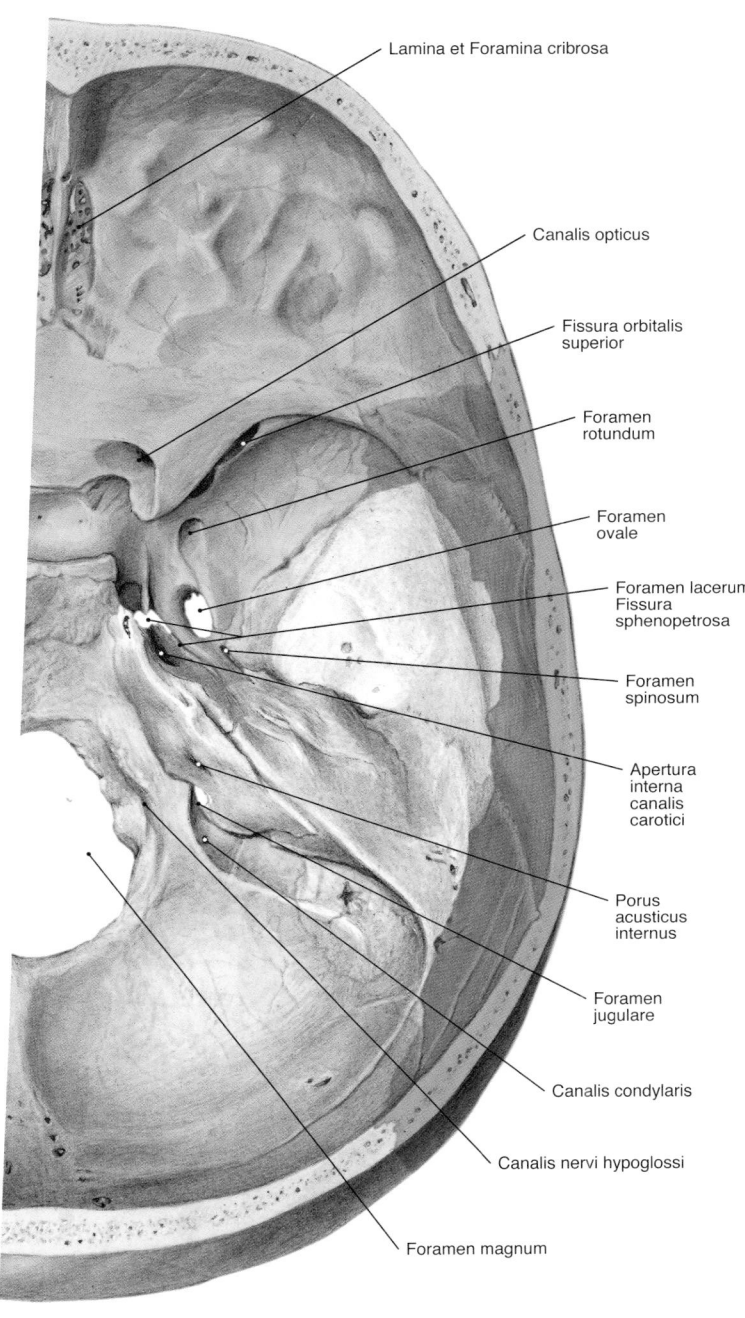

Lamina et Foramina cribrosa

Canalis opticus

Fissura orbitalis superior

Foramen rotundum

Foramen ovale

Foramen lacerum; Fissura sphenopetrosa

Foramen spinosum

Apertura interna canalis carotici

Porus acusticus internus

Foramen jugulare

Canalis condylaris

Canalis nervi hypoglossi

Foramen magnum

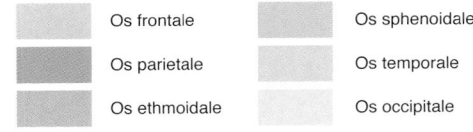

Os frontale		Os sphenoidale	
Os parietale		Os temporale	
Os ethmoidale		Os occipitale	

Fig. 1173 Internal surface of the cranial base, Basis cranii interna, and foramina.

Cranial nerves, overview

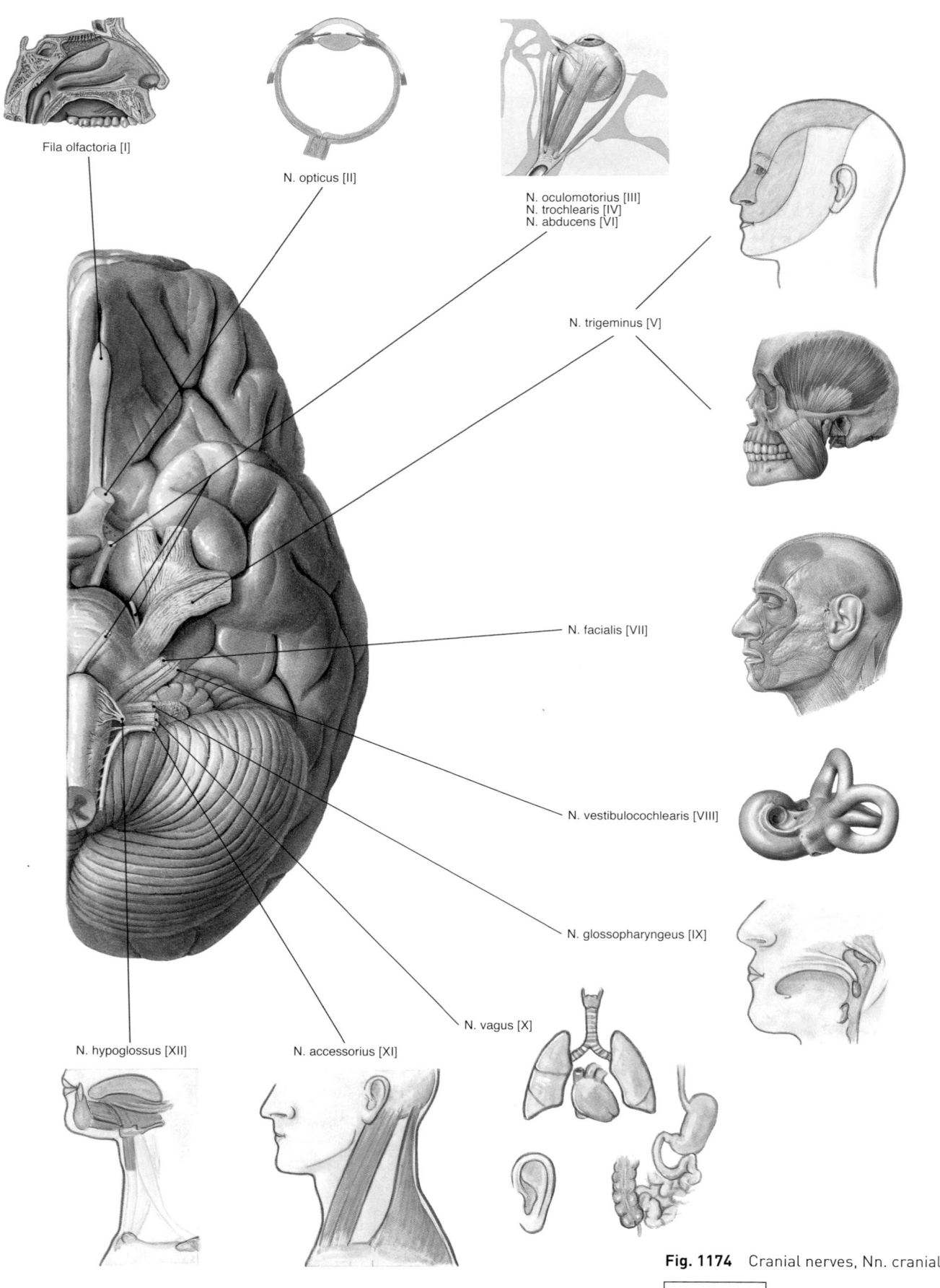

Fila olfactoria [I]

N. opticus [II]

N. oculomotorius [III]
N. trochlearis [IV]
N. abducens [VI]

N. trigeminus [V]

N. facialis [VII]

N. vestibulocochlearis [VIII]

N. glossopharyngeus [IX]

N. vagus [X]

N. hypoglossus [XII]

N. accessorius [XI]

Fig. 1174 Cranial nerves, Nn. craniales.

→ T 55, T 57

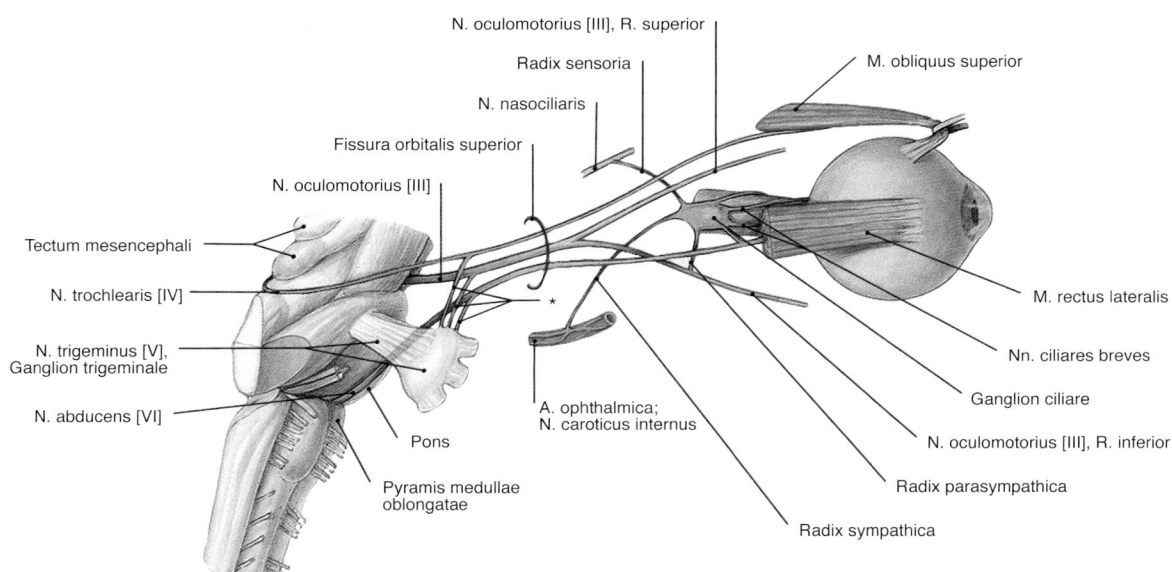

Fig. 1175 Oculomotor nerve, N. oculomotorius [III], trochlear nerve, N. trochlearis [IV], and abducens nerve, N. abducens [VI]; viewed from the right.
* Connections to the trigeminal ganglion

→ T 57 c, d, f

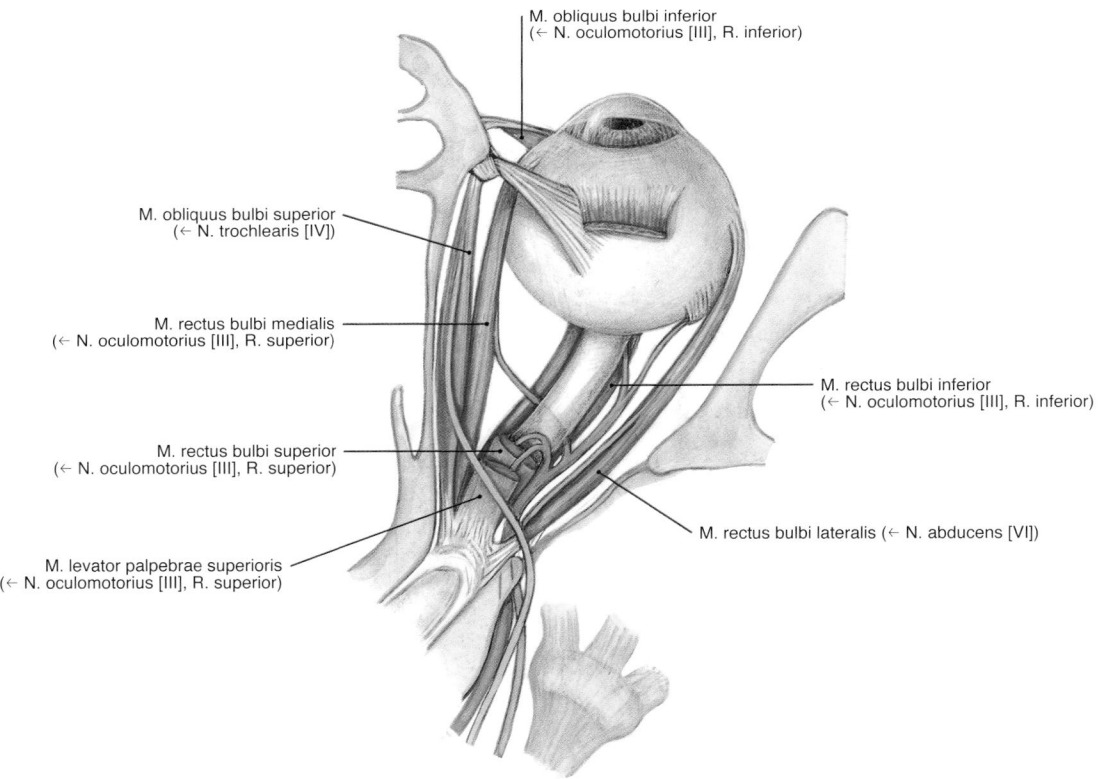

Fig. 1176 Innervation of the ocular muscles; superior view.

Cranial nerves

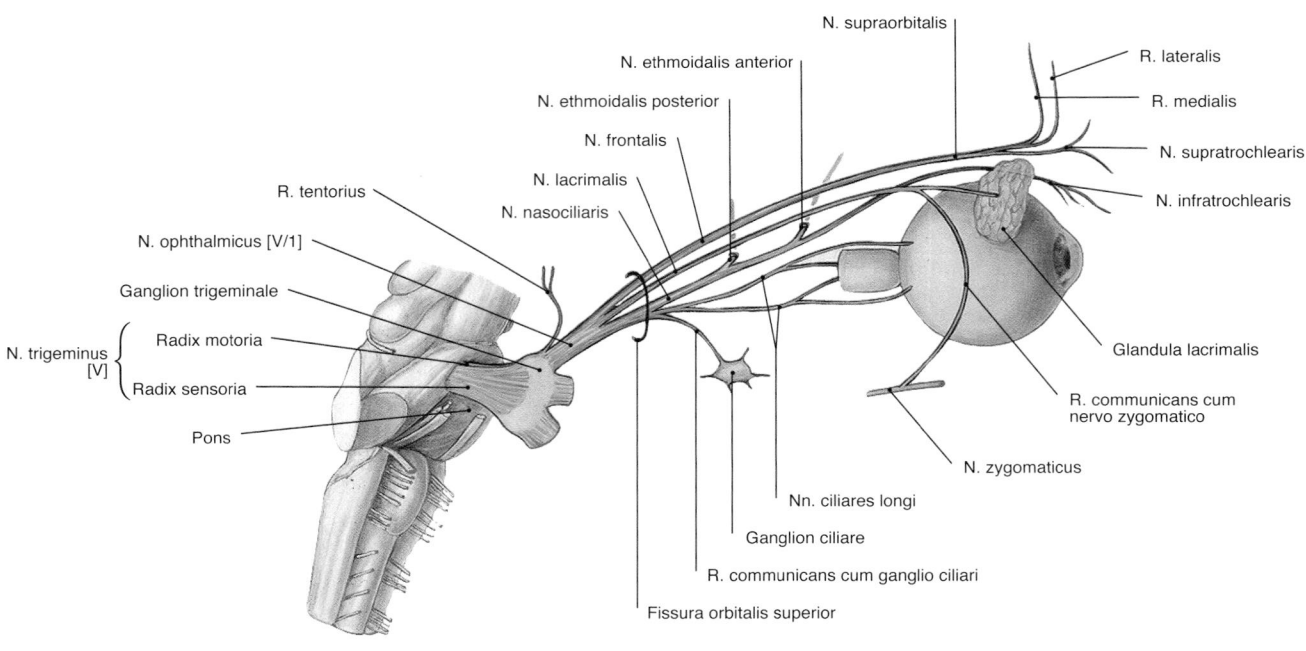

N. supraorbitalis
N. ethmoidalis anterior
N. ethmoidalis posterior
N. frontalis
N. lacrimalis
N. nasociliaris
R. tentorius
N. ophthalmicus [V/1]
Ganglion trigeminale
N. trigeminus [V]
Radix motoria
Radix sensoria
Pons
R. lateralis
R. medialis
N. supratrochlearis
N. infratrochlearis
Glandula lacrimalis
R. communicans cum nervo zygomatico
N. zygomaticus
Nn. ciliares longi
Ganglion ciliare
R. communicans cum ganglio ciliari
Fissura orbitalis superior

→ T 57 e

Fig. 1177   Ophthalmic nerve, N. ophthalmicus [V/1]; viewed from the right.

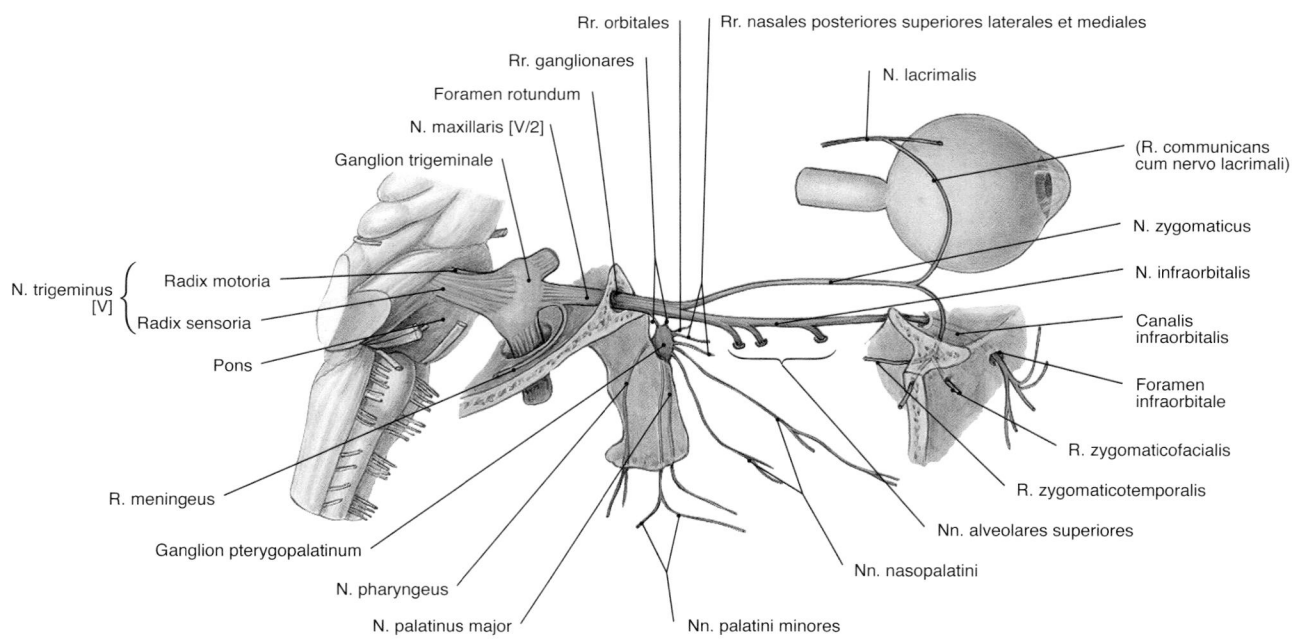

Rr. orbitales
Rr. ganglionares
Foramen rotundum
N. maxillaris [V/2]
Ganglion trigeminale
N. trigeminus [V]
Radix motoria
Radix sensoria
Pons
R. meningeus
Ganglion pterygopalatinum
N. pharyngeus
N. palatinus major
Rr. nasales posteriores superiores laterales et mediales
N. lacrimalis
(R. communicans cum nervo lacrimali)
N. zygomaticus
N. infraorbitalis
Canalis infraorbitalis
Foramen infraorbitale
R. zygomaticofacialis
R. zygomaticotemporalis
Nn. alveolares superiores
Nn. nasopalatini
Nn. palatini minores

→ T 57 e

Fig. 1178   Maxillary nerve, N. maxillaris [V/2]; viewed from the right.

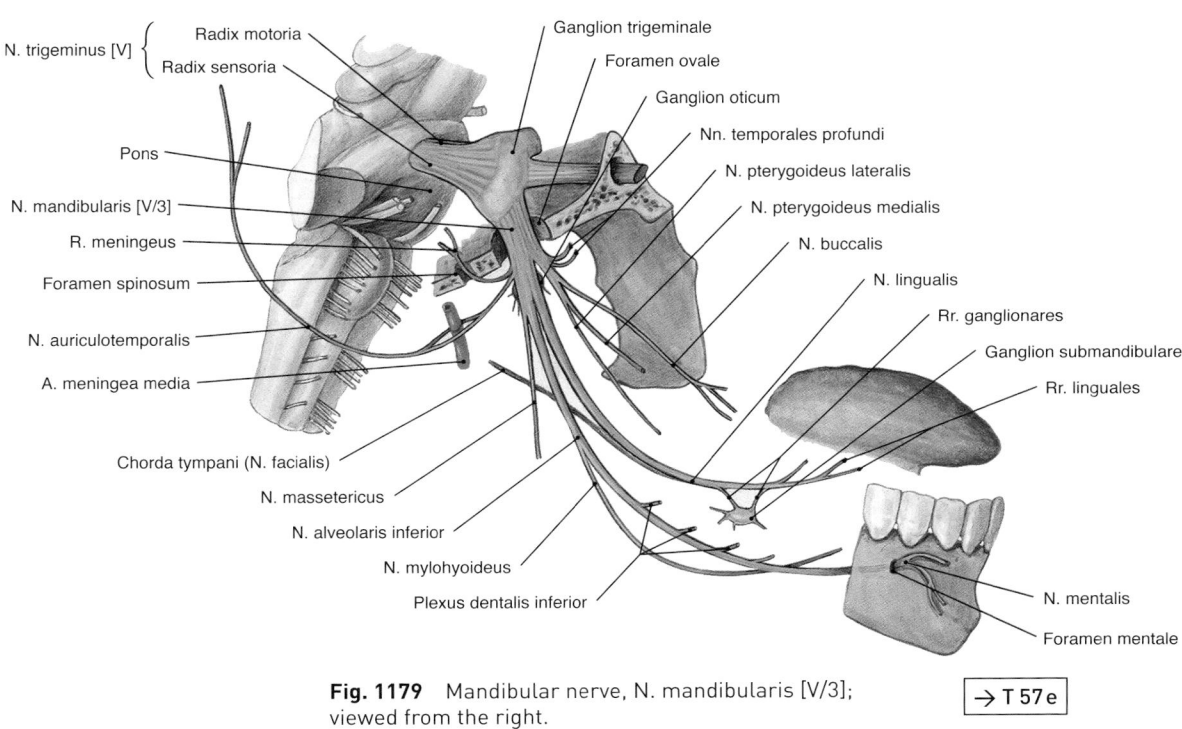

N. trigeminus [V]
Radix motoria
Radix sensoria
Ganglion trigeminale
Foramen ovale
Ganglion oticum
Pons
Nn. temporales profundi
N. mandibularis [V/3]
N. pterygoideus lateralis
R. meningeus
N. pterygoideus medialis
Foramen spinosum
N. buccalis
N. auriculotemporalis
N. lingualis
A. meningea media
Rr. ganglionares
Ganglion submandibulare
Rr. linguales
Chorda tympani (N. facialis)
N. massetericus
N. alveolaris inferior
N. mylohyoideus
Plexus dentalis inferior
N. mentalis
Foramen mentale

Fig. 1179   Mandibular nerve, N. mandibularis [V/3];
viewed from the right.

→ T 57 e

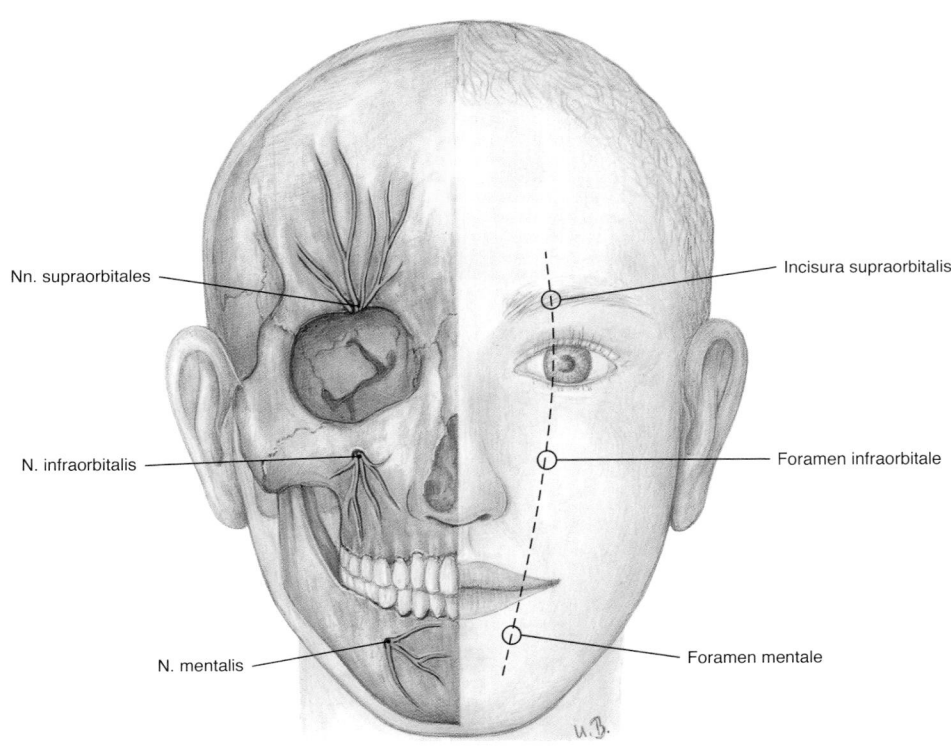

Nn. supraorbitales
Incisura supraorbitalis
N. infraorbitalis
Foramen infraorbitale
N. mentalis
Foramen mentale

Fig. 1180   Exit points of the cutaneous branches of the trigeminal nerve,
N. trigeminus [V].
Clinically, they are referred to as nerve exit points.

Cranial nerves

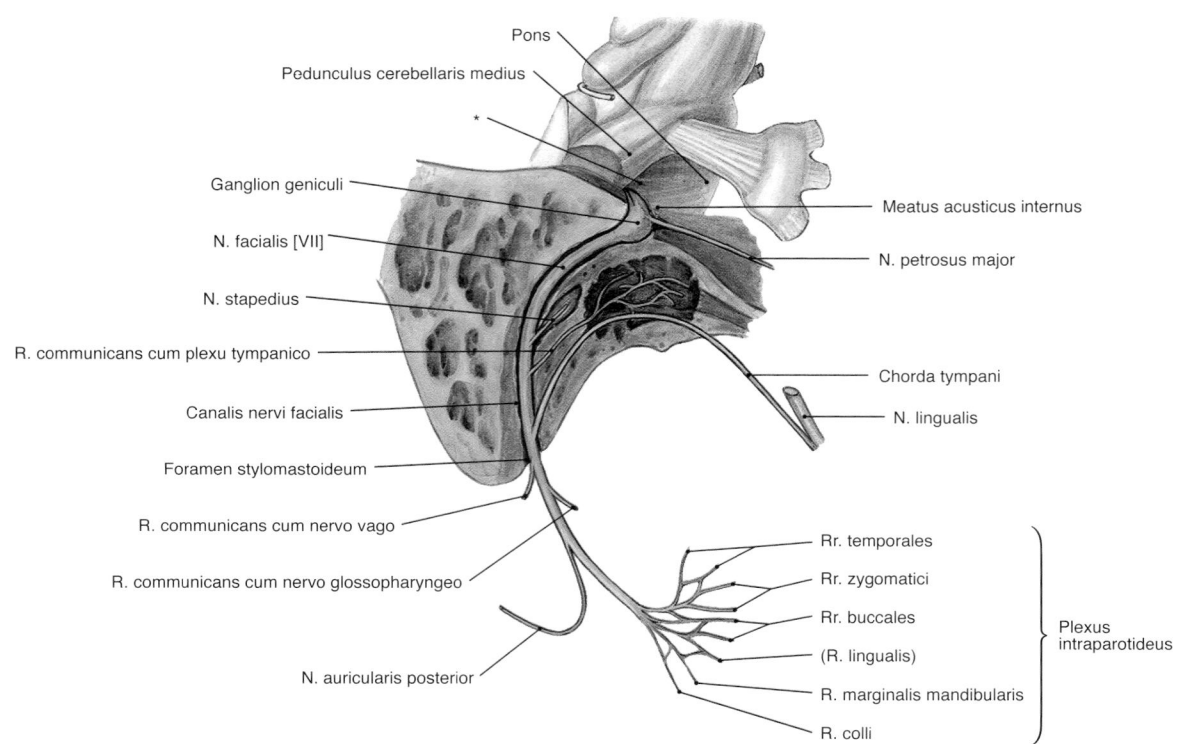

→ T 57 g

Fig. 1181 Facial nerve, N. facialis [VII];
the facial canal and the tympanic cavity have been opened;
viewed from the right.
* Clinical term: cerebellopontine angle

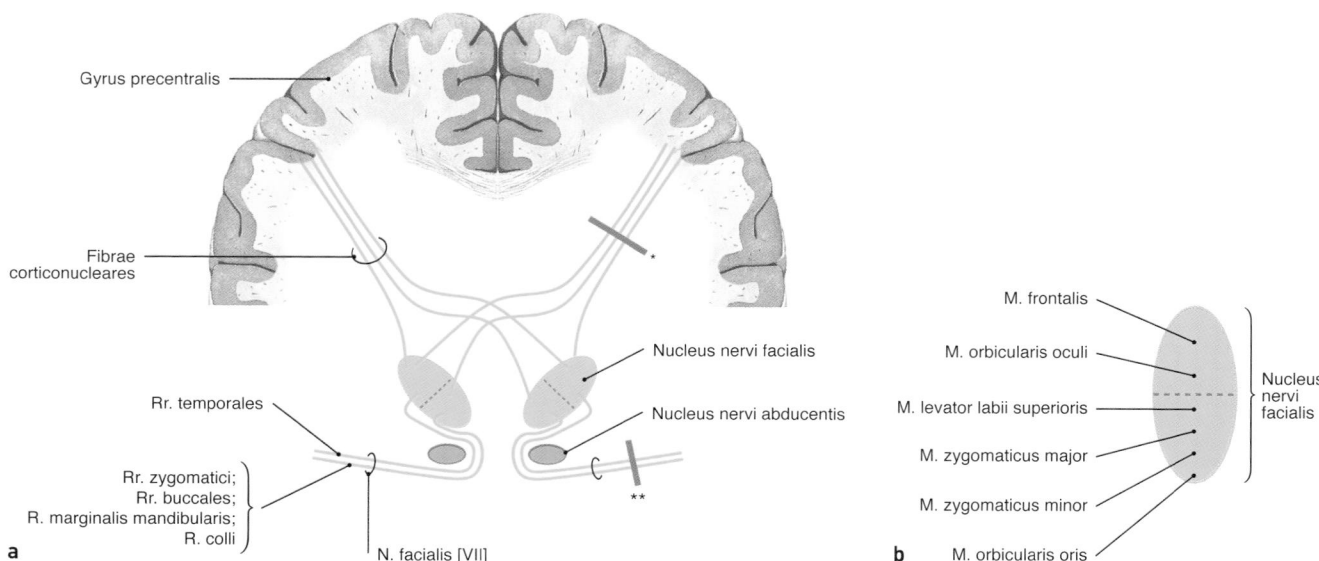

Fig. 1182 a, b Neuronal structure of the motor part
of the facial nerve, N. facialis [VII].
a Overview
b Representation of the facial muscles in the motor nucleus
of the facial nerve
Though the nuclei of the upper facial muscles receive
innervation from both hemispheres, those of the lower facial
muscles are only innervated from the contralateral side.
Therefore, patients with central palsy (*) are still able to frown
the brow and to close the eyelids just sufficiently. However, in
patients with peripheral palsy (**) all facial muscles are
paralyzed.

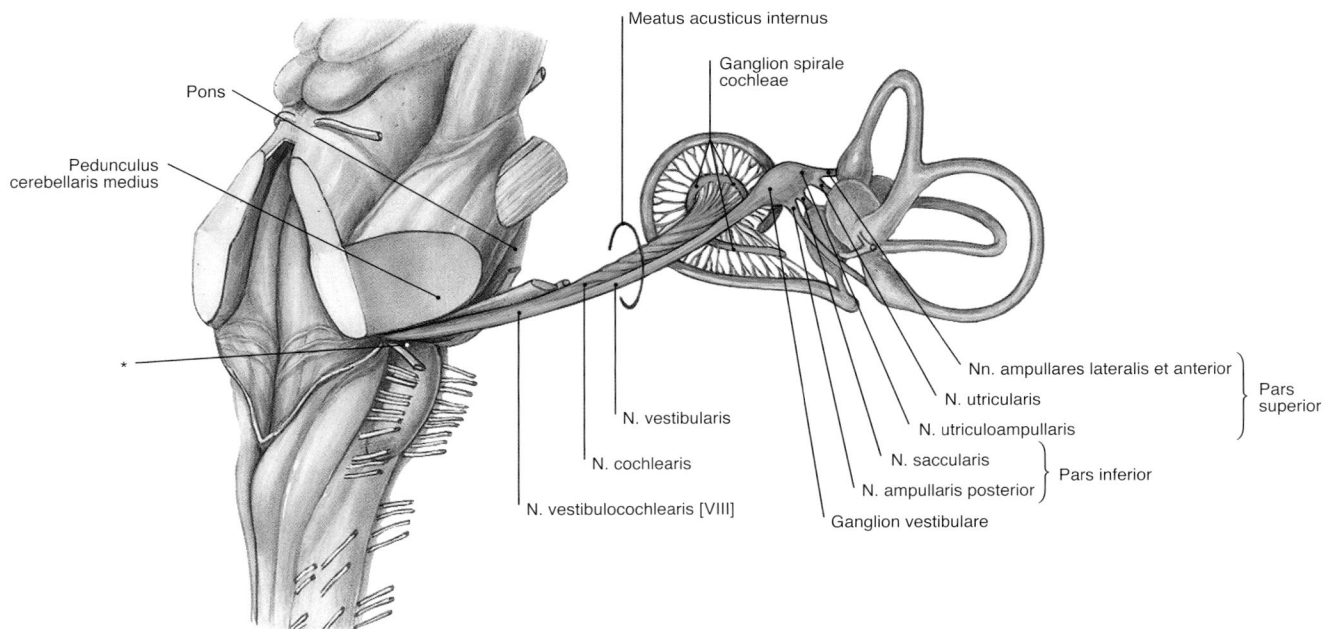

Meatus acusticus internus

Ganglion spirale cochleae

Pons

Pedunculus cerebellaris medius

Nn. ampullares lateralis et anterior

N. utricularis

N. utriculoampullaris

Pars superior

N. vestibularis

N. saccularis

N. cochlearis

N. ampullaris posterior

Pars inferior

N. vestibulocochlearis [VIII]

Ganglion vestibulare

*

Fig. 1183   Vestibulocochlear nerve, N. vestibulocochlearis [VIII]; the membranous labyrinth is greatly enlarged; posterior view from the right.
* Clinical term: cerebellopontine angle

→ T 57 h

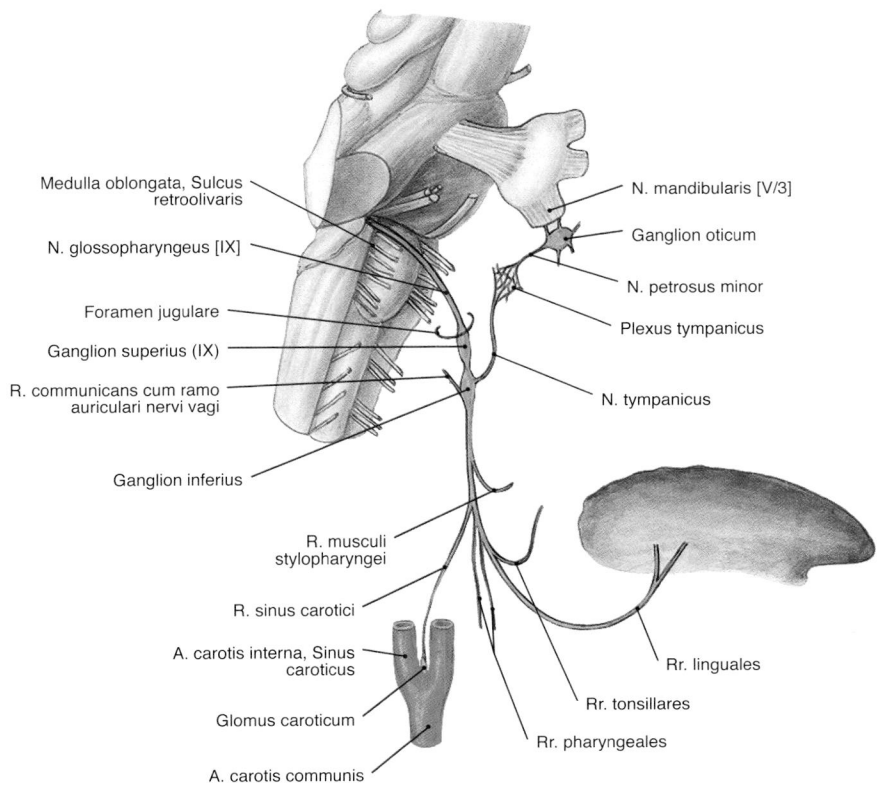

Medulla oblongata, Sulcus retroolivaris

N. mandibularis [V/3]

N. glossopharyngeus [IX]

Ganglion oticum

Foramen jugulare

N. petrosus minor

Ganglion superius (IX)

Plexus tympanicus

R. communicans cum ramo auriculari nervi vagi

Ganglion inferius

N. tympanicus

R. musculi stylopharyngei

R. sinus carotici

A. carotis interna, Sinus caroticus

Rr. linguales

Glomus caroticum

Rr. tonsillares

A. carotis communis

Rr. pharyngeales

Fig. 1184   Glossopharyngeal nerve, N. glossopharyngeus [IX]; viewed from the right.

→ T 57 i

Cranial nerves

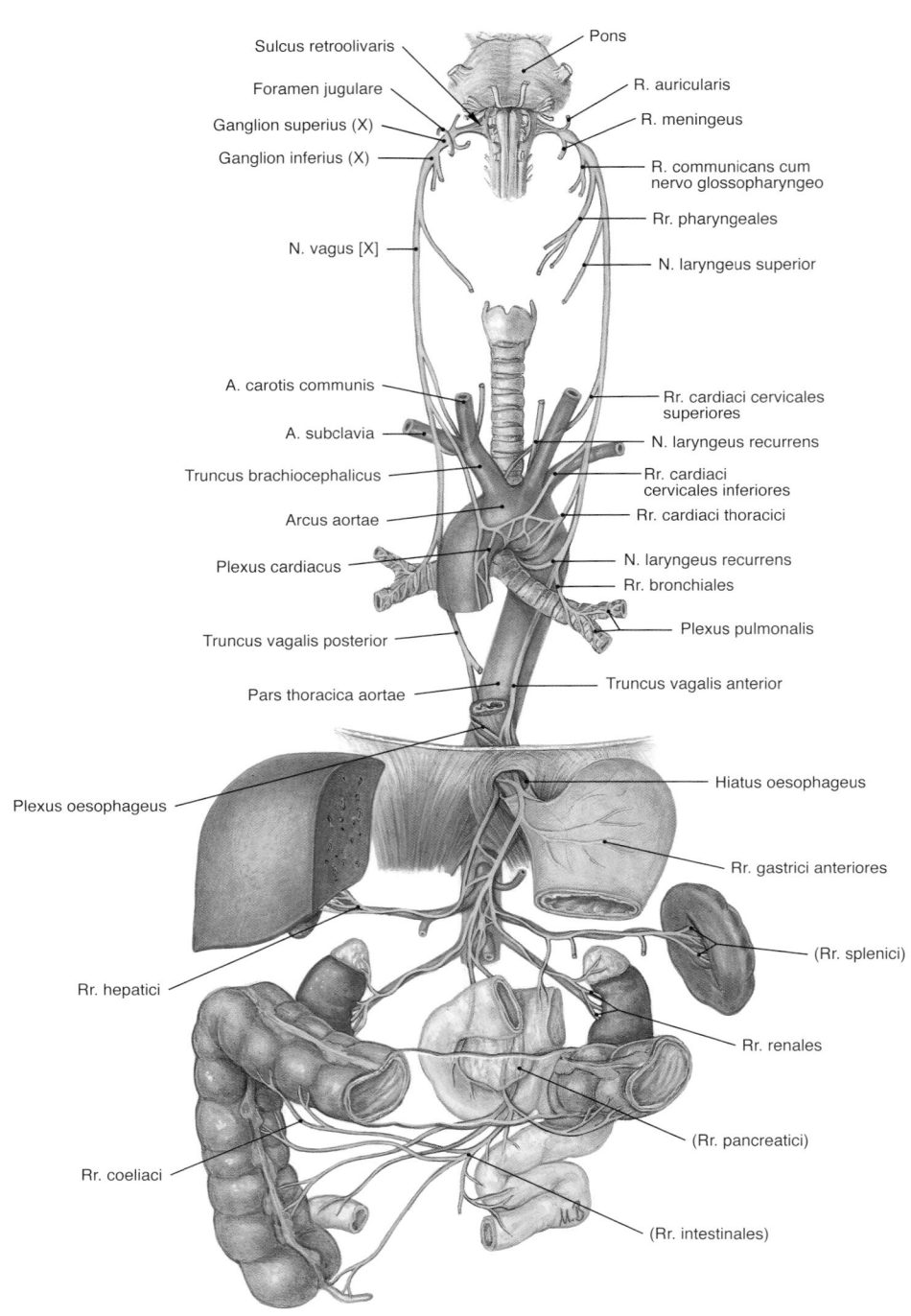

Sulcus retroolivaris

Foramen jugulare

Ganglion superius (X)

Ganglion inferius (X)

N. vagus [X]

A. carotis communis

A. subclavia

Truncus brachiocephalicus

Arcus aortae

Plexus cardiacus

Truncus vagalis posterior

Pars thoracica aortae

Plexus oesophageus

Rr. hepatici

Rr. coeliaci

Pons

R. auricularis

R. meningeus

R. communicans cum nervo glossopharyngeo

Rr. pharyngeales

N. laryngeus superior

Rr. cardiaci cervicales superiores

N. laryngeus recurrens

Rr. cardiaci cervicales inferiores

Rr. cardiaci thoracici

N. laryngeus recurrens

Rr. bronchiales

Plexus pulmonalis

Truncus vagalis anterior

Hiatus oesophageus

Rr. gastrici anteriores

(Rr. splenici)

Rr. renales

(Rr. pancreatici)

(Rr. intestinales)

→ T 57j

Fig. 1185 Vagus nerve, N. vagus [X];
both nerves;
semi-schematic;
anterior view.

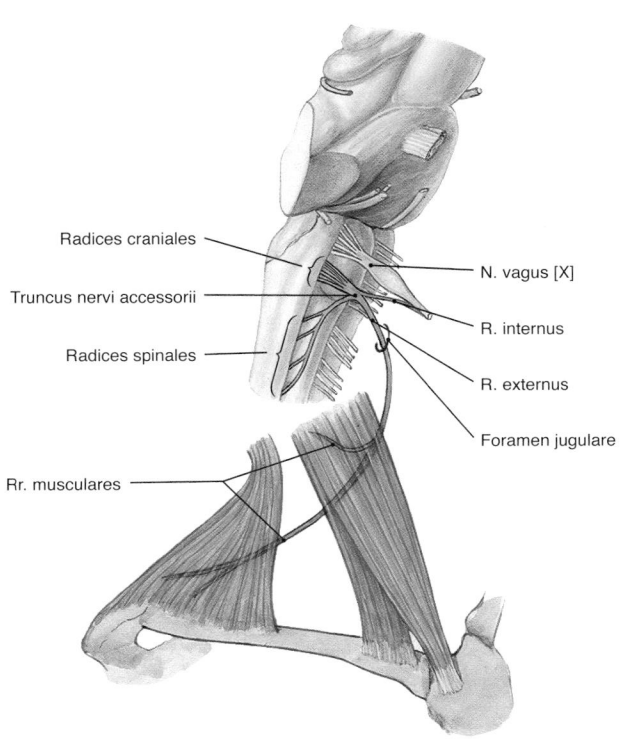

Radices craniales
Truncus nervi accessorii
Radices spinales
Rr. musculares

N. vagus [X]
R. internus
R. externus
Foramen jugulare

Fig. 1186 Accessory nerve, N. accessorius [XI]; viewed from the right. → T 57 k

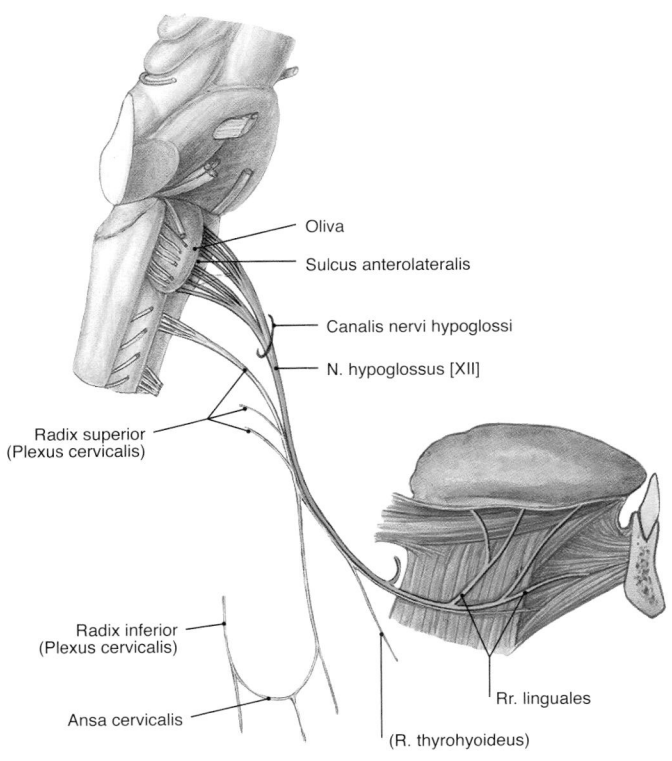

Oliva
Sulcus anterolateralis
Canalis nervi hypoglossi
N. hypoglossus [XII]
Radix superior (Plexus cervicalis)
Radix inferior (Plexus cervicalis)
Ansa cervicalis
Rr. linguales
(R. thyrohyoideus)

Fig. 1187 Hypoglossal nerve, N. hypoglossus [XII]; viewed from the right. → T 57 l

Cranial nerves

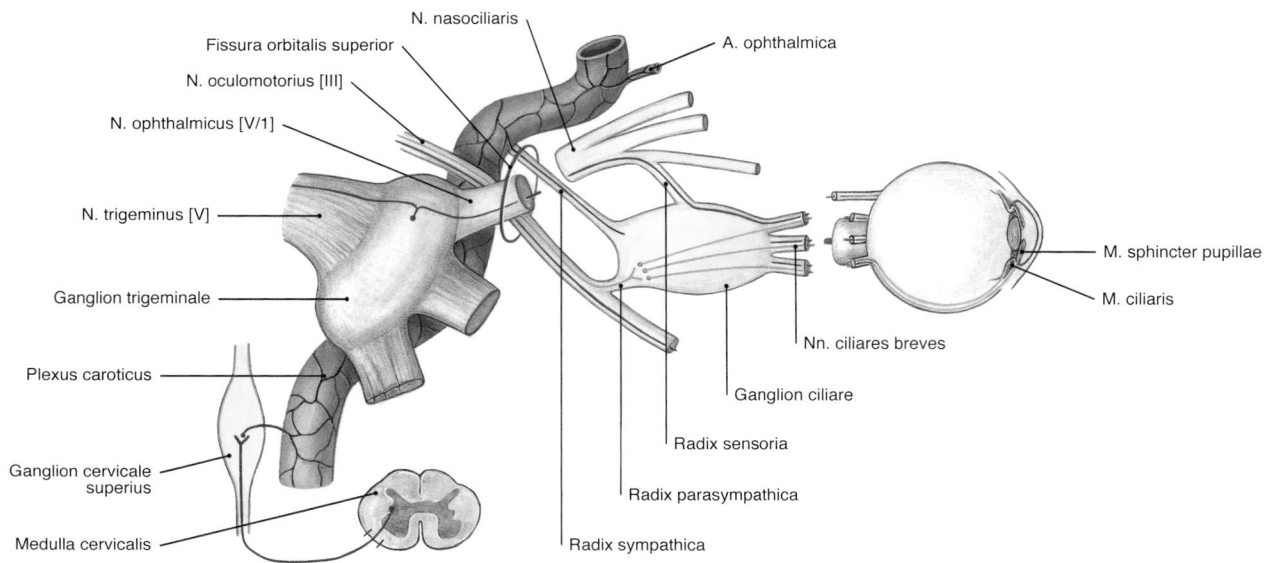

N. nasociliaris
Fissura orbitalis superior
N. oculomotorius [III]
N. ophthalmicus [V/1]
N. trigeminus [V]
Ganglion trigeminale
Plexus caroticus
Ganglion cervicale superius
Medulla cervicalis

A. ophthalmica
M. sphincter pupillae
M. ciliaris
Nn. ciliares breves
Ganglion ciliare
Radix sensoria
Radix parasympathica
Radix sympathica

Fig. 1188   Ciliary ganglion, Ganglion ciliare; overview.

Nuclear region:
Accessory nucleus of the oculomotor nerve,
Nucleus accessorius nervi oculomotorii

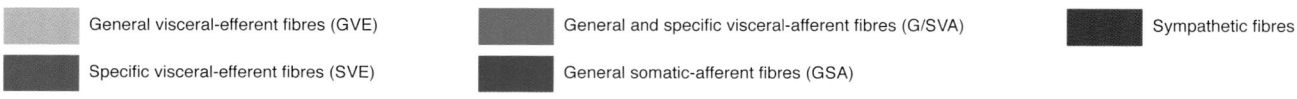

General visceral-efferent fibres (GVE)
Specific visceral-efferent fibres (SVE)
General and specific visceral-afferent fibres (G/SVA)
General somatic-afferent fibres (GSA)
Sympathetic fibres

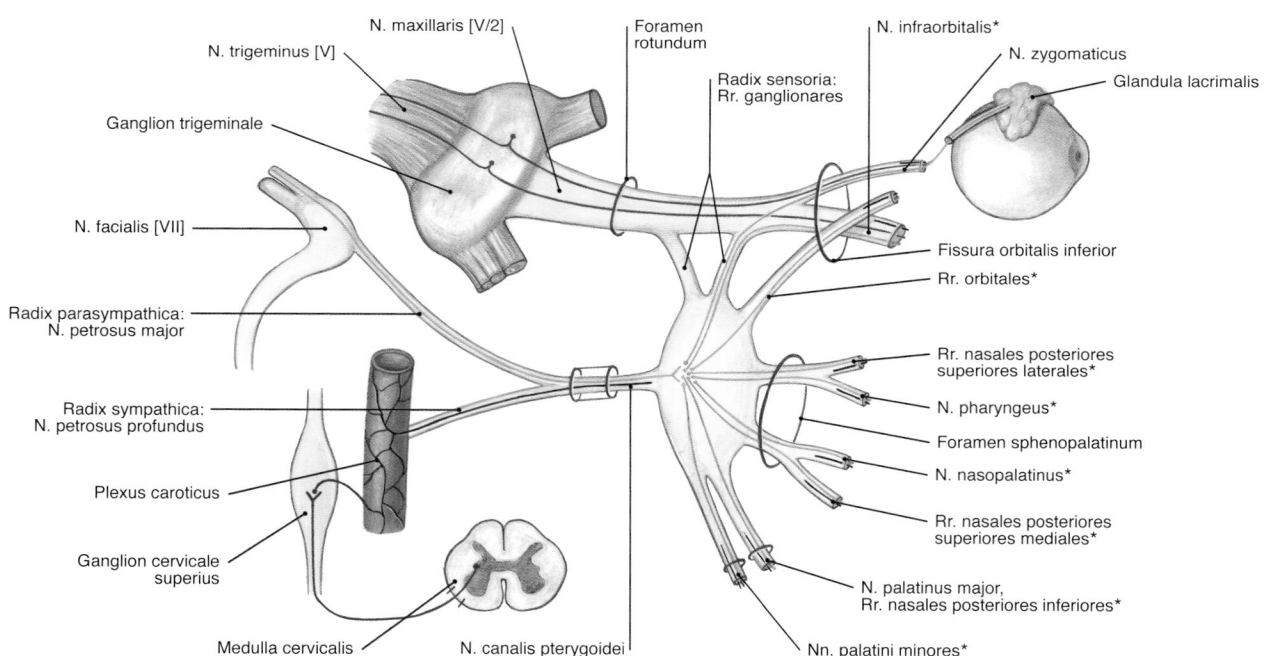

N. maxillaris [V/2]
N. trigeminus [V]
Ganglion trigeminale
N. facialis [VII]
Radix parasympathica:
N. petrosus major
Radix sympathica:
N. petrosus profundus
Plexus caroticus
Ganglion cervicale superius
Medulla cervicalis
N. canalis pterygoidei

Foramen rotundum
Radix sensoria:
Rr. ganglionares
N. infraorbitalis*
N. zygomaticus
Glandula lacrimalis
Fissura orbitalis inferior
Rr. orbitales*
Rr. nasales posteriores superiores laterales*
N. pharyngeus*
Foramen sphenopalatinum
N. nasopalatinus*
Rr. nasales posteriores superiores mediales*
N. palatinus major,
Rr. nasales posteriores inferiores*
Nn. palatini minores*

Fig. 1189   Pterygopalatine ganglion, Ganglion pterygopalatinum; overview.
* Innervation of the glands of the nose and the palate

Nuclear region:
Superior salivatory nucleus,
Nucleus salivatorius superior

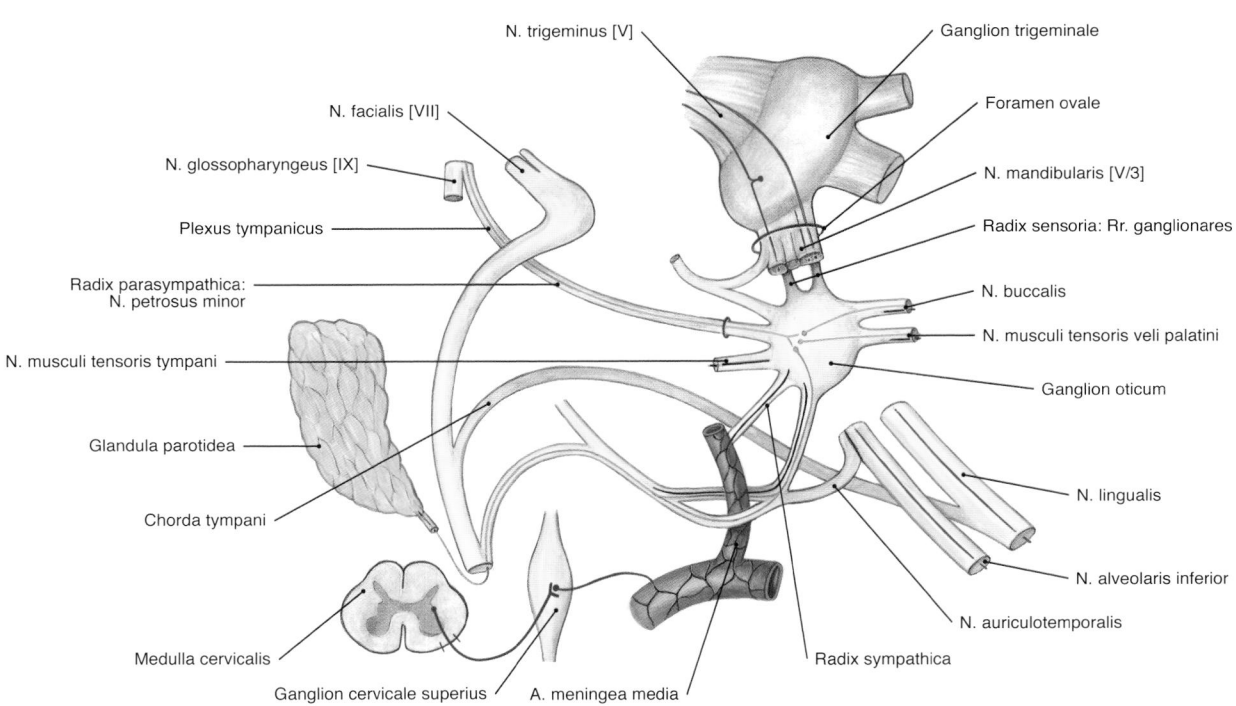

N. trigeminus [V]

Ganglion trigeminale

N. facialis [VII]

Foramen ovale

N. glossopharyngeus [IX]

N. mandibularis [V/3]

Plexus tympanicus

Radix sensoria: Rr. ganglionares

Radix parasympathica: N. petrosus minor

N. buccalis

N. musculi tensoris tympani

N. musculi tensoris veli palatini

Glandula parotidea

Ganglion oticum

Chorda tympani

N. lingualis

N. alveolaris inferior

N. auriculotemporalis

Medulla cervicalis

Radix sympathica

Ganglion cervicale superius | A. meningea media

Fig. 1190 Otic ganglion, Ganglion oticum; overview.

Nuclear region:
Inferior salivatory nucleus,
Nucleus salivatorius inferior

General visceral-efferent fibres (GVE)

General and specific visceral-afferent fibres (G/SVA)

Sympathetic fibres

Specific visceral-efferent fibres (SVE)

General somatic-afferent fibres (GSA)

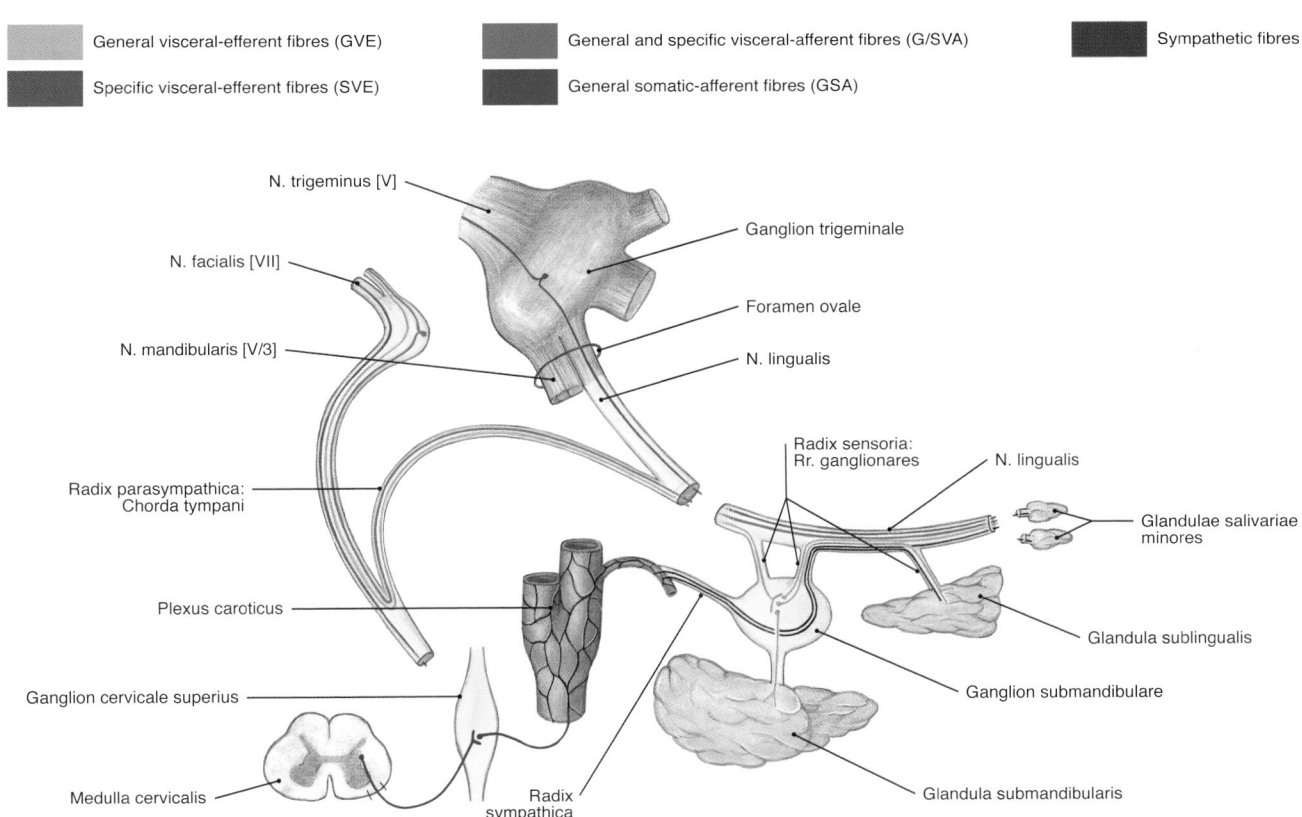

N. trigeminus [V]

Ganglion trigeminale

N. facialis [VII]

Foramen ovale

N. mandibularis [V/3]

N. lingualis

Radix sensoria: Rr. ganglionares

N. lingualis

Radix parasympathica: Chorda tympani

Glandulae salivariae minores

Plexus caroticus

Glandula sublingualis

Ganglion cervicale superius

Ganglion submandibulare

Medulla cervicalis

Radix sympathica

Glandula submandibularis

Fig. 1191 Submandibular ganglion, Ganglion submandibulare; overview.

Nuclear region:
Superior salivatory nucleus,
Nucleus salivatorius superior

Cranial nerves, topography

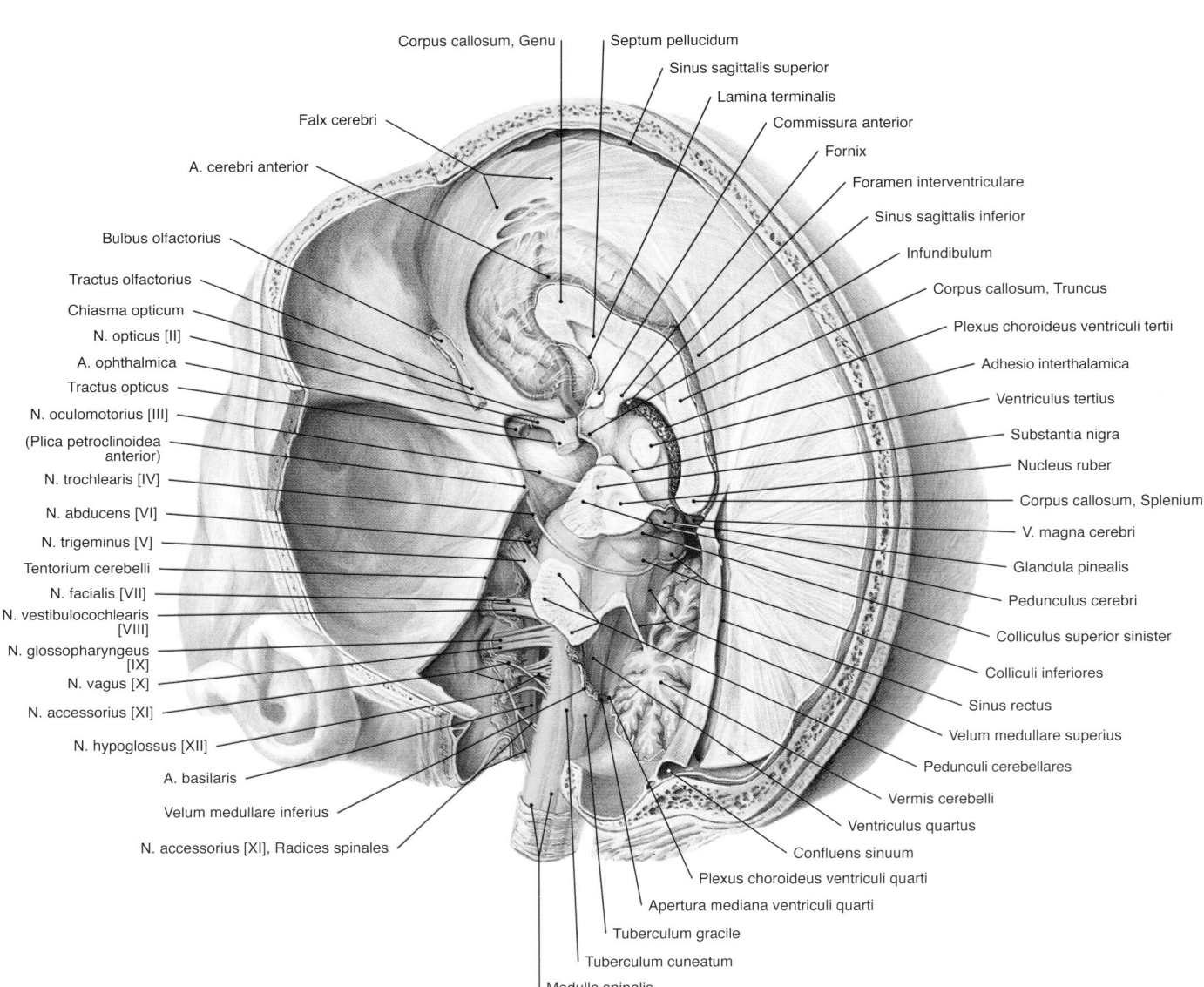

Fig. 1192 Course of the cranial nerves, Nn. craniales, in the subarachnoid space; the left hemisphere of the cerebrum and the cerebellum as well as the tentorium cerebelli have been removed.

Cranial nerves, topography

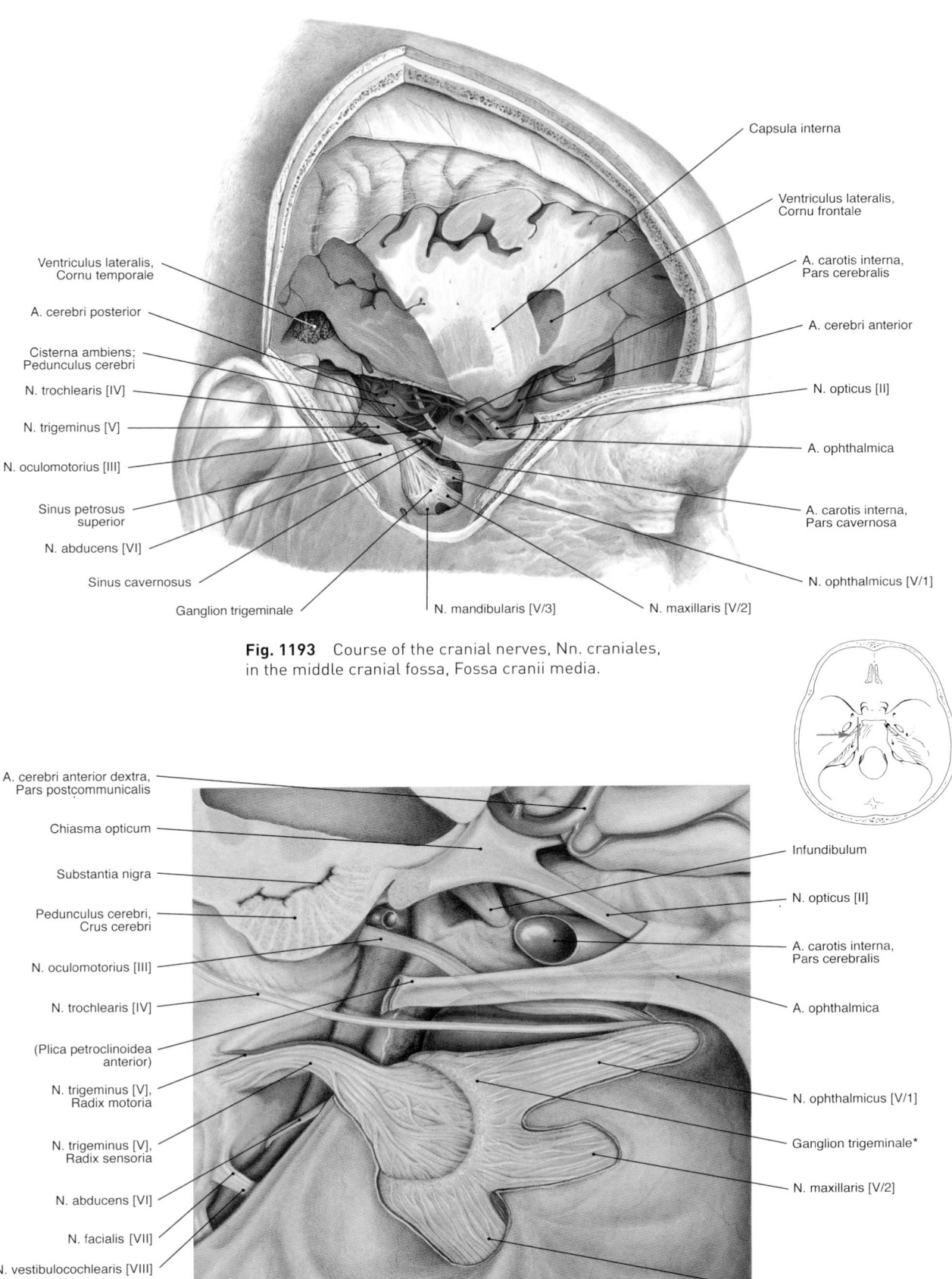

Capsula interna

Ventriculus lateralis,
Cornu frontale

A. carotis interna,
Pars cerebralis

A. cerebri anterior

N. opticus [II]

A. ophthalmica

A. carotis interna,
Pars cavernosa

N. ophthalmicus [V/1]

N. maxillaris [V/2]

Ventriculus lateralis,
Cornu temporale

A. cerebri posterior

Cisterna ambiens;
Pedunculus cerebri

N. trochlearis [IV]

N. trigeminus [V]

N. oculomotorius [III]

Sinus petrosus
superior

N. abducens [VI]

Sinus cavernosus

Ganglion trigeminale

N. mandibularis [V/3]

Fig. 1193 Course of the cranial nerves, Nn. craniales,
in the middle cranial fossa, Fossa cranii media.

A. cerebri anterior dextra,
Pars postcommunicalis

Chiasma opticum

Substantia nigra

Pedunculus cerebri,
Crus cerebri

N. oculomotorius [III]

N. trochlearis [IV]

(Plica petroclinoidea
anterior)

N. trigeminus [V],
Radix motoria

N. trigeminus [V],
Radix sensoria

N. abducens [VI]

N. facialis [VII]

N. vestibulocochlearis [VIII]

Infundibulum

N. opticus [II]

A. carotis interna,
Pars cerebralis

A. ophthalmica

N. ophthalmicus [V/1]

Ganglion trigeminale*

N. maxillaris [V/2]

N. mandibularis [V/3]

Fig. 1194 Arteries and nerves in the region of the sella turcica,
Sella turcica, and the cavernous sinus, Sinus cavernosus.
* Clinical term: GASSERian ganglion

Vessels and nerves of the cranial base

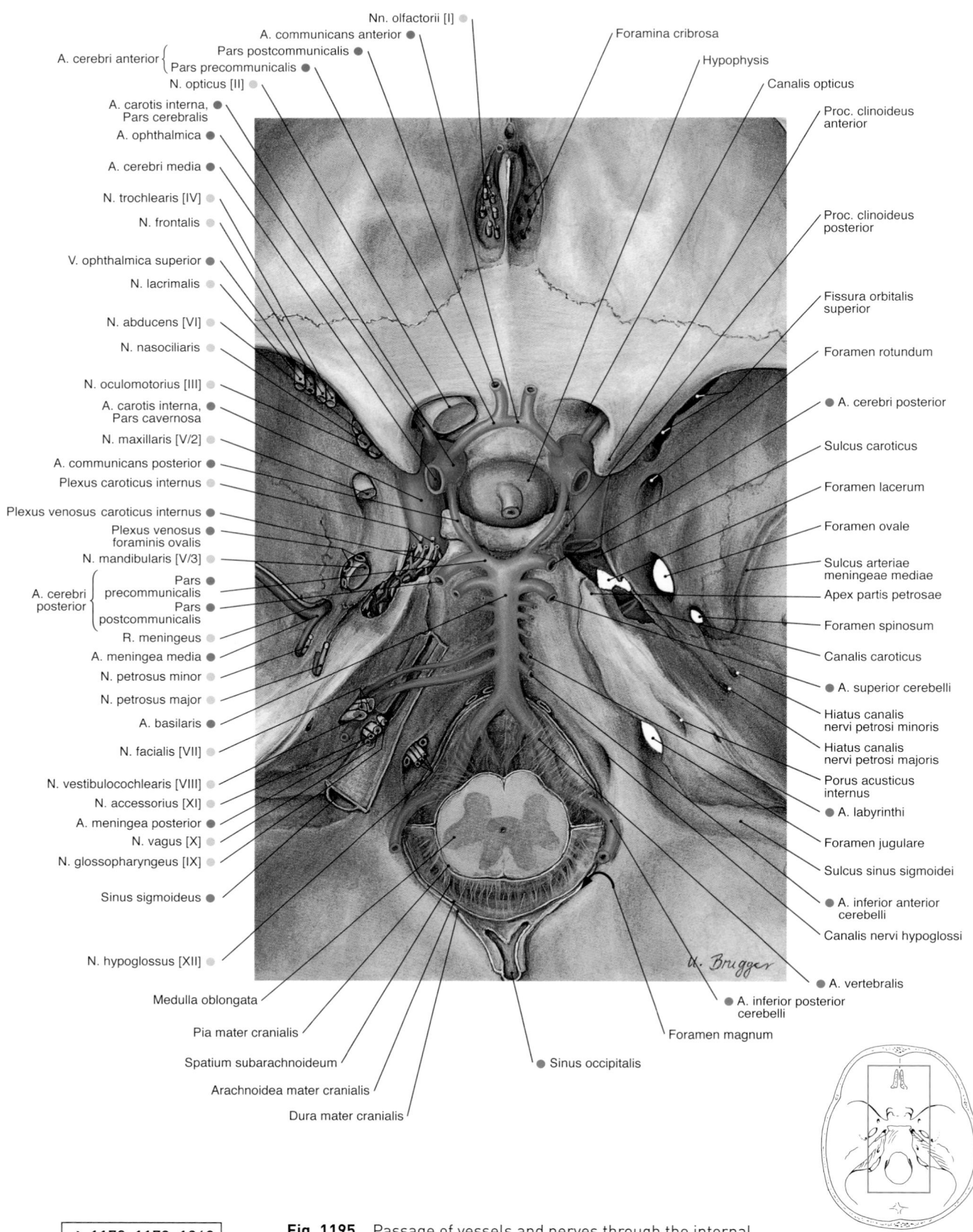

Nn. olfactorii [I] ●
A. communicans anterior ●
A. cerebri anterior { Pars postcommunicalis ●
Pars precommunicalis ●
N. opticus [II] ●
A. carotis interna, ●
Pars cerebralis
A. ophthalmica ●
A. cerebri media ●
N. trochlearis [IV] ●
N. frontalis ●
V. ophthalmica superior ●
N. lacrimalis ●
N. abducens [VI] ●
N. nasociliaris ●
N. oculomotorius [III] ●
A. carotis interna, ●
Pars cavernosa
N. maxillaris [V/2] ●
A. communicans posterior ●
Plexus caroticus internus ●
Plexus venosus caroticus internus ●
Plexus venosus ●
foraminis ovalis
N. mandibularis [V/3] ●
A. cerebri { Pars ●
posterior precommunicalis
Pars ●
postcommunicalis
R. meningeus ●
A. meningea media ●
N. petrosus minor ●
N. petrosus major ●
A. basilaris ●
N. facialis [VII] ●
N. vestibulocochlearis [VIII] ●
N. accessorius [XI] ●
A. meningea posterior ●
N. vagus [X] ●
N. glossopharyngeus [IX] ●
Sinus sigmoideus ●
N. hypoglossus [XII] ●
Medulla oblongata
Pia mater cranialis
Spatium subarachnoideum
Arachnoidea mater cranialis
Dura mater cranialis

Foramina cribrosa
Hypophysis
Canalis opticus
Proc. clinoideus anterior
Proc. clinoideus posterior
Fissura orbitalis superior
Foramen rotundum
● A. cerebri posterior
Sulcus caroticus
Foramen lacerum
Foramen ovale
Sulcus arteriae meningeae mediae
Apex partis petrosae
Foramen spinosum
Canalis caroticus
● A. superior cerebelli
Hiatus canalis nervi petrosi minoris
Hiatus canalis nervi petrosi majoris
Porus acusticus internus
● A. labyrinthi
Foramen jugulare
Sulcus sinus sigmoidei
● A. inferior anterior cerebelli
Canalis nervi hypoglossi
● A. vertebralis
● A. inferior posterior cerebelli
Foramen magnum
● Sinus occipitalis

→ 1172, 1173, 1268

Fig. 1195 Passage of vessels and nerves through the internal surface of cranial base, Basis cranii interna, and the cerebral arterial circle, Circulus arteriosus cerebri [WILLIS]; superior view.

Cavernous sinus and pituitary gland

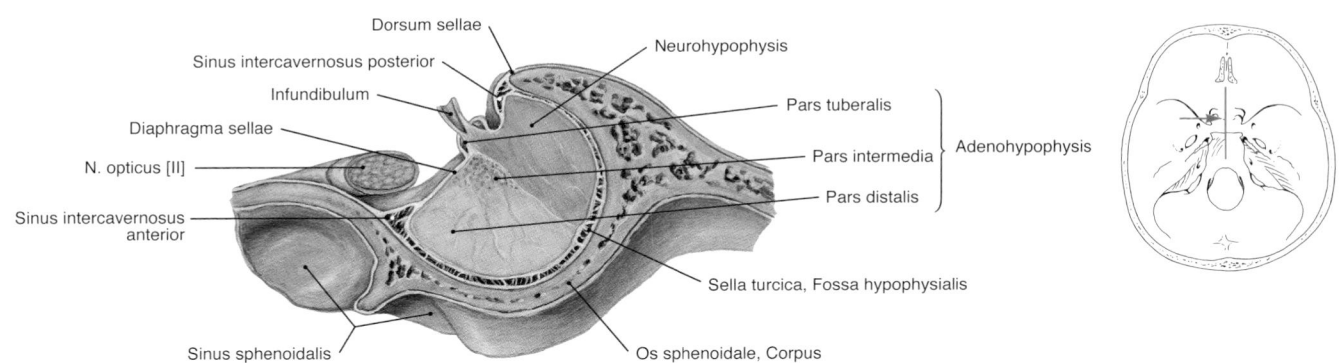

Dorsum sellae
Neurohypophysis
Sinus intercavernosus posterior
Infundibulum
Pars tuberalis
Diaphragma sellae
Pars intermedia — Adenohypophysis
N. opticus [II]
Pars distalis
Sinus intercavernosus anterior
Sella turcica, Fossa hypophysialis
Sinus sphenoidalis
Os sphenoidale, Corpus

Fig. 1196 Pituitary gland, Hypophysis [Glandula pituitaria].

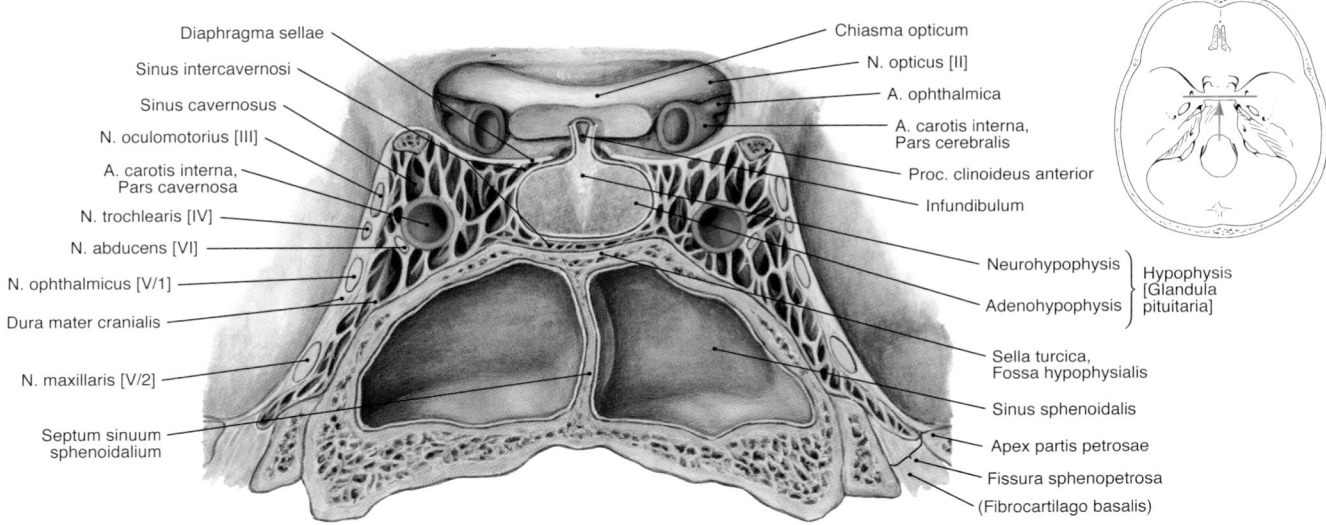

Diaphragma sellae
Chiasma opticum
Sinus intercavernosi
N. opticus [II]
Sinus cavernosus
A. ophthalmica
N. oculomotorius [III]
A. carotis interna, Pars cerebralis
A. carotis interna, Pars cavernosa
Proc. clinoideus anterior
N. trochlearis [IV]
Infundibulum
N. abducens [VI]
Neurohypophysis — Hypophysis [Glandula pituitaria]
N. ophthalmicus [V/1]
Adenohypophysis
Dura mater cranialis
Sella turcica, Fossa hypophysialis
N. maxillaris [V/2]
Sinus sphenoidalis
Apex partis petrosae
Septum sinuum sphenoidalium
Fissura sphenopetrosa
(Fibrocartilago basalis)

Fig. 1197 Pituitary gland, Hypophysis [Glandula pituitaria], and cavernous sinus, Sinus cavernosus.

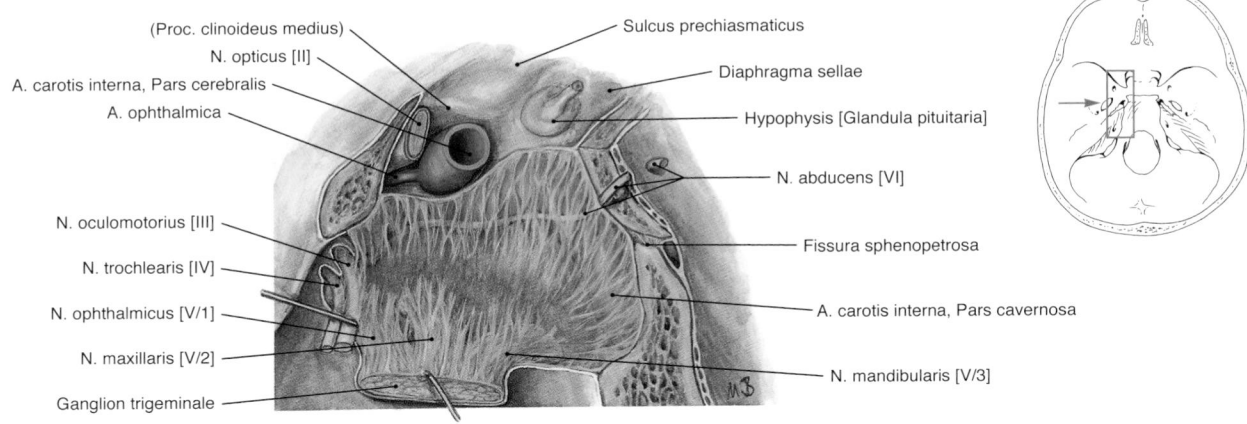

(Proc. clinoideus medius)
Sulcus prechiasmaticus
N. opticus [II]
A. carotis interna, Pars cerebralis
Diaphragma sellae
A. ophthalmica
Hypophysis [Glandula pituitaria]
N. abducens [VI]
N. oculomotorius [III]
N. trochlearis [IV]
Fissura sphenopetrosa
N. ophthalmicus [V/1]
A. carotis interna, Pars cavernosa
N. maxillaris [V/2]
N. mandibularis [V/3]
Ganglion trigeminale

Fig. 1198 Cavernous sinus, Sinus cavernosus;
the part of the cranial dura mater forming the lateral wall of the
cavernous sinus has been removed;
the trigeminal ganglion has been reflected to the side.

Cranial dura mater and superior sagittal sinus

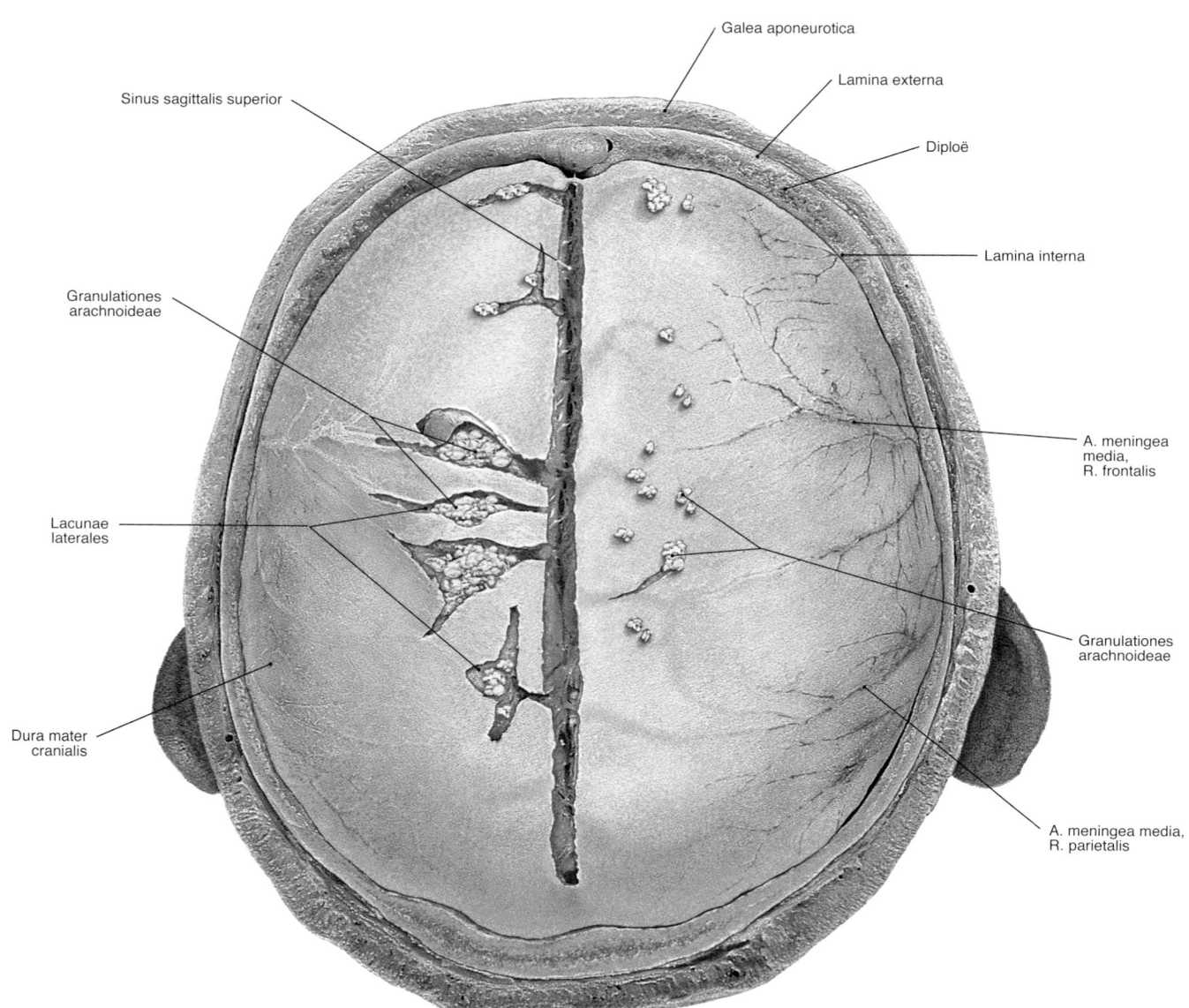

Galea aponeurotica

Lamina externa

Diploë

Lamina interna

Sinus sagittalis superior

Granulationes
arachnoideae

A. meningea
media,
R. frontalis

Lacunae
laterales

Granulationes
arachnoideae

Dura mater
cranialis

A. meningea media,
R. parietalis

Fig. 1199 Cranial dura mater, Dura mater cranialis,
and superior sagittal sinus, Sinus sagittalis superior,
with some lateral lacunae, Lacunae laterales.

Superficial vessels of the brain

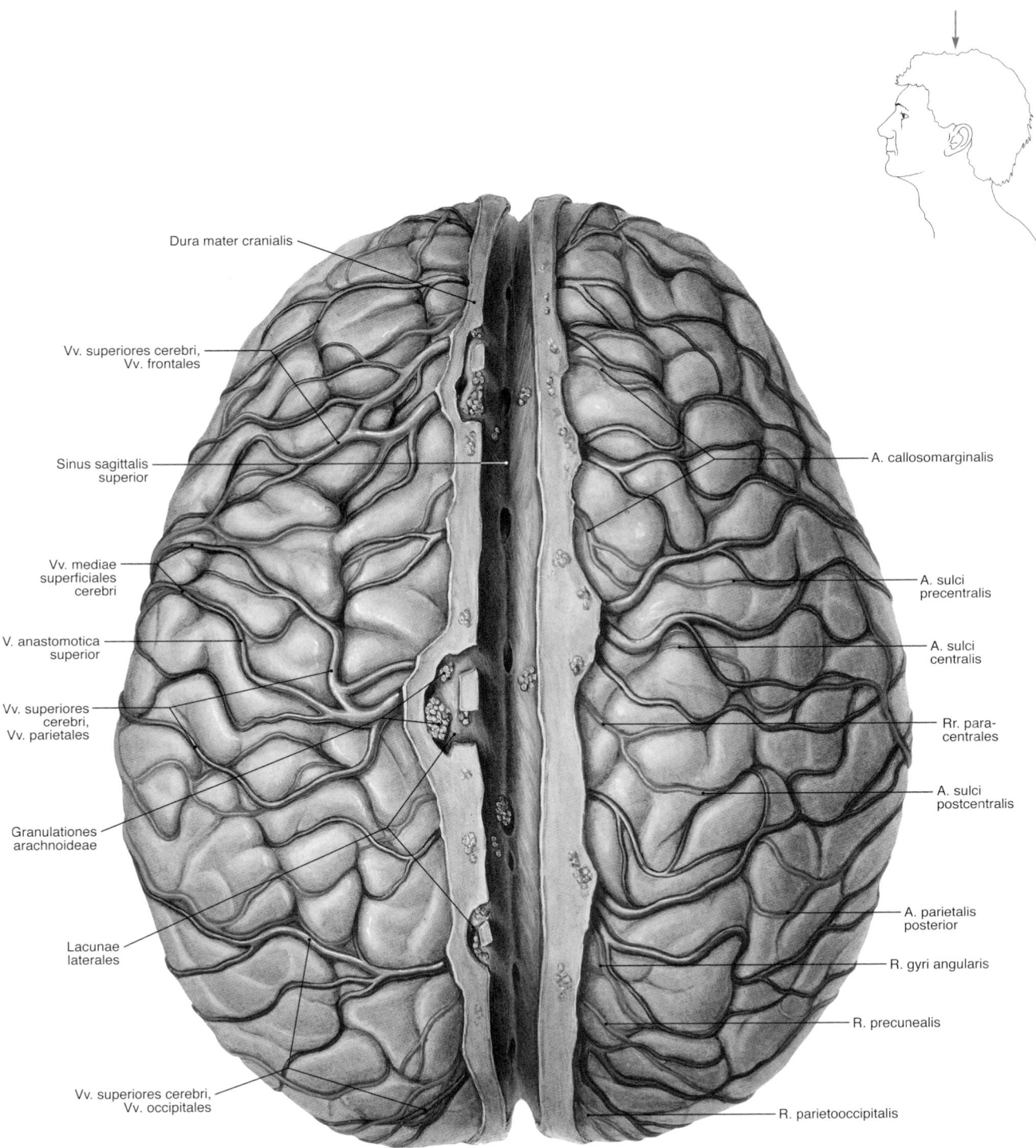

Dura mater cranialis

Vv. superiores cerebri,
Vv. frontales

Sinus sagittalis
superior

Vv. mediae
superficiales
cerebri

V. anastomotica
superior

Vv. superiores
cerebri,
Vv. parietales

Granulationes
arachnoideae

Lacunae
laterales

Vv. superiores cerebri,
Vv. occipitales

A. callosomarginalis

A. sulci
precentralis

A. sulci
centralis

Rr. para-
centrales

A. sulci
postcentralis

A. parietalis
posterior

R. gyri angularis

R. precunealis

R. parietooccipitalis

Fig. 1200 Superficial arteries and veins of the brain;
the cranial dura mater has been removed and the superior
sagittal sinus has been sectioned;
after removal of the cranial arachnoid mater.

Cranial arachnoid mater

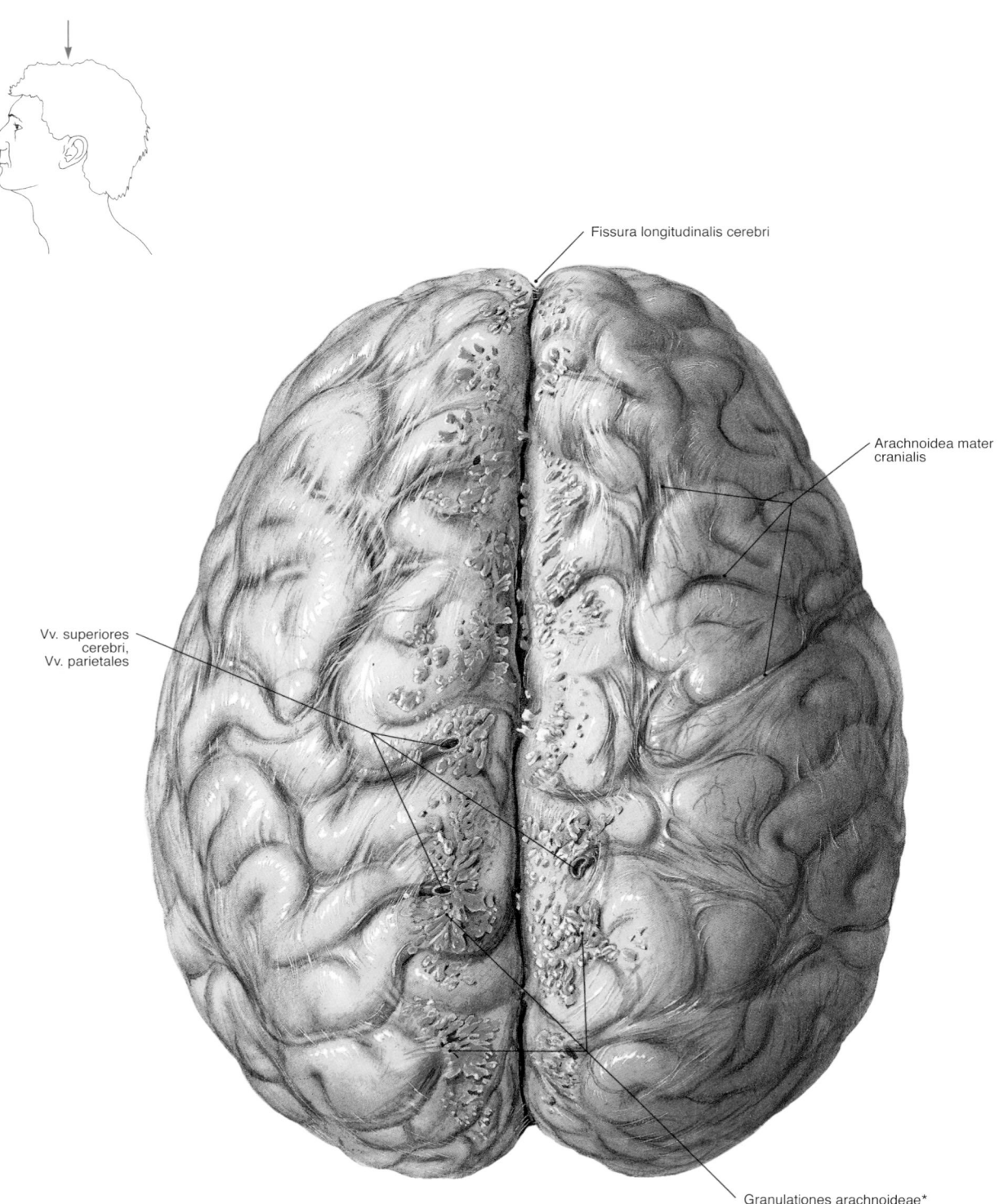

Fissura longitudinalis cerebri

Arachnoidea mater cranialis

Vv. superiores cerebri, Vv. parietales

Granulationes arachnoideae*

Fig. 1201 Brain, Encephalon, with cranial arachnoid mater, Arachnoidea mater cranialis; superior view.
* Also: PACCHIONIan granulations

Cranial arachnoid mater

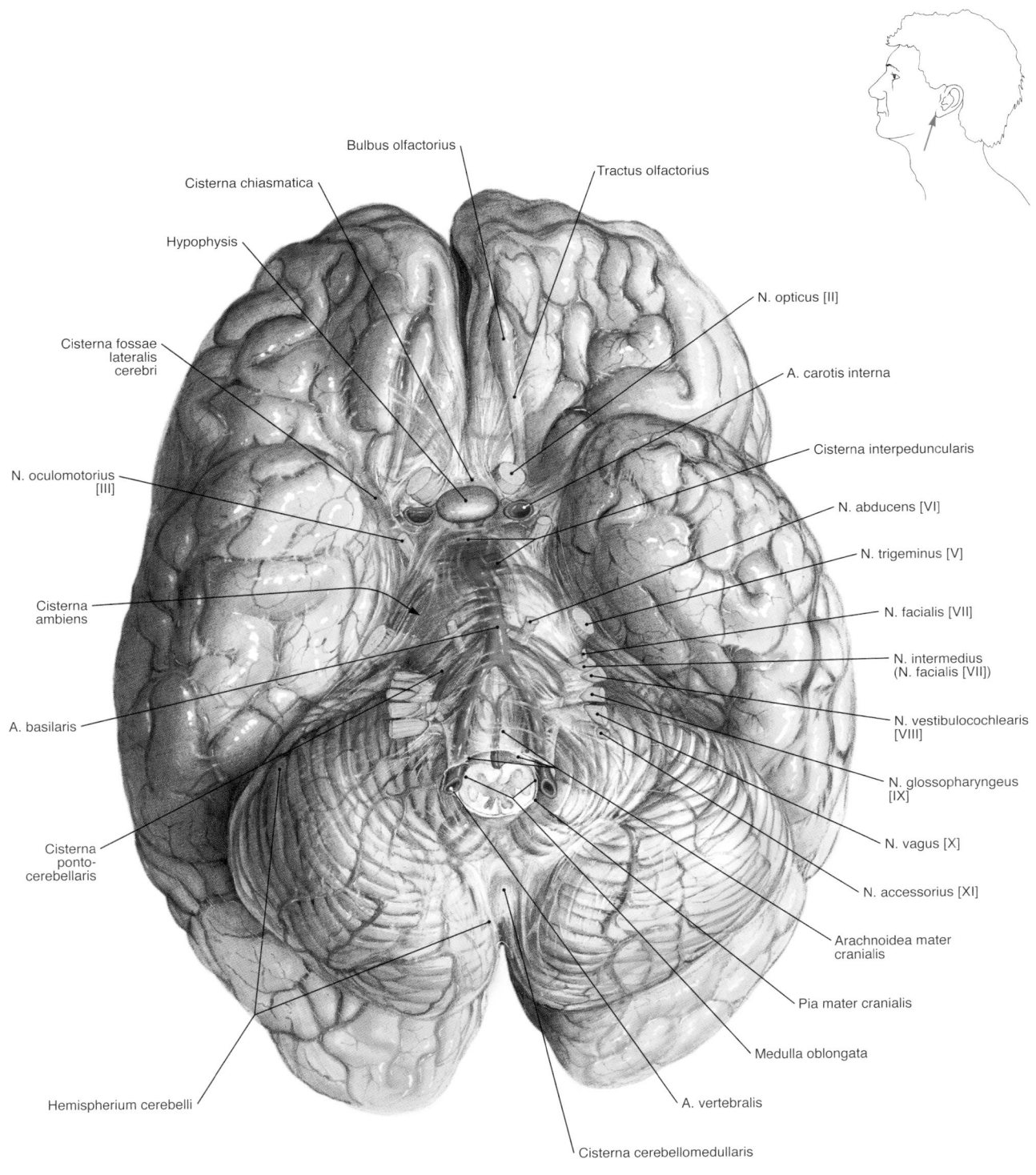

Bulbus olfactorius

Cisterna chiasmatica

Tractus olfactorius

Hypophysis

N. opticus [II]

Cisterna fossae
lateralis
cerebri

A. carotis interna

Cisterna interpeduncularis

N. oculomotorius
[III]

N. abducens [VI]

N. trigeminus [V]

N. facialis [VII]

Cisterna
ambiens

N. intermedius
(N. facialis [VII])

N. vestibulocochlearis
[VIII]

A. basilaris

N. glossopharyngeus
[IX]

N. vagus [X]

Cisterna
ponto-
cerebellaris

N. accessorius [XI]

Arachnoidea mater
cranialis

Pia mater cranialis

Medulla oblongata

Hemispherium cerebelli

A. vertebralis

Cisterna cerebellomedullaris

Fig. 1202 Brain, Encephalon, with cranial arachnoid mater,
Arachnoidea mater cranialis.

Organisation of the brain

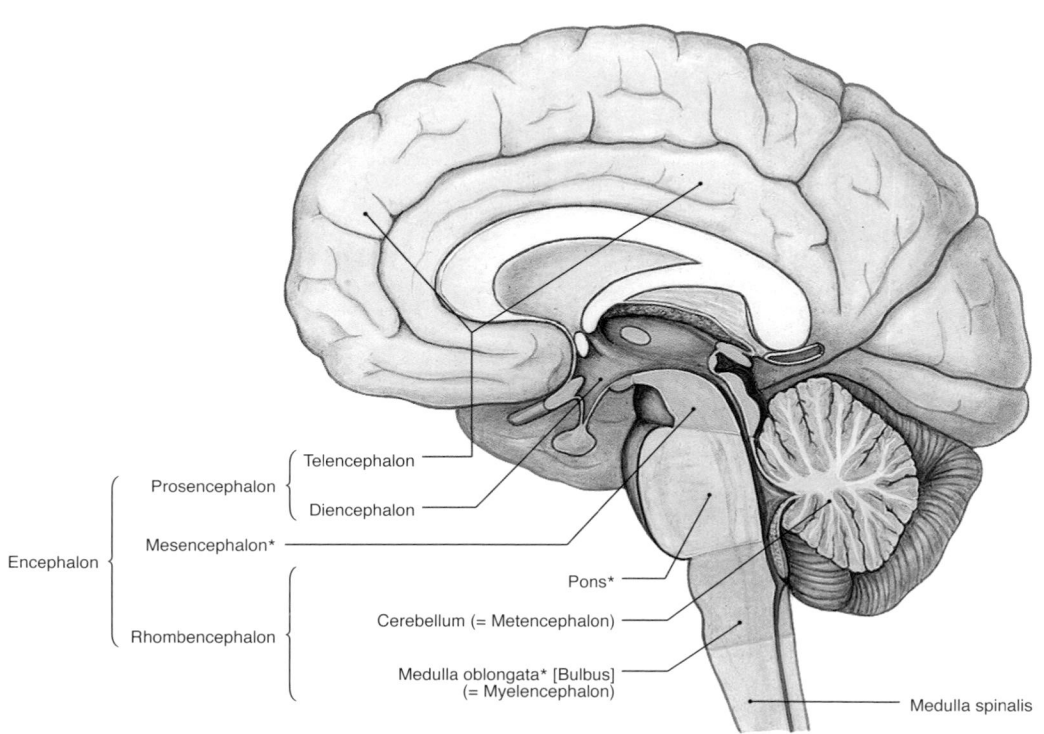

Encephalon {
- Prosencephalon {
  - Telencephalon
  - Diencephalon
}
- Mesencephalon*
- Rhombencephalon {
  - Pons*
  - Cerebellum (= Metencephalon)
  - Medulla oblongata* [Bulbus] (= Myelencephalon)
}

Medulla spinalis

Fig. 1203 Organisation of the central nervous system; median section; schema.
Parts marked with * together form the brainstem, Truncus encephali.

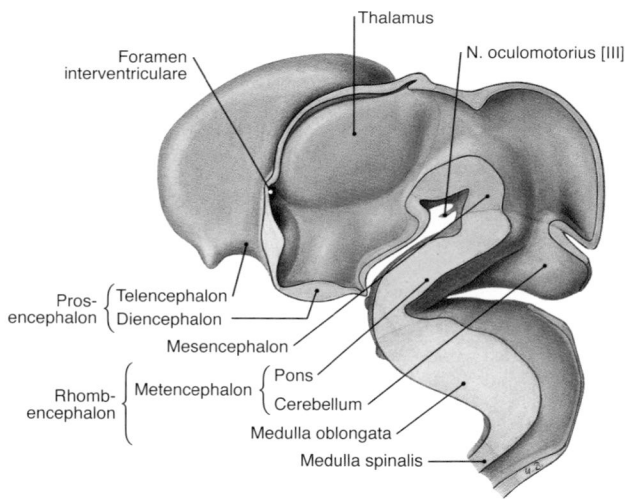

Thalamus
N. oculomotorius [III]
Foramen interventriculare

Pros-encephalon { Telencephalon / Diencephalon }
Mesencephalon
Rhomb-encephalon { Metencephalon { Pons / Cerebellum } }
Medulla oblongata
Medulla spinalis

Fig. 1204 Development of the brain; model of the brain of an approx. 2-month-old embryo; median section.

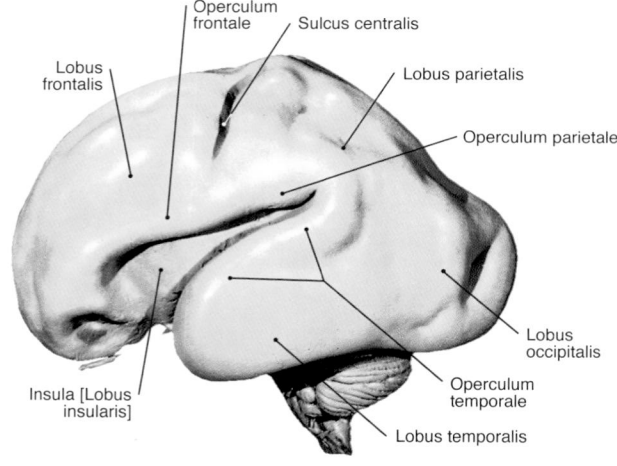

Operculum frontale
Sulcus centralis
Lobus frontalis
Lobus parietalis
Operculum parietale
Lobus occipitalis
Operculum temporale
Insula [Lobus insularis]
Lobus temporalis

Fig. 1205 Development of the brain; brain of an approx. 4-month-old foetus (crown-rump length 20 cm); viewed from the left.

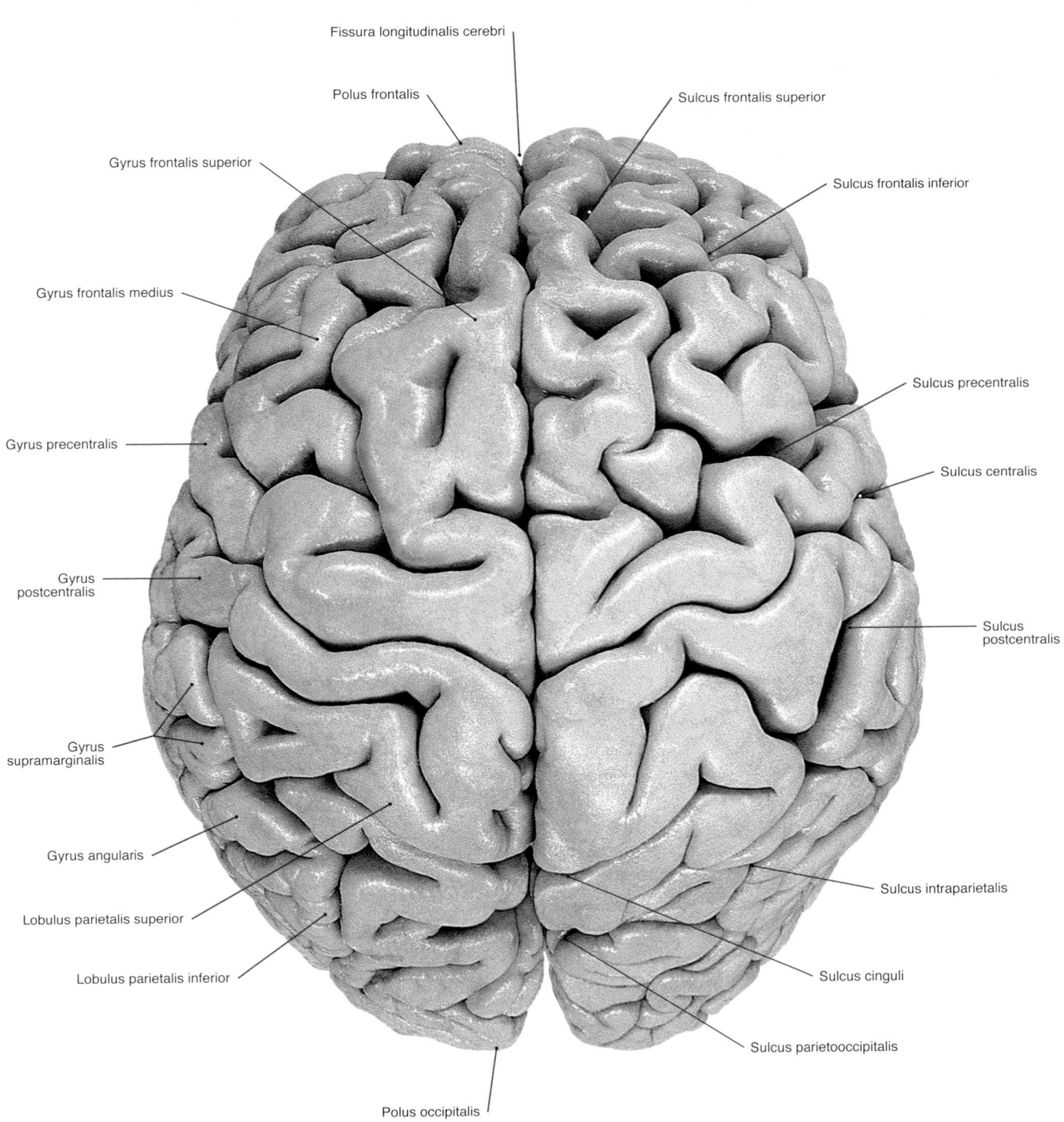

Fissura longitudinalis cerebri

Polus frontalis

Sulcus frontalis superior

Gyrus frontalis superior

Sulcus frontalis inferior

Gyrus frontalis medius

Sulcus precentralis

Gyrus precentralis

Sulcus centralis

Gyrus postcentralis

Sulcus postcentralis

Gyrus supramarginalis

Gyrus angularis

Sulcus intraparietalis

Lobulus parietalis superior

Sulcus cinguli

Lobulus parietalis inferior

Sulcus parietooccipitalis

Polus occipitalis

Fig. 1206 Cerebrum, Cerebrum;
after removal of the cranial arachnoid mater;
superior view.
Formation of the gyri varies considerably.

Base of the brain

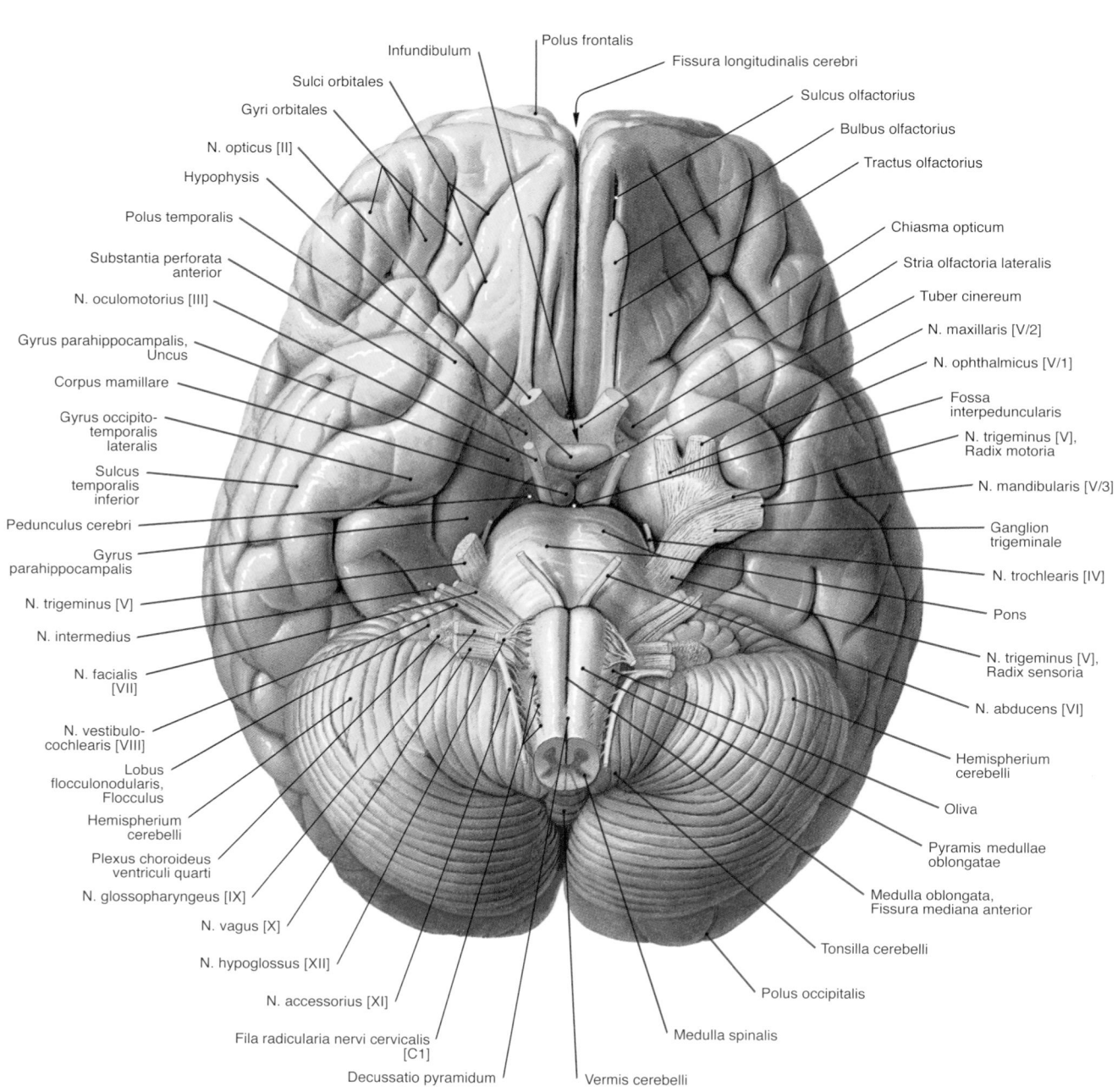

Infundibulum
Polus frontalis
Fissura longitudinalis cerebri
Sulci orbitales
Sulcus olfactorius
Gyri orbitales
Bulbus olfactorius
N. opticus [II]
Tractus olfactorius
Hypophysis
Polus temporalis
Chiasma opticum
Substantia perforata anterior
Stria olfactoria lateralis
N. oculomotorius [III]
Tuber cinereum
Gyrus parahippocampalis, Uncus
N. maxillaris [V/2]
N. ophthalmicus [V/1]
Corpus mamillare
Fossa interpeduncularis
Gyrus occipito-temporalis lateralis
N. trigeminus [V], Radix motoria
Sulcus temporalis inferior
N. mandibularis [V/3]
Pedunculus cerebri
Ganglion trigeminale
Gyrus parahippocampalis
N. trochlearis [IV]
N. trigeminus [V]
Pons
N. intermedius
N. trigeminus [V], Radix sensoria
N. facialis [VII]
N. abducens [VI]
N. vestibulo-cochlearis [VIII]
Hemispherium cerebelli
Lobus flocculonodularis, Flocculus
Oliva
Hemispherium cerebelli
Pyramis medullae oblongatae
Plexus choroideus ventriculi quarti
Medulla oblongata, Fissura mediana anterior
N. glossopharyngeus [IX]
N. vagus [X]
Tonsilla cerebelli
N. hypoglossus [XII]
N. accessorius [XI]
Polus occipitalis
Fila radicularia nervi cervicalis [C1]
Medulla spinalis
Decussatio pyramidum
Vermis cerebelli

Fig. 1207 Cerebrum, Cerebrum;
brainstem, Truncus encephali, with cerebellum,
Cerebellum, as well as cranial nerves, Nn. craniales;
inferior view.

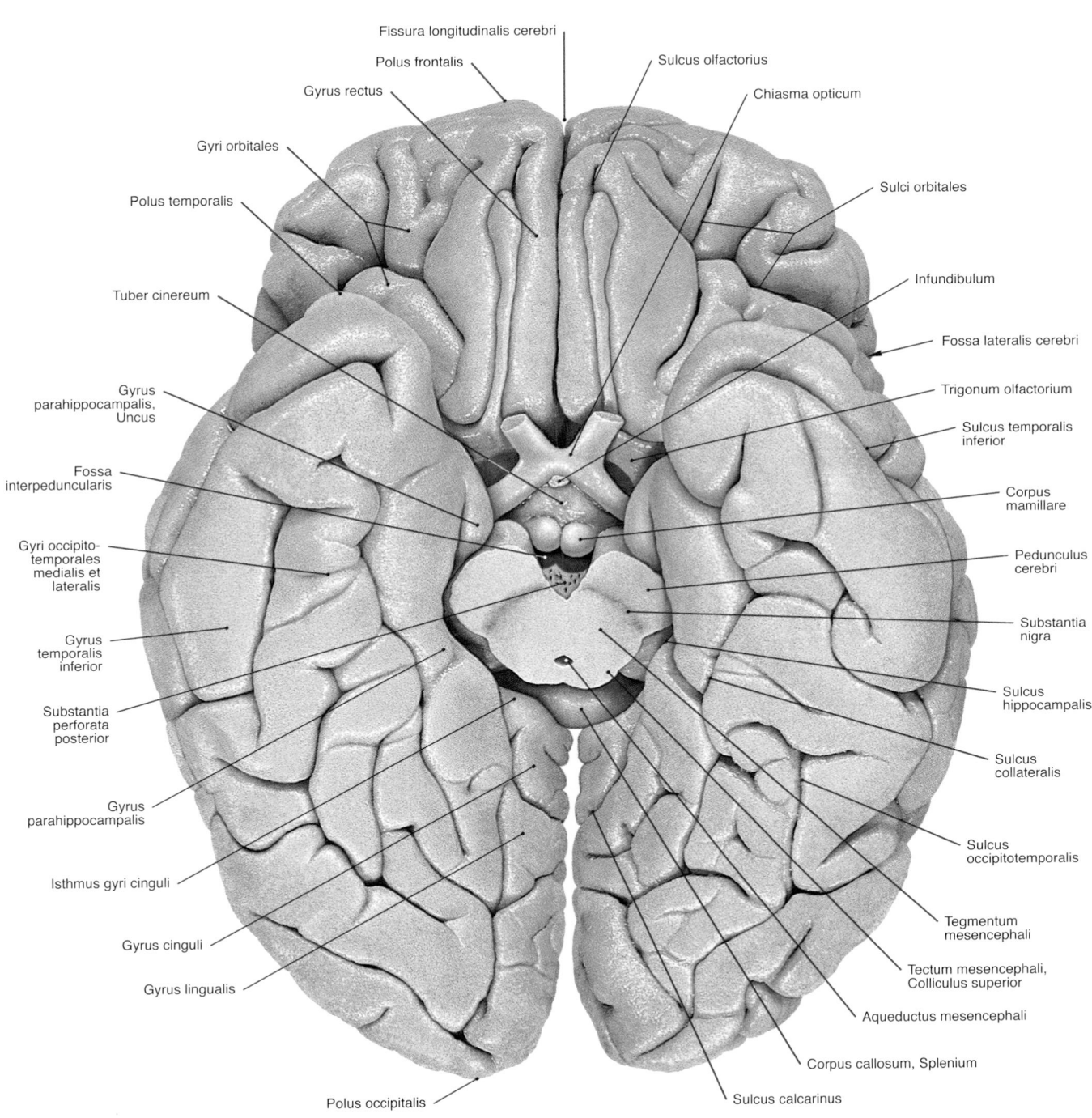

Fissura longitudinalis cerebri

Polus frontalis

Gyrus rectus

Gyri orbitales

Polus temporalis

Tuber cinereum

Gyrus parahippocampalis, Uncus

Fossa interpeduncularis

Gyri occipito-temporales medialis et lateralis

Gyrus temporalis inferior

Substantia perforata posterior

Gyrus parahippocampalis

Isthmus gyri cinguli

Gyrus cinguli

Gyrus lingualis

Polus occipitalis

Sulcus olfactorius

Chiasma opticum

Sulci orbitales

Infundibulum

Fossa lateralis cerebri

Trigonum olfactorium

Sulcus temporalis inferior

Corpus mamillare

Pedunculus cerebri

Substantia nigra

Sulcus hippocampalis

Sulcus collateralis

Sulcus occipitotemporalis

Tegmentum mesencephali

Tectum mesencephali, Colliculus superior

Aqueductus mesencephali

Corpus callosum, Splenium

Sulcus calcarinus

Fig. 1208 Gyri, Gyri, and grooves, Sulci, of the cerebral hemispheres; the midbrain has been sectioned.

Lobes of the telencephalon

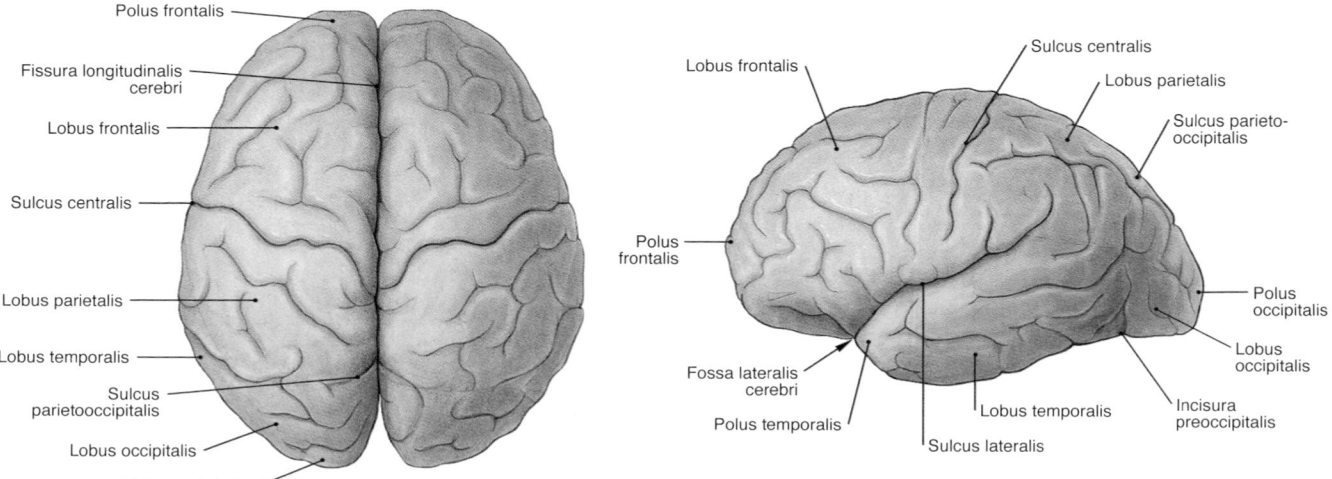

Fig. 1209 Lobes of the cerebrum, Lobi cerebri; superior view.

Fig. 1210 Lobes of the cerebrum, Lobi cerebri; viewed from the left.

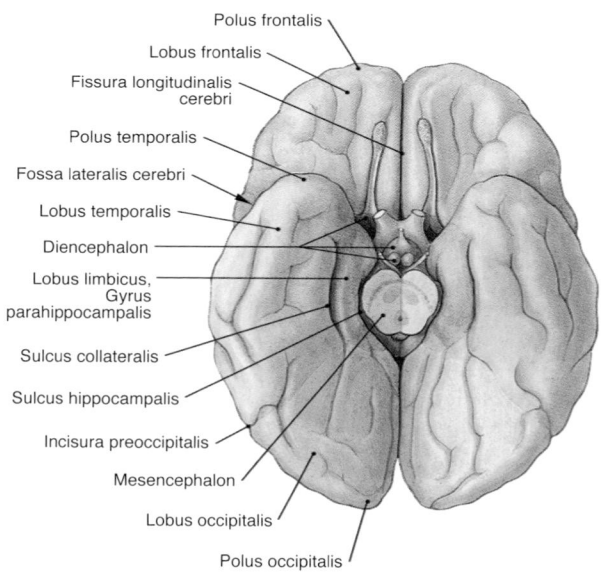

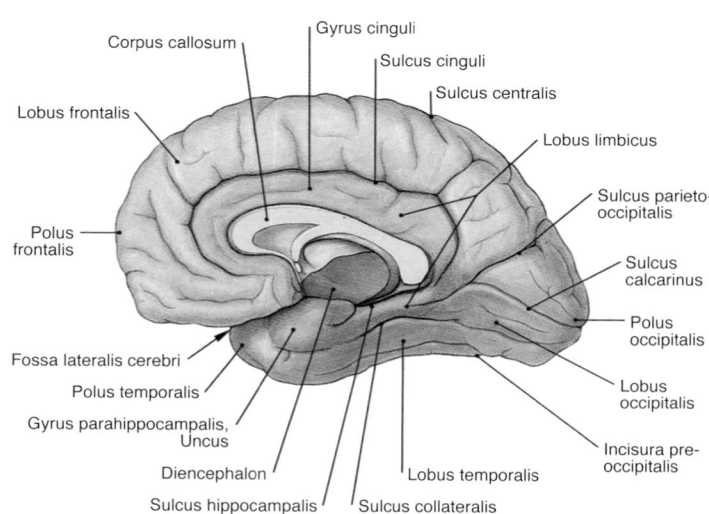

Fig. 1211 Lobes of the cerebrum, Lobi cerebri; inferior view.

Fig. 1212 Lobes of the cerebrum, Lobi cerebri; medial view.

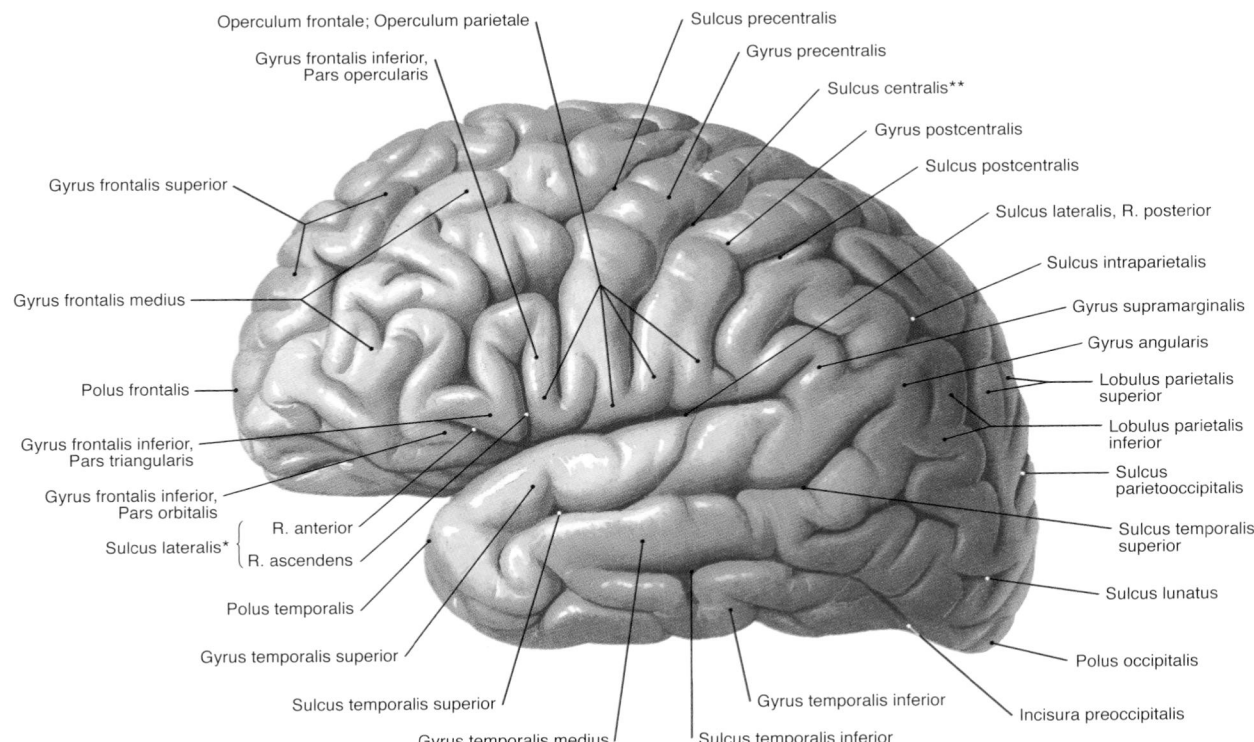

Operculum frontale; Operculum parietale
Gyrus frontalis inferior, Pars opercularis
Gyrus frontalis superior
Gyrus frontalis medius
Polus frontalis
Gyrus frontalis inferior, Pars triangularis
Gyrus frontalis inferior, Pars orbitalis
Sulcus lateralis*
R. anterior
R. ascendens
Polus temporalis
Gyrus temporalis superior
Sulcus temporalis superior
Gyrus temporalis medius

Sulcus precentralis
Gyrus precentralis
Sulcus centralis**
Gyrus postcentralis
Sulcus postcentralis
Sulcus lateralis, R. posterior
Sulcus intraparietalis
Gyrus supramarginalis
Gyrus angularis
Lobulus parietalis superior
Lobulus parietalis inferior
Sulcus parietooccipitalis
Sulcus temporalis superior
Sulcus lunatus
Polus occipitalis
Gyrus temporalis inferior
Incisura preoccipitalis
Sulcus temporalis inferior

Fig. 1213 Gyri, Gyri, and grooves, Sulci,
of the cerebral hemispheres;
viewed from the left.
* Sulcus of SYLVIUS
** Sulcus of ROLANDO

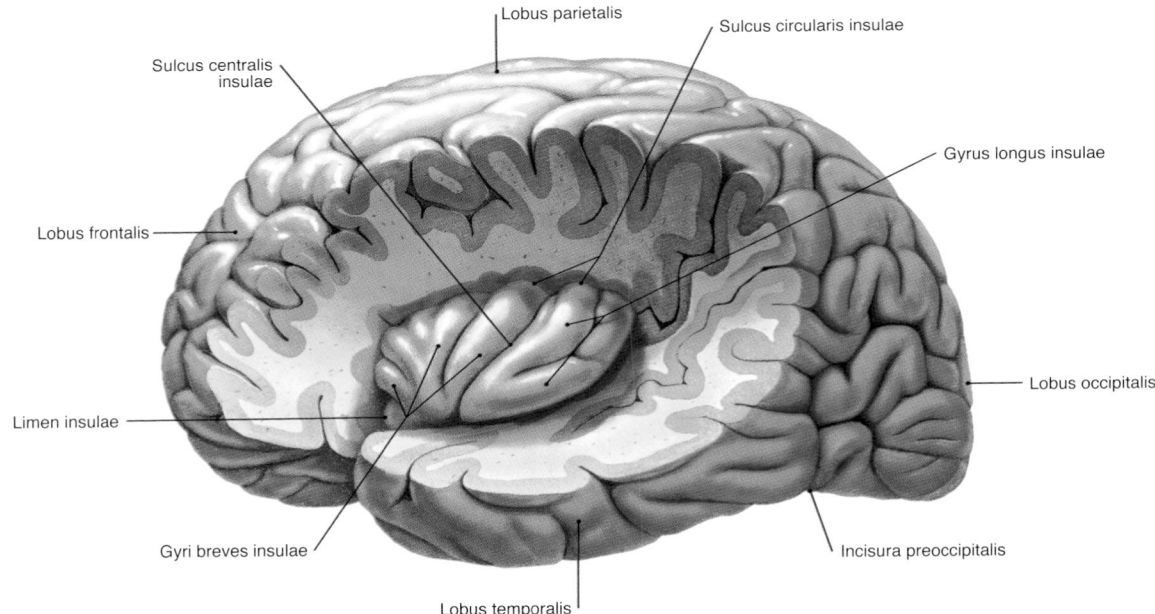

Sulcus centralis insulae
Lobus parietalis
Sulcus circularis insulae
Lobus frontalis
Gyrus longus insulae
Limen insulae
Lobus occipitalis
Gyri breves insulae
Incisura preoccipitalis
Lobus temporalis

Fig. 1214 Gyri, Gyri, and grooves, Sulci,
of the cerebral hemispheres;
exposure of the insula after removal of the frontal,
parietal and temporal opercula;
viewed from the left.

Gyri of the cerebral hemispheres

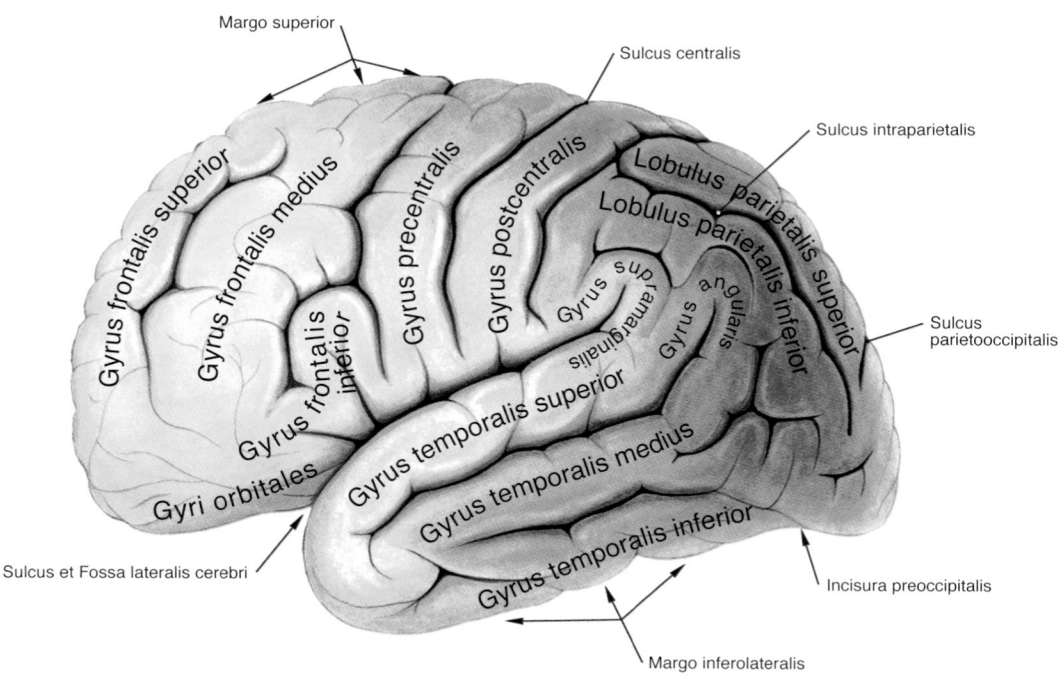

Fig. 1215 Gyri, Gyri, of the cerebral hemispheres; viewed from the left.

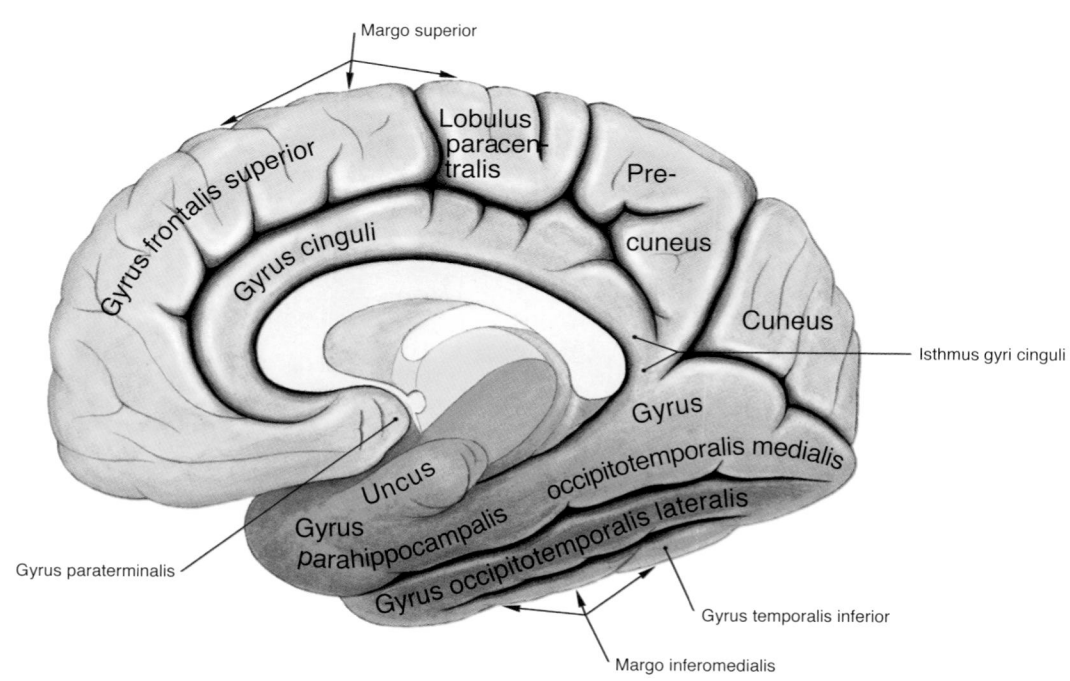

Fig. 1216 Gyri, Gyri, of the cerebral hemispheres; medial view.

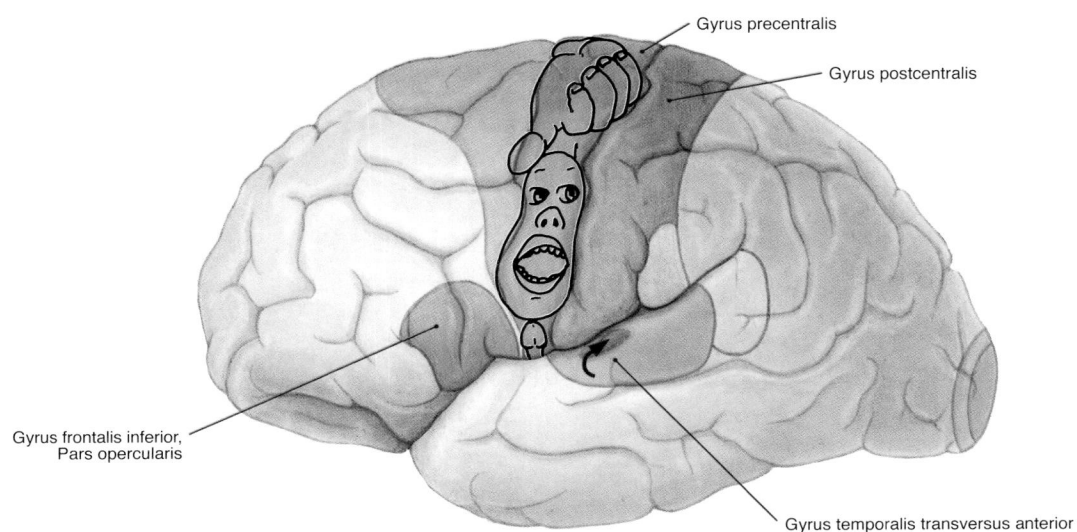

Gyrus precentralis

Gyrus postcentralis

Gyrus frontalis inferior,
Pars opercularis

Gyrus temporalis transversus anterior

Fig. 1217 Functional cortical areas of the cerebral hemispheres according to FOERSTER; viewed from the left.

The somatotopic organisation is illustrated schematically. The primary receiving area for auditory impulses (⌐) extends over the upper edge of the temporal lobe onto its inner surface.

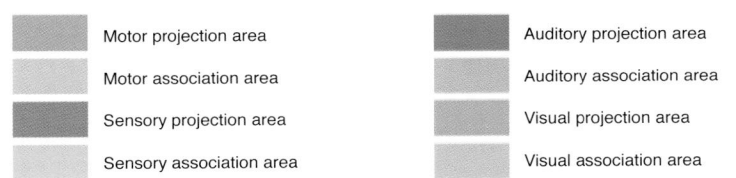

▮ Motor projection area	▮ Auditory projection area
▮ Motor association area	▮ Auditory association area
▮ Sensory projection area	▮ Visual projection area
▮ Sensory association area	▮ Visual association area

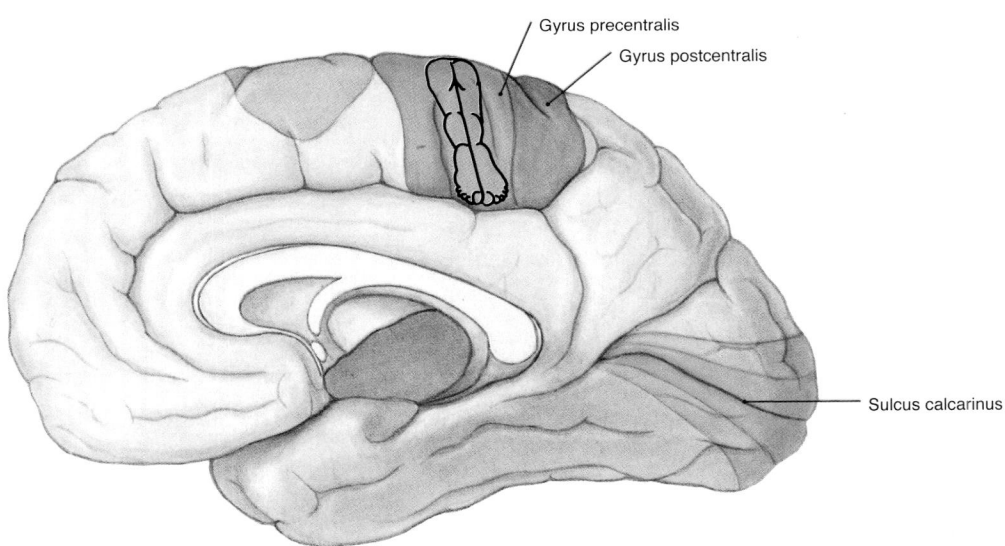

Gyrus precentralis

Gyrus postcentralis

Sulcus calcarinus

Fig. 1218 Functional cortical areas of the cerebral hemispheres according to FOERSTER; medial view.

The somatotopic organisation is illustrated schematically.

Fornix

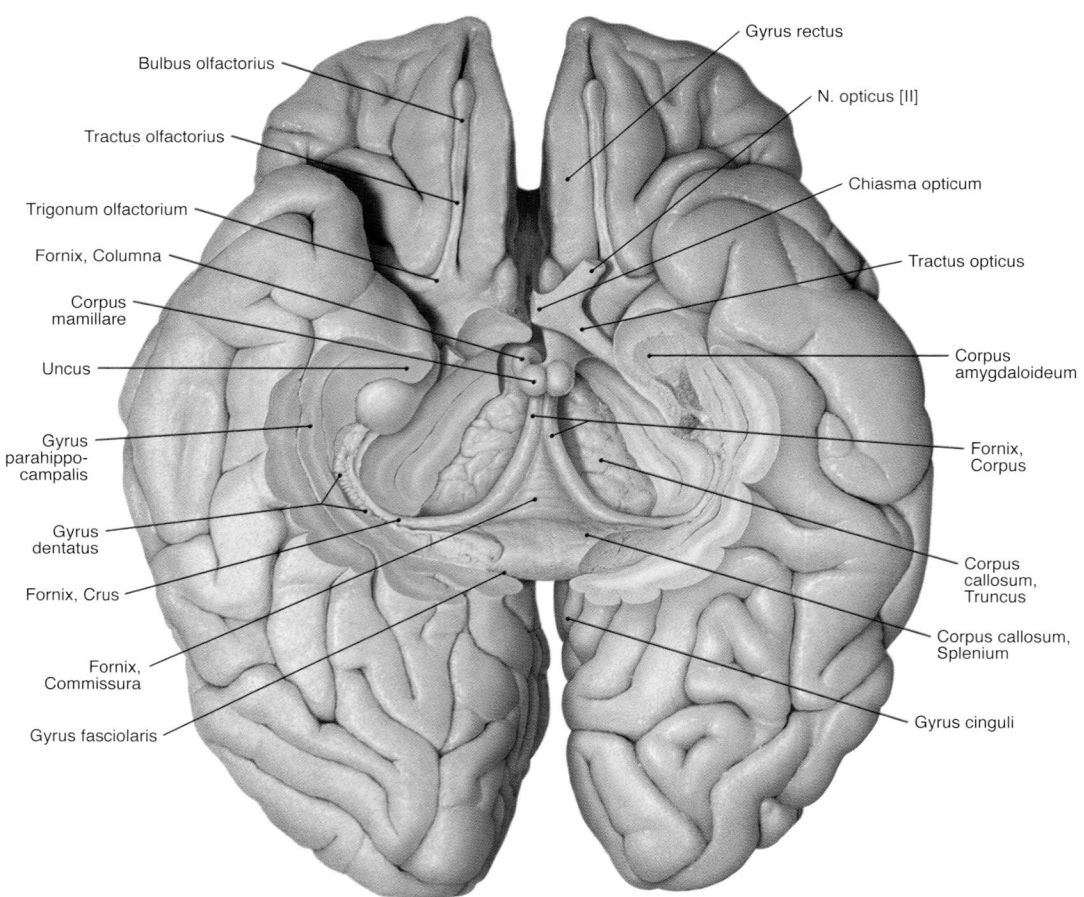

Bulbus olfactorius

Tractus olfactorius

Trigonum olfactorium

Fornix, Columna

Corpus mamillare

Uncus

Gyrus parahippo-campalis

Gyrus dentatus

Fornix, Crus

Fornix, Commissura

Gyrus fasciolaris

Gyrus rectus

N. opticus [II]

Chiasma opticum

Tractus opticus

Corpus amygdaloideum

Fornix, Corpus

Corpus callosum, Truncus

Corpus callosum, Splenium

Gyrus cinguli

Fig. 1219 Fornix, Fornix;
after removal of the basal parts of the brain;
inferior view.

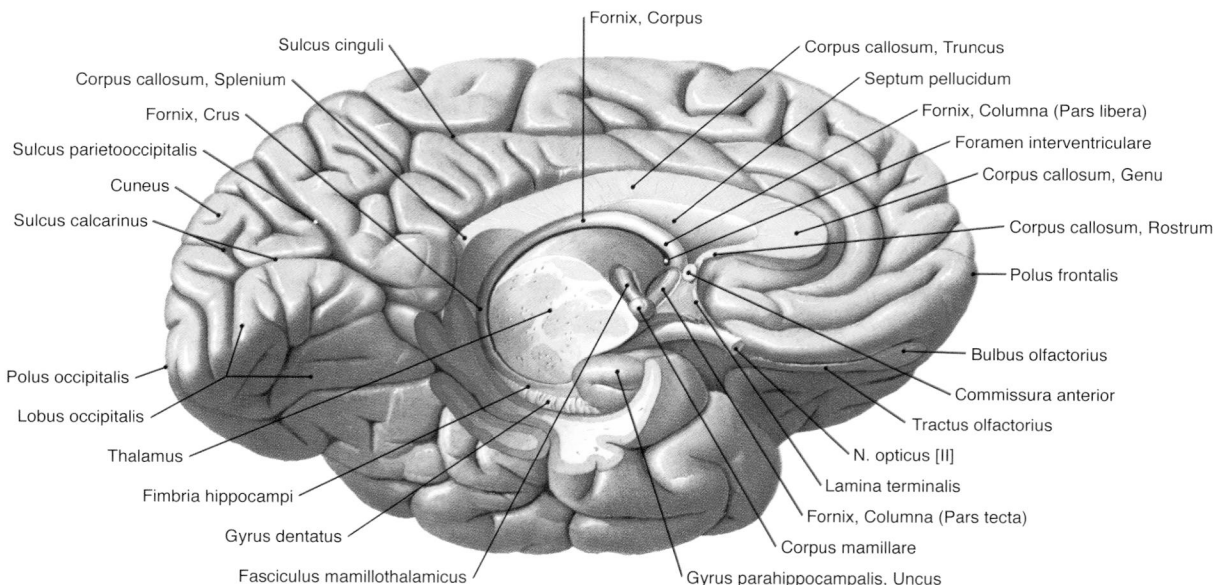

Fornix, Corpus

Sulcus cinguli

Corpus callosum, Splenium

Fornix, Crus

Sulcus parietooccipitalis

Cuneus

Sulcus calcarinus

Polus occipitalis

Lobus occipitalis

Thalamus

Fimbria hippocampi

Gyrus dentatus

Fasciculus mamillothalamicus

Corpus callosum, Truncus

Septum pellucidum

Fornix, Columna (Pars libera)

Foramen interventriculare

Corpus callosum, Genu

Corpus callosum, Rostrum

Polus frontalis

Bulbus olfactorius

Commissura anterior

Tractus olfactorius

N. opticus [II]

Lamina terminalis

Fornix, Columna (Pars tecta)

Corpus mamillare

Gyrus parahippocampalis, Uncus

Fig. 1220 Fornix, Fornix;
inferomedial view.

Fornix and anterior commissure

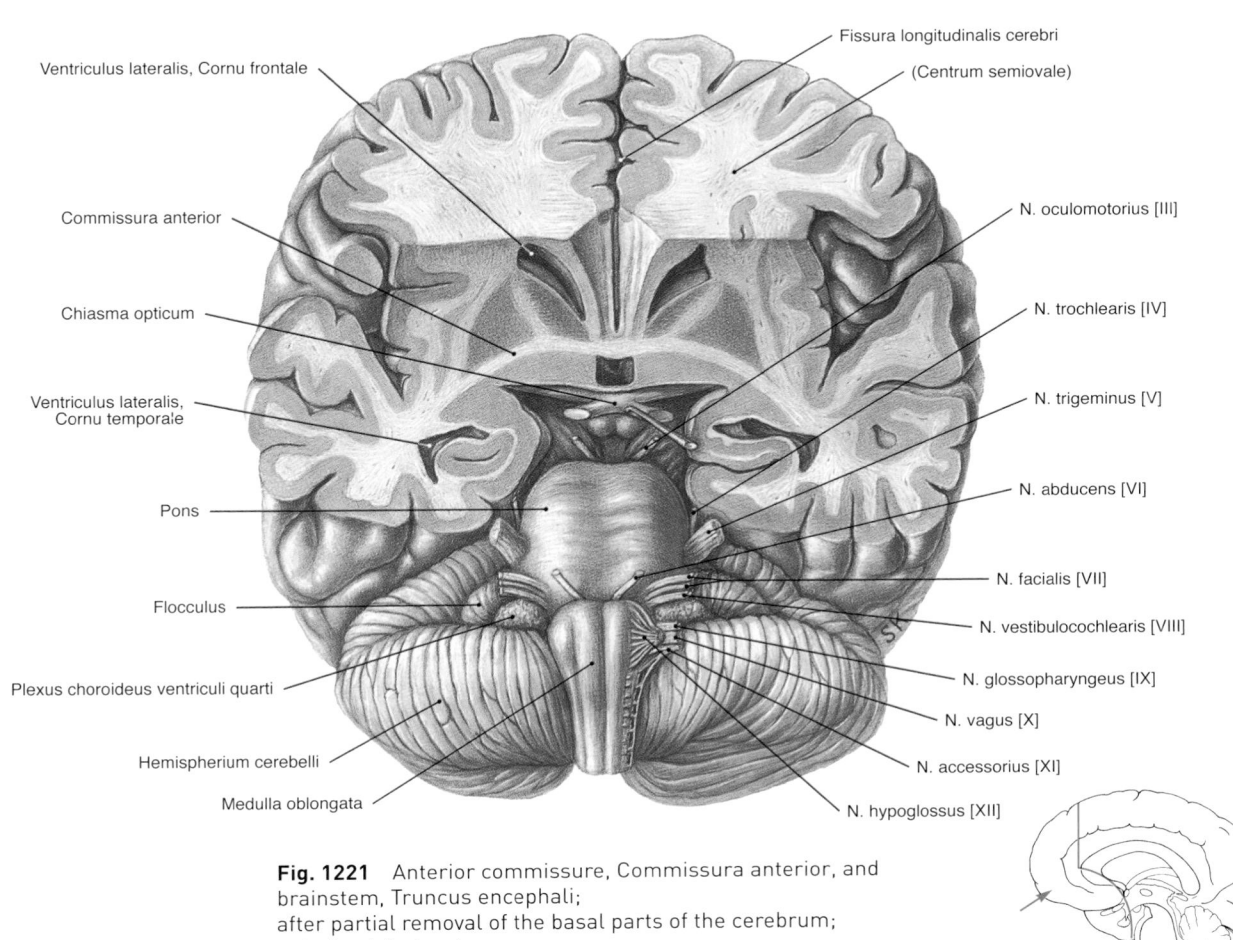

Fissura longitudinalis cerebri

(Centrum semiovale)

Ventriculus lateralis, Cornu frontale

N. oculomotorius [III]

Commissura anterior

N. trochlearis [IV]

Chiasma opticum

N. trigeminus [V]

Ventriculus lateralis, Cornu temporale

N. abducens [VI]

Pons

N. facialis [VII]

Flocculus

N. vestibulocochlearis [VIII]

N. glossopharyngeus [IX]

Plexus choroideus ventriculi quarti

N. vagus [X]

Hemispherium cerebelli

N. accessorius [XI]

Medulla oblongata

N. hypoglossus [XII]

Fig. 1221 Anterior commissure, Commissura anterior, and brainstem, Truncus encephali;
after partial removal of the basal parts of the cerebrum;
anterior-inferior view.

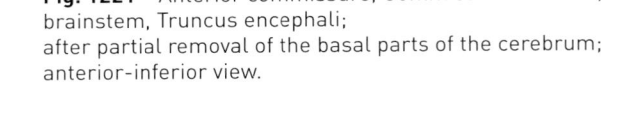
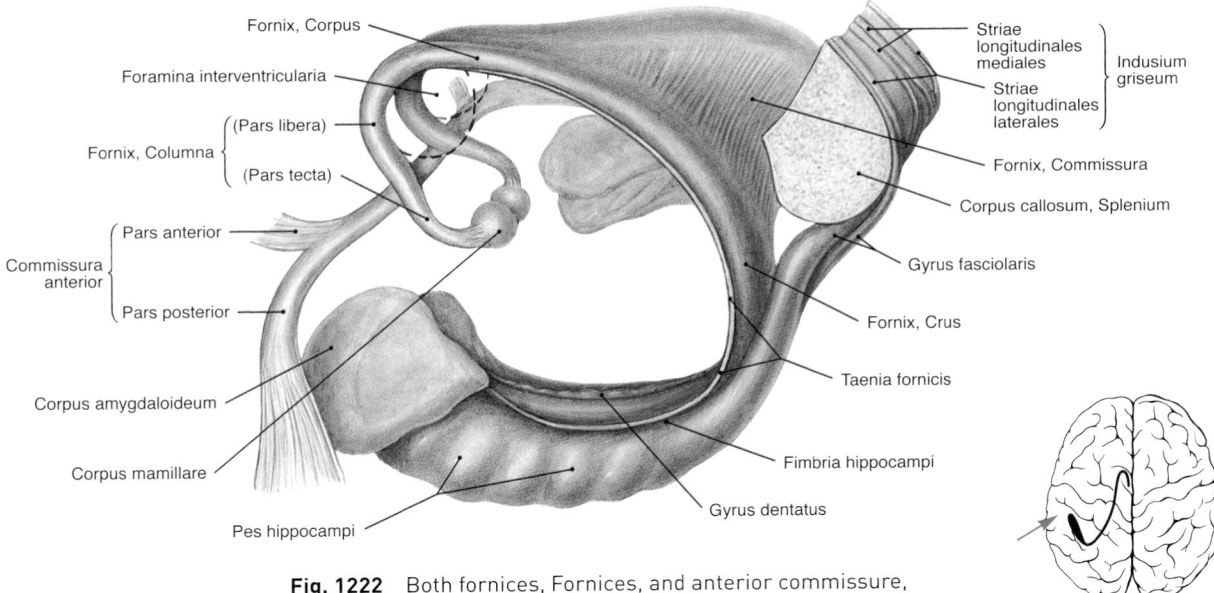

Fornix, Corpus

Striae longitudinales mediales

Foramina interventricularia

Striae longitudinales laterales

Indusium griseum

Fornix, Columna (Pars libera)

(Pars tecta)

Fornix, Commissura

Corpus callosum, Splenium

Commissura anterior — Pars anterior

Gyrus fasciolaris

Pars posterior

Fornix, Crus

Corpus amygdaloideum

Taenia fornicis

Corpus mamillare

Fimbria hippocampi

Pes hippocampi

Gyrus dentatus

Fig. 1222 Both fornices, Fornices, and anterior commissure, Commissura anterior;
viewed from the left.

Basal ganglia

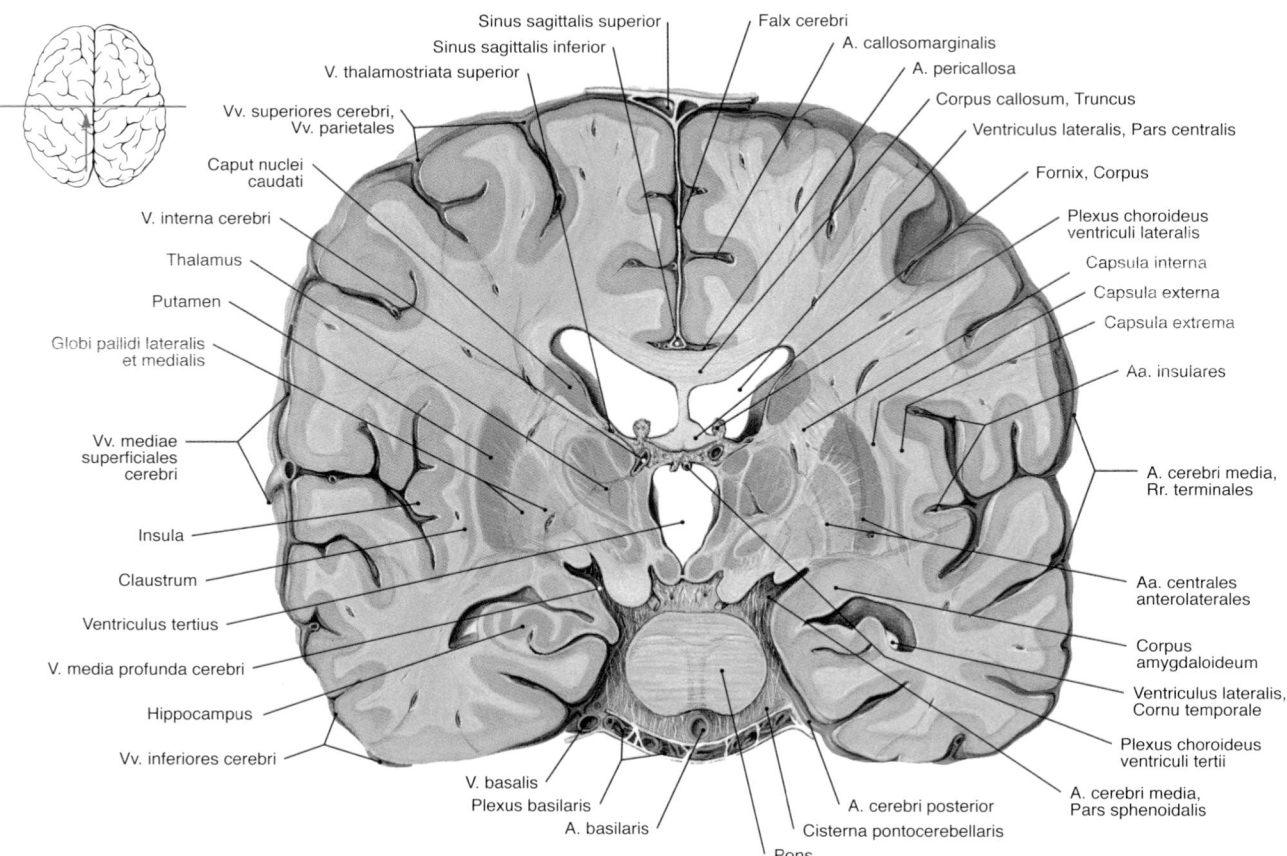

Fig. 1223 Blood supply of the basal ganglia;
frontal section;
the arteries are shown on the right and the veins on the left;
posterior view.

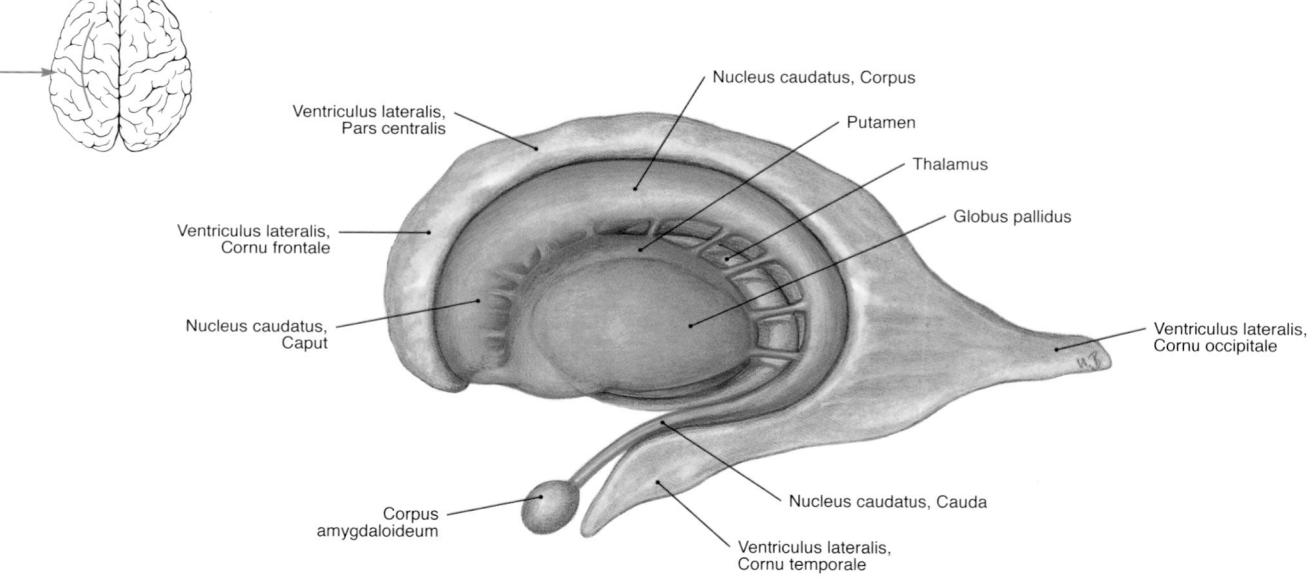

Fig. 1224 Basal ganglia and thalamus, Thalamus;
viewed from the left.

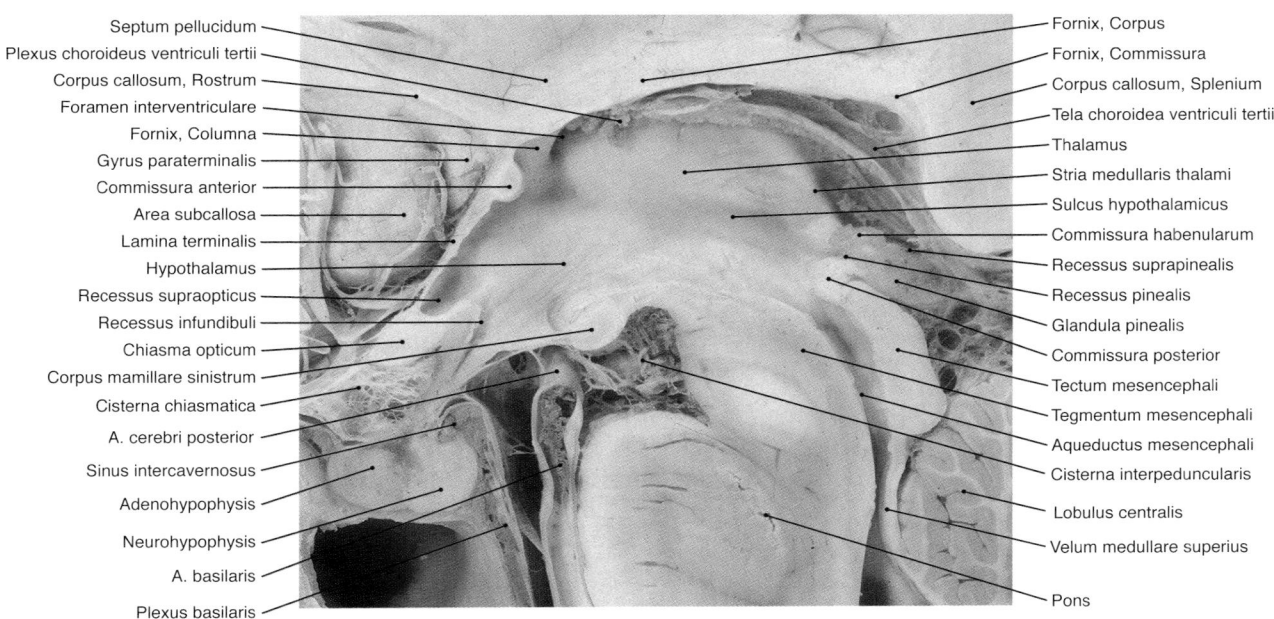

Septum pellucidum
Plexus choroideus ventriculi tertii
Corpus callosum, Rostrum
Foramen interventriculare
Fornix, Columna
Gyrus paraterminalis
Commissura anterior
Area subcallosa
Lamina terminalis
Hypothalamus
Recessus supraopticus
Recessus infundibuli
Chiasma opticum
Corpus mamillare sinistrum
Cisterna chiasmatica
A. cerebri posterior
Sinus intercavernosus
Adenohypophysis
Neurohypophysis
A. basilaris
Plexus basilaris

Fornix, Corpus
Fornix, Commissura
Corpus callosum, Splenium
Tela choroidea ventriculi tertii
Thalamus
Stria medullaris thalami
Sulcus hypothalamicus
Commissura habenularum
Recessus suprapinealis
Recessus pinealis
Glandula pinealis
Commissura posterior
Tectum mesencephali
Tegmentum mesencephali
Aqueductus mesencephali
Cisterna interpeduncularis
Lobulus centralis
Velum medullare superius
Pons

Fig. 1225 Third ventricle, Ventriculus tertius; median section.

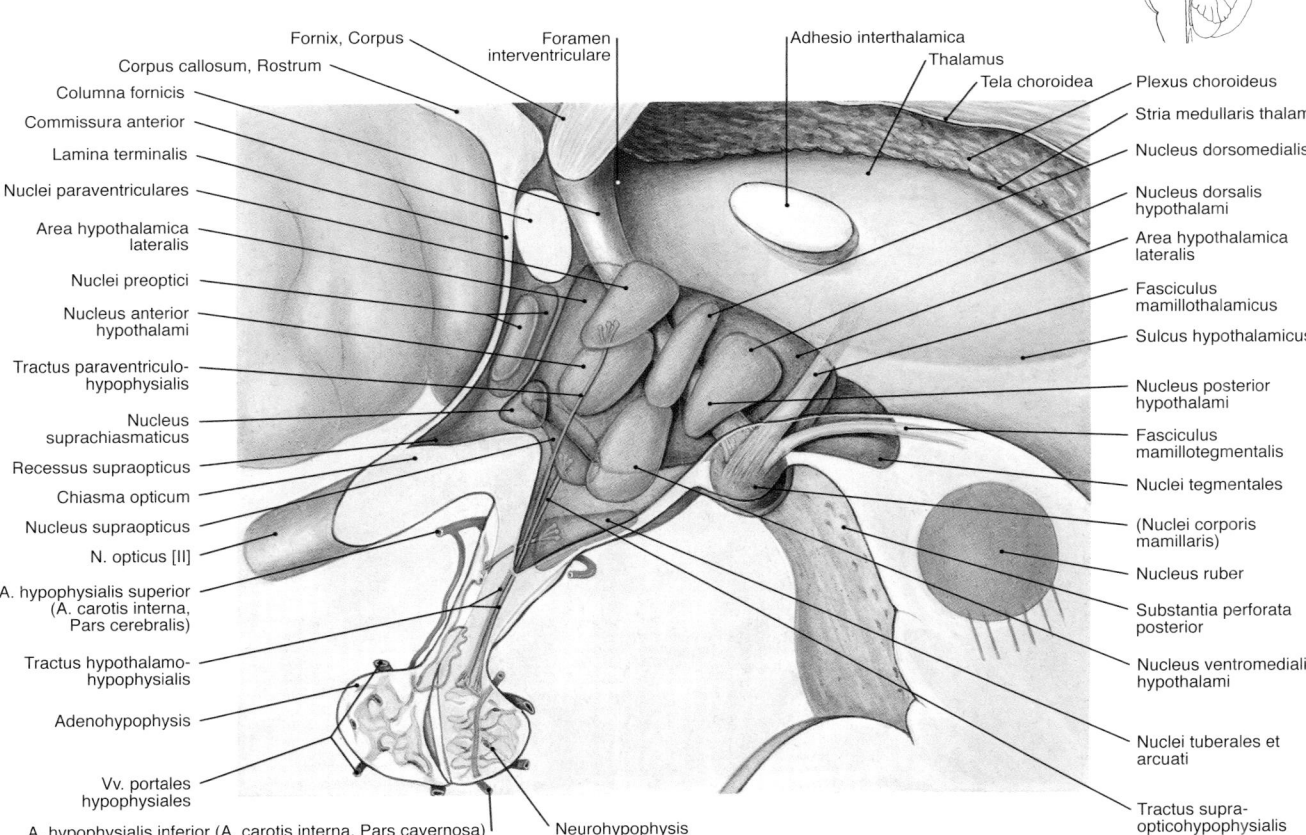

Fornix, Corpus
Corpus callosum, Rostrum
Columna fornicis
Commissura anterior
Lamina terminalis
Nuclei paraventriculares
Area hypothalamica lateralis
Nuclei preoptici
Nucleus anterior hypothalami
Tractus paraventriculo-hypophysialis
Nucleus suprachiasmaticus
Recessus supraopticus
Chiasma opticum
Nucleus supraopticus
N. opticus [II]
A. hypophysialis superior (A. carotis interna, Pars cerebralis)
Tractus hypothalamo-hypophysialis
Adenohypophysis
Vv. portales hypophysiales
A. hypophysialis inferior (A. carotis interna, Pars cavernosa)

Foramen interventriculare
Adhesio interthalamica
Thalamus
Tela choroidea

Neurohypophysis

Plexus choroideus
Stria medullaris thalami
Nucleus dorsomedialis
Nucleus dorsalis hypothalami
Area hypothalamica lateralis
Fasciculus mamillothalamicus
Sulcus hypothalamicus
Nucleus posterior hypothalami
Fasciculus mamillotegmentalis
Nuclei tegmentales
(Nuclei corporis mamillaris)
Nucleus ruber
Substantia perforata posterior
Nucleus ventromedialis hypothalami
Nuclei tuberales et arcuati
Tractus supra-opticohypophysialis

Fig. 1226 Hypothalamus, Hypothalamus; overview; nuclei are illustrated translucently; medial view.

Thalamic nuclei

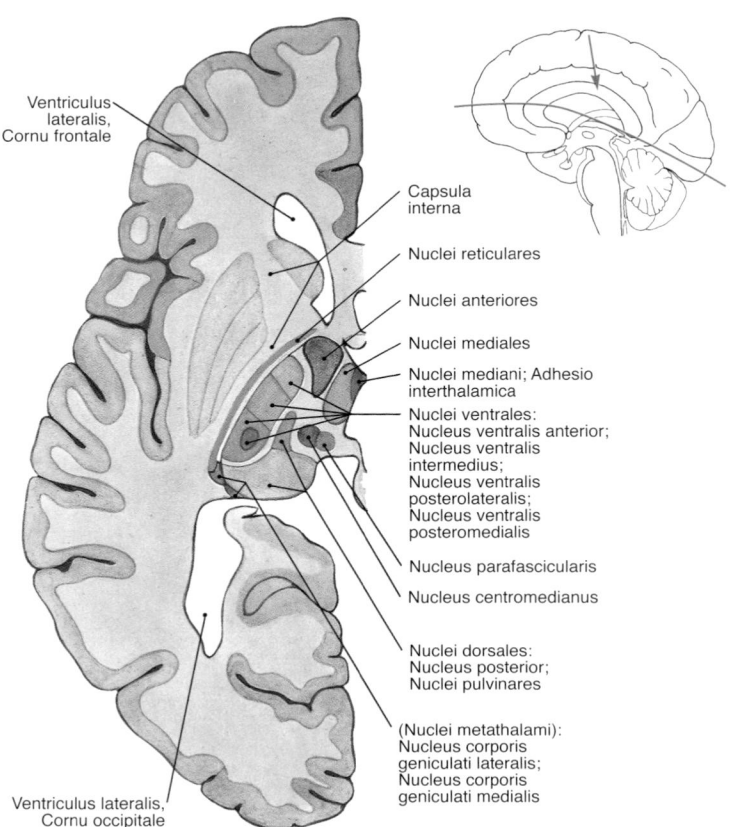

Ventriculus lateralis, Cornu frontale

Capsula interna

Nuclei reticulares

Nuclei anteriores

Nuclei mediales

Nuclei mediani; Adhesio interthalamica

Nuclei ventrales:
Nucleus ventralis anterior;
Nucleus ventralis intermedius;
Nucleus ventralis posterolateralis;
Nucleus ventralis posteromedialis

Nucleus parafascicularis

Nucleus centromedianus

Nuclei dorsales:
Nucleus posterior;
Nuclei pulvinares

(Nuclei metathalami):
Nucleus corporis geniculati lateralis;
Nucleus corporis geniculati medialis

Ventriculus lateralis, Cornu occipitale

a Horizontal section through the left cerebral hemisphere

Fig. 1227 a–c Nuclei and cortical projections of the thalamus, Thalamus.
Corresponding nuclei and cortical projections are indicated by the same colour.

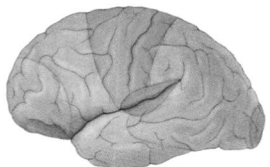

b Left cerebral hemisphere; viewed from the left

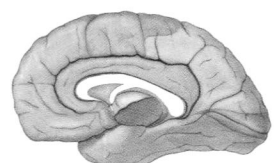

c Right cerebral hemisphere; medial view

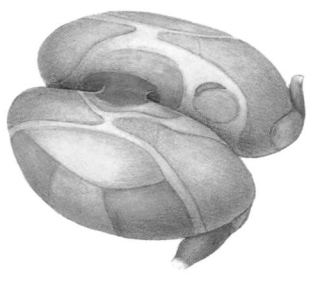

Fig. 1228 Thalamic nuclei; oblique view from posterior. For colour coding see Fig. 1227.

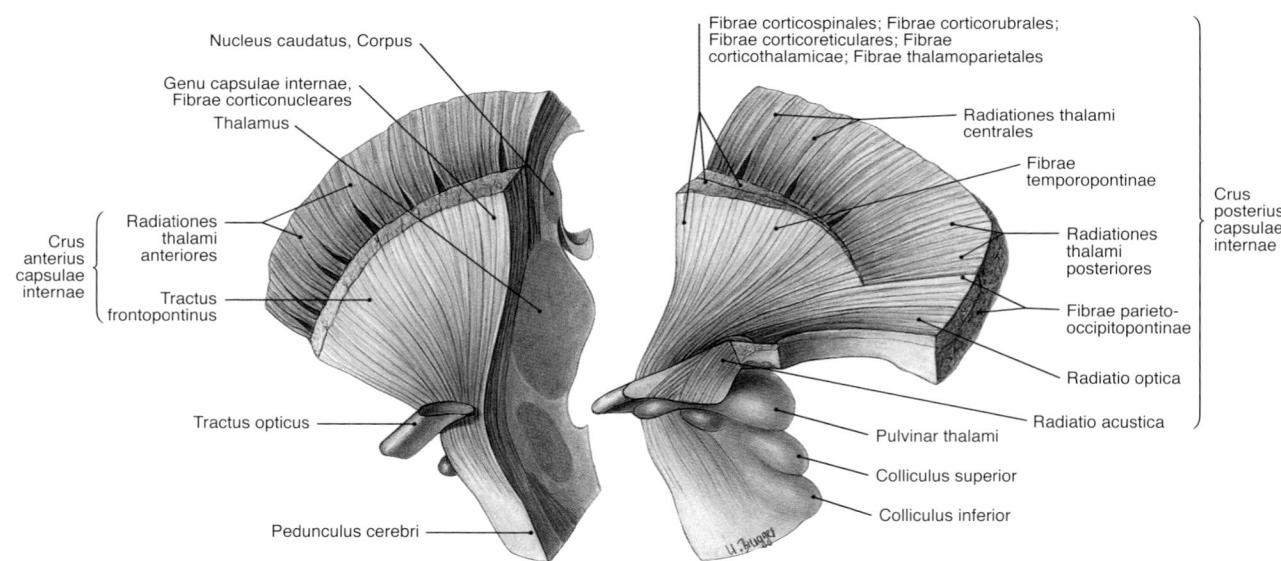

Nucleus caudatus, Corpus

Genu capsulae internae, Fibrae corticonucleares

Thalamus

Crus anterius capsulae internae

Radiationes thalami anteriores

Tractus frontopontinus

Tractus opticus

Pedunculus cerebri

Fibrae corticospinales; Fibrae corticorubrales; Fibrae corticoreticulares; Fibrae corticothalamicae; Fibrae thalamoparietales

Radiationes thalami centrales

Fibrae temporopontinae

Radiationes thalami posteriores

Fibrae parieto-occipitopontinae

Radiatio optica

Radiatio acustica

Pulvinar thalami

Colliculus superior

Colliculus inferior

Crus posterius capsulae internae

Fig. 1229 Thalamic radiation, Radiationes thalami, and internal capsule, Capsula interna, have been divided by a frontal section; viewed from the left.

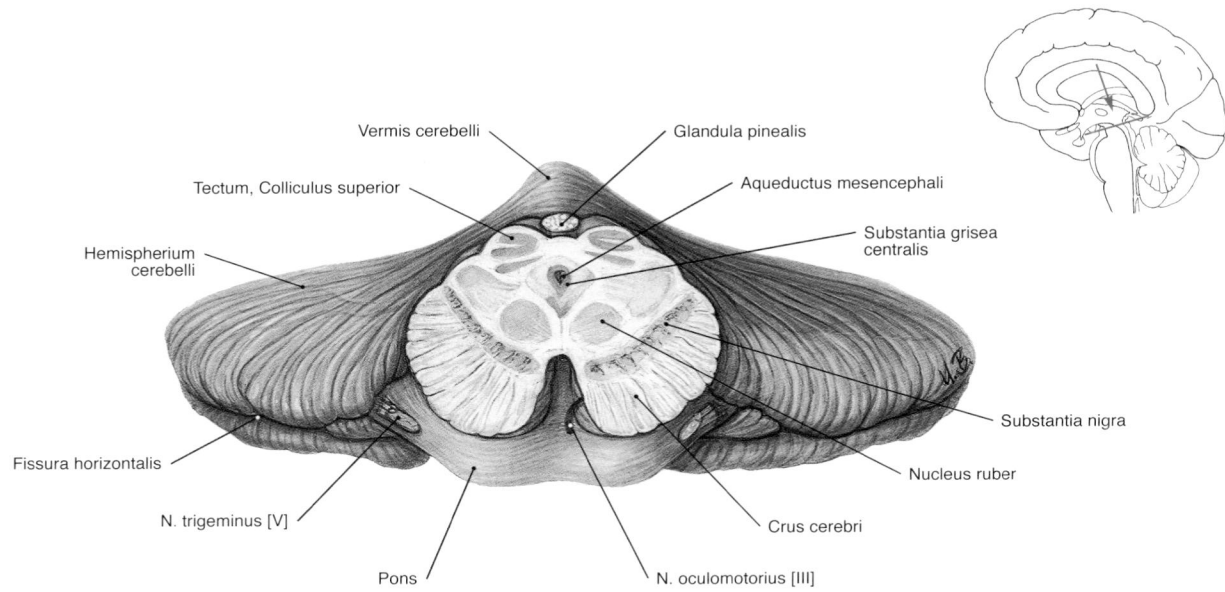

Vermis cerebelli

Tectum, Colliculus superior

Hemispherium cerebelli

Fissura horizontalis

N. trigeminus [V]

Pons

Glandula pinealis

Aqueductus mesencephali

Substantia grisea centralis

Substantia nigra

Nucleus ruber

Crus cerebri

N. oculomotorius [III]

Fig. 1230 Midbrain, Mesencephalon;
cross-section at the level of the superior colliculi;
anterior view.

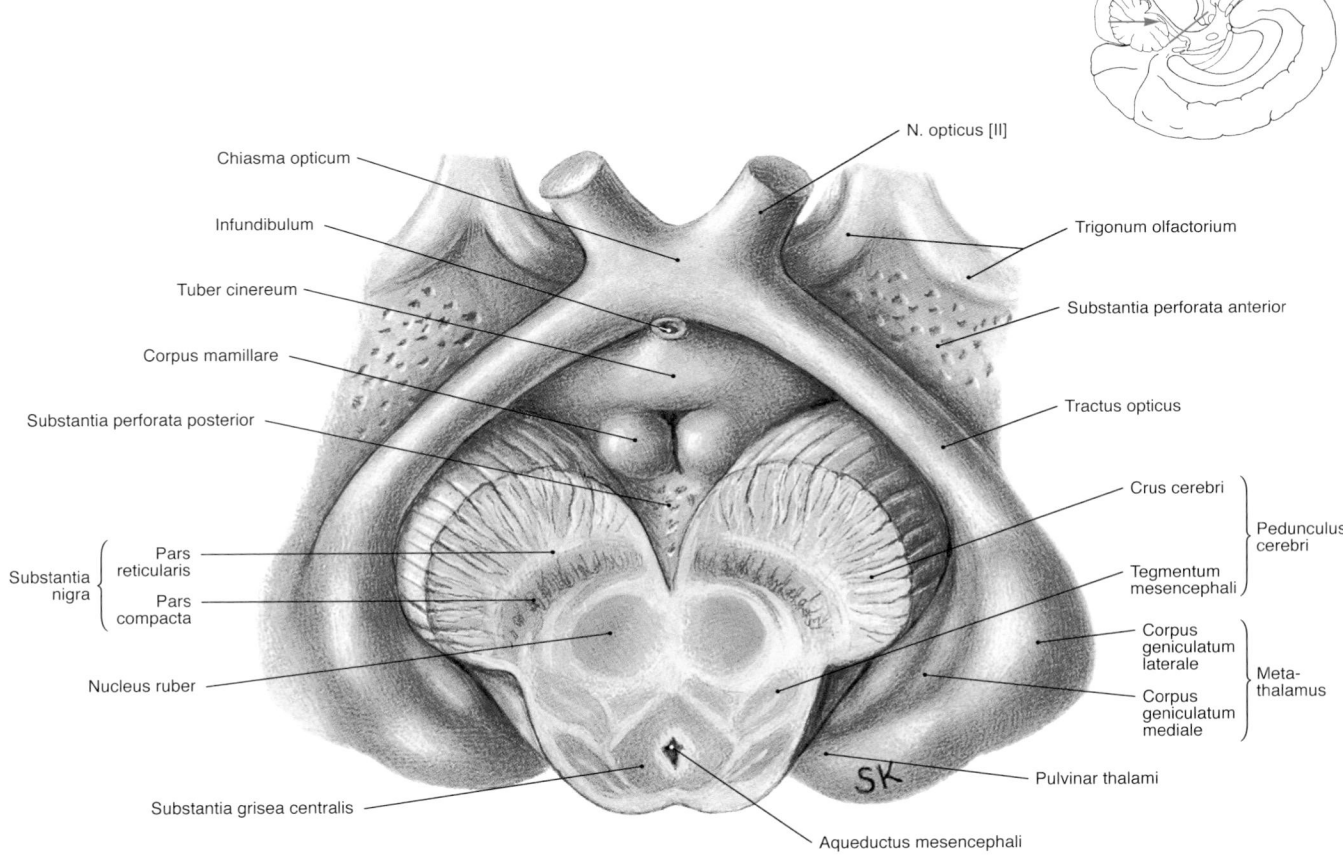

Chiasma opticum

Infundibulum

Tuber cinereum

Corpus mamillare

Substantia perforata posterior

Substantia nigra { Pars reticularis / Pars compacta }

Nucleus ruber

Substantia grisea centralis

Aqueductus mesencephali

N. opticus [II]

Trigonum olfactorium

Substantia perforata anterior

Tractus opticus

Crus cerebri

Tegmentum mesencephali

} Pedunculus cerebri

Corpus geniculatum laterale

Corpus geniculatum mediale

} Meta-thalamus

Pulvinar thalami

SK

Fig. 1231 Midbrain, Mesencephalon,
and diencephalon, Diencephalon;
after oblique section of the midbrain;
inferior view.

Midbrain and medulla oblongata

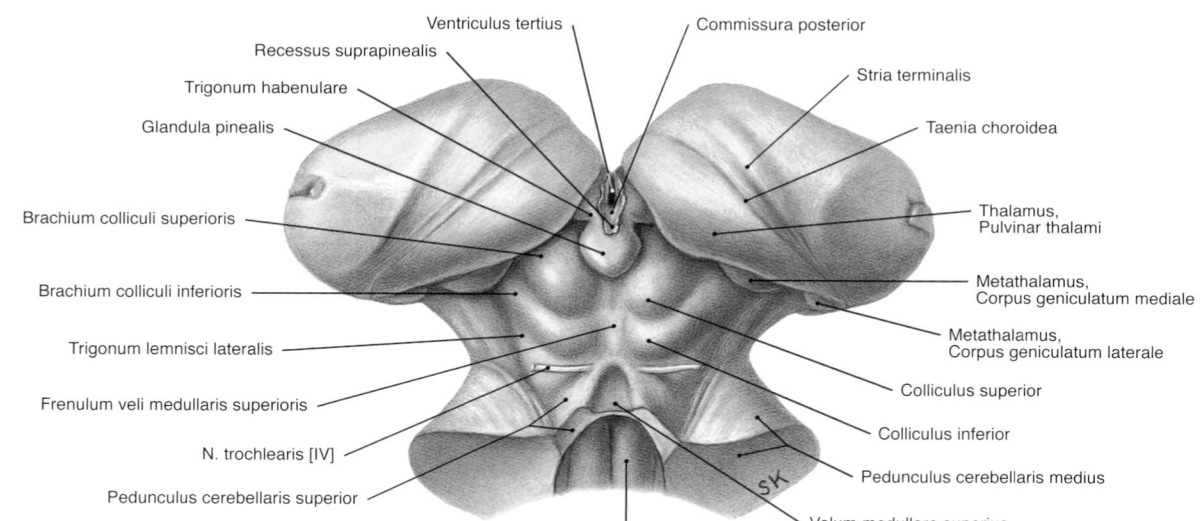

Fig. 1232 Midbrain, Mesencephalon, and pineal gland, Glandula pinealis; posterior-superior view.

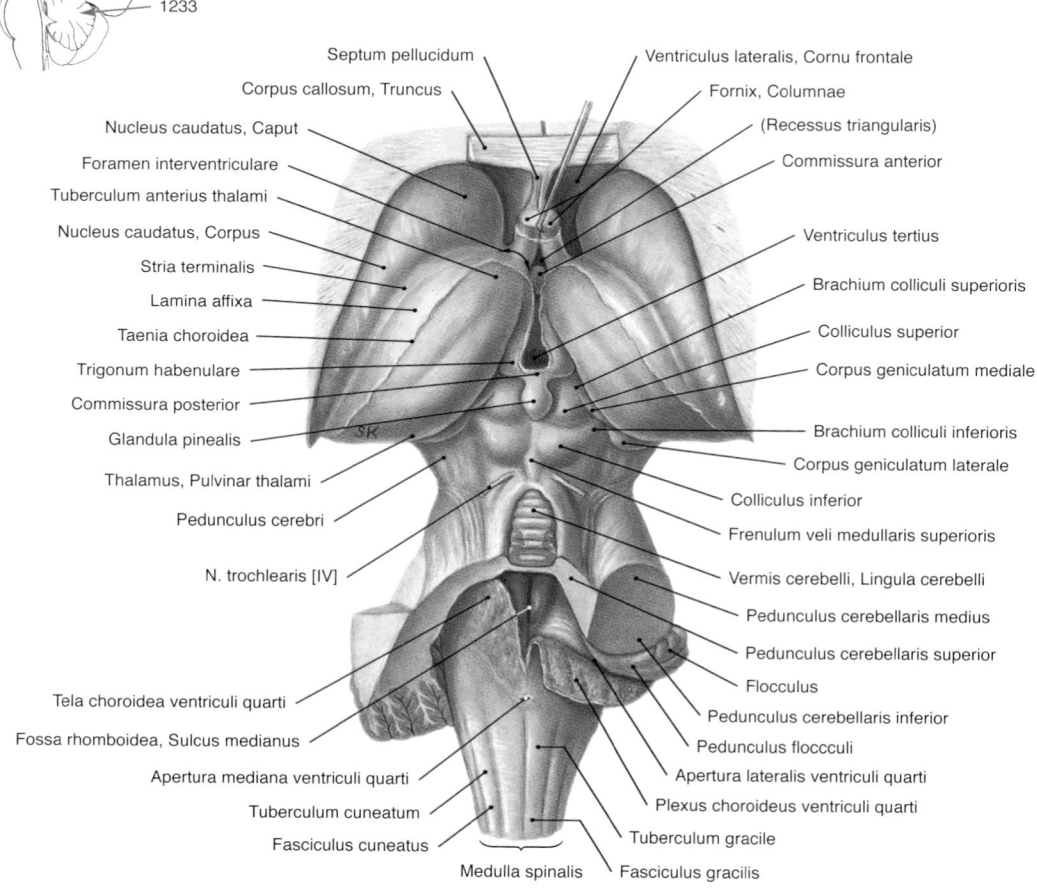

Fig. 1233 Brainstem, Truncus encephali;
the pons and major parts of the cerebellum have been removed;
the tela choroidea of the fourth ventricle has been sectioned in
the median plane and reflected to the right;
posterior-superior view.

Midbrain and medulla oblongata

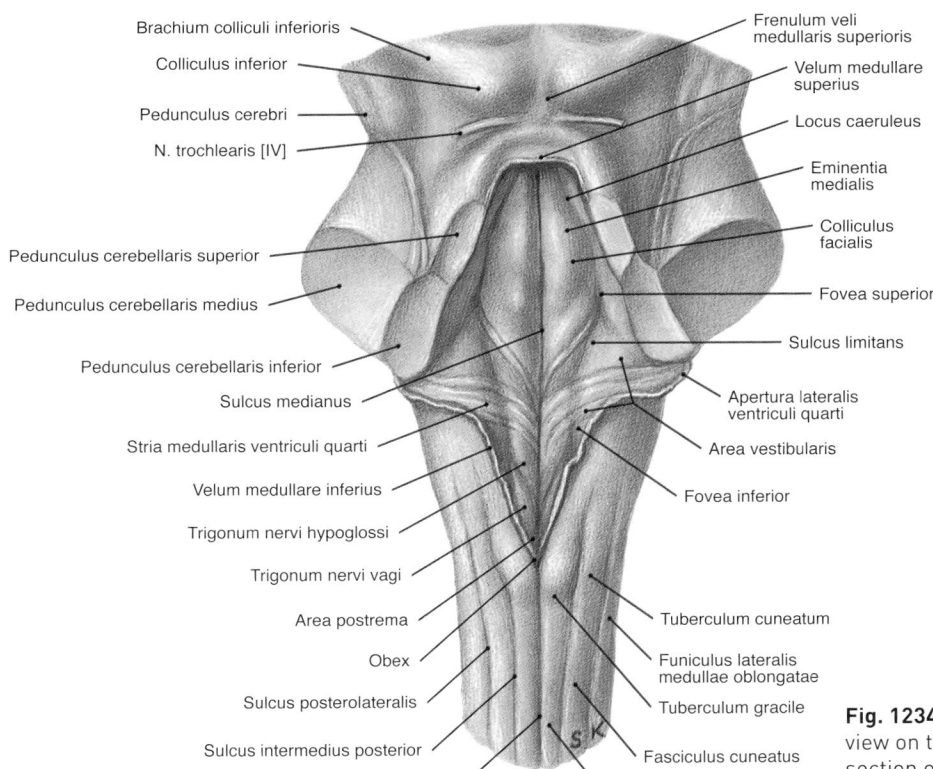

Brachium colliculi inferioris
Colliculus inferior
Pedunculus cerebri
N. trochlearis [IV]

Pedunculus cerebellaris superior
Pedunculus cerebellaris medius

Pedunculus cerebellaris inferior
Sulcus medianus
Stria medullaris ventriculi quarti
Velum medullare inferius
Trigonum nervi hypoglossi
Trigonum nervi vagi
Area postrema
Obex
Sulcus posterolateralis
Sulcus intermedius posterior
Sulcus medianus

Frenulum veli medullaris superioris
Velum medullare superius
Locus caeruleus
Eminentia medialis
Colliculus facialis
Fovea superior
Sulcus limitans
Apertura lateralis ventriculi quarti
Area vestibularis
Fovea inferior
Tuberculum cuneatum
Funiculus lateralis medullae oblongatae
Tuberculum gracile
Fasciculus cuneatus
Fasciculus gracilis

Fig. 1234 Rhomboid fossa, Fossa rhomboidea; view on the floor of the fourth ventricle after section of the cerebellar peduncles; posterior-superior view.

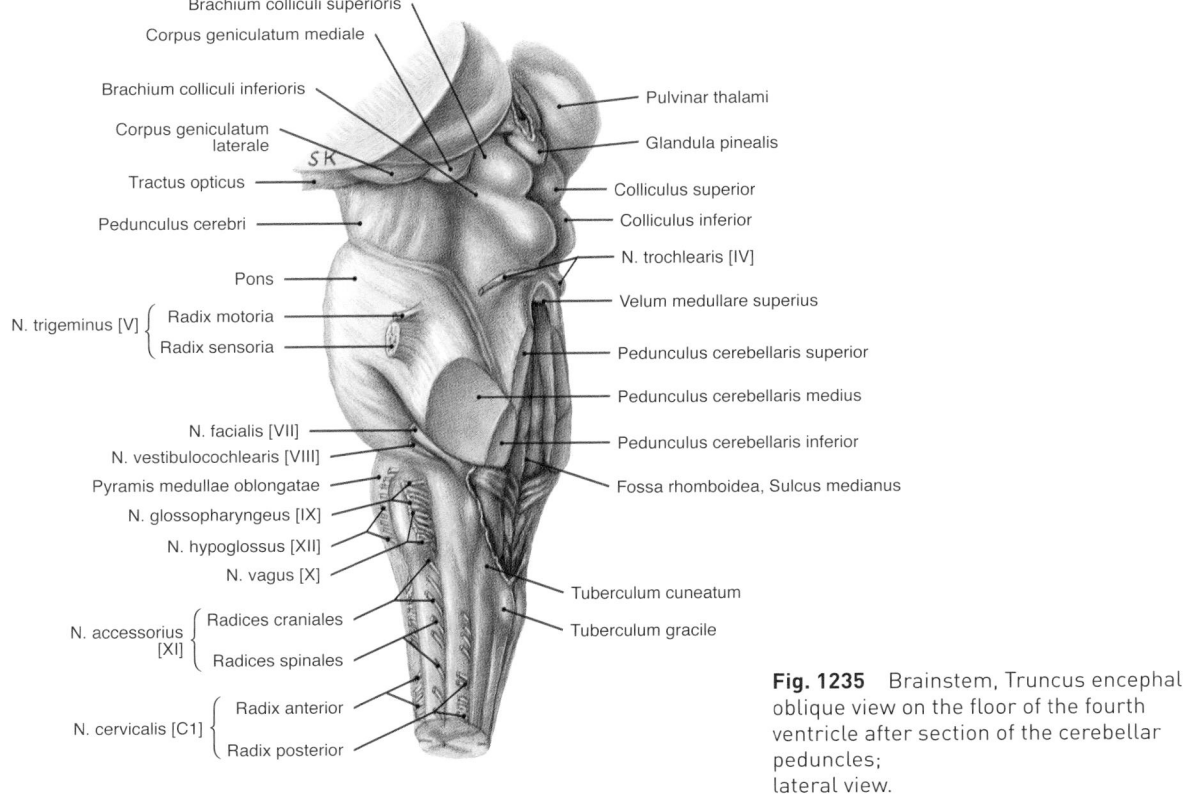

Brachium colliculi superioris
Corpus geniculatum mediale
Brachium colliculi inferioris
Corpus geniculatum laterale
Tractus opticus
Pedunculus cerebri
Pons
N. trigeminus [V] { Radix motoria
Radix sensoria

N. facialis [VII]
N. vestibulocochlearis [VIII]
Pyramis medullae oblongatae
N. glossopharyngeus [IX]
N. hypoglossus [XII]
N. vagus [X]
N. accessorius [XI] { Radices craniales
Radices spinales
N. cervicalis [C1] { Radix anterior
Radix posterior

Pulvinar thalami
Glandula pinealis
Colliculus superior
Colliculus inferior
N. trochlearis [IV]
Velum medullare superius
Pedunculus cerebellaris superior
Pedunculus cerebellaris medius
Pedunculus cerebellaris inferior
Fossa rhomboidea, Sulcus medianus

Tuberculum cuneatum
Tuberculum gracile

Fig. 1235 Brainstem, Truncus encephali; oblique view on the floor of the fourth ventricle after section of the cerebellar peduncles; lateral view.

Nuclei of the cranial nerves

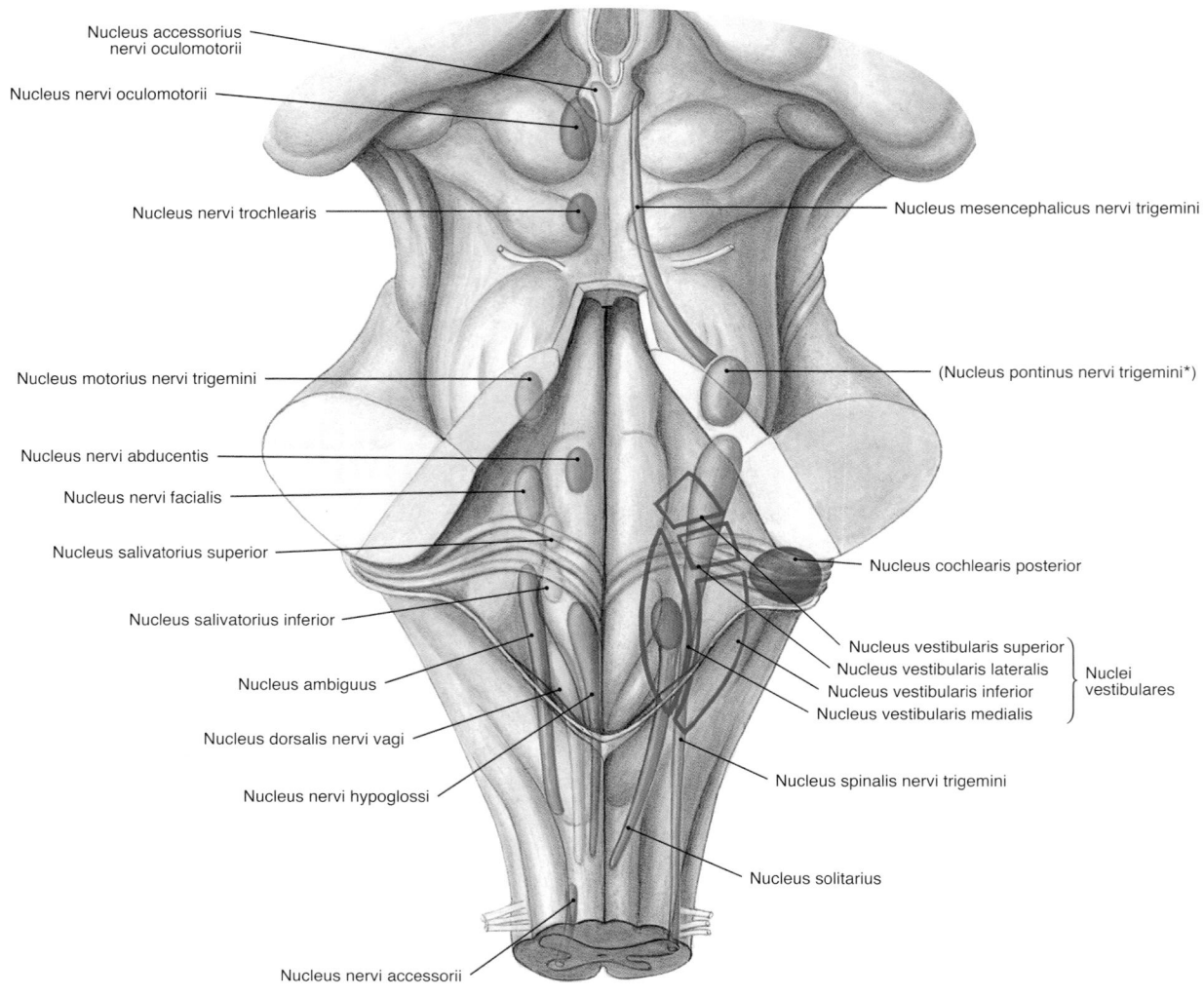

Nucleus accessorius nervi oculomotorii

Nucleus nervi oculomotorii

Nucleus nervi trochlearis

Nucleus mesencephalicus nervi trigemini

Nucleus motorius nervi trigemini

(Nucleus pontinus nervi trigemini*)

Nucleus nervi abducentis

Nucleus nervi facialis

Nucleus salivatorius superior

Nucleus cochlearis posterior

Nucleus salivatorius inferior

Nucleus vestibularis superior
Nucleus vestibularis lateralis　} Nuclei
Nucleus vestibularis inferior　　　vestibulares
Nucleus vestibularis medialis

Nucleus ambiguus

Nucleus dorsalis nervi vagi

Nucleus spinalis nervi trigemini

Nucleus nervi hypoglossi

Nucleus solitarius

Nucleus nervi accessorii

Fig. 1236　Cranial nerves, Nn. craniales; topographic overview of the nuclei; posterior view.

On the left the motor nuclei and on the right the sensory nuclei are shown.
* Clinical term: principal sensory nucleus of the trigeminal nerve

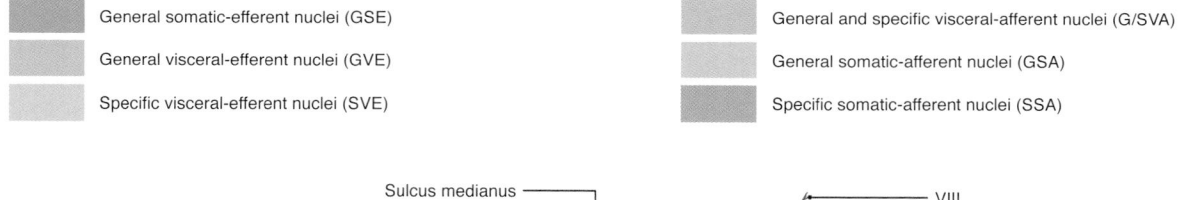

General somatic-efferent nuclei (GSE)

General visceral-efferent nuclei (GVE)

Specific visceral-efferent nuclei (SVE)

General and specific visceral-afferent nuclei (G/SVA)

General somatic-afferent nuclei (GSA)

Specific somatic-afferent nuclei (SSA)

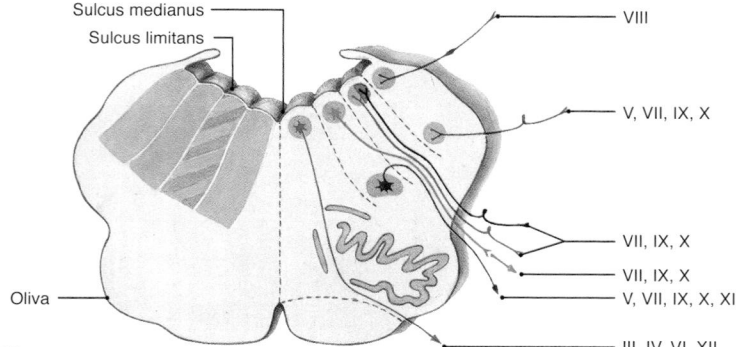

Sulcus medianus

Sulcus limitans

VIII

V, VII, IX, X

VII, IX, X

VII, IX, X

V, VII, IX, X, XI

Oliva

III, IV, VI, XII

Fig. 1237　Cranial nerves, Nn. craniales; schematic cross-section through the rhomboid fossa demonstrating the nuclei.

Nuclei of the cranial nerves

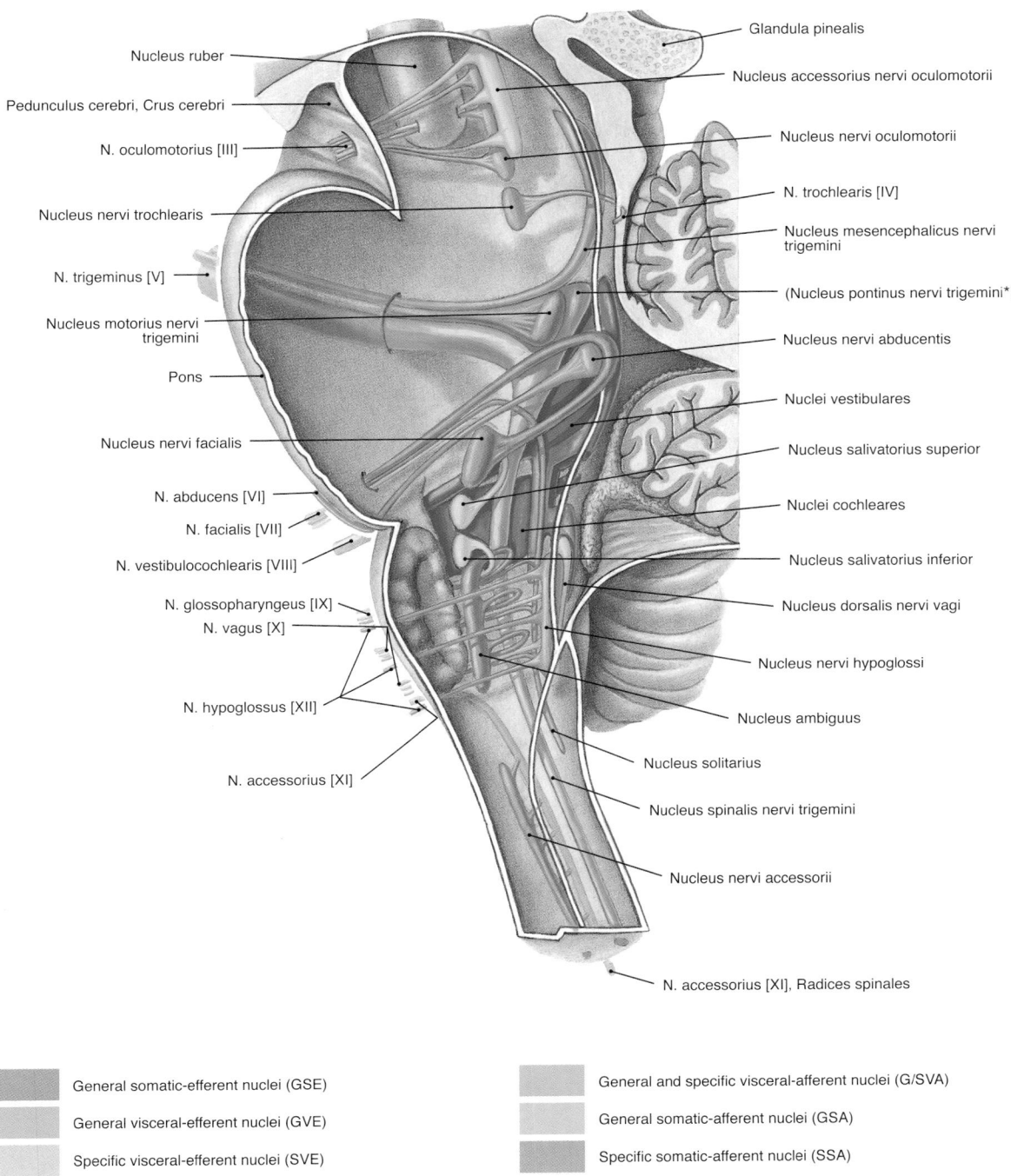

Nucleus ruber

Pedunculus cerebri, Crus cerebri

N. oculomotorius [III]

Nucleus nervi trochlearis

N. trigeminus [V]

Nucleus motorius nervi trigemini

Pons

Nucleus nervi facialis

N. abducens [VI]

N. facialis [VII]

N. vestibulocochlearis [VIII]

N. glossopharyngeus [IX]

N. vagus [X]

N. hypoglossus [XII]

N. accessorius [XI]

Glandula pinealis

Nucleus accessorius nervi oculomotorii

Nucleus nervi oculomotorii

N. trochlearis [IV]

Nucleus mesencephalicus nervi trigemini

(Nucleus pontinus nervi trigemini*)

Nucleus nervi abducentis

Nuclei vestibulares

Nucleus salivatorius superior

Nuclei cochleares

Nucleus salivatorius inferior

Nucleus dorsalis nervi vagi

Nucleus nervi hypoglossi

Nucleus ambiguus

Nucleus solitarius

Nucleus spinalis nervi trigemini

Nucleus nervi accessorii

N. accessorius [XI], Radices spinales

General somatic-efferent nuclei (GSE)

General visceral-efferent nuclei (GVE)

Specific visceral-efferent nuclei (SVE)

General and specific visceral-afferent nuclei (G/SVA)

General somatic-afferent nuclei (GSA)

Specific somatic-afferent nuclei (SSA)

Fig. 1238 Cranial nerves, Nn. craniales;
topographic overview of the nuclei in the median plane.
* Clinical term: principal sensory nucleus of the trigeminal nerve

Cerebellum

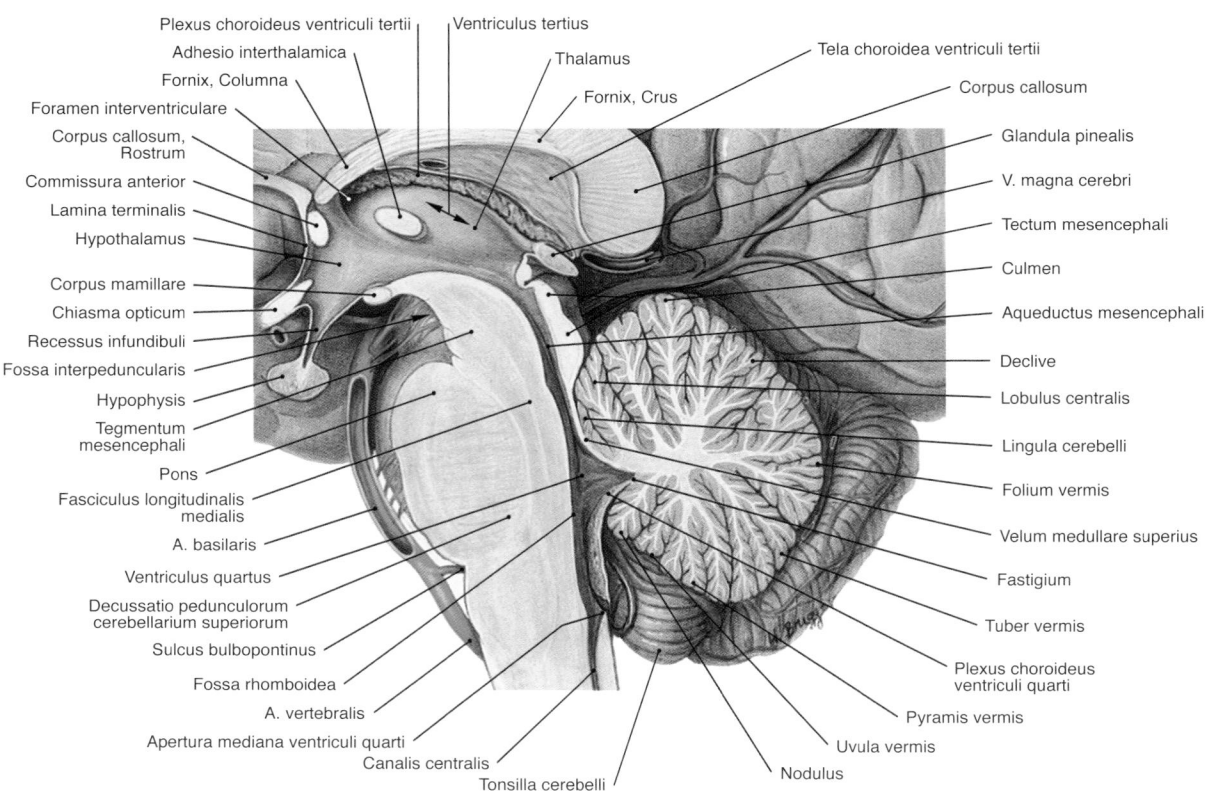

Fig. 1239 Brainstem, Truncus cerebri, with the cerebellum, Cerebellum, and the fourth ventricle, Ventriculus quartus; median section.

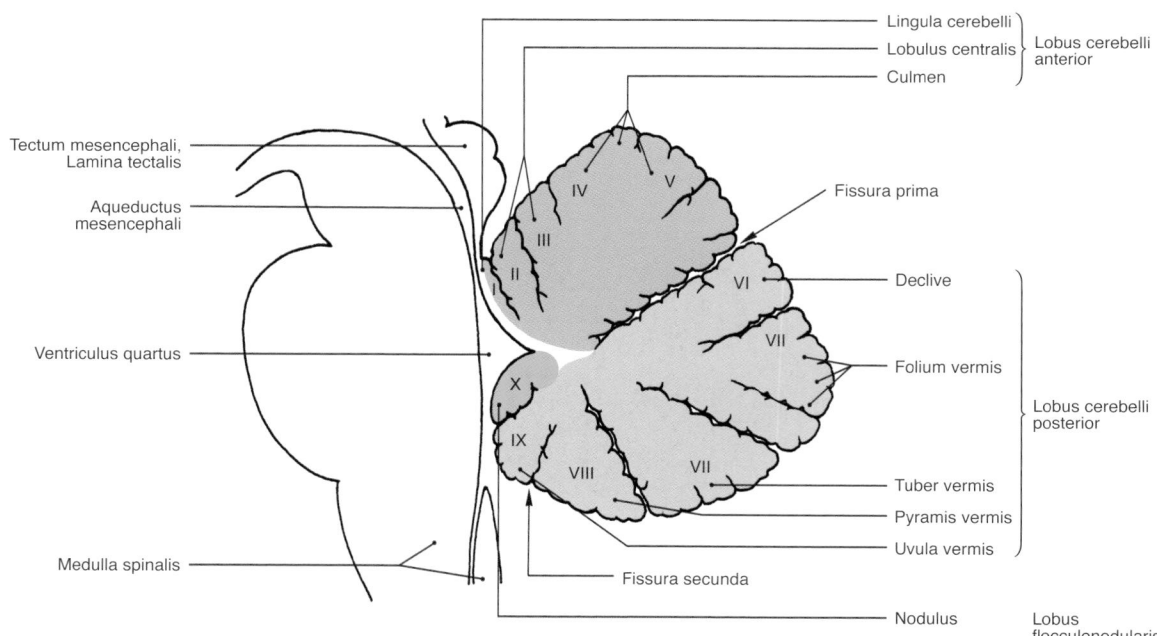

Fig. 1240 Parts of the cerebellar vermis, Vermis cerebelli; median section; overview.

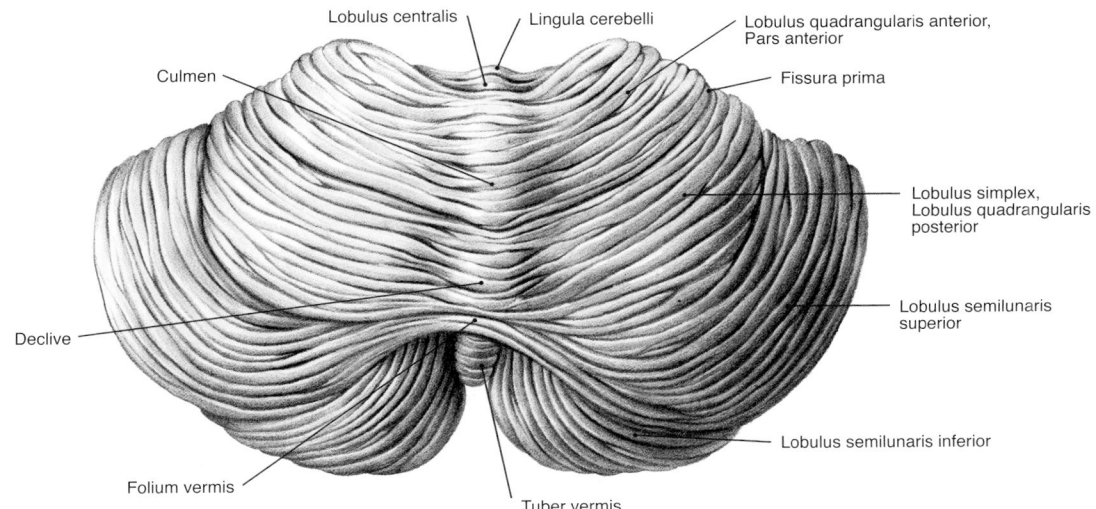

Lobulus centralis — Lingula cerebelli — Lobulus quadrangularis anterior, Pars anterior

Culmen — Fissura prima

Lobulus simplex, Lobulus quadrangularis posterior

Declive — Lobulus semilunaris superior

Lobulus semilunaris inferior

Folium vermis — Tuber vermis

Fig. 1241 Cerebellum, Cerebellum; posterior-superior view.

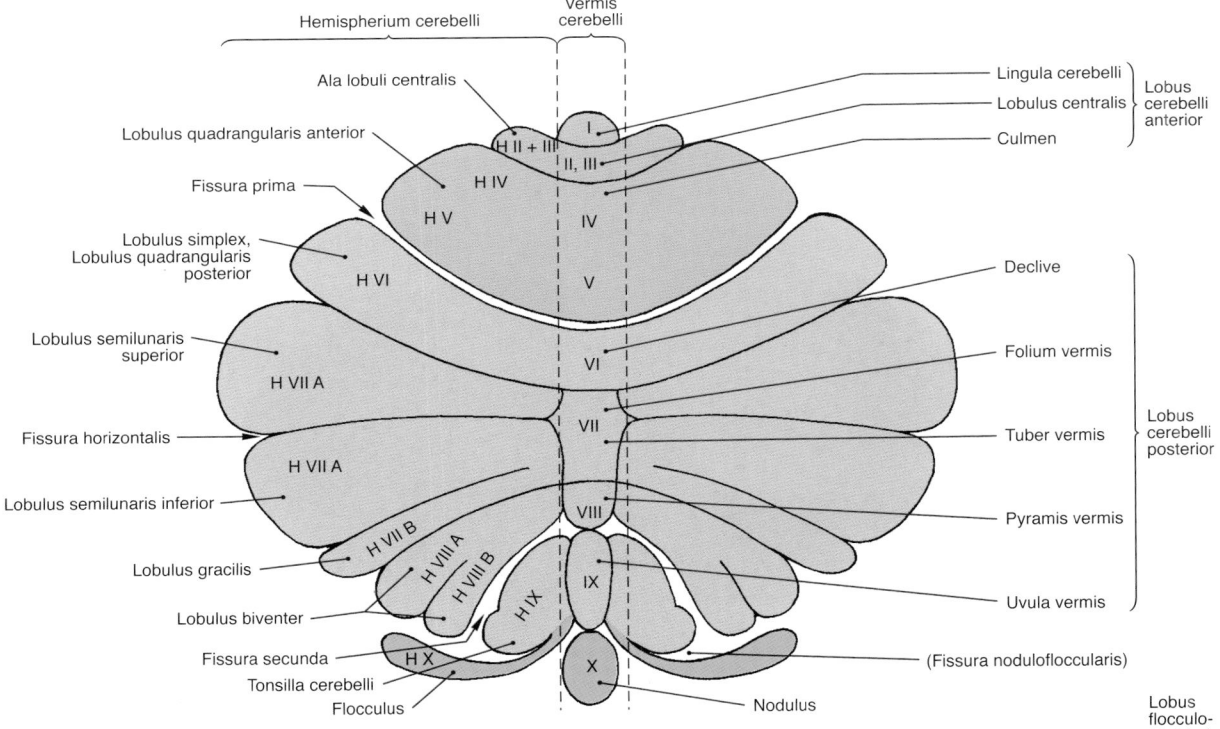

Hemispherium cerebelli — Vermis cerebelli

Ala lobuli centralis — Lingula cerebelli | Lobus cerebelli anterior

Lobulus quadrangularis anterior — H II + III — I — Lobulus centralis

H IV — II, III — Culmen

Fissura prima — H V — IV

Lobulus simplex, Lobulus quadrangularis posterior — H VI — V — Declive

Lobulus semilunaris superior — H VII A — VI — Folium vermis

Fissura horizontalis — H VII A — VII — Tuber vermis

Lobulus semilunaris inferior — VIII — Pyramis vermis

Lobulus gracilis — H VII B — H VIII A — H VIII B — H IX — IX — Uvula vermis | Lobus cerebelli posterior

Lobulus biventer — H X — X — (Fissura nodulofloccularis)

Fissura secunda — Tonsilla cerebelli — Flocculus — Nodulus | Lobus flocculo-nodularis

Fig. 1242 Cerebellum, Cerebellum; diagram of the cerebellar cortex outstretched; overview.

Cerebellum

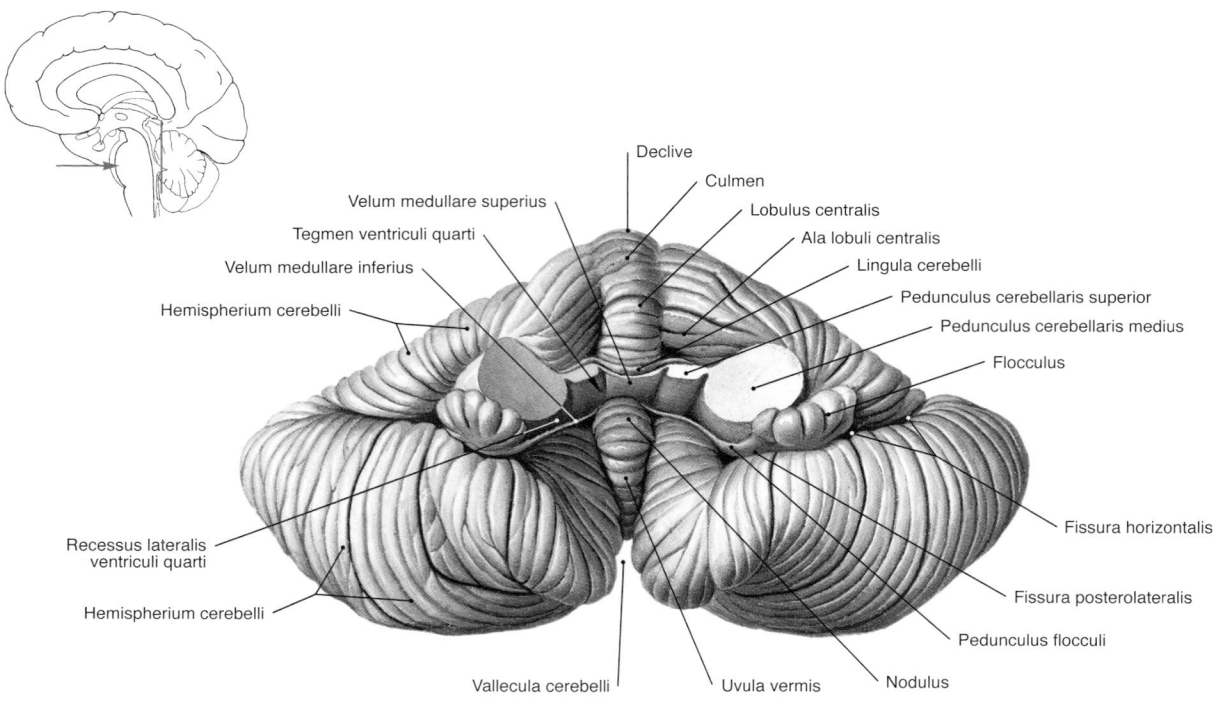

Fig. 1243 Cerebellum, Cerebellum; after section of the cerebellar peduncles; anterior view.

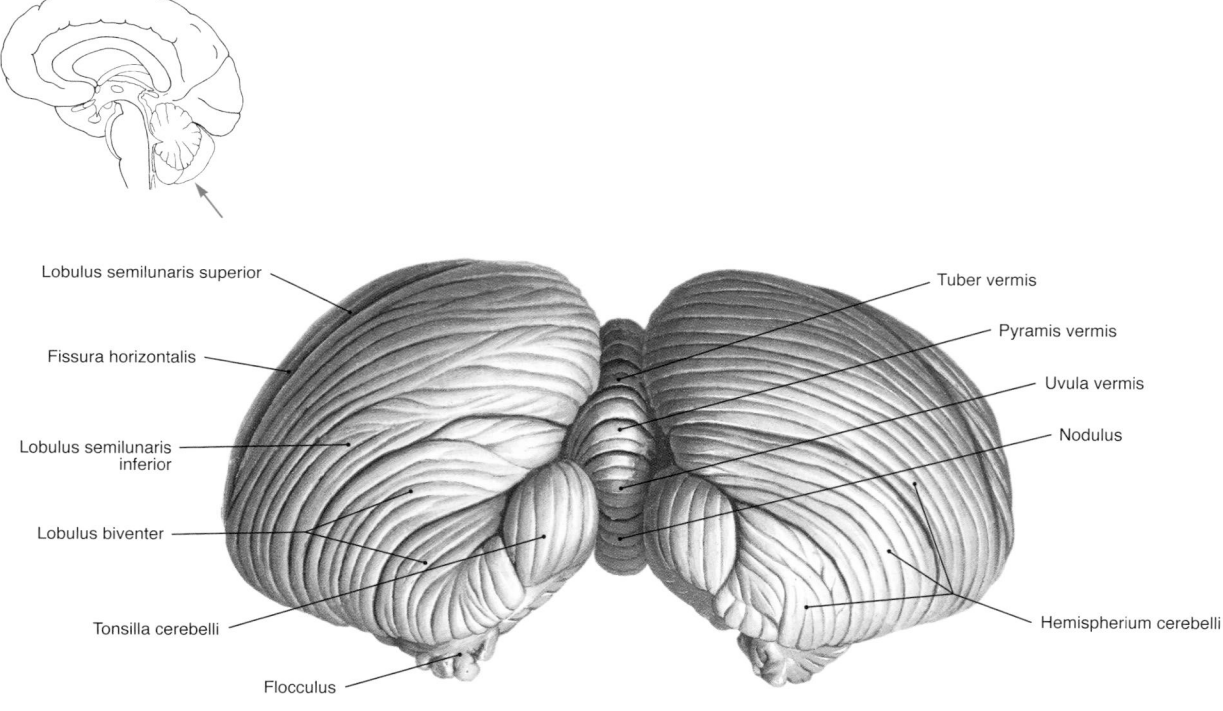

Fig. 1244 Cerebellum, Cerebellum; posterior-inferior view.

Cerebellar nuclei

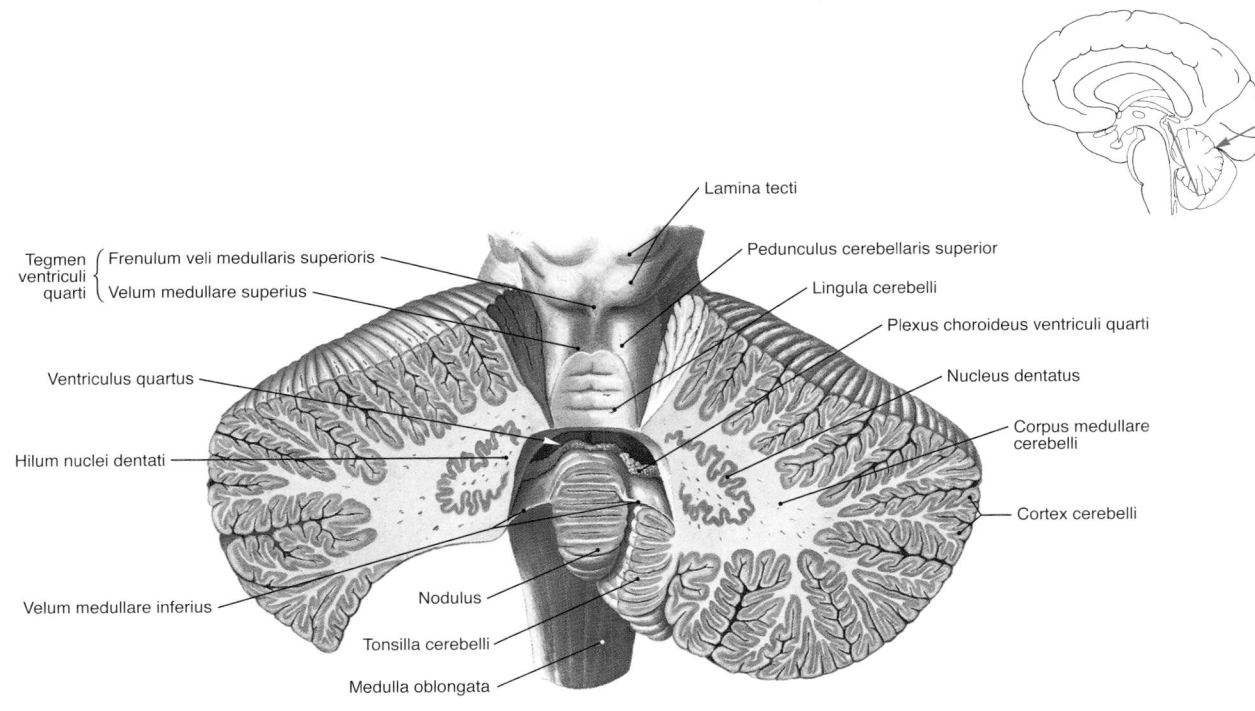

Lamina tecti

Tegmen ventriculi quarti { Frenulum veli medullaris superioris
Velum medullare superius

Pedunculus cerebellaris superior

Lingula cerebelli

Plexus choroideus ventriculi quarti

Ventriculus quartus

Nucleus dentatus

Corpus medullare cerebelli

Hilum nuclei dentati

Cortex cerebelli

Velum medullare inferius

Nodulus

Tonsilla cerebelli

Medulla oblongata

Fig. 1245 Cerebellum, Cerebellum;
oblique section;
posterior view.

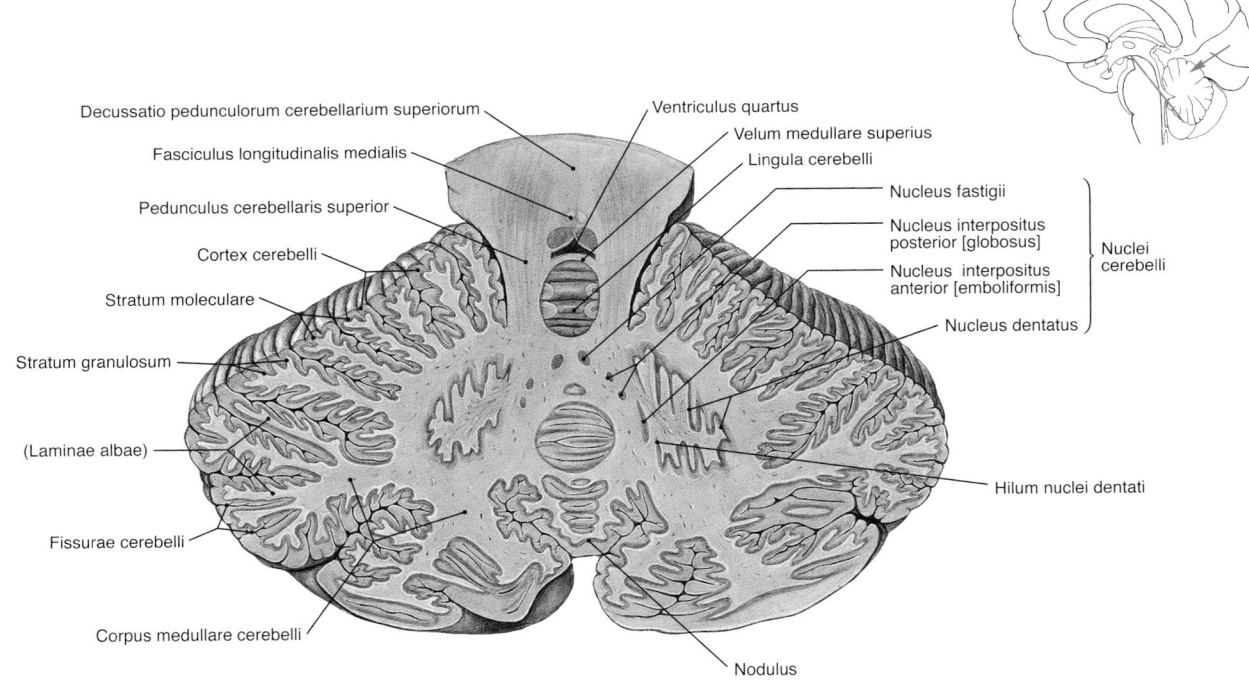

Decussatio pedunculorum cerebellarium superiorum

Ventriculus quartus

Velum medullare superius

Fasciculus longitudinalis medialis

Lingula cerebelli

Pedunculus cerebellaris superior

Nucleus fastigii

Nucleus interpositus posterior [globosus]

Nuclei cerebelli

Cortex cerebelli

Nucleus interpositus anterior [emboliformis]

Stratum moleculare

Nucleus dentatus

Stratum granulosum

(Laminae albae)

Hilum nuclei dentati

Fissurae cerebelli

Corpus medullare cerebelli

Nodulus

Fig. 1246 Cerebellum, Cerebellum;
oblique section through the upper cerebellar peduncles;
posterior view.

Association and commissural tracts

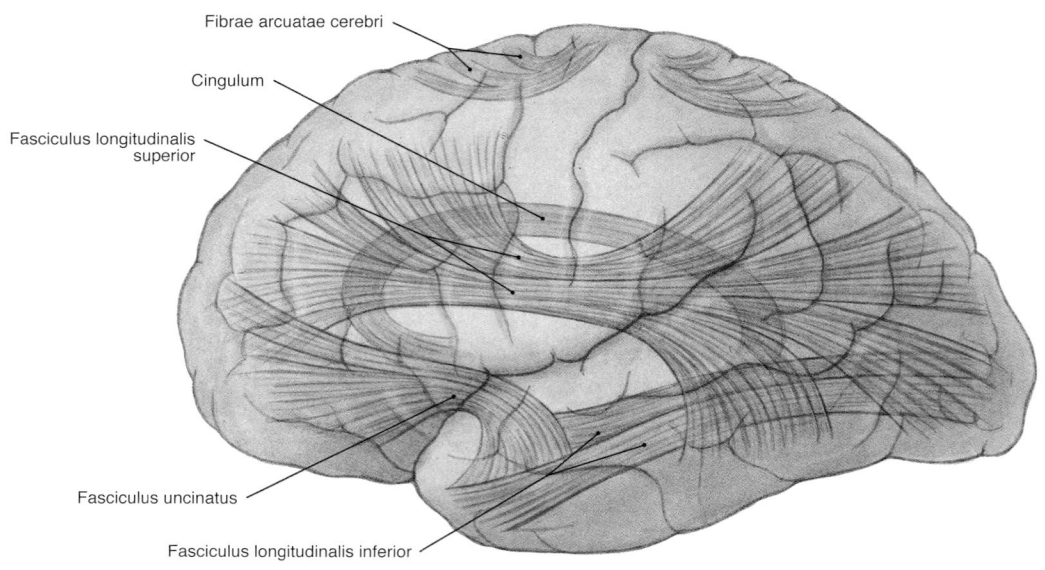

Fig. 1247 Association tracts, Neurofibrae associationis; projection onto the cerebral hemisphere; overview; viewed from the left.

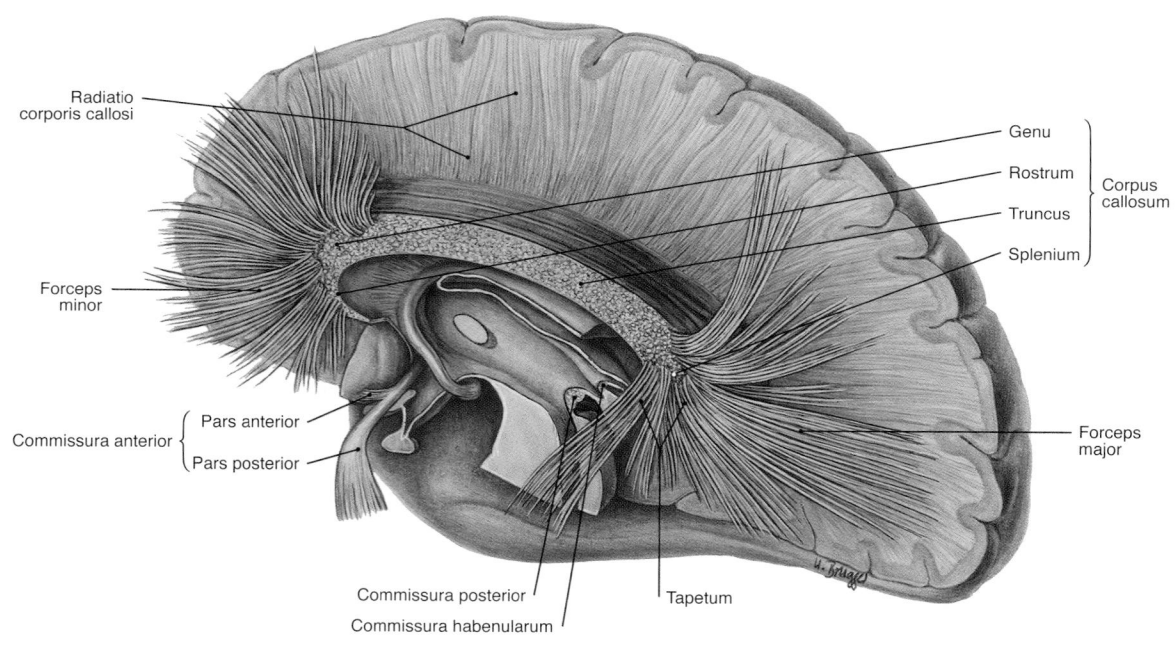

Fig. 1248 Commissural tracts, Neurofibrae commissurales; topographic overview after extensive removal of the corpus callosum in the paramedian plane; single fibres of the corpus callosum are shown; viewed from the left.

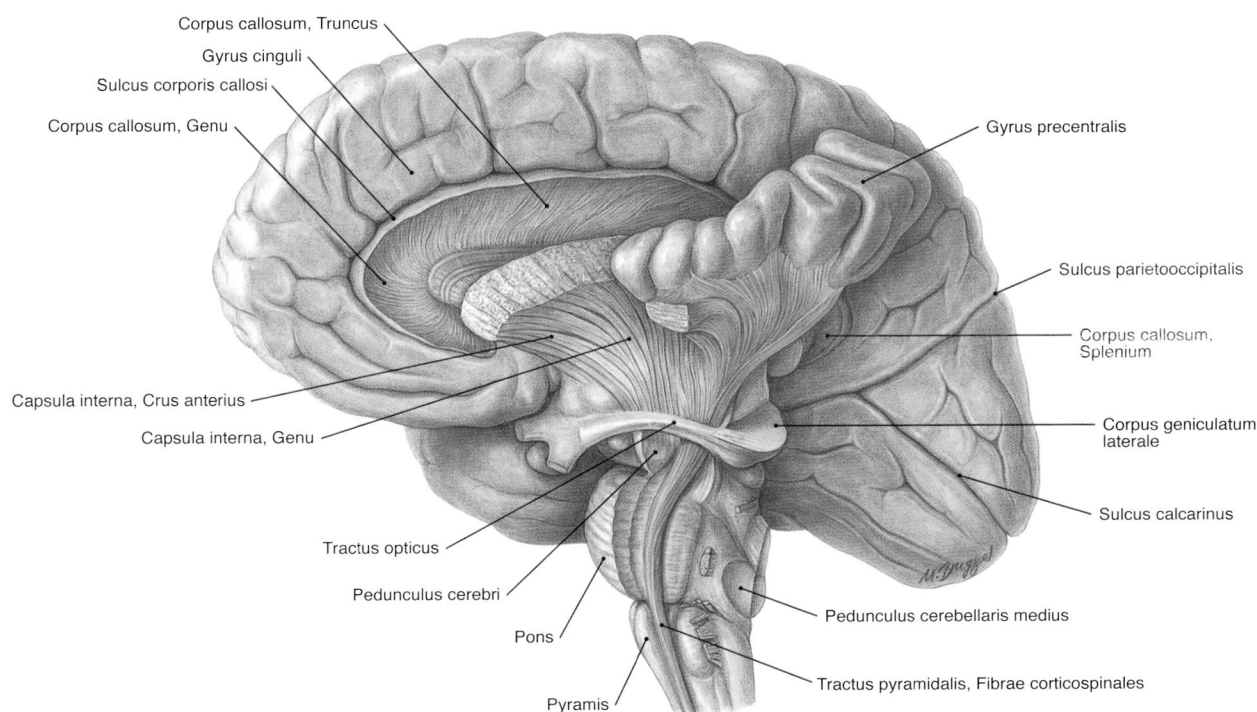

Fig. 1249 Projection tracts, Neurofibrae projectionis;
the internal capsule and the pyramidal tract have been exposed;
viewed from the left.

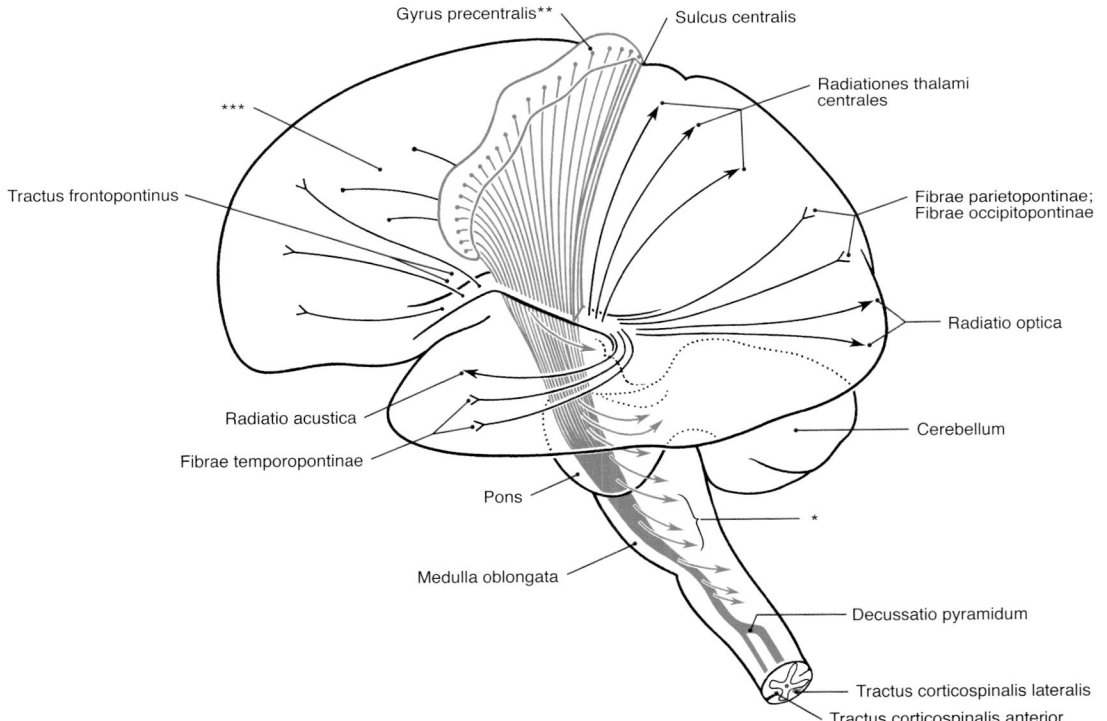

Fig. 1250 Internal capsule, Capsula interna, and pyramidal
tract, Tractus pyramidalis;
functional overview;
viewed from the left.

*   Fibres to the tectal plate and the nuclei of the hindbrain
** Perikarya of the pyramidal tract
***Perikarya of areas 6 and 8 (premotor cortex)

Internal capsule

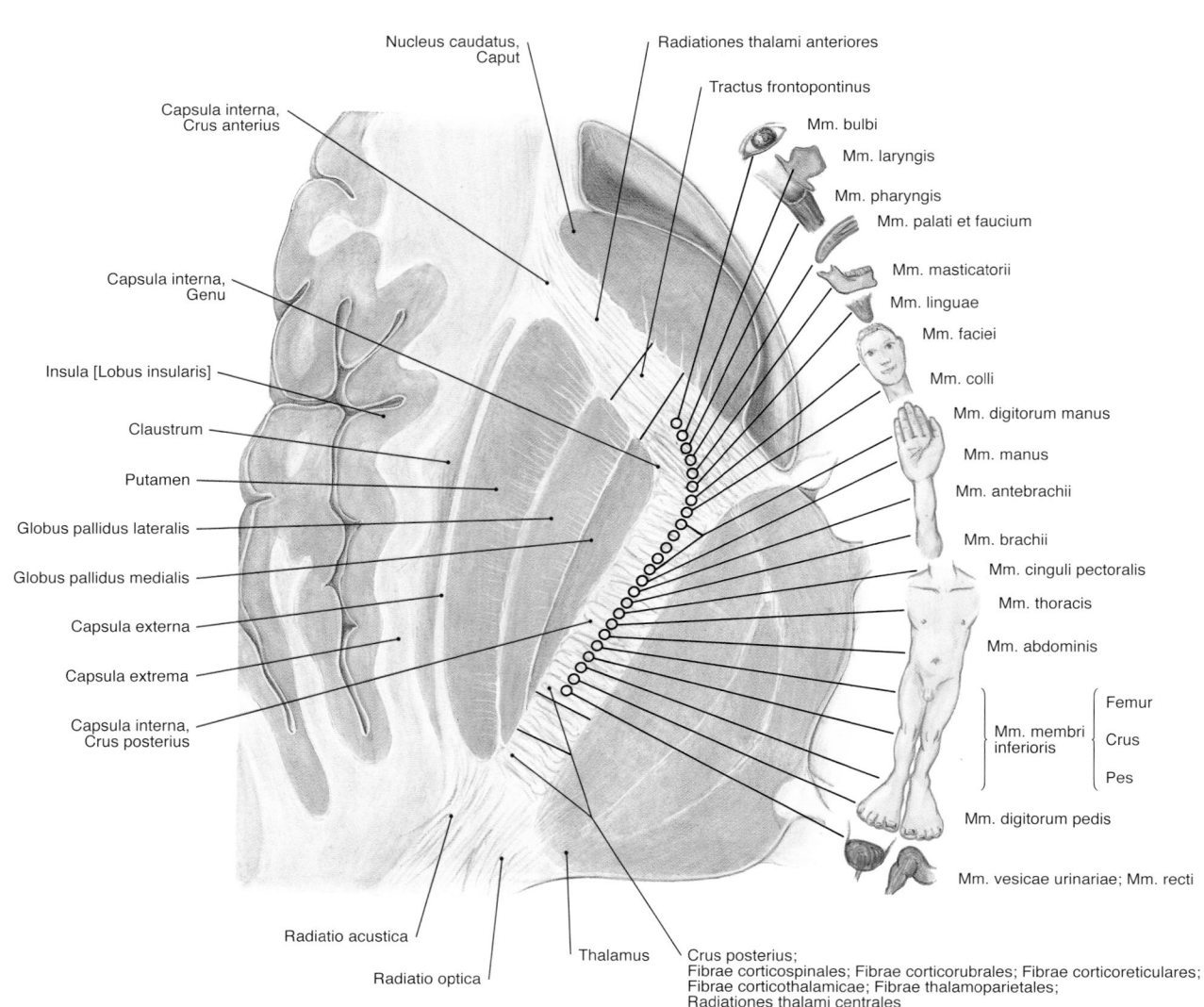

Nucleus caudatus, Caput
Radiationes thalami anteriores
Tractus frontopontinus
Capsula interna, Crus anterius
Mm. bulbi
Mm. laryngis
Mm. pharyngis
Mm. palati et faucium
Capsula interna, Genu
Mm. masticatorii
Mm. linguae
Mm. faciei
Insula [Lobus insularis]
Mm. colli
Claustrum
Mm. digitorum manus
Putamen
Mm. manus
Mm. antebrachii
Globus pallidus lateralis
Mm. brachii
Globus pallidus medialis
Mm. cinguli pectoralis
Mm. thoracis
Capsula externa
Mm. abdominis
Capsula extrema
Femur
Mm. membri inferioris
Crus
Capsula interna, Crus posterius
Pes
Mm. digitorum pedis
Mm. vesicae urinariae; Mm. recti
Radiatio acustica
Radiatio optica
Thalamus
Crus posterius;
Fibrae corticospinales; Fibrae corticorubrales; Fibrae corticoreticulares;
Fibrae corticothalamicae; Fibrae thalamoparietales;
Radiationes thalami centrales

Fig. 1251 Internal capsule, Capsula interna; functional organisation.

Pyramidal tract

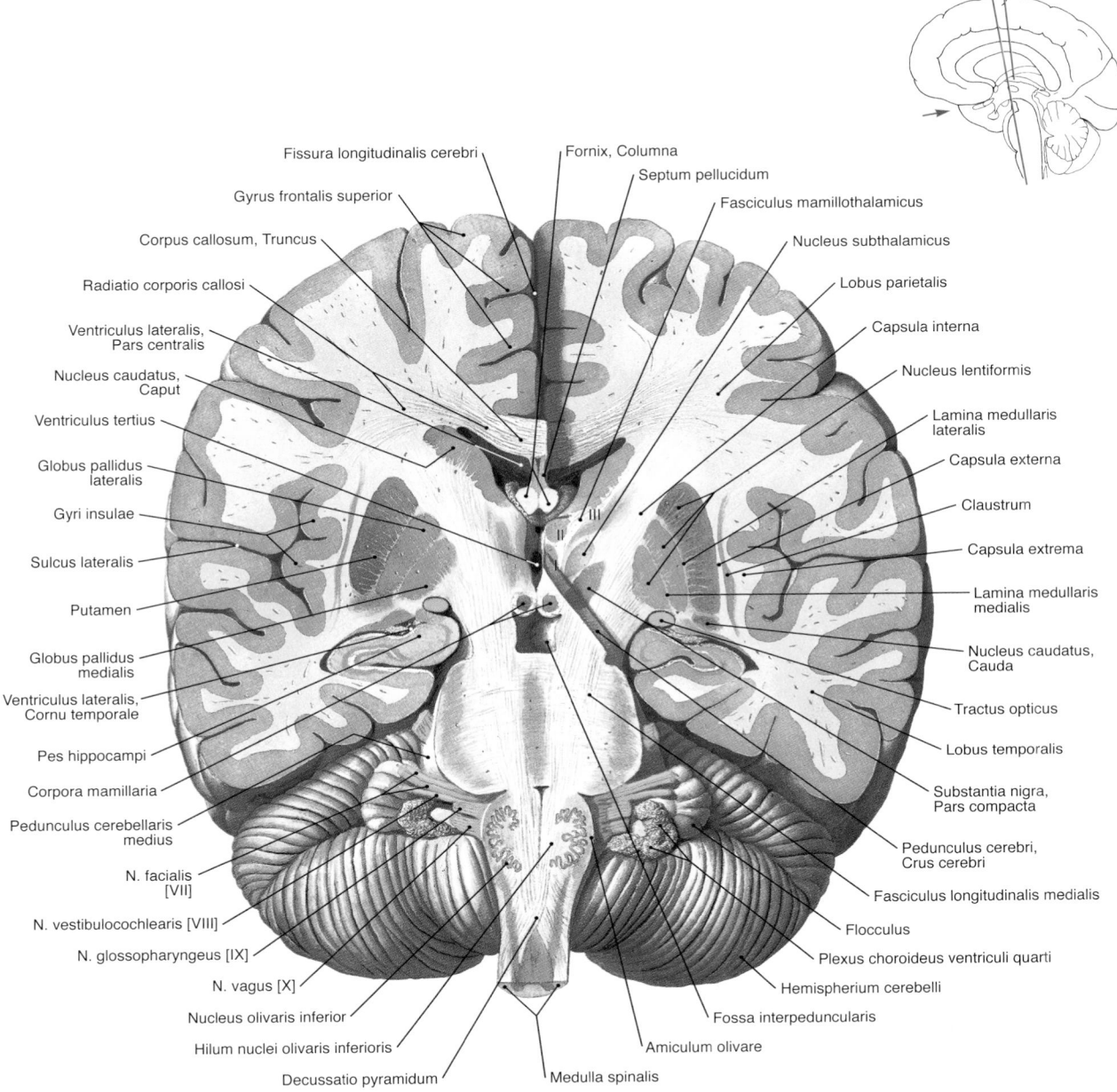

Fissura longitudinalis cerebri
Gyrus frontalis superior
Corpus callosum, Truncus
Radiatio corporis callosi
Ventriculus lateralis, Pars centralis
Nucleus caudatus, Caput
Ventriculus tertius
Globus pallidus lateralis
Gyri insulae
Sulcus lateralis
Putamen
Globus pallidus medialis
Ventriculus lateralis, Cornu temporale
Pes hippocampi
Corpora mamillaria
Pedunculus cerebellaris medius
N. facialis [VII]
N. vestibulocochlearis [VIII]
N. glossopharyngeus [IX]
N. vagus [X]
Nucleus olivaris inferior
Hilum nuclei olivaris inferioris
Decussatio pyramidum

Fornix, Columna
Septum pellucidum
Fasciculus mamillothalamicus
Nucleus subthalamicus
Lobus parietalis
Capsula interna
Nucleus lentiformis
Lamina medullaris lateralis
Capsula externa
Claustrum
Capsula extrema
Lamina medullaris medialis
Nucleus caudatus, Cauda
Tractus opticus
Lobus temporalis
Substantia nigra, Pars compacta
Pedunculus cerebri, Crus cerebri
Fasciculus longitudinalis medialis
Flocculus
Plexus choroideus ventriculi quarti
Hemispherium cerebelli
Fossa interpeduncularis
Amiculum olivare
Medulla spinalis

I–III = Thalamic nuclei, Nuclei thalami:
I   = Median nuclei, Nuclei mediani
II   = Anterior nuclei, Nuclei anteriores
III   = Ventral nuclei, Nuclei ventrales

Fig. 1252 Pyramidal tract, Tractus pyramidalis, and basal ganglia, Nuclei basales; obliquely staggered section through the posterior limb of the internal capsule, the cerebral peduncles, and the medulla oblongata.

Ventricles, projection

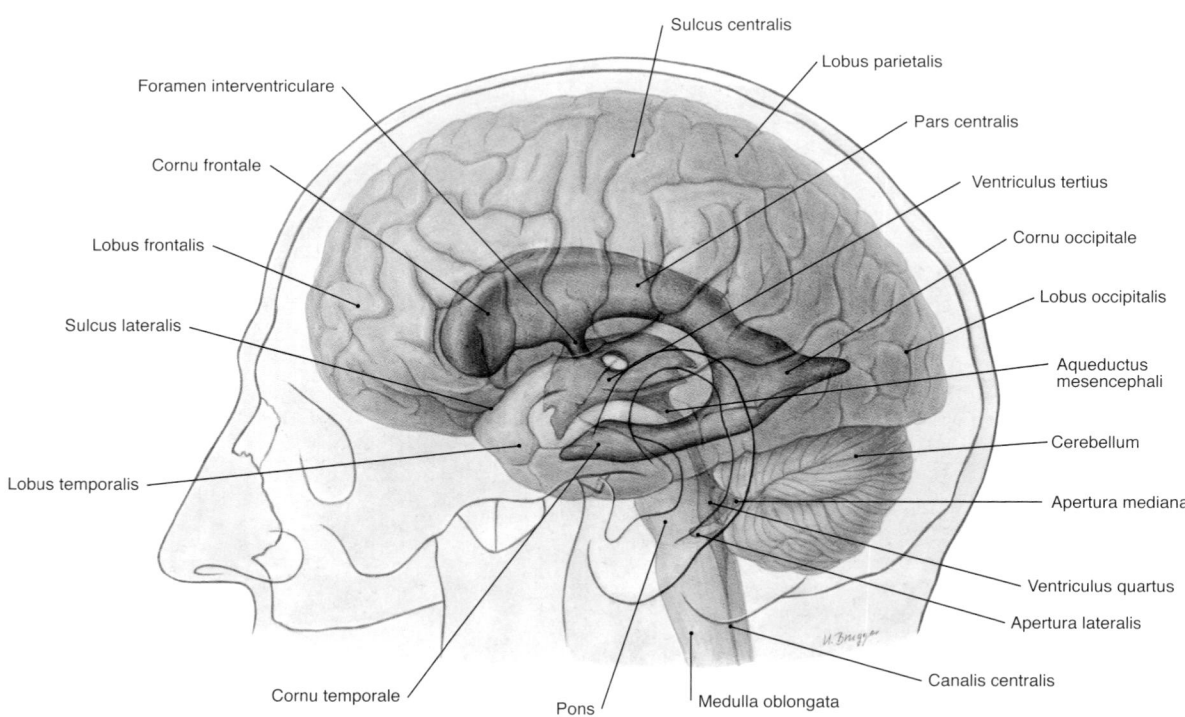

Fig. 1253 Ventricles of the brain, Ventriculi encephali.

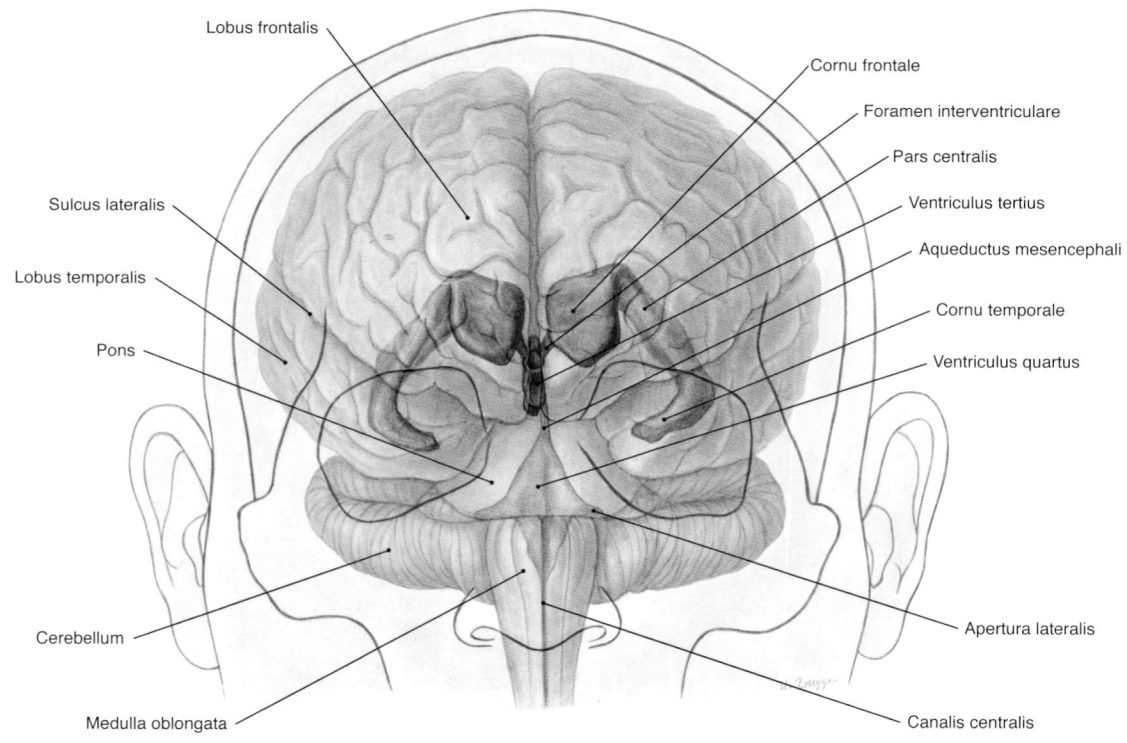

Fig. 1254 Ventricles of the brain, Ventriculi encephali; anterior view.

Inner and outer liquor spaces

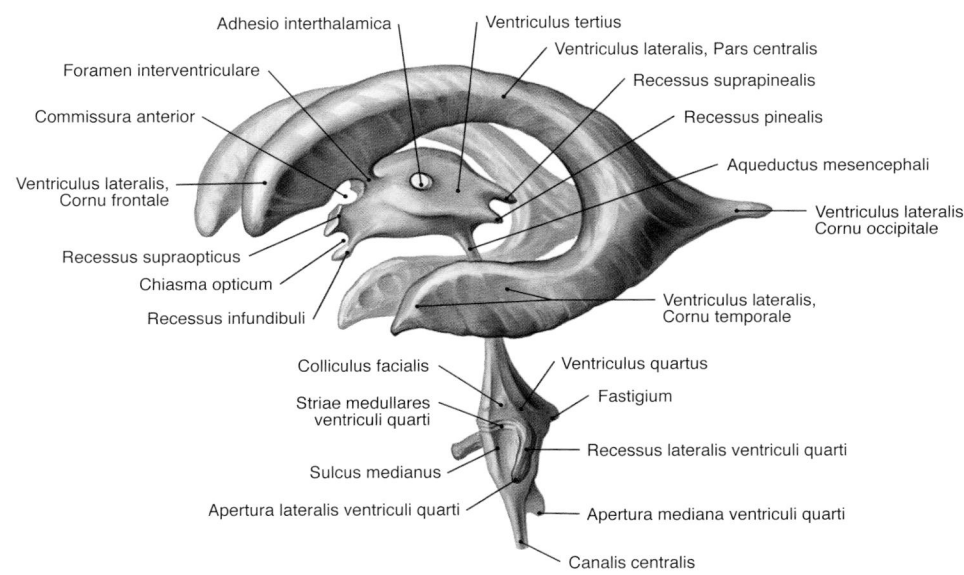

Adhesio interthalamica
Ventriculus tertius
Foramen interventriculare
Ventriculus lateralis, Pars centralis
Recessus suprapinealis
Commissura anterior
Recessus pinealis
Ventriculus lateralis,
Cornu frontale
Aqueductus mesencephali
Ventriculus lateralis,
Cornu occipitale
Recessus supraopticus
Chiasma opticum
Recessus infundibuli
Ventriculus lateralis,
Cornu temporale
Colliculus facialis
Ventriculus quartus
Striae medullares
ventriculi quarti
Fastigium
Recessus lateralis ventriculi quarti
Sulcus medianus
Apertura lateralis ventriculi quarti
Apertura mediana ventriculi quarti
Canalis centralis

Fig. 1255 Inner liquor spaces, Ventriculi encephali;
corrosion cast specimen;
oblique view from the left.

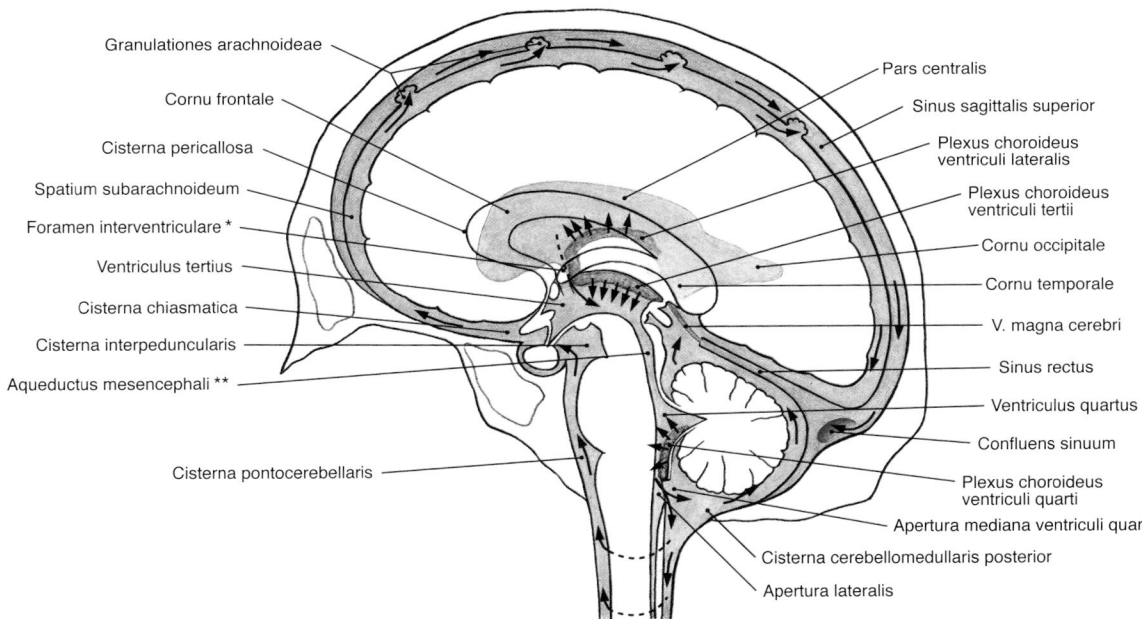

Granulationes arachnoideae
Pars centralis
Cornu frontale
Sinus sagittalis superior
Cisterna pericallosa
Plexus choroideus
ventriculi lateralis
Spatium subarachnoideum
Plexus choroideus
ventriculi tertii
Foramen interventriculare *
Cornu occipitale
Ventriculus tertius
Cornu temporale
Cisterna chiasmatica
V. magna cerebri
Cisterna interpeduncularis
Sinus rectus
Aqueductus mesencephali **
Ventriculus quartus
Confluens sinuum
Cisterna pontocerebellaris
Plexus choroideus
ventriculi quarti
Apertura mediana ventriculi quarti
Cisterna cerebellomedullaris posterior
Apertura lateralis

Fig. 1256 Ventricles of the brain, Ventriculi encephali,
and subarachnoid space, Spatium subarachnoideum;
schema of the circulation (arrows) of the cerebrospinal
fluid, Liquor cerebrospinalis, from the inner to the outer
liquor spaces.
* Clinical term: foramen of MONRO
** Clinical term: cerebral aqueduct of SYLVIUS

Brain, topography

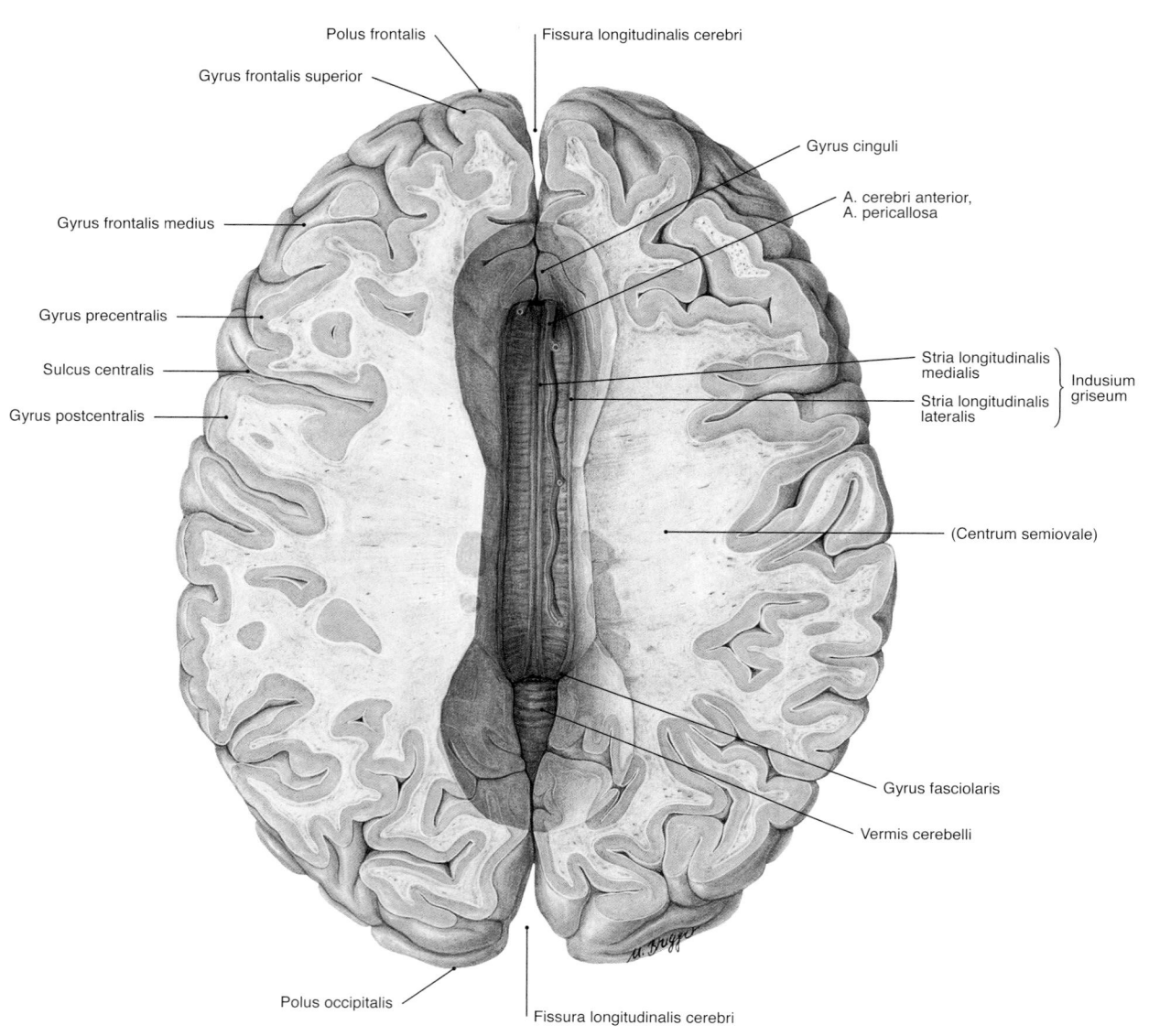

Polus frontalis

Gyrus frontalis superior

Fissura longitudinalis cerebri

Gyrus cinguli

A. cerebri anterior,
A. pericallosa

Gyrus frontalis medius

Gyrus precentralis

Sulcus centralis

Gyrus postcentralis

Stria longitudinalis
medialis

Stria longitudinalis
lateralis

Indusium
griseum

(Centrum semiovale)

Gyrus fasciolaris

Vermis cerebelli

Polus occipitalis

Fissura longitudinalis cerebri

1258

Fig. 1257 Corpus callosum, Corpus callosum;
after removal of the upper parts of the
cerebral hemispheres;
superior view.

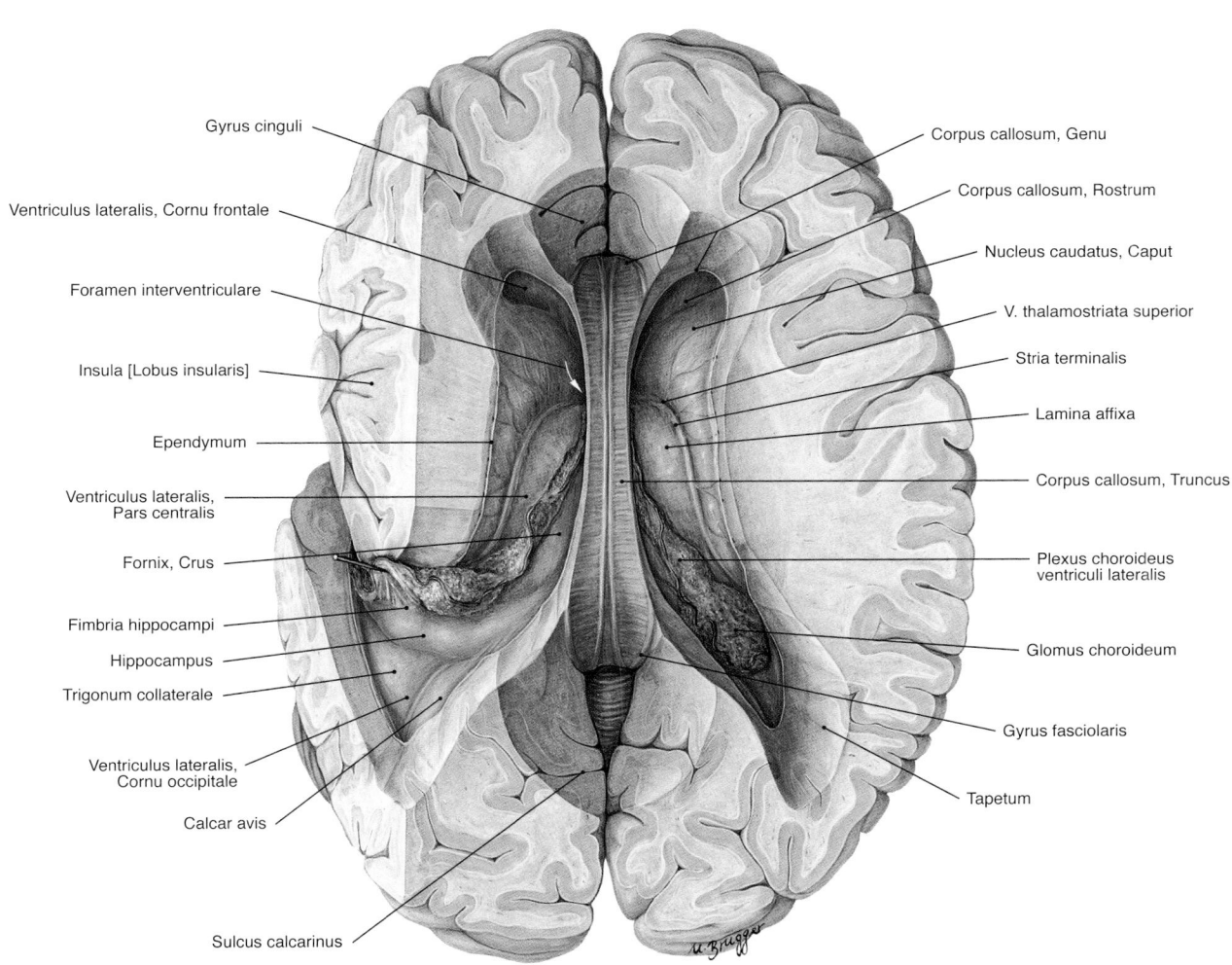

Gyrus cinguli

Ventriculus lateralis, Cornu frontale

Foramen interventriculare

Insula [Lobus insularis]

Ependymum

Ventriculus lateralis, Pars centralis

Fornix, Crus

Fimbria hippocampi

Hippocampus

Trigonum collaterale

Ventriculus lateralis, Cornu occipitale

Calcar avis

Sulcus calcarinus

Corpus callosum, Genu

Corpus callosum, Rostrum

Nucleus caudatus, Caput

V. thalamostriata superior

Stria terminalis

Lamina affixa

Corpus callosum, Truncus

Plexus choroideus ventriculi lateralis

Glomus choroideum

Gyrus fasciolaris

Tapetum

Fig. 1258   Lateral ventricles, Ventriculi laterales; after removal of the upper parts of the cerebral hemispheres; superior view.

1254

1257

Brain, topography

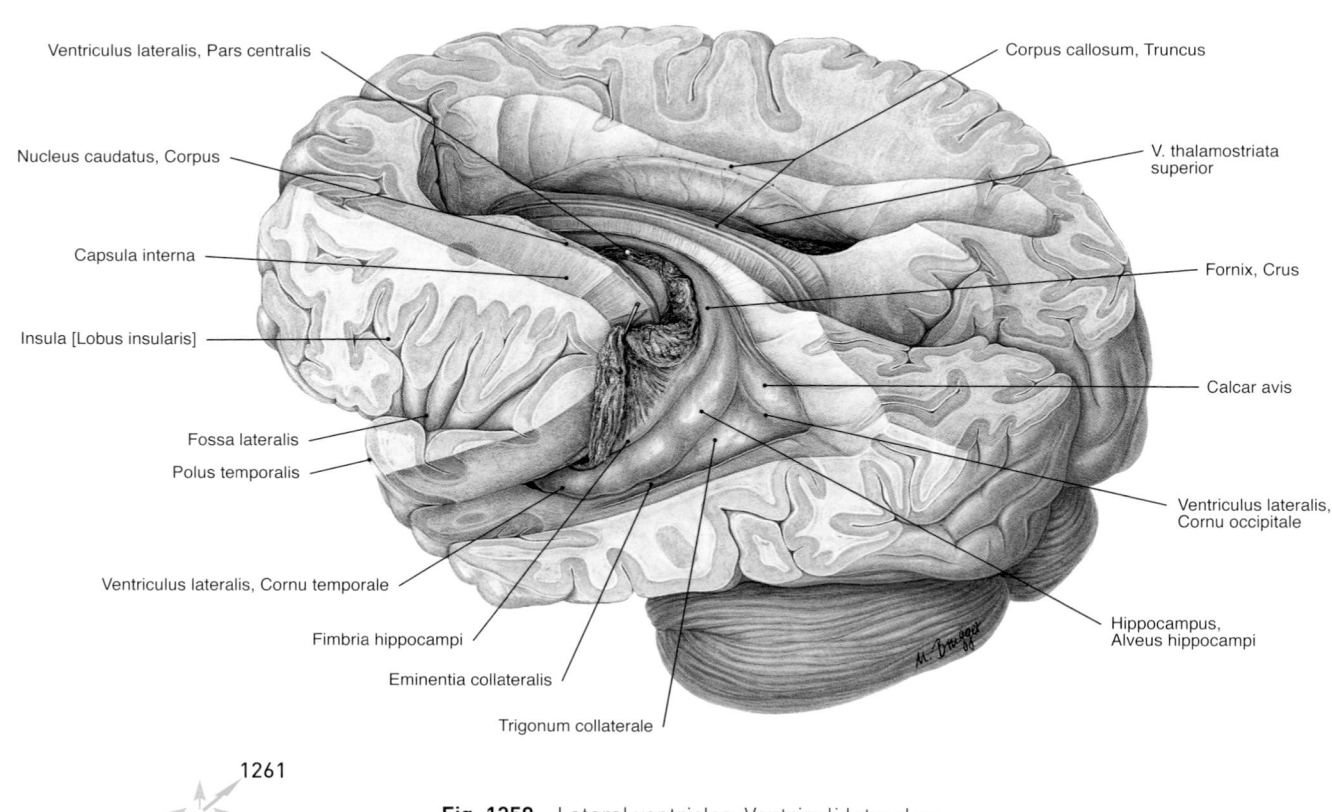

Ventriculus lateralis, Pars centralis

Nucleus caudatus, Corpus

Capsula interna

Insula [Lobus insularis]

Fossa lateralis

Polus temporalis

Ventriculus lateralis, Cornu temporale

Fimbria hippocampi

Eminentia collateralis

Trigonum collaterale

Corpus callosum, Truncus

V. thalamostriata superior

Fornix, Crus

Calcar avis

Ventriculus lateralis, Cornu occipitale

Hippocampus, Alveus hippocampi

1261

1258

Fig. 1259 Lateral ventricles, Ventriculi laterales; after removal of the upper parts of the cerebral hemispheres; posterior view from the left.

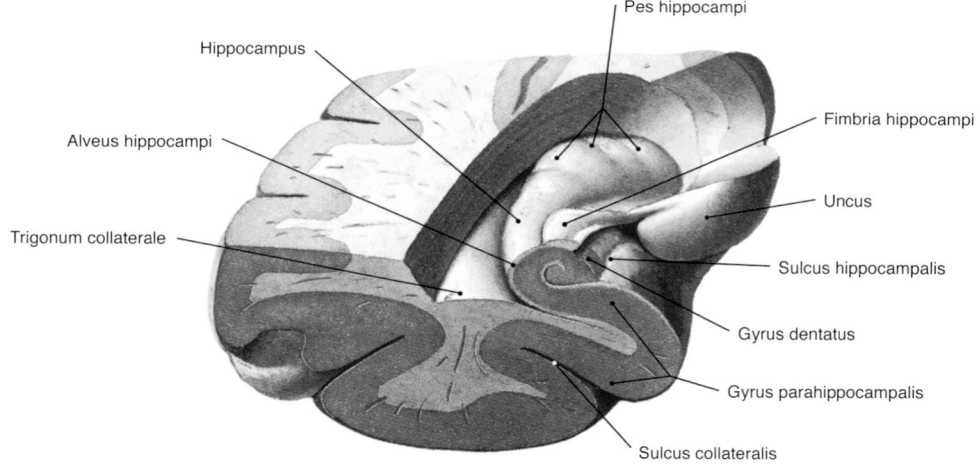

Hippocampus

Alveus hippocampi

Trigonum collaterale

Pes hippocampi

Fimbria hippocampi

Uncus

Sulcus hippocampalis

Gyrus dentatus

Gyrus parahippocampalis

Sulcus collateralis

Fig. 1260 Left temporal horn, Cornu temporale, of the lateral ventricle, Ventriculus lateralis; frontal section after removal of the temporal wall; posterior-superior view.

Brain, topography

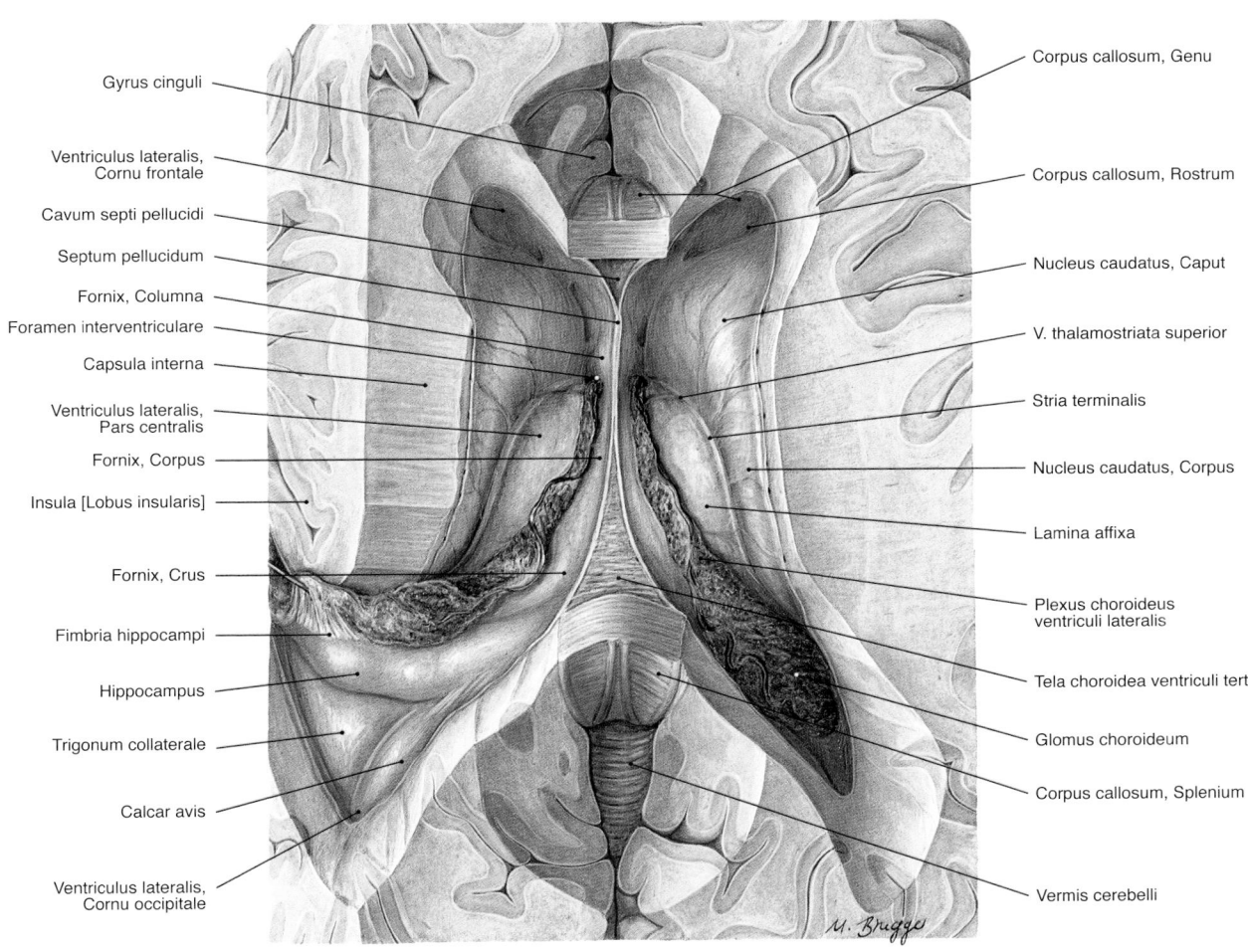

Gyrus cinguli

Ventriculus lateralis, Cornu frontale

Cavum septi pellucidi

Septum pellucidum

Fornix, Columna

Foramen interventriculare

Capsula interna

Ventriculus lateralis, Pars centralis

Fornix, Corpus

Insula [Lobus insularis]

Fornix, Crus

Fimbria hippocampi

Hippocampus

Trigonum collaterale

Calcar avis

Ventriculus lateralis, Cornu occipitale

Corpus callosum, Genu

Corpus callosum, Rostrum

Nucleus caudatus, Caput

V. thalamostriata superior

Stria terminalis

Nucleus caudatus, Corpus

Lamina affixa

Plexus choroideus ventriculi lateralis

Tela choroidea ventriculi tertii

Glomus choroideum

Corpus callosum, Splenium

Vermis cerebelli

1263

1259

Fig. 1261 Lateral ventricles, Ventriculi laterales; after removal of the upper parts of the cerebral hemispheres and the central part of the corpus callosum; superior view.

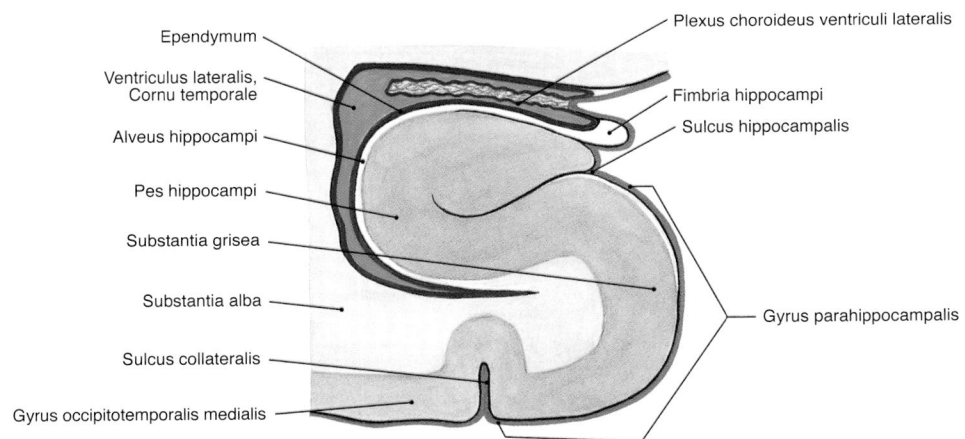

Ependymum

Ventriculus lateralis, Cornu temporale

Alveus hippocampi

Pes hippocampi

Substantia grisea

Substantia alba

Sulcus collateralis

Gyrus occipitotemporalis medialis

Plexus choroideus ventriculi lateralis

Fimbria hippocampi

Sulcus hippocampalis

Gyrus parahippocampalis

Fig. 1262 Temporal horn, Cornu temporale, of the lateral ventricle, Ventriculus lateralis; schematic frontal section.

Brain, topography

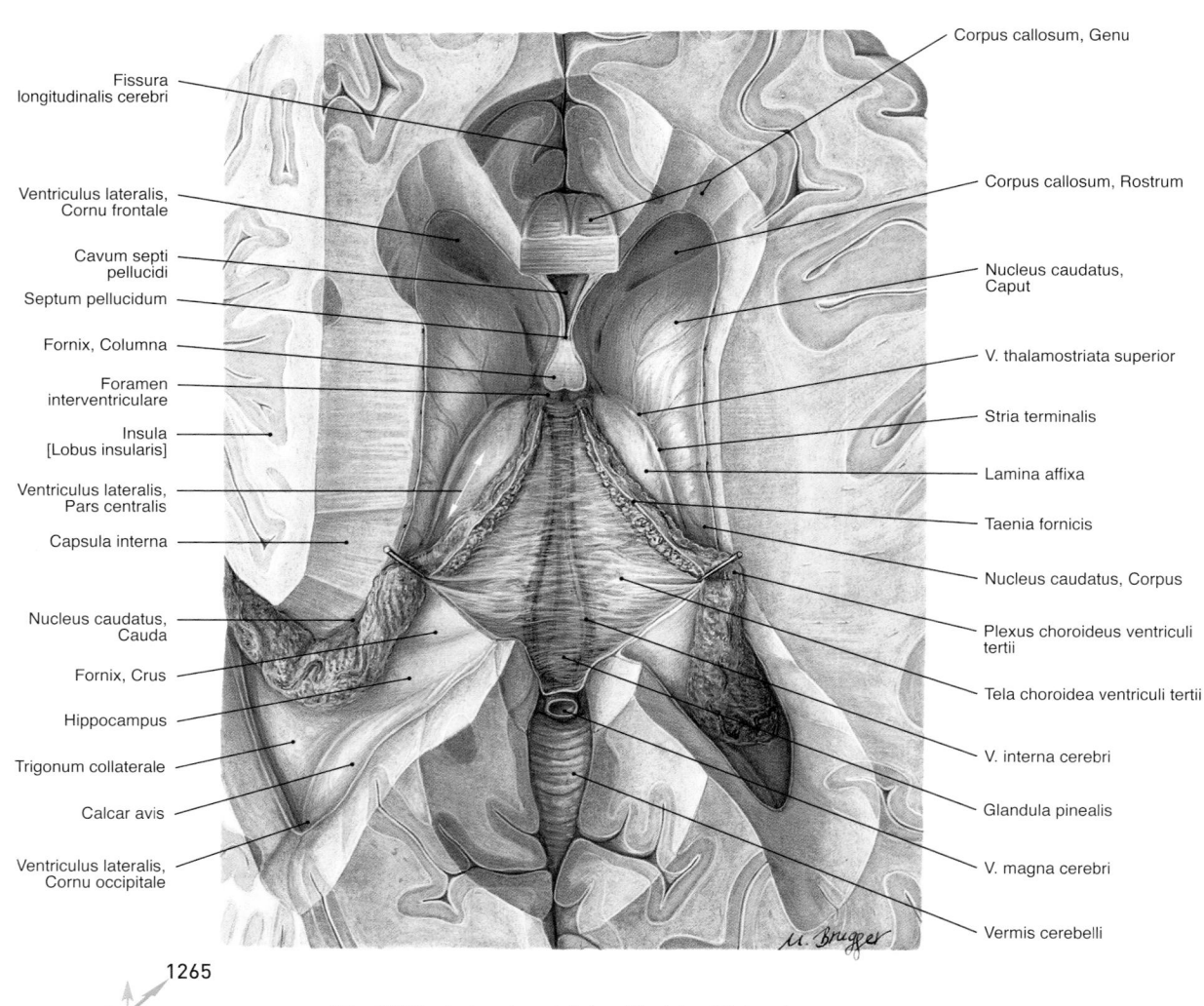

Corpus callosum, Genu

Fissura
longitudinalis cerebri

Corpus callosum, Rostrum

Ventriculus lateralis,
Cornu frontale

Nucleus caudatus,
Caput

Cavum septi
pellucidi

Septum pellucidum

V. thalamostriata superior

Fornix, Columna

Foramen
interventriculare

Stria terminalis

Insula
[Lobus insularis]

Lamina affixa

Ventriculus lateralis,
Pars centralis

Taenia fornicis

Capsula interna

Nucleus caudatus, Corpus

Nucleus caudatus,
Cauda

Plexus choroideus ventriculi
tertii

Fornix, Crus

Tela choroidea ventriculi tertii

Hippocampus

Trigonum collaterale

V. interna cerebri

Calcar avis

Glandula pinealis

Ventriculus lateralis,
Cornu occipitale

V. magna cerebri

Vermis cerebelli

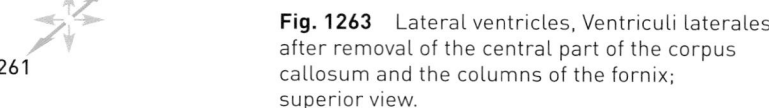

1265

1261

Fig. 1263 Lateral ventricles, Ventriculi laterales;
after removal of the central part of the corpus
callosum and the columns of the fornix;
superior view.

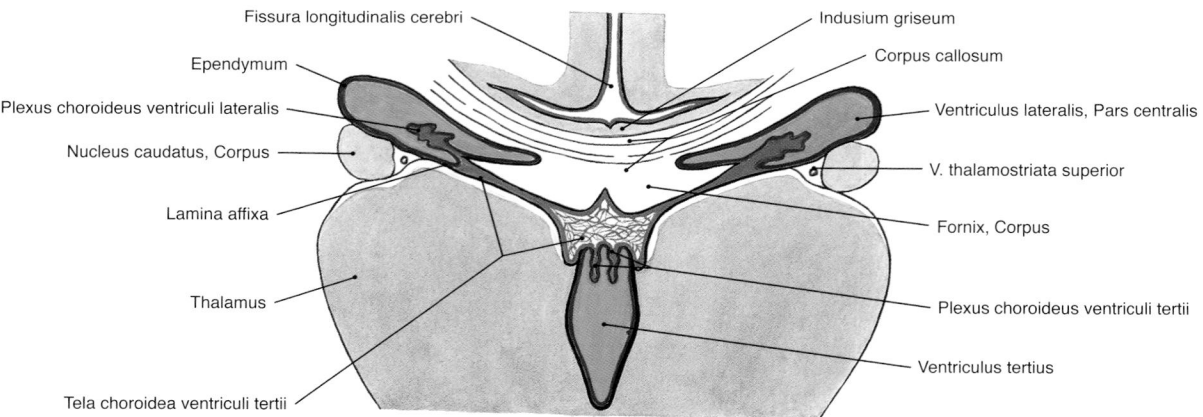

Fissura longitudinalis cerebri

Indusium griseum

Ependymum

Corpus callosum

Plexus choroideus ventriculi lateralis

Ventriculus lateralis, Pars centralis

Nucleus caudatus, Corpus

V. thalamostriata superior

Lamina affixa

Fornix, Corpus

Thalamus

Plexus choroideus ventriculi tertii

Ventriculus tertius

Tela choroidea ventriculi tertii

Fig. 1264 Central parts, Partes centrales, of the lateral ventricles
and third ventricle, Ventriculus tertius;
schematic frontal section.

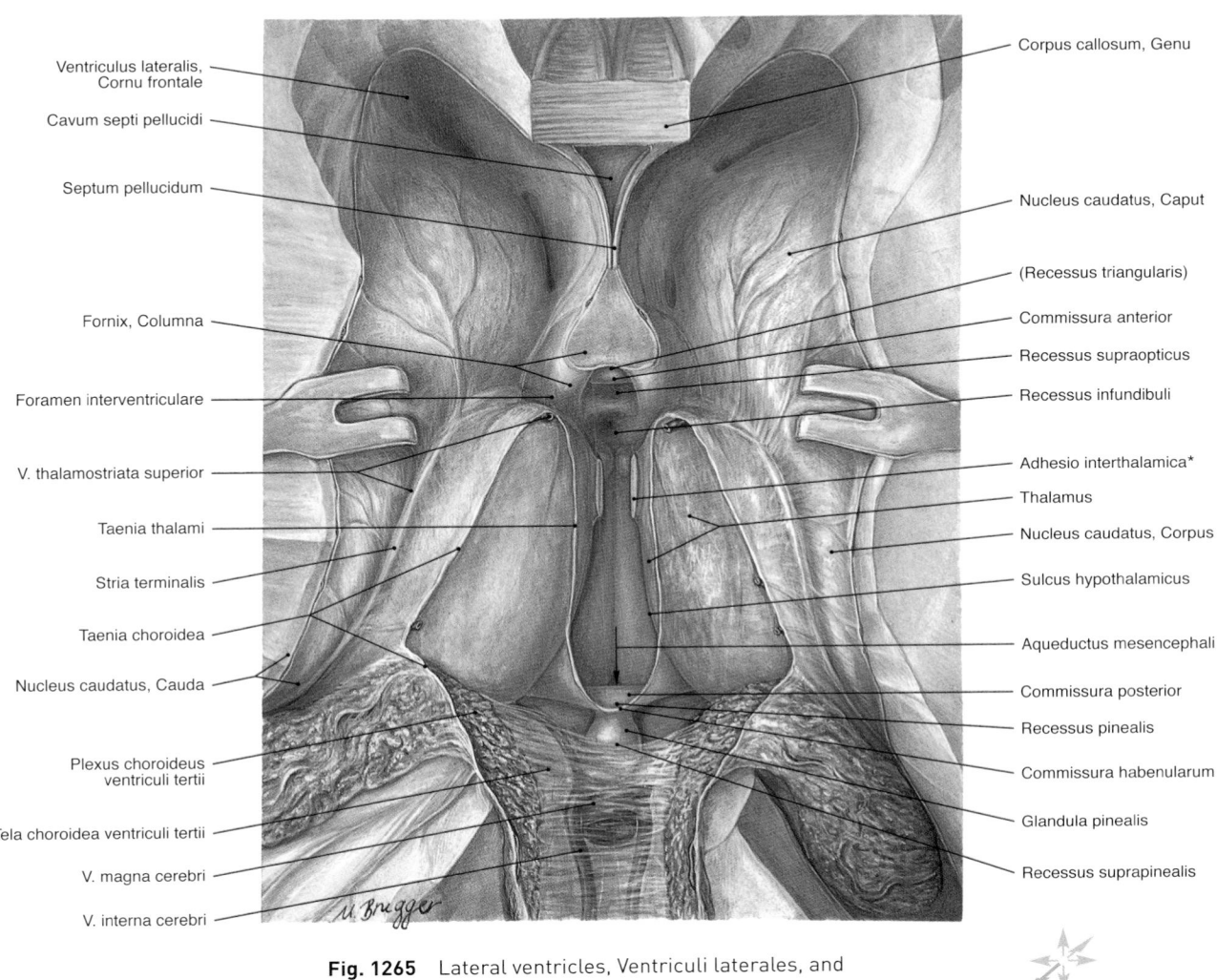

Ventriculus lateralis, Cornu frontale

Cavum septi pellucidi

Septum pellucidum

Fornix, Columna

Foramen interventriculare

V. thalamostriata superior

Taenia thalami

Stria terminalis

Taenia choroidea

Nucleus caudatus, Cauda

Plexus choroideus ventriculi tertii

Tela choroidea ventriculi tertii

V. magna cerebri

V. interna cerebri

Corpus callosum, Genu

Nucleus caudatus, Caput

(Recessus triangularis)

Commissura anterior

Recessus supraopticus

Recessus infundibuli

Adhesio interthalamica*

Thalamus

Nucleus caudatus, Corpus

Sulcus hypothalamicus

Aqueductus mesencephali

Commissura posterior

Recessus pinealis

Commissura habenularum

Glandula pinealis

Recessus suprapinealis

1263

Fig. 1265   Lateral ventricles, Ventriculi laterales, and third ventricle, Ventriculus tertius;
parts of the cerebral hemispheres, the central part of the corpus callosum as well as the fornix and the choroid plexus have been removed, the tela choroidea of the third ventricle has been reflected;
superior view.
* The interthalamic adhesion has been sectioned in the median plane.

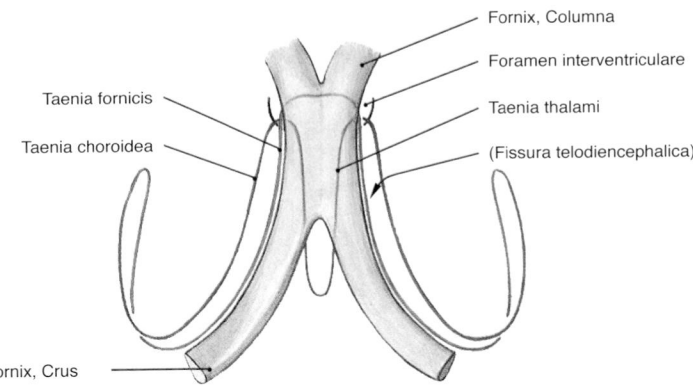

Taenia fornicis

Taenia choroidea

Fornix, Crus

Fornix, Columna

Foramen interventriculare

Taenia thalami

(Fissura telodiencephalica)

Fig. 1266   Taeniae, Taeniae, of the choroid plexus, Plexus choroideus of the cerebrum;
superior view.

Arteries of the base of the brain

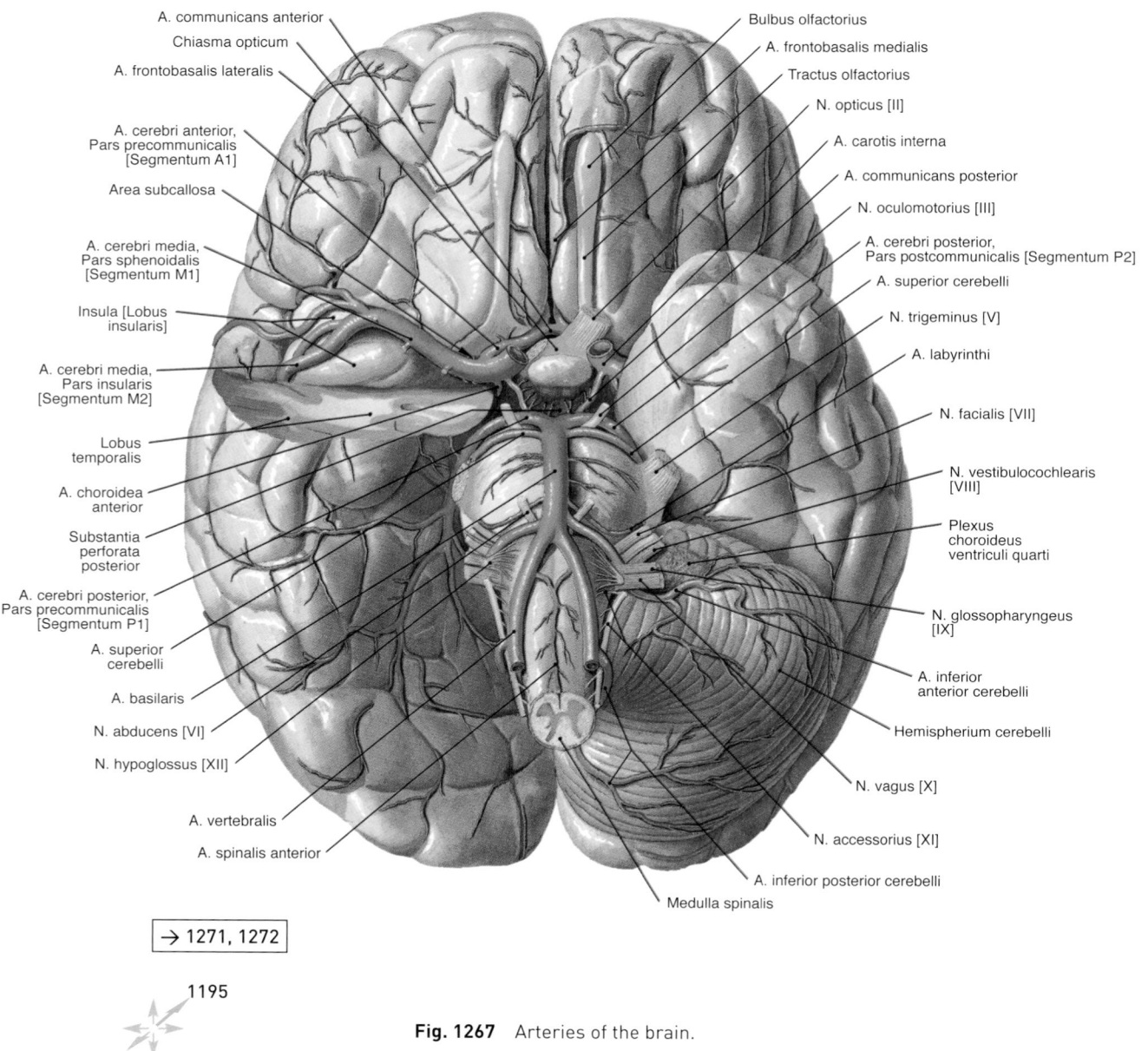

A. communicans anterior
Chiasma opticum
A. frontobasalis lateralis
A. cerebri anterior, Pars precommunicalis [Segmentum A1]
Area subcallosa
A. cerebri media, Pars sphenoidalis [Segmentum M1]
Insula [Lobus insularis]
A. cerebri media, Pars insularis [Segmentum M2]
Lobus temporalis
A. choroidea anterior
Substantia perforata posterior
A. cerebri posterior, Pars precommunicalis [Segmentum P1]
A. superior cerebelli
A. basilaris
N. abducens [VI]
N. hypoglossus [XII]
A. vertebralis
A. spinalis anterior

Bulbus olfactorius
A. frontobasalis medialis
Tractus olfactorius
N. opticus [II]
A. carotis interna
A. communicans posterior
N. oculomotorius [III]
A. cerebri posterior, Pars postcommunicalis [Segmentum P2]
A. superior cerebelli
N. trigeminus [V]
A. labyrinthi
N. facialis [VII]
N. vestibulocochlearis [VIII]
Plexus choroideus ventriculi quarti
N. glossopharyngeus [IX]
A. inferior anterior cerebelli
Hemispherium cerebelli
N. vagus [X]
N. accessorius [XI]
A. inferior posterior cerebelli
Medulla spinalis

→ 1271, 1272

1195

Fig. 1267 Arteries of the brain.

Arterial circle

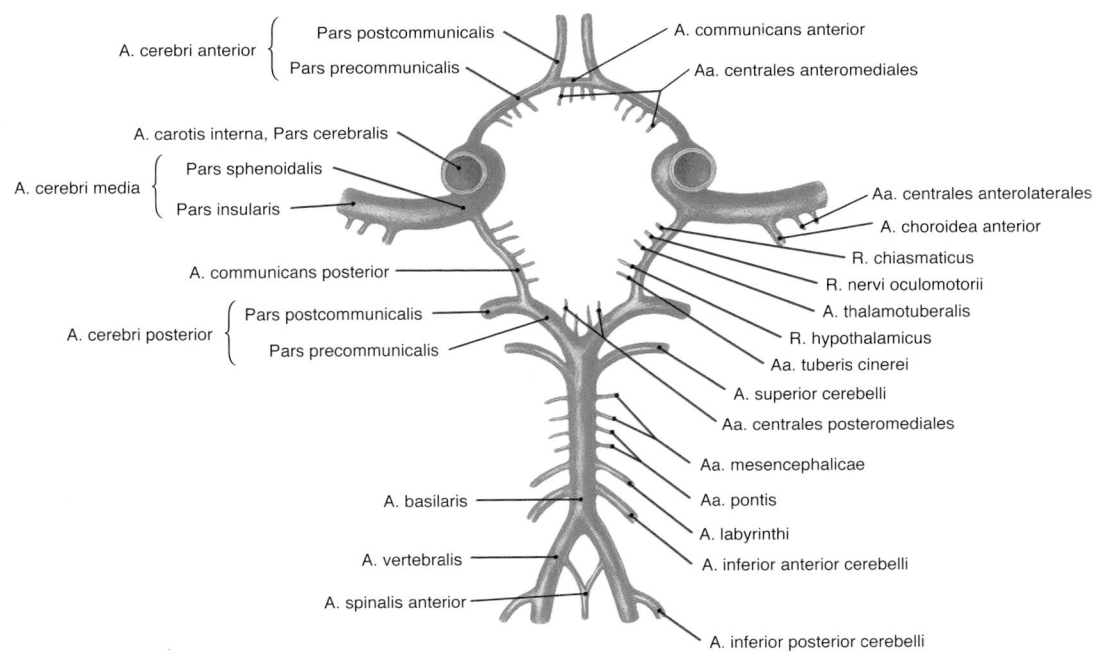

A. cerebri anterior { Pars postcommunicalis — A. communicans anterior
Pars precommunicalis — Aa. centrales anteromediales

A. carotis interna, Pars cerebralis

A. cerebri media { Pars sphenoidalis
Pars insularis

Aa. centrales anterolaterales
A. choroidea anterior
R. chiasmaticus
R. nervi oculomotorii
A. thalamotuberalis
R. hypothalamicus
Aa. tuberis cinerei
A. superior cerebelli
Aa. centrales posteromediales
Aa. mesencephalicae
Aa. pontis
A. labyrinthi
A. inferior anterior cerebelli
A. inferior posterior cerebelli

A. communicans posterior

A. cerebri posterior { Pars postcommunicalis
Pars precommunicalis

A. basilaris
A. vertebralis
A. spinalis anterior

Fig. 1268 Arterial circle of the brain,
Circulus arteriosus cerebri [WILLIS].

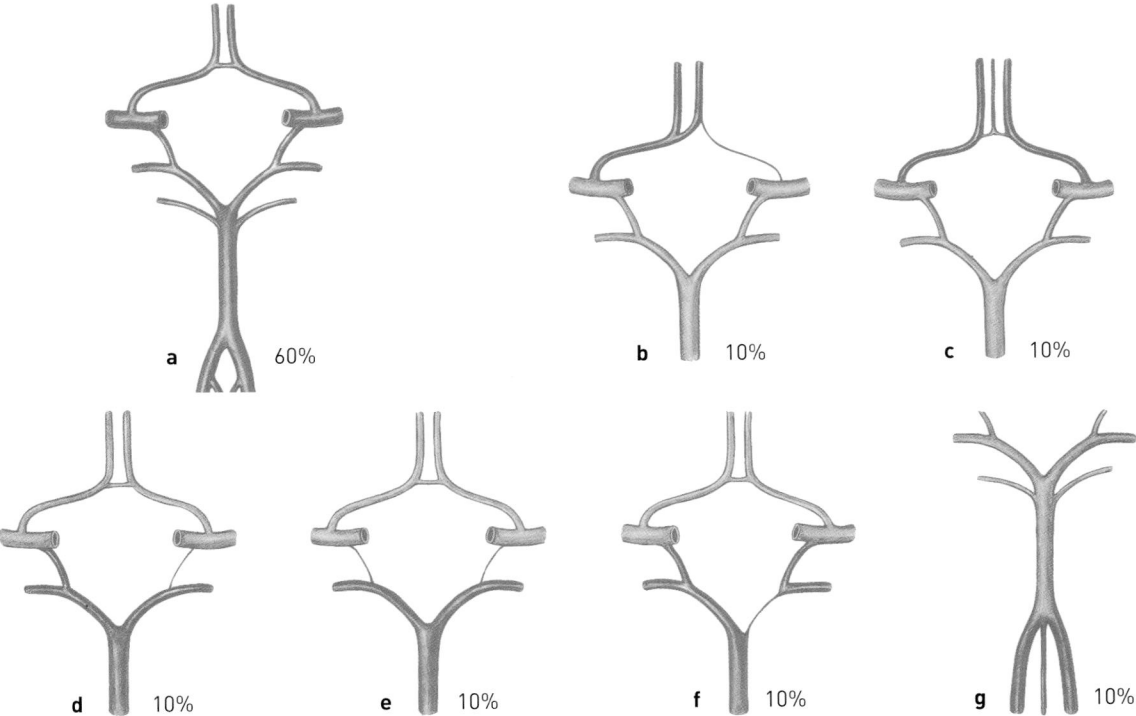

a — 60%   b — 10%   c — 10%

d — 10%   e — 10%   f — 10%   g — 10%

Fig. 1269 a–g Arterial circle of the brain,
Circulus arteriosus cerebri.
a–c Variations of the anterior portion
d–f Variations of the posterior portion
g Very far inferior union of the vertebral arteries

Arteries of the brain

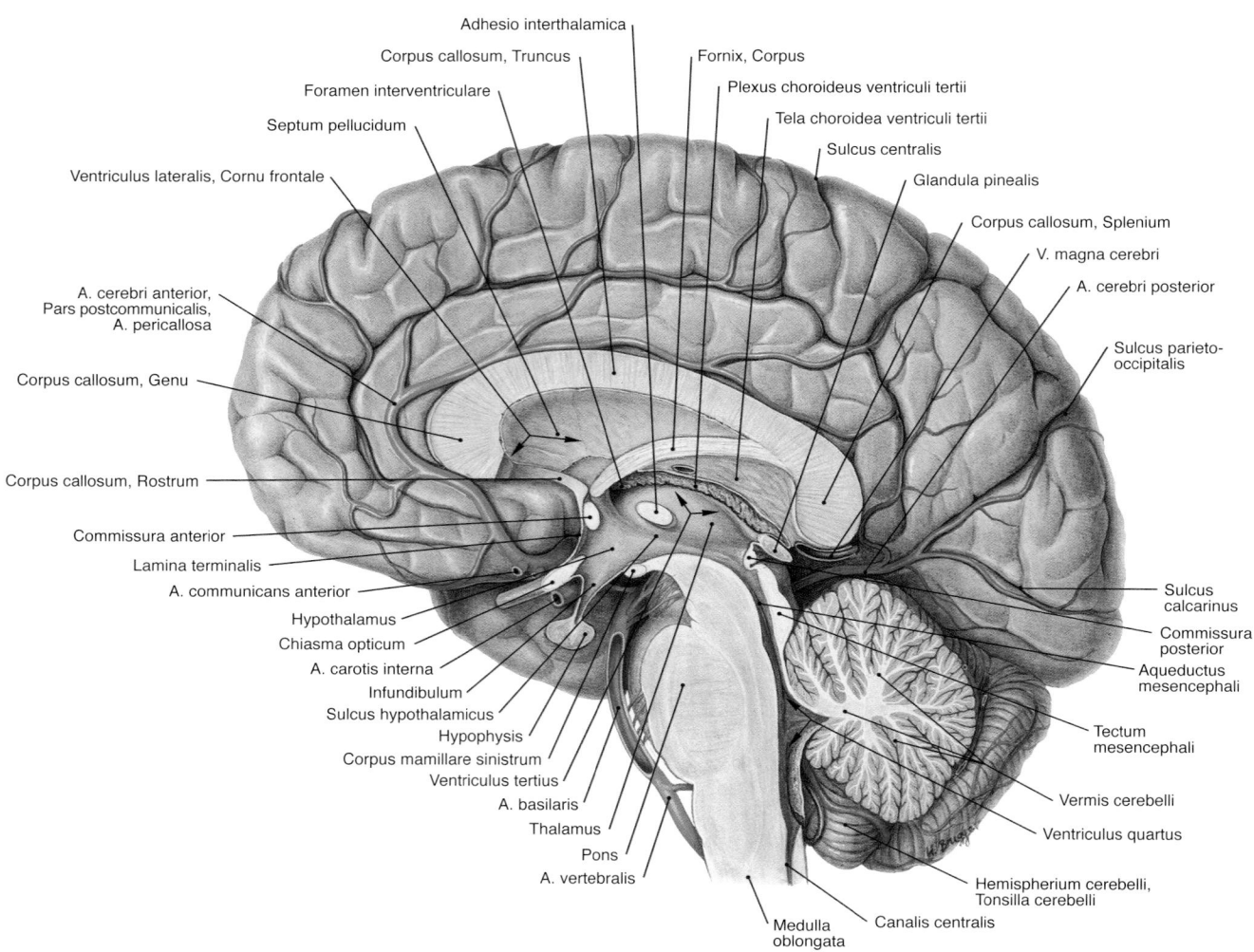

Adhesio interthalamica
Corpus callosum, Truncus
Foramen interventriculare
Septum pellucidum
Ventriculus lateralis, Cornu frontale
A. cerebri anterior, Pars postcommunicalis, A. pericallosa
Corpus callosum, Genu
Corpus callosum, Rostrum
Commissura anterior
Lamina terminalis
A. communicans anterior
Hypothalamus
Chiasma opticum
A. carotis interna
Infundibulum
Sulcus hypothalamicus
Hypophysis
Corpus mamillare sinistrum
Ventriculus tertius
A. basilaris
Thalamus
Pons
A. vertebralis
Medulla oblongata
Canalis centralis

Fornix, Corpus
Plexus choroideus ventriculi tertii
Tela choroidea ventriculi tertii
Sulcus centralis
Glandula pinealis
Corpus callosum, Splenium
V. magna cerebri
A. cerebri posterior
Sulcus parieto-occipitalis
Sulcus calcarinus
Commissura posterior
Aqueductus mesencephali
Tectum mesencephali
Vermis cerebelli
Ventriculus quartus
Hemispherium cerebelli, Tonsilla cerebelli

Fig. 1270 Medial surface of the brain, Facies medialis hemispherii cerebri; diencephalon, Diencephalon, and brainstem, Truncus encephali; staggered median section; viewed from the left.

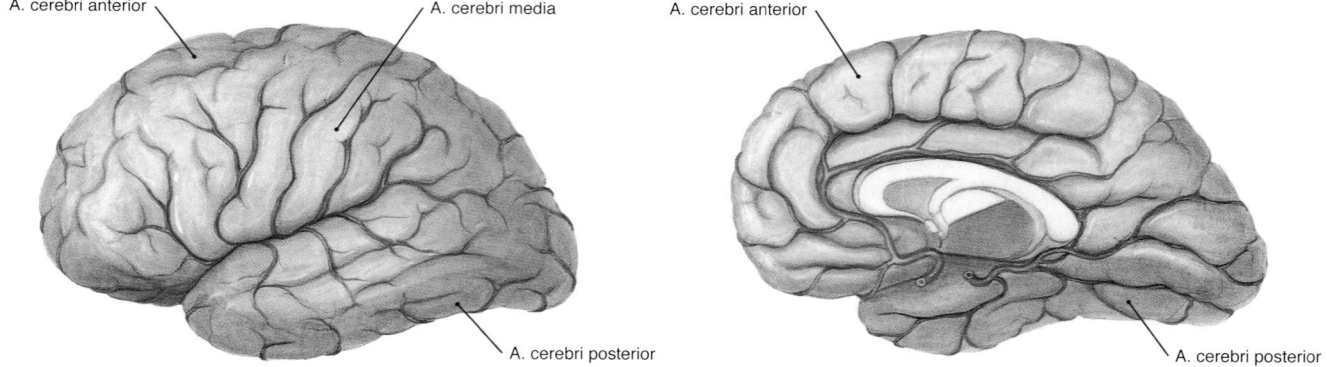

A. cerebri anterior
A. cerebri media
A. cerebri posterior

A. cerebri anterior
A. cerebri posterior

Fig. 1271 Arterial supply of the brain; viewed from the left.

Fig. 1272 Arterial supply of the brain; medial view.

Arteries and veins of the brain

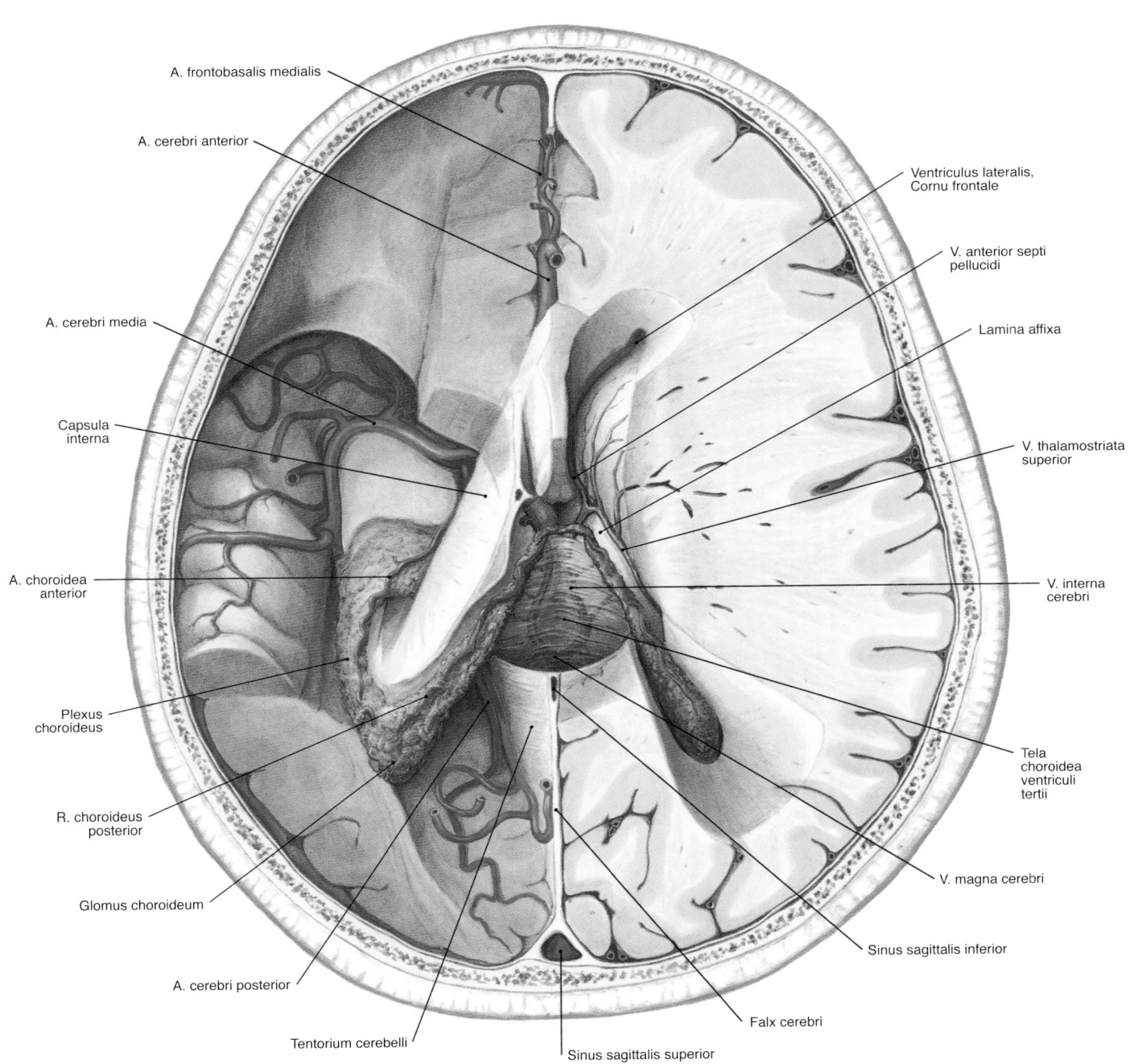

A. frontobasalis medialis

A. cerebri anterior

A. cerebri media

Capsula interna

A. choroidea anterior

Plexus choroideus

R. choroideus posterior

Glomus choroideum

A. cerebri posterior

Tentorium cerebelli

Sinus sagittalis superior

Ventriculus lateralis, Cornu frontale

V. anterior septi pellucidi

Lamina affixa

V. thalamostriata superior

V. interna cerebri

Tela choroidea ventriculi tertii

V. magna cerebri

Sinus sagittalis inferior

Falx cerebri

Fig. 1273 Arteries and veins of the brain, Arteriae et Venae cerebri.

Veins of the brain

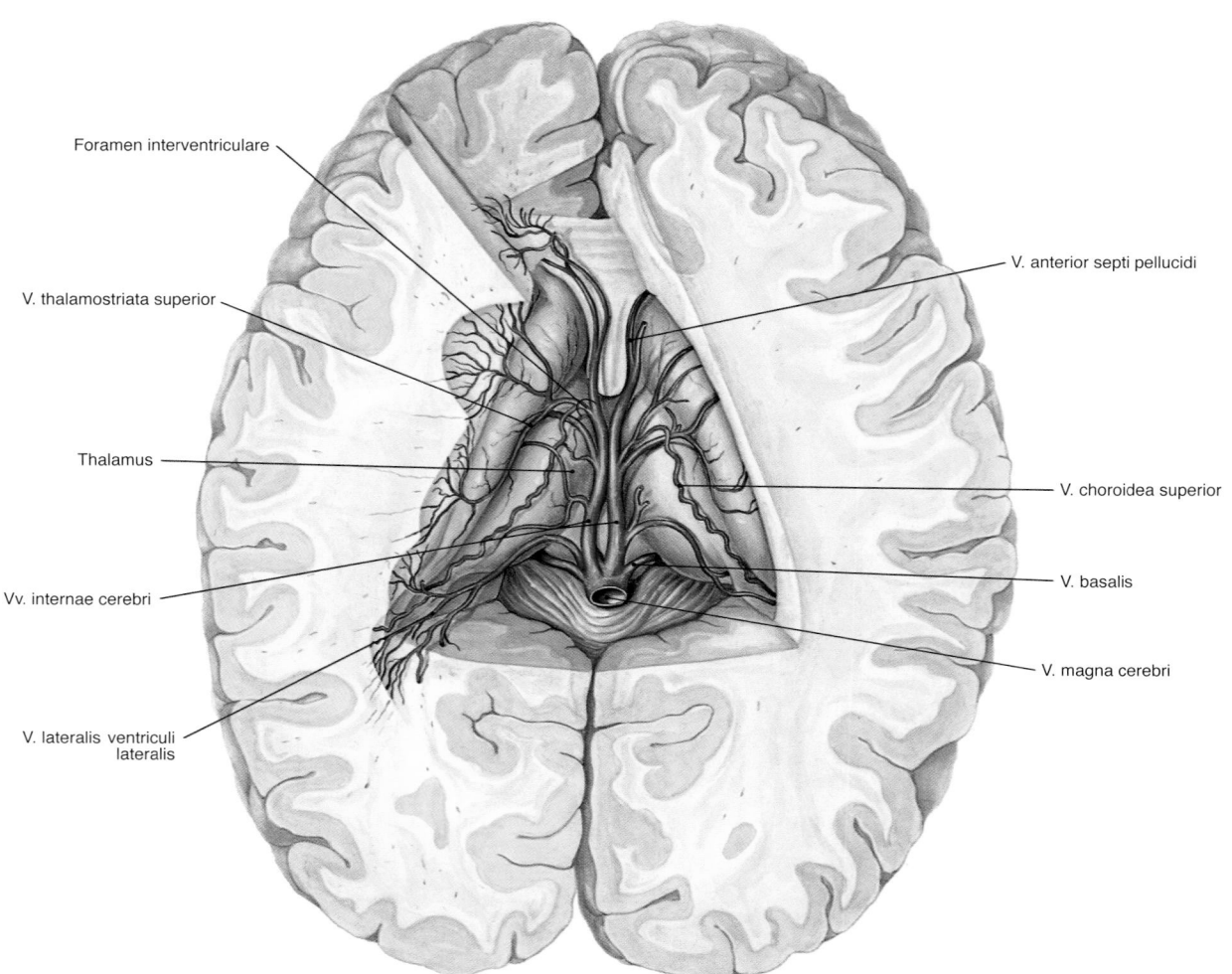

Foramen interventriculare

V. thalamostriata superior

Thalamus

Vv. internae cerebri

V. lateralis ventriculi lateralis

V. anterior septi pellucidi

V. choroidea superior

V. basalis

V. magna cerebri

Fig. 1274 Deep veins of the brain, Vv. profundae cerebri. The internal cerebral veins run within the tela choroidea of the third ventricle.

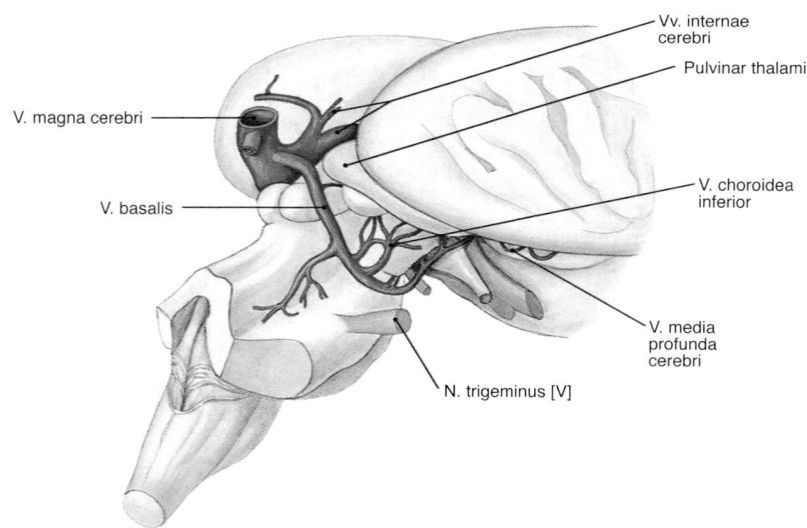

Vv. internae cerebri

Pulvinar thalami

V. magna cerebri

V. choroidea inferior

V. basalis

V. media profunda cerebri

N. trigeminus [V]

Fig. 1275 Deep veins of the brain, Vv. profundae cerebri; posterior view from the right.

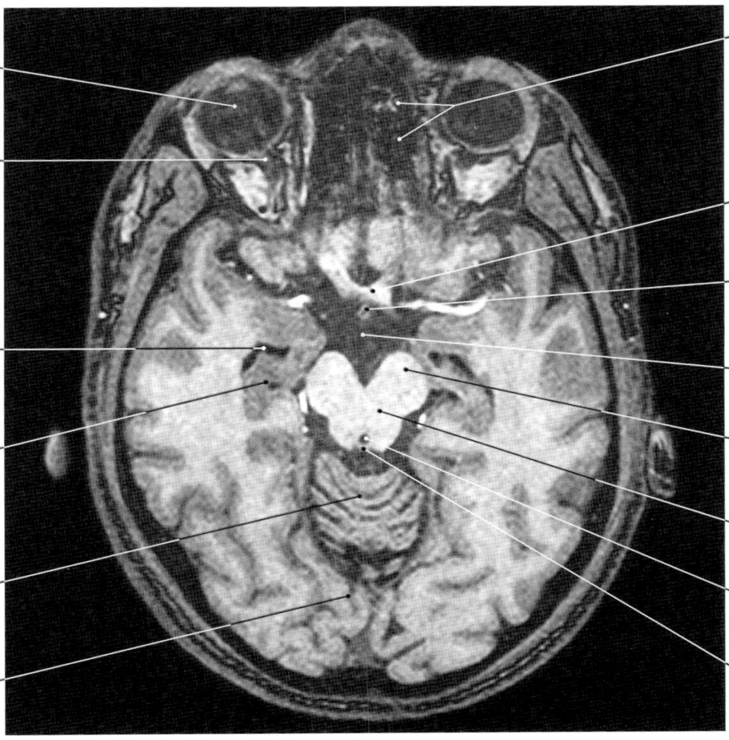

Bulbus oculi

N. opticus [II]

Ventriculus lateralis, Cornu temporale

Hippocampus

Vermis cerebelli

Sulcus calcarinus

Cellulae ethmoidales

Chiasma opticum

Infundibulum

Cisterna interpeduncularis

Pedunculus cerebri

Tegmentum mesencephali

Aqueductus mesencephali

Tectum mesencephali

Fig. 1276 Brain, Encephalon; magnetic resonance tomographic image (MRI); horizontal section at the level of the midbrain and the temporal horns of the lateral ventricles; superior view.

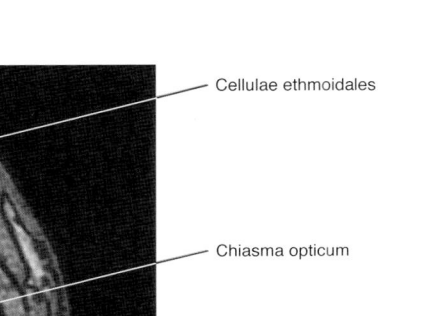

1277
1278
1276

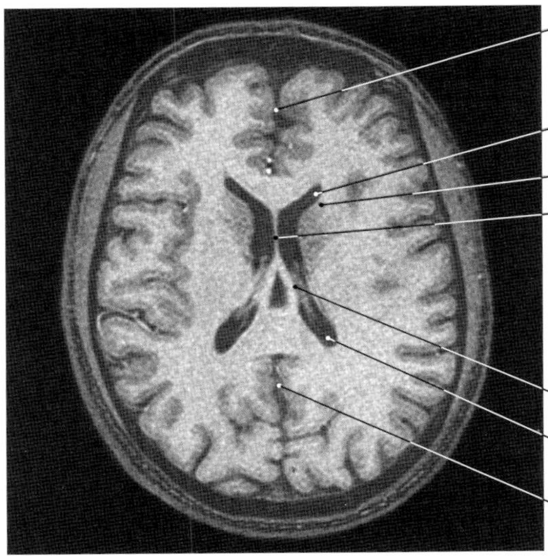

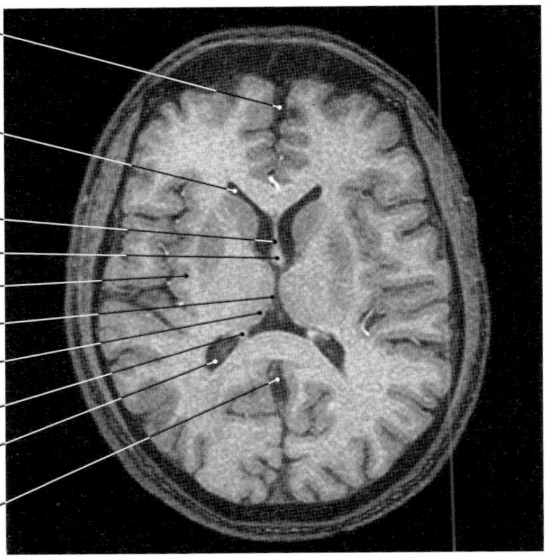

Fissura longitudinalis cerebri

Ventriculus lateralis, Cornu frontale

Nucleus caudatus, Caput

Septum pellucidum

Fornix, Columna

Insula [Lobus insularis]

Ventriculus tertius

Thalamus

Fornix, Crus

Ventriculus lateralis, Cornu occipitale

Fissura longitudinalis cerebri

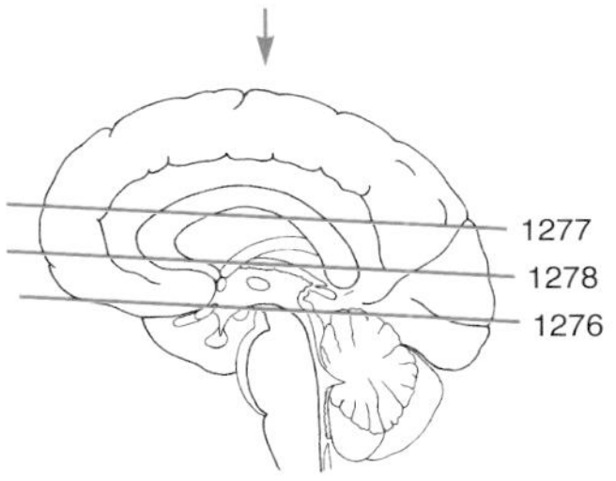

Fig. 1277 Brain, Encephalon; magnetic resonance tomographic image (MRI); horizontal section at the level of the central parts of the lateral ventricles; superior view.

Fig. 1278 Brain, Encephalon; magnetic resonance tomographic image (MRI); horizontal section at the level of the third ventricle and the opening of the temporal horns of the lateral ventricles; superior view.

Brain, sections

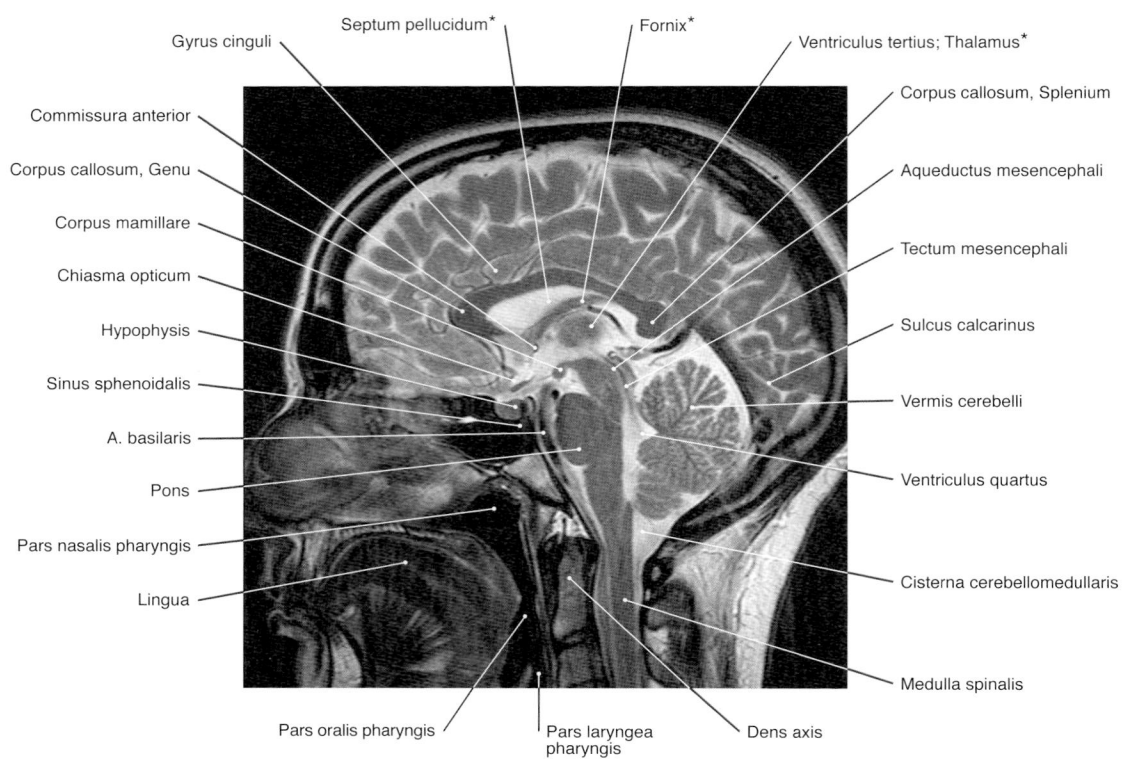

Gyrus cinguli
Commissura anterior
Corpus callosum, Genu
Corpus mamillare
Chiasma opticum
Hypophysis
Sinus sphenoidalis
A. basilaris
Pons
Pars nasalis pharyngis
Lingua

Septum pellucidum*
Fornix*
Ventriculus tertius; Thalamus*

Corpus callosum, Splenium
Aqueductus mesencephali
Tectum mesencephali
Sulcus calcarinus
Vermis cerebelli
Ventriculus quartus
Cisterna cerebellomedullaris
Medulla spinalis

Pars oralis pharyngis
Pars laryngea pharyngis
Dens axis

Fig. 1279 Brain, Encephalon;
magnetic resonance tomographic image (MRI);
median section. The structures marked with * appear
partly falsified as a consequence of the "partial-volume-
effect".

1280
1279

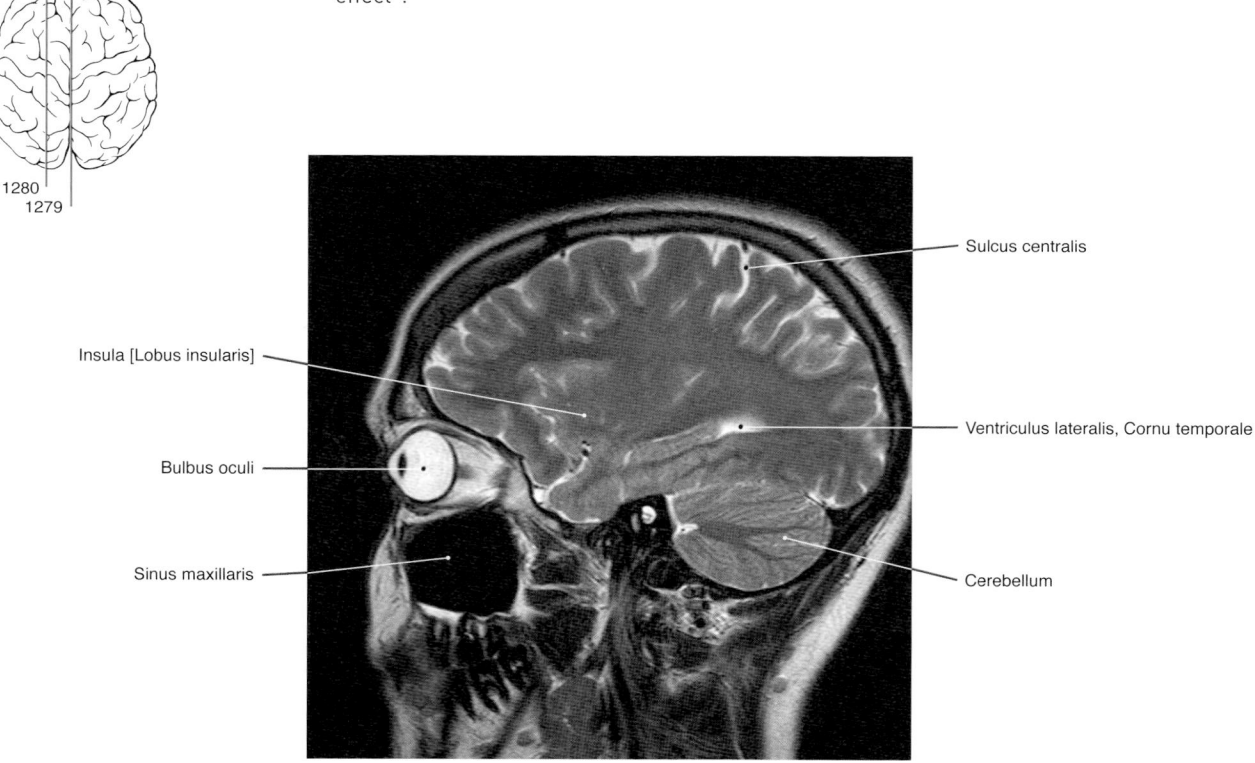

Insula [Lobus insularis]
Bulbus oculi
Sinus maxillaris

Sulcus centralis
Ventriculus lateralis, Cornu temporale
Cerebellum

Fig. 1280 Brain, Encephalon;
magnetic resonance tomographic image (MRI);
sagittal section.

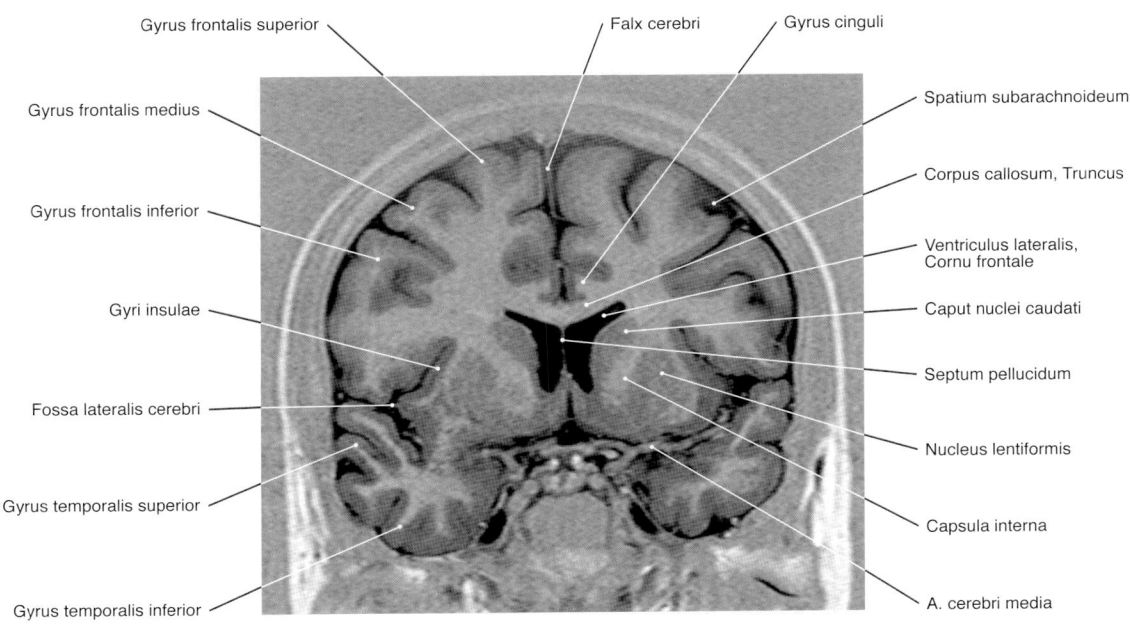

Gyrus frontalis superior

Falx cerebri

Gyrus cinguli

Gyrus frontalis medius

Gyrus frontalis inferior

Gyri insulae

Fossa lateralis cerebri

Gyrus temporalis superior

Gyrus temporalis inferior

Spatium subarachnoideum

Corpus callosum, Truncus

Ventriculus lateralis, Cornu frontale

Caput nuclei caudati

Septum pellucidum

Nucleus lentiformis

Capsula interna

A. cerebri media

Fig. 1281 Brain, Encephalon; magnetic resonance tomographic image (MRI); frontal section.

1281   1282

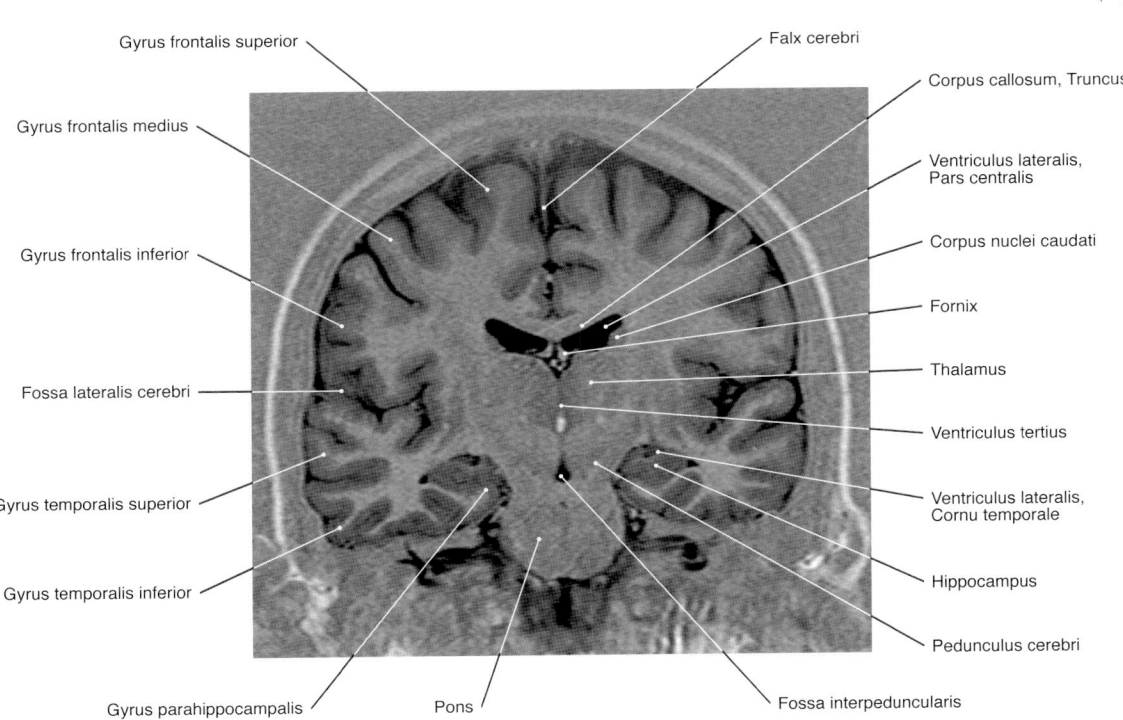

Gyrus frontalis superior

Falx cerebri

Gyrus frontalis medius

Gyrus frontalis inferior

Fossa lateralis cerebri

Gyrus temporalis superior

Gyrus temporalis inferior

Corpus callosum, Truncus

Ventriculus lateralis, Pars centralis

Corpus nuclei caudati

Fornix

Thalamus

Ventriculus tertius

Ventriculus lateralis, Cornu temporale

Hippocampus

Pedunculus cerebri

Gyrus parahippocampalis

Pons

Fossa interpeduncularis

Fig. 1282 Brain, Encephalon; magnetic resonance tomographic image (MRI); frontal section.

Brain, frontal sections

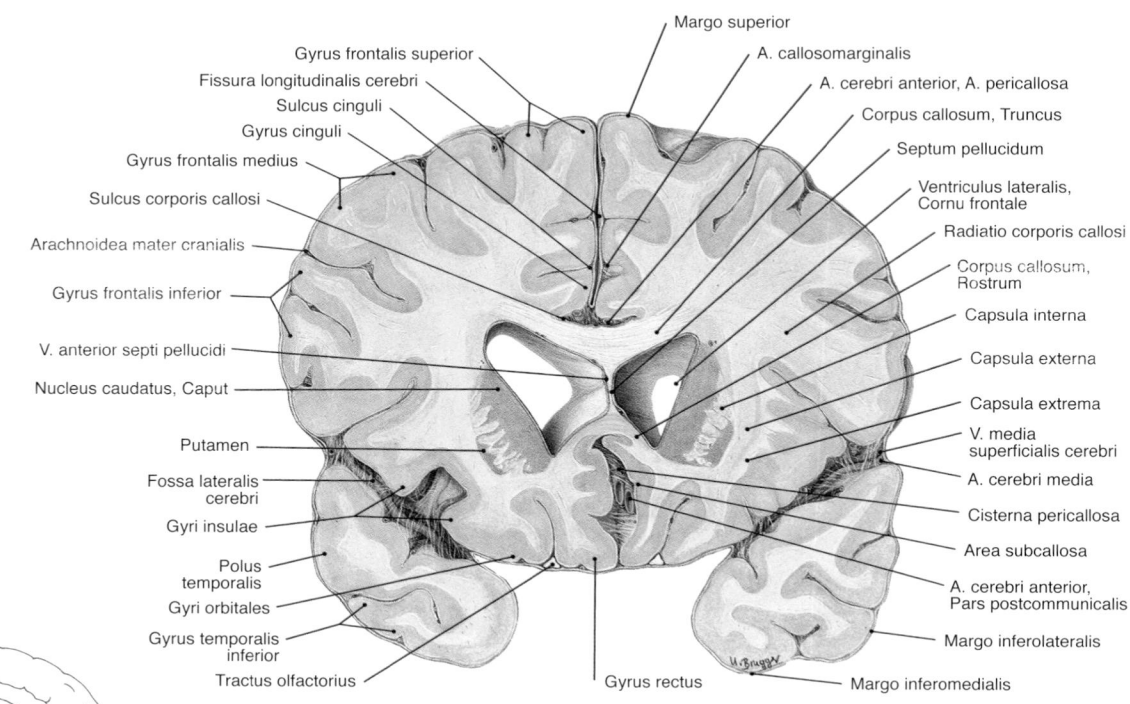

Margo superior
Gyrus frontalis superior
Fissura longitudinalis cerebri
Sulcus cinguli
Gyrus cinguli
Gyrus frontalis medius
Sulcus corporis callosi
Arachnoidea mater cranialis
Gyrus frontalis inferior
V. anterior septi pellucidi
Nucleus caudatus, Caput
Putamen
Fossa lateralis cerebri
Gyri insulae
Polus temporalis
Gyri orbitales
Gyrus temporalis inferior
Tractus olfactorius

A. callosomarginalis
A. cerebri anterior, A. pericallosa
Corpus callosum, Truncus
Septum pellucidum
Ventriculus lateralis, Cornu frontale
Radiatio corporis callosi
Corpus callosum, Rostrum
Capsula interna
Capsula externa
Capsula extrema
V. media superficialis cerebri
A. cerebri media
Cisterna pericallosa
Area subcallosa
A. cerebri anterior, Pars postcommunicalis
Margo inferolateralis
Margo inferomedialis
Gyrus rectus

Fig. 1283 Brain, Encephalon; frontal section at the level of the anterior parts of the frontal horns of the lateral ventricles.

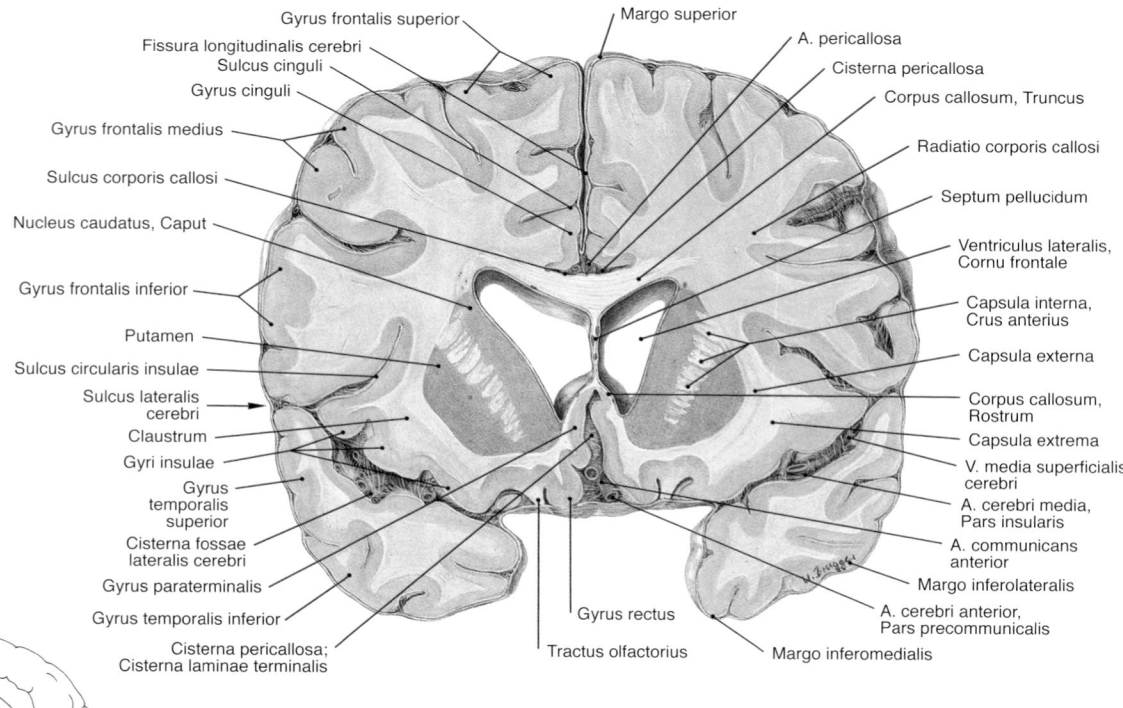

Gyrus frontalis superior
Fissura longitudinalis cerebri
Sulcus cinguli
Gyrus cinguli
Gyrus frontalis medius
Sulcus corporis callosi
Nucleus caudatus, Caput
Gyrus frontalis inferior
Putamen
Sulcus circularis insulae
Sulcus lateralis cerebri
Claustrum
Gyri insulae
Gyrus temporalis superior
Cisterna fossae lateralis cerebri
Gyrus paraterminalis
Gyrus temporalis inferior
Cisterna pericallosa; Cisterna laminae terminalis

Margo superior
A. pericallosa
Cisterna pericallosa
Corpus callosum, Truncus
Radiatio corporis callosi
Septum pellucidum
Ventriculus lateralis, Cornu frontale
Capsula interna, Crus anterius
Capsula externa
Corpus callosum, Rostrum
Capsula extrema
V. media superficialis cerebri
A. cerebri media, Pars insularis
A. communicans anterior
Margo inferolateralis
A. cerebri anterior, Pars precommunicalis
Margo inferomedialis
Gyrus rectus
Tractus olfactorius

Fig. 1284 Brain, Encephalon; frontal section at the level of the posterior parts of the frontal horns of the lateral ventricles.

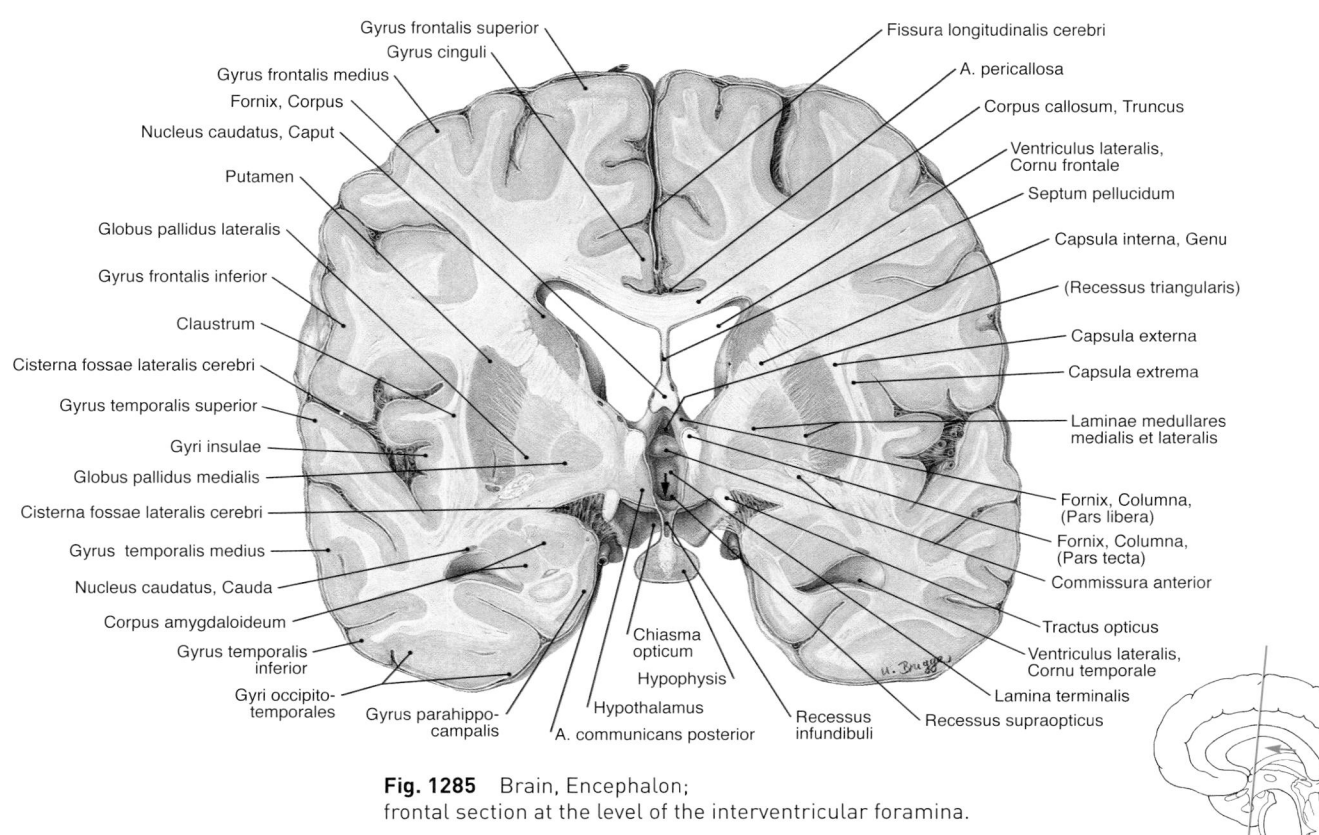

Gyrus frontalis superior
Gyrus cinguli
Gyrus frontalis medius
Fornix, Corpus
Nucleus caudatus, Caput
Putamen
Globus pallidus lateralis
Gyrus frontalis inferior
Claustrum
Cisterna fossae lateralis cerebri
Gyrus temporalis superior
Gyri insulae
Globus pallidus medialis
Cisterna fossae lateralis cerebri
Gyrus temporalis medius
Nucleus caudatus, Cauda
Corpus amygdaloideum
Gyrus temporalis inferior
Gyri occipito-temporales
Gyrus parahippo-campalis
Chiasma opticum
Hypophysis
Hypothalamus
A. communicans posterior
Recessus infundibuli

Fissura longitudinalis cerebri
A. pericallosa
Corpus callosum, Truncus
Ventriculus lateralis, Cornu frontale
Septum pellucidum
Capsula interna, Genu
(Recessus triangularis)
Capsula externa
Capsula extrema
Laminae medullares medialis et lateralis
Fornix, Columna, (Pars libera)
Fornix, Columna, (Pars tecta)
Commissura anterior
Tractus opticus
Ventriculus lateralis, Cornu temporale
Lamina terminalis
Recessus supraopticus

Fig. 1285   Brain, Encephalon;
frontal section at the level of the interventricular foramina.

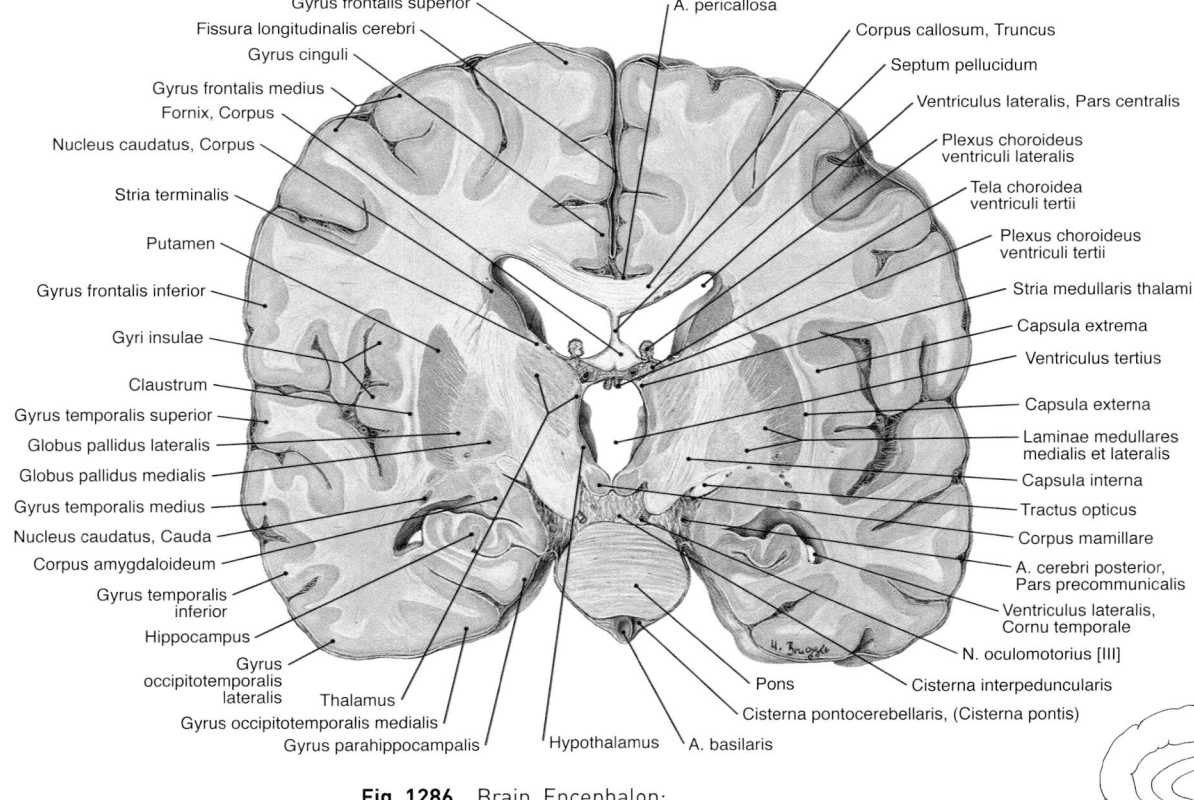

Gyrus frontalis superior
Fissura longitudinalis cerebri
Gyrus cinguli
Gyrus frontalis medius
Fornix, Corpus
Nucleus caudatus, Corpus
Stria terminalis
Putamen
Gyrus frontalis inferior
Gyri insulae
Claustrum
Gyrus temporalis superior
Globus pallidus lateralis
Globus pallidus medialis
Gyrus temporalis medius
Nucleus caudatus, Cauda
Corpus amygdaloideum
Gyrus temporalis inferior
Hippocampus
Gyrus occipitotemporalis lateralis
Thalamus
Gyrus occipitotemporalis medialis
Gyrus parahippocampalis
Hypothalamus
A. basilaris

A. pericallosa
Corpus callosum, Truncus
Septum pellucidum
Ventriculus lateralis, Pars centralis
Plexus choroideus ventriculi lateralis
Tela choroidea ventriculi tertii
Plexus choroideus ventriculi tertii
Stria medullaris thalami
Capsula extrema
Ventriculus tertius
Capsula externa
Laminae medullares medialis et lateralis
Capsula interna
Tractus opticus
Corpus mamillare
A. cerebri posterior, Pars precommunicalis
Ventriculus lateralis, Cornu temporale
N. oculomotorius [III]
Cisterna interpeduncularis
Pons
Cisterna pontocerebellaris, (Cisterna pontis)

Fig. 1286   Brain, Encephalon;
frontal section at the level of the mamillary bodies.

Brain, frontal sections

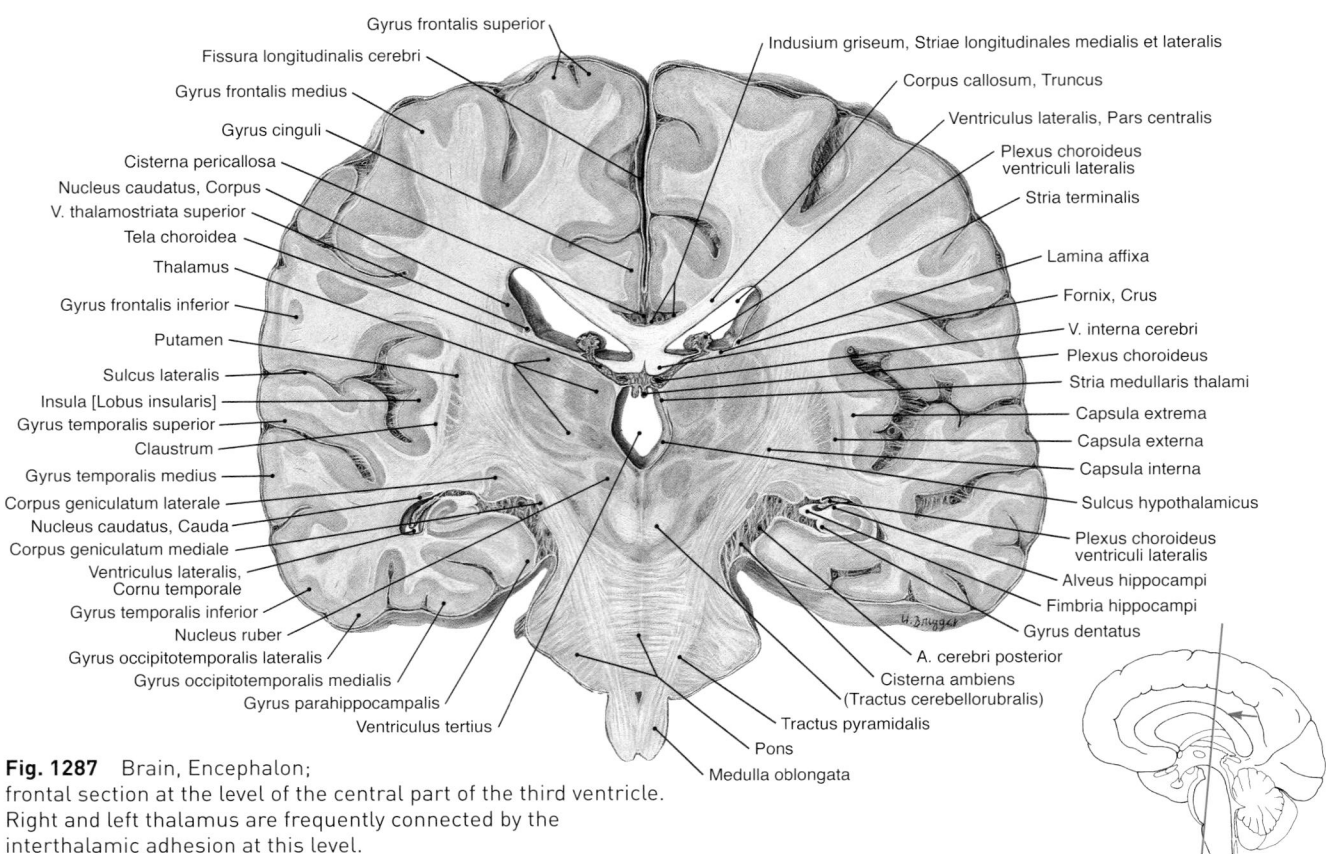

Gyrus frontalis superior
Fissura longitudinalis cerebri
Gyrus frontalis medius
Gyrus cinguli
Cisterna pericallosa
Nucleus caudatus, Corpus
V. thalamostriata superior
Tela choroidea
Thalamus
Gyrus frontalis inferior
Putamen
Sulcus lateralis
Insula [Lobus insularis]
Gyrus temporalis superior
Claustrum
Gyrus temporalis medius
Corpus geniculatum laterale
Nucleus caudatus, Cauda
Corpus geniculatum mediale
Ventriculus lateralis, Cornu temporale
Gyrus temporalis inferior
Nucleus ruber
Gyrus occipitotemporalis lateralis
Gyrus occipitotemporalis medialis
Gyrus parahippocampalis
Ventriculus tertius

Indusium griseum, Striae longitudinales medialis et lateralis
Corpus callosum, Truncus
Ventriculus lateralis, Pars centralis
Plexus choroideus ventriculi lateralis
Stria terminalis
Lamina affixa
Fornix, Crus
V. interna cerebri
Plexus choroideus
Stria medullaris thalami
Capsula extrema
Capsula externa
Capsula interna
Sulcus hypothalamicus
Plexus choroideus ventriculi lateralis
Alveus hippocampi
Fimbria hippocampi
Gyrus dentatus
A. cerebri posterior
Cisterna ambiens (Tractus cerebellorubralis)
Tractus pyramidalis
Pons
Medulla oblongata

Fig. 1287 Brain, Encephalon;
frontal section at the level of the central part of the third ventricle.
Right and left thalamus are frequently connected by the
interthalamic adhesion at this level.

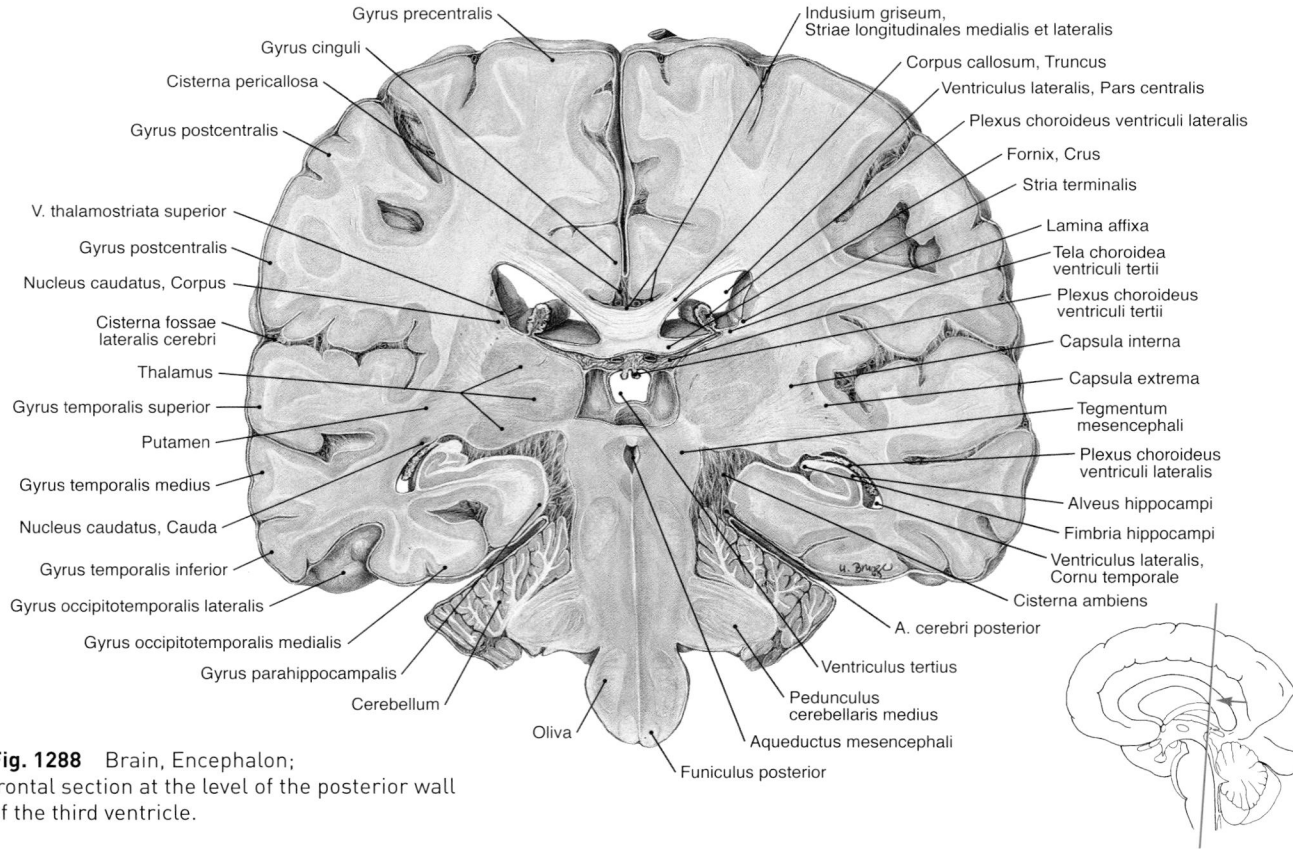

Gyrus precentralis
Gyrus cinguli
Cisterna pericallosa
Gyrus postcentralis
V. thalamostriata superior
Gyrus postcentralis
Nucleus caudatus, Corpus
Cisterna fossae lateralis cerebri
Thalamus
Gyrus temporalis superior
Putamen
Gyrus temporalis medius
Nucleus caudatus, Cauda
Gyrus temporalis inferior
Gyrus occipitotemporalis lateralis
Gyrus occipitotemporalis medialis
Gyrus parahippocampalis
Cerebellum
Oliva

Indusium griseum, Striae longitudinales medialis et lateralis
Corpus callosum, Truncus
Ventriculus lateralis, Pars centralis
Plexus choroideus ventriculi lateralis
Fornix, Crus
Stria terminalis
Lamina affixa
Tela choroidea ventriculi tertii
Plexus choroideus ventriculi tertii
Capsula interna
Capsula extrema
Tegmentum mesencephali
Plexus choroideus ventriculi lateralis
Alveus hippocampi
Fimbria hippocampi
Ventriculus lateralis, Cornu temporale
Cisterna ambiens
A. cerebri posterior
Ventriculus tertius
Pedunculus cerebellaris medius
Aqueductus mesencephali
Funiculus posterior

Fig. 1288 Brain, Encephalon;
frontal section at the level of the posterior wall
of the third ventricle.

Brain, frontal sections

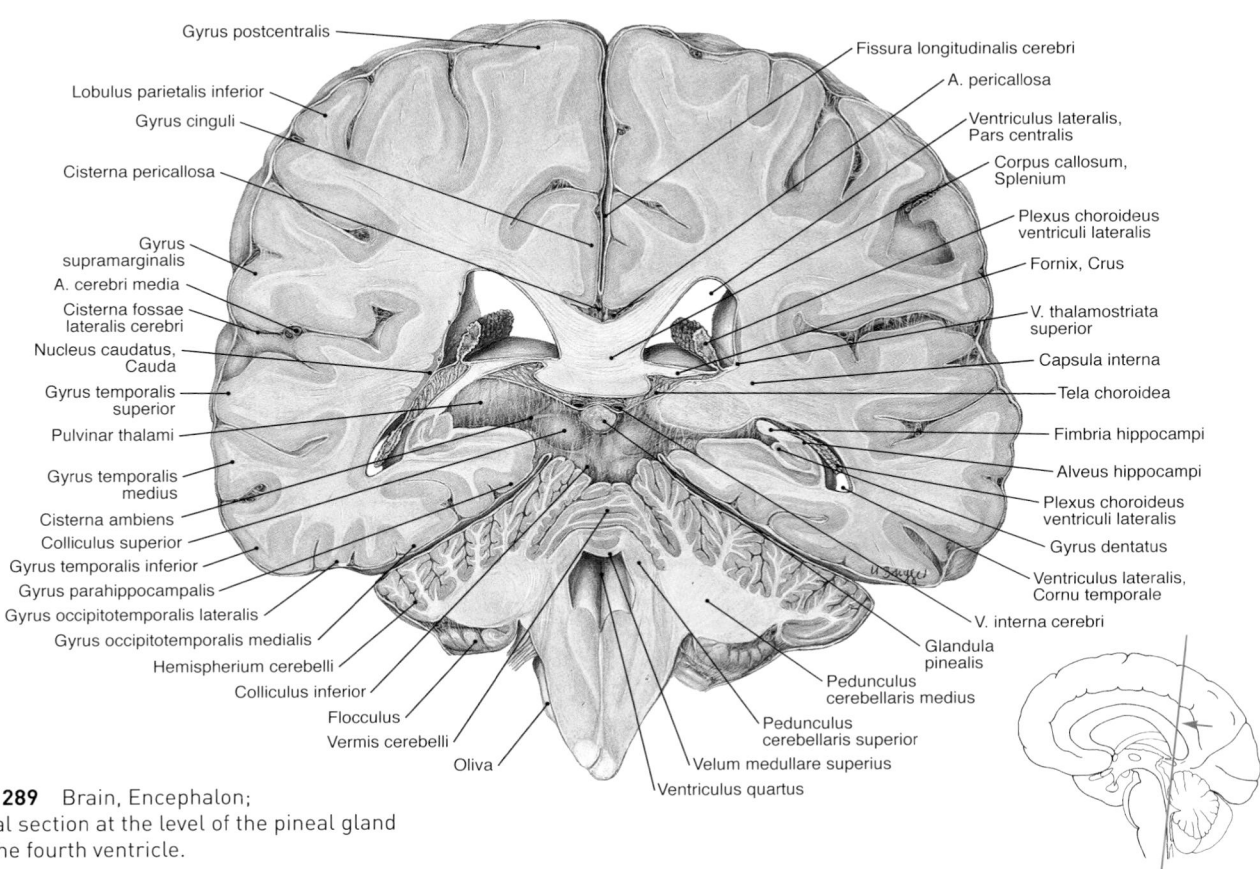

Gyrus postcentralis
Lobulus parietalis inferior
Gyrus cinguli
Cisterna pericallosa
Gyrus supramarginalis
A. cerebri media
Cisterna fossae lateralis cerebri
Nucleus caudatus, Cauda
Gyrus temporalis superior
Pulvinar thalami
Gyrus temporalis medius
Cisterna ambiens
Colliculus superior
Gyrus temporalis inferior
Gyrus parahippocampalis
Gyrus occipitotemporalis lateralis
Gyrus occipitotemporalis medialis
Hemispherium cerebelli
Colliculus inferior
Flocculus
Vermis cerebelli
Oliva

Fissura longitudinalis cerebri
A. pericallosa
Ventriculus lateralis, Pars centralis
Corpus callosum, Splenium
Plexus choroideus ventriculi lateralis
Fornix, Crus
V. thalamostriata superior
Capsula interna
Tela choroidea
Fimbria hippocampi
Alveus hippocampi
Plexus choroideus ventriculi lateralis
Gyrus dentatus
Ventriculus lateralis, Cornu temporale
V. interna cerebri
Glandula pinealis
Pedunculus cerebellaris medius
Pedunculus cerebellaris superior
Velum medullare superius
Ventriculus quartus

Fig. 1289 Brain, Encephalon;
frontal section at the level of the pineal gland
and the fourth ventricle.

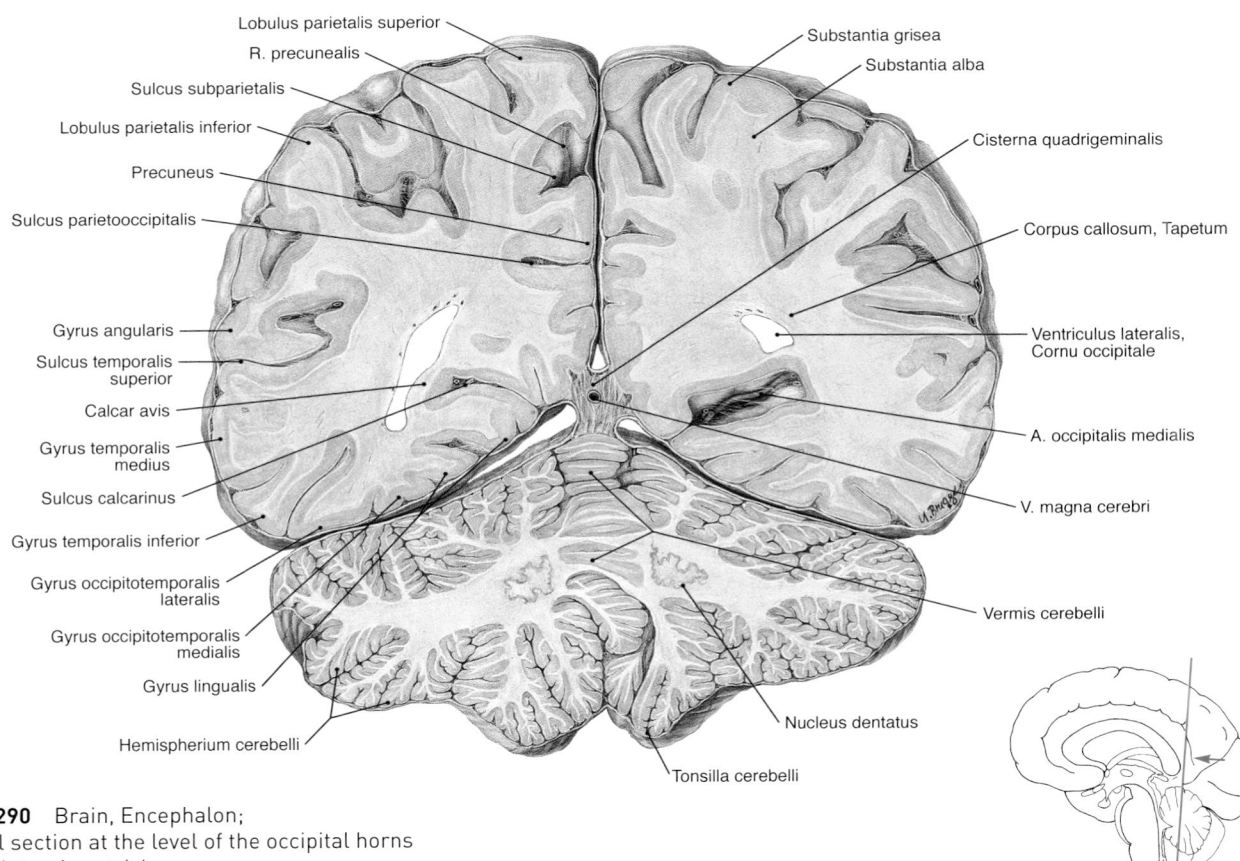

Lobulus parietalis superior
R. precunealis
Sulcus subparietalis
Lobulus parietalis inferior
Precuneus
Sulcus parietooccipitalis
Gyrus angularis
Sulcus temporalis superior
Calcar avis
Gyrus temporalis medius
Sulcus calcarinus
Gyrus temporalis inferior
Gyrus occipitotemporalis lateralis
Gyrus occipitotemporalis medialis
Gyrus lingualis
Hemispherium cerebelli

Substantia grisea
Substantia alba
Cisterna quadrigeminalis
Corpus callosum, Tapetum
Ventriculus lateralis, Cornu occipitale
A. occipitalis medialis
V. magna cerebri
Vermis cerebelli
Nucleus dentatus
Tonsilla cerebelli

Fig. 1290 Brain, Encephalon;
frontal section at the level of the occipital horns
of the lateral ventricles.

Brain, horizontal section

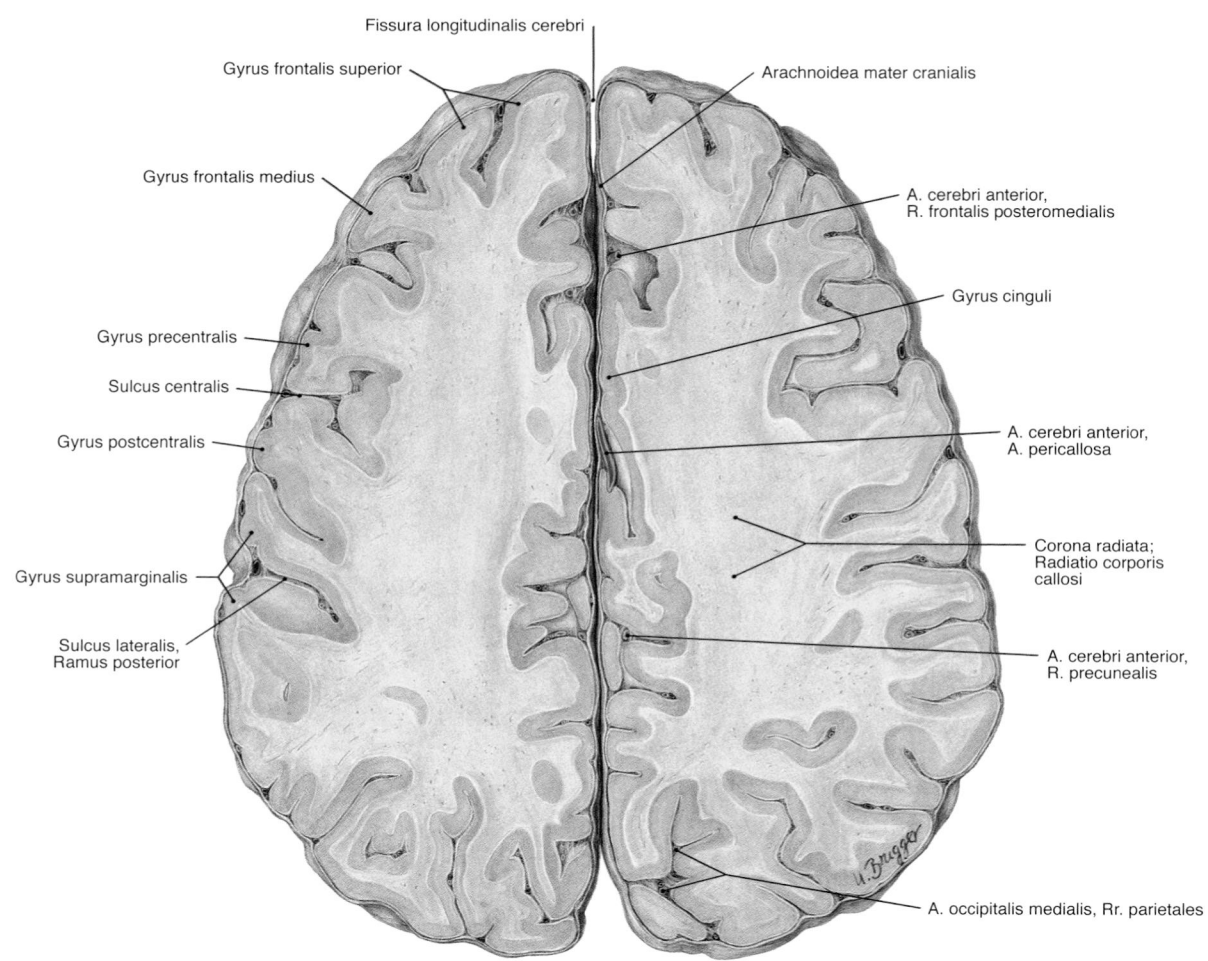

Fissura longitudinalis cerebri

Gyrus frontalis superior

Gyrus frontalis medius

Gyrus precentralis

Sulcus centralis

Gyrus postcentralis

Gyrus supramarginalis

Sulcus lateralis,
Ramus posterior

Arachnoidea mater cranialis

A. cerebri anterior,
R. frontalis posteromedialis

Gyrus cinguli

A. cerebri anterior,
A. pericallosa

Corona radiata;
Radiatio corporis
callosi

A. cerebri anterior,
R. precunealis

A. occipitalis medialis, Rr. parietales

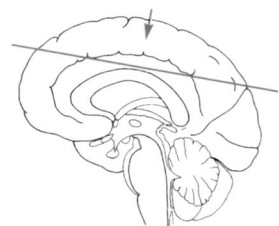

Fig. 1291 Brain, Encephalon;
horizontal section just above the corpus callosum.
In Fig. 1283–1303, the subarachnoid space appears
somewhat enlarged, particularly in the region of the
hemispheric sulci, due to the fact that these specimens
were taken from elderly individuals.

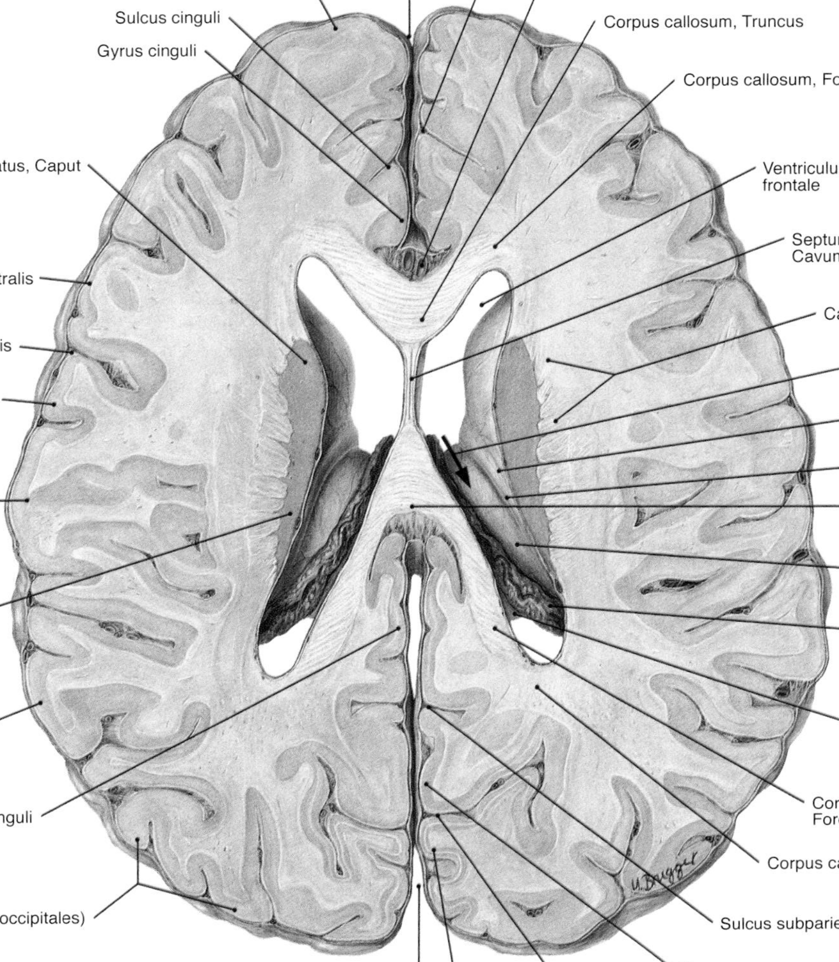

Brain, horizontal section

Fissura longitudinalis cerebri

A. cerebri anterior, A. callosomarginalis

A. pericallosa

Gyrus frontalis superior

Corpus callosum, Truncus

Sulcus cinguli

Gyrus cinguli

Corpus callosum, Forceps minor

Nucleus caudatus, Caput

Ventriculus lateralis, Cornu frontale

Septum pellucidum, Cavum septi pellucidi

Gyrus precentralis

Capsula interna

Sulcus centralis

Ventriculus lateralis, Pars centralis

Gyrus postcentralis

V. thalamostriata superior

Stria terminalis

Lobulus parietalis inferior

Corpus callosum, Truncus

Lamina affixa

Nucleus caudatus, Corpus

Plexus choroideus ventriculi lateralis

Gyrus angularis

Fornix, Crus

Gyrus cinguli

Corpus callosum, Forceps major

Corpus callosum, Tapetum

(Gyri occipitales)

Sulcus subparietalis

Precuneus

Fissura longitudinalis cerebri

Cuneus

Sulcus parietooccipitalis

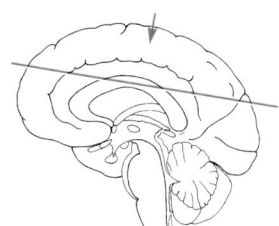

Fig. 1292 Brain, Encephalon;
horizontal section at the level of
the central part of the lateral ventricles.

Brain, horizontal section

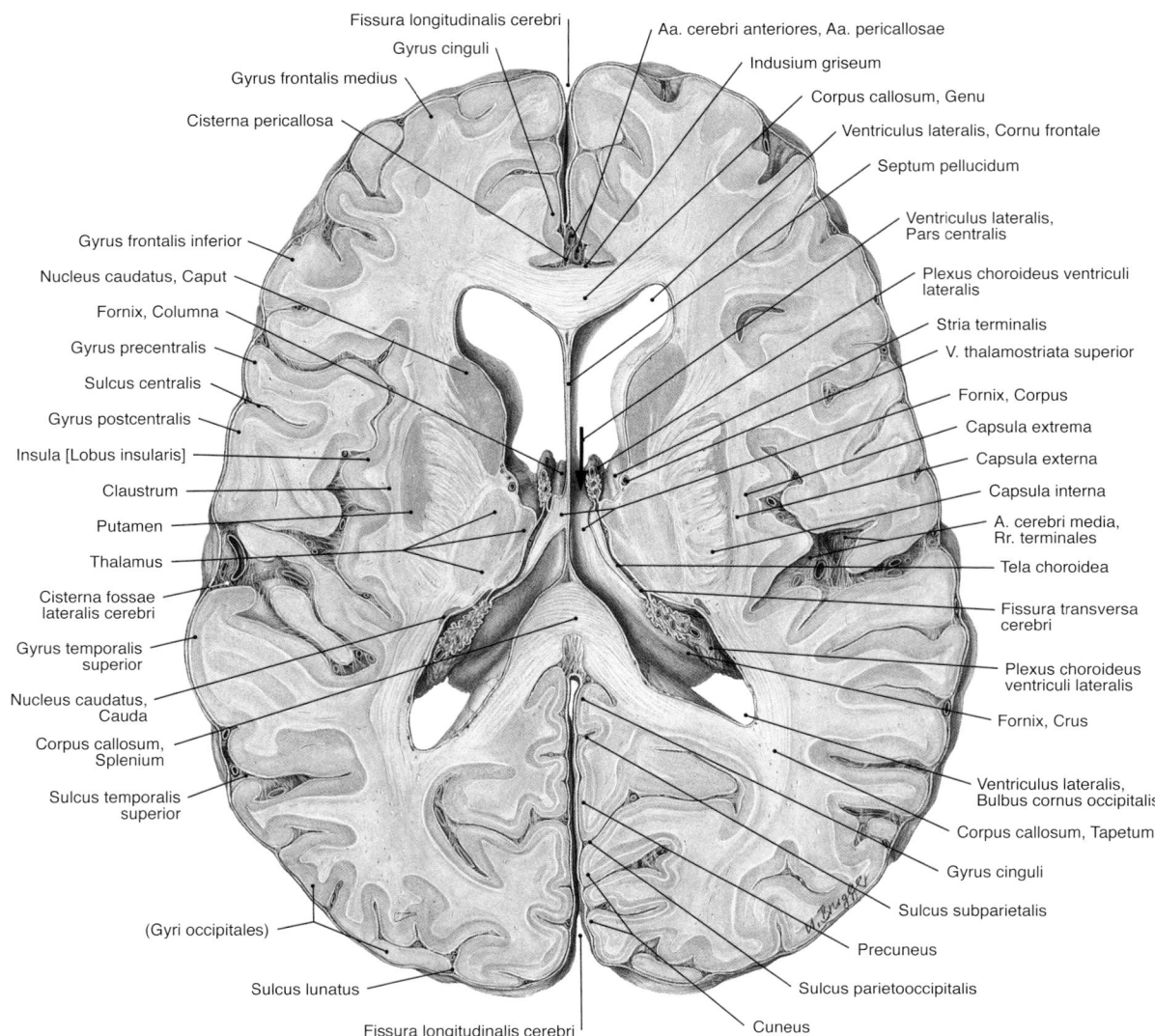

Fissura longitudinalis cerebri
Gyrus cinguli
Gyrus frontalis medius
Cisterna pericallosa

Aa. cerebri anteriores, Aa. pericallosae
Indusium griseum
Corpus callosum, Genu
Ventriculus lateralis, Cornu frontale
Septum pellucidum
Ventriculus lateralis, Pars centralis
Plexus choroideus ventriculi lateralis
Stria terminalis
V. thalamostriata superior
Fornix, Corpus
Capsula extrema
Capsula externa
Capsula interna
A. cerebri media, Rr. terminales
Tela choroidea
Fissura transversa cerebri
Plexus choroideus ventriculi lateralis
Fornix, Crus
Ventriculus lateralis, Bulbus cornus occipitalis
Corpus callosum, Tapetum
Gyrus cinguli
Sulcus subparietalis
Precuneus
Sulcus parietooccipitalis
Cuneus

Gyrus frontalis inferior
Nucleus caudatus, Caput
Fornix, Columna
Gyrus precentralis
Sulcus centralis
Gyrus postcentralis
Insula [Lobus insularis]
Claustrum
Putamen
Thalamus
Cisterna fossae lateralis cerebri
Gyrus temporalis superior
Nucleus caudatus, Cauda
Corpus callosum, Splenium
Sulcus temporalis superior
(Gyri occipitales)
Sulcus lunatus
Fissura longitudinalis cerebri

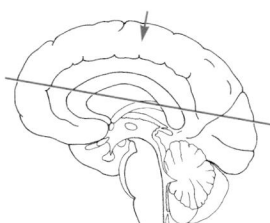

Fig. 1293 Brain, Encephalon;
horizontal section at the level of the floor of
the central part of the lateral ventricles.

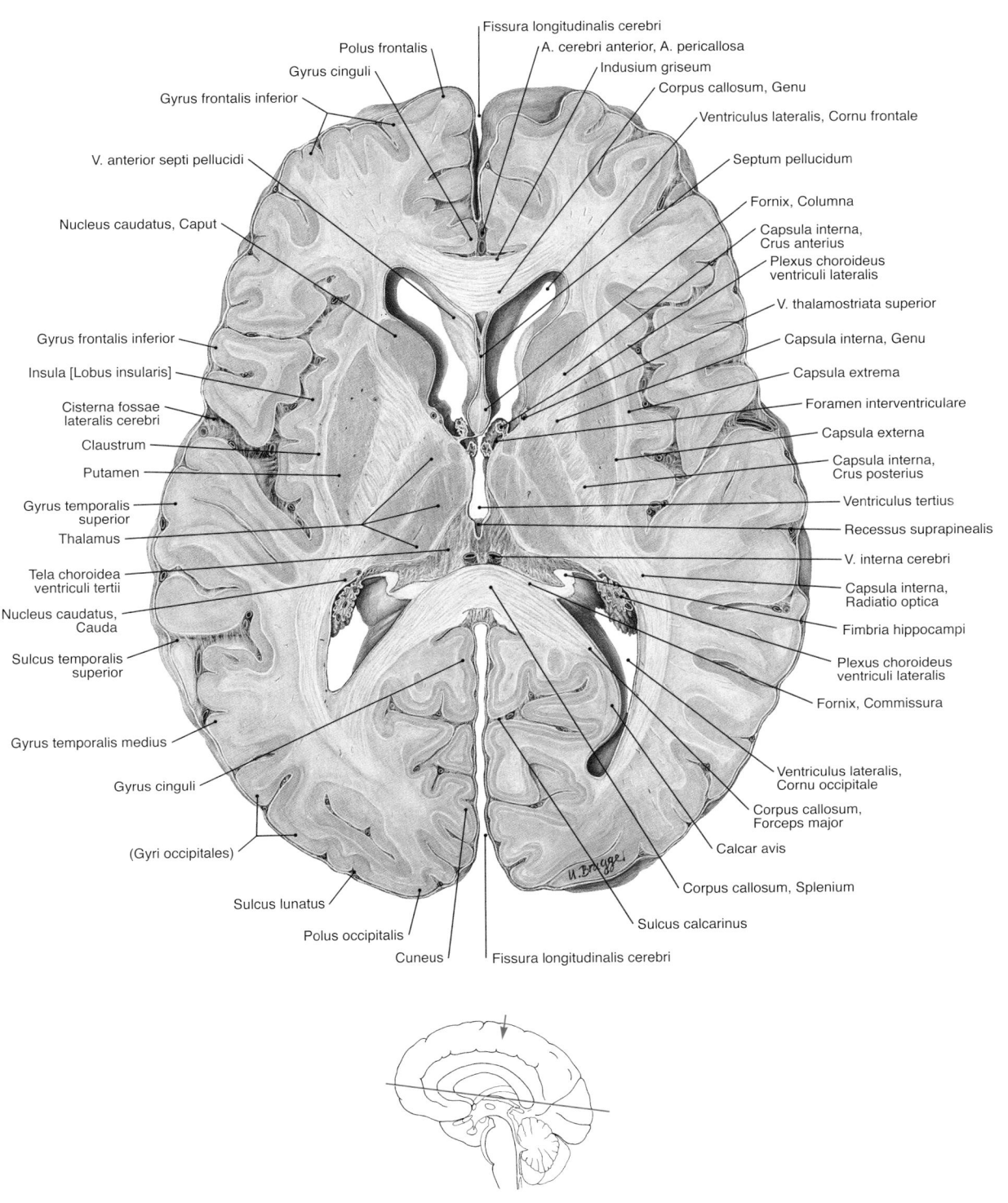

Fissura longitudinalis cerebri
Polus frontalis
Gyrus cinguli
A. cerebri anterior, A. pericallosa
Gyrus frontalis inferior
Indusium griseum
Corpus callosum, Genu
Ventriculus lateralis, Cornu frontale
V. anterior septi pellucidi
Septum pellucidum
Nucleus caudatus, Caput
Fornix, Columna
Capsula interna, Crus anterius
Plexus choroideus ventriculi lateralis
Gyrus frontalis inferior
V. thalamostriata superior
Insula [Lobus insularis]
Capsula interna, Genu
Cisterna fossae lateralis cerebri
Capsula extrema
Claustrum
Foramen interventriculare
Putamen
Capsula externa
Gyrus temporalis superior
Capsula interna, Crus posterius
Thalamus
Ventriculus tertius
Tela choroidea ventriculi tertii
Recessus suprapinealis
Nucleus caudatus, Cauda
V. interna cerebri
Sulcus temporalis superior
Capsula interna, Radiatio optica
Fimbria hippocampi
Gyrus temporalis medius
Plexus choroideus ventriculi lateralis
Gyrus cinguli
Fornix, Commissura
(Gyri occipitales)
Ventriculus lateralis, Cornu occipitale
Corpus callosum, Forceps major
Calcar avis
Sulcus lunatus
Corpus callosum, Splenium
Polus occipitalis
Sulcus calcarinus
Cuneus
Fissura longitudinalis cerebri

Fig. 1294   Brain, Encephalon;
horizontal section at the level of the upper part
of the third ventricle.

Brain, horizontal section

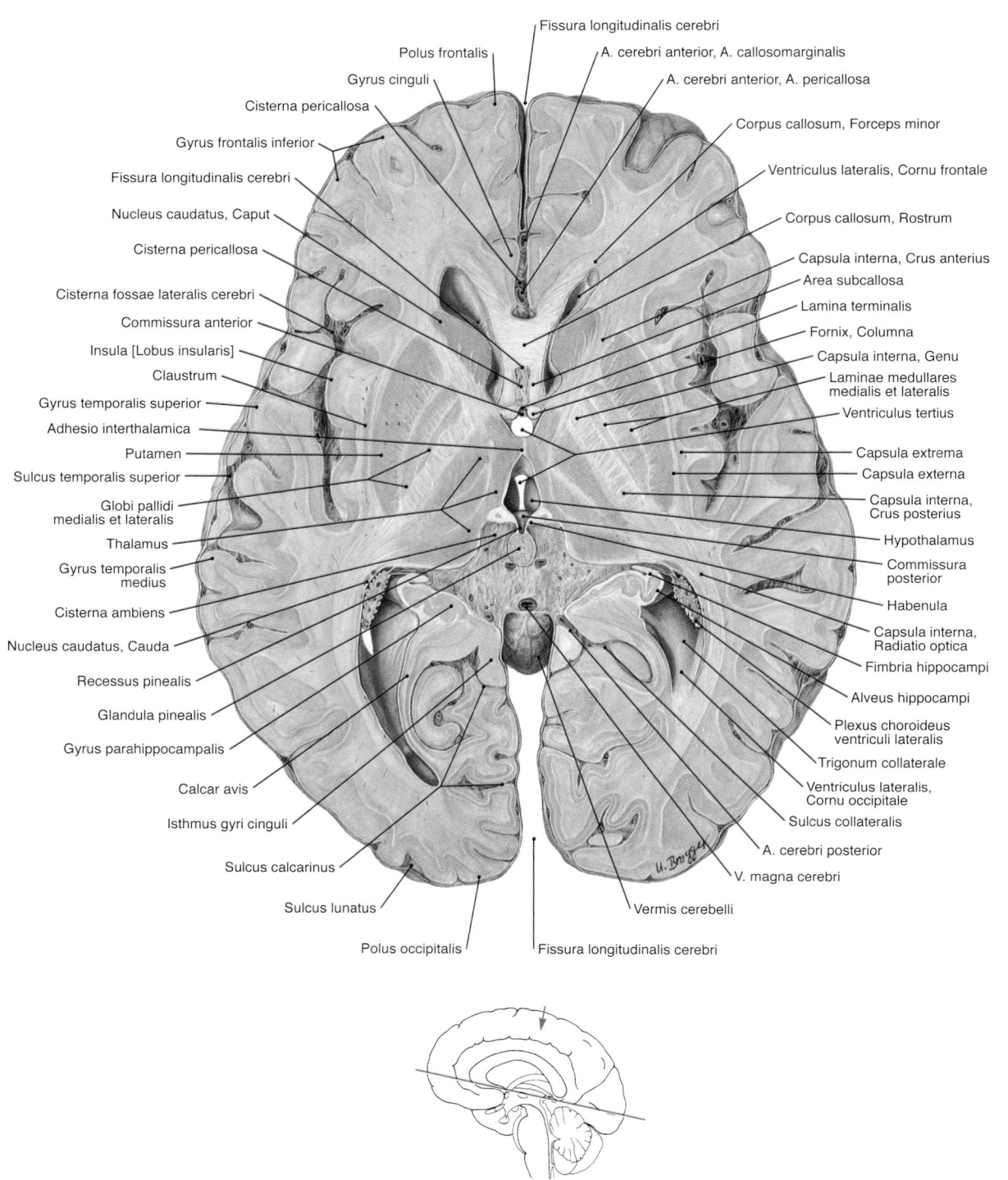

Fissura longitudinalis cerebri
Polus frontalis
A. cerebri anterior, A. callosomarginalis
Gyrus cinguli
A. cerebri anterior, A. pericallosa
Cisterna pericallosa
Gyrus frontalis inferior
Corpus callosum, Forceps minor
Fissura longitudinalis cerebri
Ventriculus lateralis, Cornu frontale
Nucleus caudatus, Caput
Corpus callosum, Rostrum
Cisterna pericallosa
Capsula interna, Crus anterius
Area subcallosa
Cisterna fossae lateralis cerebri
Lamina terminalis
Commissura anterior
Fornix, Columna
Insula [Lobus insularis]
Capsula interna, Genu
Claustrum
Laminae medullares medialis et lateralis
Gyrus temporalis superior
Ventriculus tertius
Adhesio interthalamica
Putamen
Capsula extrema
Sulcus temporalis superior
Capsula externa
Globi pallidi medialis et lateralis
Capsula interna, Crus posterius
Thalamus
Hypothalamus
Gyrus temporalis medius
Commissura posterior
Cisterna ambiens
Habenula
Nucleus caudatus, Cauda
Capsula interna, Radiatio optica
Recessus pinealis
Fimbria hippocampi
Glandula pinealis
Alveus hippocampi
Gyrus parahippocampalis
Plexus choroideus ventriculi lateralis
Calcar avis
Trigonum collaterale
Isthmus gyri cinguli
Ventriculus lateralis, Cornu occipitale
Sulcus calcarinus
Sulcus collateralis
A. cerebri posterior
Sulcus lunatus
V. magna cerebri
Polus occipitalis
Vermis cerebelli
Fissura longitudinalis cerebri

Fig. 1295 Brain, Encephalon; horizontal section through the centre of the third ventricle at the level of the interthalamic adhesion.

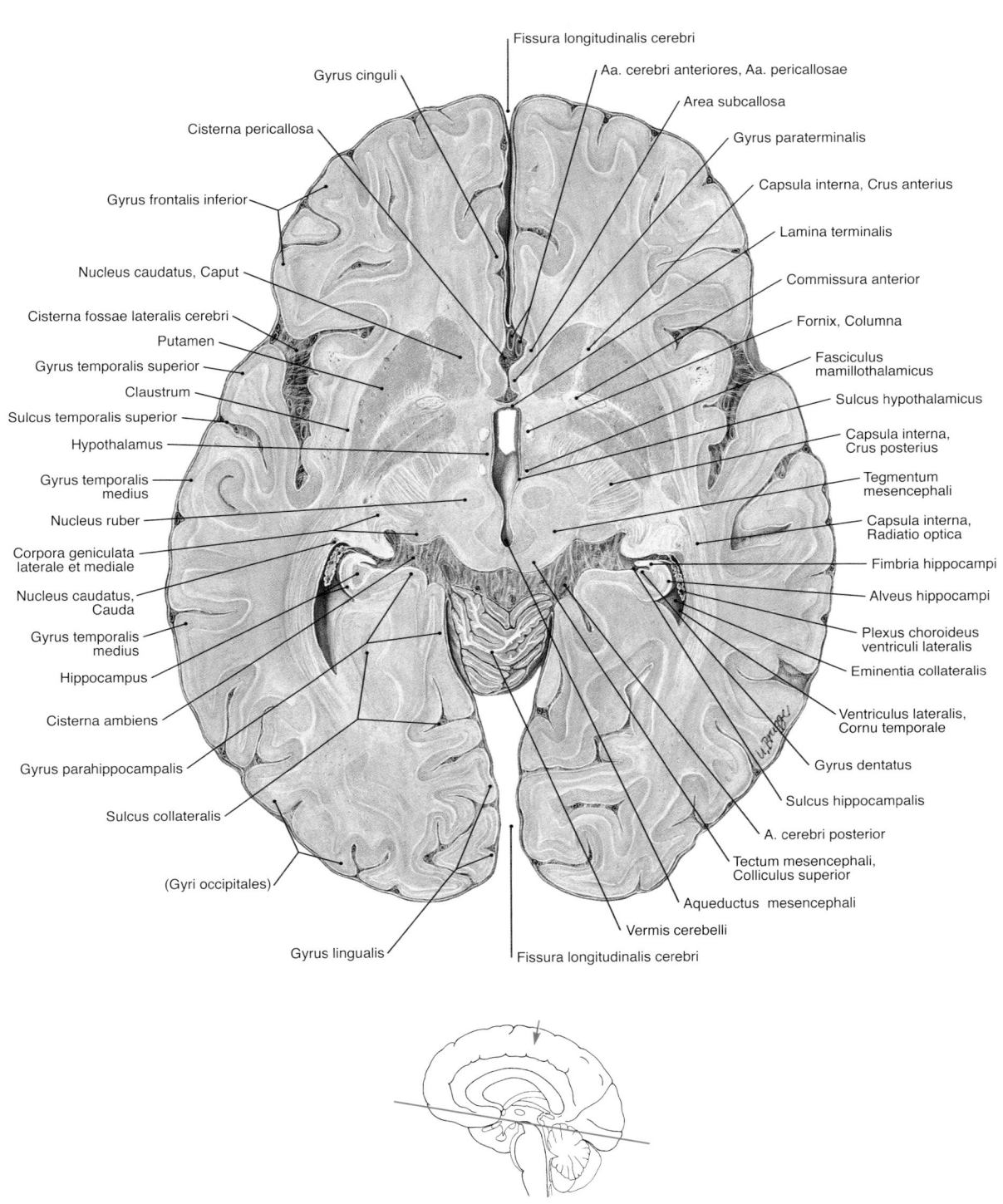

Fissura longitudinalis cerebri

Gyrus cinguli

Aa. cerebri anteriores, Aa. pericallosae

Area subcallosa

Cisterna pericallosa

Gyrus paraterminalis

Gyrus frontalis inferior

Capsula interna, Crus anterius

Lamina terminalis

Nucleus caudatus, Caput

Commissura anterior

Cisterna fossae lateralis cerebri

Fornix, Columna

Putamen

Fasciculus mamillothalamicus

Gyrus temporalis superior

Claustrum

Sulcus hypothalamicus

Sulcus temporalis superior

Capsula interna, Crus posterius

Hypothalamus

Gyrus temporalis medius

Tegmentum mesencephali

Nucleus ruber

Capsula interna, Radiatio optica

Corpora geniculata laterale et mediale

Fimbria hippocampi

Alveus hippocampi

Nucleus caudatus, Cauda

Plexus choroideus ventriculi lateralis

Gyrus temporalis medius

Eminentia collateralis

Hippocampus

Ventriculus lateralis, Cornu temporale

Cisterna ambiens

Gyrus dentatus

Gyrus parahippocampalis

Sulcus hippocampalis

Sulcus collateralis

A. cerebri posterior

Tectum mesencephali, Colliculus superior

(Gyri occipitales)

Aqueductus mesencephali

Gyrus lingualis

Vermis cerebelli

Fissura longitudinalis cerebri

Fig. 1296 Brain, Encephalon;
horizontal section through the third ventricle at the level
of the opening of the cerebral aqueduct.

Brain, horizontal section

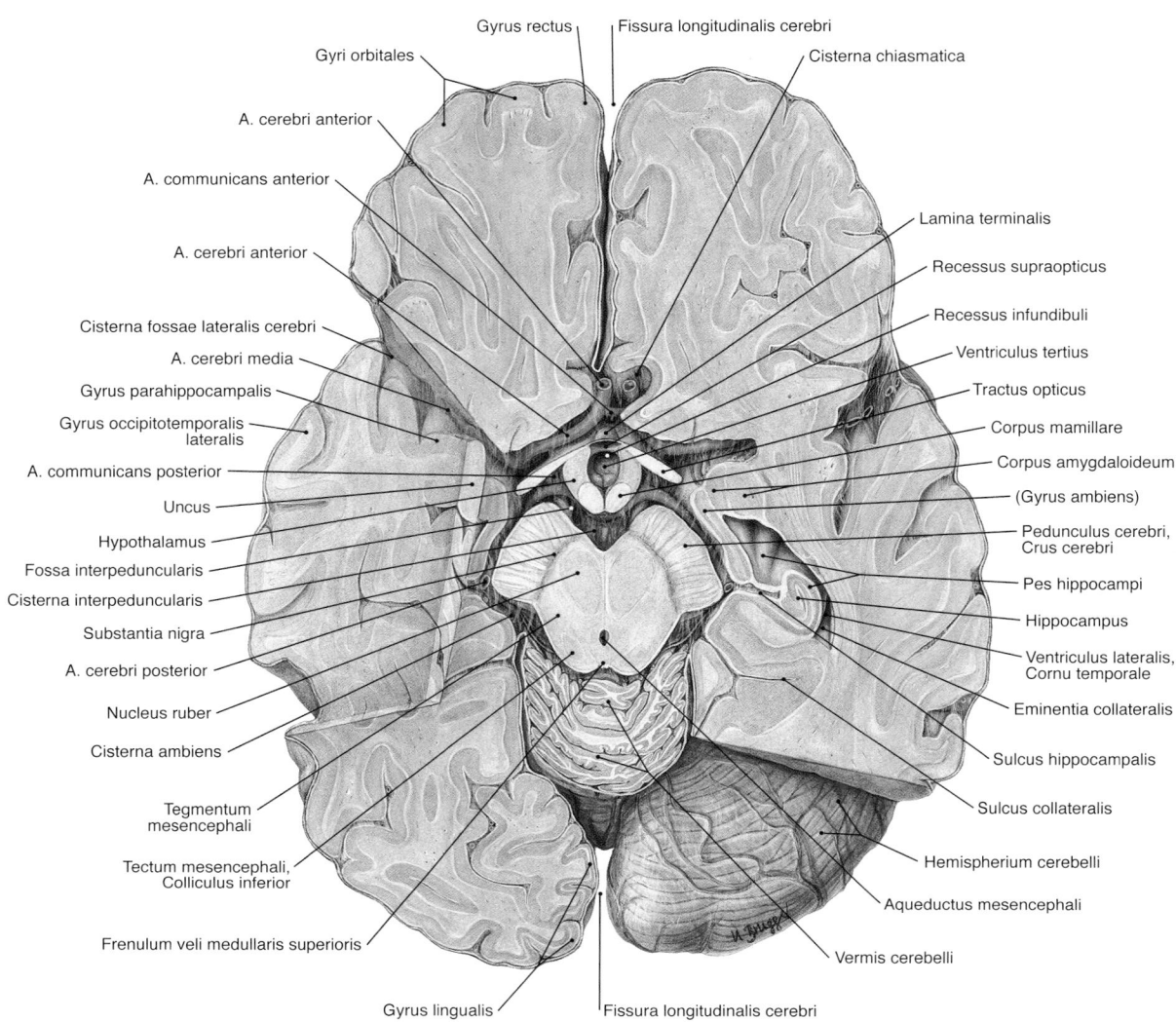

Gyrus rectus · Fissura longitudinalis cerebri
Gyri orbitales
Cisterna chiasmatica
A. cerebri anterior
A. communicans anterior
Lamina terminalis
A. cerebri anterior
Recessus supraopticus
Recessus infundibuli
Cisterna fossae lateralis cerebri
Ventriculus tertius
A. cerebri media
Gyrus parahippocampalis
Tractus opticus
Gyrus occipitotemporalis lateralis
Corpus mamillare
A. communicans posterior
Corpus amygdaloideum
Uncus
(Gyrus ambiens)
Hypothalamus
Pedunculus cerebri, Crus cerebri
Fossa interpeduncularis
Cisterna interpeduncularis
Pes hippocampi
Substantia nigra
Hippocampus
A. cerebri posterior
Ventriculus lateralis, Cornu temporale
Nucleus ruber
Eminentia collateralis
Cisterna ambiens
Sulcus hippocampalis
Tegmentum mesencephali
Sulcus collateralis
Tectum mesencephali, Colliculus inferior
Hemispherium cerebelli
Frenulum veli medullaris superioris
Aqueductus mesencephali
Vermis cerebelli
Gyrus lingualis
Fissura longitudinalis cerebri

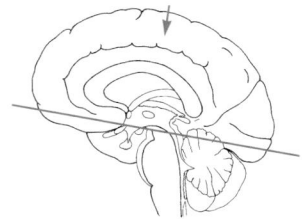

Fig. 1297   Brain, Encephalon;
staggered horizontal section through the floor of the third
ventricle at the level of the mamillary bodies.

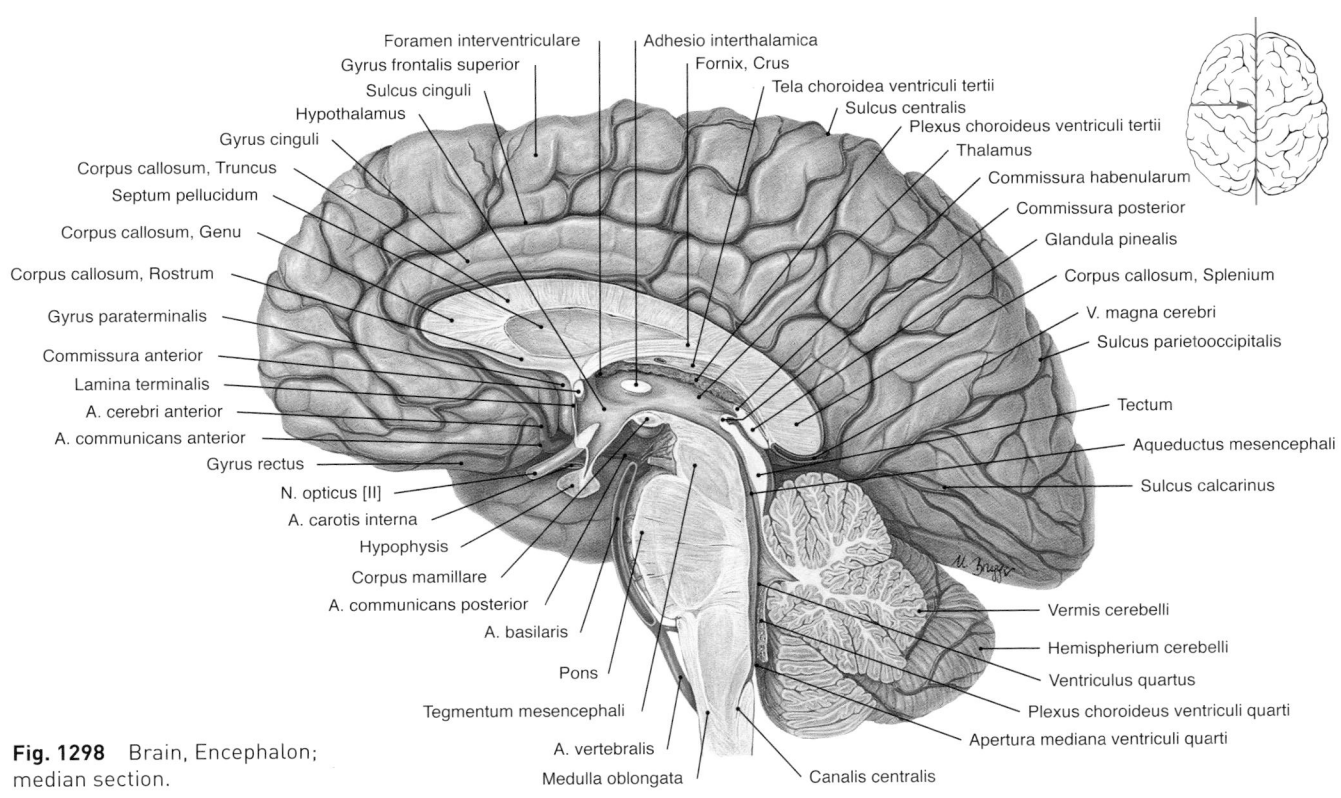

Foramen interventriculare
Gyrus frontalis superior
Sulcus cinguli
Hypothalamus
Gyrus cinguli
Corpus callosum, Truncus
Septum pellucidum
Corpus callosum, Genu
Corpus callosum, Rostrum
Gyrus parapterminalis
Commissura anterior
Lamina terminalis
A. cerebri anterior
A. communicans anterior
Gyrus rectus
N. opticus [II]
A. carotis interna
Hypophysis
Corpus mamillare
A. communicans posterior
A. basilaris
Pons
Tegmentum mesencephali
A. vertebralis
Medulla oblongata

Adhesio interthalamica
Fornix, Crus
Tela choroidea ventriculi tertii
Sulcus centralis
Plexus choroideus ventriculi tertii
Thalamus
Commissura habenularum
Commissura posterior
Glandula pinealis
Corpus callosum, Splenium
V. magna cerebri
Sulcus parietooccipitalis
Tectum
Aqueductus mesencephali
Sulcus calcarinus
Vermis cerebelli
Hemispherium cerebelli
Ventriculus quartus
Plexus choroideus ventriculi quarti
Apertura mediana ventriculi quarti
Canalis centralis

Fig. 1298 Brain, Encephalon; median section.

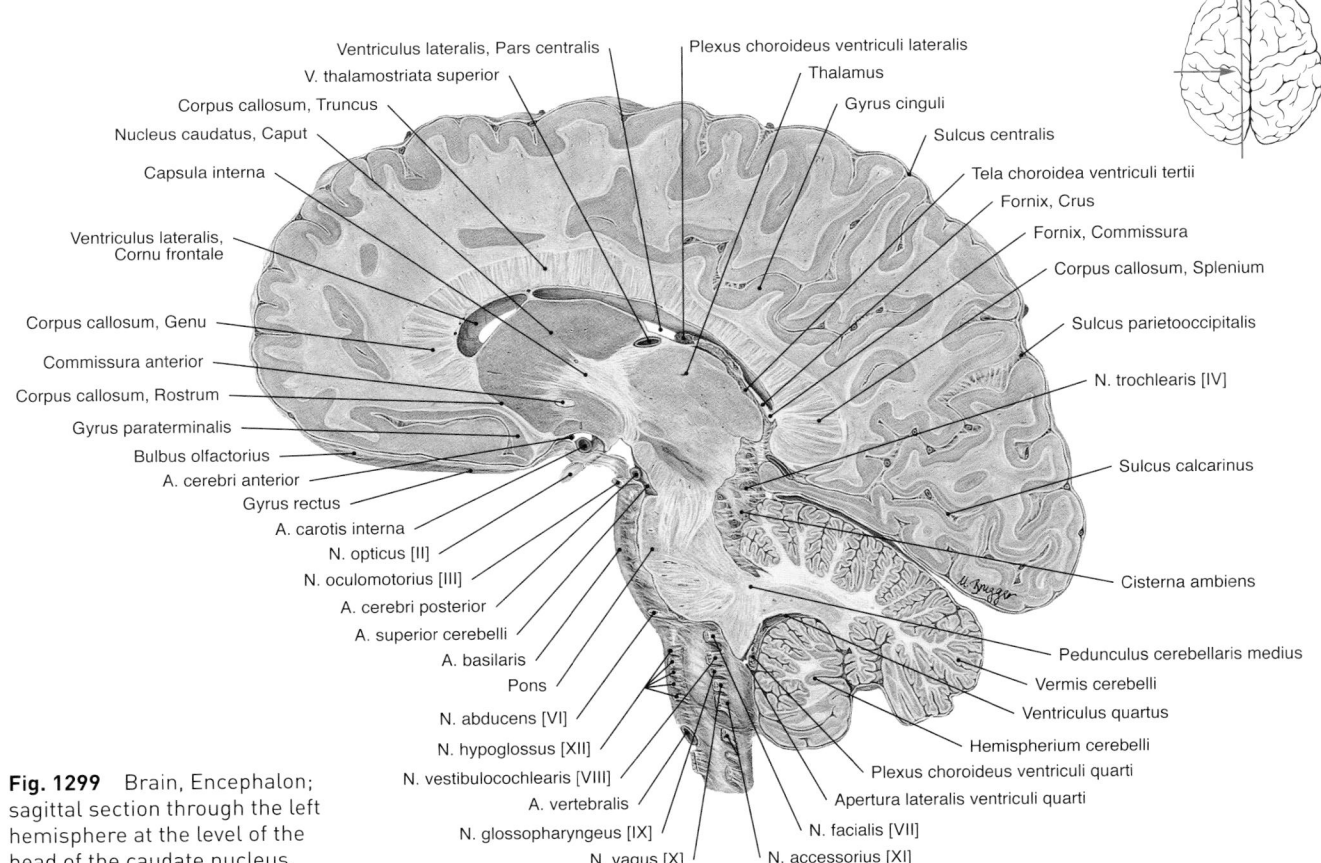

Ventriculus lateralis, Pars centralis
V. thalamostriata superior
Corpus callosum, Truncus
Nucleus caudatus, Caput
Capsula interna
Ventriculus lateralis, Cornu frontale
Corpus callosum, Genu
Commissura anterior
Corpus callosum, Rostrum
Gyrus parapterminalis
Bulbus olfactorius
A. cerebri anterior
Gyrus rectus
A. carotis interna
N. opticus [II]
N. oculomotorius [III]
A. cerebri posterior
A. superior cerebelli
A. basilaris
Pons
N. abducens [VI]
N. hypoglossus [XII]
N. vestibulocochlearis [VIII]
A. vertebralis
N. glossopharyngeus [IX]
N. vagus [X]

Plexus choroideus ventriculi lateralis
Thalamus
Gyrus cinguli
Sulcus centralis
Tela choroidea ventriculi tertii
Fornix, Crus
Fornix, Commissura
Corpus callosum, Splenium
Sulcus parietooccipitalis
N. trochlearis [IV]
Sulcus calcarinus
Cisterna ambiens
Pedunculus cerebellaris medius
Vermis cerebelli
Ventriculus quartus
Hemispherium cerebelli
Plexus choroideus ventriculi quarti
Apertura lateralis ventriculi quarti
N. facialis [VII]
N. accessorius [XI]

Fig. 1299 Brain, Encephalon; sagittal section through the left hemisphere at the level of the head of the caudate nucleus.

Brain, sagittal sections

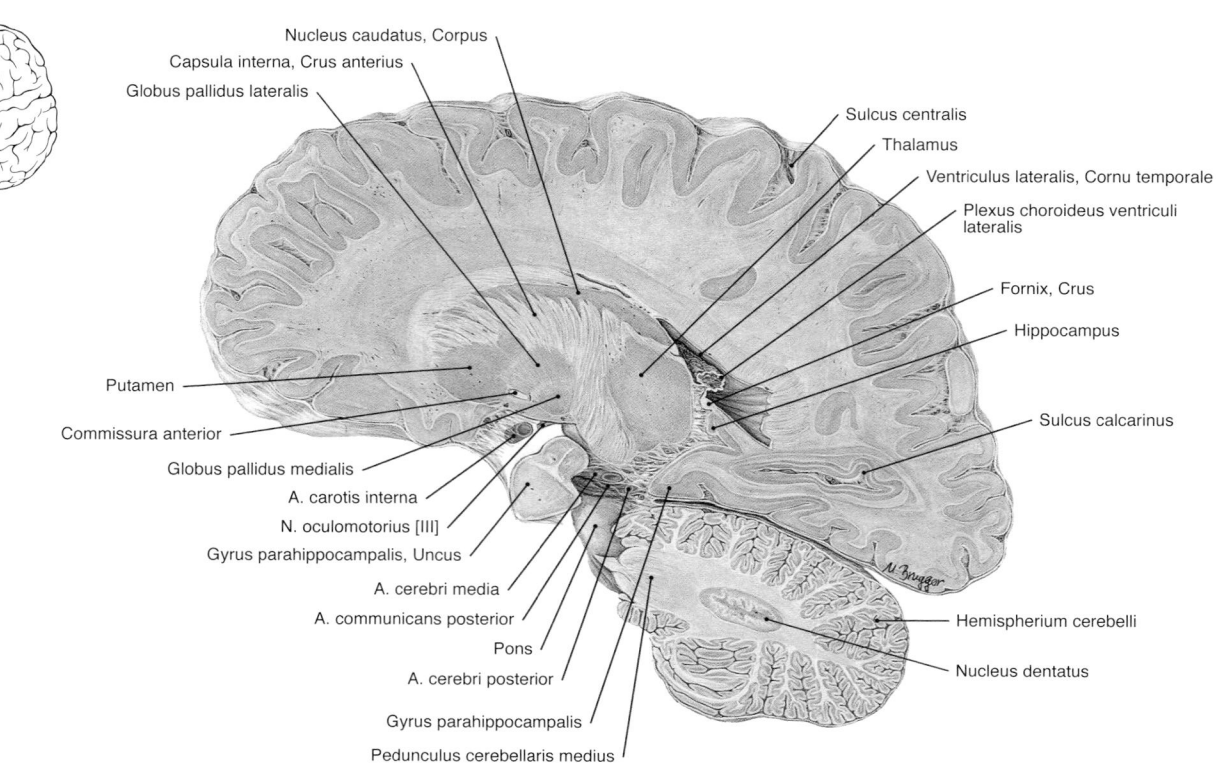

Nucleus caudatus, Corpus
Capsula interna, Crus anterius
Globus pallidus lateralis
Sulcus centralis
Thalamus
Ventriculus lateralis, Cornu temporale
Plexus choroideus ventriculi lateralis
Fornix, Crus
Hippocampus
Putamen
Commissura anterior
Sulcus calcarinus
Globus pallidus medialis
A. carotis interna
N. oculomotorius [III]
Gyrus parahippocampalis, Uncus
A. cerebri media
A. communicans posterior
Pons
A. cerebri posterior
Hemispherium cerebelli
Nucleus dentatus
Gyrus parahippocampalis
Pedunculus cerebellaris medius

Fig. 1300 Brain, Encephalon;
sagittal section through the left hemisphere
at the level of the body of the caudate nucleus.

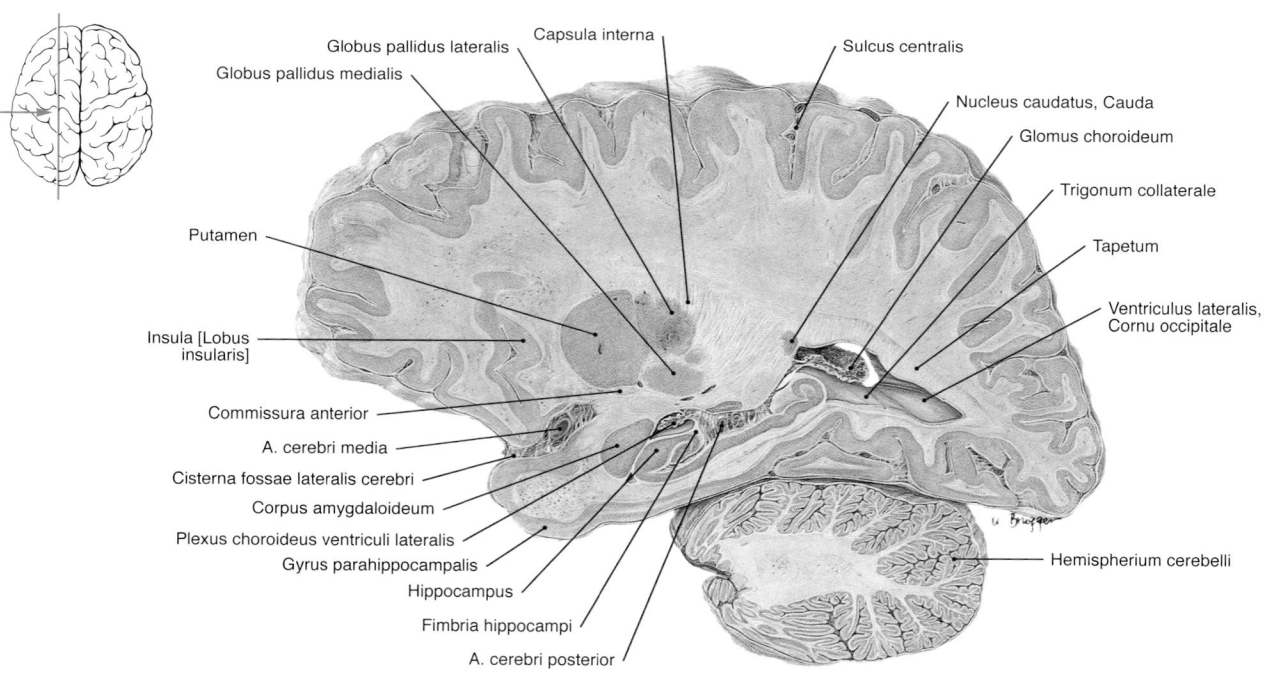

Globus pallidus lateralis
Globus pallidus medialis
Capsula interna
Sulcus centralis
Nucleus caudatus, Cauda
Glomus choroideum
Trigonum collaterale
Putamen
Tapetum
Insula [Lobus insularis]
Ventriculus lateralis, Cornu occipitale
Commissura anterior
A. cerebri media
Cisterna fossae lateralis cerebri
Corpus amygdaloideum
Plexus choroideus ventriculi lateralis
Gyrus parahippocampalis
Hemispherium cerebelli
Hippocampus
Fimbria hippocampi
A. cerebri posterior

Fig. 1301 Brain, Encephalon;
sagittal section through the left hemisphere
at the level of the amygdaloid body.

Brain, sagittal sections

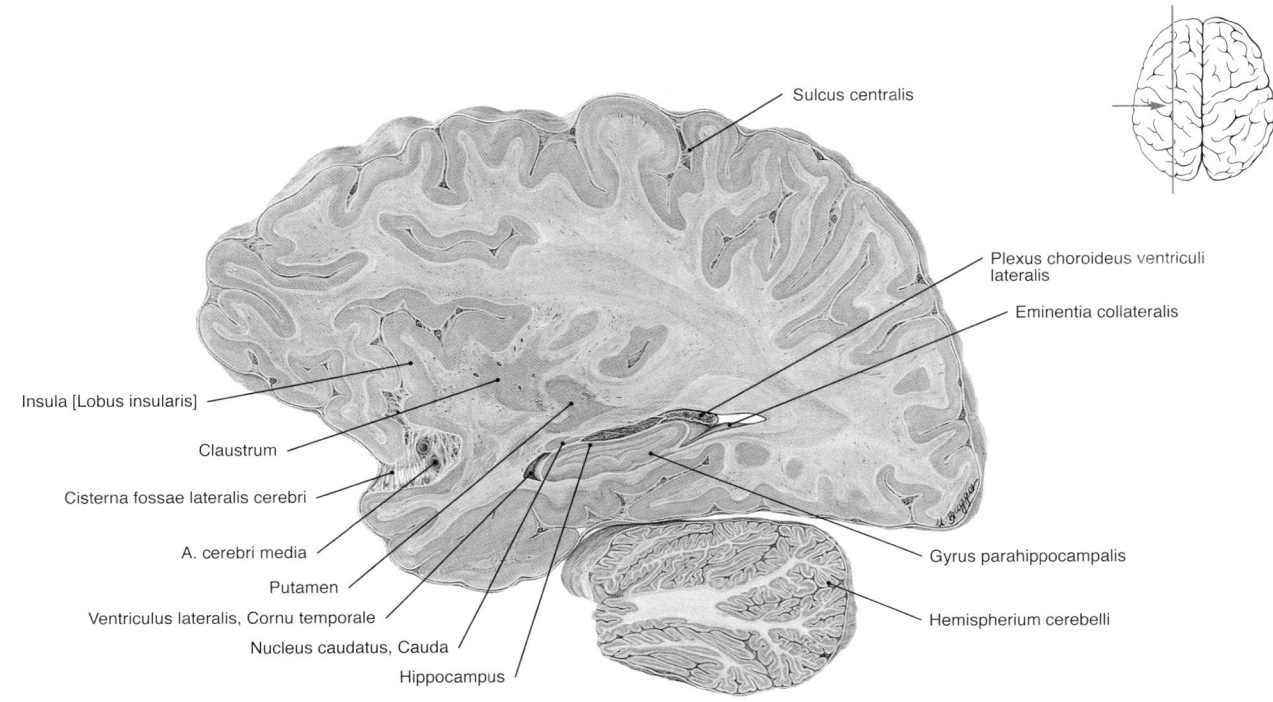

Sulcus centralis

Plexus choroideus ventriculi lateralis

Eminentia collateralis

Insula [Lobus insularis]

Claustrum

Cisterna fossae lateralis cerebri

A. cerebri media

Putamen

Ventriculus lateralis, Cornu temporale

Nucleus caudatus, Cauda

Hippocampus

Gyrus parahippocampalis

Hemispherium cerebelli

Fig. 1302 Brain, Encephalon;
sagittal section through the left hemisphere
at the level of the apex of the temporal horn.

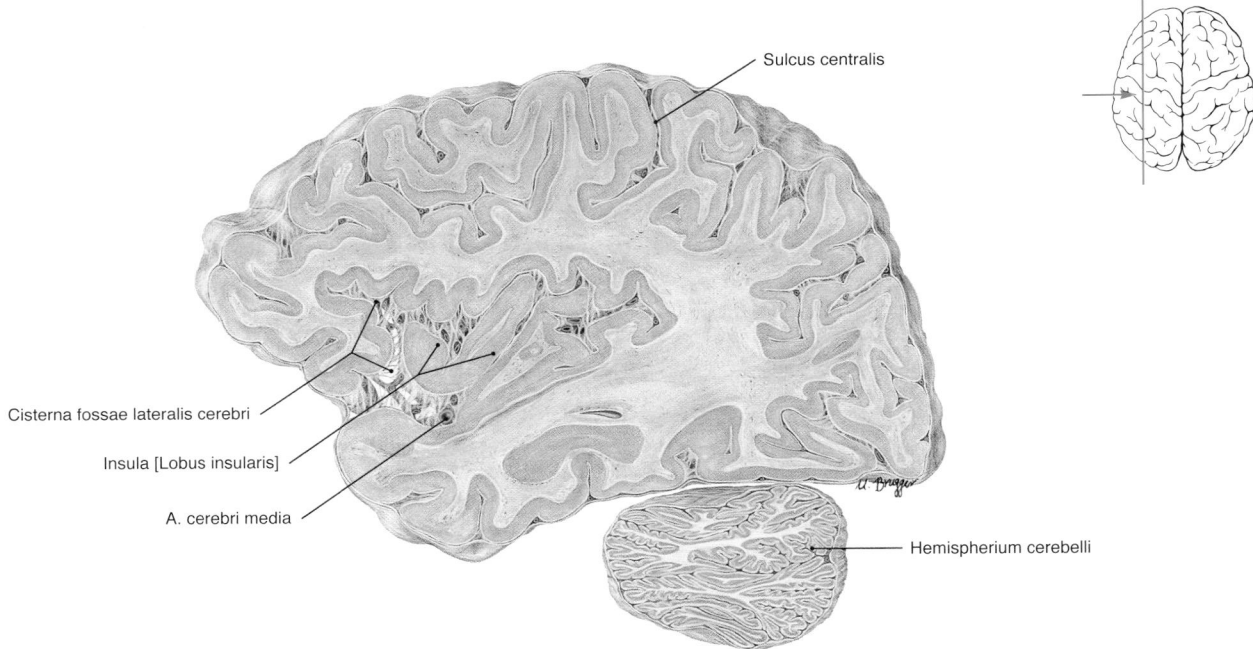

Sulcus centralis

Cisterna fossae lateralis cerebri

Insula [Lobus insularis]

A. cerebri media

Hemispherium cerebelli

Fig. 1303 Brain, Encephalon;
sagittal section through the left hemisphere
at the level of the insula.

Situs of the spinal cord

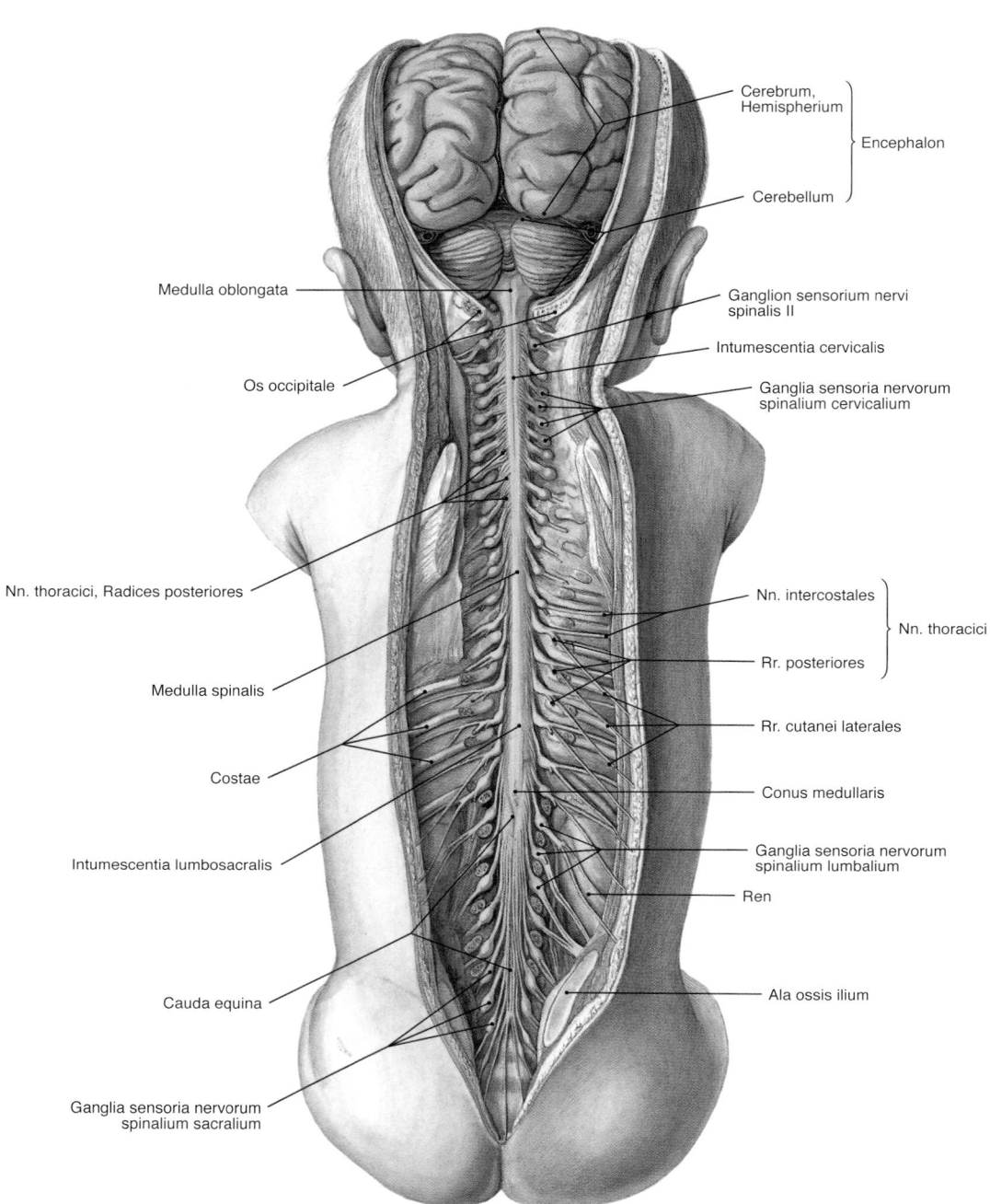

Cerebrum, Hemispherium ⎫
Cerebellum ⎬ Encephalon

Medulla oblongata

Ganglion sensorium nervi spinalis II

Intumescentia cervicalis

Os occipitale

Ganglia sensoria nervorum spinalium cervicalium

Nn. thoracici, Radices posteriores

Nn. intercostales ⎫
Rr. posteriores ⎬ Nn. thoracici

Rr. cutanei laterales

Medulla spinalis

Costae

Conus medullaris

Intumescentia lumbosacralis

Ganglia sensoria nervorum spinalium lumbalium

Ren

Cauda equina

Ala ossis ilium

Ganglia sensoria nervorum spinalium sacralium

Fig. 1304   Brain, Encephalon; spinal cord, Medulla spinalis, and spinal nerves, Nn. spinales; brain and spinal nerves in a neonate. In the neonate, the spinal cord extends two vertebral segments further caudally compared to the adult.

Segmental structure of the spinal cord

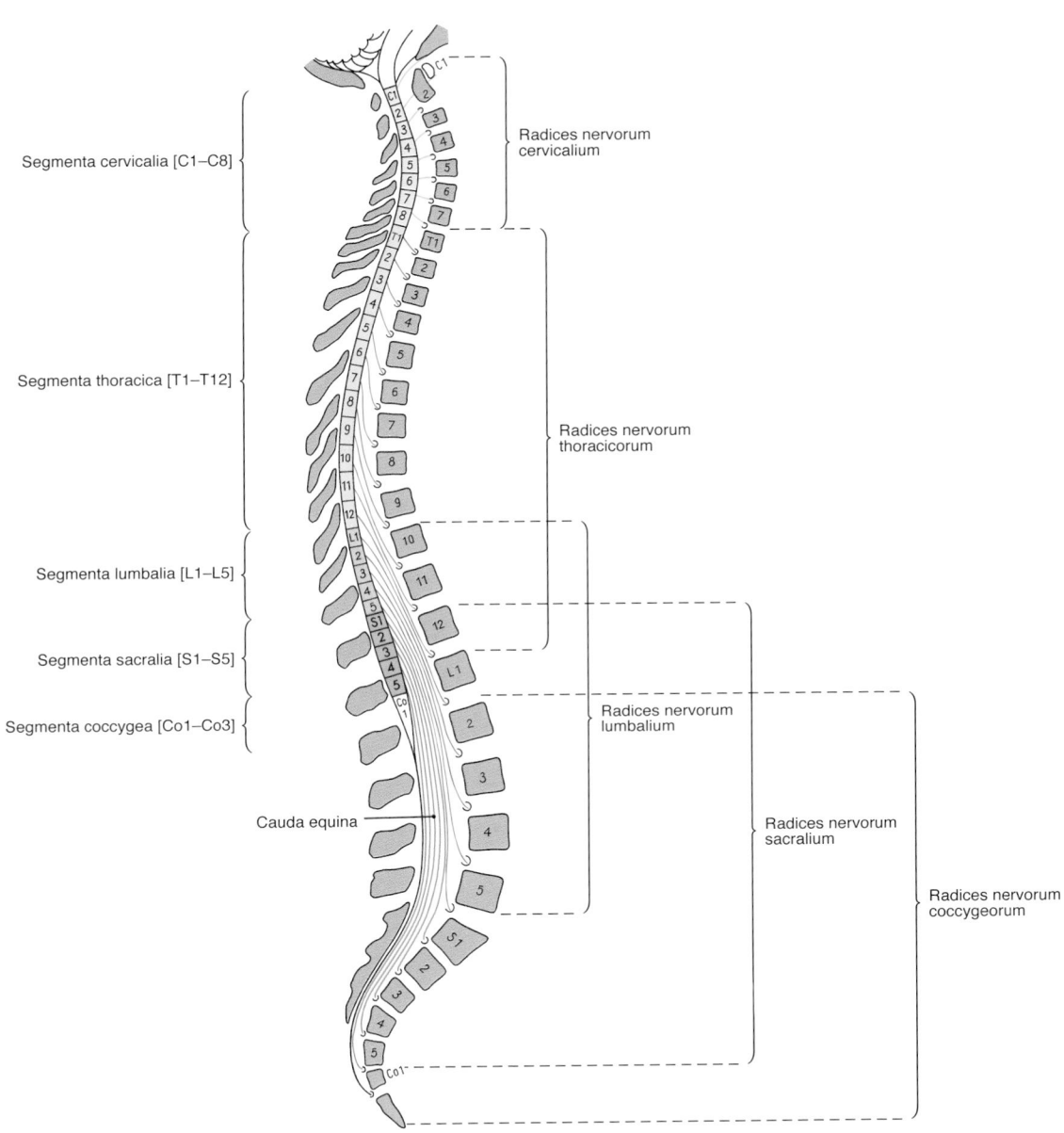

Segmenta cervicalia [C1–C8]

Segmenta thoracica [T1–T12]

Segmenta lumbalia [L1–L5]

Segmenta sacralia [S1–S5]

Segmenta coccygea [Co1–Co3]

Cauda equina

Radices nervorum cervicalium

Radices nervorum thoracicorum

Radices nervorum lumbalium

Radices nervorum sacralium

Radices nervorum coccygeorum

Fig. 1305   Spinal cord segments, Segmenta medullae spinalis, and spinal nerve roots, Radices nervorum spinalium; schematic median section.
As the spinal cord does not follow the growth of the vertebral column, the course of the spinal roots towards their corresponding segmental intervertebral foramina becomes steeper from cranial to caudal. In the neonate, the spinal cord ends at the level of the spinous process of the fourth lumbar vertebra, whereas in the adult, it extends normally only to the second lumbar vertebra.

Spinal cord

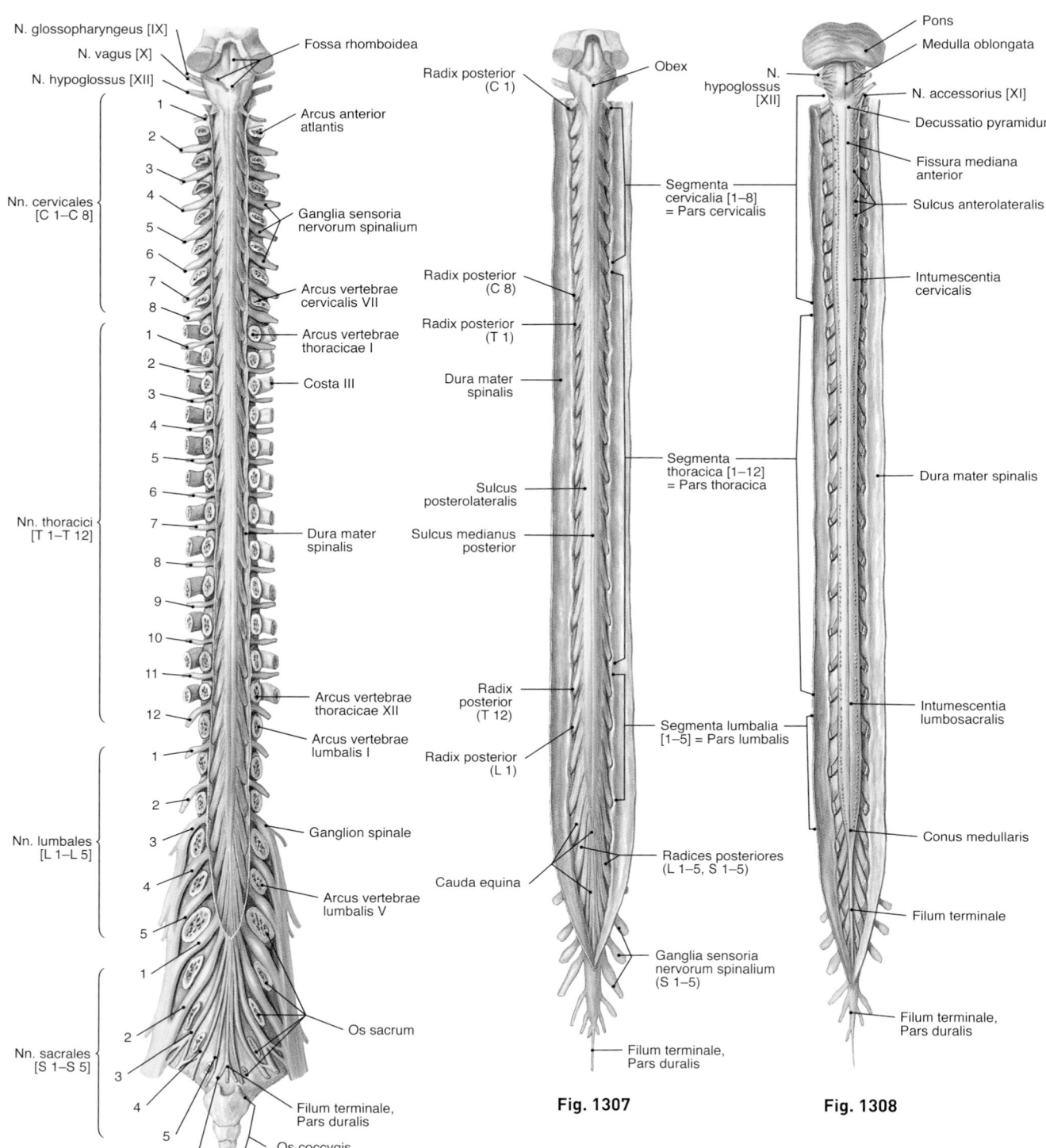

N. glossopharyngeus [IX]
N. vagus [X]
N. hypoglossus [XII]
Fossa rhomboidea
1
2
Arcus anterior atlantis
3
4
Ganglia sensoria nervorum spinalium
5
6
7
Arcus vertebrae cervicalis VII
8
Nn. cervicales [C 1–C 8]
1
Arcus vertebrae thoracicae I
2
Costa III
3
4
5
6
7
Dura mater spinalis
8
9
10
11
Arcus vertebrae thoracicae XII
12
Arcus vertebrae lumbalis I
Nn. thoracici [T 1–T 12]
1
2
3
Ganglion spinale
4
Arcus vertebrae lumbalis V
5
Nn. lumbales [L 1–L 5]
1
2
Os sacrum
3
4
Filum terminale, Pars duralis
5
Os coccygis [Vertebrae coccygeae I–IV]
N. coccygeus
Nn. sacrales [S 1–S 5]

Radix posterior (C 1)
Obex
Radix posterior (C 8)
Segmenta cervicalia [1–8] = Pars cervicalis
Radix posterior (T 1)
Dura mater spinalis
Sulcus posterolateralis
Sulcus medianus posterior
Segmenta thoracica [1–12] = Pars thoracica
Radix posterior (T 12)
Radix posterior (L 1)
Segmenta lumbalia [1–5] = Pars lumbalis
Cauda equina
Radices posteriores (L 1–5, S 1–5)
Ganglia sensoria nervorum spinalium (S 1–5)
Filum terminale, Pars duralis

Pons
Medulla oblongata
N. hypoglossus [XII]
N. accessorius [XI]
Decussatio pyramidum
Fissura mediana anterior
Sulcus anterolateralis
Intumescentia cervicalis
Dura mater spinalis
Intumescentia lumbosacralis
Conus medullaris
Filum terminale
Filum terminale, Pars duralis

Fig. 1307

Fig. 1308

Fig. 1306 Spinal cord, Medulla spinalis, and spinal nerves, Nn. spinales; situs of the spinal cord; dorsal view.
As spinal cord segments are numbered according to the spinal nerves, and the uppermost spinal nerve is counted as the first cervical nerve, there are actually eight cervical segments.

Fig. 1307 Spinal cord, Medulla spinalis, and spinal nerves, Nn. spinales; the spinal dura mater has been opened; dorsal view.

Fig. 1308 Spinal cord, Medulla spinalis, and spinal nerves, Nn. spinales; the spinal dura mater has been opened; ventral view.

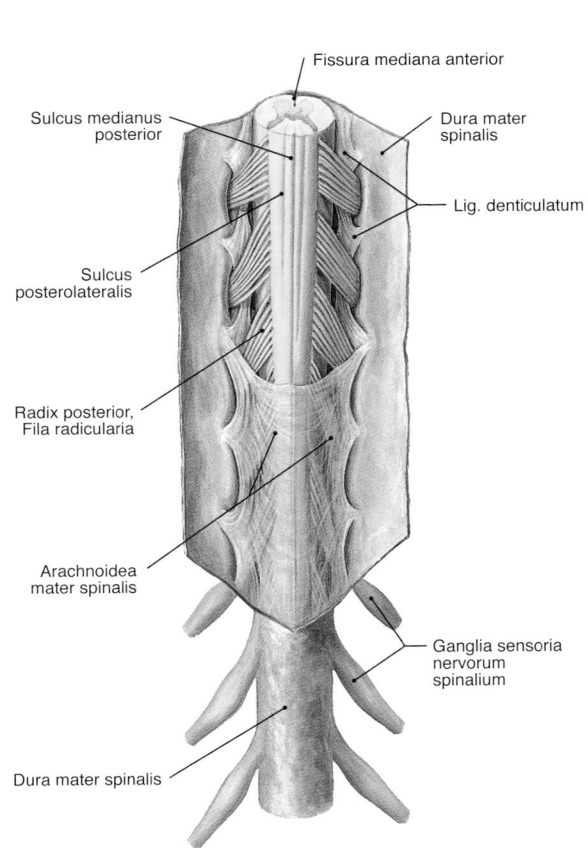

Fissura mediana anterior

Sulcus medianus posterior

Dura mater spinalis

Lig. denticulatum

Sulcus posterolateralis

Radix posterior, Fila radicularia

Arachnoidea mater spinalis

Ganglia sensoria nervorum spinalium

Dura mater spinalis

Fig. 1309 Spinal cord, Medulla spinalis, and spinal meninges, Meninges spinales; dorsal view.

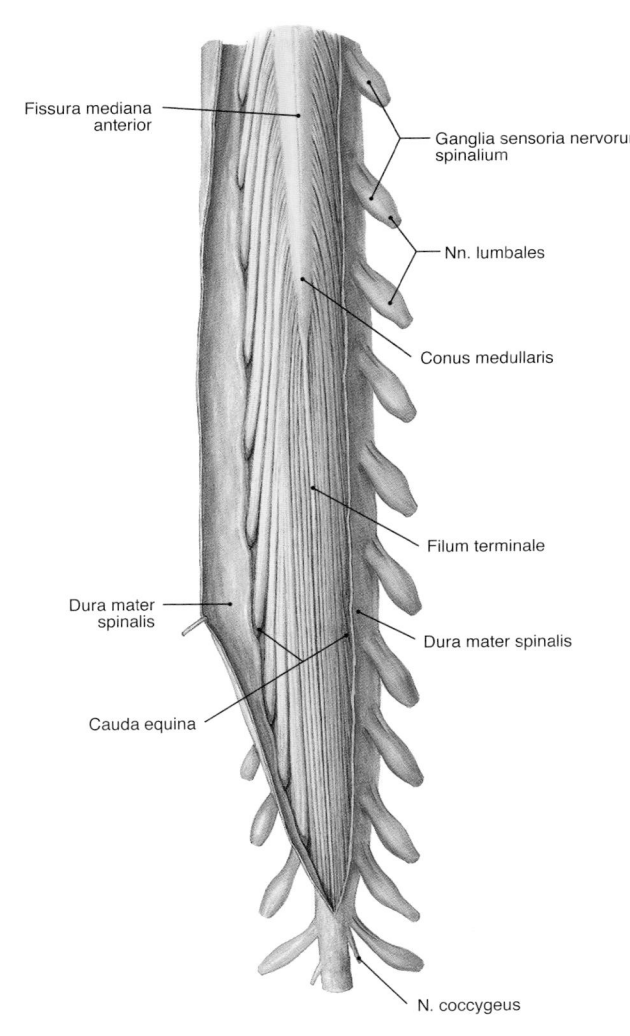

Fissura mediana anterior

Ganglia sensoria nervorum spinalium

Nn. lumbales

Conus medullaris

Filum terminale

Dura mater spinalis

Dura mater spinalis

Cauda equina

N. coccygeus

Fig. 1310 Spinal cord, Medulla spinalis; caudal part with the cauda equina, Cauda equina; ventral view.

→ 550

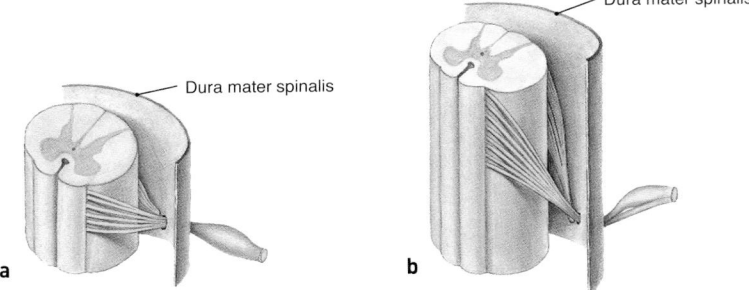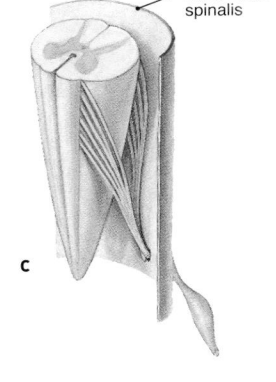

Dura mater spinalis

Dura mater spinalis

Dura mater spinalis

a

b

c

Fig. 1311 a–c Spinal nerve roots, Nn. spinales, Radices; typical course within the subarachnoid space.
a Cervical segment, Segmentum cervicale
b Thoracic segment, Segmentum thoracicum
c Lumbar segment, Segmentum lumbale

Arteries of the spinal cord

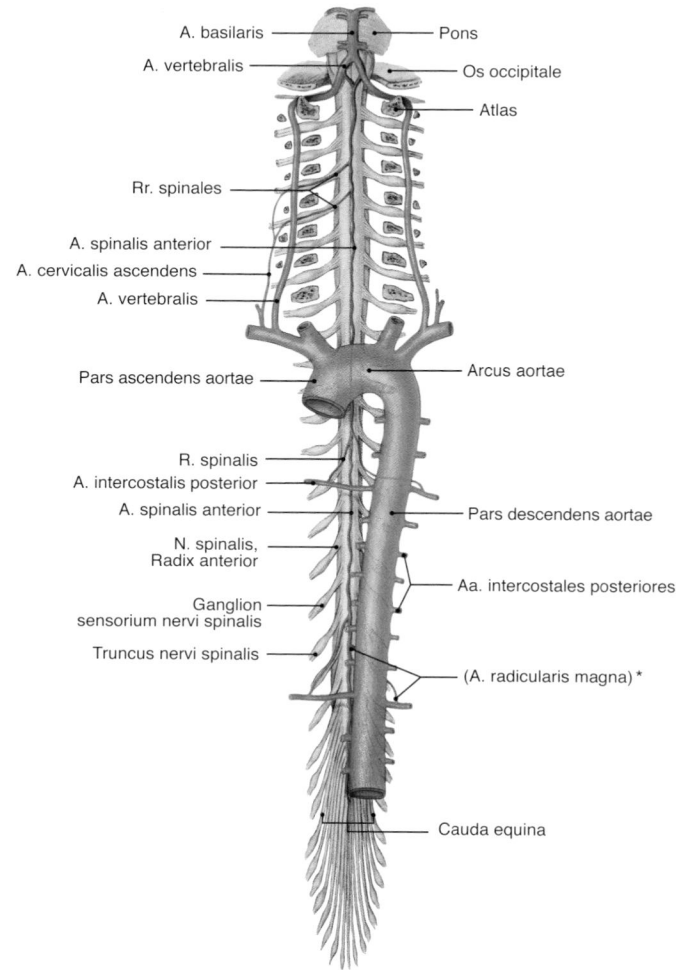

A. basilaris — Pons
A. vertebralis — Os occipitale
— Atlas
Rr. spinales —
A. spinalis anterior —
A. cervicalis ascendens —
A. vertebralis —
Pars ascendens aortae — — Arcus aortae
R. spinalis —
A. intercostalis posterior —
A. spinalis anterior — — Pars descendens aortae
N. spinalis, Radix anterior —
— Aa. intercostales posteriores
Ganglion sensorium nervi spinalis —
Truncus nervi spinalis — — (A. radicularis magna) *
— Cauda equina

Fig. 1312   Arteries of the spinal cord, Medulla spinalis.
* Clinical term: artery of ADAMKIEWICZ

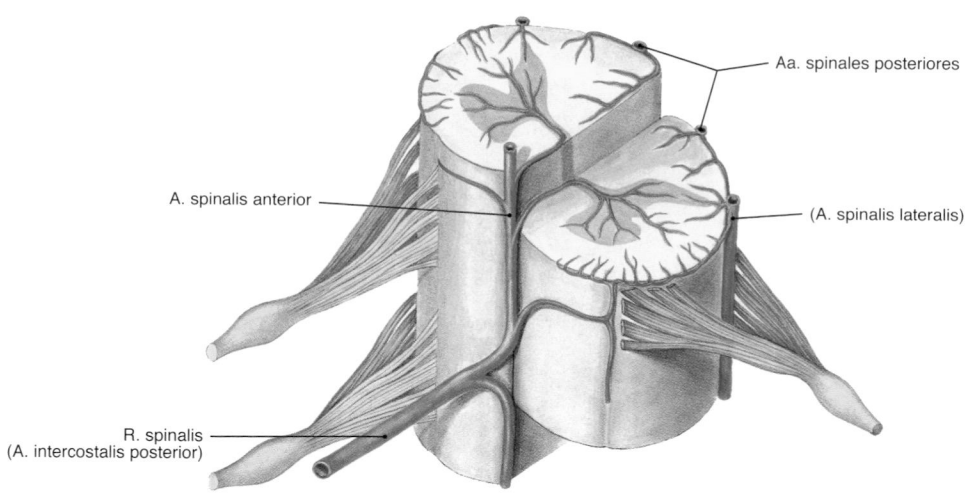

— Aa. spinales posteriores
A. spinalis anterior —
— (A. spinalis lateralis)
R. spinalis (A. intercostalis posterior) —

Fig. 1313   Arteries of the spinal cord, Medulla spinalis.

Spinal cord, structure

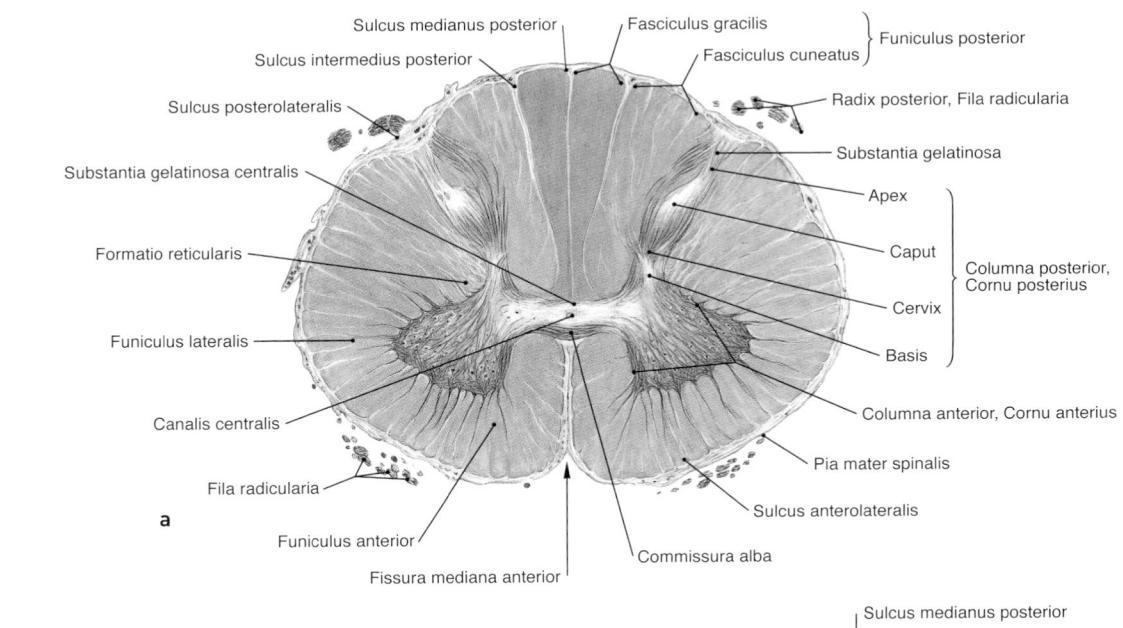

Sulcus medianus posterior
Sulcus intermedius posterior
Sulcus posterolateralis
Substantia gelatinosa centralis
Formatio reticularis
Funiculus lateralis
Canalis centralis
Fila radicularia
Funiculus anterior
Fissura mediana anterior

Fasciculus gracilis
Fasciculus cuneatus
} Funiculus posterior
Radix posterior, Fila radicularia
Substantia gelatinosa
Apex
Caput
Cervix
Basis
} Columna posterior, Cornu posterius
Columna anterior, Cornu anterius
Pia mater spinalis
Sulcus anterolateralis
Commissura alba

a

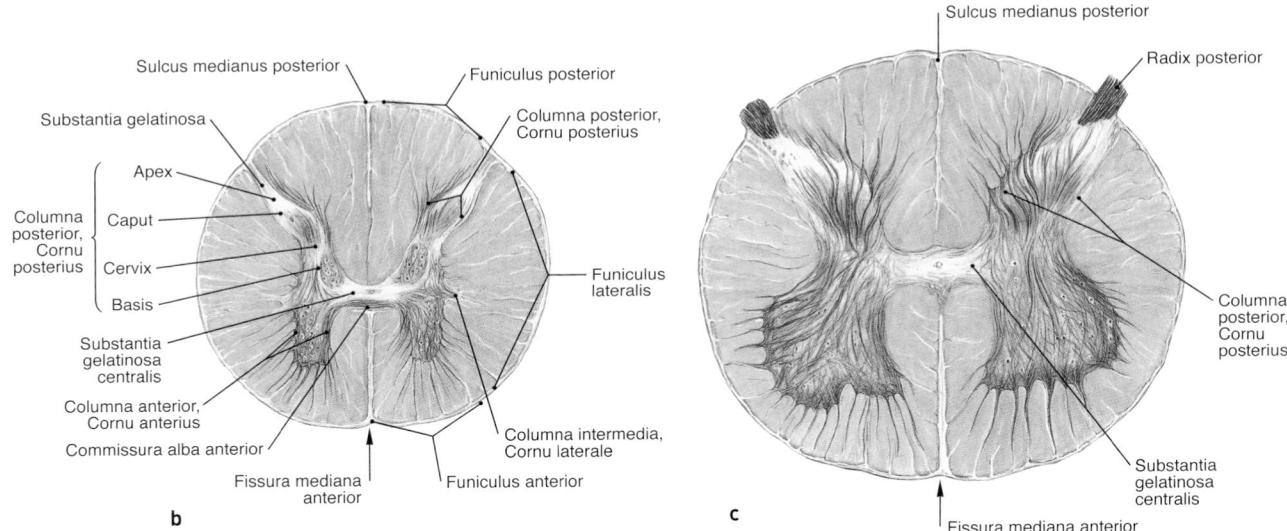

Sulcus medianus posterior
Substantia gelatinosa
Apex
Columna posterior, Cornu posterius
Caput
Cervix
Basis
Substantia gelatinosa centralis
Columna anterior, Cornu anterius
Commissura alba anterior
Fissura mediana anterior

Funiculus posterior
Columna posterior, Cornu posterius
Funiculus lateralis
Columna intermedia, Cornu laterale
Funiculus anterior

b

Sulcus medianus posterior
Radix posterior
Columna posterior, Cornu posterius
Substantia gelatinosa centralis
Fissura mediana anterior

c

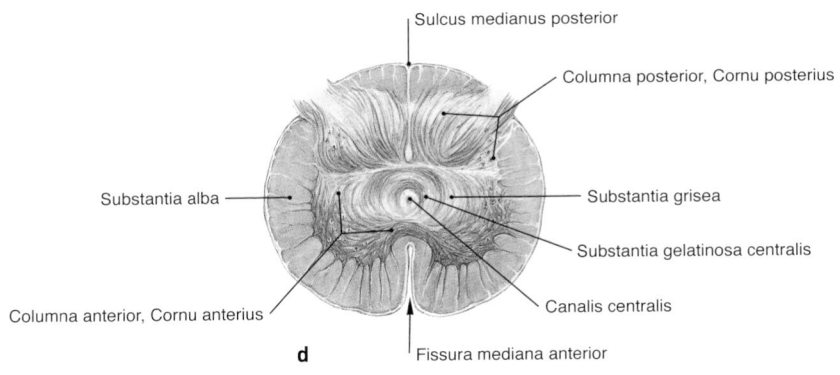

Sulcus medianus posterior
Columna posterior, Cornu posterius
Substantia alba
Substantia grisea
Substantia gelatinosa centralis
Canalis centralis
Columna anterior, Cornu anterius
Fissura mediana anterior

d

Fig. 1314 a–d Spinal cord, Medulla spinalis;
cross-sections; myelin stain; approx. 500%.
a Cervical part, Pars cervicalis
b Thoracic part, Pars thoracica
c Lumbar part, Pars lumbalis
d Sacral part, Pars sacralis

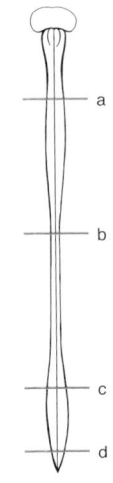

a
b
c
d

Functional organisation of the spinal cord

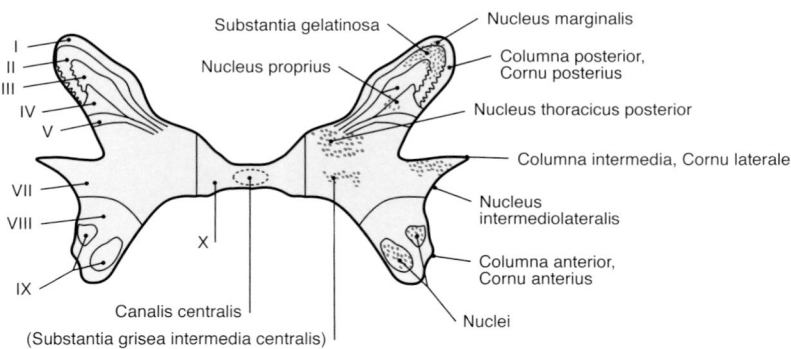

Fig. 1315 Spinal cord, Medulla spinalis;
laminar organisation of the grey matter according to its
cytoarchitecture (according to REXED, 1952), exemplified
by the tenth thoracic segment (T10).
Formation and number of the laminae vary in different
spinal cord segments.

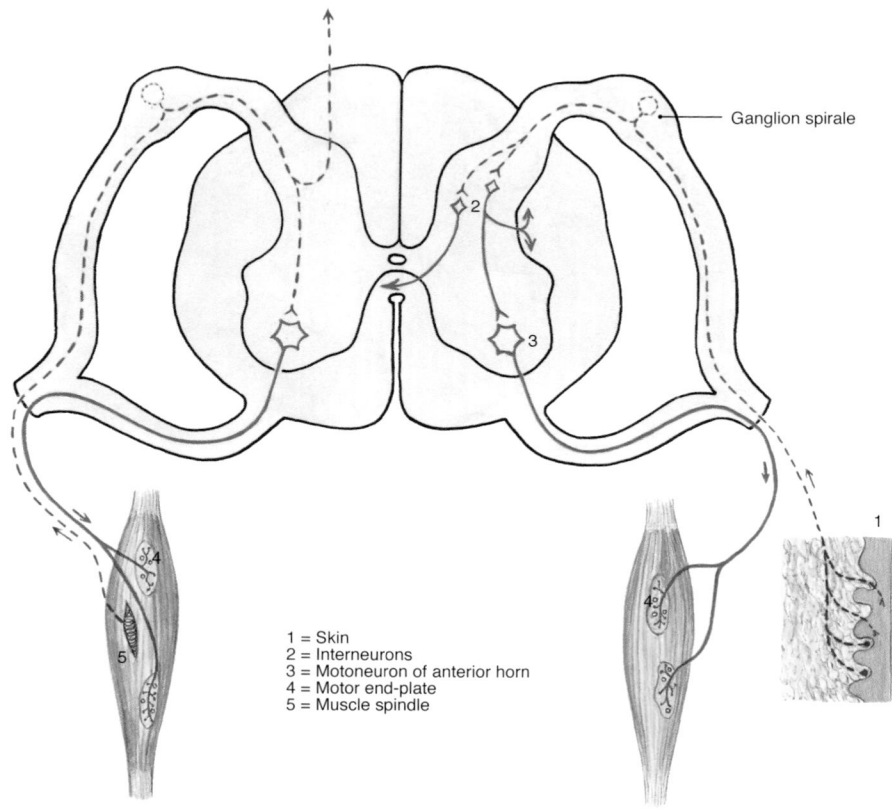

1 = Skin
2 = Interneurons
3 = Motoneuron of anterior horn
4 = Motor end-plate
5 = Muscle spindle

Fig. 1316 Reflexes at the spinal cord;
left: monosynaptic reflex (bineuronal, proprioceptive, myostatic, e.g.,
patellar tendon reflex, Achilles tendon reflex, etc.);
right: polysynaptic reflex (polyneuronal, e.g., abdominal reflex,
cremasteric reflex, plantar reflex, etc.).

Functional organisation of the spinal cord

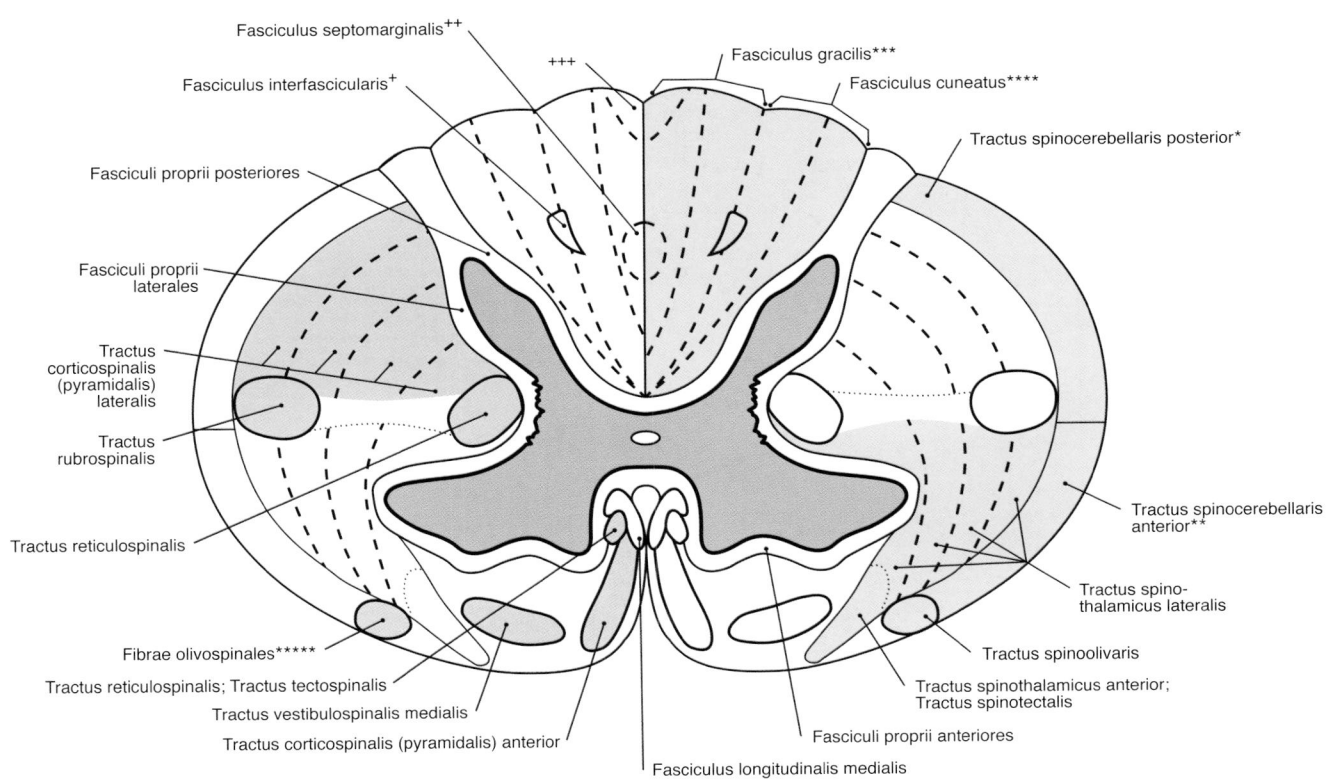

Fasciculus septomarginalis++

Fasciculus interfascicularis+

+++

Fasciculus gracilis***

Fasciculus cuneatus****

Fasciculi proprii posteriores

Tractus spinocerebellaris posterior*

Fasciculi proprii laterales

Tractus corticospinalis (pyramidalis) lateralis

Tractus rubrospinalis

Tractus reticulospinalis

Tractus spinocerebellaris anterior**

Tractus spino-thalamicus lateralis

Fibrae olivospinales*****

Tractus spinoolivaris

Tractus reticulospinalis; Tractus tectospinalis

Tractus vestibulospinalis medialis

Tractus spinothalamicus anterior; Tractus spinotectalis

Tractus corticospinalis (pyramidalis) anterior

Fasciculi proprii anteriores

Fasciculus longitudinalis medialis

Fig. 1317 Spinal cord, Medulla spinalis; schematic organisation of the white matter exemplified by a lower cervical segment.
Afferent (= ascending) pathways in blue; efferent (= descending) pathways in red.
* Clinical term: FLECHSIG's tract
** Clinical term: GOWER's tract
*** Clinical term: GOLL's tract
**** Clinical term: BURDACH's tract
***** The actual existence of these fibres has not definitely been documented.

The regions indicated by +, ++, and +++ designate descending collateral tracts of the posterior fasciculi.

+ SCHULTZE's comma tract (cervical part)
++ FLECHSIG's oval bundle (thoracic part)
+++ Triangle of PHILIPPE-GOMBAULT (lumbar and sacral parts)

Pathways of the spinal cord

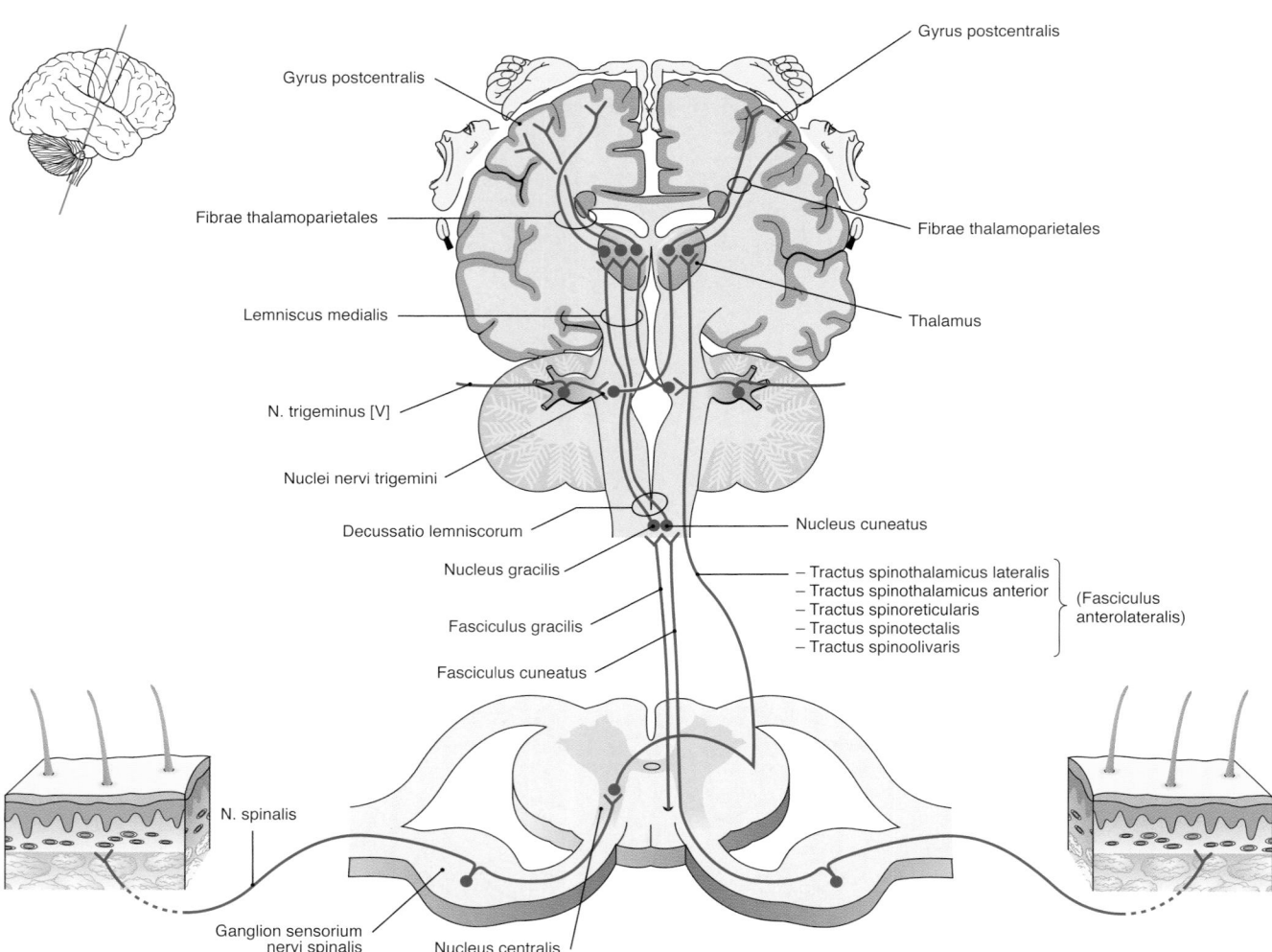

Fig. 1318   Pathways for epicritic (blue) and protopathic (green) sensibility.

Ascending pathways

Pathway for epicritic sensibility (tactile pathway)
(Precise differentiation of pressure and touch)

1. neuron (uncrossed)
    From receptors (exteroceptors) in the skin and the mucosa, as well as the periosteum, the joints and the muscle spindles etc., to the cuneate and gracile nucleus in the medulla oblongata: gracile and cuneate fasciculus (perikarya in the spinal ganglia): descending collaterals (see Fig. 1317).
2. neuron (crossed)
    From the medulla oblongata (cuneate and gracile nucleus) to the thalamus (medial lemniscus, perikarya in the cuneate and gracile nucleus).
3. neuron (uncrossed) From the thalamus to the cerebral cortex, particularly to the postcentral gyrus (thalamocortical fibres, perikarya in the thalamus).

Pathway for protopathic sensibility (pain pathway)
(Pain, temperature, general pressure sensation)

1. neuron (uncrossed)
    From receptors (exteroceptors) of the skin and the mucosa etc., to the posterior horn, laminae I–V (perikarya in the spinal ganglia).
2. neuron (crossed, some fibres possibly uncrossed)
    From the posterior horn to the thalamus, in the reticular formation and to the midbrain tectum (anterior and lateral spinothalamic tracts, spinoreticular tract, spinotectal tract; perikarya in the posterior column).
3. neuron (uncrossed)
    From the thalamus among others to the cerebral cortex, particularly to the postcentral gyrus (thalamocortical fibres, perikarya in the thalamus).

Pathways of the spinal cord

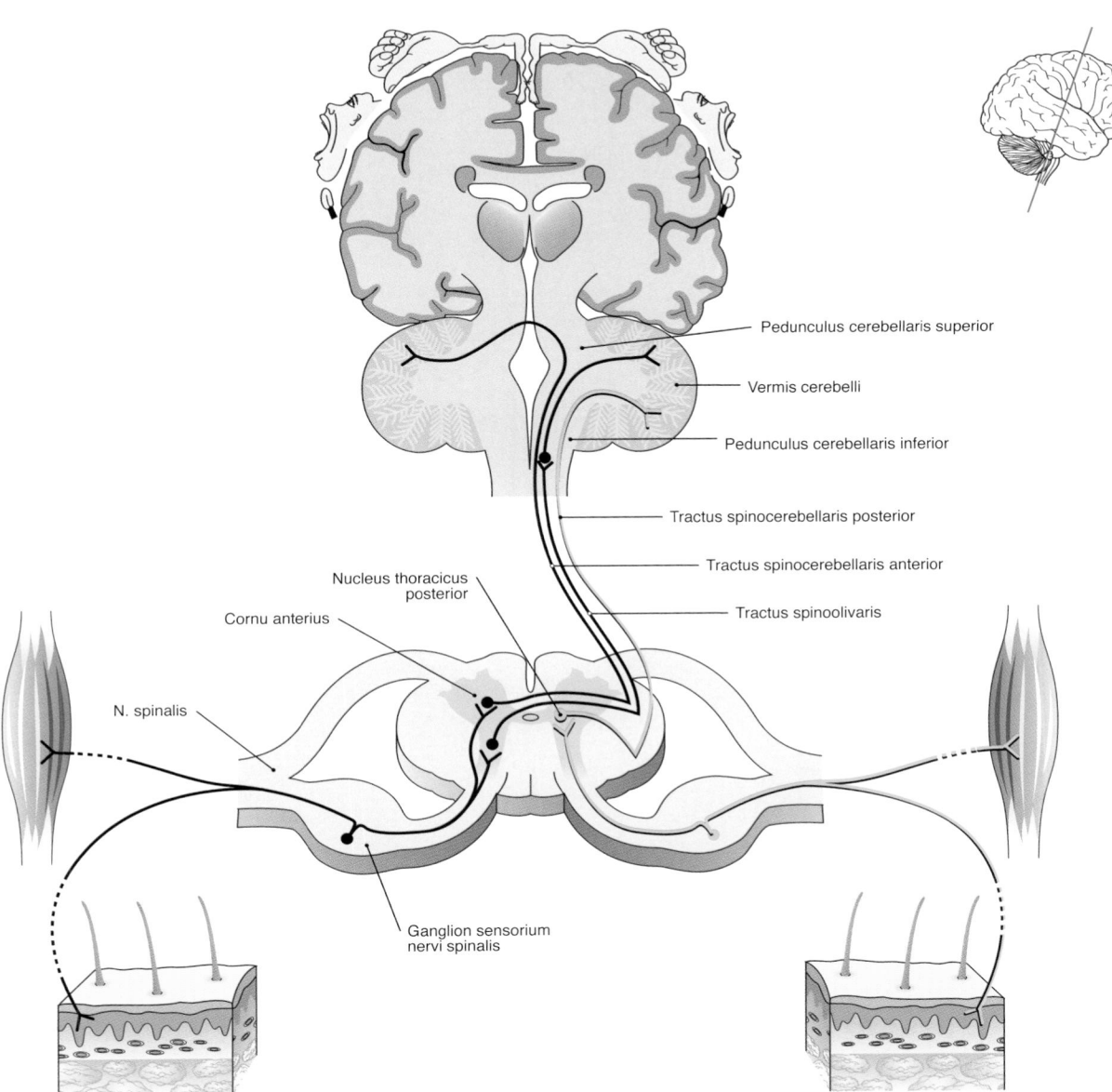

Pedunculus cerebellaris superior

Vermis cerebelli

Pedunculus cerebellaris inferior

Tractus spinocerebellaris posterior

Tractus spinocerebellaris anterior

Tractus spinoolivaris

Nucleus thoracicus posterior

Cornu anterius

N. spinalis

Ganglion sensorium nervi spinalis

Fig. 1319 Pathways for unconscious deep sensibility.

Ascending pathways

Pathway for unconscious deep sensibility
(Unconscious, but precise spatial differentiation as a prerequisite for movement coordination by the cerebellum)

Via the anterior cerebellar tract

1. neuron (uncrossed)
   From receptors (proprioceptors) in muscles, tendons, and the connective tissue to the nuclei of the intermediate zone and the anterior column (perikarya in the spinal ganglia).
2. neuron (crossed)
   From the anterior horn within the anterior spinocerebellar tract of the anterolateral tract to the cerebellum via the superior cerebellar peduncle (perikarya in the intermediate zone and the anterior horn).

Via the posterior cerebellar tract

1. neuron (uncrossed)
   From end organs (proprioceptors) in muscles, tendons, and the connective tissue to the nuclei of the posterior column and the thoracic nucleus (perikarya in the spinal ganglia).
2. neuron (uncrossed)
   From the posterior horn and the thoracic nucleus within the posterior spinocerebellar tract of the lateral tract to the cerebellum via the inferior cerebellar peduncle (perikarya in the thoracic nucleus and at the base of the posterior column).

Pathways of the spinal cord

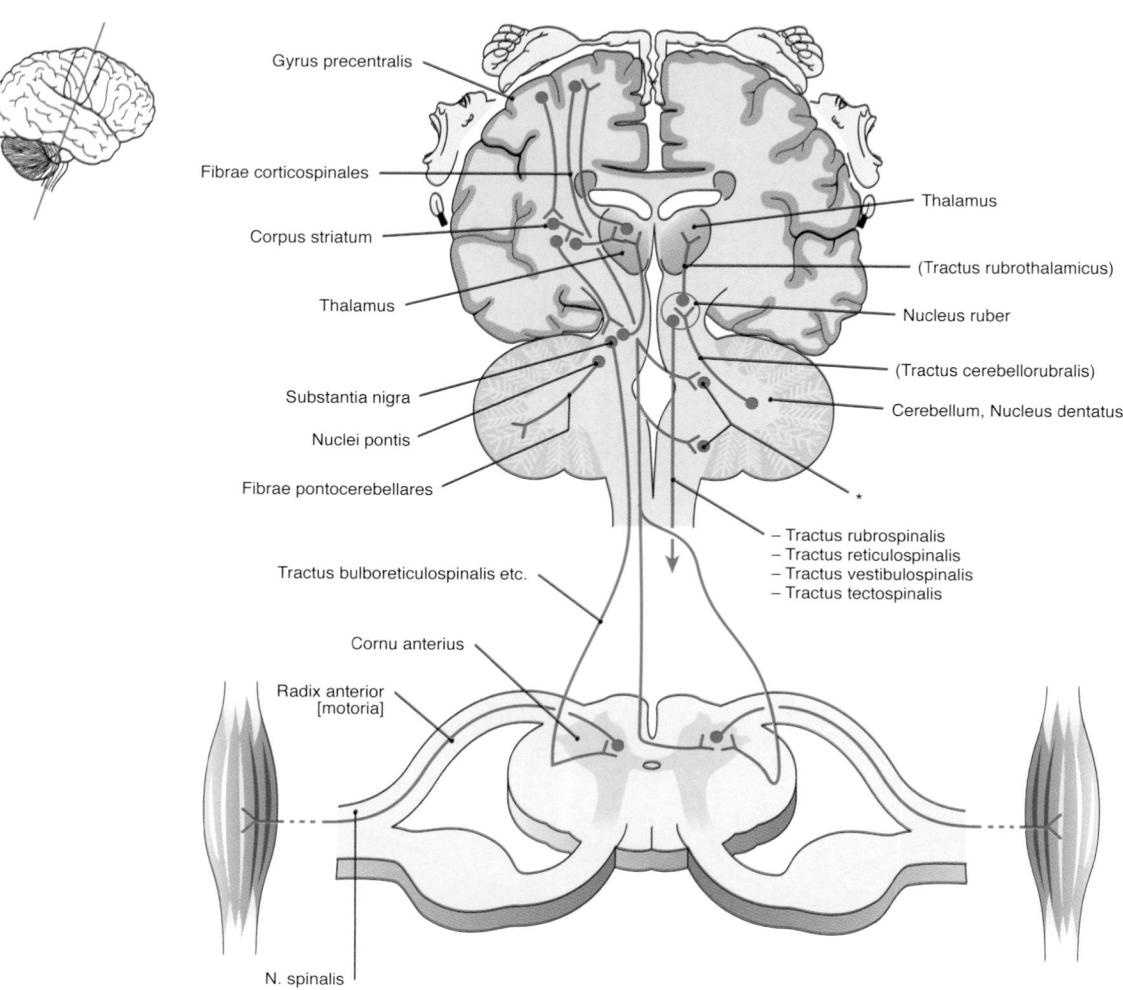

Gyrus precentralis

Fibrae corticospinales

Corpus striatum

Thalamus

Substantia nigra

Nuclei pontis

Fibrae pontocerebellares

Tractus bulboreticulospinalis etc.

Cornu anterius

Radix anterior [motoria]

N. spinalis

Thalamus

(Tractus rubrothalamicus)

Nucleus ruber

(Tractus cerebellorubralis)

Cerebellum, Nucleus dentatus

*

– Tractus rubrospinalis
– Tractus reticulospinalis
– Tractus vestibulospinalis
– Tractus tectospinalis

Fig. 1320   Pathways of the motor system.
* Motor nuclei of cranial nerves

Descending pathways

The motor system comprises a large number of nuclear regions and tracts. The "motor final path" are the motoneurons. Despite the extraordinary complexity of these circuits, the traditional organisation will be maintained for didactic reasons.

(So-called) Pyramidal tract

1. (central) neuron (crossed)
    From the cerebral cortex through the internal capsule and the cerebral peduncles to interneurons within the anterior and posterior column (lateral corticospinal tract, anterior corticospinal tract, perikarya in the precentral gyrus). Branching off of fibres to the nuclei of the cranial nerves (corticonuclear fibres and bulbar corticonuclear fibres).
2. (peripheral) neuron (motor end pathway, α-motoneurons)
    From the anterior horn to the motor end plates of the skeletal musculature (motoneurons, perikarya in the anterior horn).

(So-called) Extrapyramidal motor system

1. central neurons (crossed and uncrossed)
    From the cerebral cortex, particularly the precentral gyrus and the adjacent cortical areas including synapses to the basal ganglia, thalamus, subthalamic nucleus, red nucleus, substantia nigra, cerebellum, etc. and feedback loops to the interneurons of the anterior column (rubrospinal tract, medial and lateral vestibulospinal tract, reticulospinal tract, tectospinal tract).
2. peripheral neuron (motor end pathway, α-motoneurons)
    From the anterior horn to the motor end-plates of the skeletal muscles (motoneurons; perikarya in the anterior horn).

Lesions of the spinal cord

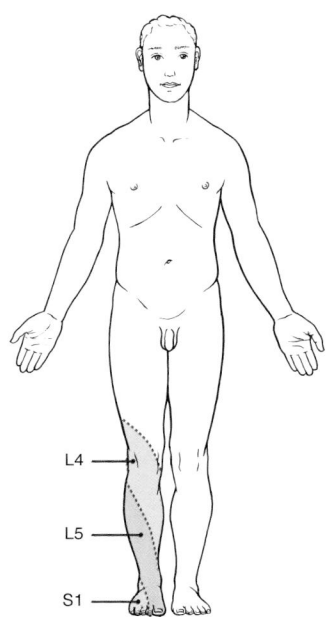

Fig. 1321 Dysfunctional cutaneous innervation due to palsy of certain, frequently affected spinal nerves.

L4
L5
S1

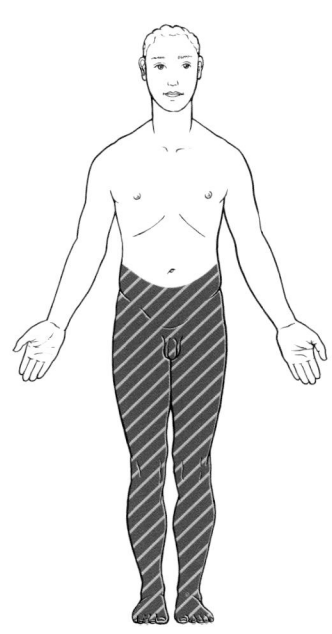

Fig. 1322 Complete paraplegia at the level of the eleventh thoracic segment.
Paralysis of the complete motor and sensory system.

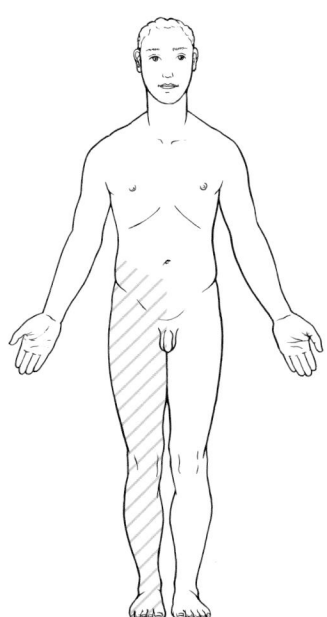

Fig. 1323 Paralysis of the tracts of the right posterior funiculus at the level of the eleventh thoracic segment.
Loss of fine tactile sensation as well as loss of sense of position and vibration (rough touch sensation remains functional).

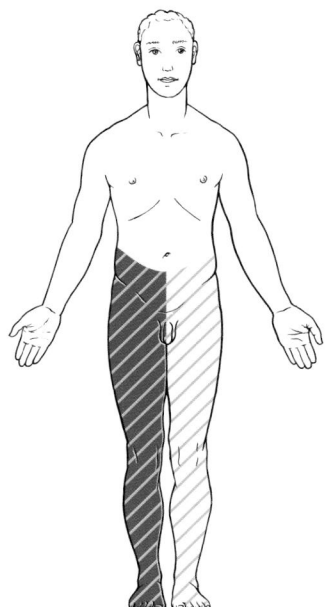

Fig. 1324 Hemiplegia (BROWN-SÉQUARD) due to disruption of the half of the spinal cord on the right side at the level of the eleventh thoracic segment.
On the right side (ipsilaterally): loss of motor function (initially flaccid, later spastic); loss of fine tactile sensation as well as loss of sense of position and vibration (rough touch sensation remains functional).
On the left side (contralaterally): loss of pain and temperature sensation.

Eyelids

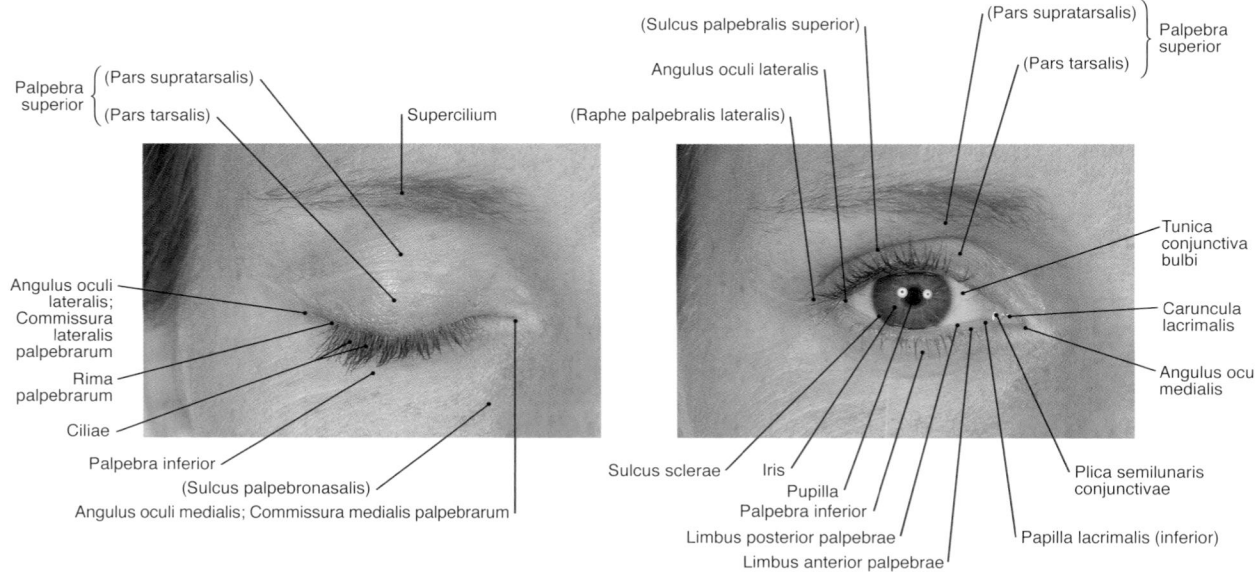

Fig. 1325 Eyelids, Palpebrae.

Fig. 1326 Eye, Oculus, and eyelids, Palpebrae.

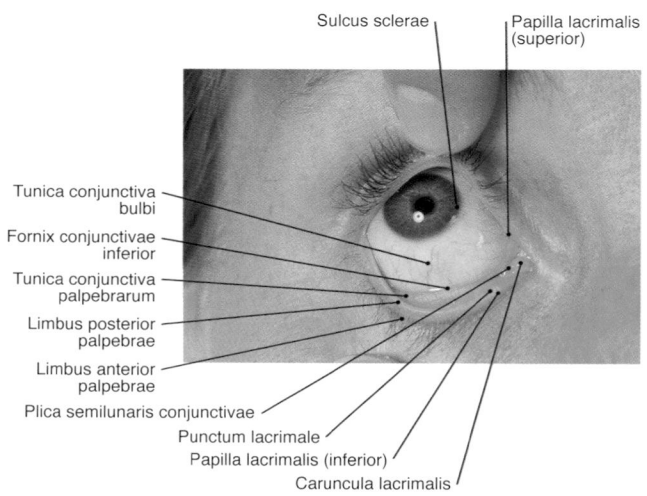

Fig. 1327 Eye, Oculus, and eyelids, Palpebrae.

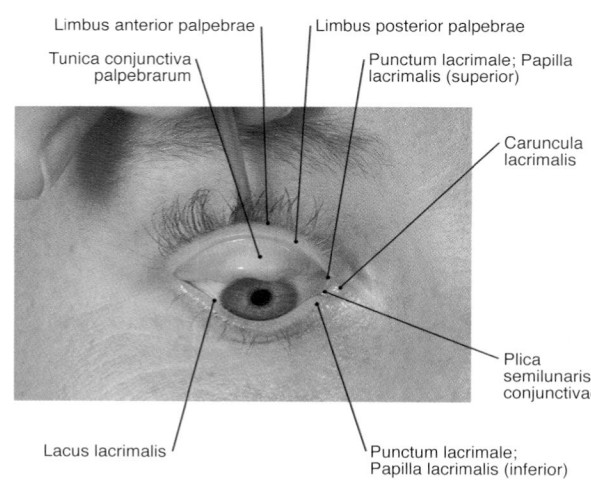

Fig. 1328 Eye, Oculus, and eyelids, Palpebrae.
Eversion of the upper eyelid (extropionisation) is hindered
by the stiffness of the tarsus, but can be facilitated with
the aid of a small hook.

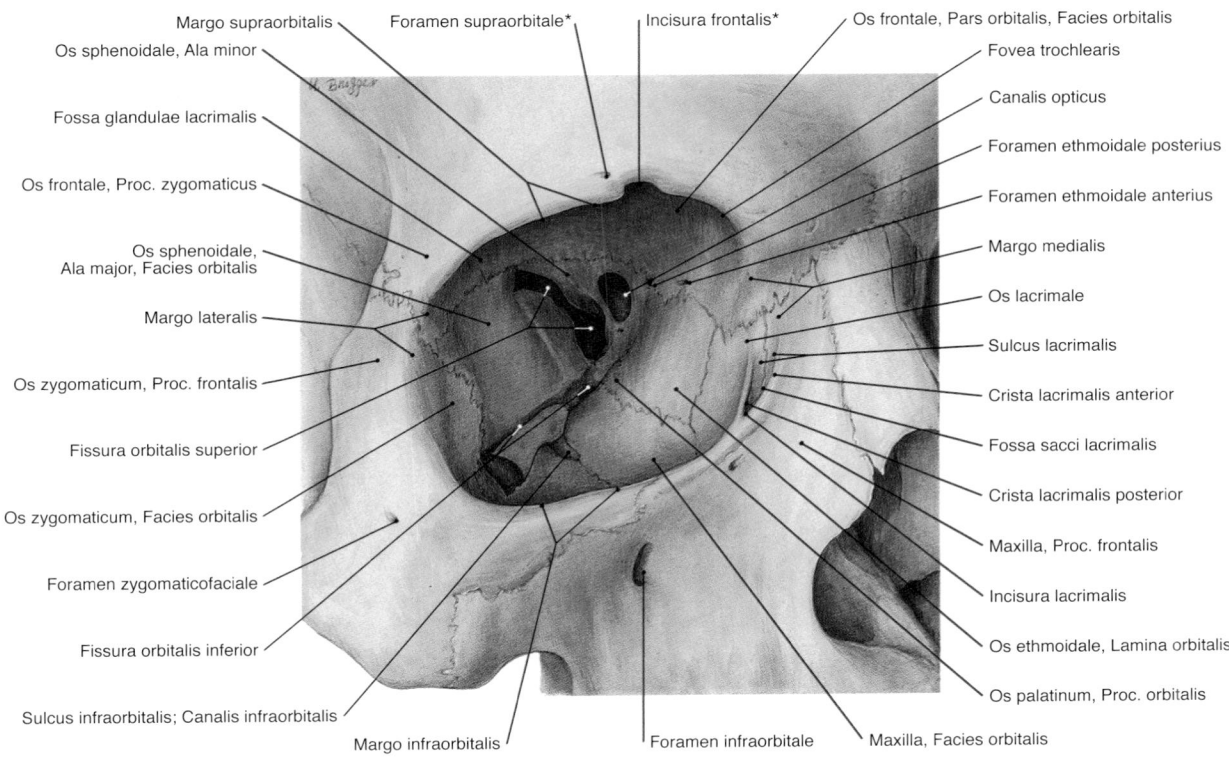

Margo supraorbitalis

Foramen supraorbitale*

Incisura frontalis*

Os frontale, Pars orbitalis, Facies orbitalis

Os sphenoidale, Ala minor

Fovea trochlearis

Fossa glandulae lacrimalis

Canalis opticus

Os frontale, Proc. zygomaticus

Foramen ethmoidale posterius

Foramen ethmoidale anterius

Os sphenoidale, Ala major, Facies orbitalis

Margo medialis

Margo lateralis

Os lacrimale

Os zygomaticum, Proc. frontalis

Sulcus lacrimalis

Fissura orbitalis superior

Crista lacrimalis anterior

Os zygomaticum, Facies orbitalis

Fossa sacci lacrimalis

Crista lacrimalis posterior

Foramen zygomaticofaciale

Maxilla, Proc. frontalis

Fissura orbitalis inferior

Incisura lacrimalis

Os ethmoidale, Lamina orbitalis

Sulcus infraorbitalis; Canalis infraorbitalis

Os palatinum, Proc. orbitalis

Margo infraorbitalis

Foramen infraorbitale

Maxilla, Facies orbitalis

Fig. 1329 Orbit, Orbita;
oblique view from lateral.
* These structures can be present as
foramina or notches.

Foramina ethmoidalia
anterius et posterius

Squama
frontalis

Os ethmoidale, Lamina orbitalis

Pars
orbitalis

Os frontale

Fissura orbitalis superior

Canalis opticus

Facies
orbitalis

Os sphenoidale,
Ala minor

Os nasale

Os sphenoidale,
Ala major

Os lacrimale

Fissura orbitalis
inferior

Maxilla,
Proc. frontalis

Canalis
nasolacrimalis

Facies
orbitalis

Maxilla

Fossa
pterygopalatina

Corpus
maxillae

Os sphenoidale,
Proc.
pterygoideus

Sinus maxillaris

Proc.
pyramidalis

Os palatinum

Proc. orbitalis

Fig. 1330 Medial wall, Paries medialis,
of the orbit, Orbita;
lateral view.

Squama frontalis

Pars orbitalis

Os frontale

Facies orbitalis

Margo lateralis

Foramen zygomaticoorbitale

Fissura orbitalis superior

Os zygomaticum,
Facies orbitalis

Ala major

Os sphenoidale

Corpus

Fissura orbitalis inferior

Fissura pterygomaxillaris

Maxilla, Facies orbitalis

Sinus maxillaris

Canalis infraorbitalis

Fig. 1331 Lateral wall, Paries lateralis,
of the orbit, Orbita;
medial view.

Eyelids

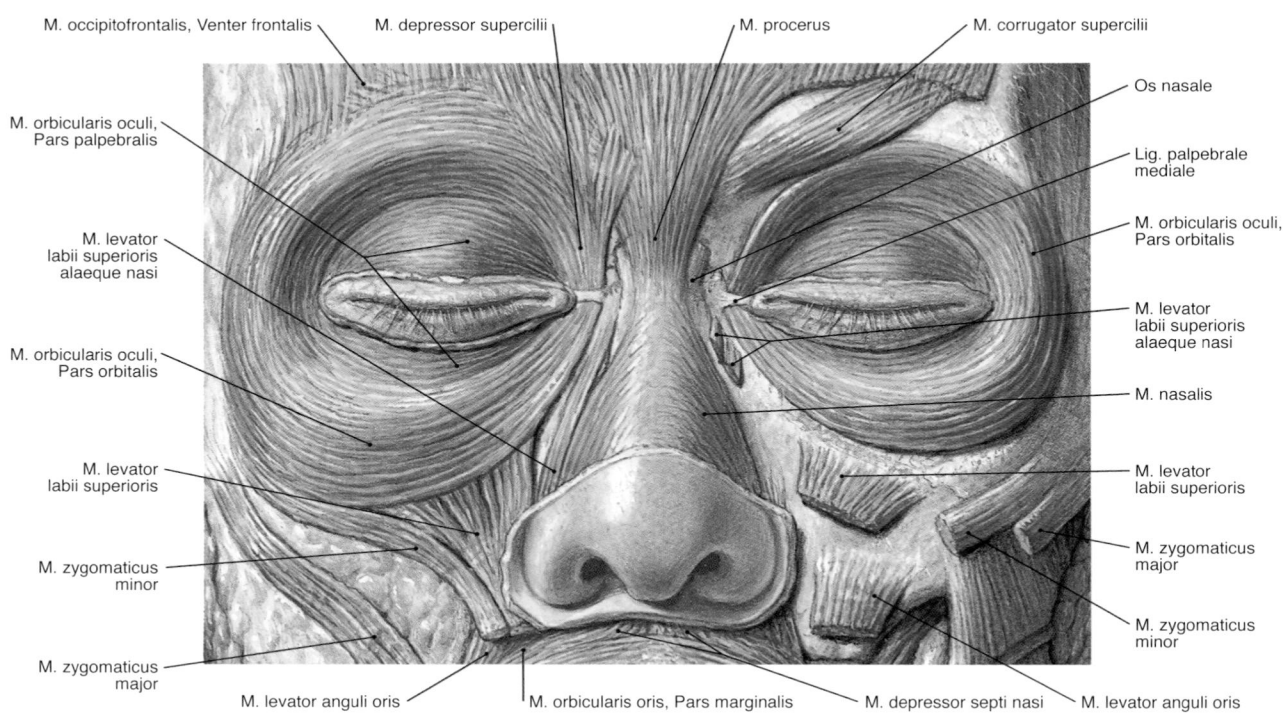

M. occipitofrontalis, Venter frontalis — M. depressor supercilii — M. procerus — M. corrugator supercilii

M. orbicularis oculi, Pars palpebralis

M. levator labii superioris alaeque nasi

M. orbicularis oculi, Pars orbitalis

M. levator labii superioris

M. zygomaticus minor

M. zygomaticus major

Os nasale

Lig. palpebrale mediale

M. orbicularis oculi, Pars orbitalis

M. levator labii superioris alaeque nasi

M. nasalis

M. levator labii superioris

M. zygomaticus major

M. zygomaticus minor

M. levator anguli oris — M. orbicularis oris, Pars marginalis — M. depressor septi nasi — M. levator anguli oris

→ 119, 120, T 1 a, c, d, e

Fig. 1332 Facial muscles, Mm. faciei.

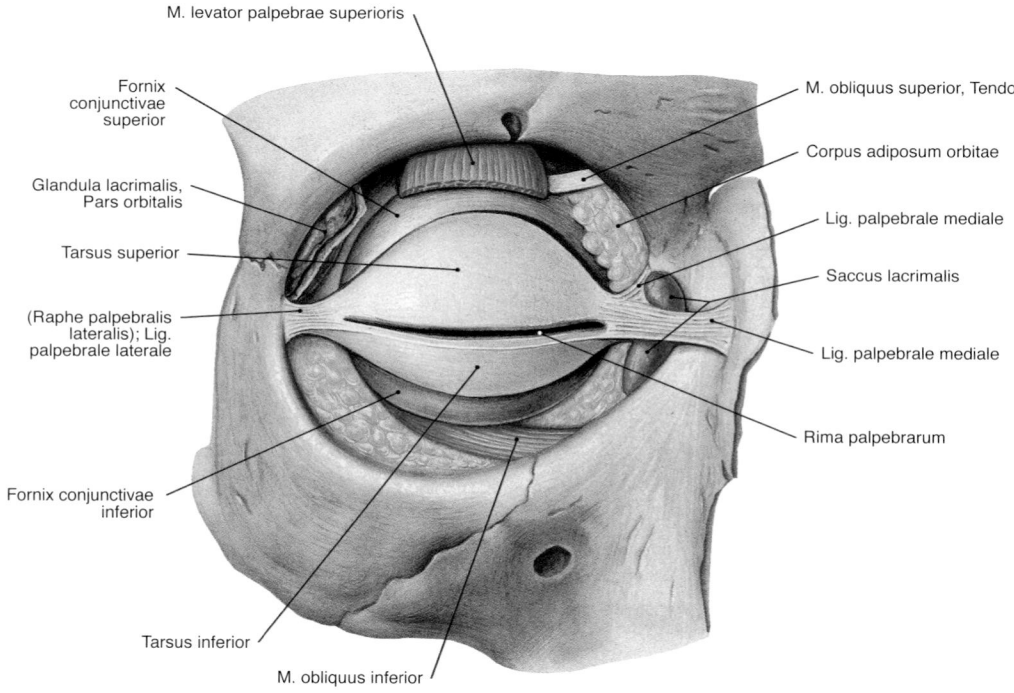

M. levator palpebrae superioris

Fornix conjunctivae superior

Glandula lacrimalis, Pars orbitalis

Tarsus superior

(Raphe palpebralis lateralis); Lig. palpebrale laterale

Fornix conjunctivae inferior

Tarsus inferior

M. obliquus inferior

M. obliquus superior, Tendo

Corpus adiposum orbitae

Lig. palpebrale mediale

Saccus lacrimalis

Lig. palpebrale mediale

Rima palpebrarum

Fig. 1333 Orbital opening, Aditus orbitalis, with eyelids, Palpebrae.

Eyelids, structure

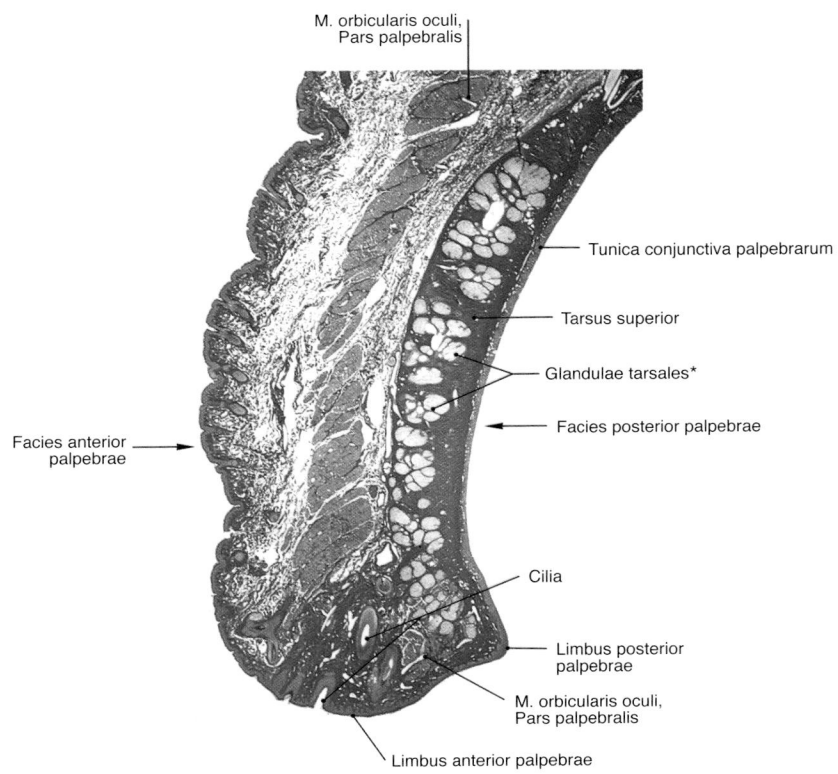

M. orbicularis oculi,
Pars palpebralis

Tunica conjunctiva palpebrarum

Tarsus superior

Glandulae tarsales*

Facies posterior palpebrae

Facies anterior
palpebrae

Cilia

Limbus posterior
palpebrae

M. orbicularis oculi,
Pars palpebralis

Limbus anterior palpebrae

Fig. 1334   Upper eyelid, Palpebra superior;
photograph of a microscopic specimen;
azan stain;
sagittal section, magnified.
* Clinical term: MEIBOMian glands

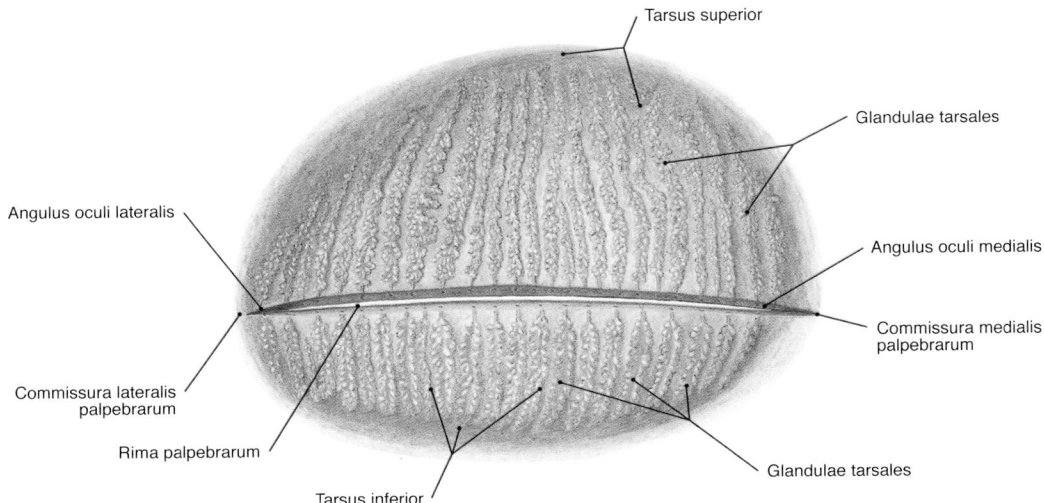

Tarsus superior

Glandulae tarsales

Angulus oculi lateralis

Angulus oculi medialis

Commissura medialis
palpebrarum

Commissura lateralis
palpebrarum

Rima palpebrarum

Glandulae tarsales

Tarsus inferior

Fig. 1335   Eyelids, Palpebrae;
translucent specimen illustrating the excretory ductules
of the tarsal glands;
posterior view.

Lacrimal apparatus

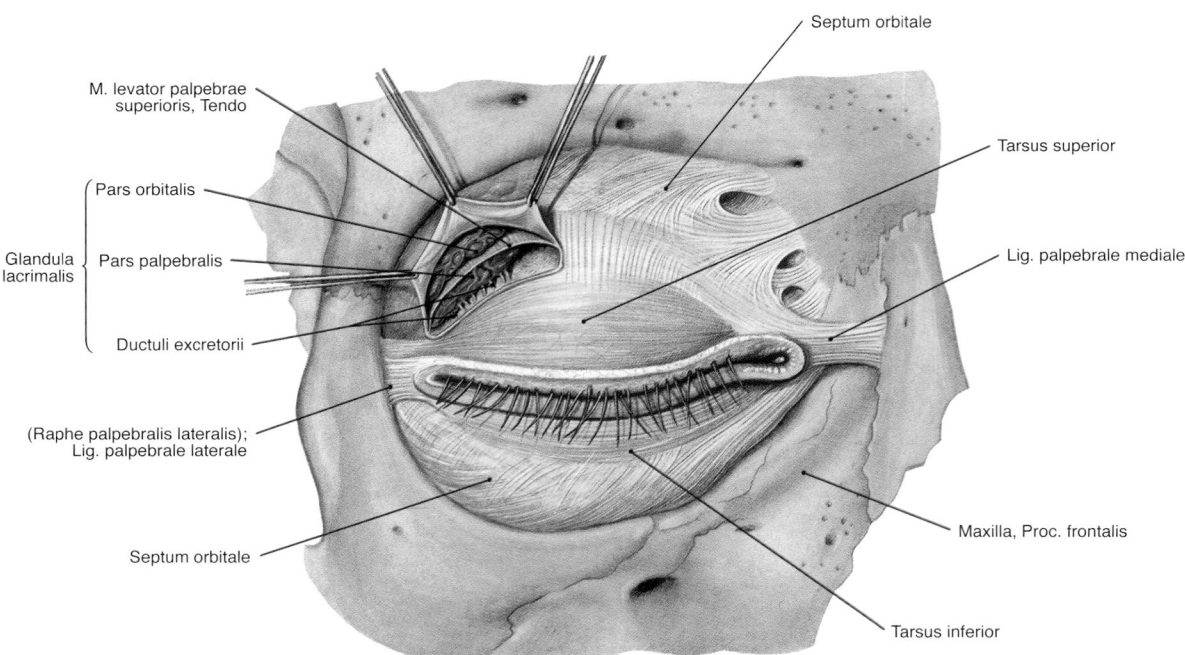

M. levator palpebrae superioris, Tendo

Pars orbitalis

Glandula lacrimalis { Pars palpebralis

Ductuli excretorii

(Raphe palpebralis lateralis); Lig. palpebrale laterale

Septum orbitale

Septum orbitale

Tarsus superior

Lig. palpebrale mediale

Maxilla, Proc. frontalis

Tarsus inferior

Fig. 1336 Orbital opening, Aditus orbitalis, with eyelids, Palpebrae, and lacrimal gland, Glandula lacrimalis.

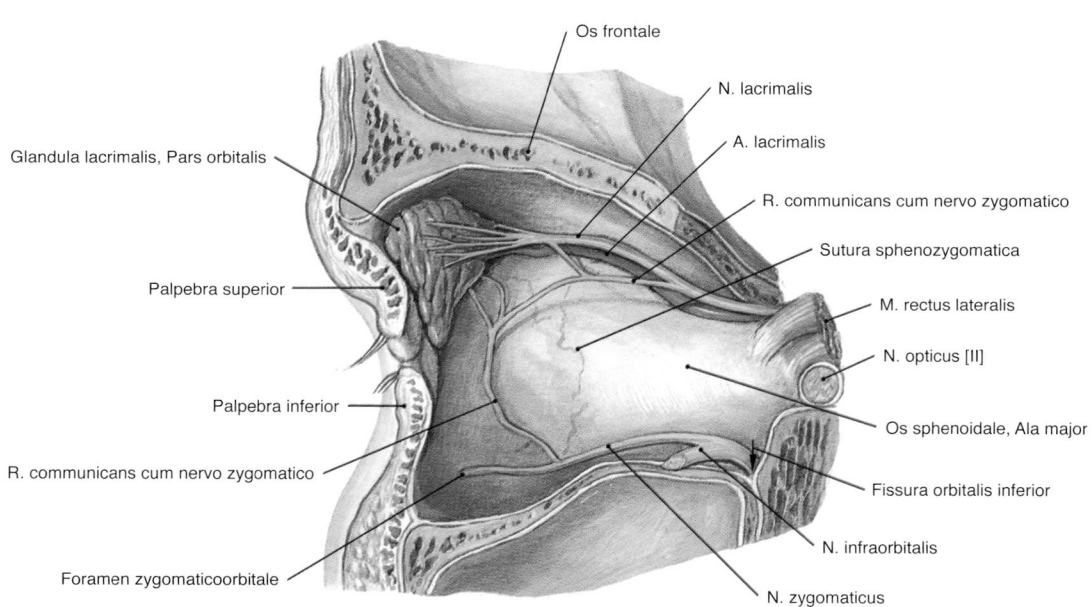

Os frontale

N. lacrimalis

A. lacrimalis

Glandula lacrimalis, Pars orbitalis

R. communicans cum nervo zygomatico

Sutura sphenozygomatica

Palpebra superior

M. rectus lateralis

N. opticus [II]

Palpebra inferior

Os sphenoidale, Ala major

R. communicans cum nervo zygomatico

Fissura orbitalis inferior

Foramen zygomaticoorbitale

N. infraorbitalis

N. zygomaticus

Fig. 1337 Innervation of the lacrimal gland, Glandula lacrimalis; medial view.

Lacrimal apparatus

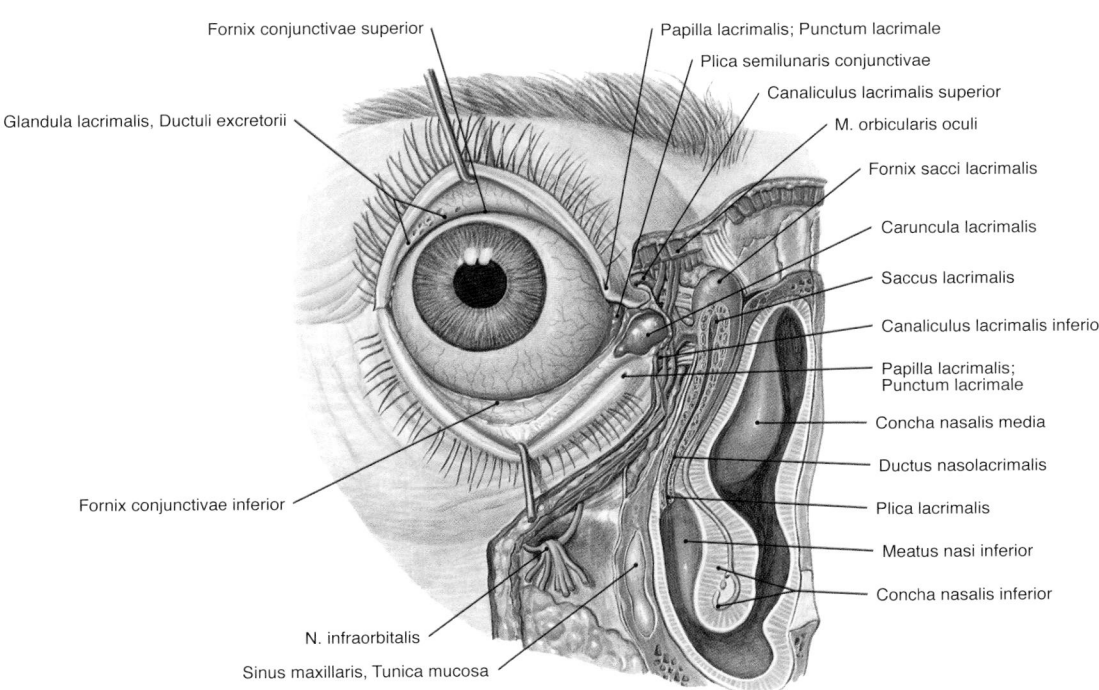

Fornix conjunctivae superior
Glandula lacrimalis, Ductuli excretorii
Papilla lacrimalis; Punctum lacrimale
Plica semilunaris conjunctivae
Canaliculus lacrimalis superior
M. orbicularis oculi
Fornix sacci lacrimalis
Caruncula lacrimalis
Saccus lacrimalis
Canaliculus lacrimalis inferior
Papilla lacrimalis; Punctum lacrimale
Concha nasalis media
Ductus nasolacrimalis
Plica lacrimalis
Meatus nasi inferior
Concha nasalis inferior
Fornix conjunctivae inferior
N. infraorbitalis
Sinus maxillaris, Tunica mucosa

Fig. 1338 Lacrimal apparatus, Apparatus lacrimalis;
the eyelids have been pulled away from the eyeball;
the nasolacrimal duct has been opened up to the inferior nasal meatus.

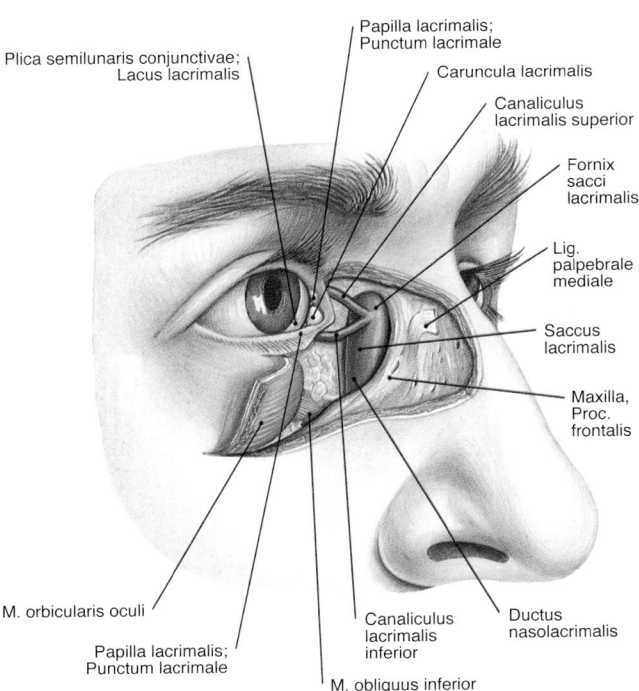

Plica semilunaris conjunctivae;
Lacus lacrimalis
Papilla lacrimalis;
Punctum lacrimale
Caruncula lacrimalis
Canaliculus lacrimalis superior
Fornix sacci lacrimalis
Lig. palpebrale mediale
Saccus lacrimalis
Maxilla, Proc. frontalis
M. orbicularis oculi
Papilla lacrimalis; Punctum lacrimale
Canaliculus lacrimalis inferior
Ductus nasolacrimalis
M. obliquus inferior

Fig. 1339 Lacrimal apparatus, Apparatus lacrimalis.

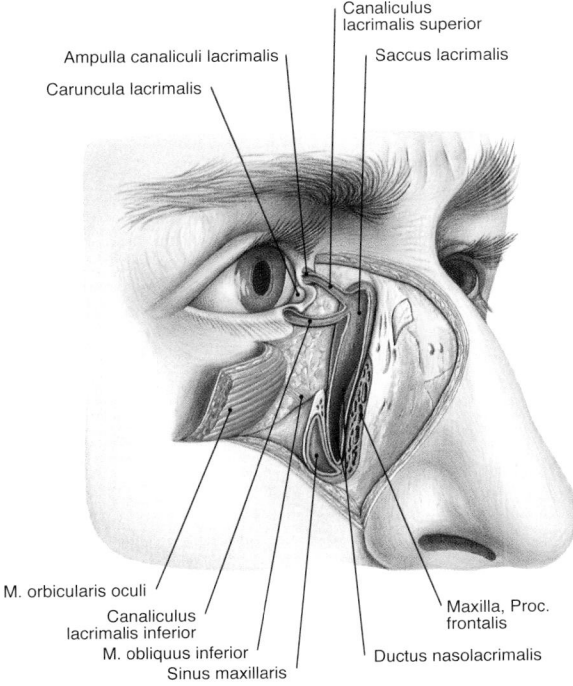

Canaliculus lacrimalis superior
Ampulla canaliculi lacrimalis
Caruncula lacrimalis
Saccus lacrimalis
M. orbicularis oculi
Canaliculus lacrimalis inferior
M. obliquus inferior
Sinus maxillaris
Maxilla, Proc. frontalis
Ductus nasolacrimalis

Fig. 1340 Lacrimal apparatus, Apparatus lacrimalis;
the nasolacrimal duct and the nasolacrimal canal
have been opened.

Extra-ocular muscles

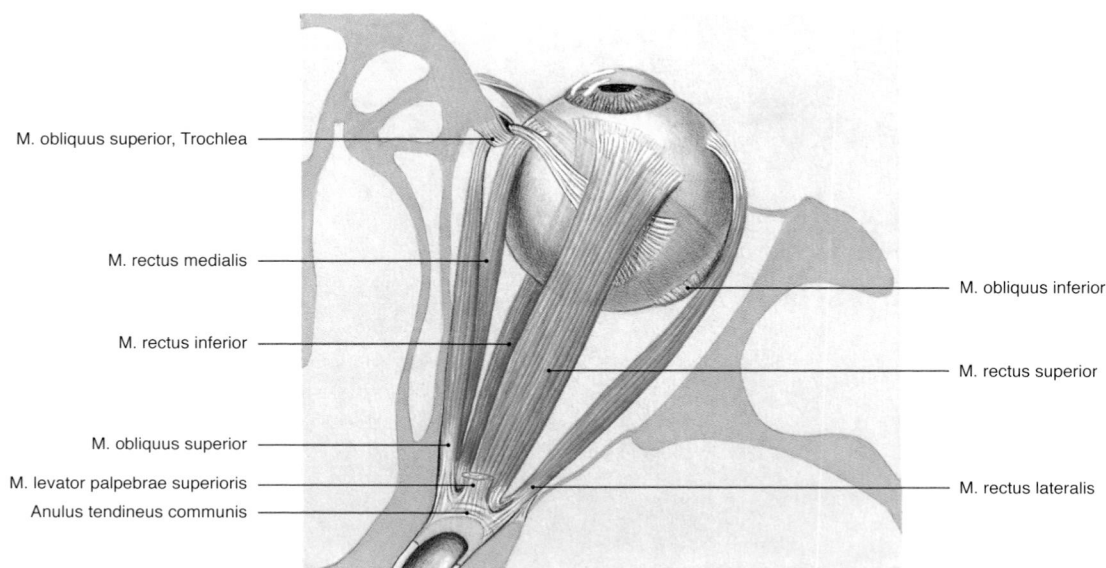

M. obliquus superior, Trochlea

M. rectus medialis

M. rectus inferior

M. obliquus superior

M. levator palpebrae superioris

Anulus tendineus communis

M. obliquus inferior

M. rectus superior

M. rectus lateralis

Fig. 1341 Extra-ocular muscles, Mm. externi bulbi; schema; superior view.

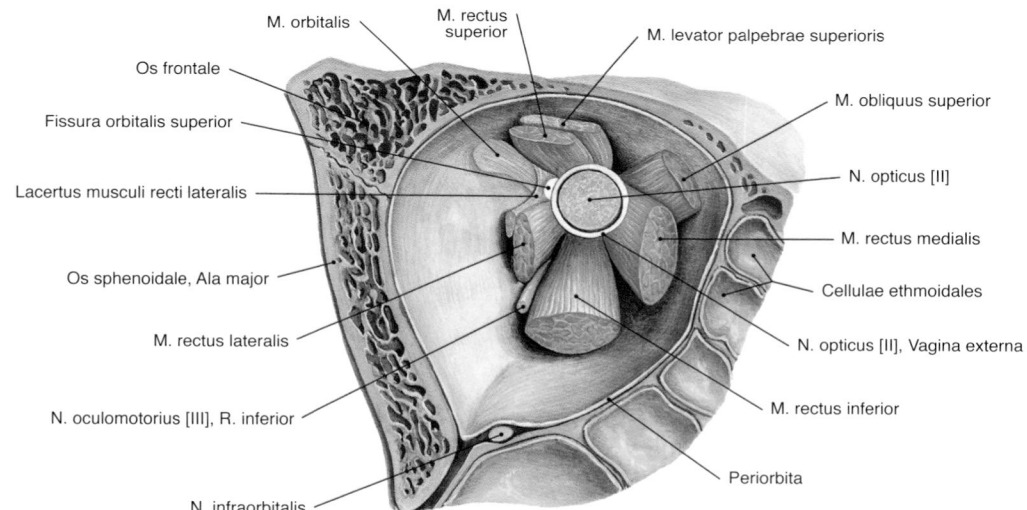

M. orbitalis

M. rectus superior

M. levator palpebrae superioris

Os frontale

Fissura orbitalis superior

Lacertus musculi recti lateralis

Os sphenoidale, Ala major

M. rectus lateralis

N. oculomotorius [III], R. inferior

N. infraorbitalis

M. obliquus superior

N. opticus [II]

M. rectus medialis

Cellulae ethmoidales

N. opticus [II], Vagina externa

M. rectus inferior

Periorbita

Fig. 1342 Extra-ocular muscles, Mm. externi bulbi; anterior view.

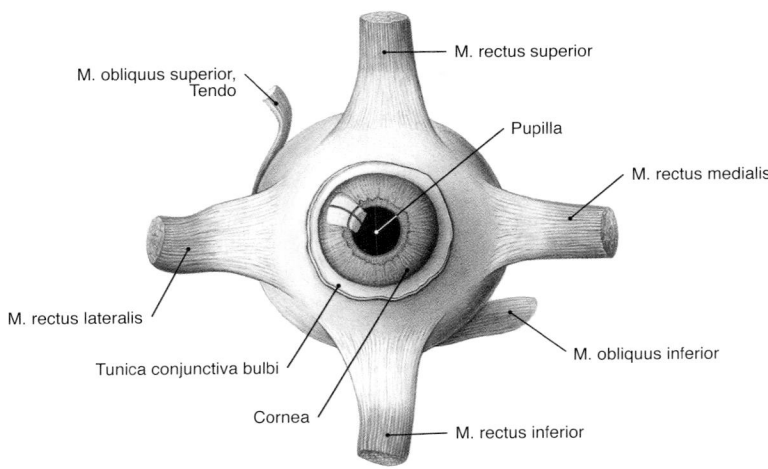

Fig. 1343 Extra-ocular muscles, Mm. externi bulbi.

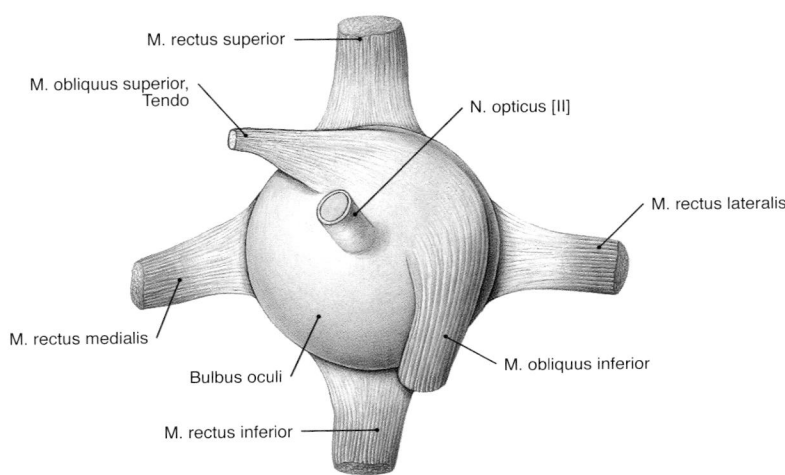

Fig. 1344 Extra-ocular muscles, Mm. externi bulbi; posterior view.

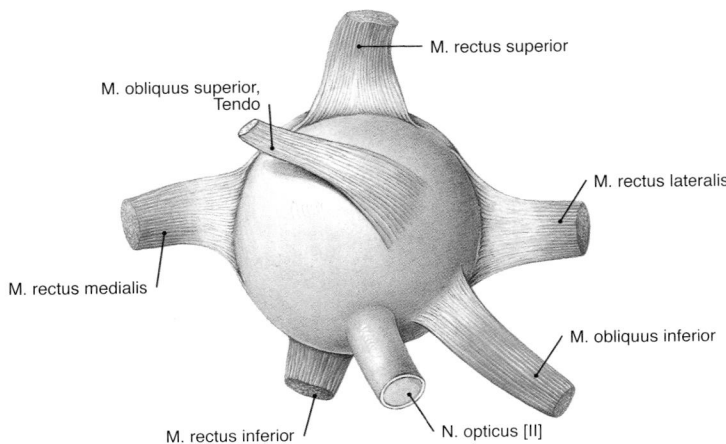

Fig. 1345 Extra-ocular muscles, Mm. externi bulbi; posterior-superior view.

Extra-ocular muscles

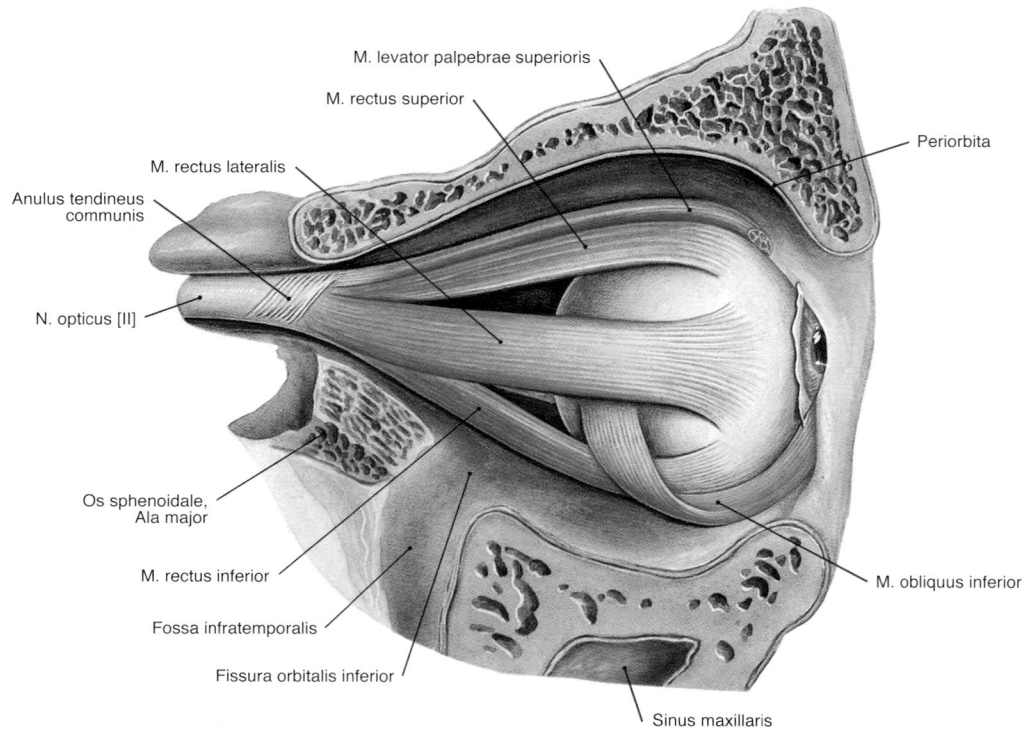

Fig. 1346 Extra-ocular muscles, Mm. externi bulbi; lateral view.

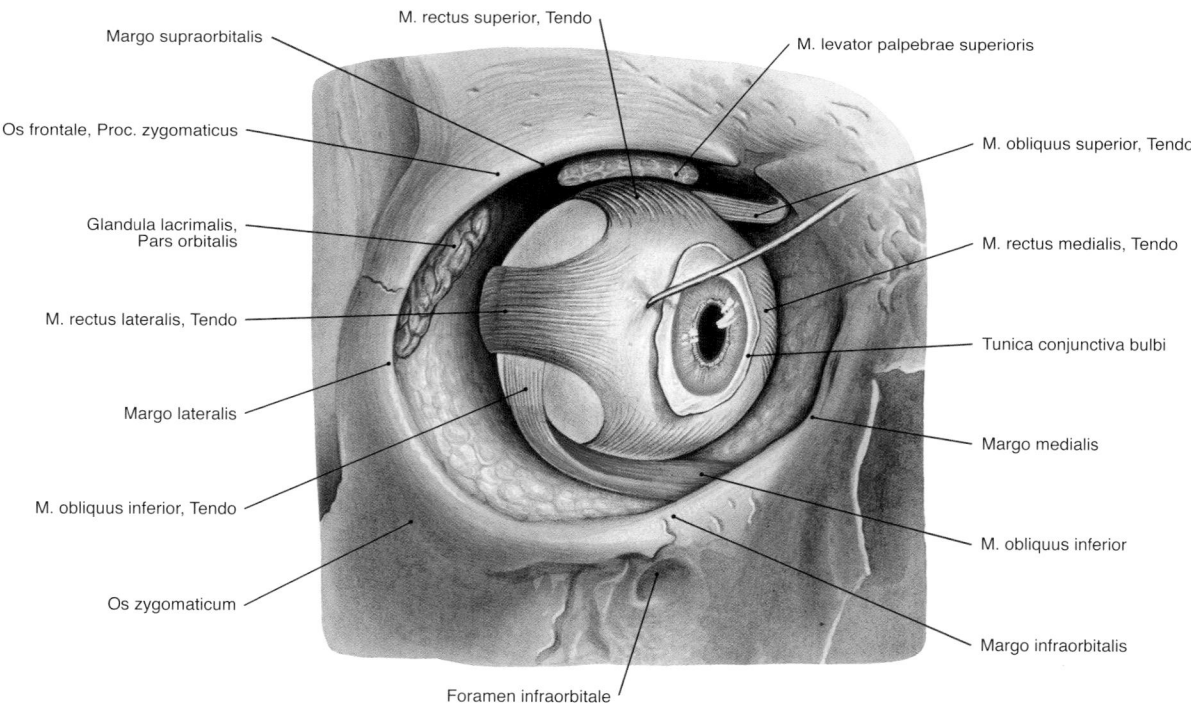

Fig. 1347 Extra-ocular muscles, Mm. externi bulbi; oblique view from anterior.

Extra-ocular muscles

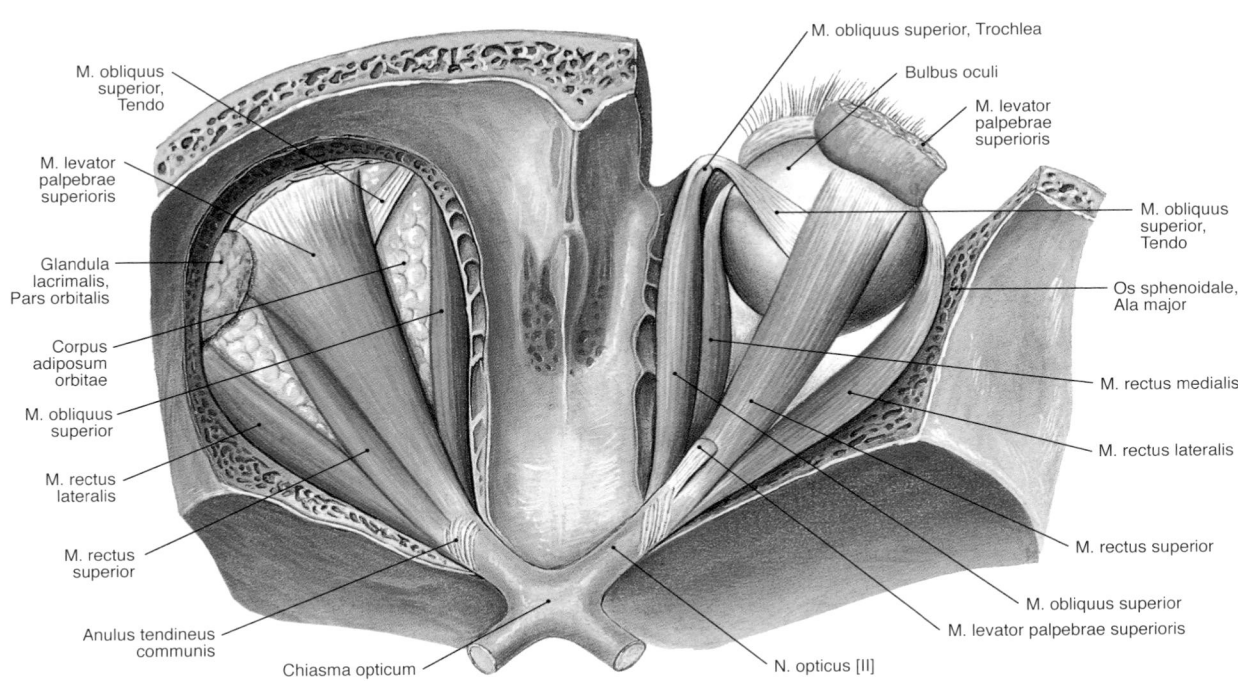

M. obliquus superior, Tendo

M. levator palpebrae superioris

Glandula lacrimalis, Pars orbitalis

Corpus adiposum orbitae

M. obliquus superior

M. rectus lateralis

M. rectus superior

Anulus tendineus communis

Chiasma opticum

M. obliquus superior, Trochlea

Bulbus oculi

M. levator palpebrae superioris

M. obliquus superior, Tendo

Os sphenoidale, Ala major

M. rectus medialis

M. rectus lateralis

M. rectus superior

M. obliquus superior

M. levator palpebrae superioris

N. opticus [II]

Fig. 1348 Extra-ocular muscles, Mm. externi bulbi; superior view.

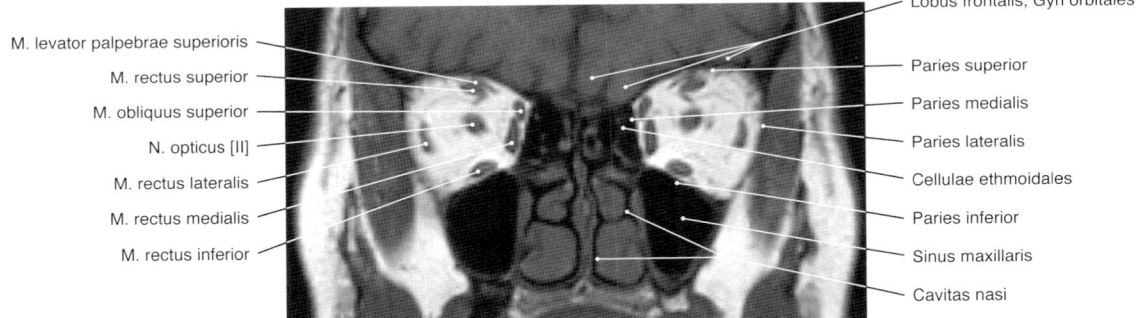

M. levator palpebrae superioris

M. rectus superior

M. obliquus superior

N. opticus [II]

M. rectus lateralis

M. rectus medialis

M. rectus inferior

Lobus frontalis, Gyri orbitales

Paries superior

Paries medialis

Paries lateralis

Cellulae ethmoidales

Paries inferior

Sinus maxillaris

Cavitas nasi

Fig. 1349 Extra-ocular muscles, Mm. externi bulbi; magnetic resonance tomographic image (MRI); frontal section through the middle of the orbit; anterior view.

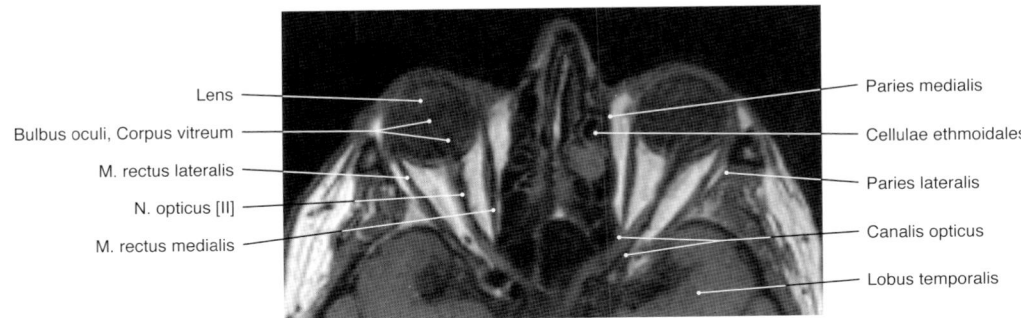

Lens

Bulbus oculi, Corpus vitreum

M. rectus lateralis

N. opticus [II]

M. rectus medialis

Paries medialis

Cellulae ethmoidales

Paries lateralis

Canalis opticus

Lobus temporalis

Fig. 1350 Eyeball, Bulbus oculi, and extra-ocular muscles, Mm. externi bulbi; magnetic resonance tomographic image (MRI); horizontal section at the level of the optic nerve; superior view.

Eyeball, structure

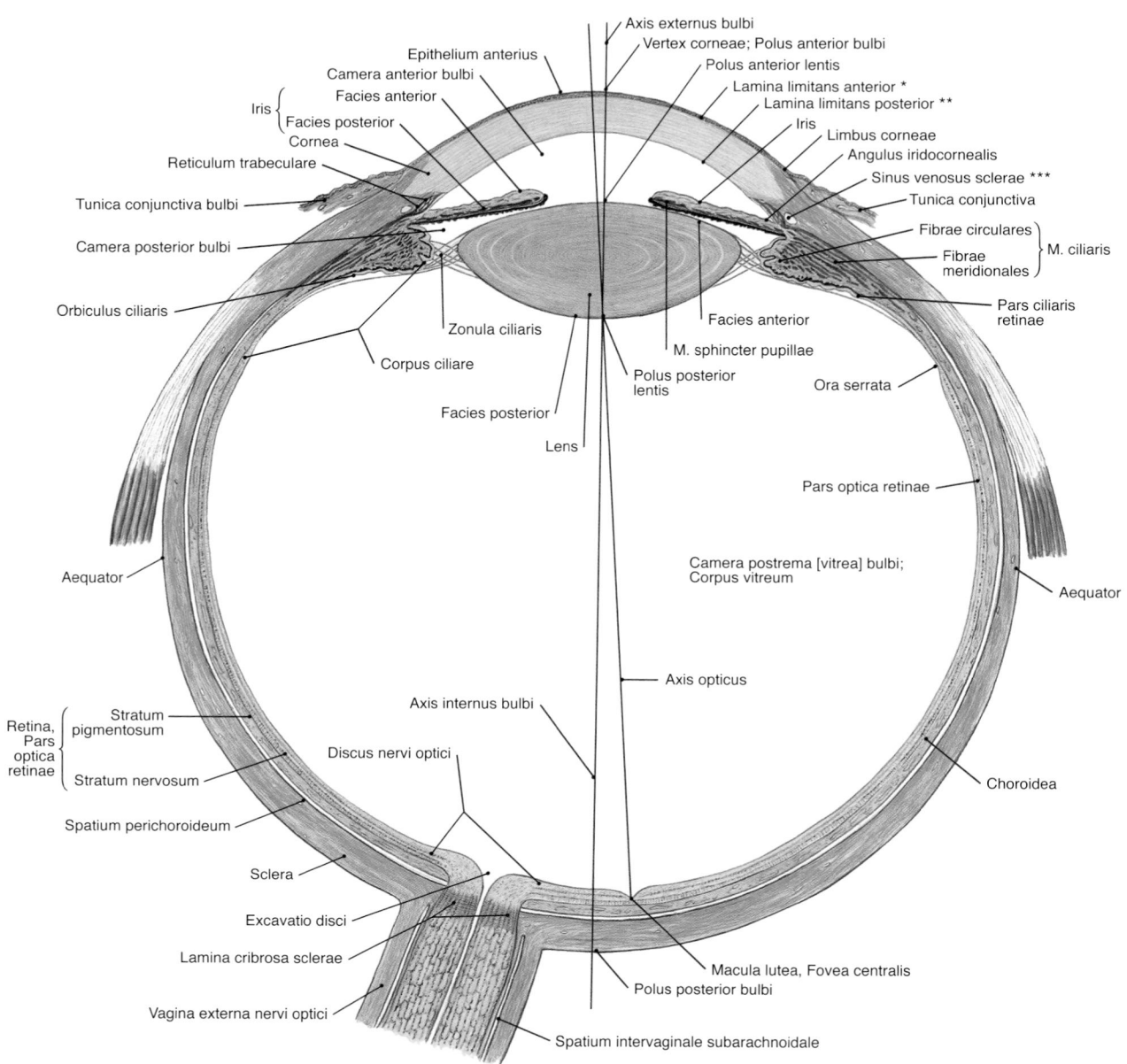

Fig. 1351 Eyeball, Bulbus oculi; schematic horizontal section at the level of the exit of the optic nerve.

* Clinical term: BOWMAN's membrane
** Clinical term: DESCEMET's membrane
*** Clinical term: canal of SCHLEMM

Dimensions of the eyeball

(Average values according to the anatomic and ophthalmologic literature)

External bulbar axis, Axis externus bulbi	24.0 mm	Radius of curvature of the sclera	13.0 mm
Internal bulbar axis, Axis internus bulbi	22.5 mm	Radius of curvature of the cornea	7.8 mm
Thickness of the cornea	0.5 mm	Power of the entire eye (distance vision)	59 dioptres
Depth of the anterior chamber	3.6 mm	Power of the cornea	43 dioptres
Thickness of the lens	3.6 mm	Power of the lens (distance vision)	19 dioptres
Distance between lens and retina	15.6 mm		
Thickness of the retina	0.3 mm	Interpupillary distance	61–69 mm

Blood vessels of the eyeball

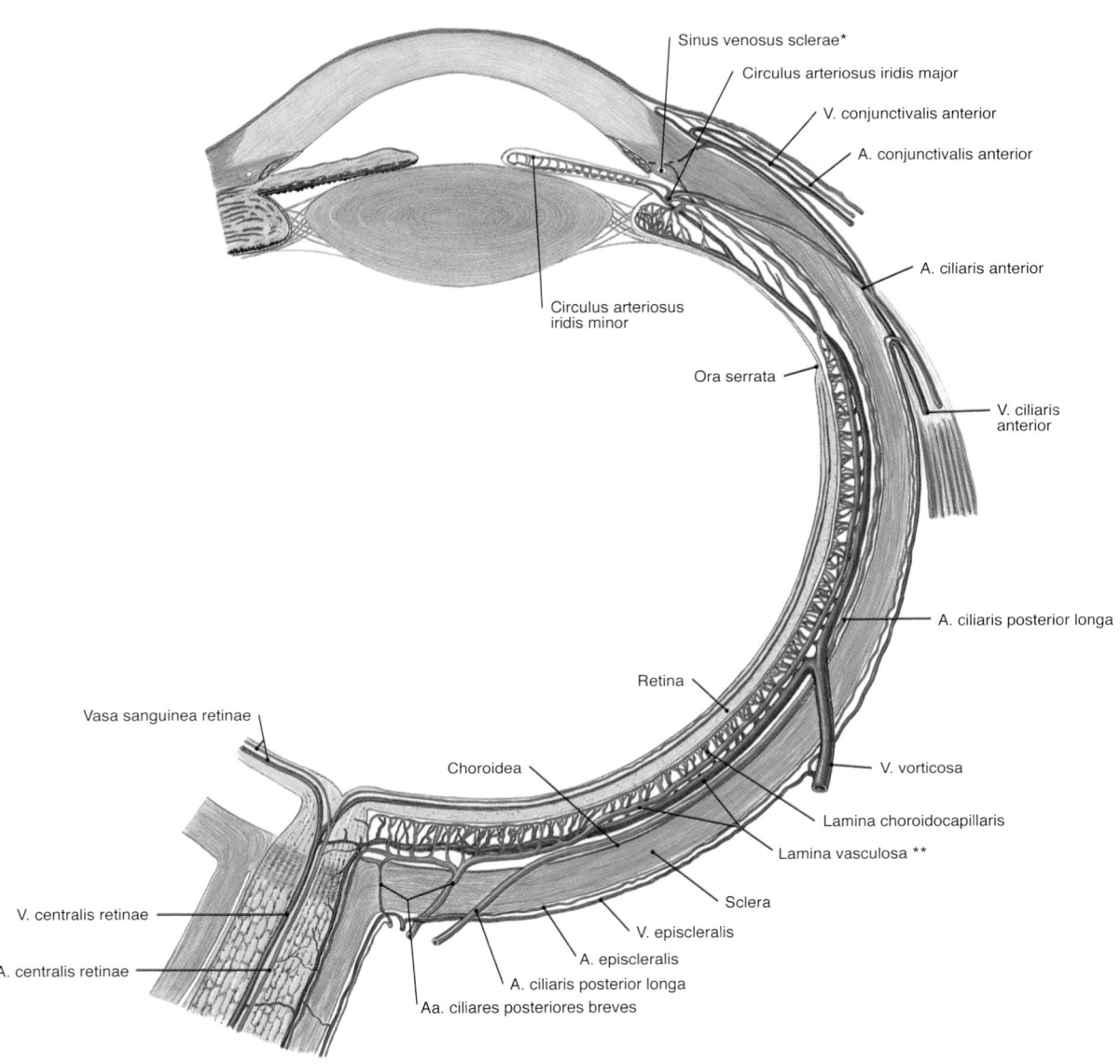

Sinus venosus sclerae*
Circulus arteriosus iridis major
V. conjunctivalis anterior
A. conjunctivalis anterior
A. ciliaris anterior
Circulus arteriosus iridis minor
V. ciliaris anterior
Ora serrata
A. ciliaris posterior longa
Retina
V. vorticosa
Vasa sanguinea retinae
Choroidea
Lamina choroidocapillaris
Lamina vasculosa **
Sclera
V. centralis retinae
V. episcleralis
A. centralis retinae
A. episcleralis
A. ciliaris posterior longa
Aa. ciliares posteriores breves

Fig. 1352 Blood vessels of the eyeball, Bulbus oculi.
* Clinical term: canal of SCHLEMM
** Clinical term: uvea

Layers of the eyeball, Tunicae bulbi

Fibrous layer of the eyeball, Tunica fibrosa bulbi
- Cornea, Cornea (pronounced curvature, translucent)
- Sclera, Sclera (lesser curvature, opaque; bluish-white in infancy, yellowish-white in senescence)

Vascular layer of the eyeball, Tunica vasculosa bulbi
- Iris, Iris, with the central circular opening, the pupil, Pupilla
- Ciliary body, Corpus ciliare, with the ciliary muscle, M. ciliaris, the ciliary process, Processus ciliaris, the ciliary zonule, Zonula ciliaris, with the zonular fibres, Fibrae zonulares, and the zonular spaces, Spatia zonularia
- Choroid, Choroidea

Inner layer of the eyeball (retina), Tunica interna bulbi (Retina)
- Nonvisual retina, Pars caeca retinae (from the pupillary-iridial margin, Margo pupillaris iridis, to the ora serrata, Ora serrata)
  Iridial part of the retina, Pars iridica retinae (single-layered, heavily pigmented), ciliary part of the retina, Pars ciliaris retinae (single-layered, unpigmented)
- Optic part of the retina, Pars optica retinae (stratified)
  1. neuron: vision cells (rod cells – brightness; cone cells – colour)
  2. neuron: bipolar ganglion cells within the retina (ganglion of the retina, Ganglion retinae)
  3. neuron: multi-polar ganglion cells (optic ganglion, Ganglion opticum), whose long axons form the optic nerve and continue in the optic tract

Ciliary body and iris

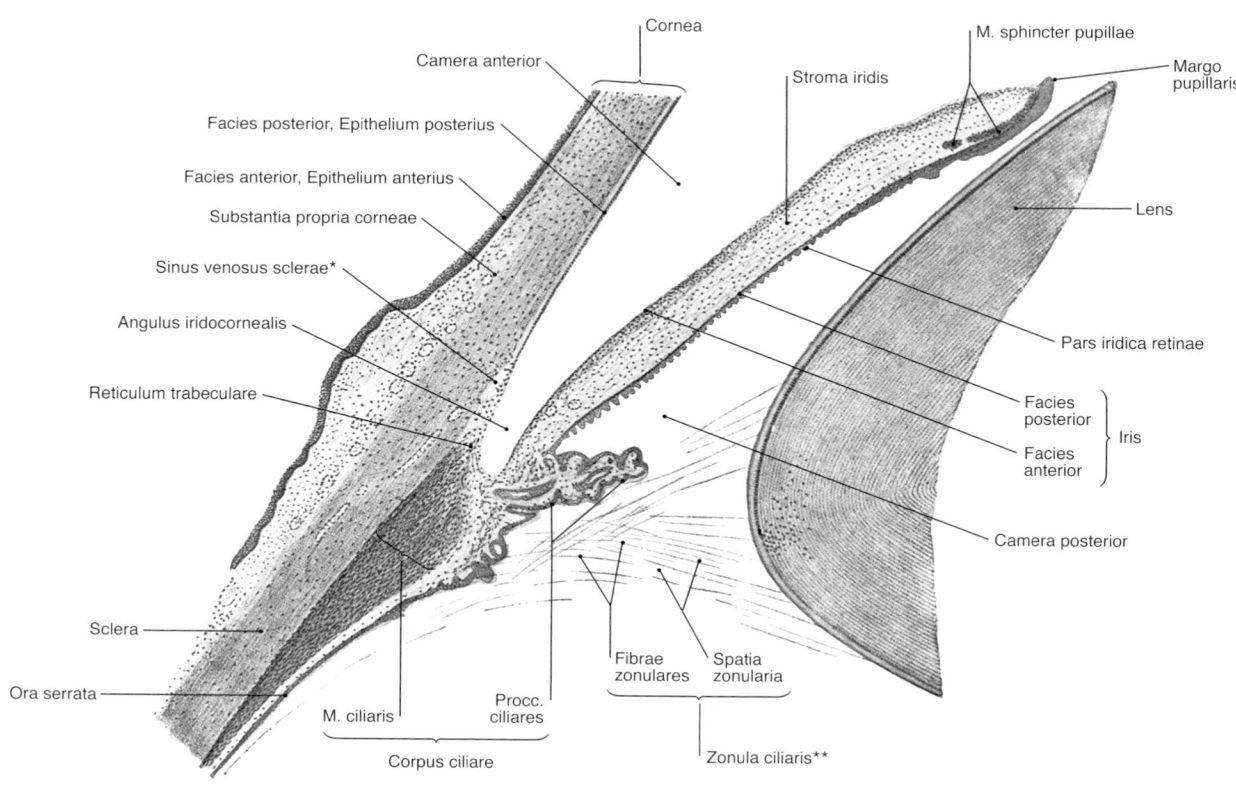

Fig. 1353   Eyeball, Bulbus oculi;
schematic horizontal section at the level of
the pupil.
* Clinical term: canal of SCHLEMM
** Clinical term: zonule of ZINN

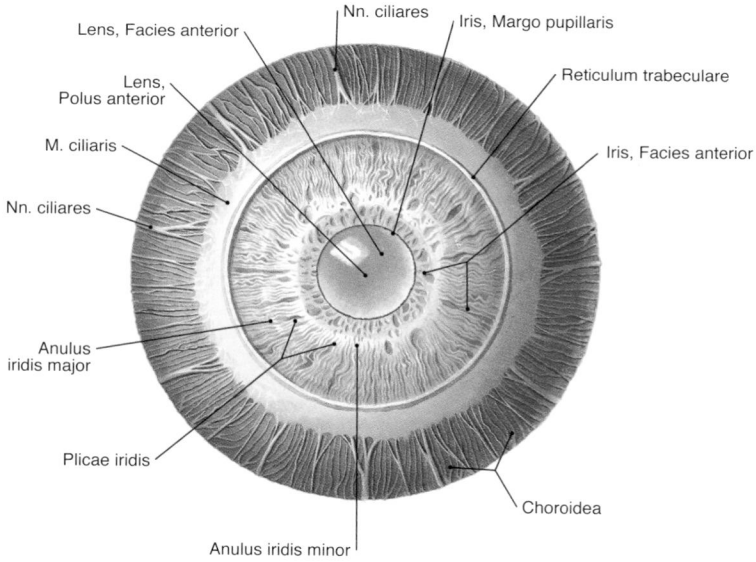

Fig. 1354   Iris, Iris, and pupil, Pupilla;
after removal of the sclera and cornea;
anterior view.

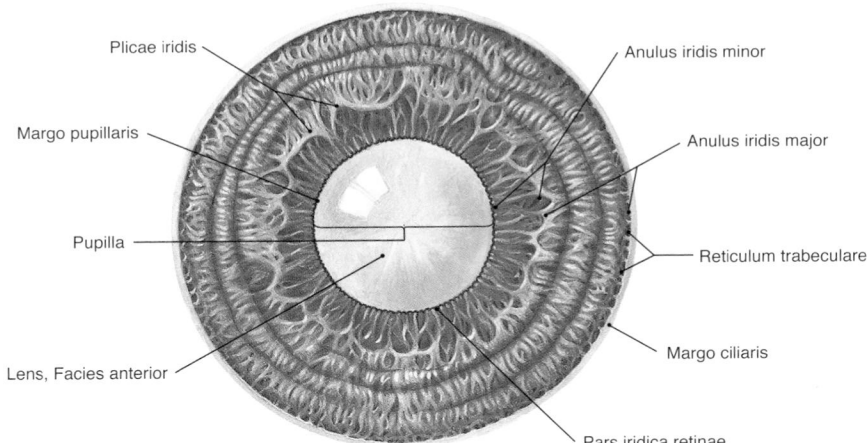

Plicae iridis

Margo pupillaris

Pupilla

Lens, Facies anterior

Anulus iridis minor

Anulus iridis major

Reticulum trabeculare

Margo ciliaris

Pars iridica retinae

Fig. 1355 Iris, Iris;
after removal of the cornea;
anterior view.

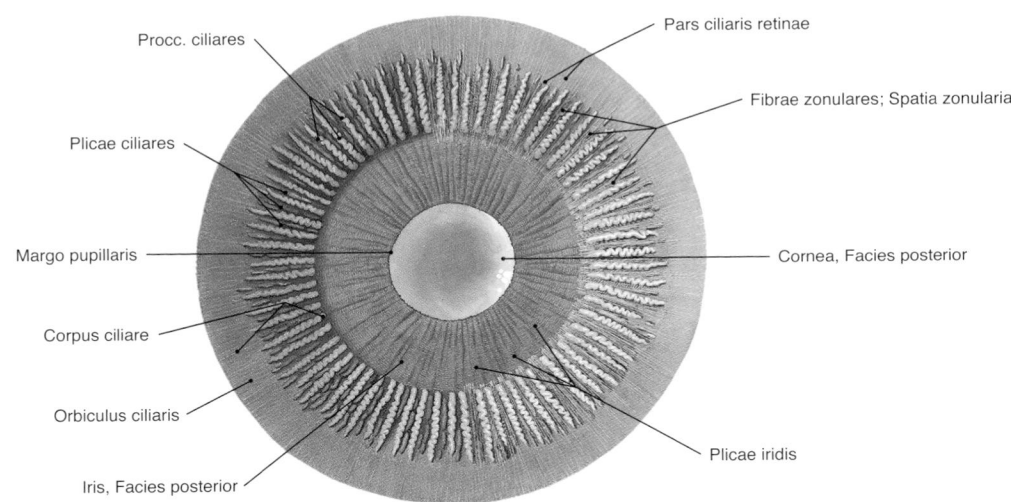

Procc. ciliares

Plicae ciliares

Margo pupillaris

Corpus ciliare

Orbiculus ciliaris

Iris, Facies posterior

Pars ciliaris retinae

Fibrae zonulares; Spatia zonularia

Cornea, Facies posterior

Plicae iridis

Fig. 1356 Iris, Iris;
posterior view.

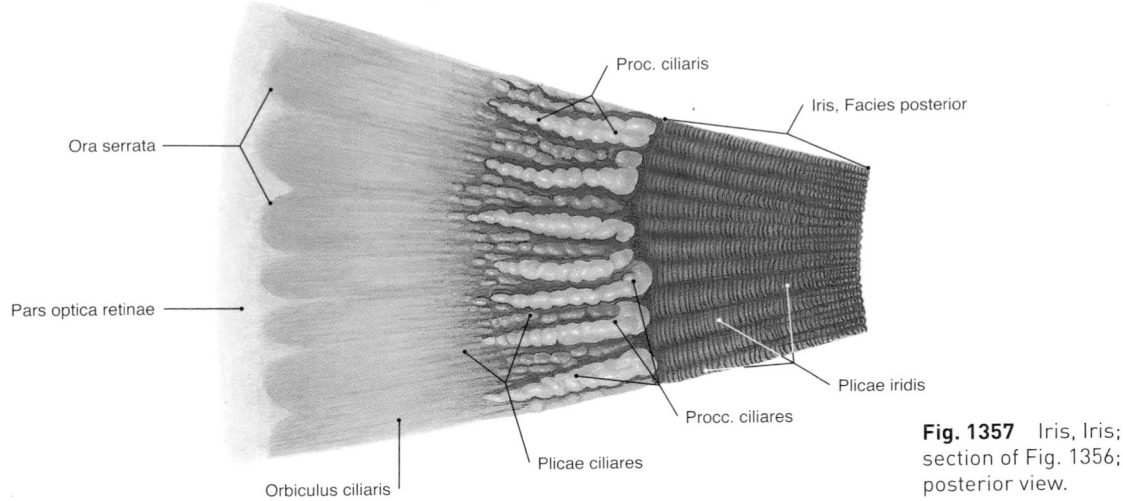

Ora serrata

Pars optica retinae

Orbiculus ciliaris

Plicae ciliares

Procc. ciliares

Proc. ciliaris

Iris, Facies posterior

Plicae iridis

Fig. 1357 Iris, Iris;
section of Fig. 1356;
posterior view.

Lens

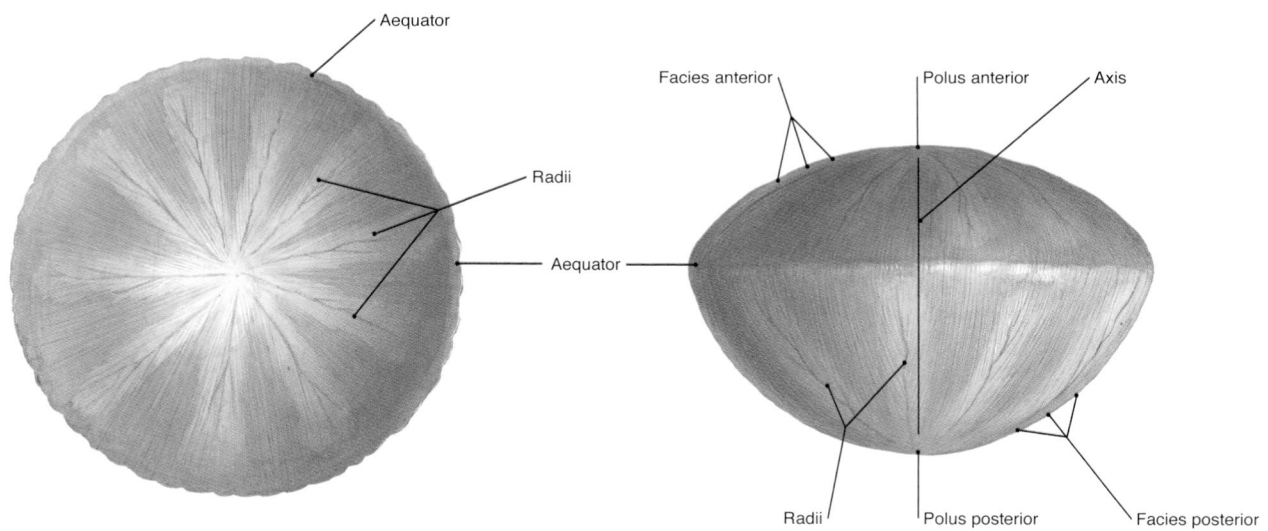

Fig. 1358 Lens, Lens;
anterior view.

Fig. 1359 Lens, Lens;
viewed from the equator.

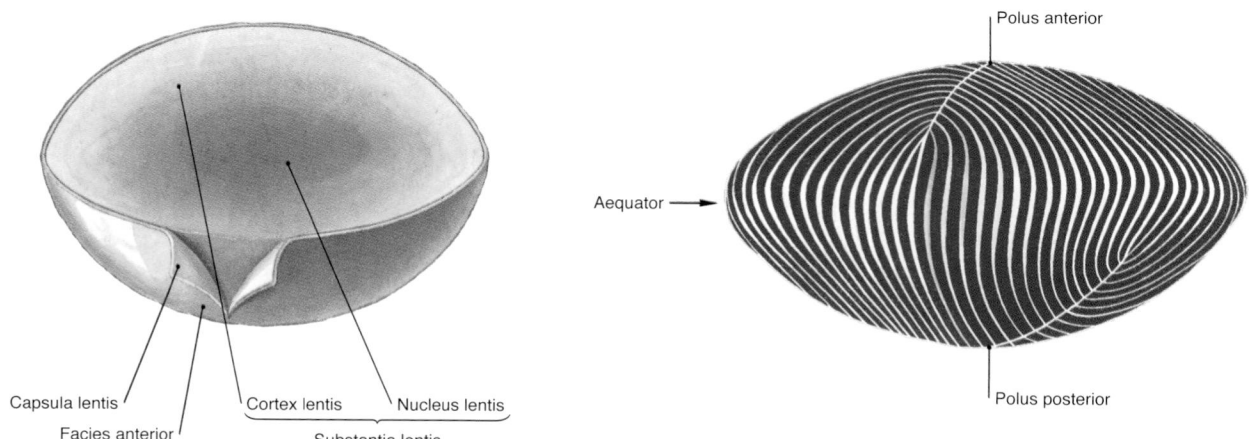

Fig. 1360 Lens, Lens;
oblique view from anterior.

Fig. 1361 Lens, Lens;
schema of the lens fibres in a neonate;
viewed from the equator.

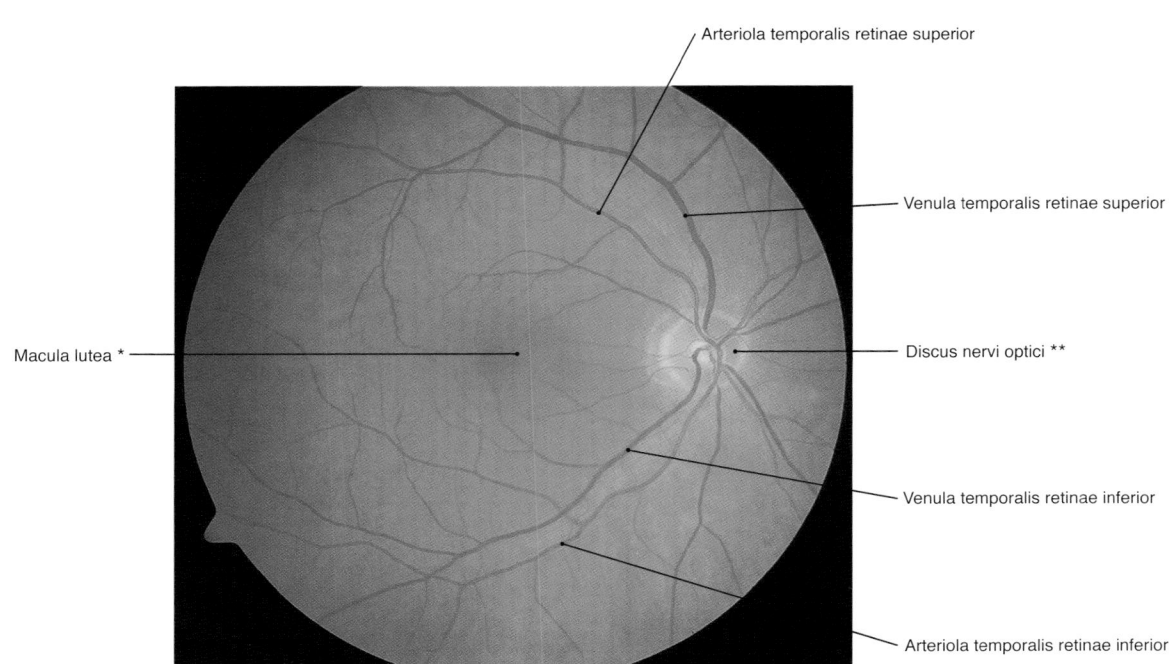

Arteriola temporalis retinae superior

Venula temporalis retinae superior

Macula lutea *

Discus nervi optici **

Venula temporalis retinae inferior

Arteriola temporalis retinae inferior

Fig. 1362   Ocular fundus, Fundus oculi;
ophthalmoscopic picture of the central region;
anterior view.
*   Clinical term: yellow spot
** Clinical term: papilla or blind spot

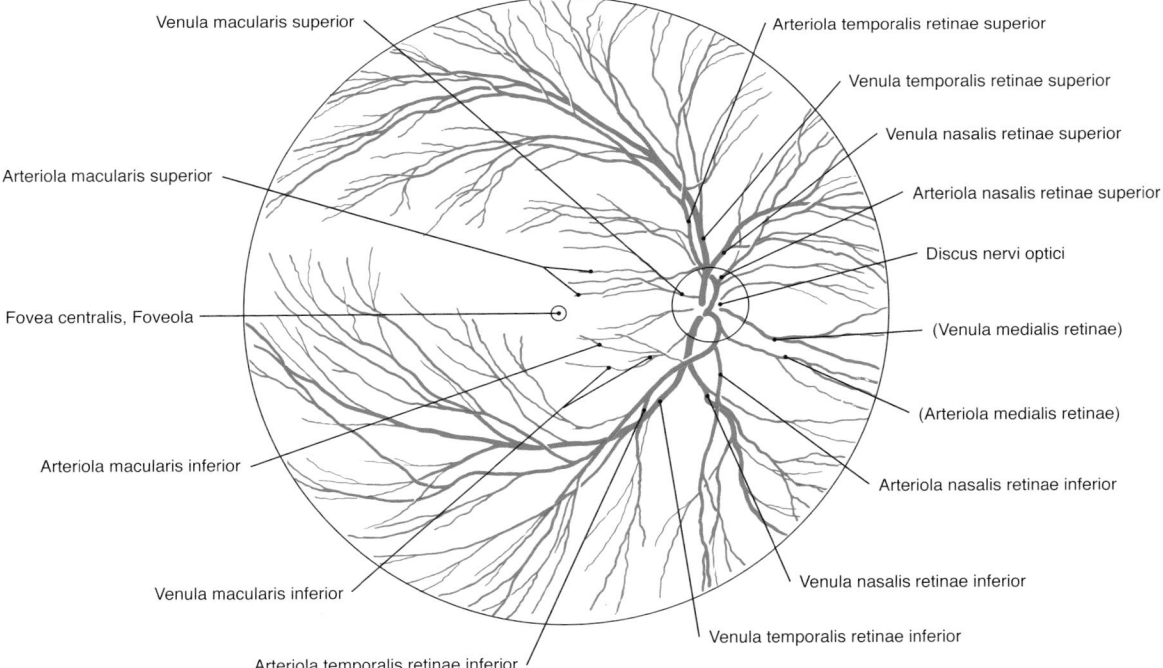

Venula macularis superior

Arteriola temporalis retinae superior

Venula temporalis retinae superior

Venula nasalis retinae superior

Arteriola nasalis retinae superior

Arteriola macularis superior

Discus nervi optici

Fovea centralis, Foveola

(Venula medialis retinae)

(Arteriola medialis retinae)

Arteriola macularis inferior

Arteriola nasalis retinae inferior

Venula nasalis retinae inferior

Venula macularis inferior

Venula temporalis retinae inferior

Arteriola temporalis retinae inferior

Fig. 1363   Blood vessels of the retina, Vasa sanguinea retinae;
schema of the course of the vessels;
anterior view.

Optic nerve

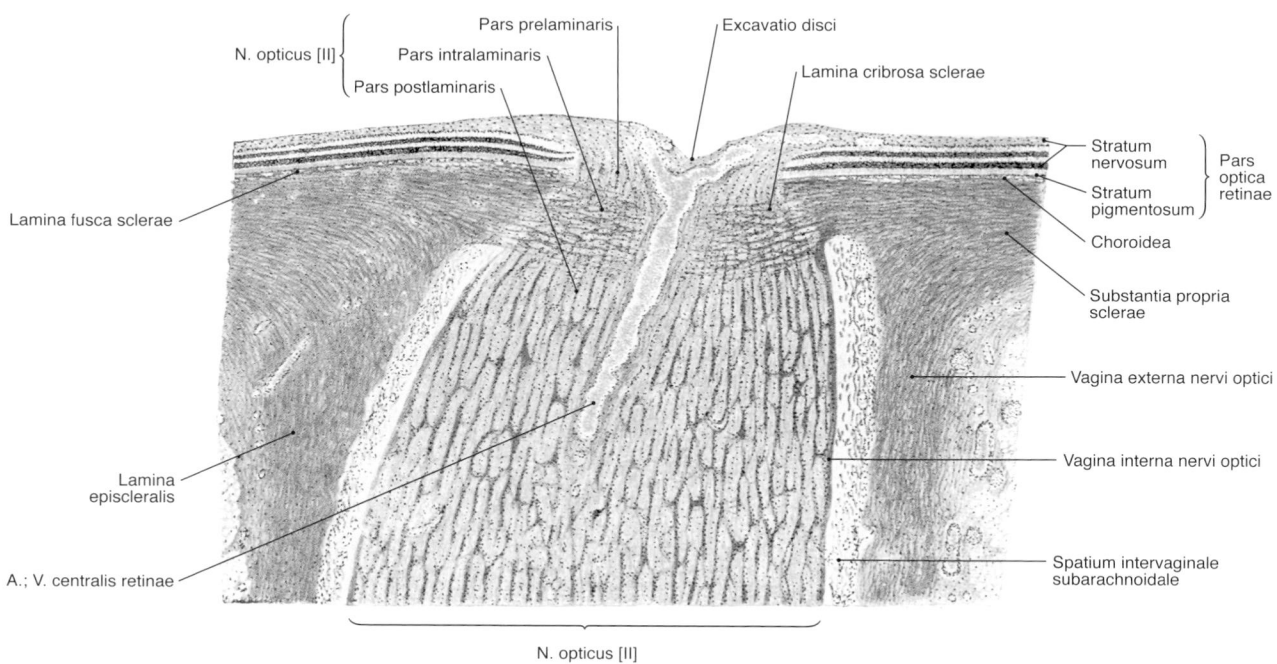

Fig. 1364 Optic nerve, N. opticus [II];
horizontal section at its exit from the eyeball.

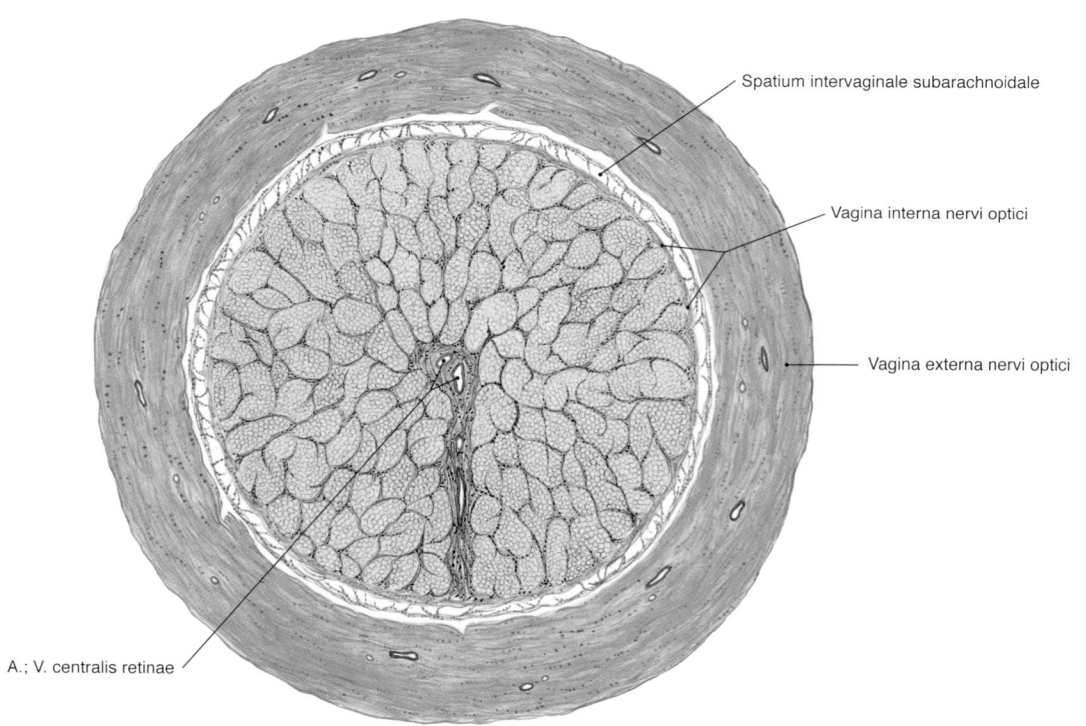

Fig. 1365 Optic nerve, N. opticus [II];
cross-section near the eyeball.

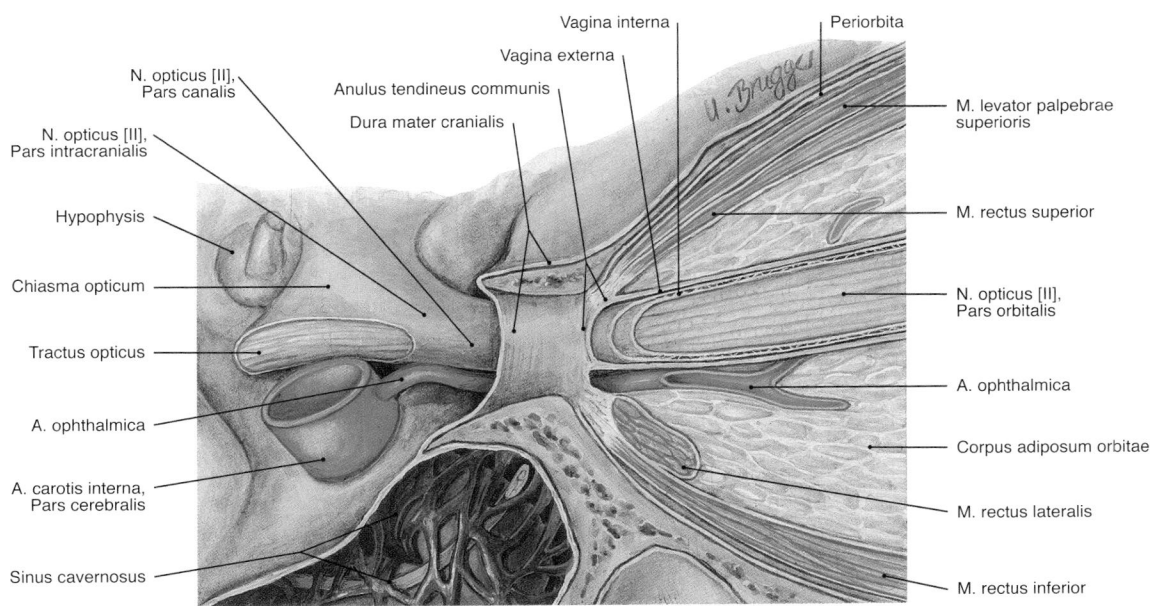

Vagina interna
Periorbita
N. opticus [II], Pars canalis
Vagina externa
Anulus tendineus communis
M. levator palpebrae superioris
N. opticus [II], Pars intracranialis
Dura mater cranialis
Hypophysis
M. rectus superior
Chiasma opticum
N. opticus [II], Pars orbitalis
Tractus opticus
A. ophthalmica
A. ophthalmica
Corpus adiposum orbitae
A. carotis interna, Pars cerebralis
M. rectus lateralis
Sinus cavernosus
M. rectus inferior

Fig. 1366   Optic nerve, N. opticus [II];
the optic canal has been opened;
viewed from the right.

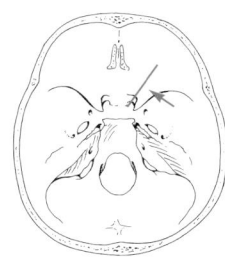

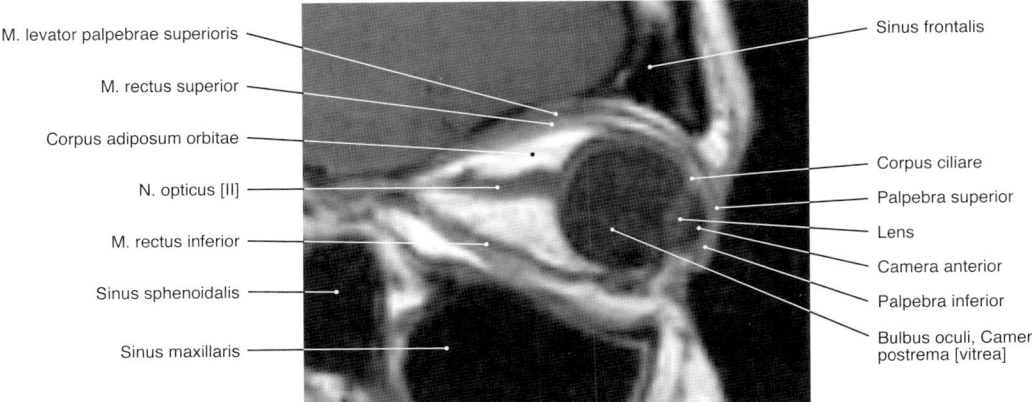

M. levator palpebrae superioris
Sinus frontalis
M. rectus superior
Corpus adiposum orbitae
N. opticus [II]
Corpus ciliare
M. rectus inferior
Palpebra superior
Sinus sphenoidalis
Lens
Camera anterior
Sinus maxillaris
Palpebra inferior
Bulbus oculi, Camera postrema [vitrea]

Fig. 1367   Orbit, Orbita;
magnetic resonance tomographic image (MRI);
vertical section along the optic nerve;
viewed from the right.

→ 1379

Optic pathway and blood vessels

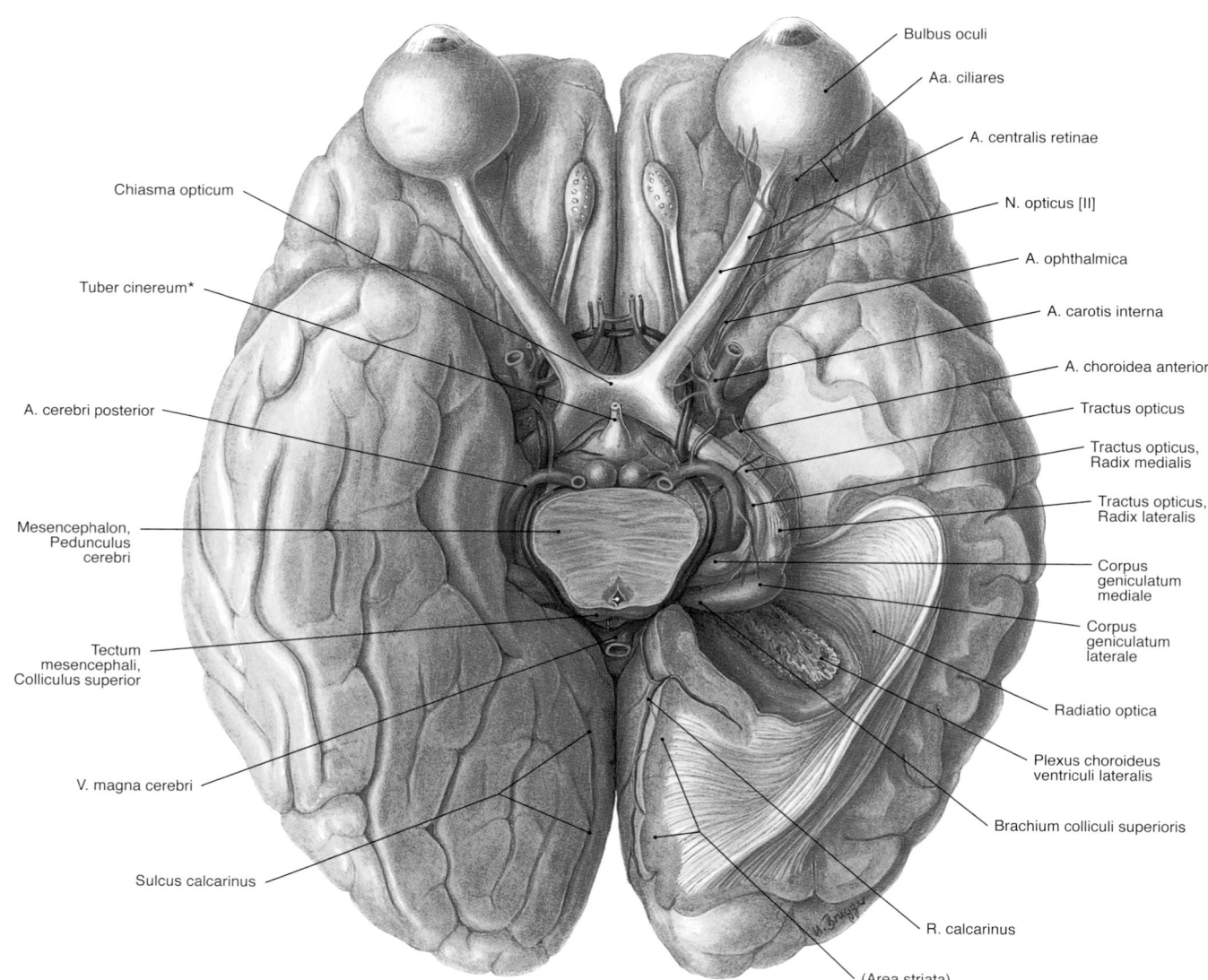

Fig. 1368 Brain, Encephalon, and blood supply of the parts of the optic pathway;
inferior view.
The pituitary gland has been removed at its infundibulum (*). Due to the close proximity of the pituitary gland and the optic chiasm, pituitary tumours can cause visual disturbances.

Optic pathway

1. neuron: rod cells and cone cells of the retina
2. neuron: bipolar ganglion cells of the retina (perikarya in the retinal ganglion)
3. neuron: multi-polar ganglion cells of the retina (perikarya in the optic ganglion)
   The axons of the optic ganglion cells extend primarily to the lateral geniculate body (lateral root), although several fibres also extend to the pretectal area and the superior colliculus (medial root), as well as to the hypothalamus.

They run within the optic nerve to the optic chiasm, where the fibres from the nasal part of the ocular fundus cross to the opposite side. Each optic tract contains fibres, which transmit information from the contralateral half of the visual field.

4. neuron: Its axons travel primarily from the lateral geniculate body to areas 17 and 18 of the cerebral cortex (striate area) in the region surrounding the calcarine sulcus.

Optic pathway

1   Common visual field
1a Visual field of the left eye
1b Visual field of the right eye
2a Projection on the left retina
2b Projection on the right retina

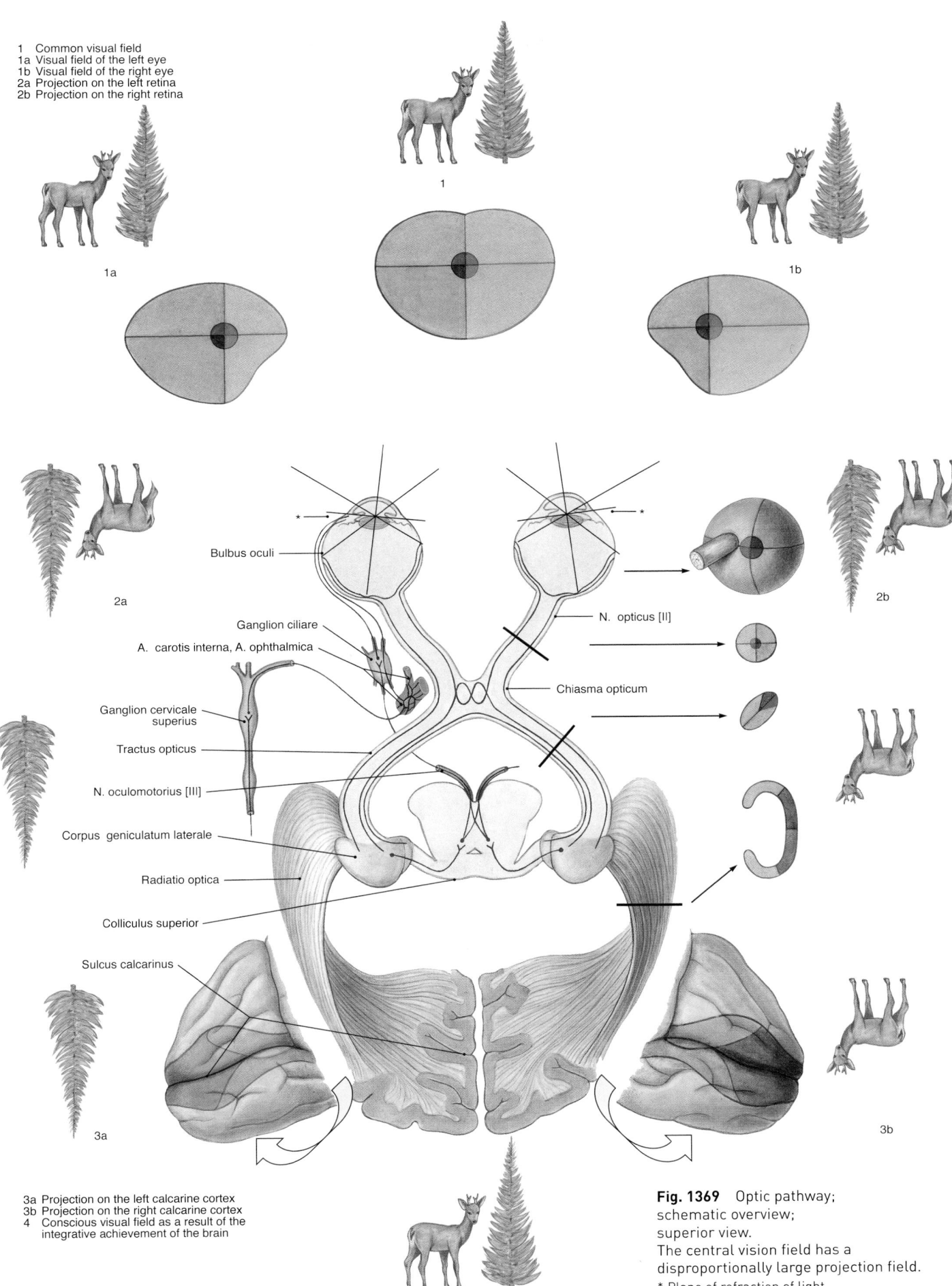

Bulbus oculi

N. opticus [II]

Ganglion ciliare

A. carotis interna, A. ophthalmica

Chiasma opticum

Ganglion cervicale superius

Tractus opticus

N. oculomotorius [III]

Corpus geniculatum laterale

Radiatio optica

Colliculus superior

Sulcus calcarinus

3a Projection on the left calcarine cortex
3b Projection on the right calcarine cortex
4 Conscious visual field as a result of the
   integrative achievement of the brain

Fig. 1369 Optic pathway;
schematic overview;
superior view.
The central vision field has a
disproportionally large projection field.
* Plane of refraction of light

Orbit, topography

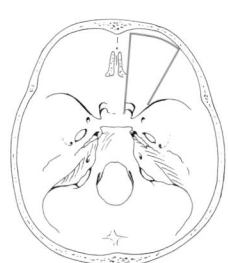

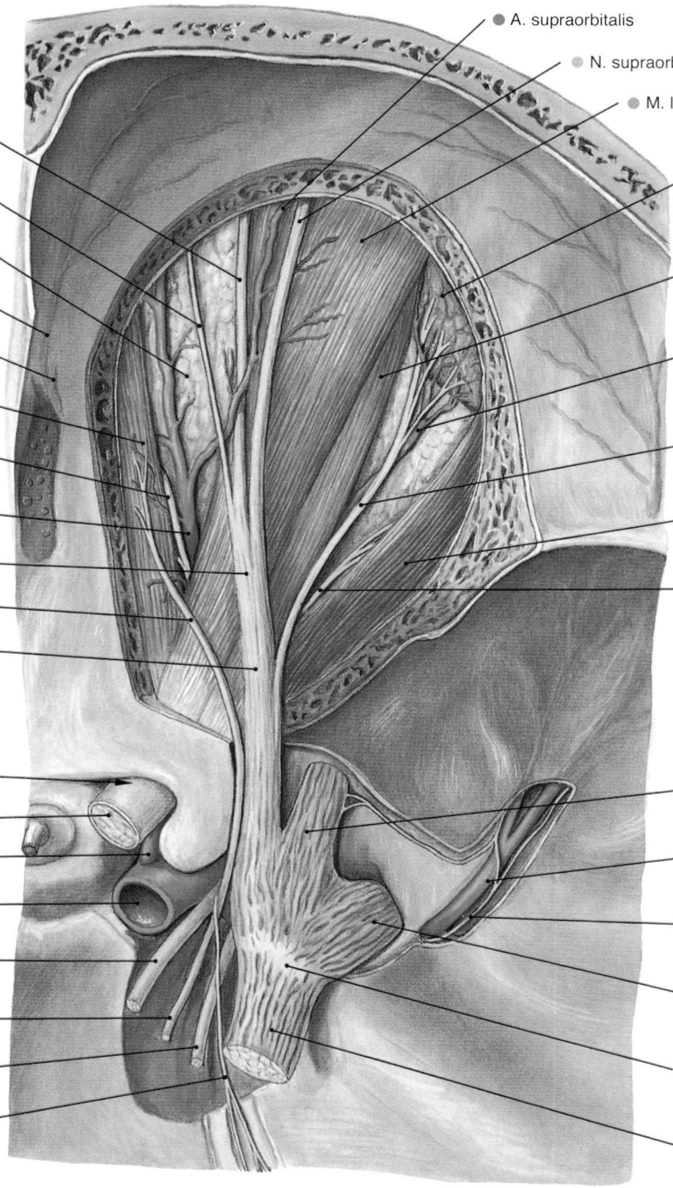

A. supraorbitalis

N. supraorbitalis, R. lateralis

M. levator palpebrae superioris

Glandula lacrimalis, Pars orbitalis

M. rectus superior

A. lacrimalis

N. lacrimalis

M. rectus lateralis

N. abducens [VI]

N. maxillaris [V/2]

A. meningea media

N. mandibularis [V/3], R. meningeus

N. mandibularis [V/3]

Ganglion trigeminale

N. trigeminus [V]

N. supraorbitalis, R. medialis

N. supratrochlearis

Corpus adiposum orbitae

R. meningeus anterior

A. ethmoidalis anterior

M. obliquus superior

N. nasociliaris

A. ophthalmica

N. frontalis

N. trochlearis [IV]

N. ophthalmicus [V/1]

Canalis opticus

N. opticus [II]

A. ophthalmica

A. carotis interna

N. oculomotorius [III]

N. trochlearis [IV]

N. abducens [VI]

R. tentorius

1371

Fig. 1370 Arteries and nerves of the orbit, Orbita; superior view.

Orbit, topography

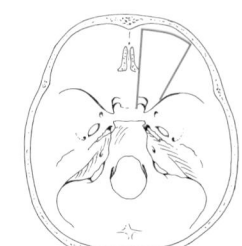

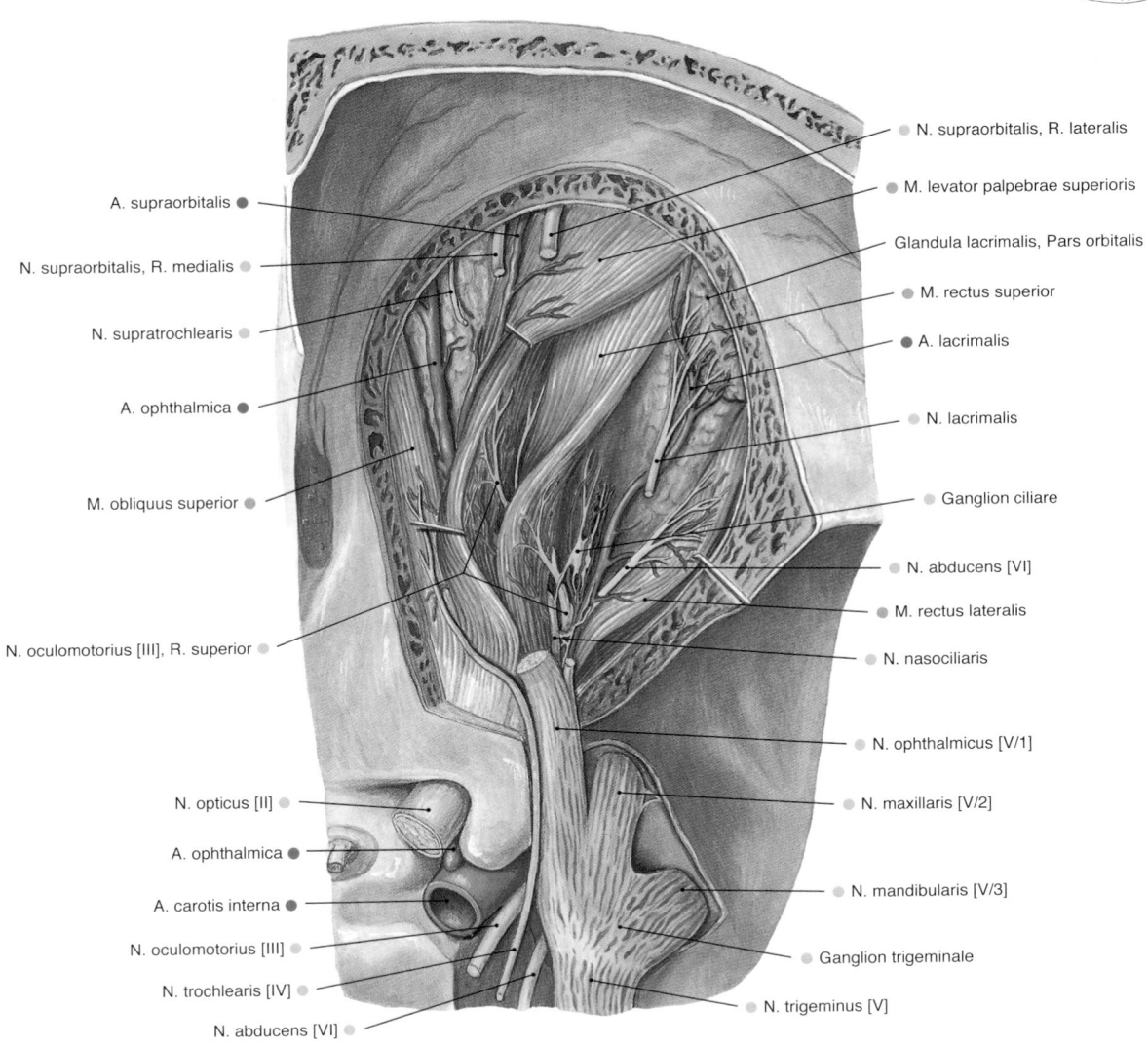

A. supraorbitalis ●

N. supraorbitalis, R. medialis ●

N. supratrochlearis ●

A. ophthalmica ●

M. obliquus superior ●

N. oculomotorius [III], R. superior ●

N. opticus [II] ●

A. ophthalmica ●

A. carotis interna ●

N. oculomotorius [III] ●

N. trochlearis [IV] ●

N. abducens [VI] ●

● N. supraorbitalis, R. lateralis

● M. levator palpebrae superioris

Glandula lacrimalis, Pars orbitalis

● M. rectus superior

● A. lacrimalis

● N. lacrimalis

● Ganglion ciliare

● N. abducens [VI]

● M. rectus lateralis

● N. nasociliaris

● N. ophthalmicus [V/1]

● N. maxillaris [V/2]

● N. mandibularis [V/3]

● Ganglion trigeminale

● N. trigeminus [V]

Fig. 1371 Arteries and nerves of the orbit, Orbita; after removal of the roof of the orbit; superior view.

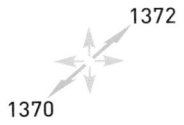

1372

1370

Orbit, topography

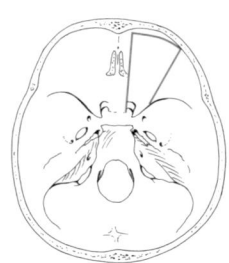

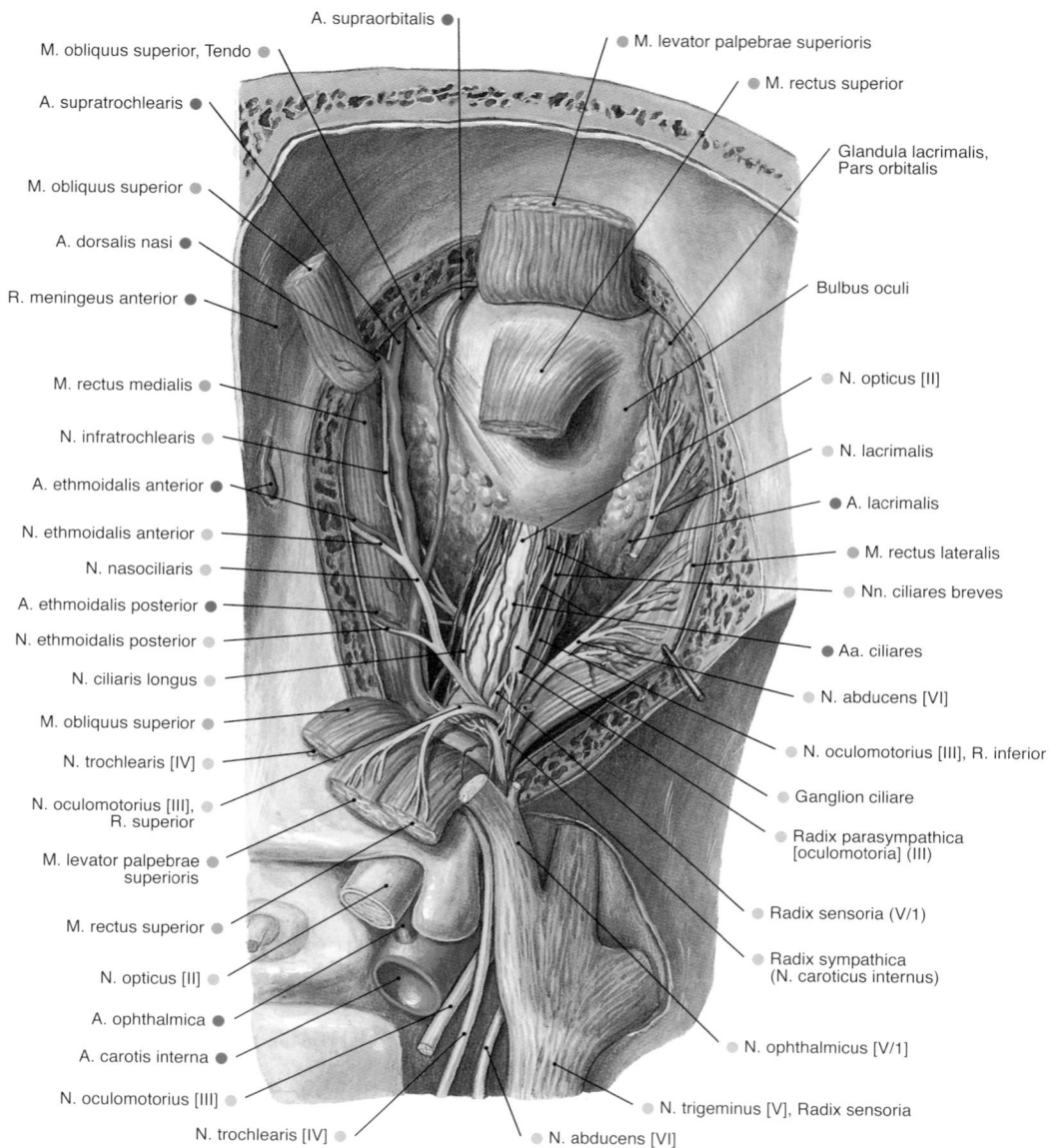

A. supraorbitalis ●

M. obliquus superior, Tendo ●

A. supratrochlearis ●

M. obliquus superior ●

A. dorsalis nasi ●

R. meningeus anterior ●

M. rectus medialis ●

N. infratrochlearis ●

A. ethmoidalis anterior ●

N. ethmoidalis anterior ●

N. nasociliaris ●

A. ethmoidalis posterior ●

N. ethmoidalis posterior ●

N. ciliaris longus ●

M. obliquus superior ●

N. trochlearis [IV] ●

N. oculomotorius [III], R. superior ●

M. levator palpebrae superioris ●

M. rectus superior ●

N. opticus [II] ●

A. ophthalmica ●

A. carotis interna ●

N. oculomotorius [III] ●

N. trochlearis [IV] ●

● M. levator palpebrae superioris

● M. rectus superior

Glandula lacrimalis, Pars orbitalis

Bulbus oculi

● N. opticus [II]

● N. lacrimalis

● A. lacrimalis

● M. rectus lateralis

● Nn. ciliares breves

● Aa. ciliares

● N. abducens [VI]

● N. oculomotorius [III], R. inferior

● Ganglion ciliare

● Radix parasympathica [oculomotoria] (III)

● Radix sensoria (V/1)

● Radix sympathica (N. caroticus internus)

● N. ophthalmicus [V/1]

● N. trigeminus [V], Radix sensoria

● N. abducens [VI]

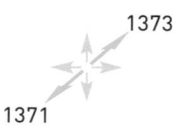

Fig. 1372 Arteries and nerves of the orbit, Orbita; after partial removal of the levator palpebrae superioris, the rectus superior and the obliquus superior muscle; superior view.

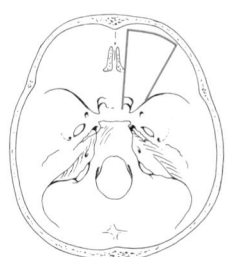

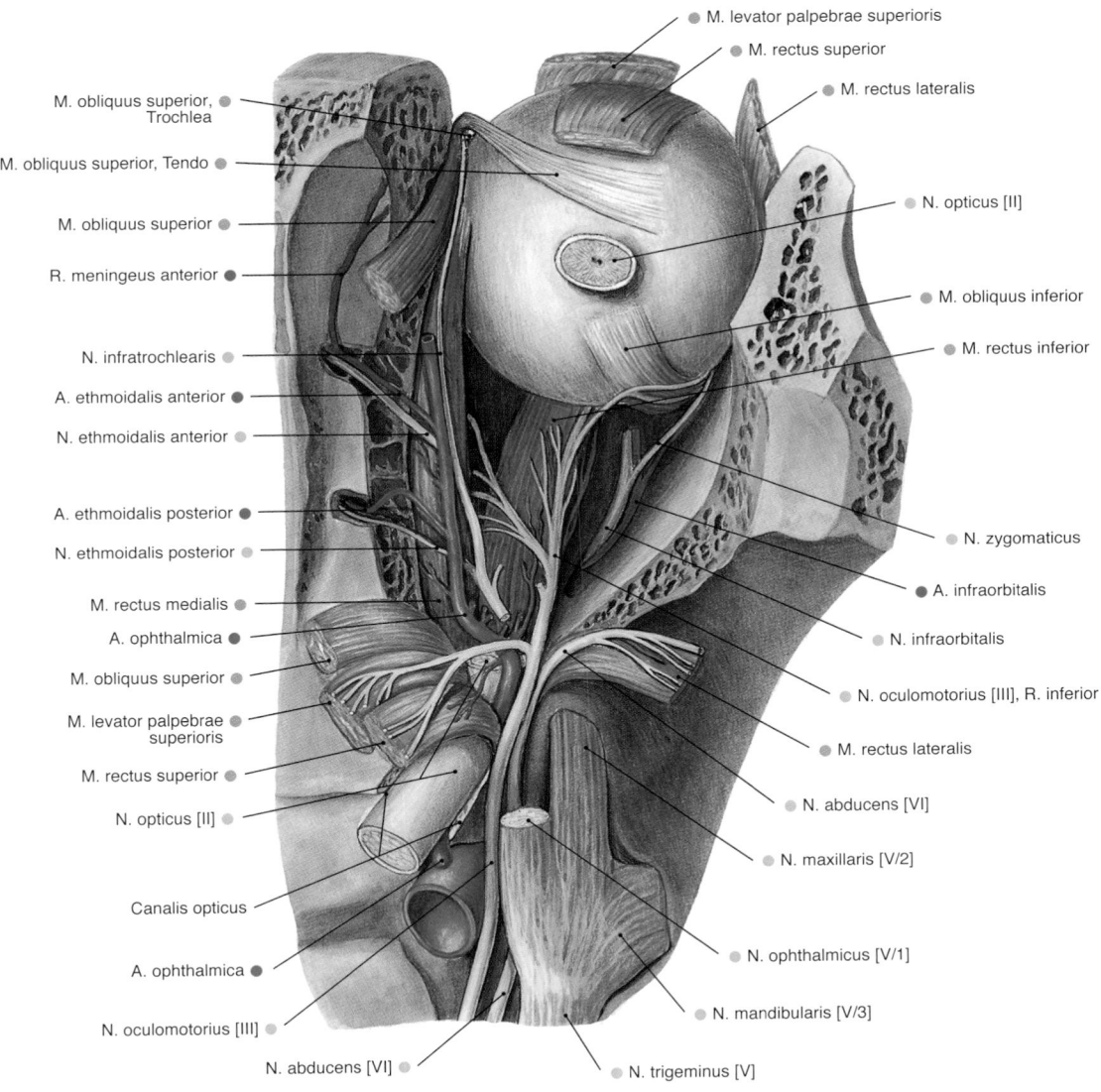

- M. levator palpebrae superioris
- M. rectus superior
- M. rectus lateralis
- M. obliquus superior, Trochlea
- M. obliquus superior, Tendo
- M. obliquus superior
- R. meningeus anterior
- N. opticus [II]
- N. infratrochlearis
- M. obliquus inferior
- A. ethmoidalis anterior
- M. rectus inferior
- N. ethmoidalis anterior
- A. ethmoidalis posterior
- N. ethmoidalis posterior
- N. zygomaticus
- A. infraorbitalis
- M. rectus medialis
- N. infraorbitalis
- A. ophthalmica
- M. obliquus superior
- N. oculomotorius [III], R. inferior
- M. levator palpebrae superioris
- M. rectus lateralis
- M. rectus superior
- N. abducens [VI]
- N. opticus [II]
- N. maxillaris [V/2]
- Canalis opticus
- N. ophthalmicus [V/1]
- A. ophthalmica
- N. mandibularis [V/3]
- N. oculomotorius [III]
- N. abducens [VI]
- N. trigeminus [V]

Fig. 1373 Arteries and nerves of the orbit, Orbita;
after section of the optic nerve;
superior view.

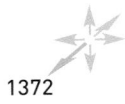

1372

Blood vessels of the orbit

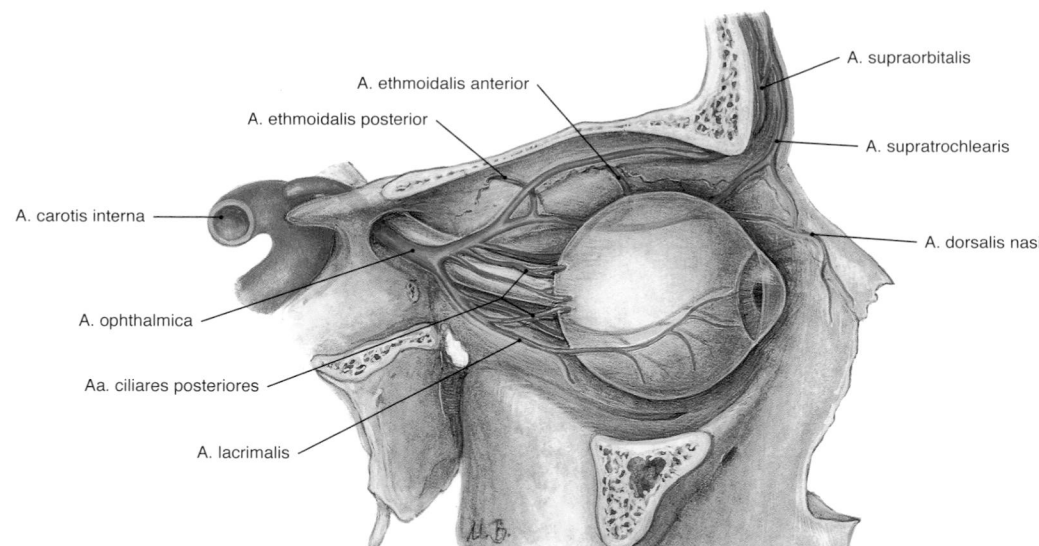

A. ethmoidalis anterior
A. ethmoidalis posterior
A. carotis interna
A. ophthalmica
Aa. ciliares posteriores
A. lacrimalis
A. supraorbitalis
A. supratrochlearis
A. dorsalis nasi

Fig. 1374   Arteries of the orbit, Orbita; lateral view.

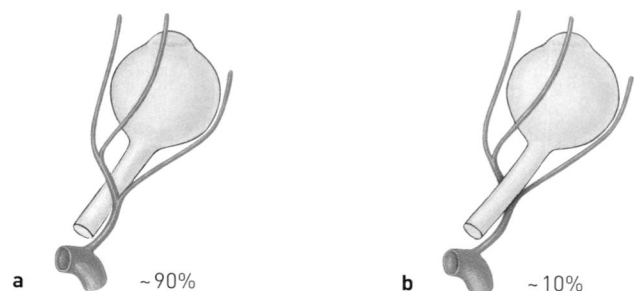

a   ~90%   b   ~10%

Fig. 1375 a, b   Variations of the ophthalmic artery, A. ophthalmica; superior view.

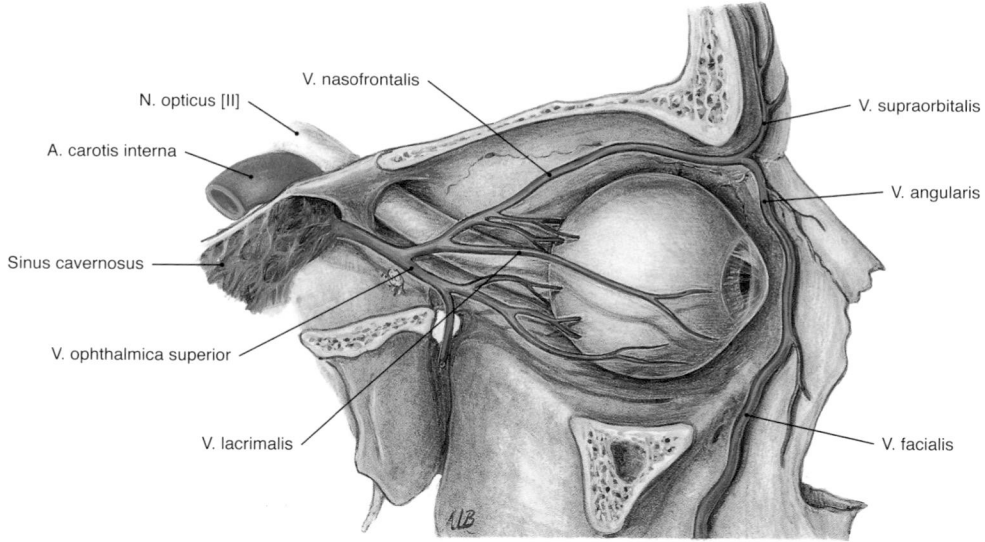

N. opticus [II]
A. carotis interna
Sinus cavernosus
V. ophthalmica superior
V. lacrimalis
V. nasofrontalis
V. supraorbitalis
V. angularis
V. facialis

Fig. 1376   Veins of the orbit, Orbita; lateral view.

Orbit, topography

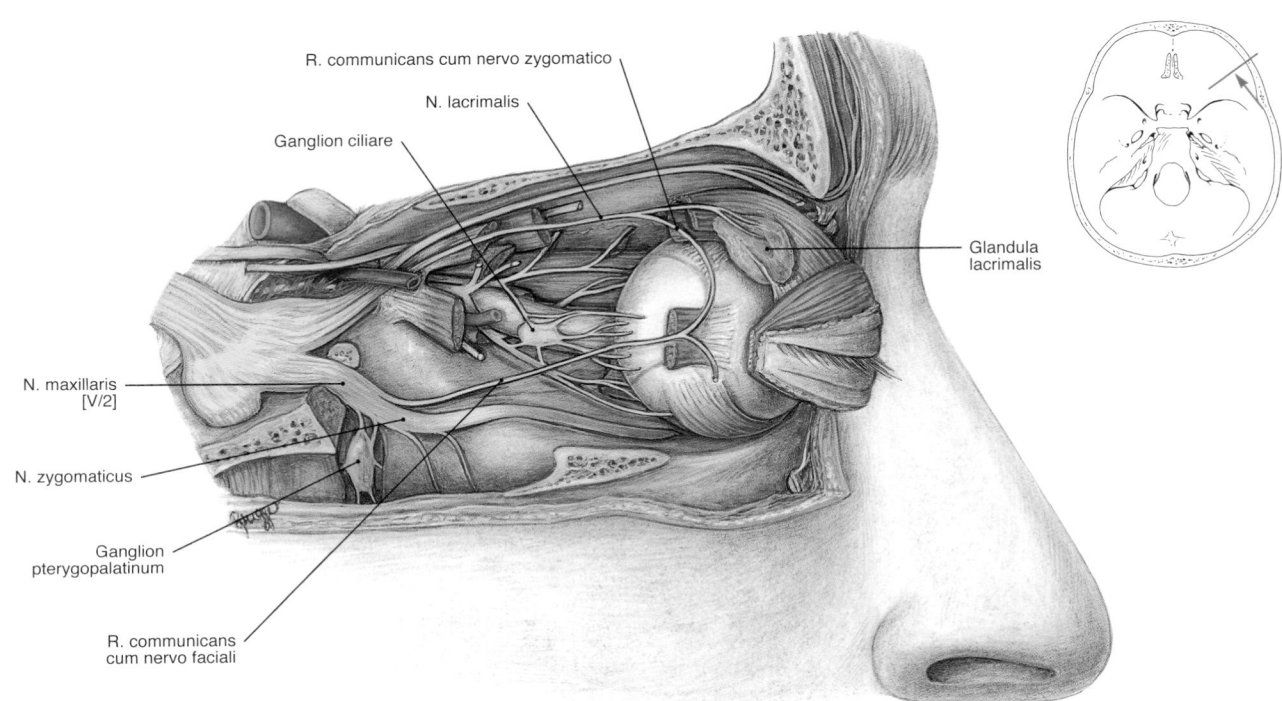

R. communicans cum nervo zygomatico

N. lacrimalis

Ganglion ciliare

Glandula lacrimalis

N. maxillaris [V/2]

N. zygomaticus

Ganglion pterygopalatinum

R. communicans cum nervo faciali

Fig. 1377 Orbit, Orbita; viewed from the right.

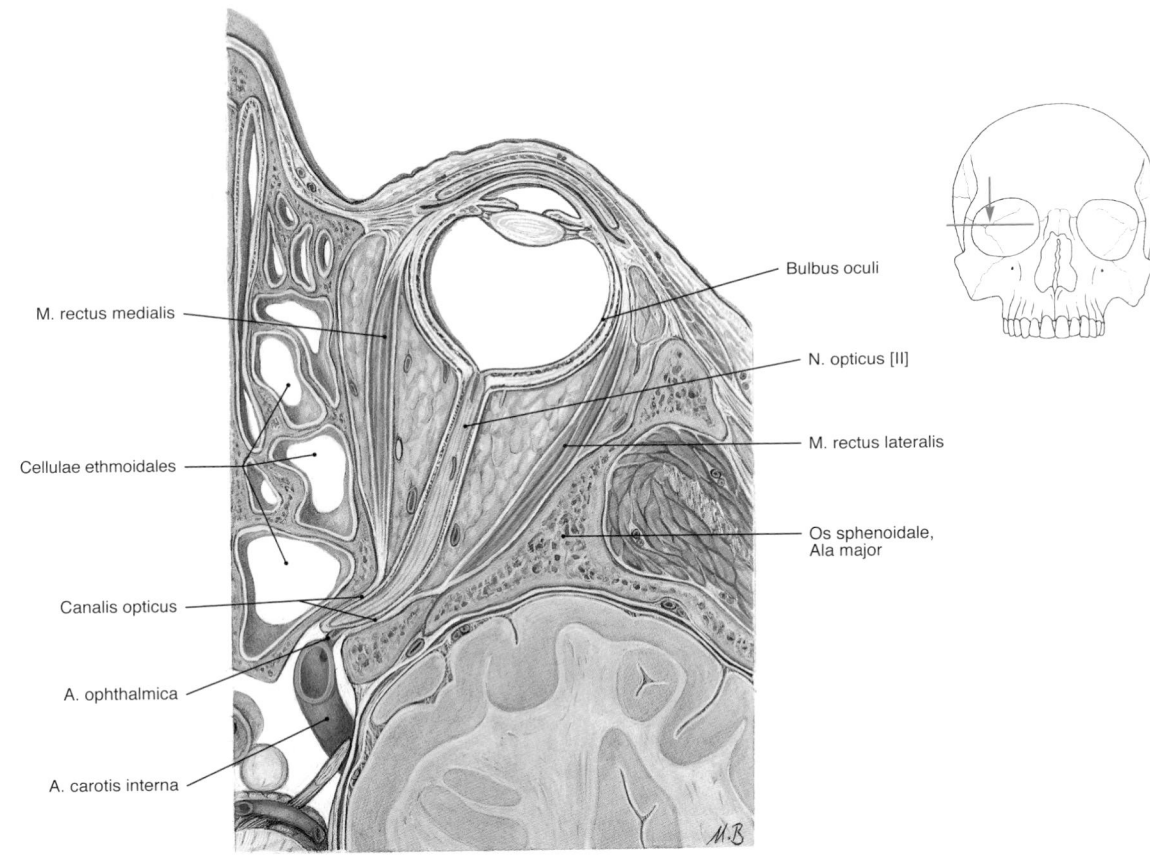

M. rectus medialis

Bulbus oculi

N. opticus [II]

Cellulae ethmoidales

M. rectus lateralis

Canalis opticus

Os sphenoidale, Ala major

A. ophthalmica

A. carotis interna

Fig. 1378 Orbit, Orbita; horizontal section; superior view.

Orbit, sections

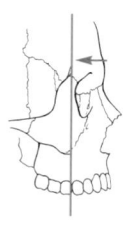

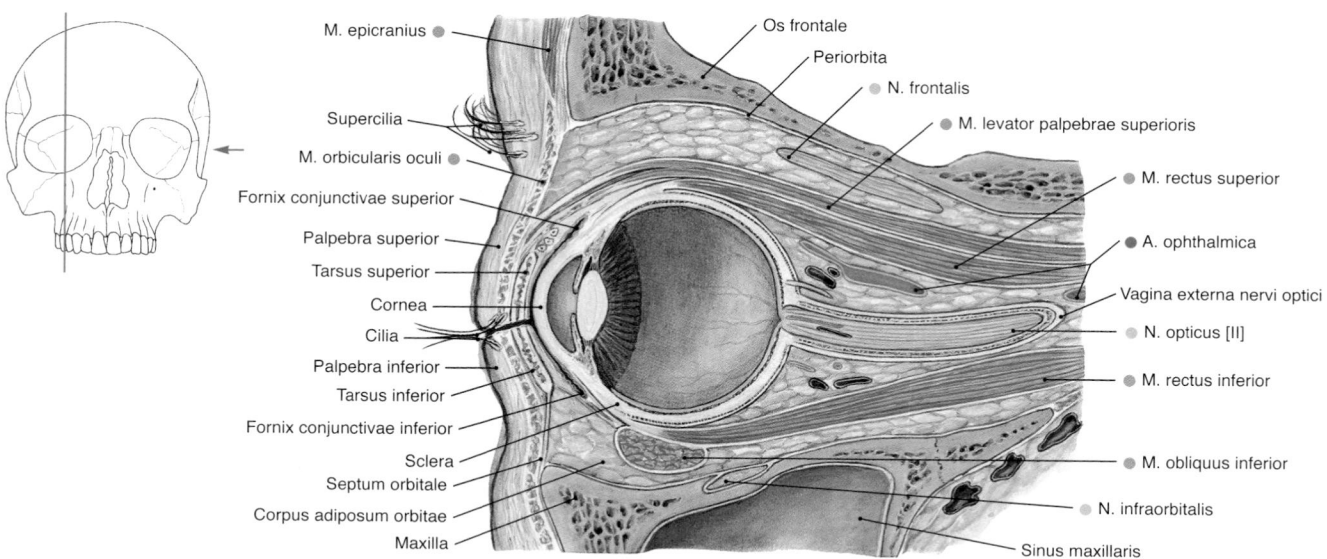

M. epicranius
Supercilia
M. orbicularis oculi
Fornix conjunctivae superior
Palpebra superior
Tarsus superior
Cornea
Cilia
Palpebra inferior
Tarsus inferior
Fornix conjunctivae inferior
Sclera
Septum orbitale
Corpus adiposum orbitae
Maxilla

Os frontale
Periorbita
N. frontalis
M. levator palpebrae superioris
M. rectus superior
A. ophthalmica
Vagina externa nervi optici
N. opticus [II]
M. rectus inferior
M. obliquus inferior
N. infraorbitalis
Sinus maxillaris

Fig. 1379 Orbit, Orbita;
vertical section through the eyeball and the optic nerve;
medial view.

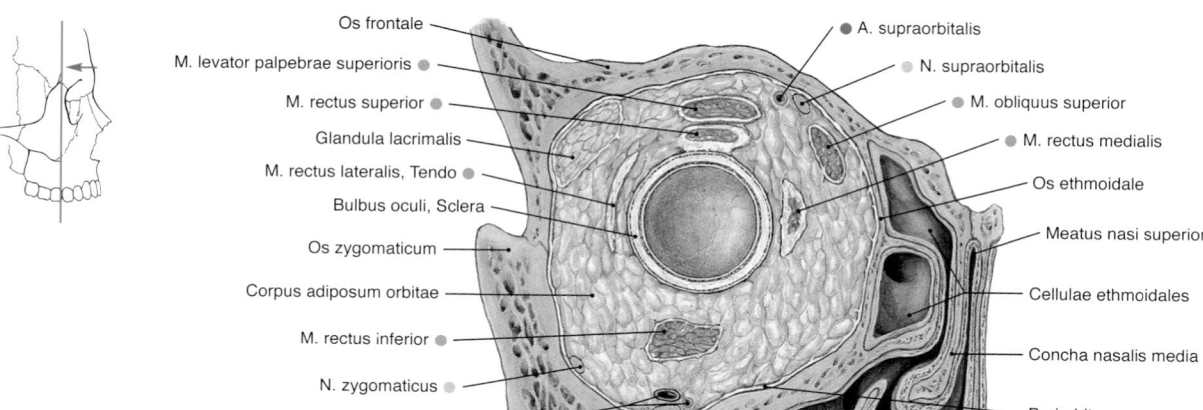

Os frontale
M. levator palpebrae superioris
M. rectus superior
Glandula lacrimalis
M. rectus lateralis, Tendo
Bulbus oculi, Sclera
Os zygomaticum
Corpus adiposum orbitae
M. rectus inferior
N. zygomaticus
(V.); A. infraorbitalis
N. infraorbitalis

A. supraorbitalis
N. supraorbitalis
M. obliquus superior
M. rectus medialis
Os ethmoidale
Meatus nasi superior
Cellulae ethmoidales
Concha nasalis media
Periorbita
Sinus maxillaris

Fig. 1380 Orbit, Orbita;
frontal section at the level of the posterior part of the eyeball;
anterior view.

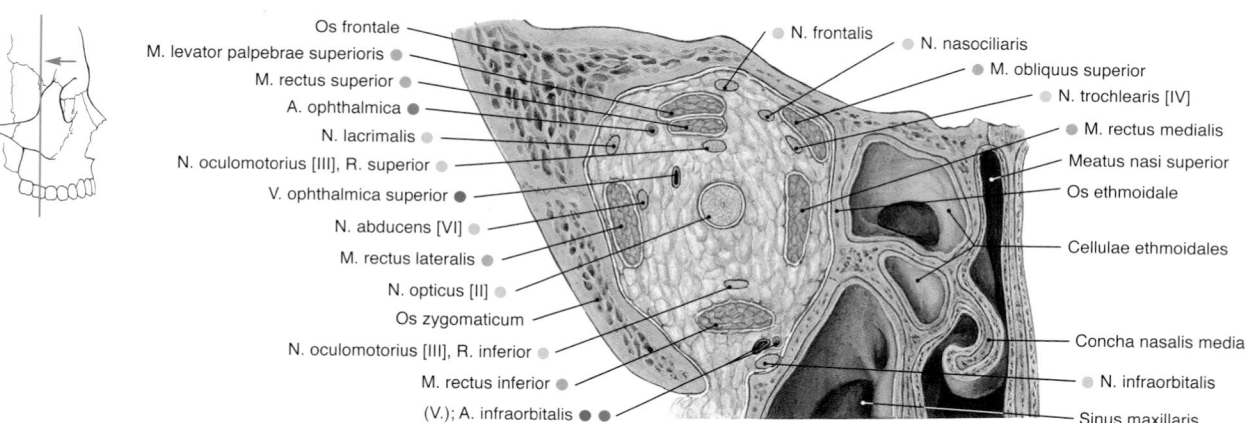

Os frontale
M. levator palpebrae superioris
M. rectus superior
A. ophthalmica
N. lacrimalis
N. oculomotorius [III], R. superior
V. ophthalmica superior
N. abducens [VI]
M. rectus lateralis
N. opticus [II]
Os zygomaticum
N. oculomotorius [III], R. inferior
M. rectus inferior
(V.); A. infraorbitalis

N. frontalis
N. nasociliaris
M. obliquus superior
N. trochlearis [IV]
M. rectus medialis
Meatus nasi superior
Os ethmoidale
Cellulae ethmoidales
Concha nasalis media
N. infraorbitalis
Sinus maxillaris

Fig. 1381 Orbit, Orbita;
frontal section at the level of the middle of the extracranial
course of the optic nerve;
anterior view.

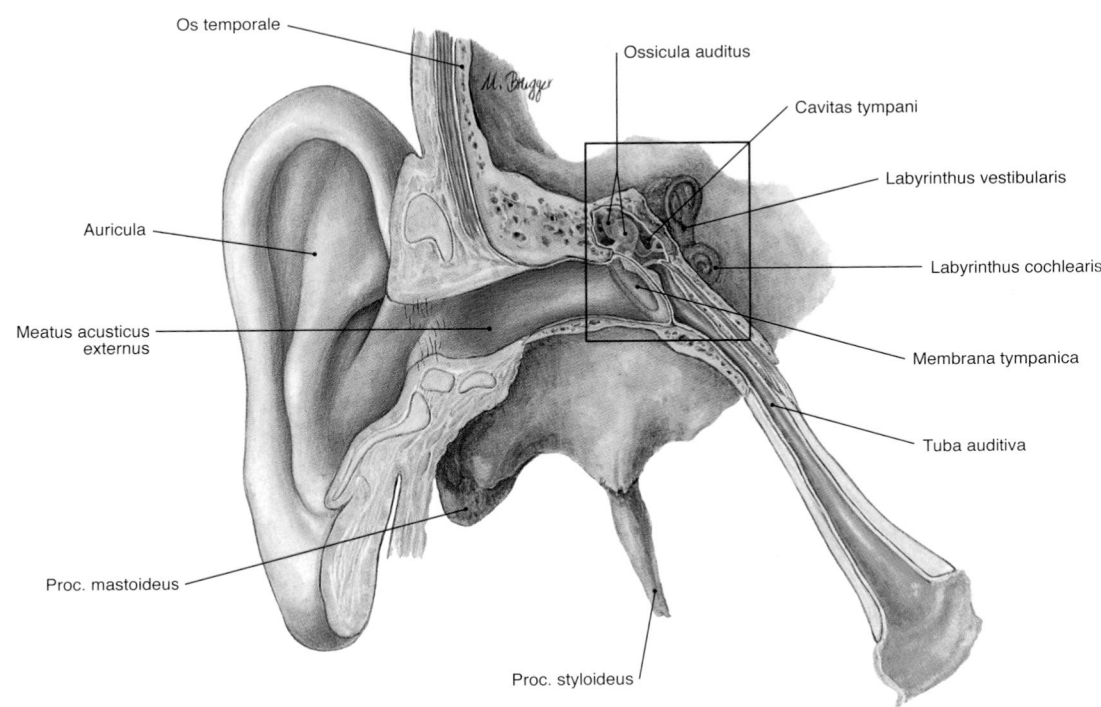

Os temporale
Ossicula auditus
Cavitas tympani
Labyrinthus vestibularis
Auricula
Labyrinthus cochlearis
Meatus acusticus externus
Membrana tympanica
Tuba auditiva
Proc. mastoideus
Proc. styloideus

Fig. 1382   Ear, Auris.

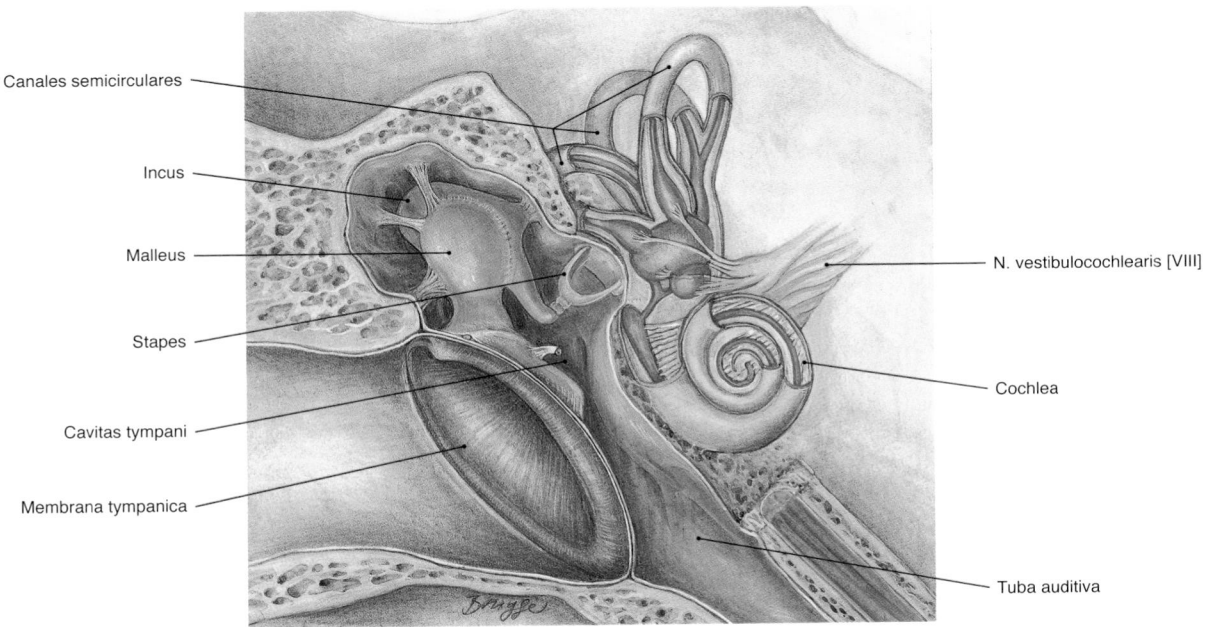

Canales semicirculares
Incus
Malleus
Stapes
Cavitas tympani
Membrana tympanica
N. vestibulocochlearis [VIII]
Cochlea
Tuba auditiva

Fig. 1383   Middle and inner ear, Auris media et interna; section from Fig. 1382; anterior view.

Auricle

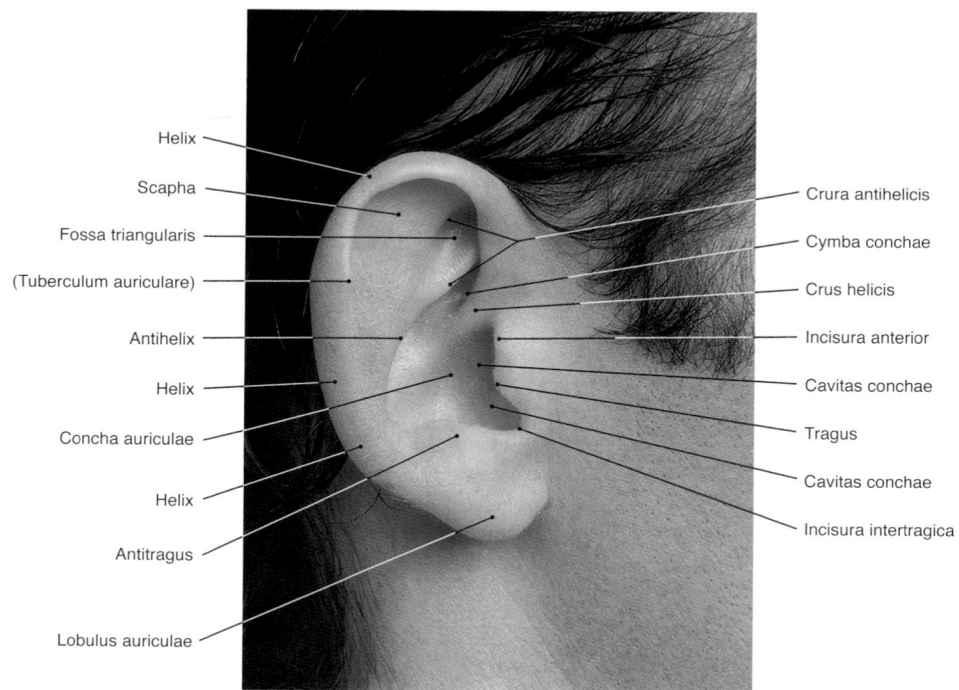

Helix
Scapha
Fossa triangularis
(Tuberculum auriculare)
Antihelix
Helix
Concha auriculae
Helix
Antitragus
Lobulus auriculae

Crura antihelicis
Cymba conchae
Crus helicis
Incisura anterior
Cavitas conchae
Tragus
Cavitas conchae
Incisura intertragica

Fig. 1384   Auricle, Auricula.

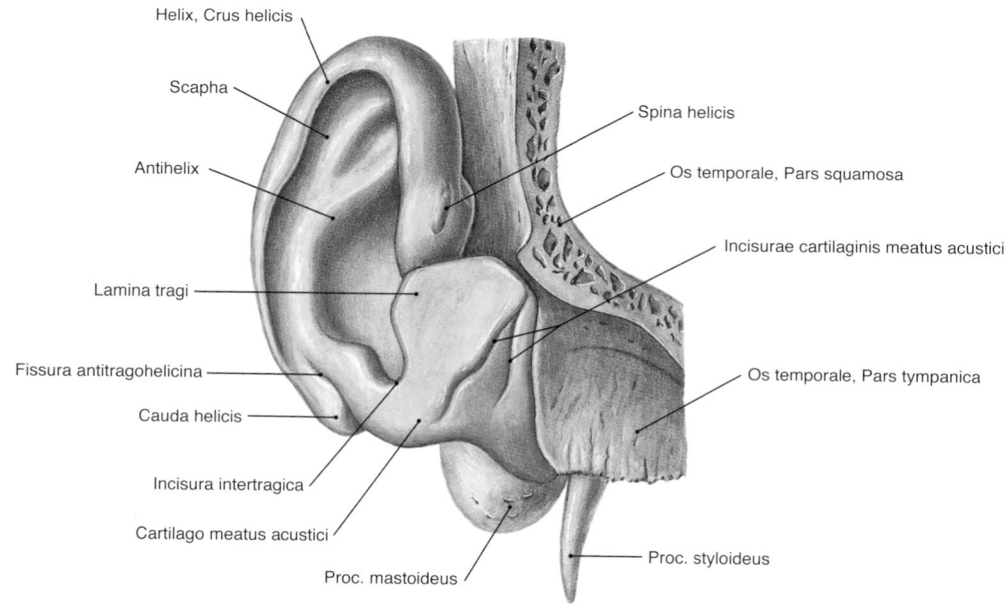

Helix, Crus helicis
Scapha
Antihelix
Lamina tragi
Fissura antitragohelicina
Cauda helicis
Incisura intertragica
Cartilago meatus acustici
Proc. mastoideus

Spina helicis
Os temporale, Pars squamosa
Incisurae cartilaginis meatus acustici
Os temporale, Pars tympanica
Proc. styloideus

Fig. 1385   Auricular cartilage, Cartilago auricularis.

Auricular muscles

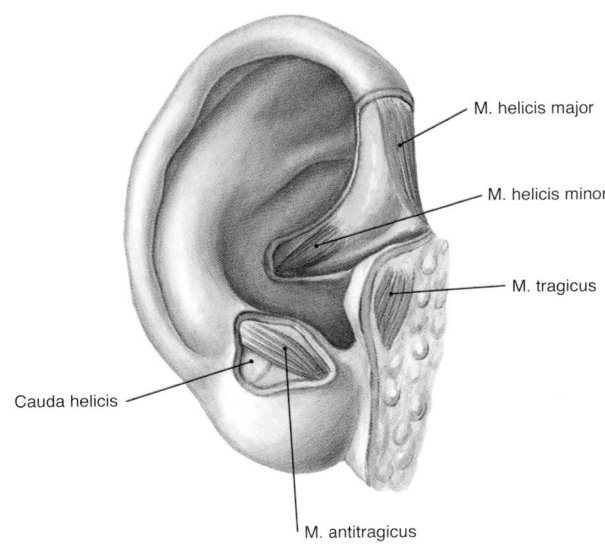

M. helicis major

M. helicis minor

M. tragicus

Cauda helicis

M. antitragicus

Fig. 1386 Auricular muscles, Mm. auriculares.

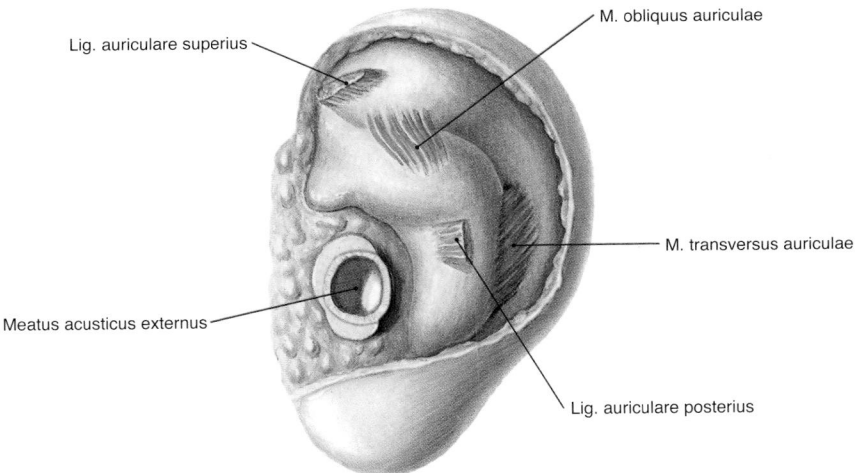

Lig. auriculare superius

M. obliquus auriculae

M. transversus auriculae

Meatus acusticus externus

Lig. auriculare posterius

Fig. 1387 Auricular muscles, Mm. auriculares.

External acoustic meatus and tympanic membrane

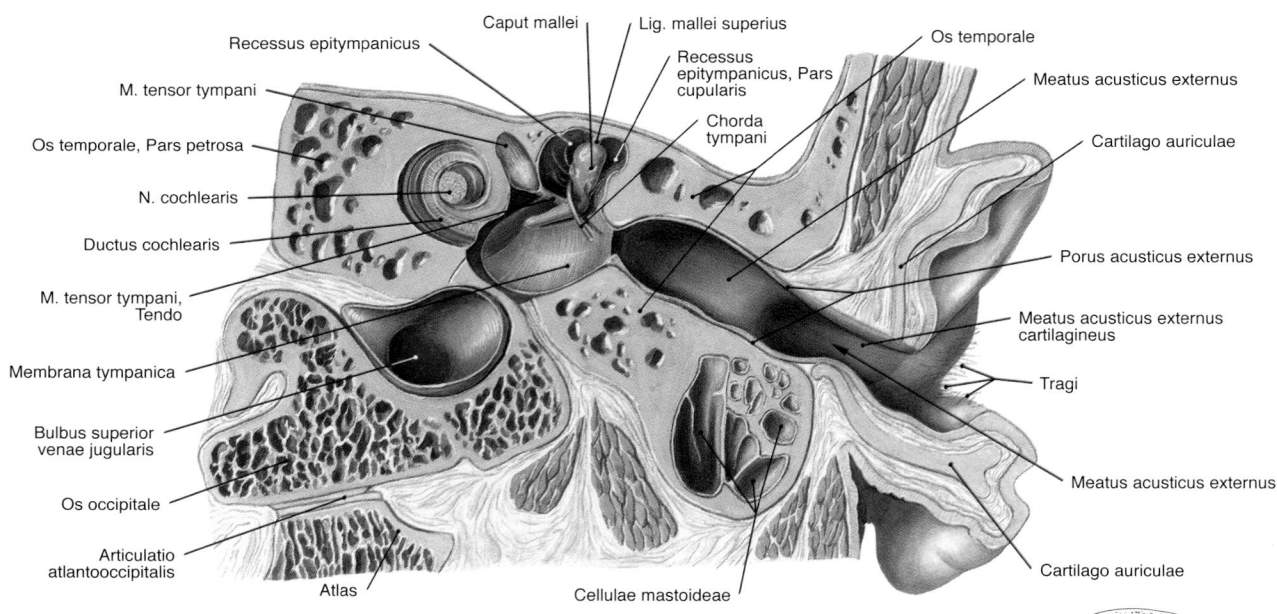

Fig. 1388 External acoustic meatus, Meatus acusticus externus; tympanic cavity, Cavitas tympani, and cochlea, Cochlea; frontal section; posterior view.

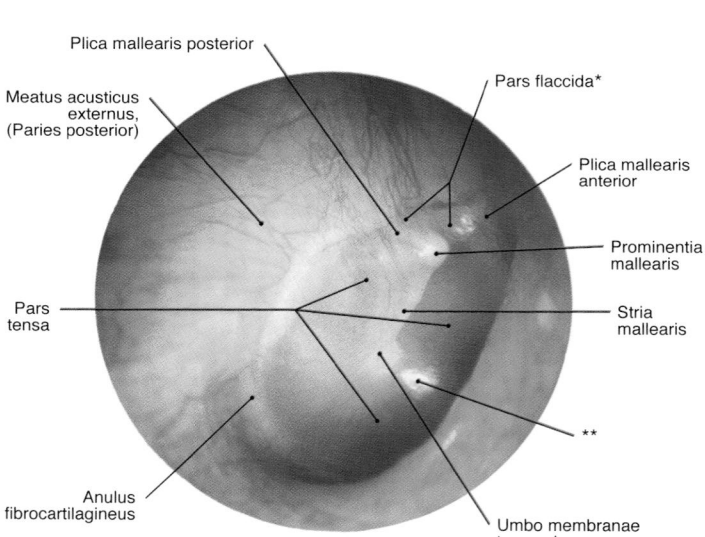

Fig. 1389 Tympanic membrane, Membrana tympanica; otoscopic image; lateral view.

* Clinical term: SHRAPNELL's membrane
** Typically occurring reflection of light

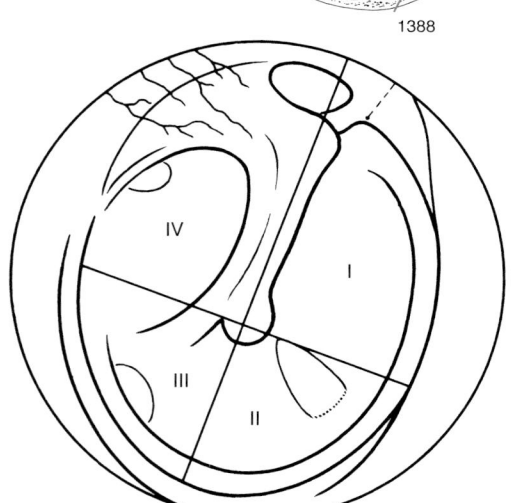

Fig. 1390 Tympanic membrane, Membrana tympanica; quadrant schema; lateral view.

In order to obtain a complete otoscopic overview of the cutaneous surface of the tympanic membrane, the external acoustic meatus must be stretched by pulling the auricle upwards and posteriorly.
To facilitate orientation, the tympanic membrane is usually divided into four quadrants (I–IV).

The longer diameter of the tympanic membrane in the adult is 10–11 mm, the shorter diameter is approx. 9 mm. The light source characteristically produces a triangular reflection of light at the umbo in the region of quadrant II.

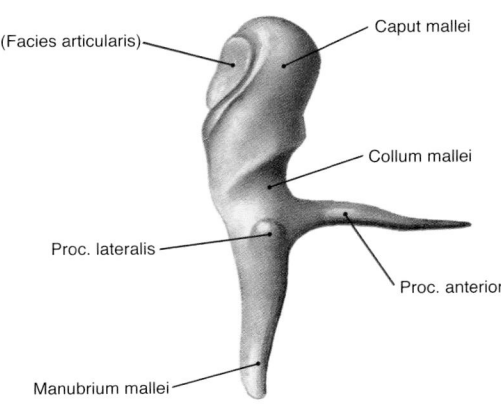

Fig. 1391 Malleus, Malleus; lateral view.

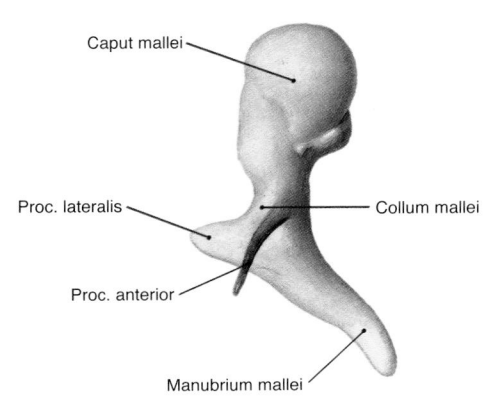

Fig. 1392 Malleus, Malleus; anterior view.

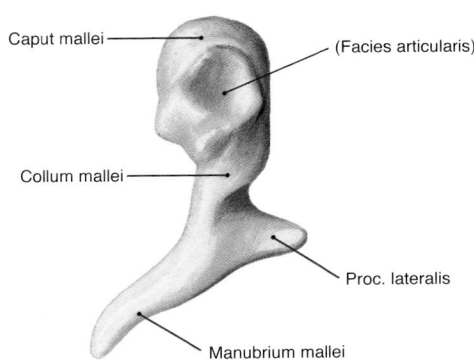

Fig. 1393 Malleus, Malleus; posterior view.

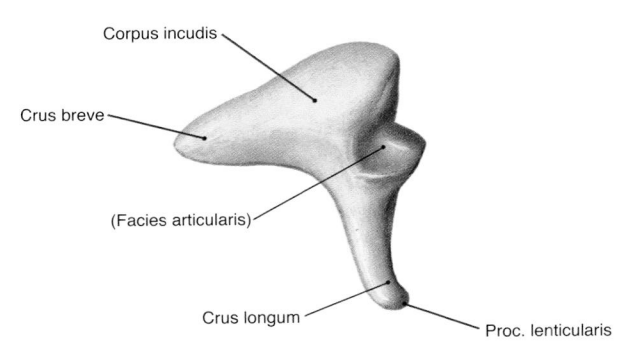

Fig. 1394 Incus, Incus; lateral view.

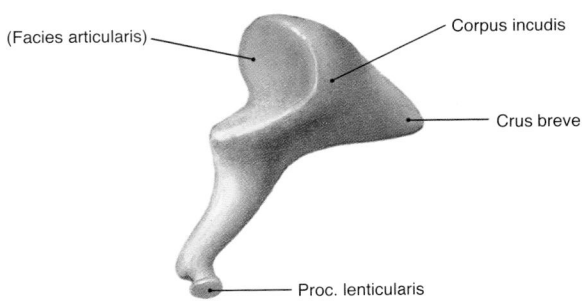

Fig. 1395 Incus, Incus; medial view.

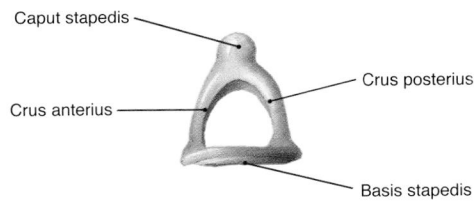

Fig. 1396 Stapes, Stapes; superior view.

Auditory ossicles

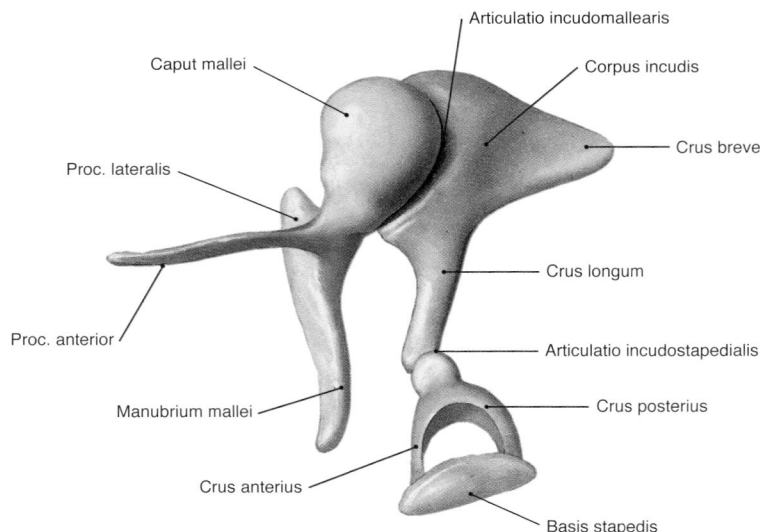

Fig. 1397 Auditory ossicles, Ossicula auditus; superomedial view.

Caput mallei
Articulatio incudomallearis
Corpus incudis
Proc. lateralis
Crus breve
Proc. anterior
Crus longum
Manubrium mallei
Articulatio incudostapedialis
Crus anterius
Crus posterius
Basis stapedis

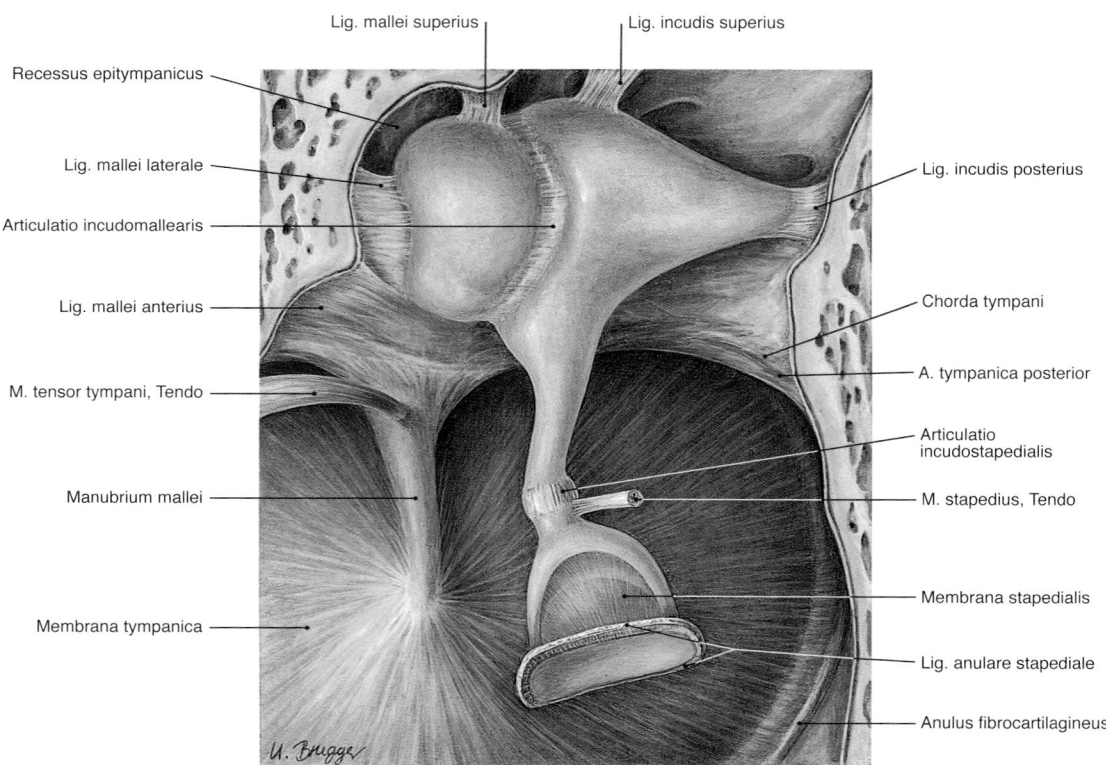

Fig. 1398 Joints and ligaments of the auditory ossicles, Articulationes et Ligamenta ossiculorum auditus; covered with mucosa; superomedial view.

Lig. mallei superius
Lig. incudis superius
Recessus epitympanicus
Lig. mallei laterale
Articulatio incudomallearis
Lig. mallei anterius
M. tensor tympani, Tendo
Manubrium mallei
Membrana tympanica
Lig. incudis posterius
Chorda tympani
A. tympanica posterior
Articulatio incudostapedialis
M. stapedius, Tendo
Membrana stapedialis
Lig. anulare stapediale
Anulus fibrocartilagineus

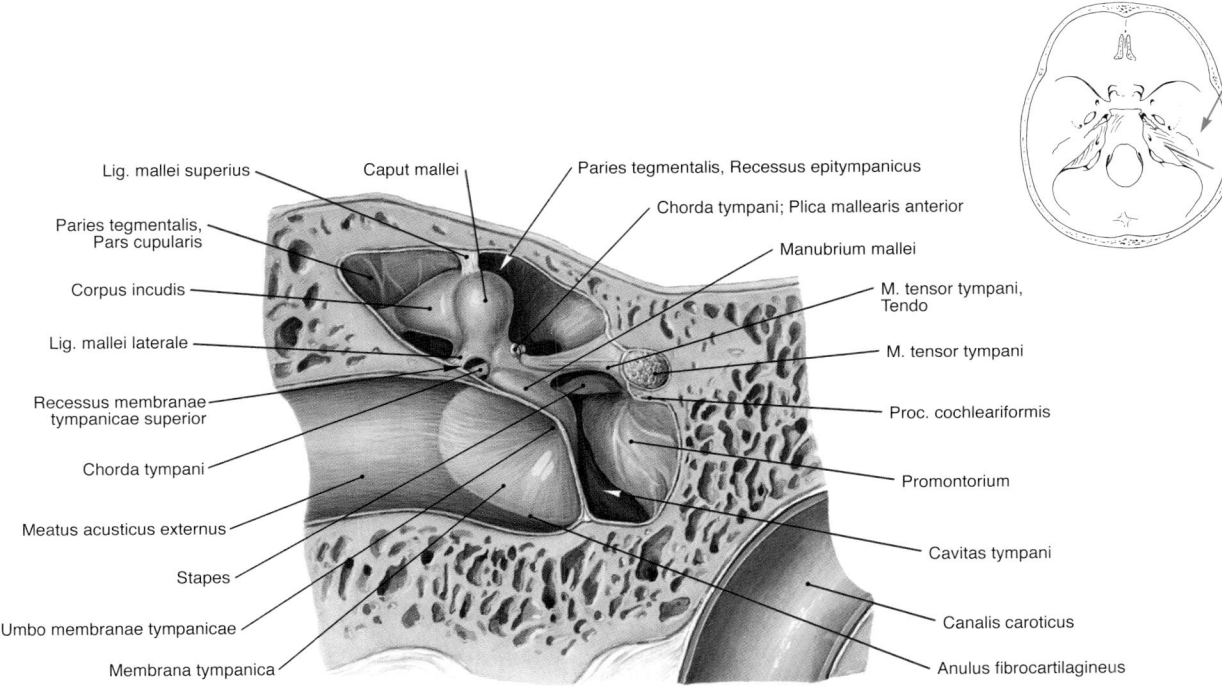

Lig. mallei superius

Caput mallei

Paries tegmentalis, Recessus epitympanicus

Chorda tympani; Plica mallearis anterior

Paries tegmentalis, Pars cupularis

Manubrium mallei

Corpus incudis

M. tensor tympani, Tendo

Lig. mallei laterale

M. tensor tympani

Recessus membranae tympanicae superior

Proc. cochleariformis

Chorda tympani

Promontorium

Meatus acusticus externus

Stapes

Cavitas tympani

Umbo membranae tympanicae

Canalis caroticus

Membrana tympanica

Anulus fibrocartilagineus

Fig. 1399 Tympanic cavity, Cavitas tympani; frontal section; anterior view.

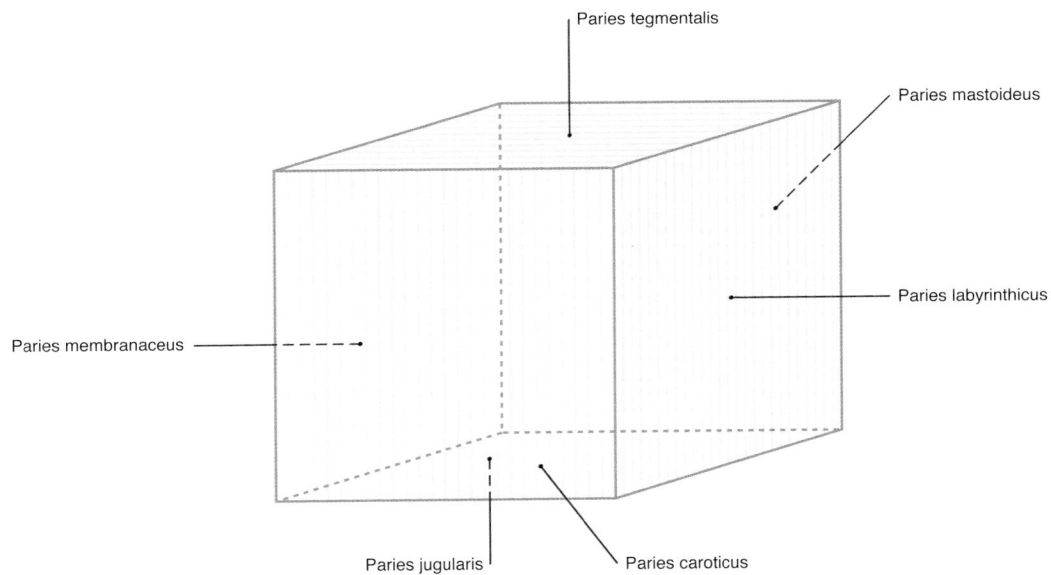

Paries tegmentalis

Paries mastoideus

Paries labyrinthicus

Paries membranaceus

Paries jugularis

Paries caroticus

Fig. 1400 Walls of the tympanic cavity, Cavitas tympani; schema for orientation.

Tympanic cavity

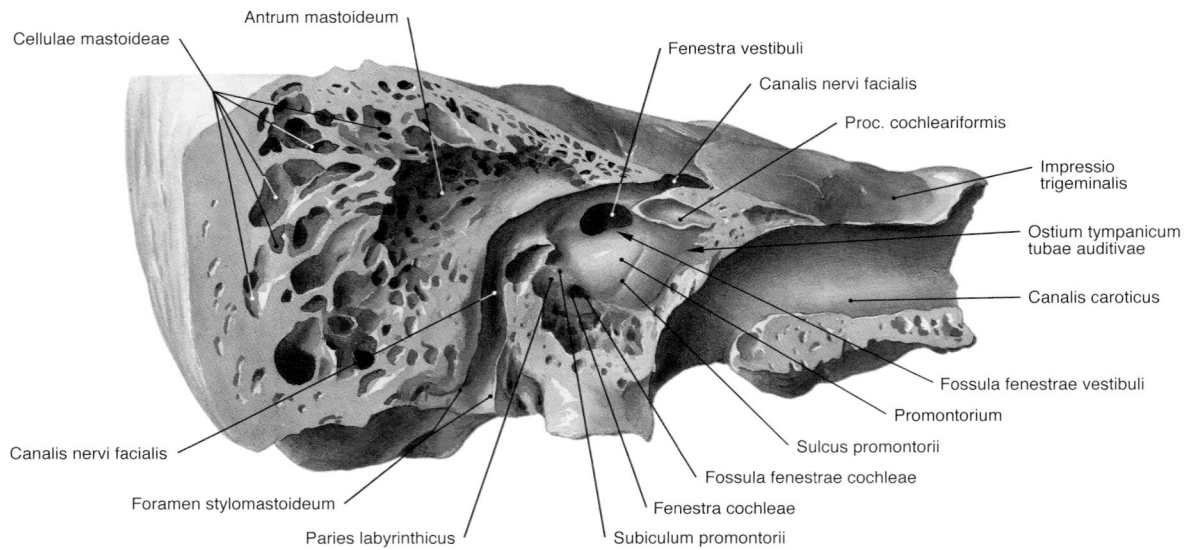

Cellulae mastoideae
Antrum mastoideum
Fenestra vestibuli
Canalis nervi facialis
Proc. cochleariformis
Impressio trigeminalis
Ostium tympanicum tubae auditivae
Canalis caroticus
Fossula fenestrae vestibuli
Promontorium
Sulcus promontorii
Fossula fenestrae cochleae
Fenestra cochleae
Subiculum promontorii
Paries labyrinthicus
Foramen stylomastoideum
Canalis nervi facialis

Fig. 1401 Medial wall, Paries labyrinthicus, of the tympanic cavity, Cavitas tympani;
after removal of the lateral wall and the adjacent parts of the anterior and superior wall;
the facial canal and the carotid canal have been opened;
anterolateral view.

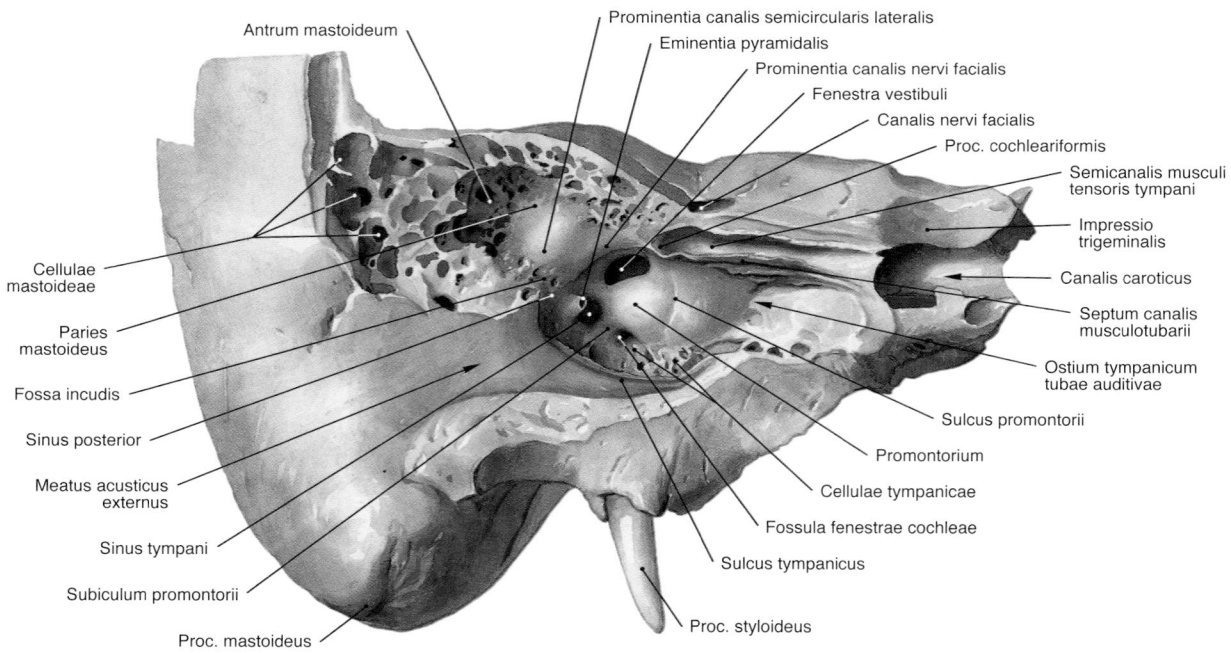

Antrum mastoideum
Prominentia canalis semicircularis lateralis
Eminentia pyramidalis
Prominentia canalis nervi facialis
Fenestra vestibuli
Canalis nervi facialis
Proc. cochleariformis
Semicanalis musculi tensoris tympani
Impressio trigeminalis
Canalis caroticus
Septum canalis musculotubarii
Ostium tympanicum tubae auditivae
Sulcus promontorii
Promontorium
Cellulae tympanicae
Fossula fenestrae cochleae
Sulcus tympanicus
Proc. styloideus
Cellulae mastoideae
Paries mastoideus
Fossa incudis
Sinus posterior
Meatus acusticus externus
Sinus tympani
Subiculum promontorii
Proc. mastoideus

Fig. 1402 Medial wall, Paries labyrinthicus, of the tympanic cavity, Cavitas tympani;
vertical section along the longitudinal axis of the petrous part of the temporal bone;
anterolateral view.

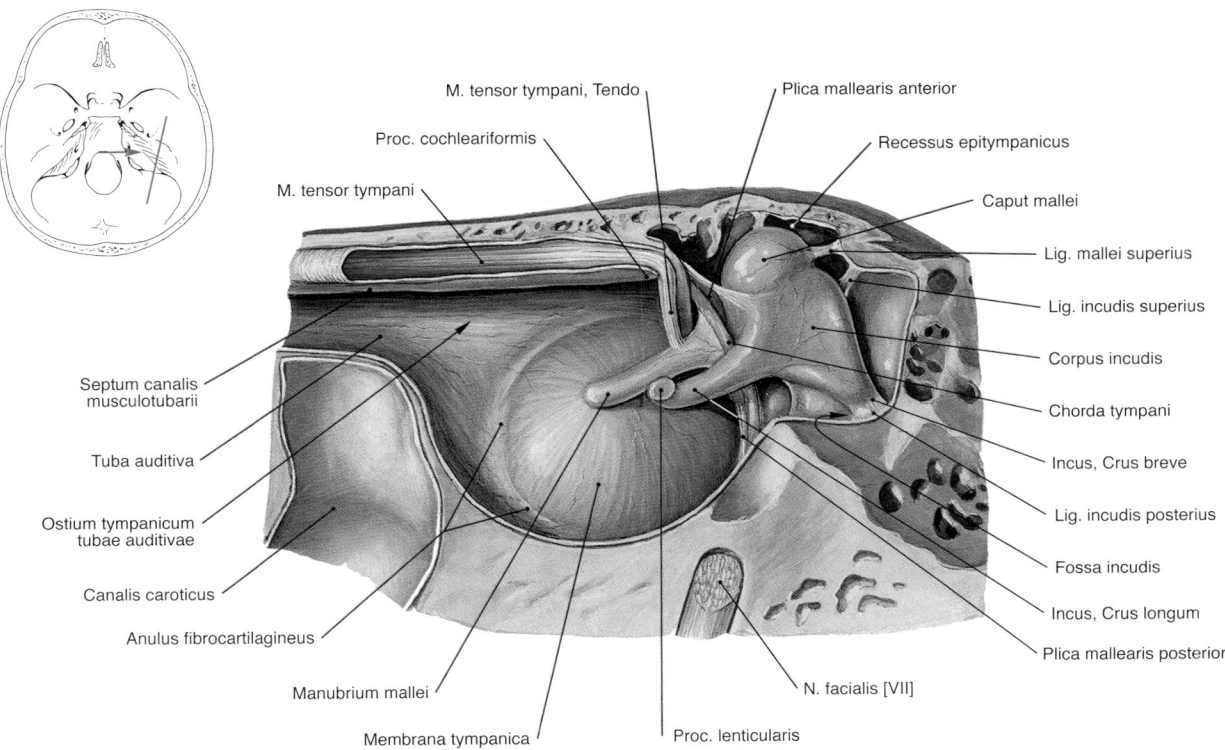

M. tensor tympani, Tendo
Proc. cochleariformis
M. tensor tympani
Plica mallearis anterior
Recessus epitympanicus
Caput mallei
Lig. mallei superius
Lig. incudis superius
Corpus incudis
Chorda tympani
Incus, Crus breve
Lig. incudis posterius
Fossa incudis
Incus, Crus longum
Plica mallearis posterior
Septum canalis musculotubarii
Tuba auditiva
Ostium tympanicum tubae auditivae
Canalis caroticus
Anulus fibrocartilagineus
Manubrium mallei
Membrana tympanica
Proc. lenticularis
N. facialis [VII]

Fig. 1403 Lateral wall, Paries membranaceus, of the tympanic cavity, Cavitas tympani; medial view.

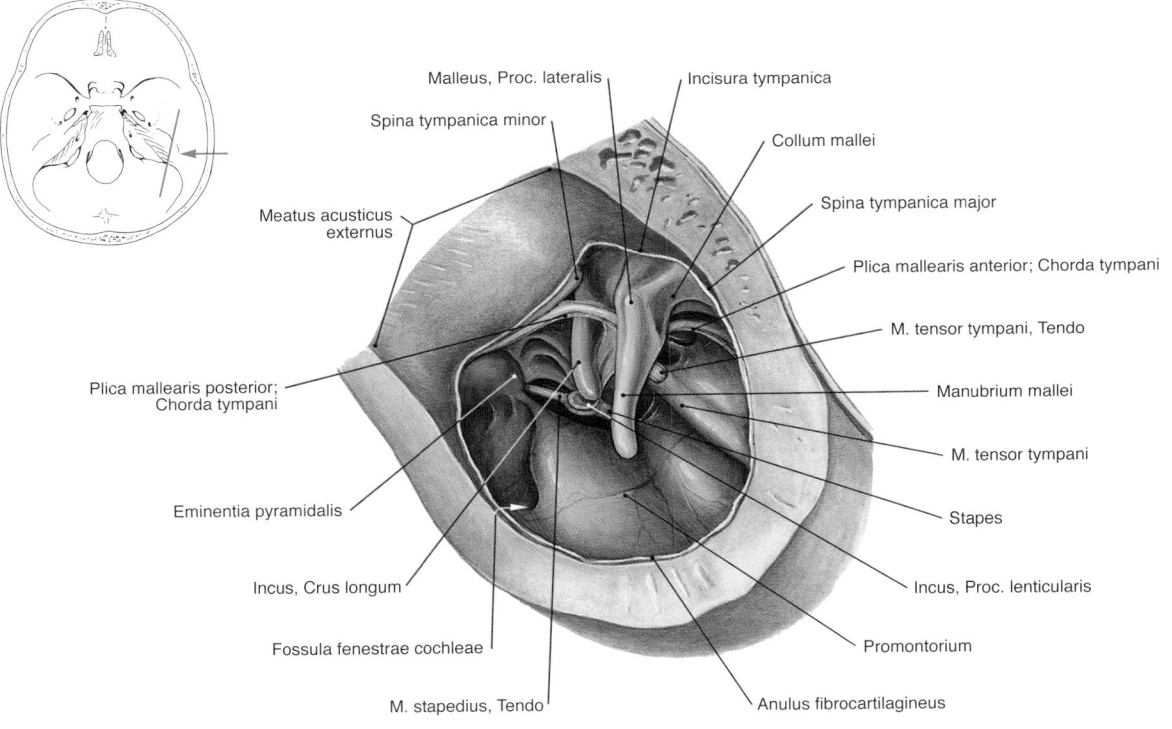

Malleus, Proc. lateralis
Spina tympanica minor
Incisura tympanica
Collum mallei
Spina tympanica major
Plica mallearis anterior; Chorda tympani
M. tensor tympani, Tendo
Manubrium mallei
M. tensor tympani
Stapes
Incus, Proc. lenticularis
Promontorium
Anulus fibrocartilagineus
Meatus acusticus externus
Plica mallearis posterior; Chorda tympani
Eminentia pyramidalis
Incus, Crus longum
Fossula fenestrae cochleae
M. stapedius, Tendo

Fig. 1404 Tympanic cavity, Cavitas tympani; after removal of the tympanic membrane; lateral view.

Auditory tube

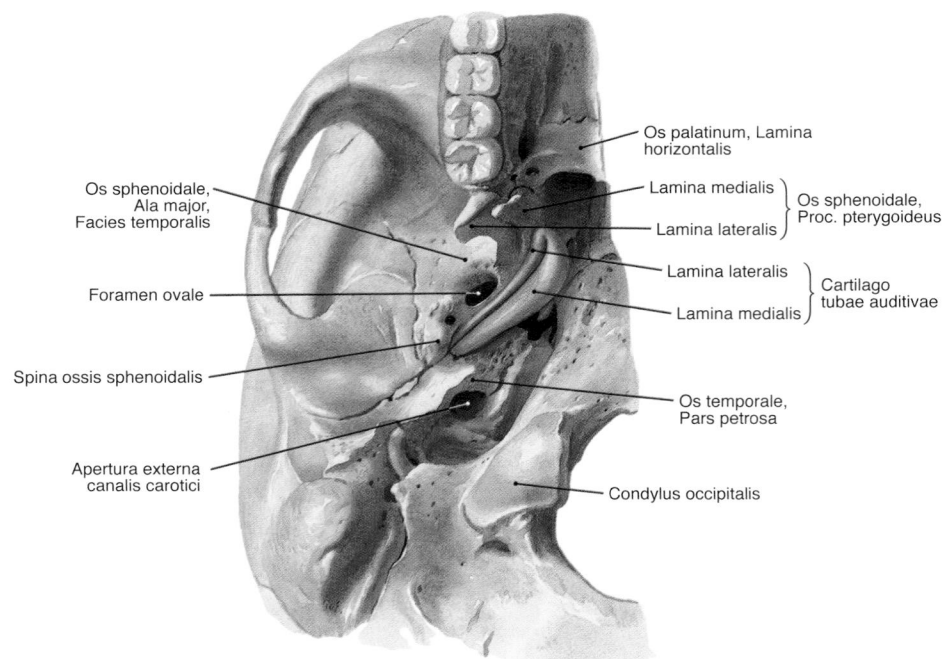

Os palatinum, Lamina horizontalis

Os sphenoidale, Ala major, Facies temporalis

Lamina medialis ⎤ Os sphenoidale,
Lamina lateralis ⎦ Proc. pterygoideus

Foramen ovale

Lamina lateralis ⎤ Cartilago
Lamina medialis ⎦ tubae auditivae

Spina ossis sphenoidalis

Os temporale, Pars petrosa

Apertura externa canalis carotici

Condylus occipitalis

Fig. 1405   Cartilage of the auditory tube, Cartilago tubae auditivae; exposed at the base of the skull; inferior view.

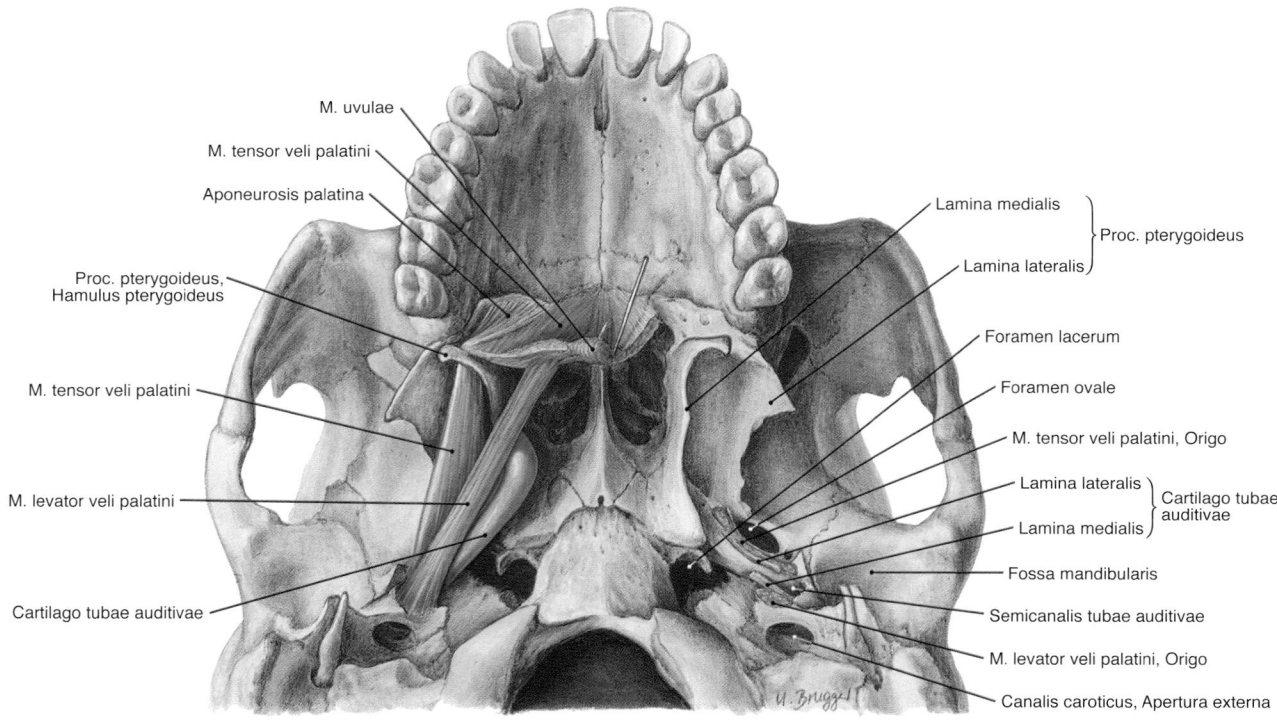

M. uvulae

M. tensor veli palatini

Aponeurosis palatina

Proc. pterygoideus, Hamulus pterygoideus

M. tensor veli palatini

M. levator veli palatini

Cartilago tubae auditivae

Lamina medialis ⎤ Proc. pterygoideus
Lamina lateralis ⎦

Foramen lacerum

Foramen ovale

M. tensor veli palatini, Origo

Lamina lateralis ⎤ Cartilago tubae
Lamina medialis ⎦ auditivae

Fossa mandibularis

Semicanalis tubae auditivae

M. levator veli palatini, Origo

Canalis caroticus, Apertura externa

→ 246, 249, T 3   **Fig. 1406**   Levator and tensor veli palatini muscles, Mm. levator et tensor veli palatini, and the cartilage of the auditory tube, Cartilago tubae auditivae.

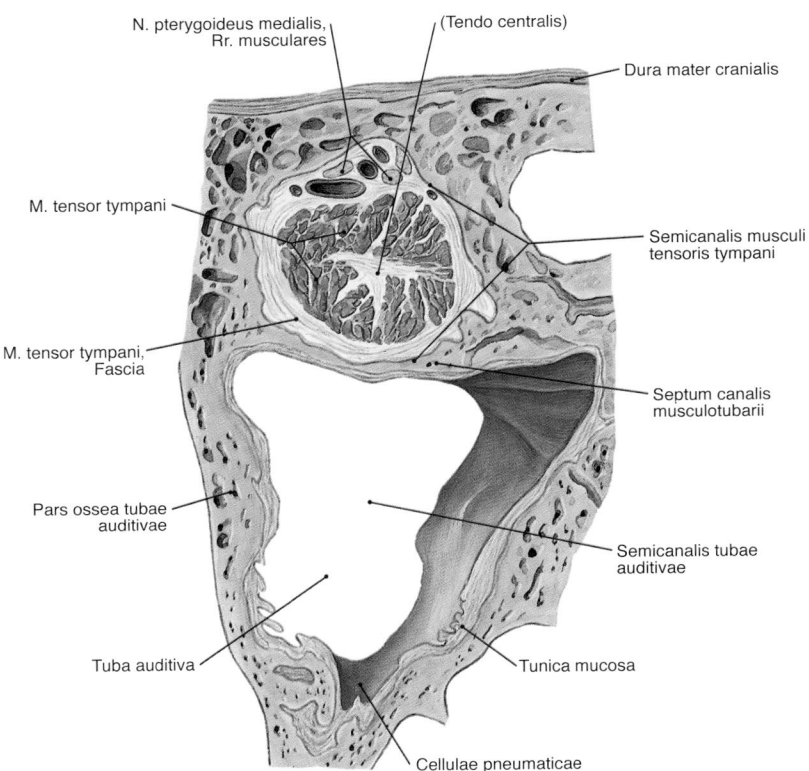

N. pterygoideus medialis, Rr. musculares
(Tendo centralis)
Dura mater cranialis
M. tensor tympani
Semicanalis musculi tensoris tympani
M. tensor tympani, Fascia
Septum canalis musculotubarii
Pars ossea tubae auditivae
Semicanalis tubae auditivae
Tuba auditiva
Tunica mucosa
Cellulae pneumaticae

Fig. 1407 Auditory tube, Tuba auditiva; cross-section at the level of the osseous part; lateral view.

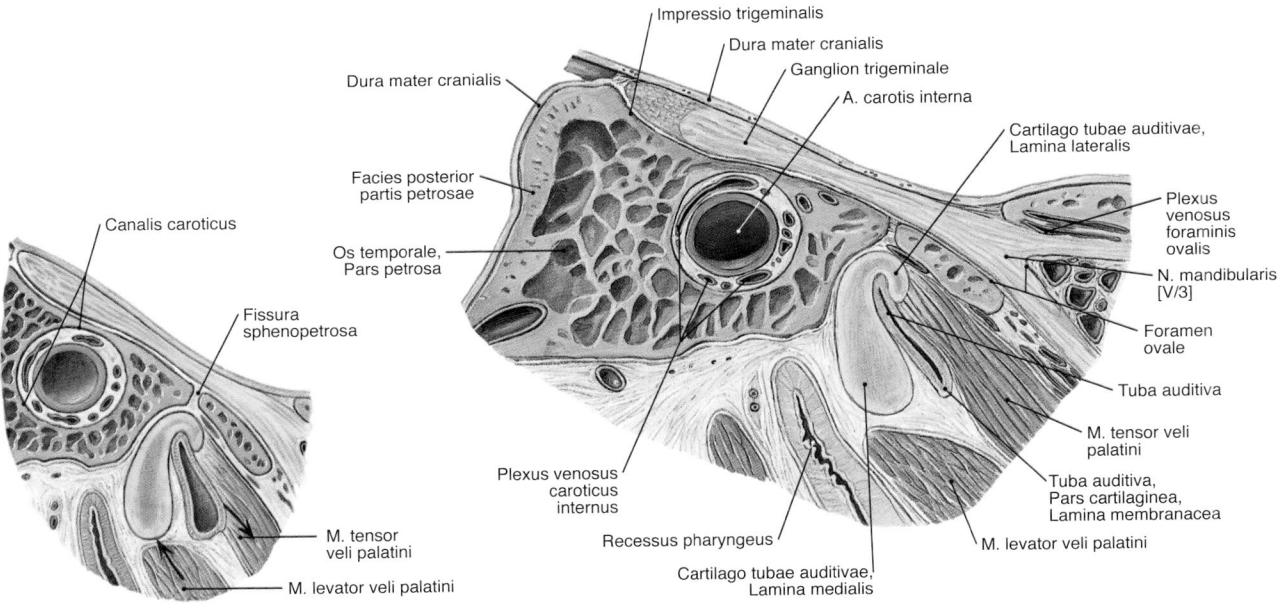

Impressio trigeminalis
Dura mater cranialis
Ganglion trigeminale
A. carotis interna
Dura mater cranialis
Cartilago tubae auditivae, Lamina lateralis
Facies posterior partis petrosae
Plexus venosus foraminis ovalis
Canalis caroticus
Os temporale, Pars petrosa
N. mandibularis [V/3]
Fissura sphenopetrosa
Foramen ovale
Tuba auditiva
M. tensor veli palatini
Plexus venosus caroticus internus
Tuba auditiva, Pars cartilaginea, Lamina membranacea
M. tensor veli palatini
Recessus pharyngeus
Cartilago tubae auditivae, Lamina medialis
M. levator veli palatini
M. levator veli palatini

Fig. 1408 Auditory tube, Tuba auditiva; cross-section at the level of the lateral aspect of the cartilaginous part; lateral view.

Fig. 1409 Auditory tube, Tuba auditiva; cross-section at the level of the medial aspect of the cartilaginous part; lateral view.

Bony labyrinth

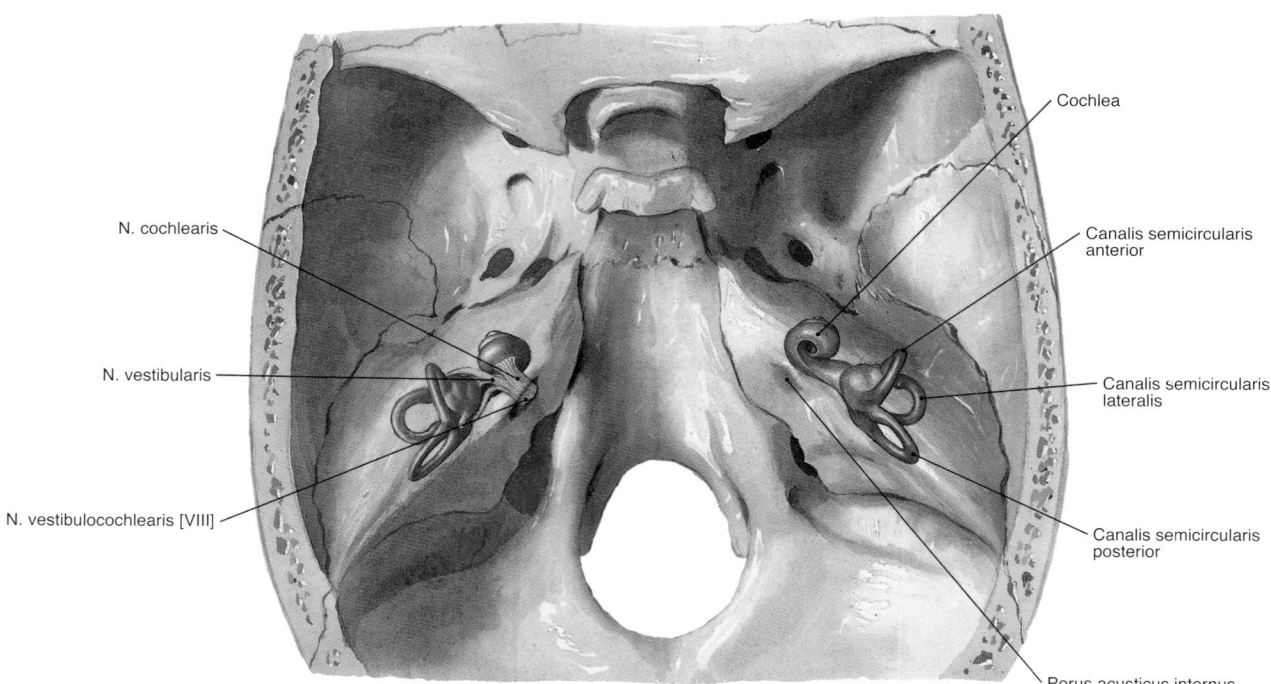

N. cochlearis

N. vestibularis

N. vestibulocochlearis [VIII]

Cochlea

Canalis semicircularis anterior

Canalis semicircularis lateralis

Canalis semicircularis posterior

Porus acusticus internus

Fig. 1410 Inner ear, Auris interna, and vestibulocochlear nerve, N. vestibulocochlearis [VIII];
cast specimen projected onto the petrous part of the temporal bone illustrating its natural position;
superior view.

Foramen rotundum

A. carotis interna, Pars cavernosa

Foramen lacerum

N. petrosus major

Cochlea

Porus acusticus internus

N. facialis [VII]

N. vestibulo-cochlearis [VIII] { N. cochlearis / N. vestibularis

Foramen jugulare

Foramen ovale

Foramen spinosum

Synchondrosis sphenopetrosa

N. facialis [VII], Ganglion geniculi

Ductus semicircularis anterior

Ductus semicircularis lateralis

Sulcus sinus sigmoidei

Ductus semicircularis posterior

→ 1173

Fig. 1411 Inner ear, Auris interna, with the facial nerve, N. facialis [VII], and the vestibulocochlear nerve, N. vestibulocochlearis [VIII];
projected onto the petrous part of the temporal bone;
superior view.

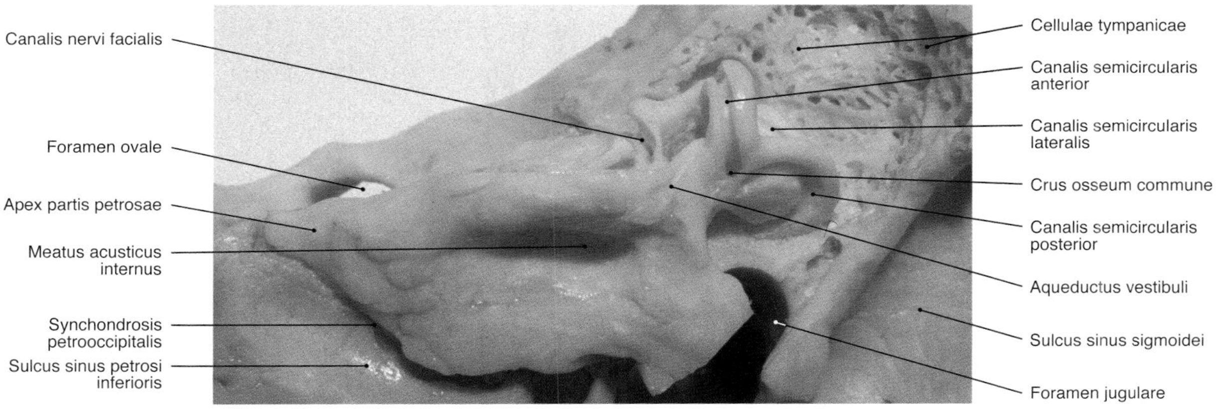

Bony labyrinth

Canalis nervi facialis

Foramen ovale

Apex partis petrosae

Meatus acusticus internus

Synchondrosis petrooccipitalis

Sulcus sinus petrosi inferioris

Cellulae tympanicae

Canalis semicircularis anterior

Canalis semicircularis lateralis

Crus osseum commune

Canalis semicircularis posterior

Aqueductus vestibuli

Sulcus sinus sigmoidei

Foramen jugulare

a

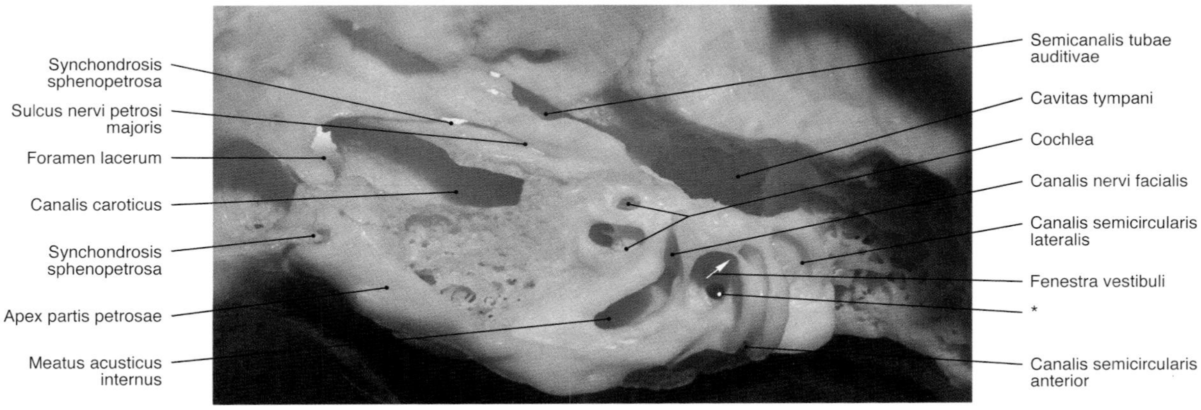

Synchondrosis sphenopetrosa

Sulcus nervi petrosi majoris

Foramen lacerum

Canalis caroticus

Synchondrosis sphenopetrosa

Apex partis petrosae

Meatus acusticus internus

Semicanalis tubae auditivae

Cavitas tympani

Cochlea

Canalis nervi facialis

Canalis semicircularis lateralis

Fenestra vestibuli

*

Canalis semicircularis anterior

b

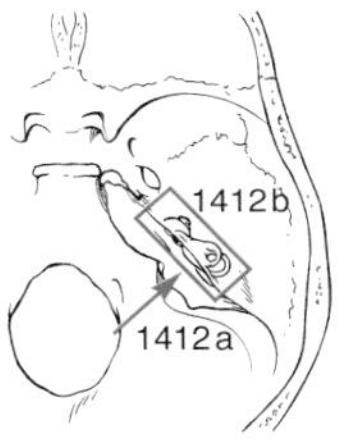

Fig. 1412a, b Bony labyrinth, Labyrinthus osseus; hollowed out of the petrous part of the temporal bone.
a Posterior-superior view
b Superior view
* Opening of the posterior canaliculus

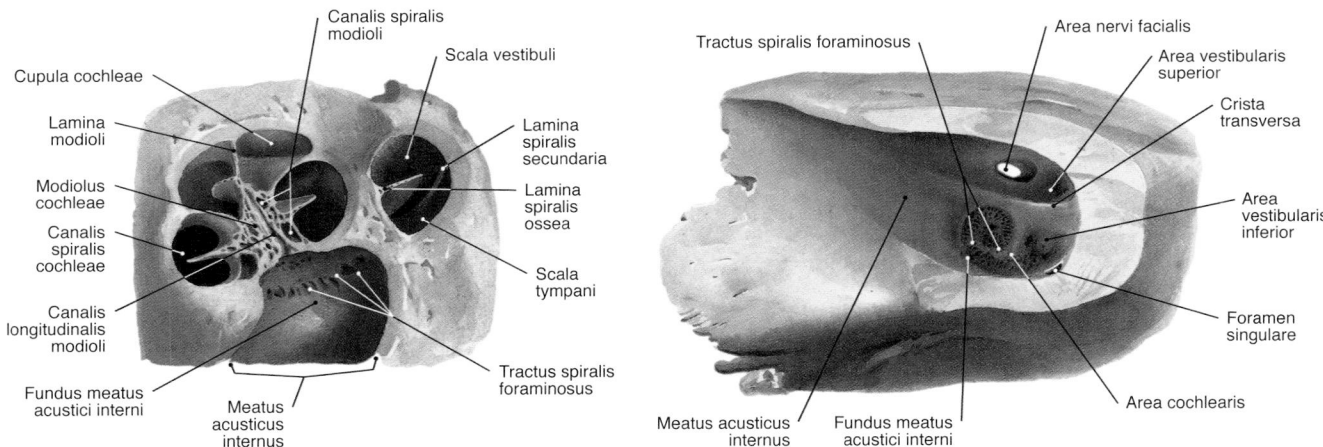

Canalis spiralis modioli

Scala vestibuli

Cupula cochleae

Lamina modioli

Modiolus cochleae

Canalis spiralis cochleae

Canalis longitudinalis modioli

Fundus meatus acustici interni

Meatus acusticus internus

Lamina spiralis secundaria

Lamina spiralis ossea

Scala tympani

Tractus spiralis foraminosus

Tractus spiralis foraminosus

Area nervi facialis

Area vestibularis superior

Crista transversa

Area vestibularis inferior

Foramen singulare

Area cochlearis

Meatus acusticus internus

Fundus meatus acustici interni

Fig. 1413 Spiral canal of the cochlea, Canalis spiralis cochleae; opened along the axis of the modiolus; superior view.

Fig. 1414 Internal acoustic meatus, Meatus acusticus internus, and fundus of the internal acoustic meatus, Fundus meatus acustici interni; after partial removal of the posterior wall; medial view.

→ 1173

Bony labyrinth

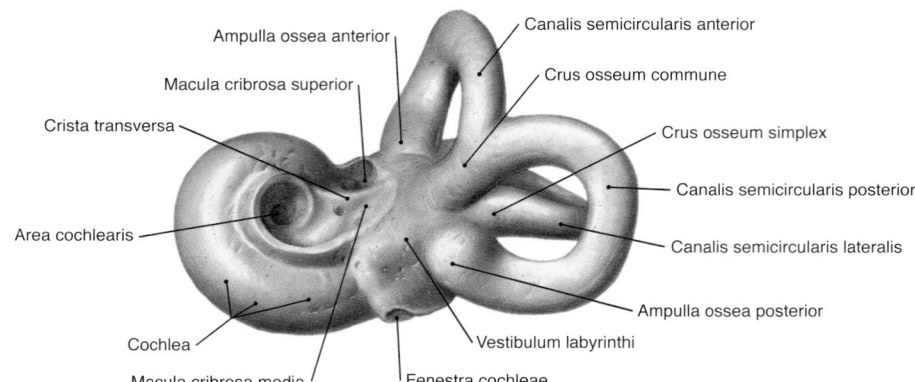

Ampulla ossea anterior
Macula cribrosa superior
Crista transversa
Area cochlearis
Cochlea
Macula cribrosa media
Canalis semicircularis anterior
Crus osseum commune
Crus osseum simplex
Canalis semicircularis posterior
Canalis semicircularis lateralis
Ampulla ossea posterior
Vestibulum labyrinthi
Fenestra cochleae

Fig. 1415 Bony labyrinth, Labyrinthus osseus;
the osseous lining of the membranous labyrinth has been
hollowed out of the petrous part of the temporal bone;
oblique view from posterior.

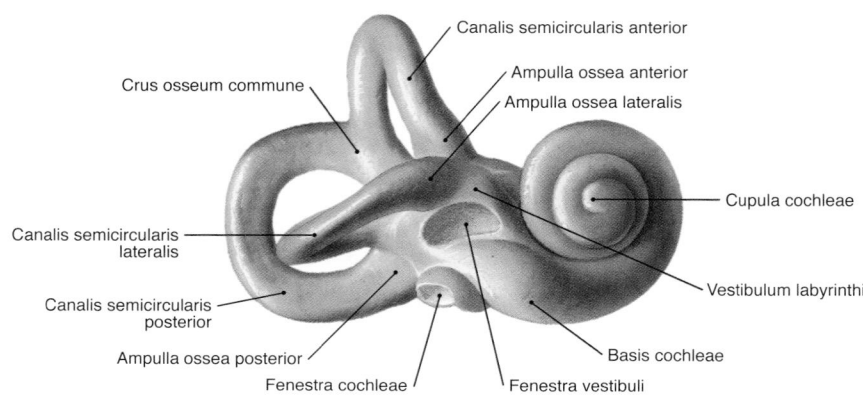

Crus osseum commune
Canalis semicircularis lateralis
Canalis semicircularis posterior
Ampulla ossea posterior
Fenestra cochleae
Canalis semicircularis anterior
Ampulla ossea anterior
Ampulla ossea lateralis
Cupula cochleae
Vestibulum labyrinthi
Basis cochleae
Fenestra vestibuli

Fig. 1416 Bony labyrinth, Labyrinthus osseus;
the osseous lining of the membranous labyrinth has been
hollowed out of the petrous part of the temporal bone;
lateral view.

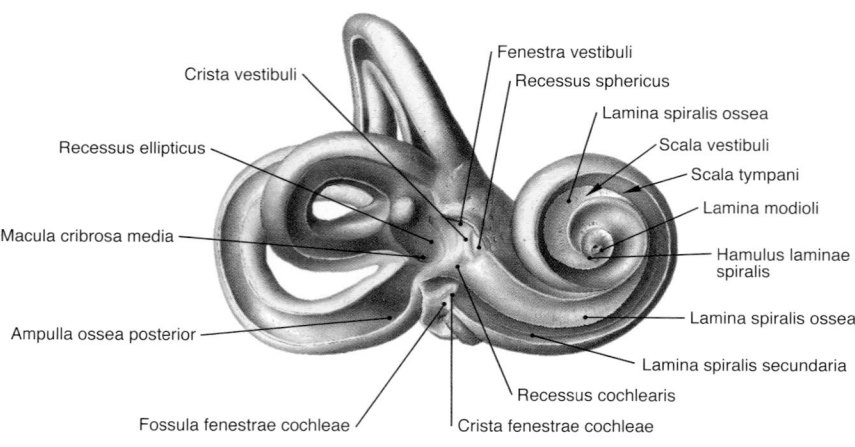

Crista vestibuli
Recessus ellipticus
Macula cribrosa media
Ampulla ossea posterior
Fossula fenestrae cochleae
Fenestra vestibuli
Recessus sphericus
Lamina spiralis ossea
Scala vestibuli
Scala tympani
Lamina modioli
Hamulus laminae spiralis
Lamina spiralis ossea
Lamina spiralis secundaria
Recessus cochlearis
Crista fenestrae cochleae

Fig. 1417 Bony labyrinth, Labyrinthus osseus;
cavities have been hollowed out;
anterolateral view.

Membranous labyrinth

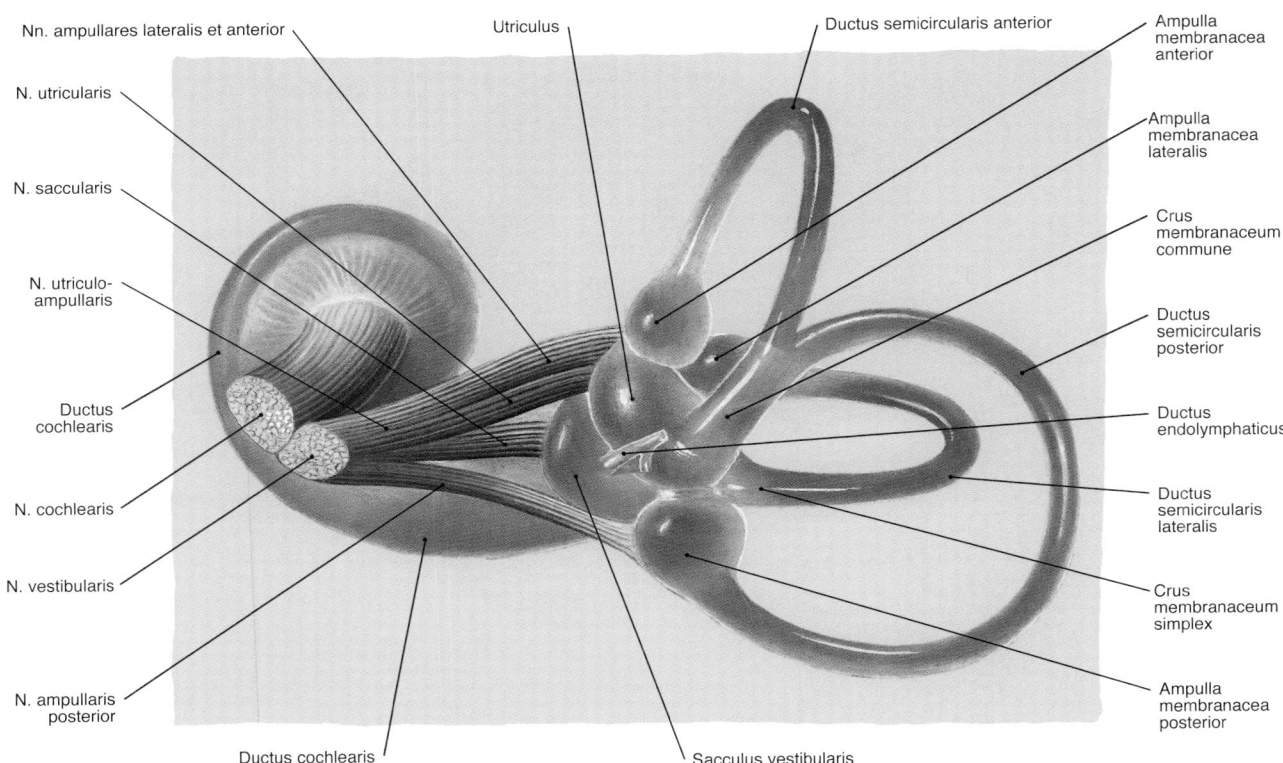

Nn. ampullares lateralis et anterior

N. utricularis

N. saccularis

N. utriculo-ampullaris

Ductus cochlearis

N. cochlearis

N. vestibularis

N. ampullaris posterior

Ductus cochlearis

Utriculus

Ductus semicircularis anterior

Ampulla membranacea anterior

Ampulla membranacea lateralis

Crus membranaceum commune

Ductus semicircularis posterior

Ductus endolymphaticus

Ductus semicircularis lateralis

Crus membranaceum simplex

Ampulla membranacea posterior

Sacculus vestibularis

Fig. 1418 Vestibulocochlear nerve, N. vestibulocochlearis [VIII], and membranous labyrinth, Labyrinthus membranaceus; semi-schematic overview; posterior view.

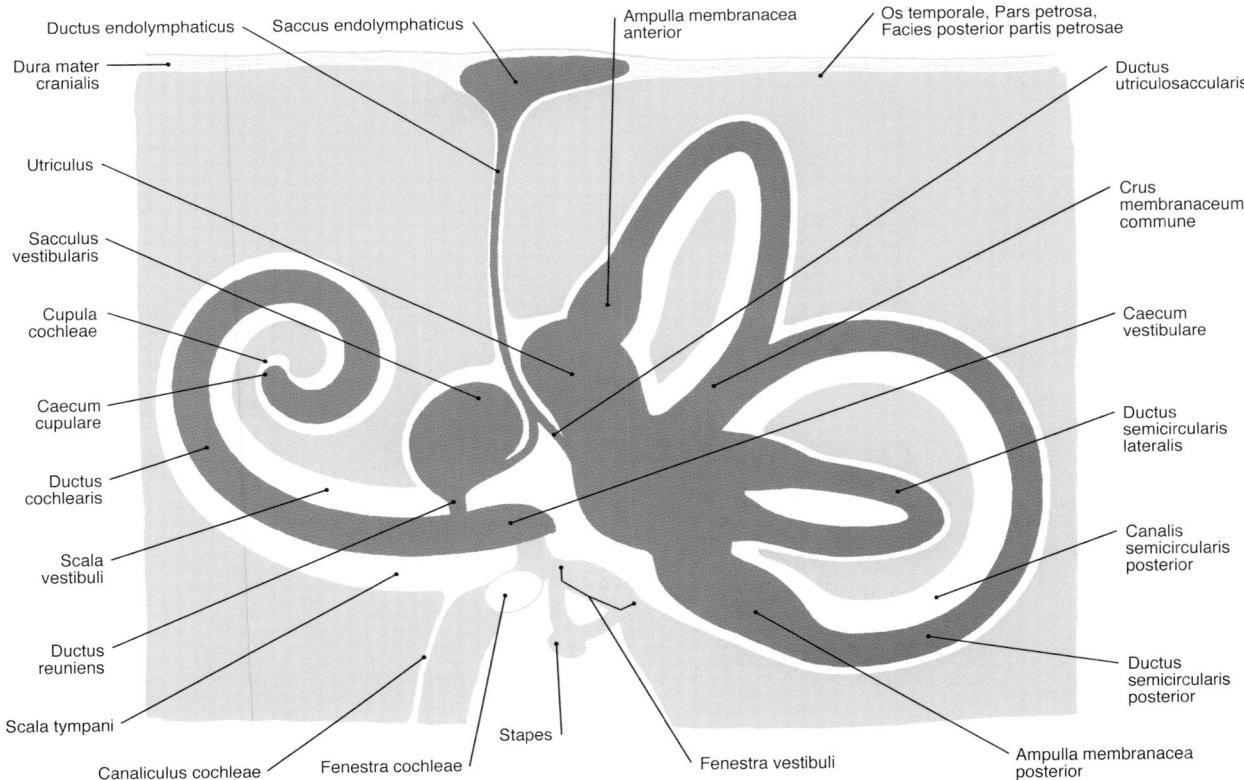

Ductus endolymphaticus

Saccus endolymphaticus

Dura mater cranialis

Utriculus

Sacculus vestibularis

Cupula cochleae

Caecum cupulare

Ductus cochlearis

Scala vestibuli

Ductus reuniens

Scala tympani

Canaliculus cochleae

Fenestra cochleae

Stapes

Ampulla membranacea anterior

Os temporale, Pars petrosa, Facies posterior partis petrosae

Ductus utriculosaccularis

Crus membranaceum commune

Caecum vestibulare

Ductus semicircularis lateralis

Canalis semicircularis posterior

Ductus semicircularis posterior

Ampulla membranacea posterior

Fenestra vestibuli

Fig. 1419 Membranous labyrinth, Labyrinthus membranaceus; overview.

Cochlea

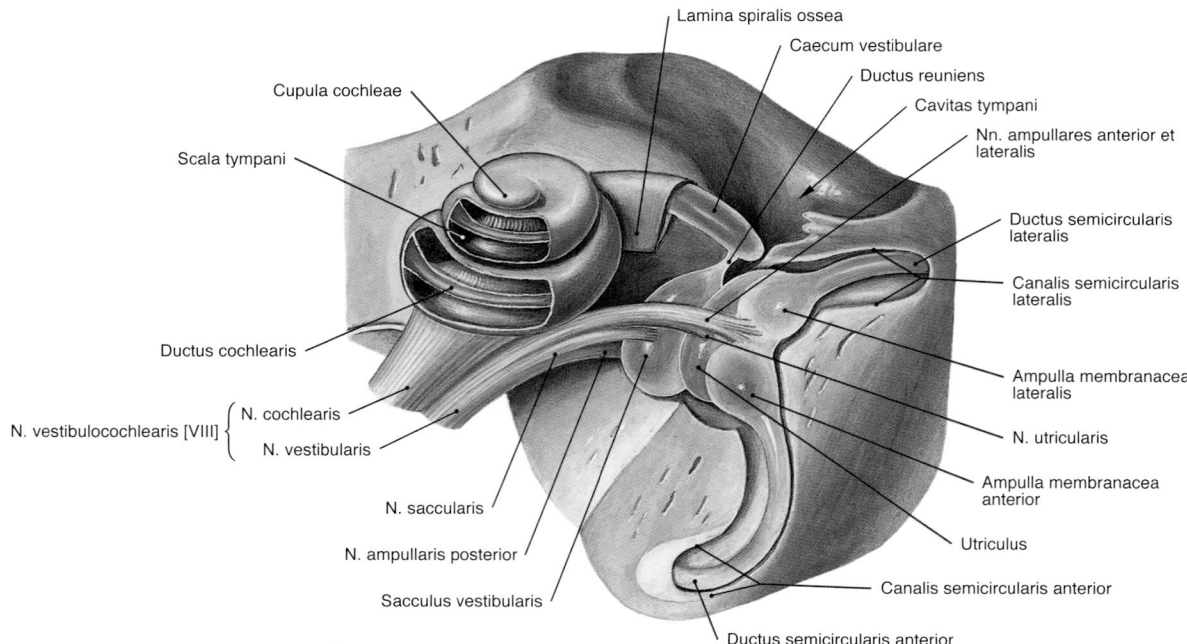

Cupula cochleae
Scala tympani
Ductus cochlearis
N. vestibulocochlearis [VIII] { N. cochlearis
N. vestibularis
N. saccularis
N. ampullaris posterior
Sacculus vestibularis

Lamina spiralis ossea
Caecum vestibulare
Ductus reuniens
Cavitas tympani
Nn. ampullares anterior et lateralis
Ductus semicircularis lateralis
Canalis semicircularis lateralis
Ampulla membranacea lateralis
N. utricularis
Ampulla membranacea anterior
Utriculus
Canalis semicircularis anterior
Ductus semicircularis anterior

Fig. 1420 Vestibulocochlear nerve, N. vestibulocochlearis [VIII], and membranous labyrinth, Labyrinthus membranaceus; superior view.

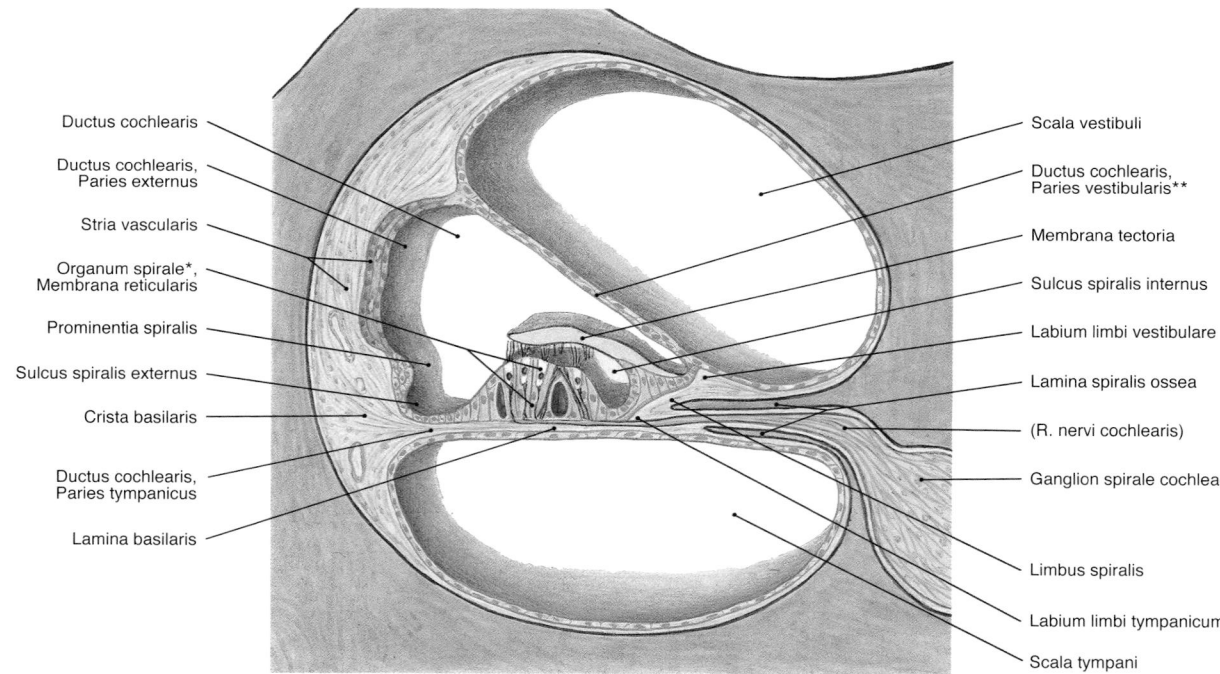

Ductus cochlearis
Ductus cochlearis, Paries externus
Stria vascularis
Organum spirale*, Membrana reticularis
Prominentia spiralis
Sulcus spiralis externus
Crista basilaris
Ductus cochlearis, Paries tympanicus
Lamina basilaris

Scala vestibuli
Ductus cochlearis, Paries vestibularis**
Membrana tectoria
Sulcus spiralis internus
Labium limbi vestibulare
Lamina spiralis ossea
(R. nervi cochlearis)
Ganglion spirale cochleae
Limbus spiralis
Labium limbi tympanicum
Scala tympani

Fig. 1421 Cochlea, Cochlea, with the spiral organ, Organum spirale.
* Clinical term: organ of CORTI
** Clinical term: REISSNER's membrane

Equilibrium organ, structure

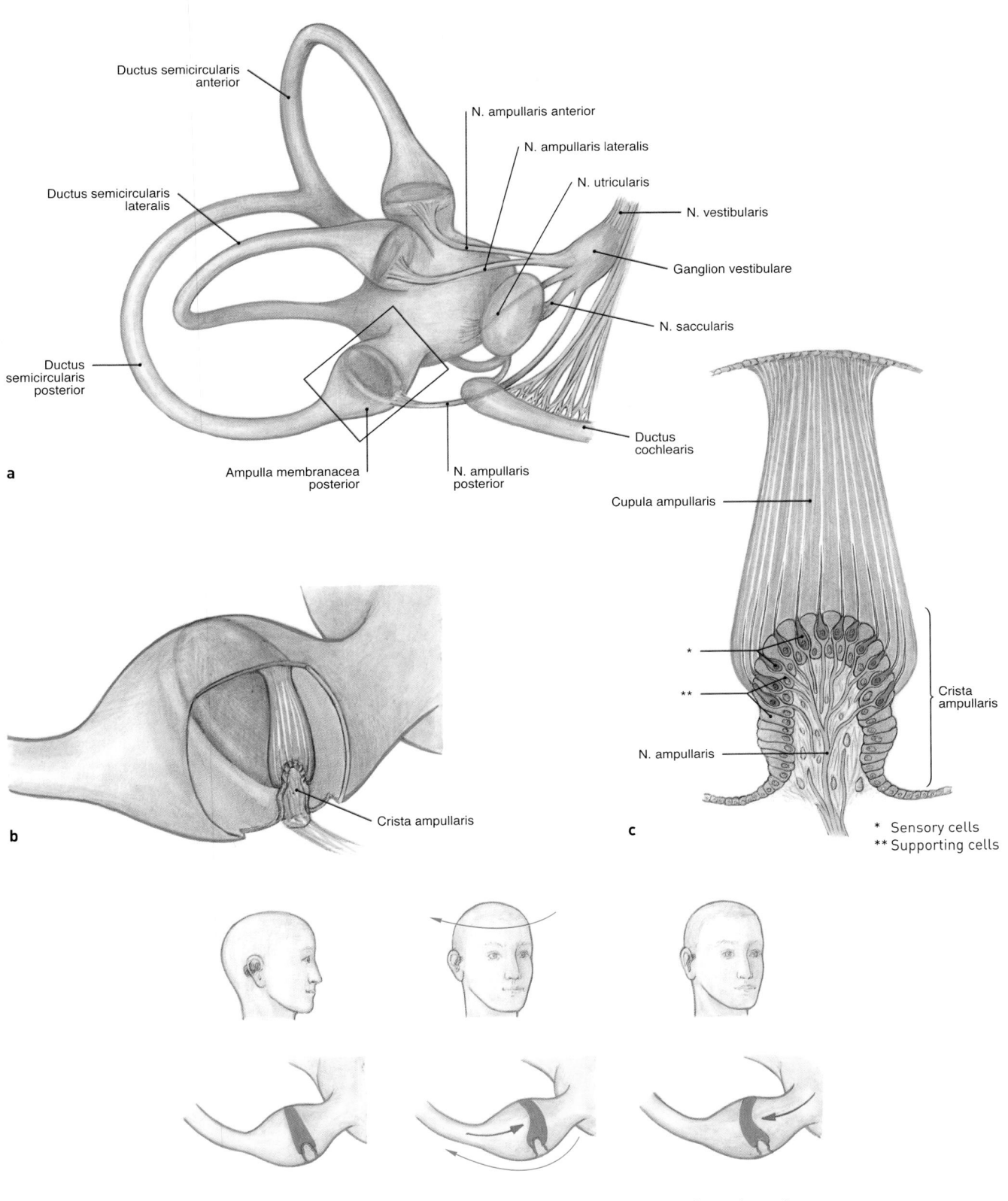

Ductus semicircularis anterior

N. ampullaris anterior

N. ampullaris lateralis

Ductus semicircularis lateralis

N. utricularis

N. vestibularis

Ganglion vestibulare

Ductus semicircularis posterior

N. saccularis

Ductus cochlearis

Cupula ampullaris

a

Ampulla membranacea posterior

N. ampullaris posterior

Crista ampullaris

N. ampullaris

Crista ampullaris

b

c

* Sensory cells
** Supporting cells

d

Resting state

Rotation of the head to the right side

Stop of rotation

Fig. 1422 a–d   Equilibrium organ; Labyrinthus vestibularis.
a Anterior view
b Higher magnification of the area indicated in **a:** the anterior part of the posterior membranous ampulla, Ampulla membranacea posterior, has been opened.

c Cross-section through the ampullary crest, Crista ampullaris
d Function of the cupula of the lateral semicircular duct, Ductus semicircularis lateralis, during rotation of the head

Hearing and equilibrium

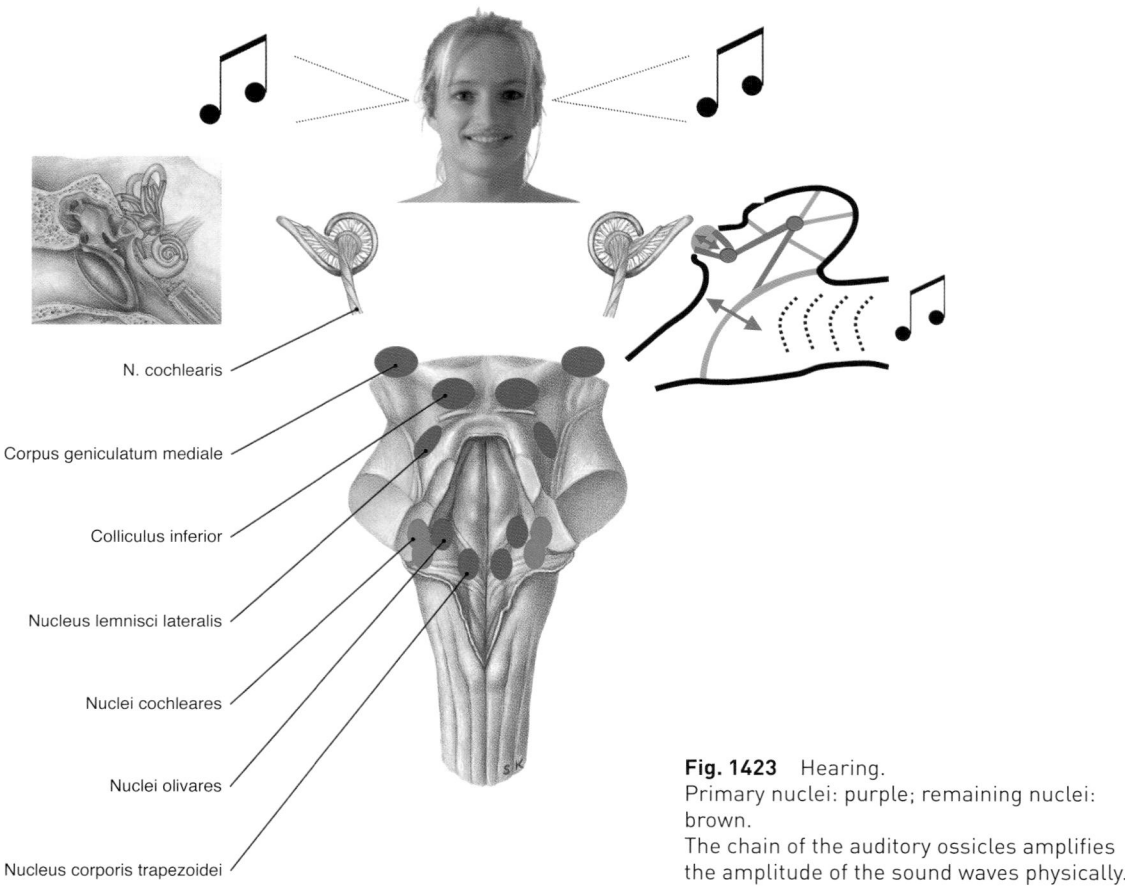

N. cochlearis

Corpus geniculatum mediale

Colliculus inferior

Nucleus lemnisci lateralis

Nuclei cochleares

Nuclei olivares

Nucleus corporis trapezoidei

Fig. 1423   Hearing.
Primary nuclei: purple; remaining nuclei: brown.
The chain of the auditory ossicles amplifies the amplitude of the sound waves physically.

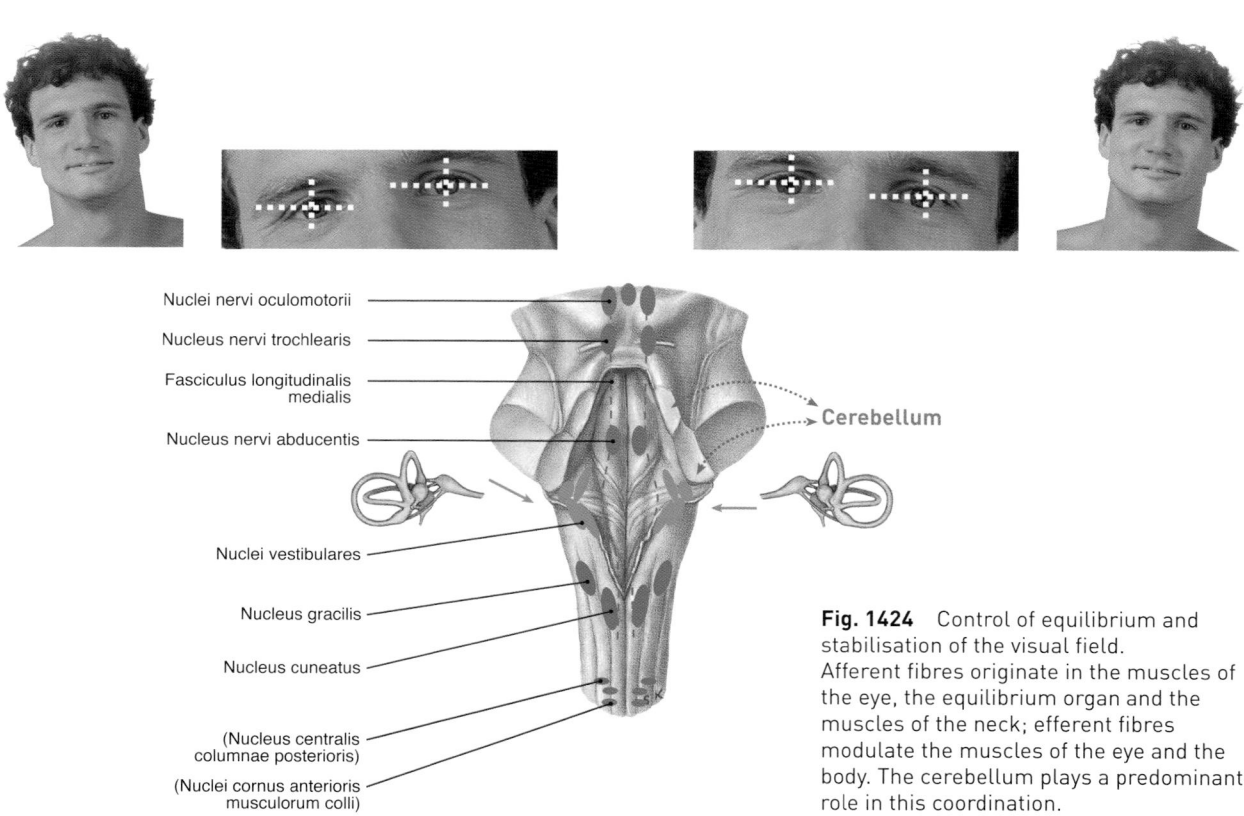

Nuclei nervi oculomotorii

Nucleus nervi trochlearis

Fasciculus longitudinalis medialis

Nucleus nervi abducentis

Cerebellum

Nuclei vestibulares

Nucleus gracilis

Nucleus cuneatus

(Nucleus centralis columnae posterioris)

(Nuclei cornus anterioris musculorum colli)

Fig. 1424   Control of equilibrium and stabilisation of the visual field.
Afferent fibres originate in the muscles of the eye, the equilibrium organ and the muscles of the neck; efferent fibres modulate the muscles of the eye and the body. The cerebellum plays a predominant role in this coordination.

Auditory and equilibrium pathway

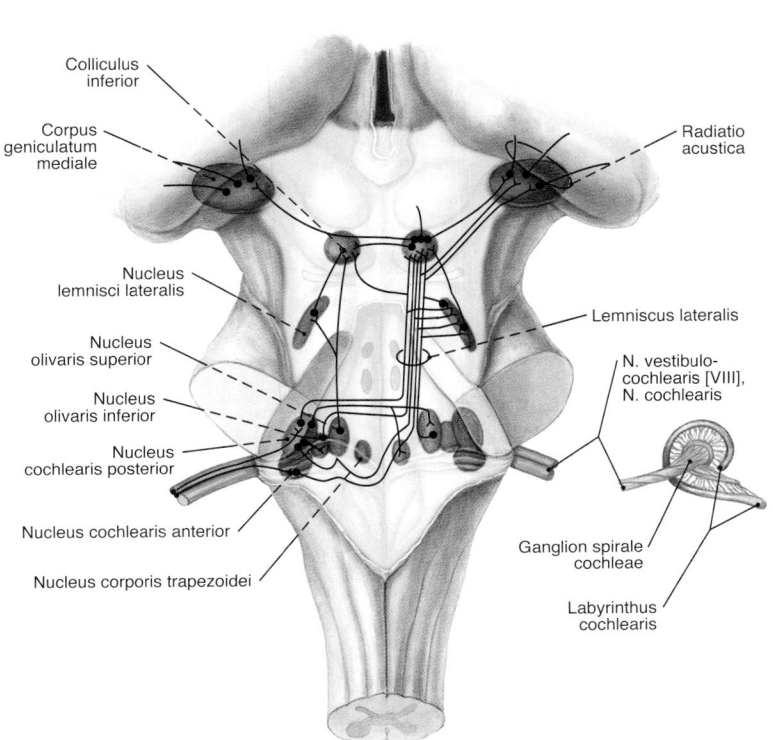

Fig. 1425 Auditory pathway; overview.

Auditory pathway

1. neuron: Bipolar cells in the spiral cochlear ganglion. After exiting the small apertures of the foraminous spiral tract within the internal acoustic meatus, the fibres form the cochlear nerve and unite with the vestibular nerve at the floor of the internal acoustic meatus to form the vestibulocochlear nerve [VIII]. Fibres from the basal cochlear parts traverse to the posterior cochlear nucleus and those from the apical parts terminate in the anterior cochlear nucleus.

2. neuron: Multi-polar ganglion cells of the cochlear nuclei. The fibres from the anterior cochlear nucleus pass mainly within the trapezoid body to the opposite side and form the lateral lemnicus, which provides a connection to the inferior colliculus. A few fibres join the lateral lemniscus of the same side. The axons of the posterior cochlear nucleus cross superficially to the rhomboid fossa and enter the lateral lemniscus of the opposite side.

3. or 4. neuron: From the inferior colliculus connections are made with the medial geniculate body.

4. or 5. neuron: The acoustic radiation connects the medial geniculate body to HESCHL's transverse gyrus and with WERNICKE's centre in the temporal lobe.

Equilibrium pathway

1. neuron: Bipolar cells in the vestibular ganglion. Their neurites pass the inferior and superior vestibular areas to form the vestibular nerve at the floor of the internal acoustic meatus, which together with the cochlear nerve then forms the vestibulocochlear nerve [VIII]. These fibres terminate at the vestibular nuclei in the lateral angle of the floor of the rhomboid fossa.

2. and subsequent neurons: Fibres originating in the lateral vestibular nucleus (DEITERS' nucleus) traverse within the lateral vestibulospinal tract to the anterior column of the spinal cord.
   Fibres originating in the superior vestibular nucleus (nucleus of BECHTEREW), the medial vestibular nucleus (SCHWALBE's nucleus) as well as the inferior vestibular nucleus (ROLLER's nucleus) traverse to the cerebellum and connect to the motor nuclei of the cranial nerves III, IV and VI, mostly via the medial longitudinal fasciculus.
   The medial vestibular nucleus and the inferior vestibular nucleus send fibres along the medial vestibulospinal tract to the anterior column of the spinal cord.

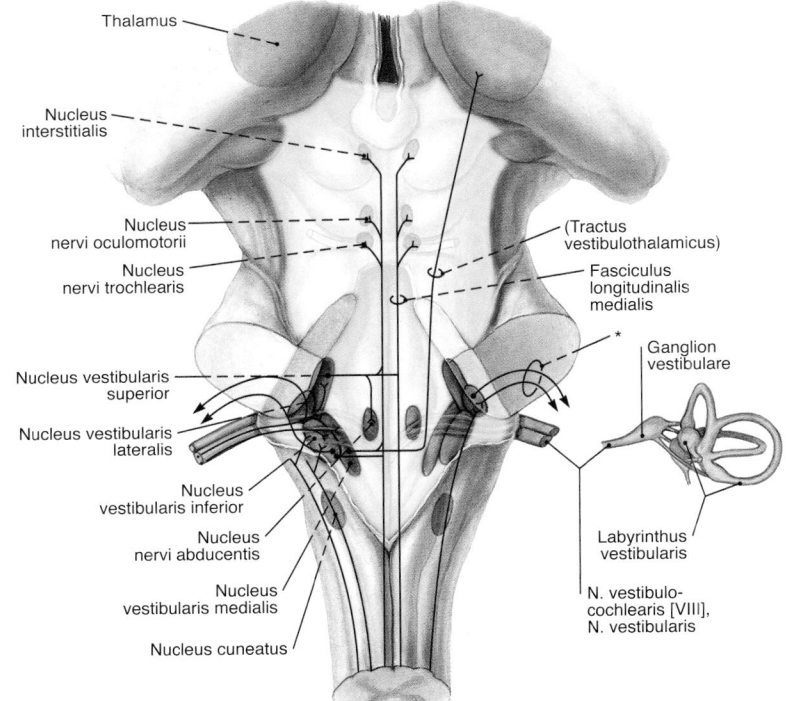

Fig. 1426 Equilibrium pathway; overview.
* Connections to the cerebellum

Nerves in the petrous part of the temporal bone

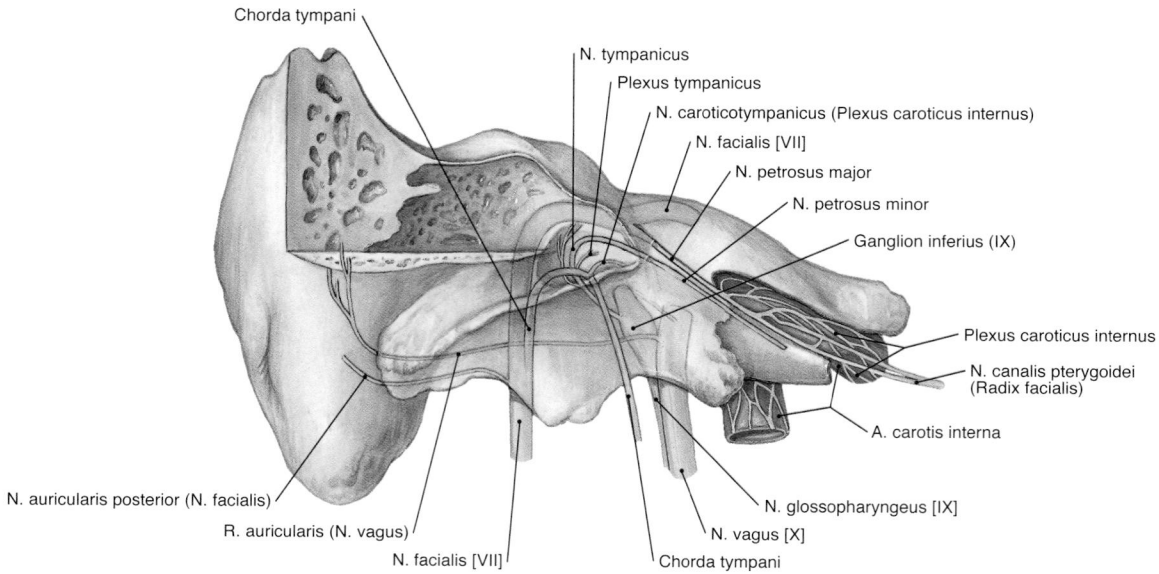

Chorda tympani
N. tympanicus
Plexus tympanicus
N. caroticotympanicus (Plexus caroticus internus)
N. facialis [VII]
N. petrosus major
N. petrosus minor
Ganglion inferius (IX)
Plexus caroticus internus
N. canalis pterygoidei (Radix facialis)
A. carotis interna
N. auricularis posterior (N. facialis)
R. auricularis (N. vagus)
N. facialis [VII]
Chorda tympani
N. glossopharyngeus [IX]
N. vagus [X]

→ 1181 **Fig. 1427** Facial nerve, N. facialis [VII];
glossopharyngeal nerve, N. glossopharyngeus [IX];
and vagus nerve, N. vagus [X];
the petrous part of the temporal bone has been partly sectioned;
the nerves are illustrated translucently;
anterior view.

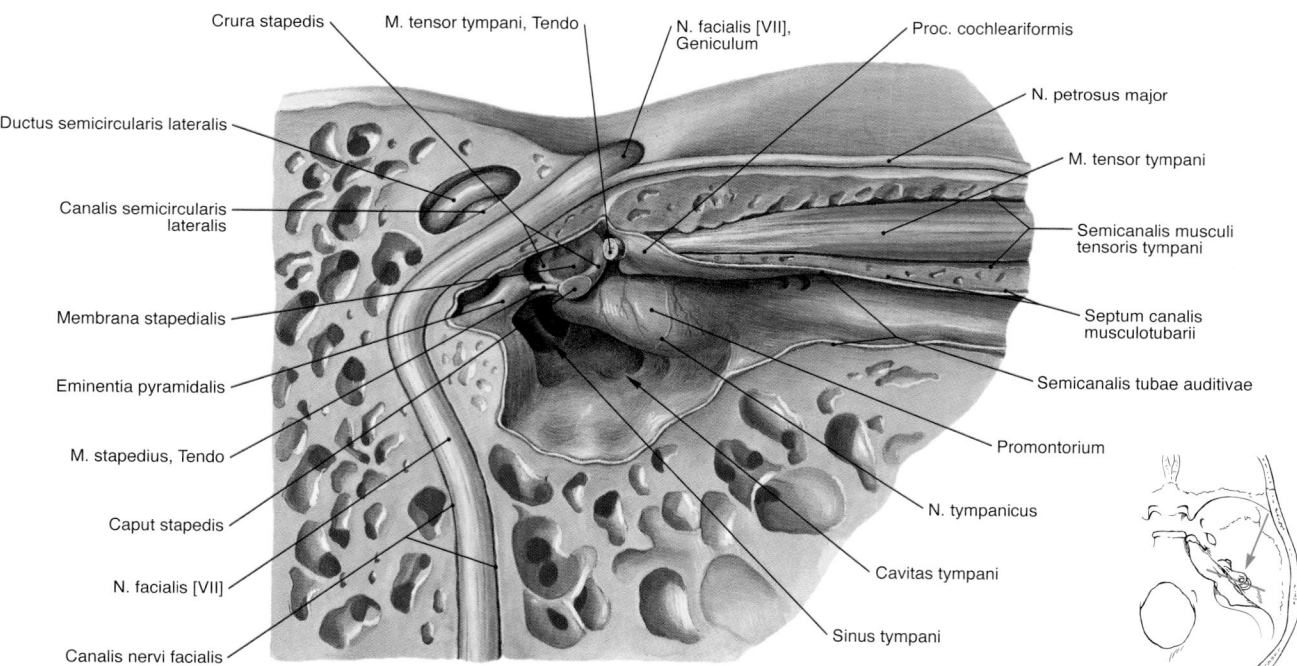

Crura stapedis
M. tensor tympani, Tendo
N. facialis [VII], Geniculum
Proc. cochleariformis
Ductus semicircularis lateralis
N. petrosus major
Canalis semicircularis lateralis
M. tensor tympani
Semicanalis musculi tensoris tympani
Membrana stapedialis
Septum canalis musculotubarii
Eminentia pyramidalis
Semicanalis tubae auditivae
M. stapedius, Tendo
Promontorium
Caput stapedis
N. tympanicus
N. facialis [VII]
Cavitas tympani
Canalis nervi facialis
Sinus tympani

Fig. 1428 Facial nerve, N. facialis [VII], and tympanic cavity, Cavitas tympani;
vertical section along the longitudinal axis of the
petrous part of the temporal bone;
the facial canal has been opened;
anterior view.

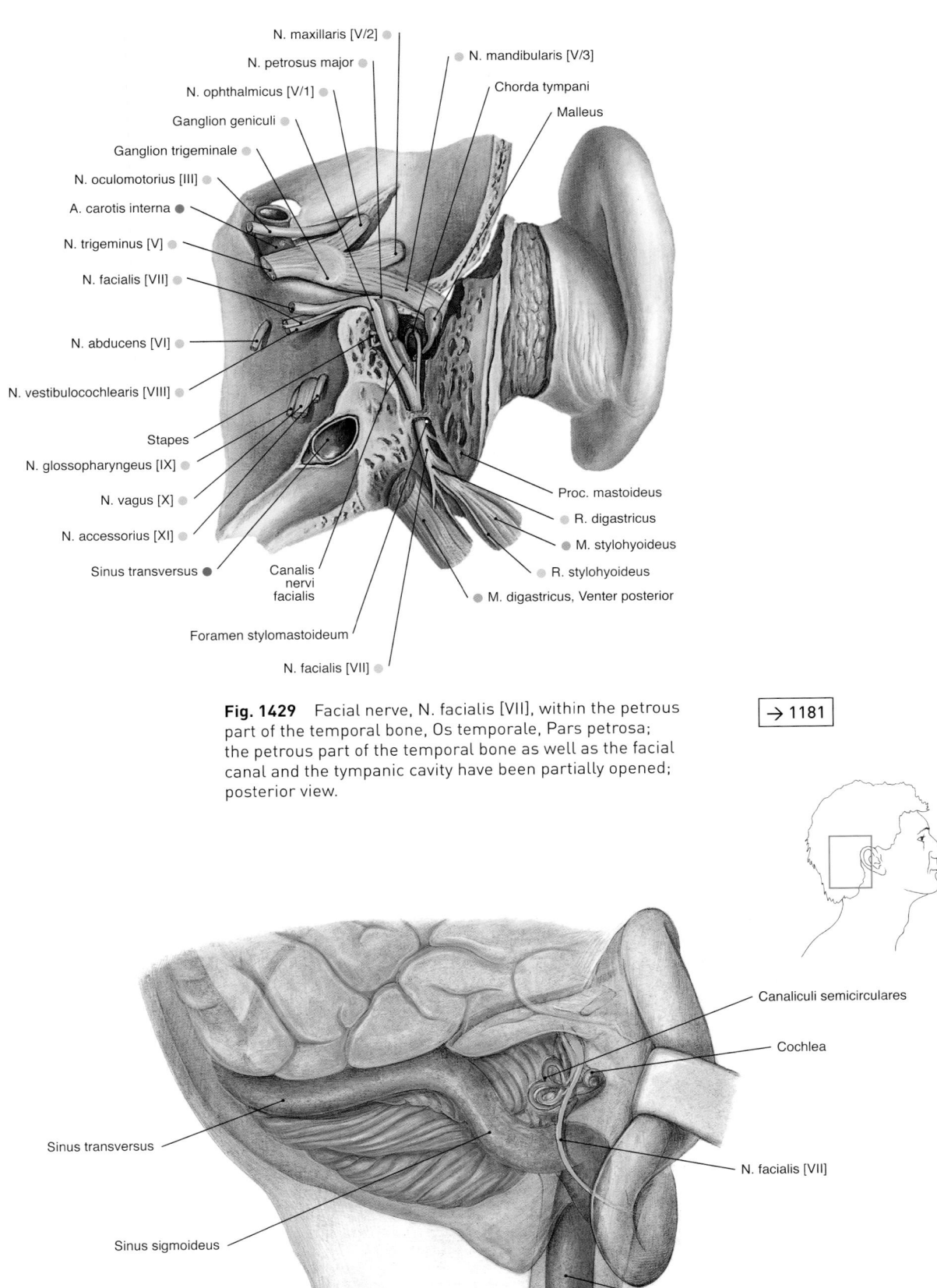

N. maxillaris [V/2]
N. petrosus major
N. ophthalmicus [V/1]
Ganglion geniculi
Ganglion trigeminale
N. oculomotorius [III]
A. carotis interna
N. trigeminus [V]
N. facialis [VII]
N. abducens [VI]
N. vestibulocochlearis [VIII]
Stapes
N. glossopharyngeus [IX]
N. vagus [X]
N. accessorius [XI]
Sinus transversus
Canalis nervi facialis
Foramen stylomastoideum
N. facialis [VII]

N. mandibularis [V/3]
Chorda tympani
Malleus
Proc. mastoideus
R. digastricus
M. stylohyoideus
R. stylohyoideus
M. digastricus, Venter posterior

Fig. 1429 Facial nerve, N. facialis [VII], within the petrous part of the temporal bone, Os temporale, Pars petrosa; the petrous part of the temporal bone as well as the facial canal and the tympanic cavity have been partially opened; posterior view.

→ 1181

Sinus transversus
Sinus sigmoideus

Canaliculi semicirculares
Cochlea
N. facialis [VII]
V. jugularis interna

Fig. 1430 Lateral projection of the inner ear.

Petrous part of the temporal bone, imaging

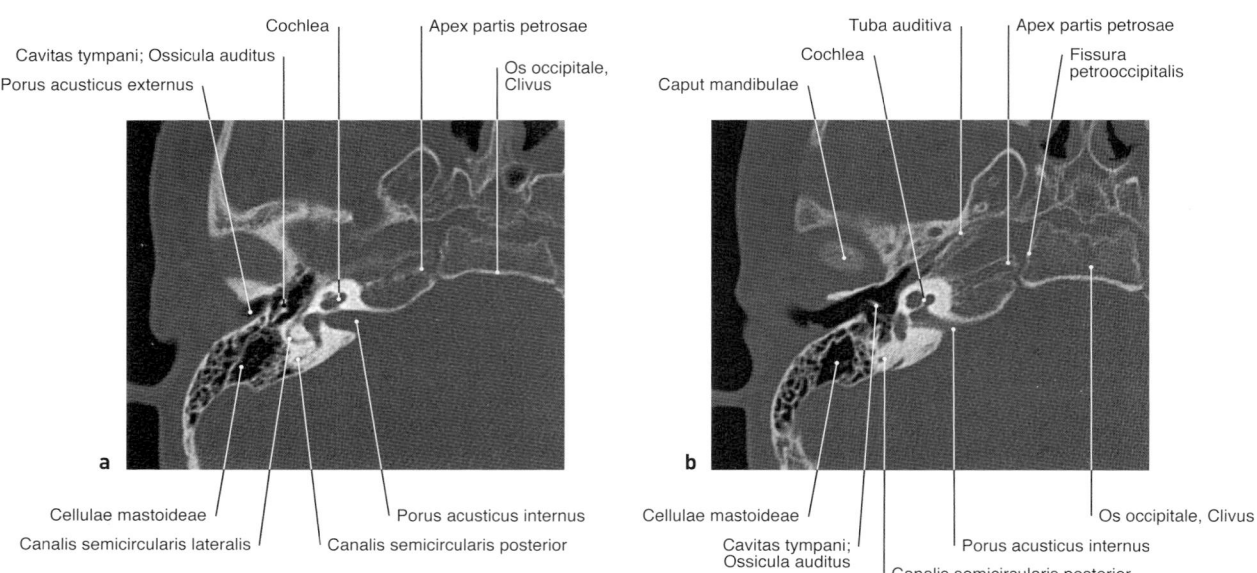

Cochlea
Cavitas tympani; Ossicula auditus
Porus acusticus externus
Apex partis petrosae
Os occipitale, Clivus

Cellulae mastoideae
Canalis semicircularis lateralis
Porus acusticus internus
Canalis semicircularis posterior

Tuba auditiva
Cochlea
Caput mandibulae
Apex partis petrosae
Fissura petrooccipitalis

Cellulae mastoideae
Cavitas tympani; Ossicula auditus
Canalis semicircularis posterior
Porus acusticus internus
Os occipitale, Clivus

Fig. 1431 a, b Petrous part of the temporal bone,
Os temporale, Pars petrosa;
high-resolution computed tomographic horizontal sections (HRCT);
inferior view.
a Through the lateral semicircular canal,
Canalis semicircularis lateralis
b Inferior to the lateral semicircular canal,
Canalis semicircularis lateralis

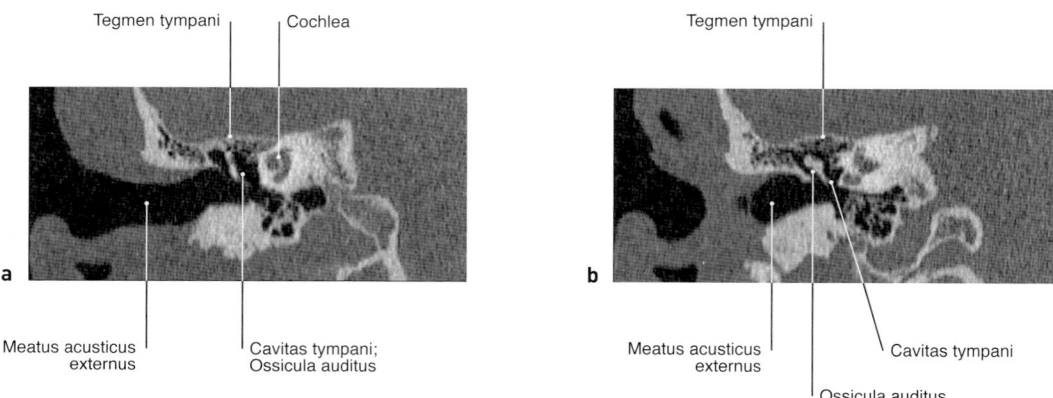

Tegmen tympani
Cochlea

Meatus acusticus externus
Cavitas tympani; Ossicula auditus

Tegmen tympani

Meatus acusticus externus
Cavitas tympani
Ossicula auditus

Fig. 1432 a, b Ear, Auris;
high-resolution computed tomographic frontal sections (HRCT);
anterior view.
a Through the base of the cochlea
b Through the external acoustic meatus

Index

The numbers refer to the page numbers.
The numbers with "T" refer to the numbers of the tables in the separate booklet.

788 Index

Area(-ae)
- vestibularis 685
- – inferior 777
- – superior 777
Areola mammae 322
Arm *See* Brachium
Arteria(-ae)
- alveolaris inferior 69, 74, 82–84, 109, 111, 116–117, 644
- – superior posterior 74, 83
- angularis 74, 80, 82–84, 644
- appendicularis 426, 432
- arcuata 441, 474, 609, 632
- ascendens 434
- auricularis posterior 19, 74, 82–84, 142, 145, 296, 644
- – profunda 83
- axillaris 18, 118, 146–147, 152, 214, 223, 226, 228, 232–233, 312, 371, 378, 380, 382
- basilaris 644–645, 662, 664, 669, 680–681, 688, 704–706, 710, 713, 723, 730
- brachialis 18, 170, 223, 227, 232–235, 238–240, 252–254
- – superficialis 237
- buccalis 74, 82–84, 644
- bulbi penis 492, 498
- – vestibuli 492
- caecalis posterior 432
- callosomarginalis 645, 667, 680, 712, 717–720
- carotis communis 18–19, 27, 73–74, 77, 84, 115, 118, 121, 133–134, 140–141, 144–155, 228, 327, 332–333, 347, 356–357, 362–365, 368–369, 371–372, 375–376, 378–382, 644–645, 657–658
- – externa 18–19, 74, 82–83, 85, 115, 134, 140, 144–147, 151, 372, 644–645
- – interna 18–19, 41, 43, 67, 69, 74, 82, 85, 101, 109, 140–141, 146–147, 372, 644–645, 648, 650–651, 657–658, 663–665, 669, 681, 704–706, 723–724, 755–760, 762–763, 775–776, 784–785
- – – angiography 645
- – – AP-radiograph 645
- – – DSA 645
- caudae pancreatis 426
- centralis(-es) anterolaterales 680, 705
- – anteromediales 705
- – posteromediales 705
- – retinae 116, 749, 754, 756
- cerebri anterior 645, 662–664, 698, 704–707, 712, 716–723
- – media 645, 664, 680, 704–707, 711–712, 715, 718, 722, 724–725
- – posterior 645, 663–664, 680–681, 704, 706–707, 713–714, 720–724, 756
- cervicalis ascendens 145–147, 152, 154–155, 730
- – profunda 152–153, 297, 373
- – superficialis 145–147, 152, 324
- choroidea anterior 704–705, 707, 756
- ciliaris(-es) 756, 760
- – anterior 749
- – posterior(-es) 762

Arteria(-ae) ciliares posterior(-es)
- – – breves 749
- – – longa 749
- circumflexa femoris lateralis 519, 609, 615–617
- – – medialis 518–519, 609, 615–617, 621–622
- – humeri anterior 223, 227, 232
- – – posterior 223, 227, 229, 231–232, 235, 295, 380
- – ilium profunda 19, 437, 479, 485, 489, 614, 617
- – – superficialis 324, 611, 617
- – scapulae 227, 235, 295, 380
- colica dextra 19, 410, 426, 432–433
- – media 19, 410, 419, 421–422, 426, 432–435
- – sinistra 19, 425–426, 433–435, 437, 475
- collateralis media 223
- – radialis 223, 234–235, 238–241
- – ulnaris inferior 223, 233–235, 238–241
- – – superior 223, 233, 238–240, 253
- comitans nervi mediani 223, 239
- communicans anterior 664, 704–706, 712, 722
- – posterior 645, 664, 704–705, 713, 722–724
- conjunctivalis anterior 749
- coronaria(-ae) 19, 342, 344
- – dextra 332–333, 336–338, 340, 342–345, 356, 377–378, 385
- – – coronary angiography 345
- – sinistra 332–333, 337–338, 340, 342–345, 356, 377–378, 385
- – – coronary angiography 345
- cremasterica 451, 483, 496
- cystica 400, 407, 426, 428,430
- descendens genus 609, 611, 614–616, 627
- digitales dorsales (Manus) 246, 250
- – – (Pes) 627, 632
- – – (Manus) 246, 250
- – palmares communes 223, 242–244, 250, 257
- – – propriae 223, 242–246, 250, 257
- – plantares communes 633, 635
- – – propriae 633–635
- dorsalis clitoridis 492
- – nasi 85, 760, 762
- – pedis 18, 609, 626, 632–633, 637, 641
- – penis 457, 485, 492, 496–498, 502
- ductus deferentis 318, 451, 455, 485
- epigastrica inferior 19, 318–319, 324, 327, 329–330, 416–417, 431, 433, 437, 454, 475, 479, 483, 485, 487, 489, 494, 511–512, 617
- – – collateral circulation 327
- – superficialis 324, 611, 617
- – superior 324, 327–328, 330
- – – collateral circulation 327
- episcleralis 749

Arteria(-ae)
- ethmoidalis anterior 41, 651, 758, 760–762
- – posterior 760–762
- facialis 19, 68, 74, 81–85, 109–110, 116–118, 140, 146–149, 151, 644
- femoralis 18, 320, 327, 331, 476, 502, 514–515, 572, 575, 609, 611, 613–617, 638–639
- – superficialis 609, 614
- fibularis 18, 609, 624, 626–630, 640–641
- frontobasalis lateralis 704
- – medialis 704, 707
- gastrica(-ae) breves 389, 424, 426, 428, 431
- – dextra 389, 426, 428, 430
- – posterior 428
- – sinistra 19, 364, 389, 410, 413, 418, 426, 428–431, 436–437, 476, 502, 505, 507
- gastroduodenalis 410, 426, 428–431, 500, 502
- gastroomentalis dextra 389, 425–426, 428–431
- – sinistra 389, 418, 426, 428–431, 505
- glutea inferior 19, 470, 482–483, 514–515, 609, 621–622, 638
- – superior 19, 470, 482–483, 512, 617, 621, 638
- helicinae 456
- hepatica communis 19, 389, 410, 426, 428–431, 436–437, 476, 507
- – – AP-radiograph 429
- – – propria 389, 400, 404, 410, 413, 425–426, 428–430, 437, 501–502, 507
- – variations 428
- hypophysialis inferior 681
- – superior 681
- ileales 19, 410, 426, 432–433, 509
- ileocolica 19, 426, 432–433, 513
- iliaca communis 18–19, 22, 27, 425, 437, 470, 472, 475–476, 479, 482–487, 489, 500–501, 512, 617
- – externa 18–19, 22, 327, 329, 437, 454, 470, 479, 482–483, 485–487, 489, 494, 511, 575, 612, 614, 616–617
- – interna 18–19, 22, 470, 475, 482–483, 485–487, 489, 612, 614, 617
- – – variations 482
- iliolumbalis 19, 475, 479, 482–483, 487
- inferior anterior cerebelli 645, 664, 704–705
- – lateralis genus 547, 609, 626–627
- – medialis genus 547, 609, 616, 627–630
- – posterior cerebelli 645, 664, 704–705
- infraorbitalis 74, 83–84, 644, 650, 761, 764
- insulares 680
- intercostalis(-es) 328, 357, 378, 385
- – posteriores 152, 303, 312, 331, 333, 362–363, 370–371, 373–374, 730
- – suprema 152, 373

Arteria(-ae)
- interlobares (Ren) 441–442, 474
- interlobulares (Hepar) 403
- interossea anterior 223, 239, 241, 248, 250
- – communis 18, 223, 239
- – posterior 197, 223, 239, 241, 250
- – recurrens 223, 240–241
- intramuscularis 31
- intraseptalis 31
- jejunales 19, 410, 426, 432–433, 435, 500, 502
- labialis inferior 74, 644
- – superior 74, 644
- labyrinthi 41, 651, 664, 704–705
- lacrimalis 116, 742, 758–760, 762
- laryngea inferior 130
- – superior 108, 114–115, 130–131, 134, 137, 141, 144–146, 151
- lienalis *See* Arteria(-ae) splenica
- lingualis 19, 74, 82, 84–85, 110, 113–117, 134, 140, 145, 151, 644
- lobaris(-es) inferiores 356–357, 359, 384
- – media 356
- – superiores 356, 383
- lobi caudati 400
- lumbales 22, 299, 437, 475, 479, 503, 617
- malleolaris anterior lateralis 609, 626, 632
- – – medialis 609, 632
- marginalis coli 426, 432–434
- masseterica 83, 85
- maxillaris 19, 69, 74, 83–85, 644
- media genus 547, 609, 627
- meningea media 41, 43, 74, 83–84, 644, 650–651, 655, 661, 664, 666, 758
- – posterior 41, 43, 140, 650–651, 664
- mesencephalicae 705
- mesenterica inferior 18–19, 22, 27, 410, 425–426, 432, 434–435, 437, 470, 472, 475, 479, 483, 485, 508–509
- – – AP-radiograph 434
- – – variations 434
- – superior 18–19, 22, 27, 373, 410–412, 425–426, 428, 431–437, 445, 475–476, 479, 500–502, 508–509, 513
- – – AP-radiograph 432
- – – variations 432
- metacarpales dorsales 246, 248, 250
- – palmares 242, 245, 250, 257
- metatarsales dorsales 609, 626, 632
- – plantares 633–634, 636
- musculophrenica 327
- nasopalatina 113
- nutricia 7
- obturatoria 19, 329, 470, 482–483, 485, 487, 489, 494–495, 514–515, 519, 575, 613, 615–617
- – variations 487
- occipitalis 19, 74, 82–84, 109, 141–144, 146–147, 295–297, 644
- – medialis 715–716

Sobotta

Atlas of Human Anatomy

Tables of Muscles, Joints and Nerves

Edited by R. Putz and R. Pabst
In collaboration with Renate Putz

Translation by S. Bedoui

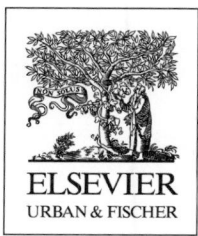

ELSEVIER
URBAN & FISCHER

URBAN & FISCHER München

Sobotta

Tables of Muscles, Joints and Nerves

Edited by R. Putz and R. Pabst
In collaboration with Renate Putz

Translation by S. Bedoui

This booklet is a supplement to Sobotta, Atlas of Human Anatomy, 14th edition. The cross-references relate to the figure numbers in the Atlas.
Abbreviations: O = Origin; I = Insertion; F = Function.

Correspondence and feedback should be addressed to:
Elsevier GmbH, Urban & Fischer Verlag, Department for Medical Student Information, Karlstraße 45, 80333 Munich, Germany
e-mail: medizinstudium@elsevier.de

Addresses of the editors:

Professor Dr. med. Reinhard Putz
Vizepräsident der
Ludwig Maximilians-Universität
Geschwister-Scholl-Platz 1
80539 München
Germany
e-mail: putz@lmu.de

Professor Dr. med. Reinhard Pabst
Leiter der Abteilung Funktionelle
und Angewandte Anatomie
Medizinische Hochschule Hannover
Carl-Neuberg-Straße 1
30625 Hannover
Germany
e-mail: pabst.reinhard@mh-hannover.de

Contents

Tables of Muscles, Joints and Nerves

1 Facial muscles (Fig. 119–122, 247, 253, 1332)

Only parts of the facial muscles actually originate from bony structures. All of them insert into the skin.

a Forehead, top of the head, temple

M. occipitofrontalis
(Together, the M. occipitofrontalis and the M. temporoparietalis are referred to as M. epicranius.)
N. facialis [VII]

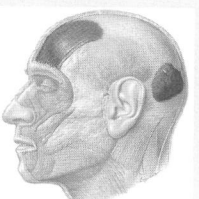

O: Venter frontalis: skin of the eyebrow and the Glabella, forms a common muscular layer with the Mm. procerus, corrugator supercilii, depressor supercilii et orbicularis oculi
Venter occipitalis: Linea nuchalis suprema

I: Galea aponeurotica

F: Moves the scalp, creates oblique wrinkle at the forehead

M. temporoparietalis
N. facialis [VII]

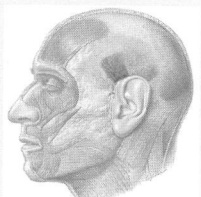

O: Temporal skin, Fascia temporalis

I: Galea aponeurotica

F: Moves the scalp

b Auricle

M. auricularis anterior
N. facialis [VII]

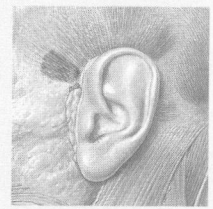

O: Fascia temporalis

I: Spina helicis

F: Moves the auricle forwards and upwards

M. auricularis superior
N. facialis [VII]

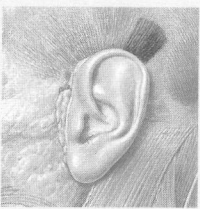

O: Galea aponeurotica

I: Dorsocranial part of the auricular root

F: Moves the auricle backwards and upwards

M. auricularis posterior
N. facialis [VII]

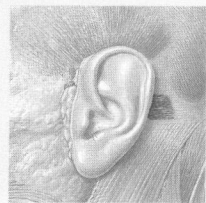

O: Proc. mastoideus, tendon of the M. sternocleido-mastoideus

I: Dorsal part of the auricular root

F: Moves the auricle backwards

2

T 1

1 Facial muscles (continuation)

c Palpebral fissure

M. orbicularis oculi (located around the Aditus orbitae in a sphincter-like fashion)
N. facialis [VII]

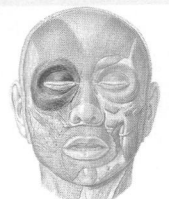

O: Pars orbitalis: Pars nasalis of the Os frontale,
Proc. frontalis of the Maxilla,
Os lacrimale,
Lig. palpebrale mediale
Pars palpebralis: Lig. palpebrale mediale,
Saccus lacrimalis
Pars lacrimalis: Crista lacrimalis posterior of the Os lacrimale,
Saccus lacrimalis

I: Pars orbitalis: Lig. palpebrale laterale, lateral transition into a circular ring-shaped muscle
Pars palpebralis: Lig. palpebrale laterale
Pars lacrimalis: Canaliculi lacrimales,
edges of the eyelids

F: Closes the eyelids, compresses the lacrimal sac, moves the eyebrows

M. depressor supercilii (branch of the Pars orbitalis of the M. orbicularis oculi)
N. facialis [VII]

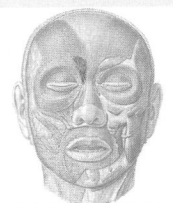

O: Pars nasalis of the Os frontale, back of the nose

I: Medial third of the skin of the eyebrow

F: Lowers the skin of the forehead and of the eyebrows,
creates an oblique wrinkle just above the root of the nose

M. corrugator supercilii
N. facialis [VII]

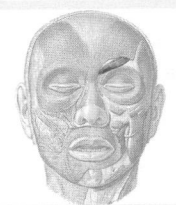

O: Pars nasalis of the Os frontale

I: Middle (lateral) third of the skin of the eyebrow,
Galea aponeurotica

F: Moves the skin of the forehead and of the eyebrows towards the root of the nose,
creates a vertical wrinkle just above the root of the nose

M. procerus
N. facialis [VII]

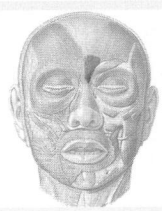

O: Os nasale,
Cartilago nasi lateralis

I: Skin of the Glabella

F: Lowers the skin of the forehead and of the eyebrows

1 Facial muscles (continuation)

d Nose

M. nasalis
N. facialis [VII]

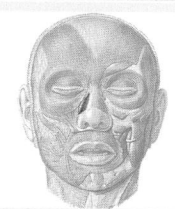

O: **Pars alaris:** Jugum alveolare of the lateral incisor tooth
Pars transversa: Jugum alveolare of the canine tooth

I: **Pars alaris:** nose wings, border of the nostril
Pars transversa: Cartilago nasi lateralis, tendinous membrane of the back of the nose

F: Moves the nose wings and thus the nose itself
Pars alaris: dilates the nostrils
Pars transversa: narrows the nostrils

M. depressor septi nasi
N. facialis [VII]

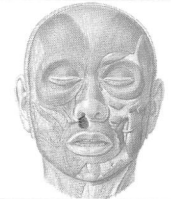

O: Jugum alveolare of the medial incisor tooth

I: Cartilago alaris major, Cartilago septi nasi

F: Moves the nose wings and thus the nose itself

e Mouth

M. orbicularis oris
N. facialis [VII]

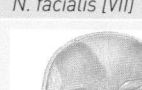

O: **Pars marginalis** and **Pars labialis:** lateral to the Angulus oris

I: Skin of the lips

F: Closes the lips, thereby also moving the nose wings, cheeks and the skin of chin

M. buccinator
N. facialis [VII]

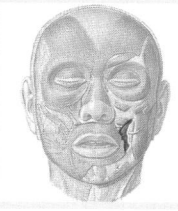

O: Posterior part of the Proc. alveolaris of the Maxilla, Raphe pterygomandibularis, posterior part of the Proc. alveolaris of the Mandibula

I: Angulus oris, upper and lower lip

F: Tenses the lips, increases the intraoral pressure (as in blowing and chewing)

M. levator labii superioris
N. facialis [VII]

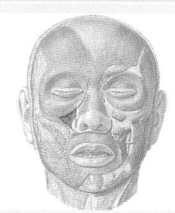

O: Margo infraorbitalis and adjacent part of the Proc. zygomaticus of the Maxilla; originates from the muscle mass of the M. orbicularis oculi

I: Upper lip

F: Draws the upper lip laterally and upwards

1 Facial muscles (continuation)

M. depressor labii inferioris
N. facialis [VII]

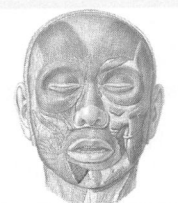

O: Basis mandibulae medial to the Foramen mentale

I: Lower lip,
chin,
deep fibres to the mucosa

F: Draws the lower lip laterally and downwards

M. mentalis
N. facialis [VII]

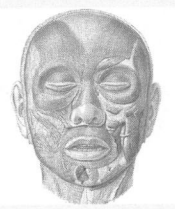

O: Jugum alveolare of the lower, lateral incisor tooth

I: Skin of the chin

F: Creates the chin's dimple, everts the lower lip (together with the M. orbicularis oris)

M. transversus menti
N. facialis [VII]

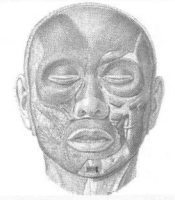

O: Oblique branch from the M. mentalis

I: Skin of the chin

F: Moves the skin of the chin

M. depressor anguli oris
N. facialis [VII]

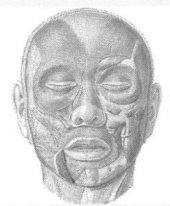

O: Basis mandibulae, just below the Foramen mentale

I: Lower lip,
cheek lateral to the Angulus oris,
upper lip

F: Pulls the angle of mouth downwards

M. risorius (frequently a part of the Platysma or the M. depressor anguli oris)
N. facialis [VII]

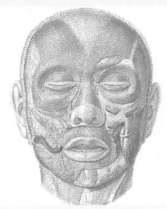

O: Fascia parotidea,
Fascia masseterica

I: Upper lip,
Angulus oris

F: Pulls the angle of mouth laterally and upwards,
creates the cheek's dimple

1 Facial muscles (continuation)

M. levator anguli oris
N. facialis [VII]

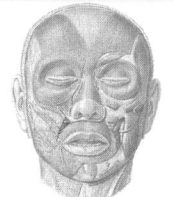

O: Fossa canina of the Maxilla

I: Angulus oris

F: Draws the angle of mouth medially and upwards

M. zygomaticus major
N. facialis [VII]

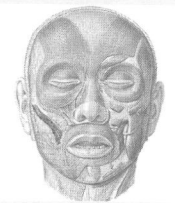

O: Os zygomaticum adjacent to the Sutura zygomaticotemporalis

I: Upper lip, Angulus oris

F: Draws the angle of mouth laterally and upwards

M. zygomaticus minor
N. facialis [VII]

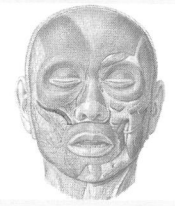

O: Os zygomaticum adjacent to the Sutura zygomaticomaxillaris

I: Upper lip, Angulus oris

F: Moves the lips, the nose wings, the cheeks and the skin of the chin, increases the nasolabial sulcus

M. levator labii superioris alaeque nasi
N. facialis [VII]

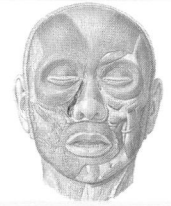

O: Proc. frontalis of the Maxilla; originates from the muscle mass of the M. orbicularis oculi

I: Nose wings, angle of mouth, upper lip, deep fibres: lateral and posterior parts of the nostril

F: Moves the lips, the nose wings, the cheeks and the skin of the chin

f Neck (Fig. 253)

Platysma
N. facialis [VII]

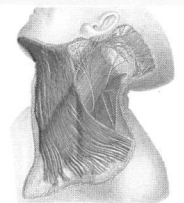

O: Basis mandibulae, Fascia parotidea

I: Skin below the Clavicula, Fascia pectoralis

F: Tenses the skin of the neck, creates vertical wrinkles

6

T 2

2 Muscles of the tongue (Fig. 178–180, 186–189)

a Internal muscles of the tongue

M. longitudinalis superior
N. hypoglossus [XII]

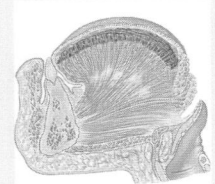

O: Radix linguae

I: Apex linguae

F: Retracts and broadens the tongue, elevates the apex of the tongue

M. longitudinalis inferior
N. hypoglossus [XII]

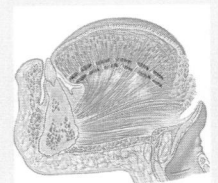

O: Radix linguae

I: Apex linguae

F: Retracts and broadens the tongue, lowers the apex of the tongue

M. transversus linguae
N. hypoglossus [XII]

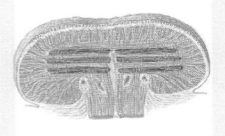

O: Lateral margin of the tongue, Septum linguae

I: Lateral margin of the tongue, Aponeurosis linguae

F: Narrows the tongue, elongates the tongue together with the M. verticalis linguae

M. verticalis linguae
N. hypoglossus [XII]

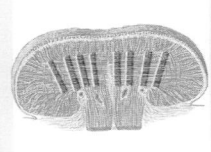

O: Radix linguae; originates from the M. genioglossus

I: Aponeurosis linguae

F: Broadens the tongue

2 Muscles of the tongue (continuation)

b External muscles of the tongue

M. genioglossus
N. hypoglossus [XII]

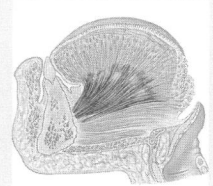

O: Spina mentalis of the Mandibula   **I:** Aponeurosis linguae   **F:** Protrudes and depresses the tongue

M. hyoglossus
N. hypoglossus [XII]

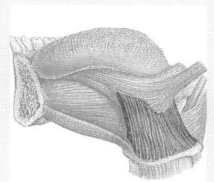

O: Cornu majus and Corpus ossis hyoidei   **I:** Lateral parts of the Aponeurosis linguae   **F:** Retracts and depresses the tongue

M. chondroglossus (variably formed)
N. hypoglossus [XII]

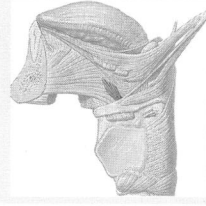

O: Cornu minus ossis hyoidei   **I:** Lateral parts of the Aponeurosis linguae   **F:** Retracts the tongue, depresses the root and the back of the tongue

M. styloglossus
N. hypoglossus [XII]

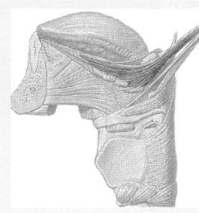

O: Anterior margin of the Proc. styloideus of the Os temporale, Lig. stylomandibulare   **I:** Enters lateral parts of the tongue from above and behind   **F:** Retracts and elevates the tongue

3 Muscles of the palate (Fig. 174, 1406)

M. levator veli palatini
Rr. pharyngeales of the N. glossopharyngeus [IX] and the N. vagus [X] (= Plexus pharyngeus)

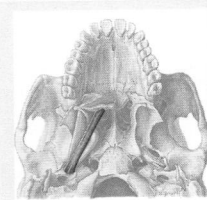

O: Inferior surface of the Pars petrosa of the Os temporale, Cartilago tubae auditivae

I: Aponeurosis palatina

F: Tenses and elevates the soft palate, expands the lumen of the auditory tube

M. tensor veli palatini (surrounds the Hamulus ossis pterygoidei as hypomochlion)
N. musculi tensoris veli palatini of the N. mandibularis [V/3]

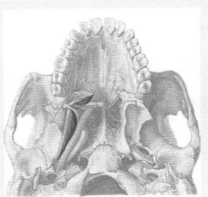

O: Fossa scaphoidea at the base of the Lamina medialis of the Proc. pterygoideus, Spina ossis sphenoidalis, membranous part of the Tuba auditiva

I: Aponeurosis palatina

F: Tenses (and elevates) the soft palate, expands the lumen of the auditory tube

M. palatoglossus
N. glossopharyngeus [IX]

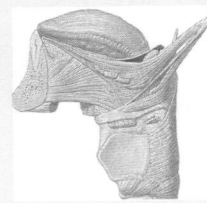

O: Aponeurosis palatina

I: Enters the internal muscles of the tongue, in particular the M. transversus linguae

F: Depresses the soft palate, elevates the root of the tongue in order to narrow the pharynx

M. uvulae (solitary muscle)
Rr. pharyngeales of the N. glossopharyngeus [IX] and the N. vagus [X] (= Plexus pharyngeus)

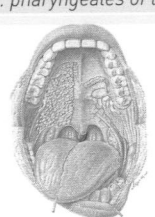

O: Aponeurosis linguae

I: Stroma of the Uvula

F: Shortens and thus thickens the uvula

4 Masticatory muscles (Fig. 111, 114–119, 121, 122)

The course of the M. masseter from the zygomatic arch to the mandibular angle may well be palpated through the skin. When clenching the teeth, the M. temporalis can be felt in the temporal fossa. The M. pterygoideus medialis inserts at the inner surface of the mandibular angle. The M. pterygoideus lateralis extends interiorely from the temporomandibular joint.

M. temporalis
Nn. temporales profundi (N. mandibularis [V/3])

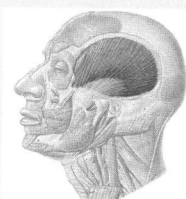

O: Os temporale below the Linea temporalis inferior, deep layer of the Fascia temporalis

I: Apex and medial surface of the Proc. coronoideus of the Mandibula

F: Anterior fibres close the jaws, posterior fibres retract the mandible (= retrusion)

M. masseter
N. massetericus (N. mandibularis [V/3])

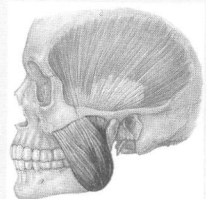

O: Pars superficialis: anterior two thirds of the inferior margin of the Arcus zygomaticus (tendinous)
Pars profunda: posterior third of the inner surface of the Arcus zygomaticus

I: Pars superficialis: Angulus mandibulae, Tuberositas masseterica
Pars profunda: inferior margin of the Mandibula

F: Closes the jaws

M. pterygoideus medialis
N. pterygoideus medialis (N. mandibularis [V/3])

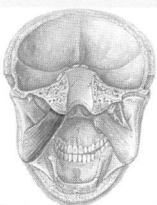

O: Fossa pterygoidea, medial surface of the Lamina lateralis of the Proc. pterygoideus, Proc. pyramidalis of the Os palatinum

I: Inferior margin of the Mandibula, Tuberositas pterygoidea

F: Closes the jaws

M. pterygoideus lateralis
N. pterygoideus lateralis (N. mandibularis [V/3])

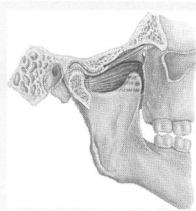

O: Caput superius: outer surface of the Lamina lateralis of the Proc. pterygoideus, Tuber maxillae (accessory)
Caput inferius: Facies temporalis of the Ala major of the Os sphenoidale

I: Caput superius: disc and capsule of the Articulatio temporomandibularis
Caput inferius: Fovea pterygoidea of the Proc. condylaris of the Mandibula

F: Caput inferius: draws the mandible interiorely (=protrusion)

5 Muscles of the pharynx (Fig. 189, 247, 248, 252)

The pharyngeal muscles are divided into the pharyngeal constrictors (Mm. constrictores pharyngis superior, medius and inferior) and the pharyngeal levator muscles (M. stylopharyngeus, M. salpingopharyngeus and M. palatopharyngeus).

a Pharyngeal constrictors

M. constrictor pharyngis superior
Rr. pharyngeales of the N. glossopharyngeus [IX] (= Plexus pharyngeus)

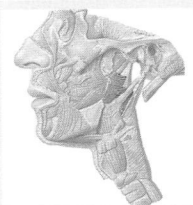

O: Pars pterygopharyngea: posterior margin of the Lamina medialis of the Proc. pterygoideus, Hamulus ossis pterygoidei
Pars buccopharyngea: Raphe pterygomandibularis
Pars mylopharyngea: Linea mylohyoidea of the Mandibula
Pars glossopharyngea: M. transversus linguae

I: Membrana pharyngobasilaris, superior third of the Raphe pharyngis

F: Constricts the pharynx, separates the Epipharynx from the Mesopharynx (together with the M. palatopharyngeus), promotes transport of food into the oesophagus by wave-like contractions (peristaltic wave)

M. constrictor pharyngis medius
Rr. pharyngeales of the N. glossopharyngeus [IX] and the N. vagus [X] (= Plexus pharyngeus)

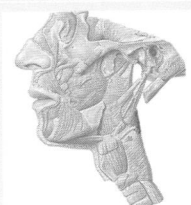

O: Pars chondropharyngea: Cornu minus ossis hyoidei
Pars ceratopharyngea: Cornu majus ossis hyoidei

I: Middle third of the Raphe pharyngis, overlaps the M. constrictor pharyngis superior

F: Constricts the pharynx from behind, promotes transport of food into the oesophagus by wave-like contractions (peristaltic wave)

M. constrictor pharyngis inferior
Rr. pharyngeales of the N. vagus [X] (= Plexus pharyngeus)

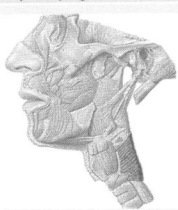

O: Pars thyropharyngea: outer surface of the Cartilago thyroidea behind the Linea obliqua
Pars cricopharyngea: lateral surface of the Cartilago cricoidea
Pars tracheopharyngea: lateral surface of the Cartilago trachealis I

I: Middle and inferior third of the Raphe pharyngis, overlaps the M. constrictor pharyngis medius

F: Constricts the pharynx from behind, promotes transport of food into the oesophagus by wave-like contractions (peristaltic wave)

b Pharyngeal levator muscles

M. palatopharyngeus (Functionally, this muscle also belongs to the muscles of the palate.)
Rr. pharyngeales of the N. glossopharyngeus [IX] (= Plexus pharyngeus)

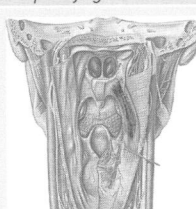

O: Aponeurosis palatina, Hamulus ossis pterygoidei

I: Cartilago thyroidea, inserts into the lateral and the posterior wall of the Pharynx

F: Constricts the isthmus of fauces, depresses the soft palate, elevates the pharyngeal wall towards the soft palate

5 Muscles of the pharynx (continuation)

M. salpingopharyngeus
Rr. pharyngeales of the N. glossopharyngeus [IX] (= Plexus pharyngeus)

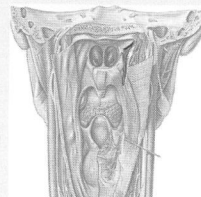

O: Free margin and inferior surface of the Cartilago tubae auditivae

I: Inserts into the lateral wall of the Pharynx

F: Elevates the pharynx

M. stylopharyngeus
R. musculi stylopharyngei of the N. glossopharyngeus [IX]

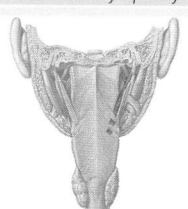

O: Proc. styloideus of the Os temporale

I: Cartilago thyroidea, inserts into the lateral wall of the Pharynx between the M. constrictor superior and the M. constrictor medius

F: Elevates the pharynx

Muscles of the larynx (Fig. 224–227)

M. cricothyroideus (Pars recta: superficial, Pars obliqua: deep)
R. externus of the N. laryngeus superior of the N. vagus [X]

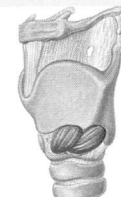

O: Outer surface of the Arcus of the Cartilago cricoidea

I: Inferior margin of the Lamina of the Cartilago thyroidea

F: Tenses the vocal cords by tilting the cricoid cartilage around a transverse axis

M. cricoarytenoideus posterior
N. laryngeus recurrens of the N. vagus [X]

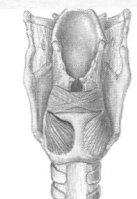

O: Posterior surface of the Lamina of the Cartilago cricoidea

I: Proc. muscularis of the Cartilago arytenoidea

F: Opens the rima glottidis by rotating the vocal process of the arytenoid cartilage outwards around a longitudinal axis, as well as by tilting the arytenoid cartilage sidewards

M. cricoarytenoideus lateralis
N. laryngeus recurrens of the N. vagus [X]

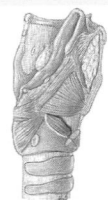

O: Lateral upper margin of the Arcus of the Cartilago cricoidea

I: Proc. muscularis of the Cartilago arytenoidea

F: Closes the intermembranous part of the rima glottidis by rotating the arytenoid cartilage inwards around a longitudinal axis

M. arytenoideus transversus
N. laryngeus recurrens of the N. vagus [X]

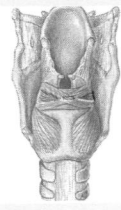

O: Lateral edge and posterior surface of the Cartilago arytenoidea

I: Lateral edge and posterior surface of the contralateral Cartilago arytenoidea

F: Closes the intercartilagenous part of the rima glottidis by approximating both arytenoid cartilages

M. arytenoideus obliquus
N. laryngeus recurrens of the N. vagus [X]

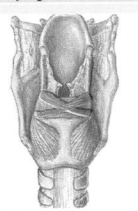

O: Base of the posterior surface of the Cartilago arytenoidea
Pars aryepiglottica: apex of the Cartilago arytenoidea

I: Apex and posterior surface of the contralateral Proc. muscularis
Pars aryepiglottica: lateral margin of the Cartilago epiglottica

F: Draws the arytenoid cartilage medially and narrows the intercartilagenous part of the rima glottidis by tilting the arytenoid cartilages inwards

6 Muscles of the larynx (continuation)

M. vocalis
N. laryngeus recurrens of the N. vagus [X]

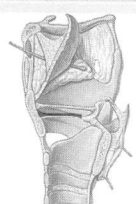

O: Inner surface of the "bow" of the Cartilago thyroidea

I: Proc. vocalis and Fovea oblonga of the Cartilago arytenoidea

F: Tenses the vocal cord and forms the edge of the rima glottidis, regulates the ability of the vocal fold to vibrate

M. thyroarytenoideus
N. laryngeus recurrens of the N. vagus [X]

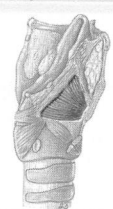

O: Inner surface of the Lamina of the Cartilago thyroidea in close proximity to the origin of the M. vocalis
Pars thyroepiglottica: Inner surface of the Lamina of the Cartilago thyroidea in close proximity to the origin of the M. thyroarytenoideus

I: Proc. muscularis and anterior surface of the Cartilago arytenoidea
Pars thyroepiglottica: lateral margin of the Cartilago epiglottica

F: Narrows the inter of the rima glottidis by rotating the arytenoid cartilage inwards around a longitudinal axis
Pars thyroepiglottica: narrows the laryngeal orifice

7 Branches and supplying areas of the cervical plexus (Fig. 253–258)

	Motor function	Sensory function
Ansa cervicalis Radix superior (= Radix anterior) Radix inferior (= Radix posterior)	Mm. infrahyoidei	
Rr. musculares	M. longus colli M. longus capitis M. rectus capitis anterior Mm. intertransversarii anteriores cervicis M. trapezius M. levator scapulae M. scalenus medius M. geniohyoideus	
Branches of the so-called Punctum nervosum N. auricularis magnus		Skin of the upper neck, the area of the mandibular angle, the anterior and posterior areas surrounding the auricle, and most of the auricle itself
N. transversus colli		Skin of the upper anterior neck
N. occipitalis minor		Skin of the occipital region
Nn. supraclaviculares mediales, intermedii, laterales		A strip of skin below the clavicle
N. phrenicus	Diaphragm	Parietal pleura, pericard, peritoneum

8 Lateral muscle of the neck (Fig. 204, 208)

The M. sternocleidomastoideus develops from the same embryonic anlage as the M. trapezius (same innervation). It traverses obliquely from the Proc. mastoideus in an anterior mediocaudal direction and is integrated in the Lamina superficialis of the Fascia cervicalis.

M. sternocleidomastoideus
N. accessorius [XI]; Plexus cervicalis

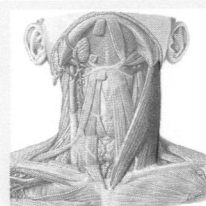

O: Caput sternale: with a long tendon from the ventral surface of the Sternum
Caput claviculare: with a short tendon from the sternal third of the Clavicula

I: Posterior area of the Proc. mastoideus,
lateral margin of the Linea nuchalis superior

F: Unilateral innervation: rotates the head contralaterally,
bilateral innervation: elevates the head and draws the head anteriorly, flexes the caudal cervical vertebrae and stretches both the cranial cervical vertebrae as well as the cranio-cervical joints

9 Suprahyoid muscles (Fig. 183–187, 204, 208)

The suprahyoid muscles form the floor of the oral cavity and function as antagonists to the infrahyoid muscles. The anterior belly of the M. digastricus is located most superficially. The next layer consists of the M. mylohyoideus, which forms a broad plate. The M. geniohyoideus is located adjacently to the interior surface of the M. mylohyoideus as a round strand. The posterior belly of the M. digastricus and the M. stylohyoideus are located dorsally.

M. mylohyoideus (The right and the left muscle together, secure the floor of the mouth in a plate-like shape.)
N. mylohyoideus (N. mandibularis [V/3])

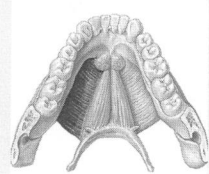

O: With a short tendon from the Linea mylohyoidea of the Mandibula

I: Raphe mylohyoidea, upper margin of the Corpus ossis hyoidei

F: Elevates the floor of the mouth and the tongue (as in swallowing), depresses the mandible, also elevates the hyoid bone, forms the muscular support for the tongue

M. digastricus (Venter posterior and Venter anterior are connected by an intertendon attached to the Cornu minus of the Os hyoideum. Venter posterior: from the origin to the intertendon; Venter anterior: from the intertendon to the insertion.)
Venter anterior: N. mylohyoideus (N. mandibularis [V/3]);
Venter posterior: R. digastricus (N. facialis [VII])

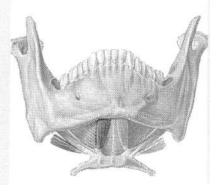

O: Incisura mastoidea of the Os temporale

I: Fossa digastrica of the Mandibula

F: Supports the M. mylohyoideus

M. stylohyoideus
R. stylohyoideus (N. facialis [VII])

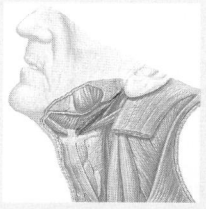

O: Proc. styloideus of the Os temporale

I: Lateral margin of the Corpus ossis hyoidei with two parts surrounding the intertendon of the M. digastricus

F: Draws the hyoid bone dorsocranially

M. geniohyoideus (The right and the left muscle are closely juxtaposed, only separated by a thin septum of connective tissue.)
Rr. ventrales from C1–C2

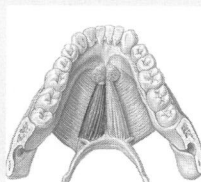

O: With a short tendon from the Spina mentalis of the Mandibula

I: Anterior surface of the Corpus ossis hyoidei

F: Supports the M. mylohyoideus in elevating the tongue, depresses the mandible, elevates the hyoid bone

10 Infrahyoid muscles (Fig. 183, 204, 208)

The infrahyoid muscles function as antagonists to the suprahyoid muscles.
The M. sternohyoideus is located superficially and is followed below by the M. sternothyroideus and the M. thyrohyoideus. The M. omohyoideus stretches most laterally.

M. sternohyoideus
Ansa cervicalis (Plexus cervicalis)

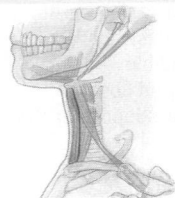

O: Cranial margin of the Cartilago costae I, inner surface of the Manubrium sterni and the capsule of the sternoclavicular joint

I: Inferior margin of the Corpus ossis hyoidei

F: Draws the hyoid bone caudally

M. sternothyroideus
Ansa cervicalis (Plexus cervicalis)

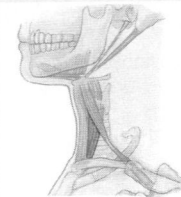

O: Inner surface of the Cartilago costae I, inner surface of the Manubrium sterni caudal to the M. sternohyoideus

I: Outer surface, Linea obliqua, of the Lamina of the Cartilago thyroidea

F: Depresses the larynx, regulates the position of the larynx between the hyoid bone and the sternum together with the M. thyrohyoideus

M. thyrohyoideus
Ansa cervicalis (Plexus cervicalis)

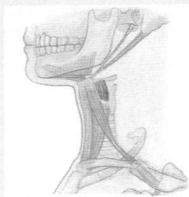

O: Outer surface, Linea obliqua, of the Lamina of the Cartilago thyroidea

I: Lateral third of the Corpus and the root of the Cornu majus of the Os hyoideum

F: Approximates the hyoid bone and the larynx, regulates the position of the larynx between the hyoid bone and the sternum together with the M. sternothyroideus

M. omohyoideus (Venter inferior and Venter superior are connected by an intertendon, which is attached to the Vagina carotica.)
Ansa cervicalis (Plexus cervicalis)

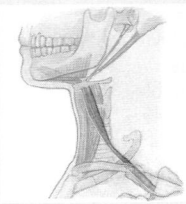

O: Venter inferior: Margo superior of the Scapula medial to the Incisura scapulae

I: Venter superior: caudal margin of the lateral outer surface of the Corpus ossis hyoidei

F: Tenses the cervical fascia due to its attachment to the carotid sheath, prevents the collapse of the V. jugularis interna

11 Scalenus muscles (Fig. 204, 208, 209, 573)

The three scalenus muscles, M. scalenus anterior, M. scalenus medius and M. scalenus posterior, traverse to the upper ribs and form a three sided muscle layer laterally of the cervical part of the vertebral column.

M. scalenus anterior
Direct branches of the Plexus cervicalis and the Plexus brachialis

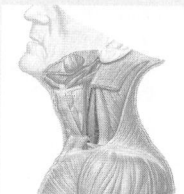

O: Tubercula anteriora of the Procc. transversi of the 3. (4.)–6. cervical vertebra

I: With a short tendon at the Tuberculum musculi scaleni anterioris of the 1. rib

F: <u>Vertebral column:</u>
flexes the cervical part of the vertebral column laterally
<u>Thorax:</u>
elevates the first rib, thereby elevating the thorax (muscle of inspiration)

M. scalenus medius
Direct branches of the Plexus cervicalis and the Plexus brachialis

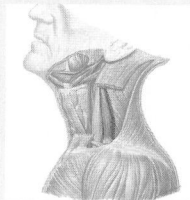

O: Tubercula of the Procc. transversi of the 3.–7. cervical vertebra

I: With a short tendon at the 1. rib, just behind the Sulcus arteriae subclaviae

F: <u>Vertebral column:</u>
flexes the cervical part of the vertebral column laterally
<u>Thorax:</u>
elevates the first rib, thereby elevating the thorax (muscle of inspiration)

M. scalenus posterior
Direct branches of the Plexus cervicalis and the Plexus brachialis

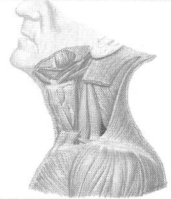

O: Tubercula posteriora of the Procc. transversi of the 5. and 6. cervical vertebra

I: With a short and flat tendon at the upper margin of the 2. (3.) rib

F: <u>Vertebral column:</u>
flexes the cervical part of the vertebral column laterally
<u>Thorax:</u>
elevates the second (and third) rib, thereby elevating the thorax (muscle of inspiration)

T 12

12 Prevertebral muscles (Fig. 209, 573)

The prevertebral muscles are located to the both sides of the bodies of the cervical and upper thoracic vertebrae, and are ensheathed by the Lamina prevertebralis of the Fascia cervicalis. The anterolateral part of the Atlas and Axis are connected by the short M. rectus capitis anterior.

M. rectus capitis anterior
Rr. ventrales of the Plexus cervicalis

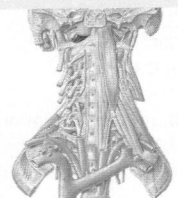

O: Proc. transversus and Massa lateralis of the Atlas

I: Pars basilaris of the Os occipitale

F: Flexes the head lateroventrally, (rotates the head ipsilaterally)

M. longus capitis
Direct branches of the Plexus cervicalis

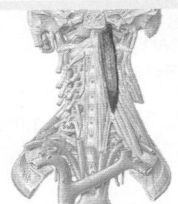

O: Tubercula anteriora of the Procc. transversi of the 3.–6. cervical vertebra

I: Outer surface of the Pars basilaris of the Os occipitale

F: Flexes the head ventrally, (rotates the head ipsilaterally)

M. longus colli
Direct branches of the Plexus cervicalis

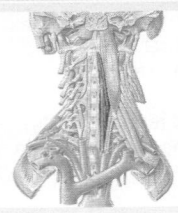

O: Bodies of the 5. cervical – 3. thoracic vertebra, Tubercula anteriora of the Procc. transversi of the 2.–5. cervical vertebra

I: Procc. transversi of the 5.–7. cervical vertebra, bodies of the 2.–4. cervical vertebra, Tuberculum anterius of the Atlas

F: Flexes the head ventrally, (rotates the head ipsilaterally)

13 Muscles of the thoracic wall (Fig. 571–577)

The M. pectoralis major moulds the surface anatomy of the anterior upper thoracic wall. The M. pectoralis minor is situated just below. Together with the M. subclavius, these muscles belong to the group of the ventral muscles of the shoulder (see Tab. 26).
The Mm. intercostales externi and interni fill the intercostal space. The Mm. subcostales and the M. transversus thoracis are located at the inner surface of the thoracic wall. Sometimes a superficially located M. sternalis can be found.

M. sternalis (inconstant muscle, in approx. 5% of the cases located on the Fascia pectoralis)
Branches of the Nn. pectorales (Plexus brachialis, Pars supraclavicularis) or Nn. intercostales (Nn. thoracici)

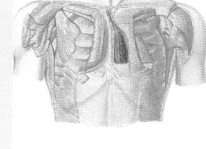

O: Edge of the Manubrium sterni

I: Inserts into the rectus sheath

F: Contracts the pectoral skin

Mm. intercostales externi
Nn. intercostales (Nn. thoracici)

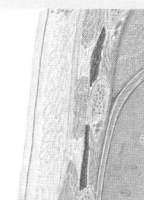

O: Inferior margin of the 1.–11. rib from the Tuberculum costae to the junction between cartilage and bone

I: Superior margin of the corresponding lower rib

F: Elevate the ribs, reinforce the intercostal space in deep inspiration

Mm. intercostales interni (Interiorly, the Vasa intercostalia posteriora and the N. intercostalis delineate the Mm. intercostales intimi.)
Nn. intercostales (Nn. thoracici)

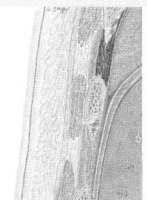

O: Superior margin of the 2.–12. rib from the sternal end of the Cartilago costalis to the Angulus costae

I: Inferior margin of the corresponding upper rib

F: Depress the ribs, reinforce the intercostal space in deep expiration

Mm. subcostales (inconstant muscles)
Nn. intercostales (Nn. thoracici)

O: Superior margin of the lower ribs between the Tuberculum and Angulus costae

I: Inferior margin of the lower ribs, always skipping one rib

F: Reinforce the thoracic wall, depress the ribs in deep expiration

M. transversus thoracis (inconstant muscle)
Nn. intercostales (Nn. thoracici)

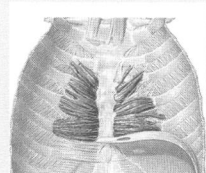

O: Corpus sterni, dorsolateral margin of the Proc. xiphoideus, Cartilago costalis of the (6.) 7. rib

I: Cartilago costalis of the 2.–6. rib close to the junction between cartilage and bone

F: Reinforces the thoracic wall in deep expiration

14 Ventral muscles of the abdominal wall (Fig. 575–578, 601)

The ventral muscles of the abdominal wall, the M. rectus abdominis and the M. pyramidalis, are located within the rectus sheath.

M. rectus abdominis
Nn. intercostales (Nn. thoracici); less frequently ventral branches of the upper Nn. lumbales

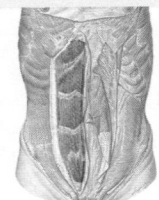

O: Outer surface of the Cartilago costalis of the 5.–7. rib, Proc. xiphoideus, Ligg. costoxiphoidea

I: Crista pubica of the Os coxae, Symphysis pubica

F: Flexes the trunk, compresses the abdomen, expiration

M. pyramidalis (inconstant muscle)
Caudal Nn. intercostales (Nn. thoracici)

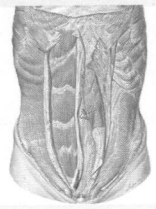

O: Crista pubica of the Os coxae, Symphysis pubica ventral to the M. rectus abdominis

I: Linea alba

F: "Tenses" the linea alba

15 Lateral muscles of the abdominal wall (Fig. 569–571, 575–578, 583, 601)

Together, the M. obliquus externus abdominis, the M. obliquus internus abdominis and the M. transversus abdominis are referred to as lateral muscles of the abdominal wall. Their tendinous layers together form the rectus sheath. In the male, parts of the M. obliquus internus abdominis and the M. transversus abdominis branch off to form the M. cremaster.

M. obliquus externus abdominis
Caudal Nn. intercostales (Nn. thoracici); N. iliohypogastricus; N. ilioinguinalis (Plexus lumbalis)

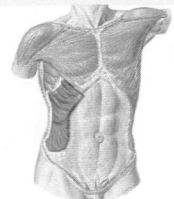

O: Outer surface of the 5.–12. rib, indented by fleshy digitations with the M. serratus anterior

I: Labium externum of the Crista iliaca, Lig. inguinale, Tuberculum pubicum, Crista pubica, Linea alba, participates in the formation of the anterior layer of the rectus sheath

F: Unilateral innervation: rotates the thorax contralaterally, flexes the vertebral column ipsilaterally, bilateral innervation: flexes the trunk, compresses the abdomen, expiration

M. obliquus internus abdominis (In the male, the most caudal fibres branch off as M. cremaster and traverse into the spermatic cord.)
Caudal Nn. intercostales (Nn. thoracici); N. iliohypogastricus; N. ilioinguinalis (Plexus lumbalis)

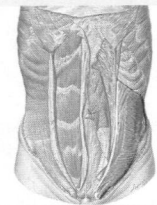

O: Superficial layer of the Fascia thoracolumbalis, Linea intermedia of the Crista iliaca, lateral two thirds of the Lig. inguinale

I: Inferior margin of the Cartilago costalis of the (9.) 10.–12. rib, Linea alba, superior to the Linea arcuata the muscle participates in the formation of both layers of the rectus sheath, whereas inferior to it all fibres insert into the anterior layer only

F: Unilateral innervation: rotates the thorax ipsilaterally, flexes the vertebral column ipsilaterally, bilateral innervation: flexes the trunk, compresses the abdomen, expiration, M. cremaster elevates the testis

15 Lateral muscles of the abdominal wall (continuation)

M. transversus abdominis (In the male, the most caudal fibres branch off as M. cremaster and traverse into the spermatic cord.)
Caudal Nn. intercostales (Nn. thoracici); N. iliohypogastricus; N. ilioinguinalis (Plexus lumbalis); N. genitofemoralis

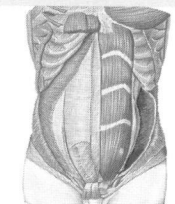

O: Inner surface of the Cartilago costalis of the (5., 6.) 7.–12. rib, Procc. costales of the lumbar vertebrae via the deep layer of the Fascia thoracolumbalis, Labium internum of the Crista iliaca, lateral third of the Lig. inguinale

I: Linea alba, superior to the Linea arcuata the muscle participates in the formation of the posterior layer of the rectus sheath, whereas inferior to it all fibres insert into the anterior layer

F: Compresses the abdomen, expiration, M. cremaster elevates the testis

16 Dorsal muscles of the abdominal wall (Fig. 583, 601)

The M. quadratus lumborum constitutes the muscular fundament of the posterior abdominal wall. Medially, this muscle is juxtaposed to the M. psoas major (see Tab. 42).

M. quadratus lumborum
N. intercostalis (N. thoracicus [T12]); Rr. musculares (Plexus lumbalis)

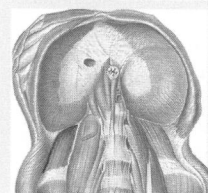

O: Posterior third of the Labium internum of the Crista iliaca, Lig. iliolumbale

I: Medial part of the 12. rib, Proc. costalis of the 4.–1. lumbar vertebra

F: Draws the ribs downwards in expiration, flexes the vertebral column ipsilaterally

17 Trunk-shoulder girdle muscles (Fig. 527, 528, 569, 570, 575, 576)

The dorsal muscles of this group, the M. trapezius, M. levator scapulae, M. rhomboideus major and M. rhomboideus minor, belong to the superficial layer according to their position. However, according to their origin and innervation they are referred to as immigrated muscles of the back. The M. serratus anterior is located at the lateral thoracic wall and traverses dorsally underneath the scapula.
The M. pectoralis minor and the M. subclavius originate from the anterior thoracic wall. They are discussed in the section of the ventral muscles of the shoulder (see Tab. 26).

M. trapezius (At the origin between the middle and lower thoracic vertebrae and at the Spina scapulae, a characteristically shaped aponeurosis is found.)
N. accessorius [XI] and branches of the Plexus cervicalis

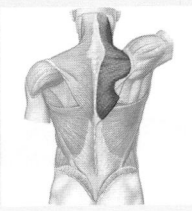

O: Pars descendens: Squama ossis occipitalis between the Linea nuchalis suprema and the Linea nuchalis superior, Procc. spinosi of the upper cervical vertebrae via the Lig. nuchae
Pars transversa: Procc. spinosi of the lower cervical and upper thoracic vertebrae
Pars ascendens: Procc. spinosi of the middle and lower thoracic vertebrae

I: Pars descendens: acromial third of the Clavicula
Pars transversa: Acromion
Pars ascendens: Spina scapulae

F: Shoulder girdle:
Pars descendens: prevents the drop of the shoulder girdle and the arm, elevates the scapula and rotates the inferior angle outwards together with the M. serratus anterior to allow for the arm to be raised over the horizontal, rotates the head contralaterally when shoulders are fixed, extends the cervical part of the vertebral column when both sides are innervated
Pars transversa: draws the scapula medially
Pars ascendens: depresses the scapula and rotates it caudally
Vertebral column:
upon bilateral innervation, flattens the kyphosis of the thoracic part of the vertebral column

M. levator scapulae
Direct branches of the Plexus cervicalis and N. dorsalis scapulae (Plexus brachialis, Pars supraclavicularis)

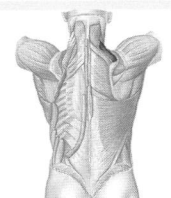

O: Tubercula posteriora of the Procc. transversi of the 1.–4. cervical vertebra

I: Angulus superior and adjacent parts of the Scapula

F: Shoulder girdle:
elevates the scapula and rotates it cranially
Vertebral column:
extends the cervical part of the vertebral column when shoulders are fixed

M. rhomboideus minor
N. dorsalis scapulae (Plexus brachialis, Pars supraclavicularis)

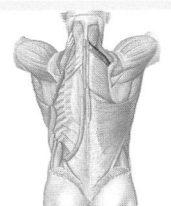

O: Proc. spinosus of the 6. and 7. cervical vertebra

I: Margo medialis of the Scapula cranially to the Spina scapulae

F: Draws the scapula medially and upwards,
holds the scapula to the trunk together with the M. serratus anterior

M. rhomboideus major
N. dorsalis scapulae (Plexus brachialis, Pars supraclavicularis)

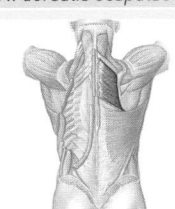

O: Proc. spinosus of the four upper thoracic vertebrae

I: Margo medialis of the Scapula caudally to the Spina scapulae

F: Draws the scapula medially and upwards,
holds the scapula to the trunk together with the M. serratus anterior

17 Trunk-shoulder girdle muscles (continuation)

M. serratus anterior (Palsy of the M. serratus anterior or the Mm. rhomboidei results in Scapula alata.)
N. thoracicus longus (Plexus brachialis, Pars supraclavicularis)

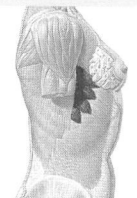

O: Pars superior: 1. and 2. rib (reasonably convergent)
Pars media: 2.–4. rib (divergent)
Pars inferior: 5.–(8.) 9. rib (strongly convergent), indented with the origin of the M. obliquus externus abdominis

I: Pars superior: Angulus superior of the Scapula
Pars media: Margo medialis of the Scapula
Pars inferior: Angulus inferior of the Scapula

F: Shoulder girdle:
draws the scapula medially, presses the scapula onto the thorax together with the Mm. rhomboidei
Pars superior: elevates the scapula
Pars media: depresses the scapula
Pars inferior: depresses the scapula and rotates the inferior angle outwards to allow for the arm to be raised over the horizontal together with the M. trapezius
Thorax:
elevates the ribs when scapula is fixed (inspiration)

18 Trunk-arm muscles (Fig. 527, 528, 569, 570)

The M. latissimus dorsi and the M. pectoralis major belong to this group. Both muscles originate from the trunk and traverse to the arm.
Due to the position of its muscular belly, and the fact that it also migrated to the back from ventrally, the M. latissimus dorsi is grouped with the superficial muscles of the back.
The M. pectoralis major originates from the thoracic wall and, accordingly, is discussed with the ventral muscles of the shoulder (see Tab. 26).

M. latissimus dorsi (Bursa subtendinea musculi latissimi dorsi at the contact area with the M. teres major)
N. thoracodorsalis (Plexus brachialis, Pars supraclavicularis)

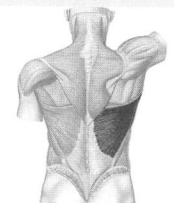

O: Proc. spinosus of the six lower thoracic and lumbar vertebrae (via Fascia thoracolumbalis), Facies dorsalis of the Os sacrum, dorsal third of the Labium externum of the Crista iliaca, (9.) 10.–12. rib, frequently with an additional indentation from the Angulus inferior of the Scapula

I: With a flat tendon surrounding the M. teres major at the Crista tuberculi minoris

F: Shoulder joint:
adduction, medial rotation, retroversion
Shoulder girdle:
draws the scapula and the arm medially and downwards

19 Spinocostal muscles (Fig. 528)

The spinocostal muscles, M. serratus posterior superior and M. serratus posterior inferior, are slim muscles with minor functional relevance, located in the depth of the muscles of the back on top of the autochthonous muscles of the back.

M. serratus posterior superior
Ventral branches of the N. cervicalis [C8] and the Nn. thoracici [T1–T4]

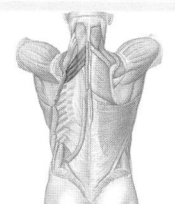

O: Proc. spinosus of the 6., 7. cervical and the 1., 2. thoracic vertebra

I: 1.–4. rib laterally to the Angulus costae

F: Elevates the 1.–4. rib (inspiration)

M. serratus posterior inferior
Ventral branches of the Nn. thoracici [T9–T12]

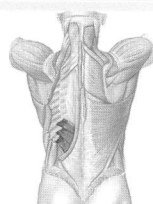

O: Proc. spinosus of the 11., 12. thoracic and 1., 2. lumbar vertebra

I: Caudal margin of the 9.–12. rib

F: Draws the 9.–12. rib downwards (expiration), with its possible antagonism to the diaphragm, it may also support forced inspiration

20 Autochthonous muscles of the back (Fig. 529, 532–538, 601)

a Autochthonous lateral muscles of the back (Fig. 529, 532, 534, 537, 601)

The lateral tract of the autochthonous muscles of the back covers the medial tract in the neck and lumbar region and is therefore also referred to as superficial part of the autochthonous muscles of the back. The following muscles with longitudinal fibres belong to this tract: M. iliocostalis, M. longissimus, Mm. intertransversarii. The oblique Mm. splenici diverge cranially (spinotransversal). The Mm. levatores costarum traverse obliquely with laterocaudal direction to the ribs.

M. iliocostalis lumborum
Rr. posteriores of the Nn. lumbales

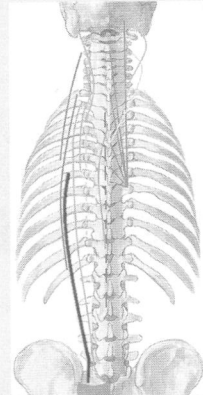

O: Together with the M. longissimus thoracis from: Procc. spinosi of the lumbar vertebrae, Facies dorsalis of the Os sacrum, dorsal third of the Crista iliaca, Fascia thoracolumbalis

I: Angulus costae of the 12.–5. rib

F: Unilateral innervation: lateral flexion, bilateral innervation: extension

M. iliocostalis thoracis
Rr. posteriores of the Nn. thoracici

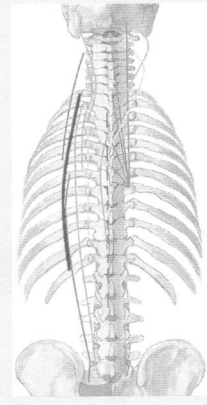

O: 12.–7. rib medially to the Angulus costae

I: Angulus costae of the (6.) 7.–1. rib

F: Unilateral innervation: lateral flexion, bilateral innervation: extension

M. iliocostalis cervicis
Rr. posteriores of the Nn. cervicales

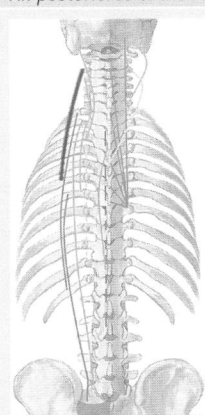

O: 7.–4. (3.) rib medially to the Angulus costae

I: Tuberculum posterius of the Proc. transversus of the 6.–(4.) 3. cervical vertebra

F: Unilateral innervation: lateral flexion, bilateral innervation: extension

20 Autochthonous muscles of the back (continuation)

M. longissimus thoracis (It is closely attached to the M. longissimus cervicis and the M. spinalis.)
Rr. posteriores of the Nn. spinales

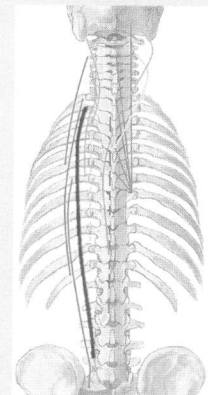

O: Together with the M. iliocostalis lumborum from: Procc. spinosi of the lumbar vertebrae, Facies dorsalis of the Os sacrum, frequently from the Proc. mamillaris of the 2. and the 1. lumbar vertebra, as well as from the Proc. transversus of the 12.–6. thoracic vertebra

I: Medial part: Proc. mamillaris of the 5. lumbar vertebra, Proc. accessorius of the 4.–1. lumbar vertebra, Procc. transversi of the thoracic vertebrae; Lateral part: Proc. costalis of the 4.–1. lumbar vertebra, deep layer of the Fascia thoracolumbalis, 12.–2. rib medially to the Angulus costae

F: Unilateral innervation: lateral flexion, bilateral innervation: extension

M. longissimus cervicis
Rr. posteriores of the Nn. spinales

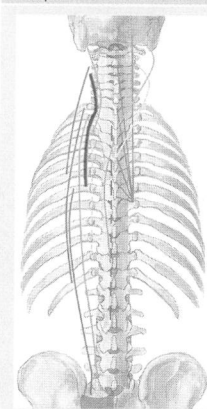

O: Proc. transversus of the 6.–1. thoracic and 7.–3. cervical vertebra

I: Tuberculum posterius of the Proc. transversus of the 5.–2. cervical vertebra

F: Unilateral innervation: lateral flexion, bilateral innervation: extension

M. longissimus capitis
Rr. posteriores of the Nn. spinales

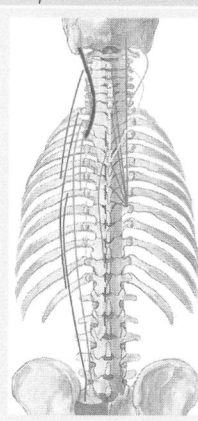

O: Proc. transversus of the 3. thoracic–3. cervical vertebra

I: Posterior margin of the Proc. mastoideus

F: Unilateral innervation: lateral flexion, bilateral innervation: extension

26

T 20

20 Autochthonous muscles of the back (continuation)

Mm. intertransversarii laterales lumborum (Strictly speaking, these muscles are of ventral descent and can therefore not be referred to as autochthonous muscles of the back.) *Rr. posteriores and anteriores of the Nn. spinales*

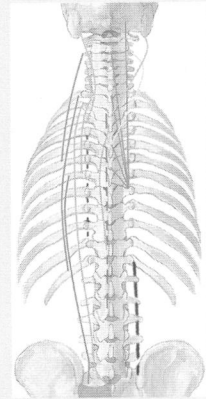

O: Tuberositas iliaca, Proc. costalis and Proc. accessorius of the 5.–1. lumbar vertebra, Proc. transversus of the 12. thoracic vertebra

I: Proc. costalis of the 5.–1. lumbar vertebra, Tuberositas iliaca

F: Unilateral innervation: lateral flexion, bilateral innervation: extension

Mm. intertransversarii mediales lumborum
Rr. posteriores and anteriores of the Nn. spinales

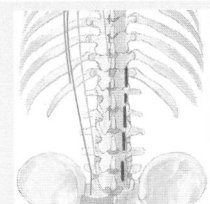

O: Proc. accessorius of the 4.–1. lumbar vertebra

I: Proc. mamillaris of the 5.–2. lumbar vertebra

F: Unilateral innervation: lateral flexion, bilateral innervation: extension

Mm. intertransversarii thoracis
Rr. posteriores and anteriores of the Nn. spinales

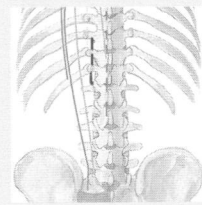

O: Proc. transversus of the 12.–10. thoracic vertebra

I: Proc. accessorius and Proc. mamillaris of the 1. lumbar vertebra up to the Proc. transversus of the 11. thoracic vertebra

F: Unilateral innervation: lateral flexion, bilateral innervation: extension

Mm. intertransversarii posteriores cervicis (Strictly speaking, these muscles are of ventral descent and can therefore not be referred to as autochthonous muscles of the back.) *Rr. posteriores and anteriores of the Nn. spinales*

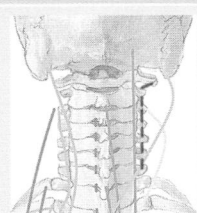

O: Tuberculum posterius of the Proc. transversus of the 6.–1. cervical vertebra

I: Tuberculum posterius of the Proc. transversus of the 7.–2. cervical vertebra

F: Unilateral innervation: lateral flexion, bilateral innervation: extension

Mm. intertransversarii anteriores cervicis (Strictly speaking, these muscles are of ventral descent and can therefore not be referred to as autochthonous muscles of the back.) *Rr. posteriores and anteriores of the Nn. spinales*

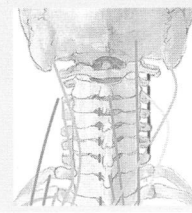

O: Tuberculum anterius of the Proc. transversus of the 6.–1. cervical vertebra

I: Tuberculum anterius of the Proc. transversus of the 7.–2. cervical vertebra

F: Unilateral innervation: lateral flexion, bilateral innervation: extension

20 Autochthonous muscles of the back (continuation)

M. splenius cervicis
Rr. posteriores of the Nn. cervicales

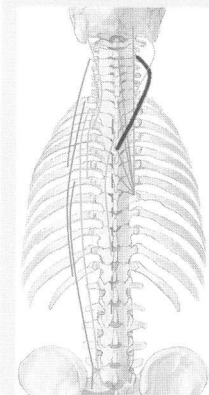

O: Proc. spinosus of the 3. thoracic –6. cervical vertebra, Lig. supraspinale

I: Tuberculum posterius of the Proc. transversus of the (3.) 2.–1. cervical vertebra

F: Unilateral innervation: lateral flexion,
rotates the cervical part of the vertebral column and the head ipsilaterally,
bilateral innervation: extends the cervical part of the vertebral column

M. splenius capitis
Rr. posteriores of the Nn. cervicales

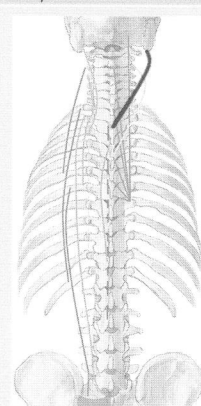

O: Proc. spinosus of the 3.–7. cervical vertebra, Lig. nuchae

I: Proc. mastoideus, (Linea nuchalis superior)

F: Unilateral innervation: lateral flexion,
rotates the cervical part of the vertebral column and the head ipsilaterally,
bilateral innervation: extends the cervical part of the vertebral column

Mm. levatores costarum (The Mm. levatores costarum longi skip one rib, whereas the Mm. levatores costarum breves traverse to the adjacent caudal rib. There are no Mm. levatores costarum longi in the mid-thoracic part.)
Rr. posteriores of the N. cervicalis [C8] and the Nn. thoracici [T1–T10]

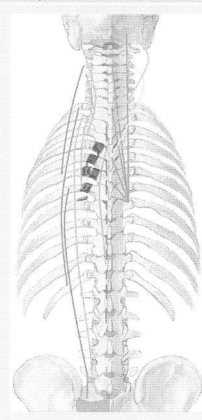

O: Proc. transversus of the 11. thoracic –7. cervical vertebra

I: 12.–1. rib laterally to the Angulus costae

F: Elevate the ribs,
lateral flexion and rotation of the vertebral column

20 Autochthonous muscles of the back (continuation)

b Autochthonous medial muscles of the back (Fig. 529, 532–535, 537, 601)

The medial tract of the autochthonous muscles is located below the lateral tract in the neck and lumbar region and is therefore also referred to as deep part of the autochthonous muscles of the back. The following muscles with longitudinal fibres belong to this tract: The Mm. interspinales and the M. spinalis. The Mm. rotatores, the Mm. multifidi and the M. semispinalis traverse obliquely converging mediocranially (transversospinal).

Mm. interspinales lumborum
Rr. posteriores of the Nn. spinales

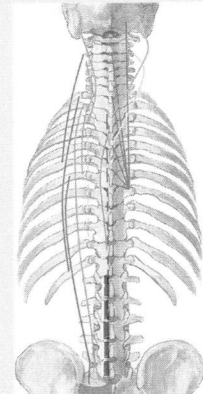

O: Proc. spinosus of the 5.–1. lumbar vertebra

I: Upper margin of the Crista sacralis mediana,
Proc. spinosus of the 5.–2. lumbar vertebra

F: Segmental extension

Mm. interspinales thoracis
Rr. posteriores of the Nn. spinales

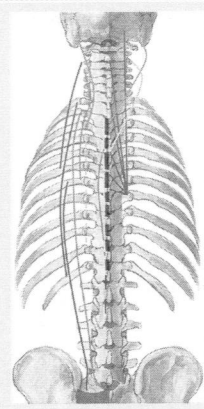

O: Proc. spinosus of the (12.) 11.–2. (1.) thoracic vertebra

I: Proc. spinosus of the (1. lumbar) 12.–3. (2.) thoracic vertebra

F: Segmental extension

Mm. interspinales cervicis
Rr. posteriores of the Nn. spinales

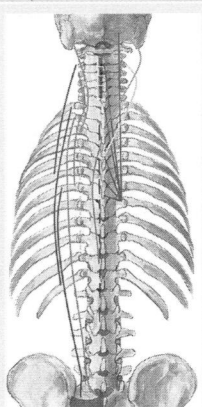

O: Proc. spinosus of the 7.–2. cervical vertebra

I: Proc. spinosus of the 1. thoracic–3. cervical vertebra

F: Segmental extension

20 Autochthonous muscles of the back (continuation)

M. spinalis thoracis [The muscle is tightly attached to the M. longissimus thoracis at its origin, and to the Mm. multifidi at its insertion.]
Rr. posteriores of the Nn. spinales

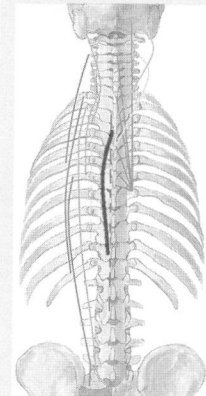

O: Proc. spinosus of the (3.) 2., 1. lumbar and the 12.–10. thoracic vertebra

I: Proc. spinosus of the (10.) 9.–2. thoracic vertebra

F: Unilateral innervation: lateral flexion, bilateral innervation: extension

M. spinalis cervicis
Rr. posteriores of the Nn. spinales

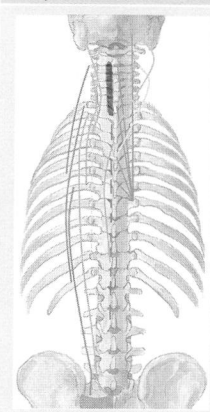

O: Proc. spinosus of the (4.) 3.–1. thoracic and the 7.–6. cervical vertebra

I: Proc. spinosus of the (6.) 5.–2. cervical vertebra

F: Unilateral innervation: lateral flexion, bilateral innervation: extension

M. spinalis capitis [inconstant muscle, tightly attached to the M. semispinalis capitis at its insertion]
Rr. posteriores of the Nn. spinales

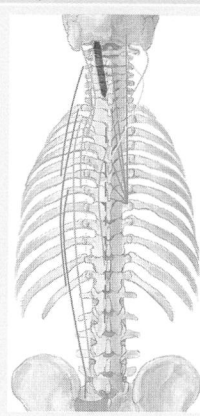

O: Proc. spinosus of the 3.–1. thoracic and the 7.–6. cervical vertebra

I: Squama ossis occipitalis between the Linea nuchalis suprema and the Linea nuchalis superior adjacent to the Protuberantia occipitalis externa

F: Unilateral innervation: lateral flexion, bilateral innervation: extension

20 Autochthonous muscles of the back (continuation)

Mm. rotatores [They are subdivided into Mm. rotatores cervicis, Mm. rotatores thoracis and the inconstant Mm. rotatores lumborum. The Mm. rotatores breves traverse to the adjacent upper vertebra, whereas the Mm. rotatores longi extend to the second next vertebra.]
Rr. posteriores of the Nn. spinales

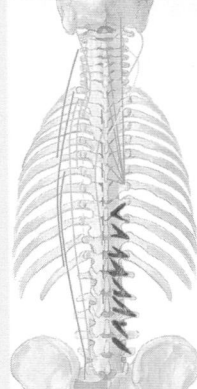

O: Procc. mamillares of the lumbar vertebrae,
Procc. transversi of the thoracic vertebrae,
Procc. articulares inferiores of the cervical vertebrae

I: Root of the Proc. spinosus of the 3.–1. lumbar, 12.–1. thoracic and 7.–2. cervical vertebra

F: Unilateral innervation: segmental lateral flexion, rotation,
bilateral innervation: segmental extension

Mm. multifidi [They are particularly well developed in the lumbar part of the vertebral column and skip two to four vertebrae.]
Rr. posteriores of the Nn. spinales

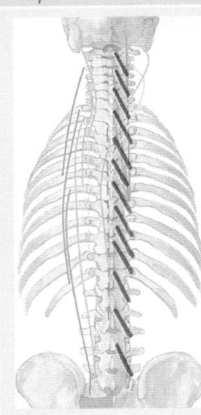

O: Facies dorsalis of the Os sacrum,
Lig. sacroiliacum posterius, dorsal part of the Crista iliaca,
Procc. mamillares of the lumbar vertebrae,
Procc. transversi of the thoracic vertebrae,
Proc. articularis inferior of the 7.–4. cervical vertebra

I: Proc. spinosus of the 5.–1. lumbar vertebra, 12.–1. thoracic and 7.–2. cervical vertebra

F: Unilateral innervation: segmental lateral flexion, rotation,
bilateral innervation: segmental extension

M. semispinalis thoracis [Its fibres skip five to seven vertebrae.]
Rr. posteriores of the Nn. spinales

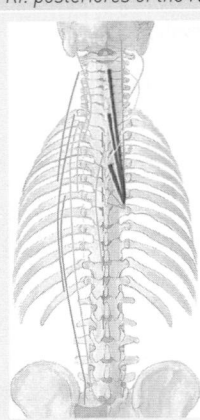

O: Proc. transversus of the (12.) 11.–7. (6.) thoracic vertebra

I: Proc. spinosus of the (4.) 3. thoracic –6. cervical vertebra

F: Unilateral innervation: rotates the vertebral column and the head contralaterally,
bilateral innervation: extension

20 Autochthonous muscles of the back (continuation)

M. semispinalis cervicis
Rr. posteriores of the Nn. spinales

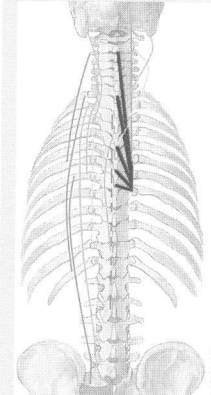

O: Proc. transversus of the (7.) 6. thoracic –7. cervical vertebra

I: Proc. spinosus of the 6.–3. cervical vertebra

F: Unilateral innervation: rotates the vertebral column and the head contralaterally, lateral flexion
bilateral innervation: extension

M. semispinalis capitis
Rr. posteriores of the Nn. spinales

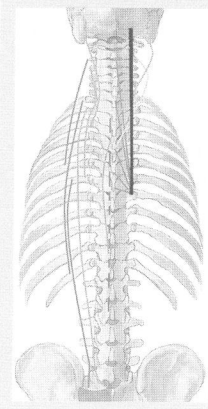

O: Proc. transversus of the (8.) 7. thoracic –3. cervical vertebra

I: Squama ossis occipitalis between Linea nuchalis suprema and Linea nuchalis superior, medial area

F: Unilateral innervation: rotates the vertebral column and the head contralaterally, lateral flexion
bilateral innervation: extension

c Autochthonous deep muscles of the neck (Fig. 532, 533, 535, 536, 538)

The Mm. recti capitis posterior minor et major and the Mm. obliqui capitis superior et inferior belong to the medial tract of the autochthonous muscles of the back, whereas the M. rectus capitis lateralis belongs to the lateral tract.

M. rectus capitis posterior major
N. suboccipitalis (dorsal branch of the N. cervicalis [C1])

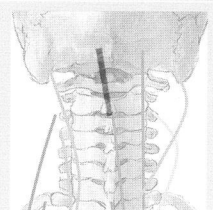

O: Proc spinosus of the Axis

I: Middle third of the Linea nuchalis inferior

F: Unilateral innervation: rotates and flexes the head ipsilaterally,
bilateral innervation: participates in the fine tuning of the position and the movement in the craniocervical joints, extension

M. rectus capitis posterior minor
N. suboccipitalis (dorsal branch of the N. cervicalis [C1])

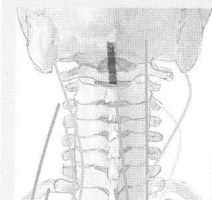

O: Tuberculum posterius of the Arcus posterior of the Atlas

I: Medial third of the Linea nuchalis inferior

F: Unilateral innervation: flexes the head ipsilaterally,
bilateral innervation: participates in the fine tuning of the position and the movement in the craniocervical joints, extension

20 Autochthonous muscles of the back (continuation)

M. obliquus capitis superior
N. suboccipitalis (dorsal branch of the N. cervicalis [C1])

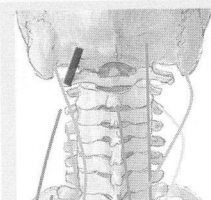

O: Tuberculum posterius of the Proc. transversus of the Atlas

I: Lateral third of the Linea nuchalis inferior

F: Unilateral innervation: flexes the head ipsilaterally,
bilateral innervation: participates in the fine tuning of the position and the movement in the craniocervical joints, extension

M. obliquus capitis inferior
N. suboccipitalis (dorsal branch of the N. cervicalis [C1])

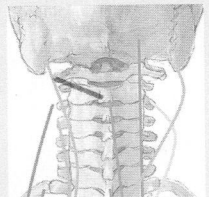

O: Proc. spinosus of the Axis

I: Posterior margin of the Proc. transversus of the Atlas

F: Unilateral innervation: rotates the Atlas (and the head) ipsilaterally,
bilateral innervation: participates in the fine tuning of the position and the movement in the craniocervical joints, extension

M. rectus capitis lateralis
Ventral branches of the N. cervicalis [C1]

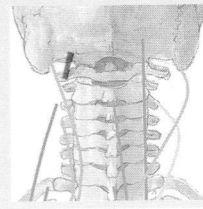

O: Anterior margin of the Proc. transversus of the Atlas

I: Proc. jugularis of the Os occipitale

F: Unilateral innervation: flexes the head ipsilaterally,
bilateral innervation: participates in the fine tuning of the position and the movement in the craniocervical joints

21 Diaphragm (Fig. 578, 583–585)

The diaphragm divides the thoracic and the abdominal cavity. Its "domes" form the floor of the right and left pleural cavity. The Pars lumbalis delineates the retroperitoneal space dorsally and constitutes a part of the dorsal abdominal wall.

Diaphragma
N. phrenicus (Plexus cervicalis)

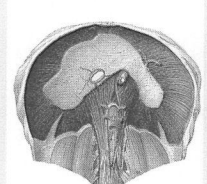

O: Pars sternalis: inner surface of the Proc. xiphoideus, rectus sheath
Pars costalis: inner surface of the Cartilago costalis of the 12.–6. rib, serrated with indentations of the M. transversus abdominis
Pars lumbalis, Crus dextrum,
– Pars medialis: Corpus of the 3.–1. lumbar vertebra, Disci intervertebrales
– Pars lateralis: Ligg. arcuata mediale (psoas arcade) and laterale (quadratus arcade)
Pars lumbalis, Crus sinistrum,
– Pars medialis: Corpus of the 4.–1. lumbar vertebra, Disci intervertebrales
– Pars lateralis: Ligg. arcuata mediale (psoas arcade) and laterale (quadratus arcade)

I: All parts merge in the Centrum tendineum.

F: Diaphragmatic breathing (Inspiration), compresses the abdomen

Passages and weak points in the diaphragm

Name	Location	Structures
Hiatus aorticus	Pars lumbalis, between Crus dextrum/sinistrum and vertebral column	Aorta; Ductus thoracicus
Hiatus oesophageus	Pars lumbalis, Crus sinistrum near the midline	Oesophagus; Nn. vagi; R. phrenicoabdominalis sinister
Foramen venae cavae	Centrum tendineum	V. cava inferior; N. phrenicus dexter, R. phrenicoabdominalis dexter
Trigonum sternocostale [LARREY's cleft]	Between Pars costalis and Pars lumbalis	A.; V. epigastrica superior
Trigonum lumbocostale	Between Pars sternalis and Pars costalis	
Unnamed	Pars lumbalis, Crus dextrum/sinistrum, (Pars medialis)	N. splanchnicus major and minor; V. azygos; V. hemiazygos
Unnamed	Pars lumbalis, between (Pars medialis) and Pars lateralis	Truncus sympathicus
Unnamed	Centrum tendineum	N. phrenicus sinister, R. phrenicoabdominalis sinister

22 Pelvic and urogenital diaphragm (Fig. 901–908, 1065)

Two partially overlapping muscle layers form the floor of the pelvic cavity. The M. levator ani, the M. ischiococcygeus and the M. sphincter ani externus, form the Diaphragma pelvis.
The Diaphragma urogenitale stretches as a triangular plate between both lower rami of the pubic bone. Its fibres are transversally orientated and support the urogenital hiatus. Among others the M. transversus perinei profundus, the M. sphincter urethrae (together they are referred to as M. compressor urethrae) and the M. transversus perinei superficialis belong to the Diaphragma urogenitale.
In the male, the Diaphragma urogenitale is only passed by the urethra, whereas in the female, both the vagina and the urethra pass through.

a Pelvic diaphragm

M. levator ani (It consists of the M. pubococcygeus and the M. iliococcygeus. The fibres of the Mm. levator prostatae, pubovaginalis and puborectalis originate from the M. pubococcygeus.)
Branches of the N. sacralis [S3 and S4]

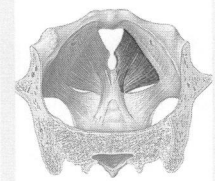

| O: **M. pubococcygeus:** inner surface of the Os pubis near the symphysis, anterior two thirds of the Arcus tendineus musculi levatoris ani, Spina ischiadica
M. iliococcygeus: posterior third of the Arcus tendineus musculi levatoris ani | I: Centrum perinei (prerectal fibres), in the male the fascia of the Prostata (M. levator prostatae), in the female the wall of the Vagina (M. pubovaginalis), radiates into the M. sphincter ani externus, forms a loop with the contralateral fibres just behind the Anus (M. puborectalis), Corpus anococcygeum, Os coccygis | F: Spans around the rectum from posterior, supports the M. sphincter ani externus to close the rectum, the medial free margin forms the urogenital hiatus, which allows the urethra in the male and both the urethra and the vagina in the female to pass through |

M. ischiococcygeus
Branches of the N. sacralis [S4 and S5]

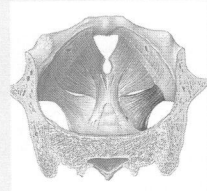

| O: Inner surface of the Spina ischiadica, predominantly attached to the Lig. sacrospinale | I: Lateral margin of the lower segments of the Os sacrum, Os coccygis | F: Supports the pelvic diaphragm |

M. sphincter ani externus (muscular loop with a ring-like shape up to the M. levator ani)
N. pudendus (Plexus sacralis)

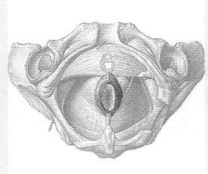

| O: **Pars subcutanea:** Dermis and subcutaneous tissues surrounding the Anus
Pars superficialis: Centrum perinei
Pars profunda: ring-like muscle | I: Dermis and subcutaneous tissues surrounding the Anus, Lig. anococcygeum | F: Closure of the anus |

22 Pelvic and urogenital diaphragm (continuation)

b Urogenital diaphragm

M. transversus perinei profundus (It is a triangular supportive muscular layer interwoven with connective tissue with openings for the urethra in the male and for both the urethra and the vagina in the female. It spans obliquely over the Arcus pubis and Angulus subpubicus, respectively, and is supplemented by the Lig. pubicum inferius and the Lig. transversum perinei profundum.)
N. pudendus (Plexus sacralis)

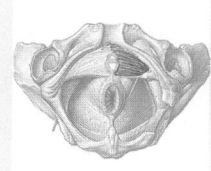

O: Ramus inferior ossis pubis, Ramus ossis ischii, connective tissue envelop of the Vasa pudenda interna

I: Centrum perinei, fasciae of the prostate and the vaginal wall

F: Supports the urogenital hiatus, seals the urethra (and the urinary bladder)

M. sphincter urethrae (muscular traction enveloping the Pars membranacea urethrae in a ring-like fashion)
N. pudendus (Plexus sacralis)

see Fig. 906, 907

O: Ring-like muscle, Lig. transversum perinei, fibres from the M. transversus perinei profundus

I: Connective tissue surrounding the Urethra (Pars membranacea), contralateral M. transversus perinei profundus, vaginal wall (M. sphincter urethrovaginalis)

F: Supports the urogenital hiatus, part of the continence organ of the Vesica urinaria, seals the urinary bladder during ejaculation

---

M. transversus perinei superficialis (inconstant muscle)
N. pudendus (Plexus sacralis)

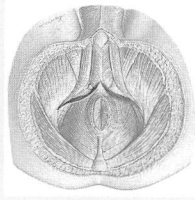

O: Superficial dicision of the M. transversus perinei profundus, Tuber ischiadicum

I: Centrum perinei

F: Supports the M. transversus perinei profundus

M. ischiocavernosus
N. pudendus (Plexus sacralis)

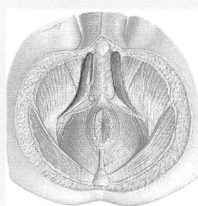

O: Ramus ossis ischii

I: Tunica albuginea corporum cavernosorum

F: Fixes the crura of penis in the male, and the crura of clitoris in the female to the inferior pubic ramus, as well as to the ramus of the ischium and the urogenital diaphragm, supports the ejaculation and the orgasm, respectively

---

M. bulbospongiosus (spans around the Bulbus penis in the male, and around the Bulbus vestibuli in the female)
N. pudendus (Plexus sacralis)

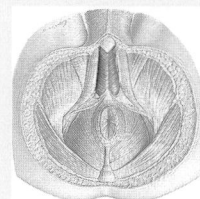

O: Centrum perinei, in the male additional origin from the Raphe penis at the lower surface of the Corpus spongiosum penis

I: In the male, it inserts laterally to the Corpus spongiosum penis into the Fascia urogenitalis inferior and the back of the Penis; in the female, the fibres are attached to the Corpus cavernosum clitoridis and the Fascia diaphragmatis urogenitalis inferior

F: In the male, it fixes the bulb of penis to the urogenital diaphragm, and is involved in the ejaculation; in the female, it fixes the bulb of vestibule to the urogenital diaphragm and supports the orgasm

23 Joints of the upper limb, Articulationes membri superioris (Fig. 276)

a Joints of the shoulder girdle, Articulationes cinguli pectoralis

Name of the joint	Type of the joint	Movements
Sternoclavicular joint, Articulatio sternoclavicularis	Irregular joint surface, Articulatio irregularis functionally: spheroideal joint (distinct feature: Discus articularis)	Rotation along a sagittal axis (as in raising the shoulder), rotation along a longitudinal axis (as in protraction and retraction of the shoulder), rotation along the longitudinal axis of the clavicle (as in swinging the arm)
Acromioclavicular joint, Articulatio acromioclavicularis	Plane joint, Articulatio plana functionally: spheroideal joint (distinct feature: variable, frequently incomplete Discus articularis	Rotation along a sagittal axis (as in raising the shoulder), rotation along a transverse axis (as in swinging the arm), rotation along a longitudinal axis (as in protraction and retraction of the shoulder)

b Joints of the free part of the upper limb, Articulationes membri superioris liberi

Name of the joint	Type of the joint	Movements
Shoulder joint, Articulatio humeri	Spheroideal joint, Articulatio spheroidea	Protraction (flexion, anteversion) Retraction (extension, retroversion) Abduction Adduction Medial rotation Lateral rotation (Circumduction: combining flexion, abduction, extension, adduction)
Elbow joint, Articulatio cubiti a) Articulatio humeroulnaris	Hinge joint, Ginglymus	Flexion Extension
b) Articulatio humeroradialis	Spheroideal joint, Articulatio spheroidea (with functional restriction: no abduction)	Flexion Extension Rotation
c) Articulatio radioulnaris proximalis	Pivot joint, Articulatio trochoidea	} Pronation and supination of the hand
Distal radioulnar joint, Articulatio radioulnaris distalis	Pivot joint, Articulatio trochoidea	
Wrist joints a) Articulatio radiocarpalis	Ellipsoid joint, Articulatio ellipsoidea	} Lateral movements of the hand (ulnar and radial abduction) Palmar flexion Dorsal flexion
b) Articulatio mediocarpalis	Hinge joint, Ginglymus	
Carpometacarpal joint of the thumb, Articulatio carpometacarpalis pollicis	Sellar joint, Articulatio sellaris	Abduction Adduction Opposition Reposition
Carpometacarpal joints (II–V), Articulationes carpometacarpales (II–V)	Plane joints, Articulationes planae	Various distinct movements
Metacarpophalangeal joints, Articulationes metacarpophalangeae	Spheroideal joints, Articulationes spheroideae (with functional restrictions)	Flexion Extension Abduction* Adduction* (*with regard to the middle finger)
Interphalangeael joints of the fingers, Articulationes interphalangeae manus	Hinge joints, Ginglymi	Flexion Extension

23 Joints of the upper limb, Articulationes membri superioris (continuation)

c Planes and axes of the movements of the joints of the upper limb

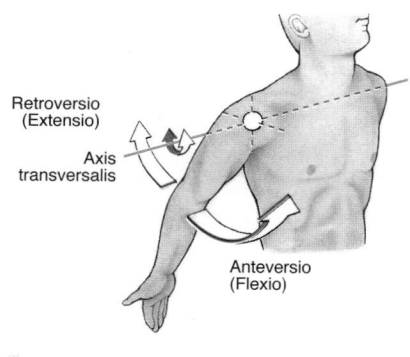

Fig. 1 Shoulder joint; movements in the sagittal plane.

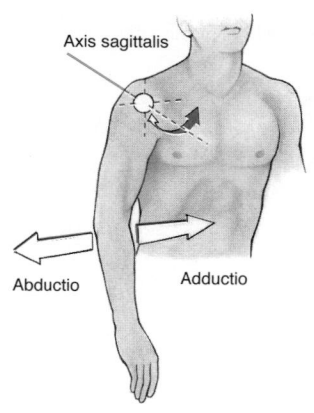

Fig. 2 Shoulder joint; movements in the frontal plane.

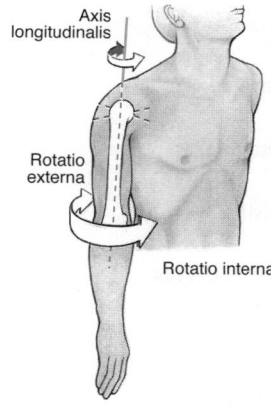

Fig. 3 Shoulder joint; movements in the transverse plane.

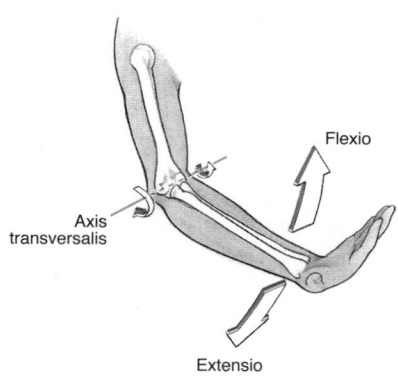

Fig. 4 Elbow joint; movements in the sagittal plane.

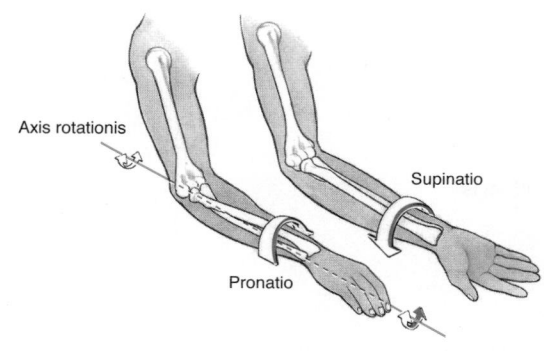

Fig. 5 Elbow joint; pronation and supination of the hand.

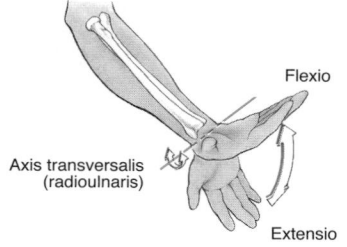

Fig. 6 Wrist joints; movements in the sagittal plane.

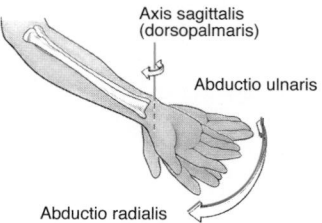

Fig. 7 Wrist joints; movements in the frontal plane.

With regard to the wrist joints, palmar flexion is also referred to as flexion and dorsal flexion as extension.

24 Branches and supplying areas of the brachial plexus (Fig. 386–395, 397, 398, 400, 401, 403, 404)

	Motor function	Sensory function
Plexus brachialis (C5) C4–T1 (T2)		
N. dorsalis scapulae (C3) C4, C5	M. levator scapulae, Mm. rhomboidei	
N. suprascapularis C4–C6	M. supraspinatus, M. infraspinatus	
Nn. subscapulares C5–C7	M. subscapularis, (M. teres major)	
N. subclavius (C4) C5, C6	M. subclavius	
N. thoracicus longus C5–C7 (C8)	M. serratus anterior	
Nn. pectorales C8–T1	M. pectoralis major, M. pectoralis minor	
N. thoracodorsalis C6–C8	M. latissimus dorsi, M. teres major	
Rr. musculares	M. longus colli, M. longus capitis	
N. musculocutaneus C5–C7	M. coracobrachialis, M. biceps brachii, M. brachialis	Skin of the radiopalmar side of the forearm
N. medianus C6–T1	M. pronator teres, M. flexor carpi radialis, M. palmaris longus, M. flexor digitorum superficialis, M. flexor pollicis longus, M. flexor digitorum profundus (radial portion), M. pronator quadratus, M. flexor pollicis brevis (Caput superficiale), M. opponens pollicis, Mm. lumbricales I, II	Skin of the radial part of the palm (3½ fingers), skin of the dorsal side of the distal phalanx (3½ fingers)
N. ulnaris C6–T1	M. flexor carpi ulnaris, M. flexor digitorum profundus (ulnar portion), M. palmaris brevis, M. flexor digiti minimi, M. opponens digiti minimi, M. abductor digiti minimi, M. flexor pollicis brevis (Caput profundum), M. adductor pollicis, Mm. lumbricales III, IV, Mm. interossei	Skin of the ulnar side of the hand (palmar: 1½ fingers, dorsal 2½ fingers), skin of the dorsal side of the distal phalanx (1½ fingers)
N. cutaneus brachii medialis C8–T1 (T2)		Skin of the mediopalmar side of the arm
N. cutaneus antebrachii medialis C8–T1		Skin of the ulnopalmar side of the forearm
N. axillaris C5–C7	M. deltoideus, M. teres minor	Skin of the shoulder
N. radialis C5–T1	M. triceps brachii, M. anconeus, M. brachioradialis, M. extensor carpi radialis longus, M. extensor carpi radialis brevis, M. supinator, M. extensor digitorum, M. extensor pollicis longus, M. abductor pollicis longus, M. extensor pollicis brevis, M. extensor indicis, M. extensor carpi ulnaris	Skin of the dorsal side of the arm, forearm and hand (2½ radial fingers with the exception of the distal phalanges)

25 Segmental innervation of the muscles of the upper limb, muscles of diagnostic importance

(According to MUMENTHALER and SCHLIACK; the indicator muscle of each segment is printed in bold.)

M. supraspinatus	C4–C5	M. abductor pollicis longus	C6–C8
M. teres minor	C4–C5	M. extensor pollicis brevis	C7–T1
M. deltoideus: C5	C5–C6	M. extensor pollicis longus	C6–C8
M. infraspinatus	C4–C6	M. extensor digitorum	C6–C8
M. subscapularis	C5–C6	M. extensor indicis	C6–C8
M. teres major	C5–C7	M. extensor carpi ulnaris	C6–C8
M. biceps brachii: C6	C5–C6	M. extensor digiti minimi	C6–C8
M. brachialis	C5–C6	M. flexor digitorum superficialis	C7–T1
M. coracobrachialis	C5–C7	M. flexor digitorum profundus	C7–T1
M. triceps brachii: C7	C6–C8	M. flexor carpi ulnaris	C7–T1
M. brachioradialis	C5–C6	M. abductor pollicis brevis	C7–T1
M. extensor carpi radialis longus	C5–C7	M. flexor pollicis brevis	C7–T1
M. extensor carpi radialis brevis	C5–C7	M. opponens pollicis	C6–C7
M. supinator	C5–C6	M. flexor digiti minimi	C7–T1
M. pronator teres	C6–C7	M. adductor pollicis	C8–T1
M. flexor carpi radialis	C6–C7	**M. abductor digiti minimi: C8**	C8–T1
M. flexor pollicis longus	C6–C8	**Mm. interossei: C8**	C8–T1

26 Ventral muscles of the shoulder (Fig. 338, 340, 341, 343, 344, 569–571)

The M. pectoralis major spans from the trunk to the upper limb and moulds the surface anatomy of the anterior upper thoracic wall. Below, the M. pectoralis minor can be found, which together with the M. subclavius belongs to the muscles spanning from the trunk to the shoulder girdle. Only the M. subscapularis is located in direct contact to the shoulder joint, spanning from the anterior surface of the scapula to the humerus.

M. pectoralis major (Its fibres converge laterally into a broad, flat tendon shaped like a bag with its opening to the top.)
Nn. pectorales medialis et lateralis (Plexus brachialis, Pars infra-/supraclavicularis)

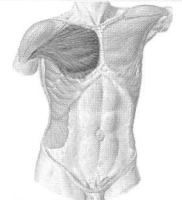

O: **Pars clavicularis:** sternal half of the Clavicula
Pars sternocostalis: Manubrium and Corpus sterni, Cartilago costalis of the 1.–7. rib
Pars abdominalis: anterior layer of the rectus sheath

I: Crista tuberculi majoris of the Humerus

F: Shoulder joint:
adduction, particularly effective when the arm is elevated,
medial rotation,
Pars clavicularis: anteversion
Shoulder girdle:
depression,
anteversion
Thorax:
elevates the sternum and the upper ribs when the shoulders are fixed (supports inspiration)

M. pectoralis minor
Nn. pectorales medialis et lateralis (Plexus brachialis, Pars infra-/supraclavicularis)

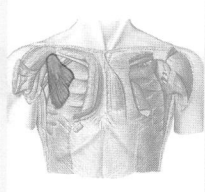

O: (2.) 3.–5. rib close to the junction between cartilage and bone

I: Tip of the Proc. coracoideus

F: Shoulder girdle:
depression
Thorax:
elevates the sternum and the upper ribs (supports inspiration)

M. subclavius (The fascia of the M. subclavius is attached to the Adventitia of the V. subclavia, thus preventing collapse of its lumen.)
N. subclavius (Plexus brachialis, Pars supraclavicularis)

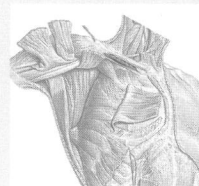

O: Junction between cartilage and bone of the 1. rib

I: Lateral third of the Clavicula

F: Shoulder girdle:
depression (with low effectiveness),
antagonizes laterally-directed traction on the clavicle

26 Ventral muscles of the shoulder (continuation)

M. subscapularis (The Bursa subtendinea musculi subscapularis lies below the muscle close to its insertion.)
Nn. subscapulares (Plexus brachialis, Pars infraclavicularis)

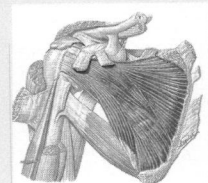

| O: Fossa subscapularis | I: Tuberculum minus and adjacent part of the Crista tuberculi minoris | F: Shoulder joint: medial rotation, abduction in the scapular plane (cranial portion), adduction in the scapular plane (caudal portion) |

27 Lateral muscles of the shoulder (Fig. 337, 340–345)

The M. deltoideus plays a major role in determining the surface contour of the shoulder. Divided by the Bursa subdeltoidea, the tendon of the M. supraspinatus is located directly below the M. deltoideus.

M. deltoideus
N. axillaris (Plexus brachialis, Pars infraclavicularis)

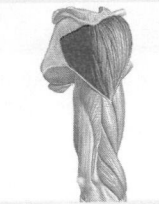

| O: **Pars clavicularis:** acromial third of the Clavicula **Pars acromialis:** Acromion **Pars spinalis:** lower margin of the Spina scapulae | I: Tuberositas deltoidea | F: Shoulder joint: **Pars clavicularis:** adduction (from about 60° increasing abduction), medial rotation, anteversion **Pars acromialis:** abduction up to the horizontal plane **Pars spinalis:** adduction (from about 60° increasing abduction), lateral rotation, retroversion **All parts:** carry the weight of the arm |

M. supraspinatus
N. suprascapularis (Plexus brachialis, Pars supraclavicularis)

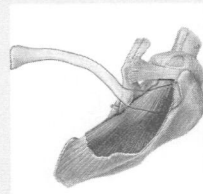

| O: Fossa supraspinata, Fascia supraspinata | I: Proximal facet of the Tuberculum majus | F: Shoulder joint: abduction in the scapular plane up to the horizontal plane, lateral rotation |

28 Dorsal muscles of the shoulder (Fig. 339–341, 343, 344)

The M. infraspinatus is located most cranially. More caudally are the M. teres minor and the M. teres major.
The M. latissimus dorsi comes from the back (see Tab. 18, trunk-arm muscles) and runs along with the M. teres major.

M. infraspinatus
N. suprascapularis (Plexus brachialis, Pars supraclavicularis)

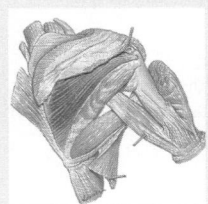

| O: Caudal margin of the Spina scapulae, Fossa infraspinata, Fascia infraspinata | I: Middle facet of the Tuberculum majus | F: Shoulder joint: cranial portion: lateral rotation, abduction in the scapular plane caudal portion: lateral rotation, adduction in the scapular plane |

28 Dorsal muscles of the shoulder (continuation)

M. teres minor
N. axillaris (Plexus brachialis, Pars infraclavicularis)

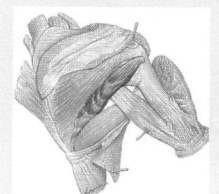

O: Caudal portion of the Fossa infraspinata, medial third of the Margo lateralis

I: Distal posterior facet of the Tuberculum majus

F: Shoulder joint: lateral rotation, adduction in the scapular plane

M. teres major (At the insertion, the M. teres major and the M. latissimus dorsi are separated by the Bursa subtendinea musculi latissimi dorsi.)
Nn. subscapulares or N. thoracodorsalis (Plexus brachialis, Pars infraclavicularis)

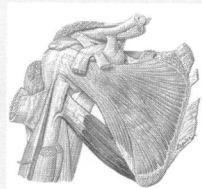

O: Margo lateralis, Angulus inferior

I: Crista tuberculi minoris medially to the M. latissimus dorsi

F: Shoulder joint: medial rotation, adduction in the scapular plane

29 Ventral muscles of the arm (Fig. 343, 344, 347–350)

The M. biceps brachii determines the surface anatomy of the ventral arm. The M. coracobrachialis is directly attached to the Caput breve of the M. biceps brachii. The M. brachialis is located most deeply.

M. biceps brachii (The tendon of the Caput longum traverses directly the shoulder joint. The Bursa bicipitoradialis is located at its insertion at the Tuberositas radii.)
N. musculocutaneus (Plexus brachialis, Pars infraclavicularis)

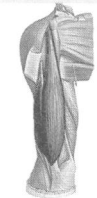

O: Caput longum: Tuberculum supraglenoidale, Labrum glenoidale
Caput breve: Tip of the Proc. coracoideus lateral to the M. coracobrachialis

I: Tuberositas radii, via the Aponeurosis musculi bicipitis brachii at the Fascia antebrachii

F: Shoulder joint:
Caput longum: abduction, anteversion, medial rotation
Caput breve: adduction, anteversion, medial rotation
Both parts: carry the weight of the arm
Elbow joint: flexion, supination

M. coracobrachialis (Normally this muscle is penetrated by the N. musculocutaneus.)
N. musculocutaneus (Plexus brachialis, Pars infraclavicularis)

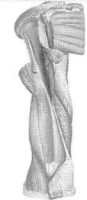

O: Tip of the Proc. coracoideus medial to the Caput breve of the M. biceps brachii

I: Facies anterior of the Humerus mediodistal to the Crista tuberculi minoris

F: Shoulder joint: medial rotation, adduction, anteversion

M. brachialis
N. musculocutaneus (Plexus brachialis, Pars infraclavicularis)

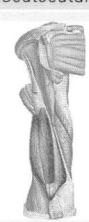

O: Facies anterior of the Humerus distal to the Tuberositas deltoidea

I: Tuberositas ulnae

F: Elbow joint: flexion

30 Dorsal muscles of the arm (Fig. 342–344, 346, 351)

The three heads of the M. triceps brachii determine the surface anatomy of the dorsal arm. The M. anconeus can be considered as a continuation of the Caput mediale of the M. triceps brachii to the forearm.

M. triceps brachii (The fibres of the Caput longum traverse in longitudinal direction, and those of the Caput mediale and Caput laterale in an oblique direction; a common broad aponeurosis is found at the insertion.)
N. radialis (Plexus brachialis, Pars infraclavicularis)

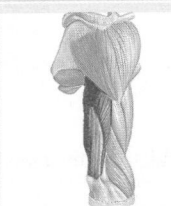

O: Caput longum: Tuberculum infraglenoidale, lower margin of the Labrum glenoidale
Caput mediale: Facies posterior of the Humerus mediodistal to the Sulcus nervi radialis, Septum intermusculare brachii mediale
Caput laterale: Facies posterior of the Humerus lateroproximal to the Sulcus nervi radialis, proximal two thirds of the Septum intermusculare brachii laterale

I: Olecranon

F: Shoulder joint:
Caput longum: adduction, support of the weight of the arm
Elbow joint:
extension

M. anconeus (It is closely positioned to the Caput mediale of the M. triceps brachii.)
N. radialis (Plexus brachialis, Pars infraclavicularis)

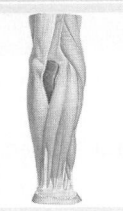

O: Epicondylus lateralis of the Humerus, capsule of the elbow joint, Lig. collaterale radiale

I: Facies posterior of the Ulna just distal to the Olecranon

F: Elbow joint:
extension

31 Superficial ventral muscles of the forearm (Fig. 352, 353, 355–359, 373)

The group of the superficial ventral muscles of the forearm consists of the following muscles in the order from radial to ulnar: M. pronator teres, M. flexor carpi radialis, M. palmaris longus, M. flexor digitorum superficialis and M. flexor carpi ulnaris.

M. pronator teres
N. medianus (Plexus brachialis, Pars infraclavicularis)

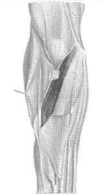

O: Caput humerale: Epicondylus medialis of the Humerus, Septum intermusculare brachii mediale
Caput ulnare: Facies medialis of the Ulna distal to the Proc. coronoideus

I: Middle third of the Facies lateralis of the Radius

F: <u>Elbow joint:</u>
Caput humerale: pronation, flexion
Caput ulnare: pronation

M. flexor carpi radialis
N. medianus (Plexus brachialis, Pars infraclavicularis)

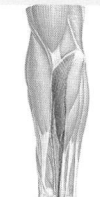

O: Epicondylus medialis of the Humerus, Fascia antebrachii

I: Palmar surface of the base of the Os metacarpi II (frequently also III)

F: <u>Elbow joint:</u>
flexion,
pronation
<u>Wrist joint:</u>
palmar flexion,
radial abduction

M. palmaris longus (inconstant muscle)
N. medianus (Plexus brachialis, Pars infraclavicularis)

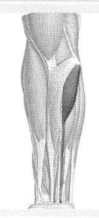

O: Epicondylus medialis of the Humerus, Fascia antebrachii

I: Aponeurosis palmaris

F: <u>Elbow joint:</u>
flexion
<u>Wrist joint:</u>
palmar flexion,
tension of the palmar aponeurosis

M. flexor digitorum superficialis (The tendons of this muscle are perforated by the tendons of the M. flexor digitorum profundus just before their insertion.)
N. medianus (Plexus brachialis, Pars infraclavicularis)

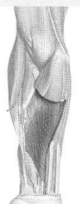

O: Caput humeroulnare:
Epicondylus medialis of the Humerus,
Proc. coronoideus
Caput radiale: Facies anterior of the Radius distal to the M. pronator teres

I: With four long tendons at the base of the Phalanx media of the 2.–5. finger

F: <u>Elbow joint:</u>
flexion
<u>Wrist joint:</u>
palmar flexion,
ulnar abduction
<u>Metacarpophalangeal joints (II–V):</u>
flexion,
adduction
<u>Proximal finger joints (II–V):</u>
flexion

M. flexor carpi ulnaris
N. ulnaris (Plexus brachialis, Pars infraclavicularis)

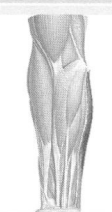

O: Caput humerale: Epicondylus medialis of the Humerus; Septum intermusculare brachii mediale
Caput ulnare: Olecranon, upper two thirds of the Margo posterior of the Ulna, Fascia antebrachii

I: Via the Os pisiforme and the Ligg. pisometacarpale and pisohamatum at the base of the Os metacarpi V and the Os hamatum

F: <u>Elbow joint:</u>
flexion
<u>Wrist joint:</u>
palmar flexion,
ulnar abduction

44

T 32

32 Deep ventral muscles of the forearm [Fig. 352, 354, 355, 359, 360, 370, 371, 374]

The M. flexor digitorum profundus is located medially with the M. flexor pollicis longus being located laterally. The M. pronator quadratus covers the distal quarter of the bones of the forearm.

M. flexor digitorum profundus
N. ulnaris for the ulnar portion, N. interosseus antebrachii anterior of the N. medianus for the radial portion (Plexus brachialis, Pars infraclavicularis)

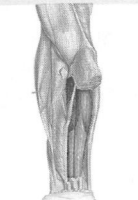

O: Proximal two thirds of the Facies anterior of the Ulna, Membrana interossea

I: Base of the Phalanx distalis of the 2.–5. finger

F: <u>Wrist joint:</u>
palmar flexion
<u>Metacarpophalangeal joints (II–V):</u>
flexion,
(adduction)
<u>Finger joints (II–V):</u>
flexion

M. flexor pollicis longus
N. interosseus antebrachii anterior of the N. medianus (Plexus brachialis, Pars infraclavicularis)

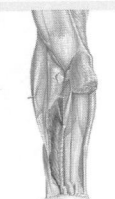

O: Facies anterior of the Radius distal to the Tuberositas radii

I: Base of the Phalanx distalis of the thumb

F: <u>Wrist joint:</u>
palmar flexion
<u>Carpometacarpal joint of the thumb:</u>
adduction,
opposition
<u>Thumb joints:</u>
flexion

M. pronator quadratus
N. interosseus antebrachii anterior (N. medianus, Plexus brachialis, Pars infraclavicularis)

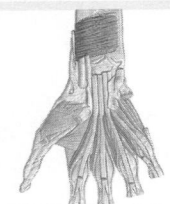

O: Distal quarter of the Margo anterior of the Ulna

I: Margo and Facies anterior of the Radius

F: <u>Radioulnar joints:</u>
pronation

33 Lateral (radial) muscles of the forearm (Fig. 352, 362, 366, 370, 371)

The group of the radial muscles of the forearm consists of the following muscles in the order from lateral to medial: M. brachioradialis, M. extensor carpi radialis longus and M. extensor carpi radialis brevis.

M. brachioradialis
N. radialis (Plexus brachialis, Pars infraclavicularis)

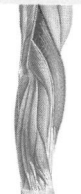

O: Margo lateralis of the Humerus, Septum intermusculare brachii laterale

I: Proc. styloideus of the Radius

F: <u>Elbow joint:</u>
flexion (particularly strong when forearm is in semipronated position), pronation or supination (from the corresponding extreme position to an intermediate one)

M. extensor carpi radialis longus
N. radialis (Plexus brachialis, Pars infraclavicularis)

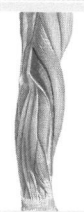

O: Distal end of the Margo lateralis of the Humerus, Epicondylus lateralis of the Humerus, Septum intermusculare brachii laterale

I: Dorsal surface of the base of the Os metacarpi II

F: <u>Elbow joint:</u>
flexion,
pronation or supination (from the corresponding extreme position to an intermediate one)
<u>Wrist joint:</u>
dorsal flexion,
radial abduction

M. extensor carpi radialis brevis
N. radialis (Plexus brachialis, Pars infraclavicularis)

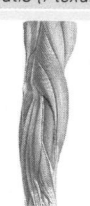

O: Epicondylus lateralis of the Humerus, Lig. anulare radii

I: Dorsal surface of the base of the Os metacarpi III

F: <u>Elbow joint:</u>
flexion,
pronation or supination (from the corresponding extreme position to an intermediate one)
<u>Wrist joint:</u>
dorsal flexion,
radial abduction

34 Superficial dorsal muscles of the forearm (Fig. 361, 363, 367, 368, 379)

The group of the superficial dorsal muscles of the forearm consists of the following muscles in the order from radial to ulnar: M. extensor digitorum, M. extensor digiti minimi and M. extensor carpi ulnaris.

M. extensor digitorum
R. profundus of the N. radialis (Plexus brachialis, Pars infraclavicularis)

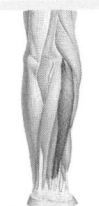

O: Epicondylus lateralis of the Humerus,
Ligg. collaterale radiale and anulare radii,
Fascia antebrachii

I: So-called dorsal aponeuroses of the 2.–5. finger

F: <u>Elbow joint:</u> extension
<u>Wrist joint:</u> dorsal flexion
<u>Metacarpophalangeal (II–V)/ finger joints (II–V):</u> extension

M. extensor digiti minimi
R. profundus of the N. radialis (Plexus brachialis, Pars infraclavicularis)

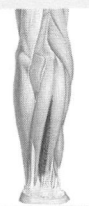

O: Epicondylus lateralis of the Humerus,
Ligg. collaterale radiale and anulare radii,
Fascia antebrachii

I: So-called dorsal aponeurosis of the 5. finger

F: <u>Elbow joint:</u> extension
<u>Wrist joint:</u> dorsal flexion, ulnar abduction
<u>Metacarpophalangeal (V)/ finger joints (V):</u> extension

M. extensor carpi ulnaris (This muscle is frequently separated from the M. extensor digitorum and the M. extensor digiti minimi by a distinct Septum intermusculare.)
R. profundus of the N. radialis (Plexus brachialis, Pars infraclavicularis)

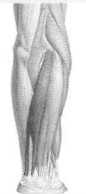

O: Caput humerale: Epicondylus lateralis of the Humerus,
Lig. collaterale radiale
Caput ulnare: proximal two thirds of the Facies posterior of the Ulna,
Fascia antebrachii

I: Dorsal surface of the base of the Os metacarpi V

F: <u>Elbow joint:</u> extension
<u>Wrist joint:</u> dorsal flexion, ulnar abduction

35 Deep dorsal muscles of the forearm (Fig. 356, 361, 364, 365, 368–371, 379)

The M. supinator enwraps the upper third of the radius laterally. Distally, the M. extensor pollicis longus, the M. extensor indicis, the M. abductor pollicis longus and the M. extensor pollicis brevis follow from lateral to medial.

M. supinator (This muscle is perforated by the R. profundus of the N. radialis in a longitudinal direction. A small tendinous arch frames the opening of the supinator canal.)
R. profundus of the N. radialis (Plexus brachialis, Pars infraclavicularis)

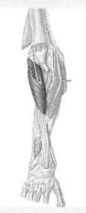

O: Epicondylus lateralis of the Humerus,
Crista musculi supinatoris of the Ulna,
Ligg. collaterale radiale and anulare radii

I: Facies anterior of the Radius between the Tuberositas radii and the insertion of the M. pronator teres

F: Radioulnar joints:
supination

M. extensor pollicis longus
R. profundus of the N. radialis (Plexus brachialis, Pars infraclavicularis)

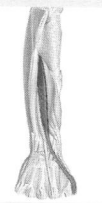

O: Distal quarter of the Facies posterior of the Ulna,
Membrana interossea

I: Phalanx distalis of the thumb

F: Wrist joint:
dorsal flexion,
radial abduction
Carpometacarpal joint of the thumb:
adduction,
reposition
Metacarpophalangeal joint of the thumb and thumb joint:
extension

M. extensor indicis
R. profundus of the N. radialis (Plexus brachialis, Pars infraclavicularis)

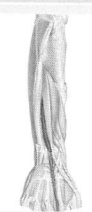

O: Distal quarter of the Facies posterior of the Ulna,
Membrana interossea

I: So-called dorsal aponeurosis of the index finger

F: Wrist joint:
dorsal flexion,
radial abduction
Metacarpophalangeal joint (II):
extension,
adduction
Finger joints (II):
extension

M. abductor pollicis longus
R. profundus of the N. radialis (Plexus brachialis, Pars infraclavicularis)

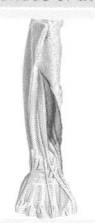

O: Facies posterior of the Ulna,
Membrana interossea,
Facies posterior of the Radius

I: Base of the Os metacarpi I

F: Radioulnar joints:
supination
Wrist joint:
dorsal flexion,
radial abduction
Carpometacarpal joint of the thumb:
extension,
reposition

M. extensor pollicis brevis
R. profundus of the N. radialis (Plexus brachialis, Pars infraclavicularis)

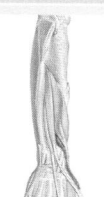

O: Facies posterior of the Radius,
Membrana interossea

I: Base of the Phalanx proximalis of the thumb

F: Wrist joint:
palmar flexion,
radial abduction
Carpometacarpal joint of the thumb:
abduction, reposition
Metacarpophalangeal joint of the thumb:
extension

36 Muscles of the thenar eminence (Fig. 372–374, 377, 378)

From superficial to deep the M. abductor pollicis brevis, the M. flexor pollicis brevis, the M. opponens pollicis and the M. adductor pollicis form the thenar eminence.

M. abductor pollicis brevis
N. medianus (Plexus brachialis, Pars infraclavicularis)

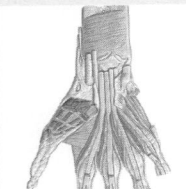

O: Retinaculum musculorum flexorum,
Tuberculum ossis scaphoidei

I: Radial sesamoid bone of the metacarpophalangeal joint of the thumb,
radial margin of the base of the Phalanx proximalis of the thumb, inserts into the dorsal aponeurosis of the thumb

F: Carpometacarpal joint of the thumb:
abduction,
opposition
Metacarpophalangeal joint of the thumb:
flexion

M. flexor pollicis brevis
Caput superficiale: *N. medianus*; Caput profundum: *R. profundus of the N. ulnaris (Plexus brachialis, Pars infraclavicularis)*

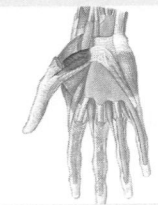

O: Caput superficiale: Retinaculum musculorum flexorum
Caput profundum: Ossa capitatum, trapezium, trapezoideum, base of the Os metacarpi I

I: Radial sesamoid bone of the metacarpophalangeal joint of the thumb,
radial margin of the base of the Phalanx proximalis of the thumb, inserts into the dorsal aponeurosis of the thumb

F: Carpometacarpal joint of the thumb:
opposition,
adduction
Metacarpophalangeal joint of the thumb:
flexion

M. opponens pollicis
N. medianus and N. ulnaris (Plexus brachialis, Pars infraclavicularis)

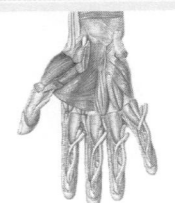

O: Retinaculum musculorum flexorum,
Tuberculum ossis trapezii

I: Entire radial margin of the Os metacarpi I

F: Carpometacarpal joint of the thumb:
opposition,
adduction

M. adductor pollicis
R. profundus of the N. ulnaris (Plexus brachialis, Pars infraclavicularis)

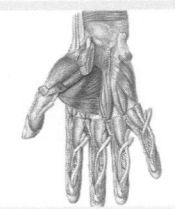

O: Caput obliquum: Os capitatum, base of the Os metacarpi II,
Lig. carpi radiatum
Caput transversum: palmar surface of the Os metacarpi III

I: Ulnar sesamoid bone of the metacarpophalangeal joint of the thumb,
ulnar margin of the base of the Phalanx proximalis of the thumb, inserts into the dorsal aponeurosis of the thumb

F: Carpometacarpal joint of the thumb:
adduction,
opposition
Metacarpophalangeal joint of the thumb:
flexion

37 Muscles of the palm (Fig. 372–374, 377–379, 382–384)

The muscles of the palm comprise a heterogeneous group. The Mm. lumbricales are tightly connected to the tendons of the M. flexor digitorum profundus. The Mm. interossei palmares and the Mm. interossei dorsales fill the spaces between the Ossa metacarpi.

Mm. lumbricales I–IV
N. medianus (I, II); N. ulnaris (III, IV) (Plexus brachialis, Pars infraclavicularis)

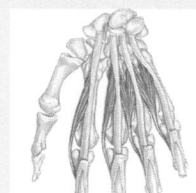

O: Radial side of the tendons I and II, as well as the facing sides of the tendons II–IV of the M. flexor digitorum profundus

I: Insert radially into the dorsal aponeurosis of the fingers II–V

F: <u>Metacarpophalangeal joints (II–V):</u> flexion, radial abduction
<u>Finger joints (II–V):</u> extension

Mm. interossei palmares I–III
N. ulnaris (Plexus brachialis, Pars infraclavicularis)

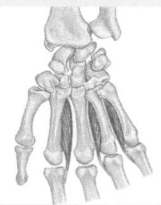

O: Ulnar side of the Os metacarpi II, radial side of the Ossa metacarpi IV and V

I: Radiate into the dorsal aponeurosis of the fingers II, IV and V

F: <u>Metacarpophalangeal joints (II, IV, V):</u> flexion, adduction (with respect to the axis of the middle finger)
<u>Finger joints (II, IV, V):</u> extension

Mm. interossei dorsales I–IV (double headed)
N. ulnaris (Plexus brachialis, Pars infraclavicularis)

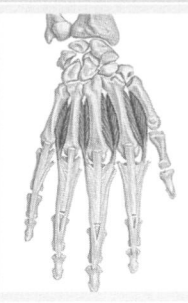

O: Facing sides of the Ossa metacarpi I–V

I: Radiate into the dorsal aponeurosis of the fingers II–IV

F: <u>Metacarpophalangeal joints (II–IV):</u> flexion, abduction (with respect to the axis of the middle finger)
<u>Finger joints (II–IV):</u> extension

38 Muscles of the hypothenar eminence (Fig. 372–374, 377)

From lateral to medial, the hypothenar eminence consists of the M. abductor digiti minimi, the M. flexor digiti minimi brevis and the M. opponens digiti minimi. The M. palmaris brevis also belongs to this group as a skin muscle.

M. palmaris brevis (consists of several separated bundles)
R. superficialis of the N. ulnaris (Plexus brachialis, Pars infraclavicularis)

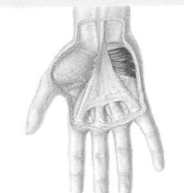

O: Medial margin of the Aponeurosis palmaris, rarely Os trapezium

I: Skin of the Hypothenar eminence

F: Tenses the skin at the hypothenar eminence

M. abductor digiti minimi
R. profundus of the N. ulnaris (Plexus brachialis, Pars infraclavicularis)

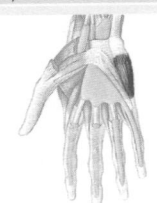

O: Os pisiforme, Lig. pisohamatum, Retinaculum musculorum flexorum

I: Ulnar margin of the Phalanx proximalis, dorsal aponeurosis of the 5. finger

F: Carpometacarpal joint (V): opposition
Metacarpophalangeal joint (V): abduction, flexion
Finger joints (V): extension

M. flexor digiti minimi brevis (inconstant muscle)
R. profundus of the N. ulnaris (Plexus brachialis, Pars infraclavicularis)

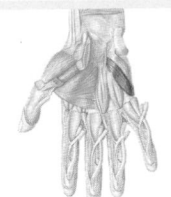

O: Retinaculum musculorum flexorum, Hamulus ossis hamati

F: Base of the Phalanx proximalis of the 5. finger, dorsal aponeurosis of the 5. finger

F: Carpometacarpal joint (V): opposition
Metacarpophalangeal joint (V): flexion, abduction
Finger joints (V): extension

M. opponens digiti minimi
R. profundus of the N. ulnaris (Plexus brachialis, Pars infraclavicularis)

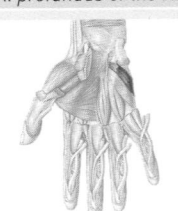

O: Retinaculum musculorum flexorum, Hamulus ossis hamati

I: Ulnar surface of the Os metacarpi V

F: Carpometacarpal joint (V): opposition

39 Joints of the lower limb, Articulationes membri inferioris (Fig. 949)

a Joints of the pelvic girdle, Juncturae cinguli pelvici

Name of the joint	Type of the joint	Movements
Sacroiliac joint, Articulatio sacroiliaca	Rigid joint, Amphiarthrosis	
Ligg. sacroiliaca anteriora Ligg. sacroiliaca posteriora Ligg. sacroiliaca interossea Lig. sacrotuberale Lig. sacrospinale	Syndesmoses, fibrous joints, Articulationes fibrosae	Limited displacement and rotation (only a few millimetres); as a consequence of the deformation of the pelvis during gait or weight-bearing
Pubic symphysis, Symphysis pubica	Cartilaginous joint, synchondrosis with interpubic disc	
Lig. pubicum superius Lig. pubicum inferius		

b Joints of the free part of the lower limb, Articulationes membri inferioris liberi

Name of the joint	Type of the joint	Movements
Hip joint, Articulatio coxae	Spheroideal joint, Articulatio spheroidea	Flexion (anteversion) extension (retroversion) adduction abduction medial and lateral rotation
Knee joint, Articulatio genus	Pivot-hinge joint, Trochoginglymus	Flexion extension medial and lateral rotation (only in flexed position)
Superior tibiofibular joint, Articulatio tibiofibularis	Rigid joint, Amphiarthrosis	Limited displacements in transverse and vertical direction, limited rotation
Inferior tibiofibular joint, Syndesmosis tibiofibularis	Syndesmosis, fibrous joint, Articulatio fibrosa	Support of the malleolar brace, which diverges slightly during dorsal extension in the ankle joint
Ankle joint, Articulatio talocruralis	Hinge joint, Ginglymus	Plantar flexion dorsal flexion
Talotarsal joint, Articulatio talotarsalis a) Articulatio talocalcaneonavicularis (= anterior part) b) Articulatio subtalaris (= posterior part)	Compound spheroideal and conoid joint Spheroideal joint Conoid joint	Lifting of the medial (supination) and lateral (pronation) margin of the foot
Transverse tarsal joint, Articulatio tarsi transversa (CHOPART's joint) a) Articulatio talocalcaneonavicularis b) Articulatio calcaneocuboidea	Rigid joints, Amphiarthroses	Minimal plantar and dorsal movements and rotation support of the longitudinal arch of the foot
Intertarsal joints a) Articulatio cuneonavicularis b) Articulationes intercuneiformes c) Articulatio cuneocuboidea	Rigid joints, Amphiarthroses	Minimal movements in the deformation of the foot during adjustment to the ground
Tarsometatarsal joints, Articulatio tarsometatarsales (LISFRANC's joint)	Rigid joints, Amphiarthroses	Minimal plantar and dorsal movements and rotation of the forefoot
Intermetatarsal joints, Articulationes intermetatarsales	Rigid joints, Amphiarthroses	Minimal movements during rotation of the forefoot
Metatarsophalangeal joints, Articulationes metatarsophalangeae	Functionally limited spheroideal joints	Flexion, extension abduction, adduction
Interphalangeal joints, Articulatio interphalangeae pedis	Hinge joints, Ginglymi	Flexion extension of the toes

39 Joints of the lower limb, Articulationes membri inferioris (continuation)

c Planes and axes of the movements of the joints of the lower limb

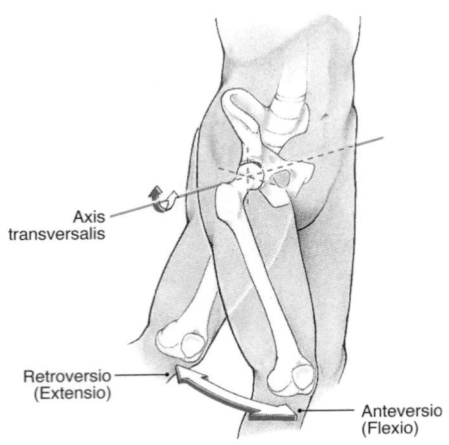

Axis transversalis

Retroversio (Extensio)

Anteversio (Flexio)

Fig. 8 Hip joint; movement in the sagittal plane.

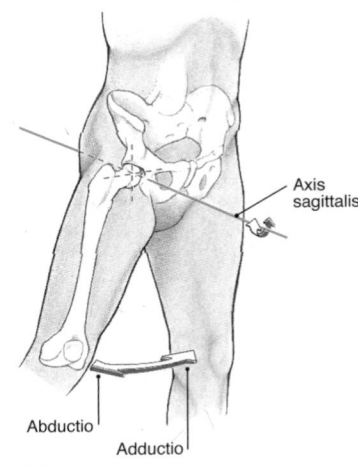

Axis sagittalis

Abductio

Adductio

Fig. 9 Hip joint; movement in the frontal plane.

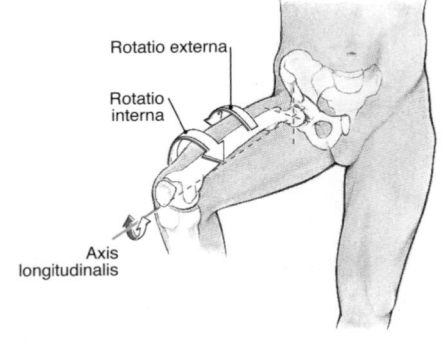

Rotatio externa

Rotatio interna

Axis longitudinalis

Fig. 10 Hip joint; movement in the transverse plane.

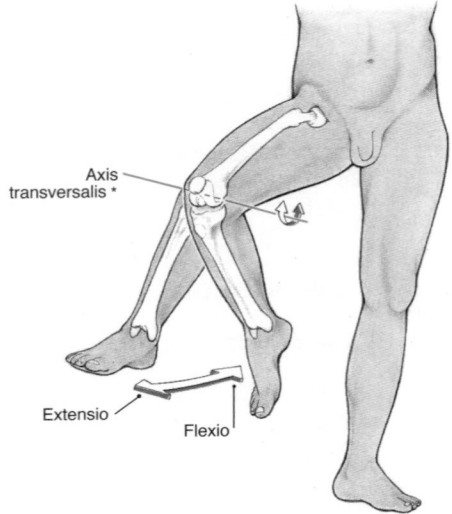

Axis transversalis *

Extensio

Flexio

Fig. 11 Knee joint; movement in the sagittal plane.

* As a consequence of the asymmetric curvature of the femoral condyles this axis, in particular, changes during the movement (inconstant axis).

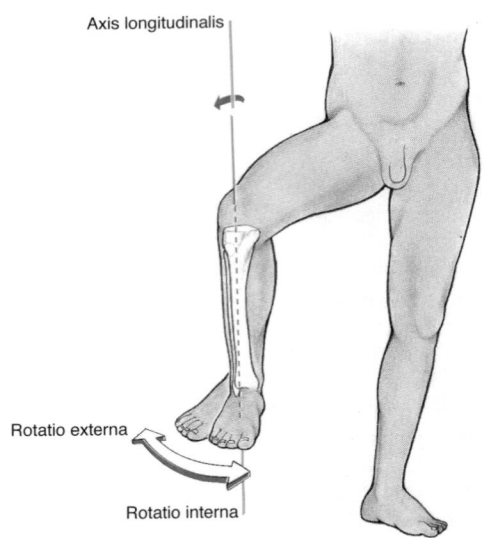

Axis longitudinalis

Rotatio externa

Rotatio interna

Fig. 12 Knee joint; movement in the transverse plane.

39 Joints of the lower limb, Articulationes membri inferioris (continuation)

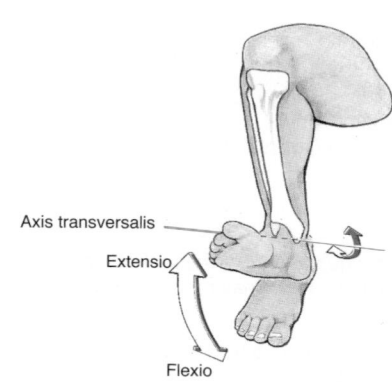

Axis transversalis

Extensio

Flexio

Fig. 13 Ankle joint;
movement in the sagittal plane.
Flexion and extension take place almost exclusively in the
ankle joint.

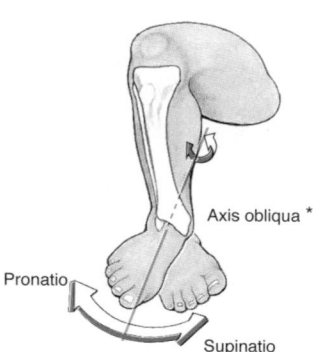

Axis obliqua *

Pronatio

Supinatio

Fig. 14 Talotarsal joint;
supination and pronation movements of the foot.
In extreme plantar flexion, pronation is also referred to as lateral
abduction, and supination as medial abduction.

* The axis runs from the inner part of the neck of the talus in a posterior
  and inferior direction to the Proc. lateralis of the Tuber calcanei and is
  actually steeper as illustrated in this figure for didactical reasons.

In the ankle joint, plantar flexion is also referred to as flexion, and dorsal flexion as extension.

40 Branches and supplying areas of the lumbosacral plexus (Fig. 595, 1105–1108)

	Motor function	Sensory function
Plexus lumbalis (T12) L1–L3 (L4)		
N. iliohypogastricus [N. iliopubicus] T12, L1 R. cutaneus lateralis R. cutaneus anterior	Mm. rectus abdominis, obliquus externus abdominis, obliquus internus abdominis, transversus abdominis, pyramidalis, cremaster	Skin covering the hip Skin above the iliac crest, the Lig. inguinale and the Mons pubis
N. ilioinguinalis (T12) L1 (L2) Nn. scrotales anteriores/ Nn. labiales anteriores	Mm. rectus abdominis, obliquus externus abdominis, obliquus internus abdominis, transversus abdominis, pyramidalis, cremaster	Skin of the inguinal region, the root of the penis, and the scrotum and the labia majora, respectively
N. genitofemoralis L 1, L 2 R. genitalis R. femoralis		Scrotal coats (including the dartos fascia) Skin at the Hiatus saphenus
N. cutaneus femoris lateralis L2, L3		Skin of the lateral and anterior side of the thigh up to the knee
N. obturatorius L2–L4 R. anterior R. cutaneus R. posterior Rr. musculares	Mm. pectineus, adductor brevis, adductor longus, gracilis M. obturatorius externus, M. adductor magnus, (M. adductor brevis), M. adductor minimus	Capsule of the hip joint Skin of the medial side of the thigh superior to the knee Capsule of the hip joint, periosteum of the posterior side of the femur
N. obturatorius accessorius L3, L4	M. pectineus	Capsule of the hip joint
N. femoralis L2–L4 Rr. musculares Rr. cutanei anteriores N. saphenus R. infrapatellaris Rr. cutanei cruris mediales	Mm. iliopsoas, pectineus, sartorius, quadriceps femoris	Capsule of the hip joint Skin of the anterior and medial side of the thigh up to the knee, periosteum of the anterior side of the femur Skin of the anterior and medial side of the knee and the medial side of the leg as well as the foot
Plexus sacralis (L4) L5–S3 (S4)		
N. m. obturatorii interni L5–S2	M. obturatorius internus	
N. m. piriformis S1, S2	M. piriformis	
N. m. quadrati femoris L5–S1 (S2)	M. quadratus femoris	
N. gluteus superior L4–S1	Mm. glutei medius and minimus, tensor fasciae latae	
N. gluteus inferior L5–S2	M. gluteus maximus	
N. cutaneus femoris posterior S1–S3 Nn. clunium inferiores Nn. perineales		Skin of the posterior side of the thigh and the proximal leg Skin of the gluteal region Perineum, scrotal skin or skin of the Labia majora, resp.
N. ischiadicus L4–S3	Ischiocrural muscles, all muscles of the leg and the foot	
N. fibularis communis L4–S2 N. cutaneus surae lateralis R. communicans fibularis	M. biceps femoris, Caput breve	Capsule of the knee joint Skin of the calf up to the lateral malleolus Connecting branch to the N. suralis

40 Branches and supplying areas of the lumbosacral plexus (continuation)

	Motor function	Sensory function
N. fibularis superficialis L4–S2 Rr. musculares	Mm. fibulares [peronei] longus and brevis	
N. cutaneus dorsalis medialis		Skin of the leg and the back of the foot up to the 1.–3. toe
N. cutaneus dorsalis intermedius Nn. digitales dorsales pedis		Skin of the lateral margin of the foot Skin of the back of the toes except for the 1. interdigital space and the lateral side of the 5. toe
N. fibularis profundus L4–S2 Rr. musculares	Mm. tibialis anterior, extensor digitorum longus, extensor hallucis longus, extensor digitorum brevis and extensor hallucis brevis	Periosteum of the bones of the leg and the capsule of the ankle joint
Nn. digitales dorsales pedis		Skin of the 1. interdigital space
N. tibialis L4–S3 Rr. musculares	Mm. triceps surae, plantaris, popliteus, tibialis posterior, flexor digitorum longus, flexor hallucis longus	Capsule of the knee joint
N. interosseus cruris		Periosteum of the bones of the leg and the capsule of the ankle joint
N. cutaneus surae medialis		Skin of the calf up to the medial malleolus, merges with the N. cutaneus surae lateralis to form the N. suralis
N. suralis N. cutaneus dorsalis lateralis		Skin of the lateral margin of the foot up to the 5. toe
Rr. calcanei laterales		Skin of the lateral heel
Rr. calcanei mediales		Skin of the medial heel
N. plantaris medialis	Mm. abductor hallucis and flexor digitorum brevis, flexor hallucis brevis (medial head), lumbricales pedis I (II)	Skin of the medial sole
Nn. digitales plantares communes Nn. digitales plantares proprii		Skin of the sole side of the medial 3½ toes and the nail areas
N. plantaris lateralis R. superficialis Nn. digitales plantares communes Nn. digitales plantares proprii R. profundus	Mm. abductor digiti minimi, quadratus plantae, Mm. flexor digiti minimi brevis, opponens digiti minimi, interossei of the 4. intermetatarsal space Mm. lumbricales pedis II–IV, adductor hallucis (Caput transversum), interossei of the 1.–4. intermetatarsal space	Skin of the plantar side of the lateral 1½ toes and the nail areas
N. pudendus (S1) S2–S4 Nn. rectales [anales] inferiores S3, S4		Skin of the anal region and the perineum
Nn. perineales Nn. scrotales posteriores/ Nn. labiales posteriores Rr. musculares	Mm. transversi perinei superficialis and profundus, bulbospongiosus and ischiocavernosus, sphincter ani externus	M. sphincter urethrae, urethral mucosa, dorsal skin of the scrotum or the Labia majora and minora, respectively, Vestibulum vaginae
N. dorsalis penis/ N. dorsalis clitoridis	M. transversus perinei profundus, M. sphincter urethrae	Skin of the penis, glans/clitoris, prepuce
N. coccygeus S4, S5 (Co1) Plexus coccygeus S4, S5 (Co1) N. anococcygeus	M. ischiococcygeus [coccygeus], M. levator ani	Skin of the coccygeal region, as well as the skin between the coccyx and the anus

41 Segmental innervation of the muscles of the lower limb, muscles of diagnostic importance

(According to MUMENTHALER and SCHLIACK; the indicator muscle of each segment is printed in bold.)

M. iliopsoas: L1, L2	T12–L3	**M. tibialis anterior: L4**	L4–L5
M. tensor fasciae latae	L4–L5	M. extensor hallucis longus	L4–S1
M. gluteus medius	L4–S1	M. popliteus	L4–S1
M. gluteus minimus	L4–S1	M. extensor digitorum longus	L4–S1
M. gluteus maximus	L4–S2	**M. soleus**	L4–S2
M. obturatorius internus	L5–S1	**M. gastrocnemius** } L5	
M. piriformis	L5–S1	M. fibularis longus	L5–S1
M. sartorius	L2–L3	M. fibularis brevis	L5–S1
M. pectineus	L2–L3	**M. tibialis posterior: S1**	L5–S2
M. adductor longus	L2–L3	M. flexor digitorum longus	L5–S3
M. quadriceps femoris: L3	L2–L4	M. flexor hallucis longus	L5–S3
M. gracilis	L2–L4	M. extensor hallucis brevis	L4–S1
M. adductor brevis	L2–L4	M. extensor digitorum brevis	L4–S1
M. obturatorius externus	L3–L4	M. flexor digitorum brevis	L5–S1
M. adductor magnus	L3–L4	M. abductor hallucis	L5–S1
M. semitendinosus	L4–S1	M. flexor hallucis brevis	L5–S3
M. semimembranosus	L4–S1	M. adductor hallucis	S1–S2
M. biceps femoris	L4–S2		

42 Ventral muscles of the hip (Fig. 583, 601, 1053, 1055, 1060–1065)

This group only comprises the M. iliacus and the M. psoas major, which together form the M. iliopsoas. These are the only ventral muscles of the hip joint, as all other ventral muscles in front of the hip joint also overstretch the knee joint and are therefore referred to as ventral muscles of the thigh.

M. iliacus
Rr. musculares (Plexus lumbalis)

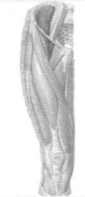

O: Fossa iliaca,
Spina iliaca anterior inferior,
anterior portion of the capsule of
the hip joint

I: Trochanter minor and adjacent
area of the Labium mediale of the
Linea aspera

F: <u>Lumbar vertebral column:</u>
lateral flexion,
extension (hyperlordosis)
<u>Hip joint:</u>
flexion,
medial rotation, (lateral rotation only
when the Mm. glutei are contracted
as well)

M. psoas major
Rr. musculares (Plexus lumbalis)

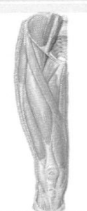

O: Superficial layer: lateral
surface of the body of the
12. thoracic –4. lumbar vertebra,
Disci intervertebrales
Deep layer: Proc. costalis of the
1.–4. lumbar vertebra

I: Trochanter minor and adjacent
area of the Labium mediale of
the Linea aspera

F: <u>Lumbar vertebral column:</u>
lateral flexion,
extension (hyperlordosis)
<u>Hip joint:</u>
flexion,
medial rotation, (lateral rotation only
when the Mm. glutei are contracted
as well)

M. psoas minor (inconstant muscle; often featuring a long tendinous plate at its insertion)
Rr. musculares (Plexus lumbalis)

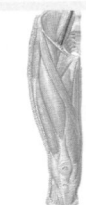

O: Lateral surface of the body of
the 12. thoracic and the 1. lumbar
vertebra

I: Fascia of the M. iliopsoas,
Arcus iliopectineus

F: <u>Lumbar vertebral column:</u>
lateral flexion,
extension (hyperlordosis)
<u>Hip joint:</u>
flexion,
medial rotation, (lateral rotation only
when the Mm. glutei are contracted
as well)

43 Dorsal muscles of the hip (Fig. 1054–1056, 1065, 1067–1074)

The M. gluteus maximus predominantly shapes the surface anatomy of the gluteal region and nearly covers all other muscles of this group. At the ventral and cranial edge, parts of the M. gluteus medius are visible, which in turn covers the M. gluteus minimus. Caudally in the deeper layer the following muscles are found: the M. piriformis, the M. gemellus superior, the M. obturatorius internus, the M. gemellus inferior and the M. quadratus femoris. The M. obturatorius internus and the Mm. gemelli superior et inferior are also called M. triceps coxae.

M. gluteus maximus (The Bursa trochanterica musculi glutei maximi is located between the Trochanter major and the Tractus iliotibialis.)
N. gluteus inferior (Plexus sacralis)

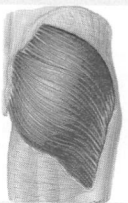

O: Facies glutea of the Ala ossis ilium dorsal to the Linea glutea posterior,
Facies posterior of the Os sacrum,
Fascia thoracolumbalis,
Lig. sacrotuberale

I: Cranial portion via the Tractus iliotibialis: Tibia just below the Condylus lateralis,
caudal portion: Tuberositas glutea,
Septum intermusculare femoris laterale

F: <u>Hip joint:</u>
cranial portion: extension, lateral rotation, abduction;
caudal portion: extension, lateral rotation, adduction
<u>Knee joint:</u>
cranial portion via Tractus iliotibialis, stabilization when the knee is extended

M. gluteus medius
N. gluteus superior (Plexus sacralis)

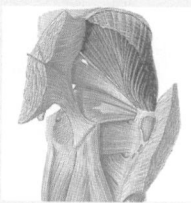

O: Facies glutea of the Ala ossis ilium between Lineae gluteae anterior and posterior

I: Tip and lateral margin of the Trochanter major

F: <u>Hip joint:</u>
ventral portion: abduction, flexion, medial rotation;
dorsal portion: abduction, extension, lateral rotation

M. gluteus minimus
N. gluteus superior (Plexus sacralis)

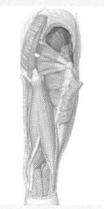

O: Facies glutea of the Ala ossis ilium between Lineae gluteae anterior and inferior

I: Tip and lateral margin of the Trochanter major

F: <u>Hip joint:</u>
ventral portion: abduction, flexion, medial rotation;
dorsal portion: abduction, extension, lateral rotation

M. piriformis
N. ischiadicus and/or N. musculi piriformis (Plexus sacralis)

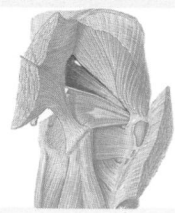

O: Laterally and between the Foramina sacralia pelvica (3.–5. sacral segment) of the Facies pelvica of the Os sacrum, Incisura ischiadica major close to the Os sacrum

I: Inner surface of the tip of the Trochanter major

F: <u>Hip joint:</u>
lateral rotation, extension, abduction

43 Dorsal muscles of the hip (continuation)

M. obturatorius internus
N. musculi obturatorii interni and Rr. musculares (Plexus sacralis)

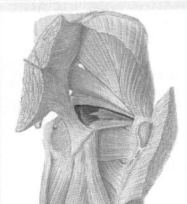

O: Circumference of the Foramen obturatum, medial surface of the Membrana obturatoria

I: Fossa trochanterica

F: <u>Hip joint:</u> lateral rotation, extension, adduction

M. gemellus superior
N. musculi obturatorii interni and Rr. musculares (Plexus sacralis)

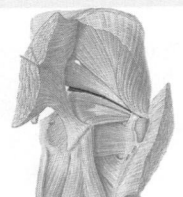

O: Spina ischiadica

I: Fossa trochanterica

F: <u>Hip joint:</u> lateral rotation, extension, adduction

M. gemellus inferior
N. musculi obturatorii interni and Rr. musculares (Plexus sacralis)

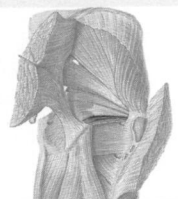

O: Tuber ischiadicum

I: Fossa trochanterica

F: <u>Hip joint:</u> lateral rotation, extension, adduction

M. quadratus femoris
N. musculi quadrati femoris (Plexus sacralis)

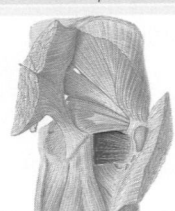

O: Lateral margin of the Tuber ischiadicum

I: Crista intertrochanterica

F: <u>Hip joint:</u> lateral rotation, adduction

44 Ventral muscles of the thigh (Fig. 1053, 1055–1058, 1061–1065, 1075–1077)

The M. sartorius stretches in a spiral-like fashion along the thigh from lateroproximal to mediodistal. With its short muscle belly, the M. tensor fasciae latae is located most laterally and passes into the Tractus iliotibialis. The major part of the ventral muscle mass of the thigh is formed by the M. quadriceps femoris.

M. quadriceps femoris
N. femoralis (Plexus lumbalis)

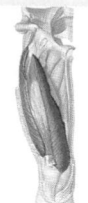

O: M. rectus femoris, Caput rectum: Spina iliaca anterior inferior
M. rectus femoris, Caput reflexum: cranial margin of the Acetabulum
M. vastus medialis: inferior two thirds of the Labium mediale of the Linea aspera
M. vastus lateralis: distal circumference of the Trochanter major, Labium laterale of the Linea aspera
M. vastus intermedius: upper two thirds of the Facies anterior and lateral aspects of the Femur
M. articularis genus: distal quarter of the Facies anterior of the Femur

I: Proximal, lateral and medial margins of the Patella, Tuberositas tibiae via the Lig. patellae, areas lateral to the Tuberositas tibiae via the Retinacula patellae

F: Hip joint (only M. rectus femoris): flexion
Knee joint: extension

M. sartorius
N. femoralis (Plexus lumbalis)

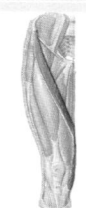

O: Spina iliaca anterior superior

I: Medial surface of the Tuberositas tibiae

F: Hip joint: flexion, lateral rotation, abduction
Knee joint: flexion, medial rotation

M. tensor fasciae latae
N. gluteus superior (Plexus lumbosacralis)

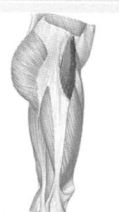

O: Spina iliaca anterior superior

I: Tibia below the Condylus lateralis (via Tractus ilitotibialis)

F: Hip joint: flexion, abduction, medial rotation
Knee joint: stabilization when the knee is extended

T 45

45 Medial muscles of the thigh (adductors)
(Fig. 1053, 1055, 1056, 1059, 1061–1065, 1071–1077)

Due to their predominant function, the muscles located at the medial side of the thigh are commonly referred to as adductors. In the ventral view, this group appears like a triangular block. The M. gracilis lies most medially. From proximal to distal follow the M. pectineus, M. adductor brevis, M. adductor longus and the M. adductor magnus. The M. obturatorius externus is covered by the M. pectineus and is juxtaposed to the neck of the femur from inferior.

M. pectineus
N. femoralis and N. obturatorius (Plexus lumbalis)

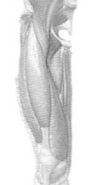

O: Pecten ossis pubis

I: Linea pectinea of the Femur

F: <u>Hip joint:</u>
adduction,
lateral rotation,
(flexion)

M. gracilis
N. obturatorius (Plexus lumbalis)

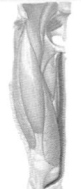

O: Medial edge of the Ramus inferior ossis pubis along the symphysis

I: Proximal end of the Tibia medial to the Tuberositas tibiae

F: <u>Hip joint:</u>
adduction,
flexion,
lateral rotation
<u>Knee joint:</u>
flexion,
medial rotation

M. adductor brevis
N. obturatorius (Plexus lumbalis)

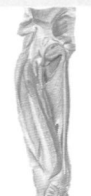

O: Ramus inferior ossis pubis closer to the Foramen obturatum than the M. adductor longus

I: Proximal third of the Labium mediale of the Linea aspera

F: <u>Hip joint:</u>
adduction,
lateral rotation,
flexion

M. adductor longus
N. obturatorius (Plexus lumbalis)

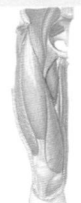

O: Os pubis below the Crista pubica up to the symphysis

I: Middle third of the Labium mediale of the Linea aspera

F: <u>Hip joint:</u>
adduction,
flexion,
lateral rotation,
(most anterior portion: medial rotation)

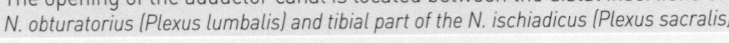

M. adductor magnus (An incomplete proximal part of the M. adductor magnus is known as M. adductor minimus. The opening of the adductor canal is located between the distal insertions of both muscles.)
N. obturatorius (Plexus lumbalis) and tibial part of the N. ischiadicus (Plexus sacralis)

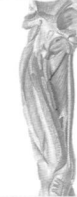

O: Medial margin of the Ramus inferior ossis pubis, Ramus and Tuber ossis ischii

I: Proximal two thirds of the Labium mediale of the Linea aspera, Tuberositas, Tuberculum adductorium, M. adductor minimus: Tuberositas glutea

F: <u>Hip joint:</u>
adduction,
lateral rotation
(anterior portion: flexion, posterior portion: extension)

45 Medial muscles of the thigh (adductors) (continuation)

M. obturatorius externus
N. obturatorius (Plexus lumbalis)

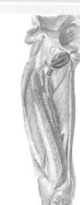

O: Circumference of the Foramen obturatum, lateral surface of the Membrana obturatoria

I: Fossa trochanterica

F: <u>Hip joint:</u> lateral rotation, adduction

46 Dorsal muscles of the thigh (ischiocrural muscles)
(Fig. 1054–1056, 1065, 1066, 1071–1078)

The ischiocrural muscles consist of the M. biceps femoris, the M. semitendinosus and the M. semimembranosus from lateral to medial.

M. biceps femoris (The Caput longum stretches over two joints, whereas the Caput breve only spans over one joint.)
Caput longum: *N. ischiadicus, tibial part (Plexus sacralis)*
Caput breve: *N. ischiadicus, fibular part (Plexus sacralis)*

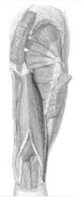

O: Caput longum: Tuber ischiadicum together with the M. semitendinosus
Caput breve: middle third of the Labium laterale of the Linea aspera

I: Caput fibulae (ensheaths the Lig. collaterale fibulare), radiates into the Fascia cruris

F: <u>Hip joint:</u> extension, adduction, (lateral rotation) <u>Knee joint:</u> flexion, lateral rotation

M. semitendinosus
N. ischiadicus, tibial part (Plexus sacralis)

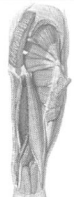

O: Tuber ischiadicum together with the Caput longum of the M. biceps femoris

I: Medial surface of the Tuberositas tibiae

F: <u>Hip joint:</u> extension, (adduction), (medial rotation) <u>Knee joint:</u> flexion, medial rotation

M. semimembranosus (The insertion of the M. semimembranosus is also referred to as Pes anserinus profundus.)
N. ischiadicus, tibial part (Plexus sacralis)

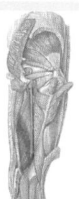

O: Tuber ischiadicum

I: Proximal end of the Tibia below the Condylus medialis, posterior capsule of the knee joint, Lig. popliteum obliquum, fascia of the M. popliteus

F: <u>Hip joint:</u> extension, (adduction), (medial rotation) <u>Knee joint:</u> flexion, medial rotation

T 47

47 Ventral muscles of the leg (Fig. 1053, 1077, 1079, 1083, 1088)

The ventral superficial and medial muscle is the M. tibialis anterior. It is followed by the M. extensor digitorum longus, from whose lateral margin the M. fibularis tertius often originates. The M. extensor hallucis longus is located most deeply.

M. tibialis anterior
N. fibularis profundus (N. ischiadicus)

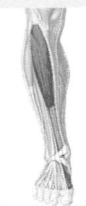

O: Proximal end of the Tibia just below the Condylus lateralis, upper two thirds of the Facies lateralis of the Tibia, Fascia cruris, (Membrana interossea)

I: Medial margin of the base of the Os metatarsi I, plantar surface of the Os cuneiforme mediale

F: <u>Ankle joint:</u> dorsal flexion
<u>Talotarsal joint:</u> supination

M. extensor hallucis longus
N. fibularis profundus (N. ischiadicus)

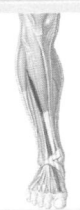

O: Distal two thirds of the Facies medialis of the Fibula, Membrana interossea, Fascia cruris

I: Base of the Phalanx distalis and the Phalanx proximalis of the Hallux

F: <u>Ankle joint:</u> dorsal flexion
<u>Talotarsal joint:</u> (supination)
<u>Joints of the great toe:</u> extension

M. extensor digitorum longus
N. fibularis profundus (N. ischiadicus)

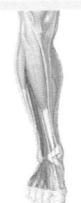

O: Proximal end of the Tibia just below the Condylus lateralis, Margo anterior of the Fibula, Membrana interossea cruris, Septum intermusculare cruris anterius, Fascia cruris

I: Dorsal aponeuroses of the 2.Ð5. toe

F: <u>Ankle joint:</u> dorsal flexion
<u>Talotarsal joint:</u> (pronation)
<u>Joints of the toes:</u> extension

M. fibularis [peroneus] tertius (inconstant muscle)
N. fibularis profundus (N. ischiadicus)

O: Distal part of the M. extensor digitorum longus

I: Base of the Os metatarsi V

F: <u>Ankle joint:</u> dorsal flexion
<u>Talotarsal joint:</u> (pronation)

See Fig. 1083

48 Lateral (fibular) muscles of the leg (Fig. 1053, 1078, 1080, 1083, 1088)

The lateral superficial muscle is the M. fibularis longus, with the M. fibularis brevis following in the next deeper layer.

M. fibularis [peroneus] longus
N. fibularis superficialis (N. ischiadicus)

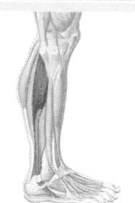

O: Caput fibulae, proximal two thirds of the Facies lateralis and the Margo posterior of the Fibula, Septa intermuscularia cruris anterius et posterius, Fascia cruris

I: Tuberositas ossis metatarsi I (II), plantar surface of the Os cuneiforme intermedium

F: Ankle joint: plantar flexion
Talotarsal joint: pronation

M. fibularis [peroneus] brevis
N. fibularis superficialis (N. ischiadicus)

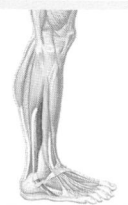

O: Distal half of the Facies lateralis and the Margo anterior of the Fibula, Septa intermuscularia cruris anterius et posterius

I: Tuberositas ossis metatarsi V, tendon strips to the little toe

F: Ankle joint: plantar flexion
Talotarsal joint: pronation

49 Superficial dorsal muscles of the leg (Fig. 1054, 1078, 1081, 1084, 1085)

The heads of the M. gastrocnemius determine the shape of the calf. It is located above the M. soleus and together these muscles form the M. triceps surae. The very small M. plantaris can be considered as a fourth head of this muscle.

M. triceps surae (Its broad tendon is also known as Achilles tendon.)
N. tibialis (N. ischiadicus)

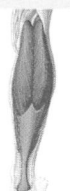

O: M. gastrocnemius, Caput mediale: Facies poplitea of the Femur proximal to the Condylus medialis
M. gastrocnemius, Caput laterale: Facies poplitea of the Femur proximal to the Condylus lateralis
M. soleus: Caput fibulae, proximal third of the Facies posterior and the Margo posterior of the Fibula, Facies posterior of the Tibia at and just below the Linea musculi solei, Arcus tendineus musculi solei
M. plantaris: Facies poplitea of the Femur proximal to the Condylus lateralis

I: Tuber calcanei (via Tendo calcaneus)

F: Knee joint: (only M. gastrocnemius and M. plantaris): flexion
Ankle joint: plantar flexion
Talotarsal joint: supination

T 50

50 Deep dorsal muscles of the leg (Fig. 1078, 1082, 1086, 1087)

The M. popliteus traverses obliquely in a lateral direction towards the knee joint. Of the muscles running towards the foot, the M. tibialis posterior is located most superficially. The muscle is followed medially by the M. flexor digitorum longus and laterally by the M. flexor hallucis longus.

M. popliteus
N. tibialis (N. ischiadicus)

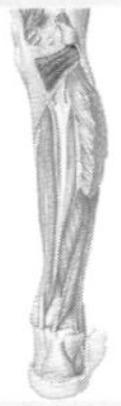	**O:** Epicondylus lateralis of the Femur	**I:** Facies posterior of the Tibia just above the Linea musculi solei	**F:** Knee joint: medial rotation, flexion

M. tibialis posterior
N. tibialis (N. ischiadicus)

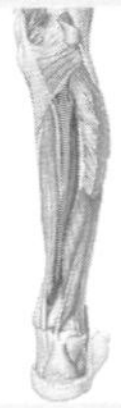	**O:** Upper three quarters of the Membrana interossea, adjacent areas of the Tibia and the Fibula	**I:** Tuberositas ossis navicularis, plantar surface of the Ossa cuneiformia I–III, base of the Ossa metatarsi II–IV	**F:** Ankle joint: plantar flexion Talotarsal joint: supination

M. flexor digitorum longus
N. tibialis (N. ischiadicus)

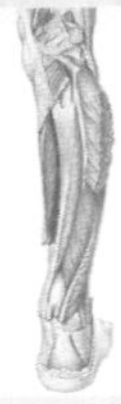	**O:** Facies posterior of the Tibia distal to the Linea musculi solei, tendon arcade between the Tibia and the Fibula proximal to the Chiasma crurale	**I:** Phalanx distalis of the 2.–5. toe	**F:** Ankle joint: plantar flexion Talotarsal joint: supination Joints of the toes: flexion

M. flexor hallucis longus
N. tibialis (N. ischiadicus)

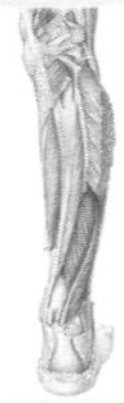	**O:** Distal two thirds of the Facies posterior of the Fibula, Membrana interossea, Septum intermusculare cruris posterius	**I:** Phalanx distalis of the great toe	**F:** Ankle joint: plantar flexion Talotarsal joint: supination Joints of the great toe: flexion

51 Muscles of the back of the foot (Fig. 1088, 1089, 1093, 1094)

Both muscles of the back of the foot only contribute insignificantly to the surface anatomy. The M. extensor hallucis brevis traverses towards the great toe, whereas the M. extensor digitorum brevis inserts at the remaining toes.

M. extensor digitorum brevis
N. fibularis profundus (N. fibularis communis)

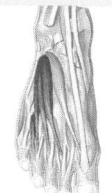

O: Dorsal and lateral surface of the Calcaneus

I: Dorsal aponeurosis of the 2.–4. toe

F: Joints of the toes: extension

M. extensor hallucis brevis
N. fibularis profundus (N. fibularis communis)

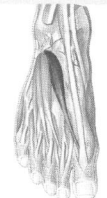

O: Dorsal surface of the Calcaneus, Sinus tarsi

I: Phalanx proximalis of the great toe

F: Metatarsophalangeal joint of the great toe: extension

52 Medial muscles of the sole (Fig. 1096–1099)

The shape of the medial margin of the foot, Eminentia plantaris medialis, is predominantly formed by the M. abductor hallucis. The M. flexor hallucis brevis is juxtaposed just lateral to the former muscle, and is followed laterally by the M. adductor hallucis.

M. abductor hallucis
N. plantaris medialis (N. tibialis)

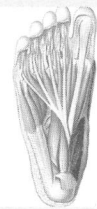

O: Proc. medialis of the Tuber calcanei, Aponeurosis plantaris, Retinaculum musculorum flexorum

I: Medial sesamoid bone of the capsule of the metatarsophalangeal joint of the great toe, medial side of the base of the Phalanx proximalis of the great toe

F: Metatarsophalangeal joint of the great toe: abduction, flexion, opposition

M. flexor hallucis brevis
Medial part (Caput mediale): *N. plantaris medialis (N. tibialis)*
Lateral part (Caput laterale): *N. plantaris lateralis (N. tibialis)*

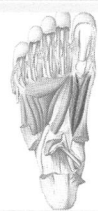

O: Plantar surface of the Ossa cuneiformia, Lig. calcaneocuboideum plantare, Lig. plantare longum, tendon of the M. tibialis posterior

I: Medial portion: medial sesamoid bone of the metatarsophalangeal joint of the great toe, base of the Phalanx proximalis I
Lateral portion: lateral sesamoid bone of the metatarsophalangeal joint of the great toe, base of the Phalanx proximalis I

F: Metatarsophalangeal joint of the great toe: flexion

52 Medial muscles of the sole (continuation)

M. adductor hallucis
N. plantaris lateralis (N. tibialis)

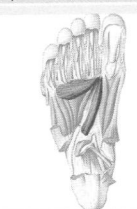

O: Caput obliquum: Os cuboideum, Os cuneiforme laterale, Lig. plantare longum, Lig. calcaneocuboideum plantare
Caput transversum: Capsules of the metatarsophalangeal joints of the toes III–V, Lig. metatarsale transversum profundum

I: Lateral sesamoid bone of the capsule of the metatarsophalangeal joint of the great toe, base of the Phalanx proximalis of the great toe

F: Metatarsophalangeal joint of the great toe: adduction towards the 2. toe, flexion

53 Muscles of the middle of the sole (Fig. 1089, 1093, 1094, 1096–1101)

Several small muscles are located deep within the plantar arch. The M. flexor digitorum brevis proximally adheres to the plantar aponeurosis. Below this muscle, the M. quadratus plantae is connected to the main tendon of the M. flexor digitorum longus, of whose four branching tendons the Mm. lumbricales pedis I–IV originate. The Mm. interossei plantares I–III and the Mm. interossei dorsales pedis I–IV fill the spaces between the Ossa metatarsi.

M. flexor digitorum brevis (Just before the insertion, its tendons are perforated by the tendons of the M. flexor digitorum longus.)
N. plantaris medialis (N. tibialis)

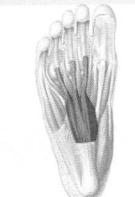

O: Plantar surface of the Tuber calcanei, Aponeurosis plantaris

I: Phalanx media of the 2.–5. toe

F: Metatarsophalangeal joints: flexion
Joints of the toes: flexion

M. quadratus plantae (This muscle is also referred to as M. flexor accessorius.)
N. plantaris lateralis (N. tibialis)

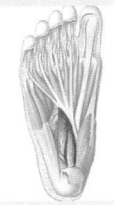

O: Plantar surface of the Calcaneus, Lig. plantare longum

I: Lateral margin of the tendon of the M. flexor digitorum longus just before its division

F: Shifts the direction of force generated by the M. flexor digitorum longus towards the longitudinal axis of the foot

Mm. lumbricales pedis I–IV
Nn. plantares medialis (I) and lateralis (II–IV) (N. tibialis)

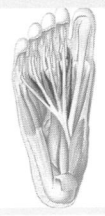

O: M. lumbricales pedis I: medial side of the tendon of the M. flexor digitorum longus to the 2. toe
Mm. lumbricales pedis II–IV: facing sides of the tendons of the M. flexor digitorum longus to the 3.–5. toe

I: Medial side of the Phalanx proximalis of the 2.–5. toe, sometimes it radiates into the dorsal aponeurosis

F: Metatarsophalangeal joints: flexion

Mm. interossei plantares pedis I–III
N. plantaris lateralis (N. tibialis)

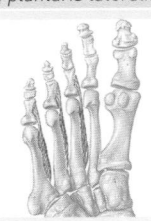

O: Plantar surface of the Ossa metatarsi III–V, Lig. plantare longum

I: Medial side of the base of the Phalanx proximalis of the 3.–5. toe

F: Metatarsophalangeal joints: flexion, adduction towards the 2. toe

53 Muscles of the middle of the sole (continuation)

Mm. interossei dorsales pedis I–IV (double headed muscles)
N. plantaris lateralis (N. tibialis)

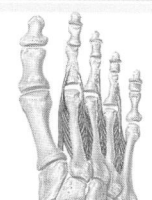

O: Facing sides of the Ossa metatarsi I–V, Lig. plantare longum

I: M. interosseus dorsalis I: medial side of the base of the Phalanx proximalis of the 2. toe
Mm. interossei dorsales II–IV: lateral side of the base of the Phalanx proximalis of the 2.–4. toe, insert into extensor aponeuroses

F: Metatarsophalangeal joints: flexion, medial abduction of the 2. toe, as well as lateral abduction of the 3. and 4. toe
Joints of the toes: (extension)

54 Lateral muscles of the sole (Fig. 1089, 1096–1099)

The M. abductor digiti minimi is located along the lateral margin of the foot, Eminentia plantaris lateralis. The M. flexor digiti minimi brevis and the M. opponens digiti minimi are situated below its plantar aspect.

M. abductor digiti minimi
N. plantaris lateralis (N. tibialis)

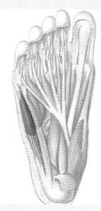

O: Proc. lateralis of the Tuber calcanei, Aponeurosis plantaris, Tuberositas ossis metatarsi V

I: Base of the Phalanx proximalis of the 5. toe

F: Metatarsophalangeal joint of the 5. toe: abduction, flexion, opposition

M. flexor digiti minimi brevis
N. plantaris lateralis (N. tibialis)

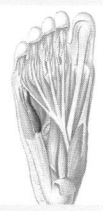

O: Base of the Os metatarsi V, Lig. plantare longum, tendon sheath of the M. fibularis longus

I: Phalanx proximalis of the 5. toe

F: Metatarsophalangeal joint of the 5. toe: abduction, flexion, (opposition)

M. opponens digiti minimi (inconstant muscle)
N. plantaris lateralis (N. tibialis)

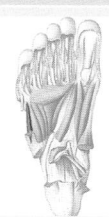

O: Lig. plantare longum, tendon sheath of the M. fibularis longus

I: Lateral margin of the Os metatarsi V

F: Metatarsophalangeal joint of the 5. toe: abduction, flexion, (opposition)

55 Cranial nerves, overview (Fig. 1174)

a	**N. olfactorius [I]**
b	**N. opticus [II]**
c	**N. oculomotorius [III]**
d	**N. trochlearis [IV]**
e	**N. trigeminus [V]** – N. ophthalmicus [V/1] – N. maxillaris [V/2] – N. mandibularis [V/3]
f	**N. abducens [VI]**
g	**N. facialis [VII]**
h	**N. vestibulocochlearis [VIII]**
i	**N. glossopharyngeus [IX]**
j	**N. vagus [X]**
k	**N. accessorius [XI]**
l	**N. hypoglossus [XII]**

56 Cranial nerves, functions (different fibre qualities) (Fig. 1188–1191, 1236, 1238)

GSE	General somatic efference: innervation of the skeletal muscles **(III, IV, VI, XII)**
GVE	General visceral efference: innervation of the muscles of the viscera and vessels, and of the glands **(III, VII, IX, X)**
SVE	Specific visceral efference: innervation of the facial muscles, the masticatory muscles, the larynx, the pharynx, the oesophagus, as well as the M. sternocleidomastoideus and M. trapezius **(V, VII, IX, X, XI)**
GVA	General visceral afference: information from the internal organs and the blood vessels **(IX, X)**
SVA	Specific visceral afference: sense of taste **(VII, IX, X)**
GSA	General somatic afference: pain, temperature, information from proprioceptive receptors in skin and locomotor system **(V, VII, IX, X)**
SSA	Specific somatic afference: sense of smell, vision, hearing, sense of balance **(I, II, VIII)**

57 Cranial nerves (Fig. 1174–1194, 1236, 1238)

a N. olfactorius [I] (Fig. 144, 1174)

All Fila olfactoria together are referred to as N. olfactorius, representing the peripheral neuron of the olfactory pathway.

Outset	Olfactory cells in the Regio olfactoria
Passage through the base of skull	Lamina cribrosa
Passage through the dura mater	Lamina cribrosa
Entry into the brain	Bulbus olfactorius
Supplying area	Mucosa (=olfactory mucosa) at the uppermost parts of the nasal cavity, the upper nasal concha and the most cranial parts of the nasal septum

b N. opticus [II] (Fig. 1174, 1368, 1369)

The N. opticus belongs to the diencephalon and is therefore not really a peripheral nerve.

Outset	Ganglion opticum of the Retina
Course within the dura mater	Vagina nervi optici
Passage through the base of skull	Canalis opticus
Further visible course	Chiasma opticum with the continuation of its fibres via the Tractus opticus to the Corpus geniculatum laterale
Supplying area	Retina

c N. oculomotorius [III] (Fig. 1175, 1176, 1236, 1238)

Nuclei (fibre quality)	• Nucleus nervi oculomotorii (double main and single accessory nucleus) (GSE) • Nucleus accessorius nervi oculomotorii (GVE) → Ganglion ciliare
Exit from the brain	Inner surface of the Pedunculus cerebri (Sulcus nervi oculomotorii)
Location in the subarachnoid space	Cisterna basalis, Cisterna interpeduncularis
Entry into the dura mater	Roof of the Sinus cavernosus
Exit from the dura mater	Fissura orbitalis superior
Passage through the base of skull	Fissura orbitalis superior (medial portion, within the Anulus tendineus)
Supplying areas	**Motor:** M. levator palpebrae superioris, Mm. recti superior, medialis and inferior, M. obliquus inferior **Parasympathetic:** M. ciliaris, M. sphincter pupillae (via Ganglion ciliare)
Attachment of other nerves	**Sensible** fibres from the N. nasociliaris (V/1) **Sympathetic** fibres from the Plexus ophthalmicus

d N. trochlearis [IV] (Fig. 1175, 1176, 1236, 1238)

Nuclei (fibre quality)	• Nucleus nervi trochlearis (GSE)
Exit from the brain	Dorsal/caudal of the Colliculus inferior (Tectum mesencephali)
Location in the subarachnoid space	Cisterna ambiens, Cisterna basalis
Entry into the dura mater	Between the Plica petroclinoidea anterior and posterior
Course within the dura mater	Lateral wall of the Sinus cavernosus
Exit from the dura mater	Fissura orbitalis superior
Passage through the base of skull	Fissura orbitalis superior (lateral portion)
Supplying area	**Motor:** M. obliquus superior

T 57

e N. trigeminus [V] (Fig. 1177–1180, 1236, 1238)

Nuclei (fibre quality)	• Nucleus mesencephalicus nervi trigemini (GSA and GVA) • Nucleus spinalis nervi trigemini (GSA and GVA) • Nucleus motorius nervi trigemini (SVE)
Exit from the brain	Lateral margin of the Pons
Location in the subarachnoid space	Cisterna basalis, Cavum trigeminale
Entry into the dura mater	Lateral wall of the Sinus cavernosus as Ganglion trigeminale
Division into three branches	– N. ophthalmicus [V/1] – N. maxillaris [V/2] – N. mandibularis [V/3]

– N. ophthalmicus [V/1]

Course within the dura mater	Lateral wall of the Sinus cavernosus
Exit from the dura mater	Fissura orbitalis superior
Exit from the base of skull	Fissura orbitalis superior – N. nasociliaris: medial portion – N. frontalis: lateral portion – N. lacrimalis: lateral portion
Supplying areas	**Sensible:** Dura mater of the anterior cranial fossa, Falx cerebri, Tentorium cerebelli, forehead, upper eyelid, back of the nose, Sclera, Cornea, Cellulae ethmoidales anteriores, Sinus sphenoidales, nasal cavity (anterior part)
Attachment of other nerves	**Parasympathetic (secretory) fibres** to the N. lacrimalis for the Glandula lacrimalis (from the Nucleus salivatorius superior via the N. facialis, N. petrosus major to the Ganglion pterygopalatinum and further on to the N. zygomaticus and R. communicans cum nervo zygomatico)

– N. maxillaris [V/2]

Course within the dura mater	Lateral wall of the Sinus cavernosus
Exit from the dura mater	Foramen rotundum
Exit from the base of skull	Foramen rotundum
Supplying areas	**Sensible:** Dura mater of the middle cranial fossa, cheek, lower eyelid, lateral parts of the nose, upper lip, teeth and gingiva of the maxilla, Cellulae ethmoidales posteriores, Sinus sphenoidalis, Sinus maxillaris, Conchae nasales superior and media, Palatum, Tonsilla palatina, Pharynx (roof)
Attachment of other nerves	**Parasympathetic (secretory) fibres** to the diverse Rr. nasales for the Glandulae nasales, to the Nn. palatini for the Glandulae palatinae as well as to the N. zygomaticus for the Glandula lacrimalis (from the Nucleus salivatorius superior via the N. facialis, N. petrosus major and the Rr. ganglionares to the Ganglion pterygopalatinum)

– N. mandibularis [V/3]

Course within the dura mater	Lateral wall of the Sinus cavernosus
Exit from the dura mater	Foramen ovale
Exit from the base of skull	Foramen ovale
Supplying areas	**Motor:** masticatory muscles, M. tensor veli palatini, M. mylohyoideus, M. digastricus (Venter anterior), M. tensor tympani **Sensible:** Dura mater of the middle cranial fossa, Cellulae mastoideae, skin of the mandible, temple, cheek, auricle (upper parts), external acoustic meatus, tympanic membrane (externally), teeth and gingiva of the mandible, anterior 2/3 of the tongue, Isthmus faucium, temporomandibular joint
Attachment of other nerves	**Sensory:** anterior 2/3 of the tongue (N. facialis [VII] via Chorda tympani to the N. lingualis) **Parasympathetic (secretory) fibres** a) to the N. lingualis for the Glandulae submandibularis and sublingualis (Nucleus salivatorius superior via the N. facialis and the Chorda tympani to the Ganglion submandibulare) b) to the N. auriculotemporalis for the Glandula parotidea (Nucleus salivatorius inferior via the N. glossopharyngeus, N. tympanicus and the N. petrosus minor to the Ganglion oticum)

f N. abducens [VI] (Fig. 1175, 1176, 1236, 1238)

Nuclei (fibre quality)	• Nucleus nervi abducentis (GSE)
Exit from the brain	Between Pons and Pyramis
Location in the subarachnoid space	Cisterna basalis
Entry into the dura mater	Upper third of the Clivus
Course within the dura mater	Via Apex partis petrosae, freely through the Sinus cavernosus, lateral to the A. carotis interna
Exit from the dura mater	Fissura orbitalis superior
Passage through the base of skull	Fissura orbitalis superior, medial portion (within the Anulus tendineus)
Supplying area	**Motor:** M. rectus lateralis

g N. facialis [VII] (Fig. 1181, 1182, 1236, 1238)

Nuclei (fibre quality)	• Nucleus nervi facialis (SVE) • Nucleus salivatorius superior (GVE) → Ganglion pterygopalatinum → Ganglion submandibulare • Nucleus solitarius (SVA)
Exit from the brain	Cerebellopontine angle
Location in the subarachnoid space	Cisterna basalis, Cisterna pontocerebellaris
Entry into the base of skull	Porus → Meatus acusticus internus
Passage through the dura mater	Fundus meatus acustici interni
Course within the base of skull	Canalis nervi facialis
Exit from the base of skull	Foramen stylomastoideum
Supplying areas	**Motor:** facial muscles, Mm. auriculares, M. digastricus (Venter posterior), M. stylohyoideus, M. stapedius **Sensory:** anterior 2/3 of the tongue (via Chorda tympani to the N. lingualis) **Parasympathetic:** Glandula lacrimalis, Glandulae nasales, Glandulae palatinae (via Ganglion pterygopalatinum), Glandula submandibularis, Glandula sublingualis (via Ganglion submandibulare)
Attachment of other nerves	**Sensible fibres** from the N. trigeminus to the facial branches of the N. facialis

h N. vestibulocochlearis [VIII] (Fig. 1183, 1236, 1238)

Nuclei (fibre quality)	• Nuclei cochleares anterior and posterior (SSA) • Nuclei vestibulares medialis, lateralis, superior and inferior (SSA)
Exit from the brain	Cerebellopontine angle
Location in the subarachnoid space	Cisterna basalis, Cisterna pontocerebellaris
Entry into the base of skull	Porus → Meatus acusticus internus
Exit from the dura mater	Fundus meatus acustici interni
Course within the base of skull	Directly to the labyrinth of the petrous part of the temporal bone
Supplying areas	**Sensory:** N. cochlearis: organ of hearing (= organ of CORTI) **Sensory:** N. vestibularis: organ of balance

i N. glossopharyngeus [IX] (Fig. 1184, 1236, 1238)

Nuclei (fibre quality)	• Nucleus ambiguus (SVE) • Nucleus spinalis nervi trigemini (GVA) • Nucleus solitarius (SVA) • Nucleus salivatorius inferior (GVE) → Ganglion oticum
Exit from the brain	Medulla oblongata, Sulcus posterolateralis (between the olive and the Tuberculum cuneatum)
Location in the subarachnoid space	Cisterna basalis
Passage through the dura mater	Foramen jugulare
Passage through the base of skull	Foramen jugulare
Supplying area	**Motor:** pharyngeal muscles (cranial parts), M. levator veli palatini, M. palatoglossus, M. palatopharyngeus, M. stylopharyngeus **Sensible:** pharyngeal mucosa (cranial parts), Tonsilla palatina, posterior third of the tongue, Plexus tympanicus, Membrana tympani (internally), Sinus caroticus **Sensory:** tongue (posterior third) **Parasympathetic:** Glandula parotidea (via Ganglion oticum), Glandulae linguales (posteriores)

j N. vagus [X] (Fig. 1185, 1236, 1238)

Nuclei (fibre quality)	• Nucleus ambiguus (SVE) • Nucleus spinalis nervi vagi (GVA) • Nucleus solitarius (SVA) • Nucleus dorsalis nervi vagi (GVE)
Exit from the brain	Medulla oblongata, Sulcus posterolateralis (dorsal to the olive)
Location in the subarachnoid space	Cisterna basalis
Passage through the dura mater	Foramen jugulare
Passage through the base of skull	Foramen jugulare
Supplying areas	**Motor:** pharyngeal muscles (caudal parts), M. levator veli palatini, M. uvulae, laryngeal muscles **Sensible:** Dura mater of the posterior cranial fossa, deep parts of the Meatus acusticus externus, Membrana tympani (externally) **Sensory:** root of the tongue **Parasympathetic:** organs of the neck, thorax and abdomen up to the point of CANNON-BÖHM

k N. accessorius [XI] (Fig. 1186, 1236, 1238)

Nuclei (fibre quality)	• Nucleus ambiguus (SVE) • Nucleus nervi accessorii (SVE)
Exit from the brain	Radices craniales: Medulla oblongata, Sulcus posterolateralis (retroolivaris) Radices spinales: Medulla cervicalis (lateral)
Location in the subarachnoid space	Cisterna basalis
Entry into the base of skull	Foramen magnum (Radices spinales)
Passage through the dura mater	Foramen jugulare
Passage through the base of skull	Foramen jugulare
Supplying area	**Motor:** M. sternocleidomastoideus, M. trapezius (together with the Plexus cervicalis)

l N. hypoglossus [XII] (Fig. 1187, 1236, 1238)

Nuclei (fibre quality)	• Nucleus nervi hypoglossi (GSE)
Exit from the brain	Medulla oblongata, Sulcus anterolateralis
Location in the subarachnoid space	Cisterna basalis
Passage through the dura mater	Canalis nervi hypoglossi
Passage through the base of skull	Canalis nervi hypoglossi
Supplying area	**Motor:** Inner muscles of the tongue, M. styloglossus, M. hyoglossus, M. genioglossus

Index

The numbers refer to the numbers of the tables.